HANDBOOK OF PHYSIOLOGY

SECTION 7: Endocrinology, VOLUME VI

HANDBOOK EDITORIAL COMMITTEE

John R. Pappenheimer, *Chairman*
Robert E. Forster
Wilfried F. H. M. Mommaerts

Handbook Editorial Committee when volume organized

Alfred P. Fishman, *Chairman*
John M. Brookhart
George F. Cahill, Jr.
Loren D. Carlson
C. Ladd Prosser

HANDBOOK OF PHYSIOLOGY

A critical, comprehensive presentation

of physiological knowledge and concepts

SECTION 7: # Endocrinology

VOLUME VI.
Adrenal Gland

Section Editors: ROY O. GREEP
EDWIN B. ASTWOOD

Volume Editors: HERMANN BLASCHKO
GEORGE SAYERS
A. DAVID SMITH

Executive Editor: STEPHEN R. GEIGER

American Physiological Society, WASHINGTON, D.C., 1975

© *Copyright 1975, American Physiological Society*

Library of Congress Catalog Card Number 60–4587

International Standard Book Number 683–03570–3

Printed in the United States of America by Waverly Press, Inc., Baltimore, Maryland 21202

Distributed by The Williams & Wilkins Company, Baltimore, Maryland 21202

Preface

The student of endocrinology always asks the question: why have two such dissimilar endocrine tissues come together in one organ, the adrenal gland? The distinction between the adrenal cortex and the adrenal medulla was recognized by the early anatomists, such as Caspar Bartholinus the Elder, who in 1611 described the adrenal gland as "capsulae atrabilariae", a capsule filled with black fluid. (This was a result of the rapid postmortem autolysis of the medulla.) Twenty years ago the editors of a volume like this would have been unable to add much more about the functional significance of the anatomic arrangement, except to point out that both parts of the adrenal gland are tissues that secrete their hormones in response to stressful conditions. Now there are, at last, clues that some of the functions of the medullary chromaffin cell are influenced by, and may even depend on, a continuous exposure to the very high concentrations of steroid hormones in adrenal venous blood. Perhaps, as our understanding increases of the fundamental processes in the chromaffin cell and of the nature and control of secretions of adrenal steroids, we shall be able to provide a better answer to the student's question.

For the time being, we hope that the reader will find in this volume much to compare and contrast between the two types of secretory tissue in the adrenal gland. Perhaps he will also be glad that, from time to time, the endocrinologist has to sit back from his research into the intricacies of hormones and reflect on the significance of his work for physiology. We hope that the material collected in this volume will not just be seen as a collection of essays but rather as a foundation upon which the physiologist can build a better understanding of the functions of the adrenal gland as a whole.

As Volume Editors we are very aware of the painstaking work done by the authors in preparing their chapters and by the American Physiological Society editorial team of Kathleen K. Lamar and Elspeth M. Root. To all these we express our gratitude.

HERMANN BLASCHKO
A. DAVID SMITH
GEORGE SAYERS
Volume Editors

Introduction

ADRENAL CORTEX

We are indeed most fortunate to have Dr. Robert Gaunt start this section of the volume with a history of the adrenal cortex. One has the feeling of being on the scene watching the pioneers build a substantial edifice of adrenocortical physiology. The dramatic moments are there, including the discovery that the secretions of the adrenal cortex ameliorate inflammatory disease.

The reader has simply to look over the list of topics covered in this part of the volume to realize the ubiquity of actions of the secretions of the adrenal cortex—all phases of organic and electrolyte metabolism—and the variety of target organs and cells involved, including the cardiovascular system, the nervous system, the lymphocyte, and connective tissue.

It is a fascinating and at the same time fundamental question as to whether many of these actions are a consequence of a single molecular "mechanism." Some of these molecular mechanisms have been considered, and we look forward to the elaboration and elucidation of this phase of adrenocortical physiology in the future.

GEORGE SAYERS

ADRENAL MEDULLA

In one respect the Editors of this part of the *Handbook* are fortunate: the importance of the secretions of the adrenal medulla for the normal functioning of the body and for pathology are well established and continue to be studied.

The enormous expansion of our knowledge of adrenergic mechanisms stems in the main from two sources. First, there are the insights that have followed upon the recognition of the catecholamines as neural transmitter substances, as well as hormones; and second, there are the enormous gains, in physiology and in medical practice, from the increased understanding of biochemical processes. All these new aspects are fully discussed in this volume.

The formation of the adrenal gland as an anatomic entity still confronts us with a challenge. The Editors have on several occasions (1, 10) drawn attention to the contrast in fundamental properties of adrenal cortex and medulla: the first a tissue continuously secreting and mainly dependent on humoral influences, the latter releasing its secretions mainly when the tissue receives nerve impulses; and there is also a difference in the presence of hormone stores, which are insignificant in the cortex and very large in the medulla. In 1960 it was pointed out that the anatomic arrangement ensured that the adrenal medulla received the cortical effluent before the latter was diluted in the systemic circulation, and in this volume we can see how the importance of this factor has been established by recent investigations. In addition to the hormonal influences that the cortex exerts on the secretory activity of the medulla, there are also new findings that show that the cortical hormones have effects on the development and structure of the chromaffin cells. This has been beautifully demonstrated by Eränkö & Eränkö (5), who have found that hydrocortisone has an effect on the number and catecholamine content of the extraadrenal chromaffin cells, both in vivo and in vitro.

However, one great problem remains unresolved—that of the formation of the adrenal gland as a circumscribed organ in higher vertebrates. How do these two different kinds of tissue, derived from such different origins, converge to find each other? No wonder that Tello, a distinguished pupil of Ramon y Cajal, long remained unconvinced that the parent cells of both the chromaffin cells and the sympathetic ganglion cells were derived from the ectodermal cells of the neural crest. These doubts have long been resolved, but the question remains: what are the factors that induce the two tissues to find each other? One is tempted to speculate that in development there are at work humoral factors also, as yet unidentified, that enable these tissues to recognize each other and to respond by growing together.

The similarities between chromaffin cells and adrenergic neurons have been underlined in recent years by a number of discoveries. First, there are the enzymes of biosynthesis, found in both types of tissue. Second, there are obvious similarities in the mode of storage and release of the chemical messengers [see (3)]. In addition, there have been interesting studies on cells intermediate between true adrenergic neurons and true chromaffin cells; these are the so-called small intensely fluorescent (SIF) cells of sympathetic ganglia. The resulting recognition, that the postganglionic sympathetic cell is not only "cholinoceptive" but also "aminoceptive," is paralleled by the presence in the adrenal medulla of amine-containing nerve endings (9). One is wondering if these medullary neurons have a function analogous to that of the aminergic structures of sympathetic ganglia, that is, to mediate a restraining influence on the chromaffin cells, an influence that can be conceived as opposed to the stimulating impulses that reach the medullary cells from the chief neurons of the splanchnic nerve. In the sympathetic ganglia the internuncial neurons are said to be dopaminergic, and one would therefore like to know if there is a connection between the amine-containing medullary neurons and the reported presence of dopamine granules in the adrenal medulla (7).

Another instance of the analogy between the postganglionic sympathetic neuron and the chromaffin cell of the adrenal medulla is seen in a recent report by Starke et al. (11), who postulate the presence on the surface of the bovine adrenal medullary cell of alpha-adrenergic receptors that mediate a reduction in catecholamine output from the stimulated chromaffin cell; this is similar to the alpha receptors present at the level of the adrenergic sympathetic nerve endings [see (6)]. If the presence of such a mechanism that regulates amine release could be established, it would be a satisfactory solution to observations that have puzzled previous workers. In 1960 Paton interpreted the effect of alpha blockers on the adrenal medullary cell as an inhibition of amine uptake. Amine uptake at the level of the adrenergic nerve endings is a phenomenon that has since been studied by many observers. However, it was pointed out some time ago (2) that in this respect the adrenal medulla and the adrenergic neurons are functionally not equivalent. At the level of the nerve endings, amine taken up may well be amine that has exerted its function as a chemical messenger. On the other hand, in the adrenal medulla it is the amine that is carried away by the way of the bloodstream that delivers the message to the effector organ. Amine uptake at the level of the chromaffin cell would thus be without a functional equivalent.

It is remarkable how biochemical studies have not only thrown light on physiological mechanisms in the adrenal medulla but have also raised entirely new questions about the functions of this gland. As the first section of the part of this volume on the medulla shows, the chromaffin cell can no longer be regarded as a cell specialized for the synthesis, storage, and secretion of catecholamines alone. The number and the variety of secretory products of the chromaffin cell is a challenge to the physiologist: why does the gland secrete adenine nucleotides, acidic glycoproteins (chromogranins), dopamine β-hydroxylase, many lysosomal enzymes, and, as recently reported (4), acetylcholinesterase? It could always be argued that those secretory products originating from the chromaffin granule are merely waste products that have to be discharged whenever the catecholamines are released. However, this is too easy a way out of the problem; it is surely more likely that the chromogranins, which are secreted weight-for-weight with the catecholamines, have some function outside the adrenal gland.

A problem such as that of the extraadrenal function of the secretory proteins will probably only be solved by looking at the overall functions of the adrenosympathetic system; these are dealt with in the last section of the part on the medulla. The challenge is, perhaps, similar to that faced by an outstanding pioneer in this field, Walter B. Cannon. His work is in no way overshadowed by the discoveries of Otto Loewi or Ulf von Euler with whose names the identification of the adrenergic transmitter is mainly associated. Cannon and his colleagues had confidence in the methods they employed: when they saw differences between the effects of sympathetic stimulation on the one hand and those of epinephrine on the other, they did not, like others, consider them as insignificant, but they made an attempt at explaining them in what we should like to call biochemical terms. However, Cannon's greatest contribution was to physiology. He gave a unifying and comprehensive interpretation to the meaning of adrenosympathetic stimulation. This work has retained its validity ever since.

Here again we see new problems that await an answer. Nothing was known in Cannon's time of the role of catecholamines in the central nervous system. Can the effects of catecholamines in the central nervous system be accounted for by Cannon's concepts? Thus we arrive at the borderline of what is strictly of interest to the readers of this volume. The presence of a blood-brain barrier for catecholamines limits the importance of the medullary hormones for the central nervous system in the main to the circulation and to certain defined areas that lie outside the blood-brain barrier.

Another question that arises from recent work is that of the nature of the general biochemical mechanism that underlies the actions of the catecholamines in the effector organs. This question follows from the discovery of the action of the catecholamines on the enzyme adenylate cyclase. It is closely linked to the discovery, by pharmacological techniques, of the different receptors for catecholamines. There seems to be general consensus that the beta receptor is situated in close juxtaposition to this enzyme, but it is not yet clear if the activating effect of the receptor on the adenylate cyclase is the only consequence of receptor activation. Moreover the biochemical counterpart of stimulation of the alpha receptors is not yet recognized. These are important problems where much can be gained from a convergence of physiological, pharmacological, and biochemical studies.

Like so many hormones, the catecholamines exert their action at the level of the cell membrane. It is still uncertain if intracellular processes are influenced only through a separate signaling system, or whether the ability of the cells of target tissues to take up catecholamines means that intracellular processes can be directly influenced by the hormones. Here is another area of study that the Editors hope will be stimulated and influenced by the contributions assembled in this volume.

REFERENCES

1. BLASCHKO, H. Chairman's opening remarks. In: *Ciba Foundation Symposium on Adrenergic Mechanisms*, edited by J. R. Vane, G. E. W. Wolstenholme, and M. O'Connor. London: Churchill, 1960, p. 61–62.
2. BLASCHKO, H. Catecholamines: metabolism and storage. In: *Recent Advances in Pharmacology*, edited by J. M. Robson and R. S. Stacey. London: Churchill, 1968, p. 135–154.
3. BLASCHKO, H., AND A. D. SMITH. A discussion on subcellular and macromolecular aspects of synaptic transmission. *Phil. Trans. Roy. Soc. London, Ser. B* 261: 273–440, 1971.
4. CHUBB, I. W., AND A. D. SMITH. Release of an isoenzyme of acetylcholinesterase from the perfused adrenal gland. *J. Physiol., London* 239: 97–98P, 1974.
5. ERÄNKÖ, O., AND L. ERÄNKÖ. Small intensely fluorescent (SIF) cells in vivo and in vitro. In: *Frontiers in Catecholamine Research*, edited by E. Usdin and S. H. Snyder. Oxford: Pergamon, 1973, p. 431–436.
6. LANGER, S. Z. Presynaptic regulation of catecholamine release. *Biochem. Pharmacol.* 23: 1793–1800, 1974.
7. LISHAJKO, F. Dopamine secretion from the isolated sheep adrenal. *Acta Physiol. Scand.* 79: 405–410, 1970.
8. PATON, W. D. M. Discussion remark. In: *Ciba Foundation Symposium on Adrenergic Mechanisms*, edited by J. R. Vane, G. E. W. Wolstenholme, and M. O'Connor. London: Churchill, 1960, p. 124–127.
9. PRENTICE, J. D. AND J. G. WOOD. Cytochemical localization of 5-hydroxydopamine in adrenergic elements of the cat adrenal medulla. *Experientia* 30: 645–648, 1974.
10. SMITH, A. D. Biochemistry of chromaffin granules. In: *The Interaction of Drugs and Subcellular Components in Animal Cells*, edited by P. N. Campbell. London: Churchill, 1968, p. 239–292.
11. STARKE, K., B-D. GÖRLITZ, H. MONTEL, AND H. J. SCHÜMANN. Local α-adrenoceptor mediated feedback inhibition of catecholamine release from the adrenal medulla? *Experientia* 30: 1170–1172, 1974.

HERMANN BLASCHKO
A. DAVID SMITH

Contents

ADRENAL CORTEX

1. History of the adrenal cortex
   ROBERT GAUNT 1

Morphology

2. Zonation of the mammalian adrenal cortex
   JOHN A. LONG 13
3. Ultrastructure of the mammalian adrenal cortex in relation to secretory function
   SASHA MALAMED 25

Biosynthesis and Function

4. Regulation of the secretory activity of the adrenal cortex: cortisol and corticosterone
   GEORGE SAYERS
   RONALD PORTANOVA 41
5. Biosynthesis of corticosteroids
   LEO T. SAMUELS
   DON H. NELSON 55
6. Theories on the mode of action of ACTH in stimulating secretory activity of the adrenal cortex
   ROBERT C. HAYNES, JR. 69
7. Regulation of aldosterone secretion
   JAMES O. DAVIS 77

Development

8. The fetal adrenal cortex
   ALFRED JOST 107

Binding to Plasma Proteins

9. Binding of corticosteroids by plasma proteins
   U. WESTPHAL 117

Circadian Rhythm

10. Circadian rhythm: man and animals
    JAMES B. ATCHESON
    FRANK H. TYLER 127

Proteins, Carbohydrates, and Fats

11. Influences of corticosteroids on protein and carbohydrate metabolism
    ROBERT STEELE 135

12. Glucocorticoid effects on lipid mobilization and adipose tissue metabolism
    JOHN N. FAIN
    MICHAEL P. CZECH 169

Electrolytes

13. Effect of corticosteroids on water and electrolyte metabolism
    BARR H. FORMAN
    PATRICK J. MULROW 179

Target Organs, Tissues, and Cells

14. Corticosteroids and circulatory function
    ALLAN M. LEFER 191
15. The role of adrenal corticosteroids in sensory processes
    ROBERT I. HENKIN 209
16. Corticosteroids and lymphoid tissue
    ALLAN MUNCK
    DONALD A. YOUNG 231
17. Corticosteroids and skeletal muscle
    ESTELLE R. RAMEY 245
18. Corticosteroids, inflammation, and connective tissue
    DAVID M. SPAIN 263

Pathophysiology

19. Pathophysiology of syndromes of cortisol excess in man
    RANDALL H. TRAVIS 271

ADRENAL MEDULLA

Morphology

20. Blood supply of the adrenal gland
    R. E. COUPLAND 283
21. Ultrastructure of the chromaffin cell
    ODILE GRYNSZPAN-WINOGRAD 295

Composition of the Chromaffin Cell

22. Physiological mechanisms controlling secretory activity of adrenal medulla
    G. P. LEWIS 309

23. The chromaffin granule and the storage of catecholamines
    HANS WINKLER
    A. DAVID SMITH 321
24. Biosynthesis of the catecholamines
    N. KIRSHNER 341
25. Control of the biosynthesis of adrenal catecholamines by the adrenal medulla
    NORMAN WEINER 357

Release of the Hormones

26. Secretomotor control of adrenal medullary secretion: synaptic, membrane, and ionic events in stimulus-secretion coupling
    W. W. DOUGLAS 367
27. Mechanism of secretion of catecholamines from adrenal medulla
    OSVALDO HUMBERTO VIVEROS 389
28. Catecholamines in blood
    B. A. CALLINGHAM 427

Physiological Role of Catecholamines

29. Adrenergic receptors
    NEIL C. MORAN 447
30. Catecholamines and the cardiovascular system
    ERIC NEIL 473
31. Reflex respiratory effects of circulating catecholamines
    N. JOELS 491

32. Action of catecholamines on bronchial smooth muscle
    J. G. WIDDICOMBE 507
33. Role of circulating catecholamines in the gastrointestinal tract
    J. B. FURNESS
    G. BURNSTOCK 515
34. Action of catecholamines on skeletal muscle
    T. TOMITA 537
35. Catecholamines in relation to the eye
    M. L. SEARS 553
36. Catecholamines and control of sweat glands
    D. ROBERTSHAW 591
37. Effects of epinephrine on glycogenolysis and myocardial contractility
    JOHN R. WILLIAMSON 605
38. Role of the adrenal medulla in adaptation to cold
    JEAN HIMMS-HAGEN 637
39. Influence of circulating catecholamines on the central nervous system
    MARTHE VOGT 667
40. Catechol-*O*-methyltransferase and other *O*-methyltransferases
    JULIUS AXELROD 669
41. Monoamine oxidase
    K. F. TIPTON 677
42. The metabolism of circulating catecholamines
    D. F. SHARMAN 699
43. Uptake of circulating catecholamines into tissues
    L. L. IVERSEN 713

Index 723

CHAPTER 1

History of the adrenal cortex[1]

ROBERT GAUNT | *Research Department, CIBA Pharmaceutical Company, Summit, New Jersey*

CHAPTER CONTENTS

Introduction and Early History
Are Adrenals Essential for Life?
Is Adrenal Cortex or Medulla Essential for Life?
Functions of Adrenal Cortex
Endocrine Role of Adrenal Cortex
Early Work with Extracts of Adrenal Cortex
Chemistry of Adrenal Cortex
Adrenal Cortex in Electrolyte and Water Metabolism
Effects on Carbohydrate Metabolism
Adrenal-Gonad-Pituitary Relations
    Adrenal-gonad
    Adrenal-pituitary
Stress
Inflammation
Obsequies for Aldosterone
Epilogue

INTRODUCTION AND EARLY HISTORY

The adrenal glands, known in the older literature as the *suprarenal bodies* or *suprarenal capsules*, led a somnolent scientific life through the Renaissance centuries. Galen was not disturbed by them, and the glands in turn were undisturbed "by the bothersome investigation of medical men" [Hyrtl, cited in (5)]. They were the legitimate but unrecognized siblings, embryologically and in steroidogenic potential, of the gonads. Unlike the adrenals, however, concern for the gonads, involving a spectrum from agricultural and advertising economics to theoretical and applied science, has been the major endocrine preoccupation of mankind throughout recorded history. This fact, exploited unscientifically in some misguided or subethical medical and pharmaceutical circles, led to an era in the first decades of the century when the emerging science of endocrinology carried an aura of unrespectability. It led one of my undergraduate professors at the University of Tulsa to mutter a disdainful "tut, tut" when I returned from the distant East in 1930 to report that I was going into endocrinology. The implication was clear that I had been lured by red lights to the wrong side of the railroad tracks. It is said (59) to have led the American pioneers of the field in 1917 to call their newborn national society The Association for the Study of Internal Secretions and thus avoid the unpleasant connotations of a word in the name of what is now The Endocrine Society. The late Henry Turner recalled that "hostility toward the fledgling specialty was such that it might have been wiser and safer to meet in secret" (77).

The adrenal cortex, however, even after unequivocal evidence of the importance of the whole adrenal was on record, was still largely ignored, in part because it operated in the shadow of the fantastically (at the time) potent humors of the adrenal medulla, which had been discovered in the early 1900s.

It would appear that Bartolomeo Eustacchio first described the adrenal glands in 1563 which he termed *glandulae Renibus incumbentes*. His Tabulae Anatomicae were left unpublished at his death and remained in various private hands for many years. They were finally published in 1714 by the great Italian clinician, Lancisi, with his own notes. Eustacchio's commentaries on his drawings have never been found (76).

Any meaningful functional studies were delayed for three centuries.

In 1716, the Academie des Sciences de Bordeaux offered a prize for an answer to the question: "Quel est l'usage des glands surrenales?" The judge was Montesquieu, then 29 years of age, who found himself unable to award the prize to any of the conflicting and, in some instances, very extraordinary theories offered in solution of the problem. He closed his searching criticism of these theories with the words: "Le hazard fera peut-être quelque jour ce que tous les soins n'ont pu faire" [2] [(5), p. 124].

The beginning of any real scientific history of the adrenal has to be dated from the concise and admirably written monograph by Thomas Addison in 1855, which

[1] In this chapter I attempt to trace the development of knowledge of the adrenal cortex to about 1950. The omissions and possible misinterpretations are self-evident. No serious attempts are made to avoid the inevitable personal slants and prejudices based on living with this subject since 1930, the first year of my graduate work. It happened that the modern history of the adrenal began in 1930, but that I attempted that year, on a morning after a party, my first adrenalectomy in a cat is highly coincidental. The martyred cat, however, is enshrined in my memory.

[2] This French idiom bothered me, too. A Frenchwoman's free translation was: "Perhaps some day chance will reveal what all of this work was unable to do."

followed an earlier short paper in 1849[3]. He described with elegant lithographs 11 fatal cases, which he and his distinguished colleagues at Guy's Hospital had observed over several preceding years, and noted:

> The leading and characteristic features of the morbid state to which I would direct attention are, anaemia[4], general languor and debility, remarkable feebleness of the heart's action, irritability of the stomach, and a peculiar change of colour in the skin, occurring in connection with a diseased condition of the "supra-renal capsules" (1).

Although there may be question in the diagnosis of some of these cases, for the first time a life-maintaining function was ascribed to the adrenals with specific description of certain important features of the symptomatology and pathology of the deficiency state.

Correct as Addison's deductions were, they did not, as noted below, lead to full acceptance or consensus. There was only a dim correlation between Addison's chronic syndrome and the quick deaths from the early attempts at adrenalectomy in animals; moreover the pigmentation of Addison's disease could not be duplicated experimentally. The approaches to these questions were long and stumbling. Prolixity, which Addison could avoid with a simple statement of a clear concept, was not avoided by his uncertain successors. For instance, it was early recognized that some "stresses" [although the word was used little in this context before Selye (64)], such as acute infections, seemed to stimulate or at least affect the adrenal as determined by its size and frequent internal hemorrhages (10). Much more widely held for nearly a century was the hypothesis, in part implied from the huge blood supply of the adrenal, that its primary role was to detoxify some one or more lethal circulating humors. Hence these two ideas were linked with superficial logic: "The suprarenals respond to many infections in such a way that it has been suggested that they exercise an important part as a detoxicating mechanism" (27).

ARE ADRENALS ESSENTIAL FOR LIFE?

The twentieth century was approached, as far as the adrenal was concerned, with few established facts and even doubts as to the necessity of the adrenal for the maintenance of life. Anyone with research experience is aware that simple biological questions are not necessarily answered in a quick and simple fashion. Although Addison's pioneering conclusions that the adrenals were essential for life were quickly verified by the experimental adrenalectomies of Brown-Sequard (8) in rabbits, dogs, cats, and guinea pigs, doubts immediately arose from numerous sources.

In 1862 Sir Samuel Wilks (78a) wrote: "It may be said, I think, with truth, that Addison's views have by no means received the support of the profession at large..." but added, "I may say at once that my own observations entirely uphold his argument" (75). Brown-Sequard's story suffered in part from the behavior of that oft-troubling rodent, the rat. In other respects, at least in retrospect, his data were less than conclusive. His experimental animals died within a few hours or at most 1 or 2 days, probably of shock. Obviously the operative technique or other factors were less than optimal. Gratiolet (25) found that extirpation of one gland only in the guinea pig similarly led to death[5]. Philipeaux (54) quickly challenged Brown-Sequard in 1856 by showing that with a two-stage operation many rats could survive total adrenalectomy indefinitely. A lively spate of papers from these and other authors considered such facts, and Brown-Sequard (9) toyed with the question whether albino animals, lacking a possibly toxic Addisonian pigment, might for this reason be able to survive adrenalectomy. This and other scattered work over the next several decades, however, gradually led to the concept that adrenalectomy in most species was fatal except in those cases, notably frequent in rats, where adrenal accessories were present. Hence the students of adrenal physiology, from 1900 to 1930, largely avoided the rat as being unsuitable for any critical adrenal studies. The controversy, however, did not die easily. In 1931 Pencharz et al. (52) revived it with an impressive report concluding that "the rat is no exception to the rule that in mammals adrenal insufficiency symptoms and death follow total adrenalectomy." It was necessary, they thought, to remove periadrenal fat and other tissues to eliminate possible offending accessories.

The question was an important one in view of the wide utility of the rat in subsequent adrenal work[6]. From various sources, however, about a century after the ques-

---

[3] The history of the adrenal is dealt with comprehensively at different stages in its development, in English, in the following especially useful literature: *The Internal Secretory Organs, Their Physiology and Pathology*, by A. Biedl, published in 1913 in New York by Wm. Woods and Co.; *Endocrinology and Metabolism*, vol. 1 and 2, edited by L. F. Barker, published in 1922 in New York by Appleton; *The Adrenal Gland*, by F. A. Hartman and K. A. Brownell, published in 1949 in Philadelphia by Lea and Febiger (the most encyclopedic review on the subject); and *Handbuch der Experimentellen Pharmakologie*, vol. xiv/2, "Adrenalcortical insufficiency," by F. G. Hofmann and E. H. Sobel, published in 1964 in Berlin by Springer Verlag.

[4] "Anemia is uncommon, although Addison considered it a cardinal sign" (29). Oligemia is more characteristic of adrenal insufficiency, but anemia, even pernicious anemia, may coexist (4).

[5] This was a finding with which I can sympathize, since my own initial attempts at right adrenalectomy in this species often led to death even before the caval-bound gland was all the way out of the body cavity.

[6] Such prolonged controversies have an unappreciated side benefit: they serve as a fine source of Ph.D. theses. In 1930 Professor W. W. Swingle, for such purposes, gave me the dictum to get some rats and "solve the problem"—an order as yet only partially fulfilled and retirement rapidly approaching. It was not made easier when I began with two false premises: *1)* an adrenal should be easier to find in a big rat than a little one; and *2)* acceptance of the then widespread notion that even in rodents, if adrenals were not removed aseptically, death from infection would quickly ensue. Hence, by ploughing through the periadrenal fat of overweight rats, draped in sterile cloth, and with instruments freshly boiled for each operation, 6 adrenalectomies per morning could be done! The work speeded up later when, from numerous duly recorded slips in technique, it became apparent that strict asepsis was not essential.

tion was first raised, a fair consensus was achieved. The essentiality of the adrenal is probably the same in rats as in other mammals. Important factors that vary survival times in rats after adrenalectomy are *a)* hereditary strain differences, possibly in part due to accessories; *b)* age of the animals; *c)* the sodium and potassium content of diet[7]; *d)* environmental conditions; and *e)* the presence or absence of temporary life-sustaining replacement therapies, which permit time for some adjustment (presumably development of accessories) and which when withdrawn frequently result in prolonged or indefinite survival. The unsolved problem concerns the location, nature, and reality of presumed adrenal accessories, which modern investigators seem to find much less frequently than did those at the turn of the century. Such accessories can be seen, particularly after temporary salt or mineralocorticoid replacement therapy, generally near the site of the left adrenal, but not necessarily in all animals that may survive indefinitely under optimal conditions (15, 19, 20, 22, 39, 52). The possibility that adrenal tissue can differentiate, given time and need, from as yet unidentified sources has not been ruled out (46).

For a much longer time, there has not been serious question that adrenalectomy leads to death in larger mammals. The problem, until replacement therapies were available for immediate postoperative use, was to accomplish the operation so as to avoid an early stress-induced death from shock and thus permit study of a gradually developing true adrenal insufficiency. Stewart and Rogoff flailed the perpetrators of sloppy technique and, using fastidious care, achieved, as did Swingle, in the late 1920s average survivals in dogs and cats of 10 days or more after total adrenalectomy (17).

IS ADRENAL CORTEX OR MEDULLA ESSENTIAL FOR LIFE?

Until the discovery of epinephrine and recognition that the medulla was its site of secretion, any distinction between the functional significance of medulla and cortex was not a question of great concern. Later preoccupation with medullary functions tended further to divert attention from the cortex. Extirpation of interrenal ("cortical") tissue in some fishes, in which it and chromaffin tissue are separate, by Biedl (5) and others, although beset by technical difficulties and uncertainties, tended to show that the interrenal organs were responsible for preventing adrenal insufficiency. Wheeler & Vincent (78) removed one adrenal and half of the other in dogs, then cauterized medullary tissue of the remaining fragment; after this the cortical portion, if itself not extensively damaged, maintained good health. Houssay & Lewis (34) in 1923 did much the same type of experiments with elasmobranchs, as had Biedl, and with dogs, as had Wheeler and Vincent. In dogs the left adrenal was exposed, its blood supply restricted, and "the gland was then opened lengthwise, with a sharp Gillette blade,

[7] It was common in early days to feed rats table scrap diets, salted to human taste.

as if it were a book and all the medulla removed with a spoon" (34). Sometime later the right adrenal was removed. Most of the dogs survived in good health, and the conclusion was that "dogs survive extirpation of all chromaphil tissue contained in the adrenals when the remaining cortex is in good state." But that future Nobel Laureates (i.e., Houssay) can, aside from making effective use of commonplace equipment, such as razor blades and spoons, suffer mundane mishaps is further recorded: "One dog (No. 1) ran away after 7 days in excellent health. Another (No. 10) did the same thing 4 days after operations, without having had symptoms" (34). The subsequent history of these animals is obscure.

At the same time Frank Hartman (27) was concluding with cautious restraint that, "from all of the evidence available we may conclude that of the two tissues the cortex is more important." Others belabored the same question on through the 1920s, and finally consensus was achieved that the adrenal cortex was essential for life and that the adrenal medulla was not.

FUNCTIONS OF ADRENAL CORTEX

The fact that the adrenal cortex was essential for life defined sharply a question of self-evident importance: what was its function? Meaningful work that began in the 1920s opened a Pandora's box of confusing information with few parallels in physiological history. As techniques slowly developed by which more and more parameters could be and were measured, it became increasingly evident that virtually no physiological process was unaffected by adrenalectomy. It was a decade in which a group of then mostly young men attacked the problem frontally, from a physiological standpoint and with the tools of "kitchen chemistry," as Pfiffner termed it. They developed a variety of working hypotheses. None was completely right, completely wrong, or, despite vehement argument[8], completely certain; but between them they set the stage for the development of one of the great chapters in endocrine and physiological history. (Among these pioneers were G. N. Stewart and his colleague J. M. Rogoff of Case Western Reserve University[9]; Frank Hartman of the University of Buffalo and later Ohio State; W. W. Swingle and his colleague J. J. Pfiffner of Princeton; Sidney Britton and H. Silvette of the University of Virginia; Robert Loeb and colleagues of Columbia University; George Harrop and co-workers of Johns Hopkins; and C. N. H. Long of the University of Pennsylvania and later Yale.) Elsewhere (18) we have detailed an impressive list of physiological facts and

[8] "... convictions and the language used to express them were strong, even if fact and theory were shaky. Like Henry Ward Beecher's ministerial friend, the early adrenal workers were not without recourse to the use of shouts to overcome doubts" (18).

[9] The tradition continues. From the same institution, an editor of this volume, George Sayers, starting under the tutelage of C. N. H. Long, became a leader of the second wave of modern adrenal workers.

measurements that were recorded by 1930—all valid but leading to no coherent or comprehensive conclusions[10].

The reasons for such confusion are now clear enough. There were no satisfactory unifying concepts to which a plethora of detailed facts could be related. There was no proof that the cortex achieved its function by secreting a hormone. The ghost of the idea that the cortex maintained life by detoxifying something hung on until the bitter end and had the superficial merit that it could explain anything. Only the multifaceted and capricious "deficiency" aspects of adrenal function were available for study without the aid of replacement or overdosage data. The tendency was for each investigator who discovered a new aspect of adrenal insufficiency to try to give it a central and unifying role in explaining the whole syndrome. To Frank Hartman's credit, it should be noted that he considered the hormone of the adrenal cortex to be a "general tissue hormone." This idea, although lacking the specificity to be of much help in designing experiments, at least obviated the need for contriving impossibly devious chains of cause-and-effect relations between all aspects of a complex syndrome.

ENDOCRINE ROLE OF ADRENAL CORTEX

Further progress was dependent on demonstrating the existence of an internal secretion from the cortex and on making such a secretory product available for appropriate study. Extraction of an active cortical principle from adrenal tissue was no easy task in the 1920s with the relatively primitive art and science available at the time. No clue as to its chemical nature was at hand, and lack of knowledge of any specific key functions required that assays of extracts be based on maintenance of life in adrenalectomized animals. A major problem was the separation of cortical principles from contaminating catecholamines of medullary tissue.

Hartman et al. (31) in 1927 prepared extracts that extended life in adrenalectomized animals, but not for indefinite periods. Rogoff & Stewart (56) probably did the same, but they recognized that their preparation was less effective than Ringer's solution, and later calculations by Hartman & Brownell (29) showed that their data lacked statistical significance. The modern and productive era in the field began, however, when lipid extracts of cortical tissue with unequivocal and relatively high potency were prepared independently in 1929–1930 by Swingle & Pfiffner (72, 73) and Hartman and co-workers (28, 30). Both groups showed that their preparations maintained adrenalectomized cats indefinitely, and, in the words of Hartman and Brownell, the animals "eat well, gain weight, play [and] fight . . . [have increased] resistance to infection and cold . . . and withstand operative or other trauma." Also, young adrenalectomized rats grew to a normal and fecund maturity on extract treatment. To prove the efficacy of their preparations, Swingle and Pfiffner maintained adrenalectomized cats in good health for 100 days, an expensive but convincing demonstration of activity. Their extracts cost about a dollar per milliliter to prepare, and 5 ml/day was necessary.

These 100-day cats, in which roughly five hundred dollars had been injected, were viewed with some economic misgiving by those of us who, as graduate students in the Princeton laboratories at the time, were not sharing in the alleged prosperity of early 1929 (18).

The first clinical trial of the Swingle-Pfiffner extracts was made, happily without any required delays for Food and Drug Administration approval of protocol, by Drs. Leonard Rountree and C. H. Greene at The Mayo Clinic in 1930. With beginners' luck, a moribund Addisonian farmer was dramatically revived:

The extract of the suprarenal cortex sent by Drs. Swingle and Pfiffner arrived on the sixth day after the patient's admission to the hospital. . . . Within thirty-six hours a marked effect on appetite and strength was apparent. The patient, who had been so nauseated as to retain water with difficulty, now asked for wieners and sauerkraut and in lieu of the latter ate a double order of beefsteak with relish (58).

Although Addison's disease is rare, it did not seem so at the time to those few who, having completely inadequate quantities of the only life-sustaining material available, had to deal with the pleas of people from around the world whose lives depended on it.

EARLY WORK WITH EXTRACTS OF ADRENAL CORTEX[11]

Since studies of adrenal insufficiency had failed to reveal a satisfactorily definable function of the adrenal cortex, Swingle's major goal, and presumably that of others, in attempts to make an active extract of the adrenal, was to be able to study the effects of overdosage of the hormone and thus perhaps pinpoint its major function. It was readily shown by those few to whom the extracts were available that the various known biochemical and pathophysiological abnormalities of adrenal insufficiency could be repaired. In this connection, it was fortunate, even if in a fashion misleading, that these extracts contained probably all the major secretory products of the adrenal. Aside from establishing the endocrine nature of the adrenal, however, this was not of great help in defining a primary function of what was presumed to

---

[10] The story of the birth of this modern era of adrenal history, particularly from the aspect of the clinicians involved, is well and delightfully told by Thorn (76) who, from youthful associations in the laboratories both of Hartman and Harrop, himself became a leading contributor to it. He in turn helped train a new generation of adrenal clinicians, which has made the study of adrenal dysfunction in man in expert hands a model of clinical precision.

[11] It was my privilege in 1942 to collaborate briefly and by long distance with E. C. Kendall, later Nobel Laureate, who supplied me and numerous others with some of the few milligrams of cortisone then available in the world. He accepted my write-up of results gracefully, except that, being a linguistic purist and foe of the adjectival noun, he forbade use of the term adrenal cortical extract —they were extracts of the adrenal cortex. With thanks for his help at the time, I honor his admonition here.

be a single hormone, lack of which obviously produced widespread physiological mayhem. No clear signs of overdosage were observed.

In an attempt to produce definite overdosage phenomena, Harrop at Johns Hopkins and Swingle at Princeton collaborated in 1931 by giving up to 100 ml of extract to dogs by intravenous and other routes. They measured some 15 metabolic and biochemical parameters. To their great disappointment nothing of consequence was seen to happen. The reluctant conclusion was that "there is no such thing as overdosage with this hormone—at any rate insofar as respiratory metabolism and the usual blood and urinary constituents are concerned" (74). Had the extracts been stronger and the experiment designed by hindsight, this discouraging result could no doubt have been avoided. As it was, however, it still took some years before convincing evidence of any overdosage effects of cortical preparations in normal animals was forthcoming. Among limiting factors were lack of knowledge that increases in blood hormone levels tended, by feedback on the pituitary, to shut off endogenous production of hormones of the cortex. Actually, by using weak preparations of short half-life, with the feedback mechanism operative, it is doubtful that sizable "overdoses" reached responsive effectors in amounts detectable except by fine measurement.

Such problems, however, excited interest and drew recruits into the field. These included competent biochemists whose role was indispensable in elucidating the nature and number of hormones involved. The subject is of such complexity that its subsequent history can only be told in terms of its individual facets, many of which developed simultaneously and interdependently.

CHEMISTRY OF ADRENAL CORTEX

The key to further physiological progress was provided in the mid 1930s by the chemical isolation and identification of numerous steroidal active principles of the cortex. Evaluation of the credits for and the subtleties of this complex but historic work, including the problems of steroidal biosynthesis involved, will be left to experts. The breakthrough was provided by the teams led by Wintersteiner and Pfiffner, by Reichstein, and by Kendall. The story of these early chemical developments has been told, although modestly, as far as their own contributions were concerned, by Pfiffner (53) and Mason (49a) and recently in great detail by Kendall (42). All involved showed that numerous steroids could be crystallized from extracts of the adrenal but that the most active life-maintaining moiety, "the amorphous fraction" (assumed to be the *one* or main long-sought adrenal hormone), remained as a water-soluble residue. This unexpected development led to much initial confusion, because serious question was raised as to whether any of the crystallized products were of physiological consequence. Clarification came as it was realized that bioassays based on the maintenance of life after adrenalectomy did not necessarily best reflect important properties of some of the compounds. In particular, Ingle's version of the muscle work test showed the unmistakable action of the compound now known as cortisone (35). Gradually it was realized that the adrenal had multiple secretions, and on this basis physiological work proceeded.

Of the numerous corticosteroids identified, 11-deoxycorticosterone, although normally secreted in trace amounts, was of particular practical importance; its partial synthesis (70) finally established the steroidal nature of the corticosteroids, and its economical production made it readily available for laboratory and clinical work. It is the "purest" prototype of the mineralocorticoids, and its study added much knowledge concerning the type of adrenal function now attributed mainly to aldosterone.

In this early work, investigators were confronted with two problems of particular difficulty. One was a practical means of synthesis of the hormones oxygenated at carbon 11 (i.e., cortisone and cortisol). Since dosage requirements were high, enough material for critical investigative work and potential clinical use could not be obtained from adrenal extracts. The second was the identification and synthesis of aldosterone, the elusive amorphous factor; this project took some 20 years. Synthesis of cortisone in the laboratories of Merck and Company resulted from the combined efforts of many workers (41, 42, 60). The final identification of aldosterone resulted from the retrospectively simple observation by Simpson and Tait that, when commercial extracts of the adrenal cortex were chromatographed on paper, the spot occupied by cortisone contained more mineralocorticoid activity than the cortisone present could possibly exert. Subsequent collaboration of Simpson and Tait with Reichstein at the University of Basle and with Wettstein and co-workers at CIBA, Ltd. in Basle, led to the identification, and soon to what was originally the enormously difficult synthesis, of aldosterone (17, 24, 68).

ADRENAL CORTEX IN ELECTROLYTE
AND WATER METABOLISM

Few ideas arise de novo, and some vague knowledge of a relation of the cortex to salt and water has long roots. For instance, unmistakable evidence of hemoconcentration in adrenal insufficiency was given in many reports before 1930 (18). In 1916 Marshall & Davis (49) had shown

a marked lowering of kidney efficiency [decreased ability to handle phenolsulfonphthalein, urea, and creatinine] in adrenalectomized cats. This may occur with a normal blood pressure, and when the animals are in excellent physical condition.

More definitively, Rogoff & Stewart (55) in 1928 had clearly extended the lives of adrenalectomized dogs by the periodic intravenous infusion of Ringer's solution— but that a toxin was being flushed out was the tentatively favored implication. In 1927 Marine & Baumann (48) and Baumann & Kurland (3) noted in adrenalectomized cats a low concentration of sodium and magnesium and elevated concentration of potassium in plasma. In addition, they showed unmistakably a prolongation of life by administration of sodium salts with the notation that "there is some indication that [the effect of] the loss of sodium is more specific than can be accounted for as a result of a possible acidosis."

The work that, by its timeliness in terms of growing interest in the field, started the bandwagon, however, was that of Loeb (43), who twice revived and then maintained an Addisonian patient in relatively good health for a long period on sodium chloride per os and per rectum. "With this report most adrenal workers rushed to their laboratories with salt shakers in hand" (18). On one point of fact, unanimity was the strange order of the day. Most investigators agreed that a high sodium intake was beneficial after adrenalectomy but that, except for the rat, it was not sufficient to maintain life indefinitely. Allers & Kendall (2), however, carefully studied the optimal combination of dietary electrolytes for use in adrenalectomized dogs. They found that indefinite maintenance could be obtained by providing food high in sodium and low in potassium. Such a regimen is without doubt the most effective nonhormonal substitute yet devised for adrenal hormones.

The interest in potassium, along with sodium, arose from numerous reports that this cation was elevated in the blood in adrenal insufficiency (3, 32) and that it was toxic to adrenalectomized animals (40, 80). That adrenal insufficiency was primarily a case of potassium intoxication and that the adrenal hormone's major function was to eliminate potassium were considered. This concept did not withstand the numerous examples that fit neither the theory nor the growing recognition that adrenalectomized animals were highly susceptible to any potentially toxic agent, including potassium. With the demise of the potassium intoxication theory went another version of the rugged old concept that the adrenal maintained life by "detoxifying" some specific substance[12].

The accumulated evidence became sufficient, however, by the mid 1930s to make mandatory the conclusion that one important function of the adrenal cortex was to maintain a homeostatic balance of sodium and potassium ions in the body. This in turn raised the questions not only of the sites and mechanisms of action involved, but also of how to correlate effects on electrolyte metabolism with pressing rival functions, the first firmly implanted one being the effect of the adrenal on carbohydrate metabolism.

A clearly defined renal tubular effect of cortical hormones, involving renal conservation of sodium and potassium extrusion, seemed to many at first to be a self-sufficient explanation of all adrenal functions. It took acrobatic logic to spread the umbrella of this one limited function wide enough to encompass all known facts about what the adrenal did; nevertheless the idea was frequently written into the reviews and even into texts of the day.

Eventually insight and perspective resulted from the demonstrations that *a*) there was more than one adrenal hormone; *b*) aldosterone had functions more or less limited to mineral metabolism; and *c*) the cortical hormones in general had widespread extrarenal, as well as renal, effects on sodium and potassium metabolism.

The mineralocorticoids with some but not complete specificity are sensitive regulators of electrolyte transport in such structures as the renal tubule, toad bladder, sweat and salivary glands, intestinal membranes, and amphibian skin. However, some related functions are more profoundly influenced by glucocorticoids. These include the distribution of water and electrolytes between internal body compartments, the integrity of terminal vascular functions, including the maintenance of blood pressure in stress, the maintenance of water diuresis, and the maintenance of blood volume during food and water deprivation. If complete specificity of function for any group of steroids exists in any such respect, it has yet to be demonstrated.

EFFECTS ON CARBOHYDRATE METABOLISM

Salt vs. sugar—these were the protagonists on the stage at the time of the six-week Cold Spring Harbor Symposium on Quantitative Biology (Endocrinology) in 1937. This meeting forced a group of investigators, who had rarely agreed on anything, to live and eat together for prolonged periods and to exchange ideas with reasonable politeness, or suffer indigestion. It did much to bring order in a chaotic field.

As noted above, an adrenal action on electrolyte metabolism, either direct or indirect, was unmistakable. From the distant past was recorded evidence that blood sugar and glycogen stores were sometimes (but not always) low in adrenal insufficiency. Cori & Cori (12), however, had shown that this occurrence depended on fasting (which due to gastrointestinal difficulties some adrenalectomized animals did spontaneously); muscle glycogen, on the other hand, was relatively unaffected. More particularly, however, Sidney Britton championed the idea that an effect on carbohydrate metabolism was the "pre-potent function" of the adrenal cortex and introduced a paper thusly: "Testimony to the profound and possibly primary involvement of the adrenal cortex in the regulation of carbohydrate metabolism is now presented" (7). He considered that adrenal involvement in the salt-water business was some side-order consequence thereof with nebulous parentage. Those of us from the saline clan used to ask with unsuspecting naivete, "If one can keep an adrenalectomized animal alive with salt but not sugar, how can the latter be pre-potent?" Britton had the following basic facts at hand: *a*) that severely reduced

---

[12] In a new dress, however, Selye thinks of a "detoxifying" role of the corticosteroids in certain stressful situations (67).

blood sugar and liver glycogen levels occurred in adrenalectomized animals; *b)* that such deficiencies were repaired with extracts of the cortex; and *c)* the highly significant fact—although one not accepted by others at the time—that overdoses of adrenal extract could build up carbohydrate stores even in normal fasting animals (6).

Also at the meeting was C. N. H. Long, who with Lukens had made the impressive demonstration that adrenalectomy, like hypophysectomy, ameliorated the glycosuria and ketonuria of pancreatic diabetes (45). Curiously, however, he found that this glycosuria was not restored by cortical extracts in what were then considered large doses.

The discussion at these meetings was spirited, although parts of it, including some of the data, never appeared in the records. Long regarded Britton's assertion that he could, with adrenal extract, make fasting rats store liver glycogen as some sort of improbable biochemical legerdemain. The only obvious difference, however, between his own experience and that of Britton was that the latter used larger doses of extract. Long went back to New Haven, used larger doses than he had before, and confirmed Britton's results! This sort of discrepancy was frequent in the field, because what in many instances was considered a large dose of extract was one that would maintain or revive adrenalectomized animals. Such effects were partly due to the amounts of aldosterone in the extracts, a steroid active in microgram quantities. Effects, such as liver glycogen deposition, resulting from cortisol or other glucocorticoids, demand manyfold greater amounts than were present in extracts then available. In any case, the continued work of Long, Fry, and their collaborators, particularly that presented in one influential and much-quoted paper (44), established in a uniformly convincing manner that some secretion of the adrenal was essential for normal gluconeogenesis from protein and for other homeostatic aspects of organic metabolism. By this time it was becoming clear also that these adrenal activities, caused primarily by the glucocorticoids, did not have to be completely linked in a direct cause-and-effect relationship with concurrent regulation of electrolyte metabolism.

ADRENAL-GONAD-PITUITARY RELATIONS

The most remarkable fact about the internal secretions is that they are correlated with one another (14).

Adrenal-Gonad

French investigators were the first to direct attention to the influence of overfunction of the cortical portion of the suprarenal upon the secondary sexual characters under the name "syndrome genito-surrenale" (47)[13].

[13] Confirmation of this statement, apparently in reference to work in the 1800s, by primary documentation was not obtained.

However, in 1902 Woolley (79) compiled all adrenal tumor cases in his own experience and in the literature available to him and tabulated "abnormally developed genitalia" in only a single instance. His text made no mention of such associated reproductive aberrations. Yet shortly thereafter, Bulloch & Sequeira (9a) and Glynn (24a) were describing classic cases of adrenogenitalism. In fact, the conspicuous features of the adrenogenital syndromes were among the factors maintaining interest in the adrenal during the early part of the century. Animal models for their study, however, were not available. One fascinating animal observation, nevertheless, was of compelling interest. Rogoff & Stewart (57) noted, and others confirmed, that, if dogs were adrenalectomized during pregnancy or estrus, instead of dying within approximately 1 week, they lived for several weeks.

Explaining these phenomena was one of the first problems attempted when active extracts of the cortex were available. In 1933 Parkins and I, working under Swingle's aegis, gave extracts of the cortex to immature rats in a totally unsuccessful effort to modify their sexual development. In view of evidence that sexual differentiation in the bird was more labile and subject to modification than that of mammals, we moved our activities to the lawn of the Cold Spring Harbor Biological Laboratory and there injected chicks for long periods beginning at an early age. All chicks grew to a handsome normal maturity. This being during the depression, we confirmed this fact by eating our specimens. A less profitable outcome was a paper, happily long forgotten by all but its authors, in which we questioned whether hyperactivity of the adrenals affected sexual development (23).

The problem of ovarian function and survival after adrenalectomy was a little easier. Working with Hays, we took advantage of the otherwise often useful and unusual reproductive cycle of the ferret. We found that follicular ovaries, like injected estrogens, reduced survival after adrenalectomy, whereas a functional corpus luteum maintained life and excellent health during the period of pseudopregnancy without cortical hormones or salt. By scrounging supplies from three sources, we obtained enough crystalline progesterone, then a new, rare, and expensive steroid, to show that it would maintain and revive ferrets through cycles of adrenal insufficiency (21). Progesterone substitutes for "standard" corticosteroids much better in some species (hamster, ferret) than others (rat, dog, man) for reasons not yet determined. That all ideas have long and devious roots, however, is again exemplified by a sentence from Biedl [(5), p. 269] written in 1913: "Mulon even regards the corpus luteum verum as a temporary suprarenal cortex."

These baffling old problems seemed much less esoteric with the subsequent finding that, among the amazing plethora of adrenal biosynthetic products, sex hormones, including androgens and progesterone, are among those normally produced. Aberrations in the normal secretory or metabolic patterns could be expected to produce the observed effects.

Adrenal-Pituitary

In 1930 Smith (69) published a paper that was a landmark in the history of endocrinology. With impressively accurate detail it described an improved technique for hypophysectomy, a documented catalogue of the now classic major resulting deficiencies (albeit ones shown not incompatible with prolonged survival), and the simple method of administering fresh pituitary implants to achieve replacement therapy. Among other things, an atrophy of the adrenal cortex, with little if any change in the medulla, was induced by the operation and repaired by implants. He wrote: "These retrogressive changes in the cortex of the adrenal seem not to have been noted by other investigators. . . . [but based on his earlier work] they are, however, in harmony with those secured in the tadpole." Although note had been made on occasion in earlier years of gross adrenal changes associated with pituitary disease or pituitary extracts, Smith's study definitively established the important basic fact of a morphological dependence of the adrenal cortex on some pituitary influence. Over the ensuing decades the volume of literature elaborating the adrenal-pituitary relationship reminds us that "great oaks from little acorns grow." Most investigators fractionating pituitary extracts looked for and generally found in them a relatively specific adrenocorticotropin (ACTH), which after much study was synthesized as a 39-amino acid polypeptide (63).

The question of physiological details, however, turned out, as usual, to have less simple answers. What was the nature and degree of functional dependence of the adrenal on pituitary factors? For one thing, Smith's survival figures showed that hypophysectomy, unlike adrenalectomy, did not lead to early death; hence, adrenal function must not be completely dependent on the pituitary. By 1937 there was considerable but not complete agreement—Arthur Grollman persistently dissented (26)—that after hypophysectomy a deficient function of the cortex was present, reparable by extracts of the cortex:

> which is in some instances hardly detectable unless one subjects the animal to physiological stress. Such deficiencies are apparent after histamine injections, after exposure to cold, after excess water, in the secretion of milk, and probably in any other physiological response for which a high level of cortical activity is necessary (16).

The specific adrenal or pituitary hormones involved could not be identified at the time because they were not available for study. Nevertheless, Ingle & Kendall (38) immediately and convincingly demonstrated the existence of a feedback system by which pituitary stimulation of the adrenal was countered by an inhibitory effect of adrenal hormones on the pituitary. It was also evident that this feedback system could not be the only regulatory mechanism involved. If it were, the enhanced adrenal secretory activity in stress, for which indirect evidence was accumulating, could not occur. These problems still constitute an area of intensive study.

The fact that all adrenal activity had to be interpreted in terms of concomitant pituitary activity added a new dimension to an already complex problem. As usual, the development of methodology was of critical importance. The finding that adrenal stimulation by ACTH could be measured by a reduction in the number of circulating eosinophils, by reduction in adrenal cholesterol, and particularly by reduction in adrenal ascorbic acid was a tool of great utility. By 1948 the ascorbic acid depletion test, developed to a high degree of precision especially by Sayers & Sayers (62), was used by them and worldwide by others not only in the bioassay of ACTH preparations, but also in the study of physiological stimuli influencing pituitary-adrenal function. Such work permitted Sayers (61) in 1950 to write comprehensively, if at times uncertainly, on the adrenal cortex and homeostasis. At least it was evident that the interaction of pituitary-adrenal hormones with other endogenous and exogenous influences was an example *par excellence* of a delicately poised homeostatic mechanism that involved virtually all organ systems.

The inference to be drawn from this early work was that the adrenal was dependent on ACTH for the secretion of hormones involved with organic metabolism (in present terminology, glucocorticoids), but not for some life-maintaining secretion (e.g., mineralocorticoids), which under optimal, but not stressful, conditions maintained life and electrolyte balance (71). As it became possible to measure the secretion rates and levels in body fluids of the hormones concerned, this concept was in general validated. The glomerulosa layer of the adrenal, the site of aldosterone secretion, is in most species relatively, but not completely, independent of the pituitary, unlike the glucocorticoid-secreting layers (13).

STRESS

It was evident to almost all who worked on adrenal problems after 1930, and to many of their predecessors, that adrenal-deficient animals were highly susceptible to a host of noxious influences (e.g., toxins, trauma, drugs, strenuous exercise, infections, environmental change, emotional stimuli). In 1946 Selye (64) summarized his own and much other work in the field[14]. He grouped the responses to such adverse stimuli generically into a syndrome resulting from nonspecific stress and in this and related publications (65) assigned a key role to the adrenal in adaptational phenomena.

[14] Along with his extensive conventional scientific work, Selye has made two individualistic contributions to endocrine and adrenal history. His flair for neologism has added many terms to the endocrine lexicon, some widely used (e.g., mineralocorticoid, glucocorticoid), some largely forgotten (e.g., testoid). He has also been a sophisticated tormentor of rats in which he has produced ingenious experimental models of disease (e.g., steroid hypertension with attendant renal and vascular pathology; granuloma pouches for the study of inflammation); he has even induced a reptilelike shedding and replacement of the skin (66), a technique as yet little used in the scientific community and one receiving no plaudits from the rat population.

The general idea that the hormones of the adrenal, in particular the glucocorticoids, secreted at homeostatically varied rates under ACTH influence, are essential for protective reactions to any stress is apparently unquestioned. Exploration of corollary matters, however, opens a beehive of questions. For instance, to what extent does the damage of long-continued stress result from chronic hypercorticism? Adrenal hyperfunction can cause disease, as witnessed in the hypertension and hypokalemia of the syndromes of Cushing and Conn, but does it do so when the hormones are produced in a regulated response to need? These open questions (36) are raised here only to note their continued existence.

INFLAMMATION

In the mid 1940s the great interest that had prevailed for over a decade in the adrenal cortex began to wane. The private granting agencies—National Institutes of Health funds not yet being available for such purposes—began to lose interest. World War II had diverted the efforts of many. Witness the thinness of the volumes of *Endocrinology* from 1943 to 1950. Problems of physiological integration of the corticosteroids, their biochemical production, and the identity of the amorphous fraction remained, but no serious evidence that adrenal steroids would be of practical value, other than in the treatment of the rare cases of adrenal insufficiency, had come to light. A counter influence intervened, however, in the form of a false report that the Germans were increasing the effective ceiling of their aviators by use of extracts of the adrenal (42).

Under governmental sponsorship, a special effort was made to prepare and study corticosteroids as a competitive military effort. In the end the chemical work, designed to make in quantity compound E (cortisone) and its 11-oxygenated relatives, was largely in the hands of teams in the biochemical laboratories of the Mayo Foundation and in those of Merck and Company; these were led by E. C. Kendall and L. Sarrett, respectively. The war was not affected by the program, because the time required for achieving goals was insufficient and the hypotheses for projected use of the steroids sought were ill-founded. Nevertheless, as in much research, the consequences to medical history were profound.

Partial synthesis of dehydrocorticosterone (compound A) was achieved in the mid 1940s (41). Unfortunately it turned out to have no striking biological activities. Sarrett's group eventually synthesized enough cortisone to permit the discovery that made the name of this steroid a byword in the language of the street.

This discovery had no strong theoretical roots. Philip Hench at The Mayo Clinic had long been seeking a cause for the ameliorating effect of pregnancy and jaundice on rheumatoid arthritis. He thought it must be due to some natural substance present in abundance in those states. "In time [after reducing the number of other possibilities], we conjectured that the antirheumatic substance X might be an adrenal hormone" (33), a conjecture fortified, but not directly suggested, by the physiological and biochemical work of his colleague and collaborator, E. C. Kendall. The decision to try compound E in rheumatic disease was made in 1941, but sufficient material was not in hand for the trial until 8 years later (42). Hench, Kendall, Slocumb, and Polley (33) accordingly in 1949 used cortisone and ACTH in 14 patients with rheumatoid arthritis. The result, which matched in its impact on medical history that of the first therapeutic use of insulin, was summarized as follows:

> Certain clinical and biochemical features of rheumatoid arthritis have been markedly improved by the daily intramuscular injection of either the adrenal cortical hormone, 17-hydroxy-11-dehydrocorticosterone (Compound E), or the pituitary adrenocorticotropic hormone, ACTH. Articular, muscular and other symptoms were lessened notably, and sedimentation rates were reduced when either hormone was employed; when the use of them was discontinued, symptoms and signs of rheumatoid arthritis usually, but not always, returned or increased promptly. Certain clinical facts and theoretic considerations combine to suggest that these adrenal and pituitary hormones may be useful against other rheumatic diseases and against certain nonrheumatic conditions which generally are relieved by pregnancy or jaundice.

The most unusual thing about this historic discovery was its unexpectedness[15]. The original hypothesis that corticosteroids were responsible for the effects of pregnancy and jaundice is still equivocal. Dwight Ingle, neither naive nor unimaginative in the field, probably bespoke what would have been said by all "authorities" when he admits:

> With some chagrin, I recalled that years earlier Gifford Upjohn had sent me a case report of a rheumatoid patient supposedly benefited by injections of adrenal cortical extract. "Do you think that adrenal hormones might be useful in arthritis?" asked Gifford. "I can't imagine anything more unlikely" was my reply (37).

Nothing in the long study of adrenal deficiency phenomena had prepared the medical world for this bizarre pharmacological overdosage effect, the like of which Swingle and Harrop searched for in vain two decades earlier.

In any case, the age of the anti-inflammatory steroids was born, and Nobel prizes went to Kendall, Hench, and Reichstein, who themselves were well aware that the grist of many mills, awaiting the luck of the observant innovator, had gone into their notable accomplishments.

Demonstration of the wide utility of cortisone in many inflammatory diseases followed the painfully slow avail-

---

[15] A decade earlier, in 1940, the basic anti-inflammatory effect of extracts of the adrenal cortex, as manifested by an inhibition of capillary permeability to trypan blue in the presence of inflammatory exudates, was clearly demonstrated by Menkin (50, 51). He related this finding, however, to a role of corticosteroids in the vascular fluid loss of secondary shock but not to rheumatoid or related diseases. Ironically, the type of test he used is in principle one used widely now to identify potentially antirheumatic compounds, but the possible connection was not recognized at the time.

ability of supplies[16]. Until the steroid was available in large quantity, its use had to be limited, and the demand was such that a black market developed for it. The use of microorganisms in the synthetic process, along with many other refinements, finally solved the problems of supply and initial excessive cost. The next chapter was the development of modified steroid molecules (e.g., prednisolone, dexamethasone) of greater potency and greater specificity than the natural hormones. Nevertheless, side effects remain a severe limiting problem in the use of all corticosteroids in inflammatory diseases. The search for more selectively active steroids continues.

OBSEQUIES FOR ALDOSTERONE

The 20-year search for the identity of the active component of the amorphous fraction was intensified by the discovery of the antirheumatic action of cortisone for reasons not entirely logical. Those of us involved were aware that no theoretical reason existed to expect that aldosterone would be of any wide therapeutic use. But cortisone, unexpectedly, developed into a therapeutic and economic jackpot. Might not the same be true of the much more potent and mysterious amorphous factor? The answer unhappily was no. The availability of aldosterone, accomplished at great expense, has indeed permitted enormous progress in physiological and pathophysiological problems and indirectly in developing antialdosterone therapies of various sorts, especially since Conn's classic description of primary aldosteronism (11). Aldosterone, like cortisone, can cause disease. For treating disease its applications are so limited that it has not been economically worthwhile to obtain Food and Drug Administration approval to market it for human use in the United States. It is cheaper for its makers to give it away. Now after 15 years it is one of the most venerable of the legally defined *investigational new drugs* (IND status), officially available only for research purposes in the United States. It is CIBA's testament to the fact that all sound research is worthwhile for some purpose, but not necessarily profitable.

EPILOGUE

The other chapters in this volume demonstrate the growing labyrinth of physiological processes with which the corticosteroids are involved. It is clear that many new chapters are still to be written as new methods and imaginative ideas are brought to bear on the problems. In the face of this plethora of current information, one looks back with some incredulity to the three main turning points in adrenal history: to 1855, when Thomas Addison looked at the diseased adrenals of his pigmented cadavers and deduced a life-maintaining function of these glands; to 1930, when the makers of the first good extracts of the adrenal cortex looked at their bottles, wondered what was in them, and speculated on the mysterious means by which they maintained life; and to 1949, when the unexpected demonstration was made, on dubious theoretical grounds, that Kendall's compound E (cortisone) alleviated the symptoms of rheumatoid disease.

REFERENCES

1. ADDISON, T. *On the Constitutional and Local Effects of Disease of the Suprarenal Capsules*. London: S. Highley, 1855.
2. ALLERS, W. D., AND E. C. KENDALL. Maintenance of adrenalectomized dogs without cortin through control of the mineral constituents of the diet. *Am. J. Physiol.* 118: 87–94, 1937.
3. BAUMAN, E. J., AND S. KURLAND. Changes in the inorganic constituents of blood in suprarenalectomized cats and rabbits. *J. Biol. Chem.* 71: 281–302, 1927.
4. BERLIN, R. Addison's disease: familial incidence and occurrence in association with pernicious anemia. *Acta Med. Scand.* 144: 1–6, 1952.
5. BIEDL, A. *The Internal Secretory Organs. Their Physiology and Pathology*. New York: Wm. Woods, 1913.
6. BRITTON, S. W., AND H. SILVETTE. Effects of cortico-adrenal extract on carbohydrate metabolism in normal animals. *Am. J. Physiol.* 100: 693–700, 1932.
7. BRITTON, S. W., AND H. SILVETTE. The apparent prepotent function of the adrenal glands. *Am. J. Physiol.* 100: 701–713, 1932.
8. BROWN-SEQUARD, C. E. Recherches experimentales sur la physiologie et la pathologie des capsules surrenales. *Compt. Rend.* 43: 422–425, 1856.
9. BROWN-SEQUARD, C. E. Recherches experimentales sur la physiologie et la pathologie des capsules surrenales. *Compt. Rend.* 45: 1036–1039, 1857.
9a. BULLOCH, W., AND J. SEQUEIRA. On the relation of the suprarenal capsules to the sexual organs. *Trans. Pathol. Soc. London* 56: 189–208, 1905.
10. COHOE, B. A. Clinical syndromes due to suprarenal disease. In: *Endocrinology and Metabolism*, edited by L. F. Barker. New York: Appleton, 1922, vol. II, p. 317.
11. CONN, J. W., AND L. H. LOUIS. Primary aldosteronism, a new clinical entity. *Ann. Internal Med.* 44: 1–15, 1956.
12. CORI, C. F., AND G. T. CORI. The fate of sugar in the animal body. VII. The carbohydrate metabolism of adrenalectomized rats and mice. *J. Biol. Chem.* 74: 473–494, 1927.
13. DEANE, H. W. The anatomy, chemistry and physiology of adrenocortical tissue. In: *The Adrenal Cortical Hormones: Their Origin, Chemistry, Physiology and Pharmacology*, edited by H. W. Deane. Berlin: Springer Verlag, 1962, part I, p. 1–185.
14. GARRISON, F. H. History of endocrine doctrine. In: *Endocrinology and Metabolism*, edited by L. F. Barker. New York: Appleton, 1922, vol. I, p. 70.
15. GAUNT, R. Adrenalectomy in the rat. *Am. J. Physiol.* 103: 494–510, 1933.
16. GAUNT, R. The adrenal-pituitary relationship. In: *Cold Spring Harbor Symposium on Quantitative Biology*, edited by the Long

---

[16] In the original report of Hench et al. (33) the following note was appended: "Merck and Company, Inc., who have supplied compound E for this study have expressed their regret that because of the exigencies of manufacture no supplies of compound E are expected for treatment or additional research until sometime in 1950 at the earliest at which time supplies still will be exceedingly small."

Island Biological Association. Long Island, N.Y.: Darwin Press, 1937, vol. v, p. 396.
17. GAUNT, R., AND J. J. CHART. Mineralocorticoid action of adrenocortical hormones. In: *Handbuch der Experimentellen Pharmakologie*, edited by H. W. Deane and B. L. Rubin. Berlin: Springer Verlag, 1962, vol. 14, part 1, p. 513.
18. GAUNT, R., AND W. J. EVERSOLE. Notes on the history of the adrenal cortical problem. *Ann. NY Acad. Sci.* 50: 511–521, 1949.
19. GAUNT, R., AND J. H. GAUNT. Survival of adrenalectomized rats after cortical hormone treatment. *Proc. Soc. Exptl. Biol. Med.* 31: 490–493, 1934.
20. GAUNT, R., J. H. GAUNT, AND C. E. TOBIN. Colony differences in survival of adrenalectomized rats. *Proc. Soc. Exptl. Biol. Med.* 32: 888–892, 1935.
21. GAUNT, R., AND H. W. HAYS. Role of progesterone and other hormones in survival of pseudopregnant adrenalectomized ferrets. *Am. J. Physiol.* 124: 767–773, 1938.
22. GAUNT, R., J. H. LEATHEM, C. HOWELL, AND N. ANTONCHAK. Some biological properties of different esters of desoxycorticosterone. *Endocrinology* 50: 521–530, 1952.
23. GAUNT, R., AND W. M. PARKINS. The alleged interrelationship of the adrenal cortical hormone and the gonads. *Am. J. Physiol.* 103: 511–516, 1933.
24. GAUNT, R., A. A. RENZI, AND J. J. CHART. Aldosterone—a review. *J. Clin. Endocrinol.* 15: 621–646, 1955.
24a. GLYNN, E. E. The adrenal cortex, its rests and tumors; its relation to the other ductless glands and especially to sex. *Quart. J. Med. Oxford* 5: 157–192, 1911–1912.
25. GRATIOLET, P. Note sur les effects qui suivent l'ablation des capsules surrenales. *Compt. Rend.* 43: 468–473, 1856.
26. GROLLMAN, A. *Essentials of Endocrinology* (2nd ed.). Philadelphia: Lippincott, 1941, p. 54.
27. HARTMAN, F. A. The general physiology and experimental pathology of the suprarenal glands. In: *Endocrinology and Metabolism*, edited by L. F. Barker. New York: Appleton, 1922, vol. 2, p. 119.
28. HARTMAN, F. A., AND K. A. BROWNELL. The hormone of the adrenal cortex. *Science* 72: 76, 1930.
29. HARTMAN, F. A., AND K. A. BROWNELL. *The Adrenal Gland*. Philadelphia: Lea and Febiger, 1949.
30. HARTMAN, F. A., K. A. BROWNELL, AND W. E. HARTMAN. A further study of the hormone of the adrenal cortex. *Am. J. Physiol.* 95: 670–680, 1930.
31. HARTMAN, F. A., C. G. MAC ARTHUR, AND W. E. HARTMAN. A substance which prolongs the life of adrenalectomized cats. *Proc. Soc. Exptl. Biol. Med.* 25: 69–70, 1927.
32. HASTINGS, A. B., AND E. L. COMPERE. Effect of bilateral suprarenalectomy on certain constituents of blood of dogs. *Proc. Soc. Exptl. Biol. Med.* 28: 376–378, 1931.
33. HENCH, P. S., E. C. KENDALL, C. H. SLOCUMB, AND H. F. POLLEY. The effect of a hormone of the adrenal cortex [17-hydroxy-11-dehydrocorticosterone (Compound E)] and of pituitary adrenocorticotropic hormone on rheumatoid arthritis. *Proc. Staff Meeting Mayo Clinic* 24: 181–197, 1949.
34. HOUSSAY, B. A., AND J. T. LEWIS. The relative importance to life of cortex and medulla of the adrenal glands. *Am. J. Physiol.* 64: 513–521, 1923.
35. INGLE, D. J. The biologic properties of cortisone: a review. *J. Clin. Endocrinol. Metab.* 10: 1312–1354, 1950.
36. INGLE, D. J. The relationship of adrenal cortex functions to disease. *Am. J. Proctol.* 12: 245–252, 1961.
37. INGLE, D. J. From A to F. *Pharos* 77–80, July 1964.
38. INGLE, D. J., AND E. C. KENDALL. Atrophy of the adrenal cortex of the rat produced by the administration of large amounts of cortin. *Science* 86: 245, 1937.
39. IWAI, J., K. D. KNUDSEN, L. K. DAHL, AND L. TASSINARI. Effect of adrenalectomy on blood pressure in salt-fed, hypertension-prone rats. *J. Exptl. Med.* 129: 663–678, 1969.
40. KENDALL, E. C. A chemical and physiological investigation of the suprarenal cortex. In: *Cold Spring Harbor Symposium on Quantitative Biology*, edited by the Long Island Biological Association. Long Island, N.Y.: Darwin Press, 1937, vol. v, p. 299–312.
41. KENDALL, E. C. The chemistry and partial synthesis of adrenal steroids. *Ann. NY Acad. Sci.* 50: 540–547, 1949.
42. KENDALL, E. C. *Cortisone*. New York: Schribner's, 1971.
43. LOEB, R. G. Effect of sodium chloride in treatment of a patient with Addison's disease. *Proc. Soc. Exptl. Biol.* 30: 808–812, 1933.
44. LONG, C. N. H., B. KATZIN, AND E. G. FRY. The adrenal cortex and carbohydrate metabolism. *Endocrinology* 26: 309–344, 1940.
45. LONG, C. N. H., AND F. D. W. LUKENS. The effects of adrenalectomy and hypophysectomy upon experimental diabetes in the cat. *J. Exptl. Med.* 63: 465–490, 1936.
46. MAC FARLAND, W. E. The vital necessity of adrenal cortical tissue in a mammal and the effects of proliferations of cortical cells from dormant coelomic mesothelium. *Anat. Record* 93: 233–249, 1945.
47. MACKENZIE, J. J. The pathological anatomy and histology of the suprarenal glands. In: *Endocrinology and Metabolism*, edited by L. F. Barker. New York: Appleton, 1922, vol. 2, p. 273.
48. MARINE, D., AND E. J. BAUMANN. Duration of life after suprarenalectomy in cats and attempts to prolong it by injections of solutions containing sodium salts, glucose and glycerol. *Am. J. Physiol.* 81: 86–100, 1927.
49. MARSHALL, E. K., AND D. M. DAVIS. Influence of adrenals on the kidneys. *J. Pharmacol. Exptl. Therap.* 8: 525–550, 1916.
49a. MASON, H. L. Only the best is good enough. *J. Clin. Endocrinol. Metab.* 24: 1214–1218, 1964.
50. MENKIN, V. Effect of adrenal cortex extract on capillary permeability. *Am. J. Physiol.* 129: 691–697, 1940.
51. MENKIN, V. Further studies on effect of adrenal cortex extract and of various steroids on capillary permeability. *Proc. Soc. Exptl. Biol. Med.* 51: 39–41, 1942.
52. PENCHARZ, R. I., J. M. D. OLMSTED, AND G. GIRAGOSSINTZ. The survival of rats after total and partial adrenalectomy and adrenal transplantation. *Physiol. Zool.* 4: 501–514, 1931.
53. PFIFFNER, J. J. The adrenal cortical hormones. *Advan. Enzymol.* 2: 325–356, 1942.
54. PHILIPEAUX, M. Note sur l'exstirpation des capsules surrenales chez les rats albinos. *Compt. Rend.* 43: 904–906, 1155–1156, 1856.
55. ROGOFF, J. M., AND G. N. STEWART. Studies on adrenal insufficiency. IV. The influence of intravenous injections of Ringer's solution upon the survival period in adrenalectomized dogs. *Am. J. Physiol.* 84: 649–659, 1928.
56. ROGOFF, J. M., AND G. N. STEWART. Studies on adrenal insufficiency in dogs. V. The influence of adrenal extracts on the survival period of adrenalectomized dogs. *Am. J. Physiol.* 84: 660–674, 1928.
57. ROGOFF, J. M., AND G. N. STEWART. Studies on adrenal insufficiency. Influence of "heat" on the survival period of dogs after adrenalectomy. *Am. J. Physiol.* 86: 20–24, 1928.
58. ROWNTREE, L. G., C. H. GREENE, W. W. SWINGLE, AND J. J. PFIFFNER. The treatment of patients with Addison's disease with the "cortical hormone" of Swingle and Pfiffner. *Science* 72: 482–483, 1930.
59. RYNEARSON, E. H. Editorial. *J. Clin. Endocrinol. Metab.* 32: 1–2, 1971.
60. SARRETT, L. H. Partial synthesis of pregnene-4-triol-17(β), 20(β),21-dione-3,11 and pregnene-4-diol-17(β),21-trione-3,11,20 monoacetate. *J. Biol. Chem.* 162: 601–632, 1946.
61. SAYERS, G. The adrenal cortex and homeostasis. *Physiol. Rev.* 30: 241–320, 1950.
62. SAYERS, G., AND M. A. SAYERS. The pituitary-adrenal system. *Recent Progr. Hormone Res.* 2: 81–115, 1948.
63. SCHWYZER, R., AND P. SIEBER. Die total synthese des β-corticotrophins (adrenocorticotropes hormon: ACTH). *Helv. Chim. Acta* 49: 134–158, 1965.
64. SELYE, H. The general adaptation syndrome and diseases of adaptation. *J. Clin. Endocrinol. Metab.* 6: 117–230, 1946.
65. SELYE, H. *The Stresses of Life*. New York: McGraw-Hill, 1956.

66. SELYE, H. *Calciphylaxis.* Chicago: Univ. of Chicago Press, 1962.
67. SELYE, H. Hormones and resistance. *J. Pharmacol. Sci.* 60: 1-27, 1971.
68. SIMPSON, S. A., AND J. F. TAIT. Recent progress in methods of isolation, chemistry, and physiology of aldosterone. *Recent Progr. Hormone Res.* 11: 183-210, 1955.
69. SMITH, P. E. Hypophysectomy and a replacement therapy in the rat. *Am. J. Anat.* 45: 205-273, 1930.
70. STEIGER, M. VON, AND T. REICHSTEIN. Desoxy-cortico-steron (21-Oxyprogesteron) aus Δ^5-3-Oxy-ätio-cholensäure. *Helv. Chim. Acta* 20: 1164-1179, 1937.
71. SWANN, H. G. The pituitary-adrenocortical relationship. *Physiol. Rev.* 20: 493-521, 1940.
72. SWINGLE, W. W., AND J. J. PFIFFNER. An aqueous extract of the suprarenal cortex which maintains the life of bilaterally adrenalectomized cats. *Science* 71: 321-322, 1930.
73. SWINGLE, W. W., AND J. J. PFIFFNER. Studies on the adrenal cortex. I. The effect of a lipid fraction upon the life span of adrenalectomized cats. *Am. J. Physiol.* 96: 153-163, 1931.
74. SWINGLE, W. W., AND J. J. PFIFFNER. The adrenal cortical hormone. *Medicine* 11: 371-433, 1932.
75. TALBOT, J. H. *A Biographical History of Medicine.* New York: Grune & Stratton, 1970, p. 416.
76. THORN, G. W. The adrenal cortex. I. Historical aspects. *Johns Hopkins Med. J.* 123: 49-77, 1968.
77. TURNER, H. H. The presidential address to The Endocrine Society. *J. Clin. Endocrinol. Metab.* 29: 290, 1969.
78. WHEELER, T. D., AND S. VINCENT. The question as to the relative importance to life of cortex and medulla of the adrenal bodies. *Trans. Roy. Soc. Can.* 11: 125-127, 1917.
78a. WILKS, S. 1862. [Cited by Talbot (75).]
79. WOOLLEY, P. G. Adrenal tumors. *Am. J. Med. Sci.* 125: 33-46, 1902.
80. ZWEMER, R. L. Electrolyte and sugar determinations as indicators of adrenal influence on normal cell activity. In: *Cold Spring Harbor Symposium on Quantitative Biology,* edited by the Long Island Biological Association. Long Island, N.Y.: Darwin Press, 1937, vol. V, p. 323-326.

CHAPTER 2

Zonation of the mammalian adrenal cortex

JOHN A. LONG | *Department of Anatomy, University of California, San Francisco, California*

CHAPTER CONTENTS

Theories of Adrenocortical Zonation
Cell Migration Theory
   Distribution of mitoses within adrenal cortex
   Origin of glomerulosa cells from capsular fibroblasts
   Migration of labeled cells
   Site of cell death
   Adrenal regeneration
Zonal Theory
   Morphological bases for considering the zona glomerulosa as distinct functional unit
   Steroid production by the zona glomerulosa
   Morphological bases for considering inner zones as distinct functional unit
   Steroid production by inner zones
   Histochemical evidence
   Role of zona reticularis in androgen secretion
   Estrogen secretion by adrenal cortex
Transformation Field Theory
Conclusion

THE DIVISION of the mammalian adrenal cortex into three concentric zones was first made by Arnold in 1866 (1). He gave these zones their now commonly used names of zona glomerulosa, zona fasciculata, and zona reticularis. Arnold based his description primarily on the arrangement of connective tissue fibers and blood vessels within the cortex. Gottschau (59) in 1883 described the structure and arrangement of the parenchymal elements of these zones. Later workers have sometimes used different terms to describe special appearances or presumed functions of one or all of the zones, but Arnold's nomenclature has withstood the test of time and is presently in general use. It should be noted that tripartite zonation is most clearly demonstrable in adrenals containing an abundance of lipid inclusions. The adrenals of man, monkey, rat, guinea pig, and rabbit are examples of this group. In so-called lipid-poor adrenals (e.g., hamster, cow, sheep, horse) the distinction between zona fasciculata and zona reticularis is less clear. The adrenals of certain species may contain special zones in addition to the classic three zones. A zona intermedia (sudanophobic zone) has been described in a number of species, including the rat, cat, dog, sheep, rabbit, and horse (23). Howard & Migeon (76) give an authoritative account of the X zone in the mouse, while Lanman (92) describes the development of the human fetal zone. The histological appearance of the adrenals from a large number of mammalian species is illustrated in the massive compilations by Kolmer (86) and Bachmann (4). The marsupials are given special attention by Bourne (17) in a valuable book that also contains an interesting historical account of research on the adrenal.

THEORIES OF ADRENOCORTICAL ZONATION

Since the existence of histologically definable zones within the cortex is not doubted, the more interesting question becomes one of the functional significance of the various zones. Gottschau (59) first proposed that adrenocortical cells arise at the periphery, migrate centripetally, and degenerate at the border between the zona reticularis and the medulla. The cell migration or "escalator" theory was supported by a great deal of work prior to World War II, including that of Hoerr (74), Zwemer and his co-workers (116, 143, 151), and Bennett (11). This theory has also been invoked to explain regeneration of the adrenal cortex after enucleation (126) or transplantation (80).

Interest in the cell migration theory waned as support for the theory of functional zonation grew. In its essentials this theory proposes that the zona glomerulosa is relatively independent of pituitary control and that this zone secretes mineralocorticoid hormones while the inner zones (fasciculata and reticularis) depend on pituitary adrenocorticotropic hormone (ACTH) and secrete steroids that influence carbohydrate and protein metabolism (i.e., glucocorticoids). This idea was proposed by Swann in his review published in 1940 (134), and initial experimental support was provided by Sarason (117) and Deane and Greep and co-workers (37, 39, 63). The notion that the zona reticularis is responsible for the secretion of adrenal androgens slightly precedes Swann's proposal (20), but this aspect is not regarded as essential by some adherents of the functional zonation hypothesis.

A third theory, the transformation field theory has been advocated by Tonutti (137) and Chester Jones (26). According to this theory, the zona fasciculata is the actively secreting part of the gland, while the zona glomerulosa and zona reticularis are areas of reserve cells (outer and inner transformation fields, respectively) that can be transformed into actively secreting fasciculata cells when stimulated by ACTH (progressive transformation). When ACTH secretion drops below a certain level the outer and inner fields undergo regressive transformation, which leaves a smaller zona fasciculata capable of being maintained by the lower level of ACTH. In addition, the histological appearance of zona glomerulosa and zona reticularis is regained.

It is the purpose of this chapter to review some of the evidence that has been used to support or refute these theories. With the exception of the complications introduced by the fact of adrenal regeneration, it appears that the notion of functional zonation provides the best working hypothesis to explain the structural zonation of the adrenal cortex.

CELL MIGRATION THEORY

Distribution of Mitoses Within Adrenal Cortex

A number of studies have been made of the distribution of mitoses within the adrenal cortex, the underlying hypothesis being that if mitotic activity were found to be confined to the outer parts of the adrenal (capsule, zona glomerulosa, outer zona fasciculata), these data would add support to the cell migration theory. Hoerr (74) has reviewed some of the older literature on this question and has added observations of his own on the occurrence of mitoses in normal guinea pigs. He also described the recovery of the adrenal after degeneration induced by chloroform anesthesia. Hoerr concluded that cells of the adrenal cortex have a short life-span and are replaced by cells arising at the border between the zona glomerulosa and the zona fasciculata. These cells then migrate centripetally to the zona reticularis where they ultimately die. Colchicine was used by Baxter (9) to arrest the mitoses in the rat adrenal. Mitoses were observed in all zones, but the greatest number were found in the zona fasciculata. This author notes that cells of the zona reticularis may be renewed in situ since a considerable number of mitoses were observed in this zone. In a study of mitotic activity during postnatal development of the rat adrenal, Mitchell (102) concluded that two regions of high mitotic activity are present after the second week of postnatal life. One is located in the glomerulosa and the other in the outer fasciculata. These two regions are separated by the mitotically inactive sudanophobic zone (zona intermedia, zone of compression), through which Mitchell believes cells of the zona glomerulosa do not pass. This author states that cells from a capsular blastema make a contribution to the cortex only during the first week or two of postnatal life. Mitchell would support a modified cell migration theory that would encompass a nonmigrating, self-sustaining zona glomerulosa and a second proliferating population of cells in the outer part of the zona fasciculata that subsequently migrates centripetally. Walker & Rennels (141) have produced strong evidence that adrenal cells labeled with tritiated thymidine do not migrate toward the inner part of the gland. They found the great majority of labeled cells in the zona glomerulosa and outermost zona fasciculata. When adrenals were examined 21 days after tritiated thymidine injection, no appreciable inward shift of labeled cells was seen even though calculations made from the observed mitotic activity of the cortex indicated that labeled cells should have moved at least one-fourth of the distance from the capsule to the medulla if they move at all. Others (77, 78, 114) have been similarly unable to demonstrate centripetal migration. On the other hand, Diderholm & Hellman (40, 41), as well as Ford & Young (50) and Brenner (18), using tritiated thymidine labeling of rat and mouse adrenocortical nuclei, have interpreted their results as supporting the cell migration theory. Wright (144) has made a careful study of the labeling indices and lengths of the various components of the cell cycle in prepubertal rat adrenals. This author concludes that the lengthening of the duration of the cell cycle in the inner zones can be interpreted as supporting inward migration of cells originating in the outer regions of the cortex. He expresses doubt that the low rate of cell proliferation measurable in the inner zones is adequate to maintain this cell population without recruitment of cells from a more actively proliferating compartment (zona glomerulosa and outer zona fasciculata). Since the time actually taken to double the volume of the zona glomerulosa of the prepubertal rat exceeds the potential doubling time (calculated from a detailed study of cell cycle kinetics), Wright et al. (145) conclude that cell loss must occur from the zona glomerulosa. They thus add support for the notion of centripetal cell migration, at least in the prepubertal rat.

A note of caution should be added to all the above data. Most researchers have worked with rodents such as rats and mice that have been sacrificed early in the working day (8 to 12 AM). Generally overlooked has been the fact that these animals exhibit a diurnal variation in the frequency of mitoses (69, 103), with the maximum number being observed during the night. The frequency of mitoses has been shown to decline with age (15), and the number of mitoses observed rises to a maximum 4–12 hr after feeding (14). The effects of these factors on the zonal distribution of mitoses have not been evaluated.

Origin of Glomerulosa Cells from Capsular Fibroblasts

A number of workers have stressed the actual or potential capacity of capsular fibroblasts to differentiate into zona glomerulosa cells and the subsequent migration of these cells through the cortex (4, 48, 49, 116, 143, 150, 151). These studies have relied on histological and cytological observation with the light microscope to construct a series of stages in the differentiation of a fibroblast into a glomerulosa cell. Recent observations utilizing electron microscopy have denied this kind of differentiation (10, 109, 149). This question is raised again in connection with observations on the regenerative capacity of the adrenal after enucleation or transplantation.

Migration of Labeled Cells

Attempts to directly demonstrate the migration of adrenocortical cells have given equivocal results. Salmon & Zwemer (116) injected trypan blue into rats of various ages (not specified) and claimed to demonstrate the centripetal movement of adrenocortical cells containing the dye marker. They did not illustrate their most important results (a band of stained cells in the inner fasciculata with an outer band of dye-free cells in the outer zones), and subsequent workers (9, 21, 96) have not been able to confirm their results.

Site of Cell Death

A basic premise of the cell migration theory is that the zona reticularis is a region of cell death and removal. One of the classic criteria of cell death is staining of nuclei after intravital administration of trypan blue. Bennett (11) observed such cells in both the outer fasciculata ("secretory zone") and the zona reticularis ("senescent zone") of the cat adrenal while Baxter (9) observed trypan blue staining of nuclei only in the zona reticularis of the rat. The latter author also observed mitotic figures in the zona reticularis. Yoffey (148) has pointed out that alkaline and acid phosphatase activity are demonstrable in cells of the zona reticularis, and he implies that since these enzymes are present, the cells containing them are viable. Current knowledge of the role of lysosomal enzymes, of which acid phosphatase is one, in intracellular degradation and cell death renders this argument less persuasive. Mikhail (98) does not find signs of degeneration in the zona reticularis of rats up to 4 months of age. Wyllie and his co-workers (146, 147) have described a process they call *apoptosis* whereby adrenocortical cells round up, undergo condensation, and are phagocytosed. Apoptosis is more frequent after ACTH withdrawal and is also described as a normal event in the adrenal of neonatal rats. In the latter case, apoptosis is more frequently seen in the deeper zones of the gland. The authors imply that this process is the mechanism of removal of effete cells in the inner zones as required by the cell migration theory. The accumulation of lipofuscin pigment in cells of the zona reticularis has been used as evidence that these cells are older than more peripheral cells (11). However, heterogenous granules with the ultrastructural characteristics of lipofuscin have been found in cells of all zones of the human adrenal cortex (J. A. Long, unpublished observations).

Adrenal Regeneration

It would appear that cell migration has not been conclusively demonstrated in the intact adrenal and that the available data can be interpreted to support local division and replacement of cells within each zone. Only in the case of regeneration of the adrenal cortex after enucleation or transplantation is it clear that cells of the capsule and adherent remnants of the zona glomerulosa can proliferate and differentiate into a histologically and functionally normal cortex. When the capsule of the adrenal is slit and the contents of the gland gently expressed (enucleation) the remaining cells can proliferate and migrate to form the cortex (62, 81, 126). Differing opinions have been expressed as to whether the new cortex arises only from adherent zona glomerulosa cells (19, 27, 62) or whether capsular fibroblasts also can differentiate into cortical parenchyma (7, 81, 142). Recent ultrastructural studies of adrenal regeneration (105, 109) provide no evidence for differentiation of fibroblasts into cortical parenchyma.

ZONAL THEORY

Even while debate on the merits of the cell migration theory was going forward, evidence for another interpretation of adrenocortical zonation was accumulating. Swann (134) tentatively suggested that the zona glomerulosa might produce hormones responsible for maintaining electrolyte balance while the inner zones might release hormones that influence carbohydrate and protein metabolism. Only the secretions of the inner zones were thought to be controlled by pituitary ACTH. Sarason (117) and Deane & Greep (37) provided support for this theory, which was named the zonal theory by Chester Jones (24). An extension of the zonal theory specifies that the zona fasciculata is responsible for the secretion of glucocorticoids, whereas the cells of the zona reticularis secrete adrenal androgens.

Morphological Bases for Considering the Zona Glomerulosa as Distinct Functional Unit

When an animal such as the rat is hypophysectomized, the inner zones (fasciculata and reticularis) undergo atrophy while the zona glomerulosa remains essentially normal in short-term experiments. After longer periods of time (2 months) the size of glomerulosa cells does decline slightly but not as drastically as the decrease in size noted in cells of the inner zones. Atrophic changes have been noted in the zona glomerulosa of dogs hypophysectomized 6–8 weeks earlier (5, 91). The absence of ACTH cannot be implicated with certainty in this decline since the effects of deficiencies of the other pituitary hormones have not been ruled out. After hypophysectomy, mitochondria of glomerulosa cells do not change and the lipid content of these cells is maintained (37). Nuclei of glomerulosa cells do not change size after hypophysectomy or ACTH injection [(75); see (138) for an opposing view] but increase in size after treatments expected to increase aldosterone secretion (spironolactone injection) and decrease in size after injection of deoxycorticosterone acetate, a treatment that decreases aldosterone secretion (131). In recently hypophysectomized animals, aldosterone secretion is in the same range as the intact controls. Moreover, hypophysectomized animals do not lose sodium in contrast to adrenalectomized animals, which will die if supplementary NaCl is not given. These animals are also capable of responding to a low-sodium diet by an increase in aldosterone secretion [see (51) for references and further discussion].

A variety of stimuli are known to cause a selective increase in aldosterone secretion, while glucocorticoid secretion remains relatively unaffected. These stimuli include low sodium intake, high potassium intake, and injections of angiotensin II, as well as a number of other maneuvers that might be expected to stimulate the release of renin from the juxtaglomerular apparatus of the kidneys [see (51) for references]. Histological evidence of selective hypertrophy of the zona glomerulosa or other criteria of increased activity of these cells has accumulated since the classic studies of Deane et al. (39) on the response of the rat's adrenal to a low-sodium diet and high doses of parenterally administered potassium. Briefly these workers found a broadening of the zona glomerulosa and a decline in the size and number of lipid droplets within the glomerulosa cells after either of the above-mentioned treatments. These changes were seen in both intact and hypophysectomized animals. No particular changes were noted in the inner zones in response to these experimental maneuvers. These results were confirmed by Hartroft & Hartroft (73), Goldman et al. (58), and Marx & Deane (94). Hartroft & Eisenstein (72) have further studied the effects of prolonged, severe sodium depletion on steroid secretion, as well as the histology and histochemistry of the adrenal gland. They again noted the hypertrophy and hyperplasia of the zona glomerulosa, but they also found a profound atrophy of the inner cortical zones. The glomerulosa cells contained lipid globules throughout the course of the experiment, which is in contrast to the lipid loss noted by other workers studying the sodium-depleted rat. Evidence has been presented for an increase in aldosterone concentration in the peripheral blood, which is accompanied by a decline in corticosterone production under these experimental conditions (43, 44).

In rats fed a diet deficient in sodium but containing elevated levels of potassium, Kovács & David (87) have noted widening of the zona glomerulosa accompanied by increased nuclear volume. The converse was true in animals given a diet containing high quantities of sodium but no potassium. These treatments did not affect the volume of zona fasciculata nuclei. Nickerson & Molteni (106) have not been able to confirm the latter result. These authors were able to cause atrophy of the zona glomerulosa in rats only by giving sodium chloride in the drinking water. Sodium chloride added to the diet was ineffective.

A common endocrinologic technique is to administer large doses of a suspected or known secretory product of an endocrine organ and to observe cytological evidence of disuse atrophy on the part of the cells that normally secrete the exogenously administered hormone. Sarason (117) and Greep & Deane (61) made good use of this technique to demonstrate that large doses of deoxycorticosterone acetate, the most powerful mineralocorticoid known before the discovery of aldosterone, caused selective atrophy of the zona glomerulosa in the rat adrenal.

For many years, the Hartrofts and their associates have noted the correlation between zona glomerulosa width, juxtaglomerular cell granularity, and renal renin content (71). It is now believed that juxtaglomerular cells release renin, an enzyme that acts on certain plasma proteins to produce angiotensin I, which is subsequently converted to angiotensin II. The latter peptide stimulates aldosterone production by the zona glomerulosa (51). Production of experimental renal hypertension or injection of renin or angiotensin increases the width of the zona glomerulosa in the rat (38, 95) but has no effect on the histology of the inner zones of the adrenal.

Shire & Spickett (123) have reported on strain differences in adrenocortical structure in five strains of mice. They also briefly review earlier studies of interspecific variation in adrenal structure and function. Globular masses of glomerulosa cells appear to be absent in the Peru strain of mice in hematoxylin- and eosin-stained sections, but this zone is prominent in CBA and other strains of mice; F1 hybrids of CBA by Peru have a distinct glomerulosa similar to that of the CBA parent. The morphological differences between these two strains of mice has been shown to be due to genetic variation at a single locus (122). There is evidence that differences in the endogenous level of ACTH may be responsible for the differences in zona glomerulosa width in these two strains (124). Thus repeated injections of ACTH caused the zona glomerulosa of CBA mice to decline in width and thus more closely resemble the zona glomerulosa of Peru mice; conversely injections of Peru mice with dexamethasone caused a widening of the zona glomerulosa. The authors suggest that Peru mice secrete higher endogenous levels of ACTH, which in turn produces the observed narrowing of the zona glomerulosa. However, no differences in the rate of aldosterone production have been detected (132). These results could be interpreted as favoring the transformation field theory.

Steroid Production by the Zona Glomerulosa

A more direct demonstration of the biosynthetic capabilities of various parts of the adrenal has been provided by in vitro incubations of capsules stripped off the adrenal. Upon histological examination, it has been found that these strippings are composed of connective tissue fibers and cells, as well as adherent zona glomerulosa cells. A variable but small number of outer fasciculata cells are also present. The remainder of the adrenal, containing cortical cells from the fasciculata and reticularis, as well as medullary cells, can also be incubated and the steroid hormones produced by each tissue compared. Giroud et al. (53), utilizing capsules and decapsulated adrenal tissue of rats, made such a comparison and found that capsules produced about 12 times as much aldosterone as did the same weight of the remaining tissue. This group subsequently reported that ACTH had little effect on aldosterone production in a similar in vitro preparation of beef adrenals while it markedly increased corticosterone production by the decapsulated tissue (129). Similar results have been obtained by Ayres et al. (3), using capsular strippings and decapsulated adrenal tissue from the cow. Baniukiewicz et al. (8) and Haning et al. (70) have performed similar experiments using adrenals separated into capsular and decapsulated parts, as well as cell suspensions derived from capsular strippings and decapsulated glands. Adrenocorticotropic hormone greatly increases the output of corticosterone by the decapsulated gland but has a much smaller effect on corticosterone and aldosterone production from capsular gland cells. Angiotensins were found to have relatively little effect on this experimental system. Similar results have been presented by Müller (104) with the exception that angiotensin II in high concentration was shown to stimulate aldosterone output from capsular tissue without a noticeable effect on steroid output from decapsulated adrenal tissue.

When the adrenal gland is sliced into thin sections parallel to the capsule, the first sections will contain mostly glomerulosa cells and deeper sections will contain successively zona fasciculata and zona reticularis cells. The slices can then be incubated in the presence of appropriate steroid precursors and the biosynthetic capacity of the several zones evaluated. This procedure has been carried out on human (2) and beef adrenal slices (84). These workers have shown that the outer slices (from the zona glomerulosa) produce the greatest quantities of aldosterone. In addition, angiotensin II stimulates the formation of aldosterone in this experimental system.

Siebenmann (125) has reported an interesting human case of subtotal necrosis of the left adrenal gland in a patient with Cushing's syndrome. At autopsy the left gland showed almost complete destruction of the zona fasciculata and reticularis while the zona glomerulosa was preserved. The right gland showed the typical hyperplasia of Cushing's syndrome. When he extracted the steroid hormones from these tissues, 95% of the steroids in the left gland were aldosterone, the remainder were identified as cortisol and corticosterone. The hyperplasic right gland contained only 3.6% aldosterone, but 81.2% of the extractable steroids were identified as cortisol and 12.8% as corticosterone.

It would thus appear that the zona glomerulosa secretes aldosterone and that the control of this secretion is relatively independent of pituitary ACTH control.

Morphological Bases For Considering Inner Zones As Distinct Functional Unit

The inner zones of the adrenal cortex, zonae fasciculata and reticularis, secrete a variety of steroids, including glucocorticoids such as cortisol and corticosterone, as well as androgens and possibly estrogens. Adrenocorticotropic hormone from the pituitary is the principal factor governing the rate of secretion of these hormones from the inner zones of the cortex. Some of the evidence for this statement is reviewed below.

It has long been appreciated that upon complete hypophysectomy, the inner zones of the cortex undergo atrophy but that the zona glomerulosa is relatively unaffected (36). The sudanophobic zone (subglomerular zone, zona intermedia) becomes broader, but the component cells become smaller (23). Cytological signs of inactivity resulting from hypophysectomy, and seen only in cells of the zonae fasciculata and reticularis, include decrease in nuclear volume (75), decline in extent of the Golgi complex (112), decrease in the number of mitochondria (37, 99), and an increase in size of lipid droplets but a decrease in number, apparently due to their fusion [see (36) for extended discussion of this topic]. Similar changes are seen in these zones when the secretory product of these zones, cortisol or corticosterone, is administered resulting in disuse atrophy. Changes in the opposite direction are seen in cells of the zonae fasciculata and reticularis when ACTH is given, that is, increase in nuclear and nucleolar volume (99, 101), dispersal of the Golgi complex (112), and increased numbers of mitochondria (100). Acute stimulation with ACTH leads to a reduction in the size and number of lipid droplets and a decrease in the amount of cholesterol contained within these droplets (36).

The adrenolytic effects of o,p'DDD [2,2-bis(2-chlorophenyl-4-chlorophenyl)-1,1-dichloroethane] are confined to the zonae fasciculata and reticularis in the dog and rat (93) and in the human (136). Cortisol secretion is greatly diminished in the dog (139a) and the human (136) after treatment with this drug, while the aldosterone secretion rate is relatively unaffected. Several cases of congenital unresponsiveness to ACTH have been reported (97). These patients have low cortisol production rates but are able to conserve sodium and show increased aldosterone secretion while receiving a low-sodium diet. In one case the adrenal gland appeared to possess a normal zona glomerulosa, while the zonae fasciculata and reticularis were atrophic. These two clinical examples again illustrate the structural and functional independence of the zona glomerulosa from the inner zones of the adrenal cortex.

Steroid Production by Inner Zones

Stachenko & Giroud (130) have provided biochemical evidence of functional zonation in the beef adrenal. The zona glomerulosa was separated from the inner zones, and each tissue fragment was incubated separately in the presence or absence of steroid precursors. Their results indicate that only the zona glomerulosa is capable of forming aldosterone; the zonae fasciculata and reticularis produce cortisol and cortisone, whereas corticosterone can be synthesized by all zones. When added to the incubation media ACTH enhanced the production of cortisol and corticosterone but had no effect on aldosterone synthesis. Sheppard et al. (120) have provided evidence of a similar zonal separation of biosynthetic capability in the rat adrenal. Shima et al. (121) have shown very clearly that ACTH stimulates cholesterol ester hydrolysis and inhibits cholesterol esterification in the decapsulated rat adrenal with no changes being observed in these parameters in the capsular gland.

Symington (135) has reviewed his own extensive studies of morphological and biochemical zonation of the human adrenal gland and has compared his results to those of others. He has concluded that the cells of the zona fasciculata (clear cells) and the zona reticularis (compact cells) are equally capable of producing glucocorticoids, androgens, and estrogens in the unstimulated state. The clear cells are most responsive to ACTH in vitro (66). After prolonged ACTH stimulation in vivo the border between clear cells and compact cells advances toward the periphery of the gland indicating that clear cells have been depleted of their precursor stores.

Histochemical Evidence

A large number of authors have used histochemical methods to detect changes in one or more zones of the adrenal cortex. Much of this evidence can be interpreted to favor the theory of functional zonation; therefore some examples of this work are reviewed here. First, some of the underlying premises of these biochemical studies are stated. Lipid inclusions in the adrenal are thought to be sites of storage of cholesterol esters, important precursors of steroid hormones (35). Decreased content of histochemically demonstrable lipid would be an indication of increased functional activity. An important enzyme in steroid biosynthesis, Δ^5-3β-hydroxysteroid dehydrogenase can be demonstrated in tissue sections by histochemical methods. Variations in the intensity of staining are interpreted as variations in the activity of the enzyme and consequently variations in rate of steroid biosynthesis. In the Haynes and Berthet hypothesis on the mechanism of action of ACTH (73a), this trophic hormone is thought to enhance adrenal phosphorylase activity via a second messenger, cyclic adenosine monophosphate. Increased phosphorylase activity results in increased glycogenolysis and glucose 6-phosphate production. The latter then enters the hexosemonophosphate shunt and is oxidized with the formation of large amounts of NADPH, an important co-factor in steroid hydroxylations. Although this theory is no longer widely supported in its original form, histochemists have taken advantage of the fact that the localization of glycogen and glucose-6-phosphate dehydrogenase can be revealed by histochemical methods.

Elema et al. (45) have succeeded in producing acute sodium depletion in rats by intraperitoneal dialysis with 5% glucose. Increases in the activities of glucose-6-phosphate dehydrogenase and isocitrate dehydrogenase were demonstrated to occur in the zona glomerulosa by histochemical methods. These results are interpreted to indicate an increased production of NADPH, an essential cofactor for steroid hydroxylations. When total nephrectomy preceded peritoneal dialysis with glucose, the increase in histochemical activity of these enzymes is partially suppressed, suggesting a role of the renin-angiotensin system in mediating the response (46, 47). In all these experiments, the stimulus selectively affected the zona glomerulosa; enzyme activities in the zona fasciculata and zona reticularis were not changed. Cohen & Crawford (32, 33) have studied the effects of low-sodium diet on glucose-6-phosphate dehydrogenase activity over long periods of time. These authors did not find an increase in glucose-6-phosphate dehydrogenase activity until about 2 weeks after beginning the experiment. This enzymatic change was accompanied by hypertrophy and hyperplasia of the zona glomerulosa and depletion of cellular lipids from glomerulosa cells. The other zones were unaffected. These results have been confirmed by others (88, 94). Sodium restriction during pregnancy in the rat enhances the increase in width of the zona glomerulosa, as well as the intensity of staining resulting from glucose-6-phosphate dehydrogenase activity (110). In rats given injections of angiotensin, there is a correlation between glucose-6-phosphate dehydrogenase activity and increased aldosterone secretion from adrenal slices (95) and the increased width of the zona glomerulosa (90).

Glick & Ochs (54) have utilized microchemical methods to quantitate cholesterol levels in the several zones of rats, cows, and monkeys. The greatest part of the cholesterol in monkey adrenal is present as the fatty acyl ester and is present in greatest quantity in the inner zones. After ACTH stimulation, total cholesterol levels decline in the inner zones, whereas administration of cortisone leads to an accumulation of cholesterol in the same zones. Griffiths & Glick (65) have assayed 11β-hydroxylase activity in the rat adrenal using tissue slices cut through the gland parallel to the capsule. The activity of this enzyme is rather uniformly distributed in unstimulated adrenals, but in adrenals stimulated with ACTH 3 hr prior to killing, a marked peak in activity is observed at the border between the fasciculata and reticularis. Similar observations have been made on glucose-6-phosphate dehydrogenase activity in man (133) and on this enzyme, as well as 6-phosphogluconic acid dehydrogenase, in the rat (60). Kuhn & Kissane (88) have been unable to confirm the latter result, although they do report that cortisone injection causes a decline in dehydrogenase activity in the inner zones without a noticeable effect on these enzymes in the zona glomerulosa. Cohen (29) was unable to visualize changes in glucose-6-phosphate dehydrogenase activity in the rat after cold stress or hypophysectomy. Glycogen and lipid content were also visualized by histochemical methods and were shown to be depleted after cold stress, the regions affected being the fasciculata and reticularis. Animals that had been hypophysectomized 3–4 weeks previously had lost their responsiveness to cold stress.

Golder & Boyns (56) have used ^{131}I-labeled ACTH to demonstrate two peaks of binding of this hormone to sections of guinea pig adrenal. The first peak of binding is at the glomerular-fascicular border, and the second peak is in the zona reticularis. For reasons not entirely clear, dexamethasone pretreatment enhanced the labeling in these peaks but did not change the zonal distribution. A similar distribution of ACTH-stimulated adenylate cyclase activity has been revealed by the same authors (57). Recently, Orenberg & Glick (108) have utilized microchemical methods to localize adenosine 3,5-monophosphate (cyclic AMP) in sections of untreated and ACTH-treated rat adrenals. In the untreated animal, a large peak of cyclic AMP concentration is found at the border between the zona reticularis and the medulla. A second peak is found at the border between the zona glomerulosa and the zona fasciculata 35 min after a large dose of ACTH. The concentration of cyclic AMP in all zones of the adrenal is higher after ACTH administration than in the untreated control animals.

Role of Zona Reticularis in Androgen Secretion

It has been customary to state that the zona reticularis is the site of synthesis and secretion of the androgenic steroids produced by the adrenal cortex. Androgens formed by the adrenal glands include dehydroepiandrosterone, testosterone, androstenedione, and 11β-hydroxyandrostenedione. The evidence that the zona reticularis is the site of synthesis of these steroids has been and remains scanty and contradictory.

Broster & Vines (20) originally suggested that the special affinity of the zona reticularis for the dye ponceau fuscin was indicative of the presence of androgenic steroids. Other workers have not been in agreement with this concept. Bennett (11) points out that steroid hormones would be removed during dehydration of the tissue in organic solvents. Bourne (17) suggests that the structures being stained are mitochondria, whereas Symington (135) tentatively proposes that RNA may be responsible for the affinity of these cells for ponceau fuscin. Blackman (13) has also denied the specificity of the staining method used by Broster and Vines but has presented histological evidence that, in several human cases where clinical signs of masculinzation or virilization were present, the zona reticularis of the adrenal was hypertrophic.

By dissecting whale adrenals along the approximate limits of the various zones and analyzing these tissue fragments for the presence of steroid hormones, Race & Wu (111) provided the first analytic results indicating that, although 17-ketosteroids (Zimmerman chromogens) were found in all three cortical zones, over 50% of the total amounts of these steroids recovered was present in the zona reticularis. Because of the conditions under which the adrenals were collected and stored, loss and redistribution of steroid seem likely.

In a case in which the zona reticularis of a human was subsequently shown to have degenerated, careful study showed abnormally low levels of 17-ketosteroids during the terminal phase of the patient's illness. Levels of 17-hydroxycorticosteroid were normal and responded well to ACTH stimulation, while the 17-ketosteroid levels did not rise in response to ACTH (107).

Griffiths et al. (66) initially reported that 11β-hydroxyandrostenedione was a secretory product of both fascicular and reticular cells (which these workers often call "clear" and "compact" cells, respectively) from slices of human adrenals incubated in vitro. They suggested that the zonae fasciculata and reticularis should be considered a functional unit with respect to this secretory capacity. Quantitative data are not given to support this particular contention. A later study (22) was carried out on human tissue prepared by cutting frozen sections parallel to the capsule such that successive sections passed through successive histological zones of the gland. The sections were incubated in tritiated dehydroepiandrosterone (DHA), and the incubation media were subsequently assayed for the presence of DHA sulfate. When the data are plotted as amount of DHA converted to the sulfate on the ordinate versus location in the cortex as the abscissa, a prominent peak of sulfation capacity is seen in the zona reticularis. Similar data were obtained by the same method utilizing the guinea pig adrenal as experimental material (82). Finally, Vinson and co-workers (140) have studied steroid production by the adrenal of the brush possum (*Trichosarus vulpecula*). The adrenal of this marsupial is of interest because a "special" zone is present within the cortex of adult females that may comprise up to 25% of the volume of the entire gland. In vitro incubation of separated normal cortex and special zone in the presence of tritiated pregnenolone or ^{14}C-progesterone revealed that both types of tissue are capable of large conversions to androstenedione but that the special zone shows a much greater capacity for reduction of this material to testosterone. However, for the purpose of this discussion, it should be noted that the special zone present in these animals is not clearly comparable to the zona reticularis in other species.

Estrogen Secretion by Adrenal Cortex

Direct evidence that estrogens are secreted by the adrenal cortex has been difficult to obtain. Baird et al. (6) have shown that estrone and estradiol-17β are secreted by the human adrenal. However, no information is available on which zone(s) of the adrenal is responsible for this capability. Therefore no further discussion is warranted [see (64)].

TRANSFORMATION FIELD THEORY

The transformation field has not been subjected to rigorous discussion here or elsewhere. This theory is essentially an interpretation of certain histological changes that are observed in adrenals during various phases of activity. It has been clearly shown, as discussed above, that the zona glomerulosa is not a "vegetative backwater" of cells held in reserve. It would be of interest to examine with the electron microscope those cases where it is claimed that the zona glomerulosa takes on the histological characteristics of the zona fasciculata. It has been observed [e.g. (119)] that mitochondria in the several zones have characteristic appearances. If it could be shown that these differences are maintained in the face of an apparent histological transformation from glomerulosa-like to fasciculata-like cells, the transformation field theory would be seriously questioned. Another point to be taken into consideration is the fact, not generally recognized, that the zona glomerulosa is locally absent in regions of the human adrenal cortex. In these areas, zona fasciculata cells, as defined by their ultrastructural characteristics, are found just beneath the capsule. This appearance may have given rise, in some cases, to an interpretation of "transformation" of zona glomerulosa into zona fasciculata.

CONCLUSION

It would appear that none of the basic assumptions of the cell migration theory, namely, formation of new cortical cells exclusively in the capsule and/or zona glomerulosa, centripetal movement of these cells, and their ultimate death in the zona reticularis, have been unequivocally established. Only in the case of adrenal regeneration is such a sequence of events seen. Recent biochemical and histochemical studies of adrenal zonation lend support to the theory of functional zonation, and it is my opinion that this body of information is the best working hypothesis on which to base further investigation.

REFERENCES

1. ARNOLD, J. Ein Beitrag zu der feineren Structur und dem Chemismus der Nebennieren. *Arch. Pathol. Anat. Physiol. Klin. Med.* 35: 64–107, 1866.
2. AYRES, P. J., O. GARROD, S. A. S. TAIT, AND J. F. TAIT. Primary aldosteronism (Conn's syndrome). In: *An International Symposium on Aldosterone*, edited by A. F. Müller and C. M. O'Connor. Boston: Little, Brown, 1958, p. 143–154.
3. AYRES, P. J., R. P. GOULD, S. A. SIMPSON, AND J. F. TAIT. The in vitro demonstration of differential corticosterone production within the ox adrenal gland. *Biochem. J.* 63: 19P, 1956.
4. BACHMANN, R. Die Nebenniere. *Handbuch Mikroskop. Anat. Mensch.* 6: 1–952, 1954.
5. BAHN, R. C., H. E. STORINO, AND R. W. SCHMIT. The mass of the zona glomerulosa following complete anterior and posterior hypophysectomy and subtotal removal of the pars tuberalis in the dog. *Endocrinology* 66: 403–408, 1960.
6. BAIRD, D. T., A. UNO, AND J. C. MELBY. Adrenal secretion of androgens and oestrogens. *J. Endocrinol.* 45: 135–136, 1969.
7. BAKER, D. D., AND R. N. BAILLIF. Role of capsule in suprarenal regeneration studied with aid of colchicine. *Proc. Soc. Exptl. Biol. Med.* 40: 117–121, 1939.
8. BANIUKIEWICZ, S., A. BRODIE, C. FLOOD, M. MOTTA, M. OKAMOTO, J. F. TAIT, S. A. S. TAIT, J. R. BLAIR-WEST, J. P. COGHLAN, D. A. DENTON, J. R. GODING, B. A. SCOGGINS, E. M. WINTOUR, AND R. D. WRIGHT. Adrenal biosynthesis of steroids in vitro and in vivo using continuous superfusion and infusion procedures. In: *Functions of the Adrenal Cortex*, edited by K. M. McKerns. New York: Appleton, 1968, vol. 1, p. 153–232.
9. BAXTER, J. S. The growth cycle of the cells of the adrenal cortex in the adult rat. *J. Anat.* 80: 139–146, 1946.
10. BELT, W. D. Electron microscopy of the adrenal cortex of the rat. *Anat. Record* 124: 258, 1956.
11. BENNETT, H. S. The life history and secretion of the cells of the adrenal cortex of the cat. *Am. J. Anat.* 67: 151–227, 1940.
12. BERGNER, G. E., AND H. W. DEANE. Effects of pituitary adrenocorticotropic hormone on the intact rat, with special reference to cytochemical changes in the adrenal cortex. *Endocrinology* 43: 240–260, 1948.
13. BLACKMAN, S. S., JR. Concerning the function and origin of the reticular zone of the adrenal cortex. *Bull. Johns Hopkins Hosp.* 78: 180–217, 1946.
14. BLUMENTHAL, H. T. The influence of time of feeding on the periodicity in activity in thyroid and adrenal gland of normal male guinea pigs. *Endocrinology* 27: 481–485, 1940.
15. BLUMENTHAL, H. T. The mitotic count in the adrenal cortex of normal guinea pigs. *Endocrinology* 27: 477–480, 1940.
16. BLUMENTHAL, H. T. The nature of cycle variation in mitotic activity: the relation of alimentation and nutrition to this phenomenon. *Growth* 14: 231–249, 1950.
17. BOURNE, G. H. *The Mammalian Adrenal Gland*. Oxford: Clarendon, 1949.
18. BRENNER, R. M. Radioautographic studies with tritiated thymidine of cell migration in the mouse adrenal after a carbon tetrachloride stress. *Am. J. Anat.* 112: 81–95, 1963.
19. BRENNER, R. M., D. I. PATT, AND L. C. WYMAN. Cellular changes during adrenocortical regeneration in the rat. *Anat. Record* 117: 759–771, 1953.
20. BROSTER, L. R., AND H. W. C. VINES. *The Adrenal Cortex*. London: Lewis, 1933.
21. CALMA, I., AND C. L. FOSTER. Trypan blue and cell migration in the adrenal cortex of rats. *Nature* 152: 536, 1943.
22. CAMERON, E. H. D., T. JONES, D. JONES, A. B. M. ANDERSON, AND K. GRIFFITHS. Further studies on the relationship between C_{19}- and C_{21}-steroid synthesis in the human adrenal gland. *J. Endocrinol.* 45: 215–230, 1969.
23. CATER, D. B., AND J. D. LEVER. The zona intermedia of the adrenal cortex. A correlation of possible functional significance with development, morphology and histochemistry. *J. Anat.* 88: 437–454, 1954.
24. CHESTER JONES, I. Variation in the mouse adrenal cortex with special reference to the zona reticularis and to brown degeneration, together with a discussion of the "cell migration" theory. *Quart. J. Microscop. Sci.* 89: 53–74, 1948.

25. CHESTER JONES, I. The relationship of the mouse adrenal cortex to the pituitary. *Endocrinology* 45: 514–536, 1949.
26. CHESTER JONES, I. *The Adrenal Cortex*. London: Cambridge Univ. Press, 1957.
27. CHESTER JONES, I., AND M. H. SPALDING. Some aspects of zonation and function of the adrenal cortex. II. The rat adrenal after enucleation. *J. Endocrinol.* 10: 251–261, 1954.
28. CHESTER JONES, I., AND A. WRIGHT. Some aspects of zonation and function of the adrenal cortex. IV. The histology of the adrenal in rats with diabetes insipidus. *J. Endocrinol.* 10: 266–272, 1954.
29. COHEN, R. B. The histochemical distribution and metabolic significance of glucose-6-phosphate dehydrogenase activity, glycogen and lipid in the stimulated adrenal cortex. *Endocrinology* 68: 710–715, 1961.
30. COHEN, R. B. Histochemical observations on carbohydrate metabolism in the adrenal cortex of the rat, with special reference to stress and sodium depletion. In: *Major Problems in Neuroendocrinology*, edited by E. Bajusz and G. Jasmin. New York: Karger, 1964, p. 379–392.
31. COHEN, R. B. Effects of long-term sodium deprivation on the adrenal cortices of rats: a histochemical study. *Endocrinology* 77: 1043–1047, 1965.
32. COHEN, R. B., AND J. D. CRAWFORD. Distribution of glycogen, lipid and glucose-6-phosphate dehydrogenase activity in the adrenal cortex of the sodium-depleted rat: a histochemical study. *Endocrinology* 71: 847–852, 1962.
33. COHEN, R. B., AND J. D. CRAWFORD. Glucose-6-phosphate dehydrogenase activity in the adrenal cortex of the sodium depleted rat: a histochemical study. *Endocrinology* 70: 288–291, 1962.
34. COHEN, R. B., AND L. A. FAGUNDES. Observations on phosphorylase activity distribution in the adrenal cortex: effect of ACTH. *Endocrinology* 78: 220–224, 1965.
35. DEANE, H. W. Intracellular lipides: their detection and significance. In: *Frontiers in Cytology*, edited by S. L. Palay. New Haven: Yale Univ. Press, 1958, p. 227–263.
36. DEANE, H. W. The anatomy, chemistry, and physiology of adrenocortical tissue. *Handbuch Exptl. Pharmakol.* 14(1): 1–185, 1962.
37. DEANE, H. W., AND R. O. GREEP. A morphological and histochemical study of the rat's adrenal cortex after hypophysectomy, with comments on the liver. *Am. J. Anat.* 79: 117–145, 1946.
38. DEANE, H. W., AND G. M. C. MASSON. Adrenal cortical changes in rats with various types of experimental hypertension. *J. Clin. Endocrinol. Metab.* 11: 193–208, 1951.
39. DEANE, H. W., J. H. SHAW, AND R. O. GREEP. The effect of altered sodium or potassium intake on the width and cytochemistry of the zona glomerulosa of the rat's adrenal cortex. *Endocrinology* 43: 133–153, 1948.
40. DIDERHOLM, H., AND B. HELLMAN. The cell renewal in the rat adrenal studied with tritiated thymidine. *Acta Pathol. Microbiol. Scand.* 49: 82–88, 1960.
41. DIDERHOLM, H., AND B. HELLMAN. The cell migration in the adrenal cortex of rats studied with tritiated thymidine. *Acta Physiol. Scand.* 50: 197–202, 1960.
42. DOERING, C. H., J. G. M. SHIRE, S. KESSLER, AND R. B. CLAYTON. Cholesterol ester concentration and corticosterone production in adrenals of the C57BL/10 and DBA/2 strains in relation to adrenal lipid depletion. *Endocrinology* 90: 93–101, 1972.
43. EISENSTEIN, A. B., AND P. M. HARTROFT. Alterations in the rat adrenal cortex induced by sodium deficiency: steroid hormone secretion. *Endocrinology* 60: 634–640, 1957.
44. EISENSTEIN, A. B., AND I. STRACK. Effect of sodium deficiency on secretion of hormones by the rat adrenal cortex. *Endocrinology* 68: 121–124, 1961.
45. ELEMA, J. D., M. J. HARDONK, J. KOUDSTAAL, AND A. ARENDS. Acute enzyme histochemical changes in the zona glomerulosa of the rat adrenal cortex. I. The effect of peritoneal dialysis with a glucose 5% solution. *Acta Endocrinol.* 59: 508–518, 1968.
46. ELEMA, J. D., M. J. HARDONK, J. KOUDSTAAL, AND A. ARENDS. Acute enzyme histochemical changes in the zona glomerulosa of the rat adrenal cortex. II. The effect of bilateral nephrectomy either alone or followed by peritoneal dialysis with 5% glucose. *Acta Endocrinol.* 59: 519–528, 1968.
47. ELEMA, J. D., M. J. HARDONK, J. KOUDSTAAL, AND A. ARENDS. Acute enzyme histochemical changes in the zona glomerulosa of the rat adrenal cortex. III. The effect of pretreatment with deoxycorticosterone acetate on the changes seen after peritoneal dialysis with 5% glucose or after total nephrectomy. *Acta Endocrinol.* 67: 117–126, 1971.
48. ELIAS, H. Growth of the adrenal cortex in domesticated Ungulata. *Am. J. Vet. Res.* 9: 173–189, 1948.
49. ELIAS, H., AND J. E. PAULY. The structure of the human adrenal cortex. *Endocrinology* 58: 714–738, 1956.
50. FORD, J. K., AND R. W. YOUNG. Cell proliferation and displacement in the adrenal cortex of young rats injected with tritiated thymidine. *Anat. Record* 146: 125–137, 1963.
51. GANONG, W. F., AND E. E. VAN BRUNT. Control of aldosterone secretion. *Handbuch Exptl. Pharmakol.* 14(3): 4–116, 1968.
52. GIROUD, C. J. P., M. SAFFRAN, A. V. SCHALLY, J. STACHENKO, AND E. H. VENNING. Production of aldosterone by rat glands in vitro. *Proc. Soc. Exptl. Biol. Med.* 92: 855–859, 1956.
53. GIROUD, C. J. P., J. STACHENKO, AND E. H. VENNING. Secretion of aldosterone by the zona glomerulosa of rat adrenal glands incubated in vitro. *Proc. Soc. Exptl. Biol. Med.* 92: 154–158, 1956.
54. GLICK, D., AND M. J. OCHS. Studies in histochemistry: quantitative histological distribution of cholesterol in adrenal glands of the cow, rat and monkey, and effects of stress conditions, ACTH, cortisone and desoxycorticosterone. *Endocrinology* 56: 285–298, 1955.
55. GOLDER, M. P., AND A. R. BOYNS. Distribution of (^{131}I)α^{1-24}-adrenocorticotrophin in the intact guinea pig. *J. Endocrinol.* 49: 649–658, 1971.
56. GOLDER, M. P., AND A. R. BOYNS. Selective uptake of radioactivity by the adrenal cortex of dexamethasone-treated guinea pigs after the administration of ^{131}I-labeled α^{1-24}-adrenocorticotrophin. *J. Endocrinol.* 53: 277–287, 1972.
57. GOLDER, M. P., AND A. R. BOYNS. Distribution of adrenocorticotrophic hormone-stimulated adenylate cyclase in the adrenal cortex. *J. Endocrinol.* 56: 471–481, 1973.
58. GOLDMAN, M. L., E. RONZONI, AND H. A. SCHROEDER. The response of the adrenal cortex of the rat to dietary salt restriction and replacement. *Endocrinology* 58: 57–61, 1956.
59. GOTTSCHAU, M. Struktur und embryonale Entwicklung der Nebennieren bei Saugetieren. *Arch. Anat. Physiol. Leipzig* 1883: 412–458, 1883.
60. GREENBERG, L. J., AND D. GLICK. Studies in histochemistry. LX. Quantitative histochemical distribution of glucose-6-phosphate and 6-phosphogluconate dehydrogenases in rat adrenal, and the influence of adrenocorticotropic hormone. *J. Biol. Chem.* 235: 3028–3031, 1960.
61. GREEP, R. O., AND H. W. DEANE. Cytochemical evidence of the cessation of hormone production in the zona glomerulosa of the rat's adrenal cortex after prolonged treatment with desoxycorticosterone acetate. *Endocrinology* 40: 417–425, 1947.
62. GREEP, R. O., AND H. W. DEANE. Histological, cytochemical and physiological observations on the regeneration of the rat's adrenal gland following enucleation. *Endocrinology* 45: 42–56, 1949.
63. GREEP, R. O., AND H. W. DEANE. The cytology and cytochemistry of the adrenal cortex. *Ann. NY Acad. Sci.* 50: 596–615, 1949.
64. GRIFFITHS, K., AND E. H. D. CAMERON. Steroid biosynthetic pathways in the human adrenal. *Advan. Steroid Biochem. Pharmacol.* 2: 223–265, 1970.
65. GRIFFITHS, K., AND D. GLICK. Determination of the 11β-

66. GRIFFITHS, K., J. K. GRANT, AND T. SYMINGTON. A biochemical investigation of the functional zonation of the adrenal cortex in man. *J. Clin. Endocrinol. Metab.* 23: 776–785, 1963.
67. GRUENWALD, P., AND W. M. KONIKOV. Cell replacement and its relation to the zona glomerulosa in the adrenal cortex of mammals. *Anat. Record* 89: 1–21, 1944.
68. HALBERG, F., M. Z. FRANTZ, AND J. J. BITTNER. Phase difference between 24-hour rhythms in cortical adrenal mitoses and blood eosinophils in the mouse. *Anat. Record* 129: 349–356, 1957.
69. HALBERG, F., R. E. PETERSON, AND R. H. SILBER. Phase relations of 24-hour periodicities in blood corticosterone, mitoses in cortical adrenal parenchyma, and total body activity. *Endocrinology* 64: 222–230, 1959.
70. HANING, R., S. A. S. TAIT, AND J. F. TAIT. In vitro effects of ACTH, angiotensins, serotonin and potassium on steroid output and conversion of corticosterone to aldosterone by isolated adrenal cells. *Endocrinology* 87: 1147–1167, 1970.
71. HARTROFT, P. M. Juxtaglomerular cells. *Circulation Res.* 12: 525–534, 1963.
72. HARTROFT, P. M., AND A. B. EISENSTEIN. Alterations in the adrenal cortex of the rat induced by sodium deficiency: correlation of histologic changes with steroid hormone secretion. *Endocrinology* 60: 641–651, 1957.
73. HARTROFT, P. M., AND W. S. HARTROFT. Studies on renal juxtaglomerular cells. II. Correlation of the degree of granulation of juxtaglomerular cells with width of the zona glomerulosa of the adrenal cortex. *J. Exptl. Med.* 102: 205–212, 1955.
73a. HAYNES, R. C., JR., AND L. BERTHET. Studies on the mechanism of action of adrenocorticotropic hormone. *J. Biol. Chem.* 225: 115–124, 1957.
74. HOERR, N. The cells of the suprarenal cortex in the guinea pig. Their reaction to injury and their replacement. *Am. J. Anat.* 48: 139–197, 1931.
75. HOLLEY, M. P. The size of nuclei in the adrenal cortex. *J. Pathol. Bacteriol.* 90: 289–299, 1965.
76. HOWARD, E., AND C. J. MIGEON. Sex hormone secretion by the adrenal cortex. *Handbuch Exptl. Pharmakol.* 14(1): 570–637, 1962.
77. HUNT, T. E., AND E. A. HUNT. The proliferative activity of the adrenal cortex using an autoradiographic technique with thymidine-H^3. *Anat. Record* 149: 387–395, 1964.
78. HUNT, T. E., AND E. A. HUNT. A radioautographic study of the proliferative activity of adrenocortical and hypophyseal cells of the rat at different periods of the estrous cycle. *Anat. Record* 156: 361–368, 1966.
79. IDELMAN, S. Contribution a la cytophysiologie infrastructurale de la corticosurrenale chez le rat albinos. *Ann. Sci. Nat. Zool.* 8: 205–362, 1966.
80. INGLE, D. J., AND G. M. HIGGINS. Autotransplantation and regeneration of the adrenal gland. *Endocrinology* 22: 458–464, 1938.
81. INGLE, D. J., AND G. M. HIGGINS. Regeneration of the adrenal gland following enucleation. *Am. J. Med. Sci.* 196: 232–239, 1938.
82. JONES, T., AND K. GRIFFITHS. Ultramicrochemical studies on the site of formation of dehydroepiandrosterone sulphate in the adrenal cortex of the guinea pig. *J. Endocrinol.* 42: 559–565, 1968.
83. JONES, T., M. GROOM, AND K. GRIFFITHS. Steroid biosynthesis by cultures of normal human adrenal tissue. *Biochem. Biophys. Res. Commun.* 38: 355–361, 1970.
84. KAPLAN, N. M., AND F. C. BARTTER. The effect of ACTH, renin, angiotensin II, and various precursors on biosynthesis of aldosterone by adrenal slices. *J. Clin. Invest.* 41: 715–724, 1962.
85. KNIGGE, K. M. The effect of hypophysectomy on the adrenal gland of the hamster (*Mesocricetus auratus*). *Am. J. Anat.* 94: 255–271, 1954.
86. KOLMER, W. Zur vergleichenden Histologie, Zytologie und Entwicklungsgeschichte der Saugernebenniere. *Arch. Mikroskop. Anat.* 91: 1–139, 1918.
87. KOVÁCS, K., AND M. A. DAVID. Effect of cortisone on the morphological reactions of the adrenal cortex due to changes in the Na/K intake. *Acta Anat.* 36: 169–181, 1959.
88. KUHN, C., III, AND J. M. KISSANE. Quantitative histochemistry of glucose-6-phosphate dehydrogenase and 6-phosphogluconate dehydrogenase in rat adrenal cortex: effect of ACTH, cortisone and sodium deprivation. *Endocrinology* 75: 741–746, 1964.
89. LAMBERG, B. A., T. PETTERSSON, A. GORDIN, AND R. KARLSSON. The effect of synthetic angiotensin-II-amide and Methopyrapone (SU 4885) on the histochemistry of the adrenal cortex of intact and hypophysectomized rats. *Acta Endocrinol.* 54: 428–438, 1967.
90. LAMBERG, B. A., T. PETTERSSON, AND R. KARLSSON. The effect of corticotropin and synthetic angiotensin on the glucose-6-phosphate and the succinic acid dehydrogenases in the adrenal cortex of the rat. *Acta Med. Scand. Suppl.* 412: 215–220, 1964.
91. LANE, N., AND R. C. DEBODO. Generalized adrenocortical atrophy in hypophysectomized dogs and correlated functional studies. *Am. J. Physiol.* 168: 1–19, 1952.
92. LANMAN, J. T. The fetal zone of the adrenal gland. Its developmental course, comparative anatomy, and possible physiologic functions. *Medicine* 32: 389–430, 1953.
93. LUSE, S. Fine structure of adrenal cortex. In: *The Adrenal Cortex*, edited by A. B. Eisenstein. Boston: Little, Brown, 1967, p. 1–59.
94. MARX, A. J., AND H. W. DEANE. Histophysiologic changes in the kidney and adrenal cortex in rats on a low-sodium diet. *Endocrinology* 73: 317–328, 1963.
95. MARX, A. J., H. W. DEANE, T. F. MOWLES, AND H. SHEPPARD. Chronic administration of angiotensin in rats: changes in blood pressure, renal and adrenal histophysiology and aldosterone production. *Endocrinology* 73: 329–337, 1963.
96. McPHAIL, M. K. Trypan blue and growth of the adrenal cortex in mice. *Nature* 153: 460, 1944.
97. MIGEON, C. J., F. M. KENNY, A. KOWARSKI, C. A. SNIPES, J. S. SPAULDING, J. W. FINKELSTEIN, AND R. M. BLIZZARD. The syndrome of congenital adrenocortical unresponsiveness to ACTH. Report of six cases. *Pediat. Res.* 2: 501–513, 1968.
98. MIKHAIL, Y. A study of some of the histological and histochemical features of the zona reticularis. *Acta Anat.* 84: 498–508, 1973.
99. MILLER, R. A. Cytological phenomena associated with experimental alterations of secretory activity in the adrenal cortex of mice. *Am. J. Anat.* 86: 405–437, 1950.
100. MILLER, R. A. The relation of mitochondria to secretory activity in the fascicular zone of the rat's adrenal. *Am. J. Anat.* 92: 329–359, 1953.
101. MILLER, R. A. Quantitative changes in the nucleolus and nucleus as indices of adrenal cortical secretory activity. *Am. J. Anat.* 95: 497–522, 1954.
102. MITCHELL, R. M. Histological changes and mitotic activity in the rat adrenal during postnatal development. *Anat. Record* 101: 161–185, 1948.
103. MÜHLEMANN, H. R., T. M. MARTHALER, AND P. LOUSTALOT. Daily variations in mitotic activity of adrenal cortex, thyroid and oral epithelium of the rat. *Proc. Soc. Exptl. Biol. Med.* 90: 467–468, 1955.
104. MÜLLER, J. Steroidogenic effect of stimulators of aldosterone biosynthesis upon separate zones of the rat adrenal cortex.

Influence of sodium and potassium deficiency. *European J. Clin. Invest.* 1: 180–187, 1970.

105. NICKERSON, P. A., A. C. BROWNIE, AND F. R. SKELTON. An electron microscopic study of the regenerating adrenal gland during the development of adrenal regeneration hypertension. *Am. J. Pathol.* 57: 335–364, 1969.

106. NICKERSON, P. A., AND A. MOLTENI. Reexamination of the relationship between high sodium and the adrenal zona glomerulosa in the rat. *Cytobiology* 5: 125–138, 1972.

107. OFSTAD, J., J. LAMVIK, K. F. STØA, AND R. EMBERLAND. Adrenal steroid synthesis in amyloid degeneration localized exclusively to the zona reticularis. *Acta Endocrinol.* 37: 321–328, 1961.

108. ORENBERG, E. K., AND D. GLICK. Quantitative histologic distribution of adenosine-3′,5′-monophosphate in the rat adrenal and effect of adrenocorticotropin. *J. Histochem. Cytochem.* 20: 923–928, 1972.

109. PENNEY, D. P., D. I. PATT, AND W. C. DIXON, JR. The fine structure of regenerating adrenocortical autotransplants in the rat. *Anat. Record* 146: 319–335, 1963.

110. POHANKA, D. G., AND R. L. PIKE. Effects of dietary sodium restriction during pregnancy on the histochemistry of the rat zona glomerulosa. *Proc. Soc. Exptl. Biol. Med.* 133: 246–251, 1970.

111. RACE, G. J., AND H. M. WU. Adrenal cortex functional zonation in the whale (*Physeter catadon*). *Endocrinology* 68: 156–158, 1961.

112. REESE, J. D., AND H. D. MOON. The Golgi apparatus of the cells of the adrenal cortex after hypophysectomy and on the administration of the adrenocorticotropic hormone. *Anat. Record* 70: 543–556, 1938.

113. REITER, R. J., AND R. A. HOFFMAN. Adrenocortical cytogenesis in the adult male golden hamster. A radioautographic study using tritiated-thymidine. *J. Anat.* 101: 723–729, 1967.

114. REITER, R. J., AND D. J. PIZZARELLO. Radioautographic study of cellular replacement in the adrenal cortex of male rats. *Texas Rep. Biol. Med.* 24: 189–194, 1966.

115. SABATINI, D. D., AND E. D. P. DE ROBERTIS. Ultrastructural zonation of adrenocortex in the rat. *J. Biophys. Biochem. Cytol.* 9: 105–119, 1961.

116. SALMON, T. N., AND R. L. ZWEMER. A study of the life history of corticoadrenal gland cells of the rat by means of trypan blue injections. *Anat. Record* 80: 421–429, 1941.

117. SARASON, E. L. Morphologic changes in the rat's adrenal cortex under various experimental conditions. *Arch. Pathol.* 35: 373–390, 1943.

118. SCHOR, N. A., AND D. GLICK. Determination of 3β-hydroxysteroid dehydrogenase system in microgram samples of tissue, quantitative histologic distribution of the enzyme in the rat adrenal and effects of adrenocorticotropin. *J. Histochem. Cytochem.* 15: 166–171, 1967.

119. SHELTON, J. H., AND A. L. JONES. The fine structure of the mouse adrenal cortex and the ultrastructural changes in the zona glomerulosa with low and high sodium diets. *Anat. Record* 170: 147–182, 1971.

120. SHEPPARD, H., R. SWENSON, AND T. F. MOWLES. Steroid biosynthesis by rat adrenal: functional zonation. *Endocrinology* 73: 819–824, 1963.

121. SHIMA, S., M. MITSUNAGA, AND T. NAKAO. Effect of ACTH on cholesterol dynamics in rat adrenal tissue. *Endocrinology* 90: 808–814, 1972.

122. SHIRE, J. G. M. A strain difference in the adrenal zona glomerulosa determined by one gene-locus. *Endocrinology* 85: 415–422, 1969.

123. SHIRE, J. G. M., AND S. G. SPICKETT. Genetic variation in adrenal structure: qualitative differences in the zona glomerulosa. *J. Endocrinol.* 39: 277–284, 1967.

124. SHIRE, J. G. M., AND J. STEWART. The zona glomerulosa and corticotrophin: a genetic study in mice. *J. Endocrinol.* 55: 185–193, 1972.

125. SIEBENMANN, R. E. Zur Lokalisation der Aldosteronbildung in der menschlichen Nebennierenrinde. *Schweiz. Med. Wochschr.* 89: 837–841, 1959.

126. SKELTON, F. R. Adrenal regeneration and adrenal-regeneration hypertension. *Physiol. Rev.* 39: 162–182, 1959.

127. SÓLYOM, J. Effect of sodium depletion and loading on the in vitro steroid production by the capsular and decapsulated adrenal gland of the rat. *Endokrinologie* 61: 92–96, 1973.

128. STACHENKO, J., AND C. J. P. GIROUD. Functional zonation of the adrenal cortex: pathways of corticosteroid biogenesis. *Endocrinology* 64: 730–742, 1959.

129. STACHENKO, J., AND C. J. P. GIROUD. Functional zonation of the adrenal cortex: site of ACTH action. *Endocrinology* 64: 743–752, 1959.

130. STACHENKO, J., AND C. J. P. GIROUD. Further observations on the functional zonation of the adrenal cortex. *Can. J. Biochem.* 42: 1777–1786, 1964.

131. STARK, E., M. PALKOVITS, J. FACHET, AND B. HAJTMAN. Adrenocortical nuclear volume and adrenocortical function. *Acta Med. Hung.* 21: 263–269, 1965.

132. STEWART, J., R. FRASER, V. K. PAPAIOANNOU, AND A. TAIT. Aldosterone production and the zona glomerulosa: a genetic study. *Endocrinology* 90: 968–972, 1972.

133. STUDZINSKI, G. P., T. SYMINGTON, AND J. K. GRANT. Triphosphopyridine-linked dehydrogenases in the adrenal cortex in man—effect of corticotrophin and distribution of enzymes. *Biochem. J.* 78: 4–5P, 1961.

134. SWANN, H. G. The pituitary-adrenocortical relationship. *Physiol. Rev.* 20: 493–521, 1940.

135. SYMINGTON, T. *Functional Pathology of the Human Adrenal Gland.* Baltimore: Williams and Wilkins, 1969.

136. TEMPLE, T. E., JR., D. J. JONES, JR., G. W. LIDDLE, AND R. N. DEXTER. Treatment of Cushing's disease. Correction of hypercortisolism by o,p'DDD without induction of aldosterone deficiency. *New Engl. J. Med.* 281: 801–805, 1969.

137. TONUTTI, E. Uber die strukturelle Funktionsanpassung der Nebennierenrinde. *Endokrinologie* 28: 1–15, 1951.

138. TONUTTI, E., F. BAHNER, AND E. MUSCHKE. Die Veranderungen der Nebennierenrinde der Maus nach Hypophysektomie und nach ACTH-Behandlung, quantitativ betrachtet am Verhalten der Zellkernvolumina. *Endokrinolgie* 31: 266–284, 1954.

139. VAN DORP, A. W. V., AND H. W. DEANE. A morphological and cytochemical study of the postnatal development of the rat's adrenal cortex. *Anat. Record* 107: 265–281, 1950.

139a. VILAR, O., AND W. W. TULLNER. Effects of o,p'DDD on histology and 17-hydroxycorticosteroid output of the dog adrenal cortex. *Endocrinology* 65: 80–86, 1959.

140. VINSON, G. P., J. G. PHILLIPS, I. CHESTER JONES, AND W. N. TSANG. Functional zonation of adrenocortical tissue in the brush possum (*Trichosurus vulpecula*). *J. Endocrinol.* 49: 131–140, 1971.

141. WALKER, B. E., AND E. G. RENNELS. Adrenal cortical cell replacement in the mouse. *Endocrinology* 68: 365–374, 1961.

142. WILLIAMS, R. G. Studies of adrenal cortex: regeneration of the transplanted gland and the vital quality of autogenous grafts. *Am. J. Anat.* 81: 199–231, 1947.

143. WOTTON, R. M., AND R. L. ZWEMER. A study of the cytogenesis of cortico-adrenal cells in the cat. *Anat. Record* 86: 409–416, 1943.

144. WRIGHT, N. A. Cell proliferation in the prepubertal male rat adrenal cortex: an autoradiographic study. *J. Endocrinol.* 49: 599–609, 1971.

145. WRIGHT, N. A., D. VONCINA, AND A. R. MORLEY. An attempt to demonstrate cell migration from the zona glomerulosa in the prepubertal male rat adrenal cortex. *J. Endocrinol.* 59: 451–459, 1973.

146. WYLLIE, A. H., J. F. R. KERR, AND A. R. CURRIE. Cell death in the normal neonatal rat adrenal cortex. *J. Pathol.* 111: 255–261, 1973.

147. Wyllie, A. H., J. F. R. Kerr, I. A. M. Macaskill, and A. R. Currie. Adrenocortical cell deletion: the role of ACTH. *J. Pathol.* 111: 85–94, 1973.
148. Yoffey, J. M. The suprarenal cortex: the structural background. In: *The Suprarenal Cortex*, edited by J. M. Yoffey. London: Butterworths, 1953, p. 31–38.
149. Zelander, T. Ultrastructure of mouse adrenal cortex. An electron microscopical study in intact and hydrocortisone-treated male adults. *J. Ultrastruct. Res. Suppl.* 2, 1959.
150. Zwemer, R. L. A study of adrenal cortex morphology. *Am. J. Pathol.* 12: 107–114, 1936.
151. Zwemer, R. L., R. M. Wotton, and M. G. Norkus. A study of corticoadrenal cells. *Anat. Record* 72: 249–263, 1938.

CHAPTER 3

Ultrastructure of the mammalian adrenal cortex in relation to secretory function

SASHA MALAMED | *College of Medicine and Dentistry of New Jersey, Rutgers Medical School, Piscataway, New Jersey*

CHAPTER CONTENTS

Adrenocortical Cell Organelles
  Smooth endoplasmic reticulum
  Mitochondria
  Lipid droplets
  Other organelles
Organelles and Steroidogenesis
Ultrastructural Changes with Functional Activity
  Zona glomerulosa
  Zona fasciculata and zona reticularis
Summary and Discussion

ADRENOCORTICAL CELL ORGANELLES

Electron microscopy reveals three outstanding ultrastructural features of mammalian parenchymal cells of the adrenal cortex (Figs. 1–3, 5, 6, 8–10) and of certain cells of other steroid-secreting glands (testicular interstitial, ovarian interstitial, theca interna, and corpora lutea cells): *1*) an abundance of smooth (nonribosome-studded) membranes of the endoplasmic reticulum and a relative lack of rough endoplasmic reticulum (with ribosomes); *2*) mitochondria differing in structure from those of most other cells; and *3*) many, large fat droplets or liposomes. In addition, septate-like cell contacts recently have been suggested as a possible distinctive characteristic of adrenocortical and other steroidogenic cells (20).

Smooth Endoplasmic Reticulum

The original electron-microscopic studies resulted in frequent reports of numerous, apparently discrete vacuoles or vesicles in the cytoplasm (30). Findings with newer preparative methods for electron microscopy (Figs. 1–3, 5, 6, 8–10) suggest that these structures are artificial modifications of an extensive network of tubules [Fig. 4; (8, 38, 40, 52)]. The agranular reticulum is generally most abundant in the cells of the zona reticularis and least abundant in those of the zona glomerulosa (18, 52), but the opposite is true for the Mongolian gerbil (49). Man is among the mammals that are the richest in adrenocortical smooth reticulum (18).

Mitochondria

Typically the mitochondria of mammalian cells, for example, liver parenchymal cells, have inner membrane infoldings that are lamellar, shelflike intrusions (cristae) into the mitochondrial matrices (Fig. 7A). In contrast, although some adrenocortical mitochondria may have cristae, characteristically they have tubular, fingerlike invaginations of their inner membranes (Figs. 3 and 5) or even vesicles that have been thought to be portions of these infoldings [Figs. 2, 6, 10; (54)]. Recent evidence (4) indicates that these seemingly "free-floating" vesicles in the mitochondrial matrix of bovine adrenocortical cells are actually sections through dilated portions of tubular infoldings of the inner mitochondrial membranes; "bottlenecks" alternate with these spheroid portions of the tubes that appear predominantly as vesicles because the plane of section seldom passes through a series of narrow bottlenecks connecting adjacent wide portions of the tubes. Other findings from the author's laboratory (unpublished observations) suggest a similar interpretation of electron micrographs of rat adrenocortical mitochondria (Fig. 6). Stereograms of these different mitochondrial forms are shown in Figure 7.

Many mammalian adrenal cortices show zonal differences in mitochondrial morphology, generally ranging from lamellar or tubular membranes in the mitochondria of the zona glomerulosa to tubular or vesicular membranes in those of the zona reticularis. The mitochondria of the zona fasciculata either are intermediate in form or resemble those of the inner zone (8, 17, 18, 30, 38–40, 49, 52, 54, 59). This zonation is so pronounced in the rat that cells of the zona glomerulosa may be identified by their tubular mitochondrial mem-

The author's electron micrographs in this chapter were produced with the partial support of National Institutes of Health Grant FR 05576.

profiles seen in such mitochondria are longitudinal sections through lamellar membrane infoldings, rather than longitudinal sections through tubular infoldings. Figure 7, *A* and *B*, shows the similarity between the two-dimensional views of longitudinal sections through either a lamellar or a tubular infolding of the inner mitochondrial membrane.)

Lipid Droplets

Spheroidal dark bodies up to a few microns in diameter are seen in all three zones of the adrenal cortex

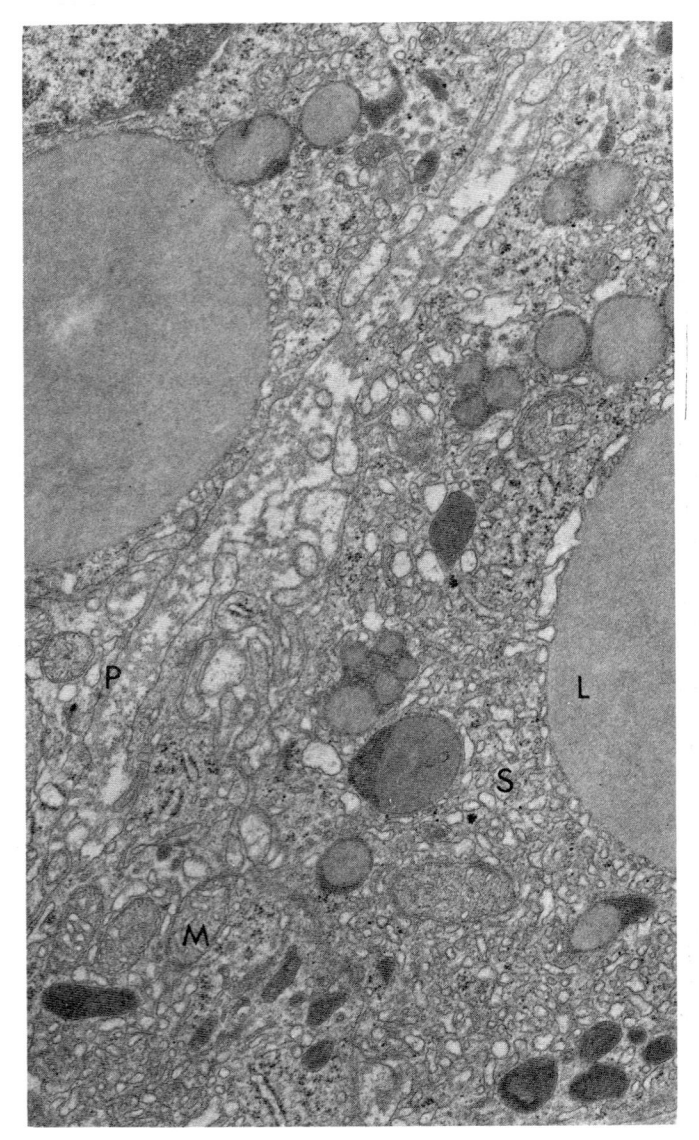

FIG. 1. Section of human adrenal cortex. Portions of 2 cells are seen, separated by connective tissue. Lipid droplets vary greatly in size. *S*, smooth endoplasmic reticulum; *M*, mitochondrion; *L*, lipid droplet; *P*, plasma membrane. × 21,100. (Electron micrograph prepared from a tissue block from the laboratory of the late Helen Wendler Deane, a friend and colleague who contributed greatly to our knowledge of the adrenal cortex.)

branes, and those of the zona fasciculata by their mitochondrial vesicles, albeit there is some disagreement about the zona reticularis (30, 52, 54). On the other hand, the mitochondria of the guinea pig adrenal cortex are similar in all its zones. Earlier work showed that these mitochondria have lamellar infoldings (60). A recent study by the author (unpublished observations) using newer methods of fixation and embedding revealed only the tubular type. (Strictly speaking, the adjective *tubular* as used in most instances above should be *tubulolamellar*, because without serial sectioning the possibility cannot be excluded that the long, U-shaped

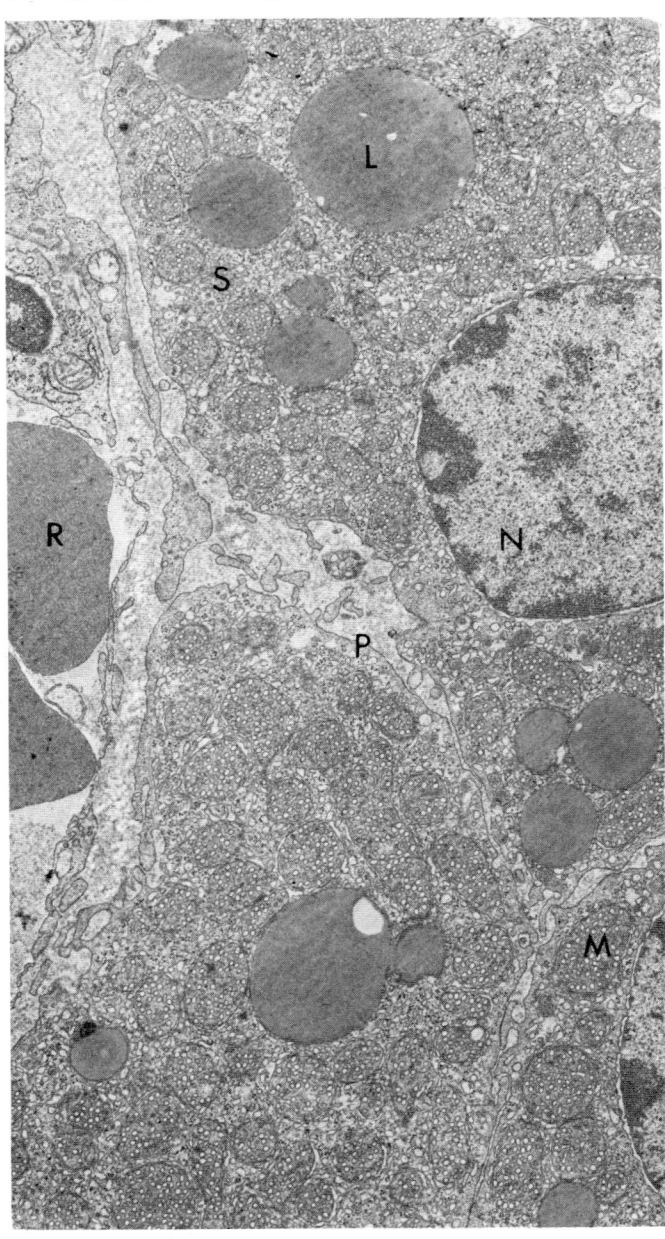

FIG. 2. Section of rat adrenal cortex. Portions of 3 cells are seen, separated by connective tissue. A portion of a capillary with red blood cells is also seen. *S*, smooth endoplasmic reticulum; *M*, mitochondrion; *L*, lipid droplet; *P*, plasma membrane; *N*, nucleus; *R*, red blood cell. × 8,780.

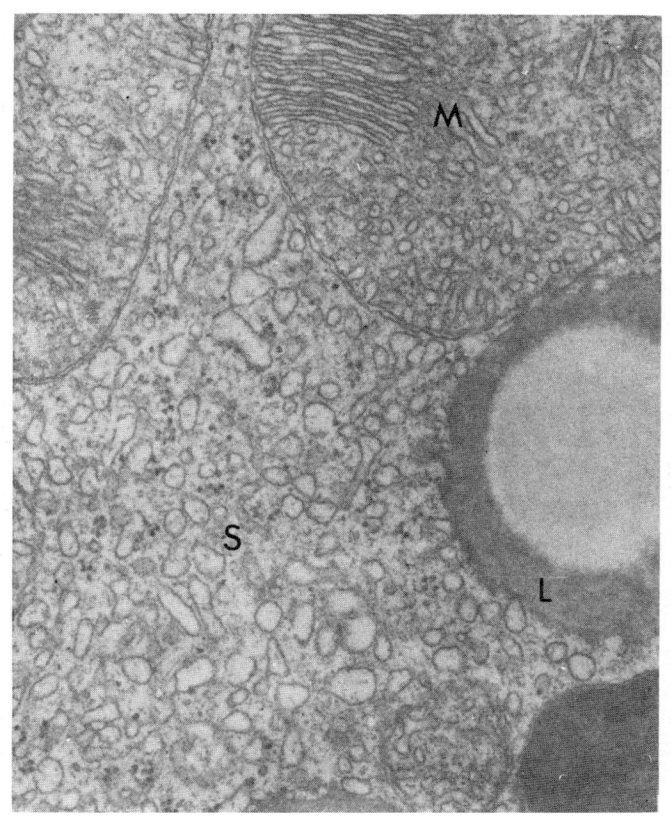

FIG. 3. Section of guinea pig adrenal cortex. Sections of the interconnecting system of tubules (see Fig. 4) termed smooth endoplasmic reticulum are seen in the center of electron micrograph. Central portion of lipid droplet has been dissolved by solvents used in preparation of tissue for electron microscopy. S, smooth endoplasmic reticulum; M, mitochondrion; L, lipid droplet. × 35,200.

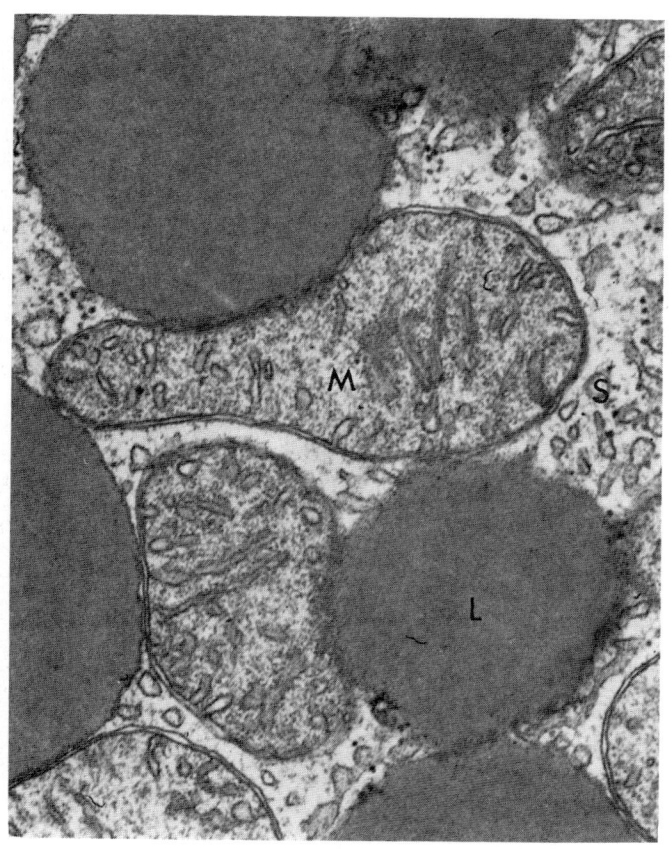

FIG. 5. Section of rat zona glomerulosa. Mitochondria here show inner membrane infoldings that may be interpreted as sections at random planes through tubules only, or through tubules and lamellae (see Fig. 7, A and B). S, smooth endoplasmic reticulum; M, mitochondrion; L, lipid droplet. × 42,700.

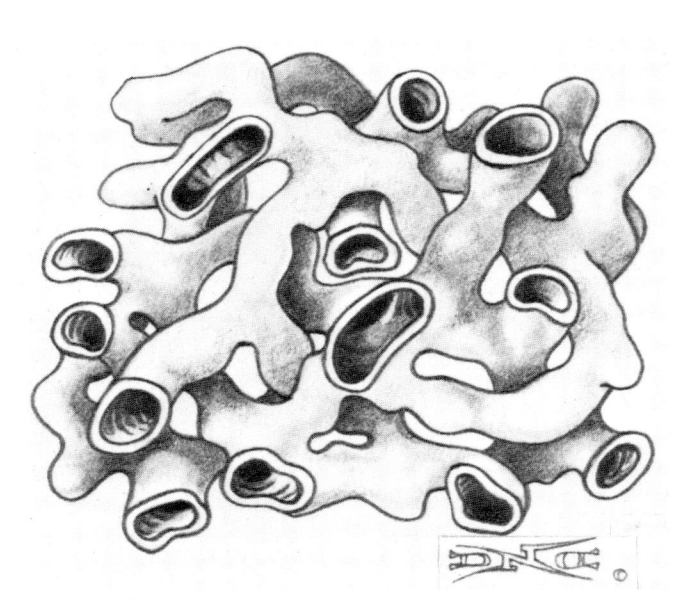

FIG. 4. Stereogram of smooth endoplasmic reticulum. Cut surface of block reveals two-dimensional profiles characteristically seen in electron micrographs (see Fig. 3).

(Figs. 1–3, 4, 8–10). They were studied extensively with the light microscope before the advent of electron microscopy. The relative frequency of these lipid droplets (liposomes) among the adrenal zones varies with the species (11, 49). They are especially abundant in both the inner and outer zones in man and the rat (18, 39, 52), but are sparse and limited to the zona glomerulosa in the hamster, spiny hedgehog, and ground squirrel (11). In contrast, the lipid droplets of the mouse, guinea pig, cat, and macaque are infrequent only in the zona glomerulosa, being relatively abundant in the inner zones (11).

Although the electron density may not be uniform within the fat droplet, a discernible substructure other than a possible limiting membrane has yet to be reported. The darkness or electron density of these bodies results from the electron-absorbing capacity of osmium tetroxide, which is commonly used in fixation and which stains the droplets. This osmiophilia is routinely used as a sign of lipid content [see (11), p. 50]. Another indication that these structures are lipid is that they frequently appear partially electron translucent or vacuolar due to the use of lipid solvents in the dehydration procedures routine in electron microscopy [Figs. 3 and

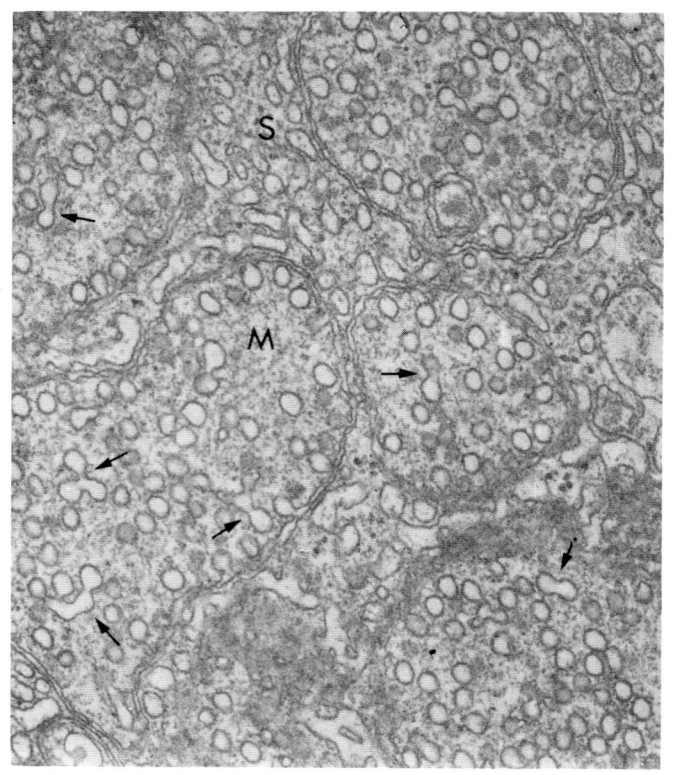

FIG. 6. Section of rat zona fasciculata. Circular profiles in mitochondrial matrices may be interpreted as sections through vesicles (see Fig. 7C) or as sections through branching tubules with bulbous portions alternating with constricted portions (see Fig. 7D). However, several profiles (*arrows*) cannot be interpreted as separate vesicles; they clearly represent sections through spheroid membranous shapes that have narrow interconnections. S, smooth endoplasmic reticulum; M, mitochondrion. × 42,700.

8; (28, 48)]. Their lipid nature is further borne out by their "washed out" appearance after methanol-chloroform (26) or acetone treatment (30). Most probably a large component of this lipid is cholesterol, the great bulk of which is esterified (11, 21, 24, 48, 51). At this time little more is known of the chemical composition of the lipid droplets. The question of whether these cell inclusions have an enveloping membrane and whether such a membrane, if seen, is real or artifact (15) is still unanswered [Fig. 8; (6, 30, 38, 39, 52)]. In any case, when the presence of a membrane is reported, it is always described as single, that is, lacking the dark-light-dark lamination of the tripartite "unit" membrane common to so many cell constituents (53).

About 75% of the total cholesterol of the rat adrenal is found in the lipid droplets (48), whether the cholesterol comes from the blood plasma or is made in the cells. In the latter case the synthesis is thought to occur in the smooth endoplasmic reticulum (see section ORGANELLES AND STEROIDOGENESIS; see also Fig. 11), and about 8% of the total cholesterol is found here (48). The close proximity of these smooth membranes to the fat droplets (Figs. 3, 5, 8–10) suggests some functional relationship (8, 30, 32, 38, 52), perhaps even that the origin of the fat droplets is within the tubules of the smooth membranes (30, 52). In this connection, laminated electron-opaque cell inclusions seen as yet only in guinea pig adrenocortical cells (Fig. 9) may represent an intermediate step in the conversion of smooth membranes to fat droplets (or vice versa) and thus may be a mechanism for the transfer of cholesterol between these cell organelles (41, 42). The concentrically arranged unit membranes of these bodies are similar to those disposed more loosely as a reticulum in the surrounding cytoplasm. The laminated bodies have an overall electron opacity similar to that of the fat droplets; indeed portions of the laminated bodies may appear as homogenous (nonlaminated) as fat droplets.

Other Organelles

Aside from the endoplasmic reticulum, mitochondria, and lipid droplets, other inclusions of adrenocortical cells have been described: Golgi complex (18, 39, 52), free ribosomes or polysomes (39, 52), glycogen (39, 52), whorled membranous bodies (52), microtubules (52), lysosomes (18, 30, 39, 52), lipofuscin bodies (18, 30, 39), microbodies (27), and dense bodies (52). Lipofuscin bodies may be a type of lysosome.

ORGANELLES AND STEROIDOGENESIS

The frequent grouping of smooth endoplasmic reticulum, mitochondria, and lipid droplets close to each other suggests some functional interaction (Figs. 3, 5, 8–10). The chemical evidence supports this view and is discussed in this section.

There is general agreement about the intracellular localization of the major steps in the synthesis of corticosteroids, despite the facts that species differences exist and that dual locations of some enzymes have been reported. Several concise summaries of the cell fractionation studies have appeared (10, 30, 40, 52). Figure 11 is a simplified scheme derived from several sources (14, 18, 19, 22, 40). Reference to this scheme shows that progesterone is a precursor of all the other corticosteroids. The mineralocorticoid hormone aldosterone is made in the cells of the zona glomerulosa. Corticosterone, the glucocorticoid hormone that is secreted by the cells of the inner adrenocortical zones of some mammals, such as the rat, is synthesized via the same, albeit shorter, pathway as the one for aldosterone. However, the chief glucocorticoid secretion of the majority of mammals, for example, the guinea pig and man, is cortisol (25, 56), which is synthesized by a pathway that deviates from the others after the production of progesterone [see (14), p. 130, 203].

Only two cell organelles, the smooth endoplasmic reticulum and the mitochondria, appear in the scheme of Figure 11. No steroidogenic enzymes are reported

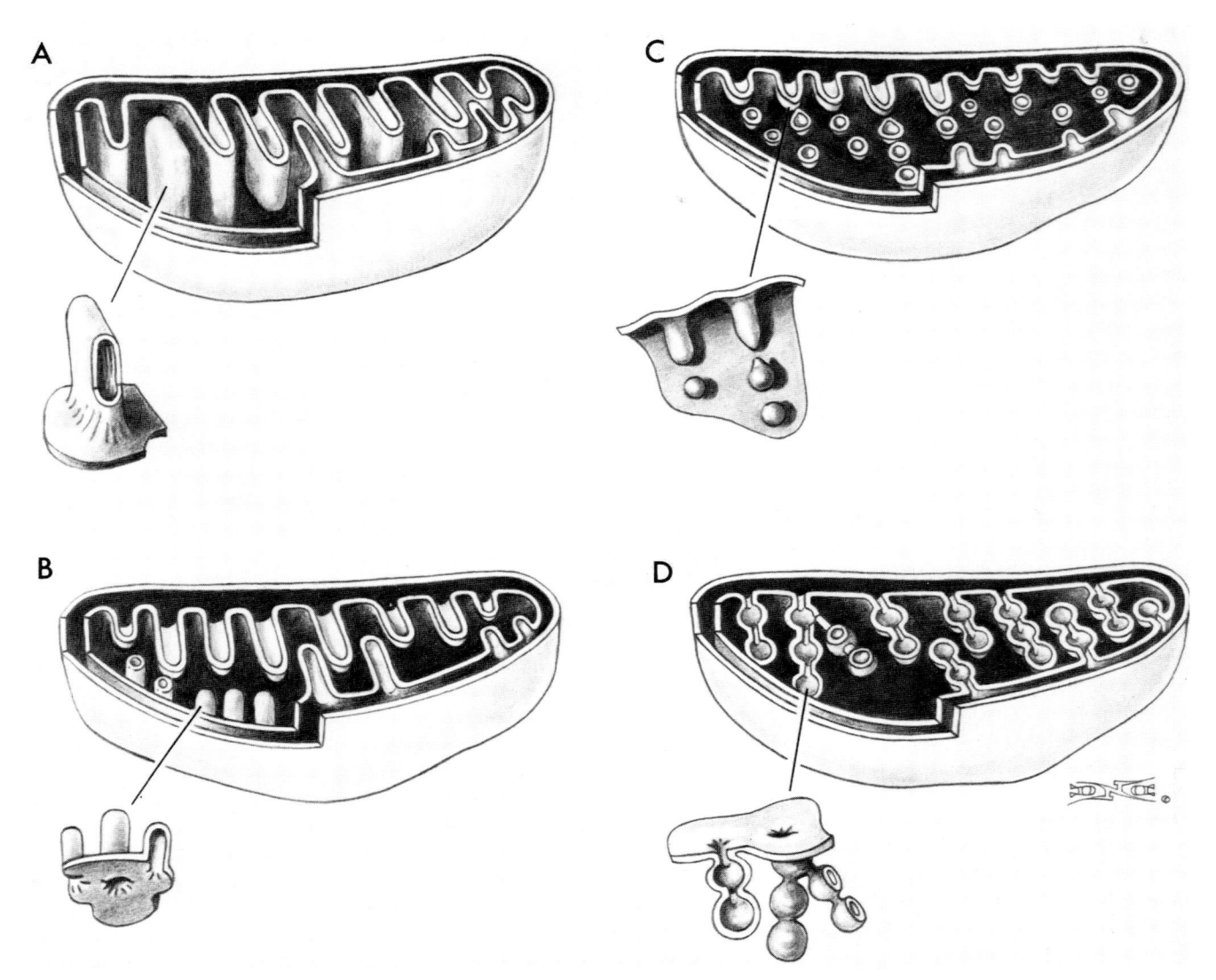

FIG. 7. Stereograms of mitochondria. Two-dimensional profiles seen on cut surfaces are characteristically seen in electron micrographs. *A*: typical liver or kidney mitochondrion, the most commonly encountered mitochondrial type. Inner membrane is thrown into lamellar or shelflike folds called cristae. These cristae may have narrowed connections with the inner membrane. *B*: typical adrenal cortex mitochondrion (except from rat inner zones and from beef). Inner membrane has tubular invaginations (see Fig. 5). *C*: typical rat zona fasciculata and reticularis mitochondrion as described by Sabatini & De Robertis (54). Free-floating vesicles presumably detached from the tubules are seen within the space surrounded by inner mitochondrial membrane. *D*: typical beef zona fasciculata mitochondrion as described by Allmann et al. (4) or rat inner zone mitochondrion as seen in Fig. 6.

in the fat droplets, which are, however, the largest intracellular depots for cholesterol, a major substrate (11, 21, 49, 51). It is not yet known whether any enzymes and substrates for steroid synthesis are in the microbodies, microtubules, and other organelles because the more sophisticated cell fractionation techniques needed for isolation of these organelles have not yet been applied to adrenocortical tissue. If any soluble steroidogenic enzymes exist in the intact cell, they would never be far from the smooth endoplasmic reticulum; indeed they might be loosely attached to these membranes (10). The assignment of certain enzymes to the smooth endoplasmic reticulum is for the most part based on indirect evidence. These enzymes are found in the high-speed microsomal fraction obtained in routine differential centrifugation, a fraction that is derived from both smooth and rough endoplasmic reticulum. Furthermore in cell fractionation studies of steroidogenic tissue the microsomal membranes have seldom been viewed in the electron microscope [see

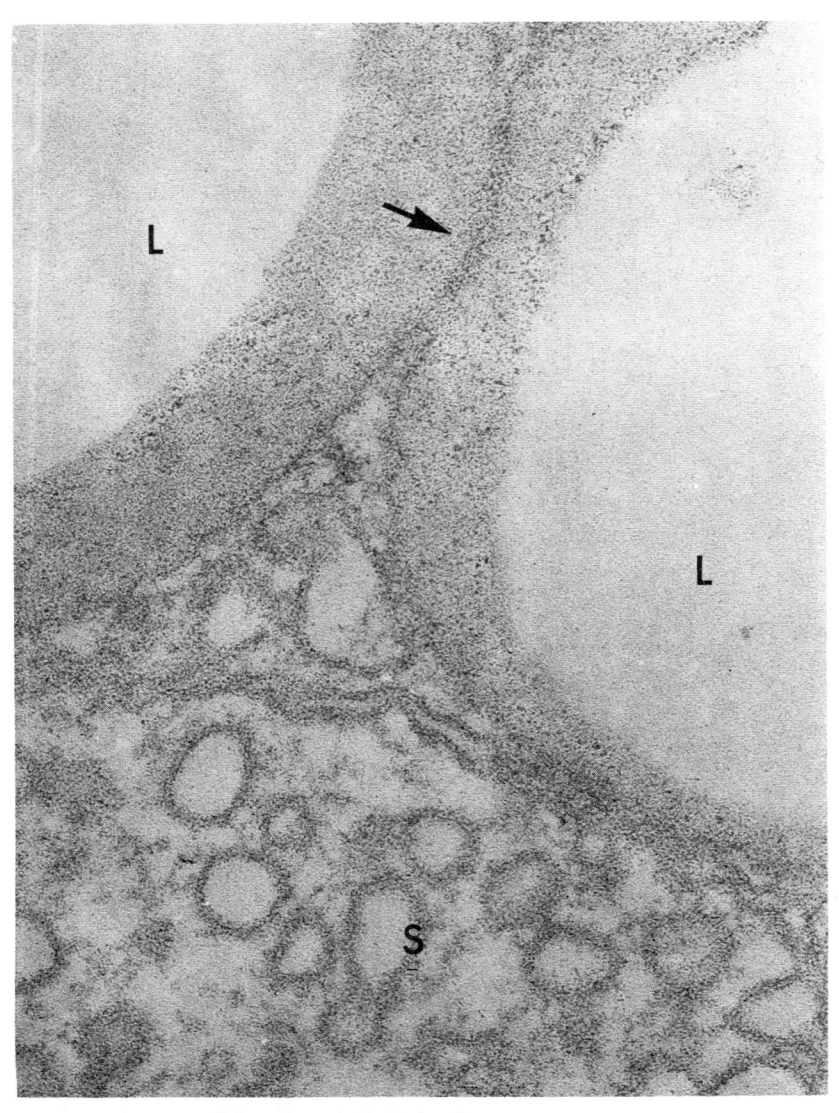

FIG. 8. Region of apposition of 2 lipid droplets in rat adrenal cortex. Although each lipid droplet has a rim that is more electron dense than its internal content, no discrete structured membrane is seen. Yet where lipid droplets are adjacent (*arrow*), their bounding regions of high electron density do not appear to permit continuity between droplets. Central portions of lipid droplets are electron translucent because they have been solubilized by lipid solvents used in preparation for electron microscopy. S, smooth endoplasmic reticulum; L, lipid droplet. × 151,000.

(10), table III; but see (31)]. Still it is generally assumed that the microsomal enzymes are mostly on smooth endoplasmic reticulum in situ, because adrenocortical cells are poor in rough membranes and rich in smooth ones.

The general lack of morphological monitoring of cell fractions makes the matching of steroidogenic enzymes and organelles less certain than it would be if possible contaminations were evaluated by electron microscopy. However, some recent studies have combined this technique with biochemistry, thus placing 3β-hydroxysteroid dehydrogenase and 21-hydroxylase mainly on smooth microsomes (31) and even pinpointing 11β-hydroxylase to the inner mitochondrial membrane (13). Other uncertainties about results of cell fractionation work stem from the possibilities of enzyme displacements, artificial reactions, heat inhibition, and artifacts due to the tissue homogenization and centrifugation [see (46) for discussion]. It is also possible that the intact intracellular spatial organization of organelles is necessary as a guide for the sequence of biosynthetic reactions; this organization is, of course, disrupted by cell fractionation. Further reason for cautious acceptance of the scheme in Figure 11 is the fact that it is based on work with adrenals from different species (mostly bovine) that generally have not had their

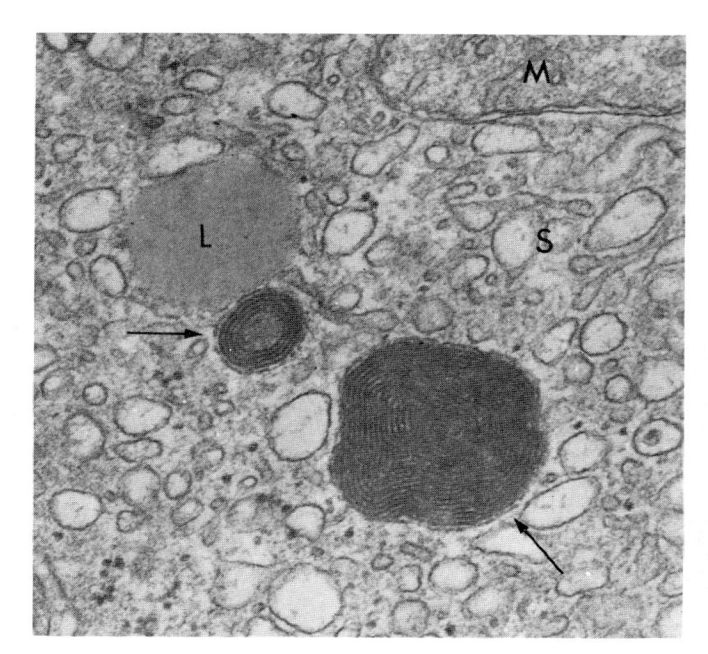

FIG. 9. Section of guinea pig adrenal cortex; 2 laminated bodies (*arrows*) are shown. S, smooth endoplasmic reticulum; M, mitochondrion; L, lipid droplet. × 58,300.

medullae removed (38) and on work with nonadrenal steroidogenic glands (10).

Putting aside these limitations for the present, certain key steps in Figure 11 are apparent. Acetate ions are built up into cholesterol with the intervention of coenzyme A in the smooth endoplasmic reticulum. (Depending on the species a varying amount of cholesterol also comes from the plasma.) The next reactions occur in the mitochondria; these hydroxylations cleave the cholesterol side chain, resulting in pregnenolone synthesis. Now the scene shifts back to the smooth endoplasmic reticulum where progesterone is formed, and further hydroxylation yields deoxycorticosterone. Then the mitochondria, in a second series of roles, produce corticosterone, cortisol, and aldosterone.

An interesting comparative approach has been used to implicate the smooth endoplasmic reticulum in the making of cholesterol from acetate. On this basis, cholesterol production seems to vary with the amount of smooth membranes in rat and guinea pig adrenal cortices and testes. However, the comparisons involve different glands and species [(9); see also (46)]; thus the differences may be due to variables other than amount of agranular reticulum.

In addition to their biosynthetic role, smooth membranes have also been implicated in the storage of cholesterol (16). In the rat adrenal, however, only about 8% of the total cholesterol is found in the microsomal fraction, whereas about 75% is found in the lipid droplets (48). Since the rat adrenal derives almost all its cholesterol from the plasma (44) similar data for adrenals that synthesize much of their cholesterol, such as those

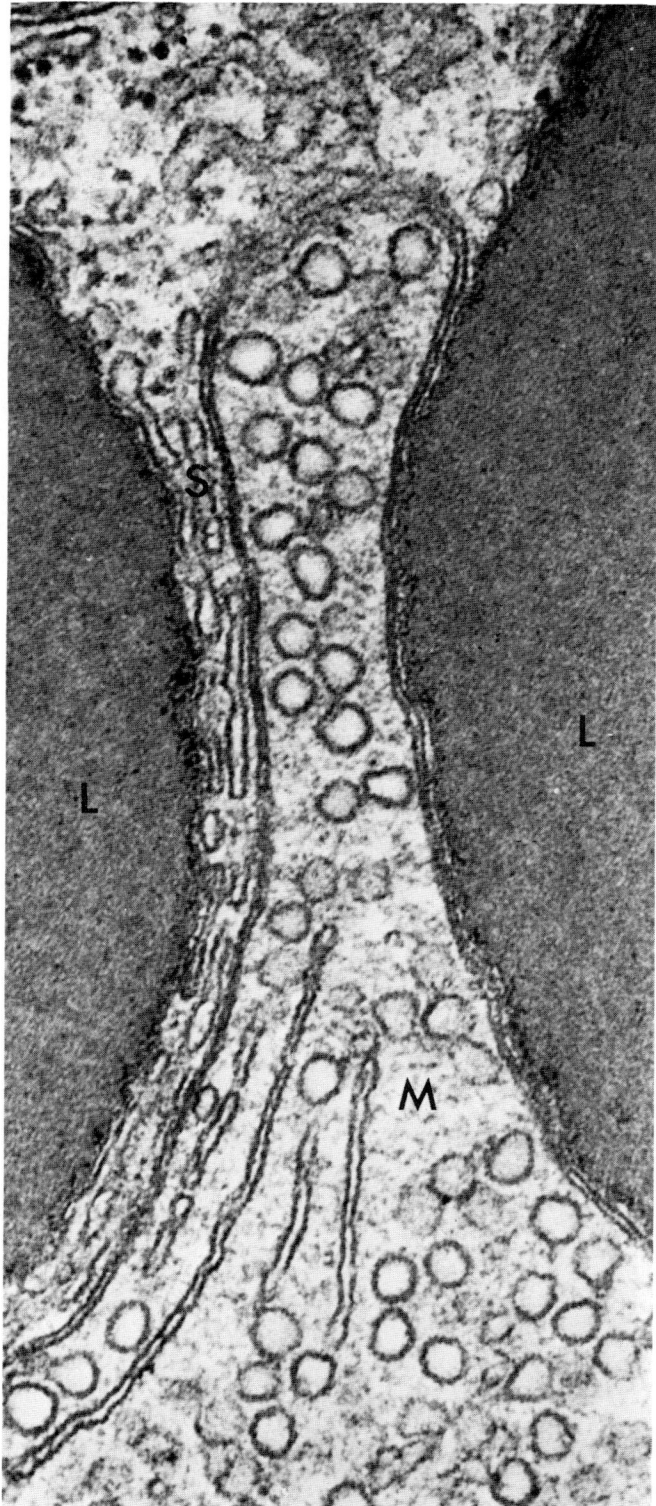

FIG. 10. Section of rat zona fasciculata. Very close to peripheries of the 2 lipid droplets, almost fusing with them, are mitochondrial and smooth endoplasmic reticulum membranes. S, smooth endoplasmic reticulum; M, mitochondrion; L, lipid droplet. × 109,000.

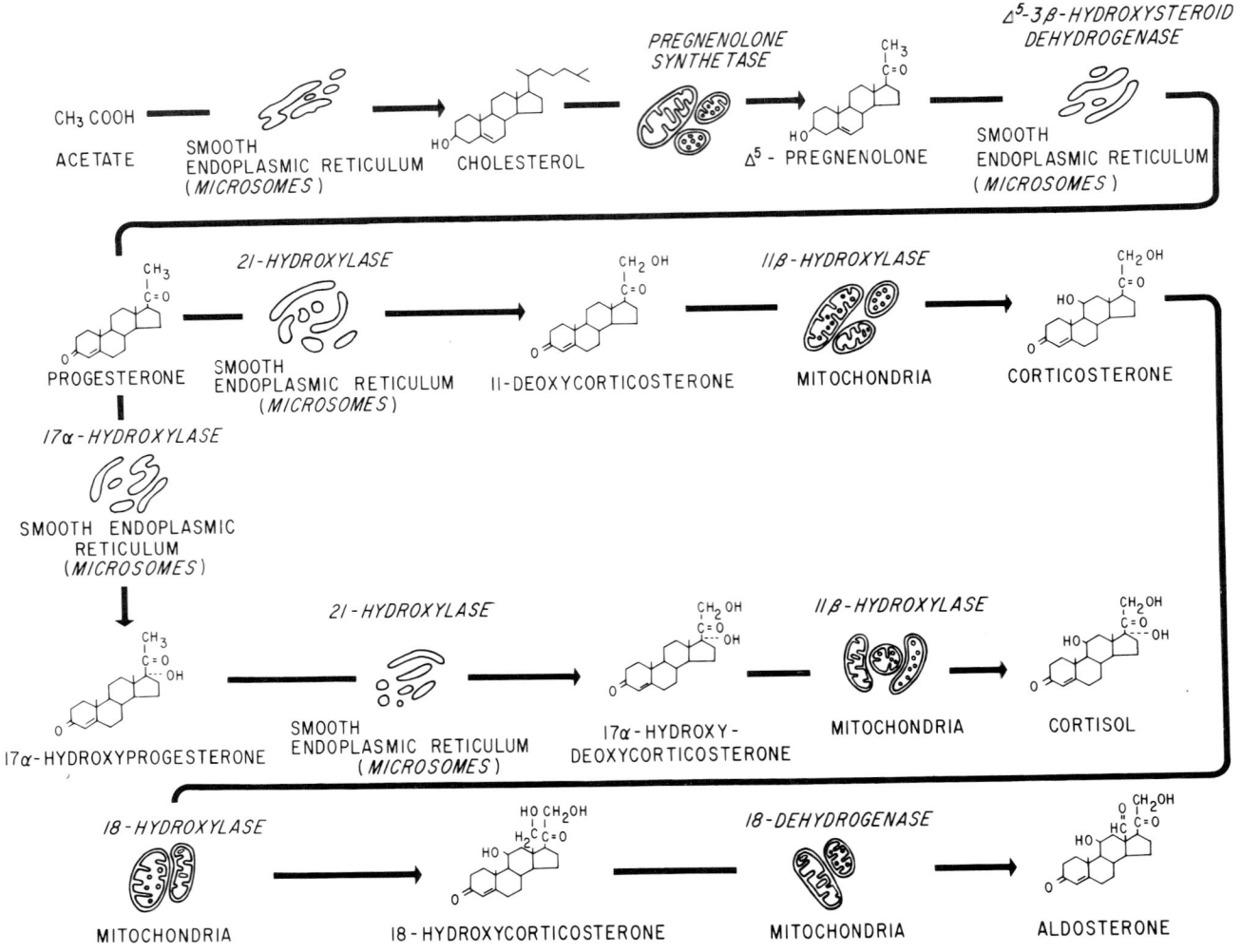

FIG. 11. Simplified scheme of steroidogenesis and its intracellular pathways. Corticosterone and cortisol are end products in the zona fasciculata and reticularis. Corticosterone produced in zona glomerulosa is converted to aldosterone.

of the guinea pig (64), would be interesting. Perhaps the storage capacity is dependent on biosynthetic activity; the two functions, after all, have been ascribed to the same organelle.

If present thinking is correct, the intracellular locale for steroidogenesis shifts twice from the agranular reticulum to the mitochondria (Fig. 11). Thus a movement of substrates or of organelle membranes or of both is implied. These possibilities are actually suggested by the ultrastructural evidence of frequent close relationships between smooth endoplasmic reticulum and lipid droplets (8, 30, 32, 38, 52) and between mitochondria and lipid droplets (32, 38, 49), wherein smooth membranes or mitochondrial membranes (Figs. 3, 5, 8–10) at times appear to be wrapped around the lipid droplets. Portions of these membranes may even appear fused with lipid droplets (Figs. 8 and 10).

The problem of charting the cytoplasmic pathway for steroid secretion in the adrenocortical cell is especially difficult because only traces of the steroid hormones are stored prior to release [(11), p. 54; (37, 61)]. The morphological expression of this lack of hormone storage is that there are as yet no cell inclusions to follow that are generally agreed to be hormone markers as are the cytoplasmic secretory granules of numerous endocrine and exocrine glands, such as the adrenal medulla, pancreas, and pituitary. However, a recent report (52) is quite provocative for it designates the abundant lipid droplets or cytoplasmic pools near them as the sites of the final products of steroidogenesis. As described, the mechanism for cellular extrusion of the steroid hormone (Fig. 12, A–D) is similar to exocytosis, the release process for a number of granules containing proteinaceous hormones, such as the chromaffin granules of the adrenal medulla and the neurosecretory granules of the neurohypophysis.

ULTRASTRUCTURAL CHANGES WITH FUNCTIONAL ACTIVITY

The experiments discussed in this section were for durations of weeks or months unless otherwise noted. The most important results are summarized in Table 1.

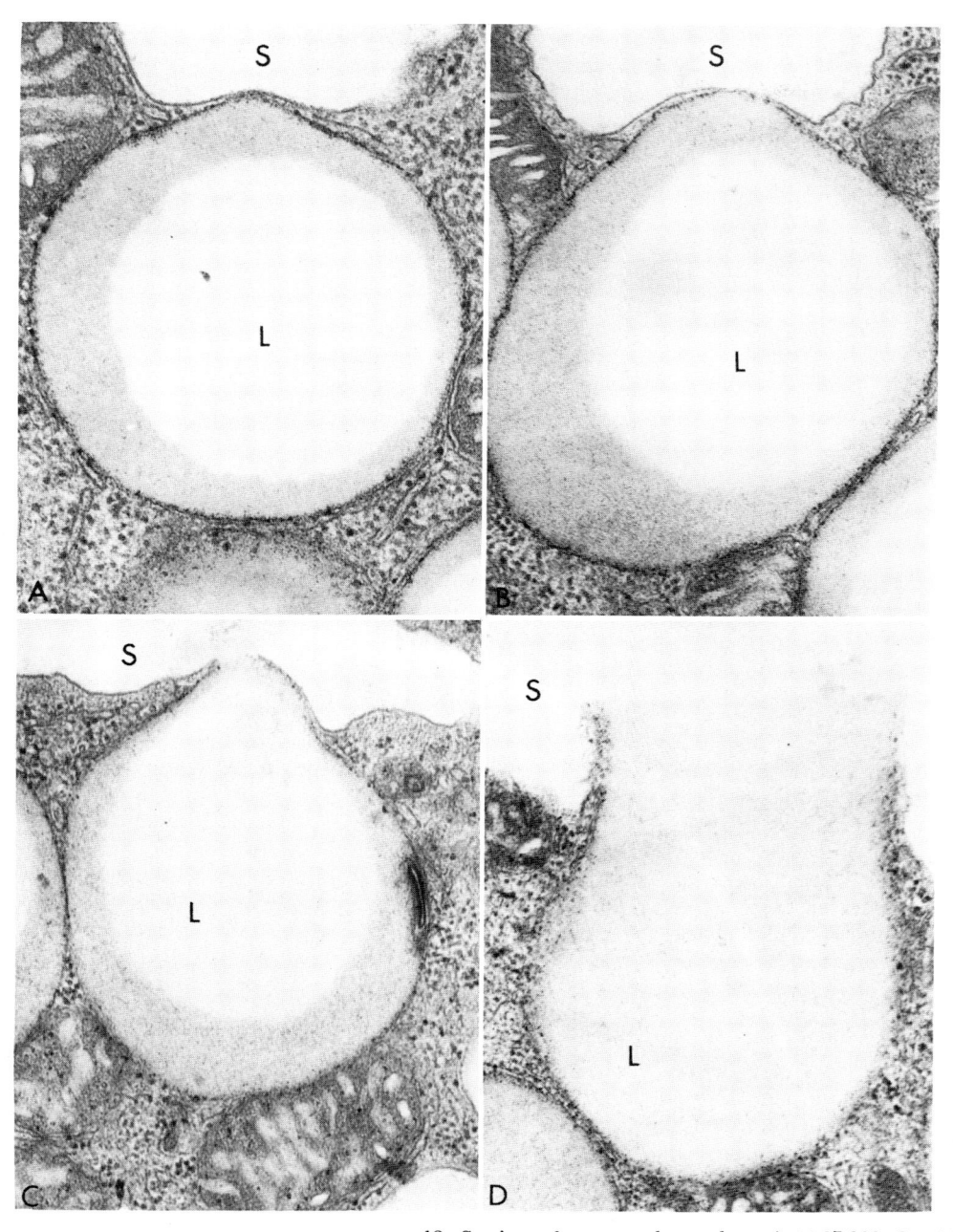

FIG. 12. Sections of rat zona glomerulosa. $A: \times 67,000$; $B: \times 52,000$; $C: \times 38,000$; $D: \times 39,500$. These views of lipid droplets are arranged to simulate a hypothetical mechanism of discharge. L, lipid droplet; S, extracellular space. [From Rhodin (52).]

Zona Glomerulosa

Decrease in the size of mouse zona glomerulosa and in concomitant hormonal activity resulting from a diet high in sodium is characterized by an increase in lipid droplets. The smooth endoplasmic reticulum and mitochondria, however, participate in a general attrition of cytoplasmic structures, which is accompanied by an increase in lysosomes, the probable agents of cytoplasmic atrophy (59).

Sodium deprivation by diet or via potassium chloride injection of the opossum (40), mouse (59), rat (23, 30), and calf (63) has been used to stimulate secretion of aldosterone, resulting in an increase of the smooth endoplasmic reticulum (23, 40, 59). Intramitochondrial deposits, possibly lipid or aldosterone precursors, have also been noted (23, 40, 63), but marked changes in mitochondrial numbers or structure have not been observed (40). There is disagreement about alterations of the lipid droplets; reports of depletions followed by restoration (23, 59) and of no quantitative change in these organelles (40) have appeared.

The generally accepted view that the cells of the zona glomerulosa are essentially independent of anterior

TABLE 1. *Summary of Long-term Quantitative Ultrastructural Changes of Adrenal Cortex in Relation to Hormone Secretion*

Secretion Level	Smooth Endoplasmic Reticulum		Mitochondria		Lipid Droplets	
	Zona glomerulosa	Zona fasciculata and reticularis	Zona glomerulosa	Zona fasciculata and reticularis	Zona glomerulosa	Zona fasciculata and reticularis
Decreased secretion by hypophysectomy or sodium loading	−	−	−	−	+	−
Increased secretion by ACTH or sodium deprivation	+	+	±	+	±	−

Decrease: −; increase: +; no change: ±.

pituitary control (12) is supported by reports that neither hypophysectomy nor ACTH administration has any marked effect on ultrastructure (29, 30, 55).

Zona Fasciculata and Zona Reticularis

In these zones, as in the zona glomerulosa, the prevalence of the smooth endoplasmic reticulum is related to secretory activity. With hypophysectomy and decreased hormone secretion of the rat the smooth endoplasmic reticulum regresses (18, 29) but then returns upon administration of ACTH (18, 30). [However, insignificant changes in these membranes after hypophysectomy have also been reported (7).] Administration of ACTH also causes a reduction of the smooth endoplasmic reticulum after 10 min (52), but after 2 hr an increase occurs (5, 30, 51).

Liposomes accumulate early after hypophysectomy (57, 58), then become depleted (12, 18); ACTH restores the liposomes (7, 29). However, the pool of liposomes is also depleted by ACTH acting acutely [10 min (52); 2 hr (30); 3 hr (58)] or over a long term [21 days (30)] on the intact animal.

After hypophysectomy of the rat, mitochondria from the inner zones diminish in number; ACTH reverses this effect of hypophysectomy (7, 18). In the intact rat ACTH increases both the number of mitochondria per cell and their mean volume [short- and long-term effect (30, 50)].

Hypophysectomy also results in qualitative alterations: rat mitochondria undergo a transformation of their internal structure such that the vesicles within their matrices are replaced by tubules. Thus they appear like mitochondria from the zona glomerulosa. This transformation is reversed by ACTH administration. The evidence for these reversible mitochondrial changes is better for cells of the zona fasciculata than for those of the zona reticularis (29, 55). Even in the case of the zona fasciculata the mitochondrial changes after hypophysectomy are described in one study as ordinary degenerative ones, that is, loss of ground substance and internal membranes, rather than as transformation of internal structure. Again these changes are reversible by ACTH (7). The differences in the experimental conditions of these studies (7, 29, 55) may explain the apparently conflicting results. Mitochondrial transformation of the sort described above seems not to occur in the ACTH-treated intact rat (65).

Intramitochondrial alterations from vesicular to tubular or tubulovesicular membranes have been reported also in cultured cells of fetal and newborn rat adrenal glands. None of these cells removed from hypophysial control and thus analogous to those in hypophysectomized animals had the appearance of zona fasciculata cells. Their mitochondria were tubular as in the zona glomerulosa or tubulovesicular as in the zona intermedia between the zona glomerulosa and the zona fasciculata. However, addition of ACTH to the culture medium resulted in cells with vesicular mitochondria typical of the zona fasciculata, as well as others typical of the zona glomerulosa. Apparently the absence of pituitary control changed the fasciculata cells toward the glomerulosa type, and then the restoration of ACTH reversed this change in ultrastructure [Fig. 13, *A* and *B*; (33)]. Actinomycin D or puromycin, suppressors of protein synthesis, inhibited the ACTH-induced reappearance of intramitochondrial vesicles (34) as did chloramphenicol, a specific inhibitor of mitochondrial protein synthesis (35). This morphological block was correlated with a steroidogenic one: 11β-hydroxylation, occurring in the mitochondria (see Fig. 11) and ordinarily increased by ACTH, was prevented by chloramphenicol (45). Human fetal adrenal cultures were affected similarly by ACTH, which induced the appearance of mitochondrial vesicles and of a marked increase in steroidogenic activity (47).

The mitochondrial transformations just discussed seem to involve the joining of vesicles to form straight tubes in the absence of ACTH and the detachment of vesicles from the straight tubes in the presence of ACTH. A simpler, more plausible interpretation is possible because of indications that the rat fasciculata mitochondria are like those of beef [Figs. 6 and 7; (4)], that is, their vesicles are actually dilated portions of tubular inner membrane infoldings. Thus the morphological effect of ACTH on these mitochondria would be simply to maintain either the series of dilations or the alternating constrictions along the tubular invaginations of the mitochondrial inner membranes.

Apart from the mitochondrial alterations just discussed, an in vitro type has been described for mitochondria isolated from cells of the bovine zona fasciculata. When isolated in a Ca^{2+}-free medium the mitochondrial vesicles disappear for the most part, the spaces between the inner and outer membranes seem expanded, and the matrices seem contracted or aggregated. The suspended mitochondria are induced by Ca^{2+} to reas-

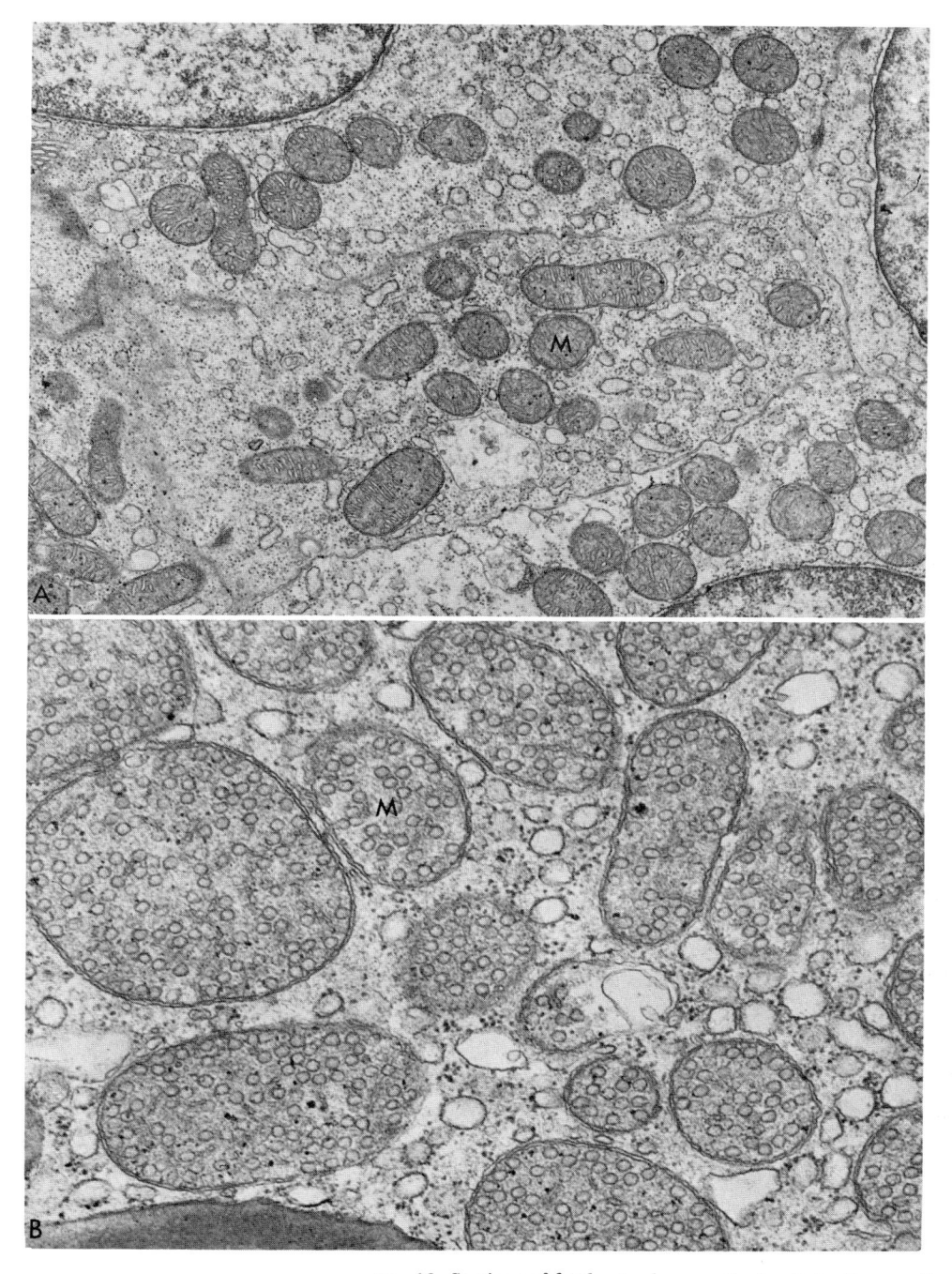

FIG. 13. Sections of fetal rat adrenocortical cells in tissue culture for 25 days. *A*: control. In the absence of ACTH, mitochondria are tubulolamellar, as are mitochondria of zona glomerulosa. × 13,800. *B*: 0.1 IU/ml ACTH added to medium on days 19 through 24. In the presence of ACTH, mitochondria are vesicular, as are mitochondria of zona fasciculata. × 37,000. *M*, mitochondrion. [From Kahri (35).]

sume an orthodox configuration so they appear as they do in situ (Fig. 14, *A* and *B*). An aggregated configuration is induced by Mg^{2+} (3). Mitochondria in the orthodox state are nonenergized or uncoupled, having lost the ability to synthesize ATP, among other properties. Those in the aggregated state are energized. However, steroidogenesis proceeds more rapidly in orthodox than in aggregated mitochondria (1). The transition from one state to the other is reversible. Thus their modulation, if present in situ, might reflect a switching from steroidogenesis (orthodox state) to ATP synthesis (aggregated state) (2).

Yet another mitochondrial change is the appearance of giant mitochondria in the rat zona fasciculata after

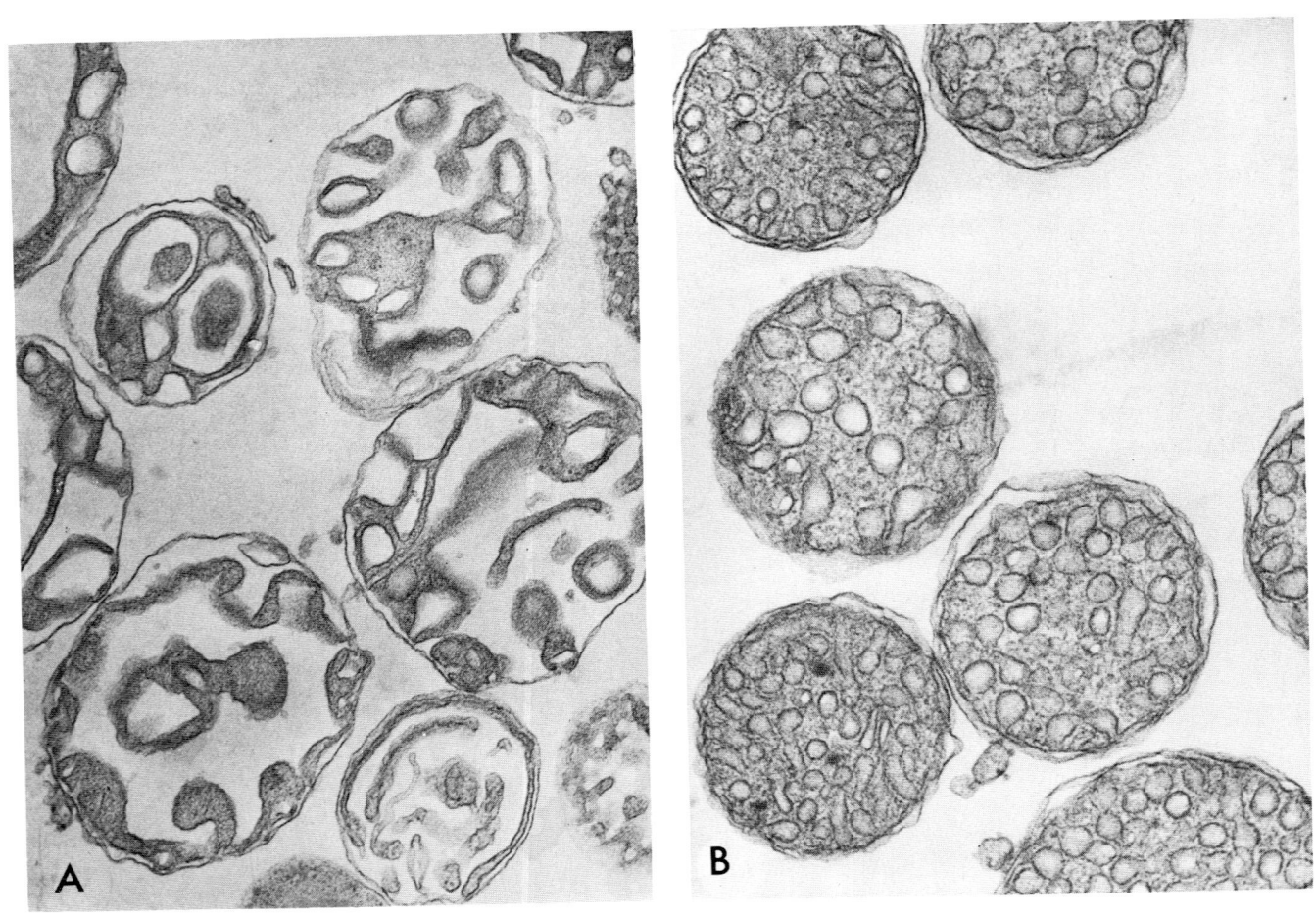

FIG. 14. Sections of isolated adrenocortical mitochondria. *A*: in the absence of Ca^{2+}, mitochondria appear aggregated. *B*: in the presence of Ca^{2+}, mitochondria assume an orthodox configuration, appearing as they do in situ. (Courtesy of Dr. D. W. Allmann.)

hypophysectomy. However, this mitochondrial gigantism has been reported only once, and its significance is obscure (62).

It should be noted that ultrastructural changes in mitochondria induced by hypophysectomy or by ACTH are not surprising if one considers the chemical evidence. These data show that ACTH specifically stimulates the steroidogenic reactions between cholesterol and pregnenolone (36), steps that have been placed in the mitochondria (see Fig. 11).

In contrast to the many ultrastructural changes that have been seen in functionally altered adrenocortical cells discussed above, no modifications of fine structure have yet been observed in trypsin-dissociated rat cells, despite stimulation to maximal secretory activity by incubation with ACTH for 2 hr (43). This may indicate that the changes seen after longer duration of treatment (several weeks or months) are delayed structural consequences of more immediate functional changes.

SUMMARY AND DISCUSSION

The ultrastructural consequences of experimental hormone imbalances described above and summarized in Table 1 are broadly predictable given the information about the intracellular sites for steroidogenic steps, which are summarized in Figure 11. Each of the organelles characteristic of adrenocortical cells (smooth endoplasmic reticulum, liposomes, mitochondria) undergoes changes after one or another experimental treatment. Yet the experimental results so far do little to elucidate the specific roles that these organelles play in hormone secretion.

Under conditions designed to decrease hormone secretion the significance of decreases in the amount of smooth endoplasmic reticulum and in the number of mitochondria is especially difficult to assess because of general cellular atrophy and because little is yet known about which changes occur first. Even more puzzling is the increase in the liposomes of the zona glomerulosa in animals on a diet high in sodium (in contrast to the decrease in liposomes of the inner zones in hypophysectomized animals). If the liposomes are cholesterol storehouses, perhaps the primary effect of a high-sodium diet on the zona glomerulosa is to inhibit mitochondrial pregnenolone synthesis, whereas the primary effect of hypophysectomy on the inner zones is on some earlier step.

When hormone secretion is stimulated, there is an increase of the smooth endoplasmic reticulum and, at least in the zona fasciculata, an increase of the mitochondria as well. Unfortunately these increases do little to confirm or deny the cell fractionation studies that assign specific biosynthetic steps to the smooth membranes and to the mitochondria. Loss of lipid droplets when secretion is enhanced by a low-sodium diet or by ACTH may indicate that these treatments stimulate pregnenolone synthesis, thus depleting cholesterol stores faster than they can be replaced.

It appears that the general message of Table 1 is that increased secretory activity results in increased steroidogenic enzymes and thus increased smooth endoplasmic reticulum and mitochondria, but decreased cholesterol and thus decreased liposomes, the organelles storing this steroid precursor. Decreased secretory activity seems to have opposite effects, except for the indication of a decrease in lipid droplets in the zona fasciculata and reticularis after hypophysectomy. This deviation, however, may be more apparent than real. Early work (57, 58) based on light microscopy has indicated that lipid droplet content of the adrenal cortex is determined by the balance between tissue cell need for corticosteroids and the mobilization of the corticosteroid precursor, cholesterol, into lipid droplets. Accordingly the lipid content of adrenocortical cells depends greatly on the time during or after stimulation when the cells are observed because of the recovery, hyperplastic, hypertrophic, and adaptive responses that may alter this balance and in turn the net values for liposome content. Thus, in contrast to the reported long-term decrease in lipid droplets after hypophysectomy (12, 18), there is evidence of a short-term increase (57, 58), and these data need not be in contradiction (57).

In contrast to the quantitative changes summarized above are the reversible qualitative changes in mitochondrial structure. These modulations from tubular to vesicular internal structure depend on the absence or presence of ACTH, respectively, thus suggesting that in the intact animal glomerular cells may be converted into fascicular cells under the influence of ACTH. However, information about possible functional modulation, that is, from glucocorticoid to mineralocorticoid secretion (and vice versa), is still not available to properly assess the significance of these structural alterations.

A cautionary note may be pertinent here. As ultrastructural studies achieve finer resolution, the unity of structure and function at the molecular level is approached. For now, however, apparent discrepancies between ultrastructure and function should be expected. One example of several discussed here and elsewhere is the ACTH reversibility of chloramphenicol's effect on mitochondrial structure (46) without similar effect on 11β-hydroxylation (63). Another is the lack of observable mitochondrial changes in the zona glomerulosa cells of sodium-depleted, and hence hypersecreting, animals that in contrast do exhibit an increase in smooth endoplasmic reticulum (40) as expected.

Besides the problems of interpretation just discussed there are a number of technical deficiencies of broad importance. They demonstrate further the need for caution in drawing conclusions from experiments done so far. The information on intracellular localization of adrenocortical steroidogenic enzymes comes largely from cell fractionation of nonadrenal bovine steroidogenic glands. Yet electron microscopy of adrenals from intact and experimental animals is limited almost exclusively to other mammals. Furthermore there has been little electron microscopy used in the cell fractionation studies. Thus there is uncertainty in the placing of individual steroidogenic enzymes specifically on either the mitochondria or the smooth endoplasmic reticulum.

The electron-microscopic work must bear its share of criticism as well. Much of our present thinking derives from studies done in the late 1950s and early 1960s when the quality of electron micrographs produced permitted rather limited conclusions. Nor have the grosser morphological identifications been as reliable as needed: positive methods of identifying the adrenocortical zones of origin of electron-microscopic specimens have been few. Quantification of morphological results has been another problem: the possibility of nonrepresentative sampling is of special concern in electron microscopy because of the small size and number of sample specimens that are usually observed. Even more troubling is the relative lack of quantitative data on changes in the numbers and sizes of cell organelles under experimental conditions.

It appears then that an understanding of how the organelles of the adrenocortical cells participate in hormone secretion must await more reliable information from new experimental studies, many of which could well be essentially refinements of what has gone before. In addition, the development of techniques for visualization and localization of substances involved in steroidogenesis, including the hormones themselves, offers a promising approach that unfortunately has been virtually absent so far.

I am grateful to Jean Gibney for her expert technical assistance and to Daniel Neil Christie for the art work of Figures 4, 7, and 11.

REFERENCES

1. ALLMANN, D. W., J. MUNROE, O. HECHTER, AND M. MATSUBA. Ultrastructural basis for the regulation of steroidogenesis in bovine adrenal cortex mitochondria. *Federation Proc.* 28: 665, 1969.
2. ALLMANN, D. W., J. MUNROE, T. WAKABAYASHI, AND D. E. GREEN. Studies on the transition of the cristal membrane from the orthodox to the aggregated configuration. III. Loss of coupling ability of adrenal cortex mitochondria in the orthodox configuration. *Bioenergetics* 1: 331–353, 1970.
3. ALLMANN, D. W., J. MUNROE, T. WAKABAYASHI, R. A. HARRIS, AND D. E. GREEN. Studies on the transition of the cristal membrane from the orthodox to the aggregated configura-

tion. II. Determinants of the orthodox-aggregated transition in adrenal cortex mitochondria. *Bioenergetics* 1: 87–101, 1970.
4. ALLMANN, D. W., T. WAKABAYASHI, E. F. KORMAN, AND D. E. GREEN. Studies on the transition of the cristal membrane from the orthodox to the aggregated configuration. I. Topology of bovine adrenal cortex mitochondria in the orthodox configuration. *Bioenergetics* 1: 73–86, 1970.
5. ASHWORTH, C. T., G. J. RACE, AND H. H. MOLLENHAUER. Study of functional activity of adrenocortical cells with electron microscopy. *Am. J. Pathol.* 35: 424–436, 1958.
6. BLOODWORTH, J. M. B., JR., AND K. L. POWERS. The ultrastructure of the normal dog adrenal. *J. Anat.* 102: 457–476, 1968.
7. BOROWICZ, J. W. Some ultrastructural changes in adrenal cortical cells of rat after hypophysectomy and following ACTH administration. *Beitr. Pathol. Anat. Allgem. Pathol.* 132: 441–468, 1965.
8. BRENNER, R. M. Fine structure of adrenocortical cells in adult male rhesus monkeys. *Am. J. Anat.* 119: 429–453, 1966.
9. CHRISTENSEN, A. K. The fine structure of testicular interstitial cells in guinea pigs. *J. Cell Biol.* 26: 911–935, 1965.
10. CHRISTENSEN, A. K., AND S. W. GILLIM. The correlation of fine structure and function in steroid secreting cells, with emphasis on those of the gonads. In: *The Gonads*, edited by W. McKerns. New York: Appleton, 1969, p. 415–488.
11. DEANE, H. W. The anatomy, chemistry, and physiology of adrenocortical tissue. In: *Handbuch der Experimentellen Pharmakologie*, edited by H. W. Deane. Berlin: Springer Verlag, 1962, part 1, p. 1–185.
12. DEANE, H. W., AND R. O. GREEP. A morphological and histochemical study of the rat adrenal cortex after hypophysectomy with comments on the liver. *Am. J. Anat.* 79: 117–145, 1946.
13. DODGE, A. H., A. K. CHRISTENSEN, AND R. B. CLAYTON. Localization of steroid 11β-hydroxylase in the inner membrane subfraction of the rat adrenal mitochondria. *Endocrinology* 87: 254–261, 1970.
14. DORFMAN, R. I., AND F. UNGAR. *Metabolism of Steroid Hormones*. New York: Acad. Press, 1965.
15. FAVARD, P. Evolution des ultrastructures cellulaires au cours de la spermatogenese de lascares. *Ann. Sci. Nat. Zool. Biol. Animale* 3: 53–152, 1961.
16. FAWCETT, D. W. Structural and functional variations in the membranes of the cytoplasm. In: *Intracellular Membranous Structure*, edited by S. Seno and E. V. Cowdry. Okayama, Japan: Chugoku Press, 1963, p. 15–40.
17. FAWCETT, D. W. *An Atlas of Fine Structure: The Cell, Its Organelles and Inclusions*. Philadelphia: Saunders, 1966.
18. FAWCETT, D. W., J. A. LONG, AND A. L. JONES. The ultrastructure of endocrine glands. *Recent Progr. Hormone Res.* 25: 315–380, 1969.
19. FORSHAM, P. H. The adrenal gland. *Clin. Symp.* 15: 3–21, 1963.
20. FRIEND, D. S., AND N. B. GILULA. A distinctive cell contact in the rat adrenal cortex. *J. Cell Biol.* 53: 148–163, 1972.
21. FRÜHLING, G. J., W. PENASSE, G. SAND, AND A. CLAUDE. Preservation du cholesterol dans la corticosurrenale du rat au cours de la preparation des tissus pour la microscopie electronique. *J. Microscopie* 8: 957–982, 1969.
22. GARREN, L. D. The mechanism of action of adrenocorticotrophic hormones. In: *Vitamins and Hormones: Advances in Research and Applications*, edited by R. S. Harris, I. G. Wool, and J. A. Loraine. New York: Acad. Press, 1968, vol. 26, p. 119–145.
23. GIACOMELLI, F., J. WIENER, AND D. SPIRO. Cytological alterations related to stimulation of the zona glomerulosa of the adrenal gland. *J. Cell Biol.* 26: 499–521, 1965.
24. GIDEZ, L. I., AND E. FELLER. Effect of the stress of unilateral adrenalectomy on the depletion of individual cholesteryl esters in the rat adrenal. *J. Lipid Res.* 10: 656–659, 1969.
25. GRANT, J. K. Biogenesis of the adrenal steroids. *Brit. Med. Bull.* 18: 99–105, 1962.
26. IDELMAN, S. Histochemie-action du methanol-chloroforme sur les liposomes des cellules cortico-surrenales. *Compt. Rend.* 257: 297–298, 1963.
27. IDELMAN, S. Mitochondries et liposomes description d'une transformation mitochondrial observee dans la corticosurrenale du rat. *J. Microscopie* 3: 437–446, 1964.
28. IDELMAN, S. Modification de la technique de Luft en vue de la conservation des lipides en microscopie electronique. *J. Microscopie* 3: 715–718, 1964.
29. IDELMAN, S. Contribution a la cytophysiologie infrastructural de la cortico-surrenale chez le rat albinos. *Ann. Sci. Nat. Zool. Biol. Animale* 8: 205–362, 1966.
30. IDELMAN, S. Ultrastructure of the mammalian adrenal cortex. *Intern. Rev. Cytol.* 27: 181–281, 1970.
31. INANO, H., A. INANO, AND B. TAMAOKI. Submicrosomal distribution of adrenal enzymes and cytochrome P-450 related to corticoidogenesis. *Biochim. Biophys. Acta* 191: 257–271, 1969.
32. KADIOGLU, D., AND R. G. HARRISON. The functional relationships of mitochondria in the rat adrenal cortex. *J. Anat.* 110: 283–296, 1971.
33. KAHRI, A. I. Histochemical and electron microscopic studies on the cells of the rat adrenal cortex in tissue culture. *Acta Endocrinol. Suppl.* 108: 1–96, 1966.
34. KAHRI, A. I. Effects of actinomycin D and puromycin on the ACTH-induced ultrastructural transformation of mitochondria of cortical cells of rat adrenals in tissue culture. *J. Cell Biol.* 36: 181–195, 1968.
35. KAHRI, A. I. Selective inhibition by chloramphenicol of ACTH-induced reorganization of inner mitochondrial membranes in fetal adrenal cortical cells in tissue culture. *Am. J. Anat.* 127: 103–129, 1970.
36. KARABOYAS, G. C., AND S. B. KORITZ. Identity of the site of action of 3',5'-adenosine monophosphate and adrenocorticotrophic hormone in corticosteroidogenesis in rat adrenal and beef adrenal cortex slices. *Biochemistry* 4: 462–468, 1965.
37. LIDDLE, G. W., D. ISLAND, AND C. K. MEADOR. Regulation of corticotrophin secretion in man. *Recent Progr. Hormone Res.* 18: 125–166, 1962.
38. LONG, J. A., AND A. L. JONES. The fine structure of the zona glomerulosa and the zona fasciculata of the adrenal cortex of the opossum. *Am. J. Anat.* 120: 463–488, 1967.
39. LONG, J. A., AND A. L. JONES. Observations on the fine structure of the adrenal cortex of man. *Lab. Invest.* 17: 355–370, 1967.
40. LONG, J. A., AND A. L. JONES. Alterations in fine structure of the opossum adrenal cortex following sodium deprivation. *Anat. Record* 166: 1–26, 1970.
41. MALAMED, S., H. KRUTH, AND G. OCHAB. Laminated lipid bodies: possible role in lipid droplet formation. *J. Cell Biol.* 55: 163a, 1972.
42. MALAMED, S., H. KRUTH, AND G. OCHAB. Possible role of lamellated lysosomes in fat droplet formation. *Anat. Record* 175: 381, 1973.
43. MALAMED, S., G. SAYERS, AND R. L. SWALLOW. Fine structure of trypsin-dissociated rat adrenal cells. *Z. Zellforsch. Mikroskop. Anat.* 107: 447–453, 1970.
44. MATSUBA, M., S. ISHIU, AND S. KOBAYASHI. Active cholesterol pool for corticoidogenesis in rat adrenal. In: *Steroid Dynamics*, edited by G. Pincus, T. Nakao, and J. F. Tact. New York: Acad. Press, 1966, p. 357–377.
45. MILNER, A. J. ACTH and the differentiation of rat adrenal cortical cells grown in primary tissue culture. *Endocrinology* 88: 66–71, 1971.
46. MILNER, A. J., AND D. W. HAMILTON. Ultrastructural criteria for assessing the functional integrity of endocrine cells in vitro. *Acta Endocrinol. Suppl.* 153: 62–80, 1971.
47. MILNER, A. J., A. I. KAHRI, AND D. B. VILLEE. Steroidogenic and morphologic effects of ACTH on human fetal adrenal cells grown in tissue culture. *Endocrine Soc. Program, 51st Meeting, 1969, Abstr. 86*, p. 73.
48. MOSES, H. L., W. W. DAVIS, A. S. ROSENTHAL, AND L. D.

Garren. Adrenal cholesterol: localization by electron microscope autoradiography. *Science* 163: 1203–1205, 1969.
49. Nickerson, P. A. Fine structure of the Mongolian gerbil adrenal cortex. *Anat. Record* 171: 443–455, 1971.
50. Nussdorfer, G., G. Mazzocchi, and L. Rebonato. Long term trophic effect of ACTH on rat adrenocortical cells—an ultrastructural morphometric and autoradiographic study. *Z. Zellforsch. Mikroskop. Anat.* 115: 30–45, 1971.
51. Okros, I. Digitonin reaction in electron microscopy. *Histochemie* 13: 91–96, 1968.
52. Rhodin, J. A. G. The ultrastructure of the adrenal cortex of the rat under normal and experimental conditions. *J. Ultrastruct. Res.* 34: 23–71, 1971.
53. Robertson, J. D. The organization of cellular membranes. In: *Molecular Organization and Biological Function*, edited by J. M. Allen. New York: Harper & Row, 1967, p. 65–106.
54. Sabatini, D. D., and E. De Robertis. Ultrastructural zonation of adrenocortex in the rat. *J. Biophys. Biochem. Cytol.* 9: 105–119, 1961.
55. Sabatini, D. D., E. De Robertis, and H. B. Bleichmar. Submicroscopic study of the pituitary action on the adrenocortex of the rat. *Endocrinology* 70: 390–406, 1962.
56. Sandor, T. A comparative survey of steroids and steroidogenic pathways throughout the vertebrates. *Gen. Comp. Endocrinol. Suppl.* 2: 284–298, 1969.
57. Sayers, G. The adrenal cortex and homeostasis. *Physiol. Rev.* 30: 241–320, 1950.
58. Sayers, G., and M. A. Sayers. The pituitary-adrenal system. *Recent Progr. Hormone Res.* 2: 81–115, 1948.
59. Shelton, J. H., and A. L. Jones. The fine structure of the mouse adrenal cortex and the ultrastructural changes in zona glomerulosa with low and high sodium diets. *Anat. Record* 170: 147–181, 1971.
60. Sheridan, M. N., and W. D. Belt. Fine structure of the guinea pig adrenal cortex. *Anat. Record* 149: 73–98, 1964.
61. Vernikos-Danellis, J., E. Anderson, and L. Trigg. Changes in adrenal corticosterone concentration in rats: method of bio-assay for ACTH. *Endocrinology* 79: 624–630, 1966.
62. Volk, T. L., and D. G. Scarpelli. Mitochondrial gigantism in the adrenal cortex following hypophysectomy. *Lab. Invest.* 15: 707–715, 1966.
63. Weber, A. F., E. A. Usenik, and S. C. Whipp. Experimental production of electron dense intramatrical bodies in adrenal zona glomerulosa cells of calves. In: *Fifth International Congress of Electron Microscopy*, edited by S. S. Breese. New York: Acad. Press, 1962, vol. 2, p. yy–7.
64. Werbin, H., and I. L. Chaikoff. Utilization of adrenal gland cholesterol for synthesis of cortisol by the intact normal and ACTH-treated guinea pig. *Arch. Biochem. Biophys.* 93: 476–482, 1961.
65. Yamori, T., S. Matsura, and S. Sakamota. An electron-microscopic study of the normal and stimulated adrenal cortex in the rat. *Z. Zellforsch. Mikroskop. Anat.* 55: 179–199, 1961.

CHAPTER 4

Regulation of the secretory activity of the adrenal cortex: cortisol and corticosterone

GEORGE SAYERS
RONALD PORTANOVA

Division of Molecular and Cellular Endocrinology, Department of Physiology, School of Medicine, Case Western Reserve University, Cleveland, Ohio

CHAPTER CONTENTS

Stimulation of Cortisol and Corticosterone Secretion by
    Adrenocorticotropic Hormone (ACTH)
  Regulatory role of adenohypophysis
  Temporal aspects of secretory response of adrenal cortex
  Mode of action of ACTH
  Receptor reserve: sensitivity
  ACTH: structure-activity relationships
  Stimulation of cortisol and/or corticosterone secretion by
    factors of questionable physiological significance
Stimulation of ACTH Secretion
  Bioassay of corticotropin-releasing factor (CRF)
  Hypothalamic CRF
  Neural paths to hypothalamic CRF release
  Neurohypophysial CRF—vasopressin
  Tissue CRF: extrahypothalamic production of CRF
Inhibition of ACTH Secretion
  Corticosteroids
    Sites of inhibitory actions of corticosteroids
    Concentration of corticosteroid and degree of
      inhibition of ACTH secretion
    Kinetics of inhibitory action of corticosteroids on ACTH
      secretion
    Relation between structure of steroid and inhibitory potency
    Mode of action expressed in biochemical terms and
      inhibition of ACTH synthesis
  Short-loop feedback of ACTH on CRF
  Central inhibitory adrenergic pathway
Concluding Remarks

IN MAN AND EXPERIMENTAL ANIMALS a great variety of stimuli ("stresses") increase levels of cortisol and corticosterone in plasma. However, even in the absence of undue disturbances in the internal or external milieu, wide fluctuations in the plasma titers of the steroids occur. The fluctuations follow a circadian rhythm with concentrations of cortisol in the plasma ranging from zero to about 20 µg/100 ml (see the chapter by Atcheson and Tyler in this volume of the *Handbook*). Hellman and his colleagues (25, 32, 106) have demonstrated that smooth curves depicting the cyclic variations of cortisol in the plasma of man over a 24-hr period are deceptive. Frequent sampling (every 20 min) combined with accurate methodology revealed that cortisol is actually secreted in episodic bursts of short duration. The secretory episodes are most frequent during the latter half of the sleep period but also occur during wakefulness. Circadian variations in plasma cortisol appear to be due to differences in the frequency and duration of the secretory episodes rather than to changes in secretory rate. During the 24-hr day there is a total of approximately 6 hr of secretory activity; the remaining 18 hr the gland is quiescent. These findings do little to justify the traditional notion of a basal or steady-state level of glucocorticoid secretion.

From the foregoing it is obvious that the goal of the regulatory mechanism, or mechanisms, is certainly not the maintenance of fixed concentrations of the corticosteroids in the plasma. We are not prepared to answer the question as to the functions served by the fluctuations (i.e., what "good" they do the organism), except in a few instances in which increased levels of glucocorticoids in the body fluids are known to help recovery from specific metabolic perturbations. We do know that these fluctuations are a result of changes in the rate of secretion of adrenocorticotropic hormone (ACTH) by the adenohypophysis.

STIMULATION OF CORTISOL AND CORTICOSTERONE
SECRETION BY ADRENOCORTICOTROPIC HORMONE

Regulatory Role of Adenohypophysis

Fluctuations in the secretory activity of the adrenal cortex are determined by fluctuations in the rate of secretion of ACTH by the adenohypophysis. After hypophysectomy the rates of secretion of cortisol and corticosterone are reduced to exceedingly low levels (26); the adrenal cortex neither responds to the great variety of stimuli (stresses) that normally activate the gland, nor does it exhibit cyclic activity. Adrenocorticotropic hormone secreted by the adenohypophysis and transported in the circulation to its target site mediates the regulatory influence (71).

Temporal Aspects of Secretory Response of Adrenal Cortex

Activation of the adrenal cortex in response to a noxious stimulus occurs by means of a multistage pathway, believed to contain both neural and humoral components. Two of the components—the adenohypophysial secretion of ACTH and the steroidogenic response of the adrenal cortex itself—are considered in some detail below. Other components, such as the peripheral and central neural mechanisms involved in the reception, transmission, and evaluation of the stimulus are also considered but only in general terms in this chapter. It is clear that each of the several components of the pathway contribute a time lag and that the total time elapsed between onset of the stimulus and activation of adrenocortical secretion can be no less than the sum of the individual time lags contributed by each component in the pathway. Since a significant increase in the secretory activity of the adrenal cortex occurs within only a few minutes after application of a noxious stimulus, each of the components involved must respond rather quickly. Experimental observations bear this out. Sydnor & Sayers (99) found that the time elapsed between application of a stimulus and increase in the rate of secretion of ACTH is exceedingly short; in the rat, plasma ACTH titers are markedly elevated within 2 min. The response time of the adrenal cortex to ACTH is also relatively short, despite the fact that the gland stores little cortisol or corticosterone, and hence enhanced secretory activity must proceed pari passu with enhanced biosynthesis of the steroids. In hypophysectomized animals (26) and in animals with adrenals transplanted to an accessible site (7, 18) the lag between the initial contact of ACTH with the adrenal cortex and the increase in secretory activity is about 3 min. Similarly, when ACTH is added to suspensions of isolated adrenal cortex cells in vitro, an increase in rate of secretion of corticosterone occurs after a lag period of 3–5 min (75).

We may conclude that the regulation of the secretory activity of the adrenal cortex involves processes that endow the gland with the capacity to quickly respond to a noxious stimulus (stress).

Mode of Action of ACTH

Intensive biochemical investigations have begun to elucidate the series of events initiated by ACTH and ending with increased secretion of steroids by a cell of the adrenal cortex (see chapters by Samuels and Nelson and by Haynes in this volume of the *Handbook*).

Adrenocorticotropic hormone interacts with a receptor on the plasma membrane of the adrenal cortex cell to generate a signal, which, after transduction and amplification within the membrane, activates adenylate cyclase. Production of cyclic AMP is enhanced and in turn increases the rate of steroidogenesis. The events occurring between cyclic AMP enhancement and the initial steroidogenic step, namely, conversion of cholesterol to pregnenolone, remain to be elucidated but probably include activation of a kinase that phosphorylates an enzyme, or enzymes, and also synthesis of a labile protein. Once pregnenolone is formed, the subsequent steps in the biosynthetic pathway occur at a rapid rate. In man and dog, cortisol and corticosterone are secreted; in the rat only corticosterone is elaborated (76).

The site of action of ACTH appears to be the outer surface of the plasma membrane. Thus ACTH, covalently linked to polymers much too large to pass through the cell membrane, exhibits steroidogenic activity upon addition to suspensions of isolated adrenal cortex cells (87, 94). If ACTH acts exclusively on the surface of the adrenal cortex cell, how is the probability that the cell will trap the few molecules of hormone that are distributed in the extracellular fluid increased?

Receptor Reserve: Sensitivity

The cells of the adrenal cortex exhibit *receptor reserve* (4, 28, 92), which is to say that ACTH need engage a very small fraction of the receptor population distributed over the outer surface of the plasma membrane to induce maximum rate of corticosteroid secretion. Seelig & Sayers (92) suggest that what may appear to be redundancy of receptors is in fact an amplification system that explains in some measure the exquisite sensitivity of the adrenal cortex to ACTH; a concentration as low as 10^{-16} M induces a significant increase in steroidogenesis. According to this view, "effective captures" are determined not only by the affinity of the ACTH molecule for receptors but also by the excess of receptors over and above that number which when activated induce maximum rate of steroidogenesis. From a teleological point of view the secretory burden on the adenohypophysis to establish a given rate of secretion of cortisol and/or corticosterone is reduced by many orders of magnitude.

ACTH: Structure-Activity Relationships

Determination of structure-activity relationships in a polypeptide the size of ACTH [39 amino acids (Fig. 1)] is a form of "molecular roulette" (102) well suited to challenge the skills of both chemist and biologist. Required of the chemist is the ability to design and synthesize potentially interesting fragments and derivatives of the native hormone. In this regard the achievements of Fujino et al. (24), Hofmann (35), Ramachandran et al. (61), Schwyzer (88), and Schwyzer & Sieber (90) have been of the greatest importance. For the biologist, the task is to devise systems that can gauge the significance of the chemical mutations. In the past, both in vivo (48, 85) and in vitro (68) techniques have been successfully applied. However, we have recently developed a new in vitro method which we believe is particularly suited to this goal. Adrenocorticotropic hormone increases the production of corticosterone when added to suspensions of isolated rat adrenal cells (84). Response and dose are related by the expression

$$B/B_{max} = A/(A + A_{50})$$

where B is the rate of corticosterone production, B_{max} is the maximum rate of corticosterone production, A is the concentration of ACTH, and A_{50} is the concentration required to induce $\frac{1}{2} B_{max}$ (92). According to the model proposed by Ariëns & Simonis (2), A_{50}, an apparent dissociation constant, is the reciprocal of the "affinity" of the hormone for its receptor and B_{max} is a measure of the effectiveness with which the hormone activates the receptor ("intrinsic activity"). In contrast to conventional methods of assay, the isolated cell technique provides measures of both affinity and intrinsic activity, information of some importance to the understanding of the relation of structure to biological action among members of a series of polypeptides related to ACTH.

The current status of investigations on the structure-activity relationship for ACTH may be summarized as follows. The 24-amino acid fragment of ACTH, ACTH$_{1-24}$, is equipotent or probably slightly more potent than the parent 39-amino acid molecule (92). The C-terminal sequence, starting with amino acid 25, has no known biological role and appears to be simply a curious vestigial appendage. Further shortening of the peptide from ACTH$_{1-24}$ to ACTH$_{1-18}$ is associated with a decrease, but by no means a drastic loss, in biological potency (36, 37, 45). When one or more of the dibasic amino acids at positions 15 through 18 are removed, a rather dramatic reduction in potency follows (36, 55). This grouping of dibasic amino acids is one of the important affinity sites of the ACTH molecule. But, despite loss of this affinity site, ACTH$_{1-10}$ if given in relatively large doses stimulates steroidogenesis when injected into hypophysectomized rats (55) or when added to a suspension of isolated adrenal cortex cells (89). The amino acids in positions 11 through 14 (the exact number as yet unknown) influence affinity but none is essential for activation of the receptor. In support of this thesis is the demonstration that ACTH$_{11-24}$ has no intrinsic activity when acting alone but is a competitive antagonist of ACTH$_{1-24}$ when the two peptides are added in combination (91).

These observations indicate that the "active center" of the ACTH molecule is in positions 1 through 10. The precise number of amino acids involved and the functional role of each in activating the receptor remain to be defined. Of interest is the demonstration by Fujino et al. (24) that ACTH$_{6-24}$ is active, whereas ACTH$_{7-23}$ is inactive in vivo. The observation of Schwyzer et al. (89) that ACTH$_{5-10}$ exhibits weak, but nevertheless significant, steroidogenic action in the isolated adrenal cortex cell system suggests that amino acids of the sequence His^6-Phe^7-Arg^8-Trp^9 are importantly involved in receptor activation. Adrenocorticotropic hormone belongs to a group of polypeptide hormones in which a single short segment of the chain activates the receptor; other regions of the chain are involved in attracting the molecule to its site of action.

Stimulation of Cortisol and/or Corticosterone Secretion by Factors of Questionable Physiological Significance

A single large dose of vasopressin increases adrenal secretory activity in the hypophysectomized dog (38) and

H-Ser-Tyr-Ser-Met-Glu-His-Phe-Arg-Trp-Gly-Lys-Pro-Val-Gly-
  1   2   3   4   5   6   7   8   9 10 11 12 13 14
                                              NH$_2$
                                               |
Lys-Lys-Arg-Arg-Pro-Val-Lys-Val-Tyr-Pro-Asp-Gly-Ala-Glu-
 15 16 17 18 19 20 21 22 23 24 25 26 27 28
Asp-Glu-Leu-Ala-Glu-Ala-Phe-Pro-Leu-Glu-Phe-OH
 29 30 31 32 33 34 35 36 37 38 39

FIG. 1. ACTH molecule. Structure shown, established by Riniker et al. (62), is that of porcine ACTH. Sequence, with minor modifications, is that first proposed by Bell and co-workers (5).

in the hypophysectomized rat (63). Both lysine vasopressin and angiotensin 5-valine stimulate cortisol secretion by the adrenal cortex of sheep but, in contrast to ACTH, fail to sustain secretory activity when infused continuously in large amounts (18). Furthermore neither vasopressin nor angiotensin II, in enormous quantities relative to an effective amount of ACTH, induces steroidogenesis when added to suspensions of isolated adrenal cortex cells (84). Under special circumstances large doses of vasopressin or angiotensin are capable of stimulating secretion of cortisol or corticosterone, but in our opinion these substances do not play a significant physiological role.

STIMULATION OF ACTH SECRETION

The thesis that stimulation of ACTH secretion is determined exclusively by a substance elaborated from neurons of the hypothalamus and transported via the portal venous system to the adenohypophysis has had a dominating influence on investigations in this field for about two decades. The accepted point of view acquired such an aura of respectability that alternative approaches were often dismissed as frivolous. But evidences to the effect that substances, arising in tissues other than the hypothalamus, stimulate ACTH release, can no longer be lightly dismissed.

A word of explanation about terminology is appropriate at this juncture. In the absence of chemical identification and assurance of biological specificity it is premature to speak of *corticotropin-releasing hormones*. We shall be content to speak of *corticotropin-releasing factors* (CRFs) a term coined by Saffran et al. (70). In the discussion to follow, we first evaluate methods of bioassay and then take up the individual CRF according to tissue source: hypothalamic median eminence CRF (HME-CRF), neurohypophysial CRF (vasopressin), and substances produced in other tissues, including liver, thymus, and cerebral cortex. Brodish (9) has used the term *tissue-CRF* for substances in this last category.

Bioassay of Corticotropin-releasing Factor

Development of a method of assay and chemical purification of biologically active substances are often interminably linked, and this appears to be the case for CRF. Lacking pure CRF we cannot be certain of the specificity of the assays, and lacking a specific assay we cannot be sure of the number and the chemical nature of CRF.

Evaluation of bioassay methods for CRF was an important section of a review by Sayers et al. (79) in 1958 on the relation between the hypothalamus and the adenohypophysis. As emphasized at that time, the intact animal is of no value for the assay of CRF. Practically any agent or tissue extract will increase the secretion of ACTH. Claims to the effect that anesthetics, analgesics, and sedatives, alone or in combination, block "nonspecific stressors" and reveal the presence of a CRF in an extract have never been backed with supporting evidence. Of perhaps special interest is the use of corticosteroids to block nonspecific stressors in an intact animal, but if the steroids block the excitatory action of CRF on the corticotrophs then the condition defeats the purpose of the assay.

If the median eminence were the sole source of CRF, then an animal with an ablative lesion in this area would be an ideal test object for CRF. McCann & Brobeck (51) reported in 1954 that a lesion in the supraopticohypophysial tract induces diabetes insipidus and inertia of the pituitary-adrenal system in rats. If the destructive lesion is not associated with impairment of the blood supply to the adenohypophysis, the adrenals remain normal in size and in sensitivity to ACTH. Acid extracts of median eminence tissue stimulate ACTH release (64), but a variety of stimuli effective in the intact animal (epinephrine, unilateral adrenalectomy, polymyxin B, serotonin, acetylsalicylic acid, histamine) fail to induce acceleration of ACTH release. However, under certain conditions noxious stimuli of relatively high intensity induce ACTH secretion in the lesioned rat (9). The evidence discussed in detail in another section supports the thesis that extrahypothalamic sites are involved in ACTH secretion.

In this connection, extracts of a number of tissues (cerebral cortex, liver, kidney, thymus) stimulate ACTH secretion in the lesioned animal. The fact that these extracts are less potent than an extract of median eminence tissue has been accepted, surprisingly enough, as evidence to support the thesis that the median eminence (hypothalamus) is the sole site of production of CRF. There can be absolutely no doubt that the lesioned animal has been and will continue to be of major importance in the assay of CRF. However, a less prejudiced assessment of the meaning of data obtained from this preparation is now possible.

Saffran & Schally (69) consider the capacity of a substance to release ACTH from anterior lobes of the pituitary in vitro to be the most direct measure of its function as a CRF. An extract of hypothalamic tissue plus norepinephrine, but neither one alone, induced an increase in the quantity of ACTH in the medium of incubated pituitary as compared to controls with no additions. An extract of cerebral cortex tissue plus norepinephrine and an extract of posterior pituitary tissue plus norepinephrine were also active.

In our laboratory, we have employed suspensions of trypsin-dispersed anterior pituitary cells of the rat for the bioassay of CRFs (59). The cells secrete ACTH when small amounts of HME extract (minimum effective dose = 0.005 HME) are added to the incubation medium, and the magnitude of the response increases as a linear function of the log-dose of extract added. The HME-induced secretion of ACTH is energy dependent, requires Ca^{2+}, and is inhibited by physiological amounts of corticosterone. Extracts of rat cerebral cortical tissue also induce significant ACTH secretion through a process inhibited by physiological amounts of corticosterone (G. Sayers and R. Portanova, unpublished data). Potency estimates, based on wet weight of tissue or total milligrams of acid-soluble protein, indicate that the cortical extracts contain approximately 30–50 times less CRF activity than extracts of HME. Acid extracts of rat heart, liver, or kidney tissue also induce ACTH release but are even less potent than the cortical extracts. Vasopressin (and several other neurohypophysial-like peptides) stimulates the release of ACTH from isolated pituitary cells through a process qualitatively similar to that of HME extract (i.e., the vasopressin-induced secretion is energy dependent, requires Ca^{2+}, and is inhibited by corticosterone). However, the CRF activity of vasopressin is quantitatively distinguished from that of HME extract in that the maximum rate of ACTH secretion induced by the polypeptide is significantly less than that induced by HME-CRF (60). These findings suggest that vasopressin is a partial agonist of ACTH secretion.

Hypothalamic CRF

The blood supply to the adenohypophysis is to a major extent carried in a portal system, although a direct arterial supply contributes to varying degrees according to species. The portal system arises in capillary loops in the median eminence; the capillaries coalesce to form veins that pass down the infundibular stem to the adenohypophysis where they break up into sinusoids. From the sinusoids, blood passes to venules that coalesce to form regular veins emptying into the cavernous sinus. On these strictly anatomic grounds, Harris (30) suggested some time ago that a chemical mediator is elaborated in the median eminence area of the hypothalamus and transported by the portal system to the adenohypophysis where it induces ACTH release. A few nerve fibers enter the adenohypophysis; their function appears to be vasomotor, and any suggestion that they may regulate ACTH secretion has long since been dismissed (79).

As pointed out above, acid extracts of median eminence tissue induce secretion of ACTH when injected into rats with lesions in the median eminence area of the hypothalamus. However, the many reports on fractionation of these extracts have in most instances led more to confusion than clarification. If one eliminates from discussion purported attempts at purification that fail to meet minimum standards of quality (acceptable bioassay, established freedom of the preparation from ACTH and from vasopressin) then exceedingly few need be mentioned. Royce & Sayers (66) concentrated HME-CRF activity in an extract of calf stalk median eminence tissue by chromatography on carboxymethyl cellulose. The purified material was free from vasopressin and ACTH; a dose of 4 µg of protein injected intravenously induced a substantial increase in rate of secretion of ACTH by the pituitary of the median eminence-lesioned rat. Biological activity was completely lost on treatment with pepsin, an enzyme that degrades neither vasopressin nor ACTH.

Neural Paths to Hypothalamic CRF Release

It is unfortunate that workers in the endocrine field have used and probably will continue to use the term *stress* to denote a stimulus effective in increasing the secretory activity of the adrenal cortex (80). Why use this jargon for the adrenal cortex? Why not use stimulus, since an effective stimulus may be beneficial, not necessarily damaging, and especially since the terminology would then be in line with that employed in other fields of physiology?

A recitation of the various stimuli that induce an increase in the secretory activity of the adrenal cortex is not delivered here [see the review by Sayers (71) and the more recent one by Allen et al. (1)]. The fact that many of these stimuli also increase the rate of secretion of aldosterone, vasopressin, growth hormone, and possibly other adenohypophysial hormones and alter blood pressure and respiration prompted the suggestion that the regulatory systems for endocrine and visceral functions employ common neuronal pathways (74). One is struck by the fact that a given stimulus may set in motion an indiscriminate number of endocrine and visceral activities. The teleological position, to the effect that these responses serve a useful purpose, must not be embraced without hesitation. Whether the indiscriminate responses are "good," "bad," or indifferent is very much an open question. Of some interest would be the establishment in time, after the initial indiscriminate responses, when more selective and appropriate responses, directed toward the mitigation of the aberrations peculiar to a given insult, come into play. Much of the work on regulation of the secretory activity of the adrenal cortex has been focused on the early period following application of a stimulus, although there have been certain notable exceptions, for example, the work of Brodish (9).

Numerous stimuli, effective in increasing ACTH secretion, evoke impulses that travel in afferents of the somatic and autonomic nervous systems into the spinal cord and brainstem (73). These impulses ascend in the spinal cord and probably traverse the brainstem via oligosynaptic and multisynaptic connections (65) to reach the hypothalamus and other brain centers. Cerebral cortex, basal ganglia, rhinencephalon, and thalamus are linked to the hypothalamus by extensive neural connections. Impulses arising in the periphery (e.g., in response to a painful stimulus) can travel fairly directly to the hypothalamus or via circuitous routes with relays at the level of cerebral cortex, thalamus, and rhinencephalon. Fear, anxiety, sorrow, and possibly joy are associated with alterations in rate of secretion of ACTH; neural pathways to hypothalamus from cerebral cortex, amygdala, and other rhinencephalic centers appear to be involved (73).

That the hypothalamus is a focal point for the various impulses is indicated by the studies of Halász (29) who devised an ingenious technique for deafferentation of the hypothalamus of the rat. Delineation of paths entering the hypothalamus and of paths within that structure leading to the median eminence has been the object of recent experimental studies [see (49)].

Neurohypophysial CRF—Vasopressin

Vasopressin induces ACTH secretion when injected intravenously into a rat with a lesion in the median eminence (51, 63), when added to the medium during incubation of pituitary fragments (22), and when added to suspensions of isolated pituitary cells (60). In considering the possible role of vasopressin, McCann (50) pointed out that many noxious stimuli that induce increased secretion of ACTH also induce vasopressin release. Furthermore, according to McCann (50), the release of vasopressin occurs rapidly enough to account for the prompt release of ACTH. Incidentally the isolation of an active factor, free from vasopressin, from median eminence tissue (HME-CRF) does not rule out vasopressin as a physiological CRF (66); the demonstration simply provides evidence that vasopressin is not the sole mediator of ACTH secretion.

Vasopressin has advantages when used in the experimental study of regulation of ACTH secretion. First, the synthetic substance is readily available. Second, vasopressin on a weight basis is by far the most potent CRF at hand. However, potency as a CRF can be deceptive. Exceedingly small quantities (less than 0.25 µg) are active in the rat with a lesion in the median eminence, but these quantities, small as they are, produce pronounced toxic effects. Finally the quantities required to induce ACTH secretion are many orders of magnitude greater than those required to induce antidiuresis.

A most intriguing, but at the same time frustrating, aspect of vasopressin is the multitude of ways in which it can bring about an increase in the secretory activity of the adrenal cortex. Mention has already been made of action in hypophysectomized animals. Sayers (72) has shown that the capacity of vasopressin to induce ACTH secretion is markedly attenuated after transection of the brainstem at the level of midbrain. Obviously the actions of injected vasopressin include, in addition to a direct one on the adenohypophysis, peripheral effects subserved by neural paths passing through the brainstem to the hypothalamus. Additionally, vasopressin appears to be able to release ACTH bound to extrapituitary sites (e.g., the kidney) (63).

The maximum rate of secretion of ACTH by isolated pituitary cells in response to vasopressin is decidedly less than that in response to HME-CRF. When added in combination with appropriate doses of HME-CRF, vasopressin inhibits ACTH secretion. Portanova & Sayers (60) suggest, on the basis of these findings, that vasopressin is a partial agonist of ACTH secretion and is related in chemical structure to the true CRF. In this connection, Saffran et al. (67) report that the ring portion of vasopressin, pressinoic acid, is a more potent CRF than the parent compound. However, Portanova and Sayers find pressinoic acid to be inactive over a wide range of concentrations in the isolated pituitary cell system (G. Sayers and R. Portanova, unpublished observations).

The physiological role of vasopressin in the regulation of ACTH secretion remains an enigma.

Tissue CRF: Extrahypothalamic Production of CRF

The studies of Brodish (9) and of Egdahl (16) have been of major importance in establishing that the hypothalamus is not the sole site of elaboration of substances that stimulate ACTH secretion. However, we should not lose sight of the fact that work reported in the late 1940s established that neither direct neural nor vascular connections with the hypothalamus are essential for the discharge of ACTH from the adenohypophysis. Transplants of the adenohypophysis in the anterior chamber of the eye discharge ACTH in response to a noxious stimulus (10, 23, 52).

Egdahl (16) devised a technique for the isolation of the pituitary from the brain. The brainstem of the dog is transected at the level of the inferior colliculus, and all brain tissue rostral to the cut, including median eminence, is removed by suction. The resultant "pituitary island" consists of anterior and posterior pituitaries. The blood supply to the anterior pituitary of the island comes from branches of the internal carotid and another vessel that passes from the posterior pituitary; the portal venous system is disrupted when the median eminence is removed. Undoubtedly blood supply to the adenohypophysis is reduced, but it is unlikely that the functional changes to be described are a consequence of leakage of ACTH from hypoxic corticotrophs.

In the absence of noxious insult, rate of secretion of corticosteroids by the adrenal cortex in dogs with a pituitary island preparation is relatively high and remains high for as long as 5 days postoperation. Burn trauma induces rapid increases in adrenal secretory activity. In an extension of these studies, Egdahl (17) has demonstrated that a pituitary island continues to secrete ACTH at relatively high basal rates and responds to noxious stimuli with an increase in ACTH secretion when all brain tissue (i.e., including brainstem and spinal cord) have been removed. These studies in the dog have been confirmed by Wise et al. (108). Furthermore in the monkey (43) and rat (109) the pituitary island exhibits the same functional capacities. The conclusion is inescapable that CRFs are produced at sites other than the central nervous system (CNS).

Witorsch & Brodish (109) have demonstrated that a noxious stimulus will increase secretion of ACTH in a rat whose entire hypothalamus has been destroyed. Furthermore extracts of liver, kidney, and thymus (tissue-CRF) induce ACTH secretion when injected into this preparation. Now a possible explanation is that the actions of noxious stimuli (including extracts of liver) are mediated by the passage of vasopressin from the posterior to the anterior pituitary (15). However, in a recent study, Brodish (9) has provided evidence that rather clearly distinguishes tissue-CRF from HME-CRF and from vasopressin. Plasma taken from hypothalamic-lesioned, hypophysectomized donor rats 5 hr after laparotomy was assayed for CRF activity in hypothalamic-lesioned recipient rats. The plasma contained a high degree of CRF activity. This CRF in the plasma (tissue-CRF), like HME-CRF and vasopressin, induced a prompt increase (peak at 20 min) in the concentration of corticosterone in the plasma of a recipient hypothalamic-lesioned rat. Tissue-CRF was distinguished by its capacity to produce a prolonged, as well as a prompt, response—plasma corticosterone remained elevated 3 hr after injection. The sites of production of tissue-CRF are yet to be defined, but the evidence is rather convincing that certain tissues, such as liver, can under certain circumstances release substances that are carried in the systemic circulation to stimulate ACTH secretion at the level of the adenohypophysis. Of additional interest is the demonstration that corticosterone administration suppresses the elaboration of tissue CRF, which otherwise develops after laparotomy.

The reader may find it difficult to reconcile reports to the effect that section of the CNS at various levels blocks the response of the adrenal cortex to numerous stimuli with reports cited to the effect that the adrenal cortex of an animal whose pituitary has been completely separated from the nervous system exhibits an increase in secretory activity when a noxious stimulus is applied. We do not pretend to be aware of all the factors entering into the complex protocols of the experimental studies that make the difference, but we do believe the following to be of some importance in the reconciliation: *a*) strength of the noxious stimulus; *b*) time after application of stimulus at which plasma level of ACTH or of corticosteroids is measured; *c*) previous exposure of the animal to trauma —referring specifically to the demonstration of Witorsch & Brodish (109) that noxious stimuli and tissue-CRF (e.g., extracts of liver, cerebral cortex) effectively increase ACTH secretion in an animal whose hypothalamus has been destroyed if the animal has been "sensitized" by prior application of a noxious stimulus.

INHIBITION OF ACTH SECRETION

Corticosteroids

Ingle (39) was the first to demonstrate an inhibitory action of corticosteroids on ACTH release. The increase in adrenal weight that normally develops during 12 hr of muscular exercise was not observed in rats treated with cortical extract during the period of activity. Furthermore cortical extract caused adrenal atrophy in normal animals but failed to inhibit increase in adrenal weight induced by ACTH administered to hypophysectomized rats, an observation interpreted to mean that the corticosteroids inhibit the secretion of the tropic hormone from the pituitary rather than interfere with its stimulatory action on the adrenal cortex (40, 83).

Introduction of adrenal ascorbic acid depletion as an index of ACTH secretion made it possible to examine stimulation and inhibition at brief intervals after application of a noxious stimulus. Administration of cortical extract prevented the decrease in adrenal ascorbic acid that otherwise accompanies exposure of the rat to cold for 1 hr; the extract did not prevent the decrease resulting from the administration of ACTH (81).

The development of methods for the assay of ACTH in the blood (98, 107) prepared the way for the accumulation of more direct evidence in support of the thesis that corticosteroids inhibit ACTH secretion. The level of ACTH in the plasma was shown to be significantly higher than normal in patients with Addison's disease (46, 100) and in adrenalectomized rats (99).

Having presented the evidences which early established that the corticosteroids play an important physiological role in the regulation of ACTH secretion, we now turn our attention to aspects of the phenomena that currently engage the attention of numerous investigators: a) the sites of inhibitory action of the corticosteroids (adenohypophysis, median eminence of the hypothalamus, brain centers); b) the influence of dose (concentration); c) the kinetics of the inhibitory action (time of onset, time for peak inhibitory effect, time of decay); d) relation of structure of steroid to inhibitory potency; and e) the mode of action expressed in biochemical terms, including inhibition of ACTH synthesis.

SITES OF INHIBITORY ACTIONS OF CORTICOSTEROIDS. A direct inhibitory action of the corticosteroids on the secretion of ACTH by the adenohypophysis is established beyond doubt. Release of ACTH into the medium was inhibited by the addition of cortisol to incubated fragments of bovine anterior pituitary tissue (57). In the instance of incubated rat pituitary fragments, basal secretion was uninfluenced, but vasopressin-induced (22) or HME-CRF-induced (3) secretion of ACTH was inhibited by adding corticosteroids to the incubation medium. Kraicer et al. (44) reported that the increase in ACTH release induced by abnormally high concentrations of potassium in the medium was inhibited by addition of corticosterone to the incubate. Fleischer et al. (20) found that dexamethasone inhibits dibutyryl cyclic AMP-induced release of ACTH from pituitary fragments in vitro.

Some have questioned the physiological significance of these results based on manipulation of pituitary fragments in vitro. However, recent observations on pituitary cells in monolayer culture and on freshly isolated anterior pituitary cells leave no doubt that the corticosteroids at physiological concentrations do suppress ACTH secretion by pituitary corticotrophs. Dexamethasone, at concentrations of 0.01–0.1 µg/ml, had no effect on ACTH synthesis but decreased secretion of ACTH by monolayer cultures of rat anterior pituitary cells. More importantly, corticosterone, at a concentration of 0.1 µg/ml, suppressed secretion of ACTH by the cultured cells (21). Isolated rat anterior pituitary cells in suspension respond to HME-CRF with secretion of ACTH into the medium (59). Corticosterone, in a concentration of 0.01 µg/ml of medium, inhibits slightly and, at a concentration of 0.1 µg/ml, markedly suppresses ACTH secretion by the isolated cells.

The evidence is clear that the adenohypophysis is an important site of the suppressive action of the corticosteroids. This does not rule out the possibility that the steroids exert an inhibitory action at other sites as well, and indeed much effort has been expended in attempting to locate such sites in the hypothalamus and other regions of the brain. In this regard, the local implantation of steroids has been a favored technique for mapping feedback sites. However, as Bogdanove (8) pointed out, the technique is prone to a fatal defect: steroids implanted at a particular brain site may diffuse or be transported to a distant site where they exert their suppressive action. Studies in Kendall's laboratory (41) support Bogdanove's suggestion. The ability of steroid implants to suppress ACTH secretion was observed to be related to the proximity of the implant to the brain ventricular system. Furthermore injection of tritiated corticosterone into the lateral ventricle was followed within minutes by the appearance of radioactivity in the adenohypophysis. These findings led Kendall (41) to conclude that steroids implanted into the brain might actually be transported in the cerebrospinal fluid to the adenohypophysis where they inhibit ACTH secretion. Kendall (41), in an illuminating historical piece, provides perspective.

> Thirty years ago, following the observations of Ingle et al. (1938) on the relationship between the pituitary and the adrenal cortex, it was assumed that the adenohypophysis was the site of feedback control of adrenocorticotropic hormone (ACTH) secretion. Twenty years ago the emphasis of feedback control moved towards the hypothalamus following Harris' observations on the significance of the hypophyseal portal system (1955). Ten years ago, virtually everyone had concluded that the hypothalamus was the site of feedback control of ACTH secretion by corticosteroids and only the proof was lacking. The pendulum has swung again and at the present time the bulk of evidence seems to favor the adenohypophysis as the primary site of feedback action and the burden of proof lies with those who claim there is hypothalamus participation.

Some evidence for the involvement of extrapituitary sites is provided by studies demonstrating an effect of the steroids on hypothalamic CRF stores. Vernikos-Danellis (104) reported that cortisol decreases the hypothalamic content of CRF and prevents the rise in CRF content normally induced by stress (ether plus sham adrenalectomy). Takebe et al. (101) also found that stress (laparotomy plus intestinal traction) increases the quantity of CRF in the hypothalamus and that dexamethasone inhibits the response. One of the many possible interpretations of these results is that the corticosteroids interfere with the production of CRF by hypothalamic neurons, a point of view espoused by Hedge & Smelik (31) on the basis of observations using an alternative, but also indirect, experimental design. If the corticosteroids do deplete hypothalamic stores of CRF by interfering with its synthesis, it might be expected that adrenalectomy would augment the quantity of CRF in the hypothalamus. The experimental findings on this point are conflicting. In chronically (2 weeks or longer) adrenalectomized animals the hypothalamic content of CRF was found by Vernikos-Danellis (104) to be increased by a factor of two, by Hiroshige (34) to be unchanged, and by Seiden & Brodish (93) to be decreased by a factor of two. The reason for these discrepancies is not apparent at this time.

Yates (110) offered the speculation that the corticosteroids inhibit the nervous system at a level above the median eminence and that the relative effectiveness or ineffectiveness of corticosteroid to inhibit a given noxious stimulus is determined by the steroid sensitivity or insensitivity of the pathway that subserved that stimulus. The inability of steroid pretreatment to completely inhibit a given type of stimulus was, in all likelihood, due to the fact that the stimulus was of relatively high intensity and that what appear to be qualitative differences among stimuli in regard to steroid inhibition are in fact quantitative differences in intensity.

For the sake of completeness we mention the work of Hill & Singer (33) and of Perón et al. (56) interpreted to mean that corticosterone at physiological concentrations can inhibit the steroidogenic action of ACTH on the adrenal cortex. However, the in vitro work of Birmingham & Kurlents (6) on rat adrenal quarters and more recent experiments on isolated adrenal cortex cells (77) clearly demonstrate that the concentration of corticosterone in the incubation media must equal 300 or more micrograms per 100 ml before significant inhibition of ACTH is observed. In conclusion, corticosteroids can exert a direct inhibitory action on the secretory activity of the adrenal cortex, but the phenomenon is of no physiological significance [see also the work in vivo (14, 97)].

CONCENTRATION OF CORTICOSTEROID AND DEGREE OF INHIBITION OF ACTH SECRETION. Important quantitative relationships were derived from the studies of Sayers & Sayers (82) who examined a variety of stimuli, including heat, cold, typhoid vaccine, and histamine administration. First, the rate of release of ACTH from the adenohypophysis is proportional to the intensity of the noxious stimulus applied. Second, the degree of inhibition of ACTH release, for any given intensity of stimulus applied, is proportional to the amount of corticosteroid administered. Third, the more intense the stimulus applied the greater the quantity of corticosteroid required to inhibit ACTH release; in the instances where the stimulus was of great intensity even large doses of cortisol (>1.0 mg) were capable of only partial blockade of the adrenal response. These observations have recently been confirmed by Kendall et al. (42) using graded doses of lysine vasopressin or epinephrine as the noxious stimuli.

KINETICS OF INHIBITORY ACTION OF CORTICOSTEROIDS ON ACTH SECRETION. That duration of exposure to steroid was an important parameter in the inhibitory process was suggested by the work of Smelik (96) who noted that, subsequent to corticosteroid administration, maximum suppression of ACTH secretion developed later than the peak of plasma steroid concentration.

In a detailed examination of the influence of length of exposure, Sirett & Gibbs (95) injected dexamethasone intraperitoneally (400 μg/100 g body wt) at various times before administration of urethane. A blood sample was withdrawn from an external jugular vein 20 min after urethane administration. In the absence of dexamethasone treatment, urethane increases the level of corticosterone in the plasma of the rat from about 10 to 50 μg/100 ml. Maximum suppression of urethane-induced ACTH secretion developed approximately 10–12 hr after the administration of dexamethasone. After 24 hr response had returned to normal. Secretion of ACTH in response to a noxious stimulus is a function of the length of time of the corticosteroid pretreatment.

Kendall et al. (42) examined the changes in the levels of corticosterone in the plasma in response to lysine vasopressin and to epinephrine at various times after injection of dexamethasone. During the interval between dexamethasone injection and injection of lysine vasopressin or epinephrine, the rats ingested dexamethasone in the drinking water (about 600 μg per rat per day). The increase in plasma corticosterone that followed administration of vasopressin or of epinephrine progressively decreased with time after initiation of dexamethasone treatment. Furthermore the more intense the noxious stimulus the larger the period required for suppression of the plasma corticosterone response.

These studies of Sirett & Gibbs (95) and of Kendall et al. (42) clearly demonstrated that optimum inhibition of ACTH secretion takes hours to develop. However, the experiments of Sayers & Sayers (82) just as clearly demonstrated that inhibitory action is manifest without significant lag; ACTH secretion was inhibited when the corticosteroids were injected subcutaneously 5 min before application of the noxious stimulus. From the results of a carefully designed and executed series of experiments, Dallman & Yates (13) arrived at the conclusion that steroid inhibition has a rapidly acting, rate-sensitive component and a slowly acting, delayed proportional component. The prompt inhibition induced by injected steroid is proportional to the rate of increase of concentration of corticosteroids in the blood. The delayed inhibition is proportional to the concentration of corticosteroids in the blood. The thesis of Dallman & Yates

(13) brings into harmony what might otherwise appear to be discrepancies among reported observations.

Corticosterone has now been shown to suppress ACTH secretion by isolated anterior pituitary cells of the rat (78). Analysis of the results are relatively simple in this in vitro system where the steroid acts directly on anterior pituitary cells. These cells in suspension respond in a dose-dependent fashion to the addition of an extract of the median eminence (HME) with secretion of ACTH into the medium. Physiological concentrations of corticosterone in the medium (0.1 and even 0.01 μg/ml) significantly depress HME-induced secretion of ACTH. The inhibition is significant in less than 15 min after addition of the steroid to the suspension. In addition to this inhibition of rapid onset is another whose imprint remains with the corticotrophs for a considerable period. Adrenalectomized rats (2 weeks postoperation) were killed at the same time of day (9 AM) but at various times after a single pulse dose of 1.0 mg of corticosterone injected subcutaneously. The anterior pituitary tissue of the animals was dispersed and the isolated cells challenged with HME-CRF. Maximum suppression of HME-CRF-induced ACTH secretion developed after 8–10 hr of steroid pretreatment; responsiveness returned to pre-steroid values after 24 hr. The results have been interpreted to mean that corticosteroids act on the corticotrophs by two separate mechanisms, one prompt in onset, the other characterized by a long lag period of onset.

One might expect the bolus of steroid secreted in response to a noxious stimulus to blunt the secretory response of the adrenal cortex to a subsequent noxious stimulus. Dallman & Jones (12) have demonstrated that such is not the case. They believe that, in the intact animal, the increase in corticosterone secretion induced by a noxious stimulus tends to inhibit ACTH secretion; however, the noxious stimulus also increases responsiveness either in the CNS or in the anterior pituitary so that subsequent stimuli tend to provoke greater than normal increase in CRF and/or ACTH secretion. The two effects of the stimulus—increased responsiveness of a central component and the suppression of ACTH secretion by the elevated titers of corticosterone—cancel, and the adrenocortical system responds to repeated stimuli with a relatively normal index of responsiveness. These observations and interpretations of Dallman & Jones (12) have rather important physiological implications.

RELATION BETWEEN STRUCTURE OF STEROID AND INHIBITORY POTENCY. Potencies, in relation to inhibition of ACTH release, have been assigned to various steroids (82). Cortisol and cortisone are equipotent; if they are arbitrarily assigned a value of 100, corticosterone, 11-deoxycorticosterone, and progesterone have potencies of 25, 12, and 0.5, respectively. These potencies parallel the gluconeogenic and anti-inflammatory potencies of the steroids. However, Cheng & Sayers (11) considered the inhibition of ACTH release by 11-deoxycorticosterone to be greater than expected if the parallelism mentioned were exact. They described insulin hypersensitivity of rats administered large doses of 11-deoxycorticosterone acetate, which they interpreted to mean that the steroid induced a relative deficiency of glucocorticoids. Furthermore they arrived at the tentative conclusion that the corticosteroids inhibit the adenohypophysis directly rather than through the mediation of a metabolite of their actions or through their deficiencies. The insulin hypersensitivity after 11-deoxycorticosterone is not unequivocally due to a relative deficiency of glucocorticoids; the phenomenon may be at least partially due to a toxic effect of 11-deoxycorticosterone on the liver.

MODE OF ACTION EXPRESSED IN BIOCHEMICAL TERMS AND INHIBITION OF ACTH SYNTHESIS. Actinomycin D inhibits the capacity of dexamethasone to suppress ACTH secretion in normal and in adrenalectomized rats (19). These observations suggest that the steroid exerts its inhibitory action by steps that include synthesis of a ribonucleic acid. Actinomycin D also blocks the suppressive action of dexamethasone on HME-induced ACTH secretion in pituitary fragments (3).

The corticosteroids reduce both ACTH secretion and the quantity of ACTH in the pituitary, indicating inhibition of synthesis of the tropic hormone. This conclusion, based on in vivo studies, is supported by the observation of Watanabe et al. (105) that ACTH synthesis by a pituitary tumor cell is suppressed when glucocorticoids are added to the culture medium. Since the pituitary normally contains relatively large stores of ACTH it is unlikely that suppression of synthesis is the sole cause of suppression of secretion. With advances in techniques for examining secretion and synthesis of ACTH in isolated cell systems (58, 105), clarification of the dynamic relations between synthesis and secretion of ACTH can be expected in the near future.

Short-loop Feedback of ACTH on CRF

Motta and co-workers (53, 54) have championed the "short-loop feedback," an inhibitory scheme whereby ACTH of the adenohypophysis acts to inhibit the elaboration of CRF by the median eminence. Indirect support comes from the demonstration that ACTH administration reduces the content of CRF in the median eminence of the hypophysectomized, adrenalectomized rat (93). Further investigation and evaluation are necessary before we can assess the physiological importance of the short-loop feedback.

Central Inhibitory Adrenergic Pathway

Experimental studies of Ganong and his colleagues (86, 103) suggest the existence of an adrenergic path in the brain that inhibits ACTH secretion. The intravenous administration of L-dihydroxyphenylalanine (L-dopa), a precursor of the catecholamines, in a dose of 50 mg/kg inhibits secretion of ACTH in the dog. That the inhibition of ACTH secretion is causally related to increased synthesis and liberation of catecholamines is suggested by the fact that the minimum effective dose (50 mg/kg) of L-dopa in inhibiting ACTH secretion is increased to 100 mg/kg by treatment of the dog with a compound that interferes with catecholamine synthesis and is reduced to 10 mg/kg by treatment of the dog with a substance that interferes with degradation of the catecholamines. Ganong (27) concludes that "these results plus the fact that there are prominent adrenergic systems in the ventral hypothalamus make it reasonable to advance the working hypothesis that in the dog a hypothalamic adrenergic system inhibits ACTH secretion." Contradictory evidence has been reported (47), and we simply must await additional reports from Ganong and his colleagues and evidences from other laboratories before making a final judgment on the physiological importance of a central inhibitory adrenergic path.

CONCLUDING REMARKS

We take this opportunity to convey our impressions and opinions status quo on regulation of the secretion of cortisol and corticosterone. Reports on the subject appear at an ever-increasing rate, placing an ever-increasing demand on the development of working hypotheses and on the building of models designed to embrace at least part of the large number of observations pertinent to regulation of ACTH secretion. We feel that it is premature to apply the sophisticated techniques of the systems control analyst to regulation of the secretion of ACTH. Recent advances in methodology have embarrassed us into the realization that we have been feeding the computers a great quantity of distorted or even incorrect information. We feel that the most pressing need is for detailed examinations of the operations of the individual parts in isolation followed by the construction of working hypotheses. Information gained from such examinations in certain instances reveals new insights into the nature of the workings in the whole animal. Of special importance is the value of these insights in the design of new experimental approaches.

We look forward to improvements of currently employed methods, developments of new and unique techniques, and greater attention to the time variable. As concrete examples of progress, we cite the isolated pituitary cell technique, the improvements in analytical methods for the analysis of steroids in the body fluids, the attention to frequency of sampling of blood for analyses, and the thorough survey of the time variable in studies designed to elucidate the role of CRFs and the inhibitory actions of the corticosteroids.

We have wondered why we still do not have pure HME-CRF. Further there is a striking contrast between the aura of respectability given the notion that HME-CRF exists and the paucity of evidence as to its chemical structure. Certainly until such time as we have more definitive chemical evidence, we must be cautious about assigning HME-CRF a major physiological role in regulating the rate of secretion of ACTH. The role of vasopressin remains an enigma. An important new development is the demonstration of CRF activity, albeit in crude extracts, in cerebral cortex, liver, and possibly other tissues. Efforts should be directed toward chemical characterization of the active substances.

Of fundamental importance to an understanding of the regulatory scheme is the demonstration that the adrenal cortex of normal undisturbed man is quiescent for the major part of the day; episodic bursts of activity account for all or at least the major fraction of the total daily secretory output of the gland. Studies should be directed to determine whether this pattern holds for dog, rat, and other species.

Finally it has given the authors a certain amount of satisfaction to see a relatively old thesis gain affirmation. The evidence is impressive that the corticosteroids exert a physiologically important inhibitory action on the corticotrophs of the adenohypophysis. Other sites of action remain to be established. Hopefully the means by which cortisol and corticosterone inhibit ACTH secretion will be expressed in biochemical terms in the near future.

REFERENCES

1. ALLEN, J. P., C. F. ALLEN, M. A. GREER, AND J. J. JACOBS. Stress-induced secretion of ACTH. In: *Brain-Pituitary-Adrenal Interrelationships*, edited by A. Brodish and E. S. Redgate. Basel: Karger, 1973, p. 99–127.
2. ARIËNS, E. J., AND A. M. SIMONIS. A molecular basis for drug action. *J. Pharm. Pharmacol.* 16: 137–157, 1964.
3. ARIMURA, A., C. Y. BOWERS, A. V. SCHALLY, M. SAITO, AND M. C. MILLER, III. Effect of corticotropin-releasing factor, dexamethasone and actinomycin D on the release of ACTH from rat pituitaries *in vivo* and *in vitro*. *Endocrinology* 85: 300–311, 1969.
4. BEALL, R., AND G. SAYERS. Isolated adrenal cells: steroidogenesis and cyclic AMP accumulation in response to ACTH. *Arch. Biochem. Biophys.* 148: 70–76, 1972.
5. BELL, P. H., K. S. HOWARD, R. G. SHEPHERD, B. M. FINN, AND J. H. MEISENHELDER. Studies with corticotrophs. II. Pepsin degradation of β-corticotropin. *J. Am. Chem. Soc.* 78: 5059–5066, 1956.
6. BIRMINGHAM, M. K., AND E. KURLENTS. Inactivation of ACTH by isolated rat adrenals and inhibition of corticoid formation by adrenocortical hormones. *Endocrinology* 62: 47–60, 1958.
7. BLAIR-WEST, J. R., J. P. COGHLAN, D. A. DENTON, B. A. SCOGGINS, E. M. WINTOUR, AND R. D. WRIGHT. The onset of effect of ACTH, angiotensin II and raised plasma potassium concentration on the adrenal cortex. *Steroids* 15: 433–448, 1970.
8. BOGDANOVE, E. M. Direct gonad-pituitary feedback: an analysis of effects of intracranial estrogenic depots on gonadotrophin secretion. *Endocrinology* 73: 696–712, 1963.
9. BRODISH, A. Hypothalamic and extrahypothalamic corticotrophin-releasing factors in peripheral blood. In: *Brain-Pituitary-Adrenal Interrelationships*, edited by A. Brodish and E. S. Redgate. Basel: Karger, 1973, p. 128–151.
10. CHENG, C. P., G. SAYERS, L. S. GOODMAN, AND C. A. SWINYARD. Discharge of adrenocorticotrophic hormone from transplanted pituitary tissue. *Am. J. Physiol.* 159: 426–432, 1949.
11. CHENG, C. P., AND G. SAYERS. Insulin hypersensitivity fol-

lowing the administration of desoxycorticosterone acetate. *Endocrinology* 44: 400–408, 1949.
12. DALLMAN, M. F., AND M. T. JONES. Corticosteroid feedback control of ACTH secretion: effect of stress-induced corticosterone secretion on subsequent stress responses in the rat. *Endocrinology* 92: 1367–1375, 1973.
13. DALLMAN, M., AND F. E. YATES. Dynamic asymmetries in the corticosteroid feedback path and distribution-metabolism-binding elements of the adrenocortical system. *Ann. NY Acad. Sci.* 156: 696–721, 1969.
14. DE WIED, D. The site of the blocking action of dexamethasone on stress-induced pituitary ACTH release. *J. Endocrinol.* 29: 29–37, 1964.
15. DUNN, J., AND V. CRITCHLOW. Vasopressin-evoked ACTH release in rats following forebrain removal. *Proc. Soc. Exptl. Biol. Med.* 136: 1284–1288, 1971.
16. EGDAHL, R. H. Adrenal cortical and medullary responses to trauma in dogs with isolated pituitaries. *Endocrinology* 66: 200–216, 1960.
17. EGDAHL, R. H. Abstract. *Program Ann. Meeting Endocrine Soc., 1962*, p. 20.
18. ESPINER, E. A., C. A. JENSEN, AND D. S. HART. Dynamics of adrenal response to sustained local ACTH infusions in conscious sheep. *Am. J. Physiol.* 222: 570–577, 1972.
19. FLEISCHER, N., AND H. BATTARBEE. Inhibition of dexamethasone suppression of ACTH secretion *in vivo* by actinomycin D. *Proc. Soc. Exptl. Biol. Med.* 126: 922–925, 1967.
20. FLEISCHER, N., R. A. DONALD, AND R. W. BUTCHER. Involvement of adenosine 3′,5′-monophosphate in release of ACTH. *Am. J. Physiol.* 217: 1287–1291, 1969.
21. FLEISCHER, N., AND W. E. RAWLS. ACTH synthesis and release in pituitary monolayer culture: effect of dexamethasone. *Am. J. Physiol.* 219: 445–448, 1970.
22. FLEISCHER, N., AND W. VALE. Inhibition of vasopressin-induced ACTH release from the pituitary by glucocorticoids *in vitro*. *Endocrinology* 83: 1232–1236, 1968.
23. FORTIER, C., AND H. SELYE. Adrenocorticotrophic effect of stress after severance of the hypothalamo-hypophyseal pathways. *Am. J. Physiol.* 159: 433–439, 1949.
24. FUJINO, M., C. HATANAKA, AND O. NISHIMURA. Synthesis of peptides related to corticotropin (ACTH). VI. Syntheses and biological activity of the peptides corresponding to the amino sequences 4–23, 5–23, 6–24, 7–23 in ACTH. *Chem. Pharm. Bull.* 19: 1066–1068, 1971.
25. GALLAGHER, T. F., K. YOSHIDA, H. D. ROFFWARG, D. K. FUKUSHIMA, E. D. WEITZMAN, AND L. HELLMAN. ACTH and cortisol secretory patterns in man. *J. Clin. Endocrinol. Metab.* 36: 1058–1068, 1973.
26. GANONG, W. F. *Review of Medical Physiology.* Los Altos: Lange Med. Publ., 1971, p. 279.
27. GANONG, W. F. Central monoaminergic systems and hypothalamic function. In: *The Hypothalamus*, edited by L. Martini, M. Motta, and F. Fraschini. New York: Acad. Press, 1971.
28. GRAHAME-SMITH, D. B., R. W. BUTCHER, R. L. NEY, AND E. W. SUTHERLAND. Adenosine-3′,5′-monophosphate as the intracellular mediator of the action of adrenocorticotropic hormone on the adrenal cortex. *J. Biol. Chem.* 242: 5535–5541, 1967.
29. HALÁSZ, B. The endocrine effects of isolation of the hypothalamus from the rest of the brain. In: *Frontiers of Neuroendocrinology*, edited by W. F. Ganong and L. Martini. London: Oxford Univ. Press, 1969, p. 307–342.
30. HARRIS, G. W. *Neural Control of the Pituitary Gland.* London: Arnold, 1955.
31. HEDGE, G. A., AND P. G. SMELIK. The action of dexamethasone and vasopressin on hypothalamic CRF production and release. *Neuroendocrinology* 4: 242–253, 1969.
32. HELLMAN, L., F. NAKADA, J. CURTI, E. D. WEITZMAN, J. KREAM, H. ROFFWARG, S. ELLMAN, D. K. FUKUSHIMA, AND T. F. GALLAGHER. Cortisol is secreted episodically by normal man. *J. Clin. Endocrinol. Metab.* 30: 411–422, 1970.
33. HILL, C. D., AND B. SINGER. Inhibition of the response to pituitary adrenocorticotrophic hormone in the hypophysectomized rat by circulatory corticosterone. *J. Endocrinol.* 42: 301–309, 1968.
34. HIROSHIGE, T. CRF assay by intrapituitary injection through the parapharyngeal approach and its physiological validation. In: *Brain-Pituitary-Adrenal Interrelationships*, edited by A. Brodish and E. S. Redgate. Basel: Karger, 1973, p. 57–78.
35. HOFMANN, K. Preliminary observations relating structure and function in some pituitary hormones. *Brookhaven Symp. Biol.* 13: 184–202, 1960.
36. HOFMANN, K., R. ANDREATTA, H. BOHN, AND L. MORODER. Studies on polypeptides. XLV. Structure-function studies in the β-corticotropin series. *J. Med. Chem.* 13: 339–345, 1970.
37. HOFMANN, K., N. YANAIHARA, S. LANDE, AND H. YAJIMA. Studies on polypeptides. XXIII. Synthesis and biological activity of a hexadecapeptide corresponding to the N-terminal sequence of the corticotropins. *J. Am. Chem. Soc.* 84: 4470–4474, 1962.
38. HUME, D. M., AND D. H. NELSON. Abstract. *Program Ann. Meeting Endocrine Soc., 1957*, p. 98.
39. INGLE, D. J. The time for the occurrence of cortico-adrenal hypertrophy in rats during continued work. *Am. J. Physiol.* 124: 627–630, 1938.
40. INGLE, D. J., G. M. HIGGINS, AND E. C. KENDALL. Atrophy of the adrenal cortex in the rat produced by administration of large amounts of cortin. *Anat. Rev.* 71: 363–372, 1938.
41. KENDALL, J. W. Feedback control of adrenocorticotropic hormone secretion. In: *Frontiers in Neuroendocrinology*, edited by W. F. Ganong and L. Martini. New York: Oxford Univ. Press, 1971.
42. KENDALL, J. W., M. L. EGANS, A. K. STOTT, R. M. KRAMER, AND J. J. JACOBS. The importance of stimulus intensity and duration of steroid administration in suppression of stress-induced ACTH secretion. *Endocrinology* 90: 525–530, 1972.
43. KENDALL, J. W., AND J. G. ROTH. Adrenocortical function in monkeys after forebrain removal or pituitary stalk section. *Endocrinology* 84: 686–691, 1969.
44. KRAICER, J., J. V. MILLIGAN, J. L. GOSBEE, R. G. CONRAD, AND C. M. BRANSON. *In vitro* release of ACTH: effect of potassium, calcium and corticosterone. *Endocrinology* 85: 1144–1153, 1969.
45. LI, C. H., J. MEIENHOFER, E. SCHNABEL, D. CHUNG, T. B. LO, AND J. RAMACHANDRAN. Synthesis of a biologically active nonadecapeptide corresponding to the first nineteen amino acid residues of adrenocorticotropins. *J. Am. Chem. Soc.* 83: 4449–4457, 1961.
46. LIDDLE, G. W., D. ISLAND, AND C. K. MEADOR. Normal and abnormal regulation of corticotropin secretion in man. *Recent Progr. Hormone Res.* 18: 125–166, 1962.
47. LIPPA, A. S., S. M. ANTELMAN, E. E. FAHRINGER, AND E. S. REDGATE. Relationship between catecholamines and ACTH: effects of 6-hydroxydopamine. *Nature New Biol.* 241: 24–25, 1973.
48. LIPSCOMB, H. S., AND D. H. NELSON. A sensitive biologic assay for ACTH. *Endocrinology* 71: 13–23, 1962.
49. MAKARA, G. B., E. STARK, J. MARTON, AND T. MÉSZÁROS. Corticotrophin release induced by surgical trauma after transection of various afferent nervous pathways to the hypothalamus. *J. Endocrinol.* 53: 389–395, 1972.
50. MCCANN, S. M. The ACTH-releasing activity of extracts of the posterior lobe of the pituitary *in vivo*. *Endocrinology* 60: 664–676, 1957.
51. MCCANN, S. M., AND J. R. BROBECK. Evidence for a role of the supraoptico-hypophyseal system in regulation of adrenocorticotrophin secretion. *Proc. Soc. Exptl. Biol. Med.* 87: 318–324, 1954.
52. MCDERMOTT, W. V., E. G. FRY, J. R. BROBECK, AND C. N. H. LONG. Mechanism of control of adrenocorticotrophic hormone. *Yale J. Biol. Med.* 23: 52–66, 1950.
53. MOTTA, M., F. FRASCHINI, F. PIVA, AND L. MARTINI. Hypothalamic and extrahypothalamic mechanisms controlling

adrenocorticotrophin secretion. *Mem. Soc. Endocrinol.* 17: 3–18, 1967.
54. MOTTA, M., B. MANGILI, AND L. MARTINI. A "short" feedback loop in the control of ACTH secretion. *Endocrinology* 77: 392–395, 1965.
55. NEY, R. L., E. OGATA, N. SHIMIZU, W. E. NICHOLSON, AND G. W. LIDDLE. Structure-function relationships of ACTH and MSH analogues. In: *Proceedings of the Second International Congress of Endocrinology*, edited by S. Taylor. Amsterdam: Excerpta Medica Foundation, 1965, p. 1184–1191.
56. PÉRON, F. G., F. MONCLOA, AND R. I. DORFMAN. Studies on the possible inhibitory effect of corticosterone on corticosteroidogenesis at the adrenal level in the rat. *Endocrinology* 67: 379–388, 1960.
57. POLLOCK, J. J., AND F. S. LABELLA. Inhibition by cortisol of ACTH release from anterior pituitary tissue in vitro. *Can. J. Physiol. Pharmacol.* 44: 549–556, 1966.
58. PORTANOVA, R. Release of ACTH from isolated pituitary cells: an energy dependent process. *Proc. Soc. Exptl. Biol. Med.* 140: 825–829, 1972.
59. PORTANOVA, R., AND G. SAYERS. An in vitro assay for corticotropin releasing factor(s) using suspensions of isolated pituitary cells. *Neuroendocrinology* 12: 236–248, 1973.
60. PORTANOVA, R., AND G. SAYERS. Isolated pituitary cells: CRF-like activity of neurohypophysial and related polypeptides. *Proc. Soc. Exptl. Biol. Med.* 143: 661–666, 1973.
61. RAMACHANDRAN, J., D. CHUNG, AND C. H. LI. Adrenocorticotropins. XXXIV. Aspects of structure-activity relationships of the ACTH molecule. Synthesis of a heptadecapeptide amide, an octadecapeptide amide, and a nonadecapeptide amide possessing high biological activities. *J. Am. Chem. Soc.* 87: 2696–2708, 1965.
62. RINIKER, B., P. SIEBER, AND W. RITTEL. Revised amino-acid sequences for porcine and human adrenocorticotrophic hormone. *Nature New Biol.* 235: 114–115, 1972.
63. ROYCE, P. C., AND G. SAYERS. Extrapituitary interaction between pitressin and ACTH. *Proc. Soc. Exptl. Biol. Med.* 98: 70–74, 1958.
64. ROYCE, P. C., AND G. SAYERS. Corticotropin releasing activity of a pepsin labile factor in the hypothalamus. *Proc. Soc. Exptl. Biol. Med.* 98: 677–680, 1958.
65. ROYCE, P. C., AND G. SAYERS. Blood ACTH: effects of ether, pentobarbital, epinephrine and pain. *Endocrinology* 63: 794–800, 1958.
66. ROYCE, P. C., AND G. SAYERS. Purification of hypothalamic corticotropin releasing factor. *Proc. Soc. Exptl. Biol. Med.* 103: 447–450, 1960.
67. SAFFRAN, M., A. F. PEARLMUTTER, AND E. RAPINO. Pressinoic acid: a peptide with potent corticotrophin-releasing activity. *Biochem. Biophys. Res. Commun.* 49: 748–751, 1972.
68. SAFFRAN, M., AND A. V. SCHALLY. In vitro bioassay of corticotropin: modification and statistical treatment. *Endocrinology* 56: 523–532, 1955.
69. SAFFRAN, M., AND A. V. SCHALLY. The release of corticotrophin by anterior pituitary tissue in vitro. *Can. J. Biochem. Physiol.* 33: 408–415, 1955.
70. SAFFRAN, M., A. V. SCHALLY, AND B. G. BENFEY. Stimulation of the release of corticotropin from the adenohypophysis by a neurohypophysial factor. *Endocrinology* 57: 439–444, 1955.
71. SAYERS, G. The adrenal cortex and homeostasis. *Physiol. Rev.* 30: 241–320, 1950.
72. SAYERS, G. Factors influencing the level of ACTH in the blood. In: *Ciba Foundation Colloquia on Endocrinology*, edited by G. E. W. Wolstenholme and E. C. P. Millar. London: Churchill, 1957, vol. 11, p. 138–149.
73. SAYERS, G. Hypothalamus and adenohypophysis: with special reference to corticotrophin release. *Proc. Intern. Congr. Endocrinol., 1st, Copenhagen, 1960*, p. 25–31.
74. SAYERS, G. Hypothalamic control of ACTH release: similarities in control systems for endocrine and visceral functions. *Physiologist* 4: 56–61, 1961.
75. SAYERS, G., R. J. BEALL, S. SEELIG, AND K. CUMMINS. Assay of ACTH: isolated adrenal cortex cells. In: *Brain-Pituitary-Adrenal Interrelationships*, edited by A. Brodish and E. S. Redgate. Basel: Karger, 1973, p. 16–35.
76. SAYERS, G., R. J. BEALL, AND S. SEELIG. Modes of action of ACTH. In: *MTP International Review of Science*. London: Butterworths, vol. 8, chapt. 7. In press.
77. SAYERS, G., AND R-M. MA. Isolated adrenal cells: Ca^{++} modified negative corticosterone feedback (Abstract). *Intern. Congr. Hormonal Steroids, 3rd, Hamburg, 1970*, p. 158–159.
78. SAYERS, G., AND R. PORTANOVA. Corticosteroids inhibit ACTH release by two separate and distinct mechanisms (Abstract). *Federation Proc.* 32: 295, 1973.
79. SAYERS, G., E. S. REDGATE, AND P. C. ROYCE. Hypothalamus, adenohypophysis and adrenal cortex. *Ann. Rev. Physiol.* 20: 243–274, 1958.
80. SAYERS, G., AND P. C. ROYCE. Regulation of the secretory activity of the adrenal cortex. *Clin. Endocrinol.* 1: 323–334, 1960.
81. SAYERS, G., AND M. SAYERS. Regulatory effect of adrenal cortical extract on elaboration of pituitary adrenotrophic hormone. *Proc. Soc. Exptl. Biol. Med.* 60: 162–163, 1945.
82. SAYERS, G., AND M. A. SAYERS. Regulation of pituitary adrenocorticotrophic activity during the response of the rat to acute stress. *Endocrinology* 40: 265–273, 1947.
83. SAYERS, G., AND M. SAYERS. The pituitary-adrenal system. In: *Recent Progress in Hormone Research*, edited by G. Pincus. New York: Acad. Press, 1948, vol. II, p. 81–116.
84. SAYERS, G., R. L. SWALLOW, AND N. D. GIORDANO. An improved technique for the preparation of isolated rat adrenal cells: a sensitive, accurate and specific method for the assay of ACTH. *Endocrinology* 88: 1063–1068, 1971.
85. SAYERS, M. A., G. SAYERS, AND L. A. WOODBURY. The assay of adrenocorticotrophic hormone by the adrenal ascorbic acid-depletion method. *Endocrinology* 42: 379–393, 1948.
86. SCAPAGNINI, U., G. R. VAN LOON, G. P. MOBERG, P. PREZIOSI, AND W. F. GANONG. Evidence for central norepinephrine-mediated inhibition of ACTH secretion in the rat. *Neuroendocrinology* 10: 155–160, 1972.
87. SCHIMMER, B. P., K. UEDA, AND G. H. SATO. Site of action of adrenocorticotropic hormone (ACTH) in adrenal cell cultures. *Biochem. Biophys. Res. Commun.* 32: 806–810, 1968.
88. SCHWYZER, R. Chemistry and metabolic action of nonsteroid hormones. *Ann. Rev. Biochem.* 33: 259–286, 1964.
89. SCHWYZER, R., P. SCHILLER, S. SEELIG, AND G. SAYERS. Isolated adrenal cells: log dose response curves for steroidogenesis induced by ACTH$_{1-24}$, ACTH$_{1-10}$, ACTH$_{4-10}$ and ACTH$_{5-10}$. *FEBS Letters* 19: 229–231, 1971.
90. SCHWYZER, R., AND P. SIEBER. Total synthesis of adrenocorticotrophic hormone. *Nature* 199: 172–174, 1963.
91. SEELIG, S., G. SAYERS, R. SCHWYZER, AND P. SCHILLER. Isolated adrenal cells: ACTH$_{11-24}$, a competitive antagonist of ACTH$_{1-39}$ and ACTH$_{1-10}$. *FEBS Letters* 19: 232–234, 1971.
92. SEELIG, S., AND G. SAYERS. Isolated adrenal cortex cells: ACTH agonists, partial agonists, antagonists; cyclic AMP and corticosterone production. *Arch. Biochem. Biophys.* 154: 230–239, 1973.
93. SEIDEN, G., AND A. BRODISH. Physiological evidence for 'short-loop' feedback effects of ACTH on hypothalamic CRF. *Neuroendocrinology* 8: 154–164, 1971.
94. SELINGER, R. C. L., AND M. CIVEN. ACTH diazotized to agarose: effects on isolated adrenal cells. *Biochem. Biophys. Res. Commun.* 43: 793–799, 1971.
95. SIRETT, N. E., AND F. P. GIBBS. Dexamethasone suppression of ACTH release: effect of the interval between steroid administration and the application of stimuli known to release ACTH. *Endocrinology* 85: 355–359, 1969.
96. SMELIK, P. G. Relation between blood level of corticoids and their inhibiting effect on the hypophyseal stress response. *Proc. Soc. Exptl. Biol. Med.* 113: 616–619, 1963.
97. STOCKHAM, M. A. Changes of plasma and adrenal corticosterone levels in the rat after repeated stimuli. *J. Physiol., London* 173: 149–159, 1964.

98. SYDNOR, K. L., AND G. SAYERS. A technic for determination of adrenocorticotrophin in blood. *Proc. Soc. Exptl. Biol. Med.* 79: 432–436, 1952.
99. SYDNOR, K. L., AND G. SAYERS. Blood and pituitary ACTH in intact and adrenalectomized rats after stress. *Endocrinology* 55: 621–636, 1954.
100. SYDNOR, K. L., G. SAYERS, H. BROWN, AND F. H. TYLER. Preliminary studies on blood ACTH in man. *J. Clin. Endocrinol. Metab.* 13: 891–897, 1953.
101. TAKEBE, K., H. KUNITA, M. SAKAKURA, Y. HORIUCHI, AND K. MASHIMO. Suppressive effect of dexamethasone on the rise of CRF activity in the median eminence induced by stress. *Endocrinology* 89: 1014–1019, 1971.
102. TEPPERMAN, J. *Metabolic and Endocrine Physiology* (2nd ed.). Chicago: Year Book Med. Publ., 1968, p. 130.
103. VAN LOON, G. R., U. SCAPAGNINI, R. COHEN, AND W. F. GANONG. Effect of intraventricular administration of adrenergic drugs on the adrenal venous 17-hydroxycorticosteroid response to surgical stress in the dog. *Neuroendocrinology* 8: 257–272, 1971.
104. VERNIKOS-DANELLIS, J. Effect of stress, adrenalectomy, hypophysectomy and hydrocortisone on the corticotropin-releasing activity of rat median eminence. *Endocrinology* 76: 122–126, 1965.
105. WATANABE, H., W. E. NICHOLSON, AND D. N. ORTH. Inhibition of adrenocorticotropic hormone production by glucocorticoids in mouse pituitary tumor cells. *Endocrinology* 93: 411–416, 1973.
106. WEITZMAN, E. D., D. FUKUSHIMA, C. NOGEIRE, H. ROFFWARG, T. F. GALLAGHER, AND L. HELLMAN. Twenty-four hour pattern of the episodic secretion of cortisol in normal subjects. *J. Clin. Endocrinol. Metab.* 33: 14–22, 1971.
107. WILLIAMS, W. C., D. ISLAND, R. A. A. OLDFIELD, AND G. W. LIDDLE. Blood corticotropin (ACTH) levels in Cushing's disease. *J. Clin. Endocrinol. Metab.* 21: 426–432, 1961.
108. WISE, B. L., E. E. VAN BRUNT, AND W. F. GANONG. Effect of removal of various parts of the brain on ACTH secretion in dogs. *Proc. Soc. Exptl. Biol. Med.* 112: 792–795, 1963.
109. WITORSCH, R. J., AND A. BRODISH. Evidence for acute ACTH release by extrahypothalamic mechanisms. *Endocrinology* 90: 1160–1167, 1972.
110. YATES, F. E. Physiological control of adrenal cortical hormone secretion. In: *The Adrenal Cortex*, edited by A. B. Eisenstein. Boston: Little, Brown, 1967, p. 133–183.

CHAPTER 5

Biosynthesis of corticosteroids

LEO T. SAMUELS | *College of Medicine, University of Utah, Salt Lake City, Utah*
DON H. NELSON | *College of Medicine, University of Utah, and L.D.S. Hospital, Salt Lake City, Utah*

CHAPTER CONTENTS

Early Steps in Biosynthesis
Conversion of Pregnenolone to Glucocorticoids and Aldosterone
Biosynthesis of C_{19} and C_{18} Steroids
Hydroxylation Pathway
Dehydrogenases
Isomerases
Distribution of Enzymes in Adrenal Cortex
Fetal-Placental Unit
Corticoid Biosynthesis in Nonmammalian Vertebrates
Genetic Blocks in Hydroxylation of Corticosteroids
Inhibitors of Biosynthesis of Corticosteroids
   Amphenone
   Metyrapone
   17α-Hydroxylase inhibitors
   18-Hydroxylase and 18-oxidase inhibitors
   Cyanoketone
   o,p'DDD
   Inhibitors of cholesterol synthesis and metabolism
   Steroids as inhibitors of corticosteroidogenesis
   Inhibitors of protein synthesis as inhibitors of corticosteroid secretion
   Ouabain
   Other inhibitors of adrenal function
Concluding Summary

EARLY STEPS IN BIOSYNTHESIS

All the known hormones of the adrenal cortex are steroids. Biosynthesis can be considered as occurring in two steps: the formation of the steroid nucleus and the modification of the substituent groups. A summary of much of the early fundamental work has been given by Hayano et al. (62).

By perfusion of acetate-^{14}C through bovine adrenals, Hechter et al. (64) first showed that the adrenal gland can synthesize cholesterol and the steroid hormones from this simple compound. Caspi et al. (21) have demonstrated that the relation of the carbons derived from the methyl and carboxyl groups of acetate in cortisol and corticosterone is the same as that found in cholesterol synthesized in the liver and other tissues, and the sequence of reactions involved in cholesterol biosynthesis appears to be identical. Acetyl coenzyme A, formed in intermediary metabolism, is converted to mevalonic acid, which is then pyrophosphorylated and decarboxylated to yield 3,3'-dimethylallyl pyrophosphate and isopentenyl pyrophosphate. These two compounds condense to form geranyl pyrophosphate, which in turn condenses with another molecule of isopentenyl pyrophosphate to form farnesyl pyrophosphate. Two molecules of farnesyl pyrophosphate interact to form presqualene pyrophosphate, which in the presence of NADPH yields squalene (3, 33, 118). The series of reactions is shown in Figure 1.

Squalene is cyclized to the 30-carbon sterol, lanosterol, which then undergoes successive oxidative demethylations, the major product being desmosterol. The C-24–C-25 double bond of desmosterol then undergoes reduction to form cholesterol. The major sequence of conversions is shown in Figure 2. The experiments of Werbin & Chaikoff (160), as well as subsequent studies (84), indicate that cholesterol is normally the only significant precursor of the adrenocortical steroids. It may originate either from synthesis in the gland or from the circulating blood, the proportion from these two sources varying with species (160). Not all the cholesterol in the gland is equally available as precursor; the mitochondrial free cholesterol appears to be more immediately utilizable by the side-chain splitting enzymes than the ester cholesterol or extramitochondrial free cholesterol (32, 47, 67, 68).

If cholesterol synthesis is blocked by metyrapone [2-methyl-1,2-bis(3-pyridyl)-1-propanone], which inhibits enzymatic reduction of the C-24–C-25 double bond in desmosterol, the levels of adrenocortical hormones first fall and then slowly return to normal as the desmosterol levels rise in the blood and the adrenal gland (139). Goodman et al. (55) have shown that desmosterol is converted to pregnenolone (3β-hydroxy-5-pregnen-20-one) at about the same rate as cholesterol, but normally the concentration of desmosterol is so low that it is unimportant as a source of adrenal steroids. The importance of cholesterol as almost the sole precursor is therefore due to its availability and not to the absolute specificity of the enzyme systems involved.

The first product of cholesterol metabolism that can

be found in the adrenal in significant amounts is pregnenolone, which has the same structure as the first 21 carbons of cholesterol; an isocaproyl side chain has simply been replaced by a ketonic oxygen. If a mixture of cholesterol-4-^{14}C and -26-^{14}C is incubated with adrenal slices or homogenates, radioactive pregnenolone and isocaproic acid can be isolated (138). More detailed study of the overall reaction has shown that a number of steps are involved.

Both NADPH and O_2 are required for pregnenolone formation (57), indicating that some of the enzymes are mixed-function oxidases (hydroxylases) which have been described by Mason (95). Because activation of the bond between C-20 and C-22 is an essential step in splitting off the isocaproyl side chain, the various possible hydroxy- and oxo-derivatives have been tested as intermediates. Of the four possible monohydroxy compounds, the 20α- and the 22R-hydroxy derivatives are readily converted to pregnenolone, whereas the 20β- and 22S-isomers are not (18, 136). 20α,22R-dihydroxycholesterol is also a precursor of pregnenolone and is formed from 20α-hydroxycholesterol (29, 129). The preferred sequences therefore seem to be those shown in Figure 3. Recently, Lieberman and co-workers (92) have introduced evidence that the intermediate hydroxy compounds may not actually exist as such during pregnenolone synthesis, but rather that the intermediates may actually be the equivalent free radicals.

Constantopoulos et al. (28) have shown that the actual moiety that is eliminated is isocaproyl aldehyde. Oxidases in the tissues then convert isocaproyl aldehyde rapidly to isocaproic acid. The entire series of reactions is catalyzed by purified adrenal mitochondria or by acetone-dried mitochondrial powders, if the incubation medium is reinforced with NADPH and O_2 is available.

CONVERSION OF PREGNENOLONE TO GLUCOCORTICOIDS AND ALDOSTERONE

Pregnenolone derived from cholesterol appears to be the precursor of all the vertebrate steroid hormones. The changes required to form the mineralocorticoid and glucocorticoid hormones involve oxidations, a shift of the Δ^5 double bond to the Δ^4 position, and the introduction of additional hydroxyl groups. In addition, to the extent that the adrenal cortex forms sex hormones or their immediate precursors the two-carbon side chain attached to C-17 must also be split off. We shall now examine the evidence pertaining to the order of these reactions.

The first question is to what extent the oxidation of the Δ^5-3β-hydroxy structure of ring A to the Δ^4-3-ketone occurs before or after 17-hydroxylation. These two possibilities are referred to as the Δ^4 and Δ^5 pathways. Present evidence indicates that the balance between the two pathways varies between species in normal adrenal tissue and may vary within species in abnormal conditions. In rodents conversion of pregnenolone to pro-

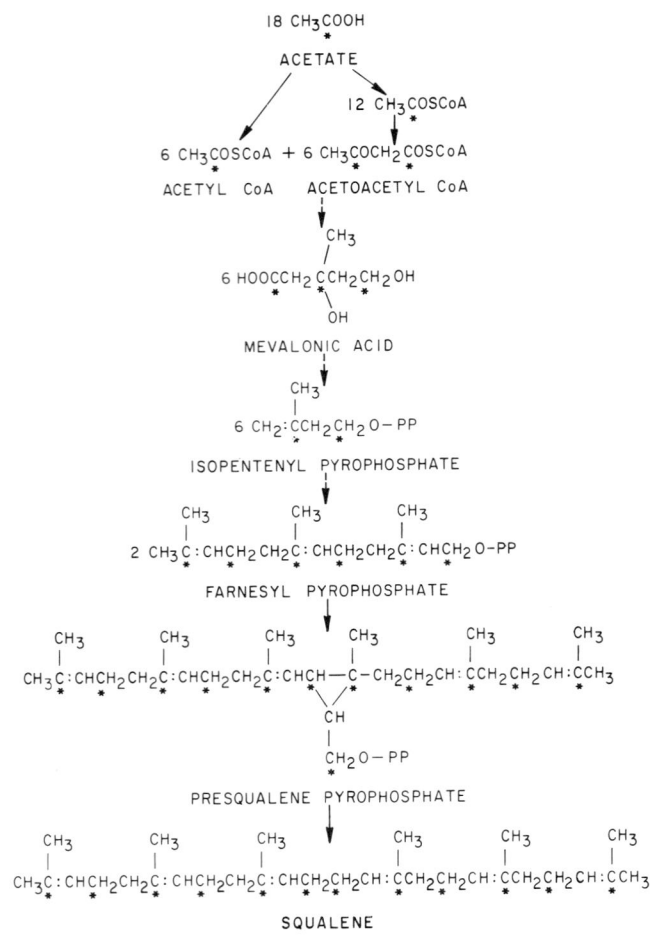

FIG. 1. Conversion of acetyl coenzyme A to squalene. *Dashed arrows* indicate that more than one step is involved in the particular conversion. *Asterisks* indicate a carbon that originated from carboxyl carbon of acetate.

FIG. 2. Biosynthesis of cholesterol from squalene. In the structures of squalene and cholesterol *asterisks* indicate position of a carbon originating from carboxyl group of acetate. Unmarked carbons in these two formulas originate from methyl groups of acetate. *Dashed arrows* indicate that conversions involve more than one step.

gesterone is the major reaction, whereas in humans and several other species there is increasing evidence that the major reaction is the conversion of pregnenolone to 17-hydroxypregnenolone [Fig. 4; (19, 20, 89, 156, 161)].

Two enzymes found in the microsomal fraction, probably in the smooth endoplasmic reticulum, are involved in the conversion of pregnenolone to progesterone: a 3β-hydroxysteroid dehydrogenase and an isomerase (39, 85). Some 3β-hydroxysteroid dehydrogenase may also be located in the mitochondria (93). The dehydrogenase utilizes NAD+ preferentially as hydrogen acceptor; NADP+ can also function but at a much lower rate (9, 79). The product of this reaction is pregn-5-ene-3,20-dione. Closely associated with the dehydrogenase is a Δ⁵-Δ⁴-isomerase that catalyzes the conversion of pregn-5-ene-3,20-dione to pregn-4-ene-3,20-dione (progesterone). The isomerase does not appear to require any coenzyme (85).

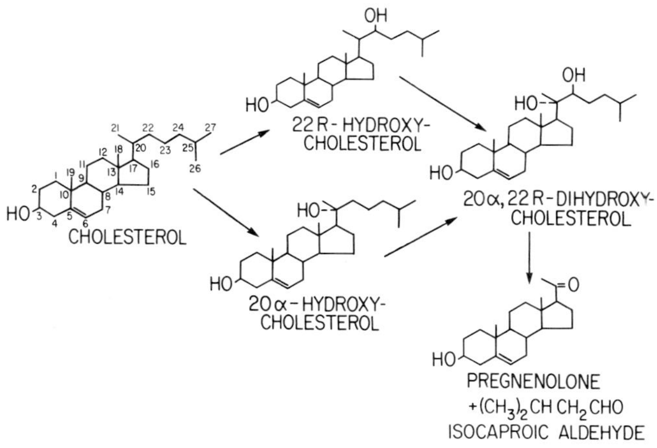

The dehydrogenation and isomerization of ring A seem to precede the introduction of hydroxyl groups in other than the 17-position in most species. As originally postulated by Hechter et al. (64) from their perfusion studies, normally 21-hydroxylation is the next step, followed by 11β-hydroxylation. Some 11β-hydroxyprogesterone can be formed first, however, which in turn can be converted to corticosterone, but this does not seem to be a major pathway (38).

There is no evidence that hydroxyl groups are ever removed in the adrenal. Thus 17-hydroxyprogesterone is a precursor of 11-deoxycortisol and cortisol but not of 11-deoxycorticosterone (DOC), corticosterone, or aldosterone; the precursor of these three compounds in all species is progesterone, which is then converted to DOC.

Aldosterone biosynthesis involves the conversion of the 18-methyl group of corticosterone to an aldehyde. The first step appears to be the formation of 18-hydroxycorticosterone, which is then oxidized to the 18-aldehyde (106, 112, 115). Aldosterone can be formed from 11-dehydrocorticosterone as well, but less efficiently (44, 128). Also DOC can undergo 18-hydroxylation, but 18-hydroxy-DOC is largely formed in cells that lack the

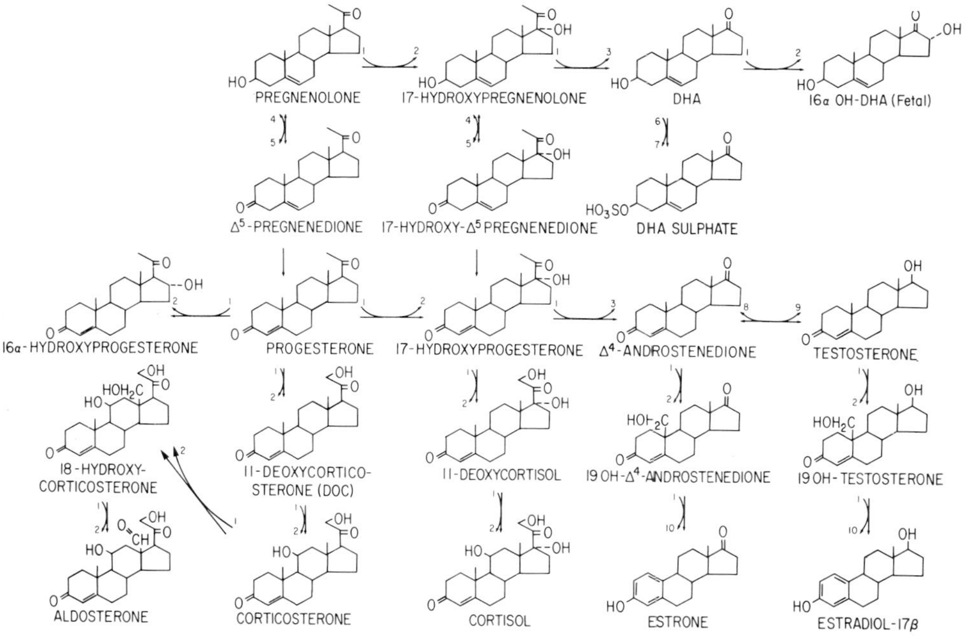

FIG. 3. Conversion of cholesterol to pregnenolone. All steps require O₂ and NADPH as cofactors.

FIG. 4. Metabolism of pregnenolone in human adrenal cortex. Cofactors involved are indicated by numbers, as follows: (1) NADPH + H+ + O₂; (2) NADP+ + H₂O; (3) NADP+ + H₂O + CH₃COOH; (4) NAD+; (5) NADH + H+; (6) adenosine 3-phosphate 5′-phosphosulfate; (7) adenosine 3′,5′-diphosphate; (8) NADPH + H+; (9) NADP+; (10) NADP+ + HCHO + 2H₂O.

enzyme oxidizing the 18-hydroxy group to the aldehyde (145).

BIOSYNTHESIS OF C_{19} AND C_{18} STEROIDS

Not only are steroids that lack the two-carbon side chain at C-17 formed during incubation of adrenal preparations, but also a number appear in the adrenal venous blood in higher concentration than in the general circulation. The most abundant is dehydroepiandrosterone (DHEA), which is largely secreted as the sulfate (8, 162). Next in amount is androstenedione, but small amounts of testosterone, estrone, and possibly estradiol-17β are also secreted (6).

These compounds, as well as 11β-hydroxytestosterone, 11β-hydroxyandrostenedione, 17-epiestriol, and 16-oxoestrone, have been identified after incubation of adrenal tissue with radioactive pregnenolone or progesterone (56, 75, 152). 17-Hydroxypregnenolone is the necessary precursor for DHEA, while most of the androstenedione and testosterone is formed from 17-hydroxyprogesterone; however, small amounts of the latter compounds can also be formed from DHEA (101).

The large production of DHEA sulfate by the adrenal glands can have significant androgenic influence, even though the ester itself is not very active. The sulfate can be metabolized to androstenedione and testosterone in the testes because of the presence of an active sulfatase and a 3β-hydroxysteroid dehydrogenase system. The prostate and seminal vesicles of the rat also contain a sulfatase that will release free DHEA in these tissues (51).

The pathways of estrogen biosynthesis in the adrenal have not been so easy to demonstrate. In 1955 Meyer (98) obtained 19-hydroxylation of androstenedione with beef adrenal homogenates, but he did not find evidence of the formation of aromatic compounds. More recently, Griffiths and co-workers (56, 87) have been able to demonstrate both high 19-hydroxylation and aromatization of testosterone by hamster adrenal homogenates. In view of evidence of secretion of small amounts of estrogens by human adrenals (6) and biological evidence of estrogenic activity originating from the adrenals in other animals, it seems probable that low levels of aromatizing activity are generally present.

HYDROXYLATION PATHWAY

The various enzymes involved in biosynthesis can be classified into three types: hydroxylases and lyases (splitting side chains), which require O_2 and NADPH; dehydrogenases, which utilize $NADP^+$ or NAD^+ as hydrogen acceptors and which are reversible; and isomerases, for which no coenzyme has been identified. Initial work with corticosteroid biogenesis indicated the presence of enzymes that carried out hydroxylations specifically at various points on the steroid molecule. These were originally assumed to be single proteins. Thus the literature commonly refers to the 11β-hydroxylase or the 20α-hydroxylase. As increased information concerning the hydroxylation process has accumulated, however, it has become apparent that there are a number of similarly constituted, multiple enzyme systems involved in the hydroxylation process, and although not definitely settled at this time, the specificity may rest in the terminal oxidase of the hydroxylation sequence, which is directly involved in the introduction of the hydroxyl radical into the steroid molecule. Studies carried out initially by Tomkins et al. (147) and Sweat & Bryson (142) suggested that a number of components might participate in the function of the various hydroxylases. Omura et al. (108) verified that three proteins were involved in the mitochondrial reaction. These have been identified by a number of workers as an FAD-containing flavoprotein, a nonheme iron protein, which has been called adrenodoxin, and a protoporphyrin hemoprotein, cytochrome P-450 (49, 76, 109, 131, 141).

The presence of a hemoprotein or similar substance that might combine directly with oxygen was suggested by the demonstration that carbon monoxide inhibited the 21-hydroxylation of 17α-hydroxyprogesterone by adrenal microsomes and the 11β-hydroxylation of DOC by adrenal mitochondria (122, 165). At the same time, the absorption band at 450 mμ appeared, indicating that cytochrome P-450 was involved (60). Evidence that molecular $^{18}O_2$ was incorporated in the 11β-hydroxylation of DOC to corticosterone gave further support to this concept (61).

Sweat & Lipscomb (143) and Ryan & Engel (122) established that the source of reducing energy for hydroxylations is NADPH. Cooper and co-workers (30) then demonstrated the stoichiometric relation of 1:1:1 for the ratio of NADPH oxidized to 17α-hydroxyprogesterone hydroxylated to oxygen reduced. It thus became apparent that the hydroxylation systems in both the microsomes and the mitochondria were similar multiple-component hydroxylation pathways.

The components of the systems in the two types of organelles differ, however. In the mitochondria the specific flavoprotein and adrenodoxin are both necessary for transfer of electrons to either cytochrome c or the cytochrome P-450, as illustrated in Figure 5. In the microsomes a different flavoprotein which reduces cytochrome c directly is the primary electron transfer agent, and a phospholipid appears to facilitate transfer to microsomal cytochrome P-450 (95a).

At the present time it is not clear whether a specific cytochrome P-450 is involved in activating each particular position on the steroid molecule, whether interaction of a specific steroid with the cytochrome P-450 causes a conformational change of the protein which determines the position activated, or if a specific protein activating the particular position on the steroid molecule is so firmly bound to the cytochrome molecule that the two have not been dissociated. Definitive answers should be forthcoming.

Conversion of cholesterol to Δ^5-pregnenolone is generally accepted as the limiting reaction in corticoid biosynthesis (81). Thus it seems likely that the effect of adrenocorticotropic hormone (ACTH) in stimulating hydroxylation is centered on those factors limiting this reaction. Haynes, McKerns, and colleagues (63, 94) have suggested that the limiting enzyme in steroid biosynthesis is phosphorylase or glucose-6-phosphate dehydrogenase, which makes reduced $NADP^+$ available to the hydroxylation pathway. Koritz (80), on the other hand, has hypothesized permeability of the mitochondrion to pregnenolone as the limiting factor and considers that ACTH mediated by 3',5'-cyclic AMP may affect secretion of pregnenolone by the mitochondrion, which releases the inhibitory effect of pregnenolone on cholesterol side-chain cleavage and results in increased pregnenolone synthesis (81).

Studies on mitochondria from normal and hypophysectomized rats receiving ACTH have demonstrated that within 15 min ACTH alters the mitochondrion's ability to synthesize increased quantities of pregnenolone (72). These studies have also shown that reducing energy may be produced by the mitochondrion from a variety of substrates, including malate, succinate, α-ketoglutarate, and β-hydroxybutyrate. Other investigators have failed to find an effect of hypophysectomy upon a number of NADPH-generating enzymes, thus suggesting that the limiting factor in the hydroxylation may be some component of the hydroxylation pathway itself (59). Fazekas & Sandor (43) have suggested that this effect may be on the stimulation of FAD pyrophosphorylase; an increase in FAD in the hydroxylation pathway might then result in increased steroid hydroxylation. Brownie et al. (16) have presented evidence that spin state changes in cytochrome P-450 correlate with the administration of ACTH. An increase in high spin state P-450 is associated with increased cholesterol binding to P-450 following stress. The mechanism of ACTH action is discussed more fully elsewhere, but at this time it appears that the limiting step in steroid biosynthesis is either availability of reducing energy to the cytochrome P-450, a limitation of some component of the hydroxylation pathway, or, somewhat less likely, permeability of the mitochondrion to pregnenolone.

Simpson & Estabrook (132) have made a strong case for malic enzyme as a prime supplier of reducing energy in bovine mitochondria. Studies carried out in the rat, however, have failed to find much malic enzyme activity (113). In the bovine adrenal the cytoplasmic malic enzyme might operate in a reverse direction to produce malate from pyruvate, bicarbonate, and extramitochondrial NADPH. This malate would then enter the mitochondria to generate NADPH through the action of mitochondrial malic enzyme. Through this mechanism the extramitochondrial glucose-6-phosphate dehydrogenase might generate NADPH by the pentose-phosphate shunt, which would then become available to the hydroxylation pathway through this malate shuttle.

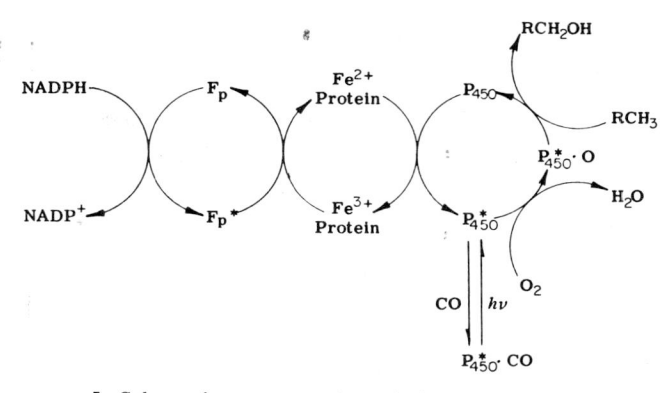

FIG. 5. Schematic representation of the pathway of electron transport for cytochrome P-450 reduction and activation of oxygen for hydroxylation reactions. F_p, flavoprotein; Fe protein, iron-containing nonheme protein; P_{450}, cytochrome P-450; R, substrate; *asterisk* indicates reduced form. [From Omura et al. (109a).]

DEHYDROGENASES

The Δ^5-3β-hydroxysteroid dehydrogenases and isomerases in the adrenal glands are closely associated in the smooth endoplasmic reticulum (9, 70). About 10% of the total activity in the tissue remains associated with the mitochondrial fraction, and the question of whether this represents reticulum strongly associated with the mitochondria or an enzyme incorporated in the mitochondrial membrane has not been fully resolved (82, 93).

Apparently dehydrogenation occurs before isomerization; the Δ^4-3-hydroxy allylic alcohols are not intermediates in the reaction (153). Because the rates of isomerization are faster than those of dehydrogenation at all substrate concentrations, the reaction catalyzed by 3β-hydroxysteroid dehydrogenase seems to be the rate-limiting step in the formation of Δ^4-3-ketosteroids (103, 104).

The question of the number and substrate specificity of 3β-hydroxysteroid dehydrogenases is still unanswered. Indirect evidence has been obtained favoring the identity (104) or nonidentity (58) of the enzymes acting on C_{27} and C_{19} steroids. Evidence obtained with the soluble dehydrogenases and isomerases induced in bacteria cannot be applied to mammalian systems because the enzymes are quite different (48).

The overall reaction from Δ^5-3β-hydroxysteroids to Δ^4-3-ketosteroids can be reversed, but only if conditions greatly favor the reduction reaction (90, 120, 153), because the conversion of the conjugated Δ^4-3-ketone to the single double bond alcohol involves a large decrease in free energy; consequently such a reversal probably has little physiological significance.

Adrenal 17β-hydroxysteroid dehydrogenase, in contrast to the 3β-hydroxysteroid dehydrogenases, is found in the cytosol. Furthermore it does not show nucleotide cofactor specificity, either NAD^+ or $NADP^+$ serving equally well. The K_m is 9.8×10^{-4}, which probably indicates a relatively weak association between enzyme and substrate. This most likely accounts for the very small proportion of testosterone secreted compared with androstenedione unless, as in congenital adrenal hyperplasia or some adrenal carcinomas, androstenedione accumulates (15).

ISOMERASES

Ewald et al. (39, 41) were able to achieve separation of extracts from beef adrenal homogenates into three fractions, each showing greatest activity with either Δ^5-pregnene-3,20-dione, 17-hydroxy-Δ^5-pregnene-3,20-dione, or Δ^5-androstene-3,17-dione. This indicates the probability of three distinct isomerases and raises the question of whether evidence of difference in order of activity of microsomal 3β-dehydrogenase-isomerase systems toward various substrates is due to a difference in dehydrogenase or isomerase.

The isomerases appear to be quite unstable when separated from the endoplasmic reticulum, being destroyed by freezing and similar mild treatment (40).

While the Δ^5-Δ^4-isomerases do not appear to involve a cofactor, NAD$^+$ and NADH seem to be activators through stabilization of the enzyme at some locus other than the active site; nucleotides therefore probably play a role under physiological conditions (107). Cyclic 3′,5′-AMP, on the other hand, seems to inhibit both the 3β-dehydrogenase and isomerase (80, 90).

DISTRIBUTION OF ENZYMES IN ADRENAL CORTEX

The enzymes involved in biosynthesis of the adrenal steroids show distinctive patterns of distribution among both intracellular components and the cells of the different zones of the cortex. The terminal hydroxylation reactions involved in splitting the cholesterol side chain are associated with the inner membrane of the adrenal mitochondrion. The same is true of the 11β-hydroxylase and 18-hydroxylase systems. The NADPH-linked flavoprotein also appears to remain associated with this membrane fraction, but the adrenodoxin is apparently in solution in the inner matrix (36, 166).

The 17α- and 21-hydroxylase systems are localized in the smooth endoplasmic reticulum. Since a washed microsomal fraction will carry out these hydroxylations, the necessary proteins for electron transfer from NADPH must also be present within the endoplasmic vesicle. As already mentioned, the 3α- and 17α-hydroxysteroid dehydrogenase-isomerase systems also appear to be associated largely with the smooth endoplasmic reticulum (9, 70).

Obviously, with this spatial arrangement of the enzymes within the cell the synthesis of both the glucocorticoids and aldosterone involves a circulation of intermediates between mitochondria and endoplasmic reticulum. The question of the forces that lead to this circulation of intermediates then arises. The transfer of pregnenolone from mitochondria to the endoplasmic reticulum does not depend on binding to a protein in the cytosol, since this seems to be lacking, but rather on a strong association with some molecule in the endoplasmic reticulum. This leads at equilibrium to a high concentration of pregnenolone in the endoplasmic reticulum compared to the cytosol (96). This transfer to the reticulum maintains a concentration differential between mitochondria and cytosol that would lead to continuous diffusion from the mitochondria. Dehydrogenation and 17α- and 21-hydroxylations take place in the endoplasmic vesicle without the intermediates coming into equilibrium with the general cytosol (K. Matsumoto, L. Bussmann, and L. T. Samuels, unpublished observations). How the DOC and 11-deoxycortisol are again transferred to the mitochondrion is not yet determined.

Cells of the glomerular, fascicular, and reticular zones of the adrenal cortex contain different enzymes. All three zones seem to have 3β-hydroxysteroid dehydrogenase and 21- and 11β-hydroxylase activities, although the production of DOC and corticosterone appears to be greatest in the fascicular zone. 18-Hydroxylases appear to be present in all, but the substrate specificity may be different. 18-Hydroxycorticosterone is formed largely in the zona glomerulosa, whereas 18-hydroxy-DOC is synthesized primarily in the other zones, as is also 19-hydroxy-DOC (91). The oxidase required to form aldosterone from 18-hydroxycorticosterone is found only in the glomerulosa. 17α-Hydroxylase activity is lacking in this zone; cortisol is therefore formed only in the fasciculata and reticularis (137, 145).

FETAL-PLACENTAL UNIT

The role of the adrenal gland in the mammalian fetus is quite different from its function in the organism after birth. During the early development of the embryo the major mass differentiating as the adrenal cortex is composed of cells that are known in later fetal life as the "fetal zone," because they involute during the latter part of pregnancy and particularly rapidly immediately after birth. They are gradually enveloped during early embryogenesis by darker cells that seem destined to become the definitive cortex of postuterine life. While this development and involution of the fetal zone is particularly striking in humans, a similar process takes place in other placental mammals. Studies of enzymes of steroid biosynthesis in the placenta and fetal adrenal cortex together with measurements of steroid concentrations in the cord blood flowing to and from the fetus have shown that there is an essential collaborative relationship between the two [Fig. 6; (34, 150)].

The placenta can synthesize cholesterol from acetate and form large amounts of pregnenolone and progesterone from both endogenous and plasma cholesterol, apparently by enzymes in the cytotrophoblastic cells (12, 46, 99, 168), but 17-hydroxylase and 17,20-lyase activities are very low (134). The only enzyme in the human placenta acting on progesterone is a reversible 20α-hydroxysteroid dehydrogenase, the product being 20α-dihydroprogesterone, a very weak progestin (111). The pregnenolone and progesterone formed, however, readily diffuse into the umbilical venous blood and the maternal circulation.

In addition to the cholesterol side-chain splitting system and 3β-hydroxysteroid dehydrogenase-isomerase activities, the placenta also has very active dehydrogenase and aromatization systems (121) for which C_{19} steroids are required as substrates; these compounds, however, are not formed in the absence of the 17α-hydroxylase and 17,20-lyase. Also present is a very active sulfatase (114, 154).

Conversely the fetal adrenal cortex has high 16α-hydroxylase, 17α-hydroxylase, and 17,20-lyase activities (151), but the fetal zone, which makes up the larger mass, lacks 3β-hydroxysteroid dehydrogenase activity (54). A very active sulfokinase, which can transfer sulfate from 3'-phosphoadenosine 5'-phosphosulfate to form steroid ester sulfates (158), is also located primarily in the fetal zone (130).

Infusion and perfusion studies with radioactive precursors confirm a sequence that could be inferred from the above data. The placenta forms large amounts of pregnenolone and progesterone, chiefly from maternal plasma cholesterol, and secretes these into the tributaries of the umbilical vein. The fetal adrenal utilizes progesterone to form DOC, corticosterone, and cortisol. The pregnenolone is sulfated, 17-hydroxylated, and converted into DHEA sulfate, the latter being largely metabolized to 16α-hydroxy-DHEA sulfate by the fetal liver (135, 167). This organ also converts estrogens to sulfates. Estrone is also 15α-hydroxylated (127). The hydroxylations at positions 16α and 15α, as well as esterification with sulfate, greatly decrease the hormonal potency of these compounds and prevent excessive progestational and estrogenic action in the fetus.

When the blood returning from the fetus reaches the placenta, the very active sulfatases present split the ester linkages. Oxidation of DHEA results in androstenedione and testosterone, which are rapidly aromatized to estrone and estradiol (133). The 16α-hydroxy-DHEA sulfate, which is present in greater concentration, is desulfated and converted by way of 16α-hydroxy-testosterone to estriol. This step accounts for the large amounts of estriol in the urine during the last trimester of pregnancy.

The free progesterone and estrogens enter both the fetal and the maternal circulation and account for the high levels of these compounds and their metabolites in the urine during pregnancy. The cooperative relationship between placenta, fetal adrenal, and fetal liver means that any disturbance of either fetal or placental function is reflected in the maternal levels of those compounds that depend on biosynthetic steps in both the placenta and fetus. Estriol is the most abundant of these in human urine and therefore has diagnostic and prognostic significance (78).

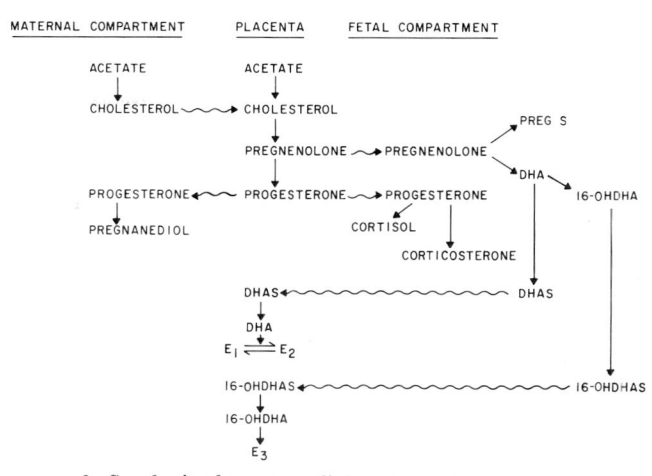

FIG. 6. Synthesis of pregnanediol and estriol in human placenta and fetal tissues. *Straight arrow* indicates an enzymatically catalyzed conversion step; *wavy arrow* indicates passage of the substance from one compartment to another; *S*, sulfate ester. [From Villee (149a).]

CORTICOID BIOSYNTHESIS IN NONMAMMALIAN VERTEBRATES

The adrenal or interrenal tissue of all vertebrates appears to contain the enzymes necessary to convert cholesterol to corticoids; the balance between the activities seems, however, to vary with family and species. Also, along the evolutionary path certain enzymes that play a major role in more primitive species have become much less important or have disappeared.

The Elasmobranchii are unique in having an active 1α-hydroxylase in their interrenal bodies, 1α-hydroxycorticosterone being a major secretory product (148). The two other classes of cartilaginous fish, the Ganoidei and Cyclostomata, do not produce this substance, however, and resemble the Teleostei in having cortisol as their major secretory product (100, 126). The routes of biosynthesis from acetate via cholesterol seem to be those common to mammals, except that both Δ^5 and Δ^4 paths are utilized in the same tissue (4, 69). 18-Hydroxy-DOC is formed in trout (5); small amounts of aldosterone are also synthesized, but it is not a major product.

In amphibians and reptiles 18-hydroxylation and aldehyde formation become important processes. Aldosterone and 18-hydroxycorticosterone are major products, together with corticosterone (22, 125). The enzymatic activity of the interrenal tissue of these orders closely resembles that of the mammalian adrenal glomerulus. The important pathway appears to be pregnenolone → progesterone → DOC → corticosterone → 18-hydroxycorticosterone → aldosterone.

The avian adrenal resembles that of the reptile and amphibian in secreting primarily corticosterone, 18-hydroxycorticosterone, and aldosterone (124). It appears to differ, however, in hydroxylating much of the progesterone formed to 11β-hydroxyprogesterone so that both the classical pathway of corticosterone formation by way of DOC and that via 11β-hydroxyprogesterone play important roles (123).

Marsupials seem to show only one major difference from the higher orders of mammals, the secretion of 21-deoxycortisol in addition to cortisol in most species examined. There are also minor variations between species, as there are in higher mammals (155).

The phylogenetic significance of the high levels of aldosterone in amphibians, reptiles, and birds is not clear. If it were related to evolution from a marine environment, fish would be expected to have the highest levels; yet the amounts present in the body fluids and the ability to synthesize this compound appear to be lower in Elasmobranchii and Teleostei than in mammals. The role of such high levels in birds and nonaquatic reptiles has not been determined. Whatever the reason, the definite zonation of the adrenals in mammals apparently is associated with the limitation of the critical 18-dehydrogenase to the glomerulus.

GENETIC BLOCKS IN HYDROXYLATION OF CORTICOSTEROIDS

Clinicians have become aware of a number of forms of congenital adrenal hyperplasia that result from deficiencies of hydroxylation reactions within the adrenal cortex. Suppression of androgen secretion by the adrenal cortex following administration of cortisone suggested that there is an apparent insufficient secretion of cortisol in these individuals, resulting in increased production of ACTH (7, 163). Elevated ACTH then leads to excessive production of androgens by the adrenal gland. The clinical forms of this condition that are recognized include 21-hydroxylase deficiency, which is most common, 21-hydroxylase deficiency associated with 18-hydroxylase deficiency, 11-hydroxylase deficiency, and 17-hydroxylase deficiency. Two other forms of adrenal hyperplasia are due to deficiencies of either 3β-hydroxysteroid dehydrogenase (14) or 18-hydroxysteroid dehydrogenase (149) and are not hydroxylase deficiencies.

In each case the deficiency results in overproduction of those compounds that are not involved in the particular enzymatic reaction. Thus in 21-hydroxylase deficiency there is an oversecretion of 17-hydroxyprogesterone, $11\beta,17$-dihydroxyprogesterone, and to a lesser degree progesterone and 11β-hydroxyprogesterone. There is also a marked increase in secretion of the adrenal androgens, DHEA, and Δ^4-androstenedione. In marked 21-hydroxylase deficiency there is insufficient secretion of aldosterone as well and thus increased loss of salt by the individual (83). When 11β-hydroxylation is interfered with, there is a considerable increase in production of DOC, leading to hypertension (14). Complete deficiency of 3β-hydroxysteroid dehydrogenase leads to failure to produce either cortisol or aldosterone and is not long compatible with life. All of these enzymatic defects are thought to result from a recessive autosomal mutation that is expressed only in those who are homozygous for the mutant gene (26).

Loss of 17-hydroxylation is not limited to the adrenal cortex but affects the gonads as well (10). Thus neither estrogens nor testosterone are produced in subjects with this defect, and they are characterized by gonadal insufficiency, as well as overproduction of adrenal steroids of the non-17-hydroxylated types, such as corticosterone and DOC.

The presence of enzymatic defects with such obvious specificity has been given as evidence that the various mixed-function oxidases involved in hydroxylation are of different types and that there may be more than one type of cytochrome P-450. Although this is a logical assumption, it is unproven at this time; failure of the development of the pathway in a specific subcellular compartment is another possible explanation that might be given. If the latter were true, then one must conclude that the hydroxylations, such as those at C-17 and C-21, both of which occur in the endoplasmic reticulum, are further compartmentalized.

INHIBITORS OF BIOSYNTHESIS OF CORTICOSTEROIDS

Inhibitors of the synthesis of the corticosteroids may work at a number of levels, including affecting the release of corticotropin-releasing factor and ACTH, in addition to acting directly on the adrenal cortex. In this section a brief account is presented of some of those substances that act directly on the gland and thereby limit synthesis of the corticosteroids.

Amphenone

The first compound to be studied in detail is the substance 2-methyl-1,2-di-3-pyridil-1-propenone, which was first described as having only progestational activity but was later noted by Hertz and co-workers (65) to result in marked hypertrophy of the adrenals, as well as the thyroid gland; this hypertrophy could be prevented by hypophysectomy (2). In collaboration with Hume and Nelson, these authors (65) then demonstrated that infusions of amphenone into the hypophysectomized dog suppress corticosteroid secretion by the adrenal. Studies on the perfused calf adrenals have shown inhibition of 11β-, 17α-, and 21-hydroxylations, as well as of oxidation of the Δ^5-3β-hydroxyl group to Δ^4-3-ketone (119). Amphenone has also been demonstrated to have an effect on the testis, as well as the thyroid and adrenal glands.

Metyrapone

Chart et al. (24) found that a derivative of amphenone, 2-methyl-1,2-bis(3-pyridyl)-1-propanone (methopyrapone, metyrapone, or SU-4885), reduces or abolishes 17-hydroxycorticosteroid secretion in the dog. It was then demonstrated independently by two groups of workers that metyrapone suppresses 11β-hydroxylation and produces an increased output of DOC and 11-deoxycortisol (71, 88). Increased secretion of these steroids from the gland was demonstrated to result from inhibition of cortisol output with resultant compensatory increase in ACTH secretion. Dominguez & Samuels (37), working with rat adrenal homogenates, have demonstrated that metyrapone is a specific 11β-hydroxylase competitive inhibitor. In the doses these workers used, metyrapone did not inhibit 21-hydroxylation, although in larger doses inhibition of this and other hydroxylations occurs. In rat adrenal mitochondrial preparations the DOC-induced shift in the cytochrome spectrum is markedly decreased by metyrapone treatment, and a characteristic spectral change is produced by metyrapone, suggesting a direct interaction between the drug and cytochrome P-450 (144, 164).

17α-Hydroxylase Inhibitors

A number of compounds have been demonstrated by Chart et al. (25) to be 17α-hydroxylase inhibitors. The one that has been studied to the greatest extent, SU-9055 [3-(1,2,3,4-tetrahydro-1-oxo-2-naphthyl)pyridine], has been shown to reduce the secretion of cortisol and 11-deoxycortisol but to cause a compensatory rise of corticosterone and DOC in the adrenal effluent of dogs.

18-Hydroxylase and 18-Oxidase Inhibitors

A number of other compounds that act in a similar manner have been described, but they differ in the relative sensitivities of the enzyme systems affected (73). The conversion of corticosterone to the aldosterone precursor, 18-hydroxycorticosterone, is inhibited by SU-9055, while another of the inhibitors, SU-8000 [3-(chlorol-3-methyl-2-indenyl)pyridine], inhibits the conversion of 18-hydroxycorticosterone to aldosterone (116). Heparin and a number of related heparinoids have been shown to affect the synthesis of aldosterone. This effect, which is apparently upon 18-hydroxylation, takes some days to become apparent when the drug is administered to animals but does not occur in vitro (1, 86).

Cyanoketone

2α-Cyano-4,4,17α-trimethylandrost-5-en-17β-ol-3-one inhibits 3β-hydroxysteroid dehydrogenase activity and blocks the conversion of pregnenolone to progesterone (53). This substance appears therefore to specifically block the 3β-ol-dehydrogenase.

o,p′DDD

Among the first agents studied, 2,2-bis(2-chlorophenyl-4-chlorophenyl)-1,1-dichloralethane was shown to have a fairly specific effect on the adrenal cortex (102). This substance, which is highly toxic in dogs, causes degenerative changes in the adrenal mitochondria with resultant decrease in adrenocortical secretion. The drug is relatively ineffective in the rat and the guinea pig but does have an effect in humans (27, 50, 146).

Inhibitors of Cholesterol Synthesis and Metabolism

Triparanol [MER-29,(p-β-diethylaminoethoxyphenyl)-1-(p-tolyl)-2-(p-chlorophenyl)ethanol] has been shown to inhibit the formation of cholesterol by preventing the saturation of the double bond in the side chain of desmosterol. Because cholesterol is a primary precursor of the adrenal corticoids, triparanol results therefore in an inhibition of corticosteroidogenesis (66). Blohm et al. (13) have demonstrated a reduction in adrenal cholesterol and production of adrenal hypertrophy in rats, whereas Melby et al. (97) have found reduction in secretion of cortisol, aldosterone, and 17-ketosteroids (66). Some authors have suggested, however, that the chief effect on adrenal function in humans is to interfere with the extraadrenal metabolism of the corticosteroids (105). A number of other inhibitors of cholesterol synthesis have been shown to interfere also with corticoid synthesis. These include *trans*-1,4-bis(2-chlorobenzylaminomethyl)cyclohexane dihydrochloride (AY9944), an inhibitor of the conversion of cholestanone (7-dihydrocholesterol) to cholesterol, a dimethylamino derivative of DHEA, and hepatocatalase (23, 110, 140).

Aminoglutethamide (Eliptin, α-ethyl-α-p-aminophenylgluteramide) inhibits the conversion of cholesterol to 20α-hydroxycholesterol (74), which results in an excessive accumulation of cholesterol in the adrenal cortex, as well as an inhibition of the synthesis of the corticoids.

Steroids as Inhibitors of Corticosteroidogenesis

A number of studies have demonstrated inhibition of corticosteroidogenesis by corticosteroids. A direct effect of corticosterone on corticoid production in vitro has been observed, in addition to the indirect effect in vivo on ACTH secretion (11). Other studies have demonstrated an effect of testosterone as a competitive inhibitor in the conversion of corticosterone to aldosterone and of DOC to corticosterone (17, 117, 159). In the latter studies competition of testosterone and DOC to combine with cytochrome P-450 has been demonstrated. Effects of the estrogens on corticosteroidogenesis have also been extensively studied (52, 77).

Inhibitors of Protein Synthesis as Inhibitors of Corticosteroid Secretion

A number of inhibitors of protein synthesis have been shown to interfere with the action of ACTH in stimulating corticosteroidogenesis, suggesting an action of ACTH through protein synthetic mechanisms. Puromycin, chloramphenicol, and cycloheximide block corticosteroid synthesis (35, 45). Cycloheximide does not block the primary action of ACTH but inhibits subsequent enzymatic process in the mitochondria. This finding is in accordance with studies demonstrating increase in cyclic AMP following combined ACTH and cycloheximide administration, although corticosteroidogenesis is blocked. Actinomycin D does not block the response of rat adrenals in vitro to ACTH, although it does block the effect of ACTH on corticosteroid production by cow adrenal slices (42).

Ouabain

Ouabain significantly inhibits aldosterone production by slices of dog adrenal cortex and prevents the stimulating effect of increased potassium in vitro (31). Ouabain markedly inhibits production of corticosterone by slices of calf adrenals but is not effective in a mitochondrial preparation of the same tissue (157).

Other Inhibitors of Adrenal Function

A number of other substances, many of which are closely related chemically to those already described, have been shown to have an inhibitory effect on adrenal secretion either in vivo or in vitro. Some of these are referred to in reviews previously cited (50, 65, 146).

CONCLUDING SUMMARY

In this chapter the development of evidence that the biosynthesis of the adrenal steroids involves a coordinated series of reactions catalyzed largely by membrane-bound enzymes that have a definite distribution both intracellularly and among the different cellular types in the adrenal cortex has been traced. Cholesterol, probably the nonesterified fraction in the mitochondria, is the primary substrate in the normal gland, although desmosterol can serve as precursor under certain abnormal conditions. Although the major products of biosynthesis are the C_{21} $11\beta,21$-hydroxysteroids corticosterone, cortisol, and aldosterone, as well as the C_{19} steroid DHEA sulfate, small amounts of all the other steroid hormones are also formed. It is not surprising therefore that when certain enzymes of the normal pathway are absent or blocked, or when the enzyme-synthesizing apparatus is disorganized, as in tumors, the production of these other hormones may become great enough to cause pathological changes.

In higher mammals in which the hormonal environment during pregnancy becomes independent of ovarian function, the fetal adrenal plays a collaborative role in the synthesis of the estrogens by the placenta. The compounds that are produced in large quantity during this period become only minor secretory products soon after birth. Thus the adrenal is a life-preserving gland even before birth.

Adrenocortical steroids are produced by all vertebrates. While there are marked quantitative variations between species and orders, the same triumvirate of corticosterone, cortisol, and aldosterone is the major secretory product, and there seems to be no discernible relation between the pattern of steroids produced and the type of environment. The mechanisms by which these steroids exert their hormonal effects are discussed in subsequent chapters in this volume.

REFERENCES

1. ABBOTT, E. C., A. G. GOWALL, D. J. A. SUTHERLAND, M. STIEFEL, AND J. C. LAIDLAW. The influence of a heparin-like compound on hypertension, electrolytes, and aldosterone in man. *J. Can. Med. Assoc.* 94: 1155–1164, 1966.
2. ALLEN, M. J., AND A. H. CORWIN. Chemical studies on pinacols obtained from *p*-aminoacetophenone and *p*-aminopropriophenone. *J. Am. Chem. Soc.* 72: 117–121, 1950.
3. ALTMAN, L. J., R. C. KOWERSKI, AND H. C. RILLING. Synthesis and conversion of presqualene alcohol to squalene. *J. Am. Chem. Soc.* 93: 1782–1783, 1971.
4. ARAI, R., H. TAJIMA, AND B. TAMAOKI. *In vitro* transformation of steroids by the head kidney, the body kidney, and the corpuscles of stannius of the rainbow trout (*Salmo gairdneri*). *Gen. Comp. Endocrinol.* 12: 99–109, 1969.
5. ARAI, R., AND B. TAMAOKI. Biosynthesis *in vitro* of 18-hydroxy-11-deoxycorticosterone by the interrenal tissue of the rainbow trout. *J. Endocrinol.* 39: 453–454, 1967.
6. BAIRD, D. T., A. UNO, AND J. C. MELBY. Adrenal secretion of androgens and oestrogens. *J. Endocrinol.* 45: 135–136, 1969.
7. BARTTER, F. C., F. ALBRIGHT, A. P. FORBES, A. LEAF, E. DEMPSEY, AND E. CARROLL. Effects of adrenocorticotropic hormone and cortisone in the adrenogenital syndrome associated with congenital adrenal hyperplasia: an attempt to explain and connect its disordered hormonal pattern. *J. Clin. Invest.* 30: 237–251, 1951.
8. BAULIEU, E-E. Studies of conjugated 17-ketosteroids in a case of adrenal tumour. *J. Clin. Endocrinol. Metab.* 22: 501–510, 1962.
9. BEYER, K. F., AND L. T. SAMUELS. Distribution of steroid-3β-ol-dehydrogenase in cellular structures of the adrenal gland. *J. Biol. Chem.* 219: 69–76, 1956.
10. BIGLIERI, E. G., M. A. HERRON, AND N. BRUST. 17-Hydroxylation deficiency in man. *J. Clin. Invest.* 45: 1946–1954, 1966.
11. BIRMINGHAM, M. K., AND E. KURLENTS. Inactivation of ACTH by isolated rat adrenals and inhibition of corticoid formation by adrenocortical hormones. *Endocrinology* 62: 47–60, 1958.
12. BLOCH, K. The biological conversion of cholesterol to pregnanediol. *J. Biol. Chem.* 157: 661–666, 1945.
13. BLOHM, T. R., T. KARIYA, AND M. W. LAUGHLIN. Effects of MER-29, a cholesterol synthesis inhibitor, on mammalian tissue lipids. *Arch. Biochem. Biophys.* 85: 250–263, 1959.
14. BONGIOVANNI, A. M., AND A. W. ROOT. The adrenogenital syndrome. *New Engl. J. Med.* 268: 1283–1289, 1963.
15. BREUER, H., AND K. DAHM. Studies of the 17β-hydroxysteroid dehydrogenase of human adrenal cortex. *Acta Endocrinol.* 45: 47–54, 1964.
16. BROWNIE, A. C., E. R. SIMPSON, C. R. JEFCOATE, AND G. S. BOYD. Effect of ACTH on cholesterol side-chain cleavage in rat adrenal mitochondria. *Biochem. Biophys. Res. Commun.* 46: 483–490, 1972.
17. BURROW, G. N. A steroid inhibitory effect on adrenal mitochondria. *Endocrinology* 84: 979–985, 1969.
18. BURSTEIN, S., AND M. GUT. Biosynthesis of pregnenolone. *Recent Progr. Hormone Res.* 27: 303–349, 1971.
19. CAMERON, E. H. D., M. A. BEYNON, AND K. GRIFFITHS. The role of progesterone in the biosynthesis of cortisol in human adrenal tissue. *J. Endocrinol.* 41: 319–326, 1968.
20. CARSTENSEN, H., G. W. OERTEL, AND K. B. EIK-NES. Secretion of 17α-hydroxy-Δ⁵-pregnenolone by the canine adrenal gland during stimulation with adrenocorticotropin. *J. Biol. Chem.* 234: 2570–2577, 1959.

21. CASPI, E., R. I. DORFMAN, B. T. KHAN, G. ROSENFELD, AND W. SCHMID. Degradation of corticosteroids. VI. Origin of the carbon atoms of steroid hormone biosynthesides in vitro in the bovine adrenal from acetate-1-C^{14}. *J. Biol. Chem.* 237: 2085–2088, 1962.
22. CHAN, S. W. C., D. P. HUANG, G. P. VINSON, AND J. G. PHILLIPS. Pathways of corticosteroid biosynthesis in snake (*Naja naja*) and frog (*Rana rugulosa*) adrenal glands. *Acta Endocrinol. Suppl.* 119: 70, 1967.
23. CHAPPEL, C. I., D. DVORNIK, P. HILL, M. KRAML, AND R. GAUDRY. *Trans*-1,4-bis(2-chlorobenzylaminomethyl)cyclohexane dihydrochloride (AY 9944): a novel inhibitor of cholesterol biosynthesis. *Circulation* 28: 651–652, 1963.
24. CHART, J. J., M. J. ALLEN, W. T. BENCZE, AND R. GAUNT. New amphenone analogs as adrenocortical inhibitors. *Experientia* 14: 151–152, 1958.
25. CHART, J. J., H. SHEPPARD, T. MOWLES, AND N. HOWIE. Inhibitors of adrenal corticosteroid 17α-hydroxylation. *Endocrinology* 71: 479–486, 1962.
26. CHILDS, B., M. M. GRUMBACH, AND J. J. VAN WYK. Virilizing adrenal hyperplasia; a genetic and hormonal study. *J. Clin. Invest.* 35: 213–222, 1956.
27. COBEY, F. A., I. TALIAFERRO, AND H. B. HAAG. Effect of DDD and some of its derivatives on plasma 17-OH-corticosterone in the dog. *Science* 123: 140–141, 1956.
28. CONSTANTOPOULOS, G., A. CARPENTER, P. S. SATOH, AND T. T. TCHEN. Formation of isocaproaldehyde in the enzymatic cleavage of cholesterol side chain by adrenal extract. *Biochemistry* 5: 1650–1652, 1966.
29. CONSTANTOPOULOS, G., P. S. SATOH, AND T. T. TCHEN. Cleavage of cholesterol side chain by adrenal cortex. III. Identification of 20α,22ξ-dihydroxycholesterol as an intermediate. *Biochem. Biophys. Res. Commun.* 8: 50–55, 1962.
30. COOPER, D. Y., R. W. ESTABROOK, AND O. ROSENTHAL. The stoichiometry of C_{21} hydroxylation of steroids by adrenocortical microsomes. *J. Biol. Chem.* 238: 1320–1323, 1962.
31. CUSHMAN, P., JR. Inhibition of aldosterone secretion by ouabain in dog adrenal tissue. *Endocrinology* 84: 808–813, 1969.
32. DAILEY, R. E., L. SWELL, AND C. R. TREADWELL. Utilization of free and esterified cholesterol-4-C^{14} for corticoid biosynthesis by hog adrenal homogenates. *Proc. Soc. Exptl. Biol. Med.* 110: 571–574, 1962.
33. DANIELSSON, H., AND T. T. TCHEN. Steroid metabolism. In: *Metabolic Pathways* (3rd ed.), edited by D. M. Greenberg. New York: Acad. Press, 1968, vol. II, p. 117–168.
34. DAVIES, I. J., K. J. RYAN, AND Z. PETRO. Estrogen synthesis by adrenal-placental tissues of the sheep and the iris monkey in vitro. *Endocrinology* 86: 1457–1459, 1970.
35. DAVIS, W. W., AND L. D. GARREN. On the mechanism of action of adrenocorticotropic hormone. The inhibitory site of cycloheximide in the pathway of steroid biosynthesis. *J. Biol. Chem.* 243: 5153–5157, 1968.
36. DODGE, A. H., A. K. CHRISTENSEN, AND R. B. CLAYTON. Localization of a steroid 11β-hydroxylase in the inner membrane subfraction of rat adrenal mitochondria. *Endocrinology* 87: 254–261, 1970.
37. DOMINGUEZ, O. V., AND L. T. SAMUELS. Mechanism of inhibition of adrenal steroid 11β-hydroxylase by methopyrapone (Metopirone). *Endocrinology* 73: 304–309, 1963.
38. EICHHORN, J., AND O. HECHTER. Role of 11β-hydroxyprogesterone as intermediary in the biosynthesis of cortisol and corticosterone. *Proc. Soc. Exptl. Biol. Med.* 97: 614–619, 1958.
39. EWALD, W., H. WERBIN, AND I. L. CHAIKOFF. Evidence for two substrate-specific Δ⁵-3-ketosteroid isomerases in beef adrenal glands, and their separation from 3β-hydroxysteroid dehydrogenase. *Biochim. Biophys. Acta* 81: 199–201, 1964.
40. EWALD, W., H. WERBIN, AND I. L. CHAIKOFF. Δ⁵-3-Ketosteroid isomerase: solubilization and stabilization in beef adrenal gland preparations. *Steroids* 3: 505–522, 1964.
41. EWALD, W., H. WERBIN, AND I. L. CHAIKOFF. Evidence for the presence of 17-hydroxypregnenedione isomerase in beef adrenal cortex. *Biochim. Biophys. Acta* 111: 306–312, 1965.
42. FARESE, R. V. Effects of actinomycin D on ACTH-induced corticosteroidogenesis. *Endocrinology* 78: 929–936, 1966.
43. FAZEKAS, A. G., AND T. SANDOR. Flavin nucleotide coenzyme biosynthesis and its relation to corticosteroidogenesis in the rat adrenal. *Endocrinology* 89: 397–407, 1971.
44. FAZEKAS, A. G., AND J. L. WEBB. Conversion of [1,2-³H]-11-dehydrocorticosterone to 18-hydroxy-11-dehydrocorticosterone and aldosterone by rabbit adrenal slices. *European J. Steroids* 1: 389–390, 1966.
45. FERGUSON, J. J., JR. Metabolic inhibitors and adrenal function. In: *Functions of the Adrenal Cortex*, edited by K. W. McKerns. New York: Appleton, 1968, vol. 1, p. 463–478.
46. FERGUSON, M. M., AND A. G. CHRISTIE. Distribution of hydroxysteroid dehydrogenases in the placentae and foetal membranes of various mammals. *J. Endocrinol.* 38: 291–306, 1967.
47. FLINT, A. P. F., AND D. T. ARMSTRONG. The compartmentation of non-esterified and esterified cholesterol in the superovulated rat ovary. *Biochem. J.* 123: 143–152, 1971.
48. FUKUSHIMA, D. K., H. L. BRADLOW, T. YAMAUCHI, A. YAGI, AND D. KOERNER. Fate of 4β-hydrogen in Δ⁵-androstene-3,17-dione on isomerization with mammalian enzyme preparation. *Steroids* 11: 541–554, 1968.
49. GARFINKEL, D. Studies on pig liver microsomes. I. Enzymic and pigment composition of different microsomal fractions. *Arch. Biochem. Biophys.* 77: 493–509, 1958.
50. GAUNT, R., J. J. CHART, AND A. A. RENZI. Inhibitors of adrenal cortical function. *Rev. Physiol.* 56: 114–172, 1965.
51. GILL, W., AND C. CHEN. Dehydroepiandrosterone sulfatase in the prostate and seminal vesicles of the rat. *Biochim. Biophys. Acta* 218: 148–154, 1970.
52. GOLDMAN, A. S. Inhibition of 3β-hydroxysteroid dehydrogenase from *Pseudomonas testosteroni* by various estrogenic and progestinic steroids. *J. Clin. Endocrinol. Metab.* 27: 320–324, 1967.
53. GOLDMAN, A. S. Further studies of steroidal inhibitors of Δ⁵,3β-hydroxysteroid dehydrogenase and Δ⁵-Δ⁴,3-ketosteroid isomerase in *Pseudomonas testosteroni* and in bovine adrenals. *J. Clin. Endocrinol. Metab.* 28: 1539–1546, 1968.
54. GOLDMAN, A. S., W. C. YAKOVA, AND A. M. BONGIOVANNI. Development of activity of 3β-hydroxysteroid dehydrogenase in human fetal tissues and in two anencephalic newborns. *J. Clin. Endocrinol. Metab.* 26: 14–22, 1969.
55. GOODMAN, D. S., J. AVIGAN, AND H. WILSON. The in vitro metabolism of desmosterol with adrenal and liver preparations. *J. Clin. Invest.* 41: 2135–2141, 1962.
56. GRIFFITHS, K., AND C. A. GILES. Metabolism of testosterone by adrenal tissue of the golden hamster and identification of 19-hydroxylated steroids. *J. Endocrinol.* 33: 333–334, 1965.
57. HALKERSTON, I. D. K., J. EICHHORN, AND O. HECHTER. A requirement for reduced triphosphopyridine nucleotide for cholesterol side chain cleavage by mitochondrial fractions of bovine adrenal cortex. *J. Biol. Chem.* 236: 374–380, 1961.
58. HANDLER, R. P., AND E. D. BRANSOME, JR. Guinea pig adrenal 3β-hydroxysteroid dehydrogenase: is there more than one enzyme? *J. Clin. Endocrinol. Metab.* 29: 1117–1119, 1969.
59. HARDING, B. W., AND D. H. NELSON. Effect of hypophysectomy on several rat adrenal NADPH-generating and oxidizing systems. *Endocrinology* 75: 506–513, 1964.
60. HARDING, B. W., S. W. WONG, AND D. H. NELSON. Carbon monoxide-combining substances in rat adrenal. *Biochim. Biophys. Acta* 92: 415–417, 1964.
61. HAYANO, M., M. C. LINDBERG, R. I. DORFMAN, J. E. H. HANCOCK, AND E. W. DOERING. On the mechanism of the C-11β-hydroxylation of steroids: a study with H_2O^{18} and O_2^{18}. *Arch. Biochem. Biophys.* 59: 529–553, 1955.
62. HAYANO, M., H. SABA, R. I. DORFMAN, AND O. HECHTER. Some aspects of the biogenesis of adrenal steroid hormones. *Recent Progr. Hormone Res.* 12: 79–124, 1956.
63. HAYNES, R. C., JR., AND T. BERTHET. Studies on the mechanism of action of the adrenocorticotropic hormone. *J. Biol. Chem.* 225: 115–124, 1957.

64. HECHTER, O., M. M. SOLOMON, A. ZAFFARONI, AND G. PINCUS. Transformation of cholesterol and acetate to adrenal cortical hormones. *Arch. Biochem. Biophys.* 46: 201–214, 1953.
65. HERTZ, R., M. J. ALLEN, J. A. SCHRICHER, F. G. DOYSE, AND L. F. HALLMAN. Studies on amphenone and related compounds. *Recent Progr. Hormone Res.* 11: 119–147, 1955.
66. HOLLOSZY, J., AND A. B. EISENSTEIN. Effect of triparanol (MER-29) on corticosterone secretion by rat adrenals. *Proc. Soc. Exptl. Biol. Med.* 107: 347–349, 1961.
67. ICHII, S., AND S. KOBAYASHI. Studies on the biosynthesis of sterol and corticosterone in rat adrenal gland. *Endocrinol. Japon.* 13: 371–377, 1966.
68. ICHII, S., S. KOBAYASHI, AND M. MATSUBA. Effect of ACTH *in vivo* on the cholesterol side-chain cleaving enzyme and on steroid hormone precursor cholesterol in rat adrenal gland. *Steroids* 5: 663–678, 1965.
69. IDLER, D. R., AND G. B. SOMGALANG. Steroids of a chondrostean: *in vitro* steroidogenesis in yellow bodies isolated from kidneys and along the posterior cardinal veins of the American Atlantic sturgeon, *Acipenser oxyrhynchus* Mitchill. *J. Endocrinol.* 48: 627–637, 1970.
70. INANO, H., A. MACHINO, AND B. TAMAOKI. Localization of the Δ^5-3β-hydroxysteroid dehydrogenase and 21-hydroxylase activities in smooth surfaced microsomes of adrenals. *Steroids* 13: 357–363, 1969.
71. JENKINS, J. S., J. W. MEAKIN, D. H. NELSON, AND G. W. THORN. Inhibition of adrenal steroid 11-oxygenation in the dog. *Science* 128: 478–479, 1958.
72. JOHNSON, L. R., A. RUHMANN-WENNHOLD, AND D. H. NELSON. The *in vivo* effect of ACTH on utilization of reducing energy for pregnenolone synthesis by adrenal mitochondria. *Ann. NY Acad. Sci.* 212: 307–318, 1973.
73. KAHNT, F. W., AND R. NEHER. On the specific inhibition of adrenal steroid biosynthesis. *Experientia* 18: 499–501, 1962.
74. KAHNT, F. W., AND R. NEHER. Adrenal steroid biosynthesis *in vitro*. III. Selective inhibition of adrenocortical function. *Helv. Chim. Acta* 49: 725–732, 1966.
75. KASE, N., AND J. KOWAL. *In vitro* production of testosterone in a human adrenal homogenate. *J. Clin. Endocrinol. Metab.* 22: 925–928, 1962.
76. KIMURA, T., AND K. SUZUKI. Components of the electron transport system in adrenal steroid hydroxylase. Isolation and properties of non-heme iron protein (adrenodoxin). *J. Biol. Chem.* 242: 485–491, 1967.
77. KITAY, J. I., M. D. COYNE, W. NEWSOM, AND R. NELSON. Relation of the ovary to adrenal corticosterone production and adrenal enzyme activity in the rat. *Endocrinology* 77: 902–908, 1965.
78. KLOPPER, A. Assessment of fetoplacental function by hormone assay. *Am. J. Obstet. Gynecol.* 107: 807–827, 1970.
79. KORITZ, S. B. The conversion of pregnenolone to progesterone by small particles from rat adrenal. *Biochemistry* 3: 1098–1102, 1964.
80. KORITZ, S. B. Feedback inhibition by pregnenolone: a possible mechanism. *Biochim. Biophys. Acta* 93: 215–217, 1964.
81. KORITZ, S. B., AND A. M. KUMAR. On the mechanism of action of the adrenocorticotrophic hormone. The stimulation of the activity of enzymes involved in pregnenolone synthesis. *J. Biol. Chem.* 245: 152–159, 1970.
82. KORITZ, S. B., J. YUN, AND J. J. FERGUSON, JR. Inhibition of adrenal progesterone biosynthesis by 3',5'-cyclic AMP. *Endocrinology* 82: 620–622, 1968.
83. KOWARSKI, A., J. W. FINKELSTEIN, J. S. SPAULDING, G. H. HOLMAN, AND C. J. MIGEON. Aldosterone secretion rate in congenital adrenal hyperplasia. A discussion of the theories on the pathogenesis of the salt-losing form of syndrome. *J. Clin. Invest.* 44: 1505–1513, 1965.
84. KRUM, A. A., M. D. MORRIS, AND L. L. BENNETT. Role of cholesterol in the *in vivo* biosynthesis of adrenal steroids by the dog. *Endocrinology* 74: 543–547, 1964.
85. KRUSKEMPER, H. L., E. FORCHIELLI, AND H. J. RINGOLD. Δ^5-3-Keto isomerases: specificity and inhibition studies in bovine adrenal homogenate fractions and distribution in rat tissue. *Steroids* 3: 295–309, 1964.
86. LAIDLAW, J. C., E. C. ABBOTT, D. J. SUTHERLAND, AND A. STEIFEL. The influence of a heparin-like compound on hypertension, electrolytes, and aldosterone in man. *Am. Clin. Climatological Assoc.* 77: 111–124, 1965.
87. LAWRENCE, J. R., AND K. GRIFFITHS. Oestrogen biosynthesis *in vitro* by adrenal tissue from the golden hamster. *Biochem. J.* 99: 27–28c, 1966.
88. LIDDLE, G. W., E. M. LOWE, AND A. P. HARRIS. Alterations of adrenal steroid patterns in man resulting from treatment with a chemical inhibitor of 11β-hydroxylation. *J. Clin. Endocrinol. Metab.* 18: 906–912, 1958.
89. LIPSETT, M. B., AND B. HOKFELT. Conversion of 17α-hydroxypregnenolone to cortisol. *Experientia* 17: 449–450, 1961.
90. LOMMER, D., R. I. DORFMAN, AND E. FORCHIELLI. Reversal of the 3β-hydroxysteroid dehydrogenase-isomerase reactions in rat adrenals. *Steroidologia* 1: 175–182, 1970.
91. LUCIS, R., A. CARBALLEIRA, AND E. H. VENNING. Biotransformation of progesterone-4-^{14}C and 11-deoxycorticosterone-4-^{14}C by rat adrenal glands *in vitro*. *Steroids* 6: 737–756, 1965.
92. LUTTRELL, B., R. B. HOCHBERG, W. R. DIXON, P. D. MCDONALD, AND S. LIEBERMAN. Studies on the biosynthetic conversion of cholesterol into pregnenolone. Side chain cleavage of a *t*-butyl analog of 20α-hydroxycholesterol, (20R)-20-*t*-butyl-5-pregnene-3β,20-diol, a compound completely substituted at C-22. *J. Biol. Chem.* 247: 1462–1472, 1972.
93. MCCUNE, R. W., S. ROBERTS, AND P. L. YOUNG. Competitive inhibition of adrenal Δ^5-3β-hydroxysteroid dehydrogenase and Δ^5-3-ketosteroid isomerase activities by adenosine 3',5'-monophosphate. *J. Biol. Chem.* 245: 3859–3867, 1970.
94. MCKERNS, K. W. Hormone regulation of the genetic potential through the pentose phosphate pathway. *Biochim. Biophys. Acta* 121: 207–209, 1966.
95. MASON, H. S. Mechanisms of oxygen metabolism. *Advan. Enzymol.* 19: 79–233, 1957.
95a. MASTERS, B. S. S., W. E. TAYLOR, AND E. I. ISAACSON. Studies on the function of adrenodoxin and TPNH-cytochrome c reductase in the mitochondria and microsomes of adrenal cortex, utilizing immunochemical techniques. *Ann. NY Acad Sci.* 212: 76–88, 1973.
96. MATSUMOTO, K., AND L. T. SAMUELS. Influence of steroid distribution between microsomes and soluble fraction on steroid metabolism by microsomal enzymes. *Endocrinology* 85: 402–409, 1969.
97. MELBY, J. C., M. ST. CYR, AND S. L. DALE. Reduction of adrenal-steroid production by an inhibitor of cholesterol biosynthesis. *New Engl. J. Med.* 264: 583–587, 1961.
98. MEYER, A. S. 19-Hydroxylation of Δ^4-androstene-3,17-dione and dehydroepiandrosterone by bovine adrenals. *Experientia* 11: 99–102, 1955.
99. MORRISON, G., R. A. MEIGS, AND K. J. RYAN. Biosynthesis of progesterone by the human placenta. *Steroids Suppl.* 2: 177–188, 1965.
100. NANDI, J., AND H. A. BERN. Corticosteroid production by interrenal tissue of teleost fishes. *Endocrinology* 66: 295–303, 1960.
101. NEHER, R., AND A. WETTSTEIN. Occurrence of Δ^5-3β-hydroxysteroids in adrenal and testicular tissue. *Acta Endocrinol.* 35: 1–7, 1960.
102. NELSON, A. A., AND G. WOODARD. Severe adrenal cortical atrophy (cytotoxic) and hepatic damage produced in dogs by feeding 2,2-bis(parachlorophenyl)-1,1-dichlorethane (DDD or TDE). *Arch. Pathol.* 48: 387–394, 1949.
103. NEVILLE, A. M., AND L. L. ENGEL. Steroid Δ-isomerase of the bovine adrenal gland: kinetics, activation by NAD and attempted solubilization. *Endocrinology* 83: 864–872, 1968.
104. NEVILLE, A. M., J. C. ORR, AND L. L. ENGEL. The Δ^5-3β-hydroxysteroid dehydrogenase of bovine adrenal microsomes. *J. Endocrinol.* 43: 599–608, 1969.

105. NEY, R. L., W. S. COPPAGE, JR., N. SHIMIZU, D. P. ISLAND, C. F. ZUKOSKI, AND G. W. LIDDLE. Effects of triparanol on the secretion and metabolism of adrenal corticosteroids. *J. Cin. Endocrinol. Metab.* 22: 1057–1064, 1962.
106. NICOLIS, G. L., AND S. ULICK. Role of 18-hydroxylation in the biosynthesis of aldosterone. *Endocrinology* 76: 514–521, 1965.
107. OLEINICK, N. L., AND S. B. KORITZ. The activation of the Δ[5]-3-ketosteroid isomerase in rat adrenal small particles by diphosphopyridine nucleotides. *Biochemistry* 5: 715–724, 1966.
108. OMURA, T., E. SANDERS, R. W. ESTABROOK, D. Y. COOPER, AND O. ROSENTHAL. Isolation from adrenal cortex of a nonheme iron protein and a flavoprotein functional as a reduced triphosphopyridine nucleotide-cytochrome P-450 reductase. *Arch. Biochem. Biophys.* 117: 660–673, 1966.
109. OMURA, T., AND R. SATO. The carbon monoxide-binding pigment of liver microsomes. I. Evidence for its hemoprotein nature. *J. Biol. Chem.* 239: 2370–2378, 1964.
109a. OMURA, T., R. SATO, D. Y. COOPER, O. ROSENTHAL, AND R. W. ESTABROOK. Function of cytochrome P-450 of microsomes. *Federation Proc.* 24: 1181–1189, 1965.
110. ORIOL-BOSCH, A., AND K. B. EIK-NES. Effect of a hepatocatalase preparation (caperase) on adrenal function in the guinea pig. *Metab. Clin. Exptl.* 13: 319–327, 1964.
111. PALMER, R., J. A. BLAIR, G. ERIKSSON, AND E. DICZFALUSY. Studies on the metabolism of C-21 steroids in human foetoplacental unit. 3. Metabolism of progesterone and 20α- and 20β-dihydroprogesterone by midterm placentas perfused in situ. *Acta Endocrinol.* 53: 407–419, 1966.
112. PASQUALINI, J. R. Conversion of tritiated 18-hydroxycorticosterone to aldosterone by slices of human cortico-adrenal gland and adrenal tumor. *Nature* 201: 501, 1964.
113. PERON, F. G., AND C. P. W. TSANG. Further studies on corticosteroidogenesis. VI. Pyruvate and malate supported steroid 11β-hydroxylation in rat adrenal gland mitochondria. *Biochim. Biophys. Acta* 180: 445–458, 1969.
114. PULKKINEN, M. O. Arylsulphatase and the hydrolysis of some steroid sulphates in developing organism and placenta. *Acta Physiol. Scand. Suppl.* 180: 1–92, 1961.
115. RAMAN, P. B., R. J. ERTEL, AND F. UNGAR. Conversion of progesterone-4-^{14}C to 18-hydroxycorticosterone and aldosterone by mouse adrenals in vitro. *Endocrinology* 74: 865–869, 1964.
116. RAMAN, P. B., D. C. SHARMA, AND R. I. DORFMAN. Studies on aldosterone biosynthesis in vitro. *Biochemistry* 5: 1795–1804, 1966.
117. REMBIESA, R., AND M. MARCHUT. Suppression of adrenal metabolism of 4-^{14}C-progesterone by testosterone-oxime and 17α-methyltestosterone-oxime in vitro. *Biochem. Pharmacol.* 18: 701–706, 1969.
118. RILLING, H. C., C. D. POULTER, W. W. EPSTEIN, AND B. LARSEN. Studies on the mechanism of squalene biosynthesis. Presqualene pyrophosphate, stereochemistry and a mechanism of its conversion to squalene. *J. Am. Chem. Soc.* 93: 1783–1785, 1971.
119. ROSENFELD, G., AND W. D. BASCOM. The inhibition of steroidogenesis by amphenone B: studies in vitro with the perfused calf adrenal. *J. Biol. Chem.* 222: 565–580, 1956.
120. ROSNER, J. M., P. F. HALL, AND K. B. EIK-NES. Conversion of progesterone to pregnenolone by rabbit testis. *Steroids* 5: 199–210, 1965.
121. RYAN, K. J. Biological aromatization of steroids. *J. Biol. Chem.* 234: 268–272, 1959.
122. RYAN, K. J., AND L. L. ENGEL. Hydroxylation of steroids at carbon 21. *J. Biol. Chem.* 225: 103–114, 1957.
123. SANDOR, T. A detailed study of the biogenesis of corticosteroids in the avian adrenal by in vitro techniques. In: *Progress in Endocrinology.* Amsterdam: Excerpta Medica Foundation, 1969, p. 730–737. (Intern. Congr. Ser. 184.)
124. SANDOR, T. A comparative survey of steroid and steroidogenesis through the vertebrates. *Gen. Comp. Endocrinol. Suppl.* 2: 284–298, 1969.
125. SANDOR, T., J. LAMOUREUX, AND A. LANTHIER. Adrenal cortical function in reptiles. The in vitro biosynthesis of adrenal cortical steroids by adrenal slices of two common North American turtles, the slider turtle (*Pseudemys scripta elegans*) and the painted turtle (*Chrysemys picta picta*). *Steroids* 4: 213–227, 1964.
126. SANDOR, T., G. P. VINSON, I. C. JONES, I. W. HENDERSON, AND B. J. WHITEHOUSE. Biogenesis of corticosteroids in the European eel *Anguilla anguilla* L. *J. Endocrinol.* 34: 105–115, 1966.
127. SCHWERS, J., G. ERIKSSON, AND E. DICZFALUSY. Metabolism of oestrone and oestradiol in the human foeto-placental unit in midpregnancy. *Acta Endocrinol.* 49: 65–82, 1965.
128. SHARMA, D. C. Studies on aldosterone biosynthesis in vitro. *Acta Endocrinol.* 63: 299–312, 1970.
129. SHIMIZU, K., M. HAYANO, M. GUT, AND R. I. DORFMAN. The transformation of 20α-hydroxycholesterol to 17α,20α-dihydroxycholesterol by human fetal adrenals. *Steroids Suppl.* 1: 85–95, 1965.
130. SHIRLEY, I. M., AND B. A. COOKE. Sulphokinase and 3β-hydroxysteroid dehydrogenase activities in the separated zones of the human foetal and newborn adrenal cortex. *Biochem. J.* 112: 29–30P, 1969.
131. SIMPSON, E. R., D. Y. COOPER, AND R. W. ESTABROOK. Metabolic events associated with steroid hydroxylation by the adrenal cortex. *Recent Progr. Hormone Res.* 25: 523–562, 1969.
132. SIMPSON, E. R., AND R. W. ESTABROOK. Mitochondrial malic enzyme. The source of reduced nicotinamide adenine dinucleotide phosphate for steroid hydroxylation in bovine adrenal cortex mitochondria. *Arch. Biochem. Biophys.* 129: 384–395, 1969.
133. SMITH, S. W., AND L. R. AXELROD. Studies on the metabolism of steroid hormones and their precursors by the human placenta at various ages of gestation. II. In vitro metabolism of 3β-hydroxyandrost-5-en-17-one. *J. Clin. Endocrinol. Metab.* 29: 1182–1190, 1969.
134. SOBREVILLA, L., D. HAGERMAN, AND C. VILLEE. The metabolism of pregnenolone and 17α-hydroxyprogesterone by homogenates of human term placentas. *Biochim. Biophys. Acta* 93: 665–667, 1964.
135. SOLOMON, S. Formation and metabolism of neutral steroids in the human placenta and fetus. *J. Clin. Endocrinol. Metab.* 26: 762–772, 1966.
136. SOLOMON, S., P. LEVITAN, AND S. LIEBERMAN. Possible intermediates between cholesterol and pregnenolone in corticosteroidogenesis. *Rev. Can. Biol.* 15: 282, 1956.
137. STACHENKO, J., AND C. J. P. GIROUD. Functional zonation of the adrenal cortex pathways of corticosteroid biogenesis. *Endocrinology* 64: 730–742, 1959.
138. STAPLE, W., W. S. LYNN, JR., AND S. GURIN. An enzymatic cleavage of the cholesterol side chain. *J. Biol. Chem.* 219: 845–851, 1956.
139. STEINBERG, D., J. AVIGAN, AND E. B. FEIGELSON. Effects of triparanol (MER-29) on cholesterol biosynthesis and on blood sterol levels in man. *J. Clin. Invest.* 40: 884–893, 1961.
140. STEINBERG, D., AND D. S. FREDRICKSON. Inhibitors of cholesterol biosynthesis and the problem of hypercholesterolemia. *Ann. NY Acad. Sci.* 64: 579–589, 1956.
141. SUZUKI, K., AND T. KIMURA. An iron protein as a component of steroid 11β-hydroxylase complex. *Biochem. Biophys. Res. Commun.* 19: 340–345, 1965.
142. SWEAT, M. L., AND M. J. BRYSON. Separation of two components of the steroid 11β-hydroxylating system. *Arch. Biochem. Biophys.* 96: 186–187, 1962.
143. SWEAT, M. L., AND M. D. LIPSCOMB. A transhydrogenase and reduced triphosphopyridinenucleotide involved in the oxidation of desoxycorticosterone to corticosterone by adrenal tissue. *J. Am. Chem. Soc.* 77: 5185–5187, 1955.
144. SWEAT, M. L., R. B. YOUNG, AND M. J. BRYSON. Studies of the oxidation state of partially purified adrenal cortex mitochondrial cytochrome P-450 and difference spectra induced

by deoxycorticosterone and metopirone. *Arch. Biochem. Biophys.* 130: 60–69, 1969.
145. TAIT, S. A. S., D. SCHULSTER, M. OKAMOTO, C. FLOOD, AND J. F. TAIT. Production of steroids by *in vitro* superfusion of endocrine tissue. II. Steroid output from bisected whole, capsular and decapsulated adrenals of normal intact, hypophysectomized and hypophysectomized nephrectomized rats as a function of time of superfusion. *Endocrinology* 86: 360–382, 1970.
146. TEMPLE, T. E., AND G. W. LIDDLE. Inhibitors of adrenal steroid biosynthesis. *Ann. Rev. Pharmacol.* 10: 199–218, 1970.
147. TOMKINS, G. M., J. F. CURRAN, AND P. J. MICHAEL. Further studies on enzymic adrenal 11β-hydroxylation. *Biochim. Biophys. Acta* 28: 449–450, 1958.
148. TRUSCOTT, B., AND D. R. IDLER. The widespread occurrence of a corticosteroid 1α-hydroxylase in the interrenals of elasmobranchii. *J. Endocrinol.* 40: 515–526, 1968.
149. ULICK, S., E. GAUTIER, K. K. VETTER, J. R. MACHELLO, S. JAFFE, AND C. V. LOWE. An aldosterone biosynthetic defect in a salt-losing disorder. *J. Clin. Endocrinol. Metab.* 24: 669–672, 1968.
149a. VILLEE, C. A. Placenta and fetal tissues: a biphasic system for the synthesis of steroids. *Am. J. Obstet. Gynecol.* 104: 406–415, 1969.
150. VILLEE, D. B. Development of endocrine function in the human placenta and fetus. *New Engl. J. Med.* 281: 533–541, 1969.
151. VILLEE, D. B., L. L. ENGEL, J. M. LORING, AND C. A. VILLEE. Steroid hydroxylation in human fetal adrenals: formation of 16-hydroxyprogesterone, 17-hydroxyprogesterone and deoxycorticosterone. *Endocrinology* 69: 354–372, 1961.
152. VINSON, G. P., AND I. C. JONES. The *in vitro* production of oestrogens from progesterone by mouse adrenal glands. *J. Endocrinol.* 29: 185–191, 1964.
153. WARD, M. G., AND L. L. ENGEL. Reversibility of steroid Δ-isomerase. II. The reaction sequence in the conversion of androst-4-ene-3,17-dione to 3β-hydroxyandrost-5-en-17-one by sheep adrenal microsomes. *J. Biol. Chem.* 241: 3147–3153, 1966.
154. WARREN, J. G., AND C. E. TIMBERLAKE. Steroid sulfatase in human placenta. *J. Clin. Endocrinol. Metab.* 22: 1148–1151, 1962.
155. WEISS, M., AND P. G. RICHARDS. Adrenal steroid secretion in the Tasmanian devil (*Sarcophilus harisii*) and the Eastern native cat (*Dasyurus viverrinus*). A comparison of adrenocortical activity of different Australian marsupials. *J. Endocrinol.* 39: 263–275, 1971.
156. WELIKY, I., AND L. L. ENGEL. Metabolism of progesterone-4-C^{14} and pregnenolone-7α-H^3 by human adrenal tissue. Formation of 16α-hydroxyprogesterone-C^{14}, corticosterone-C^{14} and cortisol-C^{14}-H^3. *J. Biol. Chem.* 238: 1302–1307, 1963.
157. WELLEN, J. J., AND T. J. BENRAAD. Effect of ouabain on corticosterone biosynthesis and on potassium and sodium concentration in calf adrenal tissue *in vitro*. *Biochim. Biophys. Acta* 183: 110–117, 1969.
158. WENGLE, B. Distribution of some steroid sulphokinases in foetal human tissue. *Acta Endocrinol.* 52: 607–618, 1966.
159. WENNHOLD, A. R., AND D. H. NELSON. Testosterone inhibition of estradiol-induced stimulation of adrenal 11β- and 18-hydroxylation. *Proc. Soc. Exptl. Biol. Med.* 133: 493–496, 1970.
160. WERBIN, H., AND I. L. CHAIKOFF. Utilization of adrenal gland cholesterol for synthesis of cortisol by the intact normal and the ACTH-treated guinea pig. *Arch. Biochem. Biophys.* 93: 476–482, 1961.
161. WHITEHOUSE, B. J., AND G. P. VINSON. Corticosteroid biosynthesis from pregnenolone and progesterone by human adrenal tissue *in vitro*. A kinetic study. *Steroids* 11: 245–264, 1968.
162. WIELAND, R. G., R. P. LEVY, D. KATZ, AND H. HIRSCHMANN. Evidence for secretion of 3β-hydroxyandrost-5-en-17-one sulfate by measurement in normal human adrenal venous blood. *Biochim. Biophys. Acta* 78: 566–568, 1963.
163. WILKINS, L., R. A. LEWIS, R. KLEIN, AND E. ROSEMBERG. The suppression of androgen secretion by cortisone in a case of congenital adrenal hyperplasia. *Bull. Johns Hopkins Hosp.* 86: 249–252, 1950.
164. WILLIAMSON, D. G., AND V. J. O'DONNELL. The interaction of metopirone with adrenal mitochondrial cytochrome P-450. A mechanism for the inhibition of adrenal steroid 11β-hydroxylation. *Biochemistry* 8: 1306–1311, 1969.
165. WILSON, L. D., D. H. NELSON, AND B. W. HARDING. A mitochondrial electron carrier involved in steroid hydroxylations. *Biochim. Biophys. Acta* 99: 391–393, 1965.
166. YAGO, N., AND S. ICHII. Submitochondrial distribution of components of the steroid 11β-hydroxylase and cholesterol side chain-cleaving enzyme systems in hog adrenal cortex. *J. Biochem., Tokyo* 65: 215–224, 1969.
167. YOUNGLAI, E. V., AND S. SOLOMON. The *in vivo* metabolism of 16α-hydroxylated C_{19} steroids in late pregnancy. *Biochemistry* 7: 1881–1888, 1968.
168. ZELEWSKI, L., AND C. A. VILLEE. The biosynthesis of squalene, lanosterol and cholesterol by minced human placenta. *Biochemistry* 5: 1805–1814, 1966.

CHAPTER 6

Theories on the mode of action of ACTH in stimulating secretory activity of the adrenal cortex

ROBERT C. HAYNES, JR. | *Department of Pharmacology, School of Medicine, University of Virginia, Charlottesville, Virginia*

CHAPTER CONTENTS

Hypotheses of Action of ACTH
    Availability of energy
        Phosphorylase activation
        Increased permeability of cells to glucose
        Activation of glucose-6-phosphate dehydrogenase
        Substrate utilization by mitochondria
    Increased permeability of mitochondria
        Control of substrate entrance
        Control of cofactor entrance
        Control of product removal
    Synthesis of protein related to stimulation of secretion by ACTH
    Direct activation of mitochondrial enzymes by cyclic adenylic acid
Conclusions

WHEN HECHTER, in 1949, showed that ACTH rapidly stimulates the synthesis and release of steroid hormones in perfused bovine adrenal glands, a new era began in the study of the action of ACTH (23). For the first time investigators were free from the limitations imposed by whole animal studies, and the discovery, soon after, that ACTH will stimulate fragments of rat adrenals (46) and slices of bovine cortical tissue (21) further simplified the experimental systems required for studies on the action of ACTH.

From the great flood of work that followed the development of convenient and efficient experimental systems, a number of hypotheses designed to describe the action of ACTH have emerged. Unfortunately none of these is completely satisfactory, and despite the large investment of effort in this area, the definitive theory of action of ACTH has yet to be constructed.

Nevertheless, progress has been made so that now certain constraints must shape and restrain any hypothesis that may be proposed to explain how ACTH acts. One of these constraints is the speed of action of ACTH. From the early work of the Worcester group (23), as well as that of many other investigators, it is known that ACTH stimulates a remarkable increase in steroidogenesis within a few minutes after it reaches adrenal cortical tissue. Any ACTH-induced alteration in the adrenal that is imputed to be part of the biological machinery by which ACTH stimulates steroidogenesis must take place within the first 2 to 3 min after ACTH is administered. Otherwise it follows, rather than precedes, the enhanced synthesis of steroid hormones and therefore need not be considered as a necessary link in the chain of events set in motion by ACTH that culminates in increased steroidogenesis.

Another concept to be considered in any hypothesis is that the rate-limiting process in the synthesis of steroid hormones is centered in the group of reactions concerned with cleavage of the side chain of cholesterol to yield pregnenolone (48). This particular step must be accelerated for steroidogenesis from endogenous precursors to be stimulated. An acceptable theory of action of ACTH must account for an increased rate of formation of pregnenolone from cholesterol, regardless of what other sites of action may be proposed.

Another constraint now generally accepted is that ACTH acts through the agency of cyclic adenylic acid. It was shown in the late 1950s that ACTH increases the level of this nucleotide within adrenal tissue and that the nucleotide can mimic ACTH in stimulating steroidogenesis (17, 20). It is now evident that ACTH activates adenyl cyclase of the adrenal cortex and probably does not affect the rate of hydrolysis of cyclic adenylic acid (13, 51). Most important, the elevation in level of cyclic adenylic acid that follows administration of ACTH precedes the acceleration in rate of steroidogenesis (13). Furthermore in the rat the doses of ACTH that produce a graded response in the secretion of corticosterone also elicit a graded response in the level of cyclic adenylic acid.

The first event of the sequence set in motion by ACTH has thus been established to be the activation of adenyl cyclase. All subsequent effects on secretion are thought to derive from the action of cyclic adenylic acid itself, and the problem of how ACTH stimulates steroidogenesis has become the problem of how cyclic adenylic acid stimulates steroidogenesis.

HYPOTHESES OF ACTION OF ACTH

Availability of Energy

Several hypotheses in which availability of energy is considered the controlling factor for the reactions of steroid synthesis have been developed. They are built on the supposition that the rate of steroidogenesis in the adrenal cortex, in general, is limited neither by enzymatic capacity nor by availability of steroid precursors, but by the level of NADPH present in the region of the enzymes.

These hypotheses have their roots in the discovery by Sweat & Lipscomb (49) and Grant & Brownie (14) that NADPH is required for hydroxylation reactions of the steroid nucleus; such hypotheses also relate to the demonstration that the same cofactor is needed for the removal of the cholesterol side chain in the formation of pregnenolone (16). Broken cell preparations of adrenal tissue provide a model of control by NADPH because such preparations as crude homogenates or purified mitochondria require supplementation with NADPH or substrates that generate NADPH as they are metabolized. The rate of steroidogenesis in these highly artificial systems is consequently a function of the level of substrates supplied. It is therefore not surprising to find hypotheses proposing that a similar situation exists within the intact adrenal cell.

Another finding that argues for control by energy supply is the observation made by various workers that, under certain conditions, ACTH stimulates hydroxylation reactions other than those associated with side-chain cleavage (1, 22, 34, 36, 47). Since all hydroxylation reactions require NADPH, a unifying explanation for the ability of ACTH to regulate several different reactions is that it facilitates these reactions by increasing the concentration of NADPH.

There are several ways in which ACTH could act to bring about an increase in the NADPH available to drive the reactions of steroid biosynthesis. Some of the hypotheses that have been proposed are discussed below.

PHOSPHORYLASE ACTIVATION. Haynes and Berthet (17, 19) found that ACTH activates glycogen phosphorylase via cyclic adenylic acid; this activation occurs in beef adrenal slices within 1 to 2 min after ACTH is added. It was proposed that the elevated phosphorylase activity in turn causes an acceleration in glycogenolysis and thereby increases the rate of formation of glucose 1-phosphate. The enzyme phosphoglucomutase is present in sufficient abundance so that there is no impediment to the formation of glucose 6-phosphate. This ester can be metabolized by the glycolytic pathway or by the pentose-phosphate route. The adrenal cortex is rich in the enzymes of the pentose-phosphate pathway, so an appreciable fraction of glucose 6-phosphate would be metabolized in this fashion; this would lead to an enhanced formation of NADPH since this compound is a product of the dehydrogenase reactions of the pentose-phosphate pathway.

The activation of phosphorylase by ACTH in the bovine adrenal cortex has been confirmed. Therefore there is reason to believe that in this species ACTH increases glycogenolysis and probably stimulates production of NADPH. However, this cannot account for the stimulation of steroidogenesis induced by ACTH, although it may help support it. The most compelling reason to look elsewhere for an explanation of the action of ACTH is that the activation of phosphorylase in the adrenal cortex is not a generalized phenomenon; the rat gland, in responding to ACTH with accelerated steroidogenesis, does not exhibit an activation of phosphorylase or evidence of increased glycogenolysis (11, 28, 54). Another serious objection to this hypothesis is that increased NADPH resulting from activity of the pentose-phosphate pathway would be located in the cytoplasm of the adrenal cell rather than within the mitochondria where it is needed for the rate-limiting steps of steroid synthesis.

INCREASED PERMEABILITY OF CELLS TO GLUCOSE. On the basis of studies with nonutilizable sugars, Eichhorn et al. (4) proposed that ACTH acts to increase the permeability of the adrenal cell to glucose. He found that ACTH increased the amount of D-xylose partitioning from the plasma into the adrenal of the rat. Other workers subsequently demonstrated that cyclic adenylic acid also allows certain sugars to enter adrenal cells more readily (50). If penetration of glucose were a rate-limiting process, the increased formation of glucose 6-phosphate that results from ACTH-increased permeability could be a stimulant to steroidogenesis, as was proposed in the phosphorylase hypothesis.

ACTIVATION OF GLUCOSE-6-PHOSPHATE DEHYDROGENASE. McKerns (38) found that a number of preparations of ACTH added directly to solutions of glucose-6-phosphate dehydrogenase prepared from beef adrenal glands stimulate the activity of the enzyme. This stimulation was characterized in kinetic studies as an increase in V_{max}, which is the velocity of an enzyme-catalyzed reaction when the enzyme itself is saturated with its substrates. McKerns proposed that this activation of glucose-6-phosphate dehydrogenase is the principal mechanism by which ACTH accelerates steroidogenesis. He suggested that the activation of the enzyme results in an increased rate of reduction of $NADP^+$ as increased quantities of glucose 6-phosphate are metabolized by the pentose pathway. As depicted in the phosphorylase hypothesis, the elevated level of NADPH would drive the reactions of steroidogenesis at an increased rate.

In support of this hypothesis, data indicating that other polypeptide hormones and cyclic adenylic acid did not activate glucose-6-phosphate dehydrogenase of the adrenal were presented. In addition, ACTH added to homogenates of rat adrenals fortified with $NADP^+$, calcium, glucose-6-phosphate dehydrogenase, and glucose 6-phosphate stimulated the synthesis of corticosterone as predicted by the hypothesis. This is the only major hypothesis of action of ACTH that excludes cyclic adenylic acid as a mediator of ACTH action.

SUBSTRATE UTILIZATION BY MITOCHONDRIA. Tsang & Peron (52) have found that pyruvate, in the presence of catalytic concentrations of acids of the tricarboxylic acid cycle, supports a rapid rate of 11β-hydroxylation of steroids in adrenal mitochondria. They concluded that oxidation of pyruvate by the tricarboxylic acid cycle may provide NADPH for steroidogenesis; reduction of this nucleotide would occur at the $NADP^+$-linked isocitrate dehydrogenase reaction and via the energy-linked transhydrogenase. Tsang and Peron suggested that ACTH might control pyruvate oxidation, production of NADPH, and ultimately steroidogenesis by regulation of malate levels in some unknown manner.

Laury & McCarthy (36) have shown that mitochondria isolated from rats treated with ACTH exhibit an accelerated rate of 11β-hydroxylation of deoxycorticosterone when supplied with malate or succinate as an energy source. Isocitrate supported a much greater rate of hydroxylation than did the other two substrates, but no effect of prior treatment with ACTH was observed when isocitrate was used. It therefore appeared that NADPH, rather than enzyme or steroid substrate levels, was rate limiting for the hydroxylation reaction and that ACTH controlled NADPH formation when succinate or malate was the energy source. These workers concluded that ACTH treatment increased the "capacity to utilize substrate, particularly malate, to support *in vitro* 11β-hydroxylation." They did not speculate in greater detail how ACTH might do this.

Unfortunately the experiments of these workers included no treatment with ACTH for less than 1 hr. It will be important to see if these mitochondrial changes occur within the first few minutes after treatment with ACTH. If they are found to take place within 1 to 2 min after ACTH administration, the hypothesis that ACTH acts by enhancing utilization of certain substrates by mitochondria will certainly assume a position of importance and will elicit intensive study.

Experiments that raise the question of the generality of the Laury-McCarthy hypothesis are those of Koritz & Kumar (31). These workers used mitochondria prepared from adrenals of rats treated in vivo with ACTH. In preparation for the experiment they incubated the mitochondria for 20 min in water. They then added calcium ions, a NADPH-generating system, and microsomes and carried out a second incubation. During the second incubation of the mitochondria, which were by then certainly swollen and highly permeable to NADPH, the fortified mitochondria (and microsomes) from ACTH-treated rats produced corticosterone more rapidly than did mitochondria from control animals.

The effect of ACTH in this experiment could hardly be on substrate metabolism in the mitochondria since NADPH was generated outside the mitochondria and supplied to the enzymes of the mitochondria through the damaged mitochondrial membrane. Furthermore no substrate, such as malate or succinate, was added in these experiments. From this one must conclude either that ACTH has multiple actions on the mitochondria with different facets becoming evident as experimental conditions are changed or that somewhere in the execution of the experiments or in their analysis some artifact of data or reasoning is present that distorts our view of the situation. It is difficult to understand why the apparent generation of NADPH by the addition of isocitrate obliterates the effect of ACTH on 11β-hydroxylation, yet the introduction of what must be very large quantities of NADPH through swollen membranes permits the effect of ACTH on corticosterone synthesis to be manifest.

Increased Permeability of Mitochondria

When it became evident that the rate-limiting reactions of steroidogenesis take place in the mitochondria, it was understandable that investigators would begin to be concerned about the double-walled membrane that surrounds these organelles and wonder if the membrane might serve as a gating mechanism under the control of ACTH. By variation in the degree of tightness of the barrier, an effective regulation of entrance or egress of substrates, cofactors, or products could in turn control the entire sequence of reactions that constitute steroidogenesis in the adrenal cortex.

The findings of several electron microscopists directed attention to the mitochondrial membrane as a potential site of control by ACTH. Lever (37) noted that mitochondria of the adrenal cortex frequently had discontinuities in their membranes so that there was no separation between cytoplasm and matrix of the organelle. This was confirmed by later workers (39, 45) who also noted that treatment with ACTH increased the number of "open form" mitochondria. In addition, ACTH caused the mitochondria to become filled with numerous small vesicles giving them a honeycomb appearance. In some instances it looked as if vesicles were in the process of being excreted through the mitochondrial membrane.

Another series of observations, in this case biochemical rather than anatomic, also focused attention on the mitochondrial membrane. This line of investigation originated with the work of Birmingham et al. (2) who observed that calcium ions were required in the incubation medium for ACTH to stimulate rat adrenal tissue in vitro.

Koritz & Peron (33), in following up this effect of calcium, found that added calcium ions stimulated steroidogenesis in adrenal homogenates, as did freezing and the addition of proteolytic enzymes. These observations were pulled together in a conceptual framework several years later as it became evident that calcium ions lead to swelling of the adrenal mitochondria (40) and that there is a correlation between the degree of swelling and the rate of 11β-hydroxylation in isolated mitochondria. This concept was reinforced by the finding that, in addition to calcium ions, a number of other agents that cause swelling also stimulate the formation of pregnenolone in adrenal particles (25). These swelling agents include fatty acids, detergents, and proteolytic enzymes.

Swelling, by stretching the mitochondrial membrane, most certainly increases the permeability of the membrane, and since swelling stimulates 11β-hydroxylation and pregnenolone synthesis it was natural that attention would be increasingly directed to the possible control of mitochondrial permeability as a regulatory mechanism.

Further support for this idea has come from the discovery (31) that ACTH treatment in vivo resulted in mitochondria that were more responsive to various swelling agents in vitro.

On the basis of these and other observations, several hypotheses of action of ACTH have been developed in which ACTH is described as altering mitochondrial permeability. The major distinction among these hypotheses is the different material (i.e., substrate, cofactor, or product) believed to be facilitated in its movement across the mitochondrial membrane.

CONTROL OF SUBSTRATE ENTRANCE. In 1955 Hechter suggested that ACTH may enhance the rate of transport of cholesterol into adrenal mitochondria (24). If the concentration of cholesterol within mitochondria limits the rate of side-chain cleavage, this accelerated entrance would stimulate the formation of pregnenolone. The basis for this concept was the observation that the method of preparation of mitochondria and the ionic composition of the incubation medium made a significant difference in the ability of isolated mitochondria to metabolize added [^{14}C]cholesterol.

Development and testing of this particular hypothesis have not been extensive. Several years after Hechter made this proposal, Koritz & Peron (32) noted that ACTH stimulates additional corticosterone synthesis in rat adrenal glands incubated with "maximally stimulating" amounts of NADPH. It is now generally considered that exogenous NADPH stimulates steroidogenesis only in damaged cells of incubated tissue, and ACTH added in addition to NADPH stimulates steroidogenesis in the healthy cells of the preparation. However, at the time of the Koritz-Peron experiments the data were interpreted as indicating that ACTH acts to make more substrate available. Although the specific substrate and mechanism of increase in its availability were not specified, one can assume that this hypothesis would include Hechter's idea of increased mitochondrial permeability to cholesterol among the various ways in which ACTH might increase availability of substrate.

Recently this hypothesis of increased cholesterol transport has been revived in a more sophisticated form. Kowal (35), studying the effect of inhibitors of protein synthesis on steroidogenesis in cultured adrenal cells, developed a model of action of ACTH in which a "regulatory" protein facilitates cholesterol transport through mitochondrial membranes. In this scheme, ACTH would "increase the level" of this protein and thereby stimulate entrance of cholesterol into the mitochondria.

The cholesterol supply hypothesis has not been tested in definitive experiments. This is not for lack of interest in such testing but rather the difficulty in devising appropriate experiments. The demonstration (26) that mitochondria prepared from ACTH-treated rats synthesize more pregnenolone than do mitochondria from control animals seems to argue against control of the rate of the cholesterol side-chain cleavage by adjustment of the influx of cholesterol into the mitochondria, since the isolated mitochondria do not have an exogenous pool of cholesterol that can feed into the mitochondria during the incubation period. However, one can anticipate a counter argument to the effect that ACTH, during the period of treatment in vivo, permitted cholesterol to enter the mitochondria at an accelerated rate, indeed so rapidly that excess cholesterol was deposited in the mitochondria. During the in vitro incubation this extra cholesterol supplied the enzymes catalyzing the first of the side-chain cleavage reactions with additional substrate, and the enzymes ordinarily operating at less than saturating levels of substrate now produced more pregnenolone as they encountered elevated concentrations of substrate. Perhaps careful analysis of cholesterol levels of mitochondria isolated from ACTH-treated rats could resolve this problem. The hypothesis of increased mitochondrial penetration of cholesterol predicts a higher level of cholesterol in the mitochondria from treated animals; this would certainly be true if the enhanced synthesis of pregnenolone in vitro is ascribed to an enlarged pool of cholesterol in these organelles.

CONTROL OF COFACTOR ENTRANCE. Hirshfield & Koritz (26) found that mitochondria from rats treated with ACTH for 15 min formed more pregnenolone during incubation than did mitochondria from rats serving as controls. This stimulation of synthesis of pregnenolone was similar to that resulting from the presence of swelling agents in that it was largely inhibited by the addition of ATP. These investigators, struck by the parallel between swelling agents and ACTH treatment, proposed that ACTH acts by altering the permeability of the mitochondria either to NADPH (in these experiments generated outside the mitochondria) or to pregnenolone itself. The latter possibility is considered in the subsection CONTROL OF PRODUCT REMOVAL.

To test the hypothesis that the mitochondria may be made more permeable to NADPH by swelling agents and ACTH, Koritz (29) performed two experiments. The first experiment was based on the assumption that oxidation of NADPH by mitochondria is a measure of its entry into the mitochondria. The mitochondria were stimulated by various swelling agents and by incubation in a KCl medium. There was "little or no" correlation between the rates of pregnenolone synthesis and the oxidation of NADPH, a result that did not favor the NADPH permeation hypothesis.

The second approach was to measure pregnenolone synthesis as a function of NADPH and calcium ion concentration. This was based on the premise that, as a greater stimulation of pregnenolone synthesis occurs with increasing levels of calcium ions, additional NADPH enters the mitochondria. The consequences of this would be an increased sensitivity to lower levels of NADPH at higher concentrations of calcium ion. It was found that there was no significant shift in the NADPH dose-response curve with different calcium ion levels.

On the basis of these experiments the authors of this hypothesis rejected it. However, the two experiments that led these workers to discard their own hypothesis are subject to some criticism.

In the first experiment it was assumed that oxidation of NADPH in the mitochondria was a measure of increase of NADPH. This, of course, would be so only if entry is rate limiting. In the swollen mitochondria used in this study, the entry of NADPH might not be rate limiting for oxidation. Under these conditions the rate of entry might well exceed some slow step in the process of oxidation. Since this possibility exists, the negative outcome cannot be considered a sufficient reason to discard the hypothesis.

In the second experiment, there is again an assumption that may not be justified. The authors believed that stimulation of pregnenolone synthesis by increased levels of calcium ions should lead to an increased sensitivity to NADPH if higher levels of calcium ions accelerate the entry of NADPH into the mitochondria. On the other hand, if additional amounts of swelling agents merely expose more and more enzymes to the contents of the incubation medium (e.g., by rupturing more mitochondria), a greater rate of enzyme activity will result at any effective level of NADPH; in other words there is an increase in V_{max}. In this model, as calcium ions are added, more enzyme molecules would encounter the NADPH of the external medium, but their sensitivity to NADPH would not be altered. The results of this second experiment, as the results of the first, are not entirely convincing; both results are negative, and the interpretation of each is highly dependent on what model of the system one believes in.

CONTROL OF PRODUCT REMOVAL. Koritz & Hall (30), in studies on the reactions involved in cleavage of the side chain of cholesterol, found that the product of the series of reactions, pregnenolone, inhibited the overall sequence carried out by extracts of mitochondria. The inhibition did not appear to be a simple product inhibition because additional cholesterol, the substrate, did not overcome the inhibition. These investigators also were able to demonstrate that pregnenolone affected only the first of the three major reactions involved in the formation of pregnenolone, that is, the hydroxylation of cholesterol to 20α-cholesterol. They concluded that pregnenolone produces a feedback or end-product type of inhibition.

Koritz and Hall proposed that ACTH acts by increasing mitochondrial permeability to pregnenolone and thereby permits pregnenolone to leave the mitochondria more rapidly after it is synthesized. Removal of pregnenolone would release the feedback inhibition of its own synthesis and would permit pregnenolone to be synthesized at a more rapid rate. This ingenious hypothesis offers a rational model for the action of ACTH and also provides an explanation for the ability of various swelling agents to stimulate pregnenolone synthesis in adrenal mitochondria (25).

Koritz and his colleagues have continued to explore the action of ACTH from the conceptual viewpoint of this hypothesis. Many of the arguments marshaled to support the hypothesis have already been discussed. They include the following observations: a) ACTH appears to sensitize mitochondrial membranes to swelling agents (31); b) swelling agents mimic ACTH in stimulating pregnenolone synthesis in isolated mitochondria, and ATP inhibits the effects of both ACTH and swelling agents (25); c) experiments designed to test an alternative hypothesis—that changes in permeability to NADPH stimulate pregnenolone synthesis—were judged to warrant rejection of this competing hypothesis (29); and d) an analysis of the dynamic relation between doses of ACTH and cortisol secretion rates in the dog adrenal was judged to be consistent with the Koritz-Hall hypothesis, provided certain new assumptions were made regarding the degree of inhibition that pregnenolone is capable of producing (53).

The necessity of introducing new assumptions to make the Koritz-Hall hypothesis compatible with the dynamics of adrenal responses may be considered one serious criticism of the hypothesis. No published data indicate that pregnenolone is capable of inhibiting its own synthesis more than about 50%. This means that between the most extreme concentrations of pregnenolone, that is, maximally inhibiting concentrations and zero concentration, there would be a range of only about a singlefold difference in rate of synthesis. This is in contrast to the ability of ACTH to increase the rate of secretion manyfold. In adrenal mitochondria producing pregnenolone and simultaneously losing it through the membrane, the change in level of pregnenolone that would result from increased permeability would be far less than a hypothetical jump from maximally inhibiting to zero concentration. This then makes it even more difficult to explain control by ACTH over a wide range of secretion rates. The counter argument to this line of reasoning is that the degree of pregnenolone inhibition of extracted enzymes may be artificially low; preparation of the enzymes may damage some of their allosteric sites of control.

Another observation that does not support the Koritz-Hall hypothesis was pointed out by Koritz & Kumar

(31). They found that, even after swelling of mitochondria in water and incubation with calcium ion, there was still a significantly greater rate of pregnenolone synthesis in mitochondria from ACTH-treated rats.

This hypothesis needs a direct experimental test. Perhaps modern techniques for rapid separation of mitochondria will permit satisfactory analysis of pregnenolone content under conditions of increased rates of synthesis. A clear demonstration of depressed pregnenolone levels in mitochondria during accelerated synthesis would provide strong support for this hypothesis.

Synthesis of Protein Related to Stimulation of Secretion by ACTH

In 1963 Ferguson (9) inaugurated an entirely new approach to the study of ACTH when he demonstrated that the protein synthesis inhibitor, puromycin, blocked ACTH- or cyclic adenylic acid-stimulated secretion by the adrenal cortex in the rat. Subsequently other investigators have confirmed these findings and have demonstrated that other inhibitors of protein synthesis also block or greatly inhibit the effect of ACTH on steroidogenesis. These agents include cycloheximide (12), acetoxycycloheximide (10), and chloramphenicol (5). Actinomycin D does not inhibit most systems, but it has been reported to block ACTH stimulation of bovine slices (6). The data of Ferguson indicated that puromycin inhibited only the response of ACTH and not the basal production of steroid. His experiments also indicated that, once the effect of ACTH had been established, the addition of puromycin was no longer inhibitory.

This latter discovery that, once established, the effect of ACTH persists, despite the addition of puromycin, prompted Ferguson to propose that the effect of ACTH "involved" the synthesis of a specific protein; once this protein is synthesized, inhibitors of protein synthesis are no longer effective.

Davis & Garren (3) have found that cycloheximide affects steroidogenesis at a step between cholesterol and pregnenolone. A block in the synthesis of the enzymes catalyzing these reactions is presumably not the cause of the inhibition since removal of the inhibitor leads to a rapid restoration of responsiveness to ACTH, and extracts of inhibited adrenal tissue have normal rates of formation of steroid from cholesterol (9, 35).

In support of the role of protein synthesis in the action of ACTH, Grower & Bransome (15) found that ACTH and cyclic adenylic acid increased incorporation of radioactivity from labeled leucine into a single electrophoretic fraction of protein obtained from cultured adrenal tumor cells treated for 15 min. The same treatment with ACTH depressed incorporation into another protein fraction. After 60 min of treatment these changes in labeling were no longer present, which suggested that protein synthesis is involved in initiation, but not maintenance, of increased steroidogenesis.

Additional support for the concept of protein synthesis as a component of ACTH action was advanced by Farese (7) whose studies suggested that ACTH treatment for 30 min produces an increase in a soluble protein that facilitates cholesterol side-chain cleavage.

The same investigator and his colleagues have studied the rates of decay of steroidogenesis after ACTH or cyclic adenylic acid are removed from contact with adrenal tissue. They have concluded that the rather slow decay points to a "third factor," a protein, as an intermediary in the action of these agents.

Criticisms of the experiments supporting the protein synthesis hypothesis have arisen as contradictory findings have appeared in the literature. For example, the observation of Ferguson, that base-line rates of steroidogenesis are not affected by the inhibitors, has been challenged in a number of experiments. This is particularly important, inasmuch as depression of adrenal function by inhibitors of protein synthesis in the absence of ACTH would take away considerable force from the argument that it is activation by ACTH that involves protein synthesis; depression of control levels of steroidogenesis would suggest the possibility that the inhibitors might be acting in a toxic manner on the process of steroidogenesis itself. Kittinger (27), using incubation periods somewhat longer than those employed by Ferguson, noted that puromycin does decrease control levels of steroid synthesis. Farese et al. (8) and Garren et al. (12) present, but do not comment on, data that show inhibition of steroidogenesis below the base-line levels of the control. Kowal (35) has demonstrated that cycloheximide inhibits basal rates of steroidogenesis within 15 min after addition to cultured adrenal cells; puromycin also inhibits steroidogenesis in this system. The meaning of these contradictory results is not clear; they do, however, raise serious questions for workers in this area.

Another observation of Ferguson—that, once established, the stimulatory effect of ACTH was not inhibited by puromycin—shaped the original hypothesis. In contrast to this, it was noted (12) that cycloheximide given in vivo caused a rapid (within 20 min), complete reversal of the previously established stimulation of ACTH; and Farese et al. (8) found that cycloheximide and chloramphenicol, added to tissue stimulated previously for 30 min with cyclic adenylic acid and incubated in the continued presence of the nucleotide, caused a progressive decrease in steroid production beginning noticeably after a 30-min contact with the inhibitors.

A final point of disagreement has been in relation to the rates of decay of steroidogenesis after removal of ACTH or cyclic adenylic acid. The experiments of Garren et al. (12) and Kowal (35) indicate that removal of ACTH leads to a rapid decline of steroidogenesis to basal levels with a half-time of about 8 min. The experiments of those workers who reported prolonged residual stimulation after removal of ACTH have been criticized in that relatively high concentrations of ACTH were used (35). The time of persistence of stimulation after removal of a stimulating agent is actually a weak argument for the involvement of protein synthesis in the action of the stimulating agent. One can conceive of many covalent changes within a tissue induced by hormones (e.g., alterations in membrane structure) that might be reversed slowly after the stimulating agent is removed.

It appears that direct experiments of the type described by Farese (7) and Grower & Bransome (15) will be the most likely to resolve the questions that surround this hypothesis of ACTH action.

Direct Activation of Mitochondrial Enzymes by Cyclic Adenylic Acid

In a series of papers Roberts and his colleagues (42–44) have demonstrated that cyclic adenylic acid directly stimulates steroid hydroxylation reactions of the mitochondria, so that with appropriate conditions an increased accumulation of pregnenolone or 11β-hydroxylated derivatives of steroids can be observed. The precise mechanism by which cyclic adenylic acid stimulates the mitochondria has not been clarified; a speculative suggestion by Roberts & Creange (41) was that the nucleotide may activate enzymes allosterically.

This hypothesis that cyclic adenylic acid activates mitochondrial enzymes directly is attractive in its simplicity and logic. It has been criticized in that levels of cyclic adenylic acid required are generally higher than needed for activation of other enzymes in broken cell preparations. Also adenylic acid itself was found in some cases to be nearly as effective as the cyclic derivative. Finally, the metabolism of pregnenolone is partially inhibited by cyclic adenylic acid; thus an accumulation of pregnenolone might be the result of inhibited metabolism rather than accelerated synthesis. These criticisms were discussed by Roberts & Creange (41), but only additional investigations will make a final evaluation possible.

CONCLUSIONS

As we have pointed out, the quest for the mechanism of action of ACTH may be misleading, for it may be that, by evolutionary adaptation, multiple chains of sequential events have evolved as the consequence of ACTH activation of the adrenal cortex (18). If there are, indeed, multiple actions of ACTH, investigators in the field may well resemble the proverbial blind men examining the elephant. As yet the big picture, if there is one, has not become obvious from an attempt to assemble the separate observations and hypotheses of the various research groups. Unfortunately, neither is any single hypothesis completely satisfactory. Even though the expression, *theories on the mode of action of ACTH*, occurs in the title of this chapter, in fact we have yet no hypothesis that has reached a stage of development so secure and satisfying that it can be dignified by the name *theory*.

REFERENCES

1. BILLIAR, R. B., AND K. B. EIK-NES. Biosynthesis of corticoids in guinea pig adrenal slices. The effect of ACTH on [1-¹⁴C] acetate incorporation into adrenal steroids. *Biochim. Biophys. Acta* 104: 503–514, 1965.
2. BIRMINGHAM, M. K., F. H. ELLIOT, AND P. H. L. VALERE. The need for the presence of calcium for the stimulation *in vitro* of rat adrenal glands by adrenocorticotropic hormone. *Endocrinology* 53: 687–689, 1953.
3. DAVIS, W. W., AND L. D. GARREN. On the mechanism of action of adrenocorticotropic hormone. The inhibitory site of cycloheximide in the pathway of steroid biosynthesis. *J. Biol. Chem.* 243: 5153–5157, 1968.
4. EICHHORN, J., I. D. K. HALKERSTON, M. FEINSTEIN, AND O. HECHTER. Effect of ACTH on permeability of adrenal cells to sugar. *Proc. Soc. Exptl. Biol. Med.* 103: 515–517, 1960.
5. FARESE, R. V. Inhibition of the steroidogenic effect of ACTH and incorporation of amino acid into rat protein *in vitro* by chloramphenicol. *Biochim. Biophys. Acta* 87: 701–703, 1964.
6. FARESE, R. V. Effects of actinomycin D on ACTH-induced corticosteroidogenesis. *Endocrinology* 78: 929–936, 1966.
7. FARESE, R. V. Adrenocorticotrophin-induced changes in the steroidogenic activity of cell-free preparations. *Biochemistry* 6: 2052–2065, 1967.
8. FARESE, R. V., L. G. LINARELLI, W. H. GLINSMANN, B. R. DITZION, M. I. PAUL, AND G. L. PAUK. Persistence of the steroidogenic effect of adenosine-3',5'-monophosphate *in vitro*: evidence for a third factor during the steroidogenic effect of ACTH. *Endocrinology* 85: 867–874, 1969.
9. FERGUSON, J. J. Protein synthesis and adrenocorticotropin responsiveness. *J. Biol. Chem.* 238: 2754–2759, 1963.
10. FERGUSON, J. J. Metabolic inhibitors and adrenal function. In: *Functions of the Adrenal Cortex*, edited by K. W. McKerns. New York: Appleton, 1968, vol. 1, p. 463–478.
11. FIELD, J. B., I. PASTAN, B. HERRING, AND P. JOHNSON. Studies on the pathways of glucose metabolism of endocrine tissues. *Endocrinology* 67: 801–806, 1960.
12. GARREN, L. D., R. L. NEY, AND W. W. DAVIS. Studies on the role of protein synthesis in the regulation of corticosterone production by adrenocorticotropic hormone *in vivo*. *Proc. Natl. Acad. Sci. US* 53: 1443–1450, 1965.
13. GRAHAME-SMITH, D. G., R. W. BUTCHER, R. L. NEY, AND E. W. SUTHERLAND. Adenosine 3',5'-monophosphate as the intracellular mediator of the action of adrenocorticotropic hormone on the adrenal cortex. *J. Biol. Chem.* 242: 5535–5541, 1967.
14. GRANT, J. K., AND A. C. BROWNIE. The role of fumarate and TPN in steroid enzymic 11β-hydroxylation. *Biochim. Biophys. Acta* 18: 433–434, 1955.
15. GROWER, M. F., AND E. D. BRANSOME, JR. Adenosine 3',5'-monophosphate, adrenocorticotropic hormone, and adrenocortical cytosol protein synthesis. *Science* 168: 483–485, 1970.
16. HALKERSTON, I. D. K., J. EICHHORN AND O. HECHTER. TPNH requirement for cholesterol side chain cleavage in adrenal cortex. *Arch. Biochem.* 85: 287–289, 1959.
17. HAYNES, R. C., JR. The activation of adrenal phosphorylase by the adrenocorticotropic hormone. *J. Biol. Chem.* 233: 1220–1222, 1958.
18. HAYNES, R. C., JR. ACTH action: the direction of future research. In: *Functions of the Adrenal Cortex*, edited by K. W. McKerns. New York: Appleton, 1968, vol. 1, p. 583–600.
19. HAYNES, R. C., JR., AND L. BERTHET. Studies on the mechanism of action of adrenocorticotropic hormone. *J. Biol. Chem.* 225: 115–124, 1957.
20. HAYNES, R. C., JR., S. B. KORITZ, AND F. G. PERON. Influence of adenosine-3',5'-monophosphate on corticoid production by rat adrenal glands. *J. Biol. Chem.* 234: 1421–1423, 1959.

21. HAYNES, R., K. SAVARD, AND R. I. DORFMAN. An action of ACTH on adrenal slices. *Science* 116: 690–691, 1952.
22. HEARD, R. D. H., E. G. BLIGH, M. C. CANN, P. H. JELLINCK, V. J. O'DONNELL, B. G. RAO, AND J. L. WEBB. Biogenesis of the sterols and steroid hormones. *Recent Progr. Hormone Res.* 12: 45–71, 1956.
23. HECHTER, O. Corticosteroid release from the isolated adrenal gland. *Federation Proc.* 8: 70–71, 1949.
24. HECHTER, O. Concerning possible mechanisms of hormone action. *Vitamins Hormones* 13: 293–346, 1955.
25. HIRSHFIELD, I. N., AND S. B. KORITZ. The stimulation of pregnenolone synthesis in the large particles from rat adrenals by some agents which cause mitochondrial swelling. *Biochemistry* 3: 1994–1998, 1964.
26. HIRSHFIELD, I. N., AND S. B. KORITZ. The stimulation of pregnenolone synthesis in the large particles from the adrenals of rats administered adrenocorticotropin *in vivo*. *Biochim. Biophys. Acta* 111: 313–317, 1965.
27. KITTINGER, G. W. Puromycin inhibition of *in vitro* cortical hormone production by the rat adrenal gland. *Steroids* 4: 539–545, 1964.
28. KOBAYASHI, S., N. YAGO, M. MORISAKI, S. ICHII, AND M. MATSUBA. *In vitro* effect of corticotropin on the activity of the phosphorylase of rat adrenal. *Steroids* 2: 167–174, 1963.
29. KORITZ, S. B. On the regulation of pregnenolone synthesis. In: *Functions of the Adrenal Cortex*, edited by K. W. McKerns. New York: Appleton, 1968, vol. 1, p. 27–48.
30. KORITZ, S. B., AND P. F. HALL. End-product inhibition of the conversion of cholesterol to pregnenolone in an adrenal extract. *Biochemistry* 3: 1298–1304, 1964.
31. KORITZ, S. B., AND A. M. KUMAR. On the mechanism of action of the adrenocorticotropic hormone. *J. Biol. Chem.* 245: 152–159, 1970.
32. KORITZ, S. B., AND F. G. PERON. Studies on the mode of action of the adrenocorticotropic hormone. *J. Biol. Chem.* 230: 343–352, 1958.
33. KORITZ, S. B., AND F. G. PERON. The stimulation *in vitro* by Ca^{++}, freezing, and proteolysis of corticoid production by rat adrenal tissue. *J. Biol. Chem.* 234: 3122–3125, 1959.
34. KOWAL, J. Adrenal cells in tissue culture. III. Effect of adrenocorticotropin and 3',5'-cyclic adenosine monophosphate on 11β-hydroxylase and other steroidogenic enzymes. *Biochemistry* 8: 1821–1831, 1969.
35. KOWAL, J. Adrenal cells in tissue culture. VII. Effect of inhibitors of protein synthesis on steroidogenesis and glycolysis. *Endocrinology* 87: 951–965, 1970.
36. LAURY, L. W., AND J. L. MCCARTHY. *In vitro* adrenal mitochondrial 11β-hydroxylation following *in vivo* adrenal stimulation or inhibition: enhanced substrate utilization. *Endocrinology* 87: 1380–1385, 1970.
37. LEVER, J. D. Physiologically induced changes in adrenocortical mitochondria. *J. Biophys. Biochem. Cytol. Suppl.* 2: 313–316, 1956.
38. MCKERNS, K. W. Mechanism of action of adrenocorticotropic hormone through activation of glucose-6-phosphate dehydrogenase. *Biochim. Biophys. Acta* 90: 357–371, 1964.
39. NISHIKAWA, M., I. MURONE, AND T. SATO. Electron microscopic investigation of the adrenal cortex. *Endocrinology* 72: 197–209, 1963.
40. PERON, F. G., F. GUERRA, AND J. L. MCCARTHY. Further studies on the effect of calcium ions and corticosteroidogenesis. II. Adrenal mitochondrial swelling by calcium ions. *Biochim. Biophys. Acta* 110: 277–289, 1965.
41. ROBERTS, S., AND J. E. CREANGE. The role of 3',5'-adenosine phosphate in the subcellular localization of regulatory processes in corticosteroidogenesis. In: *Functions of the Adrenal Cortex*, edited by K. W. McKerns. New York: Appleton, 1968, vol. 1, p. 339–398.
42. ROBERTS, S., J. E. CREANGE, AND P. L. YOUNG. Stimulation of steroid C-11β-hydroxylation in adrenal mitochondria by cyclic 3',5'-adenosine monophosphate. *Nature* 207: 188–190, 1965.
43. ROBERTS, S., J. E. CREANGE, AND P. L. YOUNG. Stimulation of steroid transformations in adrenal mitochondria by cyclic 3',5'-adenosine phosphate. *Biochem. Biophys. Res. Commun.* 20: 446–451, 1965.
44. ROBERTS, S., R. W. MCCUNE, J. E. CREANGE, AND P. L. YOUNG. Adenosine 3',5'-cyclic phosphate: stimulation of steroidogenesis in sonically disrupted adrenal mitochondria. *Science* 158: 372–374, 1967.
45. SABATINI, D. D., E. D. P. DE ROBERTIS, AND H. BLEICHMAR. Submicroscopic study of the pituitary action on the adrenocortex of the rat. *Endocrinology* 70: 390–405, 1962.
46. SAFFRAN, M., B. GRAD, AND M. J. BAYLISS. Production of corticoids by rat adrenals *in vitro*. *Endocrinology* 50: 639–643, 1952.
47. SHEPPARD, H., R. SWENSON, AND T. F. MOWLES. Steroid biogenesis by rat adrenal. Functional zonation. *Endocrinology* 73: 819–824, 1963.
48. STONE, D., AND O. HECHTER. Studies on ACTH action in perfused bovine adrenals. The site of action of ACTH in corticosteroidogenesis. *Arch. Biochem. Biophys.* 51: 457–469, 1954.
49. SWEAT, M. L., AND M. D. LIPSCOMB. A transhydrogenase and reduced triphosphopyridinenucleotide involved in the oxidation of desoxycorticosterone to corticosterone by adrenal tissue. *J. Am. Chem. Soc.* 77: 5185–5186, 1955.
50. TARUI, S., K. NONAKA, Y. IKURA, AND K. SHIMA. Stereospecific sugar transport caused by thyroid stimulating hormone and adenosine 3',5'-monophosphate in the thyroid gland and other tissues. *Biochem. Biophys. Res. Commun.* 13: 329–333, 1963.
51. TAUNTON, O. D., J. ROTH, AND I. PASTAN. ACTH stimulation of adenyl cyclase in adrenal homogenates. *Biochem. Biophys. Res. Commun.* 29: 1–7, 1967.
52. TSANG, C. P. W., AND F. G. PERON. Factors influencing the utilization of pyruvate for steroid 11β-hydroxylation by rat adrenal mitochondria. *Steroids* 15: 251–265, 1970.
53. URQUHART, J., R. L. KRALL, AND C. C. LI. Analysis of the Koritz-Hall hypothesis for the regulation of steroidogenesis by ACTH. *Endocrinology* 83: 390–394, 1968.
54. VANCE, V. K., F. GIRARD, AND G. F. CAHILL, JR. Effect of ACTH on glucose metabolism in rat adrenal *in vitro*. *Endocrinology* 71: 113–119, 1962.

CHAPTER 7

Regulation of aldosterone secretion

JAMES O. DAVIS | *Department of Physiology, University of Missouri, School of Medicine, Columbia, Missouri*

CHAPTER CONTENTS

Evidence for Humoral Mechanism in Control of Aldosterone Secretion
Role of Renin-Angiotensin System
    Locus of secretion and chemical nature of aldosterone-stimulating hormone
    Early evidence of relation of adrenal cortex to kidney
    Evidence for renin-angiotensin system as a primary control mechanism
    Renin-angiotensin-aldosterone system in lower vertebrates
    Juxtaglomerular apparatus
    Origin of renin from juxtaglomerular cells
    Factors regulating renin secretion
    Negative feedback mechanism in control of aldosterone secretion
Altered Electrolyte Metabolism and Aldosterone Secretion
    Effects of sodium intake and depletion
    Altered plasma sodium concentration
    Effects of potassium intake and altered plasma potassium concentration
    Effects of magnesium deficiency
Anterior Pituitary Gland and Aldosterone Secretion
    Effects of hypophysectomy
    Role of ACTH
    Possible role of adenohypophysial hormones other than ACTH
Other Possible Modes of Control of Aldosterone Secretion
    Effects of estrogens, progesterone, oral contraceptives, and erythropoietin
    Possible hepatic hormone
    Possible neural regulatory mechanisms
Summary and Conclusions

WITH THE DISCOVERY of aldosterone in 1953 and the development of methods for analysis of the hormone in biological fluids, extensive studies were begun to define the mechanisms that control the rate of secretion of this potent, sodium-retaining steroid. It was clear from the studies of Levy & Blalock (182) in 1939 that neural connections to the adrenal gland are unnecessary for the regulation of aldosterone secretion; they transplanted one adrenal gland to the neck of the animal and removed the other adrenal. Several of their animals lived for months in a normal, healthy condition. Consequently in the early work, from 1955 to 1960, attention was focused on humoral factors (70); the role of the anterior pituitary and of the adrenocorticotropic hormone, ACTH, and of alterations in electrolyte metabolism were considered. These were logical approaches since the trophic influence of ACTH on the adrenal cortex had been known for many years and the primary function of aldosterone is to control the excretion of salt and water. It was soon recognized (64, 93, 281) that neither ACTH nor changes in electrolyte metabolism constitute the primary mechanism for the control of aldosterone secretion. In 1959 cross-circulation experiments in dogs (281) and sheep (93) provided convincing evidence that a humoral mechanism other than ACTH or plasma electrolyte concentrations provides the primary control for the rate of aldosterone secretion.

In 1960 two findings, which were reported almost simultaneously, suggested that this other humoral mechanism in the control of aldosterone secretion is the renin-angiotensin system. First, in 1960 it was observed that a potent aldosterone-stimulating hormone (ASH) is secreted by the kidney [J. O. Davis, unpublished observations; (65)], and second, it was reported that synthetic angiotensin II increases the rate of aldosterone secretion (174) and excretion (129). In the decade that followed, extensive studies demonstrated the renin-angiotensin system to be a primary mechanism in the control of aldosterone secretion. There was also increasing evidence of the importance of the plasma level of potassium: potassium has a direct influence on the adrenal cortex in the control of aldosterone secretion (28, 85), and indirectly, potassium regulates aldosterone secretion through its influence on the release of renin by the kidney (1, 47, 271). Also infusion of synthetic angiotensin II, Na depletion, administration of ACTH, and hyperkalemia increase the potassium content of the cells of the adrenal cortex (17). The plasma level of sodium influences aldosterone secretion by a direct action on the adrenal cortex (28, 85). The other well-known factor in the control of aldosterone secretion is the plasma level of ACTH. It is the purpose of this chapter to report the observations and to describe the concepts that have developed on the control of aldosterone secretion and to synthesize this information into a meaningful body of knowledge.

EVIDENCE FOR HUMORAL MECHANISM IN CONTROL OF ALDOSTERONE SECRETION

In the early attempts to elucidate the control mechanisms for aldosterone secretion, it was recognized that the immediate stimulus might be mediated by nervous or humoral factors, or both. The discovery (182) that dogs with only one adrenal gland transplanted to the neck lived for months in a normal, healthy condition demonstrated that the sympathetic nerves to the adrenals are unnecessary for control of aldosterone production. Later, several independent observers demonstrated that the nerves to the adrenals are not essential for hypersecretion of aldosterone in response to different stimuli in the dog and in sheep. An elevated rate of aldosterone secretion was observed in dogs with an acutely transplanted adrenal gland (115). In studies (54) of dogs with only one adrenal gland that was transplanted to the neck to denervate it, a striking increase in aldosterone secretion occurred in response to chronic thoracic inferior vena cava constriction and to acute hemorrhage. In conscious sheep with only one adrenal transplanted to the neck, a striking drop in the sodium-to-potassium ratio in saliva occurred with sodium depletion (93); this finding provided indirect evidence for an increased level of aldosterone in plasma. Subsequently actual determinations of the rate of aldosterone secretion by the denervated adrenal in conscious sheep revealed hypersecretion following sodium depletion (34). These findings in both dog and sheep show that the nerves to the adrenal are unnecessary for increased aldosterone secretion, and the observations suggest that the primary control mechanisms are humoral.

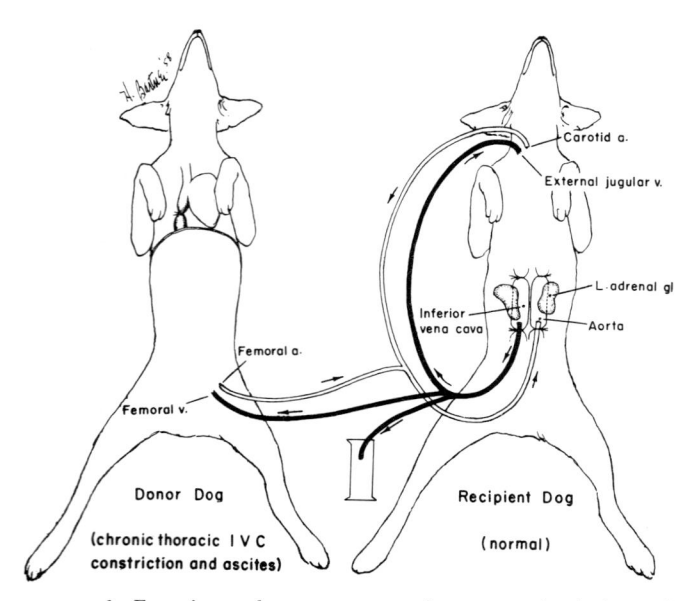

FIG. 1. Experimental arrangement for cross circulation of blood from a donor dog with chronic hyperaldosteronism secondary to thoracic inferior vena cava (*IVC*) constriction (*left*) through the isolated adrenals of a normal recipient dog (*right*). L, left; a, artery; v, vein; gl, gland. [From Yankopoulos et al. (281).]

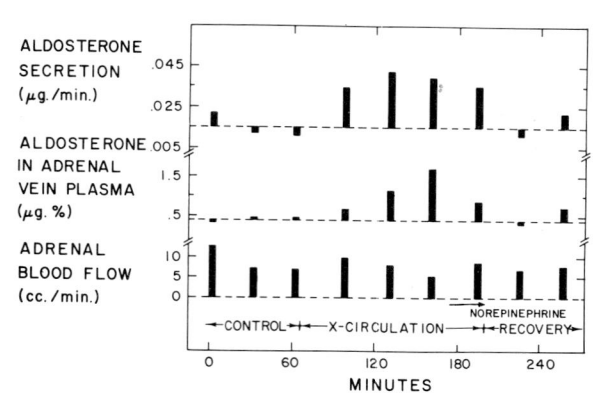

FIG. 2. A typical response in aldosterone secretion and adrenal blood flow in the recipient dog's adrenals during the control, cross-circulation (*X-circulation*), and recovery periods. A striking increase in aldosterone secretion occurred during the period of cross circulation, and there was no change in adrenal blood flow. [From Yankopoulos et al. (281).]

Direct evidence for a humoral agent was provided from cross-circulation studies in dogs (281) and sheep (93). Donor dogs with hyperaldosteronism secondary to chronic thoracic inferior caval constriction were used to cross-circulate blood through isolated adrenals of normal recipient animals [Fig. 1; (281)]. The rate of aldosterone secretion increased markedly in the isolated adrenals during cross circulation and returned to the control level during recovery observations (Fig. 2). In a control experiment, blood was circulated from normal donor dogs through normal isolated adrenals of a recipient but aldosterone secretion was unchanged. Concurrent independent observations in conscious sheep (93) provided similar evidence from cross-circulation studies for a humoral agent that stimulates the adrenal to secrete aldosterone in response to sodium depletion. In these studies in both dogs and sheep, plasma sodium and potassium concentrations were not altered and no evidence was obtained for a role for ACTH. Both groups of workers, who used different stimuli in different species, suggested that a humoral agent other than ACTH stimulated the adrenals to secrete increased amounts of aldosterone. It was proposed that this humoral agent is a hormone, and the term aldosterone-stimulating hormone (ASH) was suggested (64). Also, at the Laurentian Hormone Conference in 1958 (64), it was reported that ASH is a specific aldosterone-stimulating agent for the control of aldosterone secretion.

ROLE OF RENIN-ANGIOTENSIN SYSTEM

Locus of Secretion and Chemical Nature of Aldosterone-stimulating Hormone

Recognition that an important humoral agent regulates the rate of aldosterone secretion was followed by determination of its site of secretion and subsequently of the chemical nature of the substance. The possible loci of secretion included the hypothalamus, other brainstem regions, the pineal gland or an associated structure, the adenohypophysis, the liver, and the kidneys (65, 72, 74, 75, 78, 88, 105–108, 110, 207). The approach used was a classic endocrinologic one of removal of an organ or specific area of the body and study of the subsequent effect on aldosterone secretion, or after ablation of an organ the response to a stimulus adequate to increase aldosterone output in the animal was studied. The rationale was to locate the organ or region that when removed would block the response in aldosterone production during adequate stimulation. Acute hemorrhage, chronic thoracic caval constriction, and sodium depletion were used most extensively as stimuli to increase aldosterone secretion. In addition, extracts of various organs (65, 78, 105, 106, 207), urine (208, 218, 225, 234), lymph (152), and synthetic substances, including angiotensin II, were examined for aldosterone-stimulating activity.

Simultaneously with the recognition, from cross-circulation studies (93, 281), of the existence of an important aldosterone-stimulating agent, Farrell (106) proposed that the pineal gland or some structure closely associated with it secretes an aldosterone-stimulating substance. He suggested the name *glomerulotrophin* (106) for this substance, and later the term *adrenoglomerulotrophin* (107) was proposed. In 1959 Farrell (106) reported that extracts of the pineal gland selectively stimulated aldosterone secretion with little effect on cortisol production. These early reports of Farrell were followed by attempts to identify chemically an aldosterone-stimulating factor (108). In 1961 Farrell & McIsaac (108) reported that the active agent in pineal extracts had "colorimetric, chromatographic and fluorometric characteristics" identical with 1-methyl-6-methoxy-1,2,3,4-tetrahydro-2-carboline. Although they reported that this synthetic carboline derivative stimulated aldosterone secretion, others (34) were unable to confirm this finding. Also evidence from ablation studies (65) failed to support this hypothesis; removal of the pineal gland and associated structures had no effect on aldosterone secretion or on the increase in aldosterone production that followed chronic thoracic caval constriction or sodium depletion (Fig. 3). It seems likely that the aldosterone response to pineal extracts reported by Farrell (106) was apparent rather than real or that the aldosterone-stimulating activity reflected the presence of a substance isolated from pineal tissue during the extraction process rather than a physiological substance that is secreted. It is clear from the subsequent studies of aldosterone secretion in the following years that neither the pineal gland nor an associated structure is involved in the regulation of aldosterone secretion.

In 1960 it was discovered that the kidney is the source of a potent aldosterone-stimulating agent (65). In a series of experiments in dogs (65, 78), successive ablation of the anterior pituitary, the head, the liver, and finally the kidneys was performed; the rate of aldosterone secretion

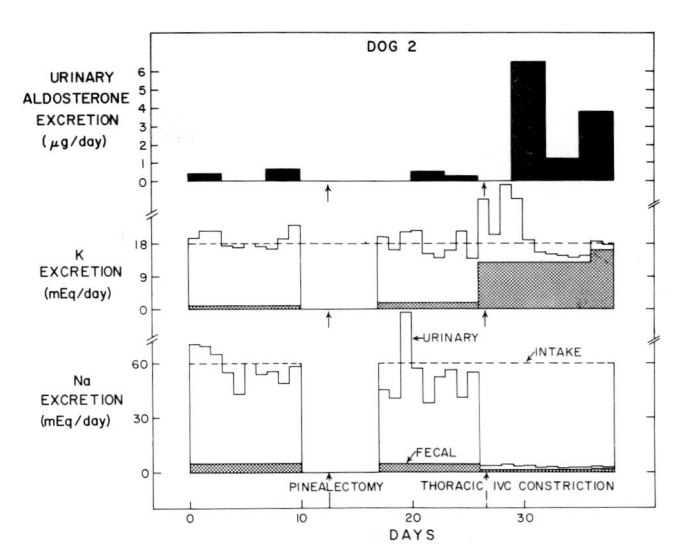

FIG. 3. Failure of pinealectomy to influence urinary aldosterone, sodium, and potassium excretion. Subsequently the animal was subjected to thoracic inferior vena cava (*IVC*) constriction, which resulted in production of hyperaldosteronism and a low sodium and high potassium ratio of fecal excretion; there was marked renal sodium retention and ascites formation. Subcommissural organ, habenular nuclei, and posterior commissure were also destroyed in this animal. [From Davis (65), by permission of Academic Press, Inc.]

was measured after removal of the region and again after acute hemorrhage. Removal of the anterior pituitary gland produced a decrease in the rate of aldosterone secretion (88, 207), but acute hemorrhage of hypophysectomized dogs resulted in a significant increase in aldosterone output (65, 78, 123). This observation demonstrated an extrapituitary source of ASH, and several subsequent studies (66–68, 73, 86) revealed that hypersecretion of aldosterone occurred in the absence of the anterior pituitary. Hyperaldosteronism has been found in sodium-depleted, hypophysectomized dogs (73) and in hypophysectomized dogs with thoracic caval constriction (73), low-output heart failure (66–68), or high-output heart failure (86).

The effects of decapitation, hepatectomy, and nephrectomy were studied in hypophysectomized dogs (65, 78) because the stress of the surgical procedure for adrenal vein cannulation results in ACTH release; a high level of ACTH in plasma might have maintained aldosterone production at a high rate even after a specific aldosterone-stimulating factor was eliminated by removal of its locus of secretion. Removal of the head or ablation of the liver from hypophysectomized dogs failed to decrease aldosterone secretion, and aldosterone output increased in response to acute blood loss (65, 78) in both experiments. In contrast, removal of the kidneys in hypophysectomized dogs produced a 50% fall in aldosterone secretion (65, 78), and acute hemorrhage failed to increase the rate of aldosterone secretion [(65, 78, 123); Fig. 4]. Injection of saline extracts from the kidneys of these hypophysectomized dogs produced a marked increase in aldosterone secretion [see Fig. 4; (65, 78, 123)], whereas similarly prepared saline extracts of liver were without effect (65, 78). It should be emphasized that the negative evidence from failure to detect an aldosterone-stimulating agent in the anterior pituitary (other than ACTH), the pineal area, the brainstem, and the liver provided important indirect evidence supporting the theory that the kidney secretes ASH.

Almost simultaneously with the discovery of ASH in 1960, Genest and associates (129) reported that the intravenous injection of synthetic angiotensin II in man augmented urinary aldosterone excretion, and Laragh and co-workers (174) found an increased rate of aldosterone secretion during infusion of angiotensin II in man. These observations on angiotensin II and the clear-cut evidence for a renal aldosterone-stimulating hormone (65, 78, 123) led to a search for the active agent in kidney extracts (79). Crude saline extracts of kidney were fractionated by ammonium sulfate precipitation; the two most active fractions for both aldosterone-stimulating and pressor activity were the 1.7 and 2.5 M ammonium sulfate fractions (Fig. 5). These two fractions are known to precipitate renin. Also heating the kidney extracts to 80 C for 10 min denatured renin and destroyed all aldosterone-stimulating and pressor activity. These observations strongly suggested the identity of ASH and renin. Since completion of these fractionation studies in 1962 (79), extensive observations from many laboratories have provided convincing evidence for the fundamental role of the renin-angiotensin system in the control of aldosterone secretion, and it is now clear that the humoral aldosterone-stimulating agent (ASH) detected from the early cross-circulation experiments was angiotensin II and that the steroidogenic response by isolated adrenals reflected increased activity of the renin-angiotensin system.

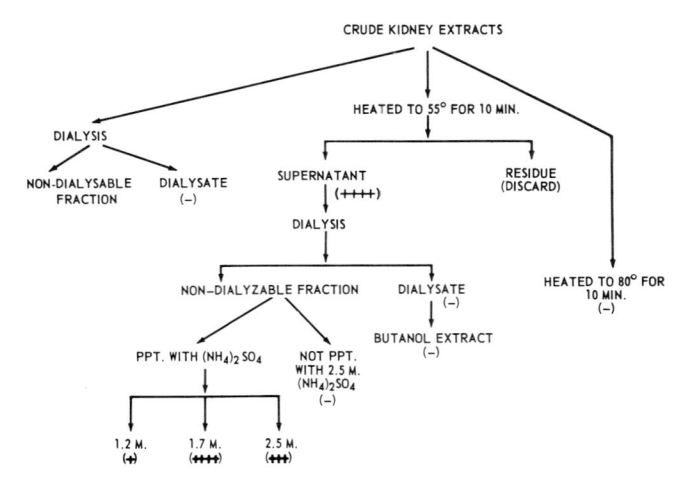

FIG. 5. Scheme for fractionation of crude kidney extracts for aldosterone-stimulating and pressor activity. *Plus* indicates presence of both types of biological activity, which parallel each other; *minus* indicates absence of either type of biological activity. Non-dialyzable fraction of heated extracts was subjected to $(NH_4)_2SO_4$ fractionation. Fractions precipitated (*PPT.*) with 1.2–2.5 M $(NH_4)_2SO_4$ were active; 1.7 and 2.5 M fractions were most active. Of this nondialyzable component, other fractions not precipitated with 2.5 M $(NH_4)_2SO_4$ were inactive. Temperatures expressed in degrees C. [From Davis et al. (79).]

Early Evidence of Relation of Adrenal Cortex to Kidney

A close functional relationship between the kidney and the adrenal cortex was suggested from many of the early studies in the 1950s. In 1951 Deane & Masson (90) found that in rats *a*) encapsulation of one kidney led to hypertrophy of the zona glomerulosa of the adrenal cortex, and *b*) injection of partially purified extracts of kidney produced enlargement of the adrenal zona glomerulosa. In 1953 Hartroft & Hartroft (143) gave rats a low-sodium diet and observed increased granulation of the renal juxtaglomerular (JG) cells. Subsequently, Hartroft and collaborators (140, 141, 145) have provided convincing evidence in both the rat and the dog that renin is secreted by the JG cells and that renin has a trophic influence on the zona glomerulosa. In 1957 Dunihue & Robertson (100) found an inverse relationship between the amount of deoxycorticosterone acetate given and the degree of JG cell granulation in rats. In 1958 Pasqualino & Bourne (222) reported that unilateral renal artery constriction in the rat led to hypertrophy of the zona glomerulosa within a few days. Also in 1958 Gross (137) postulated an inverse relationship between sodium balance and the secretion of aldosterone from studies of the renin content of the kidney in rats. In 1960 Tobian et al. (257) called attention to the large amount of evidence on the close functional interrelationships of the renal JG cells, renin, and the zona glomerulosa.

Evidence for Renin-Angiotensin System as a Primary Control Mechanism

Since 1960 an overwhelming body of evidence has indicated that angiotensin II plays an important and

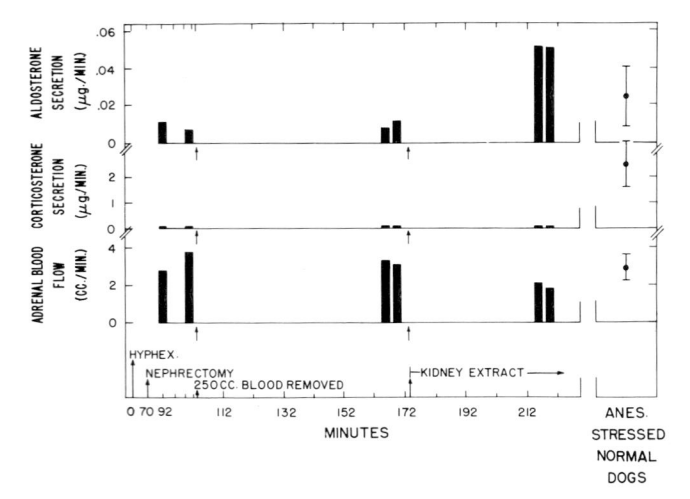

FIG. 4. Effects of acute hemorrhage on steroid secretion and adrenal blood flow in a hypophysectomized (*HYPHEX.*), nephrectomized dog and the subsequent response to a saline extract of this dog's kidneys. For comparison, mean and SEM for functions studied are presented on *right* for anesthetized (*ANES.*), stressed normal dogs. [From Davis et al. (78).]

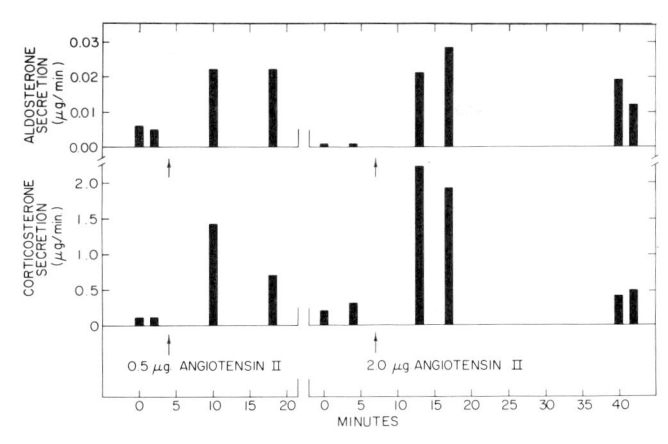

FIG. 6. Effects of single injection of synthetic angiotensin II (at 2 dose levels) on steroid secretion into the arterial supply of isolated adrenals in a hypophysectomized, nephrectomized dog. [From Davis (67).]

primary role in the regulation of aldosterone secretion. One of the first pieces of evidence was the finding that intravenous infusion of partially purified preparations of renin (28, 48, 53, 123) increased aldosterone secretion, and many investigators confirmed the work of Genest et al. (129) and Laragh et al. (174) who found that synthetic angiotensin II given intravenously stimulates aldosterone secretion. It was soon observed (67, 124) that angiotensin II acts directly on the adrenal cortex to promote aldosterone biosynthesis by infusion of the octapeptide into the arterial supply of isolated adrenals (Fig. 6), and it has been repeatedly demonstrated that angiotensin stimulates the synthesis of aldosterone in vitro. The pattern of steroid response to renin and to synthetic angiotensin II is essentially the same as that observed earlier with crude kidney extracts (53, 247). A striking increase in aldosterone secretion occurred with doses of renin (53) and angiotensin II (53) that produced only slight increments in corticosterone and cortisol secretion, and these changes in glucocorticoid secretion were physiologically insignificant; in Figure 7 the pattern of steroid response to renin is shown. These effects of angiotensin II on several steroids suggest that it has a biosynthetic action at an early stage in steroidogenesis (165, 166), and subsequent work (203) indicates that angiotensin II converts cholesterol to Δ^5-pregnenolone. Also the steroid response to angiotensin II is distinctly different from that observed with ACTH; low doses of ACTH produced a prominent effect on 17-hydroxycorticoid output but considerably less influence on aldosterone secretion [Fig. 8; (205)].

Despite the many indirect lines of evidence to suggest a renin-angiotensin-aldosterone system in the rat, the early attempts to increase aldosterone secretion during intravenous infusion of renin and angiotensin II yielded conflicting results. Some workers (188, 243) found that intravenous infusion of angiotensin II increased aldosterone secretion in hypophysectomized rats, whereas others (50, 103) failed to obtain a response. Further, intravenous infusion of renin was reported to be ineffective in augmenting aldosterone production (103, 188).

The explanation for these apparent discrepancies remains obscure, but subsequent observations (98, 168) make it clear that angiotensin II will stimulate the biosynthesis of aldosterone by the rat adrenal. In 1968 Dufau & Kliman (98) found that large doses of angiotensin II given to rats selectively increased aldosterone secretion without changing corticosterone production. At about the same time, Kinson & Singer (168) also observed a selective increase in aldosterone secretion in response to angiotensin II in rats subjected to dietary salt restriction for 1 week; the increment in aldosterone output was observed with doses of angiotensin II that produced only a slight increase in arterial pressure.

In sheep, Blair-West and associates (28) reported that during infusion of angiotensin II tachyphylaxis developed in the response in aldosterone synthesis within 3 to 10 hr, but in the dog (264) increased urinary aldosterone excretion occurred for 11 days of angiotensin infusion even with nonpressor doses. Also, Laragh and associates

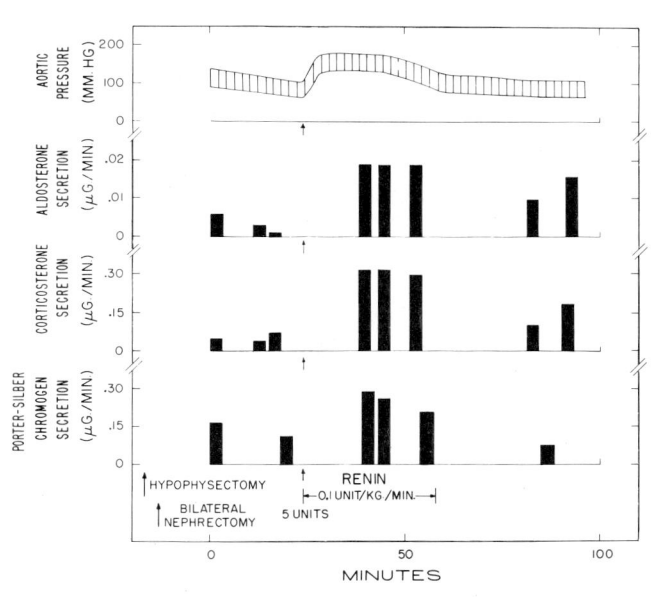

FIG. 7. Effects of renin preparation on arterial pressure and steroid secretion in a hypophysectomized, nephrectomized dog. [From Carpenter et al. (53).]

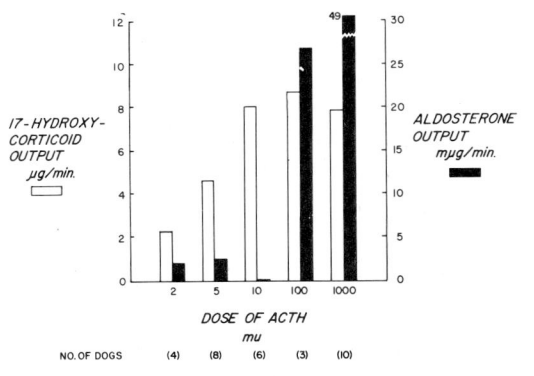

FIG. 8. Effects of ACTH on 17-hydroxycorticoid output and aldosterone secretion in hypophysectomized, nephrectomized dogs. [From Mulrow & Ganong (205).]

(172, 175) have repeatedly demonstrated that infusions of angiotensin II increased aldosterone secretion in man without evidence of tachyphylaxis, and some subjects received angiotensin II for as long as 11 days. Finally, Urquhart (263) gave a constant intravenous infusion of angiotensin II to normal conscious dogs for 8 days and observed a selective increase in aldosterone secretion without hypersecretion of corticosterone or cortisol. Apparently glucocorticoid secretion is maintained at a low basal level by the negative corticosteroid feedback mechanism mediated by the anterior pituitary (23). These results from chronic infusion studies in dog and man support the view that angiotensin II is a specific aldosterone-stimulating hormone, and they are consistent with an important homeostatic role for the renin-angiotensin system in fluid volume control (11).

Studies in several chronic experimental animal preparations with secondary aldosteronism provided evidence that increased activity of the renin-angiotensin system augments aldosterone production (65). Removal of the kidneys in hypophysectomized dogs with hyperaldosteronism secondary to thoracic caval constriction [Fig. 9; (73)], experimental low-output heart failure (65), experimental high-output heart failure (86), and chronic sodium depletion (73) produced a marked fall in aldosterone secretion, and intravenous injection of saline extracts from the kidneys of these animals into the same dogs produced a striking increase in aldosterone secretion with considerably less percentage increase in corticosterone production [see Fig. 9; (66, 73, 86)].

Early studies of the renin content of the kidneys showed a marked increase in dogs with hyperaldosteronism secondary to thoracic caval constriction (79), and the renal JG cells were found to be hypergranulated and hyperplastic. In rats with nephrosis produced by amino-nucleoside, a high positive correlation was observed between the degree of JG cell granulation and the degree of sodium retention (258). The response in arterial pressure to an intravenous injection of synthetic angiotensin II was markedly reduced in patients with cirrhosis of the liver (176) and in dogs with thoracic caval constriction (79), sodium-depletion (79), or high-output failure from an arteriovenous fistula (86), in comparison with the effect in normal human beings or dogs. In patients with hypertensive disease, a decreased pressor response has been used as a screening test for the presence of increased activity of the renin-angiotensin system.

One of the crucial lines of evidence for the pathogenic role of the renin-angiotensin system in secondary hyperaldosteronism was obtained by actual measurements of renin or angiotensin II in the renal vein or peripheral venous plasma or in lymph. In 1946 Merrill et al. (194) catheterized the renal vein in patients with congestive heart failure and reported a high concentration of renin in renal vein blood. In recent years, many reports on a variety of types of secondary aldosteronism have demonstrated either increased plasma renin activity or an increased plasma level of angiotensin II. These situations with secondary aldosteronism include *a*) acute and chronic low-sodium intake or sodium depletion (2, 23, 42–44, 46, 237, 272), *b*) thoracic caval constriction and ascites (38, 153, 239), *c*) decompensated hepatic cirrhosis and ascites (43, 44, 111, 128, 279, 280), *d*) patients or experimental animals with low-output (111, 128, 161, 194) and high-output heart failure (161), *e*) the nephrotic syndrome (128), *f*) pregnancy (43, 44, 111), *g*) some patients with renal artery stenosis and hypertensive disease (43, 44, 111, 139, 200), *h*) some cases of severe hypertensive disease without renal artery stenosis (43, 44, 111, 148, 173), *i*) acute experimental renal hypertension (46, 233), *j*) experimental hypertension secondary to constriction of one renal artery but in the presence of both kidneys in rats (138), and *k*) that following acute hemorrhage (96, 138). Although the data on plasma renin activity in these situations with secondary aldosteronism suggest the likelihood of an increased rate of renin secretion, actual measurements of renin secretion were made by Shade, Davis, and co-workers (240) in experimental aldosteronism secondary to thoracic caval constriction. Also increased amounts of renin were found in renal lymph after acute renal artery stenosis (181, 245) and in thoracic duct lymph in dogs with chronic thoracic caval constriction (152). Recently the angiotensin II concentration has been reported to be consistently higher in renal lymph than in renal arterial or renal venous plasma (7).

An important piece of evidence linking the renin-angiotensin system and the adrenal cortex was provided by in vivo studies (49) of the metabolism of ^{3}H-angiotensin II. After ^{3}H-angiotensin II was intravenously injected, it was taken up more rapidly by the adrenals than by any other organ tested. However, the kidneys and uterus were also high in ^{3}H-angiotensin II activity.

Studies with renin antibodies are also consistent with the view that the renin-angiotensin system is important

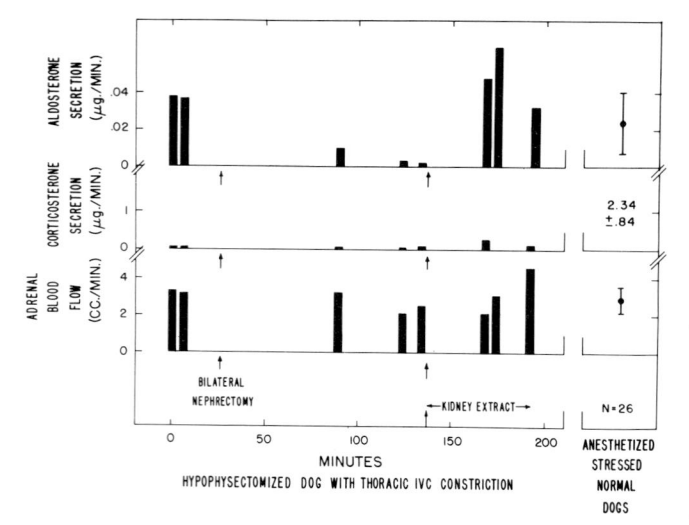

FIG. 9. Effects of bilateral nephrectomy on steroid secretion and adrenal blood flow in a hypophysectomized dog with thoracic inferior vena cava (*IVC*) constriction. Saline extract of this dog's kidneys was infused in the last part of the experiment. For comparison, average values and SEM are presented at *right* for 26 anesthetized, stressed normal dogs. [From Davis et al. (73).]

in the regulation of aldosterone secretion. Hartroft (140) observed that passive transfer of antirenin was followed by an increase in sodium excretion by the kidney in sodium-depleted dogs. Ganong and co-workers (126) found that the aldosterone-stimulating and pressor activities of both dog and hog renin were inhibited by incubation with plasma from dogs immunized with hog renin. Also dogs immunized with hog renin showed a partially blocked response in aldosterone secretion to constriction of the aorta above the kidneys (180). This evidence on the partial blocking effects of antirenin on aldosterone secretion is in contrast to earlier reports (95, 147, 272) on the reduction in blood pressure to normal levels after immunization of renal hypertensive dogs with crude preparations of renin.

Renin-Angiotensin-Aldosterone System in Lower Vertebrates

One of the important lines of evidence for the homeostatic role of the renin-angiotensin-aldosterone system in man was obtained from studies in the field of comparative physiology (83). If the renin-angiotensin system controls aldosterone secretion in primitive mammals and lower vertebrates and therefore is deeply seated phylogenetically—and, indeed, there is strong evidence for this—then surely this system is of fundamental importance in homeostasis in higher animals, including man.

The presence of renin has been reported in eight species of marine teleosts by both biochemical and histochemical techniques (197, 216, 248). The observations revealed that the renin content of the kidney of the Japanese eel was responsive to changes in the salinity of the aquatic environment: a change from fresh water to seawater led to a decrease in renal renin. Kaley and associates (58, 163) have studied the renal JG cells in fish and found intracellular granules that appear comparable to those observed in higher vertebrates. By use of Sephadex column chromatography, Sokabe et al. (249) found a number of pressor peptides in incubates of renal tissue from several species of fish. Convincing evidence for a renal-pressor system in fish has also been provided by the recent studies in the eel by Chester-Jones et al. (56). They reported that extracts of the corpuscles of Stannius from the silver eel contained a substance with a powerful pressor action. Characterization of this material showed that it resembles mammalian renin—that is, it is nondiffusible through a cellophane membrane and is heat labile. Pressor activity was also observed from studies of kidney extracts from these freshwater eels. Removal of the corpuscles of Stannius from freshwater eels was followed by a drop in arterial pressure to a level normally observed in eels adapted to seawater. These observations suggest that a renal-pressor system exists in the eel and that it is analogous to the renin-angiotensin system present in higher vertebrates. The relation of this renal-pressor system in the eel to aldosterone secretion has not been defined.

Preliminary attempts to show that adrenal cortical tissue from the eel contains enzymes for synthesis of aldosterone have yielded negative results (235). However, Bern et al. (18) found aldosterone to be present in incubates of intrarenal tissue from three species of chondrichthyean fish (dogfish, skate, ratfish). The most extensive data on the steroidogenic potency of fish renin was obtained by Taylor & Davis (252). They found that intravenous infusion of the product formed by incubation of carp kidney and carp plasma into the circulation of the American bullfrog produced a striking increase in both aldosterone and corticosterone secretion. This substance also produced a marked increase in arterial pressure in the bullfrog. Additional studies are needed to determine if a functional renin-angiotensin-aldosterone system is present in fish.

In Amphibia, aldosterone was first identified in incubates of interrenal tissue from the American bullfrog by Carstensen et al. (55). By use of the double isotope dilution procedure, Ulick & Feinholtz (262) demonstrated aldosterone secretion in the American bullfrog and measured the rate of aldosterone production. They also found that sodium depletion stimulated aldosterone secretion, but injection of synthetic angiotensin II amide 5-valine failed to alter aldosterone secretion.

The first direct evidence for a renin-angiotensin-aldosterone system in the bullfrog was provided by Johnston, Davis, and associates (162). They measured adrenal steroids in bullfrog plasma by the double isotope derivative assay procedure and found a higher concentration of both steroids in the adrenal venous effluent plasma than in peripheral venous plasma, which showed that both aldosterone and corticosterone are secreted. Intravenous infusion of a renin preparation from bullfrog kidneys into hypophysectomized frogs produced a highly significant elevation in aldosterone secretion, but corticosterone output was unchanged; this observation shows a selective action for the active agent. Infusion of renin also increased arterial pressure. The renin preparation used has several characteristics common to mammalian renin, including *a*) a pressor response in the frog similar in onset and duration to that observed with dog renin in the dog, and *b*) the active agent that is nondialyzable, stable at pH 2.6, destroyed by heat, and digested by trypsin. No pressor response to frog renin could be elicited in either the dog or rat, but frog renin incubated with frog plasma for 1 hr at 37 C formed a dialyzable pressor agent that is active in the rat. In 1966 Hartroft (142) demonstrated the presence of granules in the renal JG cells of the American bullfrog.

In two reptiles, the freshwater turtle (*Pseudemys sueanniensis*) and the crocodilian (*Caiman sclerops*), adrenal steroids have been studied by the double isotope derivative assay procedure in postcaval vein plasma and secretion rates have been calculated (215). The concentrations of steroids were so low that only corticosterone was detected in turtle plasma, but aldosterone, corticosterone, and cortisol were present in crocodilian plasma. Infusion of unincubated turtle kidney extracts into turtles increased both pressor activity and corticosterone secretion;

the active agent had characteristics similar to those of mammalian renin. Furthermore incubation of kidney extracts and plasma from turtles produced a dialyzable, heat-stable, angiotensin-like substance with pressor activity. These findings in the turtle provide evidence for a reptilian renal-pressor system with characteristics similar to the renin-angiotensin system in mammals, but no evidence for such a system was obtained from similar studies in the crocodilian.

In birds, aldosterone has been identified (253) in the adrenal venous effluent in the chicken (*Gallus domesticus*), but the level of aldosterone was so low that meaningful studies of the response to renin could not be made. There is evidence for a renal-pressor system in the chicken in that reninlike preparations produced an increase in blood pressure and, upon incubation of tissue extracts of kidney with chicken plasma, a dialyzable pressor agent that was heat stable was formed (253). Also sodium depletion in the chicken increased the renal renin content, the renal juxtaglomerular index of granulation, and the thickness of the peripheral zone of the adrenal cortex.

In a primitive mammal, the North American opossum, there is evidence for a renin-angiotensin-aldosterone system (71, 160). Intravenous infusion of renin made from opossum kidneys into hypophysectomized opossums increased both steroid secretion and arterial pressure. The most striking effect on steroidogenesis was the marked and selective increase in aldosterone secretion during the first 30 min. Later, during the infusion of renin, an accompanying increment in both corticosterone and cortisol occurred. The increase in aldosterone production was not accompanied by a change in plasma sodium or potassium concentration, and the infusion of renin did not produce an increase in sodium excretion. The opossum renin preparation, which was similar to other mammalian renin preparations in heat and pH stability, produced a slow, prolonged pressor response. Also sodium depletion in the opossum increased the renal juxtaglomerular index of granulation.

There is evidence therefore, from studies of vertebrates from Amphibia to man, for a functional renin-angiotensin-aldosterone system. These observations add support to the evidence from studies of a low-sodium intake, postural changes, and pregnancy that the renin-angiotensin-aldosterone system is an important homeostatic mechanism in human beings (70, 71). The indirect evidence for the deep-seated phylogenetic origin of the renin-angiotensin system suggests that the renin-angiotensin system is a primary control mechanism for aldosterone secretion in nearly all vertebrates. The situation in sheep and in rats seems more complex and may reflect the evolutionary emergence of unusual species.

Juxtaglomerular Apparatus

There is now convincing evidence that the JG cells of the renal afferent arterioles secrete renin and that these cells are the primary source of the enzyme. The JG cells are specialized and highly differentiated myoepitheloid cells (Fig. 10). The cytoplasm of the JG cells contains granules that are revealed by special techniques, such as the Bowie stain. The degree of granulation of the JG cells varies greatly among species. An index of JG granulation (JGI) has been formulated (145) for comparison of the degree of granulation under different conditions. After acute hemorrhage an increase in renin secretion has been found to be associated with depletion of JG cell granules, whereas in chronic states with hypersecretion of renin there is almost invariably hypergranulation of the JG cells. Studies of the JG granules by electron microscopy have demonstrated that their morphology is characteristic of true secretory bodies (145).

These specialized granular cells are most abundant in the walls of the renal afferent arterioles; however, similar cells with granules have been reported in rare instances in the efferent arterioles (8, 9), but their extent here is relatively meager compared with that in the afferent arterioles. The granular JG cells lie in close juxtaposition to the macula densa, the first segment of the distal tubule. Indeed, the JG cells and the cells of the macula densa occasionally appear inseparable and actually interdigitate with one another. This relation is uniformly present in the dog. In contrast, in the rat, Barajas & Latta (8, 9) have recently found a much closer relation between the macula densa and the efferent arteriole or mesangial cells of the glomerulus than between the macula densa and afferent arteriole. Also, Dunihue & Boldosser (99) have reported that the mesangial cells in

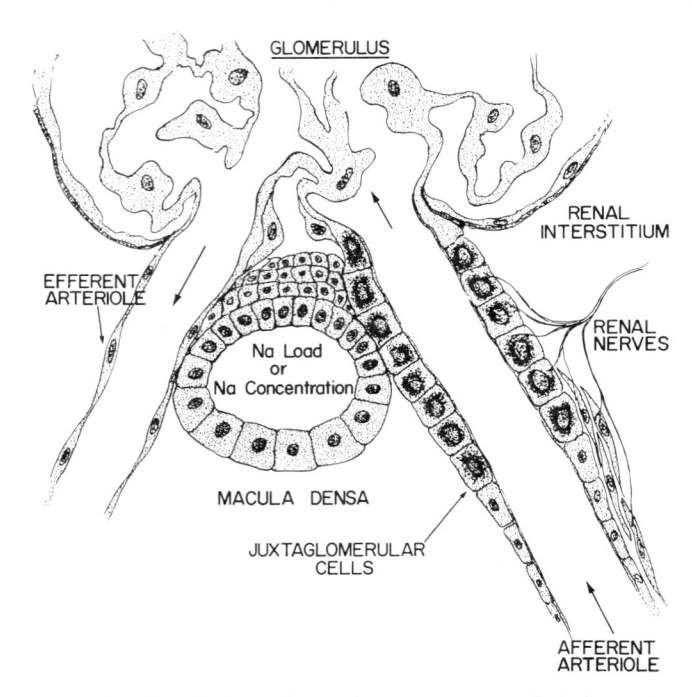

FIG. 10. Renal juxtaglomerular apparatus depicting the highly differentiated juxtaglomerular (JG) cells in the wall of the renal afferent arteriole and the adjacent macula densa. Renal sympathetic nerves end in the JG cells and in the smooth muscle cells. *Stippled areas* around the nuclei in JG cells represent granules containing renin or a precursor of renin. [From Davis (70).]

the rat respond to stimuli which increase renin secretion with changes in granulation in a way similar to the JG cells. Thus true species differences in the relation of the granular cells to the macula densa appear to exist, and this might help explain the failure to find as close functional relations in the renin-angiotensin system of the rat as in that of the dog and man. Unfortunately, similar observations on the JG apparatus in sheep have not been made.

Changes in enzyme activity in the macula densa cells have been reported to occur in association with changes in secretory activity of the JG cells (151). Also the cells of the macula densa are taller and contain specialized organelles in comparison with other renal tubular cells (9, 231). This striking degree of structural differentiation of the macula densa cells and their juxtaposition to the JG cells are highly suggestive of a close functional relation in those species, such as dog and man, in which it occurs. Indeed, in these species the two structures could function as an integrated unit, which has been called the juxtaglomerular apparatus.

Origin of Renin from Juxtaglomerular Cells

In 1939 Goormaghtigh (136) suggested that the JG cells possess endocrine activity and that they are the source of a potent pressor agent in renal hypertension. The basis for this suggestion came from Goormaghtigh's observations [see (145)] of an increase in size and degree of granulation of the JG cells in kidneys from patients with hypoxic renal disease and from patients with malignant hypertension. A decade later, Dunihue [see (145)] reported an increase in size and number of the JG granules in adrenalectomized rats, and he ascribed these changes to a fall in blood pressure.

Many different lines of evidence show that renin is secreted by the JG cells.

1. The correlation between the degree of JG cell granulation and the renin content of the kidney in a variety of circumstances in the rat is striking [see (256)]. After constriction of only one renal artery in the rat, the amount of renin extracted and the JG cell granulation increased in the "ischemic" kidney, whereas the JG granules almost disappeared and the renin content decreased in the contralateral kidney. When the kidney with renal artery constriction was excised, the JGI and kidney renin content returned to normal in the remaining kidney. Administration of deoxycorticosterone acetate (DCA) and salt to rats resulted in a reduction in JG granules and renal renin content, whereas a low-sodium diet produced hypergranulation of the JG cells and increased the renin content of the kidney. In metacorticoid hypertension in rats, both the JGI and renal renin content were reduced. Finally adrenalectomized rats exhibited a high JGI and an elevation in the renin content of the kidney. Thus in nearly all the chronic situations examined in the rat there is an excellent correlation between the degree of JG granulation and the amount of renin extractable from the kidney. This correlation strongly suggests that, under these chronic conditions, kidney renin content reflects the rate of renin secretion. Additional support for this interpretation is the finding of hyperplasia of the JG cells in the presence of a high JGI and large amounts of kidney renin.

2. Brown et al. (41), from studies in the rabbit, have isolated single glomeruli and determined their renin content. The glomeruli deep in the renal cortex contained less renin than the superficial ones, and the JG cell granules were less frequent in the afferent arterioles associated with deep juxtamedullary glomeruli. The distinct partition of renin-rich glomeruli in the superficial renal cortex and the renin-poor glomeruli in the deep cortex suggests a functional relation of renin to specific kidney functions (116).

3. Microdissection studies point to the localization of renin in the vascular pole of the glomerulus. With a clever technique, Cook (59) injected magnetic iron particles into the renal artery in rabbits to isolate glomeruli with the attached vascular pole, which included the JG cells. The vascular pole and JG cells were analyzed for pressor activity that appeared to be referrable to renin. Bing & Kazimierczak (22) also dissected out the JG apparatus in both rabbits and cats, but they concluded that the macula densa, rather than the afferent arteriole, is the source of renin. It should be pointed out that the macula densa is relatively free of granules of the type present in the highly specialized JG cells.

4. Edelman & Hartroft (102) provided the most convincing evidence for the origin of renin from the granules of the JG cells by use of the fluorescent-antibody technique. Antirenin made by injection of hog renin into dogs was conjugated with fluorescein-isothiocyanate. The fluorescein-labeled antirenin combined with and stained only the JG granules in sections of renal cortex. There is a problem with the impurity of the antigen, but this limitation was partially overcome by use of known species' cross reactions of antibodies to renin (102, 140). In other words, hog antirenin neutralizes not only hog renin but also rabbit and dog renin, so kidney from all three species was studied. This experiment localizes the JG cell granules as the specific site for renin storage.

Hypergranulation and hyperplasia of the JG cells have been observed in a variety of conditions with secondary aldosteronism, including *a*) experimental and human renal hypertension (113, 133, 138, 145, 156, 258, 260), *b*) malignant hypertension (145), *c*) thoracic inferior vena cava constriction (79), *d*) experimental high-output heart failure (86), *e*) sodium depletion (140, 141, 144), *f*) decompensated hepatic cirrhosis (145, 231, 260), *g*) experimental nephrosis (114, 258), and *h*) a syndrome of undetermined etiology with JG cell hyperplasia (16).

Factors Regulating Renin Secretion

The specific signals perceived by the JG cells to secrete renin are unknown. It has been recognized for several years that there are two intrarenal receptors that lead to renin release; these are the so-called baroreceptor in the

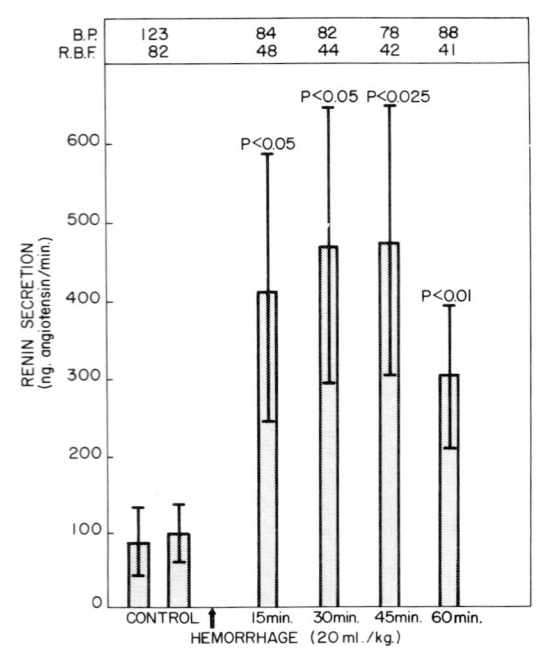

FIG. 11. Effects of hemorrhage on renin secretion; arterial pressure (B.P.), expressed as mmHg; and renal blood flow (R.B.F.), expressed as ml/min in adrenalectomized dogs with a denervated, nonfiltering kidney. N = 6. [From Blaine et al. (25).]

renal afferent arterioles and the macula densa. Considerable difficulty has occurred in attempts to relate a given stimulus to a specific receptor since most experimental maneuvers can conceivably influence both receptors.

According to the baroreceptor hypothesis, the JG cells respond to changes in the degree of "stretch" of the wall of the renal afferent arteriole with a resultant alteration in renin release. This hypothesis was first proposed by Tobian (256) in 1959 to explain his observation that a decrease in JG cell granulation occurred in association with increased mean renal perfusion pressure. This view received support from the experiments of Skinner et al. (246) who found that suprarenal aortic constriction increased renin release without a detectable change in renal blood flow. No measurements of the rate of glomerular filtration or renal sodium excretion were made, so a change in sodium concentration of renal tubular fluid and its influence on the macula densa were not considered.

A new approach to this problem has been provided by Blaine, Davis, and associates (24–26) in studies with the denervated, nonfiltering kidney in adrenalectomized dogs. In this preparation the macula densa was rendered nonfunctional by preventing glomerular filtration so that changes in renal tubular sodium load or concentration could not occur after application of a stimulus, such as hemorrhage or aortic constriction. The kidneys were denervated to exclude a direct influence of the renal nerves on the JG cells, and the dogs were adrenalectomized to eliminate a major portion of circulating catecholamines. In this denervated, nonfiltering kidney of adrenalectomized dogs, a striking increase in renin secretion occurred in response to either hemorrhage (Fig. 11) or suprarenal aortic constriction (Fig. 12). The data emphasize the importance of an intrarenal vascular receptor in the control of renin release. It seems likely that the receptor is located in the renal afferent arterioles since intrarenal arterial infusion of papaverine completely blocked the response in renin release to hemorrhage [Fig. 13; (278)] and papaverine is known to abolish renal autoregulation, which is an afferent arteriolar function. Since the observed increases in renin secretion in the nonfiltering kidney were associated with decreased renal perfusion pressure, and renal blood flow during hemorrhage and reinfusion of blood during a recovery period decreased plasma renin activity to the control level, the findings are consistent with a baroreceptor or stretch mechanism.

However, the precise nature of this afferent arteriolar receptor remains unknown. The receptor does not appear to respond only to changes in distending pressure. After hemorrhage or thoracic caval constriction there is a striking decrease in renal blood flow and arteriolar constriction associated with renin release in the nonfiltering kidney, whereas with suprarenal aortic constriction in this kidney model the initial increase in renin release is associated with renal arteriolar dilatation. This vascular receptor probably operates from a set point determined by several different inputs that regulate wall tension in the renal afferent arterioles. These inputs include not only the distending pressure of the blood but renal interstitial pressure, elastic components of the vessel wall, nervous influences, and myogenic and autoregulatory mechanisms within the vessels. Changes in afferent arteriolar wall tension as a consequence of alterations of any of these variables can conceivably occur and thereby alter the rate of renin release.

Additional support for the vascular receptor mechan-

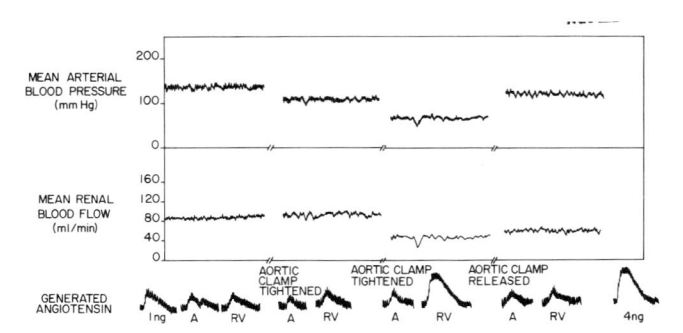

FIG. 12. Changes in arterial pressure, renal blood flow, and generated angiotensin, which was formed by incubation of renal vein (RV) and arterial plasma (A) in an adrenalectomized dog with a denervated, nonfiltering kidney during tightening of the aortic clamp. Initially, arterial pressure fell; there was no change in renal blood flow, and renin secretion increased as indicated by an increase in the amount of angiotensin generated by renal vein plasma. Further tightening of the aortic clamp produced a more marked increase in renin secretion. [From Blaine & Davis (24), by permission of The American Heart Association, Inc.]

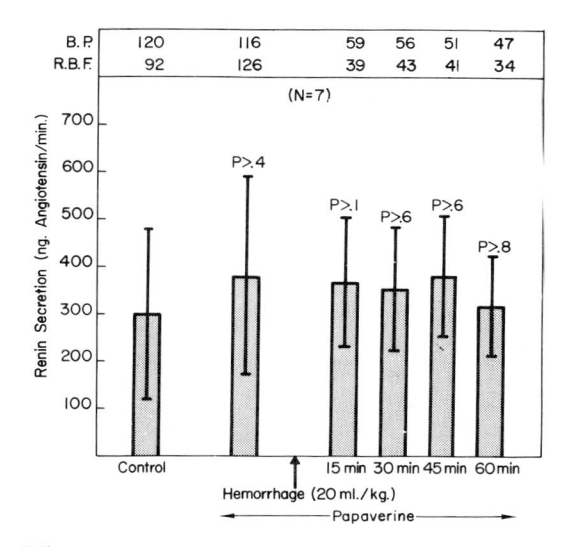

FIG. 13. Effect of intrarenal arterial papaverine on renin secretion in response to acute hemorrhage in dogs with denervated, nonfiltering kidney. B.P., blood pressure; R.B.F., renal blood flow. [From Witty et al. (278).]

ism was obtained from studies of the effects of an intrarenal papaverine infusion on renin secretion in dogs with thoracic caval constriction and ascites (240). In this chronic animal preparation with a single nonfiltering kidney, intrarenal papaverine produced a striking fall in renin secretion. Also the rate of renin secretion in dogs with caval constriction and a nonfiltering kidney was fivefold greater than in dogs with a nonfiltering kidney but otherwise normal.

Numerous experiments have been conducted in an attempt to relate the macula densa to the control of renin release. Investigators have pointed out the close anatomic relationship of the macula densa and JG cells, and certain cytological changes suggest that these two structures are intimately related. Indeed, in observations with both light and electron microscopes, morphological cellular changes consistent with a close functional relationship of these structures are shown. Vander & Miller (268) were first to provide experimental evidence for a macula densa theory of renin release. They gave diuretics to dogs subjected to aortic constriction, which alone increased renin release; the diuretics prevented a rise in renin secretion. Their interpretation of these findings was that the diuretics increased sodium load at the macula densa and prevented renin release. More recently, Vander & Carlson (267) have been more specific in suggesting that increased renin release is mediated by decreased sodium transport by the macula densa cells. Another school of thought originated with the micropuncture experiments of Thurau and associates (255) who increased the sodium concentration in the early distal tubule by injecting saline in a retrograde manner; they observed collapse of the proximal tubule and suggested that a resultant decrease in glomerular filtration rate (GFR) occurred for that nephron. Thurau and co-workers reasoned that an increased concentration of the sodium ion is perceived by the macula densa, which influences the JG cells to produce renin; they proposed that increased amounts of angiotensin II are formed within the JG cells and lead to constriction of the efferent arteriole and decreased GFR. It was further suggested that the decrease in GFR is part of a negative feedback mechanism whereby a decrease in sodium concentration at the macula densa decreases renin release. The observations of Meyer et al. (195) in the rabbit and of Cooke and associates (60) in the dog have supported the view that increased sodium concentration rather than decreased sodium load at the macula densa increases renin release. After diuretic administration (either furosemide or ethacrynic acid) but in the absence of volume depletion (reinfusion of ureteral urine into the femoral veins prevented volume depletion) renin release increased, presumably secondary to an increase in sodium delivery to the macula densa; both furosemide and ethacrynic acid act on the ascending limb of Henle's loop to decrease sodium reabsorption. Also, in the studies by Cooke et al. (60) in the dog, ureteral occlusion increased renal vein renin activity but ethacrynic acid failed to increase renin release during ureteral occlusion. When the ureter was reopened in these animals and a sodium-rich urine flowed by the macula densa, renal vein renin activity increased. More direct observations are needed to assess precisely what does occur in sodium transport in the macula densa cells under various experimental conditions. Available methodology has not been adequate to provide this information, so our knowledge of the precise signal perceived by the macula densa cells is incomplete.

It is clear that the renal nerves are involved in the control of renin secretion, but they are not essential for hypersecretion of renin to occur. Electrical stimulation of the renal nerves increased renin secretion (159, 266), and certain observations (158) have demonstrated that the response is mediated, at least in part, by a direct action of the renal nerves on the JG cells. Mogil et al. (198) failed to find an increase in renin secretion in response to sodium depletion in dogs with renal denervation, but recently, bilateral renal denervation of dogs with chronic thoracic caval constriction reduced plasma renin activity (PRA) by 50% in studies of chronic conscious dogs (240); however, the postdenervation level was still eight times the level of PRA in normal dogs. Completeness of denervation was demonstrated by analysis of renal cortical norepinephrine and by findings of barely discernible amounts (240).

The role of adrenergic receptors in renin release has been studied extensively by Winer and associates (276, 277) and more recently by Assaykeen and co-workers (4, 5). Winer and associates (276, 277) have data to support the involvement of both α and β receptors, and they have proposed that cyclic AMP is an intracellular mediator of renin release. Assaykeen and co-workers (4, 5) presented evidence for β-receptor mediation only in renin secretion. Johnson, Davis, and Witty (159) obtained evidence that norepinephrine acts directly on the JG cells, whereas in similar experiments with epinephrine, evidence for such a direct action was lacking. Both hormones do, of course, act on the renal arterioles (159) to influence renal perfusion pressure and renal blood flow, and in large enough doses GFR is decreased. Thus the adrenal medullary hormones have several loci and mechanisms of action.

Several other humoral agents are now known to influence renin secretion. Blair-West et al. (31) have reported that angiotensin II, even at physiological levels, leads to decreased renin secretion by an action on the renin secretory mechanism and thereby forms a short feedback loop in the control system. Vasopressin, at physiological levels in plasma, has been reported to decrease renin secretion (250). The concentration of plasma potassium is also a determinant of the rate of renin secretion (1, 47, 271); hyperkalemia decreases renin release, and hypokalemia augments renin secretion. Potassium appears to exert its action through an effect on the renal tubules, since an intrarenal arterial infusion of potassium with an increase in renal venous potassium from 4.5 to as high as 8.3 mEq/liter failed to influence renin secretion in the nonfiltering kidney, whereas in the filtering kidney with a similar increase of potassium concentration in renal venous plasma a striking decrease in renin secretion occurred (240). Similarly, intrarenal arterial infusion of sodium chloride decreased renin secretion (209), and the response appears to be mediated primarily by an action on the renal tubular system and possibly through the macula densa (240).

In summary, there is evidence that two intrarenal receptors, a vascular receptor located at the level of the JG cells in the renal afferent arterioles and the macula densa, are involved in renin release. It is suggested that the extent of dominance of these receptors varies with different physiological and pathophysiological situations. The important role of the renal vascular receptor has been emphasized from studies of the nonfiltering kidney, and these observations point to a fundamental mechanism that possesses functional autonomy. The renal nerves influence renin release but are not essential for hypersecretion of renin. Finally a number of humoral agents, including epinephrine, norepinephrine, sodium and potassium ions, angiotensin II, and antidiuretic hormone, influence renin secretion.

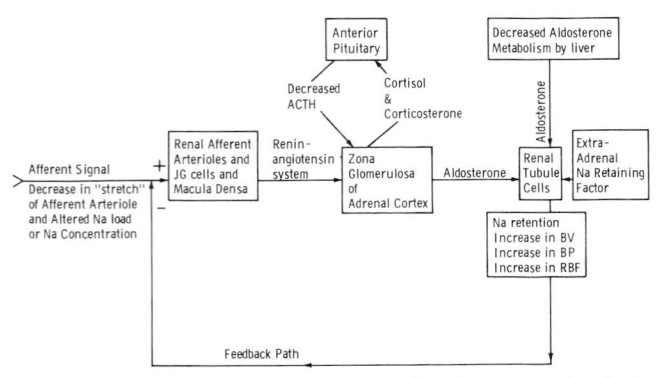

FIG. 14. Control of aldosterone secretion by a negative feedback mechanism. *BV*, blood volume; *BP*, blood pressure; *RBF*, renal blood flow.

Negative Feedback Mechanism in Control of Aldosterone Secretion

The early observations on the renin-angiotensin-aldosterone system led to the formulation of a negative feedback hypothesis for the control of aldosterone secretion (67), and evidence continues to accumulate in support of this concept. The principal components of this renin-aldosterone system are presented in Figure 14. Two intrarenal receptors, the so-called baroreceptor in the renal afferent arterioles and the macula densa, perceive signals that lead to renin release by the JG cells. As indicated earlier in this review, the precise nature of the signals perceived by these two receptors remains unknown. Renin is secreted into renal afferent arteriolar blood and probably into renal lymph, since increased amounts of renin have been found in renal (181) and thoracic duct lymph (152) during increased renin release. In blood and lymph, renin acts on angiotensinogen or renin substrate, a tetradecapeptide secreted by the liver, to produce angiotensin I, a decapeptide. Angiotensin I is converted almost quantitatively to angiotensin II by converting enzyme as blood passes through the lungs and, to a lesser extent, in the general circulation and lymphatic system. Angiotensin II acts directly on the zona glomerulosa to stimulate the biosynthesis of aldosterone. Initially an acute increase in cortisol and corticosterone secretion also occurs if the angiotensin level in blood is high (13, 23, 53). It has been proposed (23) that the initial increase in cortisol and corticosterone output is reduced by a negative corticosteroid feedback mechanism via the anterior pituitary so that the plasma level of these glucocorticoids returns to normal. According to this view, the mechanism controlling ACTH release is adjusted so that less circulating ACTH is present. Thus, in chronic secondary aldosteronism, an increased plasma level of aldosterone results from increased aldosterone secretion, whereas glucocorticoid output is normal. It should be pointed out that angiotensin II may lead to release, as well as synthesis, of aldosterone since an action of angiotensin is demonstrable within 5 min in the isolated adrenal preparation (67, 124, 152).

Another important mechanism that contributes to the level of aldosterone in plasma in both homeostasis and disease is the rate of metabolism of the hormone. The liver is the principal site for metabolism of aldosterone, and the rate of hepatic blood flow is the primary determinant of aldosterone metabolism (39, 84). A change in posture from supine to upright position reduced hepatic blood flow (63) and the rate of aldosterone metabolism (39) by approximately 50%, and consequently the plasma level of aldosterone doubled. The recent observations (269) that the plasma aldosterone level increases with standing in anephric patients are probably explicable on the basis of decreased aldosterone metabolism by the liver secondary to a decrease in hepatic blood flow. In several experimental and clinical situations, aldosterone metabolism is decreased with a resultant increase in the plasma level of aldosterone; these include acute hemorrhage (84), experimental (84) and naturally occurring low-output heart failure (39, 51, 187, 251, 280), experimental hepatic venous congestion (6), and decompensated hepatic cirrhosis (279, 280). In all these conditions, hepatic blood flow is reduced, and the observations indicate that the rate of aldosterone metabolism is controlled by a flow-limited system (39, 84, 251).

The possibility that aldosterone acts directly on the adrenal cortex [(27); J. O. Davis, unpublished data] or on the renin-releasing mechanism (127) to decrease the rate of aldosterone secretion has been examined. The results were negative; intravenous infusion of aldosterone with a substantial elevation in the plasma level of the hormone failed to influence the rate of aldosterone secretion. It has been concluded therefore that aldosterone acts via the renal tubules to promote sodium reabsorption, which leads to a sequence of changes that indirectly regulate aldosterone production.

Aldosterone acts on the renal tubules to promote sodium transport and retention of salt and water by the kidneys. This response is, however, dependent on an additional factor that acts in association with aldosterone to influence sodium reabsorption. This factor has been referred to as the extraadrenal, sodium-retaining factor (80) since the factor is essential for chronic salt and water retention in edematous states. The normal animal escapes from the sodium-retaining action of aldosterone in the absence of this factor (81).

These experimental findings could be due to changes in the rate of elaboration of a separate and distinct factor that actually decreases, rather than increases, sodium reabsorption. Thus a decrease in the plasma level of the factor would produce the net result of sodium retention. In other words, if less of a sodium-excreting factor, possibly the so-called natriuretic factor (238), is present in edematous states with hyperaldosteronemia, aldosterone might manifest itself by producing chronic sodium retention. Also physical factors may act in association with a mineralocorticoid hormone (101). Regardless of the exact nature of this factor, or factors, it is clear that experimental animals with pulmonic stenosis (82), thoracic caval constriction (80), or a large arteriovenous fistula (80) are unusually responsive to large doses of DCA or aldosterone or to angiotensin II via production of aldosterone (Fig. 15); consequently these animals possess the additional sodium-retaining factor. In addition, many patients with heart and circulatory disorders or with liver disease show evidence of the so-called extraadrenal, sodium-retaining factor.

Aldosterone, in association with this additional factor, leads to retention of salt and water by the kidney. In normal animals, including man, such retained fluid increases the circulating blood volume, arterial pressure, renal blood flow, and the rate of glomerular filtration. Bartter (11) has been one of the chief enthusiasts for the role of body fluid volume in the control of aldosterone secretion. Thus changes secondary to fluid retention could decrease renin release by the negative feedback loop depicted in Figure 14. Either or both intrarenal receptors—the vascular receptor or the macula densa—

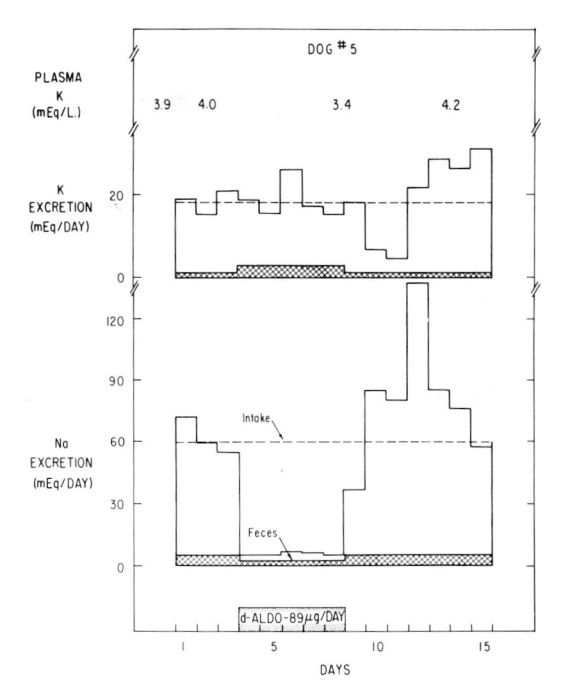

FIG. 15. Effect of intravenous infusion of d-aldosterone (d-ALDO) on sodium and potassium excretion and plasma potassium concentration in a dog with a large aortic-caval fistula. [From Davis et al. (80), by permission of The American Heart Association, Inc.]

might be involved. In congestive heart failure or in experimental thoracic caval constriction, most of the retained fluid is filtered as edema into tissue spaces or as an effusion into a serous cavity; thus the retained fluid is prevented from restoring renal arteriolar hemodynamics and macula densa sodium load or concentration to normal. Under these circumstances, the feedback loop is opened and hypersecretion of renin and aldosterone continues.

ALTERED ELECTROLYTE METABOLISM
AND ALDOSTERONE SECRETION

Effects of Sodium Intake and Depletion

The observation that a low-sodium diet increases aldosterone production in normal human beings was first made by Luetscher & Axelrad (186) from measurements of the rate of urinary aldosterone excretion. This finding was soon confirmed by others (14, 150). Extensive studies of the mechanisms involved in the increase in aldosterone biosynthesis during changes in the state of total body sodium have been made in several species. It is now established that sodium depletion increases aldosterone secretion in man (173, 223, 275), sheep (28, 30, 37, 91, 93, 94), dogs (23, 46, 73, 89), and rats (50, 57, 76, 103, 104, 188), and recently this response was observed in an amphibian, the American bullfrog [(262); J. O. Davis, unpublished observations].

Studies of the temporal changes show that the onset of

the steroidogenic response occurs rapidly in both sheep and dogs (46, 93). In sheep loss of sodium through a parotid fistula increased aldosterone output within 15 to 30 min, and in dogs both Mercuhydrin and chlorothiazide increased renin and aldosterone output within 1 to 2 hr (46).

The mechanisms whereby sodium depletion increases aldosterone secretion have been the subject of discussion and even debate. There is increased activity of the renin-angiotensin system in close association with hypersecretion of aldosterone during a low-sodium intake or sodium depletion in both man and dog, and most workers (23, 42, 43, 46, 73, 79, 138, 173, 223, 273) agree that the renin-angiotensin system is the primary control mechanism. In sheep and rats, which have also been studied extensively, there is evidence for increased activity of the renin-angiotensin system and of increased aldosterone production during sodium depletion. However, mechanisms other than the renin-angiotensin system may be more important in the overall control of aldosterone in these two species than in man and dog.

One of the first observations to show that the kidney plays an important role in the regulation of aldosterone production during sodium depletion was made in dogs (73). A marked fall in both aldosterone and corticosterone secretion occurred after sodium-depleted, hypophysectomized dogs were nephrectomized (Fig. 16). In a more recent study (76) conscious, sodium-depleted, hypophysectomized dogs were observed; again a striking drop in aldosterone secretion occurred after nephrectomy. In the early studies in sheep (36), nephrectomy of anesthetized, sodium-depleted, hypophysectomized animals failed to demonstrate a fall in aldosterone secretion, but recently (35) nephrectomy was found to reduce aldosterone production in conscious, hypophysectomized,

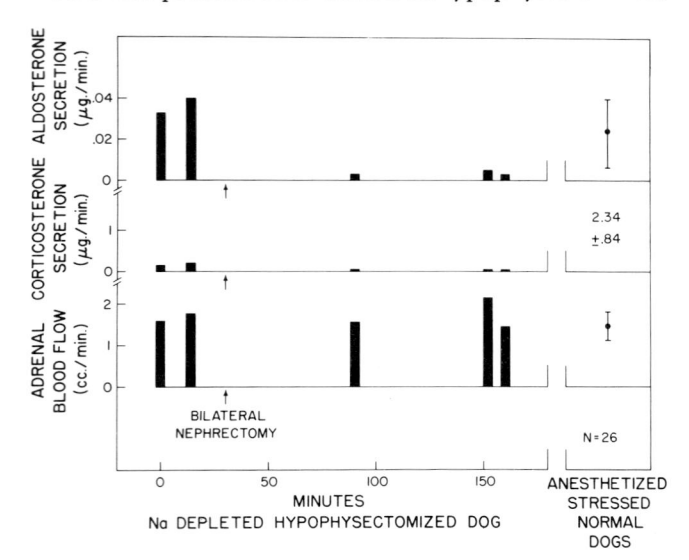

FIG. 16. Effects of bilateral nephrectomy on steroid secretion and adrenal blood flow in a sodium-depleted, hypophysectomized dog. For comparison, data on steroid secretion and adrenal blood flow for anesthetized, stressed, normal dogs are presented at *right*. [From Davis et al. (73).]

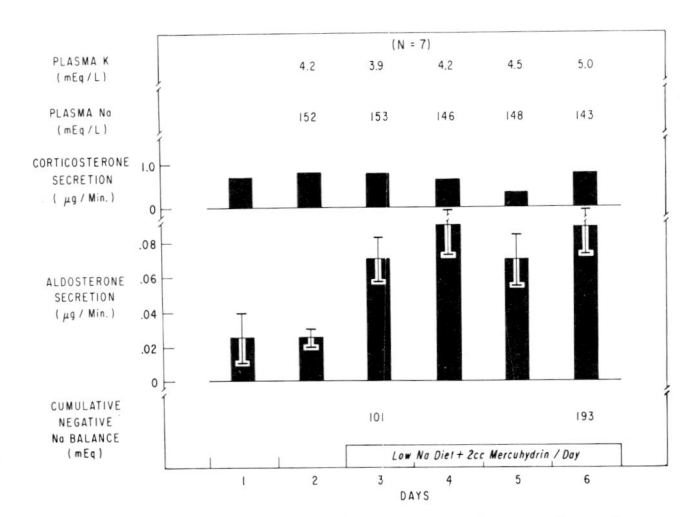

FIG. 17. Effects of sodium depletion on steroid secretion, plasma electrolytes, and cumulative sodium balance. [From Binnion et al. (23).]

sodium-depleted sheep; aldosterone secretion fell to the level observed in sodium-repleted animals, but the change did not occur until 10–12 hr after nephrectomy. In the rat (103) no difference was found in the rate of aldosterone secretion in seven sodium-depleted, hypophysectomized rats and in four sodium-depleted, hypophysectomized, nephrectomized animals. A more definitive study of the rat is needed in which the response to nephrectomy in the same animals is evaluated.

More direct evidence on the relation of the kidney and, specifically, of the renin-angiotensin system to aldosterone secretion during sodium depletion has been obtained from measurements of plasma renin activity and plasma angiotensin II levels. In the dog, plasma renin activity was measured during sodium depletion by three different procedures in conscious animals (23) and found to be markedly elevated. A fourfold increase in plasma renin activity was observed after only 1 day of sodium depletion, whereas after 4 days an eightfold increase occurred; plasma renin substrate levels were unaltered. Concurrent measurements of aldosterone secretion showed a striking elevation [Fig. 17; (23)] in association with increased plasma renin activity. No data are available on the plasma level of angiotensin II as measured by radioimmunoassay during sodium depletion in the dog. In man, Brown et al. (42) found a highly significant increase in plasma renin concentration in six medical students during salt deprivation. Also five normal subjects given a high-sodium diet showed a fall in the plasma renin level in all cases and a rise in plasma renin concentration upon resumption of a normal diet (42). Similar results were obtained in normal human beings by Winer (275), Aida et al. (2), and Fasciolo et al. (111). Veyrat et al. (271) observed an excellent inverse correlation between the level of plasma renin activity and the state of sodium balance in man. Plasma angiotensin II, as measured by radioimmunoassay (132, 265), is elevated during a low-sodium intake in man. In sheep the Australian group (37) observed increases in both plasma renin activity and plasma angiotensin II with the development of sodium depletion secondary to loss of saliva from a parotid fistula. In the rat there has been considerable indirect evidence (138) and, more recently, direct evidence (76, 135) for increased activity of the renin-angiotensin system in the sodium-depleted animal. By use of a cross-circulation assay, Gross et al. (138) obtained evidence for a high plasma renin concentration in the sodium-depleted rat. The observation [see (71)] of a decreased pressor response to the intravenous injection of synthetic angiotensin II in sodium-depleted rats is also indirect evidence of a high plasma level of angiotensin II. Finally actual measurements of plasma renin activity during sodium depletion in the rat show an increase (71, 135); the concentration of renin substrate in plasma was unchanged.

In sheep, Denton and co-workers (30, 32, 33, 92) have performed an extensive series of experiments in search of factors other than the renin-angiotensin system, ACTH, and altered plasma sodium and potassium concentrations that influence aldosterone biosynthesis during sodium depletion. As pointed out earlier in this review, the effects of nephrectomy on aldosterone secretion in sheep are delayed and less pronounced than in man and dog. Also several other observations have led these investigators to postulate the existence of "an unidentified factor in the control of aldosterone secretion" (30, 92). Among these observations, they reported the failure of clear-cut concurrent directional changes in either plasma renin activity or angiotensin II to occur consistently with altered aldosterone secretion during correction of sodium deficiency. Also the finding that an infusion of synthetic angiotensin II did not mimic completely the biosynthetic events in sodium deficiency was offered as evidence for the involvement of other factors. This is understandable, however, since chronic sodium depletion increases the cell mass of the zona glomerulosa, so that on this basis alone a greater aldosterone response would be expected with sodium depletion than with acute angiotensin II infusion.

Recently, during studies of sodium depletion, emphasis has been placed by the Australians (37, 92) on the possible involvement of some "unidentified factor" in the late stage of biosynthesis that involves conversion of corticosterone to aldosterone. They studied the in vivo production of aldosterone during adrenal arterial infusion of ^{3}H-corticosterone in sheep. With sodium deficiency up to the middle range of the aldosterone response, the percentage conversion of ^{3}H-corticosterone to aldosterone increased, and this was independent of an increase in plasma potassium concentration. When aldosterone secretion was stimulated by adrenal arterial infusion of angiotensin II, the increase in aldosterone secretion to the levels observed with sodium depletion was not associated with the increased percentage conversion of ^{3}H-corticosterone to aldosterone. This finding led these researchers to postulate that some unidentified factor is involved in this late step of the biosynthetic process during sodium depletion.

It should be pointed out that changes in plasma sodium and potassium are important in severe sodium depletion, and an increase in adrenocortical potassium might be the additional unidentified factor operative in this conversion of corticosterone to aldosterone. Binnion, Davis, and associates (23) found that severe sodium deficiency was accompanied by hyponatremia and hyperkalemia, both of which increase aldosterone secretion by a direct action on the adrenal cortex. The importance of adrenocortical potassium in aldosterone biosynthesis has been recently emphasized (17, 40), and this factor might be operative and explain these unusual findings of Blair-West and associates (30, 32, 33) and Denton (92). Indeed, it is crucial to exclude changes in potassium before postulating an "unidentified factor."

In a recent preliminary report, McCaa et al. (192) were unable to explain changes in plasma aldosterone in anephric patients after dialysis, on the basis of altered plasma sodium or potassium and ACTH; they suggested that the response was secondary to sodium depletion. In this event sodium depletion might have decreased the metabolic clearance rate of aldosterone since sodium depletion is known to decrease hepatic blood flow and aldosterone metabolism in the dog (84, 158).

Also, in the rat, several findings have been interpreted to suggest that the renin-angiotensin system is not of primary importance in the control of aldosterone secretion. This is somewhat surprising since our first evidence for the close functional relation between the kidney and the adrenal cortex was provided by studies in the rat. Deane & Masson (90) found that injection of partially purified solutions of renin produced enlargement of the zona glomerulosa in rats. Hartroft & Hartroft (143) demonstrated increased granulation of the renal JG cells in rats on a low-sodium diet. More recently, Hartroft and collaborators (145) and others (189, 190) have provided strong evidence in the rat that renin is secreted by the JG cells and that renin has a trophic action on the zona glomerulosa. In a review, Tobian (256) called attention to the vast evidence, much of which was obtained in the rat, for the close functional interrelationships of the renal JG cells, renin, and the zona glomerulosa.

Since plasma renin activity is increased in sodium-depleted rats the problem becomes one of assessing the influence of increased plasma renin activity or angiotensin II on the biosynthesis of aldosterone. This problem has been studied extensively both in vitro and in vivo. Glaz & Sugar (131) reported that the adrenals of rats injected with angiotensin II showed increased synthesis of aldosterone in vitro. Müller in 1965 (201) and again in 1971 (204) used large doses of angiotensin II in in vitro studies and found an increase in aldosterone synthesis. It should be pointed out that the concentration of angiotensin II was not measured in any of the in vitro studies. Consequently the actual concentration of angiotensin II associated with aldosterone biosynthesis is unknown; since adrenal tissue peptidases could have destroyed some of the angiotensin II the actual effective concentration might not have been high.

The early studies on the response to injection of angiotensin II on aldosterone secretion in the rat yielded conflicting results; Marx and co-workers (189, 190), Marieb & Mulrow (188), and Singer et al. (243) reported an increase in aldosterone secretion, whereas Eilers & Peterson (103) and Cade & Perenich (50) failed to observe such a change. It is now clear from more recent work that intravenous infusion of angiotensin II increases aldosterone secretion in the rat. Dufau & Kliman (98) reported that large doses of angiotensin II increased aldosterone secretion selectively without a change in corticosterone production in the rat. During sodium deficiency in rats, Kinson & Singer (168) found that intravenous infusion of angiotensin II increased aldosterone production selectively; the increase in aldosterone secretion occurred with only a slight increase in arterial pressure. However, when they (168) studied sodium-repleted rats similarly infused with angiotensin II, aldosterone secretion failed to increase, and the explanation for this lack of response is not clear. These results of Kinson and Singer support the view that angiotensin II is involved in the adrenal response to sodium depletion in the rat since an aldosterone-stimulating action of angiotensin II occurred with only slightly pressor doses and was unique to the sodium-deficient animals.

Studies on the effects of renin on aldosterone secretion have also been made in the rat. These observations are important since it is possible that the endogenous peptide differs structurally from synthetic angiotensin II. Again conflicting results have been reported. Both Eilers & Peterson (103) and Marieb & Mulrow (188) found that intravenous infusion of rat renin was ineffective in increasing aldosterone production. In contrast, Singer et al. (242) found increased concentration of kidney renin and elevated aldosterone secretion in experimental renal hypertension in the rat. Also, as noted earlier in this review, injection of renin preparations produced hypertrophy of the zona glomerulosa in rats (90). It should be pointed out that an increase in zona glomerulosa cells would increase aldosterone secretion. Finally, Masson & Travis (191) gave single doses of renin (40 units) subcutaneously to uninephrectomized rats and aldosterone secretion tripled. Although this subcutaneous dose of renin was large, the pressor effect was only moderate; perhaps only small amounts of renin were absorbed from the injection site. Masson and Travis pointed out that intravenous infusion of crude renin often produces only a transient increase in pressure, which is followed by circulatory collapse; in this event, decreased adrenal blood flow might prevent an adrenal response in aldosterone from occurring.

The question of the mechanisms involved in hypersecretion of aldosterone in the sodium-deficient rat has not been resolved to the satisfaction of all investigators, but it is clear *a*) that plasma renin activity is high in sodium-depleted rats (76, 135), and *b*) that both endogenously formed angiotensin (191, 242) and the synthetic angiotensin II amide will increase aldosterone production in the rat.

The two other well-known modes of control of aldosterone secretion, namely, the concentrations of plasma sodium and potassium and the plasma level of ACTH, are involved in the increased aldosterone secretion characteristic of sodium depletion. During sodium depletion in dogs, Binnion, Davis, and co-workers (23) found that plasma sodium and potassium were not significantly altered until the fourth day of sodium deficiency. At this time, plasma sodium decreased and potassium increased (see Fig. 17) so that both factors could have contributed to the observed increase in aldosterone secretion. Similarly in sheep, plasma electrolytes do not change until moderately severe sodium deficiency occurs (34) and then these factors influence steroidogenesis.

The importance of the adenohypophysis in the hyperaldosteronism of sodium depletion is evident from the comparative data of Binnion, Davis, and associates (23) on the responses to sodium depletion in normal and in hypophysectomized dogs (Fig. 18). They (23) found that the rate of aldosterone secretion during both the control period and during sodium depletion was three times higher in the presence than in the absence of the anterior pituitary. Net sodium loss and plasma electrolyte changes were essentially the same in the two groups of dogs.

Another piece of evidence on the role of the anterior pituitary during sodium depletion is provided by observations on simultaneous aldosterone and corticosterone secretion rates (45). Within 2 hr after the injection of Mercuhydrin, both aldosterone and corticosterone secretion increased; during the next 2 hr aldosterone secretion continued to increase, whereas corticosterone output returned to the normal control level; this situation persisted for the next 4 days of sodium depletion (45). In contrast, in hypophysectomized dogs the rates of aldosterone and corticosterone secretion increased but the levels of both hormones remained elevated throughout the 4-day period of sodium depletion (23). Binnion,

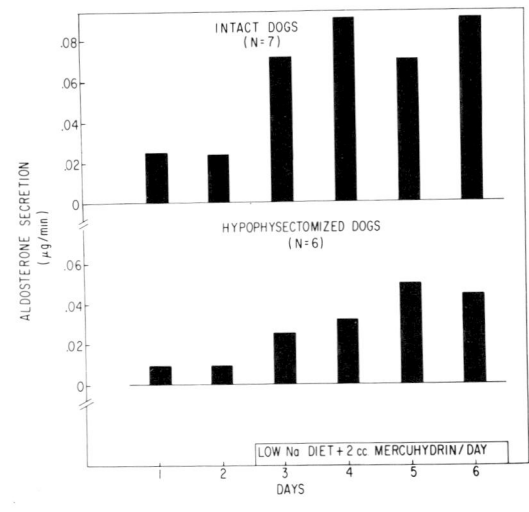

FIG. 18. Comparative data on response in aldosterone secretion to standard sodium depletion procedure in normal, conscious dogs and in conscious, hypophysectomized animals. [From Binnion et al. (23).]

Davis, and co-workers (23) suggested that the normal rate of glucocorticoid output during sodium depletion is maintained by a negative corticosteroid feedback mechanism since corticosterone output was consistently increased in sodium-depleted, hypophysectomized dogs.

As mentioned earlier, one additional mechanism may be operative in the increased aldosterone production of sodium depletion. Studies in both dogs (23) and sheep (34) have suggested that adrenocortical, intracellular sodium is changed during sodium depletion. Actual data on intracellular electrolytes of the adrenal cortex are not available, but tissue electrolyte changes have been measured and expressed in terms of fat-free tissue solids (FFTS). Studies in dogs (23) and sheep (34) have also provided evidence during sodium depletion for a decrease in adrenocortical sodium in terms of FFTS.

The most extensive observations, however, on adrenocortical electrolytes were made by Baumber, Davis, and associates (17). They found that the adrenocortical potassium, expressed as FFTS, increased under all conditions studied in dogs, including a) a pressor infusion of angiotensin II, b) a nonpressor infusion of angiotensin II, c) sodium depletion, d) injection of ACTH, and e) infusion of potassium chloride and hyperkalemia. Since all these situations are known to increase aldosterone biosynthesis, Baumber, Davis, and associates (17) suggested that increased adrenocortical potassium promotes an increase in aldosterone secretion. Also they (17) confirmed the finding of Binnion that adrenocortical sodium was decreased during sodium depletion in the dog. These observations are consistent with the recent report by Boyd et al. (40) that potassium plays a key role in the mediation of the response of the zona glomerulosa to sodium depletion in the rat. Indeed, it appears that the increase in adrenocortical potassium may be a final common pathway for mediation of increased aldosterone synthesis.

Finally, as Ganong and associates (121) have pointed out, the interaction of the various factors involved in the steroidogenesis of sodium depletion is to be considered. Sodium-depleted dogs have been reported to show increased sensitivity to angiotensin II and ACTH (121), and this unusual response has been attributed, at least in part, to the larger cell mass in the hypertrophied zona glomerulosa.

Thus the regulation of aldosterone secretion during altered sodium intake or sodium depletion appears to be complex and to involve many factors. Increased activity of the renin-angiotensin system seems to be the most important mechanism in man and dog; the extent of its involvement in sheep and rats is less well defined. A very important homeostatic control mechanism for aldosterone secretion appears to be mediated by alterations in sodium intake, which manifest themselves by way of the renin-angiotensin system.

Altered Plasma Sodium Concentration

In their early studies in sheep, Denton and associates (93, 94) observed that a combined decrease in plasma

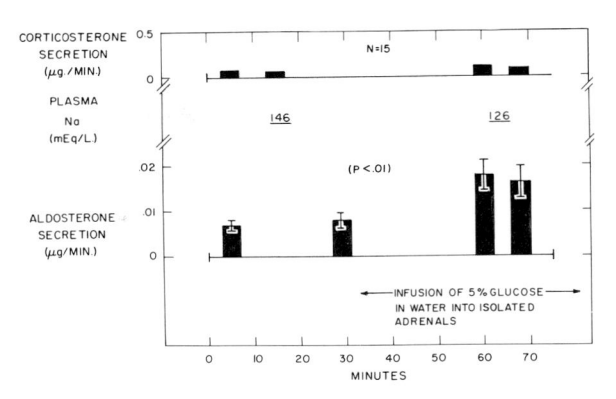

FIG. 19. Effects of hyponatremia produced by infusion of 5% glucose into arterial supply of isolated adrenals on steroid secretion. [From Davis et al. (85).]

sodium and increase in plasma potassium concentration augmented aldosterone output. Subsequently the Australian workers (28) found that a low plasma sodium level alone increased aldosterone production. These observations were confirmed in dogs (85) when aldosterone secretion was found to increase in an isolated adrenal preparation in hypophysectomized, nephrectomized dogs during perfusion with 5% glucose and a drop in plasma sodium concentration (Fig. 19). The results raise the question about the well-known observation that chronic pitressin administration during water loading leads to hyponatremia and decreased aldosterone output; this response probably reflects the overriding influence of a decrease in plasma renin activity. Other forms of overhydration in man (211) decrease plasma sodium concentration but concurrently decrease aldosterone secretion. Hyponatremia is clearly not a primary mechanism leading to hyperaldosteronism in edematous states since the plasma sodium level is usually normal in patients with uncomplicated heart failure or decompensated hepatic cirrhosis [see (85)].

Effects of Potassium Intake and Altered Plasma Potassium Concentration

The first observations on the effects of potassium loading on aldosterone production were made in 1957 by Laragh & Stoerk (178). They found that urinary aldosterone excretion increased during potassium loading in man while consuming a low-sodium diet, and they suggested that the response was mediated by an elevation in plasma potassium concentration. Other workers (14, 119) confirmed the finding of hyperaldosteronuria during potassium loading even during a normal sodium intake in human beings. Conversely a reduction in urinary aldosterone output occurred with potassium restriction (157).

In acute experiments in dogs, Moran et al. (199) obtained evidence suggesting that intravenous infusion of potassium chloride increased aldosterone secretion. The secretory response in aldosterone was blunted because the experiments were done in laparotomized dogs with a high plasma level of ACTH secondary to the surgical stress resulting from adrenal vein cannulation, and a consequent high initial rate of aldosterone secretion was present. In similar studies, Gann et al. (118) failed to detect an increase in aldosterone output with plasma potassium levels as high as 10 mEq/liter. When observations were made in hypophysectomized dogs (85), intravenous infusion of potassium chloride increased aldosterone secretion consistently with increments in plasma potassium as low as 1.3 mEq/liter. This response in hypophysectomized dogs (Fig. 20) was present after removal of the kidneys (85), which suggested a direct action of a high plasma potassium on the adrenal cortex. Local perfusion of isolated adrenals in hypophysectomized, nephrectomized dogs with either potassium chloride or potassium sulfate increased aldosterone output [(85); Fig. 21]; this result demonstrated a direct action of the potassium ion on the adrenal cortex. In studies in conscious sheep, Blair-West et al. (28) also found that an increase in the plasma potassium level without an alteration in plasma sodium concentration increased aldosterone secretion. More recently, the Australians (117) have reported that very small increases (0.5 mEq/liter) of plasma potassium concentration increase aldosterone production in sheep. Finally, in vitro studies of beef adrenal slices [see (203)] and rat adrenal tissue [see (203)] have also demonstrated that the potassium ion increases aldosterone biosynthesis.

The mechanisms by which a high potassium intake or potassium loading increase aldosterone production include *a*) the direct action of the potassium ion on the adrenal cortex, and *b*) sodium loss secondary to potassium loading with resultant activation of the renin-angiotensin system. As pointed out earlier in this review, hyperkalemia increases adrenocortical potassium, and since this change is a feature common to many factors that increase aldosterone biosynthesis it is possible that the direct action of the potassium ion is mediated through

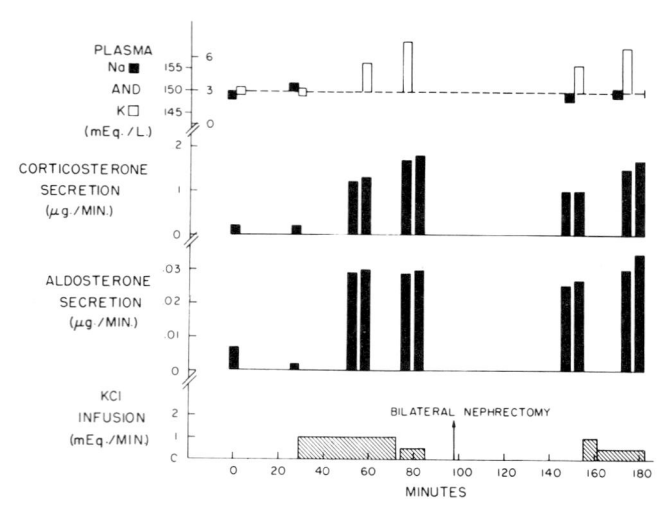

FIG. 20. Effects of hyperkalemia on steroid secretion in a hypophysectomized dog; in latter part of the experiment, response to hyperkalemia was evaluated after bilateral nephrectomy. [From Davis et al. (85).]

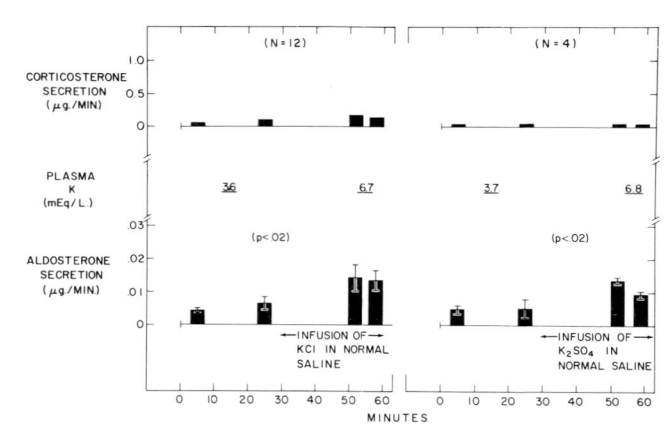

FIG. 21. Effects of infusion of potassium chloride and potassium sulfate into the arterial supply of isolated adrenals on steroid secretion and plasma potassium concentration. [From Davis et al. (85).]

an increase in intracellular potassium in the adrenal cortex. Hyperkalemia also decreases plasma renin activity (1, 47, 271), but the acute response to intravenous infusion of potassium is dominated apparently by a direct action of the potassium ion on the adrenal cortex since even small increases in plasma potassium concentration augment aldosterone output. Under chronic conditions the response of potassium loading on aldosterone secretion reflects the resultant effects of potassium *a*) to decrease plasma renin activity by a direct renal action, and *b*) to increase plasma renin activity secondary to renal sodium loss and volume depletion. In the dog, sodium excretion does not increase in response to potassium loading (85) as it does in man so the dominant mechanism in the dog appears to be secondary to hyperkalemia with an action to increase adrenocortical potassium.

The results from studies with potassium indicate that alterations in intake play a role in the physiological regulation of aldosterone secretion. It seems plausible that ingestion of foods rich in potassium, such as meat, and the subsequent transient rise in plasma potassium concentration constitute a physiological mechanism for control of aldosterone biosynthesis. Possibly an intricate feedback mechanism exists since increased circulating aldosterone promotes renal and fecal potassium loss and helps to return the plasma potassium concentration to the normal level.

The role of hyperkalemia in the aldosteronism associated with clinical and experimental states with edema must be considered. After acute constriction of the thoracic inferior vena cava (68, 70), marked increments in aldosterone secretion occurred before the plasma potassium level increased or in the absence of hyperkalemia. Also, in dogs with hyperaldosteronism secondary to chronic thoracic caval constriction or chronic experimental heart failure, the concentration of plasma potassium was frequently normal. Similarly, in patients with congestive heart failure or with cirrhosis of the liver and ascites, the concentration of plasma potassium was usually normal [see (85)]. These findings exclude a primary role of hyperkalemia in the pathogenesis of secondary aldosteronism.

In summarizing this section, it should be pointed out that an increasing amount of evidence has accumulated on the importance of the potassium ion in the control of aldosterone secretion. The potassium ion exerts a direct action on the adrenal cortex, possibly by increasing the intracellular concentration of potassium in the zona glomerulosa. In man, potassium loading results in renal loss of sodium, which stimulates the renin-angiotensin system, but this effect is partly counterbalanced by a direct influence of hyperkalemia to decrease renin secretion.

Effects of Magnesium Deficiency

Magnesium-deficient rats secreted excessive amounts of aldosterone, but corticosterone output was unaltered (130). In these animals the plasma magnesium concentration was decreased and urinary sodium excretion was low, whereas urinary potassium output was increased.

In contrast, Cope (61) failed to detect an alteration in aldosterone secretion in two patients with "almost pure magnesium deficiency," and a slight increment in aldosterone production occurred after replenishment of magnesium stores. In this study, analysis of biopsy material demonstrated that an intracellular magnesium deficiency existed; neither sodium nor potassium metabolism was detectably altered.

ANTERIOR PITUITARY GLAND AND
ALDOSTERONE SECRETION

Effects of Hypophysectomy

It has been known for many years that the adenohypophysis exerts a trophic influence on the adrenal cortex. It seemed likely therefore that anterior pituitary hormones and, specifically, ACTH might have an important role in the regulation of aldosterone secretion. Accordingly the effects of hypophysectomy on the rate of aldosterone production have been studied extensively by several investigators. Singer & Stack-Dunne (244) observed the rat, and Rauschkolb et al. (228) were first to study the dog. Both groups of workers observed a decrease in aldosterone secretion after hypophysectomy; an 83% fall in aldosterone output occurred in the rat, but the decrease in the dog was considerably less. That loss of anterior pituitary function decreases aldosterone secretion was confirmed by others (36, 75, 122, 234), and subsequent observers found an 80–90% fall in aldosterone secretion after acute hypophysectomy in the dog. Blair-West and associates (36) demonstrated a fall in aldosterone output after hypophysectomy in sheep, and Ross et al. (234) found that urinary aldosterone excretion was significantly below normal in patients with long-standing hypopituitarism. In hypophysectomized human subjects a low rate of urinary aldosterone excretion has been observed (97, 169), and measurements of the average daily rate of aldosterone production by the isotope dilution technique have revealed a reduced rate of secretion of aldosterone by hypophysectomized human beings. Finally, even in an amphibian such as the American bullfrog, hypophysectomy decreased aldosterone secretion (162).

Some confusion on the effects of hypophysectomy on aldosterone secretion exists in the early literature because of the experimental conditions under which the studies were conducted. Some workers failed to recognize that laparotomy increases ACTH output and that the acute effects of hypophysectomy in stressed animals were exaggerated. Also, in some of the early studies (228) large amounts of blood were needed for analysis of aldosterone so that the effects of hemorrhage, which stimulates renin release and aldosterone production, were superimposed upon the stimulus of laparotomy. Furthermore, since hemorrhage augments aldosterone output via the renin-angiotensin system (54, 205) the fall in aldosterone output in response to hypophysectomy was blunted (228). In one report (247) it is clear from the simultaneous measurements of the secretion rates of cortisol along with aldosterone that hypophysectomy was incomplete, which is another factor that contributed to the difficulties encountered in evaluation of anterior pituitary function. Slater et al. (247) concluded that hypophysectomy failed to decrease aldosterone secretion in sodium-depleted dogs, but the simultaneous secretion rates of cortisol of 70, 74, and 233 mg/min revealed that hypophysectomy was incomplete. These considerations account, at least in part, for the erroneous statement in the early literature that aldosterone production is independent of anterior pituitary function.

The importance of the anterior pituitary in various types of chronic experimental secondary aldosteronism is evident from observations of aldosterone secretion in hypophysectomized dogs during the responses to various stimuli. In trained, conscious dogs with aldosteronism secondary to thoracic caval constriction (77), aldosterone secretion was measured by means of a chronic indwelling adrenal venous catheter; after acute hypophysectomy an 80–90% fall in aldosterone secretion occurred (Fig. 22). Also, as pointed out earlier, the response in aldosterone secretion to a standard sodium depletion regimen was threefold greater in intact dogs when compared to hypophysectomized dogs [see Fig. 18; (23)].

Role of ACTH

The striking effect of hypophysectomy on aldosterone secretion raises the question of the specific adenohypophysial hormones involved. Many workers (14, 88, 110, 183, 205) have demonstrated an acute response in aldosterone secretion to different corticotropin preparations. The relative effects of different doses of ACTH on aldosterone and 17-hydroxycorticoid output were studied by Mulrow & Ganong [(205); see Fig. 8]. The response in aldosterone biosynthesis to ACTH is striking in every

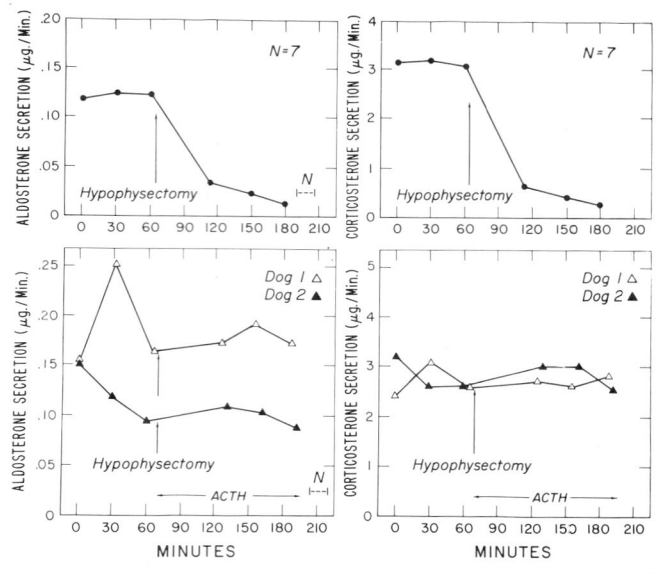

FIG. 22. Effects of hypophysectomy alone and hypophysectomy with simultaneous infusion of ACTH on steroid secretion in dogs with hyperaldosteronism secondary to thoracic caval constriction. [From Davis et al. (88).]

mammalian species studied, with the exception of the rat; in this mammal, ACTH does promote steroidogenesis, but the reported increase in aldosterone production was less than in other species. Porcine ACTH has been found to increase aldosterone secretion in the American opossum (160), one of the most primitive mammals, and in the American bullfrog (162).

The response in aldosterone production to ACTH can be modified experimentally by pretreatment with renin or by alterations in sodium or potassium balance. A low-sodium diet or sodium depletion augmented the response to ACTH (183) probably by production of hypertrophy of the zona glomerulosa. Injection of renin into dogs also produced an increase in sensitivity to ACTH (121). A similar phenomenon has been noted from studies of adrenals in rats receiving a sodium-deficient diet [see (203)]. On the other hand, a potassium-deficient diet reportedly blocked the response of rat adrenals to ACTH during in vitro studies. In this connection, the recent work of Baumber et al. (17) on the importance of adrenocortical potassium has an important bearing; as mentioned earlier, increased adrenocortical potassium may constitute a final common pathway for mediation of aldosterone biosynthesis.

In contrast to the acute response in aldosterone secretion to ACTH, the response to the chronic daily administration of ACTH is self-limited (212, 213, 260a). After 2-4 days of ACTH injection and an initial increase in aldosterone production, aldosterone secretion returned to normal or below; furthermore, after cessation of ACTH injection, aldosterone secretion became subnormal. Apparently this limited response in aldosterone secretion was partly the result of sodium retention (213, 260a). The decrease in aldosterone secretion during prolonged ACTH administration occurred on a low-sodium intake and consequently without expansion of the extracellular fluid volume (213, 260a). Also, Newton & Laragh (213) observed this response to ACTH in patients with primary aldosteronism and low plasma renin activity and suggested that reduced levels of aldosterone during ACTH treatment resulted from intraadrenal inhibition of its production.

Another approach used to evaluate the role of ACTH in the production of aldosterone was to give a glucocorticoid hormone to depress ACTH release. In dogs with thoracic caval constriction and aldosteronism (88), daily injection of cortisone produced a striking reduction in both aldosterone and corticosterone secretion. Also the ACTH content of the adenohypophysis was markedly decreased during treatment of dogs with cortisone or cortisol (109). It seems likely therefore that the observed drop in steroid production that occurred during glucocorticoid administration was secondary to decreased ACTH secretion.

In some conditions a high level of ACTH in plasma seems to initiate and maintain a high rate of aldosterone secretion, whereas in other situations the role of ACTH appears to be only supportive. After laparotomy (75, 88, 154) and after acute blood loss (54, 154, 205) the striking elevation in the rates of secretion of cortisol and corticosterone, as well as of aldosterone, suggests the presence of a high concentration of ACTH in plasma and an initiative role for the hormone. Also in both situations the pattern of steroid response is very similar to the increments in aldosterone, corticosterone, and cortisol secretion that occur after ACTH administration. Holzbauer (154) has investigated the part played by ACTH in the increased aldosterone secretion resulting from surgical stress. Her findings clearly indicate that a high level of circulating ACTH is responsible for the high rate of aldosterone secretion in acutely laparotomized dogs. After acute blood loss, renin, as well as ACTH, is released (96) so that increased amounts of angiotensin II also augment aldosterone secretion. Nevertheless the greater response to acute hemorrhage in the intact animal than in the hypophysectomized dog (78, 205) makes it clear that ACTH contributes substantially to the increased steroid production after acute blood loss.

Another situation in which ACTH plays an initiative role in aldosterone production is during acute carotid arterial constriction (20, 69, 87). During this maneuver an elevation in cortisol and corticosterone secretion was a frequent finding, and the occasional increase in aldosterone production appeared to result from increased plasma concentration of ACTH. In these experiments (20, 69, 87), nothing suggested that carotid constriction increased aldosterone output by activation of a central nervous mechanism other than ACTH, as Gann & Travis (120) have proposed. It seems likely that their finding (120) of an increased rate of aldosterone secretion in the absence of a change in cortisol after 30 min of carotid constriction was apparent rather than real; the change was significant only at the 5% level, and both the

10- and 60-min values for aldosterone secretion were unchanged. In experiments (20, 87) in which an increase in aldosterone output was associated with an elevation in cortisol and corticosterone secretion, the increase in aldosterone production was clearly evident after 60 min of carotid constriction.

In man, Rayyis & Horton (229) have suggested a link between the renin-angiotensin system and ACTH. They found that infusion of angiotensin II in pressor doses increased plasma concentration of ACTH, but nonpressor infusions of angiotensin II were without effect. Although their evidence failed to indicate that physiological levels of angiotensin II influenced plasma cortisol concentration, they pointed out that ACTH plays an important supportive role in the biosynthesis of aldosterone. Thus these experiments of Rayyis & Horton (229) in man support the earlier evidence (88) from studies of experimental aldosteronism for a supportive role of ACTH. In dogs with caval constriction and hyperaldosteronism (88), an 80–90% fall in aldosterone secretion occurred after hypophysectomy, and the response was blocked when ACTH was given intravenously during the post-hypophysectomy period (Fig. 22). This experiment demonstrates that ACTH has an important role in the maintenance of a high rate of aldosterone production. On the other hand, studies in conscious dogs with caval constriction and hyperaldosteronism (88) showed that only a low basal level of ACTH in plasma was necessary for maximal or near-maximal aldosterone production. When ACTH plays a supportive role in biosynthesis of aldosterone, as in secondary aldosteronism, another mechanism must be primarily responsible for hypersecretion of aldosterone. This mechanism is the increased activity of the renin-angiotensin system.

Possible Role of Adenohypophysial Hormones Other than ACTH

There are reports (179, 219, 221) that the anterior pituitary gland is essential for the aldosterone response to sodium depletion in the rat. The in vivo observations (221) suggested that the factor is not ACTH, growth hormone, or thyrotrophin. In in vitro studies of adrenocortical tissue from hypophysectomized, sodium-depleted rats it appeared that growth hormone repaired the deficit (179, 219). These experiments are difficult to interpret. To exclude ACTH as the factor it is necessary to give rat ACTH since the ACTH molecule might differ among species. Further there is little information on the optimal dose of ACTH. In man the response to exogenous ACTH, as pointed out earlier in this review, is not understood; the initial response is an increase in aldosterone secretion, but after several days of ACTH injection, aldosterone output returns to the normal control level, and discontinuation of ACTH is followed by depression of aldosterone below the normal control level (260a). Consequently failure to achieve a steroid response during administration of exogenous commercial ACTH does not exclude an endogenous role for the hormone.

Another interesting but indirect approach to this problem was the response to ACTH and angiotensin II in hypophysectomized dogs in comparison with dogs given large doses of a glucocorticoid (125). In chronic hypophysectomized dogs, neither ACTH nor angiotensin II had a marked stimulatory action on aldosterone secretion, whereas in steroid-treated dogs the increases in aldosterone secretion with both ACTH and angiotensin II were similar to those of untreated control dogs. Ganong and associates (125) suggested that deficiency of some pituitary factor other than ACTH might be responsible for the decreased response in the hypophysectomized animals. Another interpretation of these data is that the mass and functional state of zona glomerulosa cells were reduced more by hypophysectomy than by glucocorticoid administration; in this event the difference could be quantitative rather than qualitative.

More direct negative evidence for the role of pituitary factors other than ACTH has been obtained from studies of the response to infusion of other pituitary hormones. Both synthetic melanocyte-stimulating hormone (α-MSH) (88) and highly purified β-MSH (28, 88) failed to change the rates of secretion of aldosterone and corticosterone. Evidence (185) from in vitro studies suggested that hypothalamic extracts and growth hormone augmented aldosterone production. However, observations with growth hormone in vivo (21, 112) failed to suggest any direct influence of this hormone on steroidogenesis. Apparently growth hormone is involved in the maintenance of the architecture of the adrenal cortex and thus only in this indirect manner influences steroidogenesis (W. F. Ganong, unpublished data).

OTHER POSSIBLE MODES OF CONTROL OF ALDOSTERONE SECRETION

Effects of Estrogens, Progesterone, Oral Contraceptives, and Erythropoietin

In 1962 Llaurado and associates (184) reported that an estradiol derivative increased the fecal excretion of aldosterone in rats; it is noteworthy that rats excrete corticosteroids predominantly in feces rather than in urine. At about the same time, Singer et al. (241) observed that progesterone increased aldosterone secretion in both intact and hypophysectomized rats.

During a course of estrogen therapy to patients, Laidlaw et al. (171) found that plasma 17-hydroxycorticoids increased to levels found during pregnancy but that urinary aldosterone excretion was unchanged. In contrast, aldosterone secretion increased during progesterone administration; this was accompanied by an initial natriuresis, which contributed to the onset of hyperaldosteronism. However, a prompt reversal of the progesterone-induced natriuresis occurred within a few days and sodium retention ensued, but the increased rate of aldosterone secretion continued. It appears therefore that some mechanism other than loss of sodium is responsible for the steroidogenic action of progesterone.

More recently, Katz & Kappas (167) observed that both estriol and estradiol increased aldosterone secretion in normal, nonpregnant women. At about the same time, Crane and co-workers (62) found that oral contraceptives increase plasma renin activity. Laragh and associates (177) did a thorough study on the effects of birth control pills and found increased plasma renin substrate, plasma renin activity, and aldosterone secretion. These observations have been confirmed by several groups (214, 236, 273). The changes in renin and aldosterone were occasionally associated with the development or enhancement of hypertension. One of the most impressive and consistent abnormalities in these women receiving oral contraceptives was the striking increase in plasma renin substrate. The response in plasma renin substrate to the synthetic estrogen, diethylstilbestrol, was reported in 1952 by Helmer & Griffith (149). Newton et al. (214), in serum with increased renin substrate, found marked enhancement of the rate of angiotensin II formation upon addition of renin to serum. Despite the increased renin substrate in the plasma of these patients receiving estrogens, persistent increases in plasma renin activity were observed in only about half of the patients. To explain these findings, Newton et al. (214) suggested that the true plasma renin concentration was reduced as a result of a negative feedback mechanism.

Erythropoietin has been reported to be secreted by the JG cells (230), but the locus of secretion for the intrarenal hormone is uncertain (134). An attempt (206) to demonstrate aldosterone-stimulating activity with erythropoietin yielded negative results.

Possible Hepatic Hormone

It has been known for many years that the liver plays an important pathogenic role in fluid retention. Dogs with constriction of the inferior vena cava above the liver develop chronic hyperaldosteronism with sodium retention and ascites, whereas a constricting ligature below the liver fails to produce this syndrome. In 1965 Orloff et al. (217) suggested that increased intrahepatic venous pressure leads to release of a hepatic humoral agent that stimulates the kidney to secrete an aldosterone-stimulating agent, possibly renin. Evidence for this hypothesis was obtained from complicated cross-circulation experiments. Because of the importance of such a possible mechanism, the hypothesis was reexamined by Howards, Davis, and co-workers (155) in similar cross-circulation studies. The results of Howards and associates were readily explicable on the basis of an increase in plasma ACTH as the aldosterone-stimulating agent rather than some unknown humoral agent.

Possible Neural Regulatory Mechanisms

For more than two decades there have been reports that the central nervous system may be involved in the control of renal sodium excretion. The first observations in 1950 (224) and 1952 (274) were on patients with disease of the central nervous system and with the so-called cerebral salt-wasting syndrome. The first three cases (224) had diffuse involvement of the central nervous system. In this connection it should be pointed out that no specific lesion of the central nervous system is known to cause persistent loss of sodium in man. In several experimental studies [see (75)] on animals with brain lesions, alterations in sodium excretion were observed, but in none of the reports was there evidence to implicate a mechanism other than altered renal hemodynamic function or the stress secondary to surgical trauma. Nevertheless interest developed in the possibility that aldosterone secretion might be controlled, at least in part, by a specific center in the brain, and a number of workers have made brain lesions in search of such a center.

The possibility of the existence of a regulatory center in the diencephalon for the control of aldosterone secretion was suggested by Rauschkolb & Farrell (227) in 1956. After ablation of the diencephalon in dogs, they observed a decrease in aldosterone secretion, but no mention was made of the fate of the adenohypophysis in their experiments. Cortisol secretion fell concurrently with aldosterone in their studies, and consequently a decrease in ACTH release cannot be excluded as the mechanism for decreased aldosterone secretion. In subsequent studies by Newman et al. (210) in 1958, lesions in the ventral diencephalon in cats were associated with a decrease in aldosterone output, but again injury to the pituitary gland or its blood supply could not be excluded.

In 1964 Krieger & Krieger (170) reported that four of seven patients with pretectal disease apparently failed to increase their urinary aldosterone excretion during sodium restriction, but the change was not significant statistically. From this evidence, these workers proposed that an area in or near the posterior hypothalamus is involved in the regulation of aldosterone secretion. In one of the patients who failed to respond with an increased output of aldosterone, renal sodium excretion was as great as 26 mEq/day; this might explain the lack of a response in this case. It should also be pointed out that evaluation of changes in urinary aldosterone excretion rate is difficult because the rate of urinary excretion of this hormone is only a very small percentage of the rate of secretion and urinary excretion is extremely variable.

Other attempts to locate a diencephalic center for the control of aldosterone secretion have yielded clear-cut negative results. In 1959 Ganong and collaborators (122) studied a series of dogs with hypothalamic lesions; they found a low rate of aldosterone output only in animals with damage to the median eminence. Since 17-hydroxycorticoid secretion decreased along with aldosterone and the changes occurred only with median eminence lesions, Ganong and associates concluded that the fall in aldosterone output was secondary to decreased ACTH release. Others (74, 75) have arrived at similar conclusions from studies of dogs with both acute and chronic hypothalamic lesions; damage to the hypothalamus failed to influence aldosterone secretion unless the median eminence was injured or destroyed. These results (74, 75,

122) and the earlier findings by Rauschkolb & Farrell (227) point to the lack of evidence for a hypothalamic control mechanism independent of ACTH.

In addition to the attempts to find a diencephalic center for control of aldosterone secretion, lesions were made in the midbrain, and the entire rostral part of the brain was removed in exploratory studies of this problem. Taylor & Farrell (254) reported that discrete lesions in the rostral, dorsal midbrain decreased aldosterone secretion without a fall in cortisol output. Larger lesions in this area were reported to increase both aldosterone and cortisol secretion above the level observed with discrete lesions. Blood was not collected for 4–6 hr after the lesions were placed, and then the animals were subjected to hemorrhage to obtain enough blood for assay of adrenal steroids. The variability in the data and the methodology employed make evaluation of these observations difficult.

Removal of brain tissue rostral to the superior colliculi in hypophysectomized, nephrectomized dogs has been reported to elevate the rates of secretion of aldosterone, corticosterone, and cortisol secretion (10, 12). Since the rates of secretion of glucocorticoids, as well as of aldosterone, were higher in these midcolliculate dogs than in dogs with the brain intact the data raise the question of remaining adenohypophysial tissue and of its stimulation to secrete ACTH; this would explain the increased aldosterone secretion in the midcolliculate group. No data were given on the completeness of hypophysectomy. In contrast to these reports, other workers (72) have found that midbrain transection failed to alter the rates of aldosterone and corticosterone secretion in previously normal dogs, and these animals with a midbrain transection showed an increase in aldosterone secretion in response to acute hemorrhage. Also the hyperaldosteronism present in dogs with thoracic caval constriction was present after midbrain transection unless cardiovascular function deteriorated (72), and these dogs also showed increased aldosterone secretion after acute hemorrhage. Similarly, sodium-depleted sheep failed to show a decrease in aldosterone secretion after midcollicular section (34); however, sodium repletion failed to lower aldosterone secretion in these midcolliculate animals. It is clear therefore that the central nervous system influences aldosterone secretion via regulation of ACTH release, but evidence demonstrating an additional central nervous mechanism is lacking.

On the assumption of a central nervous mechanism for the regulation of aldosterone secretion, several workers (3, 14, 15, 120, 196) have presented evidence for the possibility *a)* of peripheral nervous receptors associated with the carotid artery and in the right atrium, and *b)* of the vagus nerve as an afferent pathway in the control of aldosterone output. In contrast, Carpenter, Davis, and Ayers (52) reported that denervation of the upper arterial tree in bilaterally vagotomized dogs was without effect on aldosterone secretion and sodium excretion. Also carotid sinus denervation and aortic depressor nerve section failed to influence aldosterone secretion (87). The evidence cited for the existence of carotid arterial receptors (15, 120) was based on the finding of an increase in aldosterone secretion in response to carotid arterial constriction. As indicated in an earlier part of this review, the effect of carotid constriction appears to be mediated via ACTH. It is concluded therefore that studies of several possible nervous mechanisms have failed to demonstrate a nervous mechanism independent of ACTH for the control of aldosterone secretion.

SUMMARY AND CONCLUSIONS

The regulation of aldosterone secretion is mediated by the renin-angiotensin system, ACTH, and the plasma concentrations of sodium and potassium. There is an increasing amount of evidence to support the view that the primary control mechanism is the renin-angiotensin system, but it is also clear that the plasma potassium concentration is important. A unifying concept is that both of these control mechanisms mediate their response by increasing adrenocortical potassium. The renin-angiotensin system operates in both homeostasis and disease and is present in all species, from amphibians to man. A renal-pressor system has been identified in fish, and fish kidney extracts incubated with homologous renin substrate produced a substance with potent aldosterone-stimulating activity when it was assayed in the bullfrog. In sodium depletion the relation of the renin-angiotensin system to aldosterone secretion varies among species, and the mechanisms appear to be unusually complex in the rat and in sheep. Alterations in plasma potassium play an important role in the homeostatic control of aldosterone production. There is clear-cut evidence that alterations in plasma sodium concentration influence aldosterone secretion, but observations are needed to evaluate the significance of this mechanism. Also important in the control of aldosterone secretion is ACTH, but it is probably more involved in secondary aldosteronism than in homeostasis. In secondary aldosteronism ACTH appears to play a supportive role in the increased production of aldosterone, whereas in situations such as laparotomy and acute carotid arterial constriction ACTH seems to initiate the increase in aldosterone secretion. Evidence is lacking to demonstrate a nervous regulatory mechanism independent of ACTH.

REFERENCES

1. Abbrecht, P. H., and A. J. Vander. Effects of chronic potassium deficiency on plasma renin activity. *J. Clin. Invest.* 49: 1510–1516, 1970.

2. Aida, M., M. Maebashi, K. Yoshinaga, K. Abe, I. Miwa, and N. Watanabe. Changes in plasma renin during sodium depletion in man. *Tohoku J. Exptl. Med.* 83: 11–14, 1964.

3. ANDERSON, C. H., M. MCCALLY, AND G. L. FARRELL. The effects of atrial stretch on aldosterone secretion. *Endocrinology* 64: 202–207, 1959.
4. ASSAYKEEN, T. A., P. L. CLAYTON, A. GOLDFIEN, AND W. F. GANONG. Effect of alpha- and beta-adrenergic blocking agents on the renin response to hypoglycemia and epinephrine in dogs. *Endocrinology* 87: 1318–1322, 1970.
5. ASSAYKEEN, T. A., AND W. F. GANONG. The sympathetic nervous system and renin secretion. In: *Frontiers in Neuroendocrinology*, edited by L. Martini and W. F. Ganong. London: Oxford Univ. Press, 1971, p. 67–102.
6. AYERS, C. R., J. O. DAVIS, F. LIEBERMAN, C. C. J. CARPENTER, AND M. BERMAN. The effects of chronic hepatic venous congestion on the metabolism of d, l-aldosterone and d-aldosterone. *J. Clin. Invest.* 41: 884–895, 1962.
7. BAILIE, M. D., F. C. RECTOR, AND D. W. SELDIN. Angiotensin II in arterial and renal venous plasma and renal lymph in the dog. *J. Clin. Invest.* 50: 119–126, 1971.
8. BARAJAS, L., AND H. LATTA. A three-dimensional study of the juxtaglomerular apparatus in the rat. *Lab. Invest.* 12: 257–269, 1963.
9. BARAJAS, L., AND H. LATTA. The juxtaglomerular apparatus in adrenalectomized rats. *Lab. Invest.* 12: 1046–1059, 1963.
10. BARBOUR, B. H., J. D. H. SLATER, A. G. T. CASPER, AND F. C. BARTTER. On the role of the central nervous system in control of aldosterone secretion. *Life Sci.* 4: 1161–1170, 1965.
11. BARTTER, F. C. Regulation of the volume and composition of extracellular and intracellular fluid. *Ann. NY Acad. Sci.* 110: 682–703, 1963.
12. BARTTER, F. C., B. H. BARBOUR, A. A. CARR, C. S. DELEA, AND J. D. H. SLATER. Control of adrenocortical steroid secretion dependent upon and independent of pituitary and kidneys. *Can. Med. Assoc. J.* 90: 240–242, 1964.
13. BARTTER, F. C., A. G. T. CASPER, C. S. DELEA, AND J. D. H. SLATER. On the role of the kidney in the control of adrenal steroid production. *Metabolism* 10: 1006–1020, 1961.
14. BARTTER, F. C., I. H. MILLS, E. G. BIGLIERI, AND C. DELEA. Studies on the control and physiological action of aldosterone. *Recent Progr. Hormone Res.* 15: 311–344, 1959.
15. BARTTER, F. C., I. H. MILLS, AND D. S. GANN. Increase in aldosterone secretion by carotid artery constriction in the dog and its prevention by thyrocarotid arterial junction denervation. *J. Clin. Invest.* 39: 1330–1336, 1960.
16. BARTTER, F. C., P. PRONOVE, J. R. GILL, JR., AND R. C. MACCARDLE. Hyperplasia of the juxtaglomerular complex with hyperaldosteronism and hypokalemic alkalosis. *Am. J. Med.* 33: 811–828, 1962.
17. BAUMBER, J. S., J. O. DAVIS, J. A. JOHNSON, AND R. T. WITTY. Increased adrenocortical potassium in association with increased biosynthesis of aldosterone. *Am. J. Physiol.* 220: 1094–1099, 1971.
18. BERN, H. A., C. C. DEROOS, AND E. G. BIGLIERI. Aldosterone and other corticosteroids from chondrichthyean interrenal glands. *Gen. Comp. Endocrinol.* 2: 490–494, 1962.
20. BIGLIERI, E. G., AND W. F. GANONG. Effect of hypophysectomy on adrenocortical response to bilateral carotid constriction. *Proc. Soc. Exptl. Biol. Med.* 106: 806–809, 1961.
21. BIGLIERI, E. G., C. O. WATLINGTON, AND P. H. FORSHAM. Sodium retention with human growth hormone and its subtractions. *J. Clin. Endocrinol. Metab.* 21: 361–370, 1961.
22. BING, J., AND J. KAZIMIERCZAK. Localization of renin in the kidney. *Proc. Intern. Congr. Nephrol., 1st, Geneve/Evian, 1961*, p. 641–644.
23. BINNION, P. F., J. O. DAVIS, T. C. BROWN, AND M. J. OLICHNEY. Mechanisms regulating aldosterone secretion during sodium depletion. *Am. J. Physiol.* 208: 655–661, 1965.
24. BLAINE, E. H., AND J. O. DAVIS. Evidence for a renal vascular mechanism in renin release: new observations with graded stimulation by aortic constriction. *Circulation Res. Suppl.* 2: 118–126, 1971.
25. BLAINE, E. H., J. O. DAVIS, AND R. L. PREWITT. Evidence for a renal vascular receptor in control of renin secretion. *Am. J. Physiol.* 220: 1593–1597, 1971.
26. BLAINE, E. H., J. O. DAVIS, AND R. T. WITTY. Renin release after hemorrhage and after suprarenal aortic constriction in dogs without sodium delivery to the macula densa. *Circulation Res.* 27: 1081–1089, 1970.
27. BLAIR-WEST, J. R., J. P. COGHLAN, AND D. A. DENTON. Evidence against an aldosterone feed-back mechanism within the adrenal gland. *Acta Endocrinol.* 41: 61–66, 1962.
28. BLAIR-WEST, J. R., J. P. COGHLAN, D. A. DENTON, J. R. GODING, J. A. MUNROE, R. E. PETERSON, AND M. WINTOUR. Humoral stimulation of adrenal cortical secretion. *J. Clin. Invest.* 41: 1606–1627, 1962.
29. BLAIR-WEST, J. R., J. P. COGHLAN, D. A. DENTON, J. R. GODING, J. A. MUNROE, AND R. D. WRIGHT. The reduction of the pressor action of angiotensin II in sodium deficient conscious sheep. *Australian J. Exptl. Biol. Med. Sci.* 41: 369–376, 1963.
30. BLAIR-WEST, J. R., M. D. CAIN, K. J. CATT, J. P. COGHLAN, D. A. DENTON, J. W. FUNDER, B. A. SCOGGINS, E. M. WINTOUR, AND R. D. WRIGHT. The mode of control of aldosterone secretion. *Proc. Intern. Congr. Nephrol., 4th, Stockholm* 2: 33–44, 1970.
31. BLAIR-WEST, J. R., J. P. COGHLAN, D. A. DENTON, J. W. FUNDER, B. A. SCOGGINS, AND R. D. WRIGHT. Inhibition of renin secretion by systemic and intrarenal angiotensin infusion. *Am. J. Physiol.* 220: 1309–1315, 1971.
32. BLAIR-WEST, J. R., J. P. COGHLAN, D. A. DENTON, J. W. FUNDER, B. A. SCOGGINS, AND R. D. WRIGHT. The effect of adrenal arterial infusion of hypertonic $NaHCO_3$ solution on aldosterone secretion in sodium deficient sheep. *Acta Endocrinol.* 66: 448–461, 1971.
33. BLAIR-WEST, J. R., J. P. COGHLAN, D. A. DENTON, J. R. GODING, E. ORCHARD, B. SCOGGINS, M. WINTOUR, AND R. D. WRIGHT. Mechanisms regulating aldosterone secretion during sodium deficiency. *Proc. Intern. Congr. Nephrol., 3rd* 1: 201–214, 1966.
34. BLAIR-WEST, J. R., J. P. COGHLAN, D. A. DENTON, J. R. GODING, M. WINTOUR, AND R. D. WRIGHT. The control of aldosterone secretion. *Recent Progr. Hormone Res.* 19: 311–363, 1963.
35. BLAIR-WEST, J. R., J. P. COGHLAN, D. A. DENTON, J. R. GODING, M. WINTOUR, AND R. D. WRIGHT. The renin-angiotensin system in the control of aldosterone secretion. *Australian J. Exptl. Biol. Med. Sci.* 46: 295–318, 1968.
36. BLAIR-WEST, J. R., J. P. COGHLAN, D. A. DENTON, J. A. MUNROE, M. WINTOUR, AND R. D. WRIGHT. The effect of bilateral nephrectomy and midcollicular decerebration with pinealectomy and hypophysectomy on the corticosteroid secretion of sodium-deficient sheep. *J. Clin. Invest.* 43: 1576–1595, 1964.
37. BLAIR-WEST, J. R., J. P. COGHLAN, D. A. DENTON, B. A. SCOGGINS, AND R. D. WRIGHT. Contrived suppression of renin secretion associated with adrenalectomy, hemorrhage, renal artery constriction, and sodium depletion. In: *International Symposium on the Renin-Angiotensin-Aldosterone-Sodium System in Hypertension*. Berlin: Springer Verlag. In press.
38. BLAIR-WEST, J. R., AND J. R. GODING. Effect of temporary thoracic caval constriction on aldosterone secretion in conscious and in anesthetized sheep. *Endocrinology* 70: 822–836, 1962.
39. BOUGAS, J., C. FLOOD, B. LITTLE, J. F. TAIT, S. A. S. TAIT, AND R. UNDERWOOD. Dynamic aspects of aldosterone metabolism. In: *Aldosterone*, edited by E. E. Baulieu and P. Robel. Oxford: Blackwell, 1964, p. 25–50.
40. BOYD, J. E., W. P. PALMORE, AND P. J. MULROW. Role of potassium in the control of aldosterone secretion in the rat. *Endocrinology* 88: 556–565, 1971.
41. BROWN, J. J., D. L. DAVIES, A. F. LEVER, R. A. PARKER, AND J. I. S. ROBERTSON. Assay of renin in single glomeruli: renin distribution in the normal rabbit kidney. *Lancet* 2: 668, 1963.
42. BROWN, J. J., D. L. DAVIES, A. F. LEVER, AND J. I. S. ROBERT-

son. Influence of sodium deprivation and loading on the plasma-renin in man. *J. Physiol., London* 173: 408–419, 1964.
43. BROWN, J. J., D. L. DAVIES, A. F. LEVER, AND J. I. S. ROBERTSON. Variations in plasma renin concentration in several physiological and pathological states. *Can. Med. Assoc. J.* 90: 201–206, 1964.
44. BROWN, J. J., D. L. DAVIES, A. F. LEVER, J. I. S. ROBERTSON, AND W. S. PEART. The estimation of renin in plasma. In: *Aldosterone*, edited by E. E. Baulieu and P. Robel. Oxford: Blackwell, 1964, p. 417–426.
45. BROWN, T. C., J. O. DAVIS, AND C. I. JOHNSTON. Acute response in plasma renin and aldosterone secretion to diuretics. *Am. J. Physiol.* 211: 437–441, 1966.
46. BROWN, T. C., J. O. DAVIS, M. J. OLICHNEY, AND C. I. JOHNSTON. Relation of plasma renin to sodium balance and arterial pressure in experimental renal hypertension. *Circulation Res.* 18: 475–483, 1966.
47. BRUNNER, H. R., L. BAER, J. E. SEALEY, J. G. G. LEDINGHAM, AND J. H. LARAGH. Influence of potassium administration and of potassium deprivation on plasma renin in normal and hypertensive subjects. *J. Clin. Invest.* 49: 2128–2138, 1970.
48. BRYAN, G. T., B. KLIMAN, J. R. GILL, JR., AND F. C. BARTTER. Effect of human renin on aldosterone secretion rate in normal man and in patients with the syndrome of hyperaldosteronism, juxtaglomerular hyperplasia and normal blood pressure. *J. Clin. Endocrinol. Metab* 24: 729–732, 1964.
49. BUMPUS, F. M., R. R. SMEBY, I. H. PAGE, AND P. A. KHAIRALLAH. Distribution and metabolic fate of angiotensin II and various derivatives. *Can. Med. Assoc. J.* 90: 190–193, 1964.
50. CADE, R., AND T. PERENICH. Secretion of aldosterone by rats. *Am. J. Physiol.* 208: 1026–1030, 1965.
51. CAMARGO, C. A., A. J. DOWDY, E. W. HANCOCK, AND J. A. LUETSCHER. Decreased plasma clearance and hepatic extraction of aldosterone in patients with heart failure. *J. Clin. Invest.* 44: 356–365, 1965.
52. CARPENTER, C. C. J., J. O. DAVIS, AND C. R. AYERS. Concerning the role of arterial baroreceptors in the control of aldosterone secretion. *J. Clin. Invest.* 40: 1160–1171, 1961.
53. CARPENTER, C. C. J., J. O. DAVIS, AND C. R. AYERS. Relation of renin, angiotensin II, and experimental renal hypertension to aldosterone secretion. *J. Clin. Invest.* 40: 2026–2042, 1961.
54. CARPENTER, C. C. J., J. O. DAVIS, J. E. HOLMAN, C. R. AYERS, AND R. C. BAHN. Studies on the response of the transplanted kidney and the transplanted adrenal gland to thoracic inferior vena caval constriction. *J. Clin. Invest.* 40: 196–204, 1961.
55. CARSTENSEN, H., A. C. J. BURGERS, AND C. H. LI. Demonstration of aldosterone and corticosterone as the principal steroids formed in incubates of adrenals of the American bullfrog (*Rana catesbeiana*) and stimulation of their production by mammalian adrenocorticotropin. *Gen. Comp. Endocrinol.* 1: 37–50, 1961.
56. CHESTER-JONES, I., I. W. HENDERSON, D. K. O. CHAN, J. C. RANKIN, W. MOSLEY, J. J. BROWN, A. F. LEVER, J. I. S. ROBERTSON, AND M. TREE. Pressor activity in extracts of the corpuscles of Stannius from the European eel (*Anguilla anguilla* L.). *J. Endocrinol.* 34: 393–408, 1966.
57. COHEN, R. B., AND J. D. CRAWFORD. Glucose-6-phosphate dehydrogenase activity in the adrenal cortex of the sodium depleted rat: a histochemical study. *Endocrinology* 70: 288–290, 1962.
58. CONNELL, G. M., AND G. KALEY. Evidence for the presence of "renin" in the kidneys of marine fish and amphibia. *Biol. Bull.* 127: 366–367, 1964.
59. COOK, W. F. Renin and the juxtaglomerular apparatus. In: *Hormones and the Kidney*, edited by P. C. Williams. New York: Acad. Press, 1963, p. 247–254.
60. COOKE, C. R., T. C. BROWN, B. J. ZACHERLE, AND W. G. WALKER. Effect of altered sodium concentration in the distal nephron segments on renin release. *J. Clin. Invest.* 49: 1630–1638, 1970.
61. COPE, C. Discussion on the regulation and biological effects of aldosterone. In: *Aldosterone*, edited by E. E. Baulieu and P. Robel. Oxford: Blackwell, 1964, p. 281.
62. CRANE, M. G., J. HEITSCH, J. J. HARRIS, AND V. J. JONES, JR. Effect of ethinyl estradiol (estinyl) on plasma renin activity. *J. Clin. Endocrinol. Metab.* 26: 1403–1406, 1966.
63. CULBERTSON, J. W., R. W. WILKINS, F. J. INGELFINGER, AND S. E. BRADLEY. The effect of the upright position upon hepatic blood flow in normotensive and hypertensive subjects. *J. Clin. Invest.* 30: 305–311, 1951.
64. DAVIS, J. O. Discussion remarks. *Recent Progr. Hormone Res.* 15: 298–304, 1959.
65. DAVIS, J. O. Mechanisms regulating the secretion and metabolism of aldosterone in experimental secondary hyperaldosteronism. *Recent Progr. Hormone Res.* 17: 293–352, 1961.
66. DAVIS, J. O. Adrenocortical and renal hormonal function in experimental cardiac failure. *Circulation* 25: 1002–1014, 1962.
67. DAVIS, J. O. The control of aldosterone secretion. *Physiologist* 5: 65–86, 1962.
68. DAVIS, J. O. The role of the adrenal cortex and the kidney in the pathogenesis of cardiac edema. *Yale J. Biol. Med.* 35: 402–428, 1963.
69. DAVIS, J. O. Discussion of aldosterone secretion in the rat. In: *Aldosterone*, edited by E. E. Baulieu and P. Robel. Oxford: Blackwell, 1964, p. 290.
70. DAVIS, J. O. The regulation of aldosterone secretion. In: *The Adrenal Cortex*, edited by A. B. Eisenstein. Boston: Little, Brown, 1967, p. 203–247.
71. DAVIS, J. O. The renin-angiotensin system in the control of aldosterone secretion. In: *Kidney Hormones*, edited by J. W. Fisher. New York: Acad. Press, 1971, p. 173–205.
72. DAVIS, J. O., E. ANDERSON, C. C. J. CARPENTER, C. R. AYERS, W. HAYMAKER, AND W. T. SPENCE. Aldosterone and corticosterone secretion following midbrain transection. *Am. J. Physiol.* 200: 437–443, 1961.
73. DAVIS, J. O., C. R. AYERS, AND C. C. J. CARPENTER. Renal origin of an aldosterone-stimulating hormone in dogs with thoracic caval constriction and in sodium-depleted dogs. *J. Clin. Invest.* 40: 1466–1474, 1961.
74. DAVIS, J. O., R. C. BAHN, AND W. C. BALL, JR. Subacute and chronic effects of hypothalamic lesions on aldosterone and sodium excretion. *Am. J. Physiol.* 197: 387–390, 1959.
75. DAVIS, J. O., R. C. BAHN, N. A. YANKOPOULOS, B. KLIMAN, AND R. E. PETERSON. Acute effects of hypophysectomy and subsequent diencephalic lesions on aldosterone secretion. *Am. J. Physiol.* 197: 380–386, 1959.
76. DAVIS, J. O., P. F. BINNION, T. C. BROWN, AND C. I. JOHNSTON. Mechanisms involved in the hypersecretion of aldosterone during sodium depletion. *Circulation Res.* 18: 143–157, 1966.
77. DAVIS, J. O., C. C. J. CARPENTER, C. R. AYERS, AND R. C. BAHN. Relation of anterior pituitary function to aldosterone and corticosterone secretion in conscious dogs. *Am. J. Physiol.* 199: 212–216, 1960.
78. DAVIS, J. O., C. C. J. CARPENTER, C. R. AYERS, J. E. HOLMAN, AND R. C. BAHN. Evidence for secretion of an aldosterone-stimulating hormone by the kidney. *J. Clin. Invest.* 40: 684–696, 1961.
79. DAVIS, J. O., P. M. HARTROFT, E. O. TITUS, C. C. J. CARPENTER, C. R. AYERS, AND H. E. SPIEGEL. The role of the renin-angiotensin system in the control of aldosterone secretion. *J. Clin. Invest.* 41: 378–389, 1962.
80. DAVIS, J. O., J. E. HOLMAN, C. C. J. CARPENTER, J. URQUHART, AND J. T. HIGGINS, JR. An extra-adrenal factor essential for renal sodium retention in the presence of increased sodium-retaining hormone. *Circulation Res.* 14: 17–31, 1964.
81. DAVIS, J. O., AND D. S. HOWELL. Comparative effect of

ACTH, cortisone and DCA on renal function, electrolyte excretion and water exchange in normal dogs. *Endocrinology* 52: 245–255, 1953.
82. Davis, J. O., D. S. Howell, and R. E. Hyatt. Sodium excretion in adrenalectomized dogs with chronic cardiac failure produced by pulmonary artery constriction. *Am. J. Physiol.* 183: 263–268, 1955.
83. Davis, J. O., C. I. Johnston, P. M. Hartroft, S. S. Howards, and F. S. Wright. The phylogenetic and physiologic importance of the renin-angiotensin-aldosterone system. *Proc. Intern. Congr. Nephrol.*, 3rd 1: 215–225, 1966.
84. Davis, J. O., M. J. Olichney, T. C. Brown, and P. F. Binnion. Metabolism of aldosterone in several experimental situations with altered aldosterone secretion. *J. Clin. Invest.* 44: 1433–1441, 1965.
85. Davis, J. O., J. Urquhart, and J. T. Higgins, Jr. The effects of alterations of plasma sodium and potassium concentration on aldosterone secretion. *J. Clin. Invest.* 42: 597–609, 1963.
86. Davis, J. O., J. Urquhart, J. T. Higgins, Jr., E. C. Rubin, and P. M. Hartroft. Hypersecretion of aldosterone in dogs with a chronic aortic-caval fistula and high output heart failure. *Circulation Res.* 14: 471–485, 1964.
87. Davis, J. O., N. A. Yankopoulos, and J. Holman. Chronic effects of carotid sinus denervation, cervical vagotomy, and aortic depressor nerve section on aldosterone and sodium excretion. *Am. J. Physiol.* 197: 207–210, 1959.
88. Davis, J. O., N. A. Yankopoulos, F. Lieberman, J. Holman, and R. C. Bahn. The role of the anterior pituitary in the control of aldosterone secretion in experimental secondary hyperaldosteronism. *J. Clin. Invest.* 39: 765–775, 1960.
89. Davis, W. W., L. R. Burwell, A. G. T. Casper, and F. C. Bartter. Sites of action of sodium depletion on aldosterone biosynthesis in the dog. *J. Clin. Invest.* 47: 1425–1434, 1968.
90. Deane, H. W., and G. M. C. Masson. Adrenal cortical changes in rats with various types of experimental hypertension. *J. Clin. Endocrinol. Metab.* 11: 193–208, 1951.
91. Denton, D. A. Angiotensin, electrolytes and aldosterone. *Australian Ann. Med.* 13: 121–135, 1964.
92. Denton, D. A. The role of renin in control of aldosterone secretion. In: *Control of Renin Secretion*, edited by T. A. Assaykeen. New York: Plenum Press, 1972, p. 167–188.
93. Denton, D. A., J. R. Goding, and R. D. Wright. Control of adrenal secretion of electrolyte-active steroids. *Brit. Med. J.* 2: 447, 522, 1959.
94. Denton, D. A., J. R. Goding, and R. D. Wright. The control of aldosterone secretion. *Clin. Endocrinol.* 1: 373–396, 1960.
95. Deodhar, S. D., E. Haas, and H. Goldblatt. Production of antirenin to homologous renin and its effect on experimental renal hypertension. *J. Exptl. Med.* 119: 425–432, 1964.
96. Dexter, L., H. A. Frank, F. W. Haynes, and M. D. Altschule. Traumatic shock. VI. The effect of hemorrhagic shock on the concentration of renin and hypertensinogen in the plasma in unanesthetized dogs. *J. Clin. Invest.* 22: 847–852, 1943.
97. Dingman, J. G., E. Gaitan, M. C. Staub, A. Arimura, and R. E. Peterson. Hypoaldosterone in panhypopituitarism (Abstract). *J. Clin. Invest.* 39: 981, 1960.
98. Dufau, M. L., and B. Kliman. Acute effects of angiotensin-II-amide on aldosterone and corticosterone secretion by morphine-pentobarbital treated rats. *Endocrinology* 83: 180–183, 1968.
99. Dunihue, F. W., and W. G. Boldosser. Observations on the similarity of mesangial to juxtaglomerular cells. *Lab. Invest.* 12: 1228–1240, 1963.
100. Dunihue, F. W., and W. V. B. Robertson. The effect of desoxycorticosterone acetate and of sodium on the juxtaglomerular apparatus. *Endocrinology* 61: 293–299, 1957.
101. Earley, L. E., and R. M. Friedler. The effects of combined renal vasodilatation and pressor agents on hemodynamics and the tubular reabsorption of sodium. *J. Clin. Invest.* 45: 542–551, 1966.
102. Edelman, R., and P. M. Hartroft. Localization of renin in juxtaglomerular cells of rabbit and dog through the use of the fluorescent-antibody technique. *Circulation Res.* 9: 1069–1077, 1961.
103. Eilers, E. A., and R. E. Peterson. Aldosterone secretion in the rat. In: *Aldosterone*, edited by E. E. Baulieu and P. Robel. Oxford: Blackwell, 1964, p. 251–305.
104. Eisenstein, A. B., and I. Strack. Effect of sodium deficiency on secretion of hormones by the rat adrenal cortex. *Endocrinology* 68: 121–124, 1961.
105. Farrell, G. Steroidogenic properties of extracts of beef diencephalon. *Endocrinology* 65: 29–33, 1959.
106. Farrell, G. The physiological factors which influence the secretion of aldosterone. *Recent Progr. Hormone Res.* 15: 275–310, 1959.
107. Farrell, G. Adrenoglomerulotropin. *Circulation* 21: 1009–1015, 1960.
108. Farrell, G., and W. M. McIsaac. Adrenoglomerulotropin. *Arch. Biochem.* 94: 543–544, 1961.
109. Farrell, G. L., R. C. Banks, and S. Koletsky. The effect of corticosteroid injection on aldosterone secretion. *Endocrinology* 58: 104–108, 1956.
110. Farrell, G. L., R. B. Fleming, E. W. Rauschkolb, F. M. Yatsu, M. McCally, and C. H. Anderson. Steroidogenic properties of purified corticotropins. *Endocrinology* 62: 506–512, 1958.
111. Fasciolo, J. C., E. De Vito, J. C. Romero, and J. N. Cucchi. The renin content of the blood of humans and dogs under several conditions. *Can. Med. Assoc. J.* 90: 206–209, 1964.
112. Finkelstein, J. W., A. Kowarski, J. S. Spaulding, and C. J. Migeon. Effect of various preparations of human growth hormone on aldosterone secretion rate of hypopituitary dwarfs. *Am. J. Med.* 38: 517–521, 1965.
113. Fisher, E. R. Correlation of juxtaglomerular granulation, pressor activity and enzymes of macula densa in experimental hypertension. *Lab. Invest.* 10: 707–718, 1961.
114. Fisher, E. R., and H. Z. Klein. Effect of sodium on juxtaglomerular index and zona glomerulosa in experimental nephrosis. *Proc. Soc. Exptl. Biol. Med.* 114: 541–544, 1963.
115. Fleming, R., and G. Farrell. Aldosterone and hydrocortisone secretion by the denervated adrenal. *Endocrinology* 59: 360–363, 1956.
116. Friedberg, E. C. The distribution of the juxtaglomerular granules and the macula densa in the renal cortex of the mouse. *Lab. Invest.* 13: 1003–1013, 1964.
117. Funder, J. W., J. R. Blair-West, J. P. Coghlan, D. A. Denton, B. A. Scoggins, and R. D. Wright. Effect of plasma (K^+) on the secretion of aldosterone. *Endocrinology* 85: 381–384, 1969.
118. Gann, D. S., J. F. Cruz, A. G. T. Casper, and F. C. Bartter. Mechanism by which potassium increases aldosterone secretion in the dog. *Am. J. Physiol.* 202: 991–996, 1962.
119. Gann, D. S., C. S. Delea, J. R. Gill, Jr., J. P. Thomas, and F. C. Bartter. Control of aldosterone secretion by change of body potassium in normal man. *Am. J. Physiol.* 207: 104–108, 1964.
120. Gann, D. S., and R. H. Travis. Mechanisms of hemodynamic control of secretion of aldosterone in the dog. *Am. J. Physiol.* 207: 1095–1101, 1964.
121. Ganong, W. F., A. T. Boryczka, and R. Shackelford. Effect of renin on adrenocortical sensitivity to ACTH and angiotensin II in dogs. *Endocrinology* 80: 703–706, 1967.
122. Ganong, W. F., A. H. Lieberman, W. J. R. Daily, V. S. Yuen, P. J. Mulrow, J. A. Luetscher, Jr., and R. E. Bailey. Aldosterone secretion in dogs with hypothalamic lesions. *Endocrinology* 65: 18–28, 1959.
123. Ganong, W. F., and P. J. Mulrow. Evidence of secretion of an aldosterone-stimulating substance by the kidney. *Nature* 190: 1115–1116, 1961.

124. Ganong, W. F., P. J. Mulrow, A. Boryczka, and A. Cera. Evidence for a direct effect of angiotensin II on adrenal cortex of the dog. *Proc. Soc. Exptl. Biol. Med.* 109: 381–384, 1962.
125. Ganong, W. F., D. L. Pemberton, and E. E. Van Brunt. Adrenocortical responsiveness to ACTH and angiotensin II in hypophysectomized dogs and dogs treated with large doses of glucocorticoids. *Endocrinology* 81: 1147–1150, 1967.
126. Ganong, W. F., E. E. Van Brunt, T. C. Lee, and P. J. Mulrow. Inhibition of aldosterone-stimulating activity of hog and dog renin by the plasma of dogs immunized with hog renin. *Proc. Soc. Exptl. Biol. Med.* 112: 1062–1064, 1963.
127. Geelhoed, G. W., and A. J. Vander. The role of aldosterone in renin secretion. *Life Sci.* 6: 525–535, 1967.
128. Genest, J. E., R. Boucher, W. Nowaczynski, E. Koiw, J. De Champlain, P. Biron, M. Chretien, and J. Marc-Aurele. Studies on the relationship of aldosterone and angiotensin to human hypertensive disease. In: *Aldosterone*, edited by E. E. Baulieu and P. Robel. Oxford: Blackwell, 1964, p. 393–416.
129. Genest, J. E., E. Koiw, W. Nowaczynski, and T. Sandor. Study of urinary adrenocortical hormones in human arterial hypertension (Abstract). *Proc. Intern. Congr. Endocrinol.*, 1st, Copenhagen, 1960, p. 173.
130. Ginn, H. E., and R. Cade. Aldosterone secretion in magnesium deficient rats. *Physiologist* 4: 40, 1961.
131. Glaz, E., and K. Sugar. The effect of synthetic angiotensin II on synthesis of aldosterone by the adrenals. *J. Endocrinol.* 24: 299–302, 1962.
132. Gocke, D. J., J. Gerten, L. M. Sherwood, and J. H. Laragh. Physiological and pathological variations of plasma angiotensin II in man. Correlation with renin activity and sodium balance. *Circulation Res. Suppl.* 1: 131–146, 1969.
133. Goldberg, M., and D. K. McCurdy. Hyperaldosteronism and hypergranularity of the juxtaglomerular cells in renal hypertension. *Ann. Internal Med.* 59: 24–36, 1963.
134. Goldfarb, B., and L. Tobian. The interrelationship of hypoxia, erythropoietin, and the renal juxtaglomerular cell. *Proc. Soc. Exptl. Biol. Med.* 8: 510–511, 1962.
135. Goodwin, F. J., J. D. Kirshman, J. E. Sealey, and J. H. Laragh. Influence of the pituitary gland on sodium conservation, plasma renin and renin substrate concentrations in the rat. *Endocrinology* 86: 824–834, 1970.
136. Goormaghtigh, N. Existence of an endocrine gland in the media of the renal arterioles. *Proc. Soc. Exptl. Biol. Med.* 42: 688–689, 1939.
137. Gross, F. Renin and Hypertension, physiologische oder pathologische Wirkstoffe? *Klin. Wochschr.* 36: 693–705, 1958.
138. Gross, F., H. Brunner, and M. Ziegler. Renin-angiotensin system, aldosterone and sodium balance. *Recent Progr. Hormone Res.* 21: 119–177, 1965.
139. Gunnells, J. C., Jr. Circulating vasoconstrictor material in hypertension (Abstract). *Circulation* 30, Suppl. III: 90, 1964.
140. Hartroft, P. Histological and functional aspects of juxtaglomerular cells. In: *Angiotensin Systems and Experimental Renal Diseases*, edited by J. Metcoff. Boston: Little, Brown, 1963, p. 5–16.
141. Hartroft, P. M. Juxtaglomerular cells. *Circulation Res.* 12: 525–538, 1963.
142. Hartroft, P. M. "Juxtaglomerular" JG cells of the American bullfrog as seen by light and electron microscopy (Abstract). *Federation Proc.* 25: 238, 1966.
143. Hartroft, P. M., and W. S. Hartroft. Studies on renal juxtaglomerular cells. I. Variations produced by sodium chloride, and desoxycorticosterone acetate. *J. Exptl. Med.* 97: 415–428, 1953.
144. Hartroft, P. M., L. N. Newmark, and J. A. Pitcock. Relationship of renal juxtaglomerular cells to sodium intake, adrenal cortex and hypertension. In: *Hypertension*, edited by J. Moyer. Philadelphia: Saunders, 1959, p. 24–32.
145. Hartroft, W. S., and P. M. Hartroft. New approaches in the study of cardiovascular disease: aldosterone, renin, hypertension, and juxtaglomerular cells. *Federation Proc.* 20: 845–854, 1961.
146. Haynes, R. C., Jr., and L. Berthet. Studies on the mechanism of action of the adrenocorticotropic hormone. *J. Biol. Chem.* 225: 115–124, 1957.
147. Helmer, O. M. Studies on renin antibodies. *Circulation* 17: 648–652, 1958.
148. Helmer, O. M. Renin activity in blood from patients with hypertension. *Can. Med. Assoc. J.* 90: 221–225, 1964.
149. Helmer, O. M., and R. S. Griffith. The effect of the administration of estrogens on the renin-substrate (Hypertensinogen) content of rat plasma. *Endocrinology* 51: 421–426, 1952.
150. Hernando-Avendano, L., J. Crabbé, E. J. Ross, W. J. Reddy, A. E. Renold, D. H. Nelson, and G. W. Thorn. Clinical experience with a physicochemical method for estimation of aldosterone in urine. *Metabolism* 6: 518–543, 1957.
151. Hess, R., and A. G. E. Pearse. Mitochondrial α-glycerophosphate dehydrogenase activity of juxtaglomerular cells in experimental hypertension and adrenal insufficiency. *Proc. Soc. Exptl. Biol. Med.* 106: 895–898, 1961.
152. Higgins, J. T., Jr., J. O. Davis, and J. Urquhart. Demonstration by pressor and steroidogenic assays of increased renin in lymph of dogs with secondary hyperaldosteronism. *Circulation Res.* 14: 218–227, 1964.
153. Higgins, J. T., Jr., J. O. Davis, and J. Urquhart. Increased plasma level of renin in experimental secondary hyperaldosteronism. *Am. J. Physiol.* 207: 814–820, 1964.
154. Holzbauer, M. The part played by ACTH in determining the rate of aldosterone secretion during operative stress. *J. Physiol., London* 172: 138–149, 1964.
155. Howards, S. S., J. O. Davis, C. I. Johnston, and F. W. Wright. The renin-angiotensin system in the control of aldosterone secretion. *Am. J. Physiol.* 214: 990–996, 1968.
156. Itskovitz, H. D., E. A. Hildreth, A. M. Sellers, and W. S. Blakemore. The granularity of the juxtaglomerular cells in human hypertension. *Ann. Internal Med.* 59: 8–22, 1963.
157. Johnson, B. B., A. H. Lieberman, and P. J. Mulrow. Aldosterone excretion in normal subjects depleted of sodium and potassium. *J. Clin. Invest.* 36: 757–766, 1957.
158. Johnson, J. A., J. O. Davis, J. S. Baumber, and E. G. Schneider. Effects of hemorrhage and chronic sodium depletion on hepatic clearance of renin. *Am. J. Physiol.* 220: 1677–1682, 1971.
159. Johnson, J. A., J. O. Davis, and R. T. Witty. Effects of catecholamines and renal nerve stimulation on renin release in the non-filtering kidney. *Circulation Res.* 29: 646–653, 1971.
160. Johnston, C. I., J. O. Davis, and P. M. Hartroft. Renin-angiotensin system, adrenal steroids and sodium depletion in a primitive mammal, the American opossum. *Endocrinology* 81: 633–642, 1967.
161. Johnston, C. I., J. O. Davis, C. A. Robb, and J. W. Mackenzie. Plasma renin in chronic experimental heart failure and during renal sodium "escape" from mineralocorticoids. *Circulation Res.* 22: 113–125, 1968.
162. Johnston, C. I., J. O. Davis, F. W. Wright, and S. S. Howards. Effects of renin and ACTH on adrenal steroid secretion in the American bullfrog. *Am. J. Physiol.* 213: 393–399, 1967.
163. Kaley, G., G. A. Robison, and B. Lubben. Comparative aspects of the renin-angiotensin system (Abstract). *Biol. Bull.* 125: 381, 1963.
164. Kaplan, N. M. The biosynthesis of adrenal steroids: effects of angiotensin II, adrenocorticotropin, and potassium. *J. Clin. Invest.* 44: 2029–2039, 1965.
165. Kaplan, N. M. The effect of ACTH and angiotensin II upon adrenal steroid synthesis. In: *Angiotensin Systems and Experimental Renal Diseases*, edited by J. Metcoff. Boston: Little, Brown, 1963, p. 97–107.
166. Kaplan, N. M., and J. G. Silah. The effect of angiotensin

II on the blood pressure in humans with hypertensive disease. *J. Clin. Invest.* 43: 659–669, 1964.
167. KATZ, F. H., AND A. KAPPAS. The effects of estradiol and estriol on plasma levels of cortisol and thyroid hormone-binding globulins and on aldosterone and cortisol secretion rates in man. *J. Clin. Invest.* 46: 1768–1777, 1967.
168. KINSON, G. A., AND B. SINGER. Sensitivity to angiotensin and adrenocorticotrophin hormone in the sodium deficient rat. *Endocrinology* 83: 1108–1116, 1968.
169. KLIMAN, B., AND R. E. PETERSON. Double isotope derivative assay of aldosterone in biological extracts. *J. Biol. Chem.* 235: 1639–1649, 1960.
170. KRIEGER, D. T., AND H. P. KRIEGER. Aldosterone excretion in pretectal disease. *J. Clin. Endocrinol. Metab.* 24: 1055–1066, 1964.
171. LAIDLAW, J. C., J. L. RUSE, AND A. G. GORNALL. The influence of estrogen and progesterone on aldosterone excretion. *J. Clin. Endocrinol. Metab.* 22: 161–171, 1962.
172. LARAGH, J. H. Interrelationships between angiotensin, norepinephrine, epinephrine, aldosterone secretion, and electrolyte metabolism in man. *Circulation* 25: 203–211, 1962.
173. LARAGH, J. H. Hormones and pathogenesis of congestive heart failure: vasopressin, aldosterone and angiotensin II. Further evidence for renal-adrenal interaction from studies in hypertension and cirrhosis. *Circulation* 25: 1015–1023, 1962.
174. LARAGH, J. H., M. ANGERS, W. G. KELLY, AND S. LIEBERMAN. The effect of epinephrine, norepinephrine, angiotensin II, and others on the secretory rate of aldosterone in man. *J. Am. Med. Assoc.* 174: 234–240, 1960.
175. LARAGH, J. H., P. J. CANNON, AND R. P. AMES. Interaction between aldosterone secretion, sodium and potassium balance, and angiotensin activity in man: studies in hypertension and cirrhosis. *Can. Med. Assoc. J.* 90: 248–256, 1964.
176. LARAGH, J. H., P. J. CANNON, C. J. BENTZEL, A. M. SICINSKI, AND J. I. MELTZER. Angiotensin II, norepinephrine, and renal transport of electrolytes and water in normal man and in cirrhosis with ascites. *J. Clin. Invest.* 42: 1179–1192, 1963.
177. LARAGH, J. H., J. E. SEALEY, J. G. G. LEDINGHAM, AND M. A. NEWTON. Oral contraceptives, renin, aldosterone, and high blood pressure. *J. Am. Med. Assoc.* 201: 918–922, 1967.
178. LARAGH, J. H., AND H. C. STOERK. A study of the mechanism of secretion of the sodium-retaining hormone (aldosterone). *J. Clin. Invest.* 36: 383–392, 1957.
179. LEE, T. C., AND D. DE WIED. Somatotropin as the non-ACTH factor of anterior pituitary origin for the maintenance of enhanced aldosterone secretory responsiveness of dietary sodium restriction in chronically hypophysectomized rats. *Life Sci.* 7: 35–45, 1968.
180. LEE, T. C., E. E. VAN BRUNT, E. G. BIGLIERI, AND W. F. GANONG. Aldosterone secretion in dogs treated with hog renin (Abstract). *Federation Proc.* 23: 301, 1964.
181. LEVER, A. F., AND W. S. PEART. Renin and angiotensin-like activity in renal lymph. *J. Physiol., London* 160: 548–563, 1962.
182. LEVY, L. E., AND A. BLALOCK. A method for transplanting the adrenal gland of the dog with reestablishment of its blood supply. *Ann. Surg.* 109: 84–98, 1939.
183. LIDDLE, G. W., L. E. DUNCAN, JR., AND F. C. BARTTER. Dual mechanism regulating adrenocortical function in man. *Am. J. Med.* 21: 380–386, 1956.
184. LLAURADO, J. G., J. L. CLAUS, AND J. B. TRUNNELL. Aldosterone excretion in feces of rats treated with estradiol. *Endocrinology* 71: 598–604, 1962.
185. LUCIS, O. J., I. DYRENFURTH, AND E. H. VENNING. Effect of various preparations of pituitary and diencephalon on the in vitro secretion of aldosterone and corticosterone by the rat adrenal gland. *Can. J. Biochem. Physiol.* 39: 901–913, 1961.
186. LUETSCHER, J. A., JR., AND B. J. AXELRAD. Increased aldosterone output during sodium deprivation in normal men. *Proc. Soc. Exptl. Biol. Med.* 87: 650–653, 1954.
187. LUETSCHER, J. A., A. J. DOWDY, A. M. CALLAGHAN, AND A. P. COHN. Studies of secretion and metabolism of aldosterone and cortisol. *Trans. Assoc. Am. Physicians* 75: 293–300, 1962.
188. MARIEB, N. J., AND P. J. MULROW. Regulation of aldosterone secretion in the rat (Abstract). *Clin. Res.* December, 1964.
189. MARX, A. J., AND H. W. DEANE. Histophysiological changes in the kidney and adrenal cortex in rats on a low-sodium diet. *Endocrinology* 73: 317–328, 1963.
190. MARX, A. J., H. W. DEANE, T. F. MOWLES, AND H. SHEPPARD. Chronic administration of angiotensin in rats: changes in blood pressure, renal and adrenal histophysiology and aldosterone production. *Endocrinology* 73: 329–337, 1963.
191. MASSON, G. M. C., AND R. H. TRAVIS. The renin-angiotensin system in the control of aldosterone secretion. *Can. J. Physiol. Pharmacol.* 46: 11–14, 1968.
192. McCAA, R. E., V. H. READ, J. D. BOWER, C. S. McCAA, AND A. C. GUYTON. Adrenal cortical response to hemodialysis, ACTH and angiotensin II in anephric man (Abstract). *Circulation* 44, Suppl. II: 67, 1971.
193. McKERNS, K. W. Mechanism of action of adrenocorticotropic hormone through activation of glucose-6-phosphate dehydrogenase. *Biochem. Biophys. Acta* 90: 357–371, 1964.
194. MERRILL, A. J., J. L. MORRISON, AND E. S. BRANNON. Concentration of renin in renal venous blood in patients with chronic heart failure. *Am. J. Med.* 1: 468–472, 1946.
195. MEYER, P., J. MENARD, N. PAPANICOLAOU, J. M. ALEXANDRE, C. deVAUX, AND P. MILLIEZ. Mechanism of renin release following furosemide diuresis in rabbit. *Am. J. Physiol.* 215: 908–915, 1968.
196. MILLS, I. H., A. CASPER, AND F. C. BARTTER. On the role of the vagus in the control of aldosterone secretion. *Science* 128: 1140–1141, 1958.
197. MIZOGAMI, S., M. OGURI, H. SOKABE, AND H. HISHIMURA. The renin-angiotensin system in the control of aldosterone secretion. *Am. J. Physiol.* 215: 991–994, 1968.
198. MOGIL, R. A., H. D. ITSKOVITZ, J. H. RUSSELL, AND J. J. MURPHY. Renal innervation and renin activity in salt metabolism and hypertension. *Am. J. Physiol.* 216: 693–697, 1969.
199. MORAN, W. H., JR., J. C. ROSENBERG, AND B. ZIMMERMAN. The regulation of aldosterone output: significance of potassium ion. *Surg. Forum* 9: 120–122, 1959.
200. MORRIS, R. C., JR., P. R. ROBINSON, AND G. A. SCHULE. The relation of angiotensin to renal hypertension. *Can. Med. Assoc. J.* 90: 272–276, 1964.
201. MÜLLER, J. Aldosterone stimulation in vitro. *Acta Endocrinol.* 48: 283–296, 1965.
202. MÜLLER, J. Aldosterone stimulation in vitro. I. Evaluation of assay procedure and determination of aldosterone-stimulating activity in a human urine extract. *Acta Endocrinol.* 48: 283–296, 1965.
203. MÜLLER, J. *Regulation of Aldosterone Biosynthesis.* New York: Springer Verlag, 1971.
204. MÜLLER, J., AND W. H. ZIEGLER. Steroidogenic effect of stimulators of aldosterone biosynthesis upon separate zones of the rat adrenal cortex. Influence of sodium and potassium deficiency. *European J. Clin. Invest.* 1: 180–187, 1970.
205. MULROW, P. J., AND W. F. GANONG. The effect of hemorrhage upon aldosterone secretion in normal and hypophysectomized dogs. *J. Clin. Invest.* 40: 579–585, 1961.
206. MULROW, P. J., W. F. GANONG, AND A. BORYCZKA. Further evidence for a role of the renin-angiotensin system in regulation of aldosterone secretion. *Proc. Soc. Exptl. Biol. Med.* 112: 7–10, 1963.
207. MULROW, P. J., W. F. GANONG, G. CERA, AND A. KULJIAN. The nature of the aldosterone-stimulating factor in dog kidneys. *J. Clin. Invest.* 41: 505–518, 1962.
208. MULROW, P. J., G. L. SHMAGRANOFF, A. H. LIEBERMAN, C. I. SLADE, AND J. A. LUETSCHER, JR. Stimulation of rat adrenocortical secretion by a factor present in human urine. *Endocrinology* 64: 631–637, 1959.
209. NASH, F. D., H. H. ROSTORFER, M. D. BAILIE, R. L. WATHEN, AND E. G. SCHNEIDER. Relation to renal sodium load and

dissociation from hemodynamic changes. *Circulation Res.* 22: 473–487, 1968.
210. NEWMAN, A. E., E. S. REDGATE, AND G. FARRELL. The effects of diencephalic-mesencephalic lesions on aldosterone and hydrocortisone secretion. *Endocrinology* 63: 723–736, 1958.
211. NEWSOME, H. H., AND F. C. BARTTER. Plasma renin activity in relation to serum sodium concentration and body fluid balance. *J. Clin. Endocrinol. Metab.* 28: 1704–1711, 1968.
212. NEWTON, M. A., AND J. H. LARAGH. Effect of corticotropin on aldosterone excretion and plasma renin in normal subjects, in essential hypertension and in primary aldosteronism. *J. Clin. Endocrinol. Metab.* 28: 1006–1013, 1968.
213. NEWTON, M. A., AND J. H. LARAGH. Effects of glucocorticoid administration on aldosterone excretion and plasma renin in normal subjects, in essential hypertension and in primary aldosteronism. *J. Clin. Endocrinol. Metab.* 28: 1014–1022, 1968.
214. NEWTON, M. A., J. E. SEALEY, J. G. G. LEDINGHAM, AND J. H. LARAGH. High blood pressure and oral contraceptives. *Am. J. Obstet. Gynecol.* 101: 1037–1045, 1968.
215. NOTHSTINE, S. A., J. O. DAVIS, AND R. M. DEROOS. Kidney extracts and ACTH on adrenal secretion in a turtle and a crocodilian. *Am. J. Physiol.* 221: 726–732, 1971.
216. OGURI, M., AND H. SOKABE. The renin-angiotensin system in the control of aldosterone secretion. *Japan. Soc. Sci. Fisheries Bull.* 34: 882–888, 1968.
217. ORLOFF, M. J., C. A. LIPMAN, S. M. NOEL, N. A. HALASZ, AND T. NEESBY. The renin-angiotensin system in the control of aldosterone secretion. *Surgery* 58: 225–247, 1965.
218. ORTI, E., E. P. RALLI, B. LAKEN, AND M. E. DUMM. Presence of an aldosterone stimulating substance in the urine of rats deprived of salt. *Am. J. Physiol.* 191: 323–328, 1957.
219. PALKOVITS, M., W. DE JONG, B. VAN DER WAL, AND D. DE WIED. The aldosterone secretory response to sodium restriction in chronically hypophysectomized corticotrophin-maintained rats as a function of duration and amount of growth hormone treatment. *J. Endocrinol.* 50: 407–411, 1970.
220. PALMORE, L. B., M. B. VALLOTTON, AND E. HABER. The renin-angiotensin system in the control of aldosterone secretion. *Science* 158: 1482–1484, 1967.
221. PALMORE, W. P., N. J. MARIEB, AND P. J. MULROW. Stimulation of aldosterone secretion by sodium depletion in nephrectomized rats. *Endocrinology* 84: 1342–1351, 1969.
222. PASQUALINO, A., AND G. H. BOURNE. Chemical changes in kidneys and adrenals of rats made hypertensive by the Goldblatt method. *Nature* 182: 1425–1427, 1958.
223. PEART, W. S. Renin and angiotensin in relation to aldosterone. *Am. J. Clin. Pathol.* 54: 324–330, 1970.
224. PETERS, J. P., L. G. WELT, E. A. N. SIMS, J. ORLOFF, AND J. NEEDHAM. Salt wasting syndrome associated with cerebral diseases. *Trans. Assoc. Am. Physicians* 63: 57–64, 1950.
225. PETERSON, R. E., AND J. MÜLLER. Aldosterone-stimulating material in urine. *Endocrinology* 71: 174–175, 1962.
226. PINCUS, G. The biosynthesis of adrenal cortical steroids. *Bull. NY Acad. Med.* 33: 587–598, 1957.
227. RAUSCHKOLB, E. W., AND G. L. FARRELL. Evidence for diencephalic regulation of aldosterone secretion. *Endocrinology* 59: 526–531, 1956.
228. RAUSCHKOLB, E. W., G. L. FARRELL, AND S. KOLETSKY. Aldosterone secretion after hypophysectomy. *Am. J. Physiol.* 184: 55–58, 1956.
229. RAYYIS, S. S., AND R. HORTON. Effect of angiotensin II on adrenal and pituitary function in man. *J. Clin. Endocrinol. Metab.* 32: 539–546, 1971.
230. REEVES, G., L. LOWENSTEIN, AND S. C. SOMMERS. A suggested mechanism of erythropoietic control by juxtaglomerular cells. *Am. J. Med. Sci.* 245: 184–188, 1963.
231. REEVES, G., L. M. LOWENSTEIN, AND S. C. SOMMERS. The macula densa and juxtaglomerular body in cirrhosis. *Arch. Internal Med.* 112: 708–715, 1963.
232. ROBB, C. A., J. O. DAVIS, J. A. JOHNSON, E. H. BLAINE, E. H. SCHNEIDER, AND J. S. BAUMBER. Mechanisms regulating the renal excretion of sodium during pregnancy. *J. Clin. Invest.* 49: 871–880, 1970.
233. ROBERTSON, J. I. S. Renin in plasma of normal and hypertensive rabbits (Abstract). *J. Physiol., London* 166: 27, 1963.
234. Ross, E. J., W. VAN'T HOFF, J. CRABBÉ, AND G. W. THORN. Aldosterone excretion in hypopituitarism and after hypophysectomy in man. *Am. J. Med.* 28: 229–238, 1960.
235. SANDOR, T., G. P. VINSON, I. C. JONES, I. W. HENDERSON, AND B. J. WHITEHOUSE. Biogenesis of corticosteroids in the European eel (*Anguilla anguilla* L.). *J. Endocrinol.* 34: 105–115, 1966.
236. SARUTA, T., G. A. SAADE, AND N. M. KAPLAN. A possible mechanism for hypertension induced by oral contraceptives. *Arch. Internal Med.* 126: 621–626, 1970.
237. SCORNIK, O. A., AND A. C. PALADINI. Significance of blood angiotensin levels in different experimental conditions. *Can. Med. Assoc. J.* 90: 269–271, 1964.
238. SEALEY, J. E., J. D. KIRSHMAN, AND J. H. LARAGH. Natriuretic activity in plasma and urine of salt-loaded man and sheep. *J. Clin. Invest.* 48: 2210–2224, 1969.
239. SHADE, R. E., J. O. DAVIS, J. A. JOHNSON, R. T. WITTY, AND B. BRAVERMAN. Effects of renal intra-arterial infusion of sodium and potassium on renin secretion in the non-filtering kidney (Abstract). *Ann. Meeting, Am. Soc. Nephrol., 5th, 1971*, p. 71.
240. SHADE, R. E., J. O. DAVIS, R. T. WITTY, J. A. JOHNSON, AND B. BRAVERMAN. Mechanisms regulating renin release in dogs with thoracic caval constriction. *Physiologist* 14: 228, 1971.
241. SINGER, B., C. LOSITO, AND S. SALMON. Effect of progesterone on adrenocortical hormone secretion in normal and hypophysectomized rats. *J. Endocrinol.* 28: 65–72, 1963.
242. SINGER, B., C. LOSITO, AND S. SALMON. Aldosterone and corticosterone secretion rates in rats with experimental renal hypertension. *Acta Endocrinol.* 44: 505–518, 1963.
243. SINGER, B., C. LOSITO, AND S. SALMON. Some studies on the effect of angiotensin II on adrenocortical hormone secretion in hypophysectomized rats with renal pedicle ligation. *Endocrinology* 74: 325–332, 1964.
244. SINGER, B., AND M. P. STACK-DUNNE. The secretion of aldosterone and corticosterone by the rat adrenal. *J. Endocrinol.* 12: 130–145, 1955.
245. SKINNER, S. L., J. W. MCCUBBIN, AND I. H. PAGE. Angiotensin in blood and lymph following reduction in renal arterial perfusion pressure in dogs. *Circulation Res.* 13: 336–345, 1963.
246. SKINNER, S. L., J. W. MCCUBBIN, AND I. H. PAGE. Control of renin secretion. *Circulation Res.* 15: 64–76, 1964.
247. SLATER, J. D., H. B. H. BARBOUR, H. H. HENDERSON, A. G. T. CASPER, AND F. C. BARTTER. Influence of the pituitary and the renin-angiotensin system on the secretion of aldosterone, cortisol, and corticosterone. *J. Clin. Invest.* 42: 1504–1520, 1963.
248. SOKABE, H. The renin-angiotensin system in the control of aldosterone secretion. *J. Japan. Med. Assoc.* 59: 502–512, 1968.
249. SOKABE, H., T. NAKAJAMA, AND T. NAKAYAMA. Differentiation of the angiotensin-like substances of nonmammalian and extrarenal origins (Abstract). *Proc. Intern. Union Physiol. Sci., Munich* 9: 525, 1971.
250. TAGAWA, H., A. J. VANDER, J. BONJOUR, AND R. L. MALVIN. Inhibition of renin secretion by vasopressin in unanesthetized sodium-deprived dogs. *Am. J. Physiol.* 220: 949–951, 1971.
251. TAIT, J. F., J. BOUGAS, B. LITTLE, S. A. S. TAIT, AND C. FLOOD. Splanchnic extraction and clearance of aldosterone in subjects with minimal and marked cardiac dysfunction. *J. Clin. Endocrinol. Metab.* 25: 219–228, 1965.
252. TAYLOR, A. A., AND J. O. DAVIS. Effects of carp kidney extracts and angiotensin II on adrenal steroid secretion. *Am. J. Physiol.* 221: 652–657, 1971.
253. TAYLOR, A. A., J. O. DAVIS, R. P. BREITENBACH, AND P. M. HARTROFT. Adrenal steroid secretion and a renal-pressor

system in the chicken (*Gallus domesticus*). *Gen. Comp. Endocrinol.* 14: 321–333, 1970.
254. TAYLOR, A. N., AND G. FARRELL. Effects of brain stem lesions on aldosterone and cortisol secretion. *Endocrinology* 70: 556–566, 1962.
255. THURAU, K., J. SCHNERMANN, W. NAGEL, M. HORSTER, AND M. WOHL. Composition of tubular fluid in the macula densa segment as a factor regulating the function of the juxtaglomerular apparatus. *Circulation Res. Suppl.* 2: 79–89, 1967.
256. TOBIAN, L. Interrelationship of electrolytes, juxtaglomerular cells and hypertension. *Physiol. Rev.* 40: 280–312, 1960.
257. TOBIAN, L., J. JANECEK, AND A. TOMBOULIAN. Correlation between granulation of juxtaglomerular cells and extractable renin in rats with experimental hypertension. *Proc. Soc. Exptl. Biol. Med.* 100: 94–96, 1959.
258. TOBIAN, L., S. PERRY, AND J. MORK. The relationship of the juxtaglomerular apparatus to sodium retention in experimental nephrosis. *Ann. Internal Med.* 57: 382–388, 1962.
259. TOBIAN, L., J. THOMPSON, R. TWEDT, AND J. JANECEK. The granulation of juxtaglomerular cells in renal hypertension, desoxycorticosterone and post-desoxycorticosterone hypertension, adrenal regeneration hypertension, and adrenal insufficiency. *J. Clin. Invest.* 37: 660–671, 1958.
260. TORIKAI, T., S. FUKUCHI, M. HANATA, H. TAKAHASHI, AND H. DEMURA. The juxtaglomerular apparatus and aldosterone in hyperaldosteronism. *Tohoku J. Exptl. Med.* 82: 74–86, 1964.
260a. TUCCI, J. R., E. A. ESPINER, P. I. JAGGER, G. L. PAUK, AND D. P. LAULER. ACTH stimulation of aldosterone secretion in normal subjects and in patients with chronic adrenocortical insufficiency. *J. Clin. Endocrinol. Metab.* 27: 568–575, 1967.
261. UEDA, H., H. YASUDA, Y. TAKABATAKE, M. IIZUKA, T. IIZUKA, M. IHORI, AND Y. SAKAMOTO. Observations on the mechanism of renin release by catecholamines. *Circulation Res. Suppl.* 2: 195–200, 1970.
262. ULICK, S., AND E. FEINHOLTZ. Metabolism and rate of secretion of aldosterone in the bullfrog. *J. Clin. Invest.* 47: 2523–2529, 1968.
263. URQUHART, J. Selective stimulation of aldosterone secretion by angiotensin II in intact dogs (Abstract). *Program Endocrine Soc. Meeting, 47th, 1965*, p. 62.
264. URQUHART, J., J. O. DAVIS, AND J. T. HIGGINS, JR. Effects of prolonged infusion of angiotensin II in normal dogs. *Am. J. Physiol.* 205: 1241–1246, 1963.
265. VALLOTON, M. B., L. B. PAGE, AND E. HABER. Radioimmunoassay of angiotensin in human plasma. *Nature* 215: 714–715, 1967.
266. VANDER, A. J. Effect of catecholamines and the renal nerves on renin secretion in anesthetized dogs. *Am. J. Physiol.* 209: 659–662, 1965.
267. VANDER, A. J., AND J. CARLSON. Mechanism of the effects of furosemide on renin secretion in anesthetized dogs. *Circulation Res.* 25: 145–152, 1969.
268. VANDER, A. J., AND R. MILLER. Control of renin secretion in the anesthetized dog. *Am. J. Physiol.* 207: 537–546, 1964.
269. VERTES, V., L. BERMAN, AND S. MITRA. The kidney and adrenal gland in hypertension (Abstract). *Circulation* 44, Suppl. II: 12, 1971.
270. VEYRAT, R., H. R. BRUNNER, E. L. MANNING, AND A. F. MULLER. Inhibition de l'activite de la renine plasmatique par le potassium. *J. Urol. Nephrol.* 73: 271–275, 1967.
271. VEYRAT, R., J. DE CHAMPLAIN, R. BOUCHER, AND J. GENEST. Measurement of human arterial renin activity in some physiological and pathological states. *Can. Med. Assoc. J.* 90: 215–220, 1964.
272. WAKERLIN, G. E. Antibodies to renin as proof of the pathogenesis of sustained renal hypertension. *Circulation* 17: 653–657, 1958.
273. WEINBERGER, M. H., R. D. COLLINS, A. J. DOWDY, G. W. NOKES, AND J. A. LUETSCHER. Hypertension induced by oral contraceptives containing estrogen and gestagen. *Ann. Internal Med.* 71: 891–902, 1969.
274. WELT, L. G., D. W. SELDIN, W. P. NELSON, III, W. J. GERMAN, AND J. P. PETERS. Role of the central nervous system in metabolism of electrolytes and water. *Arch. Internal Med.* 90: 355–378, 1952.
275. WINER, B. M. A humoral vasoconstrictor effect of salt depletion. *Proc. New Engl. Cardiovascular Soc.* 21: 43–44, 1963.
276. WINER, N., D. S. CHOKSHI, AND W. G. WALKENHORST. Effects of cyclic AMP, sympathomimetic amines, and adrenergic receptor antagonists on renin secretion. *Circulation Res.* 29: 239–248, 1971.
277. WINER, N., D. S. CHOKSHI, M. S. YOON, AND A. D. FREEDMAN. Adrenergic receptor mediation of renin secretion. *J. Clin. Endocrinol. Metab.* 29: 1168–1175, 1969.
278. WITTY, R. T., J. O. DAVIS, J. A. JOHNSON, AND R. L. PREWITT. Effects of papaverine and hemorrhage on renin secretion in the non-filtering kidney. *Am. J. Physiol.* 221: 1666–1671, 1971.
279. WOLFF, H. P. Aldosterone in clinical medicine. *Acta Endocrinol.* 124: 65–86, 1967.
280. WOLFF, H. P., D. LOMMER, J. JAHNECKE, AND M. TORBICA. Hyperaldosteronism in oedema. In: *Aldosterone*, edited by E. E. Baulieu and P. Robel. Oxford: Blackwell, 1964, p. 471–486.
281. YANKOPOULOS, N. A., J. O. DAVIS, B. KLIMAN, AND R. E. PETERSON. Evidence that a humoral agent stimulates the adrenal cortex to secrete aldosterone in experimental secondary hyperaldosteronism. *J. Clin. Invest.* 38: 1278–1289, 1959.

CHAPTER 8

The fetal adrenal cortex

ALFRED JOST | *Faculty of Sciences, University Paris VI, Paris, France*

CHAPTER CONTENTS

Functional Development of Fetal Adrenal Cortex
    Maturational changes
    Hypophysial control of adrenal development and function
    Hypothalamic control of hypophysial corticostimulating
        activity
    Fetal stress
    Human anencephals
Problem of Human Fetal Adrenal Cortex
Functions of Fetal Adrenal Cortex
    Effects on fetal organs
        Glycogen deposition in fetal liver
        Effects on maturation of adrenal medulla
        Effects on thymus and hematopoietic tissue
    Effect on parturition
    Fetal adrenocortical insufficiency and postnatal survival

FETAL ENDOCRINOLOGY deals with the functioning and physiological role of fetal endocrine glands during fetal development and delivery. However, the word fetal does not connote a steady state; it covers a series of successive physiological stages that should be distinguished. Problems concerning the adrenal cortex are multifarious: *a*) how is the specialization of the early embryonic cells into specialized adrenocortical cells controlled—this question remains unsolved; *b*) when does the release of hormones into the circulation begin and under which influence; information can be gathered from hormonal determinations in fetal blood and from studies of target organs under different conditions; *c*) on which target organs do fetal adrenocortical hormones exert physiological effects; *d*) how is the secretion rate of hormones or of related steroids controlled at different developmental stages; the peculiar steroidogenetic activity of the human fetal adrenal cortex deserves special consideration.

Only the fetal adrenal cortex of the mammal is discussed in this chapter. Although the number of publications has become very large (exhaustive quotation is impossible), information remains scattered: sustained efforts were made only in man and a few other species; different species may obey different developmental patterns and raise different problems; and finally many studies were devoted, for technical reasons, to selected developmental periods, thus leaving other periods in shadow.

Different developmental patterns are seen in three groups of species that are frequently referred to:

1. Small laboratory animals, with a short gestation period (e.g., rats, mice, rabbits): maturation of the adrenal cortex and effects on target organs occur within a few days. Intrauterine surgery permits physiological exploration.

2. Man, whose gestation period is long: the fetal endocrine processes are protracted over several months. Moreover the human placenta is a very active endocrine tissue producing steroids and pituitary-like hormones. Information has been obtained from the study of cord blood in term or premature deliveries, from experimental perfusion in vitro or in vivo of midterm (14–20 weeks) fetuses in cases of legal abortion, or from in vitro incubation with labeled precursors of adrenocortical tissue at various developmental stages. Other important clues are given by infants afflicted with congenital defects.

3. Lamb fetuses (research on goats and cows is less advanced): born heavier and more mature than human fetuses and after a shorter gestation period. Surgical procedures (i.e., hypophysectomy or adrenalectomy) and catheterization of fetal blood vessels for days or even weeks were practiced on fetuses from 90 days' gestation (25 cm, 500 g) until term (147 days). By day 90 many endocrine glands have already been functioning for a month or so. The discovery that in sheep the fetal endocrine system initiates parturition (72) has aroused deep interest in fetal endocrinology in this species.

The chronological profile of the fetal adrenocortical function throughout development remains to be explored in additional species. It should be kept in mind that comparing developmental chronology from one species to the other in terms of percentage of the gestation period has no physiological meaning.

FUNCTIONAL DEVELOPMENT OF FETAL ADRENAL CORTEX

Maturational Changes

During prenatal development the fetal adrenal cortex undergoes changes that need further elucidation. Growth of adrenal glands in rat, sheep, and human fetuses is illustrated in Figures 1–3. In the rat fetus the adrenals stop growing the day before birth (12), and this probably corresponds to diminished physiological activity; on the other hand, in the lamb fetus there is a spurt in adrenal growth before birth (see Fig. 2).

During the first part of development, the adrenals grow more rapidly than the whole body; their weight (relative to the weight of the whole fetus) increases until it reaches a maximum, between the 12th and the 17th week (75–150 g) in the human fetus (27) and on day 18 in the rat (12). Thereafter their relative weight decreases, even in the human fetus, in which they remain exceedingly large until birth.

In the rat, day 18 coincides with a maximum in adrenal corticosterone content (60), which probably precedes a spurt in hormone release (36). In the human fetal adrenals, a shift in cellular differentiation occurs after the third month, as revealed by the electron microscope (43, 74) and by biochemical analyses. The younger glands contain mainly C-19 steroids; cortisol was detected after the 16th week (7). In adrenal tissue incubated in vitro with labeled progesterone, the 21-hydroxylase activity (103) and the percentage of conversion of progesterone to cortisol (73) increase during the same period. There is a parallel change in the histochemically detectable 3β-hydroxysteroid dehydrogenase activity (34). It is not unlikely that the aforementioned changes coincide with increased hypophysial corticostimulating activity (99).

Hypophysial Control of Adrenal Development and Function

Many experiments initiated in the late 1940s on small laboratory animals [rats (104), mice (93), rabbits (44)] showed that removal of the pituitary by fetal decapitation or by destruction of the head by X-rays (93)

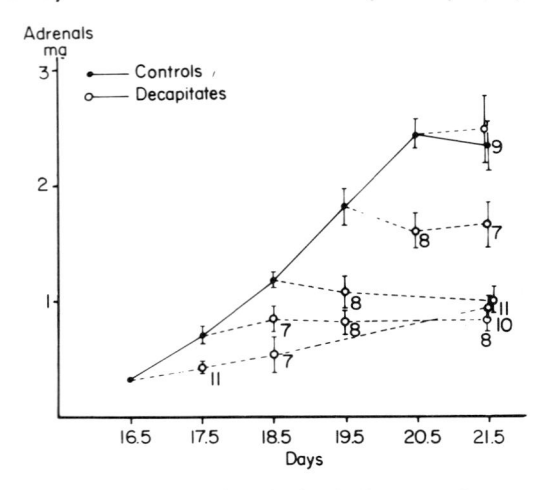

FIG. 1. Weight of 1 pair of adrenal glands from rat fetuses, according to age. *Closed circles*, controls (i.e., unoperated mothers). *Open circles*, decapitates. In each case decapitation was done at the stage corresponding to the *closed circle* at which *dashed line* begins. After day 20, growth of adrenals is stopped in controls and decapitates. Number of decapitates and confidence intervals (*vertical bars*) as indicated. [From Jost (49).]

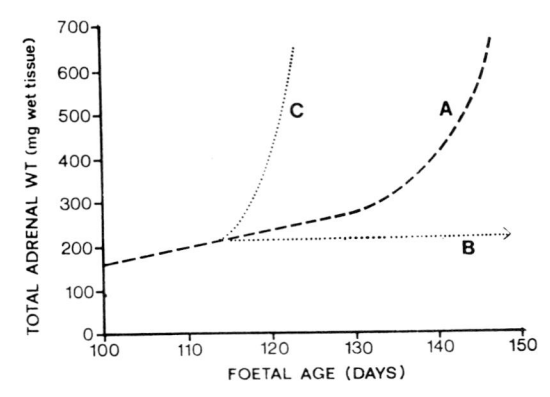

FIG. 2. Patterns of fetal adrenal growth in experimental lambs compared with pattern in normal fetuses. A, normal fetuses. B, fetal adrenal hypoplasia after fetal hypophysectomy, which led to prolonged gestation. C, adrenal hyperplasia after infusion of ACTH into a fetus, which led to premature parturition. [Adapted from Liggins (70).]

provokes stunted growth of the fetal adrenal glands. This change can be reversed by giving ACTH to the headless fetus. It should be noticed that maternal ACTH does not prevent adrenocortical atrophy in fetuses deprived of their pituitary gland [for reviews of earlier experiments, see (45, 48, 57, 58)].

An insight into the real significance of the hypophysial action on adrenal growth is given by a comparative study of the growth of the rat adrenals in the presence or absence of the pituitary gland [Fig. 1; (49)]. In control fetuses the adrenals grow steadily between day 16.5 and 20.5, whereas in fetuses decapitated on day 16.5, the adrenals are atrophic on day 21.5. However, in the absence of the pituitary they do not lose weight—they continue to grow at a very slow rate. The comparison of the growth curve of the adrenals in controls and in pituitary-less fetuses gives a measure of the significance of the pituitary stimulus for adrenal growth. In fetuses decapitated before or on day 18, approximately the same final adrenal weight is obtained on day 21.5. This weight is gained more rapidly in the presence of the pituitary than in its absence. In those fetuses decapitated later (i.e., on days 19.5 and 20.5) the initial adrenal weight is maintained until day 21.5. Some benefit from the pituitary stimulation obtained on the day of decapitation is retained for the succeeding days. However, despite maintained weight, histological changes still take place, particularly a reduction in size of the individual cortical cells (50). A similar type of pituitary control of adrenal growth was observed in rabbit fetuses (49). In Figure 2 termination of adrenal growth in lamb fetuses hypophysectomized by Liggins (70) on day 115 [confirmed by Comline et al. (16)] is illustrated; the anticipated adrenal growth under the influence of a large dose of adrenocorticotropic hormone (ACTH) is also shown.

In human newborns lacking a pituitary gland the adrenal glands are very small [cases of cyclopia (9, 25, 84) or of pituitary absence (5, 9, 94)]. It is likely that, in these infants, growth of the adrenals became insignificant from a certain stage, as in decapitated rat fetuses (Fig. 1) or in anencephalic monsters (Fig. 3).

Adrenal underdevelopment resulting from defective hypophysial stimulation is accompanied with decreased or absent endocrine function and is discussed in the section devoted to adrenal function.

Functional relations between fetal pituitary and adrenal cortex are substantiated by many feedback effects observed in the fetus [for review, see (48, 57)]. Many experiments were made on rat fetuses: an excess of corticosteroids in the fetus produced by giving hormones to the mother rat (17, 18), by submitting it to a stress (12, 88), or by injecting hormones into the fetus (56) depresses the size of the fetal adrenals. This is prevented if ACTH is injected into the fetus with the steroid (45). The excess of corticoids decreases the ACTH content of the fetal pituitary (99). Conversely, adrenalectomizing the pregnant female rat results in adrenal hypertrophy of the young at term (38, 56). This fetal adrenal hypertrophy in an adrenalectomized female does not occur if the fetus is injected with cortisone or deprived of its pituitary by decapitation (56, 57); it evidently involves the fetal pituitary. Unilateral fetal adrenalectomy is followed by enlargement of the remaining gland, unless the fetus is given cortisone (63) or is decapitated (80). Adrenal hypertrophy is produced by inhibitors of steroid hydroxylases (33).

Similar observations have been made only on a limited number of animals so far. Maternal adrenalectomy results in increased size of fetal adrenals also in mice (26). Overloading the mother with adrenocortical hormones has been reported to decrease the size of the fetal adrenals in some women given corticosteroids (37, 82) or suffering from Cushing's syndrome (66) and in monkeys given ACTH (96). The last observation indicates that, in this species, corticosteroids are more readily transferred from mother to fetus than is ACTH; this seems to be a rather general rule. Transplacental transfer of corticosteroids has been demonstrated in a few species, including man, at definite gestational stages, but differences from species to species and according to gestational age are likely to occur. For instance, in the rat, cortisol seems not to be as readily transferred from mother to fetus on day 17 as on day 21 (47).

Hypothalamic Control of Hypophysial Corticostimulating Activity

Jost et al. (51) have reviewed evidence for the hypothalamic control of the corticostimulating activity of the fetal pituitary. The hypothalamus of rat fetuses was removed with the whole brain ("encephalectomy"), leaving the pituitary in situ in the sella turcica (48, 49, 52). In fetuses encephalectomized on day 19.5, the adrenals are practically as reduced on day 21.5 as in pituitary-less fetuses; corticotropin-releasing factor (CRF) administered at the time of surgery permits a subnormal adrenal growth in the former, but not in the latter, fetuses (49, 52). These results indicate a hypothalamic control of the pituitary adrenocorticotropic function. However, there is evidence that the pituitary is capable of some activity independently from the hypothalamus: in adrenalectomized females the adrenals of the encephalectomized fetuses increase in size, as do (to a larger extent) the adrenals of intact fetuses (23); this increase is absent in decapitates (56). Similarly the adrenals of encephalectomized fetuses slightly increase in size after metyrapone administration to the mother, whereas those of pituitary-less fetuses do not (21).

Reduced adrenals were also observed in rat fetuses with electrocoagulated hypothalamus (31) and in lamb fetuses with sectioned pituitary stalk (70).

FETAL STRESS. The pituitary-adrenal system of rat fetuses responds to stresses, such as an injection of epinephrine (76, 77) or of formaldehyde solution (13), by a depletion of the adrenal ascorbic acid; this stress reaction is absent in encephalectomized fetuses (13). Liggins (70) observed an adrenal hypertrophy in lamb fetuses injected with Clostridium toxin, at 110–140 days of age.

HUMAN ANENCEPHALS. In human anencephalic monsters the adrenal cortex is strikingly smaller at term than in normal infants, although usually some more or less abnormal anterior pituitary tissue is present (2). The hypothalamicohypophysial relations are either profoundly disturbed or absent. It has been suggested that the defect of hypothalamic influence on the adenohypophysis causes deficient hypophysial corticostimulating activity (100). This interpretation is supported by the experiments on rats and is strengthened by the fact that in newborn anencephalic infants ACTH induces adrenal hypertrophy (68).

Data on the weight of adrenal glands in control and in

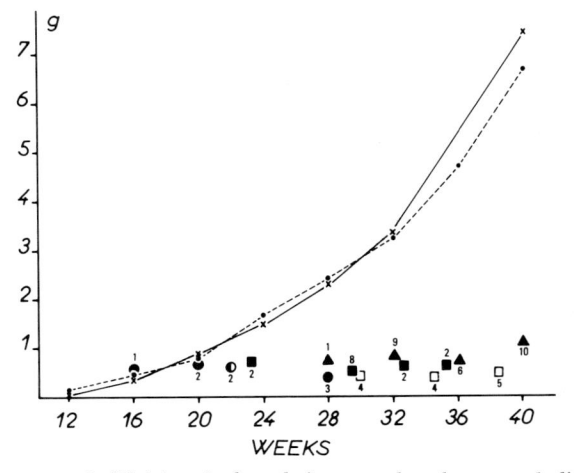

FIG. 3. Weight of adrenals in normal and anencephalic American and Japanese human fetuses. *Solid line*, normal American fetuses, weights recalculated from Jackson's data (39). *Dashed line*, normal Japanese fetuses (65). Individual values or average weight of several cases (*number* indicated) of anencephalic fetuses: *open squares*, data from Ch'in (10); *closed squares*, data from Kind (62); *closed circles*, data from Kiyono (64); *half-open circles*, data from Nichols (79); and *triangles*, data from Vaclav (101).

anencephalic fetuses are plotted in Figure 3. It appears that the hypothalamic defect impairs growth of the adrenals after the 20th week rather than producing any marked decrease in weight (compare adrenal growth curves of decapitated rat fetuses in Fig. 1 with those of human anencephals in Fig. 3). In normal human fetuses the amount of ACTH present in the pituitary increases after the 19th week (87).

PROBLEM OF HUMAN FETAL ADRENAL CORTEX

The adrenal gland of the human fetus is extremely large because of the huge development of an internal zone ("fetal zone") that regresses after birth. The outer zone, which makes up most of the postnatal cortex, is sometimes called the "adult cortex." It is much less developed than the inner part in the human fetus. The structure of the human fetal cortex, and probably also its intense biochemical activity, is rather exceptional. A similar fetal zone is present in the chimpanzee and a few other primates (67).

There is little doubt that in some way the extreme development of the human fetal adrenal cortex is linked with the intense steroid metabolism in the "fetoplacental unit" (19), which accompanies and perhaps hinders the production of adrenocortical hormones. Therefore a glance at some major aspects of this metabolism is necessary, the biochemical details being dealt with in another chapter in this volume of the *Handbook*.

The fetal adrenal cortex has a very large spectrum of enzymes capable of metabolizing steroids, but some important enzymatic systems are almost inactive (e.g., the 3β-hydroxysteroid dehydrogenase system and the aromatizing system permitting the synthesis of estrogens), whereas other systems (e.g., C-17–20 desmolase for Δ^5-17α-hydroxysteroids and sulfokinases) are very active. For several enzymes the reverse situation prevails in the placenta (e.g., very active sulfatases and aromatizing systems). Thus the adrenal gland largely uses precursors made by the placenta and releases steroids [mainly dehydroepiandrosterone sulfate or androst-5-ene-17-one-3β-yl sulfate (DHAS)], which are transformed again by the placenta (19).

At midterm the human fetal adrenal cortex is capable of making steroids from acetate and of converting cholesterol into pregnenolone. Actually the major precursors for adrenal steroids seem to be placental progesterone and pregnenolone. These two precursors correspond to two distinct metabolic pathways (Figs. 4 and 5) because little pregnenolone is converted to progesterone. The 3β-hydroxydehydrogenase-$\Delta^5 \rightarrow \Delta^4$-isomerase system is almost inactive on pregnenolone, but it has been recently shown to have some activity on Δ^5-3β,21-dihydroxy- or on Δ^5-3β,17α,21-trihydroxysteroids [Fig. 4; (85)]. The quantitative importance of this pathway probably is limited, because C-17–21 desmolase actively removes the side chain from Δ^5-steroids [Fig. 4; (90)], whereas it does not seem to do so with Δ^4-steroids (Fig. 5). Moreover many steroids are extensively sulfated in the fetal adrenals. Thus dehydroepiandrosterone (DHA) and its sulfate (DHAS) are abundant secretory products that serve as precursors for placental synthesis of estrone and estradiol.

The fetal adrenal also has a very active 16α-hydroxylating activity, and several 16α-hydroxylated compounds (e.g., 16α-hydroxy-DHA and its sulfate) are substrates for estriol synthesis in the placenta.

The role of the fetal adrenal in providing precursors for placental synthesis of estrogens is reflected in the low estrogen (mainly in the form of estriol) excretion in pregnancies with anencephalic infants whose adrenals are very reduced in size (29, 30). In the cord blood of

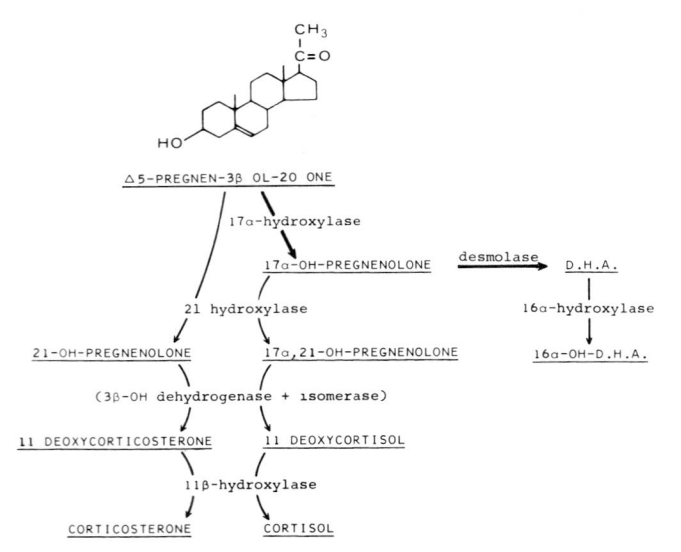

FIG. 4. Some metabolic pathways of pregnenolone in human fetal adrenal. *D.H.A.*, dehydroepiandrosterone. Sulfatation has been omitted. *Heavy line*, preferential pathway.

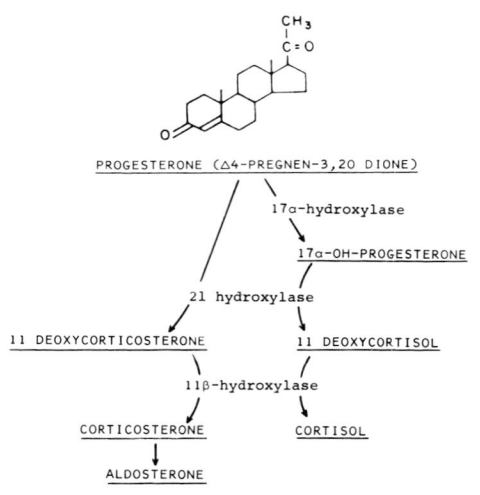

FIG. 5. Some metabolic pathways of progesterone in human fetal adrenal. Sulfatation has been omitted.

such infants, DHA, 16α-hydroxy-DHA, and their sulfates are present in very small amounts (24). A parallelism exists between the growth curve of the fetal adrenals (Fig. 3) and the curve of estrogen excretion during pregnancy.

The reason the human fetal adrenals are so exceedingly large and active still is difficult to explain in a straightforward way. A possible functional difference between the outer and the inner (fetal) cortex has been suggested, but the difference seems to be more quantitative than strictly qualitative; this question is still under investigation (97). In the past, human chorionic gonadotrophin (HCG) has been held responsible for the adrenal hypertrophy, but the adrenals still increase in size when HCG secretion decreases during the third month, and HCG levels are not lowered in pregnancies with anencephalic infants (29, 30). However, Johannisson (43) observed morphological changes reminiscent of those produced by ACTH in the adrenals of midterm fetuses given HCG.

To some extent the human fetal adrenals, for their huge volume and high rate of production of C-19 steroids, resemble the postnatal hypertrophied adrenals present in cases of congenital defect of 21- or 11β-hydroxylase, but androgens virilizing the female infant are produced only in the latter. In the adrenogenital syndrome the shortage of cortisol is responsible for an excessive ACTH release. In the normal fetus, feedback mechanisms already exist, as shown, for instance, by adrenal atrophy and diminished DHAS and 16α-hydroxy-DHAS in cord blood (98) in infants of women overloaded with corticosteroids; the fetal adrenal changes result in a decreased maternal estriol excretion. The strong stimulation of the adrenals in the normal fetus might result from a shortage of cortisol, either because the rate of synthesis is low or because the synthesized cortisol rapidly disappears (81). The high maternal concentration of plasma transcortin could be one factor; a rapid inactivation of adrenocortical hormones by sulfatation or hydrogenation, in the liver and other fetal organs, and the irreversible conversion of cortisol to cortisone in the fetus (86) could be other factors.

FUNCTIONS OF FETAL ADRENAL CORTEX

Information about the function of the fetal adrenal glands remains scattered, and the subject needs more research. Data have been gathered for different species at different developmental periods, and information concerning the human fetus—except for that related to estrogen metabolism—remains rare. Production of adrenocortical hormones by the fetus has been shown in several species [e.g., lamb (1, 3, 15) and dog (40) fetus in vivo; mouse, rabbit, calf (11), rat, and guinea pig (6) adrenal tissue in vitro], but the curve of secretion throughout pregnancy has not yet been established.

So far the physiological role of aldosterone in the fetus is not clearly understood.

Effects on Fetal Organs

Adrenal hormones are not indispensable for the survival of the rat fetus, since fetuses adrenalectomized on day 18.5 survived and developed to term in adrenalectomized mothers (41). Cases of hormonal synthetic block in humans or of fetal adrenalectomy in sheep are not as conclusive, since maternal hormones could have reached the young.

GLYCOGEN DEPOSITION IN FETAL LIVER. The role of adrenocortical hormones in glycogen deposition in the fetal liver has been mainly studied in rabbit and rat fetuses, after the initial observation of Jost & Hatey (53) that early decapitation of the rabbit fetus prevents the storage of glycogen in the liver [for review, see (58)]. In the decapitated rabbit fetus, corticosteroids given alone do not suffice to induce liver glycogen storage: addition of growth hormone, prolactin, or rat placental extracts is necessary; glycogen storage seems to obey a dual control involving a pituitary or a pituitary-like hormone and corticosteroids (46, 58). In the rat fetus the system is easier to explore, perhaps because placental prolactin-like material reaches the fetus (46, 55). Depriving the rat fetus of corticosteroids by maternal adrenalectomy, in addition to either fetal decapitation, which impairs adrenocortical function (41, 54), or fetal adrenalectomy (41), prevents glycogen deposition (Fig. 6); corticosteroids given either to the mother or to the fetus permit glycogen storage (41). In nonadrenalectomized mother rats, the maternal corticosteroids also permit subnormal glycogen deposition in decapitated fetuses (41). Corticosteroids can induce either

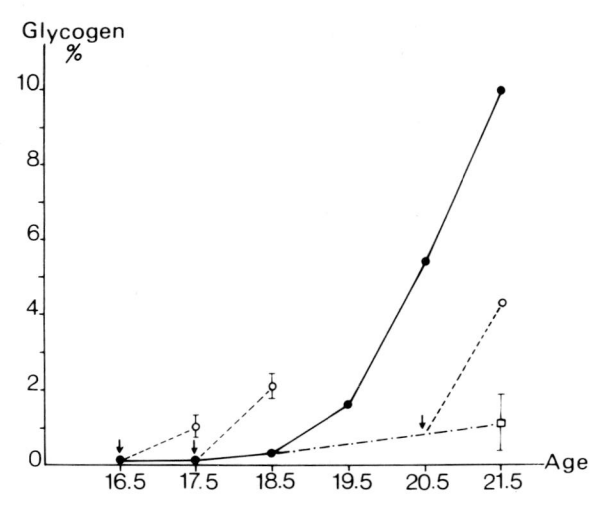

FIG. 6. Glycogen content in liver of rat fetuses, according to age in days and under various experimental conditions (i.e., percentage of fresh tissue). *Closed circles*, controls (i.e., normal mothers); *squares*, fetuses, in adrenalectomized females, decapitated on day 18.5; *open circles*, fetuses injected with 100 μg cortisol (*arrow*) 24 hr before killing. Early glycogen storage occurs in the entire fetus given cortisol on day 16.5 or 17.5. Delayed glycogen storage occurs after a cortisol injection on day 20 in decapitates of adrenalectomized females. [From Jost & Picon (58).]

delayed glycogen storage, when injected into corticosteroid-deprived fetuses, or anticipated glycogen storage, when given to the fetus prior to normal glycogen accumulation [(49); see Fig. 6]. Glycogen synthesis can also be induced in isolated fetal hepatocytes treated with cortisol in vitro (91).

Several aspects of the action of corticosteroids on fetal liver glycogen were studied in the rat: *a*) the enzymes involved and their hormonal control (42, 58, 92); *b*) electron-microscopic aspect of hepatocytes and glycogen particles: in fetuses deprived of corticosteroids from day 17 on, the hepatocytes do not differentiate much beyond the state obtained on day 18 in control fetuses (28); an early injection of cortisol anticipates the maturation of the hepatocytes in young fetuses (22); *c*) effects of corticosteroids on the size of the glycogen particles extracted from the liver by mercuric chloride: rapid glycogen accumulation results mainly from an increased number of small particles (102); this also appears in the electron-microscopic studies; *d*) early effects of cortisol on nuclei and nucleoli of the hepatocytes and on uridine incorporation (32) during the 12 hr preceding the increase in UDP-glucose-glycogen glucosyltransferase activity (92) and glycogen storage.

In hypophysectomized sheep fetuses the concentration of liver glycogen was reduced (70). In the rat fetus, corticosteroids seem to control glycogen storage in the heart (89).

EFFECTS ON MATURATION OF ADRENAL MEDULLA. Jost & Roffi (59) found very small amounts of medullary hormones in adrenals of decapitated rat or rabbit fetuses in which the cortex was very reduced in size; actually the amount of epinephrine is extremely reduced, whereas norepinephrine is rather increased (49, 95). Adrenocorticotropic hormone or large doses of cortisol given to the fetus repair these changes. This is due to the control exerted by the fetal adrenocortical hormones on the activity of phenylethanolamine *N*-methyltransferase (75), the enzyme responsible for the methylation of norepinephrine into epinephrine (Fig. 7). The activity of this enzyme is also controlled by corticosteroids in adult rats (105). Extremely small amounts of epinephrine were also present in the adrenals of hypophysectomized lamb fetuses (16).

These results demonstrate the role of the fetal adrenal cortex in the maturation of the adrenal medulla and its full ability to produce epinephrine. It is noteworthy that, in the rat fetus, maternal hormones do not reach the fetus in amounts sufficient to act on the adrenal medulla. For this effect the fetus must rely on its own adrenocortical hormones.

EFFECTS ON THYMUS AND HEMATOPOIETIC TISSUE. Fetal adrenocortical hormones seem to decrease the size of the thymus and the number of the hematopoietic cells in the liver, since these tissues are abnormally well developed in decapitated rabbit or rat fetuses. Adrenocorticotropic hormone decreases the size of the thymus (4), and cortisol decreases the amount of hematopoietic tissue in the liver (22, 78). The thymus of human anencephals is excessively large (10).

Effect on Parturition

For a long time the fetus has been considered to play no role in the termination of pregnancy and in delivery, on the basis of experiments made on rats, mice, and monkeys. When the fetuses were surgically removed, the placentas left in situ were delivered at normal term. An active part played by the fetal endocrine glands, especially by the pituitary and adrenal cortex, in determining delivery was discovered in sheep fetuses by Liggins et al. (72) and probably holds true for other ruminants (goat, cow). Lamb fetuses hypophysectomized (70, 72) or adrenalectomized (20) in utero fail to be delivered and finally die in utero. On the contrary, premature delivery can be induced in the ewe within about 4 days by infusing ACTH or glucocorticoids into the fetus; the same doses given to the mother remain inefficient (69, 71). During the 4 days preceding normal parturition, a pronounced rise in fetal plasma cortisol content and turnover occurs [(3, 15); Fig. 8]. The mechanism of action of the fetal hormone on the maternal uterus is currently under investigation.

Premature delivery is also produced in goats by infusing synthetic ACTH for 6 days into the fetus (G. D. Thorburn, D. H. Nicol, and J. M. Bassett, personal communication). Failure of parturition has been reported in Guernsey cows carrying fetuses with pituitary aplasia and hypocorticism (35, 61), but so far there is little indication that participation of the fetal adrenals in delivery is a general rule for all mammals. It has been reported that human pregnancies with anencephalic fetuses are

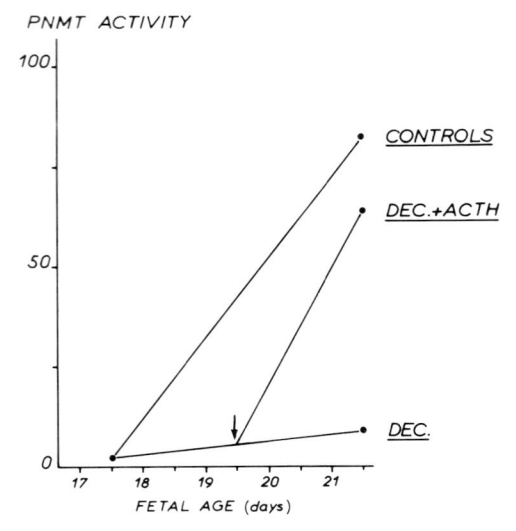

FIG. 7. Activity of phenylethanolamine *N*-methyltransferase (*PNMT*) in adrenals of rat fetuses, expressed per pair of adrenals. Increase between days 17.5 and 21.5 in controls; low values in fetuses decapitated on day 17.5 (*DEC.*); increased values in similarly decapitated fetuses given 1 IU of ACTH on day 19.5 (*arrow*). [Adapted from Margolis et al. (75).]

usually prolonged (14). Pregnancy is also prolonged in Addisonian mothers (83). The causative mechanisms remain to be explored.

Fetal Adrenocortical Insufficiency and Postnatal Survival

The survival of newborn infants suffering from severe adrenocortical deficiency (e.g., 3β-hydroxysteroid dehydrogenase deficiency or absence of a pituitary gland) is usually very short (8). Similarly, calves born with a congenital adrenal deficiency survive only briefly unless they are immediately treated (35). An unsolved question concerning such cases is whether maternal hormones reaching the fetus through the placenta could replace the effects of the adrenocortical glands on target tissues, or whether in these newborns there are physiological defects, as well as adrenal insufficiency, at birth.

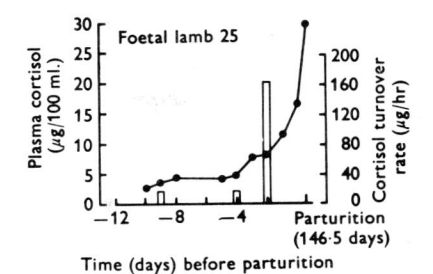

FIG. 8. Plasma cortisol concentration (*circles*) and turnover (*squares*) in fetal lamb during days preceding parturition. [From Comline et al. (15).]

REFERENCES

1. ALEXANDER, D. P., H. G. BRITTON, V. T. H. JAMES, D. A. NIXON, R. A. PARKER, E. M. WINTOUR, AND R. D. WRIGHT. Steroid secretion by the adrenal gland of foetal and neonatal sheep. *J. Endocrinol.* 40: 1–13, 1968.
2. ANGEVINE, D. M. Pathologic anatomy of hypophysis and adrenals in anencephaly. *Arch. Pathol.* 26: 507–518, 1938.
3. BASSETT, J. M., AND D. B. THORBURN. Foetal plasma corticosteroids and the initiation of parturition in sheep. *J. Endocrinol.* 44: 285–286, 1968.
4. BEARN, J. G. Hormonal control of the development of the thymus of the fetal rabbit. *Nature* 192: 875–876, 1961.
5. BLIZZARD, R. M., AND M. ALBERTS. Hypopituitarism, hypoadrenalism, and hypogonadism in the newborn infant. *J. Pediat.* 48: 783–792, 1956.
6. BLOCH, E. The metabolism of 7-³H-pregnenolone and 4-¹⁴C-progesterone by adrenal homogenates of fetal guinea-pigs and other mammalian fetuses. *Steroids* 14: 598–603, 1969.
7. BLOCH, E., K. BENIRSCHKE, AND E. ROSEMBERG. C₁₉ steroid, 17α-hydroxycorticosterone and a sodium retaining factor in human fetal adrenal glands. *Endocrinology* 58: 626–633, 1956.
8. BONGIOVANNI, A. M., W. R. EBERLEIN, A. S. GOLDMAN, AND M. NEW. Disorders of adrenal steroid biogenesis. *Recent Progr. Hormone Res.* 23: 375–479, 1967.
9. BREWER, D. B. Congenital absence of the pituitary gland and its consequences. *J. Pathol. Bacteriol.* 73: 59–67, 1957.
10. CH'IN, K. Y. The endocrine glands of anencephalic foetuses: a quantitative and morphological study of 15 cases. *Chinese Med. J. Suppl.* 2: 63–90, 1938.
11. CHOURAQUI, J., AND J. P. WENIGER. Identification des corticostéroides sécrétés par les surrénales embryonnaires de veau, lapin et souris cultivées in vitro. *Acta Endocrinol.* 65: 650–662, 1970.
12. COHEN, A. Corrélations entre l'hypophyse et le cortex surrénal chez le foetus de rat. Le cortex surrénal du nouveau-né. *Arch. Anat. Microscop. Morphol. Exptl.* 52: 277–407, 1963.
13. COHEN, A., J-C. PERNOD, AND A. JOST. Rôle de l'hypothalamus dans la réponse des surrénales du foetus de rat à une agression par le formol. *Compt. Rend. Soc. Biol.* 162: 2070–2073, 1968.
14. COMERFORD, J. B. Pregnancy with anencephaly. *Lancet* 1: 679–680, 1965.
15. COMLINE, R. S., P. W. NATHANIELSZ, R. B. PAISEY, AND M. SILVER. Cortisol turnover in the sheep foetus immediately prior to parturition. *J. Physiol., London* 210: 141–142P, 1970.
16. COMLINE, R. S., M. SILVER, AND I. A. SILVER. Effect of foetal hypophysectomy on catecholamine levels in the lamb adrenal during prolonged gestation. *Nature* 225: 739–740, 1970.
17. COURRIER, R., A. COLONGE, AND M. BACLESSE. Action de la cortisone administrée à la mère sur la surrénale du foetus de rat. *Compt. Rend.* 233: 333–336, 1951.
18. DAVIS, M. E., AND E. J. PLOTZ. The effects of cortisone acetate on intact and adrenalectomized rats during pregnancy. *Endocrinology* 54: 384–395, 1954.
19. DICZFALUSY, E., R. PION, AND J. SCHWERS. Steroid biogenesis and metabolism in the human foeto-placental unit at midpregnancy. *Arch. Anat. Microscop. Morphol. Exptl.* 54: 67–84, 1965.
20. DROST, M., AND L. W. HOLM. Prolonged gestation in ewes after foetal adrenalectomy. *J. Endocrinol.* 40: 293–296, 1968.
21. DUPOUY, J. P. Réponse du complexe hypothalamo-hypophysaire du foetus de rat à un blocage de la biosynthèse des corticostéroides par la metopirone. Influence du cortisol. *Compt. Rend.* 273: 962–965, 1971.
22. DUPOUY, J. P., AND A. JOST. Aspect ultrastructural de l'accumulation anticipée de glycogène dans le foie du foetus de rat soumis au cortisol. *Arch. Anat. Microscop. Morphol. Exptl.* 58: 183–202, 1969.
23. DUPOUY, J. P., AND A. JOST. Activité corticotrope de l'hypos physe foetale du rat: influence de l'hypothalamus et decorticostéroides. *Compt. Rend. Soc. Biol.* 164: 2422–2427, 1970.
24. EASTERLING, W. E., JR., H. H. SIMMER, W. J. DIGNAM, M. W. FRANKLAND, AND F. NATFOLIN. Neutral C 19 steroid sulfates in human pregnancy. II. Dehydroepiandrosterone sulfate, 16α hydroxy-dehydroepiandrosterone and 16α hydroxy-dehydroepiandrosterone sulfate in maternal and fetal blood of pregnancies with anencephalic and normal fetuses. *Steroids* 8: 157–178, 1966.
25. EDMONDS, H. W. Pituitary, adrenal and thyroid in cyclopia. *Arch. Pathol.* 50: 727–735, 1950.
26. EGUCHI, Y. Experimental studies on the adrenal cortex of the mouse fetus. I. Effects of maternal adrenalectomy on the adrenal of the fetus based on histology and volume determination. *Embryologia* 5: 206–218, 1960.
27. EKHOLM, E., AND K. NIEMINEVA. On prenatal changes in relative weights of human adrenals, thymus and thyroid gland. *Acta Paediat.* 39: 67–86, 1950.
28. FAVARD, P., AND A. JOST. Différenciation et charge en glycogène de l'hépatocyte du foetus de rat normal ou décapité (étude au microscope électronique). *Arch. Anat. Microscop. Morphol. Exptl.* 55: 603–632, 1966.
29. FRANDSEN, V. A., AND G. STAKEMANN. The site of production of oestrogenic hormones in human pregnancy. Hormone

excretion in pregnancy with anencephalic fetus. *Acta Endocrinol.* 38: 383–391, 1961.
30. FRANDSEN, V. A., AND G. STAKEMANN. The site of production of oestrogenic hormones in human pregnancy. III. Further observations on the hormone excretion in pregnancy with anencephalic foetus. *Acta Endocrinol.* 47: 265–276, 1964.
31. FUJITA, T., Y. EGUCHI, Y. MORIKAWA, AND Y. HASHIMOTO. Hypothalamic-hypophysial adrenal and thyroid systems: observations on fetal rats subjected to hypothalamic destruction, brain compression and hypervitaminosis A. *Anat. Record* 166: 659–672, 1970.
32. GIRARD, J., AND A. JOST. Action du cortisol sur le noyau et les nucléoles des hépatocytes de foetus de rats privés de corticostéroides. *Arch. Anat. Microscop. Morphol. Exptl.* 59: 319–330, 1970.
33. GOLDMAN, A. S. Experimental model of congenital adrenal cortical hyperplasia produced in utero with an inhibitor of 11β-steroid hydroxylase. *J. Clin. Endocrinol. Metab.* 27: 1390–1394, 1967.
34. GOLDMAN, A. S., W. C. YAKOVAC, AND A. M. BONGIOVANNI. Development of activity of 3β-hydroxysteroid dehydrogenase in human fetal tissues and in two anencephalic newborns. *J. Clin. Endocrinol. Metab.* 26: 14–22, 1966.
35. HOLM, L. W., H. R. PARKER, AND S. J. GALLIGAN. Adrenal insufficiency in postmature Holstein calves. *Am. J. Obstet. Gynecol.* 81: 1000–1008, 1961.
36. HOLT, P. G., AND I. T. OLIVER. Plasma corticosterone concentration in the perinatal rat. *Biochem. J.* 108: 339–341, 1968.
37. HOTTINGER, A. Vorübergehende passive nebennieren Insuffizienz beim Neugeborenen. *Schweiz. Med. Wochschr.* 89: 419–422, 1959.
38. INGLE, D. J., AND G. T. FISHER. Effects of adrenalectomy during gestation on the size of the adrenal glands of newborn rats. *Proc. Soc. Exptl. Biol. Med.* 39: 149–150, 1938.
39. JACKSON, C. M. On the prenatal growth of the human body and the relative growth of the various organs and parts. *Am. J. Anat.* 9: 119–165, 1909.
40. JACKSON, B. T., AND G. J. PIASECKI. Fetal secretion of glucocorticoids. *Endocrinology* 85: 875–880, 1969.
41. JACQUOT, R. Recherches sur le contrôle endocrinien de l'accumulation de glycogène dans le foie chez le foetus de rat. *J. Physiol., Paris* 51: 655–721, 1959.
42. JACQUOT, R., AND N. KRETCHMER. Effect of fetal decapitation on enzymes of glycogen metabolism. *J. Biol. Chem.* 239: 1301–1304, 1964.
43. JOHANNISSON, E. The foetal adrenal cortex in the human. Its ultrastructure at different stages of development and in different functional states. *Acta Endocrinol. Suppl.* 130, 1968.
44. JOST, A. Influence de la décapitation sur le développement du tractus génital et des surrénales de l'embryon de lapin. *Compt. Rend. Soc. Biol.* 142: 273–275, 1948.
45. JOST, A. La physiologie du cortex surrénal foetal et les interrelations endocriniennes entre la mère et le foetus. *Bull. Soc. Roy. Belg. Gynecol. Obstet.* 27: 1–16, 1957.
46. JOST, A. The role of fetal hormones in prenatal development. *Harvey Lectures Ser.* 55: 201–226, 1961.
47. JOST, A. Désordres hormonaux et tératogenèse. *Bull. Acad. Suisse Sci. Med.* 20: 460–469, 1964.
48. JOST, A. Anterior pituitary function in foetal life. In: *The Pituitary Gland*, edited by G. W. Harris and B. T. Donavan. London: Butterworths, 1966, chapt. 9, p. 299–323.
49. JOST, A. Problems of fetal endocrinology: the adrenal glands. *Recent Progr. Hormone Res.* 22: 541–569, 1966.
50. JOST, A., AND A. COHEN. Signification de l' "atrophie" des surrénales foetales du rat provoquée par l'hypophysectomie (décapitation). *Develop. Biol.* 14: 154–168, 1966.
51. JOST, A., J. P. DUPOUY, AND A. GELOSO-MEYER. Hypothalamo-hypophyseal relationships in the fetus. In: *The Hypothalamus*, edited by L. Martini, M. Motta, and F. Fraschini. New York: Acad. Press, 1970, p. 605–615.
52. JOST, A., J. P. DUPOUY, AND A. MONCHAMP. Fonction corticotrope de l'hypophyse et hypothalamus chez le foetus de rat. *Compt. Rend.* 262: 147–150, 1966.
53. JOST, A., AND J. HATEY. Influence de la décapitation sur la teneur en glycogène du foie du foetus de lapin. *Compt. Rend. Soc. Biol.* 143: 146–147, 1949.
54. JOST, A., AND R. JACQUOT. Recherches sur le contrôle hormonal de la charge en glycogène du foie foetal du lapin et du rat. *Compt. Rend.* 239: 98–100, 1954.
55. JOST, A., AND R. JACQUOT. Sur le rôle de l'hypophyse, des surrénales et du placenta dans la synthèse de glycogène par le foie foetal du lapin et du rat. *Compt. Rend.* 247: 2459–2462, 1958.
56. JOST, A., R. JACQUOT, AND A. COHEN. Sur les interrelations entre les hormones cortico-surrénaliennes maternelles et la surrénale du foetus de rat. *Compt. Rend. Soc. Biol.* 149: 1319–1322, 1955.
57. JOST, A., R. JACQUOT, AND A. COHEN. The pituitary control of the foetal adrenal cortex. In: *Human Adrenal Cortex*, edited by A. R. Currie, T. Symington, and J. K. Grant. Edinburgh: Livingstone, 1962, p. 569–579.
58. JOST, A., AND L. PICON. Hormonal control of fetal development and metabolism. *Advan. Metab. Disorders* 4: 123–184, 1970.
59. JOST, A., AND J. ROFFI. Action de la cortisone et de l'hydrocortisone sur la teneur de la surrénale du rat et de la souris en substances hypertensives. *Compt. Rend.* 246: 163–165, 1958.
60. KAMOUN, A., C. MIALHE-VOLOSS, AND F. STUTINSKY. Evolution de la teneur en corticostérone de la surrénale foetale du rat. *Compt. Rend. Soc. Biol.* 158: 828–832, 1964.
61. KENNEDY, P. C., J. W. KENDRICK, AND C. STORMONT. Adenohypophyseal aplasia, an inherited defect associated with abnormal gestation in Guernesey cattle. *Cornell Vet.* 47: 160–178, 1957.
62. KIND, C. Das endokrine System der Anencephalen mit besonderer Berücksichtung der Schilddrüse. *Helv. Paediat. Acta* 3: 244–258, 1962.
63. KITCHELL, R. L., AND L. J. WELLS. Reciprocal relation between the hypophysis and adrenals in fetal rats: effects of unilateral adrenalectomy and of implanted cortisone, DOCA and sex hormones. *Endocrinology* 50: 83–93, 1952.
64. KIYONO, H. Die pathologische Anatomie der endokrinen Organe bei Anencephalie. *Arch. Pathol. Anat. Physiol.* 257: 441–476, 1925.
65. KONDO, S. Developmental studies on the Japanese human adrenals. I. Ponderal growth. *Bull. Exptl. Biol.* 9: 51–56, 1959.
66. KREINES, K., AND W. D. DE VAUX. Neonatal adrenal insufficiency associated with maternal Cushing's syndrome. *Pediatrics* 47: 516, 1971.
67. LANMAN, J. T. The adrenal fetal zone: its occurrence in primates and a possible relationship to chorionic gonadotropin. *Endocrinology* 61: 684–691, 1957.
68. LANMAN, J. Interpretation of human foetal adrenal structure and function. In: *Human Adrenal Cortex*, edited by A. R. Currie, T. Symington, and J. K. Grant. Edinburgh: Livingstone, 1962, p. 547–558.
69. LIGGINS, C. G. Premature parturition after infusion of corticotrophin or cortisol into foetal lambs. *J. Endocrinol.* 42: 323–329, 1968.
70. LIGGINS, G. C. The foetal role in the initiation of parturition in the ewe. In: *Foetal Autonomy*, edited by G. E. W. Wolstenholme and M. O'Connor. London: Churchill, 1969, p. 218–244.
71. LIGGINS, C. G. Premature delivery of foetal lambs infused with glucocorticoids. *J. Endocrinol.* 45: 515–523, 1969.
72. LIGGINS, C. G., P. C. KENNEDY, AND L. W. HOLM. Failure of initiation of parturition after electrocoagulation of the pituitary of the fetal lamb. *Am. J. Obstet. Gynecol.* 98: 1080–1086, 1967.
73. LONGCHAMPT, J., AND R. L. AXELROD. Contribution to

steroid biosynthesis in human adrenals. *Trans. Intern. Study Group Steroid Hormones, Roma, 1963*, p. 269-277.
74. McNutt, S. N., and A. L. Jones. Observations on the ultrastructure of cytodifferentiation in the human fetal adrenal cortex. *Lab. Invest.* 22: 513-527, 1970.
75. Margolis, F. L., J. Roffi, and A. Jost. Norepinephrine methylation in fetal rat adrenals. *Science* 154: 275-276, 1966.
76. Milkovic, K., and S. Milkovic. The reactivity of the rat fetal pituitary-adrenal system during the last days of pregnancy. *Arch. Intern. Physiol. Biochim.* 66: 534-539, 1958.
77. Milkovic, K., and S. Milkovic. Studies of the pituitary-adrenocortical system in the fetal rat. *Endocrinology* 71: 799-802, 1962.
78. Nagel, J., and R. Jacquot. Le tissu hématopoïétique dans le foie foetal du rat en fin de gestation. III. Influence de l'hypophysectomie foetale. *Arch. Anat. Microscop. Morphol. Exptl.* 58: 97-104, 1969.
79. Nichols, J. Observations on the adrenal of the premature anencephalic fetus. *Arch. Pathol.* 62: 312-317, 1956.
80. Noumura, T. Development of the hypophyseal-adrenocortical system in the rat embryo in relation to the maternal system. *Japan. J. Zool.* 12: 279-299, 1959.
81. Oakey, R. E. The progressive increase in estrogen production in human pregnancy: an appraisal of the factors responsible. *Vitamins Hormones* 28: 1-36, 1970.
82. Oppenheimer, E. H. Lesions in the adrenals of an infant following maternal corticosteroid therapy. *Bull. Johns Hopkins Hosp.* 114: 146-151, 1964.
83. Osler, M. Addison's disease and pregnancy. *Acta Endocrinol.* 41: 67-78, 1962.
84. Ozawa, M. Ein Sektionsfall von Zyklopie. Zur Einteilung des 4. und 5. Typus Bocks. *Japan. J. Med. Sci.* 4: 189-195, 1939.
85. Pasqualini, J. R., J. Lowy, T. Albepart, N. Wiqvist, and E. Diczfaluzy. Studies on the metabolism of corticosteroids in the human foeto-placental unit. 3. Role of 21-hydroxy-pregnenolone in the biosynthesis of corticosteroids. *Acta Endocrinol.* 63: 11-20, 1970.
86. Pasqualini, J. R., B. L. Nguyen, F. Ubrich, N. Wiqvist, and E. Diczfalusy. Cortisol and cortisone metabolism, in the human foeto-placental unit at midgestation. *J. Steroid Biochem.* 1: 209-219, 1970.
87. Pavlova, E. B., T. S. Pronina, and Y. B. Skebelskaya. Histostructure of adenohypophysis of human fetuses and contents of somatotropic and adrenocorticotropic hormones. *Gen. Comp. Endocrinol.* 10: 269-276, 1968.
88. Picon, L. Influence de l'hyperfonctionnement des surrénales maternelles sur le développement des surrénales foetales chez le rat. *Compt. Rend. Soc. Biol.* 151: 1104-1106, 1957.
89. Picon, L., and J. Bouhnik. Action de la cortico-surrénale sur la teneur du coeur en glycogène chez le foetus de rat et de rat nouveau-né. *Compt. Rend. Soc. Biol.* 160: 288-291, 1966.
90. Pion, R. J., R. B. Jaffe, N. Wiqvist, and E. Diczfalusy. Formation of dehydro-epiandrosterone sulfate by previable human foetuses. *Biochim. Biophys. Acta* 137: 584, 1967.

91. Plas, C., F. Chapeville, and R. Jacquot. Recherches sur la différenciation fonctionnelle du foie chez le foetus de rat. Influence de l'hydrocortisone sur la synthèse du glycogène par les hépatocytes foetaux en culture. *Compt. Rend.* 270: 2846-2849, 1970.
92. Plas, C., and R. Jacquot. Recherches sur la différenciation fonctionnelle du foie chez le foetus de rat. Activité UPDG-transglucosylasique et teneur en glycogène après administration d'hydrocortisone. *Compt. Rend.* 264: 374, 1967.
93. Raynaud, A., and M. Friley. Développement intra-utérin des embryons dont les ébauches de l'hypophyse ont été détruites au moyen de rayons X au 13e jour de la gestation. II. Développement des capsules surrénales. *Compt. Rend.* 230: 331, 1950.
94. Reid, J. D. Congenital absence of the pituitary gland. *J. Pediat.* 56: 658-664, 1960.
95. Roffi, J. Influence de la cortico-surrénale sur le contenu en adrénaline et noradrénaline de la surrénale chez le foetus de rat. *Compt. Rend.* 260: 1267-1270, 1965.
96. Schmidt, I. G., and R. A. Hoffmann. Effects of ACTH on pregnant monkeys and their offspring. *Endocrinology* 55: 125-141, 1954.
97. Shirley, I. M., and B. A. Cooke. Metabolism of dehydro-epiandrosterone by the separated zones of the human foetal and newborn adrenal cortex. *J. Endocrinol.* 44: 411-419, 1969.
98. Simmer, H. H., W. J. Dignam, W. E. Easterling, M. V. Frankland, and F. Naftolin. Neutral C19-steroids and steroid sulfates in human pregnancy. III. Dehydroepiandrosterone sulfate, 16α-hydroxydehydroepiandrosterone, and 16α-hydroxydehydroepiandrosterone sulfate in cord blood and blood of pregnant women with and without treatment with corticoids. *Steroids* 8: 179-193, 1966.
99. Skebelskaya, Y. B. The effect of corticosteroid concentrations in the blood of gravid rats on the adrenocorticotropic function of hypophysis of the fetus. *Gen. Comp. Endocrinol.* 10: 263-268, 1968.
100. Tuchmann-Duplessis, H., and M. Gabe. Absence de produit de neuro-sécrétion dans la post-hypophyse des anencéphales. *Bull. Acad. Natl. Med.* 144: 102-104, 1960.
101. Vaclav, J. Aparat endokrinni u anencefalu. (L'appareil des glandes à sécrétion interne chez les anencéphales.) *S. Lékar.* 28: 399-513, 1927.
102. Vaillant, R., and A. Jost. Influence des corticostéroïdes sur le glycogène particulaire du foie foetal de rat. *Biochimie* 53: 797-806, 1971.
103. Villee, D. B., L. L. Engel, J. M. Loring, and C. A. Villee. Steroid hydroxylation in human fetal adrenals: formation of 16α-hydroxyprogesterone, 17-hydroxyprogesterone and deoxycorticosterone. *Endocrinology* 69: 354-372, 1961.
104. Wells, L. J. Some experimental evidence of production of adrenotrophin by the fetal hypophysis. *Proc. Soc. Exptl. Biol. Med.* 68: 487-488, 1948.
105. Wurtman, R. J., and J. Axelrod. Adrenaline synthesis: control by the pituitary gland and adrenal glucocorticoids. *Science* 150: 1464-1465, 1965.

CHAPTER 9

Binding of corticosteroids by plasma proteins

U. WESTPHAL | *University of Louisville, School of Medicine, Louisville, Kentucky*

CHAPTER CONTENTS

Binding Phenomenon
Binding Proteins
   General aspects
   Corticosteroid-binding globulin
      Properties
      Development
      Endocrine influences
Significance of Binding

BINDING PHENOMENON

It has been known for almost 40 years that steroid hormones form complexes with proteins of the blood serum. This association is spontaneous. The bonds are noncovalent and therefore of lower energy than the covalent chemical bonds. As a consequence the complexes dissociate readily; the unbound components and the steroid-protein complex are in a dissociation equilibrium governed by the law of mass action. Detailed discussion and references to this and other aspects of this chapter appear in a recent monograph (34).

The binding affinity between steroid and protein varies with the chemical nature of either of the two components; the association constants of the complexes may differ by several orders of magnitude. The strength of binding also depends on temperature. Generally, increase of temperature results in a decrease of binding affinity, so that at 37 C the percentage of unbound hormone is considerably greater than at 2 C or 4 C, temperatures frequently used in the biochemical investigation of the binding proteins. For example, about 99% of cortisol in human plasma is bound at 4 C versus approximately 90% at 37 C. In comparison with this temperature effect, the influence of pH on the association is small, within the pH range of general protein stability. Maximum binding affinity has been observed at neutral or slightly higher than neutral pH. Effects of pH on the strength of association are therefore negligible under physiological conditions.

The forces of association in the steroid-protein complexes are hydrophobic bonds and hydrogen bonds. The basic steroid structure, exemplified by pregnane (Fig. 1, I), is a nonpolar (hydrophobic, lipophilic) molecule. Entrance of polar substituents, such as hydroxyl or oxo groups, together with double bonds forms the different steroid hormones. The corticosteroids possess increasing numbers of oxygen functions in a C_{21}-steroid structure (see Fig. 1, I); the hormone of highest biological activity, cortisol (Fig. 1, II), has two oxo and three hydroxy groups. Samuels and co-workers (10) recognized early that the binding affinity of a steroid to serum albumin decreases in proportion to the increasing number of polar groups present in the steroid molecule. This relationship between the "polarity" of a steroid hormone and the strength of protein association is known as the "polarity rule"; it has been confirmed for the interactions of many steroids with a variety of proteins.

The polarity rule is illustrated in Figure 2. It shows the association constants for the complexes of human α_1-acid glycoprotein (AAG; orosomucoid) with three corticosteroid hormones and with their precursor progesterone from which they are derived by entrance of one, two, and three hydroxy groups. This increase in polar character results in an almost 50-fold reduction of the binding affinity. Evidently the hydrophobic forces of binding predominate over hydrogen bonding in this system, which is another way of stating that steroid and protein associate according to the polarity rule. This rule is valid in steroid interactions with albumin and various other proteins.

The methods used to study steroid-protein interactions are based on the distinction between the bound and unbound form of the steroid (ligand). This can be accomplished either by physical separation of the two forms, so that each may then be analyzed, or by investigation of specific properties of the complex, usually in solution. Requirement for the latter case is the appearance of physicochemical or bioactivity changes in the steroid hormones on binding to the protein. Alterations in the ultraviolet absorption spectrum and suppression

FIG. 1. Nonpolar (I) and "polar" (II) steroid molecules.

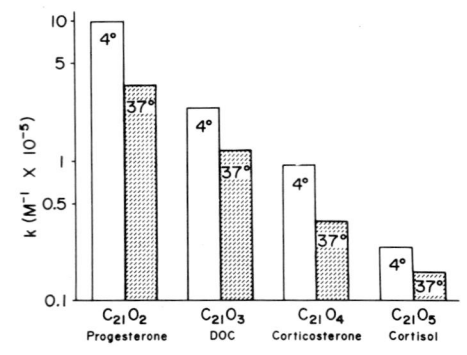

FIG. 2. Apparent association constants, k, of steroid hormone complexes with AAG, at pH 7.4. Temperatures expressed in degrees centigrade. *DOC*, deoxycorticosterone. [From data by Ganguly & Westphal (15).]

of hormonal activity by the complex formation are examples of such changes.

The steroid-protein complex is in a state of dynamic equilibrium; it dissociates readily and reversibly in the physiological environment. This equilibrium must not be disturbed if the binding analysis of the complex is to give thermodynamically valid results. Such condition is fulfilled for all methods that do not separate the bound and unbound species as long as the measuring process does not interfere with the equilibrium. In contrast, the binding equilibrium is not maintained in various procedures based on actual separation of the bound and unbound steroid molecule, such as ultrafiltration and electrophoresis. Methods that assure complete equilibration with separation of unbound ligand and protein complex are equilibrium dialysis and related techniques that apply similar principles.

BINDING PROTEINS

General Aspects

The serum proteins known to form dissociable complexes with the corticosteroid hormones are albumin (HSA, human serum albumin), α_1-acid glycoprotein (AAG), and corticosteroid-binding globulin (CBG, transcortin). These proteins have molecular weights of a similar order of magnitude, but their concentrations in the blood differ greatly. These points are illustrated in Table 1. Pertinent data for three corticosteroid hormones are also shown to facilitate comparison of the approximate molar ratios at which these steroids occur in relation to the proteins.

As further indicated in Table 1, these proteins show great differences in their binding affinity for the corticoids. Albumin has the lowest and CBG the highest affinity. A certain inverse proportionality exists between the concentration of the proteins in serum and their strength of association with the steroids. Corticosteroid-binding globulin is the major corticoid binder. Its high affinity constants indicate highly specific interactions. The concentration of CBG is low compared to that of other serum proteins; but the molar ratio of CBG : cortisol is still more than 2 : 1 under normal conditions; thus some reserve capacity of binding is provided. On the other hand, the abundant albumin takes a greater share of corticoid binding than would be expected from the association constant alone, which is four orders of magnitude smaller than that of the CBG complexes. In accordance with these considerations, Sandberg et al. (21) have found experimentally that the normal cortisol content of 12 μg/100 ml in human plasma is distributed as follows: bound to CBG, 76.0%; bound to HSA, 13.5%; unbound, 10.5%. The portion bound to AAG, approximately 2% of the total cortisol, is so small as to be negligible.

The cortisol molecule differs from corticosterone by the possession of one more hydroxy group. In accordance with the polarity rule, the affinity constants for the cortisol complexes are generally smaller than those of the corresponding corticosterone complexes (see

TABLE 1. *Corticosteroid-Protein Complexes in Human Serum*

Component	Molecular Weight	Approximate Concentration, mg/liter	Approximate Concentration, 10^{-7} M	Apparent Association Constants[a], $M^{-1} \times 10^{-5}$					
				Cortisol		Corticosterone		Aldosterone	
				4 C	37 C	4 C	37 C	4 C	37 C
HSA[b]	69,000	38,000	5,500	0.1	0.03	0.1		0.03	0.02
AAG[c]	41,000	750	180	0.20	0.15	1.0	0.37	0.30	0.05
CBG[d]	52,000	36	7	5,200	240	8,300	300	260	65
Cortisol	362	0.1	2.8						
Corticosterone	346	0.01	0.3						
Aldosterone	360	0.0006	0.02						

[a] Expressed as nk, the product of the number of binding sites, n, and the intrinsic association constant, k. [b] Human serum albumin. [c] α_1-Acid glycoprotein. [d] Corticosteroid-binding globulin. [Compiled from published data (34).]

Table 1). Aldosterone, which is bound with lower affinity to the same site in CBG as corticosterone and cortisol, is not directly comparable with the two glucocorticoids because of its predominant hemiacetal structure. The decreased binding affinity at the higher temperature is also shown in Table 1.

The interaction of the corticosteroid hormones with serum albumin is an example of the nonspecific binding typical of this protein. All other steroids investigated so far associate with albumin; the affinity varies according to their structure. The interaction is predominantly hydrophobic, as the validity of the polarity rule indicates. Serum albumin is readily available and well characterized; it has been extensively used in steroid interaction studies. For highest steroid-binding affinity it is necessary to remove the small amounts of fatty acids and possibly other lipids that adhere tenaciously to the albumin molecule during the usual purification procedures.

The biological significance of corticosteroid binding to α_1-acid glycoprotein is negligible—at least as far as we know today. This protein is important for other reasons: whereas the low concentration in serum and the chemical instability of CBG make it difficult to obtain this protein in sufficient amounts for physicochemical investigation, AAG can be readily prepared in pure form. More significantly, AAG in many respects resembles CBG, which is also a glycoprotein. The steroid complexes of the two proteins have common characteristics, such as pH and temperature dependency. Both AAG and CBG contain sialic acid, which may be removed enzymatically from either protein without impairment of the steroid-binding affinity.

Corticosteroid-binding Globulin

PROPERTIES. The major portion of the circulating corticoid hormones is associated with the corticosteroid-binding globulin (CBG, transcortin). The discovery of this binding system, characterized by high affinity and low capacity for the steroid and thus differing from steroid-albumin interaction, was first published by Daughaday (6) and by Bush (2). At the same time, Sandberg et al. (24) reported data on binding of corticosteroids to plasma and plasma fractions (obtained by Cohn fractionation) that indicated binding affinities greater than those known for albumin; the high affinities were interpreted to indicate binding to transcortin (22). These important findings and additional results of the early CBG studies have been reviewed (34).

The binding affinity of human CBG is not limited to the corticosteroids (Table 2). Progesterone interacts strongly at the same binding site, as evidenced by competitive displacement. At 37 C the association constant of the progesterone-CBG complex is about three times greater than that of the cortisol-CBG complex, in accordance with the polarity rule. Table 2 shows that testosterone is also bound, although with a somewhat

TABLE 2. *Apparent Association Constants of Steroid Complexes with Human CBG*

Steroid	Association Constant, k	
	4 C, M^{-1}	37 C, M^{-1}
Progesterone	3×10^8	8×10^7
Testosterone		1.4×10^6
Estradiol		2×10^4
Corticosterone sulfate	4×10^8	

Data from Westphal (34).

lower affinity; recent electrophoretic evidence (5) confirms by displacement studies that testosterone is bound to the cortisol-binding site. The affinity constant of the CBG complex with corticosterone sulfate is about half that of the corticosterone complex.

Chemical modification of the cortisol molecule (see Fig. 1, II) to form dexamethasone (16α-methyl-9α-fluoro-11β,17,21-trihydroxypregna-1,4-diene-3,20-dione) eliminates the binding affinity to CBG. This distinguishes CBG from the corticosteroid receptor proteins of target tissues that have a high affinity for dexamethasone as a very potent glucocortical agent.

The first preparation of a highly purified human CBG from serum of estrogen-treated males was reported by Seal & Doe (26) who characterized the binder as a glycoprotein with the electrophoretic mobility of an α_1-globulin. Several years later, the isolation of human CBG was described by other investigators (18, 31). The CBG preparation obtained in our laboratory was homogeneous by electrophoretic and immunoelectrophoretic criteria. Ultracentrifugation resulted in a symmetrical sedimentation peak. Diffusion patterns, as well as the evaluation of sedimentation coefficients at different CBG concentrations, indicated homogeneity of the protein.

Homogeneous CBG preparations were also obtained from the serum of rabbit (3) and rat (4), and more recently from guinea pig plasma (19, 25). In Table 3 the general similarity of the CBGs from these four species is shown. The molecular weights are of the order of 50,000. The absorption coefficients in ultraviolet light are similar. The CBGs are glycoproteins with a total carbohydrate content of between 25 and 29%. About 16–40% of this carbohydrate consists of sialic acid; this residue can be removed by neuraminidase without loss of binding affinity. The amino acid and carbohydrate compositions have been determined for the CBGs of the four species; again a general similarity is found, despite distinct differences in individual residues (34).

The CBG molecules of man, rat, and rabbit possess one binding site for the corticosteroids. Progesterone is bound to the same site in these three species, in contrast to the guinea pig, which produces a CBG distinct from its progesterone-binding globulin (1). The association constants of the corticosteroid-CBG complexes in the serum of several species are shown in Table 4. Values

TABLE 3. *Physicochemical Properties of the Corticosteroid Complexes of Human, Rabbit, Rat, and Guinea Pig CBG*

Parameter	Human CBG[a]	Rabbit CBG[b]	Rat CBG[c]	Cavian CBG[d]
Sedimentation coefficient, $s^0_{20,w}$ (S)	3.79	3.55	3.56	3.25[e]
Diffusion coefficient, $D_{20,w}$ (cm^2 sec^{-1}) $\times 10^7$	6.15	7.02		7.34[f]
Partial specific volume, $\bar{v}$ (ml/g)	0.708	0.695	0.711	0.703
Molecular weight	51,700[g]	40,700[h] 34,700[i]	52,600 ±3,000[j] 61,000 ±1,100[k]	~60,000 48,600[f,l]
Frictional ratio, f/fo	1.42	1.37		
$E^{1\%}_{1\,cm}$ at 279 nm	6.45	8.4	6.2	7.1[m]
$A_{280} : A_{260}$, corticosteroid complex	1.13	1.38	1.58	1.24[f]
$A_{280} : A_{260}$, complex stripped	1.57		1.71	1.46
Electrophoretic mobility at pH 8.6 (cm^2 volt^{-1} sec^{-1}) $\times 10^5$	−4.9	−5.1		
Carbohydrate, %	26.1[n]	29.2	27.8	25
Nitrogen, %	12.7	12.1		

[a] Data from Muldoon & Westphal (18). [b] Data from Chader & Westphal (3). [c] Data from Chader & Westphal (4). [d] Data from Schneider & Slaunwhite (25). [e] In 0.85% solution. Rozen (19) observed 3.65 in 0.5% solution. [f] Value reported by Rozen (19). [g] Molecular weights of 52,000 (28) and 55,700 (25) were reported from other laboratories. [h] This molecular weight includes some tetramer. [i] Molecular weight of monomer (2a). [j] From corticosterone content of complex. [k] From approach to sedimentation equilibrium. [l] Burton et al. (1) determined about 48,000 by gel filtration. [m] Rozen (19) reported 8.8. [n] Schneider & Slaunwhite (25) reported 18%.

for progesterone are included to characterize the steroid interactions in relation to the polarity rule. Evidently, human CBG follows this rule, in that progesterone is bound more firmly than cortisol. In contrast, the relative binding affinities for these two steroid hormones are reversed in rabbit CBG. The normal serum concentrations of CBG (mole/liter) are also shown in Table 4.

A characteristic property of the CBG molecule is its tendency to aggregate. This was first observed with rat CBG which forms dimeric, tetrameric, and octameric species after removal of corticosterone from the protein complex (4). This polymerization is reversible: recombination of the steroid-free aggregates with 1 mole corticosterone per mole CBG results in re-formation of the monomer. Rabbit CBG polymerizes spontaneously on gel filtration to a tetramer with loss of cortisol-binding affinity; partial recovery of the binding affinity can be obtained under certain conditions (2a). Self-association has also been reported for guinea pig CBG (25). In this case, the aggregation is accompanied by complete loss of binding affinity for cortisol; reactivation has not been achieved.

The biological significance of the polymerization is unknown. Rat CBG provides the first example of the control of the conformational structure of a carrier protein by the steroid hormone with which it forms a specific complex of high affinity. The question of whether the molecular size of the hormone-binding protein has an influence on transport or membrane permeation at the target cell is open to analysis.

DEVELOPMENT. Seal & Doe (28) have shown in studies with more than 130 vertebrate species that corticosteroid-binding macromolecules are common blood constituents. The authors (27) concluded that the fundamental mechanism of serum protein binding of corticoid hormones appeared early in the history of the vertebrates and was mediated by specific proteins of unique conformational structure. In Table 5 a few examples of high-affinity binding capacity for cortisol (μg cortisol per 100 ml serum) in the different species are given; the values selected emphasize extremes of high and

TABLE 4. *Concentration of Binding Sites and Apparent Association Constants of Steroid-CBG Complexes in Mammalian Sera*

Species	[CBG]* in 10^{-7} M	Cortisol 4 C	Cortisol 37 C	Corticosterone 4 C	Corticosterone 37 C	Progesterone 4 C	Progesterone 37 C
		\multicolumn{6}{c}{k† in 10^8 M^{-1}}
Human	7.2	6	0.3	10	0.3	7	0.9
Monkey	9.3	3	0.3		1.4		
Rat	11.3	3	0.1	5	0.3	3	
Rabbit	3.4	10	0.4	8	0.2	4	
Guinea pig	5.7	0.5	0.04	1.1	0.14	48‡	3.9‡

Determined by equilibrium dialysis in 0.05 M phosphate, pH 7.4. Sera had been stripped of endogenous steroids by gel filtration at 45 C. * Concentrations of binding sites for corticosteroids were approximately the same as those for progesterone. † Apparent association constant. ‡ Binding to progesterone-binding globulin (1). [Data from Westphal (32).]

TABLE 5. *High-affinity Binding of Cortisol in Sera of Different Species*

Species	Binding Capacity*
Lamprey	0.5
Bass	6.8
Bullfrog	1.0
Marine toad	18.0
Painted turtle	2.7
Alligator	43.0
Iguana (green)	110.0
Pelican	0.9
Pigeon	19.2
Whale	2.9
Horse	10.0
Man	22.0
Squirrel	92.0

* Values expressed as μg/100 ml. [Adapted from Seal & Doe (28).]

low binding levels. Most of the sera examined also form complexes with corticosterone, but no relation has been found between the binding capacities for these two corticoids and their relative serum concentrations.

Fetal serum has less than half the cortisol-binding activity of the adult human being (8); low values have been reported for newborn infants (20). The CBG activity in human serum remains about the same between ages 1 and 60, and the values of males do not differ significantly from those of females. No diurnal variation has been established for human serum.

A hereditary deficiency in CBG concentration has been observed in members of a family that was studied over four generations (17). The CBG level was reduced to about half normal; this was not caused by any disease state. The total 17-hydroxycorticosteroid concentration in the serum was significantly decreased, whereas the unbound 17-hydroxycorticoid concentration was in the normal range. This would suggest that the unbound hormone is the active form responsible for the regulation of corticoid biosynthesis in the feedback mechanism. De Moor et al. (9) assume from the analysis of similar cases of familial decrease of cortisol-binding capacity that an X-linked gene may be partly responsible for the control of plasma CBG. The genetically controlled abnormality of the CBG level is analogous to familial decrease and increase of the thyroxin-binding globulin, to familial absence of serum albumin and decrease in ceruloplasmin concentration, and to other hereditary serum protein deviations (34).

The gradual increase of CBG activity in the growing organism has been studied in the rat (12). In Figure 3 this development from day 12 to 57, expressed as combining affinity (C) for corticosterone, is shown in the serum of male and female animals. The C value (7) is defined as

$$C = \frac{[S_{bd}]}{[S] \times [P_t]}$$

where $[S_{bd}]$, $[S]$, and $[P_t]$ are the concentrations of bound steroid, of unbound steroid, and of total protein, respectively; it is used as a convenient term to assess the steroid-binding activity, which is a resultant of binding affinity and concentration of binding sites. The C value is closely related to the association constant

$$k = \frac{[S_{bd}]}{[S] \times [P]}$$

which differs only by the use of $[P]$, the molar concentration of unbound protein, rather than $[P_t]$. The C value becomes practically indistinguishable from the association constant (k) when $[P_t] \gg [S_{bd}]$. These relations and the measurement of various binding parameters have been discussed elsewhere (33, 34).

The low CBG activity seen on day 12 (see Fig. 3) is preceded by a significantly higher value at day 3, which suggests that the control of the CBG synthesis in the postnatal rat still reflects the influence of the maternal

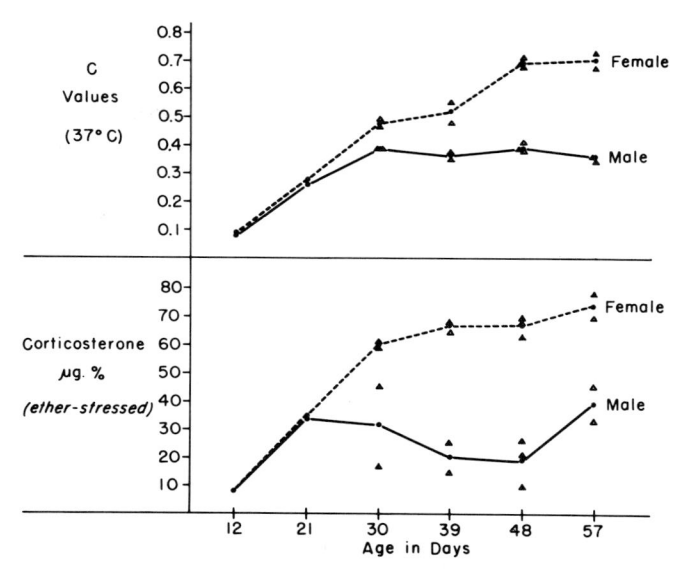

FIG. 3. Corticosterone-binding activity (C Values) and corticosterone levels (µg/100 ml) in developing rat. Each *triangle* represents average of duplicate values from one of several serum pools; *points* indicate overall averages. C value of female rats at 66 days of age equaled those at 48 and 57 days. Vaginal patency at ages 30, 39, 48, and 57 days was 0, 17, 82, and 100%, respectively, of all female rats in the group. [From Gala & Westphal (12).]

hormones (see subsection *Gonadal hormones*). Male and female rats show parallel increase of CBG activity from day 12 to about day 30 when the values in the male animals have reached their normal adult level. The C values in the females continue to rise and level off at about day 48 when they exceed those of the males by 85%; no further change was seen at days 57 and 66. Numerous determinations in our laboratory and reports by other investigators confirm the CBG activity of the adult female rat to be about twice that of the male.

The peripheral corticosterone concentration reflects the changes in the CBG level. Although the corticoid values in Figure 3 were obtained from ether-stressed rather than resting animals and show considerable fluctuations, the general similarity of the parallel changes in C values and corticosterone level in the female and male rat is evident. A calculation utilizing the average "unstressed" corticosterone values obtained in a large number of normal adult rats showed that the concentration of unbound corticosterone of the male rats (0.33 ± 0.06 µg/100 ml) was not significantly different from that of the females (0.39 ± 0.06 µg/100 ml), despite a threefold higher level of total corticosterone in the female animals (12). In accordance, the average thymus weights per 100 g body weight of the male rats (128 ± 4 mg) were not markedly different from those of the females (116 ± 5 mg).

ENDOCRINE INFLUENCES. *Gonadal hormones.* The differences in CBG activity between the male and female adult rat suggested a possible influence of the sex steroid hormones. Orchidectomy resulted in increased CBG levels. This was not yet apparent 4 days after the operation;

however, on days 14, 24, and 45 after castration the CBG activities of the male rats were increased by 41, 68, and 70%, respectively (12). This result was in agreement with the assumption of a suppressing effect of the androgenic hormone on CBG.

Direct proof was given by injection of testosterone into gonadectomized male rats. The CBG level, which by day 24 after castration had risen to 78% over the control value, was brought back to normal by injection of 5 mg testosterone per day for 10 days. A corresponding effect was seen in normal female rats: similar treatment with testosterone resulted in a 30% decrease of the CBG activity.

The same testosterone administration to normal male animals did not affect their CBG level. Presumably the normal testosterone concentration of the male rat is congruent with maximal suppression of CBG obtainable under these conditions.

The influence of estrogenic hormones on the CBG concentration in blood serum has been known for many years. Slaunwhite & Sandberg (30) observed a doubling of the transcortin capacity in human pregnancy and could mimic this increase by injection of estrogens (23). As a consequence of the high CBG concentration, the 17-hydroxycorticosteroid level rose to twice normal or higher. However, no signs of hypercorticism were observed, because the transcortin-bound corticosteroid hormone is biologically inert. Indeed, this physiological inactivity is the explanation for the rise of the peripheral corticoid with increasing CBG level during pregnancy and after estrogen administration, in the course of negative feedback regulation. The changes in the serum levels of CBG and 17-hydroxycorticosteroids in human pregnancy have been illustrated [(29); for additional details and references, see (34)].

Injection of estradiol into adult male rats, 1 and 10 μg/day for 10 days, raised the CBG activity by 56 and 72%, respectively (12). The peripheral corticosterone concentration increased slightly. The same estrogen treatment of female rats did not affect their C values, a result analogous to the experiment described earlier,

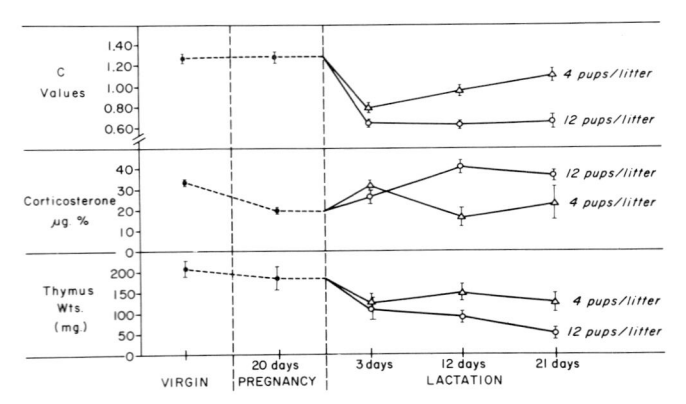

FIG. 4. Corticosterone-binding activity (*C Values*), resting corticosterone levels (μg/100 ml), and thymus weights of virgin, pregnant, and lactating rats. [From Gala & Westphal (11).]

in which male hormone did not influence the CBG activity of adult male rats.

In an effort to shed light on the mechanism of the apparently similar increase of CBG activity in the male rat after estrogen and after castration, a combination of the experimental conditions was applied in order to test for possible additive effects. It was found that the increased C values resulting from orchidectomy were not further raised by estradiol injection into the castrated animal. Failure to observe an additive effect would suggest that the elevated CBG activity in the male rat after gonadectomy and after estrogen administration is mediated by a similar mechanism.

Injection of progesterone in daily doses of 2 mg and 10 mg into adult male rats for 10 days resulted in CBG levels that were increased by 30 and 90%, respectively. The effect was smaller in female rats; the treatment with 10 mg progesterone raised the CBG activity only 22% over the female control value. In all cases, the peripheral corticosterone concentration was reduced in proportion to the increasing amounts of progesterone injected. This is in contrast to the changes of CBG and corticoid level after estrogen administration and may result from competitive displacement of corticosterone from CBG by progesterone. The increased fraction of unbound corticosteroid hormone would bring about, by negative feedback, a reduction of the total corticoid concentration, in accordance with partial occupation of the CBG binding sites by progesterone. Confirmatory reports from other laboratories for the progesterone effect on CBG and corticosterone level in the male rat, as well as for other results discussed in this section, have been reviewed (34).

In contrast to the findings in human pregnancy, the CBG activity in the pregnant rat does not increase significantly (11). A sharp decline occurs, however, shortly after parturition. Figure 4 shows that the subsequent trend of the C values depends on the number of pups nursed: a relatively fast return to nonpregnant values occurs when the litter is small, whereas mothers nursing 12 pups continue to have low transcortin activity for at least 3 weeks. In this case, the usual relationship of CBG activity and corticosteroid level is reversed: low CBG values are connected with high corticosterone and vice versa. The result is the availability of a relatively high concentration of unbound corticoid to the mother nursing the large litter, in accordance with the need for corticosteroid hormone in lactation. The thymus weights in the two groups reflect the different concentrations of unbound, physiologically active corticoid hormone. The gradual return of the three parameters to levels found in virgin animals is shown in Figure 5.

Corticosteroid hormones. An influence of corticosteroid hormones on the CBG level was suggested by the observation of increased corticosterone-binding activity in the adrenalectomized rat (35). The rise became significant between 24 and 48 hr after the operation; a maximal C value of approximately twice normal was reached on the third or fourth postoperative day. The CBG activity remained at this high level for at least 3 weeks.

A similar effect of corticoid elimination on CBG activity was seen in a human subject given dexamethasone. This treatment decreases the cortisol level to an unmeasurable value; at the same time, the CBG activity was significantly increased. This result is in accordance with the observation of elevated CBG capacity in some cases of untreated adrenal insufficiency.

The increase of CBG activity in the adrenalectomized rat can be suppressed or reversed by administration of corticosterone or cortisol. Injection of the massive dose of 5 mg daily for 4 days not only suppresses the increase of the C value in the adrenalectomized rat, but reduces it to half the normal level. This low C value is nearly the same as that obtained with intact rats after the above corticosterone treatment (i.e., half the CBG activity of the normal, saline-injected control). After cessation of the corticosteroid injections, the C values return gradually to normal levels.

The marked elevation of CBG activity in the rat after adrenalectomy presumably results from the removal of the CBG-suppressing effect of the corticosteroid hormones. This is analogous to the influence of gonadectomy in the male rat. However, the sex steroid-mediated stimuli appear to be controlled by a mechanism different from that following adrenalectomy. This conclusion is based on studies of additivity of the various endocrine influences on rat CBG that have been reviewed recently (34) in connection with the interrelations of the endocrine effects.

Thyroid-stimulating hormone and thyroxine. In view of the close relation between the CBG-affecting steroid hormones and the hypophysis, the involvement of this gland in the control of CBG activity is of interest. Rat studies showed that hypophysectomy prevents the increase in the CBG level seen after adrenalectomy and after estrogen administration (13). In the female rat, extirpation of the pituitary gland results in a marked reduction of the corticosterone-binding activity, which continues for several weeks. This is in contrast to the male rat whose lower CBG value does not decrease after hypophysectomy.

In an effort to define the cause of the reduced CBG activity after extirpation of the pituitary gland, replacement studies were performed. An anterior lobe suspension was injected into hypophysectomized female rats that had only 55% of their normal corticosterone-binding activity. This resulted in an increase of CBG to 83% of the normal level.

Further analysis showed that adrenocorticotropin, growth hormone, prolactin, luteinizing hormone, and a human pituitary gonadotrophin preparation containing predominantly follicle-stimulating hormone did not alter the CBG activity of the hypophysectomized female rats from that of the saline-injected hypophysectomized controls. The thyroid-stimulating hormone,

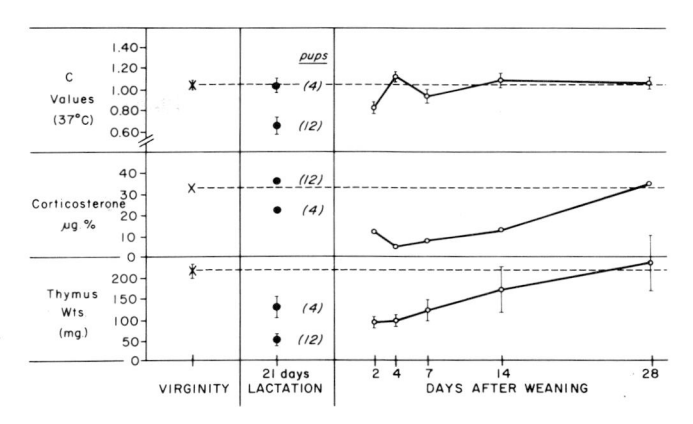

FIG. 5. Corticosterone-binding activity (*C Values*), resting corticosterone levels (μg/100 ml), and thymus weights of virgin and lactating rats and mother rats after weaning 7–9 pups per litter. [From Gala & Westphal (11).]

alone of the pituitary hormones tested, restored the normal CBG level; the value obtained was even slightly above that of the sham-hypophysectomized controls (14).

The effect of the thyroid-stimulating hormone on CBG is assumed to be mediated through increased production of thyroid hormone, which in turn enhances the CBG level. Support for such mechanism was provided by Labrie et al. (16) who found, independently of our results, that thyroidectomy decreases, and thyroxine administration increases, the CBG activity of the rat. These observations are in accordance with our conclusion that the pituitary factor involved in the control of CBG is the thyroid-stimulating hormone.

SIGNIFICANCE OF BINDING

Early interpretations of the significance of steroid hormone binding to serum proteins emphasized the transport function of the complexes. Facilitation of solubility of the water-insoluble steroids by association with proteins was part of this concept. However, a closer look at steroid solubilities in water and aqueous buffer systems shows that such solubilization is not required for most steroid hormones, least of all for the hydroxyl-rich corticosteroids. They are water soluble at their physiological concentrations. Association with the large protein molecules would hinder rather than facilitate their transport, particularly through structures of limited permeability, such as cellular membranes.

More plausible was the suggestion that the protein interaction alters some basic properties of the steroid hormones. Most importantly the biological activity is suppressed by the association, so that the protein-bound hormone circulates in the blood in an inactive form; only the unbound steroid can exert biological function. Protein binding thus provides a buffer or storage function: relatively large quantities of hormone are being circulated in the form of a biologically inert reservoir from which the active species can be rapidly produced by dissociation. The usefulness of such immediate availability of corticosteroid hormones without the effects of hypercorticism is obvious.

There are other beneficial consequences of the complex formation. Some steroid hormones (e.g., cortisol) are sensitive to chemical attack and degradation. Association with proteins provides protection against these reactions. The protection extends toward enzymatic alterations that may lead to inactivation and excretion. Accordingly metabolic clearance is reduced and the half-time of disappearance prolonged. Binding to the large protein molecules may also counteract possible permeation of the steroid hormones through capillary walls.

Unanswered is the question whether the association of the steroid hormones with specific high-affinity binders provides a mechanism for the interaction with specific target sites. No definite relation of a functional or structural nature has been established so far between the high-affinity serum binders and the specific receptor proteins of target cells.

Quantitative regulation of hormonal activity, provision of a large storage capacity of biologically inert hormone coupled with immediate availability of active hormone, protection from chemical and enzymatic attack, prevention or retardation of steroid loss through capillary walls, reduction of hepatic clearance and renal excretion—these are the logical functions of steroid hormone-binding proteins, based on the physicochemical characteristics of the interactions.

REFERENCES

1. Burton, R. M., G. B. Harding, N. Rust, and U. Westphal. Steroid-protein interactions. xxiii. Nonidentity of cortisol-binding globulin and progesterone-binding globulin in guinea pig serum. *Steroids* 17: 1–16, 1971.
2. Bush, I. E. The physicochemical state of cortisol in blood. In: *Hormones in Blood. Ciba Foundation Colloquium on Endocrinology*, edited by G. E. W. Wolstenholme and E. C. P. Millar. Boston: Little, Brown, 1957, vol. 11, p. 263–285.
2a. Chader, G. J., N. Rust, R. M. Burton, and U. Westphal. Steroid-protein interactions. xxvi. Studies on the polymeric nature of the corticosteroid-binding globulin of the rabbit. *J. Biol. Chem.* 247: 6581–6588, 1972.
3. Chader, G. J., and U. Westphal. Steroid-protein interactions. xvi. Isolation and characterization of the corticosteroid-binding globulin of the rabbit. *J. Biol. Chem.* 243: 928–939, 1968.
4. Chader, G. J., and U. Westphal. Steroid-protein interactions. xviii. Isolation and observations on the polymeric nature of the corticosteroid-binding globulin of the rat. *Biochemistry* 7: 4272–4282, 1968.
5. Corvol, P. L., A. Chrambach, D. Rodbard, and C. W. Bardin. Physical properties and binding capacity of testosterone-estradiol-binding globulin in human plasma, determined by polyacrylamide gel electrophoresis. *J. Biol. Chem.* 246: 3435–3443, 1971.
6. Daughaday, W. H. Evidence for two corticosteroid binding systems in human plasma. *J. Lab. Clin. Med.* 48: 799–800, 1956.
7. Daughaday, W. H. Binding of corticosteroids by plasma proteins. iii. The binding of corticosteroid and related hormones by human plasma and plasma protein fractions as measured by equilibrium dialysis. *J. Clin. Invest.* 37: 511–518, 1958.
8. De Moor, P., K. Heirwegh, J. Heremans, and M. Declerck-Raskin. Protein binding of corticoids studied by gel filtration. *J. Clin. Invest.* 41: 816–827, 1962.
9. De Moor, P., E. Meulepas, A. Hendrikx, W. Heyns, and H. G. Vandenschrieck. Cortisol-binding capacity of plasma transcortin: a sex-linked trait? *J. Clin. Endocrinol. Metab.* 27: 959–965, 1967.
10. Eik-Nes, K. B., J. A. Schellman, R. Lumry, and L. T. Samuels. The binding of steroids to protein. i. Solubility determinations. *J. Biol. Chem.* 206: 411–419, 1954.
11. Gala, R. R., and U. Westphal. Corticosteroid-binding globulin in the rat: possible role in the initiation of lactation. *Endocrinology* 76: 1079–1088, 1965.
12. Gala, R. R., and U. Westphal. Corticosteroid-binding globulin in the rat: studies on the sex difference. *Endocrinology* 77: 841–851, 1965.
13. Gala, R. R., and U. Westphal. Relationship between the pituitary gland and the corticosteroid-binding globulin in the rat. *Endocrinology* 78: 277–285, 1966.
14. Gala, R. R., and U. Westphal. Influence of anterior pituitary hormones on the corticosteroid-binding globulin in the rat. *Endocrinology* 79: 55–66, 1966.
15. Ganguly, M., and U. Westphal. Steroid-protein interactions. xvii. Influence of solvent environment on interaction between human α_1-acid glycoprotein and progesterone. *J. Biol. Chem.* 243: 6130–6139, 1968.
16. Labrie, F., G. Pelletier, R. Labrie, M. A. Ho-Kim, A. Delgado, B. MacIntosh, and C. Fortier. Liaison transcortine-corticostérone et contrôle de l'activité hypophyso-surrénalienne chez le rat. Interactions hypophyse-thyroide-surrénales-gonades. *Ann. Endocrinol.* 29: 29–43, 1968.
17. Lohrenz, F. N., U. S. Seal, and R. P. Doe. Adrenal function and serum concentrations in a kindred with decreased corticosteroid-binding globulin (CBG) concentration. *J. Clin. Endocrinol. Metab.* 27: 966–972, 1967.
18. Muldoon, T. G., and U. Westphal. Steroid-protein interactions. xv. Isolation and characterization of corticosteroid-binding globulin from human plasma. *J. Biol. Chem.* 242: 5636–5643, 1967.
19. Rozen, V. B., and A. G. Volchek. Isolation and study of physicochemical properties of transcortin of a guinea pig. *Probl. Endokrinol., Mosk.* 16: 81–85, 1970.
20. Sandberg, A. A., H. Rosenthal, S. L. Schneider, and W. R. Slaunwhite, Jr. Protein-steroid interactions and their role in the transport and metabolism of steroids. In: *Steroid Dynamics*, edited by G. Pincus, T. Nakao, and J. F. Tait. New York: Acad. Press, 1966, p. 1–61.
21. Sandberg, A. A., H. Rosenthal, and W. R. Slaunwhite, Jr. Transcortin: a corticosteroid-binding protein of plasma. viii. Parameters affecting cortisol metabolism. In: *Proceedings of the Second International Congress on Hormonal Steroids*, edited by L. Martini, F. Fraschini, and M. Motta. Amsterdam: Excerpta Medica Foundation, 1967, p. 707–716.
22. Sandberg, A. A., and W. R. Slaunwhite, Jr. Transcortin: a corticosteroid-binding plasma protein. *J. Clin. Invest.* 37: 928, 1958.
23. Sandberg, A. A., and W. R. Slaunwhite, Jr. Transcortin: a corticosteroid-binding protein of plasma. ii. Levels in various conditions and the effects of estrogens. *J. Clin. Invest.* 38: 1290–1297, 1959.
24. Sandberg, A. A., W. R. Slaunwhite, Jr., and H. N. Antoniades. The binding of steroids and steroid conjugates to

human plasma proteins. *Recent Progr. Hormone Res.* 13: 209–267, 1957.
25. SCHNEIDER, S. L., AND W. R. SLAUNWHITE, JR. Transcortin. A comparison of the cortisol-binding globulin from human and cavian plasma. *Biochemistry* 10: 2086–2093, 1971.
26. SEAL, U. S., AND R. P. DOE. Corticosteroid-binding globulin. I. Isolation from plasma of diethylstilbestrol-treated men. *J. Biol. Chem.* 237: 3136–3140, 1962.
27. SEAL, U. S., AND R. P. DOE. Corticosteroid-binding globulin: species distribution and small-scale purification. *Endocrinology* 73: 371–376, 1963.
28. SEAL, U. S., AND R. P. DOE. Corticosteroid-binding globulin: biochemistry, physiology, and phylogeny. In: *Steroid Dynamics*, edited by G. Pincus, T. Nakao, and J. F. Tait. New York: Acad. Press, 1966, p. 63–90.
29. SEAL, U. S., AND R. P. DOE. The role of corticosteroid-binding globulin in mammalian pregnancy. In: *Proceedings of the Second International Congress on Hormonal Steroids*, edited by L. Martini, F. Fraschini, and M. Motta. Amsterdam: Excerpta Medica Foundation, 1967, p. 697–706.
30. SLAUNWHITE, W. R., JR., AND A. A. SANDBERG. Transcortin: a corticosteroid-binding protein of plasma. *J. Clin. Invest.* 38: 384–391, 1959.
31. SLAUNWHITE, W. R., JR., S. SCHNEIDER, F. C. WISSLER, AND A. A. SANDBERG. Transcortin: a corticosteroid-binding protein of plasma. IX. Isolation and characterization. *Biochemistry* 5: 3527–3532, 1966.
32. WESTPHAL, U. Steroid-protein interactions. XIII. Concentrations and binding affinities of corticosteroid-binding globulins in sera of man, monkey, rat, rabbit, and guinea pig. *Arch. Biochem. Biophys.* 118: 556–567, 1967.
33. WESTPHAL, U. Assay and properties of corticosteroid-binding globulin and other steroid-binding serum proteins. *Methods Enzymol.* 15: 761–796, 1969.
34. WESTPHAL, U. *Steroid-Protein Interactions*. New York: Springer Verlag, 1971.
35. WESTPHAL, U., W. C. WILLIAMS, JR., B. D. ASHLEY, AND F. DEVENUTO. Steroid-protein interactions. X. Proteinbindung der Corticosteroide im Serum adrenalektomierter und hypophysektomierter Ratten. *Z. Physiol. Chem.* 332: 54–69, 1963.

CHAPTER 10

Circadian rhythm: man and animals

JAMES B. ATCHESON | *Laboratory for the Study of Hereditary and Metabolic Disorders,*
FRANK H. TYLER | *and the Department of Medicine, University of Utah*
                  | *College of Medicine, Salt Lake City, Utah*

CHAPTER CONTENTS

Cortisol
    Rhythm of cortisol secretion
    Pituitary-adrenal secretion
    Regulation of adrenocorticotropic hormone secretion
    Feedback regulation of cortisol secretion
    Alterations in circadian rhythm
        Activity-sleep cycle
        Stress
        Exogenously administered substances
Aldosterone
Testosterone; Estrogen

CLAUDE BERNARD'S CONCEPT of "la fixeté du milieu intérieur" and Cannon's concept of homeostasis imply a rather tightly controlled constancy of the internal environment. This concept is still entrenched to some degree in scientific thinking and may be perfectly appropriate for some physiological systems. However, activity in a number of biologically important functions varies rhythmically, and therefore related measurements are constantly changing, although usually in an orderly and controlled fashion. A great number of biological rhythms with vastly different periodicities (i.e., hours to years) have been identified. The term *circadian* (circa, about; dies, day) was introduced by Halberg et al. (16), for describing rhythms with periods of about 24 hr, and has gained general acceptance. Circadian is more appropriate for this purpose than "diurnal" (occurrences of the day), which is best used in contrast to "nocturnal" (occurrences of the night).

The study of circadian rhythms is fraught with difficulties. Establishing the actual existence of a presumed biological rhythm is a very real problem. The experimental situation itself may introduce additional external cues (*Zeitgeber*) that might alter an established rhythm or even create an entirely new "artificial" cycle. For example, such cyclic occurrences as laboratory noise, feeding times, specimen collections, light-dark periods, temperature, and subject anxiety may produce rhythms unlike those occurring under natural conditions.

Beyond these considerations is the statistical handling of the data collected and the determination of a valid or reasonable conclusion. The frequency of measurements within a 24-hr period is obviously an important factor, as illustrated later in this chapter. All these problems are dealt with in detail in recent publications (3, 17).

A major consideration, after the identification of such a rhythm, is determining whether it is purely endogenously controlled or dependent on periodic external factors. Even under the most strictly controlled circumstances, this can never be done with certainty. Usually several factors combine in varying degrees to determine the actual period and amplitude of the rhythm. For example, a rhythm may be endogenously determined, but its exact period might be "set" by some aspect of the environment. For example, the period of the cortisol cycle may be changed by varying the total length of the sleep-activity cycle.

Under experimental conditions, when several environmental factors (e.g., light, dark, feeding) can be kept constant, very often the period of the rhythm will change to some degree (free-running periods). Other intercurrent factors may obliterate or drastically change an established rhythm, as with stress and cortisol secretion. Still other rhythms may be predominantly, if not entirely, determined by external cues, as appears to be the case with aldosterone secretion. In addition, perhaps more subtle geophysical influences may have a very fundamental role in the genesis of some rhythms, particularly in lower animals (3).

Several excellent reviews of biological rhythms in general (17) and of a variety of circadian rhythms have appeared in recent years (1–3, 16, 18, 19, 32, 38).

CORTISOL

Rhythm of Cortisol Secretion

The possibility of circadian variation in adrenocortical function was first suggested by Pincus (42) in 1943 and later documented by study of 17-ketosteroid (17-KS)

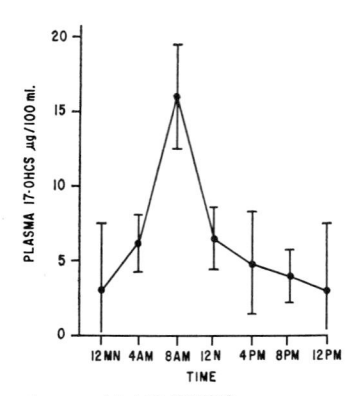

FIG. 1. Plasma 17-hydroxycorticosteroid (*17-OHCS*) concentrations from 12 normal subjects. Mean values are depicted by *points*. *Vertical bars* represent ± 1 SD. [From Nichols & Tyler (38).]

excretion in his laboratory (43). Since these initial observations a large body of data has accumulated, primarily from normal human subjects, which clearly depicts the circadian rhythm of cortisol secretion (5, 25, 31, 40, 41, 44).

When the urinary metabolites of cortisol are measured during a 24-hr period, the pattern of excretion is relatively consistent. The major excretion occurs during the morning hours, with the initial rise beginning at about 3 to 4 AM. The levels then decline during the afternoon and reach a nadir around midnight (25, 45).

Several laboratories have since observed a similar variation in plasma 17-hydroxycorticosteroids (17-OHCS), principally cortisol (35), during a 24-hr period (31, 38, 40, 41). In Figure 1 the mean cortisol values in plasma for a group of healthy human subjects studied during routine activities are depicted (38). As illustrated in the figure, the normal pattern of plasma cortisol concentration is one of rapidly rising levels shortly after midnight, with maximal levels regularly occurring at about 6 to 8 AM. Thereafter the mean level drops rapidly between 8 AM and noon and then more slowly until after midnight.

Pituitary-Adrenal Secretion

That adrenocorticotropic hormone (ACTH) could stimulate the secretion of glucocorticoids has been known for some time (43). When graded doses of ACTH are given, one sees coresoponding graded adrenal cortical responses, as illustrated in Figure 2 (27). An ACTH potentiator substance of pituitary origin in plasma, termed *adrenal weight-maintaining activity*, has been suggested. It is found in some patients with increased ACTH secretion, specifically in patients with Addison's disease and Cushing's syndrome associated with bilateral adrenal hyperplasia. The nature of this substance is entirely unknown, if indeed it is different from ACTH itself. Evidence to date indicates that it has no significant role in normal physiological processes (46, 47). Thus ACTH is presumed to be the major, if not sole, stimulus for cortisol secretion.

The administration of exogenous glucocorticoid will suppress both adrenal cortical activity and ACTH secretion. When exogenous ACTH and cortisol are administered together, adrenal function is not suppressed (27). Administration of metyrapone (SU 4885), a substance that interferes with the synthesis of cortisol, results in increased ACTH secretion in an effort to compensate for the decrease in blood cortisol (21). When sufficient exogenous cortisol is administered with metyrapone, there is no increase in ACTH secretion (21, 27). These considerations indicate that cortisol exerts feedback control over its own production through changes in ACTH secretion.

Precise documentation of this relationship in normal humans, however, has had to await the development of a relatively sensitive assay for ACTH. By using a radioimmunoassay, the direct relationship between plasma ACTH and plasma corticosteroid fluctuations has been demonstrated (8, 30, 51), as illustrated in Figure 3. A diurnal variation in ACTH levels that coincides with plasma corticosteroid levels is seen, with maximum values obtained at 4 and 6 AM. Furthermore the rise and fall of ACTH slightly precede similar changes in plasma cortisol.

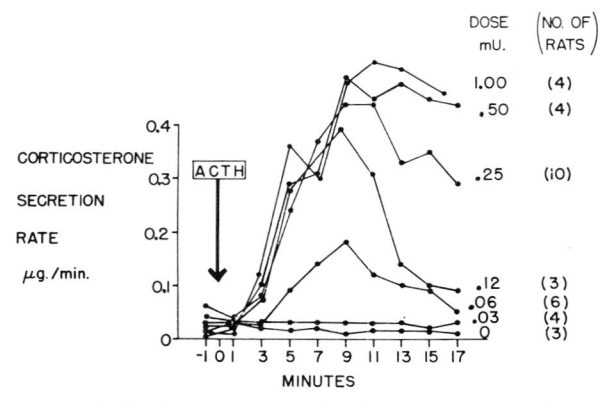

FIG. 2. Corticosterone secretion in response to graded doses of adrenocorticotropic hormone (*ACTH*), represented as a function of time between injection of ACTH and withdrawal of blood from adrenal vein. [From Liddle et al. (27).]

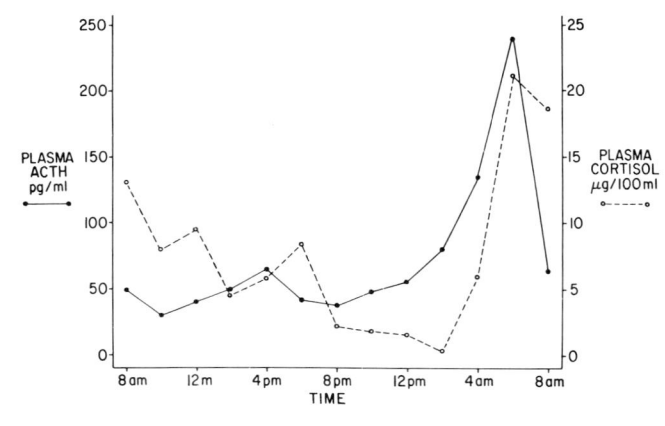

FIG. 3. Diurnal variation of plasma adrenocorticotropic hormone (*ACTH*) and cortisol in normal subject. [From Matsukura et al. (30).]

It had been assumed generally that, under normal resting conditions, plasma cortisol levels described a circadian pattern characterized by a relatively smooth rise and decline. By sampling normal human subjects as often as every 20–30 min for extended periods, several investigators have now demonstrated quite marked short-term fluctuations in plasma cortisol (17-OHCS) and plasma ACTH (4, 20, 22, 40, 49). Although the number of subjects tested in this fashion has been relatively small, the same general observations have been made by investigators working independently.

The episodic nature of this secretion is depicted in Figure 4 and is comparable to data reported by others in limited numbers of subjects (22). Plasma cortisol specific activities determined every 20 min in a single subject indicated brief episodes of brisk cortisol secretion followed by periods of essentially no cortisol secretion (20). Plasma cortisol determinations every 20 min in another individual suggested that cortisol was secreted in eight separate bursts of adrenal activity occupying only a small portion of the 24-hr period. It was estimated that nearly half of the total cortisol secreted during the 24-hr period was produced during the early morning hours during sleep (20).

The concept is evolving that the pituitary-adrenal axis is "active," in terms of ACTH and cortisol secretion, throughout only a part of a given 24-hr period. A surprisingly large proportion of the time, there may be no ACTH or cortisol secretion whatever. Additional periods of secretion may occur as the result of stimuli not related to the circadian rhythm, which makes interpretation of studies of a single subject during a 24-hr period difficult to interpret and sometimes misleading.

Despite the probably episodic nature of ACTH and cortisol secretion and their consequent fluctuating concentrations in blood, the concept of a consistent circadian rhythm of glucocorticoid secretion is still tenable. The major secretory activity of the pituitary-adrenal axis appears to occur in several acute episodes in the early morning hours, and concentration of cortisol in plasma peaks at roughly 6 to 8 AM. After these episodes of brisk secretion, the level in plasma falls as the result of distribution and metabolism of the steroid (20). A less consistent and shorter period of activity occurs during late afternoon at about 4 PM. There is also a suggestion of additional activity around noon in a few subjects, but others have not demonstrated this. Finally, a relatively consistent lack of activity occurs during the late evening hours, especially the hours on either side of midnight. These data are in keeping with a vast number of previous measurements in plasma and urine about the circadian rhythm of cortisol secretion.

However, if these recent observations are substantiated in larger numbers of subjects, they imply that there is not a "basal" or "minimal" level of continuous pituitary-adrenal activity. Rather, the system is turned off and on multiple times during a 24-hr period. This concept has important implications with respect to the study of normal subjects and those with a wide range of diseases.

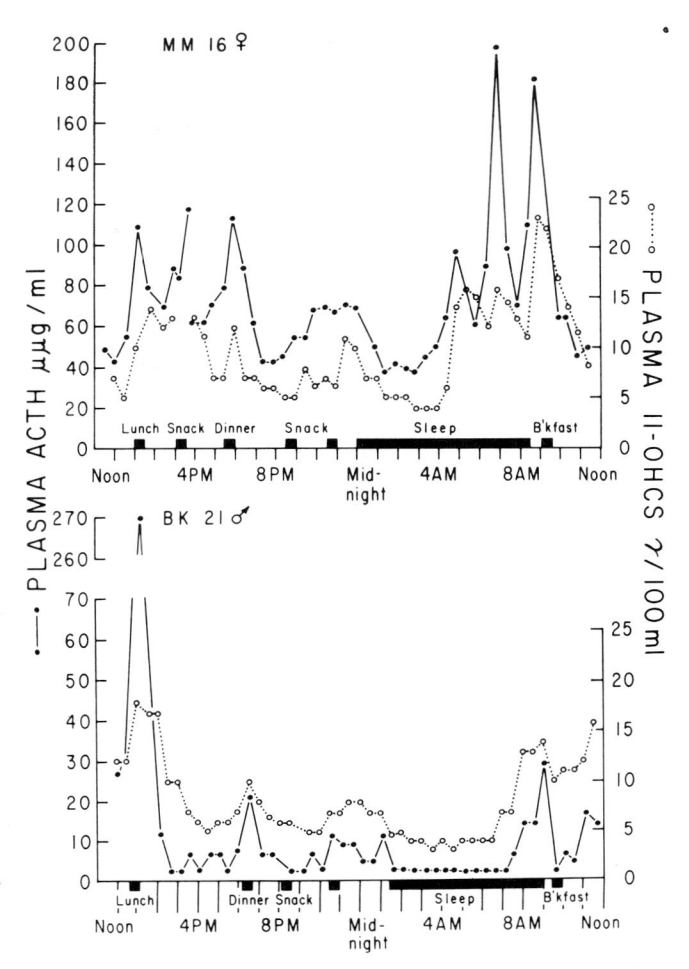

FIG. 4. Circadian periodicity of plasma 11-hydroxycorticosteroid (*11-OHCS*) and plasma adrenocorticotropic hormone (*ACTH*) levels over 24-hr period, as determined by half-hourly sampling. Meal times and sleep as indicated. *Symbols* in upper *left* corners of graphs refer to initials, age, and sex of subjects. [From Krieger et al. (22).]

Obviously, conclusions drawn from infrequent sampling are necessarily limited.

Regulation of Adrenocorticotropic Hormone Secretion

Undoubtedly the higher central nervous system exerts control over the pituitary-adrenal axis. Precise data concerning these relations are difficult to come by in experimental animals and almost impossible in man when current methods are used. Available evidence suggests that a hypothalamic polypeptide neurohumor, corticotropin-releasing factor (CRF), exerts primary control over ACTH secretion. In rats CRF is found localized primarily in the median eminence of the hypothalamus and is at least partly granule bound within nerve endings (34).

The CRF-ACTH system is probably influenced by higher nervous centers. It is generally presumed that impulses from several areas of the brain converge in or near the hypothalamus to exert a modulating influence on the hypothalamus-pituitary-adrenal system. Although there is currently much interest and activity in this area of investigation, there is not yet enough information to be precise about these very complex interactions (9, 29). A circadian or episodic variation in CRF similar to that seen in ACTH and cortisol has not yet been shown, although it is reasonable to assume its existence.

Feedback Regulation of Cortisol Secretion

For many years the control of cortisol secretion was explained solely in terms of a negative feedback mechanism. Undoubtedly this sort of mechanism must be operative under normal circumstances, and there are many kinds of evidence for it. The inhibition of ACTH release by exogenous glucocorticoid, stimulation of ACTH release by metyrapone blockade, and other such manipulations have already been described. Prior to these observations it was known, for example, that adrenal cortical atrophy was associated with hypopituitarism. An adrenal tumor producing cortisol in one gland causes atrophy of the remaining adrenal gland. Removal of one adrenal gland results in a compensatory hypertrophy of the opposite gland. In Cushing's syndrome associated with bilateral adrenal hyperplasia, there is presumably a failure of the feedback suppression of ACTH release with resultant loss of diurnal variation in ACTH levels and overproduction of glucocorticoid (12).

According to the traditional view of such a system, the level for basal blood cortisol concentration is set in the hypothalamus. When blood cortisol concentration falls below this level, the system is activated: CRF is released from storage granules in hypothalamic nerve endings and is carried via the hypophysial portal system to the adenohypophysis where it stimulates ACTH secretion. Adrenocorticotropic hormone is then carried via the circulation to the adrenal glands where cortisol is produced and secreted. Cortisol then "feeds back" via the circulation to the hypothalamus where the activating system is again suppressed. The cortisol concentration in plasma necessary to suppress this system could change rhythmically throughout the 24-hr period and account for the circadian variation in its secretion.

In addition to the "long feedback loop" just described, there is probably a "short feedback loop" as well (33). In this "internal control" system, ACTH may directly influence the regulation of its own secretion.

Over the past several years it has become obvious that a simple negative feedback control system does not entirely explain the regulation of the pituitary-adrenal axis. In such a system the end point is a given level of circulating cortisol preset by the hypothalamus. If such a system were the sole regulator, one would have to presume that the hypothalamic-pituitary system has an inherent tendency to always be maximally active. There are considerable clinical data suggesting that this is not the case. For example, in untreated Addison's disease the circulating ACTH is not constantly maximally elevated. Here ACTH varies rhythmically in a fashion similar to its normal circadian rhythm, but at higher than normal levels (14). This would not be predicted by a simple negative feedback mechanism. Similarly there is a variable ACTH response to metyrapone blockade of cortisol production, depending on time of day (see subsection EXOGENOUSLY ADMINISTERED SUBSTANCES), that is not explainable solely by a negative feedback mechanism (21).

Under conditions of severe stress, such as major surgery, adrenal corticoid output is increased considerably. Yet, when such patients are pretreated with glucocorticoids in amounts far exceeding maximal adrenal production capacity, ACTH secretion is not suppressed (10). Obviously in this situation a negative feedback system is not controlling ACTH secretion.

The studies in which ACTH and plasma cortisol have been measured simultaneously at frequent intervals (see Fig. 4) will sometimes suggest that ACTH will be secreted at a time when cortisol levels in plasma are apparently not decreasing. These recent observations of marked fluctuations in plasma ACTH and cortisol levels already described do not negate these traditional views of the feedback regulation of cortisol secretion. They do serve to point out that there are other important mechanisms, at present poorly understood, that are superimposed on the basic circadian rhythm and operate with considerable frequency.

Current data are consistent with a regulating system that operates like a variably set turn-on switch activated at different cortisol concentrations in plasma (or tissue) at different times of the day. During the evening and early postmidnight hours, only very low concentrations are activating. Between 4 and about 7 AM higher levels (about 7 μg/100 ml) activate CRF-ACTH release (21). It is not clear whether there is also a turn-off setting. The data available at present would fit equally well with a "quantum" release that is self-limiting at the time of each effective stimulus. Such a system could account for the short-term fluctuations in ACTH and cortisol levels that are superimposed on an underlying circadian rhythm. It also explains the diurnal variation of ACTH seen in untreated Addison's disease and the circadian variation in ACTH response to metyrapone.

In addition to this hypothetical mechanism that would operate under normal circumstances, there must be modulating influences from higher nervous system areas that override this basic rhythm under a variety of circumstances.

Alterations in Circadian Rhythm

ACTIVITY-SLEEP CYCLE. It is now firmly established that the normal circadian variation is closely linked to daily routine, since reversing the usual times of activity and sleep leads to a reversal of the timing of circadian variation in plasma 17-OHCS (40, 41). Maximal cortisol levels in plasma are not consistently related to the time of awakening, although the two events usually roughly coincide. Peak cortisol values are observed frequently before awakening, and the initial increase in cortisol secretion usually occurs 2–4 hr before (41). It has been postulated that cortisol secretion is related to the stage of sleep during which rapid eye movement (REM) occurs. More recently sleep stage and plasma 17-OHCS were measured at frequent intervals in two subjects. There was a rough correlation between some REM periods and some cortisol secretory periods; however, the relation seems less than perfect from the data gathered to date (20). Furthermore failure to sleep at all on a single night does not disturb the usual circadian rhythm (40, 41).

The normal circadian variation is not a response to change in posture, such as arising after sleep, since subjects kept supine exhibit the usual circadian rhythm (31). Cortisol secretion does not correlate with growth hormone release or blood glucose or insulin levels under normal resting conditions (48). However, hypoglycemia (blood glucose values below 50 mg/100 ml) regularly induces prompt ACTH and cortisol secretion. Cortisol secretion may be stimulated less consistently by a pronounced fall in the concentration of blood glucose even though hypoglycemic levels are not reached (4).

Normal human subjects in a constant light environment exhibit a typical circadian rhythm when activity and sleep are carried out during the usual hours. When the same subjects reverse their hours of sleep and activity but remain in the constant light environment, the circadian rhythm is reversed. Infants do not have a well-established circadian rhythm of cortisol secretion. This is not established until 1–3 years of age. The delay may reflect the irregular pattern of sleep and activity of young children (11).

Nocturnal animals, such as the rat, normally have a circadian rhythm just the reverse of diurnal animals (15). When rats are kept in constant light they lose their circadian periodicity (7). Similar studies in humans conducted in constant darkness would perhaps be revealing in this respect. Studies done in totally blind individuals have yielded conflicting information (24, 31). It is possible that nocturnal animals require a period of darkness as an external cue to maintain circadian periodicity. Similarly, diurnal animals may require a period of light as the synchronizing cue (23).

Humans in a somewhat isolated environment (e.g., a deep cave without time or day-night cues) will usually lengthen their circadian period by 2–3 hr, if they are allowed to select their own periods of sleep and activity (3). Subjectively they tend to underestimate the number of days spent in such a situation.

Acute alterations in the sleep-activity pattern do not change the normal circadian rhythm during that 24-hr period (40). Several 24-hr periods of altered activity and sleep in succession are required to change the circadian rhythm of cortisol secretion. Sleep-wake cycles have been altered in several subjects to coincide with 12-, 19-, and 33-hr periods. In each instance, after several days of irregular and relatively low levels of cortisol in plasma, a new rhythm developed that was synchronous with the new 12-, 19-, or 33-hr period. In general, the plasma 17-OHCS level was lowest during the initial period of sleep, rose rapidly during sleep, peaked at about the time of awakening, and thereafter fell irregularly until after the subjects were again asleep (40). These studies strongly suggest that habitual sleep-activity schedules are a primary determinant in the periodicity of cortisol secretion. However, the pituitary-adrenal system is not immediately responsive to such cues as light, arousal, posture, state of sleep, or anticipation of sleep, since the normal pattern cannot be changed acutely.

STRESS. Stresses, such as severe trauma, major surgery, psychiatric stress, and electroshock therapy, regularly result in release of ACTH and increased cortisol secretion (36). In this circumstance the negative feedback mechanism no longer functions as such. When stress is severe, exogenous glucocorticoid will not suppress ACTH secretion (10). This response continues as long as the stress operates and can become quite chronic. Thus the circadian rhythm is obliterated in this circumstance. There is no reliable way to predict a degree of stress that will result in a given amount of cortisol secretion. However, in a very general way, lesser degrees of stress cause lesser degrees of alteration in cortisol secretion and more easily suppressible ACTH release.

EXOGENOUSLY ADMINISTERED SUBSTANCES. Glucocorticoid, as already indicated, suppresses cortisol secretion indirectly by modifying ACTH release. Dexamethasone is a synthetic glucocorticoid and potent suppressor of ACTH. As indicated in Figure 5, adrenal suppression following dexamethasone treatment varies considerably, depending on the time of day a single dose is administered. A single oral dose of 0.5 mg dexamethasone given at midnight completely obliterates the early morning rise in plasma cortisol, and plasma cortisol levels remain relatively low during the ensuing 24 hr. The next expected increase in cortisol secretion occurs 24 hr later in normal fashion. If the same dose of dexamethasone is given at 8 AM, cortisol secretion is suppressed for the next 16 hr and the next early morning rise is blunted but not abolished. Similarly, when it is given at 4 PM, the early morning rise in cortisol secretion is blunted but not abolished. During the following 24-hr period the circadian rhythm again returns to normal (22).

Recent reports suggest that constant infusion of small amounts of dexamethasone may more easily suppress the early morning cortisol secretory period than that occurring later in the day (6). This was determined by urinary 17-OHCS measurements at 2-hr intervals and is in direct conflict with the work of others (21, 22) who used corticoid determinations in plasma. Perhaps the urinary data are at variance because of infrequent sampling and delay in metabolism and excretion of cortisol. Similar studies in which simultaneous plasma and urinary corticoid levels are determined at frequent intervals will be required to resolve this.

Metyrapone blocks 11β-hydroxylation in the adrenal cortex and thereby inhibits the production of cortisol. As plasma cortisol levels fall, the release of ACTH stimulates the production of a cortisol precursor, 11-

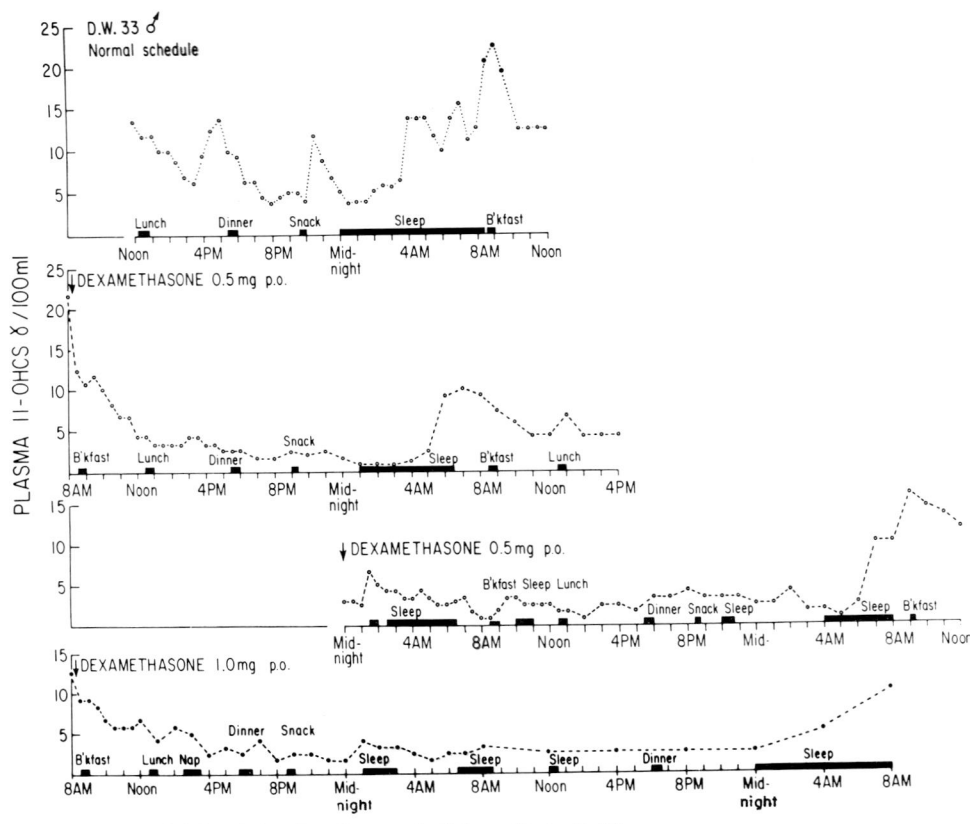

FIG. 5. Plasma 11-hydroxycorticosteroid (*11-OHCS*) levels in circadian periodicity: effect of different doses and times of dexamethasone administration. [From Krieger et al. (22).]

deoxycortisol (compound S), which is a biologically inactive steroid. When metyrapone is infused at a constant rate or given at short intervals throughout the day, the adrenal steroid production varies according to the time of day. More compound S is produced during the early morning hours than in the late afternoon and evening (21). This corresponds to the expected circadian rhythm in ACTH secretion and, in this situation, is not directly related to cortisol levels in plasma.

Circadian variation in adrenal responsiveness to ACTH is real but probably not very significant. When maximal ACTH stimulation is administered before midnight, adrenal response is less than that obtained when a similar stimulus is given in the morning. This difference is abolished by pretreatment with minimally steroidogenic doses of ACTH (41). Furthermore a constant ACTH infusion results in relatively stable 17-OHCS concentration in plasma (39). Thus the varying adrenal responsiveness to ACTH seems to relate to prior stimulation and readiness of the biochemical mechanisms for cortisol synthesis. When ACTH secretion is at a low level or absent for a few hours, as usually occurs during the late evening hours, the adrenal cortex becomes less than maximally responsive. This phenomenon is of relatively small magnitude and of course cannot account even in part for the circadian variation of plasma cortisol. However, it can be an important consideration in certain experimental situations.

ALDOSTERONE

A distinct circadian (perhaps more properly, diurnal) variation occurs in aldosterone secretion, as depicted in Figure 6 (50). Normal human subjects during their usual daily activity typically exhibit an increase in urinary aldosterone values in the morning after arising (50). Despite remaining upright during the remainder of the day, aldosterone values then decrease again late in the day. When subjects remain recumbent, the aldosterone levels do not show this variation, but remain at the usual base-line supine level. When the upright-recumbency pattern is altered such that one remains supine during the day (8 AM to 8 PM) and upright during the night (8 PM to 8 AM), the pattern of aldosterone excretion is also reversed. That is, the increase in aldosterone excretion is greatest early in the upright period no matter when this occurs. This variation is unrelated to ACTH secretion, since it is unaltered in the dexamethasone-suppressed subject. Therefore the primary determinant of aldosterone variation seems to be change in posture.

The control of the renin-angiotensin system over aldosterone secretion is well known and will not be detailed here. In normal subjects changes in plasma renin activity (PRA) have been shown to parallel changes in aldosterone levels. However, when diet and recumbent posture are held constant, plasma renin activity, unlike aldosterone level, falls during late afternoon. This fall in PRA while the subject is continuously supine is not as marked as that following upright posture since the midmorning rise does not occur in this situation. If a person remains supine and then assumes an upright position, plasma renin activity remains low until the change in posture, and then rises, but not to the extent that usually occurs during the morning (13).

Present assays are far more sensitive in detecting small changes in circulating PRA levels than they are in determining urinary excretion of aldosterone. Perhaps sensitive measurements of aldosterone in plasma would reveal a diurnal variation in plasma aldosterone similar to that in PRA.

Nonetheless, plasma renin activity does have a diurnal variation unrelated to changes in posture and diet. On the other hand, these factors plus circulating levels of mineralocorticoid obviously do have a prominent influence on PRA. Depending on the timing of such factors, the basic PRA diurnal rhythm can either be augmented or negated. These same considerations have to be taken into account with respect to changes in aldosterone secretion as well. For example, volume depletion would tend to exaggerate the usual increase in aldosterone secretion associated with upright posture but would tend to counteract the usual fall later in the day.

Exactly why PRA and aldosterone decrease during the course of the day, despite maintenance of the upright posture, is unclear but is most likely related to changes in effective plasma volume and renal blood flow. It is fairly certain that the initial rise in PRA and aldosterone concentration is due to changes in renal blood flow since it can be obliterated by bandaging the lower extremities before arising (13). The fall later in the day probably reflects the action of aldosterone on volume expansion and consequent increased renal blood flow.

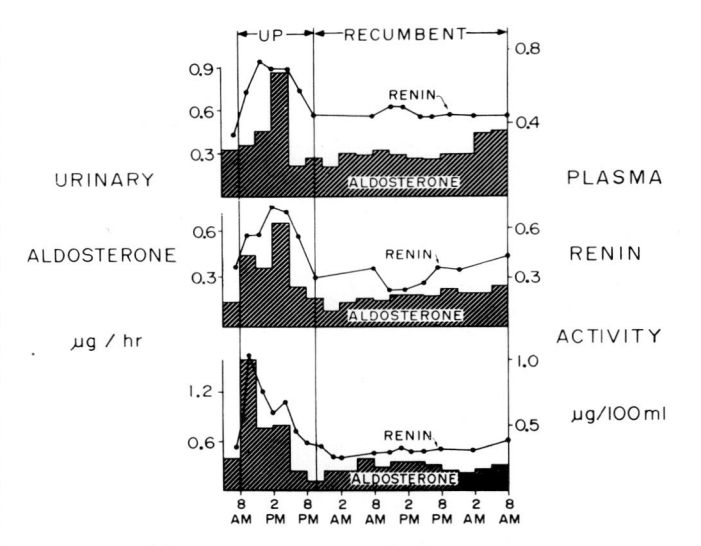

FIG. 6. Aldosterone excretion and plasma renin activity of 3 normal subjects during 12 hr of normal upright activity, followed by 36 hr of continuous recumbency. Each subject was maintained on sodium intake of 100 mEq/day. [From Wolfe et al. (50).]

Renal blood flow is known to be higher in the afternoon than in the morning in normal humans, which is in keeping with this concept.

TESTOSTERONE; ESTROGEN

There are limited data available suggesting that circulating testosterone in males has some circadian variation, with evening levels roughly 65% of morning values. Since 95% of the circulating testosterone in males originates from the testes, the adrenal contribution to this variation is not likely to be significant (28). Similarly most circulating estrogen in males originates from the testes, but even less information is available on this subject (26). Little information exists about a possible circadian variation of androgen or estrogen in females.

This investigation was supported in part by National Institutes of Health Grant TI-AM-5214.

REFERENCES

1. Aschoff, J. Comparative physiology: diurnal rhythms. *Ann. Rev. Physiol.* 25: 581–600, 1963.
2. Aschoff, J. Circadian rhythms in man. *Science* 148: 1427–1432, 1965.
3. Aschoff, J. Circadian clocks. In: *Proceedings of the Feldafing Summer School, September 1964*, edited by J. Aschoff. Amsterdam: North-Holland, 1965.
4. Berson, S. A., and R. S. Yalow. Radioimmunoassay of ACTH in plasma. *J. Clin. Invest.* 47: 2725–2751, 1968.
5. Bliss, E. L., A. A. Sandberg, D. A. Nelson, and K. Eik-Nes. The normal levels of 17-hydroxycorticosteroids in the peripheral blood of man. *J. Clin. Invest.* 32: 818–823, 1953.
6. Ceresa, F., A. Angeli, G. Boccuzzi, and L. Perotti. Impulsive and basal ACTH secretion phases in normal subjects, in obese subjects with signs of adrenocortical hyperfunction and in hyperthyroid patients. *J. Clin. Endocrinol. Metab.* 31: 491–501, 1970.
7. Cheifetz, D., N. Gaffred, and J. F. Dingman. The effect of bilateral adrenalectomy and continuous light on the circadian rhythm of corticotropin in female rats. *Endocrinology* 82: 1117–1124, 1968.
8. Demura, H., C. D. West, C. A. Nugent, K. Nakagawa, and F. H. Tyler. A sensitive radioimmunoassay for plasma ACTH levels. *J. Clin. Endocrinol. Metab.* 26: 1297–1302, 1966.
9. De Wied, D., and J. A. W. M. Weijnen. Pituitary adrenal and the brain. In: *Progress in Brain Research*, edited by D. De Wied and J. A. W. M. Weijnen. Amsterdam: Elsevier, 1970, vol. 32.
10. Estep, H. L., D. P. Island, R. L. Ney, and G. W. Liddle. Pituitary-adrenal dynamics during surgical stress. *J. Clin. Endocrinol. Metab.* 23: 419–425, 1963.

11. FRANKS, R. C. Diurnal variation of plasma 17-hydroxycorticosteroids in children. *J. Clin. Endocrinol. Metab.* 27: 75–78, 1967.
12. GIVENS, J. R., R. L. NEY, W. E. NICHOLS, A. L. GRABER, AND G. W. LIDDLE. Absence of a normal diurnal variation of plasma ACTH in Cushing's disease. *Clin. Res.* 12: 267, 1964.
13. GORDON, R. D., L. K. WOLFE, D. P. ISLAND, AND G. W. LIDDLE. A diurnal rhythm in plasma renin activity in man. *J. Clin. Invest.* 45: 1587–1592, 1966.
14. GRABER, A. L., J. R. GIVENS, W. E. NICHOLSON, D. P. ISLAND, AND G. W. LIDDLE. Persistence of diurnal rhythmicity in plasma ACTH concentration in cortisol deficient patient. *J. Clin. Endocrinol. Metab.* 25: 804–807, 1965.
15. GUILLEMIN, R., W. E. DEAR, AND R. A. LIEBETT. Nychthemeral variations in plasma free corticosteroid levels of the rat. *Proc. Soc. Exptl. Biol. Med.* 101: 394–395, 1959.
16. HALBERG, F., E. HALBERG, C. D. BARNUM, AND J. J. BITTNER. Physiologic 24-hour periodicity in human beings and mice, photoperiodism and related phenomena in plants and animals. *Am. Assoc. Advan. Sci. Publ.* 55: 803–878, 1959.
17. HALBERG, F. Chronobiology. *Ann. Rev. Physiol.* 31: 675–725, 1969.
18. HARKER, J. E. Diurnal rhythms in the animal kingdom. *Biol. Rev.* 33: 1–52, 1958.
19. HASTINGS, J. W. The biology of circadian rhythms from man to microorganism. *New Engl. J. Med.* 282: 435–441, 1970.
20. HELLMAN, L., F. NAKADA, J. CURTIS, E. D. WEITZMAN, J. KREAM, H. ROFFWARG, S. ELLMAN, D. K. FUKUSHIMA, AND T. F. GALLAGHER. Cortisol is secreted episodically by normal man. *J. Clin. Endocrinol. Metab.* 30: 411–422, 1970.
21. JUBIZ, W., S. MATSUKURA, A. W. MEILKE, G. HARADA, C. D. WEST, AND F. H. TYLER. Plasma metyrapone, adrenocorticotropic hormone, cortisol and deoxycortisol levels. *Arch. Internal Med.* 125: 468–471, 1970.
22. KRIEGER, D. T., W. ALLEN, F. RIZZO, AND H. P. KRIEGER. Characterization of the normal temporal pattern of plasma corticosteroid levels. *J. Clin. Endocrinol. Metab.* 32: 266–284, 1971.
23. KRIEGER, D. T., J. KREUZER, AND F. A. RIZZO. Constant light: effect on circadian pattern and phase reversal of steroid and electrolyte levels in man. *J. Clin. Endocrinol. Metab.* 29: 1634–1638, 1969.
24. KRIEGER, D. T., F. RIZZO, AND A. J. SILVERBERG. Circadian periodicity of plasma 17-hydroxycorticosteroids in blind subjects. *Clin. Res.* 16: 523, 1968.
25. LAIDLAW, J. C., D. JENKINS, W. J. REDDY, AND T. JAKDOSON. The diurnal variation in adrenocortical secretion. *J. Clin. Invest.* 33: 950, 1954.
26. LEACH, R. B., W. O. MADDOCK, I. TOKUYAMA, C. A. PAULSEN, AND W. O. NELSON. Clinical studies of testicular hormone production. *Recent Progr. Hormone Res.* 12: 377–398, 1956.
27. LIDDLE, G. W., D. ISLAND, AND C. K. MEADOR. Normal and abnormal regulation of corticotropin secretion in man. *Recent Progr. Hormone Res.* 18: 125–166, 1962.
28. LIPSETT, M. B., AND C. W. BARDIN. Production and metabolism of androgens in man. In: *International Encyclopedia of Pharmacology and Therapeutics*, edited by Z. Laron. London: Pergamon Press, 1968, sect. 47.
29. MARTINI, L., AND W. F. GANONG. *Neuroendocrinology*. New York: Acad. Press, 1966.
30. MATSUKURA, S., C. D. WEST, Y. ICHIKAWA, W. JUBIZ, G. HARADA, AND F. H. TYLER. A new phenomenon of usefulness in the radioimmunoassay of plasma adrenocorticotropic hormone. *J. Lab. Clin. Med.* 77: 490–500, 1971.
31. MIGEON, C. J., F. J. TYLER, J. P. MAHONEY, A. A. FLORENTIN, H. CASTLE, E. L. BLISS, AND L. T. SAMUELS. The diurnal variation of plasma levels and urinary excretion of 17-hydroxycorticosteroids in normal subjects, night workers and blind subjects. *J. Clin. Endocrinol. Metab.* 16: 622–633, 1956.
32. MILLS, J. N. Human circadian rhythm. *Physiol. Rev.* 46: 128–171, 1966.
33. MOTTA, M., F. PIVA, AND L. MARTINI. The role of "short" feedback mechanisms in the regulation of adrenocorticotropin secretion. In: *Progress in Brain Research*, edited by D. De Wied and J. A. W. M. Weijnen. Amsterdam: Elsevier, 1970, vol. 32, p. 25–32.
34. MULDER, A. H. On the subcellular localization of corticotrophin releasing factor (CRF) in the rat median eminence. In: *Progress in Brain Research*, edited by D. De Wied and J. A. W. M. Weijnen. Amsterdam: Elsevier, 1970, p. 33–41.
35. NELSON, D. H., AND L. T. SAMUELS. A method for the determination of 17-hydroxycorticosteroids in blood: 17-hydroxycorticosterone in the peripheral circulation. *J. Clin. Endocrinol. Metab.* 12: 519–526, 1952.
36. NEY, R. L., N. SHIMIZU, W. E. NICHOLSON, D. P. ISLAND, AND G. W. LIDDLE. Correlation of plasma ACTH concentration with adrenocortical response in normal human subjects, surgical patients and patients with Cushing's disease. *J. Clin. Invest.* 42: 1669–1677, 1963.
37. NICHOLS, C. T., C. A. NUGENT, AND F. H. TYLER. Diurnal variation in suppression of adrenal function by glucocorticoids. *J. Clin. Endocrinol. Metab.* 25: 343–349, 1965.
38. NICHOLS, C. T., AND F. H. TYLER. Diurnal variation in adrenal cortical function. *Ann. Rev. Med.* 18: 313–324, 1967.
39. NUGENT, C. A., K. EIK-NES, H. S. KENT, L. T. SAMUELS, AND F. H. TYLER. A possible explanation for Cushing's syndrome associated with adrenal hyperplasia. *J. Clin. Endocrinol. Metab.* 20: 1259–1268, 1960.
40. ORTH, D. N., D. P. ISLAND, AND G. W. LIDDLE. Experimental alteration of the circadian rhythm in plasma cortisol (17-OHCS) concentration in man. *J. Clin. Endocrinol. Metab.* 27: 549–555, 1967.
41. PERKOFF, G. T., K. EIK-NES, C. A. NUGENT, H. L. FRED, R. A. NIMER, L. RUSH, L. T. SAMUELS, AND F. H. TYLER. Studies of the diurnal variation of plasma 17-hydroxycorticosteroids in man. *J. Clin. Endocrinol. Metab.* 19: 432–443, 1959.
42. PINCUS, G. A diurnal rhythm in the excretion of urinary ketosteroids by young men. *J. Clin. Endocrinol. Metab.* 3: 195–199, 1943.
43. ROMANOFF, L. P., J. PLAGER, AND G. PINCUS. The determination of adrenocortical steroids in human urine. *Endocrinology* 45: 10–20, 1949.
44. SANDBERG, A. A., D. H. NELSON, J. G. PALMER, L. T. SAMUELS, AND F. H. TYLER. The effects of epinephrine on the metabolism of 17-hydroxycorticosteroids in the human. *J. Clin. Endocrinol. Metab.* 13: 629–647, 1953.
45. SANDBERG, A. A., D. H. NELSON, E. M. GLENN, F. H. TYLER, AND L. T. SAMUELS. 17-Hydroxycorticosteroids and 17-ketosteroids in urine of human subjects: clinical application of a method employing β-glucuronidase hydrolysis. *J. Clin. Endocrinol. Metab.* 13: 1445–1464, 1953.
46. SEGAL, B. M., AND N. D. CHRISTY. Potentiation of the biologic activity of ACTH by human plasma. A preliminary study. *J. Clin. Endocrinol. Metab.* 28: 1465–1472, 1968.
47. SEGAL, B. M., W. D. DRUCKER, H. BENOVITZ, A. L. VERDE, AND N. P. CHRISTY. Further studies of adrenal weight-maintaining activity in the plasma of patients with Cushing's disease. *Am. J. Med.* 49: 34–41, 1970.
48. TAKAHASHI, T., D. M. KIPNIS, AND W. H. DAUGHADAY. Growth hormone secretion during sleep. *J. Clin. Invest.* 47: 2079–2090, 1968.
49. TOURNIARE, J., J. ORGIAZZI, J. F. RIVIERE, AND H. ROUSSET. Repeated plasma cortisol determinations in Cushing's syndrome due to adrenocortical adenoma. *J. Clin. Endocrinol. Metab.* 32: 666–668, 1971.
50. WOLFE, L. K., R. D. GORDON, R. P. ISLAND, AND G. W. LIDDLE. An analysis of factors determining the circadian pattern of aldosterone excretion. *J. Clin. Endocrinol. Metab.* 26: 1261–1266, 1966.
51. YALOW, R. S., S. M. GLICK, J. ROTH, AND S. BERSON. Radioimmunoassay of human plasma ACTH. *J. Clin. Endocrinol. Metab.* 24: 1219–1225, 1964.

CHAPTER 11

Influences of corticosteroids on protein and carbohydrate metabolism

ROBERT STEELE[1] | *Biology Department, Brookhaven National Laboratory, Upton, New York*

CHAPTER CONTENTS

Corticosteroids that Influence Carbohydrate and Protein Metabolism
Vital Functions Disturbed by Adrenalectomy, and Replacement of Adrenal Secretion by Administered Corticosteroids
Effect on Carbohydrate Metabolism Utilized in Bioassay of Glucocorticoids
Resting Rate of Glucocorticoid Secretion, and Meaning of Hypercorticalism
Gross Interrelationship of Whole-animal Carbohydrate and Protein Metabolism in Glucocorticoid Effects
Physiological Mechanisms for Modifications of Carbohydrate and Protein Metabolism Caused by Glucocorticoid Deficiency and Excess
  Consequences of decreased appetite in glucocorticoid deficiency
  Changes in secretion rates of other relevant hormones
    Epinephrine
    Insulin
  Net transfer of amino acids from peripheral tissues to liver in glucocorticoid excess
    Protein metabolism in peripheral tissues
    Protein metabolism in liver
  Changes in rate of gluconeogenesis
    Early effects of glucocorticoid administration in steroid-deficient rat
    Later effects of glucocorticoid administration
  Changes in rates of glycogen breakdown and deposition
    Glycogenolysis
    Glucose uptake and glycogen synthesis by liver
  Altered facility for glucose utilization by peripheral tissues
    Glucose uptake and phosphorylation
    Oxidative decarboxylation of pyruvate

A CLASSIC METHOD for the bioassay of the glucocorticoid activity of a steroid compound utilizes the enhancement of liver glycogen deposition in the fasting adrenalectomized rat. In this particular animal an elevation of blood glucose concentration is one of the earliest manifestations of glucocorticoid action (57, 113, 129). Evidence for an important influence of these compounds on glucose metabolism led to the designation *glucocorti-*

Research described in this chapter was carried out at Brookhaven National Laboratory under the auspices of the U. S. Atomic Energy Commission.
[1] Dr. Steele died on January 18, 1974.

coid. The corticosteroids produced by the adrenal gland that have glucocorticoid activity are also those that influence protein metabolism and increase the capacity of skeletal muscle to perform long-sustained work (76).

I. CORTICOSTEROIDS THAT INFLUENCE CARBOHYDRATE AND PROTEIN METABOLISM

The skeletal structure of adrenocortical steroids and the necessary modifications to form some well-known glucocorticoids are shown in Figure 1. Modification of the basic structure in Figure 1 by the insertion of an oxygen atom at ring carbon 11 is essential for glucocorticoid activity. In addition, many of the glucocorticoids have a hydroxyl group at carbon atom 17; thus the term *11,17-oxycorticosteroids* has sometimes been used for the glucocorticoids. Note, however, that corticosterone has no oxygen at carbon atom 17; nonetheless it has glucocorticoid activity and is a known constituent, along with the glucocorticoid, cortisol, and the mineralocorticoid, aldosterone, of normal adrenal secretion.

The basic structure in Figure 1 is deoxycorticosterone (DOC), a synthetic mineralocorticoid or salt-retaining hormone, which is commonly injected as the 21-acetate ester (DOCA) for the maintenance of adrenalectomized animals when their deficient glucocorticoid function is to be preserved. Both DOC and DOCA have negligible glucocorticoid action.

Prednisolone, triamcinolone, and dexamethasone (Fig. 1) are potent synthetic compounds sometimes used in therapy, as well as in investigation of the metabolic effects of the glucocorticoids.

When more is known about the mechanism of action of the corticosteroids, the classification of these into glucocorticoids and mineralocorticoids may seem arbitrary. Many glucocorticoids have mineralocorticoid activity, for example, and aldosterone administered at very high doses has glucocorticoid activity. At present, however, the distinction is useful. This chapter deals primarily with the glucocorticoids, because it is their influence on carbohydrate and protein metabolism that has been investigated extensively.

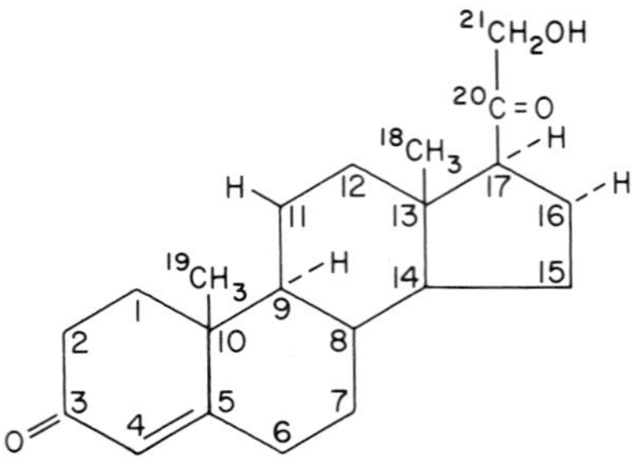

FIG. 1. Skeletal structure common to adrenocortical steroids. Ring hydrogen is shown only when its configuration is the same as that of a replacing group in one of the glucocorticoids listed; *dashed line*, α orientation; *solid line*, β orientation.

Glucocorticoid	Modification of basic structure
a) 11-Dehydrocorticosterone	11-Keto
b) Corticosterone	11β-Hydroxy
c) Cortisone	11-Keto, 17α-hydroxy
d) Cortisol (hydrocortisone)	11β-Hydroxy, 17α-hydroxy
e) Prednisolone	$\Delta^{1,2}$-11β-hydroxy, 17α-hydroxy*
f) Triamcinolone	$\Delta^{1,2}$-11β-hydroxy, 17α-hydroxy, 16α-hydroxy, 9α-fluoro*
g) Dexamethasone	$\Delta^{1,2}$-11β-hydroxy, 17α-hydroxy, 16α-methyl, 9α-fluoro*

* $\Delta^{1,2}$ indicates an additional double bond between carbons 1 and 2 in ring A.

II. VITAL FUNCTIONS DISTURBED BY ADRENALECTOMY, AND REPLACEMENT OF ADRENAL SECRETION BY ADMINISTERED CORTICOSTEROIDS

Britton & Silvette (19) restored normal vigor in moribund adrenalectomized cats by injection of the then novel bovine adrenal cortical extract prepared by Swingle and Pfiffner. The cats had refused food for a number of days following adrenalectomy, had extremely low levels of blood sugar, and were depleted of liver glycogen. After treatment with the cortical extract for 12–48 hr, the cats were found to have near-normal levels of blood sugar and significant stores of liver glycogen even though no food had been supplied to them. It was necessary then (i.e., 1932) to demonstrate that the small residue of medullary epinephrine present in the cortical extract was incapable of causing the effects seen, and this was done by control experiments.

Britton and Silvette judged correctly that the restoration of carbohydrate metabolism was a primary action of the cortical extract distinct from the restoration of electrolyte and water balance. They were aided in their judgment by the results they obtained by injecting cortical extract into intact, fasting rats and rabbits (18). Injections of the extract resulted in elevated blood sugar levels and prevented the usual fall in concentration of liver glycogen that occurs in rats after 7 hr of fasting. A dose dependency of this effect was established for use as a biological assay for adrenocortical extracts. It was also shown that the adrenocortical extract elevated blood sugar and liver glycogen levels 3 hr after its administration to rabbits fasted for 17 hr. These investigators also made preliminary observations on the amelioration, by adrenalectomy, of extreme hyperglycemia of depancreatized cats (19).

Subsequent development of procedures for sustaining properly fed adrenalectomized rats in good condition for weeks by administration of sodium chloride allowed the separate effects of glucocorticoid deficiency to be demonstrated more convincingly.

Long et al. (111) reported in 1940 that adrenalectomized animals suffered severe hypoglycemia during a 48-hr fast, but the normal glucose concentration could be restored by glucose administration and refeeding. Observations were made of the concentrations of liver and muscle glycogen and of blood glucose during fasting in normal and adrenalectomized rats and mice. This enabled adrenocortical extract to be administered when liver glycogen had been reduced to a negligible amount. Long et al. (111) reported the restoration of blood glucose and liver glycogen to normal levels by injections of adrenocortical extract over a 12-hr period while fasting was continued but found little effect during this period on levels of muscle glycogen. These investigators used increased glucose excretion in the urine by the partially depancreatized rat and the adrenalectomized, depancreatized rat to demonstrate the parallel glucosuric effects of adrenocortical extract and of several crystalline glucocorticoids. These preparations were furnished to them in small amounts by Kendall, Wintersteiner, and Pfiffner. They also demonstrated the ineffectiveness of the salt-retaining steroid, deoxycorticosterone, in increasing glucose excretion by such animals.

III. EFFECT ON CARBOHYDRATE METABOLISM UTILIZED IN BIOASSAY OF GLUCOCORTICOIDS

The effects of injection of an excess of cortisol (Table 1) on the carbohydrate stores of fasted adrenalectomized rats were summarized in 1960 by Long et al. (113).

> When adrenalectomized rats, previously fasted for 18 to 24 hours, are injected subcutaneously with 10 mg of cortisol there occurs over the next 48 hours a continuous and remarkable accumulation of carbohydrate in the bodies of the animals. The features of this effect are (a) a rise in blood glucose of about 40–50 mg per 100 ml which is evident from one to two hours after the injection, and which is sustained at this level for 48 hours; (b) an elevation of the liver glycogen, which begins somewhat later than the rise in blood glucose, but is continued for at least 24 hours and is maintained at a very high level (150–200 mg per 100 g body weight) for another 24 hours; (c) a much slower rise in muscle glycogen which is not significant until 8 to 12 hours after the injection of cortisol; (d) a total accumulation of carbohydrate ... which increases the total carbohydrate content of the body to levels usually found in glucose-fed normal animals.

Glucocorticoid secretion is increased during fasting by the superimposition of conditions more stressful than mere fasting. After such stresses the concentration

TABLE 1. *Carbohydrate Stores of Fasted Adrenalectomized Rats at Various Times After Treatment with Cortisol*

Treatment	Body Glucose[a]	Liver Glycogen	Muscle Glycogen[b]	Total Carbohydrate	Increase in Total Carbohydrate
	Mg glucose per 100 g body wt				
Control	14	2	196	212	
Cortisol[c]					
1 hour	16[d]	1[d]	210[d]	227	15
2 hours	18	3[d]	205[d]	236	24
3 hours	24	14	234[d]	272	60
4 hours	23	18	198[d]	239	27
6 hours	22	32	215[d]	269	57
12 hours	24	82	255	361	159
24 hours	25	179	284	488	276
48 hours	25	200	286	511	299
Fed, normal	21	238	368	627	

[a] Calculated on glucose space of 25 % of body wt. [b] Calculated on muscle mass of 50 % of body wt. [c] Subcutaneous injection of 10 mg. [d] No significant change from control. [Data from Long et al. (113).]

of liver glycogen increases in normal (but not in adrenalectomized) rats even though fasting is continued. This effect was described by Evans (41) in 1934, using hypoxia as the superimposed stress and comparing intact rats with adrenalectomized rats maintained on salt. The glycogen bioassay procedure mimics this stress response involving the sudden influx of a larger amount of glucocorticoid.

Figure 2 demonstrates a bioassay procedure (134) for glucocorticoids reported in 1947, when a number of pure steroids were available to establish dose-response curves in fasted adrenalectomized rats maintained on NaCl. A number of similar bioassays (9, 133, 146) were the basis for development of this procedure.

IV. RESTING RATE OF GLUCOCORTICOID SECRETION, AND MEANING OF HYPERCORTICALISM

Ingle & Baker (76) noted that the adrenalectomized male rat of 200 g body wt requires 0.25–0.50 mg cortisone per day to support life under nonstressful conditions, whereas when such animals are subjected to the exhausting muscle-work test, 2.0–4.0 mg cortisone per day is required to support optimal work output.

Glenister & Yates (56) used [^{14}C]corticosterone to measure the short-term secretion rate of corticosterone in the undisturbed male rat. The rate in the morning was 0.114 μg/min per 100-g rat, whereas in the afternoon the rate was about 1.5 times as great. These findings suggest a secretion rate of 0.33–0.5 mg/day for the 200-g rat. The authors noted that secretion rates about five times those they had observed had been found by other workers in rats in the stressful situation involving the collection of adrenal vein blood for direct measurement of corticosteroid output.

In adrenalectomized dogs, administration of 0.16–0.30 mg cortisone per 200-g body wt (0.8–1.5 mg/kg) per day for 8–16 days was an adequate replacement dose. Such a dose restored to normal the responses of the adrenalectomized dog to the injection of insulin or glucose in the resting postabsorptive state, as shown by deBodo et al. (32).

The hypophysectomized animal is severely deficient in glucocorticoid secretion, as well as in pituitary growth hormone secretion. This is due to the absence of pituitary adrenocorticotropic hormone (ACTH), which exerts minute-by-minute control over the rate of adrenal cortex secretion [see (183)]. In the continued absence of ACTH the adrenal cortex becomes atrophic and secretes little glucocorticoid.

The administration (or pathological secretion) of more glucocorticoid than is called for results in *hypercorticalism*. The intact animal is not brought into hypercorticalism by administration of glucocorticoid at less than its own unstressed physiological secretion rate because it lowers its own secretion rate when exogenous glucocorticoid is given. Administration of ACTH at a rate higher than the endogenous secretion rate leads to hypercorticalism as excess glucocorticoid is secreted in response. Ingle et al. (79) demonstrated that hyperglycemia and glucosuria could be induced in intact rats by large doses of ACTH, as well as by large amounts of glucocorticoid.

The most dramatic manifestation of hypercorticalism is *steroid diabetes*, a condition in which blood glucose

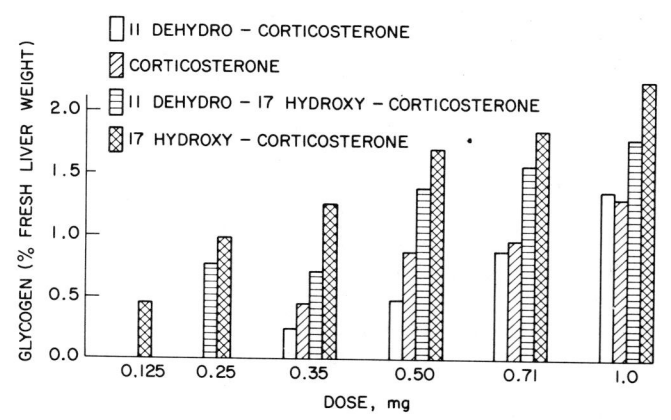

FIG. 2. Glycogen deposition obtained with pure adrenal steroids in fasted adrenalectomized rats. The assay was conducted on bilaterally adrenalectomized rats of 140–160 g body wt fasted for 1 day. These were maintained on drinking water containing 1% NaCl and on a high-protein diet the first 4 days after adrenalectomy. Indicated dose of hormone was injected subcutaneously at 2-hr intervals in 4 equal parts, each in 0.2 ml cottonseed oil, beginning the morning of the fifth day after adrenalectomy. Two hours after the last injection the whole liver was analyzed for glycogen by the method of Good et al. (59); the liver was removed to KOH solution 30 sec or less after the abdomen was opened under cyclopal anesthesia. Adrenalectomized rats given cottonseed oil alone had negligible liver glycogen (0.014%). Identification of compounds: 11-dehydrocorticosterone is (a) of Fig. 1; 11-dehydro-17-hydroxycorticosterone is (c) of Fig. 1; 17-hydroxycorticosterone is (d) of Fig. 1. [From Pabst et al. (134).]

TABLE 2. *Decrease in Urinary Glucose and Urinary Nitrogen Excretions Caused by Adrenalectomy in Fasting Depancreatized Cats*

Condition	Urinary Glucose, g/kg per day	Urinary Nitrogen, g/kg per day	Fasting Blood Sugar, mg/100 ml
Normal	0	0.5 (0.4–0.8)	
Depancreatized	3.9 (2.4–5.5)	1.6 (1.2–2.4)	346 (226–788)
Adrenalectomized and depancreatized	0.4 (0.0–1.2)	0.6 (0.2–1.0)	218 (80–342)

Range of values indicated in parentheses. [Data from Long & Lukens (112).]

concentration rises high enough so that glucose appears in the urine. This condition has been produced in the rat (79, 81), hamster (21), guinea pig (88), mouse (141), and rabbit (170). It cannot be induced in the intact dog (20, 158) or in the normal human. A small fraction of the human population predisposed to the development of diabetes is susceptible to steroid-induced glycosuria. In all the above species the removal of a large portion of the pancreas makes the animal more susceptible to this effect of excess glucocorticoid. In the susceptible species studied, histological changes in pancreatic β cells indicate increased secretory activity (88, 170, 179).

The effects of administering excess glucocorticoid do not always represent simply an increase in the effects produced by raising the glucocorticoid supply from a deficient rate to the normal secretion rate. It is believed that the primary action of the hormone remains the same but that the added amount of steroid, acting at a different balance of secretion rates of other hormones and of substrates for metabolism in the various tissues, so often produces different effects. Useful information is acquired in either case when the other influences are understood. Useful data about specific hormonal action are not acquired, however, when isolated tissues are exposed to concentrations of glucocorticoids much higher than the concentrations encountered in vivo. Nonspecific associations of steroids with numerous cell constituents (127) are common under these circumstances, and effects on cell metabolism are produced that are produced also by nonglucocorticoids.

V. GROSS INTERRELATIONSHIP OF WHOLE-ANIMAL CARBOHYDRATE AND PROTEIN METABOLISM IN GLUCOCORTICOID EFFECTS

The effects of adrenalectomy and of cortical extract administration on protein metabolism were studied initially because of interest in the then newly discovered effects of hypophysectomy on the excretion of glucose and nitrogen in the urine of animals in the fasting diabetic state. The absence of growth hormone and the deficiency in glucocorticoid secretion both contribute to the ameliorating effects of hypophysectomy on the diabetes of the depancreatized animal.

Long & Lukens (112) described in 1935 the effectiveness of adrenalectomy in causing decreases of the urinary glucose and nitrogen excretion of the fasting depancreatized cat (Table 2).

Long et al. (111) demonstrated (Table 3) that the fasting urinary nitrogen excretion of the adrenalectomized, salt-maintained rat was elevated by administration of adrenocortical extract. Cortical extract also raised the urinary nitrogen excretion of fasting normal and hypophysectomized rats. The latter result showed that the effect was not dependent on the presence of the pituitary gland.

Evans (42) showed that prior adrenalectomy, but not prior adrenal demedullation, decreased the urinary glucose and nitrogen excretion of phlorizinized fasting rats and eliminated the increased nitrogen excretion that occurs after superimposed stress during fasting in the normal rat.

In many early investigations, rats were fed ad libitum before starvation periods in which effects on nitrogen excretion were recorded; since the adrenalectomized rats ate less, they began starvation in a nutritional state that dictated a lesser fasting nitrogen excretion. Also most of the early experiments involving the effects of excess glucocorticoids on nitrogen excretion in intact rats were carried out for only a few days. The involution of lymphoid tissues that occurs in such animals very soon after excess glucocorticoid administration (35, 116, 175) liberates a large amount of protein, which acts as if it represented a temporary additional intake of fed protein and may be a major contributing factor to increased nitrogen excretion occurring over the next several days. During starvation, net nitrogen loss occurs, larger at first; nitrogen balance can be maintained

TABLE 3. *Effects of Injected Adrenocortical Extract on Nitrogen Excretion of Rats Fasted for 12 Hr Before Treatment*

	Normal Rats			Adrenalectomized Rats			Hypophysectomized Rats		
	Control*	Injected*, 1 ml/hr per 12 hr	Increase	Control*	Injected*, 1 ml/hr per 12 hr	Increase	Control*	Injected*, 1 ml/hr per 12 hr	Increase
Urine nitrogen, mg/100 g body wt per 12 hr	54±4 (12)	81±4 (6)	27	37±4 (4)	64±7 (4)	27	66±3 (6)	99±1 (11)	33

Figure in parentheses is number of rats. *Mean ± SEM. [Data from Long et al. (111).]

corticoid occurs in animals on a low-protein diet just as strongly as in animals on a high-protein diet.

Ingle (75) also demonstrated that an increased amount of glucocorticoid is not required before stress brings forth increased nitrogen excretion in force-fed adrenalectomized rats. A daily maintenance dose of cortical extract administered to adrenalectomized rats allowed the response to stress to occur. Nevertheless, as summarized by Cuthbertson (29), increased glucocorticoid secretion does occur after severe injury, such as a fracture or burn. In this case the protein-depleted animal fails to respond with increased urinary nitrogen excretion, whereas this does occur after excess glucocorticoid administration. This suggests that in the severely injured animal the increased amount of glucocorticoid secreted does not represent an excess of glucocorticoid.

Wells & Kendall (174) showed in 1940 that salt-

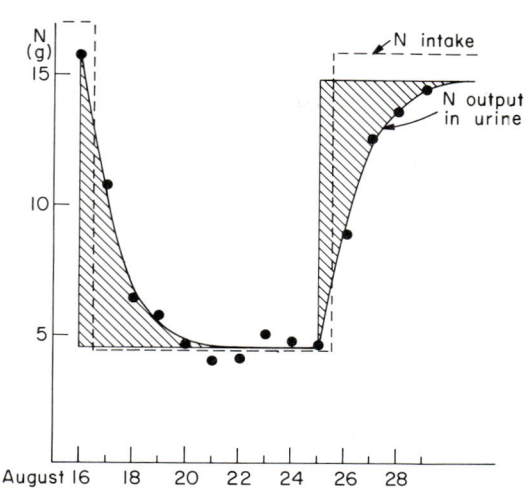

FIG. 3. Daily nitrogen excretion of human subject at 2 levels of protein intake. *Left shaded area*, stored nitrogen (N) gradually lost from body after decrease in protein intake from 17 to 4.4 g N per day; *right shaded area*, nitrogen storage in the body after protein intake was increased again to 16 g N per day. [From Martin & Robison (121).]

over a wide range of absolute values of protein nitrogen intake and excretion. Figure 3 shows the time course of changes in nitrogen excretion after changes in protein intake.

The following experiments of Ingle and his collaborators were attempts to control the effects of such perturbing factors. Figure 4 shows an experiment reported by Ingle (75) in which a 24-day regimen of cortisone just large enough to cause negative nitrogen balance was imposed on a force-fed normal rat that had been growing and had been excreting less nitrogen than it was taking in. Weight loss began immediately, and a peak in nitrogen excretion occurred after 5 days. After another 5 days, slow growth began and nitrogen excretion was less than intake. When the regimen was terminated, rapid growth resumed immediately and nitrogen excretion decreased sharply after 3 more days. The effect of excess cortisone in impeding the retention of fed nitrogen was evident throughout this experiment, whether net nitrogen balance was in a positive phase or a negative phase.

Ingle & Oberle (77) showed that a lessened excretion of urinary nitrogen does not occur in the salt-maintained, adrenalectomized rat when it is force-fed on a medium-carbohydrate (48% by dry wt) diet (Fig. 5). Nitrogen excretion of force-fed adrenalectomized and of sham-operated animals was similar up to the 14th day of forced feeding and also during a subsequent 10-day fasting period. Fasting did not cause lessened nitrogen excretion in adrenalectomized rats as compared with normal rats when both groups had been well nourished by being force-fed a standard diet for the several weeks before fasting. Silber & Porter (157) and Goodlad & Munro (60) showed that the increased urinary nitrogen excretion caused by the administration of excess gluco-

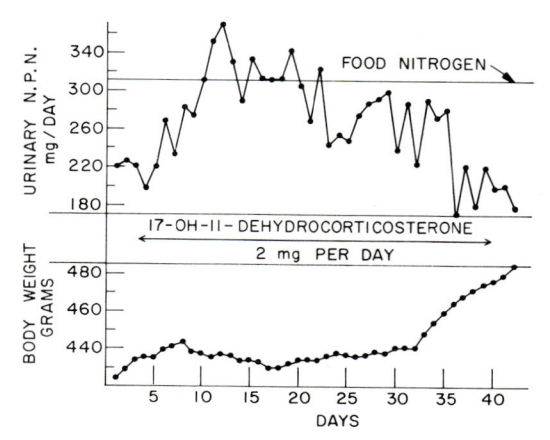

FIG. 4. Nitrogen excretion and body weight of normal, force-fed, growing rat before, during, and after regimen of cortisone just large enough to cause, at first, a negative nitrogen balance. N.P.N., nonprotein nitrogen. [Adapted from Ingle (75).]

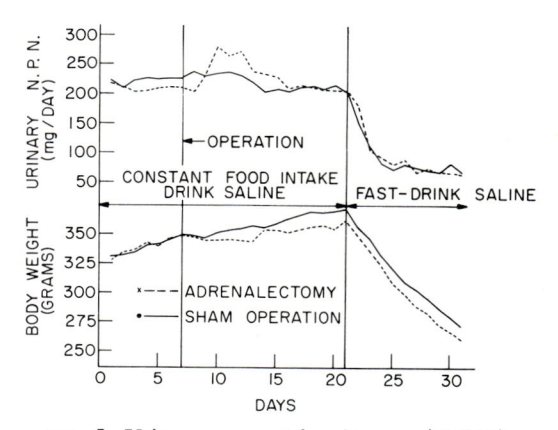

FIG. 5. Urinary nonprotein nitrogen (N.P.N.) excretions and body weights of male rats force-fed a measured amount of a medium carbohydrate (48% by dry wt) diet starting on day 0. Adrenalectomy or sham operation was done on day 7, and fasting was imposed on day 21. Lines show mean values for adrenalectomized (8) and sham operated (7) rats. [Adapted from Ingle & Oberle (77).]

maintained, adrenalectomized rats are quite capable of metabolizing large amounts of fed protein with consequent urea nitrogen excretion; this suggested that the severe hypoglycemia that develops in these animals during fasting is not due to their inability to deaminate amino acids presented to their tissues by way of the circulating blood, but rather to their inability to mobilize body protein.

Ingle & Thorn (82) then demonstrated in 1941 that adrenalectomy could abolish mild glucosuria in partially depancreatized rats on a constant food intake without causing any decrease in urinary nitrogen excretion and that continued administration of cortisone led to the excretion of more glucose carbon than could be accounted for by the carbon of the extra protein degraded, the latter amount of carbon being measured by the additional urinary nitrogen excreted. They concluded that glucocorticoids must inhibit glucose utilization by the tissues.

Glenn et al. (57) and Munck & Koritz (130) returned to this same concept at a later date, finding that glucocorticoid administration in the fasted adrenalectomized rat elevates the blood sugar concentration beginning at 30–60 min, whereas the liver glycogen increase begins only after 2 hr (Fig. 6), and no change is seen in plasma urea, plasma protein, or plasma α-amino nitrogen in the first 4 hr. Engel (40) had shown earlier that injection of adrenocortical extract into nephrectomized rats fails to accelerate the rise in plasma urea concentration until after the rise in liver glycogen concentration begins, whereas infusion of an amino acid mixture gave no evidence of such a delay in urea accumulation. The timing of the increase in urea accumulation after steroid injection parallels lysis of lymphocytes in thymus, lymph nodes, and spleen, which also occurs within a few hours (35, 116).

Initially it seemed reasonable that one should be able to account quantitatively for the urinary glucose excreted in the diabetic state in terms of the fed carbohydrate plus the conversion to glucose of the glycerol of disappearing body fat and certain amino acids of disappearing body protein, these latter amino acids being known to increase the urinary glucose and nitrogen excretion when given to the phlorizinized or diabetic animal. A reason for this was that the fatty acids of ingested fat had been found incapable of increasing the amount of glucose excreted in the phlorizinized animal or in diabetic animals, whereas dietary carbohydrate or protein did. Also it was believed, on the basis of quite inapplicable evidence (the whole-animal respiratory quotient), that absolutely no carbohydrate, once formed, was converted to CO_2 in the diabetic or phlorizinized state, and in fact that no glucose was taken up from the blood for use by the tissues in such states.

Later evidence on the metabolic pathways supported the concept that fatty acids and some of the carbon of protein cannot be converted to glucose carbon in net yield; that is, no metabolic pathway was found in mammalian tissues (contrary to the situation in some plant and bacterial cells) by which such a net conversion can occur. However, later evidence demonstrated that the conversion of pyruvate to acetyl moieties and CO_2 (the conversion of glucogenic to nonglucogenic material) does occur in the diabetic state, as well as in the normal state, and that glucose uptake by peripheral tissues from blood occurs in the diabetic state (albeit at elevated blood glucose levels) at nearly the same rate as in the normal state. These findings make it even more difficult to correlate the excreted glucose and the net increments in the total glucose and glycogen present in the body during the fasting diabetic state with the amount of nitrogen excreted.

Conversely knowledge of the metabolic pathways suggested a means by which an increased net conversion of fatty acids to CO_2 can replace, as an energy source, part of the net conversion of potentially glucogenic material to CO_2. At a given level of O_2 consumption, less pyruvate need be decarboxylated to acetyl moieties when these are already being supplied in an amount sufficient to fuel the tricarboxylic acid cycle; the pyruvate carbon so spared is available for conversion to glucose in net yield.

Knowledge that such a sparing mechanism exists shows up the weakness of the old interpretation of the failure of fatty acids to increase the urinary glucose excretion of the fasted phlorizinized or diabetic animal. The sparing mechanism is already saturated with acetyl residues, so supplying more is not effective; if a net conversion pathway from fatty acids to glucose does exist, this too may be saturated with fatty acid substrate under the conditions that are used to demonstrate the net gluconeogenic na-

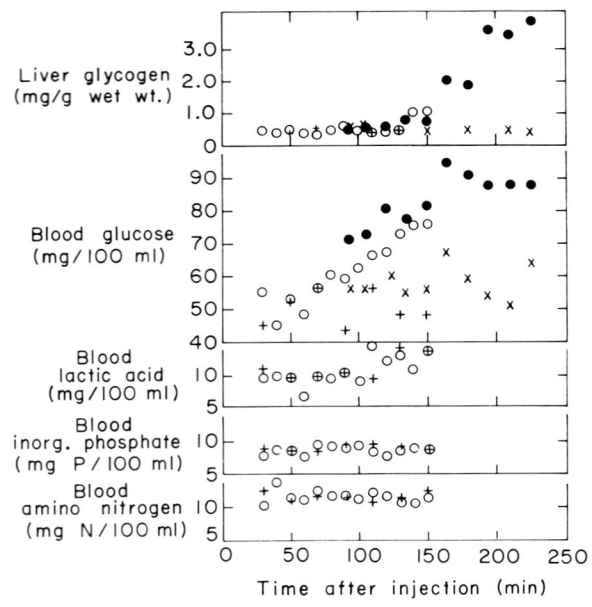

FIG. 6. Early changes in blood glucose and liver glycogen concentrations after cortisol injection in fasted, salt-maintained adrenalectomized rat. ○, cortisol injected and +, control rats, in one set of animals; ●, cortisol injected and ×, control rats in a similar separate experiment. Cortisol (2.5 mg) was injected subcutaneously into 155–220-g rats. [From Munck & Koritz (129).]

ture of administered material. The concept that there is no net conversion of fatty acids to glucose depends solely on the fact that no pathway for such a conversion has been found in mammalian tissues; however, this negative evidence must be taken seriously, because such a pathway has been pursued intensively.

Because of the sparing effects of fatty acid-derived acetyl residues (consumed in lieu of acetyl residues derived from pyruvate decarboxylation) the total carbon of all the protein catabolized, as indicated by total nitrogen excretion, has often been suggested as the basis for calculation in seeking the source for observed glucose increments. This is in contrast with the older custom of considering only part of the carbon of protein as available and counting only the increase in protein degradation as indicated by the increase in urinary nitrogen excretion. When this modified treatment of the data (together with the assumption of near zero pyruvate decarboxylation) fails to account for the amount of urinary glucose excreted or an observed increase in total body glucose and glycogen, other explanations are possible, as summarized by Landau (102). These include the assumptions: *a*) that degradation of glycoproteins, rather than normal proteins, has occurred; *b*) that the nitrogen removed from some of the protein degraded has been stored in the body in another form; and *c*) that a significant amount of the nitrogen removed from protein has been excreted in an unmeasured form, such as expired N_2.

Because of the difficulties in interpretation just described, efforts to account completely for the increments in glucose or glycogen caused by the glucocorticoids on the basis of inhibition of overall carbohydrate catabolism were inconclusive; however, it was believed that such glucocorticoid effects could not be ascribed solely to a primary action of the steroid to increase net protein degradation in the whole animal.

VI. PHYSIOLOGICAL MECHANISMS FOR MODIFICATIONS OF CARBOHYDRATE AND PROTEIN METABOLISM CAUSED BY GLUCOCORTICOID DEFICIENCY AND EXCESS

A. Consequences of Decreased Appetite in Glucocorticoid Deficiency

Leathem (105) has summarized the work describing the deficient growth of ad libitum-fed, adrenalectomized rats maintained on saline.

Ingle & Prestrud (78) found that the failure of saline-maintained, adrenalectomized rats to grow and accumulate nitrogen could be reversed by force-feeding. Cohn et al. (27) later found no defect in growth and nitrogen retention of adrenalectomized rats that were force-fed (Table 4).

Using kidney tissue in vitro, Yoshida et al. (184) investigated the part played by the amount and timing of food consumption in modifying the rate of gluconeogenesis from several precursors. Pair-feeding, with the daily ration presented all at once, eliminated the defi-

TABLE 4. *Changes in Body Composition of Normal and Adrenalectomized Rats Fed ad Libitum or Force-Fed*

Component	Normal Fed ad libitum	Normal Force-fed	Adrenalectomized Fed ad libitum	Adrenalectomized Force-fed
*Original body composition**				
Wt, g	148	159	152	157
N, g/rat†	4.83	5.03	4.96	4.97
N, % body wt‡	3.11–3.42	3.12–3.22	3.11–3.42	3.12–3.22
Fat, g/rat†	20.1	15.3	20.6	15.1
Fat, % body wt‡	12.8–14.1	9.24–9.90	12.8–14.1	9.24–9.90
Final body composition				
Wt, g	212	222	189	228
N, g/rat†	6.25	6.85	5.95	6.72
N, % body wt‡	2.80–3.08	3.02–3.13	2.97–3.29	2.83–3.07
Fat, g/rat†	20.4	39.0	14.2	35.8
Fat, % body wt‡	9.19–11.6	16.2–18.6	6.00–8.26	14.7–17.5
Change in body composition				
Wt, g	64	63	37	71
N, g/rat†	1.42	1.82	0.99	1.75
Fat, g/rat†	0.3	23.7	−6.4	20.7

* Based on analysis of rats from same groups killed at beginning of experiment. † Values are mean values of the group. ‡ Range of values. [Data from Cohn et al. (27).]

cient gluconeogenesis of the salt-maintained, adrenalectomized rat from some precursors, but not from all. The remaining differences were attributed to the fact that adrenalectomized rats spread their food consumption over a longer period than did normal rats. Force-feeding, or special pair-feeding, with 1/24 of the daily ration being presented to the rats each hour, eliminated the significant differences (Table 5). Few investigations of the effects of adrenalectomy on the enzyme activities or the metabolic functions of isolated tissues have been done with carefully controlled food intakes of the kind just described.

B. Changes in Secretion Rates of Other Relevant Hormones

1. EPINEPHRINE. Adrenalectomy removes the adrenal medulla, as well as the adrenal cortex, and so eliminates the principal source of circulating epinephrine.

Hypophysectomy reduces glucocorticoid production to low levels, because of the absence of pituitary ACTH secretion. Pohorecky & Wurtman (138) found, by assay of adrenal vein blood, that epinephrine secretion rates in dogs hypophysectomized for a long time were about 60% of normal. In response to insulin-induced hypoglycemia, epinephrine secretion rates increased about fourfold in both control and adrenalectomized dogs; the peak secretion rate in hypophysectomized dogs was about half that in control animals. Replacement therapy with ACTH sufficient to restore resting epinephrine secretion to normal resulted in responses of epinephrine secretion to insulin-induced hypoglycemia that

TABLE 5. *Influence of Manner of Feeding on Gluconeogenesis in Vitro by Kidneys of Normal and Adrenalectomized Rats*

Substrate for Gluconeogenesis	Fed ad Libitum[a]			Pair-fed[b]			Pair-fed 24 Times per Day[b]		
	Normal[c]	Adrenalectomized[d]	P value[e]	Normal[d]	Adrenalectomized[d]	P value	Normal[d]	Adrenalectomized[d]	P value
	Glucose formed, μmoles/g dried kidney per hour[f]								
None	19.5±0.9	15.6±1.0	<0.01	21.1±1.6	18.5±1.1	NS	17.7±1.5	16.6±1.6	NS
Glycerol	142.3±6.1	126.6±5.8	NS	154.8±9.5	136.2±9.1	NS	116.1±10.1	123.3±15.8	NS
Pyruvate	280.1±14.6	287.0±13.5	NS	285.5±11.6	255.9±8.3	NS	230.6±15.6	228.0±12.9	NS
α-Ketoglutarate	207.8±7.0	179.5±9.2	<0.02	200.9±13.5	181.4±13.7	NS	164.4±15.6	153.0±12.9	NS
Succinate	218.9±9.9	192.3±9.1	NS	252.4±9.4	211.8±14.4	<0.05	205.7±13.8	194.3±14.9	NS
Malate	231.4±8.7	193.3±11.6	<0.01	263.8±11.3	224.8±6.8	<0.01	207.8±12.5	184.6±16.3	NS
Glutamate	155.7±6.1	130.5±5.1	<0.01	158.1±9.2	130.5±8.8	<0.05	140.2±10.6	159.6±12.8	NS

[a] Twenty-four rats per group. [b] Twelve rats per group. [c] Mean food intake per day, 11.5 g. [d] Mean food intake per day, 10 g. [e] Paired comparison made. [f] Values expressed as means ± SE. [Data from Yoshida et al. (184).]

were about twice the peak levels in the control dogs. These experiments and the mechanisms involved in the restoration of epinephrine secretion in hypophysectomized animals by ACTH and glucocorticoids have been summarized recently by Pohorecky & Wurtman (138). Interestingly the accepted replacement dose of hydrocortisone (2 mg/kg body wt per day) in the hypophysectomized rat is ineffective in raising the level of phenylethanolamine N-methyltransferase in the adrenal gland, which is responsible for the synthesis of epinephrine from norepinephrine, whereas a replacement dose of ACTH, which restores normal glucocorticoid secretion in this animal, does elevate the level of the enzyme. This is perhaps because the blood reaching the adrenal medulla contains about 100 times as much of a particular glucocorticoid when this is being secreted by the cortex as it does when the same amount of the glucocorticoid is being delivered into the peripheral circulating blood. Deficient capacity to secrete epinephrine persists in hypophysectomized dogs when they are maintained with glucocorticoids.

The relationship between epinephrine secretion and the effects produced by glucocorticoids on glucose metabolism is under study. Rathgeb and her co-workers (142) have shown that cortisol replacement (0.8–1.2 mg/kg per day) increases the glucose turnover of the adrenalectomized dog and of the adrenal demedullated dog (I. Rathgeb, personal communication) to well above the normal rate when measured 18 hr after the last meal. In the hypophysectomized dog, which maintains its epinephrine secretion at only half the normal rate, this dose and higher doses of glucocorticoid increase the depressed rate of glucose turnover up to the normal rate but no further (33).

2. INSULIN. It is generally believed that insulin secretion is depressed in adrenalectomized animals in the postabsorptive state and that the increase in insulin secretion rate that is brought about by hyperglycemia is also less than normal. The influence of reduced dietary intake on such findings in adrenalectomized rodents has not been considered carefully.

In dogs (both control and adrenalectomized animals consuming the same daily diet in a single meal 18 hr before the observations) deBodo and co-workers (33) showed in the adrenalectomized dog (Table 6) that glucose uptake, as measured with [^{14}C]glucose, was only slightly less than normal at a slightly less-than-normal plasma glucose concentration. A small (0.25 unit/kg) intravenous injection of insulin produced a greater-than-normal increase in glucose uptake in only one of four such dogs. Considering its greater sensitivity to insulin-stimulated glucose uptake, the unusually sensitive dog must have been secreting less than a normal amount of insulin; otherwise its glucose uptake in the resting state at the then prevailing plasma glucose concentration would have been greater than was observed. For the three of four adrenalectomized dogs not sensitive to the small insulin dose, these experiments give no evidence for a depressed rate of insulin secretion in the resting postabsorptive state. Radioimmunoassayable plasma insulin is marginally decreased in the adrenalectomized dog and tends to increase during a maintenance regimen (1 mg/kg per day) of glucocorticoid (N. Altszuler, unpublished observations).

Under identical conditions of prior feeding, the hypophysectomized dog (33) is extremely sensitive to insulin-induced glucose uptake. Its reduced rate of glucose uptake in the resting postabsorptive state at its somewhat reduced plasma glucose level (Fig. 7) gives

TABLE 6. *Glucose Turnover* in the Postabsorptive State in Normal, Hypophysectomized, and Adrenalectomized Dogs*

Status	Mean Plasma Glucose, mg/100 ml	Glucose Turnover, g/m² per hr[†]
Normal (10)[‡]	107	3.80 ± 0.19[§]
Hypophysectomized (7)	90	2.59 ± 0.27
Adrenalectomized (9)	96	3.53 ± 0.16

* Release to the blood by the liver and uptake from blood by tissues. [†] Area based on area formula: m² = 0.2864 × (kg body wt)$^{0.367}$ × m (body length). Body weights at times of experiments were used. [‡] Number of experiments given in parentheses. [§] Mean ± SEM. [Data from deBodo et al. (33).]

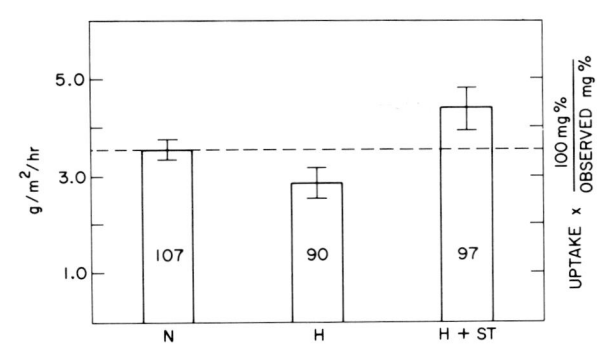

FIG. 7. Rates of glucose uptake from blood by tissues in normal (N), hypophysectomized (H), and steroid-treated (replacement regimen) hypophysectomized (H + ST) dogs. Measurements made with [^{14}C]glucose were taken 18 hr after the preceding meal in dogs that were in the unanesthetized resting state. Uptake expressed as grams of glucose per square meter of body surface area per hour. *Figures within bars*, mean plasma glucose concentrations during observations; *vertical lines*, SEM. Influence of altered plasma glucose concentration on glucose uptake has been corrected for roughly by calculation indicated on the *right* side of figure. [From deBodo et al. (33).]

evidence for a depressed insulin secretion rate, for at the normal rate of insulin secretion this animal would perish in hypoglycemia. Radioimmunoassay has confirmed the lowered plasma insulin level of this preparation (2). After a replacement regimen of cortisol (1.2–1.5 mg/kg per day, for 9–15 days), the exaggerated sensitivity of these dogs to a small dose of insulin is eliminated (Fig. 8), and they have a normal rate of glucose uptake in the resting postabsorptive state (Fig. 8) at a somewhat less-than-normal plasma glucose concentration (Fig. 7). The above facts indicate that the insulin secretion rate in the resting postabsorptive state is elevated by the replacement dose of the steroid from the depressed level seen in the untreated hypophysectomized state. Radioimmunoassayable plasma insulin levels are increased and are more responsive to administered glucose (N. Altszuler, personal communication).

Thus there is evidence in the dog that glucocorticoid administration, in doses from below normal to normal glucocorticoid secretion rate, elevates the rate of insulin secretion. Since the glucocorticoid regimen elevates the plasma glucose concentration in the postabsorptive state by a small amount (Fig. 7), part of the increase in insulin secretion rate may be explained on this basis. However, it seems likely that the responsiveness of the pancreas to glucose-stimulated insulin secretion is also increased by the glucocorticoid replacement regimen.

This effect of glucocorticoid on insulin secretion in the hypophysectomized dog takes place at a diminished level of epinephrine secretion (see section VI-B-1), and this diminished level is not elevated by the replacement dose of glucocorticoid. The relationship of epinephrine secretion to insulin secretion is being explored currently. Porte et al. (139) and Kris et al. (101) have shown that epinephrine, and to a lesser extent norepinephrine, acutely inhibits the elevation of insulin secretion brought

about by sudden hyperglycemia. On the other hand, Lerner & Porte (109) have shown more recently that epinephrine infusion does not inhibit, and may enhance, the long-continued elevated basal rate of insulin secretion brought about by prolonged glucose infusion in the human.

In the adrenalectomized rat, Sutter (165) has reported that immunoreactive insulin levels after an overnight fast are depressed. Sutter et al. (166) have also reported that insulin secretion is less responsive to increased blood glucose concentration in the adrenalectomized rat than in the normal or adrenal demedullated rat. Losert et al. (114) reported decreased serum insulin levels in adrenalectomized Chinese hamsters both in the fasting state and after an oral glucose load.

Malaisse et al. (117) found that pieces of pancreas removed from ad libitum-fed, adrenalectomized rats maintained on saline solution released less insulin in 90 min to a glucose-containing (150 mg/100 ml) incubation medium than did similar pieces removed from normal rats. Prior cortisol doses of ~1 mg/100 g per day administered to adrenalectomized rats for 3 days resulted in normal insulin release by the isolated pancreatic pieces. Methylprednisolone, at 5×10^{-5} M, incorporated in the incubation medium had no effect on insulin release by pieces of pancreas from either normal or adrenalectomized rats.

Glucocorticoids administered in excess elevate insulin secretion above normal in several species. In the experiments of Malaisse et al. (117) ~2.5 mg cortisol per 100 g per day in the normal rat, for either 2 or 5 days, raised the rate of insulin release by pancreas pieces (to the glucose-containing incubation medium) to 40 % above the control rate established for pieces from un-

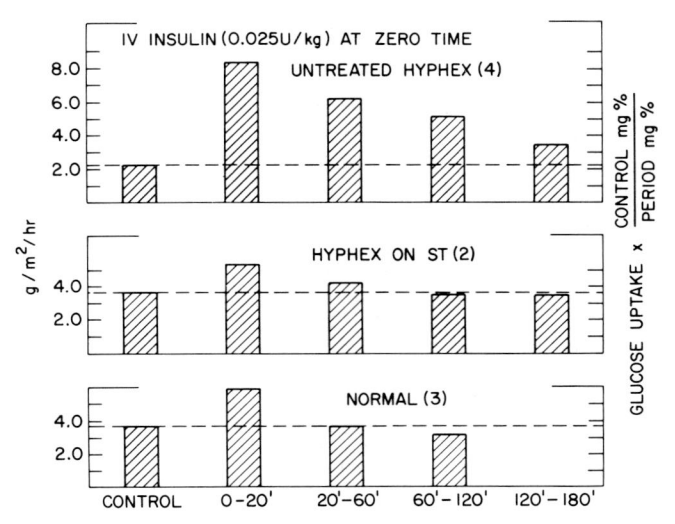

FIG. 8. Above-normal increase in glucose uptake from blood by tissues, brought about by intravenously (*IV*) injected insulin in hypophysectomized (*UNTREATED HYPHEX*) dog, and restoration to normal of the increase during replacement regimen of glucocorticoid (*HYPHEX ON ST*). See legend for Fig. 7 for explanation of units in which uptake is expressed and for calculation indicated at *right* of figure. [From deBodo et al. (33).]

TABLE 7. *Effect of Prednisolone in Excess on Insulin and Blood Glucose Concentrations in Serum of Fasting Rats*

Constituent	Days of Prednisolone Injection*			
	0	3	7	18
Blood sugar, mg/100 ml	128±4	137±3	140±3	118±4
Serum insulin, μunits/ml	21±2	48±5	59±4	54±5

Values expressed as mean ± SEM. * Dose was 10 mg/rat per day. [Data from Marco et al. (120).]

treated normal rats. With regard to observations in whole animals now to be quoted, an elevated insulin secretion rate is deduced from an elevated concentration of radioimmunoassayable insulin in serum or plasma, since it has been shown that a decrease in the rate of removal of insulin is not the causative factor under the conditions in which elevated plasma insulin levels are seen (11, 39).

Marco et al. (120) found, in rats that were fasted overnight, elevated insulin concentrations in the serum when the rats had been treated with prednisolone at ~5 mg/100 g per day for 3, 7, and 18 days (Table 7). In the first week, elevated blood glucose levels were seen, but not at 18 days at which time the serum insulin concentrations remained elevated to the same extent above normal in the absence of any stimulus for secretion provided by elevated blood glucose concentration. Under glucose-loading conditions the prednisolone-treated rats still displayed higher serum insulin levels than did the control rats. Williamson (179) has reported hyperglycemia and elevated serum insulin-like activity in normal rats given cortisone at 5 mg/100 g body wt per day for 3 days.

Bassett & Wallace (8) administered 75 mg cortisol per day to normal sheep (~1.2 mg/kg per day). This regimen, on days 4 through 15, nearly doubled the plasma glucose concentration and doubled the plasma insulin concentration measured just before the daily feeding of a standard ration (Fig. 9). The increase in immunoreactive insulin in response to the feeding or after glucose administration was also increased by the glucocorticoid.

In Chinese hamsters, Campbell et al. (21) found serum insulin levels tripled on the third day of a regimen of cortisone of 3 mg/day (15 mg/200 g body wt per day). Doses for 10–14 days maintained the elevated insulin concentration in serum at up to 40 times normal. Blood glucose values at the end of the regimen were doubled, on the average, but glucosuric levels were reached in one-third of the hamsters.

In the mouse, Rastogi & Campbell (141) found that the serum insulin concentration increased progressively during the 6- to 24-hr period after the first daily injection of 10 mg cortisone per 200 g body wt and stayed elevated during 8 days of the regimen. During the first 3 days, in which these animals were allowed continuous access to food, blood glucose values were depressed below normal rather than elevated. This indicates, perhaps, a greater-than-normal responsiveness of insulin secretion rate to blood glucose concentration in these animals. At the eighth day of the regimen the mice suffered sufficient hyperglycemia to become glycosuric, whereas serum insulin concentrations were even higher (14 times normal) than they had been at 3 days. Bovine growth hormone did not increase the concentration of serum insulin in the mice and also had little effect on the cortisone-induced hyperinsulinemia.

In the dog, Campbell & Rastogi (20) found that a new phenomenon supervenes after day 4 of a prednisolone regimen (4 mg/kg per day). At day 4 the serum insulin concentration is elevated about fourfold and the serum glucose concentration is elevated about 15 mg/100 ml in the postabsorptive state (Fig. 10). The serum insulin concentration reverts to normal on day 7, with no change in the slightly elevated serum glucose concentration, and remains normal through day 15. The insulin response to administered glucose is enhanced 24 hr after the initial prednisolone dose; on day 4 of the regimen the serum insulin concentration in response to glucose starts from a higher base-line level and rises about as much as in the control dog; on days 8 and 14 the insulin concentration starts again from the pre-prednisolone base-line level and becomes progressively less responsive to the glucose dose (Fig. 11). The changes in insulin response are such that the shapes of the curves for serum glucose concentration after the intravenous glucose load are very little altered during the 1- to 14-day period of the regimen (Fig. 11); this indicates that the varying insulin responses are being made to much the same elevations in serum glucose concentration throughout the regimen. The day 1 tolerance for glucose is elevated over the control tolerance in line with the greater insulin response on that day; this elevated tolerance for glucose is maintained during the remainder of the regimen, whereas the amount of insulin secreted in response to hyperglycemia diminishes continuously. This indicates the development of a greater sensitivity of the tissues of

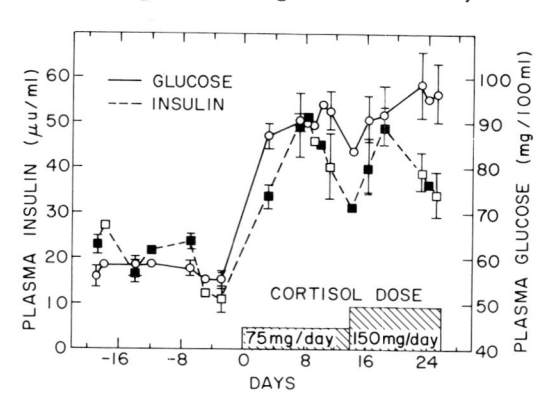

FIG. 9. Effect of cortisol on mean prefeeding plasma glucose and immunoassayable plasma insulin concentrations of 8 sheep fed once a day. Standard errors, indicated by *vertical lines*, were calculated for all points, but for the sake of clarity some have been omitted. [Adapted from Bassett & Wallace (8).]

the dog to the insulin secreted in response to hyperglycemia, which is not the expected finding (see section VI-F-1).

Man, like the dog, is resistant to severe steroid-induced hyperglycemia. Plasma insulin values apparently have not been measured in man during a prolonged glucocorticoid regimen. Perley & Kipnis (136) found, after 3 days of a dexamethasone regimen of 8 mg/day, a statistically significant elevation (from 78 ± 2 to 93 ± 3 mg/100 ml) of fasting blood sugar level in 24 men. Plasma insulin concentrations were not elevated but increased to a greater extent in response to an oral glucose load or to intravenous tolbutamide. Despite the fourfold increase in plasma insulin levels, the blood glucose levels after the glucose load declined more slowly in the dexamethasone-treated subjects. Acromegalic patients were especially responsive to the effect of dexamethasone to increase their insulin secretory responses to tolbutamide and were even more resistant to the lowering of blood sugar induced by secreted insulin.

From the above findings it may be concluded that the administration of excess glucocorticoid frequently results in elevated insulin levels in the plasma of animals after an overnight fast and also in increased increments of insulin secretion in response to hyperglycemia. Exceptions exist, notably in the dog on a prolonged regimen of excess glucocorticoid.

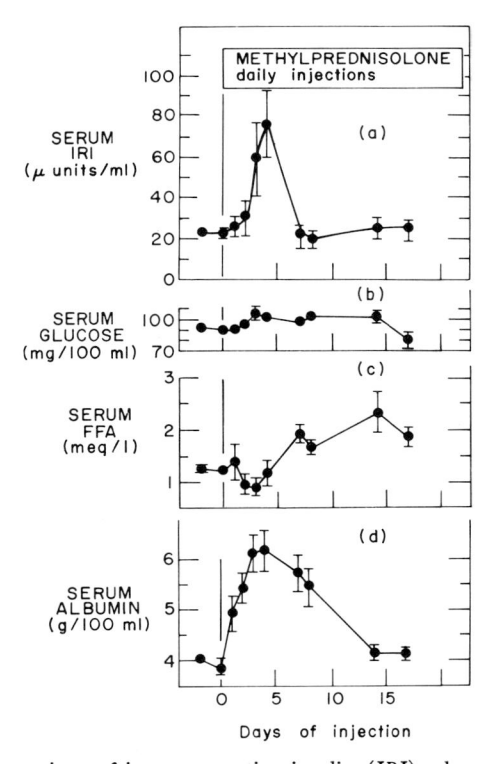

FIG. 10. Concentrations of immunoreactive insulin (*IRI*), glucose, free fatty acids (*FFA*), and serum albumin in blood sera of intact dogs in the postabsorptive state. Dogs consumed constant amount of standard diet and were injected twice daily on days indicated with 6α-methylprednisolone acetate (4 mg/kg per day) at 10 AM and 4 PM mealtimes. *Vertical lines*, SEM. [Adapted from Campbell & Rastogi (20).]

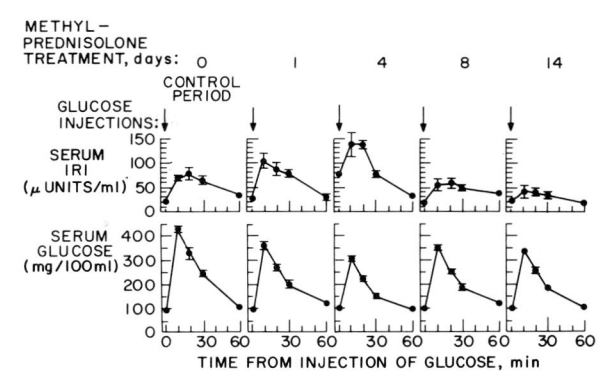

FIG. 11. Serum immunoreactive insulin (*IRI*) and serum glucose of the 4 dogs of Fig. 10 in response to intravenous glucose injection (1 g/kg body wt) in postabsorptive state on indicated day of 6α-methylprednisolone regimen. *Vertical lines*, SEM. [Adapted from Campbell & Rastogi (20).]

C. Net Transfer of Amino Acids from Peripheral Tissues to Liver in Glucocorticoid Excess

Ingle and co-workers (80) found that adrenalectomy of the rat at the time of evisceration resulted in a lessened accumulation of α-amino nitrogen in blood during the subsequent 24-hr period, the animals having been kept alive during this time by continuous glucose infusion. The interpretation of the experiment was complicated by the fact that the infusion of sufficient insulin, together with the requisite extra amount of glucose, is capable of preventing the accumulation of free amino acids in both nonadrenalectomized and adrenalectomized eviscerated rats. The effect of adrenalectomy was small but occurred at all levels of administered insulin and glucose (Fig. 12). Later investigations by Bondy et al. (17) showed that cortisone administration over 24 hr in eviscerated adrenalectomized rats reverses this effect of adrenalectomy. Other findings supporting the concept that net protein degradation in the peripheral tissues is decreased after adrenalectomy and increased by glucocorticoids have been presented (13, 40, 83, 91, 159, 164).

Silber & Porter (157) measured the distribution of total nitrogen in the body of adrenalectomized rats kept on a protein-free diet. Rats on a minimal (0.1 mg/100 g per day) cortisone replacement regimen were pair-fed with rats on 1.0 mg cortisone acetate per 100 g per day for 14 days. As shown in Table 8, nitrogen in the liver, gastrointestinal tract, and urogenital tract increased with the higher cortisone dose, whereas the carcass nitrogen decreased. Serum albumin, a protein supplied to the blood by the liver, increased in proportion to serum globulin, a protein not supplied by the liver. Total RNA of the liver and total lipid and carbohydrate of the liver increased along with liver protein and total liver weight.

Confirmatory evidence for the above has been sum-

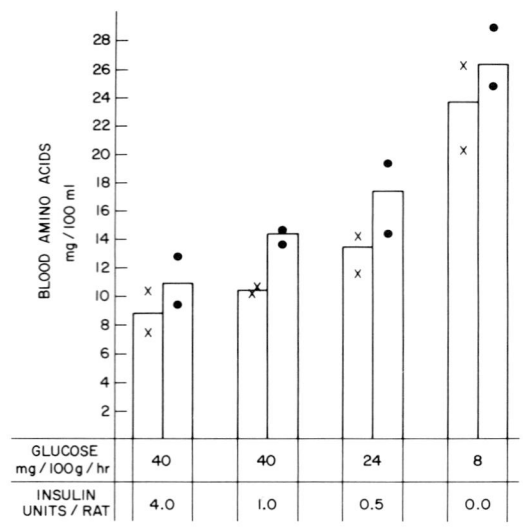

FIG. 12. Effect of adrenalectomy and evisceration on concentration of blood amino acids measured 24 hr after evisceration. Bar heights represent mean values; symbols × (adrenalectomized, eviscerated rats) and ● (eviscerated rats) show range of observed values. Insulin was injected and glucose given continuously for the 24-hr period after evisceration at rates indicated. [From Ingle et al. (80).]

marized by Munro (131) who points out that a diet rich in protein also causes deposition of both RNA and protein in the liver and concludes that cortisone acts in this way by making more amino acids, derived from carcass proteins, available to the liver. Certainly, after the steroid regimen, more amino acid is present in the liver as protein, to support a demand for gluconeogenesis.

The number of liver cells does not increase during the hepatic hypertrophy caused by glucocorticoid excess, because DNA synthesis is arrested during the regimen, as shown by Henderson et al. (68), and resumes sharply when the regimen is halted. In this respect the response of liver cells is like that of a number of somatic tissues in vivo and of mammalian cell lines maintained in tissue culture, in which cell division is inhibited by the glucocorticoids. In Henderson's study (Tables 9 and 10) growing rats failed to sustain the initial (16-hr) increased total liver RNA content (due to increased RNA synthesis) when treated for 3–16 days with excess cortisone [see also (110)]. This does not accord with the original observations of Silber & Porter (157), who reported excess cortisone was given for 14 days with elevated liver total RNA resulting (Table 8), nor with observations of Campbell and Rastogi in the hamster (21) or dog (20) treated 14 or 18 days with excess glucocorticoid, in which markedly increased liver weight and liver protein were seen at the end of the regimen. Differing amounts of glucocorticoid excess and different dietary intakes may be responsible for the discrepancy.

1. PROTEIN METABOLISM IN PERIPHERAL TISSUES. The lessened accumulation of free amino acids in the blood of the eviscerated rat after adrenalectomy and the in-

TABLE 8. *Nitrogen Distribution in Organs, and Some Blood and Liver Constituents in Adrenalectomized, Protein-depleted Rats Treated with Cortisone Acetate*

Distribution	Low Dose*	High Dose†	P
	Nitrogen, % of total‡		
Carcass	68.0±0.49	65.0±0.43	<0.01
Skin	22.1±0.45	22.6±0.32	>0.2
Liver	3.03±0.085	4.49±0.114	<0.005
Spleen	0.30±0.055	0.25±0.019	>0.2
Pleura	0.25±0.004	0.25±0.007	>0.2
Gastrointestinal	3.66±0.070	4.27±0.130	<0.01
Urogenital	2.55±0.073	2.96±0.120	<0.05
Total N, g/100 g body wt	2.79±0.061	2.67±0.037	>0.2
Total serum protein, g/100 ml	5.27±0.16	6.00±0.071	<0.005
Albumin (pooled sample), g/100 ml	1.45	2.12	
Globulin (pooled sample), g/100 ml	3.72	3.93	
Albumin:globulin ratio	0.39	0.54	
Liver wt, g/100 g body wt	2.93±0.07	4.18±0.12	<0.005
Liver protein N, mg/100 g body wt	76.5±1.31	105.5±1.86	<0.005
Liver NPN, mg/100 g body wt	9.47±0.30	13.51±0.34	<0.005
Liver carbohydrate, mg/100 g body wt	137±23.4	320±20.5	<0.005
Liver lipid (alcohol-ether solution), mg/100 g body wt	261±22.3	452±24.6	<0.005
Liver deoxyribonucleic acid, mg/100 g body wt	15.2±0.39	17.1±1.26	<0.2
Liver ribonucleic acid, mg/100 g body wt	43.8±3.56	68.4±4.10	<0.005

N, nitrogen; NPN, nonprotein nitrogen. * Low dose, 0.1 mg cortisone acetate per 100 g body wt per day. † High dose, 1.0 mg cortisone acetate per 100 g body wt per day. ‡ Skin elastin and hair omitted. [Data from Silber & Porter (157).]

TABLE 9. *Short-term Effects of Cortisone Acetate on Liver Composition of Fed Rats*

Component	Control*	Cortisone*	% Change	P Value
Liver weight, g	6.10 ± 0.12†	7.12 ± 0.11	+17	<0.001
Protein content, g	1.13 ± 0.01	1.26 ± 0.03	+12	<0.005
RNA content, mg	38.5 ± 1.0	45.8 ± 1.3	+19	<0.005
DNA content, mg	15.3 ± 0.5	14.6 ± 0.06	−5	>0.3(NS)
DNA concentration, mg/g liver	2.51 ± 0.11	2.05 ± 0.16	−18	<0.05

Effects were measured over 16 hr; 10 mg cortisone acetate, ip, was given. * Body wt for both groups of rats at time of injection was 133 ± 5 g (mean ± 1 SD). † Mean ± SEM. [Data from Henderson et al. (68).]

TABLE 10. *Long-term Effects of Cortisone Acetate Regimen on Liver Composition of Fed Rats*

Component	Initial	Final Control	Final Cortisone	% Increment Control	% Increment Cortisone
Body weight, g	136±2*	229±6	122±6	+68	−10
Liver weight, g	5.71±0.25	9.52±0.28	6.31±0.37	+67	+11
Liver DNA content, mg	10.6±0.4	17.3±0.6	10.6±0.6	+63	0
Liver RNA content, mg	32.1±1.9	53.8±2.2	33.4±1.2	+68	+4
Liver protein content, mg	737±51	1220±30	810±60	+66	+10

Effects were measured over 16 days; cortisone acetate regimen was 5 mg/day, sc. *Mean ± SEM. [Data from Henderson et al. (68).]

creased net transport of amino acids from carcass proteins to liver proteins during glucocorticoid administration both suggest that the glucocorticoids may inhibit protein synthesis in the peripheral tissues.

Early experiments, in which the net incorporation of radioactively labeled amino acids into tissue proteins in vivo over several hours was believed to indicate the rate of protein synthesis in the tissue, gave conflicting results, as noted by Lee & Williams (108). Clemens & Korner (26) have emphasized recently the care that must be exercised in the interpretation of amino acid incorporation experiments even when these are carried out using isolated pieces of tissue incubated in vitro. The difficulty in interpretation arises from uncertainty as to the specific activity (amount of label per mg free amino acid) of the labeled amino acid at the location of protein synthesis in the cell. When less label (compared with controls) is incorporated into protein over a given short period of time, the conclusion that there is less protein synthesis is valid only if there is as much label present per milligram of precursor amino acid as there is in controls.

A depressed rate of protein synthesis does not necessarily bring about a net decrement in the protein content of a tissue. Protein degradation must also not be depressed simultaneously, to the same extent or more, for then net protein loss will not occur. Measurement of the rate of degradation of the proteins of tissue cells is not possible by simple isotope techniques, such as those by which amino acid incorporation into protein is measured. In this connection, Schimke (152) demonstrated the influence of changes in degradation rate on the level of rat liver arginase. Also, Reel & Kenney (143) have shown that actinomycin D, and also cycloheximide and puromycin, causes decreased degradation of tyrosine transaminase in hepatoma cell cultures.

It is necessary to differentiate between protein synthesis in bulk, which may be changed in rate as a secondary consequence of altered cellular metabolism, and the earlier synthesis of a few specific proteins, directed via RNA synthesis, which may be induced by a glucocorticoid and which secondarily may bring about the later effects.

Wool & Weinshelbaum (182) used diaphragm muscle removed from ad libitum-fed rats adrenalectomized 4 days earlier and maintained on saline; the incorporation of [2-^{14}C]histidine into the protein of the diaphragms during 2 hr of incubation was measured. As shown in Table 11, adrenalectomy increased incorporation and cortisone maintenance decreased this toward normal; a regimen of excess cortisone decreased incorporation in diaphragms from normal and adrenalectomized rats.

Manchester et al. (119) used diaphragm muscle similar to that described above (182); the incorporation of [^{14}C]glycine into protein during 2 hr of incubation gave findings similar to those just described. In addition, the same relationships were found when the incubation medium contained no added glucose, and the increment in glycine incorporation due to the presence of insulin in the glucose-free incubation medium was found to be greater in the diaphragm of adrenalectomized rats (Table 12).

Weinshelbaum & Wool (173) repeated their observations using heart (myocardium) slices in place of diaphragm and separating the tissue after [^{14}C]phenylalanine incorporation in vitro into cell debris, mitochondria, microsomes, and the soluble fraction. Adrenalectomy increased incorporation most strongly in the microsome portion, whereas excess hydrocortisone given to the intact rat decreased incorporation equally in all portions. The latter finding led the authors to reintroduce the idea that reduced amino acid entry into the cell might be the

TABLE 11. *Incorporation of [2-^{14}C]Histidine into Protein Fraction of Diaphragms: Effect of Adrenalectomy, Steroid Replacement Therapy, and Cortisone Excess*

Experimental Condition	Protein, cpm/mg	P*
I. Normal	87 ± 2.2 (11)†	
Sham adrenalectomy	104 ± 2.8 (12)	<0.001
Adrenalectomy	150 ± 4.2 (11)	<0.001
II. Normal	96 ± 2.8 (6)	
Adrenalectomized	156 ± 5.1 (6)	<0.001
Adrenalectomized, cortisone (0.3 mg/day)	111 ± 3.5 (6)	<0.01
Adrenalectomized, DOC (0.06 mg/day)	146 ± 4.6 (6)	<0.001
III. Normal	89 ± 3.1 (6)	
Normal, cortisone (1 mg/day)	55 ± 2.1 (6)	<0.001
Normal, cortisone (2 mg/day)	48 ± 5.3 (6)	<0.001
Adrenalectomized	140 ± 3.4 (6)	
Adrenalectomized, cortisone (1 mg/day)	63 ± 4.0 (6)	<0.001
Adrenalectomized, cortisone (2 mg/day)	60 ± 2.3 (5)	<0.001

* P values are for comparison with normal control group in conditions I and II and for comparison with untreated controls in condition III. † Mean ± SEM; number of observations shown in parentheses. [Data from Wool & Weinshelbaum (182).]

TABLE 12. *Effect of Adrenalectomy and of Cortisol Administration to Rats on Incorporation of [^{14}C]Glycine into Protein of Isolated Diaphragm and on Response of This Incorporation to Insulin in the Medium*

Condition of Rat from Which Diaphragm Taken	Radioactivity in Diaphragm Protein, counts/min per disk		
	No added insulin	Insulin, 1 munit/ml	Difference
	Medium containing added glucose		
Intact + cortisol* (12)†	242 ± 3	292 ± 6 } $P < 0.001$	50 ± 6
Normal (12)	379 ± 16 } $P < 0.001$‡	448 ± 24 } $P < 0.001$	69 ± 11
Adrenalectomized (11)	433 ± 12 } $P < 0.02$	500 ± 14 } $P < 0.001$	67 ± 8
Adrenalectomized + cortisol§ (11)	311 ± 5 } $P < 0.001$	365 ± 8	54 ± 5
	Medium containing no added glucose		
Intact + cortisol (6)	250 ± 9 } $P < 0.001$	299 ± 9 } $P < 0.001$	49 ± 10
Normal (6)	349 ± 8	396 ± 10 } $P < 0.001$	47 ± 7 } $P < 0.01$
Adrenalectomized (6)	374 ± 13 } $P < 0.05$	464 ± 4 } $P < 0.001$	90 ± 11 } $P < 0.1$
Adrenalectomized + cortisol (6)	328 ± 14	401 ± 10	73 ± 9
	Pooled results		
Intact + cortisol (18)	244 ± 4 } $P < 0.001$	294 ± 5 } $P < 0.001$	50 ± 5
Normal (18)	369 ± 11 } $P < 0.01$	431 ± 16 } $P < 0.01$	62 ± 7 } $P < 0.01$
Adrenalectomized (17)	412 ± 9 } $P < 0.001$	487 ± 9 } $P < 0.001$	75 ± 6 } $P < 0.1$
Adrenalectomized + cortisol (17)	317 ± 6	378 ± 6	61 ± 4

* Treated intact rats received 5 mg cortisol per rat per day for 3 days and 5 mg 80 min before death. † Number of observations shown in parentheses. ‡ Value of P for a difference that is significant is indicated. Response to insulin is in every case significant ($P < 0.05$). § Treated adrenalectomized animals received 1 mg cortisol per rat per day for 3 days and 1 mg 80 min before death. [Data from Manchester et al. (119).]

primary mechanism for glucocorticoid depression of protein synthesis. Ferguson & Wool (52) then presented additional evidence for separate actions of glucocorticoids in natural amount rather than in excess on protein synthesis. They duplicated their original conditions but measured the incorporation of [8-^{14}C]adenine into the RNA of the diaphragm. Adrenalectomy enhanced incorporation, as it had the incorporation of amino acids into proteins, but excess cortisol in the intact rat had no effect on adenine incorporation into RNA, whereas it had depressed amino acid incorporation into proteins under the same conditions.

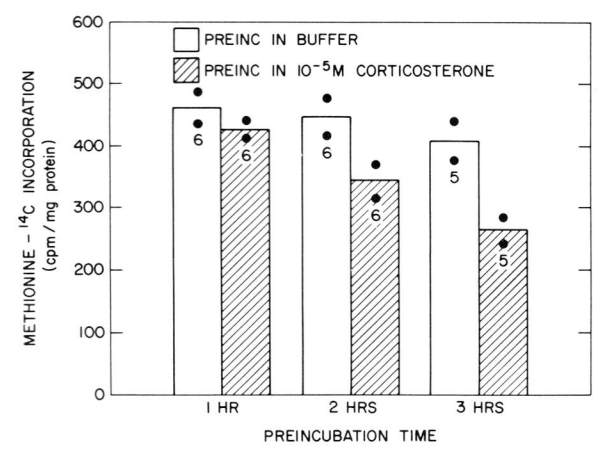

FIG. 13. Effects of various periods of preincubation (*PREINC*) with corticosterone on the subsequent incorporation of L-[^{14}C]-methionine into the protein of intact diaphragms of adrenalectomized rats. Diaphragms were incubated with L-[^{14}C]methionine for 1 hr. *Numbers in bars*, numbers of muscles used. A *bar top* represents a mean value, and distance between *dots* represents 2 SEM. [Adapted from Kostyo & Redmond (97).]

Peters et al. (137) found that isolated ribosomes of hind leg muscles taken from intact rats injected intraperitoneally 6–12 hr earlier with 20 mg triamcinolone acetonide per kilogram showed decreased incorporation of [U-^{14}C]leucine into protein.

Kostyo used diaphragms removed from normal (96) and adrenalectomized (97) rats, in such a way that muscle fibers were not cut, to demonstrate effects of adrenal steroids added to the incubation medium. After 2–3 hr preincubation with 10^{-5} M corticosterone, the cells of the diaphragms took up less [^{14}C]α-aminoisobutyric acid (an amino acid not used in protein synthesis but transported across the cell membrane by a process used by natural amino acids) from the incubation medium. Simultaneously the glucocorticoid-treated diaphragm became less able to incorporate L-[^{14}C]-methionine into tissue protein (Fig. 13). These results were interpreted to mean that the glucocorticoid inhibits the synthesis of a labile protein necessary for amino acid transport. As protein turnover in the cell eliminates the initially present labile protein, amino acid transport declines.

Munck (127) noted that with suspensions of rat thymocytes the specific receptor sites binding glucocorticoids are saturated at a glucocorticoid concentration of about 10^{-6} M. Kostyo (96), using diaphragms from normal rats, observed inhibition of α-aminoisobutyric acid uptake at 10^{-8} M dexamethasone and 10^{-7} M corticosterone.

Wool (181) demonstrated that diaphragms with uncut muscle fibers, removed from adrenalectomized rats maintained for 4 days on saline, did not accumulate increased amounts of [^{14}C]α-aminoisobutyric acid or naturally occurring [^{14}C]amino acids after 2 hr in the incubation medium. However, after the normal rat was subjected to a regimen of cortisone (2 mg/100 g per day for 3 days), depressed accumulation of all the amino acids was observed.

Eichhorn and co-workers (37) found that adrenalectomized rats maintained for 6 days with saline have a decreased ability to accumulate α-aminoisobutyric acid injected intravenously into diaphragm and gastrocnemius muscle, whereas if such rats have been kept, during this period, on a regimen of either cortisol or DOC (0.8 mg/day), the accumulation in these muscles is improved toward normal. Short-term treatment with either cortisol or DOC was found to have no effect on α-aminoisobutyrate accumulation. A depressing influence of administered mineralocorticoid (DOC) on in vivo α-aminoisobutyrate accumulation in diaphragm was noted by Blecher (16) in both normal and saline-maintained, adrenalectomized rats. Kostyo (96) also found DOC effective at 10^{-7} M in his in vitro studies.

Secondary influences operating in the intact animal, for example, the rate of insulin secretion, may influence α-aminoisobutyrate accumulation in vivo and so explain some of the conflicting findings. However, the similar mineralocorticoid effect on α-aminoisobutyrate accumulation, which is seen in both in vivo and in vitro studies, suggests that a change in α-aminoisobutyrate accumulation may not be a specific indicator for an important primary action of the glucocorticoids in their influence on protein metabolism.

Further insight into the cellular mechanisms responsible for the decreased protein synthesis brought about by glucocorticoids has been furnished by work with isolated rat thymocytes exposed to physiological concentrations of these agents in vitro or thymocytes collected after dosage of the whole animal. A working hypothesis is that the primary action of such hormones is the same in muscle, which represents the bulk of the peripheral source of protein nitrogen released during glucocorticoid excess over the long term, as it is in the lymphoid tissue. The lymphoid tissue releases its nitrogen more rapidly and probably is the major source in the rat of the extra amino acids that are made available to the liver 3-8 hr after glucocorticoid injection (35, 116, 175).

Makman et al. (116) summarized the findings up to 1966 of the group of investigators associated with A. White. Later findings by this group were cited in a paper by Makman et al. (115) that appeared in 1970. Emphasized were inhibitions of the transport and further utilization of amino acids, and of DNA and RNA precursors, by a process dependent on an energy source and on the synthesis of a specific RNA or protein, or both. Nuclear RNA polymerase activity was found decreased below control values at 3 and 6 hr of incubation of thymocytes with 10^{-6} M cortisol or with 2.5×10^{-5} M puromycin. The normal turnover of RNA polymerase, with the synthesis of new enzyme inhibited by either cortisol or puromycin, could account for the lowered polymerase activity.

The findings of Munck and his collaborators up to

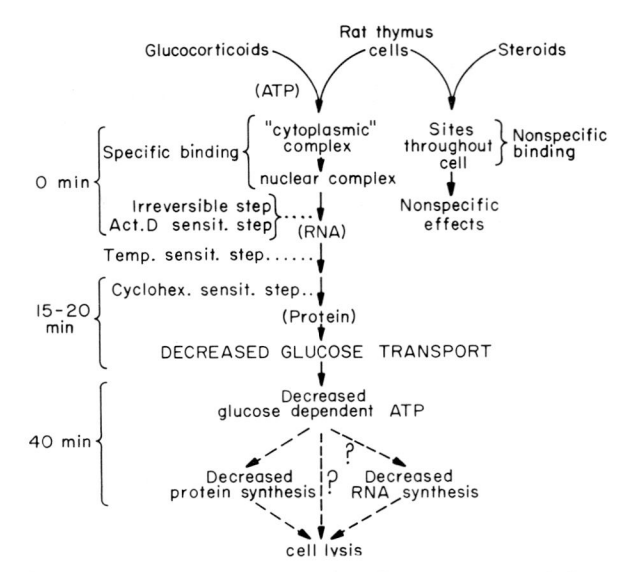

FIG. 14. Principal events that follow treatment of thymocytes with physiological amount of cortisol in vitro, and postulated relations between these events. On *left* is the time at which each event begins during incubation with cortisol at 37 C. *Brackets* and *dashed arrows*, respectively, denote substances and steps for which only indirect evidence of involvement exists. *Act. D*, actinomycin D; *temp.*, temperature; *sensit.*, sensitive; *Cyclohex.*, cycloheximide. [From Munck (127).]

1970 have been summarized by him recently (127) and are shown in Figure 14. The key finding is a block in glucose transport, which becomes detectable within 15 min after exposure of thymocytes for 5 min to cortisol at 10^{-6} M. New RNA synthesis during the initial 5-min period is indicated because this irreversible step is inhibited by actinomycin D. New protein synthesis is indicated by the fact that puromycin or cycloheximide added prior to the effect on glucose transport prevents this effect from developing. A sharp distinction is drawn between these very early effects, which appear to involve stimulation of specific RNA and specific protein synthesis, and the effects seen later, after the effect on glucose transport has occurred. These later effects are important in the net transfer of amino acids to the liver in bulk, that is, decreased overall protein and RNA synthesis. Munck (127) attributes these later effects to the earlier effect on glucose transport, because no difference could be seen between control and steroid-treated thymocytes except in the presence of glucose. This suggests that in muscle cells and adipose tissue cells, which are insulin sensitive, insulin might counteract the depressing effect of the glucocorticoids on protein synthesis, since in fat cells insulin was shown to counteract steroid-depressed glucose uptake (50). Whether the depressed glucose transport is the specific cause of the later-appearing effects of the glucocorticoids or is an early consequence of a more fundamental change, which leads also to depressed protein synthesis in the cells of peripheral tissues, remains to be proven.

2. PROTEIN METABOLISM IN LIVER. The net loss of protein from the peripheral tissues is accompanied by a net

gain of liver protein in the steroid-treated animal. This suggests that protein synthesis may be increased in liver by excess glucocorticoid.

Christensen (25) has summarized the work of his group showing the increased accumulation of α-aminoisobutyric acid in rats seen 2 hr after the administration of ⌒1.5 mg cortisol per 100 g body wt. Chambers and co-workers (24) have extended these findings to the perfused liver.

Korner (95) has presented a summary of his work relating to the amino acid-incorporating activity of rat liver microsomes from saline-maintained, adrenalectomized rats. Three days after adrenalectomy, amino acid incorporation was greatly elevated in this system and remained somewhat elevated up to 14 days; by 36 days it was somewhat below normal. Recall in this connection (Fig. 5) that extra nitrogen is excreted on days 3–8 following adrenalectomy; this suggests an increased flux of amino acids may be available to the liver at this time, due perhaps to stress during the adrenalectomy procedure and before the adrenals are actually removed. If a small dose of cortisol (0.25 or 2.0 mg/day) is given for 7 days to the adrenalectomized rat, the early-occurring elevated amino acid incorporation of the microsomal system is lowered, whereas if this same dose is given for the same time to the normal hypophysectomized or adrenalectomized hypophysectomized rat, amino acid incorporation is elevated. A larger dose of cortisol (5 mg/day) given for 7 days to the adrenalectomized rat fails to lower the supernormal amino acid incorporation of its liver microsomal fraction, so a biphasic response appears to occur as glucocorticoid dosage moves through the replacement dose to the excess dose. The changes in amino acid incorporation are brought about by changes in the ribosome fraction of the microsomes rather than by changes in the soluble fraction. The responses seen are those of a given quantity of isolated microsomes and so represent the quality of the microsomes rather than the total incorporating ability per liver cell. Total incorporation may increase because more ribosomes are present per cell. Insulin supply, growth hormone supply, and the concentration of amino acids in liver cells before killing are other important factors determining amino acid-incorporating activity of liver ribosomes (95).

Although evidence is available for very early effects of an excess of glucocorticoids on RNA and protein synthesis in thymocytes, firm evidence for such a very early effect in hepatic cells has begun to appear only recently. The problem might seem to be more straightforward for liver, where a glucocorticoid-induced increase in protein synthesis has been shown to be the mechanism that brings about increases in the amounts of several hepatic enzymes. However, a difficulty arises in that the RNA and protein effects in liver that have been studied most occur several hours after glucocorticoid administration, at a time corresponding to the secondary (inhibitory) effects on protein synthesis in thymocytes rather than to the primary (stimulatory) effect.

An effect appearing early (15 min) after ∼2.5 mg cortisol per 100 g, ip (86) was a slight inhibition (rather than an increase) in the incorporation in vivo of ^{32}P, from injected radioactive Na_2HPO_4, into the RNA of the nuclear fraction of the liver. The stimulation of ^{32}P incorporation into this fraction became marked only 45 min after cortisol injection and was then accompanied by increased synthesis of tyrosine transaminase. Drews & Brawerman (36) and Greenman, Wicks, and Kenney (61) later fractionated the RNA of liver nuclei collected 2–3 hr after cortisol injection into a ribosomal RNA precursor fraction and a messenger RNA-like fraction and found that ^{32}P incorporation had been stimulated by cortisol equally in both fractions. The incorporation of ^{32}P into transfer RNA-like material had also been increased. Agarwal et al. (1) also found no selective increases in the amount of any specific transfer RNAs.

An increase of RNA polymerase activity in rat liver nuclei, together with increased incorporation of [6-^{14}C]-orotate into nuclear RNA, was seen within 1 hr after addition of cortisol to the fluid perfusing isolated rat liver (6). Goldstein et al. (58) and Hager & Kenney (62) have also demonstrated induction of hepatic enzymes in the isolated liver and within 1 to 3 hr during perfusion with glucocorticoid-containing medium. Tomkins et al. (168) and Kenney and co-workers (107, 143, 144) demonstrated the induction of tyrosine transaminase and alanine transaminase in hepatoma cell cultures in 1–3 hr at glucocorticoid concentrations of 10^{-5} to 5×10^{-7} M.

Dahmus & Bonner (30) isolated chromatin from adrenalectomized rat livers 4 hr after cortisol injection (5 mg/100 g, ip) and found this served as a better template for DNA-dependent RNA synthesis by RNA polymerase from *Escherichia coli* than did chromatin from untreated adrenalectomized rats. Removal of proteins from the chromatin improved its template activity and eliminated the difference between the materials from the untreated and the steroid-treated rat livers. A similarly demonstrated increase in liver chromatin template activity, with a peak at 2 hr, induced in alloxan-diabetic rats by injection of insulin has been described more recently by Morgan & Bonner (124).

Feigelson and co-workers (51, 185) compared the stimulating action of cortisone (5–10 mg/kg, ip), given 2 hr earlier, on the incorporation in vivo of [^{32}P]phosphate, [2-^{14}C]glycine, and [^{3}H]orotate into rat liver RNA during a 2-hr period. Great differences in the degree of stimulation were found, and it appeared that most, if not all, of the increased incorporation was being caused by changes in the specific activity of the intracellular acid-soluble precursor purine nucleotides from which the RNA was synthesized. Cortisone, given 2 hr prior to labeling in vivo, markedly stimulated the synthesis of liver acid-soluble adenine from [2-^{14}C]glycine. Administration of ammonium bicarbonate and many amino acids produced an effect like that of cortisone, in adrenalectomized rats, on the incorporation of [2-^{14}C]-

glycine into both acid-soluble adenine and the RNA of rat liver.

The specificity of the effect of glucocorticoids on the synthesis of liver proteins has been challenged by Kenney and co-workers (85) and by others. The rapid increases in enzyme content occur when the natural fractional turnover of the enzyme is rapid; a general increase in hepatic protein synthesis might then create the erroneous impression of the specific rapid induction of these few enzymes.

It is thus evident that a primary action of glucocorticoids on the genetic apparatus of the liver cell has not yet been fully identified, nor has the mechanism been elucidated that joins such a primary effect to the increased rate of hepatic protein synthesis that follows glucocorticoid administration.

However, Yu & Feigelson (186) have presented a preliminary account indicating a very early (10-min) increase in messenger RNA synthesis in liver after cortisone acetate injection (5 mg/100 g, ip) in adrenalectomized rats. Also Hanoune & Feigelson (63) have described a cytoplasmic ribonucleoprotein component that contains more incorporated [4,5-^{3}H]leucine at the earliest time interval studied (3 hr) after cortisone injection in vivo than at any later time. This information, coupled with the knowledge that injected hydrocortisone disappears from the liver rapidly after the injection (85), suggests an early transient effect on the synthesis of a specific protein.

Korner (94, 95), Manchester (118), Weber (171, 172), and Kenney et al. (87) have reviewed aspects of the intracellular control of liver protein synthesis by the glucocorticoids.

D. Changes in Rate of Gluconeogenesis

The life-threatening consequences of deficient responses, both of glycogen breakdown and of gluconeogenesis, in response to insulin-induced hypoglycemia are shown in Figure 15. Glucose release by the liver failed to increase in this adrenalectomized dog even though the plasma glucose concentration was still at 40 mg/100 ml 2 hr after 0.08 unit/kg insulin had been injected intravenously.

The deficient gluconeogenesis of the adrenalectomized animal is also evident in fasting hypoglycemia, at a time when the extremely low levels of liver glycogen that prevail suggest the glucose being released by the liver is derived entirely from gluconeogenesis. The injection of a glucocorticoid at this time results in an increase in blood glucose concentration, which first becomes evident after about 90–120 min, and an increase in liver glycogen content, which begins about an hour later (Fig. 6 and Table 1). During this interval there is no significant increase in blood lactate, free fatty acid, or amino acid concentration (57, 129). Later, after glucocorticoid injection, many changes are seen that result in a greater response to a call for increased gluconeogenesis.

Evidence pertinent to these observations is now examined.

1. EARLY EFFECTS OF GLUCOCORTICOID ADMINISTRATION IN STEROID-DEFICIENT RAT. *a. Insignificant decrease in overall peripheral glucose uptake.* The observed rise in blood glucose concentration after cortisol treatment of the adrenalectomized rat might be caused not by increased glucose output by the liver, but by decreased uptake of glucose from the blood by the extrahepatic tissues. The evidence (67, 113, 127, 159) leads to the conclusion that the early-appearing decreased glucose uptake, which is a consequence of glucocorticoid action in thymocytes and adipose tissue cells, does not occur in muscle and that there is no significant overall decrease in glucose uptake by the peripheral tissues this early after glucocorticoid administration.

b. Message calling for increased gluconeogenesis. The message, relayed several times, directing increased gluconeogenesis to correct hypoglycemia, fails to reach the final effector mechanism in liver cells of adrenalectomized animals; the continuity of the message transmission is restored after glucocorticoid administration.

The external stimuli capable of increasing the rate of gluconeogenesis in the perfused isolated liver have been

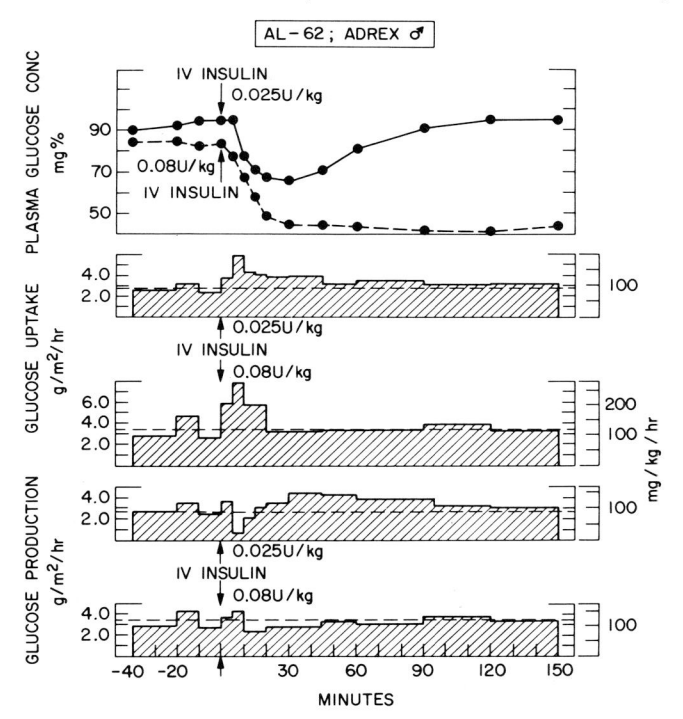

FIG. 15. Insulin hypersensitivity of adrenalectomized (*ADREX*) dog, shown as resultant of increased glucose uptake by tissues and prolonged deficient increase in glucose release by liver in response to hypoglycemia. Larger (0.8 unit/kg) dose of insulin resulted in severe hypoglycemia (*top panel*) lasting for 2 hr, during which glucose release by liver failed to increase above preinsulin level (*bottom panel*). Glucose uptake and release were measured with [^{14}C]glucose in the dog in the resting unanesthetized state 18 hr after last meal. *IV*, intravenous; *CONC*, concentration. [From deBodo et al. (33).]

dealt with recently by Exton et al. (46). Epinephrine (10^{-6} M), norepinephrine (10^{-6} M), and glucagon (10^{-8} M) increase [^{14}C]glucose production from substrate amounts of [^{14}C]alanine and [^{14}C]lactate, present in the perfusing medium (buffer, containing albumin and saline-washed erythrocytes) for the isolated perfused rat liver. Figure 16 shows the effect of the infusion of glucagon into the inflowing perfusion medium in livers taken from fed rats (48). Here the glucose and [^{14}C]-glucose contents of the effluent (not recirculated) medium are both shown to be elevated in a few minutes, and about equally, when glucagon is infused during a continued supply of [^{14}C]lactate in less than saturating substrate concentration by way of the inflowing perfusion medium. The interpretation of these findings is complicated by the facts: a) that the glycogen may become labeled to some extent in the 20 min of [^{14}C]lactate perfusion before glucagon infusion and so can furnish [^{14}C]glucose by glycogenolysis; and b) that the presence of the lactate allows gluconeogenesis to proceed from precursors other than the lactate itself, whereas gluconeogenesis from all precursors becomes inactivated in the absence of this substrate. Just prior to glucagon infusion, for example, 3 Eq of lactate carbon appear in the form of glucose for each 1 Eq of lactate carbon removed by the liver from the perfusion fluid. About one-tenth (rather than one-third) of the radioactively labeled carbon atoms of the issuing glucose are derived from the disappearing lactate carbon atoms at this moment, indicating the disappearance of the ^{14}C into side pathways without net loss of precursor carbon, as is expected in comparisons of net conversion with isotope incorporation (161).

Nevertheless the increased rate of lactate uptake (Fig. 16) and other supporting evidence leads to the conviction that glucose output is increased by an increase in gluconeogenesis from lactate within minutes after the beginning of glucagon infusion, as well as by the glycogenolysis that glucagon brings about in the perfused liver. As judged by the increased lactate uptake from the perfusing medium, the rate of gluconeogenesis is accelerated for 4 min after glucagon infusion is begun and then remains steady at the new increased rate for the next 16 min of glucagon infusion and for at least the first 12 min after glucagon infusion is terminated. The tapering off of total glucose output (but not of [^{14}C]glucose output) shown in Figure 16 is attributed by Exton & Park (48) to the exhaustion of the stored glycogen, so that glycogenolysis is no longer contributing to the total glucose release by drawing from this largely unlabeled source of glucose.

Epinephrine, norepinephrine, and glucagon operate, through different receptor sites, to increase the level of 3′,5′-adenosine monophosphate (cyclic AMP) in liver cells (46). The work of Sutherland & Rall (163) provided the foundation for understanding the intracellular mediation, by cyclic AMP, of the glycogenolytic effects of glucagon and catecholamines. It was to be expected then that an elevated level of intracellular cyclic AMP would be found during the increases in glucose release observed in perfused rat livers. What was unexpected was that cyclic AMP, when added to the perfusing fluid at 10^{-4} M, increased the rate of gluconeogenesis just as rapidly (48) and produced the same changes in the concentration of gluconeogenic intermediates (47) as did glucagon and catecholamines. Exton & Park (48) then proposed that cyclic AMP mediates, intracellularly, the action of glucagon and catecholamines on gluconeogenesis. The high concentration of cyclic AMP required in the perfusion medium to produce the increase in gluconeogenesis was expected. This intracellular hormone does not pass through the liver cell membrane readily. This is shown by the fact that the space occupied in the liver by cyclic AMP, when perfused at 10^{-4} M, is the same size as the sucrose (extracellular) space of the liver (43).

Friedmann et al. (55) explored the reason for the deficient responsiveness to glucagon of isolated perfused livers taken from adrenalectomized rats maintained on saline and fasted overnight. Exton and co-workers (44) and Eisenstein & Strack (38) had demonstrated that glucagon failed to increase gluconeogenesis from lactate or pyruvate in such perfused livers. Figure 17 shows the restoration of the normal increase in glucose release following addition of glucagon when the adrenalectomized rat has been treated with dexamethasone (~0.08 mg/100 g, sc) 30 min before the liver is removed, as well as when dexamethasone (2 μg/ml) has been included in the perfusion medium. All glucose production is from gluconeogenesis in these glycogen-deficient livers from overnight-fasted adrenalectomized rats. When dexamethasone is added at 2 μg/ml along with lactate and glucagon to the perfusion medium, glucose release is stimulated in the subsequent 80-min period, whereas in the absence of glucagon this amount of glucocorticoid

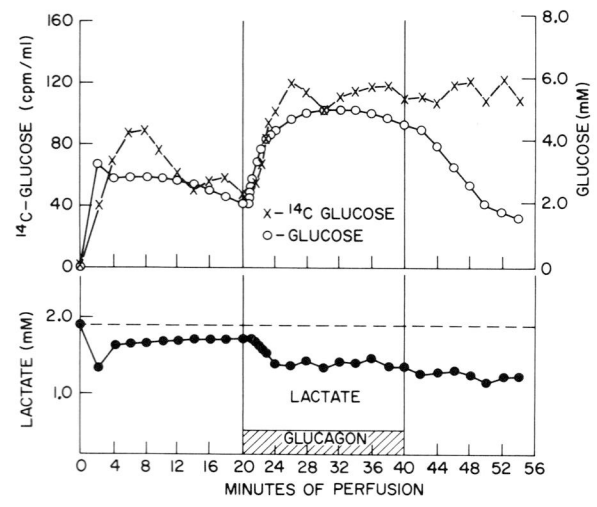

FIG. 16. Effects of glucagon added to perfusing medium on total glucose content, [^{14}C]glucose content, and lactate content of effluent medium from perfused rat liver. Inflowing perfusion medium contained [^{14}C]lactate (2.0 mM) and no glucose. [Adapted from Exton & Park (48).]

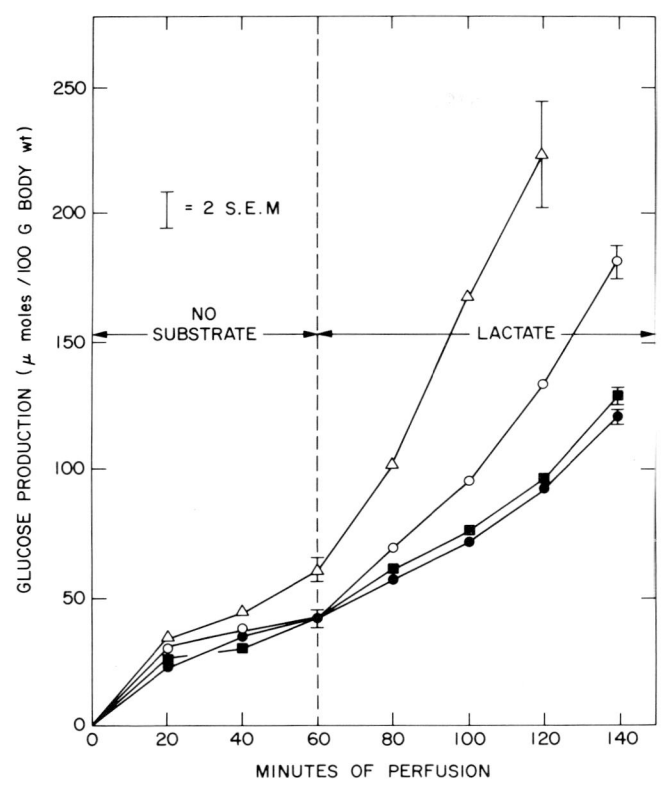

FIG. 17. Effects of dexamethasone (80 μg) injected 30 min prior to killing (△) or added 2 μg/ml in vitro at 60 min to the perfusion medium (○) on gluconeogenesis from lactate as stimulated by glucagon (0.1 μg/ml) in perfused livers taken from fasted adrenalectomized rats. All livers were perfused 60 min without substrate, then 20 mM L-lactate was supplied in perfusing medium. Control (■) livers had no other additions except lactate; dexamethasone alone (2 μg/ml) besides lactate was supplied for one group (●). [From Friedmann et al. (55).]

TABLE 13. *Effects of Dexamethasone on Incorporation of ^{14}C from [^{14}C]Lactate into Glucose by Perfused Livers from Adrenalectomized Rats*

Experimental Series*	Hormones Added	[^{14}C]Glucose Activity, cpm/100 g body wt × 10^{-3}	Significance
A†	None	123±9 (4)‡	
	Glucagon	315±25 (4)	$P < 0.0005$
B	Glucagon	266±33 (5)	
	Glucagon; dexamethasone, 2 μg/ml	492±27 (5)	$P < 0.0005$
C	None	232±20 (5)	
	Dexamethasone, 2 μg/ml	265±19 (7)	NS
D	None	292±11 (7)	
	Dexamethasone, 100 μg/ml	345±19 (7)	$P < 0.025$

* In A, DL-[2-^{14}C]lactate (20 mM, 0.45 μc) was added at 60 min and [^{14}C]glucose activity measured at 120 min; in B to D, uniformly labeled L-[^{14}C]lactate (20 mM, 0.5 μc) was added at 60 min and [^{14}C]glucose measured at 140 min.   † Livers from rats injected with 80 μg of dexamethasone 30 min prior to killing.   ‡ Mean ± SEM; figure in parentheses is number of livers.   [Data from Friedmann et al. (55).]

TABLE 14. *Effects of Glucagon and Epinephrine on Cyclic AMP Levels in Perfused Livers of Fasted, Normal and Adrenalectomized Rats*

Hormone	Cyclic AMP, nmole/g liver*	
	Normal	Adrenalectomized
None	0.9 ± 0.3†	1.2 ± 0.2
Glucagon, 3×10^{-3}M	21.2 ± 0.4	25.7 ± 1.9
Epinephrine, 5×10^{-7}M	3.4 ± 0.6	6.3 ± 1.6

* Livers were perfused for 70 min, then frozen and assayed for cyclic AMP.   † Mean ± SEM.   [Data from Exton et al. (45).]

TABLE 15. *Effects of Exogenous Cyclic AMP on Gluconeogenesis in Perfused Livers from Fasted, Normal and Adrenalectomized Rats*

Liver Donors	Cyclic AMP Added*	Gluconeogenesis, μmole/hr per 100-g rat
Normal	0	67 ± 12†
Normal	1×10^{-4}M	136 ± 23
Adrenalectomized	0	38 ± 6
Adrenalectomized	1×10^{-4}M	37 ± 4

* Concentration of cyclic AMP in perfusing medium on basis of amount of cyclic AMP added to it.   † Mean ± SEM. [Data from Exton et al. (45).]

has no effect (Fig. 17). The increase in glucose release is associated with increased conversion to glucose carbon of the ^{14}C of tagged lactate (Table 13).

Exton and co-workers (45) note that the cyclic AMP levels in the perfused livers from overnight-fasted adrenalectomized rats are increased more than usual (rather than less) by glucagon and epinephrine, whereas the effect of added cyclic AMP, at 10^{-4} M, on gluconeogenesis is not observed in these livers (Tables 14 and 15). Thus they conclude that the message for increased gluconeogenesis in livers from adrenalectomized rats passes through the elevation of intracellular cyclic AMP but then fails to produce the usual effect on gluconeogenesis. The high background level of total intracellular cyclic AMP against which the small increases are measured after addition of epinephrine and norepinephrine is bothersome. Presumably the effective cyclic AMP is confined to a particular subcellular space. Knowledge of the lack of a specific intracellular location at which the effective increase in cyclic AMP may be measured may explain why it is that glucagon elevates overall cyclic AMP in the perfused liver (fed rat) to nearly 20 times the level seen after addition of epinephrine (Table 14) while causing about the same increase in glucose output as does epinephrine.

It is hazardous to conclude that the structure of the hepatic receptor for glucagon was absolutely unimpaired in the adrenalectomized rat if one argues only from the fact that large changes still occurred in cyclic AMP level after glucagon administration. The time interval for the restoration of adrenergic receptor responsiveness in vascular smooth muscle after administration of cortisol is less than 5 min (12). If there was impairment in the response of hepatic cell receptors, in addition to impairment of the effectiveness of cyclic AMP to increase gluconeogenesis, the former might very well not be evident in the experiments described above (Fig. 17) in which dexamethasone added in vitro potentiated glucagon stimulation of gluconeogenesis only after a much longer interval.

The identity of the external message directed to the liver cell of the hypoglycemic adrenalectomized rat is not known. The source of epinephrine has been eliminated by adrenalectomy, so norepinephrine, produced in the liver in response to sympathetic nerve impulses, and circulating glucagon, secreted in greater amount because of the hypoglycemia, are the remaining known possibilities. For an account of this see Exton et al. (46) and the discussion that follows their paper. The level of glucagon during fasting probably has not been measured in adrenalectomized rats, so the possibility remains that the response of glucagon secretion to hypoglycemia is also deficient during fasting in this animal and increases rapidly after glucocorticoid administration.

Probably no impetus for increased gluconeogenesis is carried to the liver by changes in the concentration of metabolites presented to the liver by the circulating blood during the first 90 min after glucocorticoid administration to the fasted adrenalectomized rat. Exton and co-workers (46) have shown that glucose production by the perfused liver from fasted rats is responsive to changes in lactate, pyruvate, amino acid, and glycerol concentrations within the physiological range. However, as noted by Glenn et al. (57), changes in metabolite levels in the peripheral blood have not been found during the first 90 min after glucocorticoid administration to the fasted adrenalectomized rat. This does not mean that there is no change in the rate at which substrates for gluconeogenesis are being extracted from the blood by the liver. Figure 16 shows the increase in lactate extraction brought about when glucagon increases gluconeogenesis in the perfused liver. The experiments of Huckabee (73) suggest that the flow of pyruvate from peripheral tissues to the liver could be doubled without there being any change in the lactate or pyruvate concentration of the peripheral blood.

In summary, there is positive evidence in the adrenalectomized animal of a block in the chain of events leading to increased hepatic gluconeogenesis at some step beyond increased intracellular cyclic AMP concentration. There is no evidence that the hepatic cell receptors for glucagon and catecholamines are impaired by adrenalectomy, and there are indications that injected cortisol does not produce its early effect leading to increased gluconeogenesis by increasing the flow of substrates to the liver. No evidence exists on the possible impairment, by adrenalectomy, of the flow to the liver of external messages for increased gluconeogenesis (e.g., nervous impulses or increased glucagon secretion).

c. Execution of the order for increased gluconeogenesis. Figure 18 shows important steps in the formation of glucose from pyruvate. It is generally accepted that the rate of the overall process may be increased rapidly by the facilitation of a rate-controlling step between mitochondrial pyruvate and cytosol phosphoenolpyruvate [see (46, 64, 65, 98, 103, 104, 148, 155, 162, 169, 178) for pertinent observations]. The nature of the exact process that is controlled is one of the major unsolved problems of modern biochemistry, and the evidence relating to it will not be reviewed in detail. Glucagon, and catecholamines, acting by way of increased intracellular cyclic AMP, are thought to influence this control point. As shown in Figure 18, gluconeogenesis from glycerol or fructose needs not traverse the postulated control point, which is consistent with the fact that glucagon does not increase gluconeogenesis from glycerol (148) or fructose (46) by perfused rat liver.

Because the reaction catalyzed by pyruvate carboxylase is completely dependent on the presence of acetyl coenzyme A (169), an attractive hypothesis has been developed (53, 65, 70, 99, 160, 162, 178, 180), one that attributes an acceleration of gluconeogenesis to increased intracellular acetyl coenzyme A concentration brought

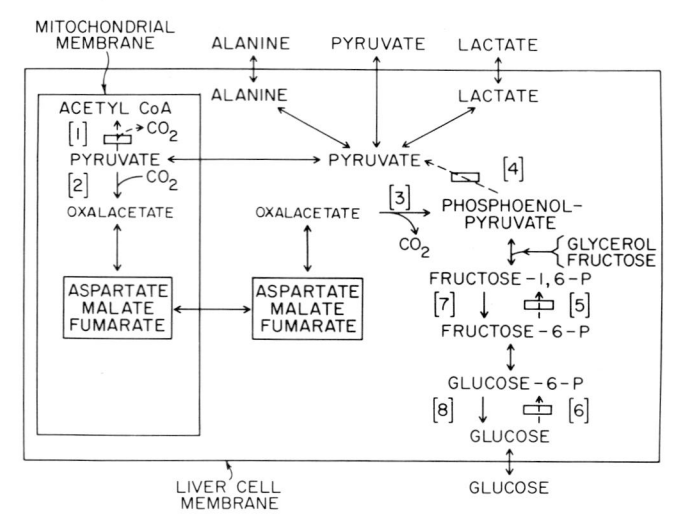

FIG. 18. Path proposed for carbon in gluconeogenesis from alanine, pyruvate, or lactate. Key steps are catalyzed by [2] pyruvate carboxylase and [3] phosphoenolpyruvate carboxykinase. Oxalacetate is believed not to penetrate the mitochondrial membrane, so is converted to and reconstituted from aspartate, malate, and fumarate which can. Reactions catalyzed by [1] pyruvate dehydrogenase (decarboxylase), [4] pyruvate kinase, [5] phosphofructokinase, and [6] glucokinase (and hexokinase) detract from the flow toward free glucose and are shown in the diagram as *dashed arrows* blocked by *rectangles*. Reactions catalyzed by [7] fructose diphosphatase and [8] glucose 6-phosphatase are potential control points not believed to operate as such. The carbon from glycerol or fructose must go through [7] and [8] on the way to glucose but need not go through [2] and [3]. [Adapted from Haynes (64) and Lardy et al. (104).]

about as a result of increased intracellular free fatty acid concentration. The catecholamines and glucagon are thought to bring about the increased intracellular free fatty acid concentration in liver cells through the cyclic AMP-mediated activation of a lipase for triglycerides, as is the case in adipose tissue. In addition, an increased flux of fatty acids from the peripheral tissues to the liver is thought to increase the free fatty acid concentration within liver cells as a later development. On the other hand, Exton and co-workers (46) have provided evidence that albumin-bound fatty acids in physiological concentration in the perfusion medium do not increase gluconeogenesis in the perfused rat liver and suggest that catecholamines and glucagon increase gluconeogenesis in another way.

Thus the way the message for increased gluconeogenesis, which is relayed by increased intracellular cyclic AMP, is finally executed is not agreed upon, and the mechanism by which the glucocorticoids facilitate the execution of the message relayed by cyclic AMP remains unknown.

d. Possibility that glucocorticoids convey a direct message for increased gluconeogenesis. Haynes (66) incubated liver slices taken from fasted adrenalectomized rats in buffer for 1 hr in the presence of 10 mM alanine or 5 mM pyruvate and 10^{-5} M triamcinolone. At the end of this time the slices were removed. Some were analyzed for glycogen content and others were incubated 2 (or 4) more hr in the same medium. At the end of the 2 (or 4) hr glucose plus glycogen was determined in the medium and slices. The production of glucose by the slices was about 1–2 μmole/100 mg tissue for a 2-hr period. At low bicarbonate concentration in the buffered medium the triamcinolone increased significantly the amount of glucose produced both in the presence of alanine and in the presence of pyruvate. It was shown that the triamcinolone did not increase alanine uptake and that increasing the rate of alanine uptake by increasing its concentration did not increase glucose production in the absence of glucocorticoid. Confirmatory evidence by other investigators and similar experiments utilizing ^{14}C-labeled substrates have been reviewed critically by Landau (102). A similar, very weak (not statistically significant) effect of dexamethasone (2 μg/ml) in the absence of added glucagon is evident in Table 13. Livers of fasted adrenalectomized rats were perfused for 80 min with 20 mM lactate plus the glucocorticoid. At 100 μg/ml a definite effect of the dexamethasone to increase glucose production in the absence of added glucagon was seen during the 80 min of this study.

The weakness of this effect and perhaps the possibility that it represents a direct rather than a permissive action of a glucocorticoid have inhibited further experimentation.

With regard to the concept of "permissive" action, Wicks et al. (177) have reported the induction of a number of hepatic enzymes in fasted adrenalectomized rats by the intraperitoneal injection of the dibutyryl derivative of cyclic AMP. The enzymes, tyrosine-α-ketoglutarate transaminase, phosphoenolpyruvate carboxykinase, and serine dehydrase, are also induced by glucagon. This is consistent with the belief that cyclic AMP is the intracellular mediator of the action of glucagon to induce hepatic enzymes. Tryptophan pyrrolase is induced by cortisol but not by either glucagon or dibutyryl cyclic AMP. Cortisol has no effect on carboxykinase or dehydrase. Furthermore combinations of cortisol and dibutyryl cyclic AMP have additive or synergistic effects on tyrosine transaminase induction. The observations of enzyme content in these experiments were made 1–4 hr after administration of the inducing agent. Later, Wicks (176) showed that glucagon and cyclic AMP, but not cortisol, could induce phosphoenolpyruvate carboxykinase in fetal rat liver (at term) that had been kept in organ culture. Lee & Kenney (107) demonstrated the induction of alanine transaminase, as well as tyrosine transaminase, by cortisol, corticosterone, and aldosterone in a hepatoma cell line in tissue culture. Reel et al. (144) demonstrated that separate mechanisms must exist for the cortisol and insulin induction of tyrosine transaminase in cultured hepatoma cells. Tomkins and co-workers (167) have discussed the induction of enzymes by the glucocorticoids and other hormones in terms of the control of gene expression.

The observations involving cultured cells are of special significance because a changed flux of metabolites or hormones originating in other tissues is eliminated as a possible cause for enzyme induction. It is evident that glucagon, insulin, and the glucocorticoids all have instant metabolic effects in one tissue or another of the body, and all have effects on the enzyme pattern of the hepatic cell that develop over a few hours. Only with glucocorticoids would the consequences of the changes in enzyme pattern be referred to as "permissive" effects.

2. LATER EFFECTS OF GLUCOCORTICOID ADMINISTRATION. Changes in liver enzyme content, which begin in the first hour after glucocorticoid administration, extend to more and more enzymes over several days. The activity of many enzymes utilized in gluconeogenesis increases.

Knox and co-workers (92, 93), Rosen & Nichol (147), and Weber and co-workers (171, 172) have summarized and described the changes of enzyme activities in tissues that occur after adrenalectomy and after glucocorticoid administration. Many of these changes follow, rather than precede, the changes in throughput in the metabolic pathways of the enzymes. Thus, in longer-term experiments, the observed changes in enzyme activities tend to serve as sensitive indicators of metabolic change (147) and may point out unexpected and unknown metabolic changes but do not elucidate the primary mechanisms responsible for the metabolic effects of glucocorticoid deficiency or excess.

The consequences of glucocorticoid excess with respect to fat mobilization are presented in section VI-*F*; the relation between the increased flux of fatty acids to the liver and increased hepatic gluconeogenesis is discussed in section VI-D-1-c.

In addition to the increased levels of enzymes concerned with gluconeogenesis (glucose 6-phosphatase, fructose 1,6-diphosphatase, phosphoenolpyruvate carboxykinase, pyruvate carboxylase), increases in the availability to the liver of amino acids for the support of gluconeogenesis augment the liver's capacity to respond to a call for increased gluconeogenesis as a later effect of glucocorticoid administration.

E. Changes in Rates of Glycogen Breakdown and Deposition

1. GLYCOGENOLYSIS. In the whole animal in the postabsorptive state and in the isolated perfused liver taken from the fed rat, hepatic glycogenolysis, as well as gluconeogenesis, contributes to the glucose output. When gluconeogenesis is assessed in terms of the incorporation of the ^{14}C of [^{14}C]lactate into the glucose released, glucagon, epinephrine, and cyclic AMP increase both gluconeogenesis and glycogenolysis in the isolated perfused liver of the fed rat (46). In such perfused livers, insulin added to the perfusion medium inhibits total glucose output and the incorporation of the ^{14}C of lactate into glucose. At the same time, it inhibits the elevation in cyclic AMP levels brought about by epinephrine and glucagon and completely prevents the increases in total glucose output brought about by cyclic AMP introduced into the perfusing medium at concentrations of 6×10^{-6} M or lower. These findings help in understanding a puzzling effect shown in Figure 15. Here a lesser hypoglycemia, produced by a lesser insulin dose, led to an increase in glucose production by the liver. The lack of such a response to the greater hypoglycemia after the greater insulin dose is very likely due to a continued inhibition of glucose output by the amount of insulin remaining in the animal at the later times. Exton and co-workers (46) favor the hypothesis that insulin acts by increasing the breakdown of cyclic AMP rather than by decreasing the rate of its formation.

Considerable increases in total glucose output in response to glucagon, epinephrine, and to larger (10^{-3} M) external concentrations of cyclic AMP occur in livers taken from fed adrenalectomized rats. The increases are one-third to one-half those that occur in livers taken from fed normal rats. Gluconeogenesis, as evaluated by incorporation of ^{14}C from [^{14}C]lactate into glucose, is increased less by these agents in livers from normal fed rats than it is in livers from normal fasted rats, and only a small difference occurs in the response between normal and adrenalectomized fed rats (Table 16). The difference occurs when the cyclic AMP concentration in the perfusion fluid is below 2×10^{-4} M (46). It can be surmised that a relative, not an absolute, refractoriness to hepatic glycogenolytic agents exists in the adrenalectomized animal with adequate liver glycogen stores.

Figures 19 and 20 illustrate the effects of glucocorticoid deficiency on epinephrine-induced elevations of blood glucose concentration, as well as the restoration of the normal response to epinephrine by a cortisone or cortisol regimen. Altszuler and co-workers (5) have demonstrated, using [^{14}C]glucose, that the initial elevation of the blood sugar level by epinephrine is due to increased release of glucose by the liver; only the persistence of the elevation in blood sugar concentration during continued epinephrine infusion is due to prevention of the usual increase in glucose uptake that is caused by hyperglycemia.

The findings illustrated in Figures 19 and 20 were summarized in 1953 by deBodo & Sinkoff (31). The refractoriness of the hypophysectomized dog to epinephrine-induced hyperglycemia was reported in 1933 by Corkill et al. (28) who suspected that adrenal cortical atrophy might play a part in this. Chaikoff and co-workers (23) confirmed the lessened hyperglycemic response of the hypophysectomized dog to epinephrine and added the observation that the rise in blood lactate was also less, indicating a lessened susceptibility of muscle glycogen to epinephrine-induced glycogenolysis. Chaikoff and co-workers (22) then demonstrated that liver glycogen and muscle glycogen levels are not depleted in the hypophysectomized dog at the time (18 hr after the last meal) their epinephrine experiments were carried out.

Schaeffer et al. (150) demonstrated that the decreased hyperglycemic effect of both intravenously administered epinephrine and intravenously administered cyclic AMP in fed, saline-maintained, adrenalectomized rats is associated with a) lowered levels of inactive liver phosphorylase prior to administration of the hyperglycemic agent, and b) a lesser increase in active phosphorylase after administration of the agent. A hydrocortisone regimen (10 mg/kg every 12 hr for 3 days) restores the level of inactive phosphorylase and the activation of phosphorylase by epinephrine and cyclic AMP. However, hydrocortisone given 15 or 30 min before epinephrine or cyclic AMP does not restore the normal hyperglycemic effect of these agents.

As shown in Figure 20, a cortisol regimen in the hypophysectomized dog restores its normal hyperglycemic response to epinephrine. It was assumed that the deficient glucocorticoid secretion of this animal was equivalent to the absent glucocorticoid secretion of the adrenalectomized dog. However, Altszuler and co-workers (3) have discovered that intravenously administered cyclic AMP produces an enhanced rather than a diminished hyperglycemic response in the hypophysectomized dog, indicating perhaps that the diminished hyperglycemic response of the hypophysectomized dog to epinephrine is due to a diminished increment in the synthesis of cyclic AMP in response to epinephrine rather than to the insensitivity of its liver cells to the cyclic AMP produced intracellularly. In this connection, deBodo and co-workers (33) have shown that a growth hormone replacement regimen in the hypophysectomized dog restores the ability of this animal to respond to hypoglycemia with a prompt in-

TABLE 16. *Effects of Adrenalectomy on Responses of Livers from Fed Rats to Gluconeogenic Agents**

Agent	Glucose Production, μmoles/100 g per hr		Gluconeogenesis, cpm [^{14}C]glucose per 100 g per hr	
	Normal	Adrenal-ectomized	Normal	Adrenal-ectomized
None	162±11†	76±7	64±7	51±5
Glucagon (4 × 10^{-8}M)	438	246±52	110	90±8
Epinephrine (1 × 10^{-5}M)	460	156±36	118	120±9
Cyclic AMP (1 × 10^{-3}M)	410±8	222±51	108±15	105±7
Cyclic AMP (2 × 10^{-4}M)	466±61	130±37	120±17	57±10
Cyclic AMP (4 × 10^{-5}M)	300	87±16	106	57±11
Cyclic AMP (2 × 10^{-5}M)	268	78	91	55

* Livers from fed rats were perfused 1 hr without substrate. Then [^{14}C]lactate was added, with the agents noted, and glucose production and [^{14}C]glucose synthesis were measured over the following hour. † Mean ± SEM. [Data from Exton et al. (45).]

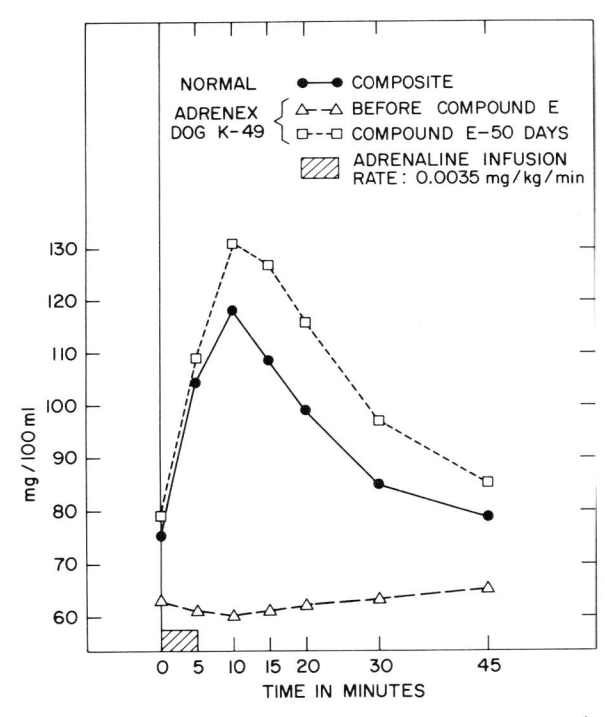

FIG. 19. Absence of normal hyperglycemic response to epinephrine (*ADRENALINE*) in the adrenalectomized (*ADRENEX*) dog and its restoration by cortisone (*COMPOUND E*) regimen. [From deBodo & Sinkoff (31).]

crease in glucose output by the liver, despite the continued absence of glucocorticoid secretion.

Schaeffer and co-workers (151) extended their observations on glycogenolysis to the gastrocnemius muscle of rat hind leg. Rats adrenalectomized 14–20 days previously, then maintained on saline and used in the fed state, were given epinephrine (1 μg/100 g, iv) or cyclic AMP (1 mg/100 g, iv), and the hind legs were frozen between 1 and 5 min later. Active phosphorylase (phosphorylase *a*; 5′-adenosine monophosphate-inde-

pendent phosphorylase) and inactive phosphorylase (phosphorylase *b*; 5′-adenosine monophosphate-dependent phosphorylase) were assayed in the isolated gastrocnemius muscles. It was found that those amounts of epinephrine or cyclic AMP did not result in the conversion of inactive to active phosphorylase in the adrenalectomized rat muscle, whereas they did in the normal rat muscle and in the muscle of adrenalectomized rats kept for 3 days on hydrocortisone (2 mg/100 g per day). Neither active nor inactive phosphorylase was diminished in the adrenalectomized rats prior to stimulation; the hydrocortisone-treated rats had twice the normal levels of total phosphorylase.

The defect in adrenalectomized rat muscle in the sequence of events leading to phosphorylase activation was explored further by Miller et al. (123) who used a perfused heart preparation. The message for increased glycogenolysis initiated both by epinephrine and by administered cyclic AMP was found unimpaired, up to and including the activation of the kinase for phosphorylase *a* activation. The reaction involving this kinase and phosphorylase *a* was impaired in the adrenalectomized rat heart and could be restored to normal by raising the calcium ion concentration in the perfusing medium. Results of preliminary experiments mentionee indicate that the hypophysectomized adrenalectomized rat loses substantially more sensitivity to phosphorylase activation by epinephrine and that this defect cannot be restored by a cortisol regimen.

2. GLUCOSE UPTAKE AND GLYCOGEN SYNTHESIS BY LIVER. Britton & Silvette (18) reported in 1932 the deficient deposition of liver glycogen following glucose injection in adrenalectomized rats. This finding was not confirmed by

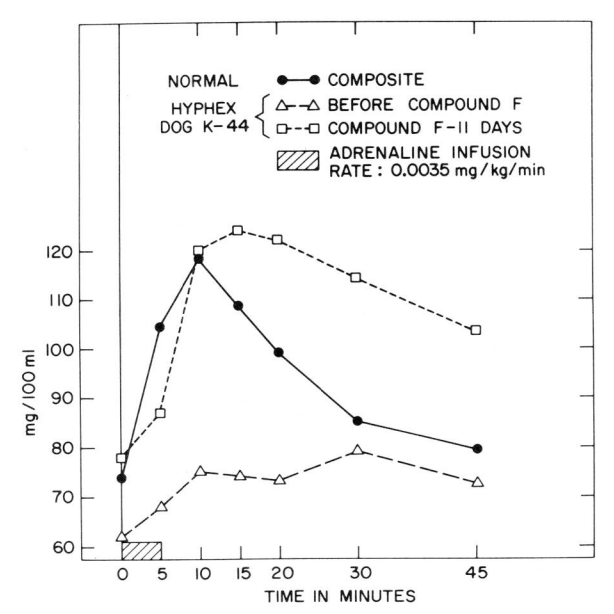

FIG. 20. Absence of normal hyperglycemic response to epinephrine (*ADRENALINE*) in the hypophysectomized (*HYPHEX*) dog and its restoration by cortisol (*COMPOUND F*) regimen. [From deBodo & Sinkoff (31).]

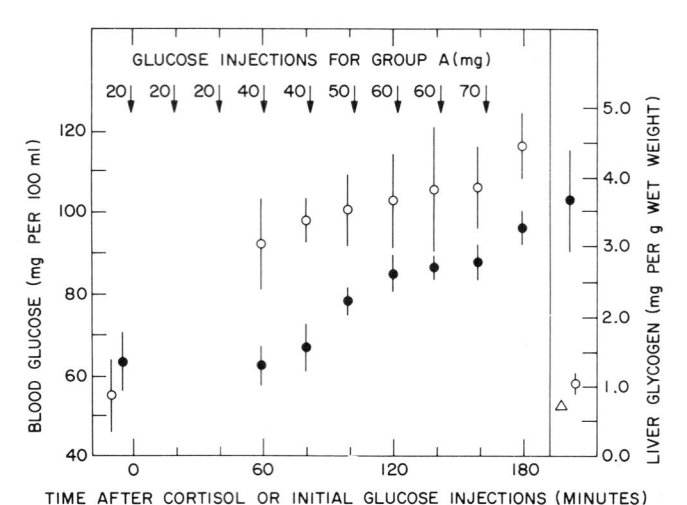

FIG. 21. Defective liver glycogen deposition of adrenalectomized rat and repair of this defect by 2.5-mg cortisol injection during the 180 min between injection and killing. Adrenalectomized rats injected repeatedly with glucose (○) to maintain their blood glucose values higher than those of cortisol-injected, adrenalectomized rats (●) were found to have deposited very little liver glycogen after 180 min, as shown by comparison with control (△) rats not injected with either cortisol or glucose. [From Dorsey & Munck (34).]

their contemporaries but was rediscovered 30 years later by Dorsey & Munck (34) and by Friedmann et al. (54). Figure 21 shows this effect of adrenalectomy and the repair of glycogen deposition, effected during 1 to 3 hr by the subcutaneous injection of cortisol (1 mg/100 g).

As shown by Bishop and co-workers (15), the incorporation of the ^{14}C of circulating [^{14}C]glucose into not only liver glycogen but also the rest of the liver constituents occurs to only a negligible extent in the postabsorptive state. The infusion of insulin along with enough extra glucose to prevent hypoglycemia results in the deposition of the ^{14}C of [^{14}C]glucose as glycogen and also accelerates its incorporation into the rest of the liver constituents.

Glycogen synthesis, which occurs primarily by the addition of glucosyl units derived from uridine diphosphate glucose to the ends of existing glycogen chains, is catalyzed by glycogen synthetase. Glycogen deposition is not a passive process governed by the availability of glucose, glucose 1-phosphate, or uridine diphosphate glucose but rather is a controlled process. Insulin promotes an increase in the I (glucose 6-phosphate-independent) form of glycogen transferase. This is due at least in part to its effect increasing the activity of a phosphatase converting the phosphorylated D (glucose 6-phosphate-dependent) form to the dephosphorylated I form (14), the latter being the "active" form for glycogen deposition. Glucagon reverses the activation of this phosphatase. Insulin also acts to decrease the activity of the kinase that reconverts the active form to the "inactive" form by catalyzing its phosphorylation. For a short review of the regulation of hepatic glycogen synthetase see Holzer & Duntze (71).

Kreutner & Goldberg (100) demonstrated that cortisol administration in the adrenalectomized rat elevates the amount of active hepatic glycogen synthetase when this is measured 2 hr later. However, cortisol fails to have this effect in the alloxan-diabetic, adrenalectomized rat, whereas injected insulin still does. The conclusion was drawn that extra insulin secreted in response to the steroid injection is responsible for the activation of glycogen synthetase and thus for the active glycogen deposition seen soon after steroid injection in the fasted adrenalectomized animal.

Hornbrook (72) found that the livers of starved, saline-maintained, adrenalectomized rats have much less of the active form of glycogen synthetase than do the livers of starved normal rats. Starved alloxan-diabetic rats also have a lowered content of the active glycogen synthetase, but not as low as adrenalectomized rats. Starved, insulin-maintained, alloxan-diabetic rats respond to cortisol in 3 hr as do normal starved rats, by increasing their levels of hepatic active glycogen synthetase, whereas initially insulin-maintained, alloxan-diabetic rats that have subsequently been adrenalectomized and then deprived of insulin for 5–7 days fail to do this. Insulin and glucocorticoid deprivation over a prolonged period prevents the response to cortisol. Bishop (14) has noted that insulin deprivation alone (alloxan-diabetic dog) prevents the acute increase in the synthetase-activating phosphatase that is brought about by insulin injection. Thus the earlier finding of Kreutner & Goldberg (100) is subject to a somewhat different interpretation. Chronic insulin deprivation, in addition to the acute absence of extra insulin secretion following glucocorticoid administration, appears to play an important role in the failure of glycogen deposition to increase after cortisol administration in the alloxan-diabetic, adrenalectomized rat. Furthermore cortisol appears to promote glycogen synthetase activation that is independent of any immediate extra insulin secretion its injection may bring about. Mersman & Segal (122) demonstrated an absence of glycogen synthetase activation during incubation of the "glycogen pellet" from homogenized livers of adrenalectomized rats fasted for 48 hr and the restoration of this activation when prednisolone acetate was given 4½ hr before the starved adrenalectomized rat was killed. They attributed this effect to the glucocorticoid and made no mention of possible changes in insulin secretion rate.

In contrast with the positive control exerted over glycogen synthesis, no direct control mechanism is known for glucose phosphorylation by liver. Salas and co-workers (149) and Sharma et al. (156) found that rat liver glucokinase is induced in 3–4 hr by insulin in the presence of glucose under conditions (alloxan diabetes, starvation) in which the prevailing glucokinase level is low. Mori (126) found that the livers of adrenalectomized rats have lowered glucokinase activity, which can be restored by cortisol administration. Since cortisol did not increase the low glucokinase levels of livers from alloxan-diabetic rats, the conclusion was drawn that the extra insulin secretion after cortisol administration was responsible for the rise in glucokinase observed in the adrenalectomized rats.

Increased glucokinase activity increases the capability of the liver to phosphorylate glucose. Evidence of another kind indicates that a glucocorticoid regimen results in an actual increase in glucose phosphorylation by liver during the fasting state. Katz & Dunn (84) introduced [2-^{3}H]glucose as a tracer for measuring the turnover of the glucose of circulating blood. They noted a much higher rate of isotope disappearance when [2-^{3}H]glucose was used and attributed this to the loss of ^{3}H from glucose 6-phosphate in liver cells during the reversible interconversion of glucose 6-phosphate and fructose 6-phosphate. The recycling of this material back to blood glucose results in an apparent influx of new, unlabeled glucose, which is included when glucose turnover is measured in this way. This cycle is not visible in experiments involving [^{14}C]glucose or [6-^{3}H]glucose, because the label is not lost or shifted in location within the glucose molecule. B. Issekutz and co-workers (personal communication) utilized this [2-^{3}H]glucose method in dogs, comparing control and long-term methylprednisolone-treated animals. The disappearance of [^{3}H]glucose from the blood, compared with the disappearance of [^{14}C]glucose from the blood in the same experiments, was increased markedly in the glucocorticoid-treated animals, indicating the more rapid operation of the cycling process through liver glucose 6-phosphate and fructose 6-phosphate in these dogs. This finding opens up the possibility of observing possible rapid increases in hepatic glucose phosphorylation in response to injected glucocorticoids or insulin independently of whether or not the carbon of the phosphorylated glucose becomes incorporated into glycogen or other liver cell constituents.

F. Altered Facility for Glucose Utilization by Peripheral Tissues

The key role of decreased glucose uptake in the sequence of events that occur shortly after the exposure of thymocytes to excess glucocorticoid has been described in section VI-C-1. On the other hand, evidence has been mentioned in section VI-D-1-a to indicate that decreased overall glucose uptake by the peripheral tissues does not play a significant part in the increased blood glucose concentration that occurs a few hours after glucocorticoid injection in the adrenalectomized rat.

A more general question is whether the glucocorticoids reduce facility for overall glucose uptake in the whole animal under any circumstances. In this connection, Lecocq et al. (106) reported an anomalous rapid effect of infused (90 min) cortisol to decrease glucose release by the liver of the anesthetized dog, an animal that had been previously altered surgically so that its portal vein blood flow had been shunted to the vena cava and no longer entered the liver. This effect was visible both by arteriovenous difference in glucose concentration across the liver and by a [^{14}C]glucose infusion technique. This observation could not be confirmed in the intact unanesthetized dog receiving the same cortisol dose and a similar [^{14}C]glucose infusion technique (N. Altszuler, personal communication). Also, Haynes & Lu (67), using a [^{14}C]glucose injection technique, found no evidence for such an acute effect of cortisol administration in the adrenalectomized rat. However, Ninomiya and co-workers (132), using a [^{14}C]glucose injection technique, observed a 20–25% reduction in glucose release by the liver during cortisol or methylprednisolone infusion in both the normal and the diabetic unanesthetized dog. In the nondiabetic animals of Lecocq and co-workers and of Ninomiya and co-workers, the decrease in glucose release by the liver was not accompanied by a substantial decrease in peripheral concentration of blood glucose, so it may be concluded a) that a decrease in overall glucose uptake had occurred simultaneously with the decrease in glucose release, and b) that this presented a lessened facility for glucose uptake by the peripheral tissues during the glucocorticoid infusion. Clearly the above findings require further examination.

An even more general question than the above is whether the glucocorticoids depress glucose "utilization." An unchanged rate of glucose uptake by peripheral tissues accompanied by an increased flow of lactate and pyruvate back to the liver for resynthesis to glucose is ordinarily considered to represent a decrease in glucose utilization.

1. GLUCOSE UPTAKE AND PHOSPHORYLATION. Ingle (74) summarizing his long experience with steroid diabetes in the rat, said:

> A daily dose of 10 mg [cortisone] per rat causes at least a temporary glycosuria in almost all of the animals tested. The rat is more likely to develop steroid diabetes when it is force fed than when it eats *ad libitum*. The twice daily force feeding of a fluid diet represents a greater dietary load per unit time than does *ad libitum* eating.
>
> In our initial studies on steroid diabetes the rats were maintained on a high carbohydrate diet. Subsequent studies showed that rats can be made to excrete glucose on any diet representing a normal calorie intake.... Steroid diabetes cannot be induced in the fasting rat by the daily injection of up to 50 mg of either cortisone or hydrocortisone per day.
>
> There is a latent period of at least three days between the beginning of administration of the steroid and the appearance of glycosuria.... With doses of 10 mg cortisone acetate per rat per day we have not seen the glycosuria disappear during periods up to six weeks.... In the rat the diabetes always disappears when the administration of the steroid is stopped.
>
> Values for glucose excretion up to 540 mg per rat per hour have been observed in steroid diabetic animals fed a high carbohydrate diet.... When these data are considered together with the finding that normal active rats can be adapted to utilize as much as 1000 mg of glucose per hour, it seems plausible that in the fed active rats having steroid

diabetes there is contribution to the glycosuria from impairment in utilization of carbohydrate.

Species, such as the rat, that are susceptible to steroid diabetes characteristically have continued hyperglycemia, hyperinsulinemia, and resistance to the blood sugar-lowering action of administered insulin during the steroid regimen. Removal of a large portion of the pancreas makes the animal more susceptible to the development of steroid diabetes. Undoubtedly the antidiabetogenic action of continued insulin secretion in intact animals of this kind is due, at least in part, to the ability of insulin to restrain the rate of glucose release by the liver. However, there is evidence indicating that fat metabolism in rats is profoundly affected by the glucocorticoids, that insulin works against these changes in fat metabolism, and finally that the deranged fat metabolism causes, by some mechanism, a decreased facility for glucose uptake by the bulk of the peripheral tissues, namely muscle.

Scow & Chernick (154) summarized in 1960 their findings with rats from which over 99% of the pancreas had been surgically removed and which had been maintained for several weeks after the operation by insulin injection and by feeding pancreatin-containing food. These rats developed severe hyperlipemia, ketosis, and fatty livers when given glucocorticoids; the effects continued to increase over the 2-day period of the study. Either insulin administration or depletion of the body fat stores prevented these effects of the glucocorticoids. Later studies by Fain and associates (49, 50), Munck (128), and others demonstrated that the release of free fatty acids by isolated rat adipose tissue, accompanied by decreased glucose uptake, was evident within a few hours after exposure of the tissue to low concentrations of glucocorticoids in vitro. These observations appear to offer a plausible explanation for the hyperlipemia, ketosis, and fatty livers seen at a longer time interval in the depancreatized, steroid-treated rat. The early decrease in glucose uptake by adipose tissue is reminiscent of the early decrease seen after exposure of thymocytes to the glucocorticoids; as mentioned in section VI-C-1 above, it is believed that the decreased glucose uptake in such tissues is insufficient to bring about a significant decrease in overall glucose uptake by the extrahepatic tissues in general. What is of present interest is the longer-term effect of fat mobilization on overall extrahepatic glucose uptake by muscle as a significant factor in steroid glycosuria.

Randle et al. (140) and Park (135) have summarized the evidence indicating that the availability of excess free fatty acids for intracellular catabolism limits the uptake and utilization of glucose by muscle. Partial inhibition is evident at the phosphorylative step catalyzed by phosphofructokinase (step 5, Fig. 18) and hexokinase (step 6, Fig. 18), and at the step of glucose transport into the cell. In the isolated perfused heart of the hypophysectomized rat, either prior growth hormone treatment or prior hydrocortisone treatment of the rat reduces the sensitivity of glucose transport to stimulation by insulin (69). The effect of hydrocortisone is additive to that of growth hormone; in both instances the effect may depend on lipid mobilization because fatty acids added in vitro diminish insulin stimulation of glucose transport (135). Glucose phosphorylation is depressed, in the isolated perfused heart of the hypophysectomized alloxan-diabetic rat, by prior treatment of the rat with either growth hormone or hydrocortisone; prior treatment with both hormones produces an additive effect (Table 17). The depressed rate of glucose phosphorylation seen in hearts taken from alloxan-diabetic rats is restored toward normal by either prior hypophysectomy or prior adrenalectomy (125).

TABLE 17. *Effect of Growth Hormone and Hydrocortisone on Uptake and Phosphorylation of Glucose[a] by Isolated Heart from Hypophysectomized, Diabetic Rats*

Treatment of Donor Rats' Hearts	Blood Plasma Glucose, mg/100 ml	Glucose Uptake, mg g^{-1} hr^{-1}	Mean Intracellular Glucose, mg/100 ml	Glucose Phosphorylation Mg g^{-1} hr^{-1}	% Normal[b]
None	379 ± 57[c]	7.2 ± 0.5 (11)[d]	37 ± 4	7.0 ± 0.5	61[e]
Growth hormone[f]	282 ± 43	5.5 ± 0.4 (9)	44 ± 5	5.3 ± 0.5	45[e]
Cortisone[i]	700 ± 53	4.1 ± 0.5 (9)	47 ± 6	3.8 ± 0.5	32[e]
Growth hormone[f] + cortisone[g]	666 ± 32	2.0 ± 0.2 (8)	66 ± 5	2.0 ± 0.2	16[e]
None	495 ± 69	9.3 ± 0.4 (9)	48 ± 6	9.0 ± 0.4	75[e]
Growth hormone[h]	362 ± 19	10.2 ± 1.0 (4)	36 ± 14	10.0 ± 1.0	88
Cortisone[i]	525 ± 71	6.1 ± 0.5 (9)	40 ± 5	5.8 ± 0.5	54[e]
Growth hormone[h] + cortisone[i]	599 ± 39	6.5 ± 0.6 (9)	27 ± 4	6.3 ± 0.6	59[e]
Growth hormone[f] + cortisone[i]	821 ± 45	3.4 ± 0.4 (7)	47 ± 4	3.1 ± 0.4	26[e]
Growth hormone[f] + cortisone[g]	785 ± 46	2.6 ± 0.2 (4)	48 ± 3	2.3 ± 0.2	19[e]

[a] Perfusion fluid consists of 3 μg insulin and 1 mg glucose per ml. [b] Comparisons made with values obtained in normal hearts at corresponding intracellular glucose concentrations. [c] Mean ± SEM. [d] Figure in parentheses is number of hearts. [e] $P < 0.01$ vs. corresponding normal control. [f] Growth hormone (0.1 mg/100 g body wt) was injected intraperitoneally at 24 and again at 12 hr before killing. [g] Hydrocortisone (2.5 mg/100 g) was injected subcutaneously at 24 hr, followed by 1.25 mg/100 g at 12 and 4 hr before killing. [h] Growth hormone (0.01 mg/100 g) was administered as above. [i] Hydrocortisone (0.25 mg/100 g) was injected at 24 hr, followed by 0.125 mg/100 g at 12 and 4 hr before killing. [Data from Morgan et al. (125).]

Kipnis and Cori (89, 90) demonstrated similar improved glucose phosphorylation by isolated rat diaphragm muscle after adrenalectomy of the alloxan-diabetic rat. Manchester et al. (119) established effects on glucose uptake by diaphragm muscle that correspond in general with the effects seen in heart muscle, as described above. These effects of hypophysectomy and adrenalectomy, and of prior growth hormone administration or prior cortisol administration on the insulin sensitivity of isolated rat diaphragm are shown in Tables 18 and 19. The effects of growth hormone and the glucocorticoids on glucose phosphorylation are thought to depend on triglyceride lipolysis. When more free fatty acids are metabolized to acetyl coenzyme A by muscle, intracellular citrate concentration rises, phosphofructokinase is inhibited, glucose 6-phosphate concentration rises, and glucose phosphorylation is depressed (135, 140).

The term *triglyceride lipolysis* is used in place of a more definite statement indicating increased free fatty acid concentration in blood for a specific reason, namely, that there are a number of instances in which the free fatty acid concentration and turnover in blood do not correlate with the intracellular free fatty acid concentration found in muscle (153). Triglyceride breakdown and fatty acid esterification within muscle cells are processes capable of altering free fatty acid concentration locally (140).

In dogs, which are not susceptible to steroid diabetes, excess growth hormone produces diabetes while causing fluctuating, poorly understood, elevations of free fatty acid concentration in plasma, as shown by

TABLE 18. *Effect of Hypophysectomy and Treatment with Growth Hormone on Uptake of Glucose During 1-Hr Incubation in Vitro, and on Response of Uptake to Different Concentrations of Insulin, by Isolated Rat Diaphragm*

Diaphragm Source and Treatment	Glucose Uptake, mg/g wet wt per hr		
	No added insulin	Insulin added	Difference
Insulin, 200 munits/ml			
Hypophysectomy (21)*	4.73 ± 0.18 } $P < 0.01$†	8.32 ± 0.21	3.59 ± 0.26 } $P < 0.01$
Normal (24)	3.83 ± 0.19 } $P < 0.05$	8.42 ± 0.19	4.59 ± 0.19 } $P < 0.1$
Intact + growth hormone‡ (24)	3.27 ± 0.14	8.48 ± 0.21	5.20 ± 0.26
Insulin, 0.5 munits/ml			
Hypophysectomy (24)	4.57 ± 0.29 } $P < 0.001$	7.83 ± 0.24 } $P < 0.001$	3.26 ± 0.21
Normal (24)	3.08 ± 0.14	6.22 ± 0.26	3.14 ± 0.19
Normal (19)	3.54 ± 0.27 } $P < 0.001$	6.32 ± 0.37 } $P < 0.001$	2.78 ± 0.52
Intact + growth hormone‡ (13)	1.98 ± 0.16	4.57 ± 0.24	2.59 ± 0.23
Insulin, 0.1 munits/ml			
Hypophysectomy (24)	4.37 ± 0.18 } $P < 0.001$	7.26 ± 0.23 } $P < 0.001$	2.89 ± 0.18 } $P = 0.01$
Normal (23)	3.11 ± 0.19	5.24 ± 0.27	2.13 ± 0.22
Normal (58)	3.04 ± 0.09	4.42 ± 0.14 } $P < 0.02$	1.38 ± 0.15 } $P < 0.05$
Intact + growth hormone‡ (54)	2.98 ± 0.07	3.95 ± 0.12	0.97 ± 0.13

* Number of observations. † Value of P for a difference that is significant is indicated. Response to insulin is in every case significant ($P < 0.01$). ‡ Treatment with growth hormone was 1 mg/rat per day for 7 days and 1 mg 80 min before the experiment. [Data from Manchester et al. (119).]

TABLE 19. *Effect of Adrenalectomy and of Treatment with Cortisol on Uptake of Glucose During 1-Hr Incubation in Vitro, and on Response of Uptake to Different Concentrations of Insulin, by Isolated Rat Diaphragm*

Diaphragm Source and Treatment	Glucose Uptake, mg/g wet wt per hr		
	No added insulin	Insulin added	Difference
Insulin, 200 munits/ml			
Adrenalectomy (8)*	2.67 ± 0.11	6.74 ± 0.24	4.07 ± 0.21
Normal (8)	2.23 ± 0.25 $P < 0.001$†	6.13 ± 0.41	3.90 ± 0.24
Normal + cortisol‡ (8)	1.84 ± 0.14	6.35 ± 0.29	4.51 ± 0.28
Insulin, 0.5 munit/ml			
Adrenalectomy (14)	3.13 ± 0.10	4.76 ± 0.11 } $P < 0.001$	1.63 ± 0.23 } $P < 0.01$
Normal (14)	3.01 ± 0.07	3.82 ± 0.10	0.81 ± 0.12
Normal (22)	3.30 ± 0.13	5.04 ± 0.22 } $P < 0.02$	1.74 ± 0.19
Intact + cortisol (22)	2.96 ± 0.17	4.35 ± 0.18	1.39 ± 0.14
Adrenalectomy (14)	2.85 ± 0.09	4.38 ± 0.19 } $P < 0.05$	1.53 ± 0.19 } $P < 0.05$
Adrenalectomy + cortisol§ (14)	2.75 ± 0.15	3.65 ± 0.24	0.90 ± 0.23

* Number of observations shown in parentheses. † Value of P for a difference that is significant is indicated. Response to insulin is in every case significant ($P < 0.01$). ‡ Treated normal animals received 5 mg cortisol per rat per day for 3 days and 5 mg 80 min before death. § Treated adrenalectomized animals received 1 mg cortisol per rat per day for 3 days and 1 mg 80 min before death. [Data from Manchester et al. (119).]

Altszuler et al. (4). Growth hormone in diabetogenic doses, just as in nondiabetogenic doses, elevates the free fatty acid concentration of plasma measured in the postabsorptive state to a peak value at day 2 of the regimen. Subsequently the value falls, but increased triglyceride lipolysis continues in effect, as evidenced by a continued high concentration of glycerol in plasma. Insulin concentration in plasma is much elevated, and glucose concentration and turnover are moderately elevated at days 2–4 of the regimen, with insulin resistance being evident. During days 5–9 of the regimen, glucose concentration and turnover and insulin concentrations in plasma remain high but are not much further elevated. During this time the diabetic state may be precipitated; when this occurs glucose concentration in plasma becomes very high and glucosuria results, with no important change having occurred in the insulin concentration of plasma or in the rate of glucose release by the liver or uptake by the tissues. The enhanced insulin resistance evidenced by these changes is accompanied by a resurgence of free fatty acid concentration in plasma (which previously had declined to far below its peak level) to a new very high level (N. Altszuler, unpublished findings).

These poorly understood relationships of fat and carbohydrate metabolism suggest that an unknown factor circulating in the blood, a factor depending for its secretion on growth hormone and the glucocorticoids, may intervene and gradually establish the diabetic state, giving rise to either steroid diabetes or growth hormone diabetes by interfering with the action of insulin on muscle cells. The history of such anti-insulin factors was reviewed in 1964 by Berson & Yalow (10).

The increased rates of glucose release and uptake brought about by a cortisol regimen in adrenalectomized and hypophysectomized dogs in the postabsorptive state were discussed in sections VI-B-1 and VI-B-2 above, in connection with changes that also occur in glucose concentration in plasma and in the rates of insulin and epinephrine secretion.

Basset and co-workers (7) have determined that, just prior to the daily feeding, sheep kept on a cortisol regimen have glucose uptakes, as measured with [^{14}C]-glucose, that are unchanged from control values but have elevated glucose concentrations in plasma. Such sheep have twice the normal values of plasma immunoreactive insulin (8), as shown in Figure 9. These findings represent evidence that a decreased facility for glucose uptake by the peripheral tissues is brought about by the glucocorticoid regimen. In contrast, Reilly et al. (145) have reported that glucose uptake from the blood is increased in fed sheep 24 hr after β-methasone injection; the sheep had elevated concentrations of blood glucose at this time, but the insulin concentrations in plasma were not measured.

Increased rates of glucose release and overall glucose uptake in the postabsorptive state were observed by Ninomiya et al. (132) at 7 and 14 days of a methylprednisolone regimen (4 mg/kg per day) in normal dogs. These dogs had only slightly elevated plasma glucose concentrations, and their plasma insulin levels, as judged by the findings of Campbell & Rastogi (20), described in section VI-B-2 above, had probably reverted to normal. These findings suggest a greater rather than a lesser sensitivity of these dogs to insulin-stimulated glucose uptake, a result consistent with the glucose tolerance tests carried out by Campbell & Rastogi (20) and described in section VI-B-2.

In summary, the prevailing rate of overall glucose uptake at any given time during a glucocorticoid regimen is a secondary phenomenon depending on *a*) the rate of glucose release by the liver (and of glucose absorption from the gut if the animal is not fasting), which tends to increase peripheral glucose uptake by elevating the blood sugar concentration, other factors being held unchanged; *b*) the rate of insulin secretion, which is increased by increased blood glucose concentration; *c*) the degree of susceptibility of certain tissues, predominantly muscle, to insulin-induced increased glucose transport; *d*) the capacity of muscle cells to phosphorylate intracellular glucose, a function not altered on a short-term basis by the insulin level in plasma; and *e*) a direct early effect of the glucocorticoids to inhibit glucose uptake by that small fraction of the total peripheral tissues, exemplified by lympoid tissue and adipose tissue. The glucocorticoid, in addition to its small direct effect, exerts pressure in some species, a pressure varying with time, toward an increase in glucose uptake. It does this by increasing the rate of glucose release by the liver and by increasing the insulin secretory response of the pancreas. On the other hand, in some species the glucocorticoid exerts an increasing pressure over a number of days toward a decrease in glucose uptake. This force is associated with increased fat mobilization and is due to a lessened capacity of muscle cells for the phosphorylation of intracellular glucose and by a lessened responsiveness of muscle cells to insulin-stimulated glucose transport. Thus the prevailing rate of glucose uptake, a value equivalent to the glucose turnover, except in the fed or the glucosuric animal, is a resultant at any given time of opposing forces created by glucocorticoid administration. The uptake varies, in its reponse to glucocorticoids, depending on the presence or absence of the pituitary and the adrenal medulla, and in the intact animal the uptake varies, in its response to the glucocorticoids, among species.

2. OXIDATIVE DECARBOXYLATION OF PYRUVATE. It has been suggested that an important feature of glucocorticoid action is a block to glucose utilization that is located subsequent to glucose transport and phosphorylation, namely, at the step by which pyruvate is converted into CO_2 and acetyl coenzyme A, just prior to the entry of the remaining two carbon atoms of pyruvate (which are contained in the latter compound) into the tricarboxylic acid cycle for conversion to CO_2. The consequence of this block during hypercorticalism is held to be an increase in the release of pyruvate-derived lactate

to the blood by the peripheral tissues. Landau (102) has reviewed critically the observations that led to the concept of a block at the pyruvate level.

Randle and associates (140) have reviewed the balance study evidence for a decreased oxidation of internally formed (i.e., by glycolysis from glucose) pyruvate in the muscle cells of the perfused heart when fatty acids are supplied in increased amounts by inclusion in the perfusing medium. The relation between intracellular fatty acid concentration and glucocorticoid action has been discussed in the preceding section. Randle and his associates also give evidence that the oxidation of externally supplied pyruvate is interfered with by the inclusion of a fatty acid in the perfusing fluid, but they note that these latter effects can be explained on the basis of decreased pyruvate transport into the muscle cell, without need to postulate decreased oxidation of intracellular pyruvate. Randle et al. (140) present evidence for inhibition of the activity of pyruvate decarboxylase (pyruvate dehydrogenase) in isolated pig heart by an increased ratio of concentrations of acetyl coenzyme A to coenzyme A, and show that this ratio is in fact increased in muscle during increased fatty acid utilization.

The link between increased fatty acid utilization and the inhibition of phosphofructokinase in muscle, mentioned in the preceding section, is by way of an increased intracellular concentration of citrate, which is an inhibitor of phosphofructokinase. An increased amount of citrate is formed in the cell as the product of the reaction between acetyl coenzyme A and oxalacetate. The increased intracellular concentration of citrate under these conditions is in interesting contrast with the decreased citrate levels in serum seen in humans after glucocorticoid administration [summarized by Landau (102)]. The finding suggests that interference with the outward transport of citrate from muscle cells may be associated with the simultaneously occurring interference with the inward transport of pyruvate into these cells when extra amounts of fatty acids are being metabolized.

The author wishes to acknowledge the valuable assistance rendered by Miss Clara Bjerknes in the preparation of this chapter.

REFERENCES

1. AGARWAL, M. K., J. HANOUNE, F. L. YU, I. B. WEINSTEIN, AND P. FEIGELSON. Studies on the effect of cortisone on rat liver transfer ribonucleic acid. *Biochemistry* 8: 4806–4812, 1969.
3. ALTSZULER, N., I. RATHGEB, R. STEELE, AND C. BJERKNES. Increased sensitivity of the hypophysectomized dog to the elevation in glucose release induced by dibutyryl 3′,5′-cyclic AMP (Abstract). *Federation Proc.* 29: 615, 1970.
4. ALTSZULER, N., I. RATHGEB, B. WINKLER, R. C. DEBODO, AND R. STEELE. The effects of growth hormone on carbohydrate and lipid metabolism in the dog. *Ann. NY Acad. Sci.* 148: 441–458, 1968.
5. ALTSZULER, N., R. STEELE, I. RATHGEB, AND R. C. DEBODO. Glucose metabolism and plasma insulin level during epinephrine infusion in the dog. *Am. J. Physiol.* 212: 677–682, 1967.
6. BARNABEI, O., AND F. SERENI. Cortisol-induced increase of tyrosine-L-ketoglutarate transaminase in the isolated perfused rat liver and its relation to ribonucleic acid synthesis. *Biochim. Biophys. Acta* 91: 239–247, 1964.
7. BASSETT, J. M., S. C. MILLS, AND R. L. REID. The influence of cortisol on glucose utilization in sheep. *Metabolism* 15: 922–932, 1966.
8. BASSETT, J. M., AND A. L. C. WALLACE. Influence of cortisol on plasma insulin in the sheep. *Diabetes* 16: 566–571, 1967.
9. BERGMAN, H. C., AND D. KLEIN. Relation of body weight to liver glycogen storage potency of adrenal cortical extracts. *Endocrinology* 33: 174–176, 1943.
10. BERSON, S. A., AND R. S. YALOW. The present status of insulin antagonists in plasma. *Diabetes* 13: 247–259, 1964.
11. BERSON, S. A., R. S. YALOW, AND B. W. VOLK. *In vivo* and *in vitro* metabolism of insulin-I[131] and glucagon-I[131] in normal and cortisone-treated rabbits. *J. Lab. Clin. Med.* 49: 331–342, 1957.
12. BESSE, J. C., AND A. D. BASS. Potentiation by hydrocortisone of responses to catecholamines in vascular smooth muscle. *J. Pharmacol. Exptl. Therap.* 154: 224–238, 1966.
13. BIRD, J. W. C., T. BERG, AND J. H. LEATHEM. Cathepsin activity of liver and muscle fractions of adrenalectomized rats. *Proc. Soc. Exptl. Biol. Med.* 127: 182–188, 1968.
14. BISHOP, J. S. Inability of insulin to activate liver glycogen transferase D phosphatase in the diabetic pancreatectomized dog. *Biochim. Biophys. Acta* 208: 208–218, 1970.
15. BISHOP, J. S., R. STEELE, N. ALTSZULER, A. DUNN, C. BJERKNES, AND R. C. DEBODO. Effects of insulin on liver glycogen synthesis and breakdown in the dog. *Am. J. Physiol.* 208: 307–316, 1965.
16. BLECHER, M. Steroid effects on permeability of rat thymic lymphocytes to α-aminoisobutyrate. *Am. J. Physiol.* 205: 446–452, 1963.
17. BONDY, P. K., D. J. INGLE, AND R. C. MEEKS. Influence of adrenal cortical hormones upon the level of plasma amino acids in eviscerated rats. *Endocrinology* 55: 354–360, 1955.
18. BRITTON, S. W., AND H. SILVETTE. Effects of cortico-adrenal extract on carbohydrate metabolism in normal animals. *Am. J. Physiol.* 100: 693–700, 1932.
19. BRITTON, S. W., AND H. SILVETTE. The apparent prepotent function of the adrenal glands. *Am. J. Physiol.* 100: 701–713, 1932.
20. CAMPBELL, J., AND K. S. RASTOGI. Elevation in serum insulin, albumin and FFA, with gains in liver lipid and protein, induced by glucocorticoid treatment in dogs. *Can. J. Physiol. Pharmacol.* 46: 421–429, 1968.
21. CAMPBELL, J., K. S. RASTOGI, AND H. R. HAUSLER. Hyperinsulinemia with diabetes induced by cortisone, and the influence of growth hormone in the Chinese hamster. *Endocrinology* 79: 749–756, 1966.
22. CHAIKOFF, I. L., G. F. HOLTOM, AND F. L. REICHERT. The glycogen content of liver and muscle in the completely hypophysectomized dog. *Am. J. Physiol.* 114: 468–472, 1936.
23. CHAIKOFF, I. L., F. L. REICHERT, L. S. READ, AND M. E. MATHES. The influence of epinephrine on the blood sugar, lactic acid and inorganic phosphorus of completely hypophysectomized dogs. *Am. J. Physiol.* 113: 306–311, 1935.
24. CHAMBERS, J. W., R. H. GEORG, AND A. D. BASS. Effect of hydrocortisone and insulin on uptake of α-aminoisobutyric acid by isolated perfused rat liver. *Biochem. Pharmacol.* 1: 66–76, 1965.
25. CHRISTENSEN, H. N. Action of cortisol on trapping of amino acids by the liver. In: *Metabolic Effects of Adrenal Hormones,*

edited by G. E. W. Wolstenholme and M. O'Connor. London: Churchill, 1960, p. 56–64.
26. CLEMENS, M. J., AND A. KORNER. Amino acid requirement for the growth-hormone stimulation of incorporation of precursors into protein and nucleic acids of liver slices. *Biochem. J.* 119: 629–634, 1970.
27. COHN, C., E. SHRAGO, AND D. JOSEPH. Effect of food administration on weight gains and body composition of normal and adrenalectomized rats. *Am. J. Physiol.* 180: 503–507, 1955.
28. CORKILL, A. B., H. P. MARKS, AND W. E. WHITE. Relation of the pituitary gland to the action of insulin and adrenalin. *J. Physiol., London* 80: 193–205, 1933.
29. CUTHBERTSON, D. P. Physical injury and its effects on protein metabolism. In: *Mammalian Protein Metabolism*, edited by H. N. Munro and J. B. Allison. New York: Acad. Press, 1964, vol. II, p. 393–397.
30. DAHMUS, M. E., AND J. BONNER. Increased template activity of liver chromatin, a result of hydrocortisone administration. *Proc. Natl. Acad. Sci. US* 54: 1370–1375, 1965.
31. DEBODO, R. C., AND M. W. SINKOFF. Anterior pituitary and adrenal hormones in the regulation of carbohydrate metabolism. *Recent Progr. Hormone Res.* 8: 511–563, 1953.
32. DEBODO, R. C., M. W. SINKOFF, M. KURTZ, N. LANE, AND S. P. KIANG. Significance of adrenocortical atrophy in the carbohydrate metabolism of hypophysectomized dogs. *Am. J. Physiol.* 173: 11–21, 1953.
33. DEBODO, R. C., R. STEELE, N. ALTSZULER, A. DUNN, AND J. S. BISHOP. On the hormonal regulation of carbohydrate metabolism; studies with C^{14} glucose. *Recent Progr. Hormone Res.* 19: 445–482, 1963.
34. DORSEY, J. L., AND A. MUNCK. Studies on the mode of action of glucocorticoids in rats: a comparison of the effects of cortisol and glucose on the formation of liver glycogen. *Endocrinology* 71: 605–608, 1962.
35. DOUGHERTY, T. F., AND A. WHITE. Functional alterations in lymphoid tissue induced by adrenal secretion. *Am. J. Anat.* 77: 81–116, 1945.
36. DREWS, J., AND G. BRAWERMAN. Alterations in the nature of ribonucleic acid synthesized in rat liver during regeneration and after cortisol administration. *J. Biol. Chem.* 242: 801–808, 1967.
37. EICHHORN, J., M. FEINSTEIN, I. D. K. HALKERSTON, AND O. HECHTER. Effects of corticoids, insulin and epinephrine on α-aminoisobutyrate accumulation in muscle of adrenalectomized rats. *Proc. Soc. Exptl. Biol. Med.* 106: 781–784, 1961.
38. EISENSTEIN, A. B., AND I. STRACK. Effect of glucagon on carbohydrate synthesis and enzyme activity in rat liver. *Endocrinology* 83: 1337–1348, 1968.
39. ELGEE, N. J., AND R. H. WILLIAMS. Pituitary and adrenal influences on insulin-I^{131} degradation. *Am. J. Physiol.* 180: 9–12, 1955.
40. ENGEL, F. L. A consideration of the roles of the adrenal cortex and stress in the regulation of protein metabolism. *Recent Progr. Hormone Res.* 6: 277–308, 1951.
41. EVANS, G. The effect of low atmospheric pressure on the glycogen content of the rat. *Am. J. Physiol.* 110: 273–277, 1934.
42. EVANS, G. The adrenal cortex and endogenous carbohydrate formation. *Am. J. Physiol.* 114: 297–308, 1936.
43. EXTON, J. H., J. G. HARDMAN, T. F. WILLIAMS, E. W. SUTHERLAND, AND C. R. PARK. Effects of guanosine 3′,5′-monophosphate on the perfused rat liver. *J. Biol. Chem.* 246: 2658–2664, 1971.
44. EXTON, J. H., L. S. JEFFERSON, R. W. BUTCHER, AND C. R. PARK. Gluconeogenesis in the perfused liver. The effects of fasting, alloxan diabetes, glucagon, epinephrine, adenosine 3′,5′-monophosphate and insulin. *Am. J. Med.* 40: 709–715, 1966.
45. EXTON, J. H., L. E. MALLETTE, L. S. JEFFERSON, E. H. A. WONG, N. FRIEDMANN, AND C. R. PARK. Role of adenosine 3′,5′-monphosphate in the control of gluconeogenesis. *Am. J. Clin. Nutr.* 23: 993–1003, 1970.

46. EXTON, J. H., L. E. MALLETTE, L. S. JEFFERSON, E. H. A. WONG, N. FRIEDMANN, T. B. MILLER, AND C. R. PARK. The hormonal control of hepatic gluconeogenesis. *Recent Progr. Hormone Res.* 26: 411–457, 1970.
47. EXTON, J. H., AND C. R. PARK. Control of gluconeogenesis in liver. III. Effects of L-lactate, pyruvate, fructose, glucagon, epinephrine, and adenosine 3′,5′-monophosphate on gluconeogenic intermediates in the perfused rat liver. *J. Biol. Chem.* 244: 1424–1433, 1969.
48. EXTON, J. H., AND C. R. PARK. Control of gluconeogenesis in liver. II. Effects of glucagon, catecholamines and adenosine 3′,5′-monophosphate on gluconeogenesis in the perfused rat liver. *J. Biol. Chem.* 243: 4189–4196, 1968.
49. FAIN, J. N. Effects of dexamethasone and growth hormone on fatty acid mobilization and glucose utilization in adrenalectomized rats. *Endocrinology* 71: 633–635, 1962.
50. FAIN, J. N., R. O. SCOW, AND S. S. CHERNICK. Effects of glucocorticoids on metabolism of adipose tissue *in vitro*. *J. Biol. Chem.* 238: 54–58, 1963.
51. FEIGELSON, M., AND P. FEIGELSON. Metabolic effects of glucocorticoids as related to enzyme induction. *Advan. Enzyme Regulation* 3: 11–27, 1965.
52. FERGUSON, L. A., AND I. G. WOOL. Adrenal cortical hormone and incorporation of radioactivity into nucleic acid of isolated rat diaphragm. *Proc. Soc. Exptl. Biol. Med.* 110: 529–532, 1962.
53. FRIEDMANN, B., E. H. GOODMAN, JR., AND S. WEINHOUSE. Effects of insulin and fatty acids on gluconeogenesis in the rat. *J. Biol. Chem.* 242: 3620–3627, 1967.
54. FRIEDMANN, B., E. H. GOODMAN, JR., AND S. WEINHOUSE. Dietary and hormonal effects on gluconeogenesis in the rat. *J. Biol. Chem.* 240: 3729–3735, 1965.
55. FRIEDMANN, N., J. H. EXTON, AND C. R. PARK. Interaction of adrenal steroids and glucagon on gluconeogenesis in perfused rat liver. *Biochem. Biophys. Res. Commun.* 29: 113–119, 1967.
56. GLENISTER, D. W., AND F. E. YATES. Sex differences in the rate of disappearance of corticosterone-4-C^{14} from plasma of intact rats: further evidence for the influence of hepatic Δ^4-steroid dehydrogenase activity on adrenal cortex function. *Endocrinology* 68: 747–758, 1961.
57. GLENN, E. M., W. L. MILLER, AND C. A. SCHLAGEL. Metabolic effects of adrenocortical steroids *in vivo* and *in vitro*: relationship to anti-inflammatory effects. *Recent Progr. Hormone Res.* 19: 107–191, 1963.
58. GOLDSTEIN, L., E. J. STELLA, AND W. E. KNOX. The effect of hydrocortisone on tyrosine-α-ketoglutarate transaminase and tryptophane pyrrolose activities in the isolated, perfused rat liver. *J. Biol. Chem.* 237: 1723–1726, 1962.
59. GOOD, C. A., H. KRAMER, AND M. SOMOGYI. The determination of glycogen. *J. Biol. Chem.* 100: 485–490, 1933.
60. GOODLAD, G. A. J., AND H. N. MUNRO. Diet and the action of cortisone on protein metabolism. *Biochem. J.* 73: 343–348, 1959.
61. GREENMAN, D. L., W. D. WICKS, AND F. T. KENNEY. Stimulation of ribonucleic acid synthesis by steroid hormones. II. High molecular weight components. *J. Biol. Chem.* 240: 4420–4426, 1965.
62. HAGER, C. B., AND F. T. KENNEY. Regulation of tyrosine-α-ketoglutarate transaminase in rat liver. VII. Hormonal effects on synthesis in the isolated perfused liver. *J. Biol. Chem.* 243: 3296–3300, 1968.
63. HANOUNE, J., AND P. FEIGELSON. Turnover of protein and RNA of liver ribosomal components in normal and cortisol-treated rats. *Biochim. Biophys. Acta* 199: 214–223, 1970.
64. HAYNES, R. C., JR. The fixation of carbon dixoide by rat liver mitochondria and its relation to gluconeogenesis. *J. Biol. Chem.* 240: 4103–4106, 1965.
65. HAYNES, R. C., JR. The control of gluconeogenesis by adrenal cortical hormones. *Advan. Enzyme Regulation* 3: 111–119, 1965.

66. HAYNES, R. C., JR. Relation of L-alanine metabolism to the action of triamcinolone in liver slices. *Endocrinology* 75: 602–607, 1964.
67. HAYNES, R. C., JR., AND Y. S. LU. Measurement of cortisol-stimulated gluconeogenesis in the rat. *Endocrinology* 85: 811–814, 1969.
68. HENDERSON, I. C., R. E. FISCHEL, AND J. N. LOEB. Suppression of liver DNA synthesis by cortisone. *Endocrinology* 88: 1471–1476, 1971.
69. HENDERSON, M. J., H. E. MORGAN, AND C. R. PARK. Regulation of glucose uptake in muscle. V. The effect of growth hormone on glucose transport in the isolated perfused rat heart. *J. Biol. Chem.* 236: 2157–2161, 1961.
70. HERRERA, M. G., D. KAMM, N. RUDERMAN, AND G. F. CAHILL, JR. Non-hormonal factors in the control of gluconeogenesis. *Advan. Enzyme Regulation* 4: 225–235, 1966.
71. HOLZER, H., AND W. DUNTZE. Metabolic regulation by chemical modification of enzymes. *Ann. Rev. Biochem.* 40: 345–374, 1971.
72. HORNBROOK, K. R. Synthesis of liver glycogen in starved alloxan diabetic rats. *Diabetes* 19: 916–923, 1970.
73. HUCKABEE, W. E. Relationships of pyruvate and lactate during anaerobic metabolism. I. Effects of infusion of pyruvate or glucose and of hyperventilation. *J. Clin. Invest.* 37: 244–254, 1958.
74. INGLE, D. J. Experimental steroid diabetes. *Diabetes* 5: 187–192, 1956.
75. INGLE, D. J. Some studies on the role of the adrenal cortex in organic metabolism. *Ann. NY Acad. Sci.* 50: 576–595, 1949.
76. INGLE, D. J., AND B. L. BAKER. *Physiological and Therapeutic Effects of Corticotropin (ACTH) and Cortisone.* Springfield, Ill.: Thomas, 1953, p. 20.
77. INGLE, D. J., AND E. A. OBERLE. The effect of adrenalectomy in rats on urinary nonprotein nitrogen during forced-feeding and during fasting. *Am. J. Physiol.* 147: 222–227, 1946.
78. INGLE, D. J., AND M. C. PRESTRUD. The effect of adrenal cortex extract upon urinary nonprotein nitrogen and change in weight in young adrenalectomized rats. *Endocrinology* 45: 143–147, 1949.
79. INGLE, D. J., M. C. PRESTRUD, AND C. H. LI. Effects of administering adrenocorticotrophic hormone by continuous injection to normal rats. *Am. J. Physiol.* 166: 165–170, 1951.
80. INGLE, D. J., M. C. PRESTRUD, AND J. E. NEZAMIS. Effect of adrenalectomy upon level of blood amino acids in the eviscerated rat. *Proc. Soc. Exptl. Biol. Med.* 67: 321–322, 1948.
81. INGLE, D. J., R. SHEPPARD, J. S. EVANS, AND M. H. KUIZENGA. A comparison of adrenal steroid diabetes and pancreatic diabetes in the rat. *Endocrinology* 37: 341–356, 1945.
82. INGLE, D. J., AND G. W. THORN. A comparison of the effects of 11-desoxycorticosterone acetate and 17-hydroxy-11-dehydrocorticosterone in partially depancreatized rats. *Am. J. Physiol.* 132: 670–678, 1941.
83. KAPLAN, S. A., AND C. S. N. SHIMIZU. Effects of cortisol on amino acids in skeletal muscle and plasma. *Endocrinology* 72: 267–272, 1963.
84. KATZ, J., AND A. DUNN. Glucose-2-t as a tracer for glucose metabolism. *Biochemistry* 6: 1–5, 1967.
85. KENNEY, F. T., D. L. GREENMAN, W. D. WICKS, AND W. L. ALBRITTON. RNA synthesis and enzyme induction by hydrocortisone. *Advan. Enzyme Regulation* 3: 1–10, 1965.
86. KENNEY, F. T., AND F. J. KULL. Hydrocortisone-stimulated synthesis of nuclear RNA in enzyme induction. *Proc. Natl. Acad. Sci. US* 50: 493–499, 1963.
87. KENNEY, F. T., J. R. REEL, C. B. HAGER, AND J. L. WITTLIFF. Hormonal induction and repression. In: *Third Kettering Symposium on Regulatory Mechanisms of Protein Synthesis in Mammalian Cells*, edited by A. San Pietro, M. R. Lamborg, and F. T. Kenney. New York: Acad. Press, 1968, p. 119–142.
88. KERN, H., AND J. LOGOTHETOPOULOS. Steroid diabetes in the guinea pig. Studies on islet-cell ultrastructure and regeneration. *Diabetes* 19: 145–154, 1970.
89. KIPNIS, D. M. Regulation of glucose uptake by muscle: functional significance of permeability and phosphorylating activity. *Ann. NY Acad. Sci.* 82: 354–365, 1959.
90. KIPNIS, D. M., AND C. F. CORI. Studies of tissue permeability. VI. The penetration and phosphorylation of 2-deoxyglucose on the diaphragm of diabetic rats. *J. Biol. Chem.* 235: 3070–3075, 1960.
91. KLINE, D. L. A procedure for the study of factors which affect the nitrogen metabolism of isolated tissues: hormonal influences. *Endocrinology* 45: 596–604, 1949.
92. KNOX, W. E., V. H. AUERBACH, AND E. C. C. LIN. Enzymatic and metabolic adaptations in animals. *Physiol. Rev.* 36: 164–254, 1956.
93. KNOX, W. E., AND O. GREENGARD. The regulation of some enzymes of nitrogen metabolism—an introduction to enzyme physiology. *Advan. Enzyme Regulation* 3: 247–311, 1965.
94. KORNER, A. The hormonal control of protein synthesis. *Biochem. J.* 115: 30–31P, 1969.
95. KORNER, A. Ribonucleic acid and hormonal control of protein synthesis. *Progr. Biophys. Mol. Biol.* 17: 61–98, 1967.
96. KOSTYO, J. L. In vitro effects of adrenal steroid hormones on amino acid transport in muscle. *Endocrinology* 76: 604–613, 1965.
97. KOSTYO, J. L., AND A. F. REDMOND. Role of protein synthesis in the inhibitory action of adrenal steroid hormones on amino acid transport by muscle. *Endocrinology* 79: 531–540, 1966.
98. KREBS, H. A. The regulation of the release of ketone bodies by the liver. *Advan. Enzyme Regulation* 4: 339–353, 1966.
99. KREBS, H. A., R. N. SPEAKE, AND R. HEMS. Acceleration of renal gluconeogenesis by ketone bodies and fatty acids. *Biochem. J.* 94: 712–720, 1965.
100. KREUTNER, W., AND N. D. GOLDBERG. Dependence on insulin of the apparent hydrocortisone activation of hepatic glycogen synthetase. *Proc. Natl. Acad. Sci. US* 58: 1515–1519, 1967.
101. KRIS, A. O., R. E. MILLER, F. E. WHERRY, AND J. W. MASON. Inhibition of insulin secretion by infused epinephrine in rhesus monkeys. *Endocrinology* 78: 87–97, 1966.
102. LANDAU, B. R. Adrenal steroids and carbohydrate metabolism. *Vitamins Hormones* 23: 1–59, 1965.
103. LARDY, H. A., D. O. FOSTER, E. SHRAGO, AND P. D. RAY. Metabolic and hormonal regulation of phosphopyruvate synthesis. *Advan. Enzyme Regulation* 2: 39–47, 1964.
104. LARDY, H. A., V. PAETKAU, AND P. WALTER. Paths of carbon in gluconeogenesis and lipogenesis: the role of mitochondria in supplying precursors of phosphoenolpyruvate. *Proc. Natl. Acad. Sci. US* 53: 1410–1415, 1965.
105. LEATHEM, J. H. Some aspects of hormone and protein metabolic interrelationships. In: *Mammalian Protein Metabolism*, edited by H. N. Munro and J. B. Allison. New York: Acad. Press, 1964, vol. I, p. 351.
106. LECOCQ, F. R., D. MEBANE, AND L. L. MADISON. The acute effect of hydrocortisone on hepatic glucose output and peripheral glucose utilization. *J. Clin. Invest.* 43: 237–246, 1964.
107. LEE, K., AND F. T. KENNY. Induction of alanine transaminase by adrenal steroids in cultured hepatoma cells. *Biochem. Biophys. Res. Commun.* 40: 469–475, 1970.
108. LEE, N. D., AND R. H. WILLIAMS. The role of the pituitary-adrenal system in cystine-S[35] incorporation into proteins. *Endocrinology* 51: 451–456, 1952.
109. LERNER, R. L., AND D. PORTE, JR. Epinephrine and insulin release: a new look (Abstract). *Diabetes* 19: 366, 1970.
110. LOEB, J. N., AND E. M. TOLENTINO. Effects of cortisone on ribosomal RNA synthesis in rat liver. *Endocrinology* 86: 1033–1040, 1970.
111. LONG, C. N. H., B. KATZIN, AND E. G. FRY. The adrenal cortex and carbohydrate metabolism. *Endocrinology* 26: 309–344, 1940.
112. LONG, C. N. H., AND F. D. W. LUKENS. Effect of adrenalectomy and hypophysectomy upon experimental diabetes in the cat. *Proc. Soc. Exptl. Biol. Med.* 32: 743–745, 1935.
113. LONG, C. N. H., O. K. SMITH, AND E. G. FRY. Actions of

cortisol and related compounds on carbohydrate and protein metabolism. In: *Metabolic Effects of Adrenal Hormones*, edited by G. E. W. Wolstenholme and M. O'Connor. London: Churchill, 1960, p. 4-19.
114. LOSERT, W., O. LOGE, AND K. D. RICHTER. Investigations on insulin secretion in normal, spontaneously diabetic, streptozotocin-diabetic and adrenalectomized Chinese hamsters (Abstract). *Diabetologia* 6: 79, 1970.
115. MAKMAN, M. H., S. NAKAGAWA, B. DVORKIN, AND A. WHITE. Inhibitory effects of cortisol and antibiotics on substrate entry and ribonucleic acid synthesis in rat thymocytes *in vitro*. *J. Biol. Chem.* 245: 2556-2563, 1970.
116. MAKMAN, M. H., S. NAKAGAWA, AND A. WHITE. Studies of the mode of action of adrenal steroids on lymphocytes. *Recen. Progr. Hormone Res.* 23: 195-219, 1967.
117. MALAISSE, W. J., F. MALAISSE-LAGAE, E. F. McGRAW, AND P. H. WRIGHT. Insulin secretion *in vitro* by pancreatic tissue from normal, adrenalectomized and cortisol treated rats. *Proc. Soc. Exptl. Biol. Med.* 124: 924-928, 1967.
118. MANCHESTER, K. L. Hormonal control of protein biosynthesis. In: *The Biological Basis of Medicine*, edited by E. E. Bittar and N. Bittar. New York: Acad. Press, 1968, vol. 2, p. 221-262.
119. MANCHESTER, K. L., P. J. RANDLE, AND F. G. YOUNG. The effect of growth hormone and of cortisol on the response of isolated rat diaphragm to the stimulating effect of insulin on glucose uptake and on incorporation of amino acids into protein. *J. Endocrinol.* 18: 395-408, 1959.
120. MARCO, J., F. MELANI, R. GOBERNA, W. H. ROLT, AND E. F. PFEIFFER, The effect of prednisolone on insulin secretion in the rat (Abstract). *Diabetologia* 5: 48, 1969.
121. MARTIN, C. J., AND R. ROBISON. The minimum nitrogen expenditure of man and the biological value of various proteins for human nutrition. *Biochem. J.* 16: 407-447, 1922.
122. MERSMAN, H. J., AND H. L. SEGAL. Glucocorticoid control of the liver glycogen synthetase-activating system. *J. Biol. Chem.* 244: 1701-1704, 1969.
123. MILLER, T. B., J. H. EXTON, AND C. R. PARK. A block in epinephrine-induced glycogenolysis in hearts from adrenalectomized rats. *J. Biol. Chem.* 246: 3672-3678, 1971.
124. MORGAN, C. R., AND J. BONNER. Template activity of liver chromatin increased by *in vivo* administration of insulin. *Proc. Natl. Acad. Sci. US* 65: 1077-1080, 1970.
125. MORGAN, H. E., D. M. REGEN, M. J. HENDERSON, T. K. SAWYER, AND C. R. PARK. Regulation of glucose uptake in muscle. VI. Effects of hypophysectomy, adrenalectomy, growth hormone, hydrocortisone and insulin on glucose transport and phosphorylation in the perfused rat heart. *J. Biol. Chem.* 236: 2162-2168, 1961.
126. MORI, N. Hexokinase and glucokinase in rat liver. I. Effects of fasting, insulin and cortisol on enzyme activity. *Nippon Naibunpi Gakkai Zasshi* 45: 968-975, 1969.
127. MUNCK, A. Glucocorticoid inhibition of glucose uptake by peripheral tissues: old and new evidence, molecular mechanisms, and physiological significance. *Perspectives Biol. Med.* 14: 265-289, 1971.
128. MUNCK, A. Studies on the mode of action of glucocorticoids in rats. II. The effects *in vivo* and *in vitro* on net glucose uptake by isolated adipose tissue. *Biochim. Biophys. Acta* 57: 318-326, 1962.
129. MUNCK, A., AND S. B. KORITZ. Studies on the mode of action of glucocorticoids in rats. I. Early effects of cortisol on blood glucose and on glucose entry into muscle, liver and adipose tissue. *Biochim. Biophys. Acta* 57: 310-317, 1962.
130. MUNCK, A., AND S. B. KORITZ. Some early effects of hydrocortisone on carbohydrate metabolism in adrenalectomized rats. *Acta Endocrinol.* 35, Suppl. 51: 821, 1960.
131. MUNRO, H. N. General aspects of the regulation of protein metabolism by diet and by hormones. In: *Mammalian Protein Metabolism*, edited by H. N. Munro and J. B. Allison. New York: Acad. Press, 1964, p. 381-481.
132. NINOMIYA, R., N. F. FORBATH, AND G. HETENYI. Effect of adrenal steroids on glucose kinetics in normal and diabetic dogs. *Diabetes* 14: 729-739, 1965.
133. OLSON, R. E., F. A. JACOBS, D. RICHERT, S. A. THAYER, L. J. KOPP, AND N. J. WADE. The comparative bioassay of several extracts of the adrenal cortex in tests employing four separate physiological responses. *Endocrinology* 35: 430-455, 1944.
134. PABST, M. L., R. SHEPPARD, AND M. H. KUIZENGA. Comparison of liver glycogen deposition and work performance tests for the bio-assay of adrenal cortex hormones. *Endocrinology* 41: 55-65, 1947.
135. PARK, C. R. Some factors regulating the utilization of carbohydrate in muscle. *Intern. Union Biochem. Ser.* 32: 711-712, 1964.
136. PERLEY, M., AND D. M. KIPNIS. Effects of glucocorticoids on plasma insulin. *New Engl. J. Med.* 274: 1237-1241, 1966.
137. PETERS, R. F., M. C. RICHARDSON, M. SMALL, AND A. M. WHITE. Some biochemical effects of triamcinolone acetonide on rat liver and muscle. *Biochem. J.* 116: 349-355, 1970.
138. POHORECKY, L. A., AND R. J. WURTMAN. Adrenocortical control of epinephrine synthesis. *Pharmacol. Rev.* 23: 1-35, 1971.
139. PORTE, D., JR., A. L. GRABER, T. KUZUYA, AND R. H. WILLIAMS. The effect of epinephrine on immunoreactive insulin levels in man. *J. Clin. Invest.* 45: 228-236, 1966.
140. RANDLE, P. J., P. B. GARLAND, C. N. HALES, E. A. NEWSHOLME, R. M. DENTON, AND C. I. POGSON. Interactions of metabolism and the physiological role of insulin. *Recent Progr. Hormone Res.* 22: 1-44, 1966.
141. RASTOGI, K. S., AND J. CAMPBELL. Effect of growth hormone on cortisone-induced hyperinsulinemia and reduction in pancreatic insulin in the mouse. *Endocrinology* 87: 226-232, 1970.
142. RATHGEB, I., R. STEELE, AND N. ALTSZULER. Effectiveness of a cortisol regimen to increase glucose turnover in the adrenalectomized dog (Abstract). *Federation Proc.* 29: 777, 1970.
143. REEL, J. R., AND F. T. KENNEY. "Superinduction" of tyrosine transaminase in hepatoma cell cultures: differential inhibition of synthesis and turnover by actinomycin D. *Proc. Natl. Acad. Sci. US* 61: 200-206, 1968.
144. REEL, J. R., K. LEE, AND F. T. KENNEY. Regulation of tyrosine α-ketoglutarate transaminase in rat liver. VIII. Inductions by hydrocortisone and insulin in cultured hepatoma cells. *J. Biol. Chem.* 245: 5800-5805, 1970.
145. REILLY, P. E. B., AND E. J. H. FORD. The effect of betamethasone on glucose utilization and oxidation by sheep. *J. Endocrinol.* 47: 19-25, 1971.
146. REINECKE, R. M., AND E. C. KENDALL. Method for bioassay of hormones of adrenal cortex which influence deposition of glycogen in the liver. *Endocrinology* 31: 573-577, 1942.
147. ROSEN, F., AND C. A. NICHOL. Corticosteroids and enzyme activity. *Vitamins Hormones* 21: 135-214, 1963.
148. ROSS, B. D., R. HEMS, AND H. A. KREBS. The rate of gluconeogenesis from various precursors in the perfused rat liver. *Biochem. J.* 102: 942-951, 1967.
149. SALAS, M., E. VIÑUELA, AND A. SOLS. Insulin-dependent synthesis of liver glucokinase in the rat. *J. Biol. Chem.* 238: 3535-3538, 1963.
150. SCHAEFFER, L. D., M. CHENOWETH, AND A. DUNN. Adrenal corticosteroid involvement in the control of liver glycogen phosphorylase activity. *Biochim. Biophys. Acta* 192: 292-303, 1969.
151. SCHAEFFER, L. D., M. CHENOWETH, AND A. DUNN. Adrenal corticosteroid involvement in the control of phosphorylase in muscle. *Biochim. Biophys. Acta* 192: 304-309, 1969.
152. SCHIMKE, R. T. The importance of both synthesis and degradation in the control of arginase levels in rat liver. *J. Biol. Chem.* 239: 3808-3817, 1964.
153. SCHONFELD, G., AND D. M. KIPNIS. Studies of extracellular and tissue fatty acid pools and glucose metabolism in striated muscle (Abstract). *J. Clin. Invest.* 45: 1071, 1966.

154. Scow, R. O., and S. S. Chernick. Hormonal control of protein and fat metabolism in the pancreatectomized rat. *Recent Progr. Hormone Res.* 16: 497–541, 1960.
155. Scrutton, M. C., and M. F. Utter. The regulation of glycolysis and gluconeogenesis in animal tissues. *Ann. Rev. Biochem.* 37: 249–302, 1968.
156. Sharma, C., R. Manjeshwar, and S. Weinhouse. Effects of diet and insulin on glucose-adenosine triphosphate phosphotransferases of rat liver. *J. Biol. Chem.* 238: 3840–3845, 1963.
157. Silber, R. H., and C. C. Porter. Nitrogen balance, liver protein repletion and body composition of cortisone treated rats. *Endocrinology* 52: 518–525, 1953.
158. Sirek, O., and C. H. Best. Intramuscular cortisone administration to dogs. *Proc. Soc. Exptl. Biol. Med.* 80: 594–598, 1952.
159. Smith, O. K. Effect of cortisol on the metabolism of glucose in eviscerated adrenalectomized-diabetic rats. *Endocrinology* 82: 447–452, 1968.
160. Soling, H. D., R. Katterman, H. Schmidt, and P. Kneer. The redox state of NAD^+-NADH systems in rat liver during ketosis, and the so-called "triosephosphate block." *Biochim. Biophys. Acta* 115: 1–14, 1966.
161. Steele, R. *Tracer Probes in Steady State Systems.* Springfield, Ill.: Thomas, 1971, p. 49–54.
162. Struck, E., J. Ashmore, and O. Wieland. Effects of glucagon and long chain fatty acids on glucose production by isolated perfused rat liver. *Advan. Enzyme Regulation* 4: 219–224, 1966.
163. Sutherland, E. W., and T. W. Rall. The relation of adenosine-3′,5′-phosphate and phosphorylase to the actions of catecholamines and other hormones. *Pharmacol. Rev.* 12: 265–299, 1960.
164. Sutherland, E. W., III, and R. C. Haynes, Jr. Increased release of amino acids from rat thymus after cortisol administration. *Endocrinology* 80: 288–296, 1967.
165. Sutter, B. C. J. Adrenals and insulinemia in the rat. II. Adrenal cortex and serum insulin. *Diabetologia* 4: 295–304, 1968.
166. Sutter, B. C. J., M. T. Strosser, and P. Mialhe. Permissive action of adrenal cortical hormones on insulin secretion in the rat (Abstract). *Diabetologia* 5: 55, 1969.
167. Tomkins, G. M., T. D. Gelehrter, D. Granner, D. Martin, Jr., H. H. Samuels, and E. B. Thompson. Control of specific gene expression in higher organisms. *Science* 166: 1474–1480, 1969.
168. Tomkins, G. M., E. B. Thompson, S. Hayashi, T. Gelehrter, D. Granner, and B. Peterkofsky. Tyrosine transaminase induction in mammalian cells in tissue culture. *Cold Spring Harbor Symp. Quant. Biol.* 31: 349–360, 1966.
169. Utter, M. F., D. B. Keech, and M. C. Scrutton. A possible role for acetyl coenzyme A in the control of gluconeogenesis. *Advan. Enzyme Regulation* 2: 49–68, 1964.
170. Volk, B. W., and S. S. Lazarus. Ultramicroscopic studies of rabbit pancreas during cortisone treatment. *Diabetes* 12: 162–172, 1963.
171. Weber, G. Hormonal control of gluconeogenesis. In: *The Biological Basis of Medicine*, edited by E. E. Bittar and N. Bittar. New York: Acad. Press, 1968, vol. 2, p. 263–307.
172. Weber, G., G. Banerjee, and S. B. Bronstein. Role of enzymes in homeostasis. III. Selective induction of increases of liver enzymes involved in carbohydrate metabolism. *J. Biol. Chem.* 236: 3106–3111, 1961.
173. Weinshelbaum, E. I., and I. G. Wool. Effect of adrenalectomy and corticosteroids on distribution of radioactivity in protein of cell fractions from myocardial slices. *Nature* 191: 1401–1402, 1961.
174. Wells, B. B., and E. C. Kendall. The influence of the adrenal cortex in phloridzin diabetes. *Proc. Staff Meetings Mayo Clinic* 15: 565–573, 1940.
175. White, A. Integration of the effects of adrenal cortical, thyroid, and growth hormones in fasting metabolism. *Recent Progr. Hormone Res.* 4: 153–181, 1949.
176. Wicks, W. D. Induction of hepatic enzymes by adenosine 3′,5′-monophosphate in organ culture. *J. Biol. Chem.* 244: 3941–3950, 1969.
177. Wicks, W. D., F. T. Kenney, and K. Lee. Induction of hepatic enzyme synthesis *in vivo* by adenosine 3′,5′-monophosphate. *J. Biol. Chem.* 244: 6008–6013, 1969.
178. Williamson, J. R. Effects of fatty acids, glucagon and anti-insulin serum on the control of gluconeogenesis and ketogenesis in rat liver. *Advan. Enzyme Regulation* 5: 229–255, 1967.
179. Williamson, J. R. Studies on the effects of steroids on adipose tissue and beta cells (Abstract). *Federation Proc.* 21: 203, 1962.
180. Williamson, J. R., E. T. Browning, and M. S. Olson. Interrelations between fatty acid oxidation and the control of gluconeogenesis in perfused rat liver. *Advan. Enzyme Regulation* 6: 67–100, 1968.
181. Wool, I. G. Corticosteroids and accumulation of C^{14}-labeled amino acids and histamine by isolated rat diaphragm. *Am. J. Physiol.* 199: 715–718, 1960.
182. Wool, I. G., and E. I. Weinshelbaum. Incorporation of C^{14}-amino acids into protein of isolated diaphragms: role of the adrenal steroids. *Am. J. Physiol.* 197: 1089–1092, 1959.
183. Yates, F. E., R. D. Brennan, and J. Urquhart. Adrenal corticoid control system. *Federation Proc.* 28: 71–83, 1969.
184. Yoshida, T., C. Cohn, and Y-H. Maa. Effects of adrenalectomy and manner of food intake on renal gluconeogenesis. *Endocrinology* 84: 417–420, 1969.
185. Yu, F., and P. Feigelson. Effects of cortisone and actinomycin D upon pyrimidine nucleotides and RNA metabolism in rat liver. *Arch. Biochem. Biophys.* 129: 152–157, 1969.
186. Yu, F., and P. Feigelson. The sequential stimulation of uracil-rich RNA species during cortisone induction of hepatic enzymes. *Biochem. Biophys. Res. Commun.* 35: 499–504, 1969.

Glucocorticoid effects on lipid mobilization and adipose tissue metabolism

JOHN N. FAIN
MICHAEL P. CZECH

Division of Biological and Medical Sciences, Brown University, Providence, Rhode Island

CHAPTER CONTENTS

Inhibition of Glucose Metabolism in Adipose Tissue
Glucocorticoids and Fatty Acid Mobilization
    Changes of lipid deposition in Cushing's syndrome
    Involvement of adrenal cortex in ketosis and fatty livers
    Stimulation of fatty acid release and lipolysis in vitro by glucocorticoids
    Adenylate cyclase, cyclic AMP, and phosphodiesterase

GLUCOCORTICOIDS increase lipid mobilization and produce ketosis in diabetic animals (68–71). However, in starved animals with an intact pancreas, glucocorticoids actually suppress ketosis (16). This may be due to a glucocorticoid-induced elevation in blood glucose concentration, which increases insulin secretion. The insulin in turn blocks the stimulatory effects of glucocorticoids on lipid mobilization. Thus whether effects of glucocorticoids on lipid mobilization and peripheral glucose utilization are seen in vivo depends on the extent to which insulin antagonizes the actions of glucocorticoids.

Our aim in this chapter is to review the available data with regard to glucocorticoid effects on lipid mobilization in vivo and in vitro. Since free fatty acid release by adipose tissue is the key site for regulation of lipid mobilization, primary emphasis is placed on the role of glucocorticoids in adipose tissue metabolism.

INHIBITION OF GLUCOSE METABOLISM IN ADIPOSE TISSUE

The early rise in blood glucose concentration that occurs about 2 hr after administration of glucocorticoids to nephrectomized (15) or intact rats (50, 51, 59) could not be accounted for by an increase in plasma urea levels. This suggested that some process other than gluconeogenesis from protein increases the concentration of glucose in blood during the early response to glucocorticoids. Hausberger (37) and Jeanrenaud & Renold (44) reported that administration of cortisone to rats resulted in impaired adipose tissue lipogenesis from radioactively labeled glucose. Administration of cortisol to rats that were injected with uniformly labeled glucose elicited a small but consistent decrease in labeled protein and lipid extracted from the epididymal fat pads (59). The recovery of label in protein and lipid from muscle and liver of treated rats was higher than that from control animals (59). These findings indicated that glucocorticoids inhibit glucose metabolism in certain extrahepatic tissues and suggested that fat was a target tissue for these hormones.

Munck (56) found that glucose uptake by fat pads in vitro from adrenalectomized, fasted rats was inhibited by cortisol administered 30 min before removal of the tissue; the effect was greater if the fat pads were excised 2.5 hr after injection. The direct addition of cortisol in vitro at concentrations as low as 9×10^{-8} M to epididymal adipose tissue decreased glucose uptake after a lag period of 2.5 hr (56). Corticosterone and deoxycorticosterone mimicked the action of cortisol, but the latter was significantly less active (56).

The inhibitory action of glucocorticoids on glucose metabolism by adipose tissue is now well established (20, 23, 27, 48) and has been extended to isolated white fat cells (4, 11). In addition to effects on epididymal adipose tissue, glucocorticoid inhibition of glucose uptake in vitro has been reported in rat dorsal subcutaneous, perirenal, inguinal, and parametrial adipose tissue (21). However, glucose uptake by brown adipose tissue of rats was unresponsive to glucocorticoids in vitro (21). Impairment of glucose utilization by glucocorticoids in vitro has been demonstrated in mouse skin (61), rat thymus cells (55, 77), and mouse lymphosarcoma cells (64) and fibroblasts (36). In these systems glucocorticoid action was associated with a delay in onset that varied from 15–20 min in thymus cells (57) to 2–4 hr in mouse fibroblasts (36).

Early increases in blood glucose concentration due to glucocorticoid administration, which cannot be accounted for in increased urea output, probably result from inhibition of peripheral utilization. However, the increased concentrations of blood glucose elicited by prolonged treatment with glucocorticoids are accompanied by increased production of urea, which can account for the appearance of virtually all the extra carbohydrate via gluconeogenesis (51). This effect may also be secondary to inhibition of peripheral glucose utilization by glucocorticoids. Young (80) found that in thymus cells the incorporation of radioactively labeled amino acids into protein was inhibited by cortisol only in the presence of glucose. The impairment of glucose metabolism in certain extrahepatic tissues may increase availability of amino acids to the liver and thus stimulate gluconeogenesis. The relation between the inhibitory effects of glucocorticoids on peripheral glucose utilization and their ability to increase blood glucose and liver glycogen have been reviewed by Munck (58) and are discussed elsewhere in this volume by Steele and Altszuler and by Munck and Young.

Whether inhibition of glucose transport by adipose tissue is the primary site at which glucocorticoids inhibit glucose metabolism remains uncertain. In thymus cells glucocorticoids appear to inhibit glucose transport since cortisol reduced the uptake of 3-O-methyl glucose, a nonmetabolizable sugar (58). Similar studies with nonmetabolizable sugars are very difficult to perform in fat cells because of their small intracellular water space.

Leboeuf et al. (48) reported that in rat adipose tissue incubated for 3 hr with 5 mM randomly labeled glucose the addition of 30 µg/ml of cortisol inhibited the conversion of glucose to carbon dioxide, glyceride-glycerol, and fatty acids. Fain et al. (27) confirmed these findings and noted that in tissue incubated for 4.5 hr with 2.8 mM glucose very low concentrations of glucocorticoids were effective (0.016 µg/ml of dexamethasone). The incorporation of radioactively labeled glucose into protein was also inhibited by glucocorticoid (20). Yorke (79) found that dexamethasone decreased lactate and pyruvate output from adipose tissue and reduced the tissue content of glycogen, glucose 6-phosphate, and α-glycerophosphate. However, pyruvate-1-^{14}C (79) and pyruvate-2-^{14}C (20) metabolism in adipose tissue was unaffected by dexamethasone in vitro. Similarly adipose tissue content of ATP, ADP, AMP, and citrate was unchanged by dexamethasone when glucose metabolism was inhibited (79).

Fructose probably does not share the transport system specific for glucose in white adipose tissue (30) but appears to be phosphorylated by the same hexokinase (40). Fain found that exposure of adipose tissue to dexamethasone did not affect the uptake or conversion of uniformly labeled fructose to CO_2, glyceride-glycerol, or fatty acid (19). This suggested that inhibition of glucose entry into fat cells may be the mechanism by which glucocorticoids inhibit glucose metabolism. Similarly, 2-deoxy-D-glucose, thought to compete with glucose for entry and phosphorylation (45), inhibited the metabolism of glucose in adipose tissue but had little effect on fructose utilization (19).

Leboeuf et al. (48) showed that cortisol reduced the concentration of glycogen in adipose tissue in vitro in the presence of 5 mM glucose. Subsequently, Jeanrenaud found that dexamethasone treatment of adipose tissue that had previously been incubated with uniformly labeled glucose for 1 hr and quickly washed free of glucose resulted in a significant decrease in labeled glycogen (43). Thus glucocorticoid-enhanced glycogen degradation appears to be independent of glucose in the medium and may represent an action on an intracellular enzyme, or enzymes.

Although the impairment of glucose metabolism in adipose tissue and fat cells caused by glucocorticoids is well documented, the reported effects on insulin-stimulated glucose utilization have varied markedly with the conditions employed. Three daily injections of cortisone into intact rats were found to reduce the glucose uptake of adipose tissue in the presence of insulin in vitro (9). Similarly, Riddick et al. (62) found that five daily injections of 5 mg of hydrocortisone per 100 g body wt inhibited the increase of glucose-1-^{14}C conversion to CO_2 in adipose tissue when a submaximal dose of insulin was administered at the same time. In contrast, several groups have reported the failure of glucocorticoids to inhibit the stimulatory effect of maximal doses of insulin on glucose metabolism of adipose tissue (19, 48, 79) and isolated fat cells (11) in vitro. However, these studies were performed with high concentrations of glucose and maximal doses of insulin, where glucose transport is no longer the rate-limiting step in glucose metabolism (10). Lundquist found that cortisol inhibited the response of adipose tissue to submaximal, but not maximal, doses of insulin (53) and suggested a competitive antagonism between insulin and glucocorticoid action. Czech & Fain (12) have studied the interaction of dexamethasone and insulin on isolated fat cells in the presence of low concentrations of glucose (0.1 mM and 0.05 mM) and found that the glucocorticoid markedly inhibits the response of fat cells to maximal doses of insulin under these conditions. Dexamethasone failed to affect the stimulatory effect of a maximal dose of insulin on glucose oxidation in fat cells in the presence of 1 mM glucose. One interpretation of these findings is that with 1 mM or more glucose and a maximal dose of insulin the intracellular enzymes involved in glucose utilization are saturated with substrate because of the large amount of sugar entering the cell, and the glucocorticoid does not reduce glucose entry below that required to maintain these saturating levels of intracellular glucose. Thus maximum amounts of CO_2 are evolved from labeled glucose by fat cells under these conditions, whether or not dexamethasone is present.

That glucocorticoids are without effect on the maximum rates of glucose oxidation induced by insulin and high concentrations of glucose supports the concept that glucocorticoids do not inhibit the enzymes involved in glucose metabolism. It is possible, however, that the Michaelis-Menten constant (K_m) of an enzyme, or enzymes, is selectively affected by these hormones in vitro Bernstein found that 0.1 mg/kg per day of dexamethasone administered to rats reduced hexokinase II activity in the epididymal fat pad to 75% of control values after 24 hr and to 50% in 48 hr (3). Stimulation of glucose-1-^{14}C conversion to CO_2 and triglyceride by insulin in vitro was proportional to the amount of hexokinase II activity in white fat cells. These late effects of glucocorticoids may differ from the in vitro effects described above.

The lag period associated with glucocorticoid action on adipose tissue and isolated white fat cells suggests a mechanism involving RNA or protein synthesis, or both. Czech & Fain (11) demonstrated that dactinomycin, an inhibitor of RNA synthesis, almost completely abolished the inhibition by dexamethasone of glucose-1-^{14}C oxidation in the white fat cell if both agents were present at the start of the incubation and labeled CO_2 production was measured over the final 2 hr of a 4-hr incubation period. When dactinomycin was added at 1 hr it inhibited the effect of dexamethasone by 32%. Addition of the antibiotic at 2 hr was without effect on the action of dexamethasone (11). No effect on basal glucose oxidation was seen after addition of dactinomycin (11).

The effects of dactinomycin on other glucocorticoid-sensitive systems are remarkably varied. Although this antibiotic inhibits cortisol action on glucose metabolism of thymus cells (81), it is without effect on the hormone's action in lymphosarcoma cells (65). In contrast, dactinomycin itself inhibited α-aminoisobutyric acid accumulation by rat diaphragm, as did corticosterone (46).

Fain found that puromycin, an inhibitor of protein synthesis, inhibited glucose utilization in adipose tissue (20). The effect was evident immediately after the start of the incubation period, whereas the inhibition by dexamethasone was delayed in onset. The aminonucleoside of puromycin mimicked the effect of puromycin, which suggested that the effect of the latter was not related to its ability to inhibit protein synthesis. More recently, Czech & Fain (11) showed that cycloheximide inhibited glucose oxidation by fat cells by a process that required a lag period of 2 hr for maximal inhibition. The similar response of glucose oxidation in white fat cells to glucocorticoid and cycloheximide suggests that the hormone may act by inhibiting the synthesis of a labile protein, or proteins, involved in glucose transport by a process dependent on RNA synthesis. In concert with this idea it has been reported that cortisol induces the removal of an inhibitor of ribonuclease activity in thymocytes (76) and promotes the degradation of trichloroacetic acid-precipitable radioactivity of newly labeled lymphocyte RNA in the presence of dactinomycin (2). Unfortunately the experiments outlined above do not allow a preference between the idea that glucocorticoids inhibit the synthesis of a protein involved in glucose transport within fat cells by an RNA-dependent process and the possibility that the action of these hormones directs the synthesis of a protein inhibitory to glucose oxidation.

Recent experiments have indicated that the inhibition by dexamethasone of glucose metabolism in the fat cell is reversible. Under controlled conditions we have found that glucose oxidation in the fat cell returns to normal levels about 2.5 hr after the glucocorticoid is washed from fat cells. The results from an experiment in which adipose tissue was incubated for 90 min in the presence of dexamethasone and collagenase and then the free fat cells washed and incubated in the absence of glucocorticoid are presented in Table 1. The conversion of uniformly labeled glucose-^{14}C to CO_2 by fat cells previously incubated with steroid was 51% lower than that by controls during the first 30 min of the recovery period, but conversion returned to control levels when CO_2 production was measured 2.5–3 hr after the start of the incubation. Dactinomycin markedly inhibited the repair processes, which occur over a 2.5-hr period after the removal of glucocorticoid from fat cells, with respect to glucose uptake. Thus both the inhibition by dexamethasone of glucose oxidation in fat cells and the recovery from this action are dependent on reactions that are blocked by dactinomycin.

The possibility that glucocorticoid inhibition of glucose metabolism was secondary to effects of the hormone on calcium metabolism was not supported in unpublished studies done in our laboratory by Dr. Paul Wieser. He found that both basal glucose-1-^{14}C oxidation to carbon dioxide and the inhibitory effect of dexamethasone were unaffected by isolation of cells in calcium-free medium followed by incubation in medium with

TABLE 1. *Effect of Dactinomycin on Recovery of Glucose Oxidation from Dexamethasone Inhibition*

Additions	Basal	Increment Due to Presence of Dexamethasone During 90 Min Prior to Experiment	Difference Due to Dexamethasone, %
	\multicolumn{3}{c}{Glucose conversion to CO_2 (μmoles/g fat cells) during first 30 min of incubation period}
None	0.57	−0.29 ± 0.03	−51 ± 6
Dactinomycin added at start of incubation	0.58	−0.32 ± 0.05	−45 ± 4
	\multicolumn{3}{c}{Glucose conversion to CO_2 (μmoles/g fat cells) during the 2.5–3-hr period}
None	0.58	−0.06 ± 0.06	−5 ± 11
Dactinomycin added at start of incubation	0.53	−0.27 ± 0.11	−51 ± 8

Fat cells from parametrial adipose tissue isolated for 90 min in Krebs-Ringer phosphate buffer containing 3% defatted serum albumin, 0.4 mg/ml crude collagenase, and 2.8 mM glucose either in the absence or presence of dexamethasone (0.032 μg/ml). Cells were washed and incubated in plastic tubes at 37 C in 3% albumin buffer. Uniformly labeled glucose-^{14}C (2.8 mM) was added at start of this incubation period or after 2.5 hr, and production of labeled CO_2 during the 30 min after glucose addition was measured. Dactinomycin (0.2 μg/ml) was added to appropriate tubes at start of incubation period. Basal values represent means of 3 experiments, and increments due to dexamethasone are the ± SEM of paired differences. Percentage differences due to dexamethasone treatment are presented ± SE of paired differences. (From M. P. Czech and J. N. Fain, unpublished observations.)

calcium content of 0–2 mM. Similar results were seen in calcium-free medium to which 0.5 mM ethylene-glycol-bis(β-aminoethyl ether)-N,N'-tetraacetic acid (EGTA) was added, except that all values were reduced by approximately 25%.

GLUCOCORTICOIDS AND FATTY ACID MOBILIZATION

Changes of Lipid Deposition in Cushing's Syndrome

Patients with Cushing's syndrome or those treated for long periods of time with large doses of glucocorticoids often exhibit an excess deposition of fat in the neck, face, and trunk, whereas the extremities have scanty deposits of fat (42). With the exception of estrogens, no known agents, other than glucocorticoids, alter the distribution of adipose tissue in man. Why some adipose tissues appear to lose lipid and others to gain lipid under the influence of glucocorticoids is not yet clear. The closest analogy in experimental animals is the finding that insulin stimulates glucose uptake and fatty acid synthesis in both brown and white adipose tissue of rats, whereas glucocorticoids only inhibit glucose metabolism by white adipose tissue (21). Chronic administration of glucocorticoids results in increased concentrations of blood glucose and increased concentrations of circulating insulin. Perhaps the adipose tissues that lose fat are those in which the stimulation of fatty acid release and inhibition of glucose uptake by glucocorticoids are not inhibited by the increased concentrations of circulating insulin. In tissues that gain lipid the effects of insulin may predominate over the effects of glucocorticoids, which would result in increased triglyceride deposition because of decreased release of fatty acids and increased synthesis. This hypothesis suggests that whether a particular adipose tissue gains or loses lipid after glucocorticoid administration will depend on whether it is more sensitive to insulin or to glucocorticoids since these agents are antagonistic to adipose tissue metabolism. Hausberger (37) originally pointed out that glucocorticoid-induced obesity in certain strains of mice was probably a result of increased insulin secretion. He (37) found that the inhibitory effect of large amounts of glucocorticoids on adipose tissue lipogenesis and lipid content in rats could be overcome by administration of large amounts of insulin. Thus whether an increase or decrease in lipid content occurs in a particular species depends on the extent to which insulin is able to antagonize glucocorticoid action on fat cells and the extent to which hyperinsulinism is induced by steroid treatment.

An antagonism between insulin and glucocorticoids with respect to lipolysis was seen by Krotkiewski et al. (47). They found an enhanced lipolysis by incubated pieces of epididymal adipose tissue removed from normal rats 4 hr after the administration of 5–11 μg dexamethasone (47). However, after treatment for 14 days with 3 or 5 μg dexamethasone daily the glycerol release by fat pads from steroid-treated rats was lower than that from controls and the concentration of plasma immunoreactive insulin was doubled. These data demonstrate that, whereas glucocorticoids acutely stimulate lipolysis in adipose tissue, this effect is more than offset by the increased secretion of insulin seen after more prolonged exposure to excess glucocorticoids.

Involvement of Adrenal Cortex in Ketosis and Fatty Livers

Wool & Goldstein (78) found that ethionine-induced fatty livers did not develop in adenalectomized female rats or after ethionine administration to adrenalectomized rats given either glucocorticoids or epinephrine. Combined treatment (glucocorticoids plus epinephrine) was required for the development of fatty livers. Levin & Farber (49) reported a similar requirement for adrenal glucocorticoids in the development of fatty livers in mice treated with growth hormone.

Houssay & Biasotti (41) in 1931 reported that hypophysectomy prevented the development of fatty livers and ketosis in diabetic dogs. Long & Lukens (52) subsequently found that adrenalectomy also prevented the development of diabetic ketosis and that, although crude extracts of anterior pituitary produced ketosis in diabetic cats that had been hypophysectomized, the extracts had no ketogenic action in adrenalectomized animals. Adrenalectomy also completely suppressed the urinary excretion of ketone bodies in normal rats after the injection of anterior pituitary extracts (31).

Scow & Chernick (69) found that glucocorticoids alone produced a marked hyperlipemia, hyperketonemia, and fatty liver in pancreatectomized rats during the first day after hypophysectomy. However, in pancreatectomized rats examined a week after hypophysectomy (68) there was little ketogenic action of glucocorticoids or of growth hormone, but combination of both hormones produced a marked ketosis (Fig. 1). Similar results have been obtained in pancreatectomized dogs; after adrenalectomy growth hormone had little ketogenic action unless the animals had also been given glucocorticoid (75).

The possibility that the ketogenic action of glucocorticoids is the result of enhanced hepatic gluconeogenesis is not supported by the data shown in Figure 1. Although glucocorticoids alone gave a maximal increase in concentration of blood glucose, only in the presence of growth hormone was ketosis produced (see Fig. 1). Since these rats were not fed the increase in concentration of blood glucose was apparently the result of hepatic gluconeogenesis.

Scow & Chernick (71) have more recently shown that glucocorticoids potentiated the ketogenic action of growth hormone in long-term hypophysectomized, pancreatectomized rats, as well as that of ACTH and thyroxine. Marked ketosis developed in response to the administration of glucocorticoids and either growth hormone, ACTH, or thyroxine, whereas these hormones alone had little effect. The data on the development of ketosis and fatty livers suggest that glucocorticoids are able to potentiate a wide variety of other lipolytic hormones, such as catecholamines, thyroid hormones, growth hormone, and ACTH. The striking ketogenic action of glucocorticoids alone seen in pancreatectomized rats shortly after hypophysectomy probably results from the inability of these animals to secrete insulin, which antagonizes the ketogenic action of glucocorticoids, and the presence of enough other lipolytic agents (such as thyroid hormones) to potentiate the action of glucocorticoids.

The major cause of diabetic ketosis is an accelerated mobilization of lipid as free fatty acids from the adipose tissue to the liver (70). The rate of hepatic ketogenesis appears to be linearly related to the concentration of free fatty acids in the plasma (7, 39, 63, 74). A combination of growth hormone and dexamethasone did not affect uptake of free fatty acids or their conversion to ketone bodies in perfused livers of hypophysectomized rats (S. S. Chernick and R. O. Scow, personal communication).

Fain & Scow (26) suggested that hypophysectomy prevents ketosis in pancreatectomized rats by decreasing free fatty acid release by adipose tissue. The elevated release of fatty acid by adipose tissue of pancreatectomized rats was reduced to very low levels after hypophysectomy (26). The high rate of free fatty acid release by adipose tissue from alloxan-induced diabetic rats was also reduced by hypophysectomy (32). These studies indicated that the ketogenic action of glucocorticoids and other lipolytic agents was probably the result of increased release of fatty acids by adipose tissue.

Glucocorticoid administration to humans increases the free fatty acids in plasma. Nayak et al. (60) found markedly elevated concentrations of free fatty acids in serum 4 hr after the administration of 100 mg cortisone. Dreiling et al. (14) gave 100 mg cortisol to normal humans and found a drop in the concentrations of free fatty acid in plasma during the first hour, which was followed by increases in the concentrations of fatty acids during the next 2 hr. The lag period in cortisol action in vivo is comparable to that required in vitro to effect fatty acid release by adipose tissue.

Adrenalectomy impairs the ability of catecholamines (38, 73) or growth hormone (35) to increase the concentrations of free fatty acids in plasma of experimental animals. The rise of concentrations of free fatty acids in plasma of rats during starvation is impaired by adrenalectomy and corrected by treatment with glucocorticoids (18, 34).

Stimulation of Fatty Acid Release and Lipolysis in Vitro by Glucocorticoids

Parametrial adipose tissue incubated for 4.5 hr in vitro, after removal from starved rats adrenalectomized 8 hr previously, released less fatty acid and utilized more glucose than did tissue from starved controls (18). Administration of 10 μg dexamethasone at the time of adrenalectomy restored these values to normal, as did the administration of growth hormone. In rats injected

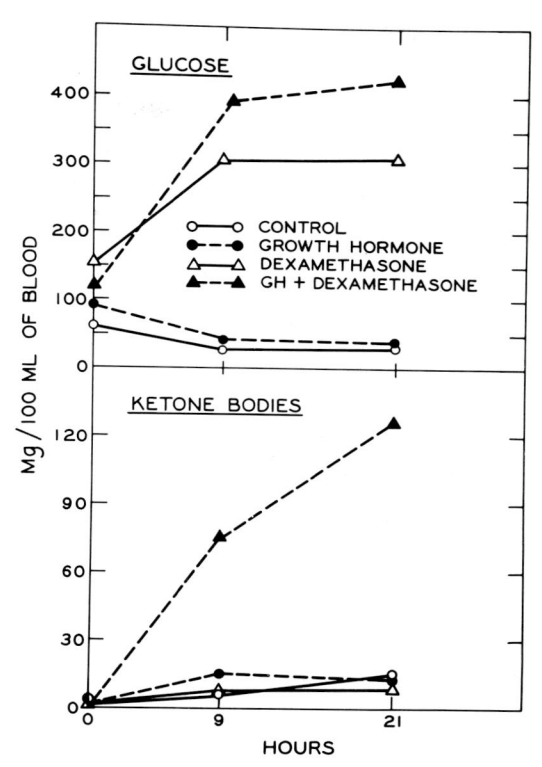

FIG. 1. Effect of 5 mg growth hormone (*GH*) and 2.5 μg dexamethasone in pancreatectomized rats hypophysectomized for 1 week. The hormones were given at 0 hr, 17 hr after the last insulin injection and feeding. [From Scow (68).]

with both hormones the subsequent rate of fatty acid release was tenfold greater than that in animals given either hormone alone (18).

The rate of fatty acid release by incubated adipose tissue was increased over a 3-hr incubation period by 3 μg or more per milliliter of cortisol in the presence of 5 mM glucose (48). Fain et al. (27) found a lag period of 1–2 hr before fatty acid release was accelerated by glucocorticoids. In adipose tissue incubated for 4.5 hr in the presence of 2.8 mM glucose the rate of fatty acid release was accelerated by corticosterone at 16–160 ng/ml and by dexamethasone at 1.6–16 ng/ml (Fig. 2). The effect of glucocorticoids on fatty acid release was specific since deoxycorticosterone had little effect at concentrations up to 3.2 μg/ml (see Fig. 2). Although 2α-methyl cortisol was effective in accelerating fatty acid release, 2α-methyl cortisone was inactive (27). The inactivity of 2α-methyl cortisone and deoxycorticosterone indicated a close relation between glucocorticoid activity in vivo and the ability to effect fatty acid release by adipose tissue.

Fain et al. (27) concluded that the increase in fatty acid release could be accounted for by a concomitant reduction in fatty acid reesterification as a result of glucocorticoid inhibition of glucose metabolism. Most agents that increase fatty acid release have been found to do so as a result of activation of triglyceride hydrolysis with the liberation of both glycerol and free fatty acids. The rate of glycerol reutilization by adipose tissue for esterifi-

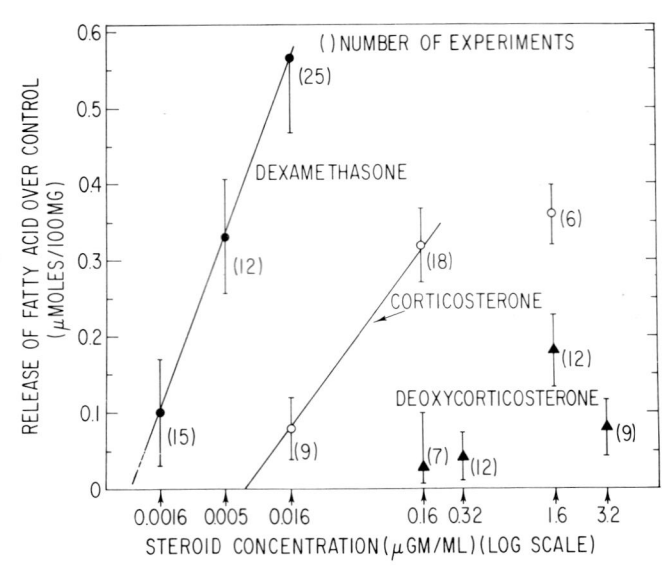

FIG. 2. Stimulation of fatty acid release by glucocorticoids in incubated pieces of parametrial adipose tissue from female rats. Steroids were added at the start of the 4.5-hr incubation period, and fatty acid release is shown as the mean ± SE of the increment due to the added steroid. [From Fain et al. (27).]

cation of fatty acids is very low, and glycerol release can be measured as a fairly accurate index of the absolute rate of lipolysis. Free fatty acid release, on the other hand, represents the net sum of the rate of lipolysis less the rate of reesterification.

In agreement with the hypothesis that the effects of glucocorticoids on fatty acid release by incubated pieces of white adipose tissue were not the result of activation of lipolysis, was the finding that glycerol release was unaffected by 16 ng/ml or less of dexamethasone (23, 43). Yorke (79) found that glycerol release was unchanged by 5 μg/ml of dexamethasone. However, Jeanrenaud (43) reported an acceleration of glycerol release when 100 ng/ml or more of dexamethasone was added during a 4-hr incubation. Mahler & Stafford (54) found that 31 μg/ml of cortisol increased both basal and norepinephrine-stimulated glycerol release by pieces of rat epididymal adipose tissue over a 90-min incubation. Goodman (33) found no effect of 16 ng/ml of dexamethasone on glycerol release from adipose tissue of normal or hypophysectomized rats but did find an enhancement of the response to catecholamines in tissue incubated for 3 hr with dexamethasone. The general consensus, from studies with incubated adipose tissue, is that the major effects of low concentrations of glucocorticoids on fatty acid release are secondary to reduced reesterification as a result of inhibition of glucose utilization, whereas direct effects on lipolysis require higher concentrations of glucocorticoids.

Although dexamethasone alone had little effect on lipolysis in white fat cells incubated in the absence of glucose, it significantly enhanced the delayed lipolytic response to growth hormone (23). Since the effect of dexamethasone occurred in the absence of glucose it is clearly not secondary to inhibition of reesterification. The potentiation of the lipolytic action of growth hormone by dexamethasone, as well as the effect of growth hormone alone, was delayed in onset and blocked by inhibitors of RNA and protein synthesis (22, 23, 25).

The mechanism by which glucocorticoids potentiate the action of growth hormone on lipolysis in free fat cells from normal rats (22, 23, 25) and the response to catecholamines by pieces of adipose tissue from hypophysectomized rats (33) appear to be similar in that they involve a dactinomycin-sensitive process.

There is a lag period of 1–3 hr before the lipolytic effect of the steroid is observed, and the effects are seen in the absence of glucose. These studies indicate that in at least two different ways glucocorticoids can increase fatty acid release—one is due to reduced reesterification as a result of inhibition of glucose metabolism, and the other is due to a permissive effect on lipolysis that is independent of glucose metabolism. Both mechanisms have a 1–3-hr lag period and appear to involve RNA and protein synthesis.

It should be noted that insulin is a potent antagonist of the lipolytic action of dexamethasone and growth hormone in vitro (23, 24). Fain et al. (24) found that an amount of insulin insufficient to stimulate glucose metabolism by isolated fat cells was able to reduce the lipolytic action of these hormones. Higher concentrations of insulin can completely block the lipolytic action of growth hormone and glucocorticoids (23, 24).

Adenylate Cyclase, Cyclic AMP, and Phosphodiesterase

Braun & Hechter (5, 6) found that adrenalectomy or prior treatment of rats with large amounts of dexamethasone over periods of up to 60 hr did not affect the ability of epinephrine, fluoride, or glucagon to stimulate the adenylate cyclase activity of fat cell ghosts. These ghosts are prepared by hypotonic lysis of fat cells and may consist primarily of plasma membrane sacs (5). However, the magnitude of the response of adenylate cyclase from ghosts to high concentrations (1 mM) of synthetic corticotropin was markedly reduced by adrenalectomy or hypophysectomy. Administration of 500 μg dexamethasone per 100 g body wt at 8, 6, or 4 hr to normal, adrenalectomized, or hypophysectomized rats prior to isolation of ghosts increased the response to ACTH. Treatment with these very large doses of dexamethasone for 40–60 hr was required for maximal effects.

Studies in our laboratory have indicated a 20% increase in adenylate cyclase activity in ghosts isolated after 3.5-hr incubation with 0.02 μg/ml of dexamethasone and then incubated with norepinephrine (Table 2). There was a similar effect on the response of adenylate cyclase from ghosts to ACTH except that the stimulation was more erratic and not statistically significant. Prior incubation of fat cells with growth hormone produced a considerably greater effect on norepinephrine-sensitive adenylate cyclase. The combination of growth hormone and glucocorticoid was no more effective than growth hormone alone (J. N. Fain, unpublished results).

The relation of the effects of dexamethasone on adenylate cyclase to its lipolytic activity is not clear. Previous reports (22, 25) indicated that after incubation of fat cells for 3 hr with dexamethasone there was no increase in the amount of cyclic AMP accumulation when catecholamines were added in the presence of theophylline. Prior incubation with growth hormone for the same period was associated with an increase in cyclic AMP accumulation. These results suggested that glucocorticoid effects on lipolysis were on some step other than the regulation of total cyclic AMP accumulation in fat cells.

It is well established that a primary effect of adrenalectomy is to reduce the response of adipose tissue to all lipolytic agents. However, Braun & Hechter (5, 6) noted an effect of adrenalectomy only on the ACTH-responsive adenylate cyclase activity of ghosts from white fat cells. The expected effect of adrenalectomy would be to diminish the sensitivity of fat cells to the lipolytic action of ACTH and catecholamines with less of an effect on the maximal rate of lipolysis. Allen & Beck (1) found that the lipolytic response of fat cells from adrenalectomized rats to epinephrine, ACTH, dibutyryl cyclic AMP, or theophylline was reduced. They found no effect of adrenalectomy on basal, epinephrine-stimulated, or fluoride-activated adenyl cyclase activity in fat cell homogenates. However, in homogenates from adrenalectomized rats the activation of adenylate cyclase by ACTH was reduced. Schönhöfer et al. (67) also found no effect of adrenalectomy or glucocorticoid treatment on the adenylate cyclase or phosphodiesterase activities in fat cell homogenates that could explain the reduced lipolytic sensitivity of fat cells to catecholamines.

The maximal accumulation of total cyclic AMP due to catecholamines in the presence of methyl xanthines was not found to be impaired in adipose tissue (8) or fat cells (1) from adrenalectomized rats. The stimulation of cyclic AMP accumulation by 50 μM epinephrine was reduced in fat cells from adrenalectomized rats, but at this high concentration of catecholamine no difference was seen in lipolysis between cells from normal and adrenalectomized rats (1).

Treatment of normal rabbits with large amounts of glucocorticoids for several days results in a marked hyperlipemia (28, 29). However, in rabbits, adrenalectomy increases the concentrations of free fatty acids and triglycerides in plasma, and these effects are abolished by the administration of glucocorticoids (13). The increased lipid mobilization seen in adrenalectomized rabbits appears to be the result of the high concentrations of ACTH in these animals coupled with the abnormal sensitivity of rabbit adipose tissue to a direct lipolytic action of ACTH (13). Rudman & di Girolamo (66) have reviewed studies indicating that rabbit adipose tissue is much more sensitive than adipose tissue from other species to the lipolytic action of ACTH and other lipolytic peptides.

TABLE 2. *Increased Norepinephrine-sensitive Adenylate Cyclase Activity in Fat Cell Ghosts After Incubation of Fat Cells With Growth Hormone and Dexamethasone*

Addition to Ghosts During Assay for Adenylate Cyclase	Value for Ghosts from Control Cells	Difference with Dexamethasone	Difference with Growth Hormone
	Adenylate cyclase activity, nmoles cyclic AMP formed per mg protein × 20 min		
None	1.1	+0.7 ± 0.60	+0.8 ± 1.10
Norepinephrine	9.5	+1.8 ± 0.42	+3.8 ± 1.20
ACTH	3.9	+1.6 ± 1.10	−1.1 ± 1.00
Fluoride	29.2	+4.6 ± 2.9	+2.0 ± 2.8

White fat cells were isolated from parametrial adipose tissue of 6 rats by incubation in 14 ml 4% albumin buffer containing 6 mg trypsin and 8 mg collagenase. After 45-min incubation, cells were isolated and then divided into 4 equal aliquots, which were incubated for 3.5 hr in 13 ml each of 4% albumin buffer. Concentration of dexamethasone was 0.02 μg/ml and of growth hormone was 0.75 μg/ml. At the end of this incubation period ghosts were prepared from each group and then incubated for 20 min (approximately 45 μg of protein per tube) in duplicate in the absence or presence of 0.2 mM norepinephrine, 2 μg/ml ACTH, or 10 mM sodium fluoride. Basal values are means of 11 experiments, and changes due to dexamethasone or growth hormone are ± SEM of paired differences. (From J. N. Fain, unpublished observations.)

Therefore it does not appear that cortisol has much, if any, effect on the lipolytic sensitivity of fat cells from rabbits to ACTH. Braun & Hechter (6) have indicated that dexamethasone administered to intact rabbits also failed to affect the stimulation of adenylate cyclase activity by ACTH in ghosts isolated from rabbit fat cells.

Our conclusion is that the effects of glucocorticoids on fatty acid release are the result of combined inhibition of fatty acid reesterification and increased sensitivity to lipolytic agents. The molecular basis for increased sensitivity to lipolytic agents remains to be elucidated, but it probably involves the ability of cyclic AMP to activate lipolysis or some mechanism unrelated to cyclic AMP. Possibly the effect of prolonged in vivo treatment of rats with large doses of dexamethasone on the ACTH sensitivity of ghosts from fat cells is not the result of a primary effect on adenylate cyclase. The only ways currently available to obtain measurable adenylate cyclase activity in particles from fat cells are mild homogenization, freezing and thawing of fat cells, or hypotonic lysis of fat cells. All these procedures result in large fragments of plasma membrane that are relatively insensitive to hormones and from which hormonal responses are easily lost. Perhaps the effects of glucocorticoids are not on adenylate cyclase or on hormonal receptors but result from an increased membrane stability that reduces the loss of hormonally sensitive adenylate cyclase during isolation of fat cell ghosts.

One suggested mechanism of glucocorticoid action involves inhibition of cyclic AMP phosphodiesterase (72). Five days after adrenalectomy it has been reported that

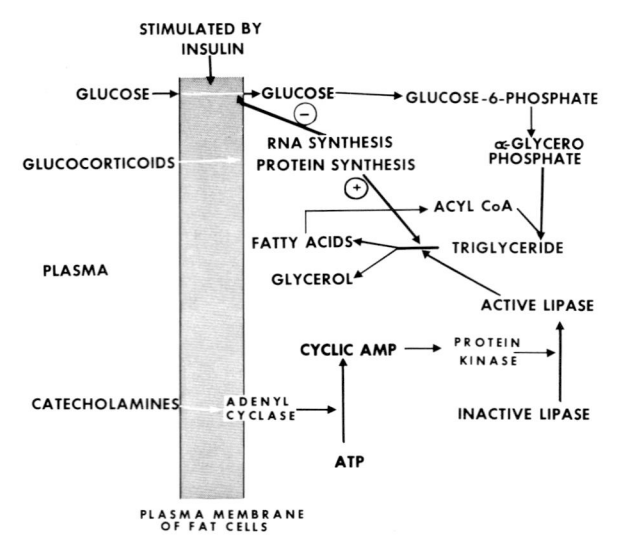

FIG. 3. Model for glucocorticoid action on adipose tissue metabolism. Glucocorticoids are postulated to act through a mechanism dependent on RNA and protein synthesis. Proteins made under the influence of the hormone activate lipolysis (+) and inhibit glucose uptake (−). Inhibition of glucose transport reduces amount of α-glycerophosphate available for fatty acid reesterification. Thus glucocorticoids increase net fatty acid release by inhibiting reesterification and also enhance lipolysis through unelucidated mechanisms.

phosphodiesterase activity of liver, kidney, and adipose, but not muscle, tissue was increased when measured in the presence of 80 μM cyclic AMP (72). Treatment with steroid for 5 days resulted in less phosphodiesterase activity in all tissues (72). The minimal time required before any effects of glucocorticoid therapy could be seen was at least 12 hr. In the same study it was also reported that insulin injection 45 min before the experiments increased hepatic phosphodiesterase activity but only in adrenalectomized, alloxan-diabetic rats that were treated with steroid (72). The relevance of the purported long-term changes in phosphodiesterase activity to the actions of glucocorticoids on lipolysis and gluconeogenesis has yet to be established. Some investigators [(1, 67); W. F. Ward and J. N. Fain, unpublished observations] have failed to see any change in phosphodiesterase activity of fat cell homogenates after previous incubation of fat cells with dexamethasone.

The main objection to the physiological relevance of steroid effects on phosphodiesterase is that inhibition of phosphodiesterase should result in increases in the accumulation of cyclic AMP. However, neither in fat cells (22, 25) nor in liver (17) have steroids been shown as yet to influence the ability of hormones to stimulate cyclic AMP accumulation.

The primary mechanism by which glucocorticoids affect lipolysis does not appear to involve changes in cyclic AMP accumulation. Similar conclusions have been reached with regard to the role of glucocorticoids in the stimulation of hepatic gluconeogenesis. The stimulation of gluconeogenesis by glucagon is markedly reduced in perfused livers from adrenalectomized rats and can be restored to normal by glucocorticoids (17). However, the stimulation of cyclic AMP accumulation seen with glucagon or catecholamines was the same in livers from adrenalectomized rats as in those from controls (17). In both liver and fat cells there is a similar lag period before effects of glucocorticoids can be demonstrated, and in both tissues the hormones whose action is potentiated act through mechanisms involving activation of adenylate cyclase.

The effects of glucocorticoids on the metabolism of adipose tissue are summarized in Figure 3. According to this scheme, glucocorticoids inhibit glucose transport into fat cells and thus reduce the availability of α-glycerophosphate for fatty acid reesterification, which results in a net increase in free fatty acid release. These steroids also increase fatty acid release by increasing the sensitivity of the processes involved in lipolysis to lipolytic agents. The scheme shown in Figure 3 suggests that the effects of glucocorticoids on lipolysis are on lipolysis itself, rather than on the ability of lipolytic agents to increase the accumulation of cyclic AMP. It should be noted that we know very little about what happens after the addition of glucocorticoids during the lag period, except that all effects of the steroids are blocked by inhibitors of RNA synthesis. The effects of inhibitors of RNA synthesis suggest that continuing RNA synthesis is a requirement for glucocorticoid inhibition of glucose uptake and stimulation of lipolysis.

ADDENDUM

The inhibition of glucose metabolism in fat cells by glucocorticoids is not secondary to activation of lipolysis. Wieser et al. (Wieser, P. B., J. A. Malgieri, W. F. Ward, R. H. Pointer, and J. N. Fain. Effects of bovine growth hormone preparations, fragments of growth hormone and pituitary anti-insulin peptide on lipolysis and glucose metabolism of isolated fat cells and adipose tissue. Endocrinology. In press.) showed that dexamethasone reduced basal and insulin-stimulated glucose oxidation by white fat cells under conditions in which lipolysis was unaffected. In fat cells glucose oxidation was depressed by lipolytic agents, but this appeared to be secondary to an increase in lipolysis. The inhibition of glucose uptake and potentiation of lipolysis due to glucocorticoids appear to be independent results of some more primary event. Inhibition of glucose uptake by glucocorticoid can be seen in the absence of any increase in lipolysis, and lipolytic effects of glucocorticoids can be seen in the total absence of glucose in the medium.

REFERENCES

1. ALLEN, D. O., AND R. BECK. Alterations in lipolysis, adenylate cyclase and adenosine 3′,5′-monophosphate levels in isolated fat cells following adrenalectomy. Endocrinology 91: 504–510, 1972.

2. AMARAL, L., AND S. WERTHAMER. Protein and RNA synthesis in human leukocytes and lymphocytes. 3. Cortisol enhanced destruction of newly synthesized RNA of cultured lymphocytes. Life Sci. Part 2 9: 661–666, 1970.

3. BERNSTEIN, R. S., AND D. M. KIPNIS. Regulation of rat hexokinase isoenzymes. II. Effects of growth hormone and dexamethasone. *Diabetes* 22: 923–931, 1973.
4. BLECHER, M. Serum protein-steroid hormone interactions. Effects of glucocorticoids on glucose metabolism in rat adipose isolated cells, and the influence of human plasma corticosteroid binding protein. *Endocrinology* 79: 541–546, 1966.
5. BRAUN, T., AND O. HECHTER. Glucocorticoid regulation of ACTH sensitivity of adenyl cyclase in rat fat cell membranes. *Proc. Natl. Acad. Sci. US* 66: 995–1001, 1970.
6. BRAUN, T., AND O. HECHTER. Comparative study of hormonal regulation of adenyl cyclase activity in rat and rabbit fat cell membranes. In: *Adipose Tissue, Regulation and Metabolic Functions*, edited by B. Jeanrenaud and D. Hepp. Stuttgart: Thieme, 1970, p. 11–19.
7. CLARK, C. M., JR., AND R. O. SCOW. Effects of fasting and hypophysectomy on FFA uptake and ketone body production by the isolated, perfused rat liver. *Diabetes* 19: 924–929, 1970.
8. CORBIN, J. D., AND C. R. PARK. Permissive effects of glucocorticoids on lipolysis in adipose tissue (Abstract). *Federation Proc.* 28: 702, 1969.
9. CORREA, P. R., E. MAGALHAES, AND M. E. KRAHL. Response of epididymal adipose tissue to small concentrations of insulin: effect of cortisone. *Proc. Soc. Exptl. Biol. Med.* 103: 704–706, 1960.
10. CROFFORD, O. B., AND A. E. RENOLD. Glucose uptake by incubated rat epididymal adipose tissue. Rate-limiting steps and site of insulin action. *J. Biol. Chem.* 240: 14–21, 1965.
11. CZECH, M. P., AND J. N. FAIN. Dactinomycin inhibition of dexamethasone action on glucose metabolism in white fat cells. *Biochim. Biophys. Acta* 230: 185–193, 1971.
12. CZECH, M. P., AND J. N. FAIN. Antagonism of insulin action on glucose metabolism in white fat cells by dexamethasone. *Endocrinology* 91: 518–522, 1972.
13. DESBALS, B., P. DESBALS, AND R. AGID. Pituitary-adrenal control of fat mobilization in rabbits. In: *Adipose Tissue, Regulation and Metabolic Functions*, edited by B. Jeanrenaud and D. Hepp. Stuttgart: Thieme, 1970, p. 28–31.
14. DREILING, D. A., E. L. BIERMAN, A. F. DEBONS, P. ELSBACH, AND I. L. SCHWARTZ. Effect of ACTH, hydrocortisone, and glucagon on plasma nonesterified fatty acid concentration (NEFA) in normal subjects and in patients with liver disease. *Metabolism* 11: 572–578, 1962.
15. ENGEL, F. L. A consideration of the roles of the adrenal cortex and stress in the regulation of protein metabolism. *Recent Progr. Hormone Res.* 6: 277–313, 1951.
16. ENGEL, F. L. The influence of the endocrine glands on fatty acid and ketone body metabolism. *Am. J. Clin. Nutr.* 5: 417–430, 1957.
17. EXTON, J. H., N. FRIEDMANN, E. H. WONG, J. P. BRINEAUX, J. D. CORBIN, AND C. R. PARK. Interaction of glucocorticoids with glucagon and epinephrine in the control of gluconeogenesis and glycogenolysis in liver and of lipolysis in adipose tissue. *J. Biol. Chem.* 247: 3579–3588, 1972.
18. FAIN, J. N. Effects of dexamethasone and growth hormone on fatty acid mobilization and glucose utilization in adrenalectomized rats. *Endocrinology* 71: 633–635, 1962.
19. FAIN, J. N. Effects of dexamethasone and 2-deoxy-D-glucose on fructose and glucose metabolism by incubated adipose tissue. *J. Biol. Chem.* 239: 958–962, 1964.
20. FAIN, J. N. Effect of puromycin on incubated adipose tissue and its response to dexamethasone, insulin, and epinephrine. *Biochim. Biophys. Acta* 84: 636–642, 1964.
21. FAIN, J. N. Comparison of glucocorticoid effects on brown and white adipose tissue of the rat. *Endocrinology* 76: 549–552, 1965.
22. FAIN, J. N., A. DODD, AND L. NOVAK. Relationship of protein synthesis and cyclic AMP to lipolytic action of growth hormone and glucocorticoids. *Metabolism* 20: 109–118, 1971.
23. FAIN, J. N., V. P. KOVACEV, AND R. O. SCOW. Effect of growth hormone and dexamethasone on lipolysis and metabolism in isolated fat cells of the rat. *J. Biol. Chem.* 240: 3522–3529, 1965.
24. FAIN, J. N., V. P. KOVACEV, AND R. O. SCOW. Antilipolytic effect of insulin in isolated fat cells of the rat. *Endocrinology* 78: 773–778, 1966.
25. FAIN, J. N., AND R. SAPERSTEIN. The involvement of RNA synthesis and cyclic AMP in the activation of fat cell lipolysis by growth hormone and glucocorticoids. In: *Adipose Tissue Regulation and Metabolic Functions*, edited by B. Jeanrenaud and D. Hepp. Stuttgart: Thieme, 1970, p. 20–27.
26. FAIN, J. N., AND R. O. SCOW. Effect of hypophysectomy on lipid metabolism in pancreatectomized rats. *Endocrinology* 77: 547–552, 1965.
27. FAIN, J. N., R. O. SCOW, AND S. S. CHERNICK. Effects of glucocorticoids on metabolism of adipose tissue in vitro. *J. Biol. Chem.* 238: 54–58, 1963.
28. FELT, V., S. RÖHLING, S. VOHNOUT, AND D. REICHL. On the mechanism of action of glucocorticoids on phospholipid metabolism in rabbits. *J. Endocrinol.* 24: 309–314, 1962.
29. FRIEDMAN, M., J. VAN DEN BOSCH, S. O. BYERS, AND S. ST. GEORGE. Effects of cortisone on lipid and cholesterol metabolism in the rabbit and rat. *Am. J. Physiol.* 208: 94–105, 1965.
30. FROESCH, E. R., AND J. L. GINSBERG. Fructose metabolism of adipose tissue. I. Comparison of fructose and glucose metabolism in epididymal adipose tissue of normal rats. *J. Biol. Chem.* 237: 3317–3324, 1962.
31. FRY, E. G. The effect of adrenalectomy and thyroidectomy on ketonuria and liver fat content of the albino rat following injections of anterior pituitary extract. *Endocrinology* 21: 283–291, 1937.
32. GARLAND, P. B., AND P. J. RANDLE. Regulation of glucose uptake by muscle. *Biochem. J.* 93: 678–687, 1964.
33. GOODMAN, M. H. Permissive effects of hormones on lipolysis. *Endocrinology* 86: 1064–1074, 1970.
34. GOODMAN, H. M., AND E. KNOBIL. Some endocrine factors in regulation of fatty acid mobilization during fasting. *Am. J. Physiol.* 201: 1–3, 1961.
35. GOODMAN, H. M., AND E. KNOBIL. Growth hormone and fatty acid mobilization: the role of the pituitary, adrenal and thyroid. *Endocrinology* 69: 187–189, 1961.
36. GRAY, J. G., W. B. PRATT, AND L. ARONOW. Effect of glucocorticoids on hexose uptake by mouse fibroblasts in vitro. *Biochemistry* 10: 277–284, 1971.
37. HAUSBERGER, F. X. Action of insulin and cortisone on adipose tissue. *Diabetes* 7: 211–220, 1958.
38. HAVEL, R. J., AND A. GOLDFIEN. The role of the sympathetic nervous system in the metabolism of free fatty acids. *J. Lipid Res.* 1: 102–108, 1959.
39. HEIMBERG, M., I. WEINSTEIN, AND M. KOHOUT. The effects of glucagon, dibutyryl cyclic adenosine 3′,5′-monophosphate, and concentration of free fatty acid on hepatic lipid metabolism. *J. Biol. Chem.* 244: 5131–5139, 1969.
40. HERNÁNDEZ, A., AND A. SOLS. Transport and phosphorylation of sugars in adipose tissue. *Biochem. J.* 86: 166–172, 1963.
41. HOUSSAY, B. A., AND A. BIASOTTI. The hypophysis, carbohydrate metabolism and diabetes. *Endocrinology* 15: 511–523, 1931.
42. INGLE, D. J. Relationship of the adrenal cortex to the metabolism of fat. *J. Clin. Endocrinol. Metab.* 3: 603–612, 1943.
43. JEANRENAUD, B. Effect of glucocorticoid hormones on fatty acid mobilization and re-esterification in rat adipose tissue. *Biochem. J.* 103: 627–633, 1967.
44. JEANRENAUD, B., AND A. E. RENOLD. Studies on rat adipose tissue in vitro. VII. Effects of adrenal cortical hormones. *J. Biol. Chem.* 235: 2217–2223, 1960.
45. KIPNIS, D. M., AND C. F. CORI. Studies of tissue permeability. VI. The penetration and phosphorylation of 2-deoxyglucose in the diaphragm of diabetic rats. *J. Biol. Chem.* 235: 3070–3075, 1960.
46. KOSTYO, J. L., AND A. F. REDMOND. Role of protein synthesis in the inhibitory action of adrenal steroid hormones on amino acid transport by muscle. *Endocrinology* 79: 531–540, 1966.
47. KROTKIEWSKI, M., J. KROTKIEWSKA, AND P. BJÖRNTORP. Effects of dexamethasone on lipid mobilization in the rat. *Acta Endocrinol.* 63: 185–192, 1970.

48. LEBOEUF, B., A. E. RENOLD, AND G. F. CAHILL, JR. Studies on rat adipose tissue *in vitro*. IX. Further effects of cortisol on glucose metabolism. *J. Biol. Chem.* 237: 988–991, 1962.
49. LEVIN, L., AND R. K. FARBER. Hormonal factors which regulate the mobilization of depot fat to the liver. *Recent Progr. Hormone Res.* 7: 399–435, 1952.
50. LONG, C. N. H., E. G. FRY, AND M. BONNYCASTLE. The effect of cortisol on carbohydrate deposition and urea nitrogen excretion in the adrenalectomized rat. *Acta Endocrinol. Suppl.* 51: 819, 1960.
51. LONG, C. N. H., B. KATZIN, AND E. G. FRY. The adrenal cortex and carbohydrate metabolism. *Endocrinology* 26: 309–344, 1940.
52. LONG, C. N. H., AND F. D. W. LUKENS. The effects of adrenalectomy and hypophysectomy upon experimental diabetes in the cat. *J. Exptl. Med.* 63: 465–490, 1936.
53. LUNDQUIST, I. On the significance of serum dilution and cortisol antagonism in the rat fat pad bioassay of insulin. *Acta Endocrinol.* 58: 11–26, 1968.
54. MAHLER, R. F., AND W. L. STAFFORD. The lipolytic effect of glucocorticoids. In: *The Control of Lipid Metabolism*, edited by J. K. Grant. New York: Acad. Press, 1963, p. 155–158.
55. MORITA, Y., AND A. MUNCK. Effect of glucocorticoids *in vivo* and *in vitro* on net glucose uptake and amino acid incorporation by rat-thymus cells. *Biochim. Biophys. Acta* 93: 150–157, 1964.
56. MUNCK, A. Studies on the mode of action of glucocorticoids in rats. II. The effects *in vivo* and *in vitro* on net glucose uptake by isolated adipose tissue. *Biochim. Biophys. Acta* 57: 318–326, 1962.
57. MUNCK, A. Metabolic site and time course of cortisol action on glucose uptake, lactic acid output, and glucose 6-phosphate levels of rat thymus cells *in vitro*. *J. Biol. Chem.* 243: 1039–1042, 1968.
58. MUNCK, A. Glucocorticoid inhibition of glucose uptake by peripheral tissues: old and new evidence, molecular mechanisms, and physiological significance. *Perspectives Biol. Med.* 14: 265–289, 1971.
59. MUNCK, A., AND S. B. KORITZ. Studies on the mode of action of glucocorticoids in rats. I. Early effects of cortisol on blood glucose and on glucose entry into muscle, liver and adipose tissue. *Biochim. Biophys. Acta* 57: 310–317, 1962.
60. NAYAK, R. V., E. B. FELDMAN, AND A. C. CARTER. Adipokinetic effect of intravenous cortisol in human subjects. *Proc. Soc. Exptl. Biol. Med.* 111: 682–686, 1962.
61. OVERELL, B. G., S. E. CONDON, AND V. PETROW. The effect of hormones and their analogues upon the uptake of glucose by mouse skin *in vitro*. *J. Pharm. Pharmacol.* 12: 150–153, 1959.
62. RIDDICK, F. A., JR., D. M. REISLER, AND D. M. KIPNIS. The sugar transport system in striated muscle. Effect of growth hormone, hydrocortisone and alloxan diabetes. *Diabetes* 11: 171–178, 1962.
63. ROSE, H., M. VAUGHAN, AND D. STEINBERG. Utilization of fatty acids by rat liver slices as a function of medium concentration. *Am. J. Physiol.* 206: 345–350, 1964.
64. ROSEN, J. M., J. J. FINA, R. J. MILHOLLAND, AND F. ROSEN. Inhibition of glucose uptake in lymphosarcoma P1798 by cortisol and its relationship to the biosynthesis of deoxyribonucleic acid. *J. Biol. Chem.* 245: 2074–2080, 1970.
65. ROSEN, J. M., J. J. FINA, R. J. MILHOLLAND, AND F. ROSEN. Studies on the inhibition of glucose uptake by cortisol (C) in cell suspensions of lymphosarcoma P1798 (Abstract). *Federation Proc.* 29: 921, 1970.
66. RUDMAN, S., AND M. DI GIROLAMO. Comparative studies on the physiology of adipose tissue. *Advan. Lipid Res.* 5: 35–117, 1967.
67. SCHÖNHÖFER, P. S., I. F. SKIDMORE, M. I. PAUL, B. R. DITZION, G. L. PAUK, AND G. KRISHNA. Effects of glucocorticoids on adenyl cyclase and phosphodiesterase activity in fat cell homogenates and the accumulation of cyclic AMP in intact fat cells. *Arch. Pharmacol.* 273: 267–282, 1972.
68. SCOW, R. O. Diabetic ketosis and fat mobilization in the hypophysectomized-pancreatectomized rat. In: *Perspectives in Biology*, edited by C. F. Cori, V. G. Foglia, L. F. Leloir, and S. Ochoa. Amsterdam: Elsevier, 1963, p. 150–157.
69. SCOW, R. O., AND S. S. CHERNICK. Hormonal control of protein and fat metabolism in the pancreatectomized rat. *Recent Progr. Hormone Res.* 16: 497–545, 1960.
70. SCOW, R. O., AND S. S. CHERNICK. Mobilization, transport and utilization of free fatty acids. In: *Comprehensive Biochemistry*, edited by M. Florkin and E. H. Stotz. Amsterdam: Elsevier, 1970, vol. 18, p. 19–50.
71. SCOW, R. O., AND S. S. CHERNICK. Action of pituitary and adrenal hormones in the development of diabetic ketosis. *Proc. Congr. Intern. Diabetes Federation, 7th, Buenos Aires. Excerpta Med. Found. Intern. Congr. Ser.* 231: 771–780, 1971.
72. SENFT, G., G. SCHULTZ, K. MUNSKE, AND M. HOFFMAN. Effects of glucocorticoids and insulin on $3',5'$-AMP phosphodiesterase activity in adrenalectomized rats. *Diabetologia* 4: 330–335, 1968.
73. SHAFRIR, E., K. E. SUSSMAN, AND D. STEINBERG. Role of the pituitary and the adrenal in the mobilization of free fatty acids and lipoproteins. *J. Lipid Res.* 1: 459–465, 1960.
74. SPITZER, J. J., AND W. T. MCELROY, JR. Some hormonal effects on uptake of free fatty acids by the liver. *Am. J. Physiol.* 199: 876–878, 1960.
75. URGOITI, E. J., B. A. HOUSSAY, AND C. T. RIETTI. Hypophyseal and adrenal factors essential for ketoacidosis of pancreatectomized dogs. *Diabetes* 12: 301–307, 1963.
76. WIERNIK, P. H., AND R. M. MACLEOD. The effect of a single large dose of 9α-fluoroprednisolone on nucleodepolymerase activity and nucleic acid content of the rat thymus. *Acta Endocrinol.* 49: 138–144, 1965.
77. WIRA, C., AND A. MUNCK. Specific glucocorticoid receptors in thymus cells. *J. Biol. Chem.* 245: 3436–3438, 1970.
78. WOOL, I. G., AND M. S. GOLDSTEIN. Role of neurohumors in the action of the adrenal cortical steroids: mobilization of fat. *Am. J. Physiol.* 175: 303–306, 1953.
79. YORKE, R. E. The influence of dexamethasone on adipose tissue metabolism *in vitro*. *J. Endocrinol.* 39: 329–343, 1967.
80. YOUNG, D. A. Glucocorticoid action on rat thymus cells. Interrelationships between carbohydrate, protein, and adenine nucleotide metabolism and cortisol effects on these functions *in vitro*. *J. Biol. Chem.* 244: 2210–2217, 1969.
81. YOUNG, D. A. 6-Min-stimulatory effects of cortisol *in vitro* on precursor incorporation into RNA and protein in rat thymus cells (Abstract). *Federation Proc.* 29: 778, 1970.

CHAPTER 13

Effect of corticosteroids on water and electrolyte metabolism

BARR H. FORMAN
PATRICK J. MULROW

Department of Internal Medicine, Yale University School of Medicine, New Haven, Connecticut

CHAPTER CONTENTS

Effect of Corticosteroids
  On kidney
    Sodium excretion
    Potassium excretion
    Magnesium, calcium, and acid-base balance
  On salivary gland
  On sweat
  On muscle
  On bone
  On gastrointestinal tract
  On salt appetite and sensitivity
  On sodium-potassium adenosine triphosphatase
Water Metabolism
Mechanism of Action of Aldosterone

A MAJOR FUNCTION of the adrenal cortex is the regulation of water and electrolyte metabolism. Aldosterone, most potent of the mineralocorticoids, is secreted by the zona glomerulosa at a rate of about 100 µg/day in normal human beings on a liberal sodium intake. The secretion rate increases severalfold in response to sodium or volume depletion. The main action of aldosterone is on electrolyte excretion by the kidney, but it also affects the electrolyte excretion of the salivary and sweat glands and the gastrointestinal tract. The glucocorticoids secreted by the adrenal cortex, chiefly cortisol in man, have some mineralocorticoid action but mainly affect water excretion.

EFFECT OF CORTICOSTEROIDS

On Kidney

SODIUM EXCRETION. In early studies it was shown that acute administration of mineralocorticoids increased sodium reabsorption and potassium excretion. The site of action within the kidney has been under investigation. From stop-flow experiments, Vander et al. (136) proposed an action of aldosterone on the distal tubule.

He demonstrated that aldosterone administration to adrenalectomized dogs lowered the high concentration of sodium in the distal tubule to normal. Using free-flow micropuncture techniques, Hierholzer et al. (71) found that sodium concentrations in the lumen of the distal tubule were elevated in adrenalectomized rats, and the ratio of sodium concentration in tubular fluid to that in plasma (TF/P$_{Na}$) of the adrenalectomized rat was reduced by administration of aldosterone (Fig. 1). No difference in similar ratios from the proximal tubule was found between normal and adrenalectomized animals either in free-flow or stationary microperfusion experiments, but an abnormally high TF/P$_{Na}$ ratio was noted at the beginning of the distal tubule. This latter finding was confirmed by Murayama et al. (109) and suggests decreased sodium reabsorption in the loop of Henle. The reduced diluting and concentrating ability in Addisonian patients indirectly supports abnormal transport of sodium by Henle's loop, but this reduced ability may be an indirect effect of volume depletion and reduced glomerular filtration rate (GFR), which would cause increased proximal reabsorption with decreased delivery of sodium to the ascending limb. Wright et al. (141), using a free-flow micropuncture technique, found no effect on the TF/P$_{Na}$ ratio in the proximal tubule when a mineralocorticoid was administered to adrenalectomized dogs (Fig. 2). Since urinary sodium excretion diminished after administration of mineralocorticoid there must have been an effect somewhere in the distal tubule. Spironolactone, an inhibitor of mineralocorticoid action, did not lower proximal tubular TF/P inulin ratios in dogs, even though the fraction of filtered sodium excreted increased by 2% (35).

There are reports that indicate a defect in proximal tubular function in adrenalectomized rats. Using the split-drop technique, Hierholzer and co-workers (72, 73) found impaired sodium reabsorption in proximal tubules that was corrected by 3–5 days of aldosterone or cortisone, but not by dexamethasone, replace-

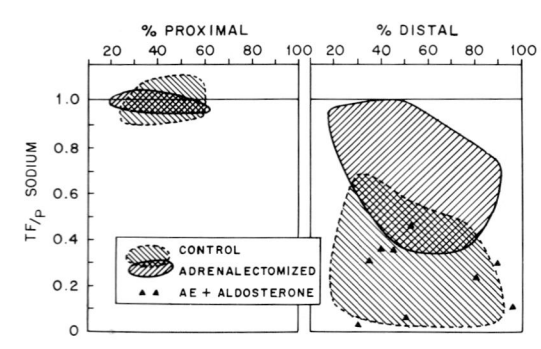

FIG. 1. Tubular fluid-to-plasma (TF/P) sodium concentration ratios in control animals, adrenalectomized rats, and adrenalectomized rats (AE) treated with d-aldosterone. Contour diagrams indicate range of values. [From Hierholzer et al. (71.)]

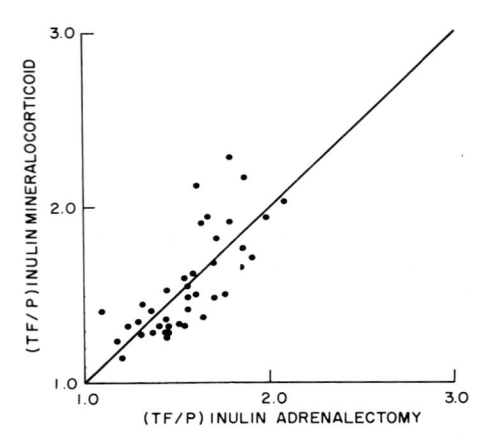

FIG. 2. Tubular fluid-to-plasma (TF/P) inulin concentration ratios measured in 7 adrenalectomized dogs before and after administration of 9α-fluorocortisol. Identity line indicates no change in TF/P inulin after steroid replacement. [From Wright et al. (141).]

ment. Since this defect was not seen in studies using free-flow techniques, it has been argued that the increased transit times in the adrenalectomized animal masked the defect by permitting tubular fluid to remain in contact with the tubular epithelium for longer periods of time (72). Stolte et al. (127), however, perfused the proximal tubule of adrenalectomized rats at a constant rate and still found diminished reabsorption of sodium. Since the diameter of the proximal tubule after adrenalectomy did not change, he contended that a defect in sodium reabsorption of the proximal tubule existed and was corrected by small doses of aldosterone. In contrast, Cortney (24) corrected these alterations in contact time and flow rate in adrenalectomized rats by a mannitol diuresis but found no change in proximal sodium reabsorption after adrenalectomy. Using split-drop technique, Lynch et al. (99) showed no change in proximal reabsorptive time after 9α-fluorocortisol was administered to adrenalectomized dogs, and found no change in free-flow sodium reabsorption of proximal tubules after adrenalectomy.

However, other kinds of evidence suggest that aldosterone may affect the proximal tubule. Tritiated aldosterone administered to rats appears in the proximal, as well as the distal, tubule (138), and actinomycin D inhibits a portion of sodium reabsorption in proximal tubules in adrenalectomized rats treated with aldosterone (137).

Therefore mineralocorticoids appear to act on the distal tubule, but a proximal effect is still unclear and has not been demonstrable by free-flow techniques.

POTASSIUM EXCRETION. Stimulation of potassium excretion by aldosterone depends to a large extent on the amount of sodium in the diet. Animals on a diet totally lacking in sodium exhibit no kaliuresis after aldosterone administration (50).

Potassium ions are reabsorbed along the proximal tubule and Henle's loop. Secretion of potassium into the distal tubule accounts for 60–90% of urinary potassium (56, 101). Adrenalectomy prevents the normal increase in the TF/P_K ratio in the late distal tubule (71). According to Giebisch et al. (56), increased concentration of sodium ions in the lumen of the distal tubule may increase the electrical negativity of the lumen in relation to the peritubular fluid. Potassium then diffuses passively down this electrical gradient. There appears to be no stoichiometric relation between the reabsorption of sodium and the secretion of potassium. Presumably aldosterone or other mineralocorticoids increase sodium reabsorption and consequently increase this electrical gradient, and thereby facilitate potassium excretion.

Adaptation to chronic hyperkalemia requires the presence of the adrenal cortex (5, 132). This adaptation remains to some degree after nephrectomy but is abolished by adrenalectomy. Whether increased aldosterone secretion is necessary is not clear. Schultze et al. (119) demonstrated adaptation to chronic potassium loading in adrenalectomized and subtotally nephrectomized dogs receiving both high and low doses of mineralocorticoid.

When a mineralocorticoid is administered for several days, the kidney escapes from the sodium-retaining, but not from the potassium-losing, effect of the hormone [(7); Fig. 3]. This escape phenomenon (i.e., the failure to retain additional sodium despite continued administration of mineralocorticoid) cannot be explained by changes in GFR, renal nerve activity, or dilution of plasma proteins. The evidence suggests that intrarenal physical factors and possibly an unidentified sodium-losing hormone play a role (15, 28, 31, 37, 77, 92, 93, 97, 120). During the escape phenomenon, sodium reabsorption by the proximal tubule is diminished and the increased delivery of sodium and water to the distal tubule may override the enhanced sodium reabsorption induced by the mineralocorticoid in the distal tubule (36, 141). Recently, however, no decrease in proximal sodium reabsorption was found during mineralocorticoid escape in dogs (87). Subjects with congestive heart failure, cirrhosis with ascites, nephrosis, and other conditions associated with edema retain sodium and water. Frequently aldosterone secretion is

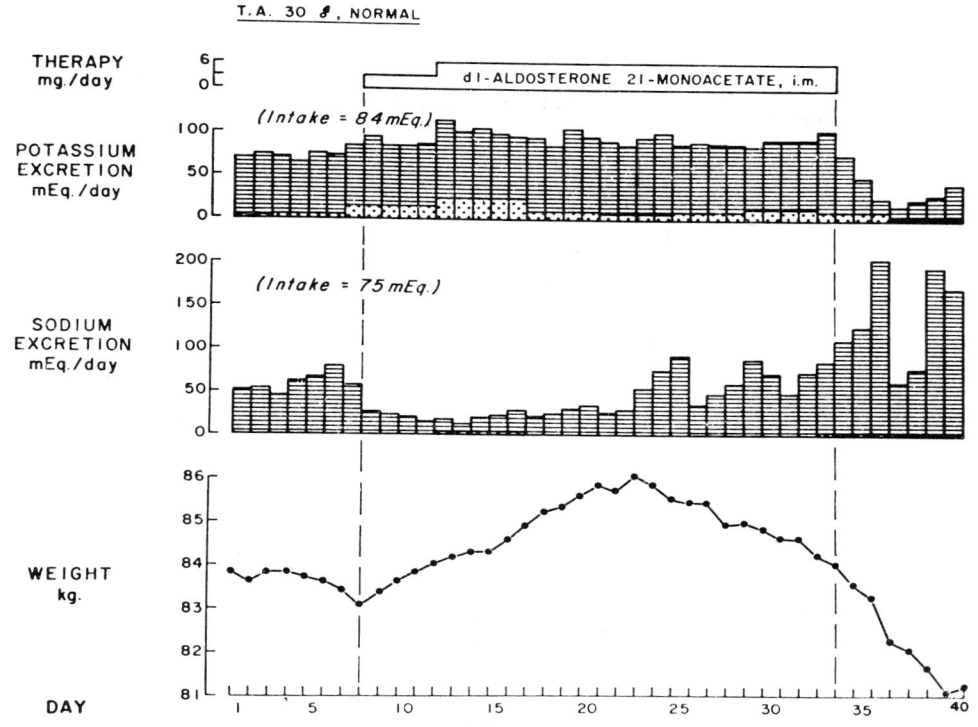

FIG. 3. Effect of aldosterone on weight and sodium and potassium excretion in normal subject (*T.A.*) receiving a constant diet. [From August et al. (7).]

elevated in these conditions, but clearly "escape" does not occur (48, 58, 74, 107).

MAGNESIUM, CALCIUM, AND ACID-BASE BALANCE. Magnesium concentrations in plasma are elevated in adrenal insufficiency (29), and hypomagnesemia has been reported in a few cases of primary aldosteronism (100, 106). Increased magnesium excretion with normal concentrations in plasma is, however, more commonly observed in these patients (75). Suki et al. (130) reported increased calcium excretion with prolonged mineralocorticoid administration, and it would therefore appear that calcium and magnesium excretion is influenced by mineralocorticoids. This effect, however, is probably indirect and secondary to volume expansion. Massry et al. (103) reported that, in dogs treated with deoxycorticosterone acetate (DCA), sodium excretion fell on the first day but calcium and magnesium excretion did not increase until the third day. Presumably sodium retention led to expansion of extracellular fluid volume and inhibited proximal tubular reabsorption of calcium and magnesium, as well as sodium (Fig. 4). Lemann et al. (91) also reported no change in calcium or magnesium excretion after administration of cortisol or aldosterone in acute human studies, despite a decrease in sodium excretion. The decreased sodium and chloride excretion after aldosterone administration was associated with increased excretion of potassium and hydrogen ions, whereas cortisol increased only potassium excretion (Figs. 5 and 6). Similarly, Bartter et al. (10) reported increased ammonia, hydrogen, and potassium ion excretion after aldosterone administration. Lindeman et al. (96), however, did show increased calcium and magnesium excretion after large doses of cortisol.

Although primary aldosteronism is associated with a metabolic alkalosis, the mechanism of the alkalosis and the role of mineralocorticoids in acid-base balance are not clear. It has been difficult to produce significant alkalosis in normal men by administration of aldosterone (78), but recently Kassirer et al. (79) produced alkalosis in normal subjects on a low-salt diet who were given sodium bicarbonate supplement. These subjects developed very large potassium deficits. The alkalosis was resistant to saline loading and dependent on aldosterone administration for maintenance. In Cushing's syndrome the hypokalemic alkalosis is more closely correlated with mineralocorticoid than with glucocorticoid production (118). An aldosterone deficiency may be associated with acidosis. Kurtzman et al. (88) reported a hyperkalemic metabolic acidosis in adrenalectomized dogs receiving only glucocorticoid replacement. Bicarbonate reabsorption was normal, but ammonium ion production was impaired. Adrenalectomized rats challenged with respiratory acidosis have impaired renal acid excretion and enhanced bicarbonate reabsorption, but the latter is not dependent on adrenal secretions (98). However, Roth & Gamble (116) have shown that chronic administration of DCA to dogs increased bicarbonate reabsorption independently of potassium levels.

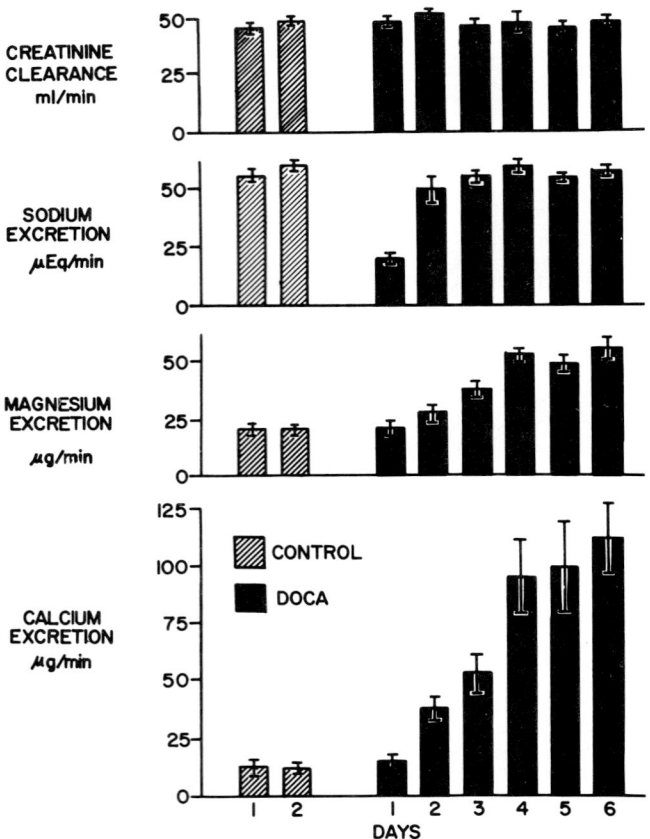

FIG. 4. Changes (mean ± SE) in excretion of sodium, magnesium, and calcium observed in 6 dogs receiving 20 mg deoxycorticosterone acetate per day over 6 successive days. [From Massry et al. (103).]

On Salivary Gland

In 1938 McCance (104) demonstrated decreased sodium and increased potassium concentrations in human saliva after sodium depletion, a physiological maneuver known to increase aldosterone production. Administration of DCA to Addisonian patients reduces the high concentration of sodium in saliva (52). The salivary gland, like the gastrointestinal tract, does not escape from prolonged mineralocorticoid administration, and a salivary Na^+/K^+ ratio of less than 0.25 is indicative of aldosteronism (90). In sheep the salivary Na^+/K^+ ratio can be used as an index of aldosterone secretion (13). Although sodium deficiency sensitizes the parotid gland of sheep to the action of aldosterone, 60–90 min elapse before the onset of aldosterone action (123), but the lag period is considerably longer in man (7). The mechanism of action of aldosterone on the salivary glands is not clear. Whether aldosterone increases sodium reabsorption or decreases sodium secretion is unknown.

On Sweat

Aldosterone and other mineralocorticoids decrease sodium concentration in sweat, and there is no escape from prolonged administration (23). During acclimatization to heat, humans excrete increased quantities of aldosterone and decreased sodium concentrations in sweat (23). Siegenthaler et al. (122) showed that spironolactone inhibited the fall in concentration of sodium in sweat. The response of the sweat gland to heat stress is sluggish (115), so it is not surprising that McConahay et al. (105) did not show an effect of a 4-hr aldosterone infusion on sweat composition. It appears that enzyme induction by aldosterone is much slower in sweat glands than in the kidney.

On Muscle

Administration of aldosterone results in decreased potassium and increased sodium content in muscle (53, 95). Presumably, this lowered potassium and increased sodium content is an indirect effect resulting from increased potassium loss and sodium reabsorption by the kidney, since administration of aldosterone to rats on a low-sodium diet, which prevents potassium loss (50),

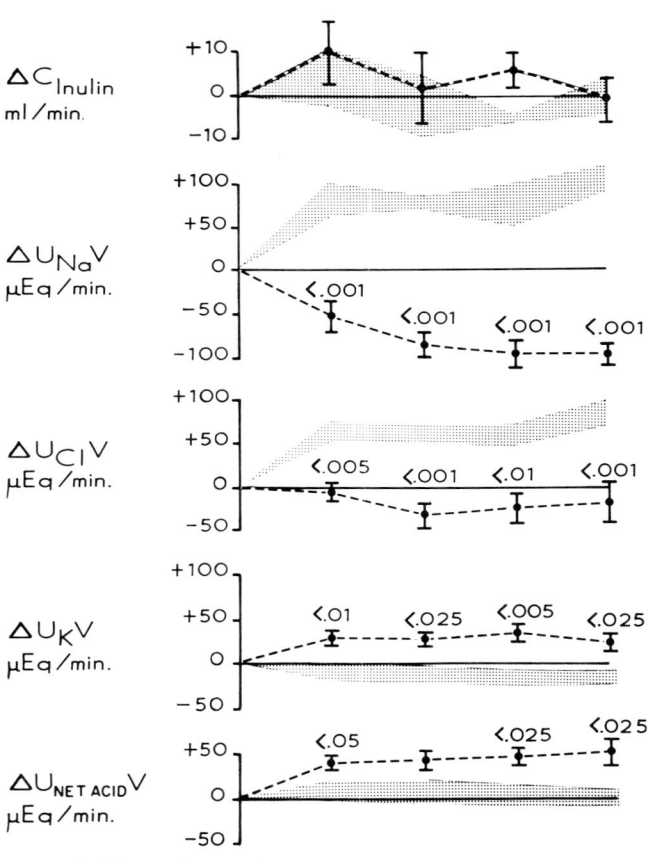

FIG. 5. Mean changes from control after aldosterone administration. *Shaded areas* enclose ± 1 SEM change after placebo. P values present likelihood that changes after cortisol did not differ from those after placebo. ΔC_{Inulin}, change in clearance of inulin from control; $\Delta U_{Na}V$, change in sodium excretion from control; $\Delta U_{Cl}V$, change in chloride excretion from control; $\Delta U_K V$, change in potassium excretion from control; $\Delta U_{net\ acid}V$, change in net acid excretion from control. [From Lemann et al. (91).]

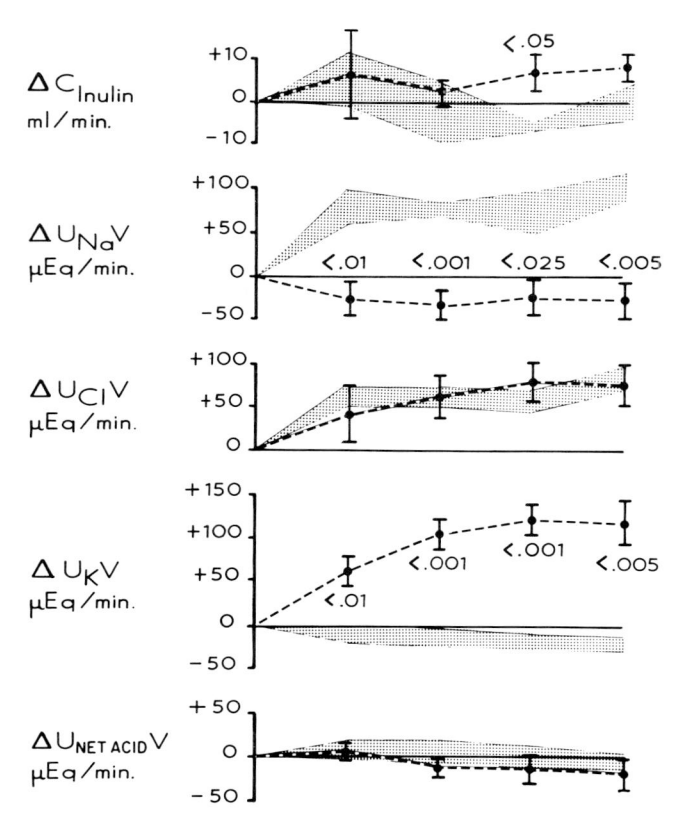

FIG. 6. Mean changes from control after cortisol administration. *Shaded areas* enclose ± 1 SEM change after placebo. *P* values present likelihood that changes after cortisol did not differ from those after placebo. See Fig. 5 for explanation of symbols. [From Lemann et al. (91).]

does not alter muscle electrolyte content. In vitro studies, however, do suggest a direct effect of aldosterone on muscle. Addition of aldosterone to a tissue culture of human laryngeal cells resulted in a lower sodium content (114). Adler (2) reported an effect of aldosterone on the rat diaphragm in vitro. When the potassium concentration in the incubation medium was 5.0 mEq/liter, aldosterone lowered tissue potassium by 2–3%, but aldosterone had no effect when the potassium concentration was higher, which seemed to offset the action of aldosterone (Fig. 7). It was not possible to study sodium concentration levels in this model.

On Bone

The effects of adrenalectomy and mineralocorticoid administration on bone sodium have yielded conflicting reports, partly because of species differences and differences in techniques, such as failure to completely remove bone marrow and periosteum before measuring the sodium content of compact bone. Green et al. (63), in analyzing whole bone, found that DCA had no effect on the uptake of ^{22}Na within 5 hr of administration. The decrease in ^{22}Na uptake was found in bone after adrenalectomy only when the animals were sodium deficient (108). It has been reported that adrenalectomy lowers sodium concentration in rat bone (113), but in these investigations whole bone (compact bone plus marrow) was analyzed. A decrease of sodium concentration in serum would contribute to a decline in bone sodium. Administration of aldosterone or DCA to rats decreased the amount of ^{22}Na and ^{40}K uptake by compact bone (117), whereas adrenalectomy or treatment with spironolactone increased the uptake. These findings suggest that aldosterone plays a role in regulating the transfer of electrolytes between bone and extracellular fluid, and studies in man support the possibility that aldosterone prevents the expansion of a radioactive sodium pool by preventing uptake of sodium by bone (129).

Glucocorticoids inhibit bone growth (16, 51), suppress formation of bone matrix proteins (17), and can result in osteoporosis (76). Dogs pretreated with radioactive calcium (^{47}Ca) release ^{47}Ca into the blood when given a glucocorticoid (55). Cortisone inhibits the hypocalcemic response to calcitonin in rats (134). Gordan (61) believes that the osteoporosis caused by cortisol is mediated by parathyroid hormone secreted in response to the induced hypocalcemia. Gordan et al. (62) and Eliel et al. (43) report that glucocorticoids conserve calcium and phosphorus in hypoparathyroid patients and rats.

On Gastrointestinal Tract

Patients with primary aldosteronism and dogs with secondary aldosteronism have increased potassium loss in the stool (30, 142, 143). Administration of DCA to Addisonian patients reduced sodium content in the stool (45). Aldosterone, 9α-fluorocortisol, and cortisol administration to normal men diminished the sodium and increased the potassium content of stools (19), whereas spironolactone prevented the potassium loss that usually results from aldosterone administration (44). The gastrointestinal (GI) tract, like the sweat and salivary

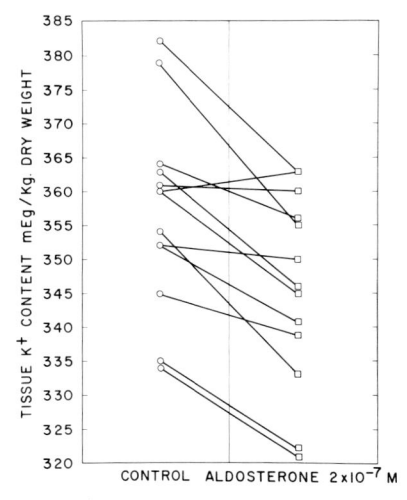

FIG. 7. Effect of aldosterone on tissue potassium content. *Lines* join values from control tissue (○) and aldosterone-treated tissue (□), which have been incubated simultaneously. [From Adler (2).]

glands, does not escape from the effect of prolonged mineralocorticoid administration.

The site of action of aldosterone on the GI tract has been the subject of several reports. Berger et al. (12) used isolated intestinal loops in dogs and found that DCA increased sodium reabsorption but did not change sodium influx. Potassium movement into and out of the loop was increased with a net increase in secretion into the colon. Levitan (94) was unable to show increased potassium loss into the colon of humans receiving aldosterone, although sodium reabsorption was increased.

Aldosterone increased short-circuit current in a rat colon preparation, a measure of net sodium transport (41), but it did not have an effect when added to the luminal side of the colon. This is similar to the in vitro effects of aldosterone on toad bladder and frog skin preparations (21, 25, 26). Thompson et al. (133) noted in man a decrease in stool sodium after aldosterone administration and correlated this sodium change with the increased potential difference across the colonic epithelium. Recently rectal potential difference (PD) has been recommended as a screening test for primary aldosteronism. The PD in man is increased by mineralocorticoid administration and decreased by spironolactone [(42); Fig. 8].

Glucorticoids decrease intestinal transport of calcium (22, 66), whereas adrenalectomy increases it (49). It is believed that glucocorticoids alter calcium transport in the gut by blocking the action of vitamin D. Avioli et al. (9) showed in man that prednisone increases tritiated vitamin D_3 turnover and decreases "peak IV" (25-hydroxycholecalciferol) (14). In rat studies, however, glucocorticoids did not alter the rate of formation of vitamin D metabolites, nor did they interfere with the localization of vitamin D in the small intestine (82). Cellular transport of calcium was decreased, and flux studies showed that the active component of the transport system was diminished by cortisone.

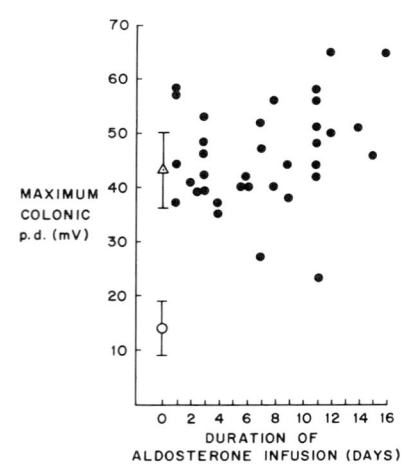

FIG. 8. Maximum colonic potential difference (p.d.) after different durations of aldosterone infusion into rats, *closed circles*; p.d. without aldosterone infusion (mean ± SD; 12 rats), *open circle*; p.d. after 6 hr aldosterone infusion (mean ± SD; 12 rats), *open triangle*. [From Thompson & Edmonds (133).]

On Salt Appetite and Sensitivity

Addisonian patients have an increased ability to detect salt (69). Large doses of DCA do not reduce this enhanced sensitivity, but replacement doses of cortisone do (68). Glucocorticoids have no effect in normal subjects. Adrenalectomy stimulates the salt appetite of rats, and small doses of DCA normalize it (140). In intact rats large doses of DCA increase salt appetite (70). It is unlikely that changes in salivary electrolyte composition mediate this response since the salt appetite is stimulated in adrenalectomized and severely sodium-deficient sheep, despite marked and opposite changes in salivary Na^+/K^+ ratios (33). Furthermore increased sodium concentration in the arterial circulation of the partoid and lingual glands did not greatly affect salt appetite (11). The mechanism by which mineralocorticoids stimulate salt appetite is unknown, although Wolf & Steinbaum (139) have shown that lesions in the dorsolateral hypothalamic region abolish the stimulatory effect of DCA on salt appetite.

On Sodium-Potasssium Adenosine Triphosphatase

Much data has accumulated indicating that the active transport of cations is linked to a magnesium-dependent, sodium-potassium adenosine triphosphatase (Na-K ATPase). This subject has recently been reviewed by Katz & Epstein (81). Landon et al. (89) showed a fall in Na-K ATPase activity in the rat kidney 5–7 days after adrenalectomy. Acute administration of aldosterone did not return the enzyme activity to normal, even though maximal sodium retention was observed, but after several days of large doses of aldosterone the Na-K ATPase levels returned to normal. Glucocorticoid administration was also effective in achieving this, as shown by Chignell et al. (20) and Katz & Epstein (80). Many factors, however, are known to affect Na-K ATPase, such as a diet high in protein or uninephrectomy and other maneuvers that increase the GFR and the work load of the kidney. Katz & Epstein (80) therefore proposed that the increased tubular sodium transport, and not a specific effect of the corticosteroids, induces the enzyme increase. The work of Hendler et al. (67) seems to bear this out. They found the highest concentration of Na-K ATPase in the outer medullary portion of the dog kidney, an area containing the ascending limb of Henle, which has an enormous capacity for sodium transport. Although this link between cation transport and Na-K ATPase is well known, the exact mechanism and the role of the corticosteroids await further elucidation.

WATER METABOLISM

The impaired ability to excrete a water load is one of the major defects of the adrenal-insufficient subject and largely accounts for the hyponatremia that is often present. Glucocorticoids, but not mineralocorticoids, correct the impaired water excretion. The mechanism of glucocorticoid action continues to be a subject of controversy. Alterations in plasma volume and renal hemodynamics, elevated antidiuretic hormone (ADH) levels in plasma, and direct glucocorticoid effects on water permeability of the distal nephron have been postulated to be involved in the decreased excretion of water. Plasma volume and GFR are reduced in adrenal insufficiency, and glucocorticoids may increase GFR (59). Studies by Kleeman and associates (27, 84–86) suggest that the normalization of solute-free water clearance in Addisonian subjects by glucocorticoids is not fully explained by increases in plasma volume or by changes in renal hemodynamics or ADH levels. In contrast, Gill et al. (57) improved free water clearance in adrenal-insufficient subjects by saline infusion. Cortisol therapy in addition to the saline infusions had no further effect on free water clearance. This study, however, showed that changes in GFR and solute excretion did not fully explain the increase in free water clearance after saline infusion.

Studies by Ackerman & Miller (1) show that glucocorticoids cannot directly improve the water excretion of hypovolemic normal subjects but can correct the impairment in Addisonian patients who are glucocorticoid deficient and normovolemic. They concluded that a defect in water excretion exists in the distal tubule as a result of either abnormal ADH levels or increased permeability of the distal tubule to water. Increased levels of circulating ADH have been reported in Addisonian subjects by Ahmed et al. (4). Hydration alone did not suppress these levels to normal, but hydration plus glucocorticoid therapy did. Glucocorticoids suppress the antidiuretic response to nicotine (34) and increase the osmotic threshold for ADH release in human subjects (6). Moreover studies of the impaired water excretion in patients with anterior pituitary insufficiency indicate that glucocorticoids are necessary to suppress the inappropriately elevated ADH levels (3). Glucocorticoids can correct the impaired water excretion of adrenalectomized rats with hereditary hypothalamic diabetes insipidus, but aldosterone is also needed to correct the dilution defect (64). This seems to exclude an obligatory role of ADH in the impaired excretion of adrenal insufficiency. Studies by Raisz et al. (112) and Kleeman et al. (85) suggest a direct effect of glucocorticoids on the permeability of the renal tubule to water.

Micropuncture studies support the increased permeability of the distal tubule to water in adrenal insufficiency with correction by glucocorticoid treatment (126). These effects of adrenalectomy and glucocorticoid replacement took several days to become evident, whereas the defect in water clearance in the intact animal is corrected by glucocorticoids more acutely. Bladders depleted of exogenous steroids by prolonged incubation have increased water permeability that is returned to normal when cortisol is added to the incubation medium (102).

A possible effect of glucocorticoids on shifts of body fluids has been suggested by Swingle et al. (131). Sodium excretion decreased in fasted, adrenalectomized dogs given aldosterone, but water loss continued. Blood pressure and blood volume fell. After glucocorticoids were given, blood volume and blood pressure increased, but serum sodium concentration fell due to dilution caused by an apparent shift of water out of the cells into the extracellular space.

In a recent study by de Bermudez & Hayslett (32), administration of glucocorticoids to intact rats on a low-sodium diet caused no acute change in GFR or sodium excretion. After 4 days of administration, glucocorticoids did increase GFR and blood flow without altering proximal tubular function. There was a disproportionate rise in innercortical blood flow. The increased GFR following chronic administration without any increase in sodium excretion indicates increased reabsorption of sodium by the tubules.

Mineralocorticoids may also influence water excretion. During water diuresis, Sonnenblick et al. (124) showed that aldosterone increased free water clearance and proposed that aldosterone must have acted at a site where sodium can be extracted without water, such as the loop of Henle. This effect is probably not important physiologically, as aldosterone alone does not correct the impairment of water excretion in adrenalectomized subjects. Moreover, Yunis et al. (144) could not demonstrate an effect of aldosterone on solute free water clearance.

MECHANISM OF ACTION OF ALDOSTERONE

The predominant biological action of aldosterone is to stimulate sodium transport by the kidney. Using the isolated toad bladder as a model system, several investigators have contributed to the understanding of the mechanism of action of aldosterone (8, 25, 38, 39, 111, 121). Recent studies involving the rat kidney extended these concepts to a mammalian species (18, 46, 137). Most of the evidence is consistent with the concept that aldosterone stimulates active sodium transport by a series of reactions, including DNA-dependent synthesis of RNA and de novo synthesis of protein. In many respects the effects of aldosterone on protein synthesis are similar to those of other steroid hormones. Presumably, specific receptors in the supernatant or cell sap transport aldosterone to the nucleus. Here it is bound to another receptor protein, which interacts with the nuclear DNA, possibly by removing histones from specific sites on the DNA. This "active" DNA then produces specific forms of RNA, which in turn regulate protein synthesis (110).

The nature of the protein synthesized through the action of aldosterone is in dispute. Edelman and co-workers believe an enzyme enhances utilization of substrates to provide the energy needed for active transport (47). Most of the energy is supplied by oxidative phosphorylation, although glycolysis can support, to a limited extent, increased sodium transport by aldosterone (65, 83). Sharp & Leaf (121) suggest that aldosterone induces the formation of a protein that acts as a permease and facilitates the entry of sodium into the cell. It is this entry of sodium that enhances utilization of substrate to supply the energy necessary for the sodium pump. Several recent studies tend to support the latter possibility. Handler et al. (65) demonstrated that the stimulation of glycolysis in the toad bladder by aldosterone is secondary to the augmentation of sodium transport since ouabain inhibits the aldosterone effect on both sodium transport and glycolysis. Furthermore removal of sodium from the medium bathing the mucosal side of the bladder suppresses the increased oxygen consumption and utilization of substrates of the tricarboxylic acid (TCA) cycle (83). However, aldosterone independently increases the activity of the TCA cycle enzymes that contribute to increased aerobic energy supply for the transport system (83). This stimulation is independent of sodium transport but dependent on protein synthesis. Goodman et al. (60) recently showed increased incorporation of phospholipids into the membrane of the toad bladder within 20 min after addition of aldosterone to the incubation medium. These results may well explain the long delay before the onset of action of aldosterone in target organs. The delay is the time required for the synthesis of a protein necessary for its action.

Although new RNA and protein synthesis is necessary for the effect of aldosterone on sodium transport, they do not appear necessary for the aldosterone effect on potassium excretion. Actinomycin D administration to rats inhibited only the antinatriuretic, and not the kaliuretic, effect of aldosterone (40).

Data indicate that aldosterone action may occur without de novo RNA or protein synthesis. Vancura et al. (135), using the toad bladder, could not demonstrate increased RNA synthesis by aldosterone and suggested that the increased RNA synthesis reported by others may be due to bacterial contamination of their preparations. The RNA turnover is extraordinarily slow in the toad bladder and slower than the latency period observed before the onset of aldosterone action.

Several investigators have demonstrated an effect of aldosterone and cortisol on sodium transport in canine and human red blood cells in vitro (54, 125, 128). These cells do not have the DNA and RNA system necessary for protein synthesis.

REFERENCES

1. ACKERMAN, G. L., AND C. L. MILLER. Role of hypovolemia in the impaired water diuresis of adrenal insufficiency. *J. Clin. Endocrinol. Metab.* 30: 252-258, 1970.
2. ADLER, S. An extrarenal action of aldosterone on mammalian skeletal muscle. *Am. J. Physiol.* 218: 616-621, 1970.
3. AGUS, Z. S., AND M. GOLDBERG. Role of antidiuretic hormone in the abnormal water diuresis of anterior hypopituitarism in man. *J. Clin. Invest.* 50 (7): 1478-1489, 1971.
4. AHMED, A. B. J., B. C. GEORGE, C. GONZALEZ-AUVERT, AND J. F. DINGMAN. Increased plasma arginine vasopressin in clinical adrenocortical insufficiency and its inhibition by glucosteroids. *J. Clin. Invest.* 46: 111-123, 1967.
5. ALEXANDER, E. A., AND N. G. LEVINSKY. An extrarenal mechanism of potassium adaptation. *J. Clin. Invest.* 47: 740-748, 1968.
6. AUBRY, R. H., H. R. NANKIN, A. M. MOSES, AND D. H. P. STREETEN. Measurement of the osmotic threshold for vasopressin release in human subjects and its modification by cortisol. *J. Clin. Endocrinol. Metab.* 25: 1481-1492, 1965.
7. AUGUST, J. T., D. H. NELSON, AND G. W. THORN. Response of normal subjects to large amounts of aldosterone. *J. Clin. Invest.* 37: 1549-1555, 1958.
8. AUSIELLO, D. A., AND G. W. G. SHARP. Localization of physiological receptor sites for aldosterone in the bladder of the toad *Bufo marinus. Endocrinology* 82: 1163-1169, 1968.
9. AVIOLI, L. V., S. J. BIRGE, AND S. W. LEE. Effects of prednisone on Vitamin D metabolism in man. *J. Clin. Endocrinol. Metab.* 28: 1341-1346, 1968.
10. BARTTER, F. C., AND P. FOURMAN. The different effects of aldosterone-like steroids and hydrocortisone-like steroids on urinary excretion of potassium and acid. *Metabolism* 11: 6-20, 1962.
11. BEILHARZ, S., D. A. DENTON, AND J. R. SABINE. The effect of concurrent deficiency of water and sodium on the sodium appetite of sheep. *J. Physiol., London* 163: 378-390, 1962.
12. BERGER, E. Y., G. KANZAKI, AND J. M. STEELE. The effect of desoxycorticosterone on the unidirectional transfers of sodium and potassium into and out of the dog intestine. *J. Physiol., London* 151: 352-362, 1960.
13. BLAIR-WEST, J. R., J. P. COGHLAN, D. A. DENTON, J. R. GODING, AND R. D. WRIGHT. The effect of adrenal cortical steroids on parotid salivary secretion. In: *Salivary Glands and Their Secretions*, edited by L. M. Streebny and J. Meyer. New York: Pergamon Press, 1964, p. 253-279.
14. BLUNT, J. W., AND H. F. DELUCA. The synthesis of 25-hydroxycholecalciferol—a biologically active metabolite of vitamin D_3. *Biochemistry* 8: 671-675, 1969.
15. BLYTHE, W. B., D. D'AVILA, H. J. GITELMAN, AND L. G. WELT. Further evidence for a humoral natriuretic factor. *Circulation Res.* 28, Suppl. II: 21-31, 1971.
16. BOHR, H. H. The influence of different hormones on bone formation in rats. *Acta Endocrinol.* 58: 116-122, 1968.
17. CANNON, P. R., L. E. FRAZIER, AND R. H. HUGHES. The influence of cortisone upon protein metabolism. *Arch. Pathol.* 61: 271-279, 1956.
18. CASTLES, T. R., AND H. E. WILLIAMSON. Mediation of aldosterone induced antinatriuresis via RNA synthesis (31834). *Proc. Soc. Exptl. Biol. Med.* 124: 717-719, 1967.
19. CHARRON, R. C., C. E. LEME, D. R. WILSON, T. S. ING, AND O. M. WRONG. The effect of adrenal steroids on stool composition, as revealed by in vivo dialysis of faeces. *Clin. Sci.* 37: 151-167, 1969.
20. CHIGNELL, C. F., P. M. RODDY, AND E. O. TITUS. Effect of adrenal steroids on Na^+-K^+-dependent adenosine triphosphate. *Life Sci.* 4: 559-566, 1965.
21. CIVAN, M. M., AND R. E. HOFFMAN. Effect of aldosterone on electrical resistance of toad bladder. *Am. J. Physiol.* 220: 324-328, 1971.
22. COLLINS, E. J., E. R. GARRETT, AND R. L. JOHNSTON. Effect of adrenal steroids on radio-calcium metabolism in dogs. *Metabolism* 11: 716-726, 1962.
23. CONN, J. W. Aldosteronism in man. 1. Some clinical and climatological aspects. *J. Am. Med. Assoc.* 183: 775-781, 1963.
24. CORTNEY, M. A. Renal tubular transfer of water and electrolytes in adrenalectomized rats. *Am. J. Physiol.* 216: 589-598, 1960.
25. CRABBE, J. Stimulation of active sodium transport by the isolated toad bladder with aldosterone in vitro. *J. Clin. Invest.* 40: 2103-2110, 1961.
26. CRABBE, J. Stimulation by aldosterone of active sodium trans-

port across the isolated ventral skin of Amphibia. *Endocrinology* 75: 809–811, 1964.
27. CUTLER, R. E., C. R. KLEEMAN, J. KOPLOWITZ, M. H. MAXWELL, AND J. T. DOWLING. Mechanisms of impaired water excretion in adrenal and pituitary insufficiency. III. *J. Clin. Invest.* 41: 1524–1530, 1962.
28. DAUGHARTY, T. M., L. J. BELLEAU, J. A. MARTINO, AND L. E. EARLEY. Interrelationship of physical factors affecting sodium reabsorption in the dog. *Am. J. Physiol.* 215: 1442–1447, 1968.
29. DAVANZO, J. P., H. C. CROSSFIELD, AND W. W. SWINGLE. Effect of various adrenal steroids on plasma magnesium and the electrocardiogram of adrenalectomized dogs. *Endocrinology* 63: 825–830, 1958.
30. DAVIS, J. O., W. C. BALL, JR., R. C. BAHN, AND M. J. GOODKIND. Relationship of adrenocortical and anterior pituitary function to fecal excretion of sodium and potassium. *Am. J. Physiol.* 196: 149–152, 1959.
31. DAVIS, J. O., J. URQUHART, J. T. HIGGINS, E. C. RUBIN, AND P. M. HARTROFT. Hypersecretion of aldosterone in dogs with a chronic aortic-caval fistula and high output heart failure. *Circulation Res.* 14: 471–485, 1964.
32. DE BERMUDEZ, L., AND J. P. HAYSLETT. Effect of methylprednisolone on sodium reabsorption and the zonal distribution of blood flow. *Abstr. Proc. Ann. Meeting Am. Soc. Nephrol., 5th, 1971*, p. 18.
33. DENTON, D. A. Salt appetite. In: *Handbook of Physiology. Alimentary Canal*, edited by C. F. Code. Washington, D. C.: Am. Physiol. Soc., 1967, sect. 6, vol. 1, chapt. 31, p. 433–459.
34. DINGMAN, J. F., AND R. H. DESPOINTES. Adrenal steroid inhibition of vasopressin release from the neurohypophysis of normal subjects and patients with Addisons disease. *J. Clin. Invest.* 39: 1851–1863, 1960.
35. DIRKS, J. H. Micropuncture study on the effect of ouabain and spironolactone on sodium reabsorption by the proximal tubule of the dog (Abstract). *Clin. Res.* 15: 356, 1967.
36. DIRKS, J. H., W. J. CIRKSENA, AND R. W. BERLINER. The effect of saline infusion on sodium reabsorption by the proximal tubule of the dog. *J. Clin. Invest.* 44: 1160–1170, 1965.
37. EARLEY, L. E. Influence of hemodynamic factors on sodium reabsorption. *Ann. NY Acad. Sci.* 139: 312–327, 1966.
38. EDELMAN, I. S., R. BOGOROCH, AND G. A. PORTER. On the mechanism of action of aldosterone on sodium transport. The role of protein synthesis. *Proc. Natl. Acad. Sci. US* 50: 1169–1177, 1963.
39. EDELMAN, I. S., R. BOGOROCH, AND G. A. PORTER. Specific action of aldosterone on RNA synthesis. *Trans. Assoc. Am. Physicians* 77: 307–316, 1964.
40. EDELMAN, I. S., AND G. M. FIMOGNARI. On the biochemical action of aldosterone. *Recent Progr. Hormone Res.* 24: 1–44, 1968.
41. EDMONDS, C. J., AND J. MARRIOTT. Sodium transport and short-circuit current in rat colon *in vivo* and the effect of aldosterone. *J. Physiol., London* 210: 1021–1039, 1970.
42. EDMONDS, C. J., AND P. RICHARDS. Measurement of rectal electrical potential difference as an instant screening test for hyperaldosteronism. *Lancet* 2: 624–627, 1970.
43. ELIEL, L. P., C. THOMSEN, AND R. CHANES. Antagonism between parathyroid extract and adrenal cortical steroids in man. *J. Clin. Endocrinol. Metab.* 25: 457–464, 1965.
44. ELMSLIE, R. G., A. T. MULHOLLAND, AND R. SHIELDS. Blocking by spironolactone (SG 9420) of the action of aldosterone upon the intestinal transport of potassium, sodium and water. *Gut* 7: 697–699, 1966.
45. EMERSON, K. E., S. S. KAHN, AND D. JENKINS. The role of the gastrointestinal tract in the adaptation of the body to the prevention of sodium depletion by cation exchange resins. *Ann. NY Acad. Sci.* 57: 280–290, 1953.
46. FANESTIL, D. D., AND I. S. EDELMAN. Characteristics of the renal nuclear receptors for aldosterone. *Proc. Natl. Acad. Sci. US* 56: 872–879, 1966.
47. FANESTIL, D. D., G. A. PORTER, AND I. S. EDELMAN. Aldosterone stimulation of sodium transport. *Biochim. Biophys. Acta* 135: 74–88, 1967.
48. FARBER, S. J., AND R. J. SOBERMAN. Total body water and total exchangeable sodium in edematous states due to cardiac, renal or hepatic disease. *J. Clin. Invest.* 35: 779–791, 1956.
49. FINKLESTEIN, J. D., AND D. SCHACHTER. Active transport of calcium by intestine: effects of hypophysectomy and growth hormone. *Am. J. Physiol.* 203: 873–880, 1962.
50. FINN, A. L., AND L. G. WELT. Effect of aldosterone administration on electrolyte excretion and glomerular filtration rate in the rat. *Am. J. Physiol.* 204: 243–244, 1963.
51. FOLLIS, R. H. Effect of cortisone on growing bones of the rat (18607). *Proc. Soc. Exptl. Biol. Med.* 76: 722–724, 1951.
52. FRAWLEY, T. F., AND G. W. THORN. The relationship of the salivary sodium-potassium ratio to adrenal cortical activity. In: *Proceedings of the Second Clinical ACTH Conference*, edited by J. R. Mote. London: Churchill, 1951, p. 115–122.
53. FRENCH, I. W., AND J. F. MANERY. The effect of aldosterone on electrolytes in muscle, kidney cortex and serum. *Can. J. Biochem.* 42: 1459–1476, 1964.
54. GALL, G., P. USHER, J. C. MELBY, AND R. KLEIN. Effects of aldosterone and cortisol on human erythrocyte Na^+ efflux. *J. Clin. Endocrinol. Metab.* 32: 555–561, 1971.
55. GARRETT, E. R., R. L. JOHNSTON, AND E. J. COLLINS. Kinetics of steroid effects on Ca^{47} dynamics in dogs with the analog computer. I. *J. Pharm. Sci.* 51: 1050–1057, 1962.
56. GIEBISCH, G., R. M. KLOSE, AND G. MALNIC. Renal tubular potassium transport. *Bull. Swiss Acad. Med. Sci.* 23: 287–312, 1967.
57. GILL, J. R., JR., D. S. GANN, AND F. C. BARTTER. Restoration of water diuresis in Addisonian patients by expansion of the volume of extracellular fluid. *J. Clin. Invest.* 41: 1078–1085, 1962.
58. GILL, J. R., JR. Edema. *Ann. Rev. Med.* 21: 269–280, 1970.
59. GOLDSMITH, C., F. C. RECTOR, JR., AND D. W. SELDIN. Evidence for a direct effect of serum sodium concentration on sodium reabsorption. *J. Clin. Invest.* 41: 850–859, 1962.
60. GOODMAN, D. B. P., J. E. ALLEN, AND H. RASMUSSEN. Studies on the mechanism of action of aldosterone hormone-induced changes in lipid metabolism. *Biochemistry* 10: 3825–3831, 1971.
61. GORDAN, G. S. Recent progress in calcium metabolism: clinical application. *Calif. Med.* 114: 28–43, 1971.
62. GORDAN, G. S., J. HANSEN, AND W. LUBICH. Effects of hormonal steroids on osteolysis. *Proc. Intern. Congr. Hormonal Steroids, 2nd. Excerpta Med. Found. Intern. Congr. Ser.* 132: 786–793, 1967.
63. GREEN, D. M., T. B. REYNOLDS, AND R. J. GIRERD. Mechanisms of desoxycorticosterone action. X. Effects on tissue sodium concentration. *Am. J. Physiol.* 181: 105–113, 1955.
64. GREEN, H. H., A. R. HARRINGTON, AND H. VALTIN. On the role of antidiuretic hormone in the inhibition of acute water diuresis in adrenal insufficiency and the effects of gluco- and mineralocorticoids in reversing the inhibition. *J. Clin. Invest.* 49: 1724–1736, 1970.
65. HANDLER, J. S., A. S. PRESTON, AND J. ORLOFF. The effect of aldosterone on glycolysis in the urinary bladder of the toad. *J. Biol. Chem.* 244: 3194–3199, 1969.
66. HARRISON, H. E., AND H. C. HARRISON. Transfer of Ca^{45} across intestinal wall in vitro in relation to action of Vitamin D and cortisol. *Am. J. Physiol.* 199: 265–271, 1960.
67. HENDLER, E. D., J. TORRETTI, AND F. H. EPSTEIN. The distribution of sodium-potassium-activated adenosine triphosphate in medulla and cortex of the kidney. *J. Clin. Invest.* 50: 1329–1337, 1971.
68. HENKIN, R. I., J. R. GILL, JR., AND F. C. BARTTER. Studies on taste thresholds in normal man and in patients with adrenal cortical insufficiency. The role of adrenal cortical steroids and of serum sodium concentration. *J. Clin. Invest.* 42: 727–735, 1963.
69. HENKIN, R. I., AND D. H. SOLOMON. Salt-taste threshold in

adrenal insufficiency in man. *J. Clin. Endocrinol. Metab.* 22: 856–858, 1962.
70. HERXHEIMER, A., AND D. M. WOODBURY. The effect of deoxycorticosterone on salt and sucrose taste preference thresholds and drinking behaviour in rats. *J. Physiol., London* 151: 253–260, 1960.
71. HIERHOLZER, K., W. WIEDERHOLT, H. HOLZGREVE, G. GIEBISCH, R. M. KLOSE, AND E. E. WINDHAGER. Micropuncture study of renal transtubular concentration gradients of sodium and potassium in adrenalectomized rats. *Arch. Ges. Physiol.* 285: 193–210, 1965.
72. HIERHOLZER, K., AND H. STOLTE. The proximal and distal tubular action of adrenal steroids on Na^+ reabsorption. *Nephron* 6: 188–204, 1969.
73. HIERHOLZER, K., W. WIEDERHOLT, AND H. STOLTE. Hemmung der Natrium-resorption im proximalen und distalen Konvolut adrenalektomierter Ratten. *Arch. Ges. Physiol.* 291: 43–62, 1966.
74. HOLUB, D. A., AND J. W. JAILER. Sodium and water diuresis in cirrhotic patients with intractable ascites following chemical inhibition of aldosterone synthesis. *Ann. Internal Med.* 53: 425–444, 1960.
75. HORTON, R., AND E. G. BIGLIERI. Effect of aldosterone on the metabolism of magnesium. *J. Clin. Endocrinol. Metab.* 22: 1187–1192, 1962.
76. IANNACONE, A., J. L. GABRILOVE, S. A. BRAHMS, AND L. J. SOFFER. Osteoporosis in Cushing's syndrome. *Ann. Internal Med.* 52: 570–586, 1960.
77. JOHNSTON, C. I., J. O. DAVIS, S. S. HOWARDS, AND F. S. WRIGHT. Cross circulation experiments on the mechanism of the natriuresis during saline loading in the dog. *Circulation Res.* 20: 1–10, 1967.
78. KASSIRER, J. P., F. M. APPLETON, J. A. CHAZAN, AND W. B. SCHWARTZ. Aldosterone in metabolic alkalosis. *J. Clin. Invest.* 46: 1558–1571, 1967.
79. KASSIRER, J. P., D. C. LOWANCE, AND W. B. SCHWARTZ. Aldosterone induced metabolic alkalosis in man. *Abstr. Ann. Meeting Am. Soc. Nephrol., 5th, 1971*, p. 36.
80. KATZ, A. I., AND F. H. EPSTEIN. The role of sodium-potassium-activated adenosine triphosphate in the reabsorption of Na^+ by the kidney. *J. Clin. Invest.* 46: 1999–2011, 1967.
81. KATZ, A. I., AND F. H. EPSTEIN. Physiologic role of sodium-potassium-activated adenosine triphosphate in the transport of cations across biologic membranes. *New Engl. J. Med.* 278: 253–261, 1968.
82. KIMBERG, D. V., R. D. BAERG, E. GERSHON, AND R. T. GRAUDUSIUS. Effect of cortisone treatment on the active transport of calcium by the small intestine. *J. Clin. Invest.* 50: 1309–1321, 1971.
83. KIRSTEN, E., R. KIRSTEN, A. LEAF, AND G. W. SHARP. Increased activity of enzymes of the tricarboxylic acid cycle in response to aldosterone in the toad bladder. *Arch. Ges. Physiol.* 300: 213–225, 1968.
84. KLEEMAN, C. R., J. W. CZACZKES, AND R. CUTLER. Mechanism of impaired water excretion in adrenal and pituitary insufficiency. IV. *J. Clin. Invest.* 43: 1641–1648, 1964.
85. KLEEMAN, C. R., J. KOPLOWITZ, M. H. MAXWELL, R. CUTLER, AND J. T. DOWLING. Mechanisms of impaired water excretion in adrenal and pituitary insufficiency. II. *J. Clin. Invest.* 39: 1472–1480, 1960.
86. KLEEMAN, C. R., M. H. MAXWELL, AND R. E. ROCKNEY. Mechanisms of impaired water excretion in adrenal and pituitary insufficiency. I. *J. Clin. Invest.* 37: 1799–1808, 1958.
87. KNOX, F. G., E. G. SCHNEIDER, T. P. DRESSER, AND R. E. LYNCH. Natriuretic effect of increased proximal delivery in dogs with salt restriction. *Am. J. Physiol.* 219: 904–910, 1970.
88. KURTZMAN, N. A., M. G. WHITE, AND P. W. ROGERS. Aldosterone deficiency and renal bicarbonate reabsorption. *J. Lab. Clin. Med.* 77: 931–940, 1971.
89. LANDON, E. J., N. JAZAB, AND L. FORTE. Aldosterone and sodium-potassium-dependent ATPase activity of rat kidney membranes. *Am. J. Physiol.* 211: 1050–1056, 1966.
90. LAULER, D. P., R. B. HICKLER, AND G. W. THORN. The salivary sodium-potassium ratio: a useful "screening test" for aldosteronism in hypertensive subjects. *New Engl. J. Med.* 267: 1136–1137, 1962.
91. LEMANN, J., JR., W. F. PIERING, AND E. J. LENNON. Studies of the acute effects of aldosterone and cortisol on the interrelationship between renal sodium, calcium and magnesium excretion in normal man. *Nephron* 7: 117–130, 1970.
92. LEVINSKY, N. G., AND R. C. LALONE. The mechanism of sodium diuresis after saline infusion in the dog. *J. Clin. Invest.* 42: 1261–1276, 1963.
93. LEVINSKY, N. G., AND R. C. LALONE. Sodium excretion during acute saline loading in dogs with vena caval constriction. *J. Clin. Invest.* 44: 565–573, 1965.
94. LEVITAN, R. Salt and water absorption from the normal human colon: effect of 9α fluorohydrocortisone administration. *J. Lab. Clin. Med.* 69: 558–564, 1967.
95. LIM, V. S., AND G. D. WEBSTER. The effect of aldosterone on water and electrolyte composition of incubated rat diaphragms. *Clin. Sci.* 33: 261–270, 1967.
96. LINDEMAN, R. D., J. HONARI, AND W. O. SMITH. Acute effects of cortisone and aldosterone on urinary divalent cation excretion. *Abstr. Ann. Meeting Am. Soc. Nephrol., 1st, Los Angeles, 1967*, p. 38.
97. LINDHEIMER, M. D., R. C. LALONE, AND N. G. LEVINSKY. Evidence that an acute increase in glomerular filtration has little effect on sodium excretion in the dog unless extracellular volume is expanded. *J. Clin. Invest.* 46: 256–265, 1967.
98. LUKE, R. G., AND H. LEVITIN. The renal and electrolyte response to respiratory acidosis in the adrenalectomized rat. *Yale J. Biol. Med.* 39: 27–37, 1966.
99. LYNCH, R. I., E. G. SCHNEIDER, L. R. WILLIS, AND F. G. KNOX. Effect of mineralocorticoids on proximal Na^+ reabsorption in dogs. *Abstr. Ann. Meeting Am. Soc. Nephrol., 5th, 1971*, p. 47.
100. MADER, I. J., AND L. T. ISERI. Spontaneous hypopotassemia, hypomagnesemia, alkalosis and tetany due to hypersecretion of corticosterone-like mineralocorticoids. *Am. J. Med.* 19: 976–988, 1955.
101. MALNIC, G., R. M. KLOSE, AND G. GIEBISCH. Micropuncture study of renal potassium excretion in the rat. *Am. J. Physiol.* 206: 674–686, 1964.
102. MARUMO, F. The effect of glucocorticoids on the water permeability of the toad bladder. *Arch. Ges. Physiol.* 299: 149–157, 1960.
103. MASSRY, S. G., J. W. COBURN, AND L. W. CHAPMAN. The effect of long-term desoxycorticosterone acetate administration on the renal excretion of calcium and magnesium. *J. Lab. Clin. Med.* 71: 212–219, 1968.
104. MCCANCE, R. A. The effect of salt deficiency in man on the volume of the extracellular fluids and on the composition of sweat, saliva, gastric juice and cerebrospinal fluid. *J. Physiol., London* 92: 208–218, 1938.
105. MCCONAHAY, T. P., S. ROBINSON, AND J. L. NEWTON. d-Aldosterone and sweat electrolytes. *J. Appl. Physiol.* 19: 575–579, 1964.
106. MILNE, M. D., R. D. MUEHRCKE, AND I. AIRD. Primary aldosteronism. *Quart. J. Med.* 26: 317–333, 1957.
107. MULROW, P. J. Aldosterone in hypertension and edema. In: *Duncan's Diseases of Metabolism* (6th ed.), edited by P. K. Bondy. Philadelphia: Saunders, 1969, p. 1083–1102.
108. MUNRO, D. S., R. S. SATOSKAR, AND G. M. WILSON. The effect of adrenalectomy on bone sodium metabolism. *J. Physiol., London* 142: 438–452, 1958.
109. MURAYAMA, Y., A. SUZUKI, M. TADOKORO, AND F. SAKAI. Microperfusion of Henle's loop in the kidney of the adrenalectomized rat. *Japan. J. Pharmacol.* 18: 518–519, 1968.
110. O'MALLEY, B. W. Unified hypothesis for early biochemical

sequence of events in steroid hormone action. *Metabolism* 20: 981–988, 1971.
111. PORTER, G. A., AND I. S. EDELMAN. The action of aldosterone and related corticosteroids on sodium transport across the toad bladder. *J. Clin. Invest.* 43: 611–620, 1964.
112. RAISZ, L. G., W. F. MCNEELY, L. SAXON, AND J. D. ROSENBAUM. The effects of cortisone and hydrocortisone on water diuresis and renal function in man. *J. Clin. Invest.* 36: 767–779, 1957.
113. REIDENBERG, M. M., AND R. W. SEVY. Effect of adrenocortical steroids on bone electrolyte metabolism (26557). *Proc. Soc. Exptl. Biol. Med.* 107: 132–134, 1961.
114. RICHARDS, P., K. SMITH, A. METCALFE-GIBSON, AND O. WRONG. Action of d-aldosterone on the electrolyte composition of human cells grown *in vitro*. *Lancet* 2: 1099–1102, 1966.
115. ROBINSON, S., J. R. NICHOLAS, J. H. SMITH, W. J. DALY, AND M. PEARCY. Time relation of renal and sweat gland adjustments to salt deficiency in man. *J. Appl. Physiol.* 8: 159–165, 1955.
116. ROTH, D. G., AND J. L. GAMBLE, JR. Deoxycorticosterone-induced alkalosis in dogs. *Am. J. Physiol.* 208: 90–93, 1965.
117. ROVNER, D. R., D. H. P. STREETEN, L. H. LOUIS, C. T. STEVENSON, AND J. W. CONN. Content and uptake of sodium and potassium in bone. *J. Clin. Endocrinol. Metab.* 23: 938–944, 1963.
118. SCHAMBELAN, M., P. E. SLATON, JR., AND E. G. BIGLIERI. Mineralocorticoid production in hyperadrenocorticism. *Am. J. Med.* 51: 299–303, 1971.
119. SCHULTZE, R. C., D. D. TAGGART, H. SHAPIRO, J. P. PENNELL, S. CAGLAR, AND N. S. BRICKER. On the adaptation in potassium excretion associated with nephron reduction in the dog. *J. Clin. Invest.* 50: 1061–1068, 1971.
120. SEALEY, J. E., AND J. H. LARAGH. Further studies of a natriuretic substance occurring in human urine and plasma. *Circulation Res.* 28, Suppl. II: 32–43, 1971.
121. SHARP, G. W. G., AND A. LEAF. Mechanism of action of aldosterone. *Physiol. Rev.* 46: 593–633, 1966.
122. SIEGENTHALER, P. P., R. DE HALLER, R. VEYRAT, AND A. F. MULLER. Influence d'un inhibiteur d'un antoganiste de l'aldosterone sur la concentration du sodium sudoral. Effet extra-renal des spirolactones. *Helv. Med. Acta* 29: 550–555, 1962.
123. SIMPSON, S. A., AND J. F. TAIT. Recent progress in methods of isolation, chemistry and physiology of aldosterone. *Recent Progr. Hormone Res.* 11: 183–219, 1955.
124. SONNENBLICK, E. H., P. J. CANNON, AND J. H. LARAGH. The nature of the action of intravenous aldosterone: evidence for a role of the hormone in urinary dilution. *J. Clin. Invest.* 40: 903–913, 1961.
125. SPACH, C., AND D. H. P. STREETEN. Retardation of sodium exchange in dog erythrocytes by physiologic concentrations of aldosterone *in vitro*. *J. Clin. Invest.* 43: 217–227, 1964.
126. STOLTE, H., J. P. BRECHT, M. WIEDERHOLT, AND K. HIERHOLZER. Influence of adrenalectomy and glucocorticoid hormones on water permeability of superficial nephron segments in the rat kidney. *Arch. Ges. Physiol.* 299: 99–127, 1968.
127. STOLTE, H., M. WIEDERHOLT, AND K. HIERHOLZER. Resorpshemmung im proximalen Konvolut der Saugetierniere nach Adrenalektomie und ihre Beeinflussung durch Steroidhormone. In: *Aktuelle Probleme der Nephrologie*, edited by H. P. Woff and F. Kruck. Berlin: Springer Verlag, 1966, p. 521–527.

128. STREETEN, D. H. P., AND A. M. MOSES. Action of cortisol on sodium transport in canine erythrocytes. *J. Gen. Physiol.* 52: 346–362, 1968.
129. STREETEN, D. H. P., A. RAPOPORT, AND J. W. CONN. Existence of a slowly exchangeable pool of body sodium in normal subjects and its diminution in patients with primary aldosteronism. *J. Clin. Endocrinol. Metab* 23: 928–937, 1963.
130. SUKI, W. N., R. S. SCHWETMANN, F. C. RECTOR, AND D. W. SELDIN. The effect of chronic mineralocorticoid administration on calcium excretion in the rat (Abstract). *Clin. Res.* 15: 372, 1967.
131. SWINGLE, W. W., J. P. DAVANZO, D. GLENISTER, H. C. CROSSFIELD, AND C. WAGLE. Role of gluco- and mineralocorticoids in salt and water metabolism of adrenalectomized dogs. *Am. J. Physiol.* 196: 283–286, 1959.
132. THATCHER, J. S., AND A. W. RADIKE. Tolerance to potassium intoxication in the albino rat. *Am. J. Physiol.* 151: 138–146, 1947.
133. THOMPSON, B. D., AND C. J. EDMONDS. Comparison of effects of prolonged aldosterone administration on rat colon and renal electrolyte excretion. *J. Endocrinol.* 50: 163–169, 1971.
134. THOMPSON, J., AND M. R. URIST. Influence of cortisone and calcitonin on bone morphogenesis. *Clin. Orthopaedics* 71: 253–270, 1970.
135. VANCURA, P., G. W. G. SHARP, AND R. A. MALT. Kinetics of RNA synthesis in toad bladder epithelium: action of aldosterone during the latent period. *J. Clin. Invest.* 50: 543–551, 1971.
136. VANDER, A. J., R. L. MALVIN, W. S. WILDE, J. LAPIDES, L. P. SULLIVAN, AND V. M. MCMURRAY. Effects of adrenalectomy and aldosterone on proximal and distal tubular sodium reabsorption (24338). *Proc. Soc. Exptl. Biol. Med.* 99: 323–325, 1958.
137. WIEDERHOLT, M. Mikropunktionsuntersuchungen am proximalen und distalen Konvolut der Ratteniere über den Einfluss von Actinomycin D auf den Mineralocorticoidabhangigen Na-transport. *Arch. Ges. Physiol.* 292: 334–342, 1966.
138. WILLIAMS, M. A., AND W. I. BABA. The localization of (^{3}H) aldosterone and (^{3}H) cortisol within renal tubular cells by electron microscope autoradiography. *J. Endocrinol.* 39: 543–554, 1967.
139. WOLF, G., AND E. A. STEINBAUM. Sodium appetite elicited by subcutaneous formalin: mechanism of action. *J. Comp. Physiol. Psychol.* 59: 335–339, 1965.
140. WOLFE, G. Sodium appetite elicited by desoxycorticosterone. *Dissertation Abstr.* 26: 2343, 1965.
141. WRIGHT, F. S., F. G. KNOX, S. S. HOWARDS, AND R. W. BERLINER. Reduced sodium reabsorption by the proximal tubule of DOCA-escaped dogs. *Am. J. Physiol.* 216: 869–875, 1969.
142. WRONG, O., A. METCALFE-GIBSON, R. B. I. MORRISON, S. T. NG, AND A. V. HOWARD. *In vivo* dialysis of faeces as a method of stool analysis. *Clin. Sci.* 28: 357–375, 1965.
143. WRONG, O., R. B. I. MORRISON, AND P. E. HURST. A method of obtaining faecal fluid by *in vivo* dialysis. *Lancet* 1: 1208–1209, 1961.
144. YUNIS, S. L., D. D. BERCOVITCH, R. M. STEIN, M. F. LEVITT, AND M. H. GOLDSTEIN. Renal tubular effects of hydrocortisone and aldosterone in normal hydropenic man: comment on sites of action. *J. Clin. Invest.* 43: 1668–1676, 1964.

CHAPTER 14

Corticosteroids and circulatory function

ALLAN M. LEFER | *Department of Physiology, University of Virginia School of Medicine, Charlottesville, Virginia*[1]

CHAPTER CONTENTS

Cardiovascular Consequences of Chronic Adrenocortical Insufficiency
   Heart
   Peripheral vasculature
   Blood volume
Cardiac Effects of Corticosteroids
   Inotropic effects in isolated cardiac tissue
     Mineralocorticoids
     Glucocorticoids
   In whole animal
     Electrocardiographic effects
     Myocardial metabolic effects
     Inotropic effects
Peripheral Vascular Effects of Corticosteroids
   Blood pressure and vascular resistance
   Microcirculation
   Isolated vascular smooth muscle
Role of Corticosteroids in Blood Volume Regulation
Interaction Between Corticosteroids and Other Agents in Regulation of Circulatory Function
   Catecholamines
   Renin and angiotensin II
   Cardiac glycosides
   Kinins
Summary and Conclusions

CORTICOSTEROIDS are ubiquitous humoral agents that influence the functional status of virtually every organ system and thus play a key role in preserving and maintaining total body homeostasis (137). Adrenal hormones have been recognized as circulatory regulating hormones since 1849, when Addison described a state of circulatory collapse to be a prominent feature of adrenal insufficiency (2). Approximately a century elapsed before the chemical structures of the corticosteroids became known. Thus it has only been in recent years that synthetic corticosteroids have been available for investigation. Cardiovascular studies of corticosteroids have received considerable attention because of the prominent hypotension observed in adrenal insufficiency and the

[1] Present address: Department of Physiology, Jefferson Medical College, Thomas Jefferson University, Philadelphia, Pennsylvania.

marked degree of hypertension resulting from hypersecretion of adrenal corticosteroids (e.g., Conn's syndrome, Cushing's syndrome). Nevertheless the basic mechanisms of the cardiovascular actions of corticosteroids are only recently emerging.

The major purposes of this review are to evaluate and define *a)* the physiological and pharmacological actions of corticosteroids on the heart and peripheral vasculature, *b)* the cardiovascular consequences of removal of the circulating corticosteroids, and *c)* the interaction between corticosteroids and other humoral agents on circulatory function.

CARDIOVASCULAR CONSEQUENCES OF CHRONIC ADRENOCORTICAL INSUFFICIENCY

The essential role of the corticosteroids in the homeostatic regulation of the cardiovascular system can be readily appreciated by the extent of the circulatory disturbances observed in their absence. Total adrenalectomy results in a marked hypotension and a severe reduction in cardiac output. The adrenalectomized animal is in a precarious hypodynamic state, so that exposure to noxious stimuli (e.g., cold, hemorrhage, infection) often results in circulatory collapse.

In Figure 1 the circulatory changes that occur 10 days after bilateral adrenalectomy in the cat are depicted. Arterial blood pressure, cardiac output, and heart rate decrease. Peripheral resistance is elevated, but left atrial pressure and blood volume are not significantly altered. These changes are very similar to those occurring in the chronically adrenalectomized dog (123).

There has been much controversy over the locus of the primary circulatory defect in chronic insufficiency. Some workers claim that the heart is the primary site of impairment (22, 43, 80, 86, 122, 172), whereas others emphasize peripheral vascular dysfunction (50, 118, 119, 176, 180) or hypovolemia (157, 158, 178) as the main factor contributing to the circulatory failure. The experimental evidence in support of each of these three major hypotheses is evaluated.

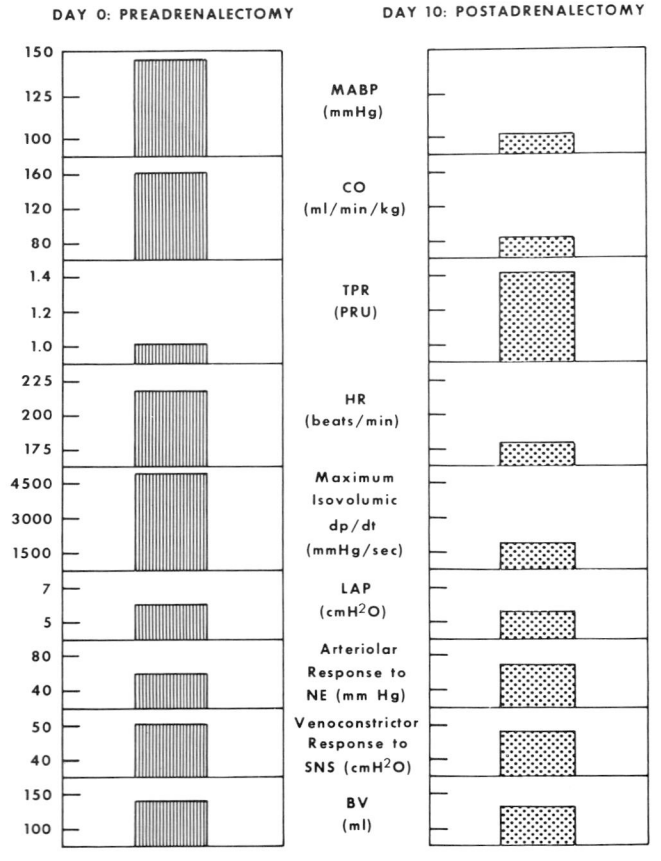

FIG. 1. Hemodynamic status of chronically adrenalectomized, anesthetized cats 10 days postadrenalectomy compared with that of preadrenalectomy controls. *MABP*, mean arterial blood pressure; *CO*, cardiac output; *TPR*, total peripheral resistance; *PRU*, peripheral resistance units; *HR*, heart rate; *LAP*, left atrial pressure; *SNS*, sympathetic nerve stimulation; *NE*, norepinephrine; *BV*, blood volume. Ten days postadrenalectomy MABP and CO are significantly reduced, whereas TPR is elevated. Maximum isovolumic dP/dt (i.e., the maximal rate of generation of pressure in the left ventricle) is reduced 40%, indicating a major cardiac impairment. However, LAP, an index of cardiac filling pressure, is essentially normal, which suggests that the defect in the heart is not due to diminished venous return. Arteriolar response to intraarterially injected norepinephrine is normal, as is response of capacitance vessels to sympathetic nerve stimulation. Blood volume is only slightly reduced. Thus the overall hemodynamic picture is one of severe cardiac impairment without any major peripheral vascular dysfunction.

Heart

Evidence is accumulating for an impairment of cardiac performance in chronic adrenal insufficiency. The alterations in a variety of anatomic, mechanical, and biochemical indices of cardiac function are summarized in Table 1. The most important single finding is that the performance of the heart as a pump is severely impaired in adrenal insufficiency. Lefer & Sutfin (85) have reported a substantial decrease in the developed tension of the heart in adrenal insufficiency. Webb et al. (172) and Lefer et al. (86) also found a large depression in cardiac contractility in adrenalectomized dogs and cats by ventricular function curve analysis. These tests assess the reserve capacity of the left ventricle. Similar degrees of depression in peak left ventricular pressure or the first derivative of pressure with respect to time (i.e., dP/dt) have also been observed (169) and indicate that the mechanical performance of the heart as muscular tissue is also impaired. Furthermore, Solomon et al. (147) found the left ventricular work index of rat heart-lung preparations obtained from chronically adrenalectomized rats to be reduced 72%, a finding that also points to a mechanical defect in cardiac muscle. These severe changes occurred, despite only a 10% reduction in dry heart weight. These modest decreases in heart weight have been found in rats (7, 64), but not in cats (134), which indicates that cardiac atrophy is only a small component of the cardiac defect.

The mechanical performance of papillary muscles isolated from adrenalectomized rats was also depressed

TABLE 1. *Summary of Cardiac Changes in Adrenal Insufficiency*

Finding	Implication	Ref.
Tension developed and dP/dt decreased, 40–60%	Impaired mechanical performance of the myocardium	85, 169
Ventricular function depressed, 50%		86, 172
Work performance decreased, 70%		147
Cardiac dry weight slightly decreased or unchanged	Atrophy of heart is not a major factor	7, 64, 133, 147
Electrophysiological properties normal when corrected for K$^+$	Membrane properties of heart are not impaired	101, 132
No consistent changes observed in myofibrils	The ultrastructural changes observed are difficult to correlate with the mechanical findings	43, 133
Cardiac glycogen decreased	Alterations in carbohydrate storage are probably not responsible for weakened cardiac performance	10, 40, 41
Cardiac catecholamine content not altered	Adrenergic mechanisms are probably normal in the heart	73, 174
Cardiac K$^+$ and H$_2$O concentration normal	Electrolyte balance and ionic pumps can function adequately although renal tubules may be performing inadequately	107
ATPase activity decreased	Rate of conversion of chemical to mechanical energy may be an important factor	133, 134

(82). Although cardiac excitability and contractility were essentially normal in freshly isolated papillary muscles from adrenalectomized rats (82, 165), 3 hr after removal from the heart these papillary muscles exhibited a 51% decline in initial developed tension compared with only an 11% decrease for controls. This latent decline in mechanical performance has recently been observed in atria isolated from adrenalectomized rats (53). No measurements of force-velocity relations are available in isolated cardiac preparations from adrenalectomized animals. Therefore a defect in the velocity of contraction that was not observed may have existed initially after isolation of cardiac tissue. Despite this gap in our understanding, considerable evidence points to an impairment of cardiac performance in chronic adrenal insufficiency, which is of sufficient magnitude to be a major contributory factor to the postadrenalectomy circulatory collapse.

The ultrastructural status of the heart in adrenal insufficiency is not clear at the present time. Sufficient high-quality electron micrographs and controls for mixing and staining artifacts are lacking, so that no consensus may be reached at present regarding the status of myocardial ultrastructure in adrenal insufficiency. It is clear, however, that sarcomere length differs among cardiac preparations, and this variation alone can cause apparent alterations in the appearance of the myofibrils (133). Thus no convincing changes in myocardial ultrastructure that could explain functional impairment of the myocardium observed in adrenalectomized animals have been reported.

Few biochemical studies on the heart in adrenal insufficiency are presently available. Russell & Bloom (135) did not detect any significant changes in cardiac glycogen of adrenalectomized rats, although others (10, 40, 41) have reported marked decreases in the same species. Diurnal rhythms can partially mask these changes if the experiments are not carefully controlled. Dexamethasone prevented the decline in cardiac concentration in adrenalectomized rats, whereas deoxycorticosterone acetate (DCA) was ineffective in this respect (40). It is unlikely that the decreased cardiac glycogen concentration initiates the profound decline in cardiac performance in the adrenalectomized animal because *a*) the heart primarily utilizes fatty acids rather than carbohydrates, and *b*) the decrease in cardiac glycogen occurs after cardiac performance is markedly impaired in the adrenalectomized cat (133).

In a promising new approach to the understanding of the cardiac defect in adrenal insufficiency, Rovetto and associates (134) demonstrated a 40% reduction in myofibrillar adenosine triphosphatase (ATPase) activity in hearts isolated from adrenalectomized cats. Comparable decreases in ATPase activity also occurred in extracted actomyosin, as well as purified myosin, which indicates that the defect probably occurs in the contractile machinery per se. Since dexamethasone prevented the decrease in myosin ATPase activity and since the myosin ATPase activity was closely correlated with peak left ventricular power development (133) the defect in myosin ATPase activity may represent a critical step in the impaired myocardial performance in the adrenalectomized animal. Further studies on the alterations of the myosin molecule may prove fruitful in explaining the cardiac impairment of adrenal insufficiency.

Webb & Degerli (171) found a decrease in cardiac oxygen consumption and CO_2 production in chronic adrenalectomy when measured in vivo. However, these changes in cardiac metabolism are probably nonspecific and may be secondary to a low arterial blood pressure and cardiac output. No changes in cardiac and plasma catecholamine levels have been reported in adrenalectomized dogs [(73); R. W. Sevy, personal communication] and rats (174) 2 or 3 weeks after adrenalectomy. Thus neither catecholamine deficiency nor an impaired rate of myocardial cellular metabolism appears to play a decisive role in the depression of ventricular performance in adrenalectomized animals.

Electrocardiographic (ECG) abnormalities frequently occur in adrenalectomized animals and progressively worsen with the severity of the adrenal insufficiency. The first ECG alteration that usually occurs is an increase in the amplitude of the T wave (129). Subsequently the T wave broadens (129, 150), the S-T segment becomes depressed (150), and the P wave progressively flattens and, in some cases, may disappear entirely (106, 129, 150). Frequently the remaining ventricular complexes may show bizarre arrhythmias (59, 106, 129). The most commonly cited hypothesis for the ECG alterations seen in adrenal insufficiency is an increase in the plasma K^+ concentration (106, 129, 150, 177). However, increased plasma K^+ does not explain the phenomenon, since several workers (36, 66) have shown that ECG changes are observed in the adrenalectomized dog after K^+ levels have been restored to normal. Moreover, intravenous addition of potassium to concentrations exceeding that observed in adrenalectomized animals did not produce the ECG abnormalities seen in adrenal insufficiency (106).

Very few quantitative electrophysiological studies have been performed on hearts from adrenalectomized animals. Monnereau-Soustre et al. (101) have observed a 15-mv decrease in the resting potential of the rat heart after chronic adrenalectomy. Rovetto & Lefer (132) have shown that the decrease in the resting potential of papillary muscles from adrenalectomized rats occurs only in the presence of an elevated extracellular K^+ concentration. Thus the resting potential of cardiac muscle cells passively coincides with the predicted value calculated from the Nernst equation (i.e., resting potential proportional to log of ratio of internal K^+ concentration over external K^+ concentration), as do cells from normal rats. Furthermore the configuration of the intracellular ventricular action potential is normal (132). Thus the hyperkalemia observed in adrenal insufficiency does not directly produce arrhythmias or alter the waveform of the cardiac action potential, but only causes a partial depolarization of the resting membrane potential.

Finally, no significant changes in myocardial intracellular water or electrolyte concentrations have been reported in adrenal insufficiency (107); this indicates that defects in cation transport probably are not of sufficient magnitude to critically alter cardiac performance.

Peripheral Vasculature

That peripheral vascular collapse is a prominent feature of the circulatory collapse observed in adrenal insufficiency has been championed by Ramey and co-workers (118, 119). This hypothesis is based on observations in adrenalectomized animals subjected to various nonspecific stimuli in which the observed circulatory collapse was attributed to a weakness of the corticosteroid-deprived vasculature to maintain its constrictor tone in the face of excessive levels of catecholamines. This hypothesis is supported by the studies of Fritz & Levine (50) who demonstrated that the mesoappendix vasculature of salt-maintained, adrenalectomized rats was not only initially less responsive to topically applied norepinephrine, but eventually became completely unresponsive to repeated applications of the drug. These observations were later confirmed by others in studies with the hamster cheek pouch (176) and rat mesoappendix (4, 180). These changes certainly provide evidence for an impaired circulatory system but do not directly implicate the peripheral vasculature since a large impairment of cardiac contractility could account for these findings.

Other investigators have failed to observe major abnormalities in the constrictor response of the splanchnic vessels after chronic adrenalectomy (22, 47, 168). Verrier et al. (168) found the resistance vessels of the mesenteric circulation to be constricted 10 days after adrenalectomy in the cat. Furthermore there was no tendency for an impaired responsiveness of this bed to intraarterially injected norepinephrine. A similar lack of vascular impairment has been reported by Fowler & Cleghorn (47), who observed a clearly discernible vasoconstriction in response to either intravenously administered catecholamines or to splanchnic nerve stimulation in the moribund adrenalectomized cat.

Several investigators observed normal pressure-flow relations in the femoral bed and showed the bed to be constricted after chronic adrenalectomy in the dog (22, 131) and cat (168, 173). No data on the properties of blood vessels from other vascular beds (e.g., renal, cerebral, and skeletal muscle beds) are presently available. However, isolated strips of renal, femoral, and carotid arteries from adrenalectomized dogs were found to exhibit normal responsiveness to norepinephrine and angiotensin II (R. W. Sevy, personal communication), which indicates that these vessels have the capacity to constrict to appropriate humoral stimuli.

Chronic adrenalectomy results in an elevated total peripheral resistance (TPR) in dogs (123, 172), cats, and rats (173). Thus the net effect of chronic adrenalectomy on the resistance vessels (i.e., small arteries and arterioles) is to produce a generalized vasoconstriction. Therefore the hypotension observed cannot be attributed to an inability of the resistance vessels to maintain their tone. Rather it would appear that the increase in TPR represents a generalized reflex vasoconstriction in response to the systemic hypotension observed in the adrenalectomized animal.

Although central venous pressure is normal in chronic adrenal insufficiency (168, 173), very little is known about the functional status of the capacitance vessels (i.e., small veins and venules) and of venous return to the heart in adrenocortical insufficiency. Recently, Verrier et al. (168) found the venomotor response of the leg bed in the chronically adrenalectomized cat to be normal, which suggested that the neuroeffector junction, as well as the venous smooth muscle, was not impaired. Further studies would be helpful in determining whether capacitance vessels in other beds contribute to a decreased venous return, which could diminish cardiac function in adrenal insufficiency, although the fact that central venous pressure is normal provides an argument against a large decrease in venomotor tone.

The concept that chronic adrenal insufficiency is associated with a large increase in capillary permeability is controversial. An increased lymphatic protein concentration has been observed in the terminal stages of adrenal insufficiency and is suggestive of an increased capillary permeability (30). This may reflect proteolysis and a generalized damage to membranes in the terminal state. Moreover, Renkin & Zaun (128) were unable to demonstrate any significant differences between control and adrenalectomized preparations with respect to capillary permeability to fluids, proteins, or sucrose. Furthermore since a major reduction in blood volume does not occur it seems unlikely that increased capillary permeability is a major factor in the postadrenalectomy circulatory collapse. Rather, the stasis in the microcirculatory beds (i.e., hamster cheek pouch and rat mesoappendix) observed during adrenal insufficiency (176, 180) can be attributed to poor cardiac performance. Direct studies, such as iontophoresis of small amounts of vasoactive agents directly on localized microvascular components correlated with quantitation of the responses of these vessels, would help to resolve this important question.

Blood Volume

There have been numerous reports of a decreased blood volume after chronic adrenalectomy (21, 157, 158, 178), and several investigators (156–158) have suggested that a reduction in blood volume is the primary event in the circulatory failure seen in adrenal insufficiency. However, postadrenalectomy circulatory collapse can occur in the normovolemic animal (25, 169). Consideration of the species, steroidal regimen, sodium intake, and stage of insufficiency (i.e., moderate vs. terminal), however, can clarify many of the apparently contradictory findings.

Wyman & tum Suden (178) found a 22 % decrease in blood volume in 30 % of their adrenalectomized rats (not steroid supported), whereas no change in blood volume was observed in the remaining 70 %. Similarly, Hechter (61) has found that adrenalectomized rats allowed free access to saline maintained a normal blood volume. Only in the terminal stages of adrenal crisis were large decreases in blood volume observed in most cases (178). The situation is comparable in adrenalectomized cats. Britton & Silvette (21) observed a 20 % decrease in blood volume in adrenalectomized cats not maintained on saline. Verrier et al. (169) have since observed a 21 % reduction in blood volume under similar conditions and have shown that saline maintenance alone, without steroid support, is sufficient to maintain a normal blood volume. Thus the rat and cat are quite resistant to hypovolemia, even in the absence of free access to dietary sodium.

In the adrenalectomized dog, blood volume has been reported to decrease only 17 % (25) in saline-maintained animals, but decreases of 33–35 % (52, 158) have been reported in a more severe degree of insufficiency, and decreases of 42–46 % (25, 157) were observed in the terminal stages. Thus a severe hypovolemia can occur in the dog, although this usually is a late or a terminal event. Although frank hypovolemia is probably not a major causative factor of the circulatory collapse observed in chronic adrenal insufficiency in some species, one cannot completely disregard even a moderate degree of hypovolemia in view of the fact that the adrenalectomized animal is quite sensitive to hemorrhage. Thus a moderate degree of hypovolemia may contribute to the post-adrenalectomy circulatory collapse since cardiac reserve is very low in these animals.

CARDIAC EFFECTS OF CORTICOSTEROIDS

Inotropic Effects in Isolated Cardiac Tissue

Many investigators have found that relatively low concentrations of a variety of corticosteroids exert cardiotonic actions on isolated heart preparations. Some preparations are more sensitive to corticosteroids than others, and other preparations are responsive to one or several corticosteroids. Only rabbit atria appear to be unresponsive to corticosteroids (20, 87, 90).

MINERALOCORTICOIDS. Aldosterone, the most potent naturally occurring mineralocorticoid present in all higher vertebrates, has been widely tested in isolated cardiac preparations. It has been shown to exert a positive inotropic effect in papillary muscles isolated from cats (80, 81, 93, 95, 138, 160), guinea pigs (138), and monkeys (104) in concentrations on the order of 10^{-9} M but was ineffective in rat trabeculae carneae under similar experimental conditions (166). Aldosterone was also found to be ineffective over a wide range of concentrations in isolated frog hearts (54, 57). This unresponsiveness is probably not due to the lower temperature of the perfusate because aldosterone was shown to exert a slightly greater positive inotropic effect in mammalian cardiac tissue at 27 than at 37 C (81). Sayers & Solomon (139) found a similar lack of temperature specificity with other corticosteroids in the rat heart-lung preparation.

In the blood-perfused rat heart-lung preparation, physiological concentrations of aldosterone enabled the heart to perform two to four times as much work as that performed without aldosterone (9). However, this effect may not have been due solely to an inotropic action since one cannot exclude beneficial effects on the pulmonary or coronary vasculature in this preparation. In contrast, aldosterone (5, 68) failed to exert a positive inotropic effect in the blood-perfused dog heart-lung preparation. This lack of response in the dog heart-lung preparation is not due to a concentration effect. However, aldosterone may exert a restorative effect only on the corticosteroid-deficient myocardium and be ineffective in the presence of normal corticosteroid concentrations, since it was ineffective when perfused with normal blood (5, 68) but was effective when perfused with corticosteroid-depleted blood (9).

It should be noted that aldosterone exerts a maximum positive inotropic effect of only 20–35 %, a value considerably less than that exerted by cardiac glycosides or catecholamines (138, 162) under comparable experimental conditions (see Fig. 2). Therefore, although aldosterone does exert a cardiotonic effect, the effect is modest and should not be considered a substitute for cardiac glycosides or a panacea for cardiac failure.

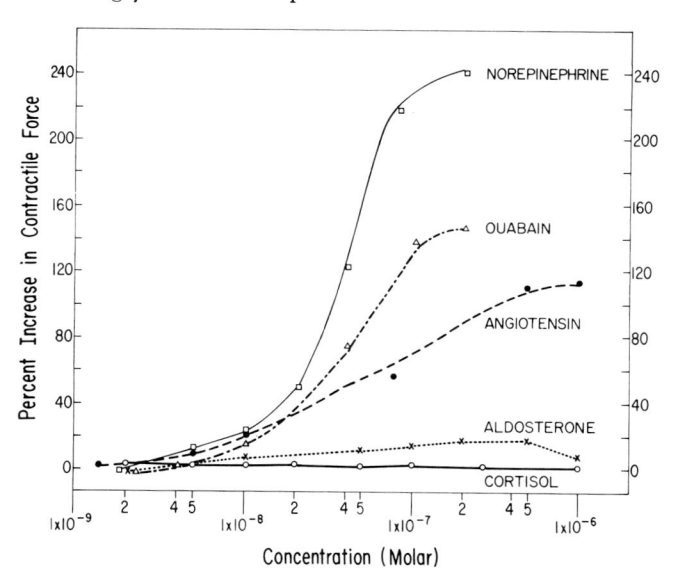

FIG. 2. Relative inotropic effects of aldosterone and cortisol compared with those of other more commonly used inotropic agents. All studies performed on isolated cat papillary muscles under identical conditions of stretch, frequency of contraction, temperature, and chemical composition of bathing solution. Aldosterone in a concentration of 10^{-8} to 5×10^{-7} M exerted a clearly discernible positive inotropic effect in this preparation. However, the magnitude of response observed is much less than that seen with norepinephrine, ouabain, or angiotensin. Inotropic activity of cortisol is negligible.

Other mineralocorticoids have been shown to exert positive inotropic effects in isolated cardiac tissue. Deoxycorticosterone (DOC) exerts a positive inotropic effect in the isolated frog heart (57, 58, 65, 96) and in the dog heart-lung preparation (5). However the β-glucoside of DOC is not as effective as the aglycone (68, 96). Low doses of DOC have been reported to stimulate beating rat and chick heart fragments in tissue culture (98), but high doses of DOC are depressant in these preparations (31, 32). Similar biphasic effects occur in isolated guinea pig hearts (65) and in the electrically driven cat papillary muscle preparation (46). In general, DOC in moderate doses exerts a small positive inotropic effect, which is slightly more effective than that of its acetate and substantially more active than that of its β-glucoside. High doses of DOC are generally depressant, although in some cases this depressant effect may be due to the steroid vehicle.

The potent synthetic mineralocorticoid, 9α-fluorocortisol (9αFF), which also has some glucocorticoid activity in high concentrations, possesses cardiotonic properties. Nayler (105) found that 9αFF increased the work and efficiency of the isolated toad heart, but to a lesser extent than did cardiac glycosides. Tanz and collaborators (161, 163) reported that 9αFF protected the cellular integrity of cardiac muscle cells, which normally degenerate after several hours of electrical stimulation in an isolated tissue bath. Another halogen-substituted steroid, 2α-methyl-9α-fluorocortisol, which has mineralocorticoid potency similar to that of aldosterone, did not exert a significant inotropic effect in isolated cat papillary muscles (81), but the ethanol vehicle may have masked a potential inotropic effect. Several of these studies emphasize the importance of careful controls for the steroid solvent or vehicle, many of which have direct effects on cardiac tissue.

Most mineralocorticoids therefore exert positive inotropic effects that are modest when compared to the much larger inotropic effects observed with cardiac glycosides or catecholamines tested under the same conditions as the mineralocorticoids (see Fig. 2). There is a relatively long latent period for the inotropic effect of mineralocorticoids (i.e., about 20–60 min for attainment of the peak effect). This latency is similar to that observed with aldosterone in the intact animal and may represent a period of enzyme induction (44) or tissue binding (67) that may be obligatory for the action of these steroids. The inotropic effect of mineralocorticoids is probably not directly mediated by sodium and potassium transport or by coronary blood flow changes since it can occur in the absence of these changes. The inotropic effect is enhanced under conditions of cardiac hypodynamia, a feature shared with many other inotropic agents (e.g., ouabain, angiotensin, norepinephrine) (13).

GLUCOCORTICOIDS. The two major naturally occurring glucocorticoids, corticosterone and cortisol, have not been shown to exert a convincing inotropic effect. Several investigators have failed to find any inotropic activity of cortisol in the isolated frog (58), cat, or guinea pig heart (138), in the dog heart-lung preparation (68), or in several papillary muscle preparations (46, 138). Depressant effects of the vehicles may have masked possible inotropic effects since the aqueous form of cortisol exerted a small, positive inotropic effect (81) at concentrations of the free base usually found to be depressant (46). Cortisol has been shown to stimulate the rate of embryonic chick heart fragments (31, 32), the endurance of rat heart-lung preparations (139), and the overall performance of acidotic dog heart-lung preparations (102), but no direct inotropic measurements were made in any of these studies. Thus cortisol may not have actually exerted a direct inotropic effect in these experiments. The beneficial or cardiotonic action of cortisol may therefore have been due to a metabolic or other cellular effect.

Corticosterone did not stimulate the frog heart (57, 58) or the dog heart-lung preparation (5), and a cardiodepressant effect of corticosterone was reported in isolated rat hearts (103) and in embryonic chick heart fragments (31). However, corticosterone was a potent cardiotonic agent in the rat heart-lung preparation (139, 147). In these experimental preparations, high doses of corticosterone clearly depressed the heart. Thus the evidence does not favor the view that corticosterone exerts a direct positive inotropic effect, although it may improve cardiac function indirectly.

Several other glucocorticoids have been tested for inotropic activity in isolated heart preparations. Cortisone, in low-to-moderate concentrations, exerts a small cardiotonic effect in several mammalian preparations (32, 65, 159, 162), but not in the isolated frog heart (58), whereas high doses of cortisone uniformly depressed the heart (46, 159). Prednisolone (5, 81, 162), methylprednisolone, dexamethasone (81), and betamethasone (81) appear to have no significant inotropic activity, and 11-dehydrocorticosterone depressed cat papillary muscles (46) under similar conditions.

Thus glucocorticoids exert small, positive inotropic effects, if at all, usually at high concentrations. The inotropic action of these steroids, when it occurs, may be partially due to the mineralocorticoid effects exerted by these steroids at high doses. In this regard, several of the more potent synthetic glucocorticoids that do not have salt-retaining properties (e.g., prednisolone and methylprednisolone) are devoid of inotropic activity. Despite the lack of prominent inotropic effects, glucocorticoids may be essential for the maintenance of normal cardiac activity by some other action since glucocorticoids appear to be necessary for completely normal cardiac function in adrenalectomized animals.

In Whole Animal

The cardiac effects of corticosteroids are more difficult to interpret in the whole animal. The rate of inactivation of corticosteroids is more rapid in the intact animal than in isolated systems because of the presence of the liver, kidneys, and other metabolic systems (e.g., plasma enzymes and blood cells). Furthermore one cannot be sure of the directness of the effect in the whole animal unless cardiac or peripheral factors are rigidly controlled. The secretory status of the animal's own adrenal cortices can present a problem if the rate of secretion is abnormal or if it varies during the course of an experiment. Because of these problems one must interpret effects in the whole animal with some degree of caution.

ELECTROCARDIOGRAPHIC EFFECTS. There have been several studies of the electrocardiographic effects of corticosteroids (1, 36, 37, 129). Cortisone in high doses (12.5 mg/kg per day) increased the amplitude of the P wave, the QRS complex, and the T wave in the rabbit; this increase was accompanied by an elevation of the S-T segment (1) in the absence of changes in serum electrolytes. These are generally the opposite of ECG changes seen in adrenalectomized animals. Roberts (129) also found that cortisone restored ECG abnormalities in adrenalectomized dogs without altering serum electrolyte concentrations. These normalizing effects were manifested as an increase in the amplitude of the P wave and a narrowing of the T wave and may indicate an enhanced velocity of conduction of the cardiac excitation wave. Similar ECG effects of cortisone have also been reported in adrenalectomized hamsters (177). Da Vanzo et al. (37) found that excess administration of a variety of mineralocorticoids was associated with a diphasic T wave, whereas excess administration of glucocorticoids induced an inverted T wave. However, these effects are probably not related to any significant hemodynamic effect. Thus corticosteroids appear to exert a general normalizing role on the electrocardiogram. Apparently high doses of most corticosteroids, in themselves, do not produce arrhythmias.

MYOCARDIAL METABOLIC EFFECTS. Little information is available on the effects of corticosteroids on myocardial metabolism. Daw et al. (40) showed that dexamethasone increased the cardiac glycogen concentration of adrenalectomized and normal rats within 4 hr (41), whereas DCA was ineffective in both conditions. The fact that dexamethasone increased the cardiac glycogen concentration above normal values suggests that the effect of the glucocorticoid is more than merely permissive, as postulated by Ingle (69). Dexamethasone simultaneously increased total glycogen transferase activity and decreased the activity of the active form of this regulatory enzyme. This alteration in glycogen transferase activity may be the mechanism for the corticosteroid-induced increase in cardiac glycogen concentration. Further work is needed to determine the physiological significance of these metabolic effects, as well as to characterize the effects of corticosteroids on the metabolism of other substrates (e.g., fatty acids, ketone bodies, amino acids) in the heart.

INOTROPIC EFFECTS. Loubatières and co-workers studied the inotropic activity of a variety of corticosteroids in intact dogs and found that almost all the steroids tested demonstrated positive inotropic effects of greater magnitude than that observed in isolated heart preparations. Dexamethasone (18, 19, 92) exerted a 70–80% increase in cardiac contractile force, whereas methylprednisolone, betamethasone, and triamcinolone exerted a 40–50% increase in contractile force (18, 19, 92) in the anesthetized dog. This same group showed that small doses of aldosterone exerted a 15–25% increase in contractile force in anesthetized (93) and in conscious dogs (95). All these steroids were injected intravenously, so that systemic pressor effects (e.g., change in outflow resistance of the heart) may have modified the cardiac effects in these studies. The large magnitude of these changes is also surprising in view of the much smaller inotropic effects usually observed in isolated cardiac tissue. However, the responses were reported in percentage increases with no absolute values reported, and if the hearts were depressed from the anesthetic or the surgery, one would expect a relatively larger response than in normal animals. Moreover these large effects have not been duplicated elsewhere (80, 81, 108), even in dogs subjected to bilateral vagotomy and carotid sinus denervation (70) in order to remove the neural regulatory mechanisms, which could mask potential myocardial or peripheral vascular effects, or both.

Cortisol, in concentrations ranging from low to massive, usually is either inactive or only very weakly inotropic in the whole animal (35, 70, 71, 80, 146). However, Bouyard (18) found that low-to-moderate doses of cortisol exerted a negative inotropic effect in the dog heart. Since the aqueous form of cortisol was used, the depressant effect obtained could not be attributed to a vehicle effect. Thus, as in isolated heart preparations, glucocorticoids are only very weakly cardiotonic or are ineffective. This, of course, does not rule out possible actions of these steroids on other aspects of cardiac function (i.e., myocardial metabolism).

PERIPHERAL VASCULAR EFFECTS OF CORTICOSTEROIDS

Blood Pressure and Vascular Resistance

Relatively little information concerning the acute effects of exogenous corticosteroid administration on systemic blood pressure in normal animals is available. Lefer and co-workers (70, 80) found physiological concentrations of a variety of corticosteroids to be ineffective in altering mean arterial blood pressure (MABP). Similarly, large doses of cortisol or methylprednisolone did not acutely alter blood pressure in normal humans (108, 112), nor did aldosterone acutely alter systemic blood pressure in normal rats (49) or dogs (70, 80).

In addition, acute administration of corticosteroids exerted no major effect on local vascular resistance. For example, topical or systemic administration of glucocorticoids had no effect on vascular tone of the rat mesoappendix circulation (4) or the perfused rabbit or dog hindquarters (71, 110). Thus the consensus is that corticosteroids do not have a prominent acute effect on systemic blood pressure or vascular resistance.

The results of chronic corticosteroid administration to normal animal and human subjects are more variable. Chronic administration of cortisone to normal animals resulted in local vasoconstriction in the rabbit ear chamber (8) and hamster cheek pouch (177). However, cortisone was without effect on the tone of the rat mesenteric vasculature (4). Furthermore other corticosteroids, such as dexamethasone, 9αFF, and DOC, failed to produce significant alterations in blood pressure, cardiac output, or TPR in dogs (80, 143) or humans (142), despite the fact that they were given in doses that potentiated the pressor response to catecholamines. Thus exogenous corticosteroids do not appear to alter systemic blood pressure in normal animals acutely or chronically, unless the animals are sensitized by salt loading or unilateral nephrectomy, or both. Nevertheless corticosteroids may play a regulatory role in the local autoregulation of blood flow in certain beds. However, additional evidence must be obtained to document this possible action.

Microcirculation

Few direct studies exist on the microcirculatory effects of corticosteroids. Schayer (141) has proposed that a dilator substance (i.e., "induced histamine") which plays a role in local regulation of microcirculatory flow is produced by a rapid one-step process from the readily available precursor, histidine, via the action of histidine decarboxylase. Schayer postulated the primary action of glucocorticoids to be the reduction of induced histamine formation; thereby the caliber of precapillary sphincters is modulated. The findings that chronic cortisone treatment produced microvascular constriction in the rabbit ear chamber (8) and hamster cheek pouch (177) are consistent with this view. However, Altura (4) has challenged Schayer's hypothesis by demonstrating that no peripheral vasodilation occurred in untreated adrenalectomized rats, despite the elevated tissue histamine content, and that either acute or long-term administration of glucocorticoids failed to alter vascular tone in the mesoappendix microvasculature. Considerably more information, preferably direct measurement of total and induced histamine levels in tissue and in blood, must be related to blood flow in a discrete vascular bed before this hypothesis can be adequately evaluated.

Some investigators (74, 179, 180) have suggested that physiological concentrations of corticosteroids are important to the maintenance of the structural integrity of the microcirculation. Kramár et al. (74) have shown that blood vessels of adrenalectomized rats and dogs rupture more readily than do those of nonadrenalectomized controls. Furthermore cortisone, but not DOC, enabled the capillaries to withstand greater external pressures. Zarem & Zweifach (179) observed a very rapid protective effect of cortisol on the microcirculation. They noted that the disruptive action of EDTA (ethylenediaminetetraacetic acid), which is thought to act at the basement membrane, in adrenalectomized rats could be reversed by cortisol in as short a time as 30 min. These workers claimed that corticosteroids may prevent the loss of vascular integrity by protecting the intercellular cement in the microcirculation. The specificity of the corticosteroids in these effects is not known at present, nor is the mechanism of such a capillary-stabilizing effect. Membrane-stabilizing effects are usually not encountered at physiological concentrations of corticosteroids; concentrations on the order of 10^{-4} to 10^{-3} M are required to stabilize lysosomal membranes (70).

Isolated Vascular Smooth Muscle

Corticosteroids, by themselves, do not induce spontaneous contraction of isolated vascular smooth muscle (48, 130). However, they significantly potentiate tension development by vasoactive agents, such as catecholamines (11, 16, 17, 48, 62, 72, 111, 130). Bohr & Cummings (17) have determined the relative steroid potencies in potentiating the epinephrine response in aortic strips and found them to be 2α-methyl-9α-fluorocortisol > cortisone > aldosterone > cortisol > DCA. Fowler & Chou (48) studied the potentiation of norepinephrine by corticosteroids and found the relative potencies to be corticosterone > cortisol > aldosterone. Thus no apparent relation exists between these relative potencies and other properties of these steroids because both glucocorticoids and mineralocorticoids potentiate catecholamines in vitro.

Several hypotheses have been proposed to explain the potentiating effect of corticosteroids on catecholamine-induced contraction of isolated vascular smooth muscle. One hypothesis is that corticosteroids potentiate catecholamines by altering the ionic gradient (i.e., Na^+, K^+, or Ca^{2+}) across the vascular smooth muscle cell. Bohr and associates (15, 17) have proposed that DCA reduces K^+ transport into the smooth muscle cells, and thus the ratio of K^+ inside the cell to K^+ outside the cell (K_i/K_o) is lowered. Presumably the altered potassium gradient leads to an increased vascular reactivity to epinephrine. Raab (115), on the other hand, has suggested that the transmembrane gradient of Na^+ is more important. The evidence cited is the well-known dependence of DCA hypertension on increased dietary salt intake accompanied by an increase in aortic wall Na^+ (164). Still others claim that adrenal steroids potentiate catecholamine effects via a more efficient calcium utilization by vascular smooth muscle cells (63). In this connection, Hinke (63) has shown that arteries from DCA-hypertensive rats were resistant to abolition of contraction in Ca^{2+}-free perfusate and that less Ca^{2+} was required to reestablish the contraction of vessels from DCA-hypertensive rats than from untreated controls. Bohr (15) has also suggested that the DOC potentiation of epinephrine may operate through mobilization of calcium ions. He has demonstrated that DOC preferentially potentiates the slow phase (S component) of aortic strip contraction, which has been shown to be directly dependent on the availability of free calcium.

Another hypothesis is based on the supposition that corticosteroids (e.g., cortisol) act at the level of the adrenergic receptors to increase their affinity for agonists such as catecholamines (11). Besse & Bass (11) concluded that cortisol alters the interaction of catecholamines with its vascular smooth muscle receptors, since cortisol potentiation occurred in reserpinized (i.e., depleted of endogenous catecholamine stores) preparations and was independent of membrane depolarization or of availability of calcium. Furthermore cortisol did not potentiate amines with one or both phenolic hydroxyl groups absent. Since the phenolic hydroxyl groups of catecholamines are thought to be associated with receptor affinity, Besse & Bass (11) proposed that cortisol exerts its potentiating effect by increasing the affinity of the adrenergic receptor for the catecholamines. Although direct proof for this mechanism is lacking, the hypothesis is intriguing and may help to elucidate corticosteroid receptor mechanisms.

A third hypothesis is that cortisol potentiates catecholamines by inhibiting the enzymatic hydrolysis of the catecholamines. Kalsner (72) found that cortisol potentiated catecholamines in cocaine- or reserpine-treated aortic strips, but not in the presence of a catechol-O-methyltransferase (COMT) inhibitor. This was interpreted as evidence for inhibitors of COMT as the primary mechanism for the cortisol-induced potentiation of catecholamines. However, direct measurement of the effects of cortisol on COMT activity would be helpful in providing more conclusive evidence for this hypothesis.

Thus, on one hand, mineralocorticoids may potentiate catecholamines via an effect on electrolytes, although the precise cation involved and the mechanism of the potentiation are prooly understood. Carefully controlled radioactive tracer experiments studying the compartmental distribution of these cations may help to resolve these questions. On the other hand, glucocorticoids act independently of electrolytes and may alter the kinetics of the catecholamine-receptor interaction or availability of the catecholamine to the receptor site. However, these mechanisms are so poorly understood that more fundamental information on receptor mechanisms must be acquired before progress can be made on this problem.

ROLE OF CORTICOSTEROIDS IN BLOOD VOLUME REGULATION

The relative efficacy of mineralocorticoids and glucocorticoids in maintaining or elevating the plasma volume in adrenal insufficiency has been the subject of considerable investigation. It is well established that adrenalectomized animals given mineralocorticoids (e.g., DOC or aldosterone), along with dietary salt, maintain a normal blood volume for periods of days or weeks (52, 155, 170). However, Swingle and co-workers (154–157) have shown that animals supported on mineralocorticoids and supplementary salt for longer periods of time eventually experience a gradual decline in blood volume. Periodic treatment with glucocorticoids prevented this latent decline in blood volume. Swingle and associates (151–153) have also shown that the plasma volume of fasted adrenalectomized animals not given salt or steroid does not increase in response to DOC or aldosterone, whereas 2α-methyl-9α-fluorocortisol or cortisone returns the plasma volume to normal. It would also be of interest to determine whether salt-excreting glucocorticoids (i.e., dexamethasone, methylprednisolone) are capable of preserving a completely normal blood volume in adrenalectomized animals to ascertain whether salt retention is the primary mechanism of the plasma volume expansion. The ability to correct or prevent the moderate hypovolemic state seen in adrenal insufficiency at the present time appears to be common to both mineralocorticoids and glucocorticoids, although no specific mechanism can be ascribed to this effect.

In contrast to the situation seen in adrenal insufficiency, mineralocorticoids, but not glucocorticoids, are capable of inducing an increase in plasma volume in animals with intact adrenals. However, it should be noted that the increase in plasma volume induced by mineralocorticoids is only a modest one (i.e., a 10% increase) (28, 29, 38, 52). Glucocorticoids, such as cortisone (14, 38, 170), cortisol, dexamethasone, and prednisolone (91), all fail to significantly alter plasma volume in normal animals.

Thus corticosteroids play a supportive role in the normal regulation of plasma volume. However, the effects of corticosteroids seem to be overridden by other homeostatic mechanisms (e.g., alterations in glomerular filtration rate, secretion rate of antidiuretic hormone, and balance of oncotic and hydrostatic pressures at the capillary level) to protect the animals against hypervolemia in the presence of excess corticosteroids and to minimize blood volume loss in adrenal insufficiency.

INTERACTION BETWEEN CORTICOSTEROIDS AND OTHER AGENTS IN REGULATION OF CIRCULATORY FUNCTION

In addition to direct effects on the circulatory system, corticosteroids may modulate the circulatory effects of other agents. In this regard, corticosteroids are important in the pathogenesis of certain types of hypertension but do not have a major direct effect on vascular smooth muscle tone. Thus the role of corticosteroids in the regulation of cardiovascular function cannot be fully determined until their interaction with other agents that profoundly alter circulatory function are known. Two basic types of interaction between chemical agents on biological systems can occur. If an agent enhances the effectiveness of another agent, *potentiation* results. If an agent diminishes the effectiveness of another agent, the phenomenon is termed *antagonism*. These terms are used in this review without any implication of receptor mech-

TABLE 2. *Interaction of Corticosteroids with Other Agents*

Agent	Mineralocorticoids Acute	Mineralocorticoids Chronic	Glucocorticoids Acute	Glucocorticoids Chronic	Cardiovascular Site of Interaction	Mechanism
Norepinephrine	0	+	0	0 or −	Predominantly heart	Probably due to increased Na$^+$ in extracellular fluid or cells perhaps via binding capacity of norepinephrine storage granules
Angiotensin	0	+	0	0	Heart and peripheral vasculature	Availability of Na$^+$ ions may play a key role inhibiting renin release or directly sensitizing receptor cells
Cardiac glycosides	−	NS	− or 0	NS	Heart and peripheral vasculature	Appears to be a competitive antagonism
Kinins	0	NS	0	NS	Unknown	Unknown

0, no effect; +, potentiation; −, antagonism; NS, not studied.

anisms. The interactions between corticosteroids and each of the major types of cardiovascular agents studied are summarized in Table 2.

Catecholamines

The adrenalectomized animal exhibits an impaired responsiveness to exogenously administered catecholamines. Also repeated application of norepinephrine or epinephrine to the adrenalectomized animal results in a progressively weakened pressor response, which eventually leads to a state of circulatory collapse (119). Thus the adrenalectomized animal is unable to increase its blood pressure in response to low or moderate concentrations of catecholamines, and high concentrations of catecholamines result in circulatory collapse. Several investigators have found an impaired pressor response to epinephrine or norepinephrine in chronic adrenal insufficiency (22, 26, 34, 45, 85, 119, 126, 127), as well as to noncatecholamine pressor agents (e.g., vasopressin, BaCl$_2$) (6, 47). However, the responsiveness to catecholamines is not impaired 2–3 days after adrenalectomy (56, 99, 122). Measurement of pressor responses alone does not allow one to distinguish between cardiac and peripheral vascular impairment. Since cardiac contractile force and cardiac output responses to catecholamines were also impaired in chronic adrenal insufficiency, a cardiac component may contribute to the overall diminished responsiveness to catecholamines (85, 131).

The influence of corticosteroids on the circulatory response to catecholamines in animals with intact adrenals has also been extensively studied. Chronic administration of mineralocorticoids potentiates the systemic pressor effect of epinephrine and norepinephrine. Deoxycorticosterone (DOC) and DCA (24, 83, 97, 114, 116, 117, 143, 148) potentiate catecholamine responses in the rat, dog, and the normal human, although considerable variation occurs in the amount of potentiation. Chronic administration of other mineralocorticoids, such as 9α-fluorocortisol (142) and aldosterone (55), also results in potentiation of the pressor effect of catecholamines, although some investigators report a prolongation of the duration of the response or a decreased threshold, rather than a potentiation of the magnitude of the pressor response (110, 124). In general, mineralocorticoids appear to potentiate the circulatory effects of both epinephrine and norepinephrine to an equal extent in the intact animal.

In contrast, acute (83, 124) or chronic administration of glucocorticoids usually does not potentiate the systemic pressor response to catecholamines (34, 83, 117, 143). However, when glucocorticoids are given in concentrations that exert mineralocorticoid effects, potentiation can occur (76, 77, 100, 124).

In an attempt to localize the site of the potentiation, Carlini et al. (24) found that chronic administration of DCA exerted a potentiating effect on the systemic pressor effects of epinephrine, but not in the isolated perfused hind limb. Verrier et al. (168) confirmed the finding of potentiation in the intact cat but failed to observe potentiation in the splanchnic bed. These findings suggest that the potentiation may be related to cardiac phenomena, rather than to changes in vascular smooth muscle alone, since the effect cannot be obtained in isolated perfused vascular beds.

Several hypotheses have been advanced to explain the corticosteroid potentiation of the pressor effect of catecholamines in the intact animal. A prolongation of catecholamine response may be explained on the basis of a longer biological half-life of the catecholamines, perhaps induced by some metabolic effect of the corticosteroids (109). Others postulate a direct sensitization of the effector cell, whether it be vascular or cardiac muscle (4, 124).

The prevailing hypothesis that explains much of the available data was proposed by Raab (115) in 1959, although modifications of this hypothesis have been advanced by other investigators over the last decade. This hypothesis is based on the well-known sodium-retaining action of mineralocorticoids, whether by increased renal tubular sodium reabsorption or extrarenal mechanisms, or both. Presumably some of the increased sodium gradually accumulates in the blood vessel wall (164) and perhaps in the myocardium. The sodium presumably accumulates in tissue sites and not in plasma because the plasma sodium pool is quite labile. However, it is not clear whether the sodium is bound intracellularly or whether it accumulates in the interstitial space. Nevertheless the additional sodium is thought to enhance the sensitivity of the effector cells without necessarily increasing its basal state of contraction (i.e., without inducing increased cardiac or vascular smooth muscle tone per se). The basic support for this hypothesis is that *a*) mineralocorticoids are more effective than glucocorticoids in potentiating catecholamines; *b*) mineralocorticoids cause sodium retention, although an escape from the renal effects of mineralocorticoids eventually occurs; *c*) a high-sodium intake enhances catecholamine pressor responses; *d*) a low-sodium intake reduces the pressor response of catecholamines; and *e*) mineralocorticoids are not very effective acutely possibly because it takes several days to accumulate enough intracellular or interstitial sodium to cause potentiation (115). Additional data on the amounts and location of the additional sodium would be helpful in assessing this hypothesis. Furthermore it is not known whether sodium directly alters the vascular smooth muscle or cardiac muscle cell contractile machinery or whether it mediates the effect through some other mechanism. In this connection, de Champlain et al. (42) have shown that sodium balance influences the capacity of cardiac norepinephrine storage granules to bind norepineprine and that the storage capacity of the granules correlates with the blood pressure. Thus sodium restriction or depletion results in an increased capacity of the sympathetic storage granules to bind norepinephrine, which makes less free norepinephrine available to react with effector sites. Conversely, DCA and NaCl decrease the capacity of the storage granules to bind norepinephrine. This would allow a greater pressor response to a given dose of exogenously administered norepinephrine. These studies were performed entirely in cardiac muscle, and thus it would be desirable to know if the same relations exist in vascular smooth muscle storage granules.

Renin and Angiotensin II

There is a marked loss of responsiveness to renin (56, 109, 127, 136) and to angiotensin II (3, 109) in adrenalectomized animals, even to the point of complete abolition of the pressor response. It appears that the impairment of the renin response occurs at an earlier time and to a more complete degree than the impairment of the angiotensin response (136). In animals with intact adrenals, chronic administration of mineralocorticoids generally potentiates the pressor response to renin (33, 55, 109) and to natural or synthetic angiotensin (55, 83). However, acute administration of mineralocorticoids or glucocorticoids fails to potentiate the pressor effect of renin or angiotensin (3, 60, 109, 145).

The mechanism for the decreased responsiveness to angiotensin in adrenal insufficiency and the increased responsiveness to angiotensin after chronic administration of mineralocorticoids also appears to be linked to the availability of sodium ions. Institution of a low-sodium diet or a regimen that depletes body sodium results in a decreased pressor response to angiotensin (12, 39, 60, 121). Conversely increasing total body sodium results in an increased pressor response to angiotensin (12, 60, 83, 121). Similarly the inotropic effect of angiotensin in isolated cardiac muscle depends on the external sodium concentration (79).

Although sodium ions may mediate the potentiation of angiotensin and renin by mineralocorticoids, the final common pathway may be via renin release. It is known that increasing the tissue or plasma sodium concentration, either by administration of exogenous mineralocorticoid or by salt loading, results in an inhibition of renin release, which decreases the endogenous angiotensin level. Under conditions of increased plasma sodium, cardiac and vascular smooth muscle can exhibit an increased responsiveness to exogenous angiotensin. Conversely in adrenal insufficiency or in sodium-depleted animals, a low plasma sodium concentration results in greater renin release with elevation of endogenous angiotensin production. Under these conditions, exogenously administered angiotensin may be less effective. The renin hypothesis, however, does not explain the potentiating effect of sodium on isolated tissues since in vitro high concentration of sodium probably acts directly on muscle cells to enhance their responsiveness to angiotensin (79). Thus the precise linkage between sodium concentration and muscle responsiveness is not completely understood. Unraveling of this mechanism would aid in the elucidation of the potentiation mechanism to angiotensin.

Cardiac Glycosides

Corticosteroids have been shown acutely to inhibit the contractile response of digitalis-like glycosides in a variety of isolated heart (51, 78, 84, 113) and vascular smooth muscle (140) preparations. Furthermore, Kunz & Wilbrandt (75) showed that several corticosteroids antagonized the cardiac glycoside-induced potassium loss from isolated guinea pig hearts. Other investigators have failed to demonstrate an antagonism of cardiac glycosides in rat ventricular strips (125) or isolated atria (88, 89); however, these preparations were unresponsive to corticosteroids alone (87, 166) and thus may be insensitive to corticosteroids. Several mineralocorticoids (e.g., aldosterone, DOC, 2α-methyl-9α-fluorocortisol, 9α-fluorocortisol) are effective in antagonizing the inotropic effect of cardiac glycosides (78), although Kunz & Wilbrandt (75) reported that several glucocorticoids also inhibited the glycoside-induced K^+ loss of isolated hearts. However, these glucocorticoids were ineffective in antagonizing the inotropic effect of ouabain (78). Thus the specificity for the antagonism of mechanical activity appears to be more rigid than that for cation transport.

Conversely adrenalectomized rats (167) and hearts obtained from adrenalectomized rats (113) are more sensitive to the cardiac effects of digitalis glycosides than are normal controls, a finding in support of the contention that myocardial failure exists in adrenal insufficiency. Mineralocorticoids are able to restore normal sensitivity more effectively than are glucocorticoids. The preponderance of data indicates that mineralocorticoids and high concentrations of some glucocorticoids acutely antagonize the effects of cardiac glycosides in isolated cardiac and vascular smooth muscle, although a precise structure-activity relation has not been defined.

The kinetics of the antagonism of cardiac glycosides by corticosteroids are suggestive of competitive antagonism (140). Read et al. (120) showed that aldosterone and ouabain compete for receptor sites in the heart and other organs. About 10 min is necessary to achieve a maximal level of tissue uptake of corticosteroids in the heart (67). In this connection Lefer & Sayers (84) showed that aldosterone required a latent period of about 20 min to fully antagonize the effects of ouabain.

Wilbrandt (175) has suggested that corticosteroids act as chelating agents and thus facilitate transport of cations across biological membranes. Bush (23) has argued against the Wilbrandt hypothesis; he claims that *a*) the corticosteroids do not have the stability or solubility to act as cation carriers, *b*) the α-ketol side chain in ring D does not possess properties that would enable it to chelate cations, and *c*) a stereochemical incompatability exists between corticosteroids and cardiac glycosides that would make their competition difficult. However, since the active binding sites are not known and since corticosteroid-glycoside antagonism does occur, one may presume that the differences in stereochemical configuration do not mask the binding sites of these two groups of steroids. Thus competition for cation receptors cannot be eliminated as a possible mechanism of the antagonism, although chelation in ring D is probably an oversimplification. Recently, Selye et al. (144) found that spironolactone, a steroidal antagonist of aldosterone action, was capable of protecting against the cardiotoxic effects of digitoxin in rats. Perhaps spironolactone, which possesses both the lactone ring and the steroid nucleus of the cardiac glycosides, is more effective in binding to the cardiac glycoside receptors and thus is a more effective antagonist than mineralocorticoids, which possess only the steroid nucleus.

Kinins

Earlier results supported the hypothesis that glucocorticoids (27, 149) antagonize the biological actions of kinins (e.g., bradykinin). In fact this antagonism was purported to be the mechanism of the anti-inflammatory action of glucocorticoids. The basic evidence to support the concept of a glucocorticoid-kinin antagonism is that *a*) adrenalectomized animals are more responsive to the effects of exogenously administered kinins (149) and *b*) cortisol appears to inhibit the release of kinin from kininogen, activated by glass contact (27). Unfortunately these criteria are not sufficiently specific to prove the glucocorticoid-kinin interaction. Thus adrenalectomized animals are more sensitive to many noxious agents in a generalized nonspecific manner. Suddick (149) reported that glucocorticoids (i.e., cortisone, cortisol) protected against the lethal effects of submaxillary gland extracts injected into adrenalectomized rats. The inference made was that bradykinin is the toxic substance in the extract; however, other substances may have contributed to the lethality. In the experiments of Cline & Melmon (27), kinin formation was not actually measured but rather plasma kininogen concentration was determined. Alterations in rate of protein synthesis, degradation, or transport of kininogen could exert alterations in the kininogen concentration unrelated to kinin formation.

More recently, several investigators have failed to obtain evidence for an inhibitory action of glucocorticoids on the kallikrein-kinin system (44a, 62a, 82a). These workers have carefully analyzed the effects of several glucocorticoids (i.e., cortisol, cortisone, dexamethasone, methylprednisolone) in well-controlled experiments and found that none of these glucocorticoids influenced the biological actions of bradykinin, the formation of bradykinin by the action of kallikrein on plasma kininogen, or the rate of inactivation of bradykinin by kininases. Thus, acutely, glucocorticoids do not appear to exert a direct inhibitory action on the kallikrein-kinin system as was earlier thought. Certainly the anti-inflammatory action of these steroids operates by some mechanism other than kinin antagonism.

SUMMARY AND CONCLUSIONS

Corticosteroids are of great importance in the regulation of circulatory function. In the absence of corticosteroids, circulatory collapse, characterized largely by an impairment of myocardial function, occurs. The view that peripheral vascular collapse is a major contributory factor to the circulatory collapse has been recently challenged in controlled, perfused vascular preparations.

There is convincing evidence for a large depression in cardiac performance after chronic adrenalectomy, but not for an anatomic impairment of the myocardium. At present it appears that defects in the contractile proteins of the heart may be important in exerting the defect in contractility.

The changes in blood volume reported in adrenal insufficiency are quite variable and depend on type of support therapy and stage of adrenal insufficiency. However, the observed reductions in blood volume are usually only moderate, except in the terminal stages, although dogs are more sensitive than other common laboratory mammals. Furthermore hypotension and circulatory collapse occur in normovolemic, adrenalectomized animals. Thus a diminished plasma volume cannot be regarded as an essential feature of the circulatory collapse phenomenon observed in chronic adrenal insufficiency, but since even a moderate degree of hypotension may potentiate the cardiac defect, one cannot completely disregard hypovolemia as a contributory factor.

Mineralocorticoids exert modest positive inotropic effects in isolated cardiac tissue, whereas glucocorticoids are either less effective or completely inactive. In the whole animal the situation is more complex. Corticosteroids, particularly mineralocorticoids, are capable of inducing ECG alterations, but little is known concerning the cardiac metabolic effects of corticosteroids. Several corticosteroids exert apparent cardiotonic effects in the whole animal, but the directness of these effects remains to be established.

The effects of corticosteroids on vascular resistance are not well established. Large changes in vascular resistance do not occur in response to acute or chronic administration of corticosteroids in normal, nonsensitized animals. Although corticosteroids may help to maintain the morphological integrity of the vessels of the microcirculation, their role in the regulation of blood flow through the microcirculation is not well understood. Corticosteroids do not directly alter the tone of isolated smooth muscle preparations, but many are capable of potentiating the contractile effects of constrictor agents, such as catecholamines.

Corticosteroids exert a regulatory role in the maintenance of a normal blood volume, but they induce only a small increase in blood volume in the normal animal. The actions of corticosteroids on blood volume may be an effect of the permissive type. The magnitude of the variations in blood volume associated with steroidal excess or deficiency are minimized by other homeostatic mechanisms involved in blood volume regulation.

Chronic administration of mineralocorticoids, but not glucocorticoids, potentiates the pressor effects of catecholamines and angiotensin. The mechanism of this potentiation may involve the accumulation of sodium ions in the vicinity of the effector cell (i.e., myocardial or vascular smooth muscle). Cardiac glycosides are antagonized by mineralocorticoids and some glucocorticoids. The mechanism of this antagonism appears to be related to the competition between corticosteroids and cardiac glycosides for receptor sites on the effector cells. Corticosteroids do not appear acutely to antagonize the effects of kinins.

Thus corticosteroids play a variety of physiological and pharmacological roles in the maintenance and protection of cardiovascular function under a wide variety of conditions. In general, corticosteroids are essential for the normal functioning of the circulatory system. It is also of interest that even extremely high doses of corticosteroids, acutely or for periods of a few days, are remarkably nontoxic and may even be of value in the amelioration of circulatory function in situations such as those existing in circulatory shock.

REFERENCES

1. ABRAMS, W. B., AND R. N. HARRIS. The effect of cortisone on the electrocardiograms of normal rabbits. *Am. Heart J.* 42: 876–883, 1951.
2. ADDISON, T. Anemia: disease of the suprarenal capsules. *London Med. Gaz.* 43: 517–518, 1849.
3. AJZEN, H., AND J. W. WOODS. Blood pressure responses to angiotensin II following aldosterone and adrenalectomy. *Acta Physiol. Latinoam.* 17: 131–136, 1967.
4. ALTURA, B. M. Role of glucocorticoids in local regulation of blood flow. *Am. J. Physiol.* 211: 1393–1397, 1966.
5. ARESKOG, N. H. The effect of catecholamines, corticosteroids and angiotensin II on the heart-lung preparation of the dog. *Acta Soc. Med. Upsalien.* 67: 164–178, 1962.
6. ARMSTRONG, C. W. J., R. A. CLEGHORN, J. L. A. FOWLER, AND G. A. McVICAR. Some effects of stimulation of sympathetic nerves and injection of pressor drugs in adrenalectomized cats. *J. Physiol., London* 96: 146–163, 1939.
7. ASCHKENASY, A. Effets de la surrénalectomie et des injections de cortisone sur le poids du coeur, du muscle gastrocnemien et du tube digestif sous-diaphragmatique. *Ann. Endocrinol.* 23: 145–163, 1962.
8. ASHTON, N., AND C. COOK. In vivo observations of the effects of cortisone upon the blood vessels in rabbit ear chambers. *Brit. J. Exptl. Pathol.* 33: 445–450, 1952.
9. BALLARD, K., A. LEFER, AND G. SAYERS. Effect of aldosterone and of plasma extracts on a rat heart-lung preparation. *Am. J. Physiol.* 199: 221–225, 1960.
10. BARTA, E., AND H. PAVLOVICÔVA. Role of adrenals in maintaining the level of carbohydrate metabolism in the failing heart. *Cor et Vasa* 7: 60–70, 1965.
11. BESSE, J. C., AND A. D. BASS. Potentiation by hydrocortisone of responses to catecholamines in vascular smooth muscle. *J. Pharmacol. Exptl. Therap.* 154: 224–238, 1966.
12. BLAIR-WEST, J. R., J. P. COGHLAN, D. A. DENTON, J. R. GODING, J. A. MUNROE, AND R. D. WRIGHT. The reduction of the pressor action of angiotensin II in sodium-deficient conscious sheep. *Australian J. Exptl. Biol. Med. Sci.* 41: 369–376, 1963.
13. BLINKS, J. R., AND J. KOCH-WESER. Physical factors in the analysis of the actions of drugs on myocardial contractility. *Pharmacol. Rev.* 15: 531–599, 1963.
14. BLOMSTEDT, B. Effect of cortisone on plasma volume, total blood volume and serum protein. *Acta Endocrinol.* 55: 472–480, 1967.
15. BOHR, D. F. Contraction of vascular smooth muscle. *Can. Med. Assoc. J.* 90: 174–179, 1964.
16. BOHR, D. F., D. C. BRODIE, AND D. H. CHEU. Effect of electrolytes on arterial muscle contraction. *Circulation* 17: 746–749, 1958.
17. BOHR, D. F., AND G. CUMMINGS. Comparative potentiating action of various steroids on the contraction of vascular smooth muscle. *Federation Proc.* 17: 17, 1958.
18. BOUYARD, P. Actions cardiovasculaires des derives steroides. *Ann. Anesthesiologie Franc.* 6: 37–49, 1965.
19. BOUYARD, P., AND M. KLEIN. Actions cardio-vasculaires de la bétaméthasone et de l'ouabaine chez le chien. *Compt. Rend. Soc. Biol.* 157: 2252–2254, 1963.
20. BRIGGS, A. H., AND W. C. HOLLAND. Antifibrillatory effects of electrolyte-regulating steroids on isolated rabbit atria. *Am. J. Physiol.* 197: 1161–1164, 1959.
21. BRITTON, S. W., AND H. SILVETTE. On the function of the adrenal cortex—general, carbohydrate and circulatory theories. *Am. J. Physiol.* 107: 190–206, 1934.
22. BROWN, F. K., AND J. W. REMINGTON. Arteriolar responsiveness in adrenal crisis in the dog. *Am. J. Physiol.* 182: 279–284, 1955.
23. BUSH, I. E. Chemical and biological factors in the activity of adrenocortical steroids. *Pharmacol. Rev.* 14: 317–445, 1962.
24. CARLINI, E. A., A. H. SAMPAIO, AND A. C. M. PAIVA. Vascular reactivity of rats with desoxycorticosterone and metacorticoid hypertension. *Acta Physiol. Latinoam.* 9: 138–142, 1959.

25. CLARKE, A. P. W., R. A. CLEGHORN, J. K. W. FERGUSON, AND J. L. A. FOWLER. Factors concerned in the circulatory failure of adrenal insufficiency. *J. Clin. Invest.* 26: 359–363, 1947.
26. CLEGHORN, R. A., J. L. A. FOWLER, W. F. GREENWOOD, AND A. P. W. CLARKE. Pressor responses in healthy adrenalectomized dogs. *Am. J. Physiol.* 161: 21–28, 1950.
27. CLINE, M. J., AND K. L. MELMON. Plasma kinins and cortisol: a possible explanation of the anti-inflammatory action of cortisol. *Science* 153: 1135–1137, 1966.
28. CLINTON, M., JR., AND G. W. THORN. Effect of desoxycorticosterone acetate administration on plasma volume and electrolyte balance of normal human subjects. *Bull. Johns Hopkins Hosp.* 72: 255–264, 1943.
29. CLINTON, M., JR., G. W. THORN, AND H. EISENBERG. Effect of synthetic desoxycorticosterone acetate therapy on plasma volume and electrolyte balance in normal dogs. *Endocrinology* 31: 578–581, 1942.
30. COPE, O., A. G. BRENIZER, JR., AND H. POLDERMAN. Capillary permeability and the adrenal cortex: studies of cervical lymph in the adrenalectomized dog. *Am. J. Physiol.* 137: 69–78, 1942.
31. CORNMAN, I., AND J. L. GARGUS. Serum and serum fractions as antagonists for desoxycorticosterone inhibition of the chick heart in tissue culture. *Am. J. Physiol.* 189: 347–349, 1957.
32. CORNMAN, I., M. MACDONALD, AND E. TRAMS. Reversal of desoxycorticosterone inhibition of heart beat by serum fractions: comparison with known substances. *Am. J. Physiol.* 189: 350–354, 1957.
33. CROXATTO, H., F. MONCKEBERG, S. JARPA, AND V. SILVA. Implantacion de desoxicorticoesterona en ratas y senibilidad a la renina, hipertensia adrenalina y vasopresina. *Bol. Soc. Biol. Concepcion, Chile* 10: 34–39, 1953.
34. D'AGOSTINO, S. A., AND E. T. SEGURA. Effect of aldosterone and corticosterone upon vasomotor reactivity in adrenalectomized rats. *Acta Physiol. Latinoam.* 14: 352–357, 1964.
35. DALTON, D. H., P. HAIRSTON, AND W. H. LEE. Influence of massive glucocorticoid administration on myocardial inotropism. *Surg. Forum* 19: 147–149, 1968.
36. DAVANZO, J. P., H. C. CROSSFIELD, AND W. W. SWINGLE. Effect of various adrenal steroids on plasma magnesium and the electrocardiogram of adrenalectomized dogs. *Endocrinology* 63: 825–830, 1958.
37. DAVANZO, J. P., H. C. CROSSFIELD, AND W. W. SWINGLE. Effect of various adrenal steroids on the electrocardiogram of adrenalectomized dogs. *Circulation Res.* 9: 48–52, 1961.
38. DAVIS, A. K., A. C. BASS, AND R. R. OVERMAN. Comparative effects of cortisone and DCA on ionic balance and fluid volumes of normal and adrenalectomized dogs. *Am. J. Physiol.* 166: 493–503, 1951.
39. DAVIS, J. O., P. M. HARTROFT, E. O. TITUS, C. C. J. CARPENTER, C. R. AYERS, AND H. E. SPIEGEL. The role of the renin-angiotensin system in the control of aldosterone secretion. *J. Clin. Invest.* 41: 378–389, 1962.
40. DAW, J. C., A. M. LEFER, AND R. M. BERNE. Influences of corticosteroids on cardiac glycogen concentration in the rat. *Circulation Res.* 22: 639–647, 1968.
41. DAW, J. C., A. M. LEFER, AND R. M. BERNE. Time course of glucocorticoid dependent changes in cardiac glycogen concentration. *Proc. Soc. Exptl. Biol. Med.* 131: 1042–1044, 1969.
42. DE CHAMPLAIN, J., L. R. KRAKOFF, AND J. AXELROD. Relationship between sodium intake and norepinephrine storage during the development of experimental hypertension. *Circulation Res.* 23: 479–491, 1968.
43. DEGERLI, I. U., W. R. WEBB, AND W. R. LOCKWOOD. The glucocorticoid deprived myocardium. *Arch. Surg.* 89: 457–461, 1964.
44. EDELMAN, I. S., R. BOGOROCH, AND G. A. PORTER. On the mechanism of action of aldosterone on sodium transport: the role of protein synthesis. *Proc. Natl. Acad. Sci. US* 50: 1169–1177, 1963.
44a. EISEN, V., L. GREENBAUM, AND G. P. LEWIS. Kinins and anti-inflammatory steroids. *Brit. J. Pharmacol.* 34: 169–176, 1968.
45. ELLIOTT, T. R. Some results of excision of the adrenal glands. *J. Physiol., London* 49: 38–53, 1914.
46. EMELE, J. R., AND D. D. BONNYCASTLE. Cardiotonic activity of some adrenal steroids. *Am. J. Physiol.* 185: 103–106, 1956.
47. FOWLER, J. L. A., AND R. A. CLEGHORN. The response of splanchnic blood vessels and the small intestine to vasoconstrictor influences in adrenal insufficiency in the cat. *Am. J. Physiol.* 137: 371–379, 1942.
48. FOWLER, N. O., AND N. H. F. CHOU. Potentiation of smooth muscle contraction by adrenal steroids. *Circulation Res.* 9: 153–156, 1961.
49. FRIEDMAN, S. M., C. L. FRIEDMAN, AND M. NAKASHIMA. Effects of aldosterone on blood pressure and electrolyte distribution in the rat. *Am. J. Physiol.* 195: 621–627, 1958.
50. FRITZ, I., AND R. LEVINE. Action of adrenal cortical steroids and norepinephrine on vascular responses of stress in adrenalectomized rats. *Am. J. Physiol.* 165: 456–465, 1951.
51. FUJINO, S., S. YOROZUYA, T. IZUMI, AND M. TANAKA. Antiouabain action of steroid hormones on twitch and potassium contracture in heart ventricle strip of frog. *Japan. J. Pharmacol.* 19: 148–156, 1969.
52. GAUDINO, M., AND M. F. LEVITT. Influence of the adrenal cortex on body water distribution and renal function. *J. Clin. Invest.* 28: 1487–1497, 1949.
53. GERLACH, A., AND P. A. VAN ZWIETEN. Mechanical performance and calcium metabolism in rat isolated heart muscle after adrenalectomy. *Arch. Ges. Physiol.* 311: 96–104, 1969.
54. GROSS, F. Renal and extrarenal actions of aldosterone and its influence on sodium transport. *Intern. Congr. Endocrinol., 1st, Copenhagen, July, 1960*, p. 61–63.
55. GROSS, F., AND P. LICHTLEN. Verstarkung der pressorischen Wirkung von Renin, drucksteigernden Peptiden und adrenergischen Wirkstoffen nach Nephrektomie und bei Uberdosierung von Cortexon und Kochsalz an der Ratte. *Arch. Exptl. Pathol. Pharmakol.* 233: 323–337, 1958.
56. GROSS, F., AND F. SULSER. Der Einfluss der Nebennieren auf die blutdrucksteigernde Wirkung von Renin und auf pressorische Substanzen in den Nieren. *Arch. Exptl. Pathol. Pharmakol.* 230: 274–283, 1957.
57. HAJDU, S. Bioassay for cardiac active principles based on the staircase phenomenon of the frog heart. *J. Pharmacol. Exptl. Therap.* 120: 90–98, 1957.
58. HADJU, S., AND A. SZENT-GYÖRGYI. Action of DOC and serum on the frog heart. *Am. J. Physiol.* 168: 159–170, 1952.
59. HALL, C. E., AND R. A. CLEGHORN. Cardiac lesions in adrenal insufficiency. *Can. Med. Assoc. J.* 39: 126–133, 1938.
60. HEALY, J. K., J. B. SUSZKIW, V. W. DENNIS, AND G. E. SCHREINER. Effect of aldosterone and salt intake on renal and pressor actions of angiotensin. *Nephron* 3: 329–343, 1966.
61. HECHTER, O. Concerning the hypersensitivity of adrenalectomized rats to vascular stress. *Endocrinology* 36: 77–87, 1945.
62. HEINEMAN, A. C., AND T. S. DANOWSKI. Potentiation and stabilization of aortic strip pressor assay by plasma and hydrocortisone: routine use in the diagnosis of pheochromocytoma. *Am. J. Med. Sci.* 239: 167–173, 1960.
62a. HENNINGSEN, S. J., AND H. ZACHARIAE. Influence of betamethasone on Hageman factor activation of human plasma kallikrein. *Scand. J. Clin. Lab. Invest. Suppl.* 107: 135–138, 1969.
63. HINKE, J. A. M. Effect of Ca^{++} upon contractility of small arteries from DCA-hypertensive rats. *Circulation Res.* 18, Suppl. I: 23–34, 1966.
64. HOELSCHER, B. Effect of adrenalectomy on cardiac output of parabiotic and single rats. *Am. J. Physiol.* 179: 171–176, 1954.
65. HOFFMANN, G. On the effect of adrenal cortical hormones on heart muscle. *Arch. Exptl. Pathol. Pharmakol.* 222: 224–226, 1954.

66. HOFMANN, F. G., AND E. H. SOBEL. Adrenocortical insufficiency. In: *The Adrenocortical Hormones: Their Origin, Chemistry, Physiology, and Pharmacology*. Berlin: Springer Verlag, 1964, part 2, p. 27–183.
67. HOLLANDER, W., D. W. KRAMSCH, A. V. CHOBANIAN, AND J. C. MELBY. Metabolism and distribution of intravenously administered d-aldosterone-1,2-H³ in the arteries, kidneys and heart of dog. *Circulation Res.* 18, Suppl. I: 35–47, 1966.
68. IMAI, S., H. MURASE, M. KATORI, M. OKADA, AND T. SHIGEI. A study on the structure-activity relationship of the cardiotonic steroids. *Japan. J. Pharmacol.* 15: 62–71, 1965.
69. INGLE, D. Permissive action of hormones. *Endocrinology* 14: 1272–1274, 1954.
70. JEFFERSON, T., T. M. GLENN, AND A. M. LEFER. Cardiovascular and lysosomal actions of corticosteroids in the intact dog. *Proc. Soc. Exptl. Biol. Med.* 136: 276–280, 1971.
71. KADOWITZ, P. J., AND A. C. YARD. Circulatory effects of hydrocortisone and protection against endotoxin shock in cats. *European J. Pharmacol.* 9: 311–318, 1970.
72. KALSNER, S. Mechanism of hydrocortisone potentiation of responses to epinephrine and norepinephrine in rabbit aorta. *Circulation Res.* 24: 383–395, 1969.
73. KAYE, M. P., M. JELLINEK, T. COOPER, AND C. R. HANLON. Effect of adrenalectomy on myocardial catecholamines. *J. Surg. Res.* 4: 257–259, 1964.
74. KRAMÁR, J., V. W. MEYERS, H. H. MCCARTHY, AND M. SIMAY-KRAMÁR. Further study on the endocrine relations of capillary resistance. *Endocrinology* 60: 589–596, 1957.
75. KUNZ, H. A., AND W. WILBRANDT. Antagonistische Wirkung zwischen Herzglykosiden und Steroiden auf die Kaliumabgabe des Herzmuskels. *Helv. Physiol. Acta* 21: 83–87, 1963.
76. LECOMTE, J., A. DRESSE, AND H. VANCAUWENBERGE. Action des hormones corticostéroïdes et de corticoïdes aparentés sur quelques effets des amines sympathicomimétiques. *Arch. Intern. Physiol. Biochim.* 68: 720–734, 1960.
77. LECOMTE, J., J. GRÉVISSE, AND M. L. BEAUMARIAGE. Potentiation par l'hydrocortisone des effects moteurs de l'adrenaline. *Arch. Intern. Pharmacodyn.* 119: 133–141, 1959.
78. LEFER, A. M. Corticosteroid antagonism of the positive inotropic effect of ouabain. *J. Pharmacol. Exptl. Therap.* 151: 294–299, 1966.
79. LEFER, A. M. Influence of mineralocorticoids and cations on the inotropic effect of angiotensin and norepinephrine in isolated cardiac muscle. *Am. Heart J.* 73: 674–680, 1967.
80. LEFER, A. M. Effects of corticosteroids on myocardial contractility. In: *Factors Influencing Myocardial Contractility*, edited by R. D. Tanz. New York: Acad. Press, 1967, p. 611–631.
81. LEFER, A. M. Factors influencing the inotropic effect of corticosteroids. *Proc. Soc. Exptl. Biol. Med.* 125: 202–205, 1967.
82. LEFER, A. M. Influence of corticosteroids on mechanical performance of isolated rat papillary muscles. *Am. J. Physiol.* 214: 518–524, 1968.
82a. LEFER, A. M., AND T. F. INGE, JR. Lack of interaction between glucocorticoids and the kallikrein-kinin system. *Proc. Soc. Exptl. Biol. Med.* 145: 658–662, 1974.
83. LEFER, A. M., J. L. MANWARING, AND R. L. VERRIER. Effect of corticosteroids on the cardiovascular responses to angiotensin and norepinephrine. *J. Pharmacol. Exptl. Therap.* 154: 83–91, 1966.
84. LEFER, A. M., AND G. SAYERS. Antagonism of the inotropic action of ouabain by aldosterone. *Am. J. Physiol.* 208: 649–654, 1965.
85. LEFER, A. M., AND D. C. SUTFIN. Cardiovascular effects of catecholamines in experimental adrenal insufficiency. *Am. J. Physiol.* 206: 1151–1155, 1964.
86. LEFER, A. M., R. L. VERRIER, AND W. W. CARSON. Cardiac performance in experimental adrenal insufficiency in cats. *Circulation Res.* 22: 817–827, 1968.
87. LEVY, J. V., AND V. RICHARDS. Effects of aldosterone on contractile and electrical properties of driven isolated rabbit atria. *Proc. Soc. Exptl. Biol. Med.* 3: 602–606, 1962.
88. LEVY, J. V., AND V. RICHARDS. Aldosterone-ouabain actions on isolated rabbit atria. *Arch. Intern. Pharmacodyn.* 146: 363–373, 1963.
89. LEVY, J. V., AND V. RICHARDS. Effect of aldosterone on ouabain-induced potassium loss from isolated rabbit atria. *Proc. Soc. Exptl. Biol. Med.* 114: 280–283, 1963.
90. LEVY, J. V., AND V. RICHARDS. Effect of aldosterone, ouabain and deoxycorticosterone on oxygen uptake of isolated cardiac muscle. *J. Pharmacol. Exptl. Therap.* 144: 104–109, 1964.
91. LIECHTY, R. D., AND R. H. OSBORNE. Blood volume response to the administration of glucocorticoids in humans. *J. Trauma* 5: 741–745, 1965.
92. LOUBATIÈRES, A., P. BOUYARD, AND M. KLEIN. Etude comparée de l'action inotrope cardiaque des 9-α-fluorocorticoides chez le chien anesthétié. *Compt. Rend. Soc. Biol.* 158: 1699–1701, 1964.
93. LOUBATIÈRES, A., P. BOUYARD, AND A. SASSINE. Mise en evidence du tropisme de la d-aldosterone pour le coeur. *Compt. Rend.* 255: 1147–1148, 1962.
94. LOUBATIÈRES, A., AND A. SASSINE. Action cardiotonique de la d-aldosterone. *Compt. Rend.* 255: 374–376, 1962.
95. LOUBATIÈRES, A., AND A. SASSINE. Le tropisme et l'action cardiotonique de la d-aldosterone peuvent être demonstrés chez le chien non anesthésie. *Compt. Rend.* 256: 781–782, 1963.
96. LOYNES, J. S., AND C. W. GOWDEY. Cardiotonic activity of certain steroids and bile salts. *Can. J. Med. Sci.* 30: 325–332, 1952.
97. MASSON, G. M. C., I. H. PAGE, AND A. C. CORCORAN. Vascular reactivity of rats and dogs treated with desoxycorticosterone acetate. *Proc. Soc. Exptl. Biol. Med.* 73: 434–436, 1950.
98. MCCARL, R. L., B. F. SZUHAJ, AND R. T. HOULIHAN. Steroid stimulation of beating of cultured rat-heart cells. *Science* 150: 1611–1613, 1965.
99. MEIER, R., AND H. J. BEIN. Der Einfluss der Nebennieren auf die Wirkung kreislaufaktiver Substanzen. *Helv. Physiol. Pharmacol. Acta* 12: 83–84c, 1954.
100. MENDLOWITZ, M., N. NAFTCHI, H. L. WEINREB, AND S. E. GITLOW. Effect of prednisolone on digital vascular reactivity in normotensive and hypertensive subjects. *J. Appl. Physiol.* 16: 89–94, 1961.
101. MONNEREAU-SOUSTRE, H., M. F. REVIAL, AND Y. M. GARGOUÏL. Distribution des électrolytes au niveau de myocarde de rat surrénalectomisé et polarisation membranaire. *Compt. Rend. Soc. Biol.* 162: 957–961, 1958.
102. NAHAS, G. G. Effect of hydrocortisone on acidotic failure of the isolated heart. *Circulation Res.* 5: 489–492, 1957.
103. NASMYTH, P. L. The effect of corticosteroids on the isolated mammalian heart and its response to adrenaline. *J. Physiol., London* 139: 323–336, 1957.
104. NAYLER, W. G. The inotropic action of d-aldosterone on papillary muscles isolated from monkeys. *J. Pharmacol. Exptl. Therap.* 148: 215–217, 1965.
105. NAYLER, W. G. Cardiac metabolism: ionic changes. Influence of calcium ions, 9-α-fluorohydrocortisone and cardiac glycosides on the isolated toad heart. *Australian J. Exptl. Biol. Med. Sci.* 35: 241–248, 1957.
106. NICHOLSON, W. M., AND L. J. SOFFER. Cardiac arrhythmia in experimental suprarenal insufficiency in dogs. *Bull. Johns Hopkins Hosp.* 56: 236–244, 1935.
107. NOBLE, R. L. Physiology of the adrenal cortex. In: *The Hormones*, edited by G. Pincus and K. V. Thimann. New York: Acad. Press, 1950, vol. II, p. 67–180.
108. NOVAK, E., S. S. STUBBS, C. E. SECKMAN, AND M. S. HERRON. Effects of a single large intravenous dose of methylprednisolone sodium succinate. *Clin. Pharmacol. Therap.* 11: 711–717, 1970.
109. OSTROVSKY, D., AND A. G. GORNALL. Effects of aldosterone and other adrenal hormones on the blood pressure responses to renin and angiotensin. *Can. Med. Assoc. J.* 90: 180–184, 1964.
110. PANISSET, J. C., P. BOIS, AND A. BEAULNES. Effet de la desoxy-

corticosterone et du methyl-fluorocortisol sur la réponse vasculaire a l'adrenaline. *Rev. Can. Biol.* 20: 71–73, 1961.
111. PANISSET, J. C., P. BOIS, AND A. BEAULNES. Effect of aldosterone and spironolactone on smooth muscle responsiveness to adrenaline. *Rev. Can. Biol.* 22: 103–105, 1963.
112. PASTORELLE, D. J., AND R. H. CLAUSS. Regulation of physiologic arteriovenous communications in man demonstrated by hydrocortisone infusion. *Ann. Surg.* 157: 433–437, 1963.
113. POLDRE, A., AND M. TAESCHLER. Einfluss von Nebennierenrinden-hormonen auf die kardiotone und toxische Wirkung des Lanatosid C. *Helv. Physiol. Pharmacol. Acta* 14: 37–38c, 1956.
114. RAAB, W. Cardiovascular effects of desoxycorticosterone acetate in man. *Am. Heart J.* 24: 365–377, 1942.
115. RAAB, W. Transmembrane cationic gradient and blood pressure regulation: interaction of corticoids, catecholamines and electrolytes on vascular cells. *Am. J. Cardiol.* 4: 752–774, 1959.
116. RAAB, W., R. J. HUMPHREYS, AND E. LEPESCHKIN. Potentiation of pressor effects of nor-epinephrine and epinephrine in man by desoxycorticosterone acetate. *J. Clin. Invest.* 29: 1397–1404, 1950.
117. RAAB, W., AND J. YAFFE. Effect of cortisone upon the pressor catecholamine-potentiating action of desoxycorticosterone acetate (DCA). *Exptl. Med. Surg.* 10: 249–253, 1952.
118. RAMEY, E. R., AND M. S. GOLDSTEIN. The adrenal cortex and the sympathetic nervous system. *Physiol. Rev.* 37: 155–195, 1957.
119. RAMEY, E. R., M. S. GOLDSTEIN, AND R. LEVINE. Action of norepinephrine and adrenal cortical steroids on blood pressure and work performance of adrenalectomized dogs. *Am. J. Physiol.* 165: 450–455, 1951.
120. READ, V. H., D. L. BOMER, D. L. SMITH, C. S. MCCAA, AND L. L. SULYA. Effects of ouabain, spirolactone and a salt-free diet on the tissue uptake of H^3 aldosterone in rats. *Proc. Intern. Congr. Biochem., 6th, New York* 7: 592, 1964.
121. REID, W. D., AND J. H. LARAGH. Sodium and potassium intake, blood pressure and pressor response to angiotensin. *Proc. Soc. Exptl. Biol. Med.* 120: 26–29, 1965.
122. REIDENBERG, M. M., E. A. OHLER, AND R. W. SEVY. Cardiovascular responses to norepinephrine in acute adrenal insufficiency. *Proc. Soc. Exptl. Biol. Med.* 97: 889–892, 1958.
123. REIDENBERG, M. M., E. A. OHLER, R. W. SEVY, AND C. HARAKAL. Hemodynamic changes in adrenalectomized dogs. *Endocrinology* 72: 918–923, 1963.
124. REIS, D. J. Potentiation of the vasoconstrictor action of topical norepinephrine on the human bulbar conjunctival vessels after topical application of certain adrenocortical hormones. *J. Clin. Endocrinol. Metab.* 20: 446–456, 1960.
125. REITER, M. Untersuchungen uber den Einfluss von Corticosteron auf die Kontraktionskraft des isolierten Herzmuskels und auf die inotrope Wirkung des g-Strophanthins. *Z. Biol.* 112: 151–155, 1960.
126. REMINGTON, J. W. Circulatory factors in adrenal crisis in the dog. *Am. J. Physiol.* 165: 306–318, 1951.
127. REMINGTON, J. W., W. D. COLLINGS, H. W. HAYNES, W. M. PARKINS, AND W. W. SWINGLE. The response of the adrenalectomized dog to renin and other pressor agents. *Am. J. Physiol.* 132: 622–628, 1941.
128. RENKIN, E. M., AND B. D. ZAUN. Effects of adrenal medullary hormones on capillary permeability in perfused rat tissue. *Am. J. Physiol.* 180: 498–502, 1955.
129. ROBERTS, K. E. Effects of cortisone on electrocardiographic changes in adrenal insufficiency. *Proc. Soc. Exptl. Biol. Med.* 79: 32–34, 1952.
130. RONDELL, P., AND F. GROSS. Method for isometric recordings from isolated vessels under various conditions. *Helv. Physiol. Pharmacol. Acta* 18: 366–375, 1960.
131. ROSENFELD, H., R. W. SEVY, AND E. A. OHLER. Vascular responses to norepinephrine in adrenal insufficiency. *Proc. Soc. Exptl. Biol. Med.* 100: 800–802, 1959.

132. ROVETTO, M. J., AND A. M. LEFER. Electrophysiologic properties of cardiac muscle in adrenal insufficiency. *Am. J. Physiol.* 218: 1015–1019, 1970.
133. ROVETTO, M. J., A. M. LEFER, AND R. A. MURPHY. Alterations in myocardial cell function in adrenal insufficiency. *Arch. Ges. Physiol.* 329: 59–71, 1971.
134. ROVETTO, M. J., R. A. MURPHY, AND A. M. LEFER. Cardiac impairment in adrenal insufficiency: reduced ATPase activity of myocardial contractile proteins. *Circulation Res.* 26: 419–428, 1970.
135. RUSSELL, J. A., AND W. BLOOM. Hormonal control of glycogen in the heart and other tissues in rats. *Endocrinology* 58: 83–94, 1956.
136. SALMOIRAGHI, G. C., AND J. W. MCCUBBIN. Effect of adrenalectomy on pressor responsiveness to angiotonin and renin. *Circulation Res.* 2: 280–283, 1954.
137. SAYERS, G. The adrenal cortex and homeostasis. *Physiol. Rev.* 30: 241–320, 1950.
138. SAYERS, G., A. M. LEFER, AND G. R. NADZAM. Aldosterone and cardiac function. *Endocrinology* 78: 211–213, 1966.
139. SAYERS, G., AND N. SOLOMON. Work performance of a rat heart-lung preparation: standardization and influence of corticosteroids. *Endocrinology* 66: 719–730, 1960.
140. SCHATZMANN, H. J. Kompetitiver Antagonismus zwischen g-Strophanthin und Corticosteron an isolierten Streifen von Rattenaorten. *Experientia* 15: 73–74, 1959.
141. SCHAYER, R. W. Induced synthesis of histamine, microcirculatory regulation and the mechanism of action of the adrenal glucocorticoid hormones. *Progr. Allergy* 7: 187–212, 1963.
142. SCHMID, P. G., J. W. ECKSTEIN, AND F. M. ABBOUD. Effect of 9-α-fluorohydrocortisone on forearm vascular responses to norepinephrine. *Circulation* 34: 620–626, 1966.
143. SCHMID, P. G., J. W. ECKSTEIN, AND F. M. ABBOUD. Comparison of effects of deoxycorticosterone and dexamethasone on cardiovascular responses to norepinephrine. *J. Clin. Invest.* 46: 590–598, 1967.
144. SELYE, H., M. KRAJNY, AND L. SAVOIE. Digitoxon poisoning: prevention by spironolactone. *Science* 164: 842–843, 1969.
145. SILVA, V., AND H. CROXATTO. Administracion de desoxicorticosterona y sensibilidad a la hipertensina y adrenalina en ratas. *Acta Physiol. Latinoam.* 1: 47–56, 1950.
146. SMALL, H. S., S. W. WEITZNER, AND G. G. NAHAS. Cardiovascular effects of levarterenol, hydrocortisone hemisuccinate and aldosterone in the dog. *Am. J. Physiol.* 196: 1025–1028, 1959.
147. SOLOMON, N., R. H. TRAVIS, AND G. SAYERS. Corticosteroids and the functional capacity of the rat heart-lung preparation. *Endocrinology* 64: 535–541, 1959.
148. STURTEVANT, F. M. The biology of metacorticoid hypertension. *Ann. Internal Med.* 49: 1281–1293, 1958.
149. SUDDICK, R. P. Glucocorticoid-kinin antagonism in the rat. *Am. J. Physiol.* 211: 844–850, 1966.
150. SWINGLE, W. W., G. BARLOW, E. COLLINS, E. J. FEDOR, W. J. WELCH, AND J. M. RAMPONA. Serum potassium and electrocardiographic changes in adrenalectomized dogs maintained on cortisone acetate. *Endocrinology* 51: 353–361, 1952.
151. SWINGLE, W. W., J. P. DAVANZO, H. C. CROSSFIELD, D. GLENISTER, M. OSBORNE, R. ROWEN, AND G. WAGLE. Glucocorticoids and maintenance of blood pressure and plasma volume of adrenalectomized dogs subjected to stress. *Proc. Soc. Exptl. Biol. Med.* 100: 617–622, 1959.
152. SWINGLE, W. W., J. P. DAVANZO, D. GLENISTER, H. C. CROSSFIELD, AND G. WAGLE. Role of gluco- and mineralocorticoids in salt and water metabolism of adrenalectomized dogs. *Am. J. Physiol.* 196: 283–286, 1959.
153. SWINGLE, W. W., J. W. REMINGTON, V. A. DRILL, AND W. KLEINBERG. Differences among adrenal steroids with respect to their efficacy in protecting the adrenalectomized dog against circulatory failure. *Am. J. Physiol.* 136: 567–576, 1942.
154. SWINGLE, W. W., AND A. M. SWINGLE. Effect of adrenal

steroids upon plasma volume of intact and adrenalectomized dogs. *Proc. Soc. Exptl. Biol. Med.* 119: 452–455, 1965.
155. SWINGLE, W. W., AND A. J. SWINGLE. Activation, inhibition and reversal of inhibition of plasma volume changes in adrenalectomized and intact dogs. *Proc. Soc. Exptl. Biol. Med.* 125: 815–818, 1967.
156. SWINGLE, W. W., AND A. J. SWINGLE. Development of chronic low plasma volumes in long-term adrenalectomized dogs. *Proc. Soc. Exptl. Biol. Med.* 125: 811–814, 1967.
157. SWINGLE, W. W., AND A. J. SWINGLE. Terminal insufficiency in adrenalectomized dogs maintained for three years on substitution therapy and the apparent absence of accessory cortical tissue in this species. *Endocrinology* 81: 406–408, 1967.
158. SWINGLE, W. W., H. M. VARS, AND W. M. PARKINS. A study of the blood volume of adrenalectomized dogs. *Am. J. Physiol.* 109: 488–501, 1934.
159. TANZ, R. D. Studies on the action of cortisone acetate on isolated cardiac tissue. *J. Pharmacol. Exptl. Therap.* 128: 168–175, 1960.
160. TANZ, R. D. Studies on the inotropic action of aldosterone on isolated cardiac tissue preparations; including the effects of pH, ouabain and SC-8109. *J. Pharmacol. Exptl. Therap.* 135: 71–78, 1962.
161. TANZ, R. D., G. M. CLARK, AND R. W. WHITEHEAD. Influence of 9-alpha fluorohydrocortisone on contractility and Na content of isolated cat papillary muscle. *Proc. Soc. Exptl. Biol. Med.* 92: 167–169, 1956.
162. TANZ, R. D., AND C. F. KERBY. The inotropic action of certain steroids upon isolated cardiac tissue; with comments on steroidal cardiotonic structure-activity relationships. *J. Pharmacol. Exptl. Therap.* 131: 56–64, 1961.
163. TANZ, R. D., R. W. WHITEHEAD, AND G. J. WEIR. Cardiotonic activity of 9-alpha fluorohydrocortisone. *Proc. Soc. Exptl. Biol. Med.* 94: 258–262, 1957.
164. TOBIAN, L., AND J. BINION. Artery wall electrolytes in renal and DCA hypertension. *J. Clin. Invest.* 33: 1407–1414, 1954.
165. ULLRICK, W. C., B. B. BRENNAN, AND W. V. WHITEHORN. Characteristics of cardiac tissue from adrenalectomized rats. *Am. J. Physiol.* 200: 117–121, 1961.
166. ULLRICK, W. C., AND R. L. HAZELWOOD. Influence of aldosterone on isometric tension development in the rat heart. *Am. J. Physiol.* 204: 1001–1004, 1963.
167. UNTERMAN, D., A. C. DEGRAFF, AND H. S. KUPPERMAN. Effect of hypoadrenalism and excessive doses of desoxycorticosterone acetate upon response of the rat to ouabain. *Circulation Res.* 3: 280–284, 1955.
168. VERRIER, R. L., T. J. O'NEILL, AND A. M. LEFER. Functional capacity of resistance and capacitance vessels in adrenal insufficiency. *Am. J. Physiol.* 217: 341–347, 1969.
169. VERRIER, R. L., M. J. ROVETTO, AND A. M. LEFER. Blood volume and myocardial function in adrenal insufficiency. *Am. J. Physiol.* 217: 1559–1564, 1969.
170. WALSER, M., D. W. SELDIN, AND C. H. BURNETT. Blood volume and extracellular fluid volume during administration of ACTH and cortisone. *Am. J. Med.* 18: 454–461, 1955.
171. WEBB, W. R., AND I. U. DEGERLI. Myocardial metabolism. Effects of adrenalectomy and acute cortisol replacement. *J. Surg. Res.* 8: 73–77, 1968.
172. WEBB, W. R., I. U. DEGERLI, J. D. HARDY, AND M. UNAL. Cardiovascular responses in adrenal insufficiency. *Surgery* 58: 273–282, 1965.
173. WEINER, D. E., R. L. VERRIER, D. T. MILLER, AND A. M. LEFER. Effect of adrenalectomy on hemodynamics and regional blood flow in the cat. *Am. J. Physiol.* 213: 473–476, 1967.
174. WESTFALL, T. C., AND H. OSADA. Influence of adrenalectomy on the synthesis of norepinephrine in the rat heart. *J. Pharmacol. Exptl. Therap.* 167: 300–308, 1969.
175. WILBRANDT, W. Permeability and transport systems in living cells. *J. Pharm. Pharmacol.* 11: 65–79, 1959.
176. WYMAN, L. C., G. P. FULTON, AND M. H. SHULMAN. Direct observations on the circulation in the hamster cheek pouch in adrenal insufficiency and experimental hypercorticalism. *Ann. NY Acad. Sci.* 56: 643–658, 1953.
177. WYMAN, L. C., G. P. FULTON, F. N. SUDAK, AND G. N. PATTERSON. Electrocardiograms and serum electrolyte levels in hamsters with adrenal insufficiency and hypercorticalism. *Proc. Soc. Exptl. Biol. Med.* 84: 280–283, 1953.
178. WYMAN, J. C., AND C. TUM SUDEN. Studies on suprarenal insufficiency. VII. The blood volume of the rat in suprarenal insufficiency, anaphylactic shock and histamine shock. *Am. J. Physiol.* 94: 579–585, 1930.
179. ZAREM, H. A., AND B. W. ZWEIFACH. Microcirculatory effects of cortisol. Protective action against Na₄EDTA damage. *Proc. Soc. Exptl. Biol. Med.* 118: 602–606, 1965.
180. ZWEIFACH, B. W., E. SHORR, AND M. M. BLACK. The influence of the adrenal cortex on behaviour of terminal vascular bed. *Ann. NY Acad. Sci.* 56: 626–633, 1953.

CHAPTER 15

The role of adrenal corticosteroids in sensory processes

ROBERT I. HENKIN | *Section on Neuroendocrinology, National Heart and Lung Institute, Bethesda, Maryland*

CHAPTER CONTENTS

Gustation
   Detection in states of adrenal cortical insufficiency
   Recognition in states of adrenal cortical insufficiency
   Recognition-detection relationships
   Detection and recognition in states of adrenal corticosteroid excess
   Other steroid hormones
Olfaction
   Detection in states of adrenal cortical insufficiency
   Detection in Cushing's syndrome
   Other steroid hormones
Audition
   Detection in states of adrenal cortical insufficiency
   Recognition in states of adrenal cortical insufficiency
   Detection and recognition in Cushing's syndrome
Other Sensory Systems
Discussion
Conclusions

ADRENAL CORTICOSTEROIDS have been shown to regulate many different processes in several organ systems in species ranging from bacteria to man. Regulation of rates of enzyme synthesis through induction or inhibition has been well studied and is an important and well-documented phenomenon. However, the role adrenal corticosteroids play in the regulation of sensory processes, although extremely important for effective tissue or organ function, has not been extensively studied and is poorly understood. Indeed the whole process of stimulus-receptor recognition, particularly at the receptor membrane, has only recently been recognized as an important initial event in biochemical processes (1, 39). Only in recent years has the role of adrenal corticosteroids as regulators of detection and recognition of sensory signals for various sensory modalities emerged. Adrenal corticosteroids appear to regulate the level at which sensory input is perceived and the manner by which this information is integrated by the central nervous system. This chapter emphasizes this regulation in the sensory processes of taste, smell, and hearing and demonstrates how these processes are affected by adrenal corticosteroids.

GUSTATION

The initial observation of the role of adrenal corticosteroids in gustation was made by Richter (70) in 1936 when he noted that adrenalectomized rats exhibited an increased preference for NaCl as measured by a two-bottle preference test. This test consisted of the rat choosing between two available fluids, one preferred, the other rejected to a measurable extent. Although the latency of the onset of this increased NaCl preference varied from 1 to 9 days after adrenalectomy, it averaged approximately 3 days (77). This effect was eliminated entirely after bilateral section of the glossopharyngeal, chorda tympani, and lingual nerves (72, 74). After these surgical procedures the adrenalectomized rat did not increase its NaCl intake and subsequently died. Section only of the glossopharyngeal and chorda tympani nerves did not eliminate this effect, and these rats exhibited the same increase in salt preference as did neurally intact adrenalectomized rats (72, 74). Treatment of the adrenalectomized rat with cortisone-like drugs, with deoxycortisone acetate (DOCA), or with transplantation of adrenal cortical tissue to the eye was associated with the return of salt preference to normal levels (71).

Findings of increased NaCl preference in adrenalectomized rats were also noted by others who suggested, as did Richter, that this preference was related to an increased need of the adrenalectomized rat for salt solutions (5, 12, 32, 96–98). The counter ion was apparently of little importance, for sodium phosphate, as well as lactate, was preferred in a manner similar to NaCl (76, 77). Only sodium iodide among the sodium salts was not preferred to water (76, 77), and this same lack of preference also extended to dextrose (73) and to the chlorides of iron, magnesium, and aluminum (76, 77). Some curious and important inconsistencies in this phenomenon were noted by Richter and others. Adrenalectomized rats exhibited an increased preference not only for sodium salts but also potassium, ammonium, and calcium salts (76, 77). In later studies, at the same time that increased salt preference was noted, adrenalectomized rats exhibited a decrease in their salt taste threshold as measured behaviorally (75). This change amounted to a 15-fold increase in sensitivity. These apparently paradoxical effects were unexplained and were understandably overlooked in view of the more easily identifiable role of sodium intake in the maintenance of sodium equilibrium.

Although salt craving in patients with adrenal cortical insufficiency had been well known for many years (87, 90), this phenomenon was dramatically emphasized in studies in adrenalectomized rats. In man only one report of a lowered salt taste threshold had been reported prior to 1962 in a patient with hypotension and pulmonary arteriolar sclerosis (17). No data on the adrenal glands were given.

Herxheimer & Woodbury (49) reported a decreased preference (increased threshold) for NaCl in rats to whom they had administered DOCA in apparent contradiction to previous studies, but they noted little if any effect on sucrose. An increased salt appetite was observed by others who administered DOCA to rats (8–10, 19, 69). This effect was noted to persist for 2–3 days after DOCA injections were discontinued (19). This effect of DOCA was also observed not only for NaCl but also for Na_2HPO_4 (9) and the nonsodium salt NH_4Cl (9). The effect of DOCA was potentiated by ACTH, cortisone, and BAL (8).

In man a lowered taste threshold for NaCl was observed during a period of excessive water intake (94) and during sodium deprivation (94). An increased taste threshold was also observed for NaCl during water deprivation (95). These results were related to decreases in intracellular Na^+ concentration, which was assumed to occur secondarily to the increased fluid intake observed with DOCA administration. These results are at variance with other studies in man in which significant expansion of the extracellular fluid volume after administration of antidiuretic hormone had no effect on salt taste thresholds (44).

In an attempt to elucidate these varying results, Pfaffman & Bare (65) measured the electrical activity of the chorda tympani nerve in normal and adrenalectomized rats after placement of various tastants on the anterior two-thirds of the tongue. They found no differences in electrical thresholds between these two groups of animals. From these studies they concluded that salt deficiency, per se, did not alter the sensitivity of the taste receptor.

These apparently contradictory studies in both man and laboratory animals remained unresolved until 1962 when a series of studies were carried out to clarify these important and provocative early studies.

To apply these studies to man new measurement techniques had to be developed to aid in the definition of taste acuity. By means of a forced-choice, three stimulus drop technique, two indicators of taste acuity, detection and recognition thresholds, were developed to obtain quantitative data. *Detection threshold*, determined operationally by a variation of the method of limits, was defined as the least concentrated solution of solute and water that could be detected as different from water (44, 47, 48). To measure this threshold one drop of each of three solutions was used as the stimulus: two solutions were water, one was water and solute. The subject was forced to select the solute-containing solution as different from the other two. The median concentration of all the subjects' responses was chosen to express the central tendency measurement of the group. Subjects were also required to state whether the solution selected as different was salty, bitter, sweet, or sour. Through this latter procedure (47), in a manner similar to that described above, a *recognition threshold*—defined as the least concentrated solution correctly identified as salt, sweet, sour, or bitter —was operationally determined. These thresholds were measured for representatives of four taste qualities: for salt, NaCl, $NaHCO_3$, and KCl were used; for sweet, sucrose; for sour, HCl; and for bitter, urea. A reciprocal relationship exists between threshold and acuity. A lowering of threshold is consistent with an increased acuity, whereas an elevation of threshold is consistent with a decreased acuity.

Detection in States of Adrenal Cortical Insufficiency

Detection thresholds in normal volunteers and in patients with untreated adrenal cortical insufficiency are compared in Figure 1. Among the normal volunteers, median detection thresholds for the three salt solutions and for sucrose were approximately the same, 12 mM. For urea, detection threshold was 120 mM. For HCl the median detection threshold was 0.8 mM, which was lower than for the salts, sucrose, or urea. These thresholds were similar to those obtained in normal volunteers by other investigators (11, 16, 33, 54, 64, 79). Median detection threshold for each salt solution among the patients with untreated adrenal cortical insufficiency was approximately 0.1 mM, which was significantly lower (detection acuity increased) than that obtained in the normal volunteers. Detection thresholds for sucrose, HCl, and urea were also significantly lower among patients with untreated adrenal cortical insufficiency than among the normal volunteers. The pattern of responsiveness for taste detection acuity among the untreated patients was similar to that noted for the normal volunteers although at a level of responsiveness approximately 150 times greater. Detection thresholds for the three salts and sucrose were the same. There was a relative increase in the median detection threshold for urea, whereas the median detection threshold for HCl was relatively lower than that for either NaCl, sucrose, or urea. This increased detection acuity in patients with untreated adrenal cortical insufficiency has also been observed by other investigators [(56, 66, 68); J. C. Beck, personal communication] and has served as an adjunctive tool in the clinical diagnosis of adrenal cortical insufficiency.

These data demonstrated that patients with untreated adrenal cortical insufficiency detected solutions of representatives of four taste qualities at significantly lower concentrations than did normal volunteers. This phe-

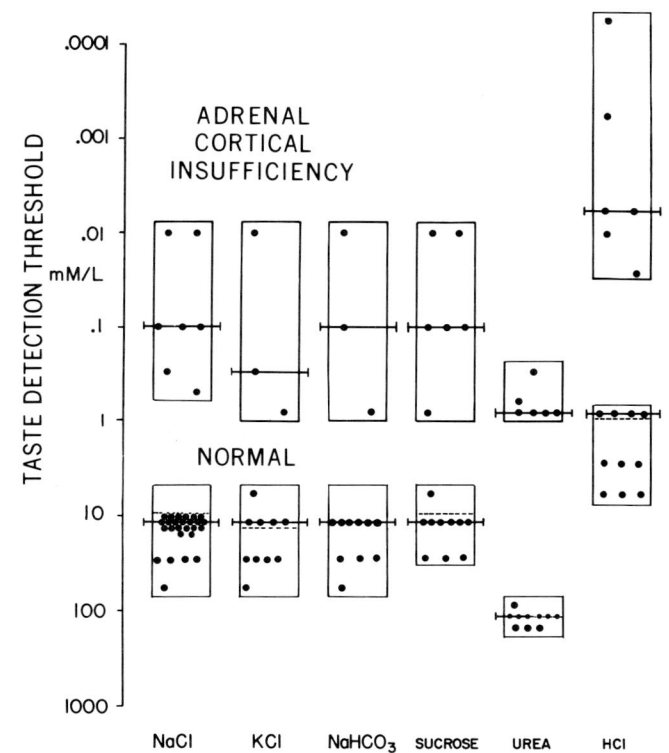

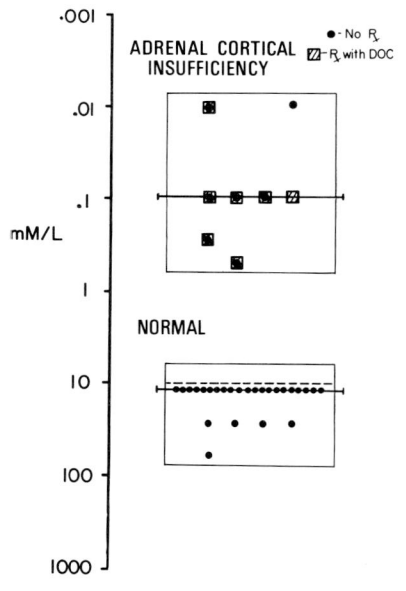

FIG. 1. Detection thresholds in normal volunteers compared with those in patients with untreated adrenal cortical insufficiency for representatives of 4 taste qualities. *Circles* in lower enclosures, individual detection thresholds for each quality in normal volunteers. *Enclosures* define upper and lower limits of range of responses of volunteers. *Lines* through enclosures represent median detection thresholds of volunteers. *Dashed lines* within lower enclosures indicate median detection thresholds determined by other investigators (11, 54, 64). *Circles* and *upper enclosures* represent, respectively, individual detection thresholds and range of response in patients with adrenal cortical insufficiency, either untreated or taken off replacement therapy. *Solid lines* through enclosures represent the median detection thresholds of untreated patients. [From Henkin et al. (44).]

detection threshold for NaCl in patients after treatment with DOCA or in the untreated state was the same, 0.1 mM (Fig. 2). Similar data were obtained for the detection of each of the other salts and for sucrose, HCl, and urea. Thus Na-K-active steroids, although they play a significant role in the control of serum sodium and potassium concentration and of extracellular fluid volume, did not return to normal the increased detection acuity observed in these patients.

In a further series of experiments, changes in detection acuity were studied in patients with adrenal cortical insufficiency before and after treatment with the carbohydrate-active steroid prednisolone [(Δ_1F), 20 mg/day for 2 or more days]. This treatment returned taste thresholds to normal in each patient (Fig. 3). In the untreated state, median detection threshold for NaCl was 0.1 mM; however, after treatment with Δ_1F for 2 days the median detection threshold was 12 mM. This threshold was not significantly different from that obtained in normal volunteers.

This return to normal was independent of the type of carbohydrate-active steroid used. Treatment with hydrocortisone, cortisone, and dexamethasone all returned taste detection acuity to normal (34, 35). This return to normal acuity was independent of the route of administration of the hormone (i.e., oral, subcutaneous, or intravenous). However, the amount of hormone administered influenced the time required to return taste detection acuity to normal. Administration of large amounts of hormone required less time to return detection acuity to normal than administration of small amounts of hormone. Patients who were maintained on adequate re-

nomenon was particularly striking because the ranges of taste detection acuity of the untreated patients and the normal volunteers did not overlap. Whereas salt craving had been observed in 10–20% of patients with untreated adrenal cortical insufficiency, virtually all these patients exhibited decreased detection thresholds for each taste quality.

To evaluate further the relationship between taste detection acuity and the various changes in adrenal cortical hormones, detection acuity for each of four taste qualities was measured daily in patients with adrenal cortical insufficiency before and after treatment with daily intramuscular injections of 20 mg DOCA for periods of 2–7 days (Fig. 2). Comparison of detection thresholds of the patients with those of normal volunteers revealed that the increased detection sensitivity (lowered thresholds) observed in patients with untreated adrenal cortical insufficiency persisted even though they were treated with DOCA for as long as 7 days; the median

FIG. 2. Detection thresholds for NaCl in normal volunteers compared with those in patients with adrenal cortical insufficiency treated with deoxycorticosterone acetate (*DOC*). *Hatched squares*, detection thresholds in each patient after treatment. Data presented here for NaCl are similar to those obtained with representatives of each of 4 taste qualities. [From Henkin (35).]

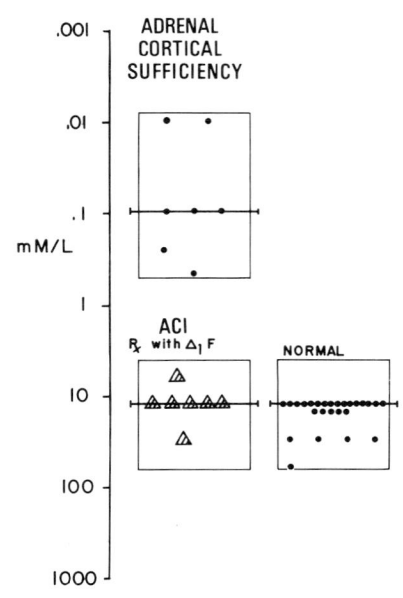

FIG. 3. Detection thresholds for NaCl in normal volunteers compared with those in patients with adrenal cortical insufficiency (ACI) treated with the carbohydrate-active steroid prednisolone ($\Delta_1 F$). *Hatched triangles*, detection thresholds in each patient after treatment. [From Henkin (35).]

placement doses of these hormones never exhibited abnormalities of taste detection.

Metabolic balance studies were carried out in several patients with adrenal cortical insufficiency to investigate further the mechanism of this phenomenon. One such study involving taste detection (shown for NaCl but also observed with each of the other taste qualities) is shown in Figure 4. A similar pattern of response occurred in each patient for each taste quality tested. Detection thresholds were first determined approximately 1 week after all replacement therapy had been withdrawn. At this time the patient's detection threshold for NaCl was 0.1 mM, a level significantly lower than normal. She weighed 42 kg, her serum potassium concentration was 5.5 mEq/liter, and her serum sodium concentration was 132 mEq/liter. After oral treatment with $\Delta_1 F$ (20 mg/day), her taste detection thresholds returned to normal within 48 hr without significant alteration in serum sodium or potassium concentrations or in extracellular fluid volume, as represented by measurements of body weight. Treatment with $\Delta_1 F$ then continued for 10 days. During this time taste detection acuity remained within normal limits. At the end of this period treatment with $\Delta_1 F$ was discontinued. Within 4 days detection thresholds for NaCl fell from a normal threshold of 30 mM to 0.1 mM, a level significantly below normal. These data demonstrate the lag period between the time that treatment with carbohydrate-active steroids was stopped and the onset of increased detection acuity. Increased detection acuity did not occur immediately after treatment was discontinued but appeared gradually over a period of 3–4 days. Additional experiments suggested that this lag period could not be shortened (34, 35). At the time this patient's taste detection sensitivity increased (thresholds were decreased) to abnormal levels, there was no significant alteration either in body weight, hyponatremia, or hyperkalemia.

Six days after treatment with $\Delta_1 F$ was discontinued DOCA was given intramuscularly (20 mg/day) for 2 days. This treatment lowered serum potassium concentration to normal (3.5 mEq/liter), raised serum sodium concentration to normal (136 mEq/liter), and produced an increase in body weight of approximately 2 kg. Despite this correction of serum electrolytes to normal and an increase in body weight, there was no alteration of increased detection acuity for the taste of NaCl or for three other taste qualities.

On the 24th day of the study 200 mg hydrocortisone acetate was given intravenously, and within 24 hr taste detection thresholds for each taste quality returned to normal. This return was not accompanied by a further increase in body weight or change in serum sodium or potassium concentration.

These data indicate a lag period between the beginning of replacement therapy with carbohydrate-active steroids and the return of taste detection acuity to normal. Approximately twice as much time was required for the increase in taste detection acuity to occur after treatment was discontinued as was required for acuity to decrease to normal after treatment with carbohydrate-active steroids was reinstituted.

These data also demonstrate that the return of taste detection acuity to normal is dose related. After treatment with 20 mg $\Delta_1 F$ each day for 2 days, taste detection acuity in the patient returned to normal, whereas it returned to normal within 24 hr after treatment with 200 mg hydrocortisone acetate (Fig. 4). In another patient, whose daily maintenance dose of $\Delta_1 F$ was 5.0 mg, treatment with 2.5 mg each day for 4 days did not return detection acuity to normal.

The mechanism by which these lag periods occur is not known. The period of 3–5 days before increased acuity occurs after withdrawl of carbohydrate-active steroids varied little among the patients studied. This lag period is long if the short half-life of most carbohydrate-active steroids (less than 24 hr) is considered. These data suggest that, even though significant carbohydrate-active steroid activity cannot be found in blood or urine of most patients 48 hr after the last dose of steroid is administered, tissue levels of this hormone are still measurable, and at least another 24–28 hr are required before some tissue stores are depleted to a level where increased detection sensitivity occurs. Indeed adrenal corticosteroid levels can be measured in some animal tissues as long as 3 weeks after adrenalectomy (42, 43a). It is also of interest to note that increased salt preference was demonstrated in rats an average of 3–4 days after they were adrenalectomized (77). By contrast, physiological effects of Na-K-active steroids, similarly evaluated, demonstrated that 24–48 hr after treatment with DOCA was discontinued in patients with adrenal cortical insufficiency some manifestations of hyperkalemia and hyponatremia could

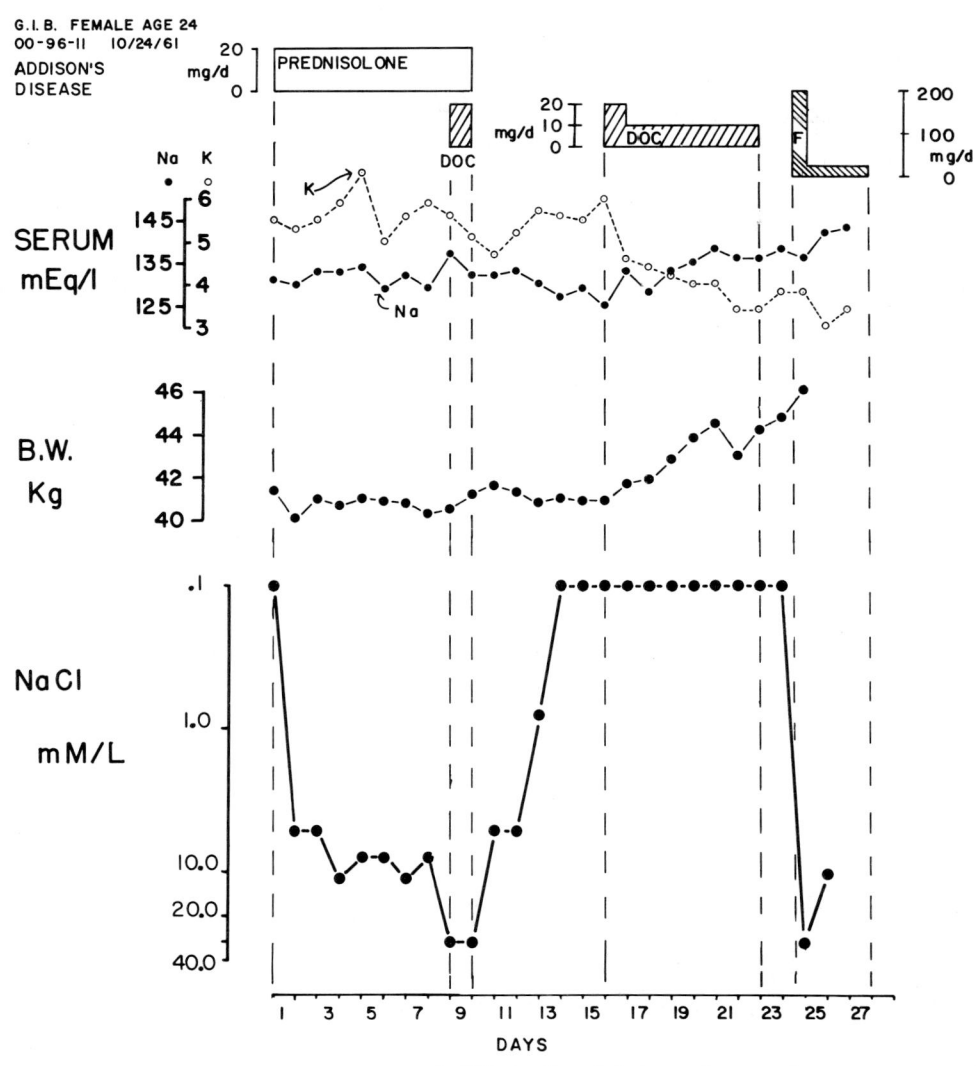

FIG. 4. Effects of prednisolone, deoxycorticosterone acetate (*DOC*), hydrocortisone acetate (*F*), and no treatment on serum sodium and potassium concentrations, body weight (*B.W.*), and taste detection thresholds for NaCl in 1 patient with adrenal cortical insufficiency. Hormone therapy is expressed in milligrams per day (mg/d). Threshold values for NaCl ranging from 6 to 60 mM are within normal limits. Serum concentration of sodium between 135 and 145 mEq/liter and of potassium between 3.5 and 4.5 mEq/liter is considered within normal limits. [From Henkin et al. (44).]

be observed. The possible differences in tissue storage and release of Na-K-active and carbohydrate-active steroids are not well known, but these observations may offer clues to some of the differences in their timing of action.

As would be expected there is a marked circadian variation in taste detection acuity that closely follows the pattern of circulating levels of cortisol in man [(36); Fig. 5]. As the circulating level of cortisol increases in normal man in the early morning hours, taste detection acuity for NaCl also increases (detection thresholds decrease), reaching peak levels at approximately similar times. The circulating level of cortisol falls abruptly thereafter, and there is a similar relatively abrupt decrease in taste detection acuity (detection thresholds increase) for NaCl; lowest levels occur between 6 and 9 AM in both parameters (36). A gradual increase in taste detection acuity then follows over the next 15–18 hr. In patients with untreated adrenal cortical insufficiency, little if any circadian pattern of variation in taste detection acuity was observed after their taste detection acuity increased 3–4 days after withdrawal of hormonal therapy. These changes occurred both in patients with adrenal cortical insufficiency due to Addison's disease and in patients with panhypopituitarism (36), which further relates the change to alterations in cortisol rather than to alterations in ACTH. However, after replacement of hormonal therapy and the return of taste detection acuity to normal levels a circadian pattern of variation was observed that could not be distinguished from that of euadrenal normal volunteers (36).

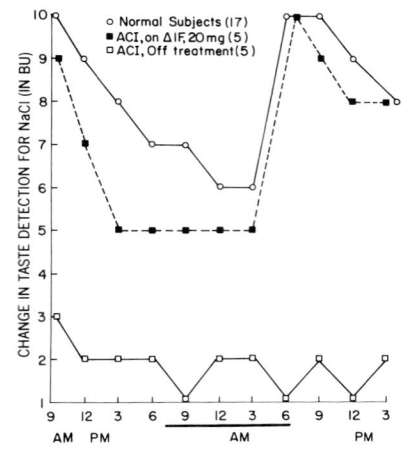

FIG. 5. Comparison of circadian pattern of variation in taste detection acuity (median detection threshold) for NaCl in normal subjects and in patients with adrenal cortical insufficiency (ACI) without treatment and after treatment with prednisolone [($\Delta_1 F$), 20 mg/day, given orally in divided doses every 6 hr for 2 days]. Numbers in parentheses, number of subjects. BU signifies a bottle unit based on the concentration of NaCl presented. 1 BU = 10^{-4} mM NaCl, 2 = 10^{-3}, 3 = 10^{-2}, 4 = 10^{-1}, 5 = 0.5, 6 = 0.8, 7 = 3, 8 = 6, 9 = 12, 10 = 30. Note increased detection acuity and absence of circadian pattern of variation in patients with untreated adrenal cortical insufficiency. Note that detection acuity decreased (detection threshold increased) to normal limits after treatment with $\Delta_1 F$ for 2 days and that the circadian pattern of variation was similar to that observed in normal volunteers. Note also increased detection acuity for NaCl in patients with ACI off treatment. *Solid black line* on ordinate indicates hours of darkness. [From Henkin (36).]

Recognition in States of Adrenal Cortical Insufficiency

Coincident with the onset of increased taste detection acuity in patients with untreated adrenal cortical insufficiency, there was a significant decrease in taste recognition acuity (increased thresholds). This manifested itself as a significant increase in median recognition threshold for each of four qualities at the same time that a significant decrease in each median detection threshold occurred. This is exemplified in one patient with adrenal cortical insufficiency in Figure 6. During treatment with carbohydrate-active steroids both detection and recognition thresholds for each taste quality were within normal limits. For convenience, this is shown only for NaCl in Figure 6. After withdrawal of therapy there was the progressive increase in detection acuity (decreased detection thresholds) as shown previously. In addition there was a concomitant, progressive decrease in recognition acuity (increased recognition threshold). Patients generally called NaCl bitter at concentrations they called salty when on treatment. Thus, at a time when detection acuity for NaCl was 1,000 or more times as sensitive as normal, recognition acuity (the ability to integrate taste information) was about one-fifth to one-tenth normal. This dichotomy in responsiveness persisted as long as carbohydrate-active steroids were withheld. Treatment with DOCA (20 mg/day for 2 days) altered neither the lowered detection threshold nor the elevated recognition threshold. However, within 24 hr after carbohydrate-active steroid therapy was resumed, detection and recognition thresholds for each taste quality had returned to normal. These results suggest that salt craving in man may be a manifestation of the decreased recognition acuity observed after withdrawal of therapy, for it was still observed after treatment with Na-K-active steroids, at a time when body electrolyte distribution was normal.

In an effort to quantitate measurements of taste recognition further, "forced scaling" judgments over the entire range of taste acuity were obtained on an absolute but subjective scale from 0 to 100 (28, 41, 47). For normal subjects taste intensity increases with increasing tastant concentration for all taste qualities and follows a curve that is essentially symmetrical about its midpoint (Fig. 7). The curves for two taste qualities (NaCl and sucrose) are nearly coincident, whereas those for HCl and urea can be superimposed on these two by displacement along the concentration axis.

Various analytical equations can be used to express the two major characteristics of these curves (i.e., their symmetry about their midpoint and their similar shape). Of the possible empirical equations, the data are best

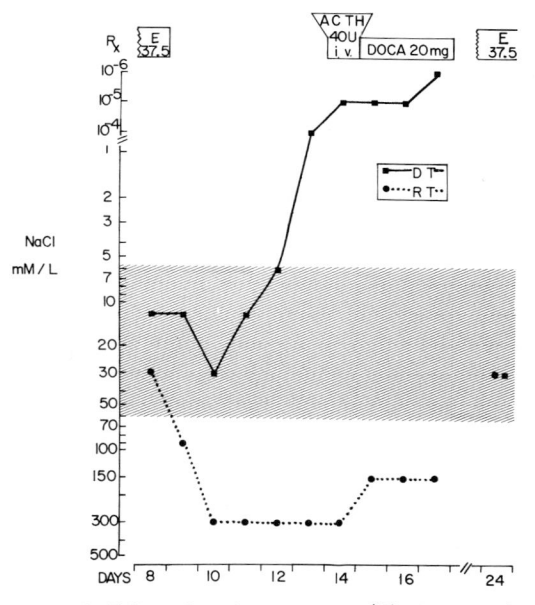

FIG. 6. Effect of cortisone acetate (E), deoxycorticosterone acetate (DOCA), ACTH, and no treatment on detection threshold (DT) and recognition threshold (RT) for NaCl in 1 patient with adrenal cortical insufficiency. Threshold values for NaCl ranging from 6 to 60 mM are within normal limits for both sensory detection (■) and recognition (●). Note that with the termination of hormonal replacement there is both an increase in sensory detection acuity (threshold decrease) and a decrease in sensory integrative capacity (threshold increase). Solutions of NaCl as concentrated as 150 mM were called either sweet, bitter, sour, or salty without specific pattern. Treatment with ACTH (40 units iv over 8 hr) altered neither serum or urinary levels of carbohydrate-active steroid, nor taste detection or recognition thresholds. [From Henkin (35).]

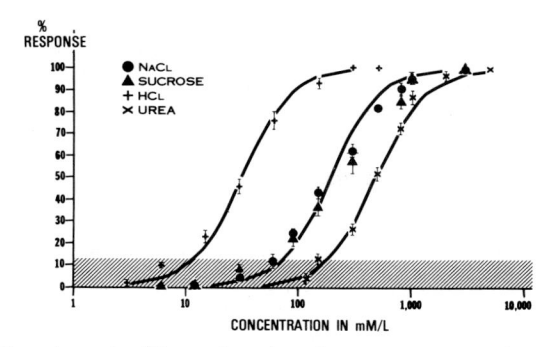

FIG. 7. Taste intensity (I) as a function of tastant concentration (T) for 4 taste qualities in normal subjects. Per cent taste response intensity (I) measured on a scale from 1 to 100 is plotted on *ordinate*. On *abscissa*, T is plotted. Each symbol represents mean ± 1 SEM of the responses of 21 normal subjects. *Hatched area*, distribution of detection thresholds for taste qualities. Threshold events comprise no more than 10% of entire dynamic taste range. [From Henkin & Bradley (41).]

represented by

$$I/I_{max} = \frac{K(T)^2}{K(T)^2 + 1} \qquad (1)$$

where I is the intensity at the concentration T, I_{max} is the maximum intensity at highest T, and K is a constant (41).

The curves in Figure 7 represent the best empirical fit of Equation *1* to the experimental points. The K values, obtained at T^{-2} where I/I_{max} is equal to 0.5, are, in decreasing order, 1.0×10^{-3} for HCl, 2.8×10^{-5} for sucrose, 2.8×10^{-5} for NaCl, and 4.5×10^{-6} for urea.

As expected, there appears to be a specific relationship between detection and recognition thresholds and intensity judgments; that is, detection and recognition thresholds lie within a narrow range at the lower end of each intensity curve. In order to demonstrate these latter interrelationships quantitatively the mean intensity judgments at detection and recognition thresholds were calculated (Table 1). On the average, normal subjects give an appropriate recognition response to tastants at recognition threshold at an intensity between 5 and 10% of the maximum response. Thus recognition and, of course, detection thresholds occur at a relatively low intensity response for all taste qualities.

Forced scaling for patients with adrenal cortical insufficiency indicates that responses retain a pattern similar to that observed in normal volunteers but are shifted to a higher concentration of tastant. This shift is essentially of the same magnitude for each taste quality (Fig. 8). There is no change in the order of intensity response for these taste qualities, for the K values retain the same rank order and relative value: 1.6×10^{-4}, 6.6×10^{-6}, 6.6×10^{-6}, and 1×10^{-6} for HCl, sucrose, NaCl, and urea, respectively.

It is difficult to determine whether or not the empirical equation that best fits these data optimally represents the data. In fact, the experimental points below $I/I_{max} = 0.5$ generally lie above the curve, whereas those above $I/I_{max} = 0.5$ generally lie below the curve. This suggests that the data may be better represented by an equation of lower order in T than T^2 (41).

Recognition thresholds for patients with adrenal cortical insufficiency, off treatment, still occur between 5 and 10% of the maximum intensity as in the case of normal subjects, albeit at relatively higher concentrations. Recognition still occurs within a relatively narrow spectrum of the total dynamic range of intensity, despite the increase in recognition threshold. Detection thresholds for patients occur at concentrations at which intensities are only a small fraction of a percent of the total intensity range. This is in marked contrast to normal subjects whose detection thresholds occur at concentrations where intensities, as calculated from Equation *1*, are about 1%, the mean measured value being 1.1% of the total dynamic range of taste responsiveness (see Table 1).

Patients with several diseases of the adrenal cortex exhibited this same pattern of alteration of tastant detection and recognition. Patients with untreated idiopathic adrenal cortical insufficiency (Addison's disease), patients in whom both adrenal glands were surgically

TABLE 1. *Ratio of Recognition Threshold to Detection Threshold and Subjective Intensity Response for Each of Four Taste Qualities*

Taste Quality	R:D Ratio	Mean Intensity at RT, %	Mean Intensity at DT, %
Sucrose	2.5	5.5 ± 1.0*	0.7 ± 0.7
NaCl	2.5	5.8 ± 0.7	0.4 ± 0.3
HCl	1.0	5.8 ± 1.1	1.7 ± 1.0
Urea	1.25	9.5 ± 1.4	1.5 ± 0.7
Mean		6.7	1.1

R:D, recognition threshold:detection threshold; RT, recognition threshold; DT, detection threshold. * Mean ± 1 SEM.

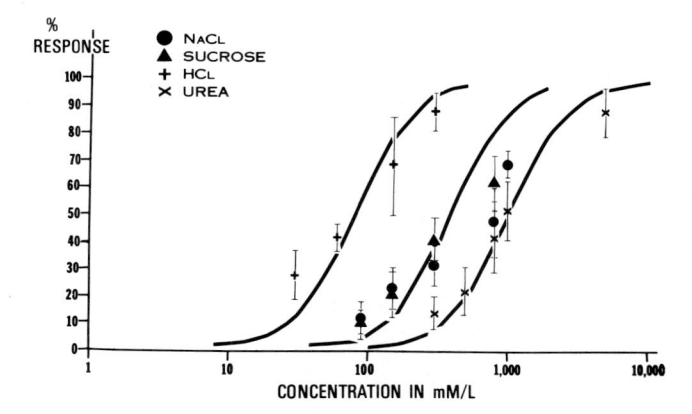

FIG. 8. Taste intensity (I, per cent response) as a function of tastant concentration (T) for four taste qualities in patients with untreated adrenal cortical insufficiency. Response patterns retain a slope similar to those observed in normal volunteers (Fig. 7), but responses are shifted to higher concentrations. Each symbol represents mean ± 1 SEM of the responses of 5 patients untreated 4 or more days. [From Henkin & Bradley (41).]

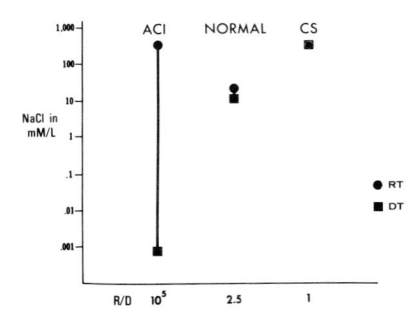

FIG. 9. Detection and recognition acuity expressed as R:D ratios for NaCl in normal subjects and in patients with untreated adrenal cortical insufficiency (*ACI*) and Cushing's syndrome (*CS*). *DT* and *RT*, detection and recognition thresholds, respectively. Results noted here for NaCl are similar for each of 3 other taste qualities. [From Henkin & Bradley (41).]

removed, and patients with untreated panhypopituitarism exhibited these responses (34, 35, 41, 48). Patients with untreated congenital virilizing adrenal cortical hyperplasia of the salt-losing or non-salt-losing types (37, 41), who were treated with carbohydrate-active steroids and then studied after removal of these hormones, also exhibited these responses. It is clear that patients with these latter conditions, studied after long-term treatment with suppressive doses of carbohydrate-active steroids, were functionally similar to patients with idiopathic or surgically produced adrenal cortical insufficiency.

Recognition-Detection Relationships

There was always a consistent relationship between the recognition and detection thresholds (R:D ratio) for the four taste qualities tested (40, 41). This ratio ranged in normal subjects from a lowest possible value of unity to a value usually not exceeding 10 (Fig. 9). Because of the increased detection acuity and decreased recognition acuity the R:D ratios for patients with untreated adrenal cortical insufficiency were markedly elevated compared to those of normal subjects. Whereas the R:D ratio for all taste qualities ranged from 1 to 10 in normal subjects, it ranged from 10^4 to 10^7 in patients with untreated adrenal cortical insufficiency. In this sense the dynamic range over which taste events occur in patients with untreated adrenal cortical insufficiency is increased by a factor of 10^3 to 10^6 over that of normal volunteers.

Detection and Recognition in States of Adrenal Corticosteroid Excess

In a reciprocal relationship taste detection acuity has been found to be lower (elevated detection thresholds) than normal in each patient with Cushing's syndrome studied in our laboratory (35, 41). Each of these patients had excessive secretion of carbohydrate-active steroid due to the presence of adrenal cortical hyperplasia, adenoma, or carcinoma. However, this aspect of taste-steroid relationships is not as well studied as that relating changes in taste acuity to the absence of adrenal corticosteroids. Treatment of normal subjects with large oral doses of various carbohydrate-active steroids, including prednisolone (50 mg/day for 5–8 days) did not lower taste detection sensitivity below normal (35, 41). Endogeneous secretion of excessive amounts of aldosterone from patients with aldosterone-secreting tumors of the adrenal cortex or with nodular adrenal cortical hyperplasia also did not significantly affect taste detection sensitivity (41). Treatment of normal volunteers with large amounts of Na-K-active steroids (20 mg DOCA per day for 2–5 days) also did not alter taste acuity in any significant manner (Table 2).

Taste recognition acuity was also significantly decreased in patients with Cushing's syndrome, as in patients with untreated adrenal cortical insufficiency. Indeed the presenting clinical symptom of several pa-

TABLE 2. *Taste Acuity in Patients with Various Diseases of Adrenal Cortex*

Condition	Untreated		Replacement Therapy	
	Detection acuity	Recognition acuity	Na-K-active steroid; D/R acuity	CAS; D/R acuity
Decreased adrenal cortical steroid secretion				
Addison's disease	High	Low	No change	Normal
Bilateral adrenalectomy	High	Low	No change	Normal
Panhypopituitarism	High	Low	No change	Normal
Congenital adrenal hyperplasia				
Salt-losing type	High	Low	No change	Normal
Non-salt-losing type	High	Low	No change	Normal
Increased adrenal cortical steroid secretion				
Cushing's syndrome	Low	Low	No change	Normal (sup)
Adrenal cortical carcinoma	Low	Low	No change	Normal (sup)
Aldosteronoma	Normal	Normal	No change	No change
Normal adrenal cortical steroid secretion				
Normal volunteers	Normal	Normal	No change	No change
Normal volunteers + metyrapone	High	Low		

CAS, carbohydrate-active steroid. D, detection; R, recognition. Sup, endogenous CAS secretion suppressed by administration of exogenous CAS or other agents.

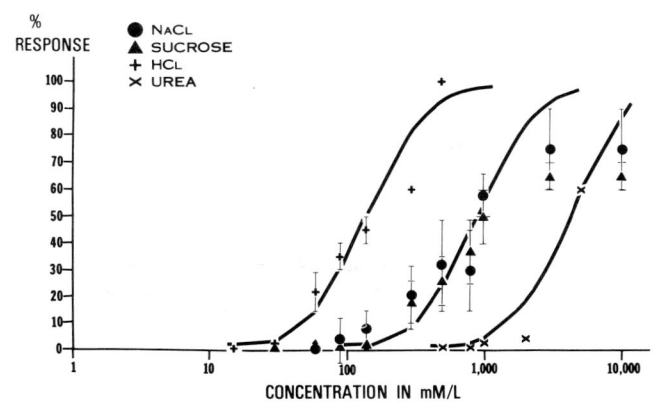

FIG. 10. Taste intensity (I, per cent response) as a function of tastant concentration (T) for 4 taste qualities in patients with untreated Cushing's syndrome. Each symbol represents the mean ± 1 SEM of the responses of 5 untreated patients. Response patterns are similar to those observed in normal volunteers or in patients with untreated adrenal cortical insufficiency but are shifted to still higher concentrations. [From Henkin & Bradley (41).]

tients with Cushing's syndrome was their inability to obtain normal taste from their food. This symptom preceded their later symptoms of hypertension, diabetes, and muscle weakness. In these patients detection and recognition thresholds were usually the same, the R:D ratios being close to unity for all taste qualities. This indicates a narrowing of the dynamic range over which tastants were appreciated in contrast to the expanded dynamic range observed in patients with untreated adrenal cortical insufficiency (see Fig. 9).

Forced-scaling responses in patients with Cushing's syndrome are shown in Figure 10. The K values (See Eq. 1) in these patients remain in the same rank order and relative value as in normal volunteers and in patients with untreated Addison's disease: 5.1×10^{-5}, 1.2×10^{-6}, 1.2×10^{-6}, and 5.7×10^{-8} for HCl, sucrose, NaCl, and urea, respectively. Each tastant curve was shifted to a higher concentration than in normal subjects or in patients with untreated adrenal cortical insufficiency. This shift was similar for each taste quality except that the urea curve was shifted to a greater extent in patients with Cushing's syndrome, shifting to a higher concentration (T) by a larger factor than any other tastant curve. This phenomenon is most easily observed upon comparison of intensity responses of the three groups of subjects to a single tastant respresentative of each taste quality (Fig. 11). These data indicate that recognition acuity for each tastant is affected to a greater extent in patients with Cushing's syndrome than in patients with adrenal cortical insufficiency.

Suppression of endogenous carbohydrate-active steroid secretion in patients with Cushing's syndrome by administration of exogenous carbohydrate-active steroid (decadron suppression), metyrapone, aminoglutethamide, or mitotane, or after surgical adrenalectomy, returned taste detection and recognition acuity and forced scaling to normal for as long as suppression was maintained [(35, 41); Table 2]. Treatment with Na-K-active steroids had no effect on abnormal taste acuity in these patients. Withdrawal of carbohydrate-active steroids from those patients with Cushing's syndrome who were successfully treated with bilateral surgical adrenalectomy resulted in changes in taste acuity similar to those observed in patients with untreated adrenal cortical insufficiency.

Other Steroid Hormones

Other steroid hormones have been reported to be related to some aspects of taste acuity in animals. Allara (2) implied that castration of male rats decreased taste sensation and that exogenous administration of testosterone propionate was implicated with a return of taste function toward normal. These studies were particularly related to changes in the structure of taste buds, castration associated with decreases in taste bud number, and administration of exogenous testosterone associated with a return of taste bud number toward normal. In other studies, Allara (2a) reported that exogenous administration of estrogen to male rats was associated with a decrease in the number of taste buds, whereas after it was stopped taste bud number returned toward normal. Valenstein (88a) noted that male and female rats differed in their preference responses for glucose and saccharin solutions. Taste acuity also appears to change systematically in women during the menstrual cycle with a greater detection acuity observed during the follicular phase of the cycle, a lesser detection acuity observed during the luteal phase, albeit all within the limits generally regarded as normal (35a). These studies in rat and man, while provocative and interesting, do not definitely implicate any specific gonadal steroid in the taste process. Further work in this area is necessary to provide these correlates, if they exist.

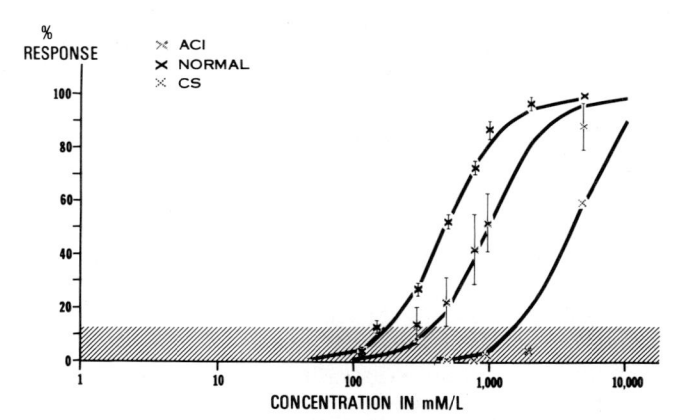

FIG. 11. Comparison of taste intensity (I, per cent response) as a function of tastant concentration (T) for patients with untreated adrenal cortical insufficiency (ACI) and patients with untreated Cushing's syndrome (CS) and in normal subjects for the taste of urea. Hatched area, distribution of detection and recognition thresholds relative to entire dynamic range over which taste events occur. Note that responses of patients with ACI and CS are uniformly shifted to higher concentrations. [From Henkin & Bradley (41).]

OLFACTION

The participation of carbohydrate-active steroids in the regulation of taste acuity has been applied to other sensory modalities. This possibility was initially suggested by studies in sheep in which olfactory cues appeared to determine NaCl preference after placement of a chronic parotid fistula and subsequent sodium depletion (6).

To study olfaction in man detection and recognition thresholds for several olfactory stimuli were obtained in a manner similar to that used to obtain these measurements for taste. Normal volunteers or patients with several diseases of the adrenal cortex were required to sniff each of three bottles, two of which contained water or mineral oil, whereas one was an aqueous solution of NaCl, KCl, NaHCO$_3$, sucrose, urea, HCl, or pyridine, or a solution of nitrobenzene or thiophene in mineral oil. The subject was required to state which one of the three solutions was different from the other two and if possible to describe the difference. Thirteen different concentrations of solutes along with two solutions of the appropriate solvent were presented in a mixed design similar to that used previously for the taste studies (38, 47, 59). In this manner, median detection and recognition thresholds were operationally obtained for the vapors above these solutions. The median detection threshold was defined as the least concentrated vapor detected as different from water or mineral oil among a given subject group; the median recognition threshold was defined as the least concentrated vapor recognized correctly as the vapor. Recognition thresholds for NaCl, KCl, NaHCO$_3$, urea, HCl, or sucrose are not particularly meaningful due to the difficulty experienced by all sub-

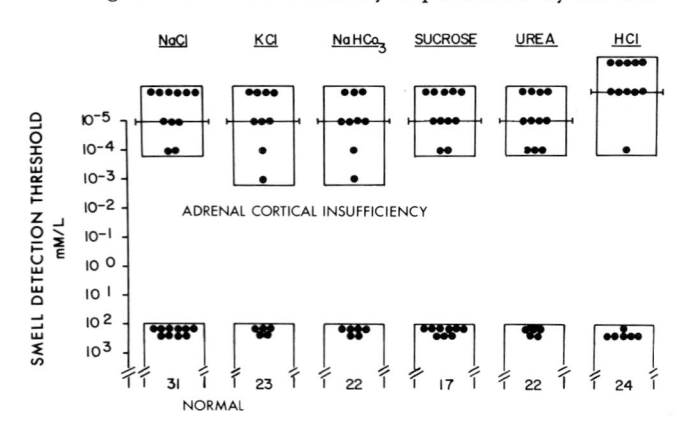

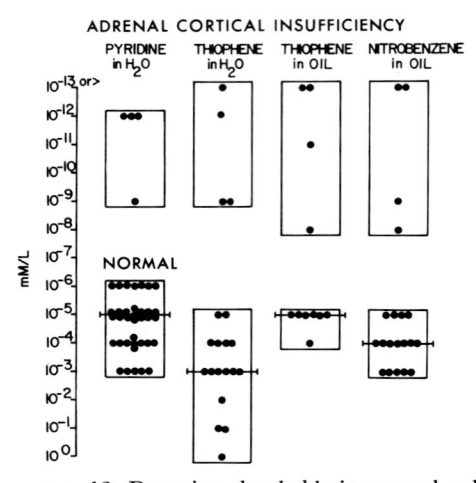

FIG. 12. Detection thresholds in normal volunteers compared with those in patients with untreated adrenal cortical insufficiency for vapor above a solution of NaCl and solutions of other solutes. *Lower circles*, individual detection thresholds; *open enclosures*, range of responsiveness in normal volunteers. *Numbers* at open end of lower enclosures indicate number of normal volunteers who could not detect any difference between water and the vapor above a solution of NaCl or other solutions of solutes as concentrated as 300 mM. *Upper circles, enclosures,* and *lines* through the enclosures represent similar data obtained in patients with untreated adrenal cortical insufficiency. *Lines* through enclosures represent median detection thresholds. [From Henkin & Bartter (38).]

FIG. 13. Detection thresholds in normal volunteers compared with those in patients with untreated adrenal cortical insufficiency for vapor above solutions of various concentrations of pyridine, thiophene, and nitrobenzene. Data in *lower portion* of figure represent responses of normal volunteers. Data in *upper portion* of the figure represent responses of patients with untreated adrenal cortical insufficiency. Detection thresholds of patients are significantly lower (detection acuity is greater) than those of normal volunteers for each vapor. There is no overlap between the responses of the groups. [From Henkin & Bartter (38).]

jects in identification of the olfactory stimulus. However, recognition thresholds for pyridine, nitrobenzene, or thiophene were obtained.

Detection in States of Adrenal Cortical Insufficiency

As with taste, patients with untreated adrenal cortical insufficiency exhibited increased detection acuity (decreased thresholds) for the vapor above solutions of NaCl, KCl, NaHCO$_3$, sucrose, urea, and HCl (Fig. 12). The responses of 43 normal subjects for these same solutes indicate that most normal subjects either could not discriminate between water and these solutions or at best could distinguish between water and solutes as concentrated as 150 mEq/liter. However, patients with untreated adrenal cortical insufficiency, using olfactory clues alone, detected differences between water and these solutes 1/10,000 as dilute as could normal subjects. There was no overlap between the responses of the normal subjects and those of the untreated patients, similar to the results shown with gustatory stimuli. The median detection threshold obtained among the untreated patients was approximately 1/100 the concentration they required to detect a difference between water and these solutes through the sense of taste.

Differences in the detection of vapors above water and pyridine, water and thiophene, mineral oil and thiophene, and mineral oil and nitrobenzene between normal subjects and patients with untreated adrenal cortical insufficiency are shown in Figure 13. As in the previous studies, patients with untreated adrenal cortical insufficiency detected each solute in significantly lower concentration than did normal volunteers, the difference in acuity being approximately 10^4, as with taste.

Demonstration of increased detection acuity in patients with adrenal cortical insufficiency has not been repeated in man by other investigators. However, they have been verified in the rat by using quite different measurement techniques with results qualitatively similar to those observed in man (P. C. Sakellaris, unpublished observations).

Increases in olfactory detection acuity (decreased thresholds) did not return to normal after treatment of patients with adrenal cortical insufficiency with Na-K-active steroids. In these studies with Na-K-active steroids, daily intramuscular injections of 20 mg DOCA were given to seven patients with adrenal cortical insufficiency for 2–10 days without any alteration in their olfactory detection acuity, although there were increases in their body weight and correction of their hyponatremia and hyperkalemia toward normal levels. Similar results occurred after presentation of other solutes, including pyridine, nitrobenzene, or thiophene. There was no overlap between the responses of the patients and those of the normal subjects.

Treatment of patients with adrenal cortical insufficiency with carbohydrate-active steroids returned olfactory detection acuity for all solutes to normal. Treatment with prednisolone (20 mg/day) returned acuity to the normal range within 24 hr. Four of the seven treated patients could no longer detect any difference between a solution of NaCl as concentrated as 300 mM and two solutions of water. Similar results were obtained after the presentation of stimuli generally considered odorous, as well as with those stimuli generally considered nonodorous.

A metabolic study was carried out in several patients with adrenal cortical insufficiency in whom changes in taste and olfaction were correlated with changes in serum electrolytes and body fluids after treatment with various adrenal steroid hormones (Fig. 14). The study presented in Figure 14 is representative of that carried out in

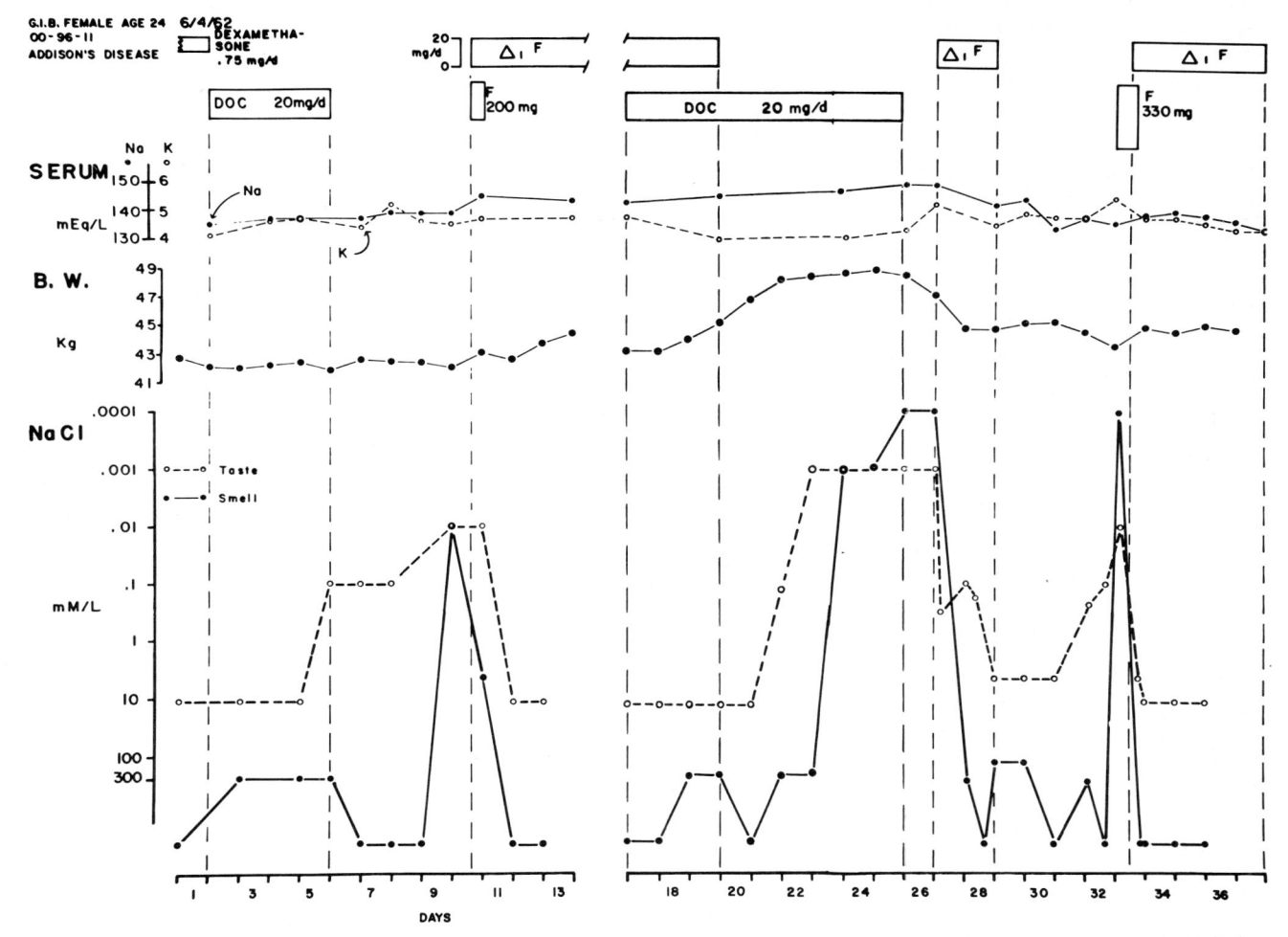

FIG. 14. Effect of dexamethasone, deoxycorticosterone acetate (DOC), prednisolone ($\Delta_1 F$), hydrocortisone (F), and no treatment on serum sodium and potassium concentrations, body weight ($B.W.$), and detection thresholds for the taste and smell of NaCl in 1 patient with adrenal cortical insufficiency. Threshold values for the vapor above a solution of NaCl equal to or greater than 150 mM are within normal limits. [From Henkin (35).]

several patients. Results were similar for all vapors studied. Taste data from a similar study previously carried out in this same patient are shown in Figure 4. For this second study (Fig. 14) she returned to the hospital so that taste and olfaction could be studied simultaneously.

Initially, after treatment with a maintenance dose of 0.75 mg dexamethasone, both taste and smell detection thresholds for NaCl were normal, as were body weight and serum concentrations of sodium and potassium. After treatment with dexamethasone was discontinued and treatment with DOCA (20 mg/day) was begun, there was no change in serum sodium or potassium concentrations or in body weight; however, within 4 days after dexamethasone was discontinued, taste detection thresholds for NaCl had decreased to the same abnormally low levels previously observed (see Fig. 4). Olfactory detection thresholds significantly decreased 7 days after treatment with carbohydrate-active steroids was discontinued. Treatment with Δ_1F (20 mg/day) returned smell sensitivity to normal within 24 hr, whereas an additional 12 hr was required before taste sensitivity returned to the normal range. This study was then repeated to document once again the timing of these changes. For convenience, only a portion of this study is illustrated (see second portion of Fig. 14). Taste and smell thresholds were both significantly lower than normal at the beginning of this portion of the study because the patient was without treatment with carbohydrate-active steroids for the preceding 9 days. Treatment with carbohydrate-active steroids once again returned taste and smell detection thresholds to normal with smell detection returning to normal first, followed by a return of taste detection to normal approximately 12 hr later. Withdrawal of carbohydrate-active steroids once again produced an increase in taste detection acuity, this time within 3 days after treatment was stopped. Subsequent treatment with carbohydrate-active steroids once again returned smell sensitivity to normal approximately 12 hr after treatment was initiated.

The basis for the differences in the timing of changes in gustatory and olfactory detection acuity is not known. However, the concentration of carbohydrate-active steroids in those tissues involved with olfaction may persist for a longer time after the hormone has decreased significantly in blood, urine, and other tissues, including those involved with taste acuity. In addition, once these stores are utilized they may be replaced more readily than tissue stores in the gustatory system when carbohydrate-active steroid becomes available again. This differential sensitivity may be related to differences in the manner by which different parts of the nervous system metabolize and bind carbohydrate-active steroid.

As with taste there is a circadian pattern of variation in normal man for olfaction that closely follows the changes in circulating levels of cortisol. Thus olfactory detection acuity is greatest in the early morning hours when circulating cortisol is highest (Fig. 15) and falls rather abruptly with the rather abrupt decrease in cortisol that occurs after this time (36). As with taste there is a subsequent gradual increase in olfactory detection acuity to higher levels over the next few hours of the day (36). As with taste, little if any circadian pattern of variation in olfactory detection acuity was observed in patients with adrenal cortical insufficiency after withdrawal of hormonal replacement therapy for sufficient time to produce increased olfactory detection acuity. These changes were observed both in patients with Addison's disease and in patients with panhypopituitarism, which again relates these changes to alterations in cortisol rather than to alterations in ACTH levels. However, after replacement of hormonal therapy, which returned olfactory detection to normal levels, a circadian pattern of variation similar to that observed in euadrenal normal volunteers was observed in the patients [(36); Fig. 15].

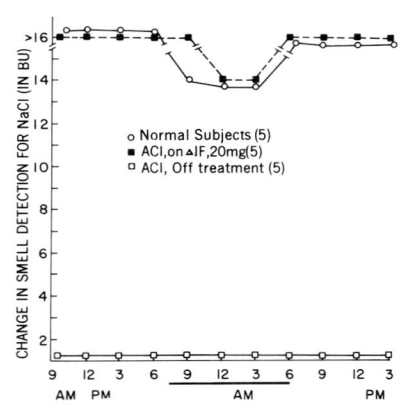

FIG. 15. Comparison of circadian pattern of variation in smell detection acuity (median detection threshold), for the vapor above a series of solutions of NaCl in normal subjects and in patients with adrenal cortical insufficiency (ACI) without treatment and after treatment with the carbohydrate-active steroid prednisolone [(Δ_1F), 20 mg/day, in divided doses orally every 6 hr for 2 days]. 1 BU = 10^{-6} mM NaCl, 2 = 10^{-5}, 3 = 10^{-4}, 4 = 10^{-3}, 5 = 10^{-2}, 6 = 10^{-1}, 7 = 0.5, 8 = 0.8, 9 = 3, 10 = 6, 11 = 12, 12 = 30, 13 = 60, 14 = 150, 15 = 300, >16 >300. Note that a circadian pattern of variation similar to that seen in normal volunteers can be observed in patients with adrenal cortical insufficiency treated with Δ_1F for 2 days. However, no circadian pattern of variation can be observed in patients with adrenal cortical insufficiency untreated for 4 or more days in whom increased detection sensitivity was observed. Note also increased detection acuity for NaCl in patients with adrenal cortical insufficiency without treatment. [From Henkin (36).]

Detection in Cushing's Syndrome

As with taste, patients with Cushing's syndrome exhibit significant elevations (decreased acuity) in both detection and recognition thresholds for each vapor tested (35, 41). Untreated patients commonly complained that foods were not flavorful, that they could not recognize bathroom odors, and that they had eaten spoiled food because they could not recognize the odor of tainted food. After successful treatment of their underlying disease these patients all exhibited a decrease in their detection and recognition thresholds toward or to normal. These objective measurements were mirrored in the subjective responses of the patients who noted a return of their olfactory acuity such that the flavor of food was once again apparent and vapors were identifiable. They exhibited no distortion of the vapors identified upon return of their acuity to normal.

Other Steroid Hormones

Other steroid hormones may play some role in olfactory acuity in both man and animals, although this role is confounded by neural and genetic factors. Patients with chromatin-negative gonadal dysgenesis may exhibit hyposmia (decreased olfactory acuity), but this condition is not significantly affected by exogenous administration of gonadal hormones (33b). Women with various types of amenorrhea also exhibit hyposmia of specific types (59); however, the specific hormonal defect either in the hypothalamic-pituitary axis, the pituitary-gonadal axis, the endocrine glands themselves, or in the relationships among these systems has not been clearly related to the observed olfactory deficit. Women with anosmia or type I hyposmia (33c) generally have been observed to exhibit unstimulated ovaries with oocytes present (59), and with appropriate therapy may become fertile. However, their olfactory acuity is not changed to any significant degree by any therapeutic measure yet applied. Women with type II hyposmia (33c) generally have been observed to exhibit streak gonads without oocytes (59) and have generally been infertile.

Men with various types of hypogonadism may also exhibit hyposmia (31a), and as noted for women, the specific type of hormonal defect has not been clearly related to the olfactory defect observed. Anosmia or type I hyposmia in hypogonadal men, in contrast to women, appears to be closely associated with hypogonadotrophic hypogonadism and a defect both in the hypothalamic-pituitary axis and in the testis as well (31a). Type II hyposmia in hypogonadal men, again in contrast to women, appears to be associated with a gonadal defect that is responsive to clomiphene administration, although this therapy does not appear to influence their olfactory acuity (31a).

Olfactory acuity, per se, in castrated animals has not been systematically studied, although gonadal function in several animal species in whom various lesions have been made in the olfactory system have been extensively studied. In these latter cases the effect of the olfactory lesions on gonadal function is time, species, and sex dependent and appears related to changes in the hypothalamic-pituitary axis, which ultimately affect the gonadal system (78a).

AUDITION

The detection and recognition of auditory stimuli are also influenced by adrenal cortical steroids, as are the senses of taste and smell. To demonstrate these interrelationships, measurements of auditory detection and recognition were compared in normal volunteers and in several patients with diseases involving the adrenal cortex.

Detection in States of Adrenal Cortical Insufficiency

Auditory detection acuity in normal subjects is compared with that in eight patients with adrenal cortical insufficiency in Figure 16. Four of the patients had adrenal cortical insufficiency caused by Addison's disease or subsequent to adrenalectomy, whereas four had adrenal cortical insufficiency secondary to panhypopituitarism. Auditory acuity was measured in the same manner in both normal volunteers and patients by each of two investigators, one of whom participated in the study without knowledge of the identity or the treatment given to the subjects or patients. Each subject was seated alone, comfortably, in an armchair, in an Industrial Acoustic Corporation Model 1204 double-walled sound chamber. Sinusoidal auditory signals were provided by a Southwestern Industrial Electronics M-2 R-C audio-oscillator attenuated by a Model 350-B Hewlett-Packard attenuator and delivered through Knight KN848 circumaural earphones. Auditory signals were delivered in a standard manner by a variation of the method of limits. Each subject raised his hand to signal when he heard the tone presented by the investigator. The details of this procedure have been previously described (43, 46).

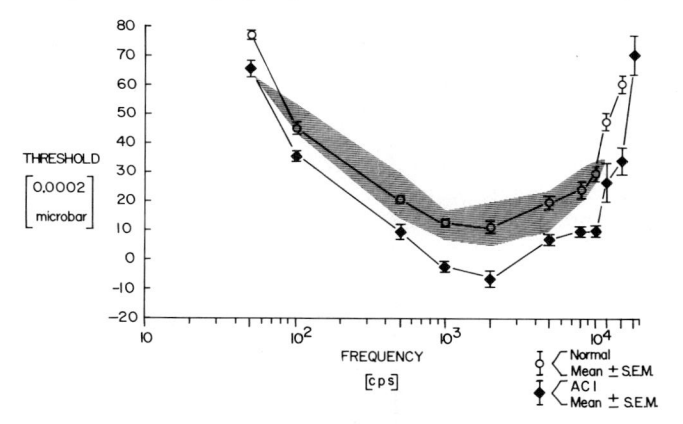

FIG. 16. Comparison of auditory detection thresholds for sinusoidal stimuli in normal volunteers with those in patients with untreated adrenal cortical insufficiency (*ACI*). *Ordinate* is scaled in absolute sound pressure units of microbars, referable to 0.0002 dynes/cm^2; *abscissa* is scaled in frequency units of cycles per second (cps or Hz). *Borders* of shaded area indicate the upper and lower limits of detection acuity of a large number of normal subjects determined by 3 groups of investigators under various conditions (84, 86, 89). *Open circles* within this shaded area illustrate mean detection thresholds obtained in a group of normal volunteers, under conditions used for the present studies. *Lines* extending above and below these circles indicate ± 1 SEM. Data obtained in normal subjects in the present studies fall within the rather large variation usually considered normal. *Black diamonds* below shaded area illustrate mean detection thresholds obtained in 8 patients with untreated adrenal cortical insufficiency and panhypopituitarism. *Lines* extending above and below these symbols indicate ± 1 SEM. Thresholds obtained in untreated patients are significantly lower than those found in normal subjects for all frequencies above 100 Hz. [From Henkin (35).]

The normal range of hearing acuity is shown in the shaded area in Figure 16 (84, 86, 89). The mean lower limit of frequency response in normal subjects under the conditions of the study was 50 Hz; the mean upper limit of responsiveness was 15,500 Hz. Most acute auditory detection for the normal subjects was between 1,000 and 4,000 Hz. The untreated patients exhibited a significant increase in the range of their frequency responsiveness compared to the normal volunteers. This increase was particularly apparent at the upper limits of the frequency range, where the patients detected a sinusoidal signal approximately 3,500 Hz higher than did the normal volunteers, dependent, of course, on the method used to determine these limits, as noted previously (43, 46). The auditory detection thresholds of the patients were significantly lower than those of the normal subjects not only in the range where hearing sensitivity is most acute, between 1,000 and 4,000 Hz, but over most of the frequency range above 5,000 Hz as well.

Figure 17 illustrates that treatment of patients with adrenal cortical insufficiency with DOCA, carried out in experiments similar to those described above for the sensory modalities of taste and olfaction, neither raised auditory detection thresholds significantly nor decreased their frequency response range, although it did return serum sodium and potassium concentration to normal and increased extracellular fluid volume.

Treatment of patients with adrenal cortical insufficiency with carbohydrate-active steroid returned auditory detection thresholds to normal limits after treatment with 20 mg prednisolone for as little as 2 days (Fig. 18). This return encompassed both a diminution of the range of frequency response to normal and an increase in the intensity required to detect the auditory signals.

A general effect of the withdrawal of carbohydrate-active steroid on the dynamic range of auditory responsiveness in normal subjects and in patients with untreated adrenal cortical insufficiency is shown in

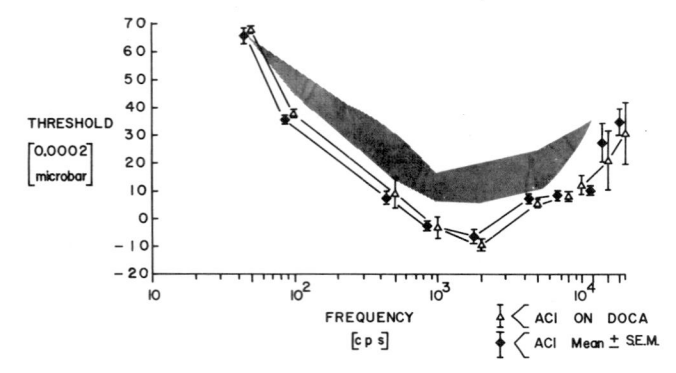

FIG. 17. Comparison of auditory detection threshold for sinusoidal stimuli in normal subjects with those in patients with adrenal cortical insufficiency (*ACI*) treated with deoxycorticosterone acetate (*DOCA*). Presentation of data is similar to that in Fig. 16. *Open triangles*, which are generally adjacent to the lower closed diamonds, indicate that treatment of the patients with DOCA does not alter the already lowered auditory detection acuity. [From Henkin (35).]

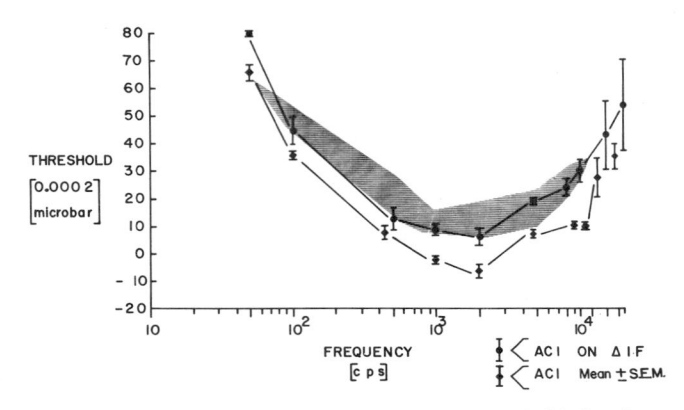

FIG. 18. Comparison of auditory detection thresholds for sinusoidal stimuli in normal subjects with those in patients with adrenal cortical insufficiency (*ACI*) treated with prednisolone ($\Delta_1 F$). Presentation of data is similar to that in Figs. 16 and 17. *Closed circles* within shaded area illustrate auditory detection thresholds obtained in patients after treatment with $\Delta_1 F$. Note that these circles are all within shaded area and mean values cannot be distinguished from those of normal subjects. [From Henkin (35).]

Figure 19. The dynamic range refers to the limits over which man responds to auditory stimuli; the upper limit refers to the intensity of auditory stimuli that produces acoustical pain [i.e., pain threshold (53)], and the lower limit refers to the auditory stimuli that can be just detected as different from silence (i.e., detection threshold). In normal subjects this range extends over approximately 80 db. Patients with untreated adrenal cortical insufficiency exhibit a compression of this dynamic range of hearing (Fig. 19). They exhibit a significant increase in hearing acuity at the lower or detection threshold end of the audible range but a more than compensatory decrease in acuity or sensitivity at the upper limit of hearing (pain threshold), which narrows their dynamic range. The increase in acuity at detection threshold is approximately 10–12 db; the decrease in sensitivity at the pain threshold is approximately 20 db. Thus the total dynamic range over which auditory events are perceived in patients with untreated adrenal cortical insufficiency is approximately 70 db. This compares to a range of 80 db in normal volunteers. Thus in the untreated patients the dynamic auditory range was decreased by approximately 10 db or a factor of 2. This indicates that, whereas auditory detection acuity is significantly greater than normal in patients with untreated adrenal cortical insufficiency, their overall responsiveness is less than normal over the entire audible range. This contrasts with the expansion of the dynamic range these patients exhibit for taste stimuli. In addition, loudness judgments of the untreated patients, including their discomfort level for speech and noise, were below those obtained in normal subjects by more than 20 db and were statistically significant (43). Judgments of the discomfort level for speech, a reliable correlate of the upper limit of audition, were, in the untreated patients, approximately 30 db below those of normal subjects. The upper limit of the comfort

sented to normal volunteers and to patients with untreated adrenal cortical insufficiency 40 and 60 db above each subject's detection threshold at 1,000 Hz under standardized conditions described elsewhere in detail (35, 43). In addition, words from which frequencies above 500 Hz had been selectively filtered out, low pass filtered speech (LPFS), were also presented 40 db and 60 db above each subject's detection threshold at 1,000 Hz in a standard manner (43). The results of these experiments were expressed in terms of the percentage of the number of words correctly recognized. These same words were also presented to the patients after treatment with DOCA and with Δ_1F.

The untreated patients correctly recognized approximately 60% of the words from the PB lists presented 40 db above threshold and only 89% when presented 60 db above threshold (Table 3). After treatment with DOCA, there was no significant change in responsiveness at either loudness level. However, after treatment with Δ_1F (20 mg/day for 48 hr) responsiveness increased to 98% and 96% for the lists presented 40 and 60 db above threshold, respectively. These responses were not significantly different from those obtained in normal subjects. Intravenous therapy for 5 days with 40 units of ACTH in two patients with panhypopituitarism and in one with a relative adrenal cortical insufficiency

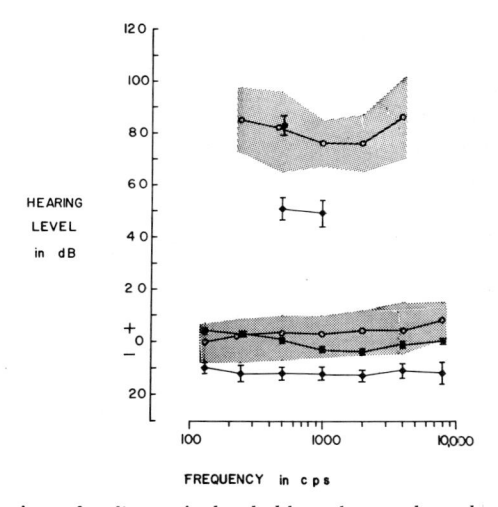

FIG. 19. Comparison of audiometric thresholds and contralateral threshold shifts (CTS) in normal subjects with those in patients with adrenal cortical insufficiency, off treatment. [From Henkin & Daly (43).]

1. *Open circles* at top of figure represent mean CTS determined in 44 normal subjects, aged 15–34, by Jepson (53); upper and lower limits of upper shaded area represent range of these responses. *Closed circle* within upper shaded area represents CTS determined in the 20 normal subjects of this study. *Lines* above and below this closed circle represent ± 1 SEM. Data for CTS at 500 cycles/sec in the subjects of this study are similar to that obtained by Jepson (53).

2. *Diamonds* directly below upper shaded area represent mean CTS obtained in this study of 12 patients with adrenal cortical insufficiency, off treatment, aged 19–57; *lines* above and below these rectangles represent ± 1 SEM.

3. *Open circles* at bottom of figure represent mean audiometric thresholds in normal subjects obtained by Jepson (53); *lower shaded area*, the range of these thresholds. *Closed points* within lower shaded area represent audiometric thresholds obtained in the normal subjects of this study, with ± 1 SEM. *Diamonds* below the lower shaded area represent audiometric thresholds obtained in patients with adrenal cortical insufficiency, off treatment. *Lines* above and below represent ± 1 SEM. At each frequency both mean audiometric threshold and CTS for patients with adrenal cortical insufficiency were significantly below those of either group of normal subjects.

level for speech in normal subjects is usually 5–10 db below the discomfort level for speech (43); in the untreated patients the upper limit of the comfort level for speech was significantly below normal but maintained the relationship of being 5–10 db below the discomfort level for speech (43). The mean contralateral threshold shift (CTS) in the untreated patients was below that of normal subjects by approximately 30 db, a statistically significant difference [Fig. 19; (43)]. In normal subjects the CTS is elicited between 75 and 90 db. The significant lowering of the CTS in the untreated patients indicates that the reflex threshold, and hence the upper limit of the auditory range in the patients, was markedly reduced.

Recognition in States of Adrenal Cortical Insufficiency

To study integration of auditory stimuli, standardized lists of 50 phonetically balanced (PB) words were pre-

TABLE 3. *Speech Discrimination Ability in Normal Volunteers and in Patients with Adrenal Cortical Insufficiency*

Subjects and Conditions	PB Words[a]		LPFS Words[b]	
	40 db	60 db	40 db	60 db
	% correct			
Normal volunteers	92 ±1.2[c]	97 ±0.6[c]	31 ±1.7	54 ±1.6
Adrenal cortical insufficiency, untreated	63 ±5.2[d]	88 ±2.8[e]	6 ±1.6[d]	23 ±2.5[d]
Adrenal cortical insufficiency, treated with DOCA	64 ±5.2[d]	89 ±1.3[e]	7 ±2.2[d]	23 ±3.6[d]
Adrenal cortical insufficiency, treated with carbohydrate-active steroid	89 ±3.0	96 ±3.1	31 ±2.0	56 ±3.3
Addison's disease (partial) or panhypopituitarism after treatment with ACTH, 40 units/day, 4th day	86 ±4.2	95 ±0.7	28 ±4.2	47 ±10.1

DOCA, deoxycorticosterone acetate; ACTH, adrenocorticotropin. [a] PB, phonetically balanced word lists presented 40 and 60 db above detection threshold determined at 1,000 cycles/sec. [b] LPFS, low pass filtered speech word lists presented 40 and 60 db above detection threshold determined at 1,000 cycles/sec. [c] Mean ± 1 SEM. [d] $P < 0.01$, with respect to results of normal volunteers or after treatment with carbohydrate-active steroids. [e] $P < 0.01$, with respect to results of normal volunteers; $P < 0.02$ with respect to results after treatment with carbohydrate-active steroids.

(i.e., unstimulated levels of urinary and plasma cortisol were below normal, but ACTH increased these levels to within normal limits) also returned word recognition and adrenal cortical function to normal. These results demonstrate that without treatment the patients were less able to recognize words than were normal subjects, that treatment with DOCA did not improve their ability, and that only treatment with carbohydrate-active steroid returned auditory integration to normal.

A response pattern even more strikingly abnormal than that for the PB words occurred after the presentation of the LPFS words. Recognition of LPFS words by patients untreated or treated with DOCA was relatively more impaired than was recognition of the PB words when compared to that of normal volunteers. Treatment of the patients with $\Delta_1 F$ returned responsiveness to normal.

The inability to recognize PB or LPFS words occurred while the patients were enclosed in a soundproof room, seated alone, receiving auditory information through earphones placed over their ears. Normally, auditory communication, as well as other modalities of sensory communication, is overdetermined by the admixture of stimuli from the several sensory modalities; for example, hand signals, facial expressions, tonal inflection, and body and eye movements comprise the total sensory context in which normal auditory communication takes place. In general, patients with untreated adrenal cortical insufficiency understand speech, follow commands, and perform reasonably well in an unrestricted environment. However, when all cues other than auditory ones are removed by isolating the patient in a soundproof room and presenting noninflected random monosyllabic words that do not have any meaningful connection with one another through a pair of earphones, these patients experience great difficulty with auditory integration. This was initially noted clinically before the performance of these experiments by the repeated failure of the untreated patients to perform tasks while in the soundproof room if the instructions were given only through the earphones. Not uncommonly the experimenters had to enter the soundproof room with the patients, remove the earphone and then vis-a-vis, with hand gestures and inflected speech, explain the required task slowly and carefully. In addition, if the patient were first studied during treatment with carbohydrate-active steroids and then studied again subsequent to the removal of these hormones, the patients would experience difficulty with test performance after steroid withdrawal. Tasks they had previously performed adequately had to be carefully and slowly reexplained. This phenomenon was also observed during the presentation of pure gustatory stimuli during which gross errors in gustatory recognition were commonly made.

In general, the patients, off treatment, experienced more difficulty with recognition of the latter portion of words than with their initial portion. Thus a word such as nip was not uncommonly confused with the word nit, and the word knee with need. The patients were not aware of this increase in their confusion or their confusability. They commonly overestimated their performance on the word recognition tasks by 10–20%, particularly so with the LPFS words. Upon questioning about their confusion they indicated that they could hear the words clearly but had difficulty in distinguishing what the specific word was. They heard only one word, and their confusion was related mainly to their inability to specify the word exactly.

This inability to recognize words occurred at the same time that other auditory recognition or "integrative" abnormalities occurred. Localization of conversational speech more than 30° away from either side of a midline presentation was in error by 15–45°; however, untreated patients were able to localize speech when presented in or very close to the midline [i.e., a direct presentation with little or no deviation using a straight line from the nose as midline (43)]. They had difficulty in judging the change in character of an amplitude modulated tone as it was amplified over a range of just noticeable increments from 1 to 5 db. The mean difference limen for the untreated patients was 3.3 db, or approximately 2.5 times greater sound energy was required by the patients to make this judgment than was required by the normal subjects (43). Their ability to judge the loudness of tones presented alternately to each ear was also severely impaired when untreated and was influenced profoundly by the previously presented stimulus. The magnitude of these errors in some patients was such that they were matching as equal tones that were four times as loud or as soft as the standard tone (43). This effect has been commonly called "anchoring" (5a). However, each of these integrative abnormalities returned to normal after treatment with carbohydrate-active steroid was resumed.

Detection and Recognition in Cushing's Syndrome

As with taste and smell, patients with Cushing's syndrome exhibit an increase in auditory detection thresholds for sinusoidal stimuli and a decrease in auditory recognition or integrative ability. The measurements of these latter deficits were quantitatively similar to those observed in patients with untreated adrenal cortical insufficiency. In addition, pain was produced by auditory signals at significantly higher intensity levels in patients with Cushing's syndrome than in either normal volunteers or in patients with untreated adrenal cortical insufficiency. These changes resulted in a shift in the dynamic auditory range to higher detection levels at both lower and upper limits rather than to a compression of the dynamic range as observed in patients with untreated adrenal cortical insufficiency. This phenomenon of increased auditory pain thresholds at the upper limit of the dynamic auditory range has been previously observed in studies during which large amounts of exogenous adrenal corticosteroids were administered to normal volunteers (23, 78). Similar increases in heat pain thresholds have also been observed after administration of exogenous adrenal corticosteroids or ACTH (15). In the rat auditory seizure threshold has been raised after administration of adrenal corticosteroids and lowered after adrenalectomy (18). Successful treatment of patients with Cushing's syndrome resulted in an increase of their auditory detection acuity toward or to normal and a return of their auditory integrative capacity to normal limits.

OTHER SENSORY SYSTEMS

The visual system may be influenced by adrenal corticosteroids in a manner similar to taste, smell, and hearing. Topical application of steroids in the eye has produced exophthalmos and increased intraocular pressure in animals (21, 91, 92), and in man, glaucoma and subsequent decreased visual acuity (24, 29, 60). In man these changes have been associated with optic atrophy (60) and related to a genetic propensity to develop glaucoma (3). Exophthalmos has also been produced in euthyroid man with local applications of steroids to the eye (85). Similarly, 6–8% of patients with untreated Cushing's syndrome have been observed to exhibit exophthalmos and increased intraocular pressure with subsequent decreases in visual acuity (61, 67, 80, 85). One patient with Cushing's syndrome had exophthalmos as the initial manifestation of his disease (61). Treatment of Cushing's syndrome generally relieved the increased pressure, and visual acuity not uncommonly returned to normal (7). It is curious, however, that adrenal corticosteroids and ACTH have been used in the treatment of the exophthalmos of Graves disease. The flicker-fusion threshold (i.e., the point at which a flickering visual stimulus is appreciated as a steady visual stimulus) also appears to be influenced by adrenal corticosteroids (62). The rate at which this integrative visual task occurs falls with the onset of adrenal cortical insufficiency and increases toward normal with adrenal hormonal steroid replacement therapy (62).

As previously noted, pain stimuli produced by acoustical means (42, 43), but also by thermal (15) or other (31, 57, 58) means, are influenced by the presence or absence of adrenal corticosteroids. Thresholds for stimuli that elicit pain on the tongue via an electrical discharge are also lower (increased pain sensitivity) in patients with adrenal cortical insufficiency in whom replacement therapy has been withdrawn (56). These thresholds increase to normal levels (sensitivity decreases) upon replacement of hormonal therapy (56).

Administration of progesterone to animals has not only been associated with the production of anesthesia (30, 51, 83) but also decreased responsiveness to pain, cold, and prick stimuli (55) presumably via a general inhibitory effect on brain activity (4, 81). Some of these effects are dose dependent, but the relationships between the production of anesthesia and the production of seizures after administration of progesterone, cortisone, ACTH, or their analogues have not always been clear (50, 88). Deoxycorticosterone acetate (DOCA) itself has been used as an anticonvulsant (1a). Similarly anesthesia has been produced by administration of exogenous adrenal corticosteroids (82), and changes in sleep patterns have been well documented in normal volunteers given exogenous adrenal corticosteroids (26) or ACTH (27a) and in patients with adrenal cortical insufficiency after replacement therapy has been withdrawn (27). It is of interest that in patients with untreated adrenal cortical insufficiency there is a significant increase in delta sleep, whereas in patients with Cushing's syndrome the converse effect occurs (56b); that is, a significant decrease in delta sleep occurs (56b). The timing of these changes in patients with adrenal cortical insufficiency follows precisely that observed in changes in taste, smell, and hearing (27). All changes return to normal within 48 hr of replacement with carbohydrate-active steroids, again in a time relation similar to that observed with the sensory modalities of taste, smell, and hearing (27). Similarly, raising thresholds to the production of seizures by auditory stimuli with carbohydrate-active steroids and the lowering of such thresholds after adrenalectomy indicate the general nature of this phenomenon (18, 93). The changes in sleep patterns observed in patients with Cushing's syndrome have been shown in some patients to revert to or toward normal after appropriate therapy for this disease (56a).

DISCUSSION

One question raised in the initial investigations of Richter was directed at the site of action of carbohydrate-active steroids. This site could be the sensory receptor itself, the nerve, the CNS, or some combination of the three. Present information suggests that effects occur at each of these sites, and it is not possible to specify any one site as more important or more critical than the other.

However, irrespective of the site of action, the data collected suggest features common to changes in each sensory modality.
1. Increased detection acuity occurs with too little carbohydrate-active steroid.
2. Decreased recognition or integrative acuity occurs with either too much or too little carbohydrate-active steroid.
3. Low recognition acuity in states of carbohydrate-active steroid excess or deficiency may be overcome by increasing the stimulus intensity.
4. Changes in taste, smell, olfactory, and pain detection and recognition can be returned to normal through the correction of the carbohydrate-active steroid excess or deficiency.

The taste system offers a useful manner of evaluating the effects of carbohydrate-active steroids on receptor events. For convenience the gustatory process can be divided into two general sets of events: preneural or receptor events, and neural events (28, 39).

Preneural molecular events involve the interaction or binding between tastant (T) and receptor molecule (R), an event that presumably takes place at the membrane of the taste receptor (28, 39, 41). The result of this specific interaction between tastant and receptor molecule is most likely the formation of a tastant-receptor complex:

$$R + 2T \xrightleftharpoons[K_{-1}]{K_1} RT_2 \qquad K = K_1/K_{-1} \qquad (2)$$

or

$$\frac{(RT)_2}{(R) + (RT_2)} = \frac{K(T)^2}{K(T^2)^2 + 1} \qquad (3)$$

From Equation 3, Equation 1 may be derived if it is assumed that the intensity (I) is proportional to the concentration of RT complexes. The single parameter K represents the binding constant for the formation of the RT_2 complex (41).

This model would explain how the intensity function would reach a maximum at high tastant concentrations; the tastant molecules would complex with all the available receptor molecules, and introduction of more tastant would not form more complexes. As the tastant concentration decreased the number of receptor molecules complexed would also decrease and at a sufficiently low concentration the signal produced would no longer be recognized, albeit detected. If tastant concentration were to be decreased further it would not be detected from background.

The signal produced by this complex formation presumably occurs at the taste receptor and is anatomically, spatially, and temporally separated from the neural events. Thus the classification of preneural and neural events has physical bases.

Carbohydrate-active steroid deficiency and excess states may affect the preneural events of taste by affecting the binding constants by which tastant-receptor molecule complexes occur or by affecting the stoichiometry of binding. In looking at the data in Figures 7–9 from the first point of view, both excessive and inadequate amounts of carbohydrate-active steroid appear to decrease the binding constants for all taste qualities because the intensity curves are all shifted to higher concentrations. From the second point of view the possible deviation of the data from Equation 1 toward an equation of a lower order (in T) would imply that the stoichiometry of binding is altered. Apparently there is a concentration of carbohydrate-active steroid at which the intensity is maximal for a given tastant concentration, and either an excess or a deficiency of carbohydrate-active steroid lowers the intensity.

The fit of Equation 1 to the data suggests that two tastants are required for the recognition process to occur normally. The equation does not specify the spatial relationships among the tastants and receptors. However, these relationships are suggestive of the existence of cooperative binding in which K would be the product of the square $[(Ki)^2]$ of the intrinsic binding constants (Ki) of the tastants and a coupling term Kc (i.e., $K = Ki^2 Kc$). According to this interpretation, states of excess or deficient carbohydrate-active steroid would shift the intensity curves by reducing the coupling constant, which would, in the limit of $Kc = 1$, also shift the binding stoichiometry to a lower order. High tastant concentrations can overcome this decoupling by sheer mass action.

However, the neural events of taste involve the depolarization of the taste nerves subsequent to the preneural events of taste. How the formation of the RT_2 complex ultimately leads to the depolarization of the taste nerve is not known. However, there is an anatomic separation between the membrane of the taste receptor, where presumably the RT_2 complex forms, and the tight junction at which the taste nerve joins the receptor. The neural events also include conduction of the impulse along the axons that mediate the taste response, transmission across the synapses of the nerves of the taste system, and integration of the taste information within the central nervous system.

In the absence of carbohydrate-active steroid there are significant changes in the manner by which neural signals are conducted along axons and transmitted across synapses in animals (13, 22, 25, 52) and in man (14, 20, 35, 45, 63). In carbohydrate-active steroid deficiency states, axonal conduction velocities are increased slightly (35, 45), whereas synaptic delay, particularly in polysynaptic sensory systems, is markedly increased (13, 22, 25, 52, 63). In patients with excessive levels of carbohydrate-active steroid, axonal conduction velocities are usually slightly below normal, although the association of other abnormalities, such as those of carbohydrate metabolism, makes interpretation of these data difficult (35). These changes in neural conduction and transmission in states of excess or deficient carbohydrate-active steroid result in gross abnormalities in the timed arrival of sensory signals in the CNS from the periphery. Since sensory recognition is critically dependent on the appropriate perception of the arrival of patterns of sensory signals in the CNS, alterations in this timing would result in a significant information loss (43). This would explain the inability of these patients to recognize tastants or other sensory stimuli at normal recognition threshold concentrations. Increasing tastant concentrations, which would result in a larger number of afferent signals per unit time, could overcome the information loss produced by the conduction and transmission abnormalities and allow sensory recognition to occur. This interpretation is analogous to the interpretation, in terms of carbohydrate-active steroid decoupling of tastant binding, described in the previous section, only here applied to the neural events of taste.

One of the most striking abnormalities among the effects of carbohydrate-active steroid on gustation is the detection of all tastants at extremely low intensities by patients with untreated adrenal cortical insufficiency. This suggests that carbohydrate-active steroid not only affects the conduction and transmission of a neural signal but also plays a significant role in controlling the base line or background level of neural activity. Although the absence of carbohydrate-active steroid, which is reflected by lowered carbohydrate-active steroid levels in neural tissue (35, 42), may produce increases in "neural excitability," it may do this simply by lowering the background level of neural activity. These incoming signals of low intensity could be more easily detected because of their higher signal-to-noise ratio. These hypotheses are consistent with the findings that patients with untreated adrenal cortical insufficiency are more sensitive to painful auditory stimuli as they are more sensitive to painful stimuli of other sensory modalities (35, 56). Conversely patients with Cushing's syndrome are less sensitive to painful auditory stimuli (23), which demonstrates once again the role of carbohydrate-active steroids in this complex system.

CONCLUSIONS

Sensory detection and integration are regulated by a complex feedback system involving the interaction of the endocrine and the nervous systems. Studies in man and in other animals have demonstrated, after removal of adrenal cortical hormone activity, a significant increase in ability to detect sensory signals through the modalities of taste, olfaction, and audition. For taste, detection of each of four qualities is increased by a factor of at least 100; for olfaction, detection of various odorants, some previously considered to be without significant vapor pressure, is increased by a factor of at least 1,000. For audition, detection of sinusoidal signals is increased by at least 13 db, particularly between 1,000 Hz and 4,000 Hz, the most sensitive region of auditory acuity. Treatment of patients with adrenal cortical insufficiency with Na-K-active steroids such as DOCA does not alter this increased sensory detection acuity, although it does reverse the abnormal electrolyte balance present. Thus the hyperkalemia, hyponatremia, and decreased extracellular fluid concentration observed in patients with untreated adrenal cortical insufficiency can return to normal without any alteration in their increased sensory acuity. Treatment with carbohydrate-active steroids alone returns sensory detection acuity to normal for each sensory modality.

Studies of patients with Cushing's syndrome, who exhibit excessive adrenal secretion of carbohydrate-active steroids, reveal a significant decrease in sensory detection acuity for the sensory modalities of taste, olfaction, and audition. Suppression of endogenous carbohydrate-active steroid secretion to normal levels by treatment with exogenous steroid hormones or aminoglutethimide or by surgical removal of the adrenal glands results in a return to normal sensory detection acuity. Excessive treatment with adrenal toxic agents or failure to adequately replace corticosteroids after surgical adrenalectomy brings about clinical changes consistent with adrenal cortical insufficiency that are reflected by sensory changes appropriate to that condition.

Coincident with the removal of carbohydrate-active steroids, sensory integration for the sensory modalities of taste and audition significantly decreases. For taste, recognition of each of four qualities is decreased by a factor of 100; for audition, recognition of various signals is markedly impaired. For audition, this impairment involves losses of ability to understand speech, changes in tonal quality, localization of tonal stimuli, and judgment of bilateral equal loudness. Treatment with Na-K-active steroids does not alter these decreases in sensory perception ability; this is similar to the failure of this treatment to alter increases in sensory detection acuity. However, treatment with this class of steroids returns the abnormal electrolyte balance to normal. Treatment with carbohydrate-active steroids returns sensory perception to normal for taste and audition at a time when sensory detection acuity also returns to normal. Excessive endogenous secretion of carbohydrate-active steroids, as in Cushing's syndrome, is also associated with a decrease in the ability to integrate sensory information. Thus not only do these latter patients exhibit decreased detection acuity but also decreased integrative capacity. Treatment of the underlying adrenal disease, which returns corticosteroid secretion to normal, is associated with a return of both detection and recognition acuity to normal. This indicates a continuum and perhaps a maximum-minimum relationship between carbohydrate-active steroid and neural activity, as well as between sensory detection and recognition acuity.

These reciprocal changes in sensory detection and perception occur in physiological, as well as pathological, conditions. There is a circadian pattern of change in taste detection acuity in normal subjects such that, when carbohydrate-active steroid secretion is at its lowest level, taste detection acuity is at its highest. When carbohydrate-active steroid secretion is at its highest level, taste detection acuity is at its lowest.

These reciprocal changes in sensory detection and recognition have been related to changes in the manner by which carbohydrate-active steroids influence the metabolism of neural tissue of which they are a normal component (35). After adrenalectomy the concentration of these steroids in tissues of the central and peripheral nervous systems decreases significantly. This decrease is associated with an alteration in the manner by which neural impulses are conducted along axons and across synapses; conduction velocity along peripheral axons is significantly increased above normal, whereas conduction across synapses is significantly prolonged. This results in a marked change in the timing by which neural stimuli from the periphery reach the higher integrative centers of the nervous system. It is this alteration in perception of the timed arrival of the sensory signals from the periphery that is the hypothetical mechanism for the loss of perceptual ability observed in adrenal cortical insufficiency and is reflected by a net loss of information. Associated with this alteration in timing is an alteration in excitability of the nervous system such that stimuli that normally would be rejected as subthreshold produce depolarization of neurons. This increase in neural excitability by which normally subthreshold stimuli are appreciated, albeit in an abnormal manner, is the hypothetical mechanism for the increase of sensory detection acuity observed in adrenal cortical insufficiency.

Normally carbohydrate-active steroids are presumed to act in an inhibitory manner in both central and peripheral nervous systems; their presence inhibits both the detection and recognition of incoming sensory signals (35). Their removal releases this inhibition, and sensory detection and recognition change in the manner described above. Reciprocal changes in detection and recognition acuity may be such that increases in detection acuity are always associated with decreases in recognition acuity. This concept may help to explain some aspects of the reciprocal changes in detection and recognition acuity observed in the absence of carbohydrate-active steroids. However, if the signal-to-noise ratio is raised such that a signal of greater intensity is required for detection, as in Cushing's syndrome, recognition thresholds are similarly raised since integration can take place only after receipt of an adequate sensory signal. Thus there is a decrease in both sensory detection and integration acuity with excessive secretion of endogenous carbohydrate-active steroids. Under these conditions, as shown for the taste R:D (recognition:detection) ratio, which is usually close to unity in patients with Cushing's syndrome, there is little if any difference in the detected or integrated signal. This concept may help to explain some aspects of the concomitant changes in detection and recognition thresholds observed in Cushing's syndrome.

REFERENCES

1. Adler, J., G. L. Hazelbauer, and M. M. Dahl. Chemotaxis toward sugars in *Escherichia coli*. *J. Bacteriol.* 115: 824–847, 1973.
1a. Aird, R. B., and G. S. Gordan. Anticonvulsant properties of desoxycorticosterone. *J. Am. Med. Assoc.* 145: 715–719, 1951.
2. Allara, E. Sull'influenza determinata della castrazione e somministrazione di propionato di testosterone sulle formazioni gustative di *Mus rattus albinus*. *Boll. Soc. Ital. Biol. Sperimentale* 28: 58–69, 1952.
2a. Allara, E. Sull'influenza esercitata dagli ormoni sessuali sulla struttura delle formazioni gustative di *Mus rattus albinus*. *Riv. Biol.* 44: 209–299, 1952.
3. Armaly, M. F. The heritable nature of dexamethasone-induced ocular hypertension. *Arch. Ophthalmol.* 75: 32–35, 1966.
4. Atkinson, R. M., B. Davis, M. A. Pratt, H. M. Sharpe, and E. G. Tomich. Action of some steroids on the central nervous system of the mouse. II. Pharmacology. *J. Med. Chem.* 8: 426–432, 1965.
5. Bare, J. K. The specific hunger for sodium chloride in normal and adrenalectomized white rats. *J. Comp. Physiol. Psychol.* 42: 242–253, 1949.
5a. Bachsbaum, M., J. Silverman, and R. I. Henkin. Contrast effects on the auditory evoked response and its relation to psychophysical judgment. *Perception Psychophysics* 9: 379–384, 1971.
6. Bott, E., D. A. Denton, and S. Wellers. The innate appetite for salt exhibited by sodium-deficient sheep. In: *Olfaction and Taste II*, edited by T. Hayashi. London: Pergamon Press, 1967, p. 415–429.
7. Boyer, J. M., and H. P. Neuner. Cushing's syndrome and raised intraocular pressure. *German Med. Monthly* 13: 205–212, 1968.
8. Braun-Menendez, E. Action of desoxycorticosterone on water exchange in the rat (Abstract). *Am. J. Physiol.* 163: 701, 1950.
9. Braun-Menendez, E. Aumento del apetito especifico para la sal provocado la desoxicorticosterona. II. Sustancias que potencian o inhiber esta accion. *Rev. Soc. Arg. Biol.* 28: 23–32, 1952.
10. Braun-Menendez, E., and P. Brandt. Aumento del apetito especifico para la sal provocado por la desoxicorticosterona. I. Caracteristicos. *Rev. Soc. Arg. Biol.* 28: 15–23, 1952.
11. Cameron, A. T. The taste sense and the relative sweetness of sugars and other sweet substances. *Sugar Res. Found. Sci. Rep. Ser.* 9, 1947.
12. Carr, W. J. The effect of adrenalectomy upon the NaCl taste threshold in rat. *J. Comp. Physiol. Psychol.* 45: 377–380, 1952.
13. Chambers, W. F., S. K. Freedman, and G. H. Sawyer. The effect of adrenal steroids on evoked reticular responses. *Exptl. Neurol.* 8: 458–469, 1963.
14. Ciganek, L. The EEG response (evoked potential) to light stimulus in man. *Electroencephal. Clin. Neurophysiol.* 13: 165–172, 1961.
15. Clark, W. C., M. W. Ropes, and W. Bauer. Changes produced by the administration of ACTH and cortisone in rheumatoid arthritis. In: *Proceedings of the First Clinical ACTH Conference*, edited by J. R. Mote. Philadelphia: Blakiston, 1950, p. 337–362.
16. Cragg, L. H. The sour taste: threshold values and accuracy, the effects of saltiness and sweetness. *Trans. Roy. Soc. Can. Sect. III* 31: 131–140, 1937.
17. Darley, W., and C. A. Doan. Primary pulmonary arteriosclerosis with polycythemia: associated with the chronic ingestion of abnormally large quantities of sodium chloride (Halophagia). *Am. J. Med. Sci.* 191: 633–647, 1936.
18. Davenport, V. D. Relation between brain and plasma electrolytes and electroshock seizure thresholds in adrenalectomized rats. *Am. J. Physiol.* 156: 322–327, 1949.
19. DeWardener, H. E., and A. Herxheimer. The effect of a high water intake on salt consumption, taste thresholds and salivary secretion in man. *J. Physiol., London* 139: 53–63, 1957.
20. Engel, G. L., and S. G. Margolin. Neuropsychiatric disturbances in Addison's disease and the role of impaired carbohydrate metabolism in production of abnormal cerebral function. *Arch. Neurol. Psychiat.* 45: 881–884, 1941.
21. Essex, H. E. Exophthalmus in hypophysectomized and cortisone-treated albino rats. *Am. J. Physiol.* 181: 375–378, 1955.
22. Feldman, S. Electrophysiological alterations in adrenalectomy. *Arch. Neurol.* 7: 460–470, 1962.
23. Feldman, S., and D. P. Kidron. Experiences with ACTH and cortisone in organic diseases of the nervous system. *Monatsschr. Psychiat. Neurol.* 132: 96–114, 1956.
24. Francois, J. Cortisone et tension oculaire. *Ann. Oculist* 187: 805–816, 1954.
25. Feldman, S., J. C. Todt, and R. W. Porter. Effect of adrenocortical hormones on evoked potentials. *Neurology* 11: 109–115, 1951.
26. Gillin, J. C., L. S. Jacobs, D. H. Fram, and F. Snyder. Acute effect of a glucocorticoid on normal human sleep. *Nature* 237: 398–399, 1972.

27. GILLIN, J. C., L. S. JACOBS, F. SNYDER, AND R. I. HENKIN. Effects of decreased adrenal corticosteroids: changes in sleep in normal subjects and patients with adrenal cortical insufficiency. *Electroencephal. Clin. Neurophysiol.* 36: 283-289, 1974.
27a. GILLIN, J. C., L. S. JACOBS, F. SNYDER, AND R. I. HENKIN. Effects of ACTH on the sleep of normal subjects and of patients with Addison's disease. *Neuroendocrinology* 15: 21-31, 1974.
28. GIROUX, E. L., AND R. I. HENKIN. Oral effects of hydrolytic enzymes on taste acuity in man. *Life Sci., Part 1* 10: 361-370, 1971.
29. GOLDMANN, H. Cortisone glaucoma. *Arch. Ophthalmol.* 68: 621-626, 1962.
30. GYERMEK, L., G. GENTHER, AND N. FLEMING. Some effects of progesterone and related steroids on the central nervous system. *Intern. J. Neuropharmacol.* 6: 191-198, 1967.
31. HABIF, D. V., C. C. HARE, AND G. H. GLASER. Perforated duodenal ulcer associated with pituitary adrenocorticotropic hormone (ACTH) therapy. *J. Am. Med. Assoc.* 144: 996, 1950.
31a. HAMILTON, C. R., JR., R. I. HENKIN, G. WEIR, AND B. KLIMAN. Olfactory status and response to clomiphene in male gonadotrophin deficiency. *Ann. Internal Med.* 78: 47-55, 1973.
32. HARRIMAN, A., AND R. B. MACLEOD. Discriminative thresholds for salt for normal and adrenalectomized rats. *Am. J. Physiol.* 66: 465-471, 1953.
33. HARRIS, H., AND H. KALMUS. Genetical differences in taste sensitivity to phenylthiourea and to anti-thyroid substances. *Nature* 163: 878, 1949.
33b. HENKIN, R. I. Abnormalities of taste and olfaction in patients with chromatin negative gonadal dysgenesis. *J. Clin. Endocrinol. Metab.* 27: 1436-1440, 1967.
33c. HENKIN, R. I. The definition of primary and accessory areas of olfaction as the basis for a classification of decreased olfactory acuity. In: *Olfaction and Taste II*, edited by T. Hayashi. London: Pergamon Press, 1967, p. 235-252.
34. HENKIN, R. I. The effects of corticosteroids and ACTH on sensory systems. In: *Progress in Brain Research*, edited by D. de Wied and J. A. W. M. Weijnen. Amsterdam: Elsevier, 1970, vol. 32, p. 270-294.
35. HENKIN, R. I. The neuroendocrine control of perception. In: *Perception and Its Disorders*, edited by D. A. Hamburg, K. H. Pribram, and A. J. Stunkard. Baltimore: Williams & Wilkins, 1970, vol. 48, p. 54-107.
35a. HENKIN, R. I. Sensory changes during the menstrual cycle. In: *Biorhythms and Human Reproduction*, edited by M. Ferin, F. Halberg, R. M. Richart, and R. L. Vande Wiele. New York: Wiley, 1974, p. 277-285.
36. HENKIN, R. I. A study of circadian variation in taste in normal man and in patients with adrenal cortical insufficiency: the role of adrenal cortical steroids. In: *Biorhythms and Human Reproduction*, edited by M. Ferin, F. Halberg, R. M. Richart, and R. L. Vande Wiele. New York: Wiley, 1974, p. 397-408.
37. HENKIN, R. I., AND F. C. BARTTER. Increased sensitivity of taste and smell in patients with congenital adrenal hyperplasia (Abstract). *Clin. Res.* 12: 270, 1964.
38. HENKIN, R. I., AND F. C. BARTTER. Studies on olfactory thresholds in normal man and in patients with adrenal cortical insufficiency: the role of adrenal cortical steroids and of serum sodium concentration. *J. Clin. Invest.* 45: 1631-1639, 1966.
39. HENKIN, R. I., AND D. F. BRADLEY. Regulation of taste acuity by thiols and metal ions. *Proc. Natl. Acad. Sci. US* 62: 30-37, 1969.
40. HENKIN, R. I., AND D. F. BRADLEY. Hypogeusia corrected by Ni^{++} and Zn^{++}. *Life Sci., Part 1* 9: 701-709, 1970.
41. HENKIN, R. I., and D. F. BRADLEY. On the mechanism of action of carbohydrate-active steroids on tastant detection and recognition. In: *Steroid, Hormones and Brain Function*, edited by C. Sawyer and R. Gorski. Los Angeles: Univ. of California Press, 1971, p. 339-353.
42. HENKIN, R. I., A. G. T. CASPER, R. BROWN, AND A. B. HARLAN. Presence of corticosterone and cortisol in the central and peripheral nervous system of the cat. *Endocrinology* 82: 1058-1061, 1968.

43. HENKIN R. I., AND R. L. DALY. Auditory detection and perception in normal man and in patients with adrenal cortical insufficiency. *J. Clin. Invest.* 47: 1269-1280, 1968.
43a. HENKIN, R. I., J. A. FONTANA, AND M. D. WALKER. On the mechanism of the presence and distribution of adrenal corticosteroids in the central and peripheral nervous system. In: *Hormonal Steroids*. Amsterdam: Excerpta Medica Foundation, 1971, p. 772-805. (Intern. Congr. Ser. 219.)
44. HENKIN, R. I., J. R. GILL, JR., AND F. C. BARTTER. Studies on taste thresholds in normal man and patients with adrenal cortical insufficiency: the effect of adrenocorticosteroids. *J. Clin. Invest.* 42: 727-735, 1963.
45. HENKIN, R. I., J. R. GILL, JR., J. R. WARMOLTS, A. A. CARR, AND F. C. BARTTER. Steroid dependent increase on nerve conduction in adrenal insufficiency (Abstract). *J. Clin. Invest.* 42: 941, 1963.
46. HENKIN, R. I., R. E. MCGLONE, R. L. DALY, AND F. C. BARTTER. Studies on auditory thresholds in normal man and in patients with adrenal cortical insufficiency: the role of adrenal cortical steroids. *J. Clin. Invest.* 46: 429-435, 1967.
47. HENKIN, R. I., P. J. SCHECHTER, R. C. HOYE, AND C. F. T. MATTERN. Idiopathic hypogeusia with dysgeusia, hyposmia and dysosmia: a new syndrome. *J. Am. Med. Assoc.* 217: 434-440, 1971.
48. HENKIN, R. I., AND D. H. SOLOMON. Salt-taste threshold in adrenal insufficiency in man. *J. Clin. Endocrinol. Metab.* 22: 856-858, 1962.
49. HERXHEIMER, A., AND D. WOODBURY. The effect of deoxycorticosterone on salt and sucrose taste preference thresholds and drinking behavior in rats. *J. Physiol., London* 151: 253-265, 1960.
50. HEUSER, G., G. M. LING, AND N. A. BUCHWALD. Sedation or seizures as dose-dependent effects of steroids. *Arch. Neurol.* 13: 195-203, 1965.
51. HEUSER, G., G. M. LING, AND M. KLUVER. Sleep induction by progesterone in the pre-optic area in cats. *Electroencephal. Clin. Neurophysiol.* 22: 122-127, 1967.
52. HOAGLAND, H. Studies of brain metabolism and electrical activity in relation to adrenocortical physiology. *Recent Progr. Hormone Res.* 10: 29-63, 1954.
53. JEPSEN, O. Middle-ear muscle reflexes in man. In: *Modern Developments in Audiology*, edited by J. Jerger. New York: Acad. Press, 1963, p. 193.
54. KNOWLES, D., AND P. E. JOHNSON. A study of the sensitivities of prospective judges to the primary tastes. *Food Res.* 6: 207, 1941.
55. KOMISARUK, B. R., P. G. MCDONALD, D. I. WHITMOYER, AND C. H. SAWYER. Effects of progesterone and sensory stimulation on EEG and neuronal activity in the rat. *Exptl. Neurol.* 19: 494-507, 1967.
56. KOSOWICZ, J., AND A. PRUSZEWICZ. The "taste" test in adrenal insufficiency. *J. Clin. Endocrinol. Metab.* 27: 214-218, 1967.
56a. KRIEGER, D. T., AND G. P. GEWIRTZ. Recovery of hypothalamic-pituitary-adrenal function, growth hormone responsiveness and sleep EEG pattern in a patient following removal of an adrenal cortical adenoma. *J. Clin. Endocrinol. Metab.* 38: 1075-1082, 1974.
56b. KRIEGER, D. T., AND S. M. GLICK. Growth hormone and cortisol responsiveness in Cushing's syndrome. *Am. J. Med.* 52: 25-40, 1972.
57. LEE, R. E., AND C. C. PFEIFFER. Effects of cortisone and 11-desoxycortisone on pain thresholds in man. *Proc. Soc. Exptl. Biol. Med.* 77: 752-754, 1951.
58. LEVINE, R., AND M. S. GOLDSTEIN. Neuro-endocrine relationships. In: *Progress in Neurology and Psychiatry*. New York: Grune & Stratton, 1951, vol. 6, p. 218-226.
59. MARSHALL, J. R., AND R. I. HENKIN. Olfactory acuity, menstrual abnormalities and oocyte status. *Ann. Internal Med.* 75: 207-211, 1971.
60. MILLER, S. J. H. Steroid glaucoma. *Trans. Ophthalmol. Soc. UK* 85: 289-294, 1965.
61. MORGAN, D. C., AND A. S. MASON. Exophthalmus in Cushing's syndrome. *Brit. Med. J.* 2: 481-483, 1958.

62. MURAWSKI, B. J., W. J. REDDY, AND H. M. FOX. Relationship of adrenal cortical function to flicker-fusion threshold. *J. Appl. Physiol.* 11: 468–474, 1957.
63. OJEMANN, G. A., AND R. I. HENKIN. Steroid dependent changes in human visual evoked potentials. *Life Sci., Part 1* 6: 327–333, 1967.
64. PFAFFMANN, C. The sense of taste. In: *Handbook of Physiology. Neurophysiology*, edited by H. W. Magoun. Washington, D.C.: Am. Physiol. Soc., 1959, sect. 1, vol. I, chapt. 20, p. 507–533.
65. PFAFFMANN, C., AND J. K. BARE. Gustatory nerve discharges in normal and adrenalectomized rats. *J. Comp. Physiol. Psychol.* 43: 320–324, 1950.
66. PITTMAN, J. A., AND R. J. BESCHI. Taste thresholds in hyper- and hypo-thyroidism. *J. Clin. Endocrinol. Metab.* 27: 895–896, 1967.
67. PLOTZ, C. M., A. I. KNOWLTON, AND C. RAGAN. The natural history of Cushing's syndrome. *Am. J. Med.* 13: 597–614, 1952.
68. PRUSZEWICZ, A., AND J. KOSOWICZ. Quantitative and qualitative studies of the taste and smell in adrenal insufficiency. *Endokrynol. Polska* 17: 321–327, 1966.
69. RICE, K. K., AND C. P. RICHTER. Increased sodium chloride and water intake of normal rats treated with desoxycorticosterone acetate. *Endocrinology* 33: 106–115, 1943.
70. RICHTER, C. P. Increased salt appetite in adrenalectomized rats. *Am. J. Physiol.* 115: 155–161, 1936.
71. RICHTER, C. P. The spontaneous activity of adrenalectomized rats treated with replacement and other therapy. *Endocrinology* 20: 657–666, 1936.
72. RICHTER, C. P. Transmission of taste sensation in animals. *Trans. Am. Neurol. Assoc.* 65: 49–50, 1939.
73. RICHTER, C. P. Salt taste thresholds for normal and adrenalectomized rats. *Endocrinology* 24: 367–371, 1939.
74. RICHTER, C. P. The internal environment and behavior. V. Internal secretions. *Am. J. Psychiat.* 97: 878–893, 1941.
75. RICHTER, C. P. Sodium chloride and dextrose appetite of untreated and treated adrenalectomized rats. *Endocrinology* 29: 115–125, 1941.
76. RICHTER, C. P. Total self regulatory functions in animals and human beings. *Harvey Lectures Ser.* 38: 63–103, 1942.
77. RICHTER, C. P., AND J. F. ECKERT. Mineral metabolism of adrenalectomized rats studied by the appetite method. *Endocrinology* 22: 214–224, 1938.
78. ROSEN, H., AND S. FELDMAN. Some observations on the effect of ACTH and cortisone in oto-rhino-laryngology. With special reference to the effect of cortisone on acoustic function. *Pract. Oto-Rhino-Laryngol.* 15: 10–19, 1953.
78a. SATO, N., E. W. HALLER, R. D. POWELL, AND R. I. HENKIN. Sexual maturation in bulbectomized female rats. *J. Reprod. Fertility* 36: 301–309, 1974.
79. SCHUTZ, H. G., AND J. F. PILGRIM. Sweetness of various compounds and its measurement. *Food Res.* 22: 206, 1957.
80. SCHWARZ, F., P. J. DER KINDEREN, AND M. HOUTSTRA-LANZ. Exophthalmus-producing activity in the serum and in the pituitary of patients with Cushing's syndrome and acromegaly. *J. Clin. Endocrinol. Metab.* 22: 718–725, 1962.
81. SELYE, H. Studies concerning the anesthetic action of steroid hormones. *J. Pharmacol. Exptl. Therap.* 73: 127–141, 1941.
82. SELYE, H. Anesthetic effect of steroid hormones. *Proc. Soc. Exptl. Biol. Med.* 46: 116–121, 1941.
83. SELYE, H. Correlation between the chemical structure and the pharmacological actions of the steroids. *Endocrinology* 30: 437–458, 1942.
84. SIVIAN, L. J., AND S. D. WHITE. On minimum audible sound fields. *J. Acoust. Soc. Am.* 4: 288–321, 1933.
85. SLANSKY, H. H., G. KOLBERT, AND S. GARTNER. Exophthalmus induced by steroids. *Arch. Ophthalmol.* 77: 579–581, 1967.
86. STEINBERG, J. C., H. C. MONTGOMERY, AND M. B. GARDNER. Results of the World's Fair hearing tests. *J. Acoust. Soc. Am.* 12: 291–301, 1940.
87. THORN, G. W. *The Diagnosis and Treatment of Adrenal Insufficiency.* Springfield, Ill.: Thomas, 1949.
88. TORDA, C., AND H. G. WOLFF. Effect of cortisone and ACTH on the threshold of convulsions induced by pentomethylene tetrozol. *Federation Proc.* 10: 137, 1951.
88a. VALENSTEIN, E. S., J. W. KAKOLEWSKI, AND W. C. COX. Sex differences in taste preference for glucose and saccharin solutions. *Science* 156: 942–943, 1967.
89. VON BEKESY, G. [Cited in: *Speech and Hearing in Communication*, edited by H. Fletcher. Princeton: Van Nostrand, 1953, p. 132.]
90. WILKINS, L., AND C. P. RICHTER. A great craving for salt by a child with corticoadrenal insufficiency. *J. Am. Med. Assoc.* 114: 866–868, 1940.
91. WILLIAMS, A. W. Exophthalmus in cortisone-treated experimental animals. *Brit. J. Exptl. Pathol.* 34: 621–624, 1953.
92. WILLIAMS, A. W. Pathogenesis of cortisone-induced exophthalmus in guinea pigs. *Brit. J. Exptl. Pathol.* 36: 245–247, 1955.
93. WOODBURY, D. M. Relation between the adrenal cortex and the central nervous system. *Pharmacol. Rev.* 10: 275–357, 1958.
94. YENSEN, R. Influence of salt deficiency on taste sensitivity in human subjects. *Nature* 181: 1472–1474, 1958.
95. YENSEN, R. Influence of water deprivation on taste sensitivity in man. *Nature* 182: 677–679, 1958.
96. YOUNG, P. T. Concerning the mechanism of appetite. *Psychol. Bull.* 35: 716–717, 1938.
97. YOUNG, P. T. The experimental analyses of appetite. *Psychol. Bull.* 38: 129–164, 1941.
98. YOUNG, P. T. Studies on food preference, appetite and dietary habit. IX. Palatability versus appetite as determinants of the critical concentrations of sucrose and sodium chloride. *Comp. Psychol. Monogr.* 19: 1–44, 1949.

CHAPTER 16

Corticosteroids and lymphoid tissue

ALLAN MUNCK
DONALD A. YOUNG[1] | *Department of Physiology, Dartmouth Medical School, Hanover, New Hampshire*

CHAPTER CONTENTS

Lymphoid System and Immune Responses
Actions of Hormones on Lymphoid Tissues: Glucocorticoid
    Specificity
Effects of Glucocorticoids on Lymphocyte Morphology and
    Lymphoid Tissue Organization and Function
Metabolic Effects of Glucocorticoids on Lymphoid Tissue
Glucocorticoid Receptors and Initial Steps in Actions of
    Glucocorticoids on Lymphoid Cells
Physiological Significance of Glucocorticoid Actions on Lymphoid
    Tissue

A RELATION between the adrenal cortex and the lymphoid system was foreshadowed as early as 1855 in the work of Thomas Addison who noted that the blood of a victim of the disease that came to bear his name had "a considerable excess of white corpuscles . . ." (1). In the cases he dealt with, Addison found no enlargement of the thymus, spleen, or lymph nodes; the first to associate Addison's disease with thymus enlargement appears to have been Star (107). Boinet (9) subsequently found hypertrophied thymus glands in rats that had been adrenalectomized, an observation established quantitatively in careful studies by Jaffe (60).

During the late nineteenth and early twentieth centuries, much confusion regarding what constituted normal lymphoid tissue was engendered by the so-called "status thymicolymphaticus," a resounding diagnosis often applied in cases of sudden and otherwise unexplained death in which the thymus and lymph nodes appeared to be hypertrophied. Considerable speculation was devoted to the role of adrenal insufficiency in the pathophysiology of status thymicolymphaticus [see, for example (60)]. This example of medical mythology, as it has been termed by Greenwood & Woods (47), redolent of ancient medicine, apparently was the creation of pathologists whose standards for normal lymphoid tissue were derived from people who died of various well-defined illnesses. Through the work of Selye (106), it eventually became clear that virtually any form of illness or stress will cause atrophy of the lymphoid organs and that what pathologists had taken to be hypertrophy was probably in most cases simply a lack of atrophy.

Selye showed that the influence of stress on lymphoid tissue is mediated by the adrenal glands, but he was unable to distinguish clearly between the role of the cortex and that of the medulla. It was left to Ingle (56, 57) and Wells & Kendall (116) to demonstrate that thymus involution in normal, adrenalectomized, or hypophysectomized rats can be produced by administering extracts or purified steroids from the adrenal cortex. These same workers showed that the ability of steroids to bring about involution is associated with what later would be called glucocorticoid, rather than mineralocorticoid, activity. Beginning in the 1940s, extensive studies were carried out by White, Dougherty, and their collaborators on the nature of the changes produced in lymphoid tissue by adrenal steroids and on the relation of those changes to the immune response (25–30, 117, 118).

At present there are three major areas of activity in the study of interactions of glucocorticoids with lymphoid tissue. One encompasses the experimental and therapeutic uses of glucocorticoids as tools for suppression of immune responses. The second includes the applications of glucocorticoids for control of neoplastic proliferation of the lymphoid system. The third, which may be called the endocrinologic area, deals with the physiological functions and molecular mechanisms of glucocorticoid actions on lymphoid tissue. Many current problems, such as that of the origin of glucocorticoid resistance in certain normal and leukemic lymphocytes, are of profound importance to workers in more than one of these areas, so although in the present review we write from an endocrinologic standpoint, we try to place some of these problems in a broader setting.

Progress has been quite uneven, as this review will show. During the last decade, with the development of systems in which the metabolic effects of glucocorticoids on lymphocytes can be studied in vitro, there have been major advances in our knowledge of the mechanisms of action of glucocorticoids on lymphoid tissue. There have also been great strides in the understanding of how the

---

[1] Present address: Department of Medicine and Radiation Biology and Biophysics, University of Rochester School of Medicine and Dentistry, Rochester, New York.

lymphoid system governs immune responses—the thymus, for example, has at last acquired a function. Developments continue apace, but so far these rich harvests of new knowledge have not provided us with answers to basic questions on the physiological role of glucocorticoid actions on lymphoid tissue either in normal homeostasis or in the response to stress.

Certain aspects of the topics we discuss have been covered in several reviews (7, 18, 28, 44, 114).

LYMPHOID SYSTEM AND IMMUNE RESPONSES

To provide a framework for discussion of hormone actions we give a brief account of present views on the relation of structure to function in the lymphoid system. We have relied heavily on a number of recent reviews and monographs (15, 45, 46, 62, 73, 74, 88), but this field is in a highly fluid state so that any survey, such as the present one, is bound to gloss over many controversial questions.

In functional terms, lymphoid tissues may be regarded as consisting of two parallel systems (Fig. 1). One system governs mainly the cell-mediated immune responses involved in rejection of transplants and in delayed hypersensitivity; the other governs the humoral responses mediated by circulating antibodies. Although the functions of these systems cannot be sharply differentiated, the first appears to serve mainly to protect the organism against internal neoplastic proliferation and the second to protect against external agents, such as viruses and bacteria. To some extent the systems are independent of each other, but in recent years it has become clear that in many cases the first system exerts important regulatory influences over the second.

In mammals, chickens, and other species, the first system is associated with the thymus. Neonatal thymectomy virtually abolishes the capacity to reject a graft. In chickens the second system is associated with the bursa of Fabricius. Bursectomy drastically reduces antibody formation but leaves intact the ability to reject a graft. Mammals undoubtedly have lymphoid tissues with functions analogous to those of the avian bursa, but the location of these tissues remains uncertain. One current suggestion, not universally accepted, identifies the mammalian equivalent of the bursa with gut-associated lymphoid tissues.

The thymus and the bursa of Fabricius and its mammalian equivalent are designated as primary lymphoid organs. Lymphocytes in these organs are derived from stem cells originating largely in fetal liver or bone marrow. Seeding from bone marrow continues in the adult, and repopulation of primary organs after depletion by irradiation or hormone treatment depends on this process. It is no longer thought that lymphocytes can develop from thymic epithelial or reticular cells.

Primary lymphoid organs appear to initiate the differentiation and multiplication of stem cells into immunocompetent cells (i.e., cells that can react with foreign antigens and initiate immune responses). In the thymus, local hormonal factors may be important in stimulating these maturation processes, which are independent of antigenic stimulation. The immunocompetent cells are mostly small lymphocytes. Large lymphocytes probably do not initiate immune responses.

Small lymphocytes from primary lymphoid organs in turn seed the peripheral lymphoid organs: lymph nodes, spleen, and various gut-associated tissues. Those derived from the thymus are referred to as thymus-derived lymphocytes, or T cells. In chickens those derived from the bursa are referred to as bursa-derived, and in mammals those derived from the mammalian equivalent of the bursa are referred to as non-thymus-derived or—somewhat confusingly—as bone marrow-derived lymphocytes. They are also commonly designated as B cells. Both T and B cells are found in peripheral lymphoid organs. In addition, T cells comprise most of the circulating pool of small lymphocytes.

In the peripheral organs, lymphocytes from the primary organs undergo the final stages of maturation necessary for their direct participation in immune responses. Antigens leading to antibody formation are trapped in lymph nodes and other peripheral organs, where, possibly after processing by macrophages or related cells, they interact with lymphocytes that may possess specific antibody-like receptors on their membranes. This interaction stimulates proliferation and differentiation of lymphocytes to form *a*) plasma cells that produce antibody to the antigen and *b*) "memory" cells that give rise to an enhanced subsequent response to the antigens. Memory cells are probably small lymphocytes similar to those that

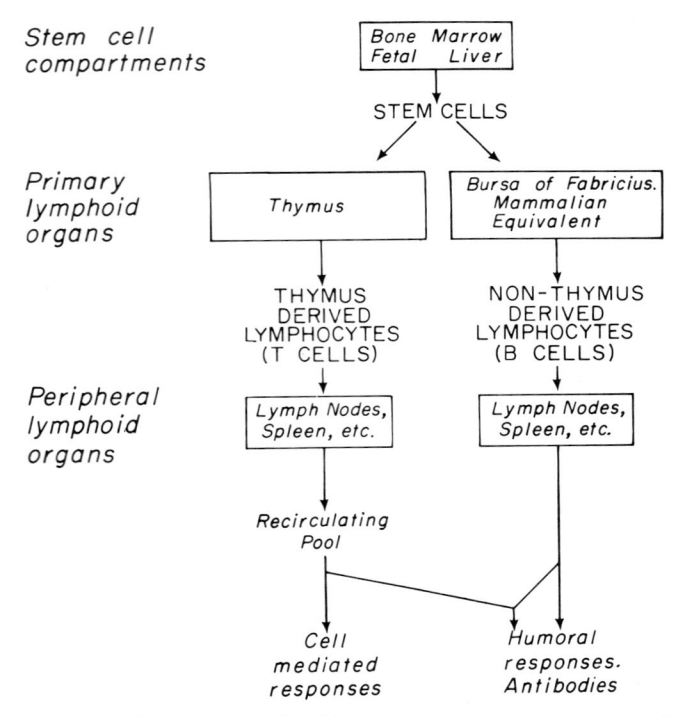

FIG. 1. Functional relationships among major compartments of lymphoid system.

interact with the antigen initially. The precursors of the antibody-producing plasma cells are undoubtedly B cells.

In cell-mediated immune responses stimulated by a foreign graft, the graft antigen is probably recognized by circulating T cells that interact directly with the graft and then find their way to regional lymph nodes where they stimulate production of memory cells and of cells (perhaps also lymphocytes) that invade and destroy the graft.

Small lymphocytes, the chief protagonists in immune responses, are a highly heterogeneous and mobile group of cells, as is evident from the many specialized roles they fulfill. Heterogeneity can be observed at a gross level in the large variations in life-spans among lymphocyte populations. Many small lymphocytes recirculate continuously and have long life-spans, up to 10 years in man. By contrast, the majority of thymus lymphocytes never leave the thymus and are destroyed after a life-span of about 3 days. The significance of this rapid turnover is not known. In the recirculating lymphocyte pool in rats, about 90% of the cells have life-spans of many months. Most of these lymphocytes are probably T cells, and their long life-span may explain the relative ineffectiveness of adult thymectomy in reducing cellular immune responses. A few of the recirculating lymphocytes, of unknown function, have life-spans of about 2 weeks. The content of long-lived small lymphocytes in various parts of the lymphoid system increases in the following order: bone marrow and thymus; spleen; blood; regional lymph nodes; thoracic duct lymph. Recirculation of lymphocytes is a process, apparently sensitive to hormones, by which lymphocytes circulate continuously from the blood to the peripheral lymphoid system and back, with a cycling time of a few hours. The purpose of recirculation may be to continuously permit interactions between lymphocytes of varied antigenic specificities and peripheral tissues, perhaps in fulfillment of the "surveillance" function proposed by Burnet (15).

ACTIONS OF HORMONES ON LYMPHOID TISSUES: GLUCOCORTICOID SPECIFICITY

Among the many hormonal actions on lymphoid tissue that have been described, the lympholytic actions of the glucocorticoids are the most pronounced and have been most extensively studied. Thyroid and growth hormones under certain conditions stimulate growth of lymphatic tissue, and androgens and estrogens suppress growth [see (25, 90)], but the sex hormones, as discussed below, have little, if any, activity compared to glucocorticoids in assays designed to measure acute involution of lymphoid tissue. Several hormones, including epinephrine, mediated perhaps by cyclic AMP, stimulate mitogenic activity in thymic lymphocytes in vitro [see (67)]. What role any of these hormones play in the widely observed involution of lymphoid tissue with increasing age of the individual remains unclear, despite much research and speculation, and it is quite possible that this phenomenon does not require hormones at all. For example, adrenalectomy, gonadectomy, and thyroidectomy, singly or in various combinations, apparently do not prevent age involution [see (25)].

All lymphoid tissues evidence some degree of atrophy in response to glucocorticoids. The morphological and metabolic characteristics of these hormone actions are discussed in detail later (see sections EFFECTS OF GLUCOCORTICOIDS ON LYMPHOCYTE MORPHOLOGY AND LYMPHOID TISSUE ORGANIZATION AND FUNCTION, and METABOLIC EFFECTS OF GLUCOCORTICOIDS ON LYMPHOID TISSUE), and for now it suffices to mention that the different tissues vary considerably in sensitivity, the thymus being the most sensitive in rodents (28). Considerable variation in sensitivity also occurs among species and even among strains of rats and mice, and within any strain, sensitivity may vary with age and sex [see (92)].

Most bioassays for activities of steroids on lymphoid tissue employ adrenalectomized rats or mice and determine thymolytic activity, which is a measure of the decrease in thymus weight that follows steroid treatment. In Table 1 the thymolytic activity of a number of steroids is compared to glycogenic activity. Glycogenic activity (i.e., the ability to stimulate deposition of liver glycogen in adrenalectomized, fasted rats or mice) is often taken as the prototypical glucocorticoid activity. The wide range of activities reported for some of these compounds may be ascribed not only to the sources of variability mentioned above, but also to variations in bioassay procedures.

Within the latitude afforded by the data in Table 1 it is clear that there is fairly close correspondence between thymolytic and glycogenic activity. This correspondence has been found to apply to a vast array of synthetic and natural steroids and justifies the inclusion of thymolytic or, more generally, lympholytic activities among those activities characteristic of glucocorticoids.

TABLE 1. *Relative Thymolytic and Glycogenic Activities of Various Steroids*

Steroid	Thymolytic	Glycogenic
Dexamethasone	16–95	20–265
Triamcinolone	4	7–47
9α-Fluoroprednisolone	8–17	13–49
Prednisolone	2–11	3–10
Cortisol	1.0	1.0
Cortisone	0.6–1.0	0.3–0.6
Corticosterone	0.2–0.5	0.3–0.8
Cortexolone (11-deoxycortisol)	0	0
11-Epicortisol		0
Deoxycorticosterone	0–0.1	0–0.1
Progesterone	0	
Testosterone**	0	0
Estradiol	0	0

Values represent range of activities and were obtained with assays in which rats or mice were employed. * Cortisol = 1.0.
** As free alcohol or propionate. [Compiled from (23, 24, 53, 92, 98).]

Thymolytic activity is not associated with mineralocorticoid activity, as represented in Table 1 by deoxycorticosterone; nor is it associated in these assays with the progestational, androgenic, and estrogenic activities represented by the last three entries in Table 1. However, deoxycorticosterone, progesterone, testosterone, and estradiol have all been found to potentiate to some degree the thymolytic activity of glucocorticoids (24) by mechanisms that are not understood. It is possible that testosterone suppresses development of primary lymphoid organs in the chicken by acting on the nonlymphoid epithelial structures in those organs (112).

In connection with the actions of steroids on lymphoid tissues, it has occasionally been suggested that the activity of a given steroid may in part be determined by metabolic transformations which the steroid undergoes within the lymphoid tissues themselves (28, 114). Plausible though such ideas may be, they have received little experimental support. For example, Dougherty et al. (28) have proposed that corticosterone, by virtue of its resistance to certain transformations to which cortisol is susceptible, may gain lympholytic activity relative to cortisol. In fact, however, corticosterone is about half as active as cortisol whether its activity is determined in vivo (Table 1) or, as discussed later (see section GLUCOCORTICOID RECEPTORS AND INITIAL STEPS IN ACTIONS OF GLUCOCORTICOIDS ON LYMPHOID CELLS), in vitro (Table 2), the in vitro determinations being carried out under conditions in which cortisol is not significantly metabolized (82). Results with thymus (16) suggest some role for 11β-hydroxysteroid dehydrogenase, the enzyme governing interconversion of cortisol and cortisone, in regulating sensitivity to glucocorticoids in mice. Similar results are not found with rats, however. Nor can the resistance of certain lymphosarcomas to glucocorticoids be ascribed to metabolism of the steroids (16); resistance may in fact be related to deficiency of glucocorticoid receptors, as mentioned later in this chapter, or to other derangements in the early steps of hormone action.

EFFECTS OF GLUCOCORTICOIDS ON LYMPHOCYTE MORPHOLOGY AND LYMPHOID TISSUE ORGANIZATION AND FUNCTION

Glucocorticoids exert suppressive effects on virtually all functions [see (44)] and elements of the lymphoid system. Decreases in size and weight of the thymus, bursa of Fabricius, lymph nodes, spleen, and Peyer's patches and decreases in number of circulating lymphocytes and bone marrow lymphocytes have been repeatedly observed in conditions of acute or chronic glucocorticoid excess brought about by administration of exogenous steroid or ACTH, Cushing's syndrome, or stress [see (25)]. Although conditions of glucocorticoid excess may be regarded as abnormal, changes in levels of circulating lymphocytes have also been observed to accompany normal diurnal variations of glucocorticoid levels in blood (12). Furthermore the entire lymphoid system hypertrophies in response to adrenalectomy [see (25)]. Thus suppression of lymphoid tissues occurs even with basal levels of glucocorticoids.

The time course of glucocorticoid effects of lymphoid tissues at the histological and cytological level has generally been studied after treatment with large doses of hormones. Because of its high sensitivity to glucocorticoids and its architectural simplicity, the thymus is the organ in which changes are most readily seen and most easily interpreted. Studies with the light microscope show that the loss in thymus mass is primarily the result of destruction of the small lymphocytes of the cortex; cells in the medulla are relatively unaffected. Differences between cortical and medullary thymocytes, with respect to a number of parameters—size, mitotic activity, mitochondrial content, development of endoplasmic reticulum, histocompatibility antigens, radiosensitivity, lifespan, and immunologic function—suggest that they are two distinct cell populations (18, 62, 74).

The response to glucocorticoids observed in the mouse thymus (29, 30, 59, 91) begins with tissue edema (at 1–3 hr) and a gradual increase in number of pyknotic cells—large numbers of cells are affected within 6 hr. By 16–24 hr lymphocytolysis is widespread and cellular debris is considerable; almost all small lymphocytes of the cortex are affected. The lytic changes are accompanied by the appearance of increasing numbers of macrophages, which ultimately contain inclusions of fragmented cells. During the next 2 days phagocytosis of disintegrated cells continues and nonphagocytized nuclear remnants accumulate. By the third day the weight of the gland has reached a minimum of less than one-third of its original weight, the cortex is nearly devoid of lymphocytes, and considerable collapse of the reticulum has occurred. Since large lymphocytes and reticulum cells are unaffected, a relative increase is seen in their numbers. During this entire period little change is seen in the medulla, which contains most of the surviving lymphocytes. After the third day, during the reconstitution phase, the number of small lymphocytes in the cortex increases, probably because of inward migration of small lymphocytes from bone marrow or bursa-equivalent tissues (74).

As seen with the electron microscope, the lymphocytolytic effects of glucocorticoids appear to originate within the nucleus. The earliest changes observed by Cowan & Sorenson (22) were coarsening and increased osmophilia of nuclear chromatin in affected cells and peripheral migration of chromatin to the nuclear membrane accompanied by formation of masses with an arc-like border (cf. the chromatin pattern in normal thymocytes in Fig. 2A, and that in thymocytes from glucocorticoid-treated mice in Fig. 2B). These chromatin abnormalities, occasionally seen as early as 2 hr after hormone injection, become widespread by 8 hr and gradually proceed (by 16 hr in most cells) to total nuclear osmophilia, with dissolution of the nuclear membrane, cell fragmentation, and phagocytosis. Apart from the fact that glucocorticoid-induced destruction is widespread and follows a characteristic time course, apparently nothing distinguishes steroid-killed cells from cells undergoing spontaneous degeneration in the normal animal.

Burton et al. (17) have shown that similar electron-microscopic changes can be induced in thymocyte cultures by direct addition of 10^{-6} M cortisol in vitro, which indicates that the lethal effects of cortisol do not require mediation by other tissues. Two lines of evidence—namely, that cells have to be metabolically healthy to display glucocorticoid sensitivity and that, in contrast to cell killing with detergents, the glucocorticoid killing does not take place at low temperatures (22 C as compared to 38 C)—suggest that glucocorticoid killing is an active process requiring cellular metabolism. These findings agree with evidence cited below on the mechanisms by which glucocorticoid effects are initiated.

Early descriptions of cytotoxic effects of glucocorticoids refer to shedding of cytoplasm by budding as a prominent feature of the lymphocytolytic response. The significance of budding is unclear. In vitro it has been produced only with very high doses of steroids (41). It has not been observed in electron-microscopic studies, possibly because of the thin sections used (22). The hypothesis that budding represents antibody release from lymphocytes (118) has not been substantiated [see (26, 44)].

In addition to their lymphocytolytic effects, glucocorticoids also exhibit actions on lymphocytes that may be reversible and occur via fundamentally different mechanisms. Glucocorticoids have been reported to both inhibit (27) and stimulate (48, 119) mitosis, to inhibit lymphocyte migration (26) and circulation (99), to influence import and export of lymphocytes from the thymus and other lymphoid tissues (35), to accelerate lymphocyte differentiation (48), and to modify the sensitization process by which antigens induce lymphocyte differentiation and proliferation (19). The direct lymphocytolytic action of glucocorticoids on small lymphocytes probably accounts for the depletion of lymphocytes seen after large doses of glucocorticoids; these other less dramatic hormone actions, however, may not only play significant roles in the response to excess hormone, but may be important in determining lymphoid tissue architecture and mass and cellular migration patterns in the normal animal.

Although small lymphocytes are the primary targets for the cytolytic effects of glucocorticoids, all small lymphocytes are not equally sensitive. The type and degree of response of a particular tissue are probably the result of complex interplay between sensitive and resistant cell lines in that tissue. The percent of nucleated cells surviving in mice 2 days after a single injection of 2.5 mg cortisol was found by Cohen et al. (19) to be 6% in the thymus, 21% in the spleen, and 79% in the marrow. Studies of lymphocyte turnover [see (38)] and function have led to the conclusion (21, 36) that glucocorticoid-sensitive cells are short lived and immunologically incompetent, whereas resistant cells are long lived and immunologically competent. For example, the 5% or so surviving thymocytes (mostly in the medulla) from mice treated with mas-

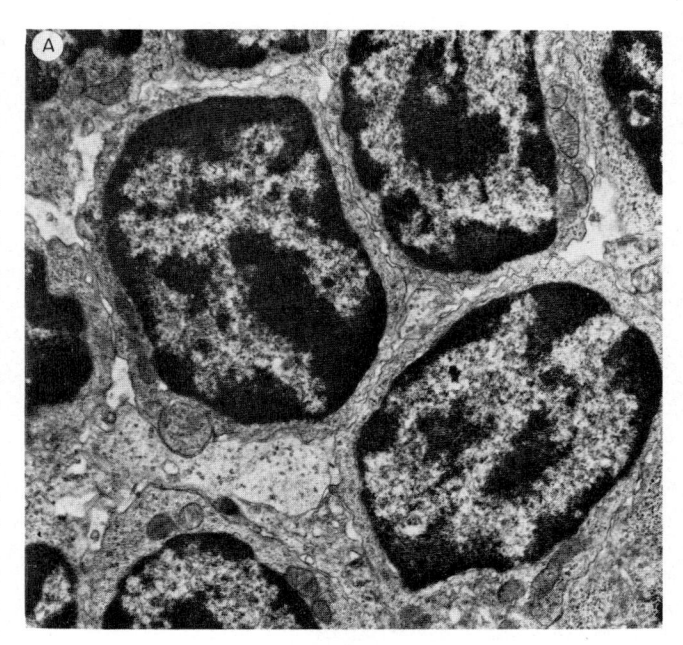

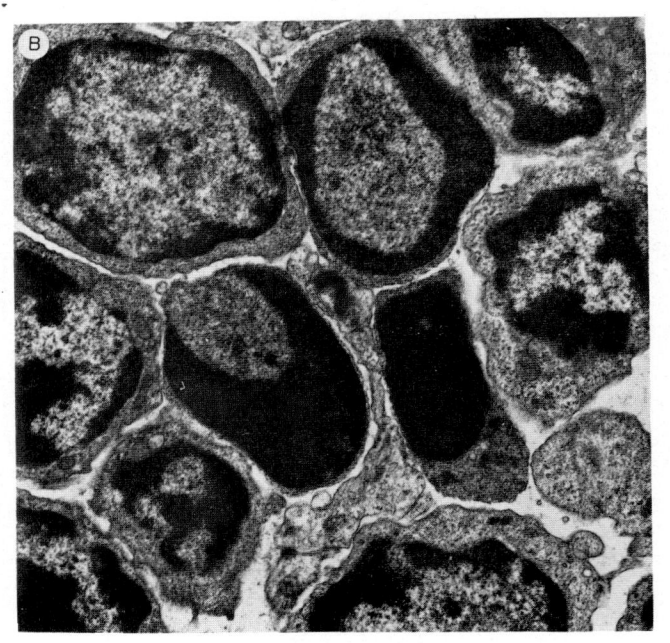

FIG. 2. *A*: portion of thymus populated with lymphocytes from 6-week-old control mice. × 7,100. *B*: portion of thymus from mice 8 hr after injection of 0.5 mg cortisol. Dense chromatin at nuclear membrane of lymphocytes is characteristic degeneration effect after glucocorticoid treatment. × 6,500. [From Cowan & Sorensen (22).]

sive doses of glucocorticoids in certain assays appear to include all the immunologically competent cells of the original intact thymus that were involved either in the graft-vs.-host reaction or in antibody formation [see (18, 20, 21)]. Immunologically competent T cells that have migrated to the periphery also display glucocorticoid resistance (18, 21). Other glucocorticoid-resistant cells are the pyroninophyllic and plasma cells in the medullary cords of lymph nodes, in Peyer's patches, and in splenic red pulp.

In addition to being found in the thymus cortex, glucocorticoid-sensitive cells are found in the cortical regions of lymph nodes, splenic white pulp, and Peyer's patches (29, 48), the germinal centers of the cortical regions of the latter three tissues being particularly sensitive. For instance, in rabbits, glucocorticoids injected several days after antigen inhibited preparation for a secondary response, apparently by interfering with germinal center production and formation of memory cells (34). Of the three components of the antibody-forming system from spleen—marrow-derived precursors of antibody-forming cells, thymus-derived helper cells (i.e., T cells that cooperate with B cells in the antibody response), and macrophages—only the first is glucocorticoid sensitive, since after large doses of glucocorticoids the immunocompetence of the spleen is restored only by the addition of bone marrow cells from untreated animals [see (18, 62)]. Curiously enough, the bone marrow lymphocytes that give rise to B cells appear to be glucocorticoid resistant (18, 21). Normal human peripheral lymphocytes, tested in culture, are resistant to glucocorticoids, but lymphocytes from patients with lymphocytic leukemia are often sensitive (105).

The picture that seems to be emerging is that, at various stages of their immunologic maturation, small lymphocytes participating in both the cellular immune response and humoral antibody formation undergo marked changes in glucocorticoid sensitivity. It is conceivable that these changes occur through alterations in glucocorticoid receptors, which, as discussed later (see section GLUCOCORTICOID RECEPTORS AND INITIAL STEPS IN ACTIONS OF GLUCOCORTICOIDS ON LYMPHOID CELLS), may account for the difference between sensitive and resistant lymphoid tumor cells. Present knowledge of the overall effects of glucocorticoids in immunosuppression is incomplete. Immunosuppression may well involve hormone actions that are not directed specifically at the lymphoid system, such as anti-inflammatory actions (7, 26). For example, doses of glucocorticoids that are effective in suppressing inflammation are often not effective in suppressing the immunologic mechanisms presumed to be operating in the disease that is being treated [see (44)].

METABOLIC EFFECTS OF GLUCOCORTICOIDS ON LYMPHOID TISSUE

Given the lympholytic effects described above, one would expect glucocorticoids to exert profound influences on cellular metabolic functions. Indeed, since the ultimate result of hormone action is cell destruction, all metabolic functions must eventually be affected. The questions we consider in this section are *a*) after exposure of lymphoid cells to glucocorticoids, what metabolic changes take place and *b*) how are these changes causally related among each other and how do they lead to cell destruction? In the next section we consider how the metabolic changes are initiated.

Administration of glucocorticoids in vivo results in the following changes: *a*) decreased rates of uptake and metabolism of glucose and other substrates in rat and mouse thymus cells (6, 75, 108, 113); *b*) decreased incorporation of precursors into protein and RNA and DNA of rat, mouse, and rabbit thymus, lymph nodes, spleen, lymphoma, and lymphosarcoma cells (11, 13, 31, 43, 55, 68, 69, 89, 96, 109, 110); *c*) decreased uptake of macromolecular precursors (amino acids and nucleosides) into intracellular pools of rat thymus, spleen, and lymph node cells (39, 69)—an early increase in protein synthesis has also been reported (108); *d*) decreased activity of certain enzymes, such as RNA polymerases (40, 86, 87); *e*) increased efflux of cellular DNA and amino acids from rat thymus (51, 111); and *f*) increased levels of free fatty acids in mouse thymus (115).

Glucocorticoid-induced increases have been observed in activities of enzymes, such as deoxyribonuclease, ribonuclease, β-glucuronidase, arylsulfatase, and cathepsins (2, 66, 85, 97). These enzymes are known to be associated with lysosomes and would be expected to be released by cell destruction [see (10)]. At late stages of tissue breakdown, lysosomal enzymes may also be contributed by infiltrating phagocytic cells (85).

Causal relationships among the many metabolic effects described have been difficult to establish from experiments in vivo, and most of our understanding has come from results obtained with thymus cell suspensions in vitro. Although Schrek (104) showed many years ago that cortisol and corticosterone at low concentrations in vitro would kill incubated rabbit thymus cells and Gabourel & Aronow (42) convincingly demonstrated glucocorticoid actions on lymphoma cells in culture and in addition developed a glucocorticoid-resistant sub line (4), until the mid 1960s attempts to produce physiologically meaningful metabolic effects in short-term incubations of lymphocytes with glucocorticoids in vitro consistently failed, leading occasionally to suggestions that lympholytic actions of glucocorticoids might be mediated through hormone actions on liver or other tissues [see (54)]. The difficulties were resolved when it was realized that gentle methods of cell preparation are necessary to preserve sufficient integrity of cellular metabolic controls so that specific glucocorticoid actions would become measurable and that use of low concentrations of steroids (10^{-6} M or less) is necessary to avoid the nonspecific effects exerted by almost all steroids at concentrations of 10^{-5} M and greater (75, 77).

With the availability of isolated cell systems, many of the effects described above have been reported in vitro. In particular, with thymus cell suspensions it has been shown that glucocorticoids inhibit glucose uptake (75); incorporation of amino acids into protein, which probably reflects both decreased cellular uptake of amino acids and decreased protein synthesis (75, 122); incorporation of precursors into RNA and DNA (68, 69, 121);

and RNA polymerase activity (71). These effects are specific for steroids with glucocorticoid structure and can be obtained with concentrations of glucocorticoids in the physiological range (61, 68, 71). Comparable results have been found with lymphoma and lymphosarcoma cells (42, 93, 94) and with human leukemic lymphocytes (5). Such changes, particularly in protein and nucleic acid metabolism, are what one would expect a priori to find in cells that are dying as a result of exposure to glucocorticoids.

Two general views appear to have guided research on the relation of these effects to the primary hormone actions. The first is that the inhibitory effects on incorporation of precursors into RNA and protein and on RNA polymerase are themselves direct expressions of the primary actions, that is, that the hormones act directly to inhibit the protein synthetic machinery of the cell [see (86)]. The second is that the inhibitory effects on protein and nucleic acid metabolism are consequences of preceding effects, particularly on glucose uptake, which in turn may depend on still earlier actions (6, 75, 78, 80).

On the whole, although the problem is still far from solved, present evidence favors the second view. Careful measurements of the time course of appearance of the various inhibitory effects after thymus cells have been treated with cortisol show that the inhibition of glucose uptake appears abruptly between 15 and 20 min, well before the inhibitory effects on protein and RNA metabolism, which do not become measurable until after about 1 hr (69, 71, 75, 78, 121–123). Furthermore, in the absence of substrates, the cortisol effects on protein and RNA metabolism are much diminished or do not appear at all, even after prolonged incubation (69, 121). The inhibitory effects therefore appear to depend at least partly on prior inhibition of glucose utilization. Lymphosarcoma cells exhibit a somewhat similar time sequence and substrate dependence for cortisol effects (94). Through what pathways the effect on glucose is transmitted to the later inhibitory effects is not clear, but ATP may be involved (122, 123). Fatty acids have been proposed as the initiators of the nuclear damage that is the first visible sign of cytolysis (17), and some recent evidence supporting this idea indicates that in lymphosarcoma cells, glucocorticoid resistance is correlated with resistance to damage by fatty acids (115).

Whether the late effects can be accounted for solely by an early effect on glucose remains an open question. There is no doubt that other substrates, such as pyruvate, can substitute for glucose, so that effects independent of glucose do occur. But among many substrates tested, glucose, which probably is the principal substrate in vivo, is by far the best in maintaining levels of protein synthesis and uridine incorporation into RNA and is also the substrate with which the largest cortisol effects are elicited (69, 121). Drews & Wagner (32) have suggested that their results on relative time courses of RNA synthesis and uridine phosphorylation demonstrate separate actions of cortisol and glucose, but their argument is weakened by the fact that they compare the effects of complete absence of glucose in vitro with the effects of prednisolone administered in vivo.

Lymphoid tissue is not the only tissue in which glucocorticoids exert rapid inhibitory actions on glucose uptake, and the general hypothesis that glucocorticoids initiate catabolic processes in peripheral tissues by decreasing glucose uptake dates back 30 years to the studies of Ingle (58) and Drury (33). Similar actions have been demonstrated with skin and adipose tissue, and for each of these tissues there is reason to suppose that the effects on glucose are at least partly responsible for catabolic effects [see (80)].

GLUCOCORTICOID RECEPTORS AND INITIAL STEPS IN ACTIONS OF GLUCOCORTICOIDS ON LYMPHOID CELLS

In the preceding section we have described the principal metabolic effects produced in lymphoid cells by glucocorticoids during the first few hours of their actions in vivo and in vitro and have summarized the evidence that a common antecedent of many of these effects may be inhibition of glucose uptake, the earliest metabolic effect observed so far. In this section we describe what has been learned so far about events preceding the effect on glucose uptake. Most of the studies we deal with have employed rat thymus cell suspension, but lymphocytes from other sources, including man, and from lymphomas and lymphosarcomas respond similarly with respect to glucose metabolism and possess similar glucocorticoid receptors (8, 37, 52, 64, 93, 94). Somewhat paradoxically, as will appear, although the ultimate actions of glucocorticoids on lymphoid tissue are catabolic, the initial steps are probably anabolic—they involve stimulation of RNA and protein synthesis.

As already remarked, the relative activities of various steroids on glucose uptake by thymus cells in vitro, given in Table 2, compare well with activities in vivo (see Table 1) when allowance is made for the absence of metabolic transformation of steroids in vitro. For example, the inactivity of cortisone in vitro is entirely consistent with the evidence that cortisone in vivo acquires activity only by transformation to cortisol, a transformation that does not take place appreciably in rat thymus cell suspensions.

Inhibition of glucose uptake is in all likelihood due to inhibition of glucose transport. This conclusion rests on the following observations: a) decreased uptake is accompanied by increased cellular levels of glucose 6-phosphate and decreased lactic acid production, which indicates a block between glucose and glucose 6-phosphate (78, 81); b) of the two steps—transport and phosphorylation—leading from extracellular glucose to glucose 6-phosphate, the latter does not appear to be rate limiting since there is little if any free glucose inside the cells, and the capacity of cell hexokinases to phosphorylate glucose far exceeds the maximal rate of glucose uptake by intact cells;

TABLE 2. *Relative Activities of Steroids in Rat Thymus Cells in Vitro*

Steroid	Inhibition of glucose uptake	Receptor binding*	Nonspecific binding**
Dexamethasone	10	4.8	3
9α-Fluoroprednisolone	18	3.6	1
Prednisolone	1.2	1.3	1
Cortisol	1.0	1.0	1
Corticosterone	0.4	0.5	2
Deoxycorticosterone	<0.2	0.5	4
Progesterone	<0.1	0.4	25
Cortexolone (11-deoxycortisol)	<0.1	0.3	3
17α-Hydroxyprogesterone	<0.1	0.1	4
Testosterone	<0.1	<0.05	3
Cortisone	<0.1	<0.05	1
11-Epicortisol	<0.1	<0.05	
Tetrahydrocortisol	<0.2	<0.05	2

All measurements were made at 37 C under similar incubation conditions. * Measured by competition with cortisol-^{3}H. ** Relative nonspecific binding is determined by dividing the amount (moles/liter packed cells) of a given steroid bound, when it is present at a concentration in the medium of 10^{-5} M, by the amount of cortisol bound under the same conditions. [After Munck & Brinck-Johnsen (82).]

c) cortisol inhibits transport of 3-*O*-methylglucose, a glucose analogue that is not phosphorylated or otherwise metabolized by thymus cells but that competes with glucose for uptake (76, 80). Transport of 2-deoxyglucose, another analogue, is similarly inhibited in lymphosarcoma cells (94, 95).

Evidence that lymphocytes possess specific glucocorticoid binding sites that are the receptors through which the hormones exert their actions has been obtained by studying binding of tritium-labeled steroids to thymus cells (81, 82, 102). Metabolic transformation of glucocorticoids is very slight under the conditions of these studies, and all evidence to date indicates that the various bound fractions of steroid that have been identified with cortisol and other glucocorticoids consist of unaltered hormone. All steroids tend to become bound to some extent. Much of this binding, even with very active glucocorticoids, is nonspecific—it is unrelated to glucocorticoid activity—as can be seen from Table 2. Nonspecific binding, in fact, is related rather to the nonspecific metabolic activity mentioned in the previous section.

With glucocorticoids such as cortisol, corticosterone, and dexamethasone, a small fraction, characterized by the fact that it dissociates and associates much more slowly than does nonspecifically bound steroid, is bound specifically to what can be shown by a number of criteria to be glucocorticoid receptors (i.e., the molecular entities through which glucocorticoids initiate their metabolic activity). These receptors, of which there are about 5,000 per cell, bind glucocorticoids reversibly with high affinity. Cortisol at 37 C has a binding constant of about 2.5 × 10^7 M^{-1}, which is about the value that would be expected for receptors that become saturated over the physiological range of concentrations of glucocorticoids in blood. The corollary to this observation is that the limit of physiological response to high concentrations of cortisol is set by the number of available receptors. Binding constants for other steroids relative to cortisol, measured by competition with cortisol, are listed in Table 2. They are in reasonable agreement with glucocorticoid activities in vitro, the largest discrepancies arising with substances such as cortexolone, which binds fairly strongly but has little or no glucocorticoid activity. As would be expected if the binding sites for which it competes are the glucocortioid receptors, cortexolone behaves as a very effective antiglucocorticoid—it blocks the metabolic activity of cortisol when it is added with cortisol to thymus cells. This antiglucocorticoid activity of cortexolone has also been observed with other systems in vitro.

Two forms of glucocorticoid-receptor complexes have been identified: *1*) a nuclear-bound form, which can be extracted from isolated nuclei with high-salt concentrations; and *2*) a form that is not bound to the nucleus, commonly referred to as "cytoplasmic," although it may or may not be in the cytoplasm (83, 84, 100, 120). When cortisol is incubated with thymus cells at 3 C, it forms almost exclusively the cytoplasmic complex. Upon warming of the cells to 37 C the cytoplasmic complex is transformed within seconds to the nuclear complex (83). Formation of the cytoplasmic complex appears to be an obligatory initial step, even when cells are exposed to cortisol at 37 C, at which temperature most, if not all, the receptor-bound cortisol is found in the nuclear form. Saturable binding of cortisol to thymus and lymph cell nuclei has also been found with hormone injected in vivo (14, 65). A hypothesis consistent with all observations so far, though it is by no means proved, is that at 37 C cortisol, to which thymus cells appear to be freely permeable, enters the cell and binds to the cytoplasmic receptor to form a complex that has high affinity for certain nuclear acceptor sites; this complex then becomes rapidly fixed in the nucleus (80, 83).

Similar receptors have recently been identified in cultured lymphoma cells and in cells of lymphosarcoma P1798. In both these systems, cells from glucocorticoid-sensitive lines appear to contain significantly more receptors than cells from glucocorticoid-insensitive lines (8, 64), which indicates that glucocorticoid sensitivity in neoplastic tissue, as in normal tissue, may be limited by the number of available receptors. Receptors for glucocorticoids have also been found in lymphocytes from patients with chronic lymphocytic leukemia (A. Munck and O. R. McIntyre, unpublished results) and in lymphocytes from the thymus, bursa, and blood of chickens (103).

Glucocorticoid receptors from thymus cells have been extracted and studied in isolation (63, 83, 84, 100, 101, 120). They are at least in part proteins since they are inactivated by proteolytic enzymes. Their affinities for various steroids are similar to those measured with intact cells, and they are greatly stabilized by bound glucocorticoids (63, 84). The isolated cytoplasmic cortisol-receptor complex, when warmed and added to isolated thymus cell nuclei, becomes rapidly bound to the nuclei; such binding apparently duplicates the process that takes place in cells (84).

A comparison of the time course of formation of cortisol-receptor complexes after addition of cortisol to thymus cells at 37 C with the time course of inhibition of glucose transport under the same conditions is of considerable importance for an understanding of the relationship between these two events. As indicated in Figure 3, formation of the nuclear complex via the cytoplasmic complex starts immediately, with little or no lag, and reaches a maximum within 10 min (82, 83). By contrast, the inhibition of glucose metabolism evidences a distinct time lag—it begins rather abruptly after 15–20 min (78) and increases thereafter to about 50% inhibition by 2 hr.

The delay of 5–10 min between formation of cortisol-receptor complexes and inhibition of glucose transport in itself suggests the existence of intermediary steps. More direct experimental approaches, schematically outlined in Figure 3, show that there are in fact at least three such steps (49, 50, 76). During the first few minutes of exposure to cortisol, almost simultaneously with formation of the nuclear cortisol-receptor complex, a step takes place that is irreversible—removal of cortisol after 5 min (by washing or by displacement with cortexolone) does not reverse the subsequent effects of cortisol on glucose transport.

Similarly, actinomycin D, which does not affect binding, blocks cortisol effects when added with cortisol, but not when added 5 min later. Therefore, coincident with the irreversible step and perhaps identical to it, there appears to be a step involving RNA synthesis, a conclusion entirely consistent with the evidence that during this initial period cortisol-receptor complexes become bound in the nucleus (76).

Cycloheximide, which stops protein synthesis in a thymus cell suspension within 5 min, influences cortisol effects in a manner quite different from actinomycin D. It blocks the cortisol effect on glucose metabolism only when it is present during the period glucose metabolism begins to be inhibited (from 15 min on). It does not block if it is added together with, or before, cortisol and is washed out within 15 min. These results strongly suggest that inhibition of glucose transport is mediated by a cortisol-induced protein, the synthesis of which begins after about 15 min (49, 50, 80).

Finally, between the actinomycin D-sensitive and cycloheximide-sensitive steps and separate from both, is a temperature-sensitive step, characterized by the fact that its rate at 20 C is much slower than at 37 C, so that cooling of a cell suspension markedly delays the appearance of the cortisol effect.

All these observations on the initial actions of glucocorticoids on glucose metabolism are consistent with the following hypothesis (49, 50, 80), which is supported by

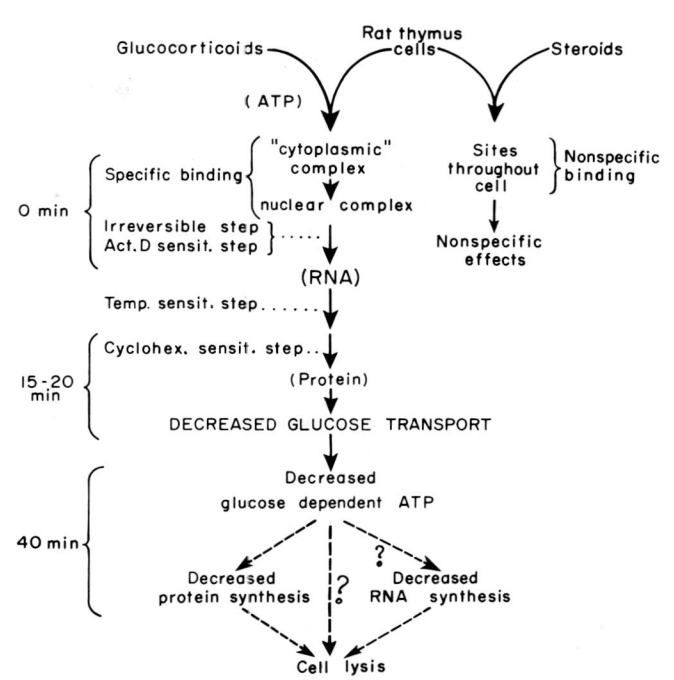

FIG. 3. Principal events identified in interactions of glucocorticoids with rat thymus cells, and postulated relations among them. Times on *left* provide rough indication of time each event begins during incubation with cortisol at 37 C. *Act. D sensit.*, actinomycin D-sensitive; *Temp. sensit.*, temperature-sensitive; *Cyclohex. sensit.*, cycloheximide-sensitive. [From Munck (80).]

other studies with thymus (70) and lymphosarcoma cells (94): the cortisol-receptor complex, upon binding in the nucleus, immediately stimulates synthesis of a particular form of RNA; this RNA, after a temperature-sensitive step that may represent its transfer from the nucleus to the cytoplasm, stimulates synthesis of a protein that rapidly inhibits glucose transport. Up to the inhibition of glucose transport, it should be noted, the early cortisol effects are all stimulatory. The catabolic nature of the ultimate glucocorticoid effects is determined by the inhibitory nature of the hypothetical protein, or proteins.

We have concentrated in this section on the genesis of glucocorticoid inhibition of glucose transport because this inhibition is the earliest clearly established effect of glucocorticoids on lymphoid cells and because there is good evidence that it is important in determining later events. There is no reason to believe, however, that it is the only early effect. Other early effects may in the future be uncovered, and may or may not be found to depend on receptor mechanisms similar to those just discussed, and on subsequent steps involving RNA and protein synthesis.

PHYSIOLOGICAL SIGNIFICANCE OF GLUCOCORTICOID ACTIONS ON LYMPHOID TISSUE

Of the many varied actions of the glucocorticoids, those on lymphoid tissue are among the most rapid and drastic. No attempts so far, however, have succeeded in conclusively establishing for them a significant physiological role. Consequently we limit ourselves here to a brief review of a few of the ideas that have been considered in this context.

The problem may be approached from two general points of view: *1*) that of the immunologist, who asks in what way, if any, glucocorticoids promote normal function of lymphoid tissue; and *2*) that of the endocrinologist, who asks how the actions on lymphoid tissue contribute to the overall function of glucocorticoids in protecting the organism against stress.

There are few indications that glucocorticoids are essential for normal immune responses. Despite reports that these hormones may be necessary for antibody production in vitro (3) and that under certain conditions they stimulate lymphocyte proliferation (48, 119), there appears to be no clear-cut evidence that in the intact organism antibody production is impaired in the absence of glucocorticoids (3, 26). High levels of glucocorticoids, as described above, cause lymphoid tissue to break down. Early suggestions that this breakdown might serve the useful function of releasing antibodies have never received convincing experimental support, however (26).

A hypothesis that dates back to the early days of adrenal physiology and that has since been thoroughly substantiated is that breakdown of peripheral tissues provides substrates for hepatic gluconeogenesis [see (80)]. An extended version of the hypothesis is that breakdown of lymphoid tissue in stress may serve to provide various substances—amino acids, nucleotides, possibly even strands of DNA—for repair and regulation of injured tissues. Although there is some evidence for this idea, it has so far not been tested adequately [see (72)]. Other proposals could also be mentioned but would add little to what has been said.

Unsatisfactory as is the state of affairs described in this section—leaving open even the possibility that the lympholytic effects serve no useful physiological purpose whatever—our lack of understanding is by no means limited to glucocorticoid actions on lymphoid tissue. In fact, it can be said of virtually all the metabolically defined actions of glucocorticoids that their relation to the protective functions of glucocorticoids in stress is unknown [see (79)]. How these problems will eventually be resolved is far from clear, but at least in the case of lymphoid tissue one may hope that when the subtleties of glucocorticoid effects on the various components of the immunologic system are better understood, both in the adult and during development, a more coherent physiological picture will emerge.

REFERENCES

1. ADDISON, T. *On the Constitutional and Local Effects of Disease of the Suprarenal Capsules.* London: Highley, 1855.
2. AMBELLAN, E., AND J. S. ROTH. Steroid effects on rat thymus acid ribonuclease. *Biochem. Biophys. Res. Commun.* 28: 244–248, 1967.
3. AMBROSE, C. T. The requirement for hydrocortisone in antibody-forming tissue cultivated in serum-free medium. *J. Exptl. Med.* 119: 1027–1049, 1964.
4. ARONOW, L., AND J. D. GABOUREL. Development of a hydrocortisone-resistant sub-line of mouse lymphoma *in vitro*. *Proc. Soc. Exptl. Biol. Med.* 111: 348–349, 1962.
5. BARAN, D. T., M. A. LICHTMAN, AND W. A. PECK. Alpha-aminoisobutyric acid transport in human leukemic lymphocytes: in vitro characteristics and inhibition by cortisol and cycloheximide. *J. Clin. Invest.* 51: 2181–2189, 1972.
6. BARTLETT, D., Y. MORITA, AND A. MUNCK. Rapid inhibition by cortisol of incorporation of glucose *in vivo* into the thymus of the rat. *Nature* 196: 897–898, 1962.
7. BAXTER, J. D., AND P. H. FORSHAM. Tissue effects of glucocorticoids. *Am. J. Med.* 53: 573–589, 1972.
8. BAXTER, J. D., A. W. HARRIS, G. M. TOMKINS, AND M. COHN. Glucocorticoid receptors in lymphoma cells in culture: relationship to glucocorticoid killing activity. *Science* 171: 189–191, 1971.
9. BOINET, E. Recherches expérimentales sur les fonctions des capsules surrénales. *Compt. Rend. Soc. Biol.* 51: 671–672, 1899.
10. BOWERS, W. E., AND C. DEDUVE. Lysosomes in lymphoid tissue. *J. Cell Biol.* 32: 349–364, 1967.
11. BRINCK-JOHNSEN, T., AND T. F. DOUGHERTY. Studies on the effect of cortisol and corticotrophin on incorporation of adenine-8-^{14}C into the lymphatic tissue nucleic acids. *Acta Endocrinol.* 49: 471–478, 1965.
12. BROWN, H. E., AND T. F. DOUGHERTY. The diurnal variation of blood leukocytes in normal and adrenalectomized mice. *Endocrinology* 58: 365–375, 1956.
13. BRUNKHORST, W. K. Effect of cortisol on amino acid incorporation by nuclear and cytoplasmic fractions of rabbit thymus. *Endocrinology* 82: 277–281, 1968.
14. BRUNKHORST, W. K. Intracellular binding of corticosterone in thymus tissue. *Biochem. Biophys. Res. Commun.* 35: 880–886, 1969.
15. BURNET, F. M. The concept of immunological surveillance. *Progr. Exptl. Tumor Res.* 13: 1–27, 1970.
16. BURTON, A. F. Inhibition of 11β-hydroxysteroid dehydrogenase activity in rat and mouse tissues *in vitro* and *in vivo*. *Endocrinology* 77: 325–331, 1965.
17. BURTON, A. F., J. M. STORR, AND W. L. DUNN. Cytolytic action of corticosteroids on thymus and lymphoma cells *in vitro*. *Can. J. Biochem.* 45: 289–297, 1967.
18. CLAMAN, H. N. Corticosteroids and lymphoid cells. *New Engl. J. Med.* 287: 388–397, 1972.
19. COHEN, I. R., L. STAVY, AND M. FELDMAN. Glucocorticoids and cellular immunity *in vitro*. Facilitation of the sensitization phase and inhibition of the effector phase of a lymphocyte anti-fibroblast reaction. *J. Exptl. Med.* 132: 1055–1070, 1970.
20. COHEN, J. J., AND H. N. CLAMAN. Thymus-marrow immunocompetence. v. Hydrocortisone-resistant cells and processes in the hemolytic antibody response of mice. *J. Exptl. Med.* 133: 1026–1034, 1971.
21. COHEN, J. J., M. FISCHBACH, AND H. N. CLAMAN. Hydrocortisone resistance of graft vs. host activity in mouse thymus, spleen, and bone marrow. *J. Immunol.* 105: 1146–1150, 1970.
22. COWAN, W. K., AND G. D. SORENSON. Electron microscopic observations of acute thymic involution produced by hydrocortisone. *Lab. Invest.* 13: 353–370, 1964.
23. DORFMAN, R. I., AND A. S. DORFMAN. The relative thymolytic activities of corticoids using the ovariectomized-adrenalectomized mouse. *Endocrinology* 69: 283–291, 1961.
24. DORFMAN, R. I., AND A. S. DORFMAN. Thymolytic activity of corticoids in combination with other steroids. *Endocrinology* 71: 271–276, 1962.
25. DOUGHERTY, T. F. Effect of hormones on lymphatic tissue. *Physiol. Rev.* 32: 379–401, 1952.
26. DOUGHERTY, T. F. The mechanisms of action of adrenocortical hormone in allergy. *Progr. Allergy* 4: 319–360, 1954.
27. DOUGHERTY, T. F. Lymphocytokaryorrhectic effects of

adrenocortical steroids. In: *The Lymphocyte and Lymphocytic Tissue*, edited by J. W. Rebuck. New York: Hoeber, 1959, p. 112–124.
28. DOUGHERTY, T. F., M. L. BERLINER, G. L. SCHNEEBELI, AND D. L. BERLINER. Hormonal control of lymphatic structure and function. *Ann. NY Acad. Sci.* 113: 825–843, 1964.
29. DOUGHERTY, T. F., AND A. WHITE. Functional alterations in lymphoid tissue induced by adrenal cortical secretion. *Am. J. Anat.* 77: 81–116, 1945.
30. DOUGHERTY, T. F., AND A. WHITE. An evaluation of alterations produced in lymphoid tissue by pituitary-adrenal cortical secretion. *J. Lab. Clin. Med.* 32: 584–605, 1947.
31. DREWS, J. The effect of prednisolone injected *in vivo* on RNA synthesis in rat thymus cells. *European J. Biochem.* 7: 200–208, 1969.
32. DREWS, J., AND L. WAGNER. Alterations in the phosphorylation of [³H]uridine and RNA synthesis in rat thymus cells after glucose depletion and treatment with prednisolone. *European J. Biochem.* 16: 541–548, 1970.
33. DRURY, D. R. Control of blood sugar. *J. Clin. Endocrinol. Metab.* 2: 421–430, 1942.
34. DURKIN, H. G., AND G. J. THORBECKE. Relationship of germinal centers in lymphoid tissue to immunologic memory. v. The effect of prednisolone administered after the peak of the primary response. *J. Immunol.* 106: 1079–1085, 1971.
35. ERNSTRÖM, U. Hormonal influences on thymic release of lymphocytes into the blood. In: *Hormones and the Immune Response*, edited by G. E. W. Wolstenholme and J. Knight. London: Churchill, 1970, p. 53–60.
36. ESTEBAN, J. N. The differential effect of hydrocortisone on the short-lived small lymphocyte. *Anat. Record* 162: 349–356, 1968.
37. EURENIUS, K., T. V. DALTON, H. J. LOKEY, AND O. R. MCINTYRE. The mechanism of glucocorticoid action on the phytohemagglutinin-stimulated lymphocyte. I. In vitro binding of corticosteroids to lymphoid tissue. *Biochim. Biophys. Acta* 177: 572–578, 1969.
38. EVERETT, N. B., AND R. W. TYLER. Lymphopoiesis in the thymus and other tissues: functional implications. *Intern. Rev. Cytol.* 22: 205–237, 1967.
39. FEILGELSON, M., AND P. FEIGELSON. Metabolic effects of glucocorticoids as related to enzyme induction. *Advan. Enzyme Regulation* 3: 11–27, 1965.
40. FOX, K. E., AND J. D. GABOUREL. Effect of cortisol on the RNA polymerase system of rat thymus. *Mol. Pharmacol.* 3: 479–486, 1967.
41. FRANK, J. A., AND T. F. DOUGHERTY. Cytoplasmic budding of human lymphocytes produced by cortisone and hydrocortisone in *in vitro* preparations. *Proc. Soc. Exptl. Biol. Med.* 82: 17–19, 1953.
42. GABOUREL, J. D., AND L. ARONOW. Growth inhibitory effects of hydrocortisone on mouse lymphoma ML-388 *in vitro*. *J. Pharmacol. Exptl. Therap.* 136: 213–221, 1962.
43. GABOUREL, J. D., AND J. P. COMSTOCK. Effect of hydrocortisone on amino acid incorporation by microsomes isolated from mouse lymphoma ML-388 cells and rat thymus. *Biochem. Pharmacol.* 13: 1369–1376, 1964.
44. GABRIELSEN, A. E., AND R. A. GOOD. Chemical suppression of adaptive immunity. *Advan. Immunol.* 6: 91–229, 1967.
45. GATTI, R. A., O. STUTMAN, AND R. A. GOOD. The lymphoid system. *Ann. Rev. Physiol.* 32: 529–546, 1970.
46. GOWANS, J. L. Lymphocytes. *Harvey Lectures Ser.* 64: 87–119, 1968.
47. GREENWOOD, M., AND H. M. WOODS. Status thymico-lymphaticus considered in the light of recent work on thymus. *J. Hyg.* 26: 305–326, 1927.
48. GYLLENSTEN, L. The cellular composition of lymphatic tissue during involution after administration of corticosteroid. A quantitative study in guinea pigs. *Acta Pathol. Microbiol. Scand.* 56: 35–45, 1962.
49. HALLAHAN, C., D. A. YOUNG, AND A. MUNCK. Evidence for a protein synthetic step in the early action of cortisol on glucose uptake in rat thymus tissue. *Federation Proc.* 30: 308, 1971.
50. HALLAHAN, C., D. A. YOUNG, AND A. MUNCK. Time-course of early events in the action of glucocorticoids on rat thymus cells *in vitro*: synthesis and turnover of a hypothetical cortisol-induced protein inhibitor of glucose metabolism and of a presumed RNA. *J. Biol. Chem.* 248: 2922–2927, 1973.
51. HAYNES, R. C., JR., AND E. W. SUTHERLAND, III. Altered metabolism of DNA in rat thymus, an early response to cortisol. *Endocrinology* 80: 297–301, 1967.
52. HEDESKOV, C. J., AND V. ESMANN. Major metabolic pathways of glucose in normal human lymphocytes and the effect of cortisol. *Biochim. Biophys. Acta* 148: 372–383, 1967.
53. HILGAR, A. G., AND L. C. TRENCH. *Thymolytic and Glycogenic Endocrine Bioassay Data*. Bethesda, Md.: National Cancer Institute, US Dept. Health, Education, and Welfare, 1968.
54. HOFERT, J. F., AND A. WHITE. Inhibition of the lymphocytolytic activity of cortisol by total hepatectomy. *Endocrinology* 77: 574–581, 1965.
55. HOLLANDER, V. P., C. GORDON, AND N. HOLLANDER. Effects of corticoid injection and of adrenalectomy on *in vitro* amino-acid incorporation into microsomes of P1798 lymphosarcoma. *Nature* 213: 1036–1037, 1967.
56. INGLE, D. J. Atrophy of the thymus in normal and hypophysectomized rats following administration of cortin. *Proc. Soc. Exptl. Biol. Med.* 38: 443–444, 1938.
57. INGLE, D. J. Effect of two steroid compounds on weight of thymus of adrenalectomized rats. *Proc. Soc. Exptl. Biol. Med.* 44: 174–175, 1940.
58. INGLE, D. J. Problems relating to the adrenal cortex. *Endocrinology* 31: 419–438, 1942.
59. ISHIDATE, M., JR., AND D. METCALF. The pattern of lymphopoiesis in the mouse thymus after cortisone administration or adrenalectomy. *Australian J. Exptl. Biol. Med. Sci.* 41: 637–649, 1963.
60. JAFFE, H. L. The influence of the suprarenal gland on the thymus. III. Stimulation of the growth of the thymus gland following double suprarenalectomy in young rats. *J. Exptl. Med.* 40: 753–760, 1924.
61. KATTWINKEL, J., AND A. MUNCK. Activities *in vitro* of glucocorticoids and related steroids on glucose uptake by rat thymus cell suspensions. *Endocrinology* 79: 387–390, 1966.
62. KATZ, D. H., AND B. BENACERRAF. The regulatory influence of activated T cells on B cell responses to antigen. *Advan. Immunol.* 15: 1–94, 1972.
63. KIRKPATRICK, A. F., N. KAISER, R. J. MILHOLLAND, AND F. ROSEN. Glucocorticoid-binding macromolecules in normal tissues and tumors. Stabilization of the specific binding component. *J. Biol. Chem.* 247: 70–74, 1972.
64. KIRKPATRICK, A. F., R. J. MILHOLLAND, AND F. ROSEN. Stereospecific glucocorticoid binding to subcellular fractions of the sensitive and resistant lymphosarcoma P1798. *Nature New Biol.* 232: 216–218, 1971.
65. LANG, R. F., AND W. STEVENS. Evidence for intranuclear receptor sites for cortisol in lymphatic tissue. *J. Reticuloendothelial Soc.* 7: 294–304, 1970.
66. MACLEOD, R. M., C. E. KING, AND V. P. HOLLANDER. Effect of corticosteroids on ribonuclease and nucleic acid content in lymphosarcoma P1798. *Cancer Res.* 23: 1045–1050, 1963.
67. MACMANUS, J. P., J. F. WHITFIELD, AND T. YOUDALE. Stimulation by epinephrine of adenyl cyclase activity, cyclic AMP formation, DNA synthesis and cell proliferation in populations of rat thymic lymphocytes. *J. Cellular Physiol.* 77: 103–116, 1971.
68. MAKMAN, M. H., B. DVORKIN, AND A. WHITE. Alterations in protein and nucleic acid metabolism of thymocytes produced by adrenal steroids *in vitro*. *J. Biol. Chem.* 241: 1646–1648, 1966.
69. MAKMAN, M. H., B. DVORKIN, AND A. WHITE. Influence of cortisol on the utilization of precursors of nucleic acids and protein by lymphoid cells *in vitro*. *J. Biol. Chem.* 243: 1485–1497, 1968.
70. MAKMAN, M. H., B. DVORKIN, AND A. WHITE. Evidence for induction by cortisol *in vitro* of a protein inhibitor of transport

and phosphorylation processes in rat thymocytes. *Proc. Natl. Acad. Sci. US* 68: 1269–1273, 1971.
71. MAKMAN, M. H., S. NAKAGAWA, B. DVORKIN, AND A. WHITE. Inhibitory effects of cortisol and antibiotics on substrate entry and ribonucleic acid synthesis in rat thymocytes *in vitro. J. Biol. Chem.* 245: 2556–2563, 1970.
72. METCALF, D. *The Thymus*. New York: Springer Verlag, 1966, p. 83.
73. MILLER, J. F. A. P., AND G. F. MITCHELL. Thymus and antigen-reactive cells. *Transplant. Rev.* 1: 3–42, 1969.
74. MILLER, J. F. A. P., AND D. OSOBA. Current concepts of the immunological function of the thymus. *Physiol. Rev.* 47: 437–520, 1967.
75. MORITA, Y., AND A. MUNCK. Effect of glucocorticoids *in vivo* and *in vitro* on net glucose uptake and amino-acid incorporation by rat-thymus cells. *Biochim. Biophys. Acta* 93: 150–157, 1964.
76. MOSHER, K. M., D. A. YOUNG, AND A. MUNCK. Evidence for irreversible, actinomycin D-sensitive, and temperature-sensitive steps following binding of cortisol to glucocorticoid receptors and preceding effects on glucose metabolism in rat thymus cells. *J. Biol. Chem.* 246: 654–659, 1971.
77. MUNCK, A. Steroid concentration and tissue integrity as factors determining the physiological significance of effects of adrenal steroids *in vitro*. *Endocrinology* 77: 356–360, 1965.
78. MUNCK, A. Metabolic site and time course of cortisol action on glucose uptake, lactic acid output, and glucose 6-phosphate levels of rat thymus cells *in vitro*. *J. Biol. Chem.* 243: 1039–1042, 1968.
79. MUNCK, A. The effects of hormones at the cellular level. In: *Recent Advances in Endocrinology* (8th ed.), edited by V. H. T. James. London: Churchill, 1968, p. 139–180.
80. MUNCK, A. Glucocorticoid inhibition of glucose uptake by peripheral tissues: old and new evidence, molecular mechanisms, and physiological significance. *Perspect. Biol. Med.* 14: 265–289, 1971.
81. MUNCK, A., AND T. BRINCK-JOHNSEN. Specific metabolic and physicochemical interactions of glucocorticoids *in vivo* and *in vitro* with rat adipose tissue and thymus cells. *Proc. Intern. Congr. Hormonal Steroids. Excerpta Med. Found. Intern. Congr. Ser.* 132: 472–481, 1967.
82. MUNCK, A., AND T. BRINCK-JOHNSEN. Specific and nonspecific physicochemical interactions of glucocorticoids and related steroids with rat thymus cells *in vitro*. *J. Biol. Chem.* 243: 5556–5565, 1968.
83. MUNCK, A., AND C. WIRA. Glucocorticoid receptors in rat thymus cells. *Advan. Biosci.* 7: 301–330, 1971.
84. MUNCK, A., C. WIRA, D. A. YOUNG, K. M. MOSHER, C. HALLAHAN, AND P. A. BELL. Glucocorticoid-receptor complexes and the earliest steps in the action of glucocorticoids on thymus cells. *J. Steroid Biochem.* 3: 567–578, 1972.
85. NAKAGAWA, S., B. DVORKIN, AND A. WHITE. Response of some hydrolases in thymus and lymphosarcoma of rats to injection of adrenal steroid hormones. *Yale J. Biol. Med.* 41: 120–132, 1968.
86. NAKAGAWA, S., AND A. WHITE. Acute decrease in RNA polymerase activity of rat thymus in response to cortisol injection. *Proc. Natl. Acad. Sci. US* 55: 900–904, 1966.
87. NAKAGAWA, S., AND A. WHITE. Properties of an aggregate ribonucleic acid polymerase from rat thymus and its response to cortisol injection. *J. Biol. Chem.* 245: 1448–1457, 1970.
88. NOSSAL, G. J. V., AND G. L. ADA. *Antigens, Lymphoid Cells, and the Immune Response*. New York: Acad. Press, 1971.
89. PRATT, W. B., S. EDELMAN, AND L. ARONOW. The effect of cortisol, administered *in vivo*, on the *in vitro* incorporation of DNA and RNA precursors by rat thymus cells. *Mol. Pharmacol.* 3: 219–224, 1967.
90. RAPELA, C. E. *Relación de la Glándula Suprarrenal Con el Timo*. Buenos Aires: Editorial El Ateneo, 1944.
91. RINGERTZ, N., A. FAGRAEUS, AND K. BERGLUND. On the action of cortisone on the thymus and lymph nodes in mice. *Acta Pathol. Microbiol. Scand. Suppl.* 93: 44–51, 1952.

92. RINGLER, I. Activities of adrenocorticosteroids in experimental animals and man. In: *Methods in Hormone Research*, edited by R. I. Dorfman. New York: Acad. Press, 1964, vol. III, p. 227–349.
93. ROSEN, J. M., J. J. FINA, R. J. MILHOLLAND, AND F. ROSEN. Inhibition of glucose uptake in lymphosarcoma P1798 by cortisol and its relationship to the biosynthesis of deoxyribonucleic acid. *J. Biol. Chem.* 245: 2074–2080, 1970.
94. ROSEN, J. M., J. J. FINA, R. J. MILHOLLAND, AND F. ROSEN. Inhibitory effect of cortisol *in vitro* on 2-deoxyglucose uptake and RNA and protein metabolism in lymphosarcoma P1798. *Cancer Res.* 32: 350–355, 1972.
95. ROSEN, J. M., R. J. MILHOLLAND, AND F. ROSEN. A comparison of the effect of glucocorticoids on glucose uptake and hexokinase activity in lymphosarcoma P1798. *Biochim. Biophys. Acta* 219: 447–454, 1970.
96. ROSEN, J. M., F. ROSEN, R. J. MILHOLLAND, AND C. A. NICHOL. Effects of cortisol on DNA metabolism in the sensitive and resistant lines of mouse lymphoma P1798. *Cancer Res.* 30: 1129–1136, 1970.
97. SACHS, G., C. DEDUVE, B. S. DVORKIN, AND A. WHITE. Effect of adrenal cortical steroid injection on lysosomal enzymic activities of rat thymus. *Exptl. Cell Res.* 28: 597–600, 1962.
98. SARETT, L. H., A. A. PATCHETT, AND S. L. STEELMAN. The effects of structural alteration on the anti-inflammatory properties of hydrocortisone. *Progr. Drug Res.* 5: 11–153, 1963.
99. SCHNAPPAUF, H., AND U. SCHNAPPAUF. Modifications de la recirculation lymphocytaire induites par stimulation antigénique, ACTH et cortisone. *Nouvelle Rev. Franc. Hematol.* 8: 555–564, 1968.
100. SCHAUMBURG, B. P. Studies of the glucocorticoid-binding protein from thymocytes. I. Localization in the cell and some properties of the protein. *Biochim. Biophys. Acta* 214: 520–532, 1970.
101. SCHAUMBURG, B. P. Studies of the glucocorticoid-binding protein from thymocytes. III. pH dependence of the binding and density-gradient centrifugation of the protein. *Biochim. Biophys. Acta* 263: 414–423, 1972.
102. SCHAUMBURG, B. P., AND E. BOJESEN. Specificity and thermodynamic properties of the corticosteroid binding to a receptor of rat thymocytes *in vitro*. *Biochim. Biophys. Acta* 170: 172–188, 1968.
103. SCHAUMBURG, B. P., AND M. CRONE. Binding of corticosterone by thymus cells, bursa cells and blood lymphocytes from the chicken. *Biochim. Biophys. Acta* 237: 494–501, 1971.
104. SCHREK, R. Cytotoxic action of hormones of the adrenal cortex according to the method of unstained cell counts. *Endocrinology* 45: 317–334, 1949.
105. SCHREK, R. Prednisolone sensitivity and cytology of viable lymphocytes as tests for chronic lymphocytic leukemia. *J. Natl. Cancer Inst.* 33: 837–847, 1964.
106. SELYE, H. Thymus and adrenals in the response of the organism to injuries and intoxications. *Brit. J. Exptl. Pathol.* 17: 234–248, 1936.
107. STAR, P. An unusual case of Addison's disease; sudden death; remarks. *Lancet* 284, 1895.
108. STEVENS, W., C. BEDKE, AND T. F. DOUGHERTY. Effects of cortisol acetate on various aspects of cellular metabolism in mouse lymphatic tissue. *J. Reticuloendothelial Soc.* 4: 254–283, 1967.
109. STEVENS, W., C. COLESSIDES, AND T. F. DOUGHERTY. Effects of cortisol on the incorporation of thymidine-2-C^{14} into nucleic acids of lymphatic tissue from adrenalectomized CBA mice. *Endocrinology* 76: 1100–1108, 1965.
110. STEVENS, W., C. COLESSIDES, AND T. F. DOUGHERTY. A time study on the effect of cortisol on the incorporation of thymidine-2-^{14}C into nucleic acids of mouse lymphatic tissue. *Endocrinology* 78: 600–604, 1966.
111. SUTHERLAND, E. W., III, AND R. C. HAYNES, JR. Increased

release of amino acids from rat thymus after cortisol administration. *Endocrinology* 80: 288–296, 1967.
112. SZENBERG, A. Influence of testosterone on the primary lymphoid organs of the chicken. In: *Hormones and the Immune Response*, edited by G. E. W. Wolstenholme and J. Knight. London: Churchill, 1970, p. 42–45.
113. TAPPAN, D. V., R. K. BOUTWELL, AND B. BOOTH. Influence of *in vivo* administration of adrenocorticoids on metabolism of thymus, liver and tumor tissues. *Proc. Soc. Exptl. Biol. Med.* 97: 52–56, 1958.
114. TIOLLAIS, P. Actions des hormones cortico-surrénales sur le tissu lymphoide. *Exposes Ann. Biochem. Med.* 28: 197–228, 1967.
115. TURNELL, R. W., L. H. CLARKE, AND A. F. BURTON. Studies on the mechanism of corticosteroid-induced lymphocytolysis. *Cancer Res.* 33: 203–212, 1973.
116. WELLS, B. B., AND E. C. KENDALL. A qualitative difference in the effect of compounds separated from the adrenal cortex on distribution of electrolytes and on atrophy of the adrenal and thymus glands of rats. *Proc. Staff Meeting Mayo Clinic* 15: 133–139, 1940.
117. WHITE, A. Influence of endocrine secretions on the structure and function of lymphoid tissue. *Harvey Lectures Ser.* 43: 43–70, 1947.
118. WHITE, A., AND T. F. DOUGHERTY. The role of lymphocytes in normal and immune globulin production, and the mode of release of globulin from lymphocytes. *Ann. NY Acad. Sci.* 46: 859–883, 1946.
119. WHITFIELD, J. F., J. P. MACMANUS, AND R. H. RIXON. Cyclic AMP-mediated stimulation of thymocyte proliferation by low concentrations of cortisol. *Proc. Soc. Exptl. Biol. Med.* 134: 1170–1174, 1970.
120. WIRA, C., AND A. MUNCK. Specific glucocorticoid receptors in thymus cells. Localization in the nucleus and extraction of the cortisol-receptor complex. *J. Biol. Chem.* 245: 3436–3438, 1970.
121. YOUNG, D. A. Glucocorticoid action on rat thymus cells. Interrelations between carbohydrate, protein, and adenine nucleotide metabolism and cortisol effects on these functions. *J. Biol. Chem.* 244: 2210–2217, 1969.
122. YOUNG, D. A. Glucocorticoid action on rat thymus cells. II. Interrelationships between ribonucleic acid and protein metabolism and between cortisol and substrate effects on these metabolic parameters *in vitro*. *J. Biol. Chem.* 245: 2747–2752, 1970.
123. YOUNG, D. A., S. GIDDINGS, A. SWONGER, G. KLURFELD, AND M. MILLER. Interrelationships among the effects of glucocorticoids on carbohydrate, adenine nucleotide, RNA, and protein metabolism in rat thymus cells. *Proc. Intern. Congr. Hormonal Steroids, 3rd, Hamburg, 1970. Excerpta Med. Found. Intern. Congr. Ser.* 210: 843–853, 1971.

CHAPTER 17

Corticosteroids and skeletal muscle

ESTELLE R. RAMEY | Department of Physiology and Biophysics, Georgetown University Medical Center, Washington, D.C.

CHAPTER CONTENTS

Mineralocorticoids and Skeletal Muscle
    Work capacity and electrolyte balance
    Direct muscle-aldosterone effects
Glucocorticoids and Skeletal Muscle
    Carbohydrate metabolism
    Protein metabolism
    Exercise and glucocorticoid levels
Steroid Myopathy
Exercise as Systemic Stress
    Lysosomes
    "Second messengers"—cyclic AMP and prostaglandins
Conclusions

THE SUGGESTION OF A RELATIONSHIP between skeletal muscle function and the adrenal gland dates from the publication of a paper by Dr. Thomas Addison in 1849 in the *London Medical Gazette:* he reported that a syndrome consisting of anemia and marked muscular weakness was found to be associated with pathological changes in the "supra-renal capsules." In 1855 Addison (1) published his classic monograph and called attention again to the pronounced muscular asthenia that characterized patients with this disease. Since Addison's time, clinicians have repeatedly confirmed his observation that one of the most consistent responses to adrenal insufficiency is an extremely low threshold of fatigue (86, 126, 171, 190). When experiments were designed to reproduce the signs and symptoms of Addison's disease in the laboratory, it was observed that laboratory animals also exhibited this marked skeletal muscle fatigue when both adrenals were surgically removed (18, 53, 110, 174, 176).

Attempts to clarify the relationship between the hormones of the adrenal gland and the complex manifestations of adrenal insufficiency were complicated, however, by the discovery of a potent physiological substance, epinephrine, elaborated by the medullary portion of the compound gland. In the early part of this century much of the published research sought to establish that the observed results of adrenalectomy, including muscular weakness, were due essentially to the lack of circulating epinephrine (22, 78).

Some investigators, however, suggested that the interrenal (cortical) tissue might play a significant role in the ability to perform muscular work (58, 93, 188). In a unique series of experiments, Biedl (18) in 1902 used Elasmobranchii in which the cortical adrenal tissue is anatomically separated from the medullary tissue. When he removed only the cortical tissue he observed that these animals died in about 3 weeks and that death was always preceded by progressive and severe muscular weakness.

Later, Wislocki & Crowe (194) observed that the degree of muscle weakness noted after adrenalectomy seemed to be a function of the amount of adrenal tissue left in the animal. If more than one-fifth of the total adrenal tissue remained, the characteristic asthenia of adrenal insufficiency did not develop. At about the same time (i.e., 1922) Mauerhofer (137) showed that rats in which residual adrenal tissue could be demonstrated did well in relatively sheltered circumstances and maintained normal cage activity but were far more easily fatigued by exercise than were intact animals.

Cannon and his co-workers (27, 43) were simultaneously investigating the physiological significance of the sympathetic nervous system and the adrenal medulla in the performance of strenuous exercise but could not demonstrate a crucial role for this system. Subsequently, while developing a work performance test, Ingle found that adrenal demedullation did not limit the ability of experimental animals to perform muscular work (83, 103, 104). More recent work has confirmed this observation (79). With their quantitative work performance technique, Ingle et al. (102) found that, if 60–80% of the adrenal tissue was destroyed in rats, their work output was only 38% of normal. It was thus established that the hormones of the adrenal cortex are critical for normal skeletal muscle function, at least during periods of high demand (68, 85, 98, 99).

When active extracts of adrenal cortical tissue became available, the restoration of work performance in adrenalectomized animals could be used as an index of the potency of the extract administered. In 1931 Hartman & Lockwood (85) showed that adrenal cortical extract administered to adrenalectomized rats prolonged the work capacity of the gastrocnemius muscle, when stimulated in situ, to six times that of gastrocnemius muscles from untreated adrenalectomized animals. Ingle used this phenomenon as the basis for a bioassay of the cortical steroids (94, 97, 100, 105, 106, 108). The most potent cortical steroids for the maintenance of skeletal muscle contraction were shown to be the C_{11}-oxycorticoids, later known as the glucocorticoids. These hormones were also shown to be critical for survival under other prolonged stress conditions (205). Concomitantly it was shown that cellular changes in the adrenal cortex were manifest within a few hours after a stress response was evoked (206). Many investigators described a significant increase in adrenal gland weight and secretion after strenuous exercise in intact animals (9, 51, 64, 94, 206). This adrenal hypertrophy did not occur in hypophysectomized animals that were forced to work (95, 106), and the hypothalamic-hypophysial-adrenal activation necessary to support homeostatic responses to stress has since been well characterized (81).

With the fact that adrenal cortical hormones are necessary for sustained skeletal muscle performance established, the obvious question is, why? Despite hundreds of experiments designed to answer this question, no satisfactory explanation of a primary site of action is yet available. Adrenal insufficiency, directly or indirectly, affects all known homeostatic systems, including electrolyte and water balance, metabolism of carbohydrate, protein, and fat, cardiovascular regulation, and neural responses (151). A primary defect in any one of these regulatory systems would ultimately impair skeletal muscle function and work performance. In addition, the corticosteroids may have a direct effect on the intrinsic structure and function of the muscle fiber itself. All these possibilities have been investigated in an attempt to identify the fundamental mechanism of fatigue in adrenal insufficiency.

MINERALOCORTICOIDS AND SKELETAL MUSCLE

The literature concerning the effects of mineralocorticoid insufficiency on the composition of body fluid compartments is confusing because many investigators have done chemical studies on nearly moribund adrenalectomized animals in severe electrolyte imbalance, marked hemoconcentration, and dehydration. In addition, dietary regimen or hormonal restoration has varied both qualitatively and quantitatively. Obviously, in circumstances where nearly all homeostatic support systems are seriously impaired, the work capacity of skeletal muscle will suffer even if the muscles themselves are intact. If the extracellular electrolyte imbalance persists, secondary effects on skeletal muscle could produce deterioration in the myofibrils without the specific involvement of the mineralocorticoids. Thus the use of an animal's overall work capacity or even the use of the contractility of isolated muscles as an index of a direct action of the mineralocorticoids on skeletal muscle must be examined with the above disclaimers in mind.

Early research showed that removal of the adrenals led to a decrease in serum sodium and an increase in serum potassium (14, 41, 78). Most of these changes can be attributed to the effects of the adrenal hormones on the kidney, but some data show that, even in the absence of the kidneys, adrenalectomy produces shifts in electrolytes and water in the extrarenal tissues (159, 195). Many of the signs and symptoms of adrenal insufficiency, including certain aspects of muscle asthenia, can be attributed to these alterations in electrolyte and water balance. With the loss of extracellular sodium, the osmotic concentration of the extracellular fluid falls and water and potassium tend to enter cells (69). This electrolyte imbalance can be ameliorated not only by administration of the mineralocorticoids, but simply by substituting 1% saline for normal drinking water (7, 10, 11, 29, 84, 177). On the other hand, the overhydration of extrarenal tissues is not entirely reversed by such a regimen (117). It can be demonstrated, for example, that the hemoconcentration of adrenalectomized dogs can be corrected even in the face of continued sodium diuresis if the 11-oxysteroids are administered. The mineralocorticoids, however, do not seem to regulate body water distribution independently of electrolyte transport (69, 175). These hormones, in effect, seem to be far more limited in their range of action than the glucocorticoids. In physiological concentrations the action of the mineralocorticoids appears limited to the regulation of sodium and potassium transport across epithelial cells (55). The net effect of their action, however, is to alter the electrolyte milieu of all tissues, including skeletal muscle.

Since the ratio of extracellular to intracellular sodium or potassium is intimately related to the electrical properties of the membrane and to the overall irritability of the system, changes in serum electrolyte patterns would be expected to alter the functional capacity of the neuromuscular apparatus, and they do. For example, in primary aldosteronism, muscle weakness and paralysis reflect the altered potassium gradient across the cell. The potassium depletion in this condition is seen both in the extracellular and intracellular fluids, but the fall in the extracellular fluid is proportionately greater. The resting membrane potential of muscle increases under these circumstances. When the muscle loses more than one-third of its normal potassium concentration, very rapid deterioration of muscle function is observed. The hyperpolarization of the muscle membrane raises the threshold for excitation at the myoneural junction, and a hypokalemic paralysis may ensue. In this situation, muscular contraction itself helps to reduce the hyperpolarization of the muscle by altering potassium movement; this phenomenon explains why patients suffering from hyperaldosteronism may prevent incipient hypokalemic paralysis by exercising (138). This is an illustration of a homeostatic adjustment of electrolyte distribution and skeletal muscle function that can be made, despite persistent abnormalities in serum aldosterone levels.

Work Capacity and Electrolyte Balance

Normal mineralocorticoid levels and the restoration of normal extracellular electrolyte levels alone do not restore the work capacity of adrenalectomized animals (96, 192). One reason for this may be that intracellular electrolyte content of skeletal muscle under these circumstances can still be abnormal. The most convincing evidence suggests, however, that the ionic composition of skeletal muscle in adrenalectomized animals largely reflects the composition of the extracellular fluid (32, 33, 195) and that resting membrane potentials are normal in salt- or mineralocorticoid-treated adrenalectomized animals (124, 125, 156).

Nevertheless, muscle fatigue ensues rapidly in adrenalectomized animals lacking glucocorticoids (96, 192). This has been interpreted by some investigators to mean that the myofibrils themselves deteriorate when only mineralocorticoids are available (193). Other evidence disputes this concept (76, 152, 164). Recently, Sexton (164), with a modification of Szent-Gyorgi's technique for obtaining extracted muscle fibers from glycerinated muscle (178), measured the isometric tension developed by fibers from the anterior tibialis muscle and the medial head of the gastrocnemius muscle in intact and adrenalectomized rats. When sodium chloride supplementation was withheld from his adrenalectomized animals for more than 48 hr before removal of the muscles, the isometric tension generated by the glycerol-extracted muscle fibers (on addition of ATP in phosphate buffer) showed a 32% decrease from normal. If, however, the adrenalectomized rats were maintained for 7 days with NaCl replacement but without adrenal steroid supplementation, the isometric tension developed by their muscles was not significantly different from intact controls. In addition, adrenalectomized animals from which both salt and carbohydrate were withheld for 48 hr did not differ markedly from animals in which only salt was removed from the diet.

These data lend support to the concept that the intrinsic structure of the resting skeletal muscle fibers of adrenalectomized animals in electrolyte balance is not markedly altered. The nature of Sexton's preparation, however, does not speak to any possible alterations in membrane properties or in synaptic transmission at the myoneural junction or in excitation-contraction coupling. The inability to sustain repetitive muscle contractions could reflect defects at any of these sites. What Sexton's preparation does show is that severe electrolyte imbalance can ultimately affect the properties of the muscle fiber itself. Ivanyuta (109) reported that under these conditions such fibers exhibit significant decreases in ATPase activity, and Sexton suggests that prolonged sodium depletion by alteration in ATPase activity and in ATPase binding sites might decrease the rate of splitting of the actin-myosin cross links formed during muscle contraction. The work of Davies (42) lends some support to such a hypothesis, and there is also some morphological evidence that structural degeneration of the myofibrils may be observed in muscle removed from animals in adrenal insufficiency and electrolyte imbalance (172).

The easy fatigability of the salt-maintained, adrenalectomized animal, however, is not explained by the above data. It is known that in situ the initial tension of the skeletal muscles of such animals is normal (77, 184). For example, Winter & Flataker (192) used a rope-climbing test to determine work capacity. Although the salt-treated, adrenalectomized animals could not perform as much work as either intact or cortisone-treated controls, they were able to sustain substantial work loads for several days before collapsing. Recently, Tipton and his group (179) have demonstrated that adrenalectomized rats maintained only on salt therapy could be trained over an 80-day period to perform repeated tests of treadmill exercises at a level well above untrained adrenalectomized rats on the same dietary regimen. No hormonal supplement was used in either group. As in other stresses, adaptation to substantial amounts of exercise may be induced slowly in the total absence of the adrenal hormones. It is of interest in the adaptation procedures described above that stimulation of individual skeletal muscles in situ showed no correlation between the contractility of these muscles and the animals' overall work capacity. The muscles of the untrained animals appeared to be as responsive as those of the trained rats, despite a marked difference in total work achieved on the treadmill. These results are reminiscent of the early work done by Hales et al. (82) who showed that repetitive contraction in situ of one gastrocnemius muscle of an adrenalectomized rat could be sustained for several hours before fatigue occurred. If at this point they tried to elicit contractions from the opposite gastrocnemius muscle in the same animal, fatigue of the previously unstimulated muscle was manifested within minutes. This speaks to a more generalized homeostatic defect than to a specific fault in the structure of the myofibrils.

Lefer (128), using rat papillary muscle in vitro, also found that the initially developed tension, the threshold of excitation, and the length-tension relations in his preparation were unchanged when adrenalectomized rats were maintained in electrolyte balance. After 30 min, differences between these muscles and those removed from intact animals were manifest. The adrenalectomized preparations showed a greater loss of intracellular potassium together with a more rapid decline in contractility. Dexamethasone-treated, adrenalectomized animals did not show this defect. It is of interest that, when the concentration of potassium ion in the external medium was doubled, Lefer found it possible to prevent the abnormal decline in tension. Changes in calcium ion concentration in the medium could also restore tension patterns to normal. Lefer proposed that, since an optimal external K^+ concentration is associated with the maximal operation of the sodium pump, subtle changes in the nature of the membrane transport system in salt-maintained, adrenalectomized animals could possibly shift the optimal K^+ ratio and thus affect membrane potentials and muscle performance. In later experiments, however, Rovetto & Lefer (156) could find no significant change in the membrane potential of the muscle if extracellular electrolytes were maintained in the normal range. In addition, normal ionic gradients could be established in papillary muscle from adrenalectomized animals at a time when functional decrements were quite apparent and changes in the membrane potential did not parallel the decline in tension. These data are similar to those reported by Laplaud & Gargouil (124, 125) who found that the resting potential of skeletal muscle is indeed reduced in adrenal insufficiency accompanied by electrolyte imbalance but that restoration of normal extracellular electrolyte patterns reestablished normal resting membrane polarity. It did not restore, however, the work capacity of the skeletal musculature.

Direct Muscle-Aldosterone Effects

There are few data on the direct cellular effects of mineralocorticoids on skeletal muscle. Adler (2) and others (63) have reported that aldosterone acts on rat diaphragm in vitro to decrease to a small degree (2–3 %) the intracellular potassium concentration. Others have been unable to confirm these data (6, 132), but the complexity of the interrelation between the concentration of intra- and extracellular potassium and of the action of aldosterone on muscle in vivo or in vitro probably accounts for the discrepancies. Adler (2) points out that chronic feeding of diets high in potassium leads to chronically elevated aldosterone levels, which in turn may lead to a slight depletion of intracellular skeletal muscle potassium. This probably represents the potassium adaptation described by Alexander & Levinsky (6). When animals so adapted are given a large dose of potassium, Adler postulates that their greater rate of survival lies in their ability to replete intracellular muscle potassium and thus remove potassium quickly from the extracellular fluid. Under these circumstances chronic aldosterone elevation is coincident with accelerated potassium entry into, rather than out of, the muscle cell. It is impossible to conclude from such data that a specific mechanism of aldosterone action on the membrane transport of potassium in skeletal muscle has been illuminated.

Most of the data available on the action of aldosterone at the cellular or subcellular level are derived from studies on the toad kidney or bladder cells. There are a few similarities between these tissues and skeletal muscle in vitro as regards responsiveness to aldosterone. For example, there is a time lag between the administration of aldosterone and its effect on the rate of sodium reabsorption by the toad bladder and kidney (62). Similarly, a latent period characterizes the reaction of the rat diaphragm to aldosterone in vitro (2); this observation is based on studies of the rate of potassium movement out of the skeletal muscle cell. The extrarenal effect of aldosterone on sodium movement, however, varies from tissue to tissue (65, 131, 196). Aldosterone has been shown to decrease the sodium content of some extrarenal tissues (159) and to increase the sodium content of others (65, 132). The sodium content of skeletal muscle in vivo does not seem to respond markedly one way or the other to mineralocorticoid administration (196).

The effect of aldosterone on rate-limiting reactions for electrolyte transport into and out of tissues may nevertheless be at similar sites in many cells, and it is of interest to examine data obtained from the more responsive tissues. Studies of toad bladder and kidney indicate that aldosterone fixes to specific binding sites on the cell membrane and is also localized in the cell nucleus (54, 166). A specific binding protein of high molecular weight has been postulated. The data further suggest that the next reaction is the synthesis of a specific DNA-dependent RNA that induces the synthesis of proteins critical for an aldosterone-responsive transport system for sodium. This system appears to be different from the mechanism that supports basal levels of ion movement through the cell membrane (28, 38, 54, 62, 149, 165). Puromycin and actinomycin block only the aldosterone-stimulated transport of sodium and have no effect on the basal rate of sodium movement, whereas ouabain has been shown to depress both transport systems (166). Similarly, substrates, such as pyruvate and acetoacetate, augment sodium transport in the toad bladder exposed to aldosterone but have no significant effect on untreated cells (166). It has also been shown (62) that injection of aldosterone into rats increases the incorporation of leucine into the proteins of the microsomal fraction of the kidney and that this effect occurs about 1 hr before the maximum antinatriuretic and kaliuretic effect of the hormone. There is evidence, however, that these two effects are not stoichiometrically related (12, 62, 191). The kaliuretic effect does not appear to be mediated by induction of RNA and protein synthesis (62), but the latency of aldosterone action is similar for both the antinatriuretic and the kaliuretic effects. It is difficult to extrapolate these data to the muscle-steroid relation since, in vivo, sodium retention under the influence of aldosterone is reflected mainly in the extracellular sodium and only secondarily and minimally in the intracellular sodium of skeletal muscle (159).

In summary, it is doubtful that mineralocorticoids in the physiological range of concentration have direct effects on skeletal muscle membrane transport of electrolytes. Correction of electrolyte imbalance by the administration of mineralocorticoids or by adequate dietary sodium chloride, however, restores to the adrenalectomized animal the ability to grow and function relatively normally in the sheltered conditions of the laboratory (10, 11). This must mean that the development of the skeletal musculature can proceed in the total absence of adrenal steroids. Considerable data also show that the resting muscle fibers in these circumstances are not significantly altered as regards internal structure or chemical composition (10, 11, 35, 37, 49, 161, 180, 196). Nor is there good evidence for abnormal resting membrane potentials or initial muscle tension. Aldosterone in vitro in nonphysiological concentrations may act directly on certain skeletal muscles to effect electrolyte shifts (2, 6, 63, 132), and in general these effects are not inconsistent with the in vivo responses of hyperaldosteronism (6, 138). But none of these data explain why the adrenalectomized animal maintained in electrolyte balance cannot perform a normal amount of muscle work. The only known way to restore muscle work capacity to normal in adrenalectomized animals is by the administration of appropriate amounts of the glucocorticoid hormones.

GLUCOCORTICOIDS AND SKELETAL MUSCLE

The term *glucocorticoid* reflects the emphasis that endocrinologists have placed on the carbohydrate-regulating function of these ubiquitous hormones. The C_{11}-oxycorticoids, however, have been shown to affect virtually all aspects of the homeostatic adjustments required in maintaining life under stressful conditions (151, 160). Vigorous muscle contraction apparently constitutes this kind of high-demand situation for the organism. There is no doubt that the glucocorticoids are an absolute requirement for sustaining not only muscular contraction, but the life of the exercising animal as well. There is no satisfactory answer to the more general question of steroid-stress-survival mechanisms. Certainly the maintenance of an adequate blood glucose level is necessary for efficient functioning of the neuromuscular apparatus, and the glucocorticoids act on both hepatic and extrahepatic systems to sustain optimal glucose levels (23, 133, 140, 187). Ingle & Nezamis (107), however, showed in 1948 that constant intravenous infusion of glucose into an adrenalectomized rat subjected to a repetitive stimulation of the gastrocnemius muscle did not prevent the characteristically rapid onset of fatigue and collapse. Like the maintenance of extracellular fluid electrolytes, the maintenance of extracellular glucose levels does not substitute for the C_{11}-oxycorticoids in restoring normal work capacity to adrenalectomized animals.

Carbohydrate Metabolism[1]

The classic experiments of Long et al. (133) demonstrated a marked increase in the formation of carbohydrate associated with an increased nitrogen excretion in animals treated with large amounts of corticosteroids. They suggested that increased extrahepatic protein catabolism supplied the liver with glucogenic amino acids, and thus gluconeogenesis was increased. The increase in nitrogen excretion was sufficient to account for the newly formed carbohydrate in fasted, intact or adrenalectomized animals given large amounts of adrenal hormones. Increased protein breakdown in muscle was clearly an end effect of hyperadrenocorticism, and the search began for the site of action of the hormones identified as the C_{11}-oxycorticoids.

The sequence of events that results in corticoid-mediated protein catabolism has not yet been clarified. One school has held that the initial effect in extrahepatic tissues is inhibition of glucose intake and utilization at the cell membrane (52). Animals given large amounts of cortical steroids show a striking accumulation of carbohydrate in the body, which is evidenced by a hyperglycemia that occurs within 1 to 2 hr after the injection of the hormone, a marked rise in liver glycogen that begins within 3 hr, and a much smaller rise in muscle glycogen that is not manifest until about 8–12 hr after administration of the steroids (134). About 70 % of the catabolized protein, as measured by urea excretion, can be accounted for in this way, but even in the fasting animal the utilization of carbohydrate for energy needs is not greatly increased. This would suggest a simultaneous depression of glucose utilization in extrahepatic tissues, but it has been difficult to demonstrate a very marked peripheral inhibition of glucose uptake or utilization in eviscerated animals treated with cortisol (8, 21, 134, 189). Since the skeletal musculature comprises the bulk of the metabolizing mass of the body, even a small inhibition of glucose utilization in skeletal muscle should manifest itself in substantial alterations in overall glucose uptake. The changes that have been observed are significant but small (140).

Studies of isolated rat diaphragm with cortisone added to the medium have not solved the problem. Glucose uptake in diaphragms from adrenalectomized rats has been variously reported to be unchanged or increased (122, 123). Herman & Ramey (90, 91) have pointed out that the selection of the medium may alter the effects observed. Pretreatment of rats with cortisol ultimately alters the uptake of glucose by the rat diaphragm. These procedures also depress the insulin responsiveness of the muscle, but the length of cortisol pretreatment required to change the metabolic behavior of the diaphragm suggests that a complex series of reactions precedes the effects on glucose metabolism (123, 182). Many effects that have been reported on the nature of cortisol inhibition of muscle carbohydrate metabolism in vivo may be quite indirect. For example, the impaired phosphorylation of glucose induced by cortisol may be explained on the basis of increased utilization of fatty acids (89, 144). In the intact organism, Randle et al. (155) suggest that cortisol stimulates fatty acid release from adipose tissue. This is followed by an increase in concentration of fatty acids and ketones in serum, which impairs glucose utilization in muscle. In the same way, Hennes et al. (89) explain the relative

---

[1] The discussion that follows is directed toward the metabolic events in muscle. For a description of the events in other tissues, see the chapters by Steele, by Fain and Czech, and by Munck and Young in this volume of the *Handbook*.

pyruvate intolerance of corticoid-treated humans as a result of enhanced utilization of fatty acids and ketone bodies by muscle with subsequent competition for coenzyme A. Thus the results obtained in the whole animal given large amounts of cortisol may present a skewed picture of the normal role of the glucocorticoids in regulating muscle metabolism in vivo. Obviously, studies with isolated rat diaphragm would eliminate liver-fat-muscle interrelations.

A specific defect in muscle carbohydrate metabolism resulting from glucocorticoid insufficiency has been suggested to account for the poor work performance, but this has been difficult to document. One finds early reports of decreased (87, 142), increased (23), and normal (34) rates of lactic acid production from contracting muscles in adrenalectomized animals of low (23, 34, 36, 136) and normal (10, 11, 37, 49) glycogen levels, and of decreased (34) and normal (92) rates of phosphorylation in skeletal muscle. Diaphragms from adrenalectomized rats when studied in vitro do show measurable differences in certain aspects of carbohydrate metabolism. For example, Wool & Weinshelbaum (202) found increased incorporation of ^{14}C-labeled glucose, carboxylic acids, or bicarbonate into the protein of diaphragms removed from adrenalectomized rats. There is also evidence that adrenalectomy increases the insulin sensitivity of some extrahepatic tissues (123) and some evidence that it does not (130). There are reports that the activation of muscle phosphorylase may be impaired by adrenal insufficiency (113, 161), but other data indicate that this response is normal (92, 127). Hess et al. (92) report that in the rat diaphragm corticosterone does not increase phosphorylase activity nor does it potentiate the epinephrine-induced rise in enzyme activity. On the other hand, Schaeffer's group (161) found that, although adrenalectomy does not result in any absolute change in phosphorylase levels of active or inactive gastrocnemius muscle, there was a significant decrease in phosphorylase activation by exogenous epinephrine or cyclic AMP (161). They could restore the response to normal by pretreatment with cortisol. It was necessary, however, to pretreat the adrenalectomized animal for 3 days before this restoration occurred. Acute cortisol administration had no effect on either the epinephrine or the cyclic AMP activation of the phosphorylase system, which suggests, as in many other similar situations, that the steroids are not immediately acting as cofactors. The differences in these reports may be due to differences in the muscles studied (i.e., diaphragm vs. gastrocnemius).

It is difficult to reconcile Schaeffer's results with the report by Ramey et al. (152) that gastrocnemii removed from adrenalectomized rats given 1% saline as drinking water did not show significant differences in the rate of glycogenolysis associated with muscle contraction. They found a defect in the response to catecholamines not in the skeletal muscle itself, but in the cardiovascular response to the amines (76, 77, 151). In Schaeffer's studies, time was required to restore muscle responsiveness to epinephrine; Ramey et al. (151), however, were able to restore immediately the pressor response to the catecholamines in adrenalectomized dogs by simultaneous intravenous infusion of the steroids and norepinephrine.

In 1960 Russell & Wilhelm (159) reviewed the evidence available and concluded that the cortical steroids in physiological concentration probably do not have direct effects on the metabolism of carbohydrate in muscle. They pointed out that well-nourished, adrenalectomized animals in electrolyte balance do not require glucocorticoids to maintain normal muscle glycogen levels. When such animals are fasted or worked their muscles respond with a decrease in glycogen concentration, and when fed a high-carbohydrate diet, muscle glycogen levels increase in a normal fashion (11, 157). Peripheral utilization of carbohydrate is only slightly altered in the eviscerated rat or dog, and the fasting respiratory quotient is normal (31, 140, 158).

Munck in 1971 also concludes that skeletal muscle is not a prime target for cortical steroid regulation of glucose utilization by extrahepatic tissue (140). He and others have been able to demonstrate that, even in vitro, physiological levels of glucocorticoids can inhibit glucose utilization by other extrahepatic tissues, such as skin, adipose tissue, and lymphoid tissue. Muscle does not appear to be affected within the time course of these studies. It is interesting that the mechanism proposed by Munck (140) to account for the inhibition of glucose utilization by the glucocorticoid-sensitive tissues (skin, adipose, and lymphoid) involves *a*) formation of a hormone-receptor complex, *b*) binding of this complex to the nucleus, and *c*) synthesis of a species of RNA, which shortly thereafter induces the synthesis of a protein that inhibits glucose transport. This proposal is reminiscent of the hypothesis described by Sharp & Leaf (166) and others (54) for the mechanism by which aldosterone alters membrane transport of electrolytes. In both instances the relatively rapid synthesis of a new protein is required to change the dynamics of the membrane transport systems.

There is much evidence to indicate that the turnover rate of protein in muscle is slower than that in other tissues (143, 181). Buchanan (24) showed that in rats and mice 63% of liver protein is replaced within 9 days, whereas only 17% of muscle protein is replaced during this time. Even in 50 days, when a turnover of 94% of liver protein has occurred, muscle protein replacement is 47%. As a corollary to this, it may be supposed that enzyme turnover rates are slow in muscle (161). If cortical steroids achieve their effects on glucose transport into the cell by inducing new protein synthesis, one would expect to find that such transport rates in muscle would be minimally affected in the usual time course of experiments in which physiological amounts of glucocorticoids are used. As Munck points out (140), a small glucocorticoid-sensitive pool of extrahepatic tissues responds with a rapid corticoid-induced inhibition of glucose utilization and provides a "trigger" for the hepatic increase of gluconeogenesis. Skeletal muscle does not belong to this pool, and therefore direct steroid inhibition of glucose utilization by muscle is probably not involved in the response to stress.

Protein Metabolism[2]

Net loss of extrahepatic protein can be induced by *a*) an increase in the rate of catabolism with no change in the rate of synthesis, *b*) a decrease in the rate of synthesis with no change in the rate of catabolism, or *c*) a combination of increased rates of catabolism and decreased rates of anabolism. It is probable that the net corticoid-induced breakdown of peripheral protein is normally regulated by the liver in intact animals (134, 145). There is no doubt, however, that glucocorticoids can affect protein turnover in the eviscerated animal (170) and in the rat diaphragm in vitro (200, 201).

Adrenalectomy has been shown to increase the incorporation of ^{14}C-labeled amino acids into the proteins of the isolated rat diaphragm (200), and Wool and Weinshelbaum conclude that this is due mainly to an acceleration of protein synthesis. Since the muscles of well-fed, adrenalectomized animals in electrolyte balance grow normally and since there is little indication of diaphragm dysfunction, the physiological significance of these data is unclear. It has been abundantly demonstrated that the opposite effects can be obtained by pretreating animals with large amounts of glucocorticoids. Diaphragms removed from such animals have an increased uptake of labeled amino acids, including the nonutilizable α-aminoisobutyric acid (AIB) (15, 116, 118, 120, 197, 198). Opinions about the effects of adding the hormone to the incubation medium itself differ. Wool & Weinshelbaum (201) and Manchester & Young (135) did not observe inhibition of labeled amino acid uptake under such conditions, but others have reported significant in vitro effects (118–120). If corticosteroids change amino acid uptake rates by decreasing the production of labile protein elements needed to maintain the functional integrity of the membrane transport system, as suggested by Kipnis & Cori (114), then a time lag should be manifest, and it is. This may account in part for the discrepancies in various in vitro studies on uptake by the cut diaphragm. Kostyo and associates have been able to demonstrate inhibitory effects of the steroids added to the incubation medium (118–120). The latency period is not unlike that observed in the eviscerate animal (170).

Support for the concept of inhibition of de novo protein production as a possible site of action of the steroids comes from other studies with substances that suppress protein synthesis, such as puromycin. Kipnis & Cori (114) showed that the inhibition of AIB uptake by puromycin required a lag time similar to that observed in the inhibition of corticosterone uptake. However, addition of puromycin or actinomycin and also of the corticosteroids to the medium often yields inconsistent results (26, 199). Another problem in interpreting data from steroids added in vitro is that in Kostyo's studies deoxycorticosterone produced virtually the same degree of inhibition of amino acid uptake by the diaphragm as did corticosterone (120). This is certainly not the situation in vivo. The possibility that deoxycorticosterone effects on potassium movement might have affected the amino acid transport in vitro is unlikely since Wool & Weinshelbaum (201) found that even large changes in intracellular potassium had no effect on amino acid (phenylalanine) incorporation into the protein of the diaphragm in normal, adrenalectomized, or cortisone-pretreated rats.

Conclusions cannot be drawn as to the effects of corticosteroids on skeletal muscle without hedging the interpretation with a description of the dose level of the hormone that is used. De Loecker and co-workers (47, 48) have shown that different amounts of cortisol may elicit opposite effects on incorporation of labeled amino acids (e.g., glycine incorporation into muscle proteins). Even in vitro their data show that, although large doses of cortisol (10 mg/day to 150-g rats) increased protein catabolism, lower dose levels did not significantly decrease the overall level of the incorporated label in long-term experiments. They did find that the mitochondrial, microsomal, and supernatant protein fractions showed some reduction in incorporated ^{14}C levels, but the protein fractions of the cell debris showed an increased specific activity at the same time. It is this latter fraction that is responsible for the highest percentage of amino acid incorporation.

Protein synthesis takes place mainly in the microsomes and soluble cell fractions. De Loecker and associates used microsomes combined with the soluble supernatant cell fractions and showed that high cortisol levels resulted in a decrease in ^{14}C-labeled glycine and leucine incorporation, whereas lower cortisol levels stimulated an increase in amino acid incorporation. These observations are consistent with the fact that glucocorticoids administered to adrenalectomized animals in physiological doses stimulate growth and development of the muscles, as well as other tissues of the organism. Only at much higher glucocorticoid levels is net tissue catabolism manifest. At such levels it is demonstrable that the glucocorticoids produce net increases in the release of amino acids from skeletal muscle (20, 116) and an increase in the muscle content of free amino acids (15). These effects have been observed in the eviscerate preparation as well (170), with a delay period comparable to the in vitro studies.

Exercise and Glucocorticoid Levels

There are striking conundrums with respect to the relationship between skeletal muscle and the cortical steroids. Both the adrenal insufficiency of Addison's disease and the adrenal excess of Cushing's syndrome are associated with muscle dysfunction (5). In the normal

---

[2] See the chapter by Steele, in this volume of the *Handbook*, for a discussion of the effects of the corticosteroids on protein metabolism in various tissues.

animal, vigorous muscle contraction requires glucocorticoids, but it is by no means clear that increased levels of these steroids in blood are always found in working animals or humans. Foss et al. (64) found that the free 11-hydroxycorticosteroid levels in working dogs were not significantly altered until the work demand was of high intensity and long duration (64). Suzuki and his associates studied the rate at which 17-hydroxycorticoids from adrenals are secreted into the lumboadrenal veins of conscious dogs under different exercise regimens and found that the secretion rate was related to the state of fatigue of the animal but not to exercise intensity or duration (173). Even in Foss' studies the elevated levels of glucocorticoids in blood were well below those observed in Cushing's syndrome or in most experiments done with exogenous steroids.

Large amounts of steroids produce net protein catabolism in resting muscle. Increased protein anabolism is observed, however, in the muscles of working animals. Work hypertrophy is an old observation. It is apparent therefore that, if glucocorticoids are indeed chronically elevated in the normal working organism, this elevation is consistent with increased, rather than decreased, synthesis of muscle protein even over long periods of time.

STEROID MYOPATHY

Cushing in 1932 reported that one of the clinical manifestations of hypercorticism was muscle wasting and weakness (39). In recent years the widespread use of anti-inflammatory agents has produced iatrogenically a large number of individuals with the signs and symptoms of Cushing's syndrome. Some of these patients develop a steroid myopathy. Others receiving the same amount of hormone for long periods of time do not (4). There is no good explanation for differences of this kind. The steroid myopathies have been intensively studied (56, 57, 60, 75, 142, 150, 165). Large doses of glucocorticoids may lead ultimately to a net loss of total body weight together with a significant redistribution of body mass (128, 141), but many aspects of steroid myopathy are not understood. The weakness exhibited by animals or humans under these circumstances might be due to at least two abnormalities: *1*) potassium depletion; and *2*) excessive protein catabolism. Studies of the total exchangeable potassium in which ^{24}K was used in humans receiving triamcinolone and other corticoids, however, have not shown significant differences from the untreated controls (13). Serum potassium is usually not significantly altered in humans or experimental animals with steroid myopathy, and feeding of supplemental potassium has no observable effects on the course of the myopathy (4).

This puts the explanation for the muscle degeneration and weakness squarely in the realm of the increased protein catabolism that has been so well documented. The results of nitrogen balance studies in humans, however, have been inconclusive in this regard. In some studies a greater nitrogen loss was shown during steroid treatment than during control periods (66), but in others no evidence of increased protein breakdown has been found (4). Also the increased incidence of myopathy with triamcinolone, as compared to prednisolone, could not be correlated with its effects on nitrogen metabolism (4).

Studies at the subcellular level have been numerous and have yielded interesting suggestions as to the sequence of events within the myofibril that accompany steroid myopathy (3, 169). Afifi & Bergman (3) removed several kinds of skeletal muscle from cortisone-treated rabbits after varying periods of daily exposure (2–58 days) to large amounts of the hormone. By using both light and electron microscopy, they correlated the chronological sequence of pathological alterations with certain chemical changes. The early response was manifested by the appearance of massive glycogen aggregates, but the architecture of the myofibrils was preserved. Continued exposure to glucocorticoids produced mitochondrial alterations, Z line changes, and evidence of active regenerative processes, despite the overall catabolic response. In the late phase of degeneration of the muscle, they observed breakdown of the contractile elements, necrosis, cellular infiltration and phagocytosis, and a reduction in glycogen accumulation.

The mechanism to account for the glycogen deposition has been explored to some degree (3, 129, 168). In Leonard's experiments the increase in muscle glycogen was not associated with a change in muscle phosphorylase (129), nor could the increase in glycogen be correlated with the level of radioactive steroid within the muscle. It has been suggested that the glucocorticoids directly or indirectly activate glycogen synthetase and thus favor the transformation of uridine diphosphoglucose (UDPG) to glycogen (168, 204). As the corticoid myopathy goes on to frank necrosis, the glycogen decrease might be due to a decrease in the activity of the UDPG glycogen synthetase that has been reported in the late stages of nonhormonally related muscle dystrophies (50). Thus the effect of cortisol on muscle enzymes seems to depend on previous alterations in the structure of the muscle fiber.

An especially interesting finding in Afifi's work is that the glucocorticoids induced a marked thickening in "basement membranes" of capillaries and to a somewhat lesser degree of the muscle fibers they supplied (3). This thickening has been observed in human steroid myopathy as well (4) and is completely reversed when steroid administration is discontinued. All other indices of steroid atrophy also disappear after sufficient recovery time. The recovery process appears to be similar to that reported for normal rat myoblasts during skeletal muscle differentiation (17). The thickening of the basement membrane may be associated with alterations in insulin secretion induced by the high steroid levels, although there is nothing in Afifi's data to support or deny such a hypothesis.

At subcellular levels the data obtained by use of a

series of anti-inflammatory drugs, such as triamcinolone acetonide, are often difficult to reconcile. Peters et al. (148) used triamcinolone in very high doses to study the effect on the incorporation of uridine into isolated muscle ribosomes from rats pretreated with the drug. They found a rapid decrease in the incorporation of labeled uridine and orthophosphate into the RNA of hind limb skeletal muscle that was accompanied by a decrease in the incorporating ability of muscle ribosomes and polysomes; there was, however, no change in the concentration of the muscle ATP or free amino acids. These results are not consistent with the previous reports of Ferguson and Wool who used cortisol in a 4-day pretreatment schedule before measuring similar parameters. They found that cortisol did not affect the rate of incorporation of labeled adenine into the RNA of the rat diaphragm (61), even though the rate of incorporation of amino acids into muscle protein was decreased by about 50% after such prolonged exposure to the hormone (200). Peters' data may explain why some of the powerful synthetic anti-inflammatory drugs (e.g., triamcinolone) are associated with a higher incidence of induced myopathies than are the naturally occurring steroids.

Another difficulty that has not been resolved in explaining steroid myopathy is that not all the skeletal muscles of the body seem to be equally affected even in the presence of large amounts of circulating glucocorticoids (40, 74). Smith (169) found that greater wasting occurred in the pale muscle fibers than in the dark fibers in the mixed muscles of rabbits treated with pharmacological amounts of corticosteroids and that the diaphragm did not appear to be markedly involved in the overall myopathy. On the other hand, D'Agostino & Chiga (40) found that the red fibers in rabbits were predominantly affected, whereas Afifi & Bergman (3), as well as Ellis (57), could find no predilection to catabolism in any one type of fiber in the rabbit under conditions of hypercorticism.

Experience with patients with Cushing's syndrome would suggest that there is, in fact, a differential muscle response to excessive endogenous glucocorticoid secretion. These individuals frequently exhibit more marked wasting in the proximal than in the distal muscles (139, 169). There is also no good evidence for deterioration of the diaphragm. This kind of myopathic distribution has also been observed in patients treated with exogenous steroids (142). Interestingly during prolonged starvation in the intact organism, when cortical steroid secretion is elevated, the soleus muscle loses proportionately less weight than the gastrocnemius muscle. Faludi and his co-workers (60) point out that the body-to-muscle weight ratio is unchanged for the pectoral muscles during prolonged cortisone treatment but is markedly decreased for the quadriceps muscles. Cardiac muscle is very resistant to the catabolic action of cortisone. In fact, Faludi's group found that the body-to-muscle weight ratio for cardiac muscle is actually increased under these circumstances.

The well-designed studies of Goldberg & Goodman (74) may elucidate the mechanism of the differential responses of the muscles to excess cortisone. By using hypophysectomized rats treated with 10 mg/day of cortisone acetate, they found that the animals lost almost a quarter of their total body weight in 10 days. Even in this state of profound negative nitrogen balance, weight loss in the dark, tonic soleus muscle was not significant, whereas the pale plantaris muscle lost 40% of its mass. This loss occurred in the protein and aqueous compartments to the same degree. Two other phasic pale muscles, the anterior tibialis and the gastrocnemius, also lost about 40% of their total mass. These investigators tested the hypothesis that muscles with the lowest rates of protein synthesis are most susceptible to the long-term catabolic effects of the corticosteroids. They reasoned that any technique producing a reduction in the rate of protein synthesis in normally cortisol-resistant muscles should then make these muscles more sensitive to the catabolic effects of the hormone. They took advantage of the facts that denervation of a skeletal muscle leads to decreased protein synthesis and that forced work leads to an increase in protein synthesis (71). The normal basal rate for protein turnover is faster in the soleus than in the plantaris (70, 72), but denervation reduced this rate and at the same time increased the sensitivity to cortisone. The increase was greater than could be accounted for by denervation alone and represented a specific response to the hormone. On the other hand, work-induced hypertrophy of the soleus and plantaris occurring after tenotomy of the gastrocnemius resulted in a decreased sensitivity to the catabolic actions of the steroid in both muscles.

These results are quite different from the effects of growth hormone on muscle size, in which the hormonally mediated increase in protein synthesis is independent of the innervation (73). Goldberg and associates make a good case for the involvement of cortisone in the regulation of both protein synthesis and protein catabolism in skeletal muscle (70, 72, 73). They point out that the cortisone-induced decrease of muscle mass in situ occurred at a much faster rate than could be accounted for from known estimates of protein turnover. Goldberg considered the slow turnover of protein in muscle and the possibility that the cortisone treatment had completely blocked amino acid incorporation into new protein, which it does not do (147), and found that the time course of atrophy of the affected muscles required simultaneous acceleration of protein catabolism and deceleration of protein synthesis. This finding is consistent with those obtained from other studies (15, 20, 116, 170).

Tonic muscle systems seem to be relatively less involved in the mobilization of muscle protein for gluconeogenesis. This is a teleologically satisfying construct because these muscles are more critical for survival during a prolonged stress than are some of the phasic muscles. The carbon skeletons provided by protein mobilization for new glucose formation (59, 133) would thus come from the more expendable tissues. Sparing of the diaphragm and cardiac muscle is obviously useful, and indeed these muscles seem to be more steroid resistant. If the house must be burned to provide heat it is wise to leave the floor and foundations to the last.

EXERCISE AS SYSTEMIC STRESS

Any satisfactory explanation of the critical requirement for glucocorticoids during muscle work must include an explanation not only for the muscle failure in adrenal insufficiency, but perhaps more fundamentally the reason for the total collapse and death of the adrenalectomized animal forced to work without these hormones. Despite reports of alterations in such parameters as mean conduction velocity of muscle afferent fibers (80) or general depression of receptor generator potentials or in repetitive response of the intrafusal fibers of the spindles (80), muscle removed from adrenalectomized animals and stimulated through the attached motor nerve does not behave very differently from normal muscle (152), nor does the nerve itself (203). This is not to say that adrenalectomized animals do not suffer neural deficits. On the sensory side, the work of Henkin et al. (88) has clearly demonstrated, for example, that the taste sensitivity of Addisonians is 100 times more acute than normal. There are, however, systemic effects attendant upon activation of the neuromuscular apparatus in the absence of the glucocorticoids that cannot be explained simply by altered sensitivity of myoneural responses.

The intimate relationship between the systemic effects of glucocorticoid insufficiency and the ultimate failure of muscle contraction is demonstrated in the work of Ramey et al. (152) in which salt-treated, adrenalectomized rats swam to exhaustion and collapse. The diaphragm and a section of abdominal muscle were then removed and suspended in a large volume of oxygenated, buffered nutrient medium. The muscles were electrically stimulated either directly or, in the case of the diaphragm, through the attached phrenic nerve. The muscles continued to contract for several hours and were indistinguishable from muscles removed from intact animals. Neither the nerve, the myoneural junction, nor the muscle appeared to be profoundly affected by the glucocorticoid insufficiency that had been well established in the animal. Other studies (182, 184) confirm this observation.

Goldstein and co-workers (76, 77) further demonstrated that, in adrenalectomized dogs in salt balance, the muscle responsiveness was closely related to the blood pressure and to the reaction of the cardiovascular system to endogenous catecholamine production. Schweitzer (162) showed, in acutely adrenalectomized cats or in intact cats, that a drop in blood pressure below certain critical levels (70 mmHg) leads to rapid failure of muscle contraction. Subsequently, Ramey et al. (153) showed that a brief restoration of gastrocnemius muscle contraction could be elicited in the exhausted adrenalectomized dog by raising his blood pressure with norepinephrine infusion. The pressor response was short lived and less than that observed in intact animals. Intravenous infusion of glucocorticoids in aqueous extract immediately restored the blood pressure response to norepinephrine and the muscles could then be made to contract normally again (153). Fritz & Levine (67) were able to demonstrate that in the absence of glucocorticoids repeated application of norepinephrine to the rat mesoappendix caused irreversible atonia and stasis in the vascular bed with actual vessel disruption. Not only are pressor responses inadequate (30, 163), but any continuous demand for homeostatic vascular adjustments that invokes sympathetic discharge leads to shock and death of the adrenally insufficient animal (151).

The strength of a unitary hypothesis regarding glucocorticoid action must depend therefore on its ability to explain the overall fragility of the animal when subjected to any stress. Ingle's imaginative concept of the permissive action of these steroids (101) identified many of the putative actions of these hormones to be supporting rather than regulatory. For example, much has been said in this review about the catabolic effect of increased amounts of glucocorticoids. Yet Ingle was able to demonstrate elegantly that under conditions of stress a variable mobilization of protein was manifest with a constant level of hormone. The work of Sayers (160) and others lends strength to this kind of formulation.

Such generalized systemic responses suggest a general involvement of the glucocorticoids in the maintenance of tissue integrity. Steroids have been said to influence cells by *a*) inducing adaptive increases in the amount of enzyme protein itself, *b*) serving as direct activators of such systems as the transhydrogenase mechanisms, or *c*) changing membrane transport systems either at the cell surface or at the surface of subcellular particles. The effect of glucocorticoids on cell free systems lends little support to the first two hypotheses. Data on cell membrane transport kinetics in muscle do not provide compelling evidence that this structure is the primary site of glucocorticoid action. This suggests that the glucocorticoids probably act at the intracellular level. There is evidence that tritiated cortisol enters most tissues with varying degrees of ease (183). In the eviscerate animal the muscle concentrates large amounts of tritiated cortisol soon after systemic injection of the hormone. Walker et al. (183) conclude that there is no significant barrier between muscle and plasma with respect to cortisol entry across the cell membrane. They found the same situation to apply to adipose tissue and to the pituitary gland but suggest a blood-brain barrier to the hormone. There is no structural problem therefore in locating the initial site of action of cortisol within the muscle cell.

Lysosomes

The intracellular compartmentation of enzymes can serve as a device for hormonal regulation of enzyme activity. As deDuve and others have pointed out (44,

46), the rate of release of enzymes from such compartments within the cell must be a primary area of metabolic regulation. The effects of glucocorticoids on subcellular particles have been observed with reference to ribosomal activity in protein synthesis and to mitochondrial changes and the oxidative capacity of the cell. Another cell fragment of great interest as a possible primary site of steroid action is the lysosome. Hypothetically the cathepsins associated with this structure would be injurious to the whole animal if they were released in abnormal quantities. This would provide a possible explanation of the stress sensitivity of the adrenally insufficient animal if it were shown that systemic levels of free acid hydrolases are elevated to a greater degree than in normal animals forced to make homeostatic adjustments. It could account for the fact that strenuous muscular exercise can induce shock in the same way that tissue trauma produces collapse in the absence of the corticoids.

One problem with respect to contracting muscle as a source of lysosomal cathepsins is some uncertainty concerning the actual presence of lysosomes in the myofibril itself. Pellegrino & Franzini (146) state categorically that with the electron microscope no lysosomes have ever been detected in normal muscle fibers. It has been suggested therefore that the lysosomal activity of muscle results from the presence of phagocytic cells, which are known to be rich in lysosomes (25). Bird et al. (19), despite the lack of electron-micrographic evidence for muscle lysosomes, were able to isolate muscle components that met all deDuve's criteria for these subcellular particles. Another problem is that, because of the nature of the myofibrillar structure, more shearing force is required to shatter the cells than is needed to shatter such tissues as the liver. This might give a false picture of the fragility of muscle lysosomes. Nevertheless, comparisons between muscle fragments from adrenalectomized and intact animals can expose differences within the limitations of the technique.

The great interest in corticoid regulation of lysosomal fragility stems from the fact that lysosomal rupture has been associated with many stress situations, such as hypervitaminosis A (186), inflammation (112), and ischemia (45); stability of the lysosome was increased by glucocorticoids (46, 185, 186). These hormones protect rabbit hepatic lysosomes both in vivo and in vitro against many potentially disruptive agents, such as streptolysins, high vitamin A concentrations, and high hydrogen ion concentrations (46, 111, 186). Consistent with this is the finding that well-nourished, adrenalectomized animals in good health and in electrolyte balance seem to have liver and muscle lysosomal structures that are more fragile than those of intact animals (16, 19). By using the classic endocrine techniques of restoring the hormone in physiological amounts, Berg & Bird (16) were able to increase the stability of liver and muscle lysosomes to normal values, as measured by the release of acid hydrolases, ribonuclease, cathepsin D, β-glucuronidase, and aryl sulfatase. Pharmacological doses of corticosterone actually increased the stability of the lysosomes beyond that characteristic of normal animals. Similarly, hydrolase levels in serum suggest a stress-induced defect in adrenalectomized animals (112, 226). Unstressed adrenalectomized rats have normal hydrolase concentrations in serum but exhibit a greater-than-normal rise in these potentially injurious substances when stressed.

These data apparently could provide a unitary hypothesis to account for the role of glucocorticoids in protecting the animal against a stress-induced acceleration of cathepsin release. There are, however, several inconsistencies in this simplified picture of the stress response. Glucocorticoids are also necessary for accelerated protein catabolism during starvation or any other period of metabolic demand. Teleologically, it makes sense for the "stress" steroids to decelerate the release of injurious cathepsins by stabilizing lysosomes, but it is necessary to account simultaneously for their acceleration of proteolytic enzyme activity in extrahepatic tissues, such as muscle.

Ingle's work suggests that it is not the absolute level of the hormones themselves that regulates the rate of protein breakdown. They seem to act to increase the accessibility of the catabolic enzymes to the primary regulators, whatever they may be. This could not be accomplished by increasing the stability of subcellular particles that sequester such enzymes. In addition, it is well known that excess corticoids are associated with necrotic changes in skeletal muscle and that necrosis is associated with increased activity of acid hydrolases. Yet the data discussed above show that glucocorticoids induce necrosis and at the same time act to decrease both specific and total hydrolase activity (16).

"Second Messengers"—Cyclic AMP and Prostaglandins

The relationship of the glucocorticoids to the cyclic AMP systems has not been clarified. Basal levels of cyclic AMP in the tissues of adrenalectomized animals are not significantly different from normal. For example, it has been shown that glucocorticoids are necessary for the glucagon and epinephrine activation of gluconeogenesis in the liver, but this lack of responsiveness does not result from impaired activation of adenyl cyclase. In the absence of the steroids, both glucagon and epinephrine increase the levels of cyclic AMP. It appears therefore that the effect of the glucocorticoids is at a step beyond cyclic AMP formation. There are reports that administration of cyclic AMP to adrenalectomized animals does not elicit a normal activation of the phosphorylase system in muscle (161) and normal gluconeogenesis in liver. This is not due to an absolute loss of sensitivity to cyclic AMP, however. There is a decrease in response to the nucleotide that can be overcome even in the absence of the steroids by increasing the concentration of the cyclic AMP used. In cardiac muscle a similar situation pertains. At low concentrations of epinephrine or cyclic AMP, there was an impaired glycogenolytic response in hearts removed from adrenalectomized animals that could be attributed to impaired activation of phosphorylase. At higher concentrations of epinephrine in the same preparations, however, it was possible to obtain a normal increase in lactate output and full activation of phosphorylase.

These data suggest that the exact relation of the glucocorticoids to the response of primary enzyme systems to "second messengers" remains vague. This seems to be the case not only in the muscle-liver gluconeogenesis interrelations, but also at the site of lipolysis in adipose tissue, where the normal lipolytic action of epinephrine requires the presence of glucocorticoids but cyclic AMP accumulation does not. Here the steroids appear to permit the nucleotide activation of a lipase.

The situation with respect to muscle is further complicated by the fact that phosphorylase activation in this tissue may occur by several different mechanisms. Activation of phosphorylase without an increase in cyclic AMP occurs in a muscle that contracts as a result of nerve stimulation. This may result from the release of calcium ions within the myofibril. In vitro the addition of calcium ions will readily activate phosphorylase. Epinephrine-induced activation of phosphorylase need not be normal therefore in order that a contracting muscle break down glycogen, and this may account for the apparent normal glycogenolysis in contracting muscles from adrenalectomized animals.

Prostaglandins are another possible mediator of overall glucocorticoid action. They seem to interact with the cyclic AMP system at several sites. For example, prostaglandin E_1 inhibits epinephrine-stimulated and nerve-stimulated lipolysis of intact adipose cells. Some membrane component seems to be necessary for these inhibitory effects (154). Prostaglandins have been shown to be released from diaphragm muscle by either neural stimulation or by use of biogenic amines. The prostaglandins so released affect smooth muscle and may therefore have generalized effects on the small blood vessels. They may act by displacing calcium ion from membranous structures. This in turn may alter the ion permeability of plasma and intracellular interfaces and the sodium flux. The relationship of the glucocorticoids to the release of the prostaglandins and to the ultimate action of the prostaglandins in the whole organism has not been explored.

On the basis of these interesting but unexplained phenomena it is possible to formulate a hypothesis. Glucocorticoids act to limit release of acid hydrolases from intracellular structures. The regulation of prostaglandin formation by such enzymes may be common to all tissues, including skeletal muscle. In the absence of the glucocorticoids the fragility of lysosomes is increased, and with the stress of strenuous muscle contraction an abnormal amount of substances such as phospholipase A is released. These in turn lead to the production of larger-than-normal amounts of prostaglandins, which lowers blood pressure. At the same time, the exercise elicits sympathetic discharge with elevated circulatory catecholamines. The adrenal insufficiency diminishes the pressor response to catecholamines and increases the toxicity of these agents at the small blood vessels. Under these circumstances the depressor prostaglandins contribute to the systemic deterioration by generally displacing membrane-bound calcium and increasing flux of sodium into cells. Such ionic changes could affect the behavior of intracellular organelles, as well as the activity of adenyl cyclase itself. The glucocorticoids in this complex system might act to regulate primarily the rate of release of prostaglandins and secondarily all the mechanisms within the cell that are related to calcium-to-magnesium ratios and sodium flux. Although the evidence to support such a relationship is fragmentary, it may provide a basis for further experimentation.

CONCLUSIONS

An interaction between the glucocorticoids and skeletal muscle can be demonstrated both in adrenal insufficiency and adrenal hyperfunction. Muscle work capacity is compromised in both instances. In Addison's disease, muscle asthenia is associated with relatively normal structure and chemistry of the resting muscle and the inability to sustain repetitive contractions for long periods of time. Strenuous work induces vascular collapse, shock, and death in the adrenalectomized animal, despite the maintenance of electrolyte balance by the appropriate administration of sodium chloride or mineralocorticoids. The maintenance of a normal blood sugar is similarly without restorative effects under these conditions. In vitro studies on muscles removed from such animals have not revealed biochemical lesions that could account for the physiological incapacity of the whole animal. The observed fragility of the small blood vessels and the toxic response to sympathetic activation that is found in adrenal insufficiency can be corrected only by the administration of adequate amounts of glucocorticoids. Some of the effects of exercise in adrenalectomized animals may be due to a decreased stability of tissue lysosomes and an increased release of acid hydrolases into the systemic circulation together with prostaglandins.

The muscle catabolism associated with Cushing's syndrome can be mimicked in the laboratory by the administration of large amounts of glucocorticoids. In vitro experiments with steroids added to the medium have yielded contradictory results. Pretreatment of the animal with large doses of hormone for long enough periods of time, however, decreases the ability of the isolated rat diaphragm to incorporate labeled amino acids into protein. Similar results have been reported for changes in ribosomes obtained from such diaphragms. Increased protein catabolism is also manifest in muscles after exposure in situ to excess glucocorticoids. It is unlikely that the initiating step in the protein catabolic process is direct inhibition of glucose uptake and utilization in skeletal muscle. The liver, because it regulates lipid metabolism, may indirectly affect the rate of glucose utilization in muscle.

In physiological states, the glucocorticoids are associated with normal growth and development of skeletal muscle not only at rest, but also during periods of exercise and muscle hypertrophy. It is difficult to conclude therefore that in the normal animal glucocorticoids produce generalized muscle catabolism. A wide range of responses to systemic hypercorticism is observed in the different muscles of the body. The soleus, for example, is far less sensitive to the catabolic actions of cortisol than is the gastrocnemius. Steroid sensitivity may be related to the intrinsic rate of protein turnover in different kinds of muscle, with phasic muscles exhibiting greater responsiveness than tonic muscles. Since it has been shown that the rate of gluconeogenesis in the whole animal cannot be related directly to absolute levels of serum glucocorticoids, the control of this system is probably not a dose-response function of cortisol. The permissive action of these steroids has not been explained at the systemic or cellular or subcellular level. The primary site of action of adrenal steroids on skeletal muscle continues to elude endocrinologists.

REFERENCES

1. ADDISON, T. *On the Constitutional and Local Effects of Disease of the Suprarenal Capsules.* London: Highley, 1855.
2. ADLER, S. An extrarenal action of aldosterone on mammalian skeletal muscle. *Am. J. Physiol.* 218: 616–621, 1970.
3. AFIFI, A. K., AND R. A. BERGMAN. Steroid myopathy, a study of the evolution of the muscle lesion in rabbits. *Johns Hopkins Med. J.* 124: 6–68, 1969.
4. AFIFI, A. K., R. A. BERGMAN, AND J. C. HARVEY. Steroid myopathy, clinical histologic and cytologic observations. *Johns Hopkins Med. J.* 123: 158–174, 1968.
5. ALBRIGHT, F. Cushing's syndrome; its pathological physiology and its connection with problems of reaction of body to injurious agents ("alarm reaction" of Selye). *Harvey Lectures Ser.* 38: 123–186, 1943.
6. ALEXANDER, E. A., AND N. G. LEVINSKY. An extrarenal mechanism of potassium adaptation. *J. Clin. Invest.* 47: 740–748, 1968.
7. ALLERS, W. D., AND E. C. KENDALL. Maintenance of adrenalectomized dogs without cortin thru control of the mineral constituents of the diet. *Am. J. Physiol.* 118: 87–92, 1934.
8. ALTSZULER, N., R. STEELE, J. S. WALL, AND R. C. DE BODO. Mechanism of the 'anti-insulin' action of 11,17-oxycorticosteroids in hypophysectomized dogs. *Am. J. Physiol.* 192: 219–226, 1958.
9. ANDERSEN, D. H. The effect of food and of exhaustion on the pituitary, thyroid, adrenal and thymus gland of the rat. *J. Physiol., London* 85: 162–167, 1935.
10. ANDERSON, E. The physiology of the salt-treated adrenalectomized animal. In: *Essays in Biology.* Berkeley: Univ. of California Press, 1943, p. 33–49.
11. ANDERSON, E., M. JOSEPH, AND V. HERRING. Growth and survival of adrenalectomized rats given various levels of NaCl. *Proc. Soc. Exptl. Biol. Med.* 44: 477–485, 1940.
12. BARGER, A. C., R. D. BERLIN, AND J. F. TULENKO. Infusion of aldosterone 9-a-fluorohydrocortisone and antidiuretic hormone into the renal artery of normal and adrenalectomized unanesthetized dogs: effect on electrolyte and water excretion. *Endocrinology* 62: 804–815, 1958.
13. BAUER, F. K., E. L. DUBOIS, AND N. TELFER. Total exchangeable potassium in SLE with reference to triamcinolone myopathy. *Proc. Soc. Exptl. Biol. Med.* 105: 671–673, 1960.
14. BAUMANN, E. J., AND S. KURLAND. Changes in the inorganic constituents of blood in suprarenalectomized cats and rabbits. *J. Biol. Chem.* 71: 281–302, 1927.
15. BEITHEIL, J. J., M. FEIGELSON, AND P. FEIGELSON. The differential effects of glucocorticoid on tissue and plasma amino acid levels. *Biochim. Biophys. Acta* 104: 91–97, 1965.
16. BERG, T., AND J. W. BIRD. Properties of muscle and liver lysosomes in adrenalectomized rats. *Acta Physiol. Scand.* 79: 335–350, 1970.
17. BERGMAN, R. A. Observations on the morphogenesis of rat skeletal muscle. *Bull. Johns Hopkins Hosp.* 110: 187–201, 1962.
18. BIEDL, A. *Internal Secretory Organs.* Baltimore: Wm. Wood, 1913.
19. BIRD, J. W. C., T. BERG, AND J. H. LEATHEM. Cathepsin activity of liver and muscle fractions of adrenalectomized rats. *Proc. Soc. Exptl. Biol. Med.* 127: 182–188, 1968.
20. BONDY, P. K. The effect of the adrenal and thyroid glands upon the rise of plasma amino acids in the eviscerated rat. *Endocrinology* 45: 605–608, 1949.
21. BONDY, P. K., D. J. INGLE, AND R. C. MEEKS. Influence of adrenal cortical hormones upon the level of plasma amino acids in eviscerate rats. *Endocrinology* 55: 354–360, 1954.
22. BRITTON, S. W. Adrenal insufficiency and related consideration. *Physiol. Rev.* 10: 617–682, 1930.
23. BRITTON, S. W., H. SILVETTE, AND R. F. KLINE. Adrenal insufficiency in American monkeys. *Am. J. Physiol.* 123: 705–711, 1938.
24. BUCHANAN, D. L. Total carbon turnover measured by feeding a uniformly labeled diet. *Arch. Biochem. Biophys.* 94: 500–511, 1961.
25. BUCHANAN, W. E., AND T. B. SCHWARTZ. Lysosomal enzyme activity in heart and skeletal muscle of cortisone treated rats. *Am. J. Physiol.* 212: 732–736, 1967.
26. BURROW, G. N., AND P. K. BONDY. Effect of puromycin on the action of insulin on sugar and amino acid transport in muscle. *Endocrinology* 75: 455–457, 1964.
27. CANNON, W. B., H. F. NEWTON, E. M. BRIGHT, V. MENKEN, AND R. M. MOORE. Some aspects of the physiology of animals surviving complete exclusion of sympathetic nerve impulses. *Am. J. Physiol.* 89: 84–107, 1929.
28. CASTLES, T. R., AND H. E. WILLIAMSON. Stimulation *in vivo* of renal RNA-synthesis by aldosterone. *Proc. Soc. Exptl. Biol. Med.* 119: 308–311, 1965.
29. CLARK, W. G. Maintenance of adrenalectomized guinea pigs. *Proc. Soc. Exptl. Biol. Med.* 46: 253–257, 1941.
30. CLEGHORN, R. A., J. L. A. FOWLER, W. F. GREENWOOD, AND A. P. W. CLARKE. Pressor responses in healthy adrenalectomized dogs. *Am. J. Physiol.* 161: 21–28, 1950.
31. COHN, C., B. KATZ, B. HUDDLESTAN, M. KOLINSKY, AND R. LEVINE. Utilization of carbohydrate by extrahepatic tissues of the adrenalectomized dog. *Am. J. Physiol.* 170: 87–93, 1952.
32. COLE, D. F. Chemical changes in the tissues of the rat after adrenalectomy. *J. Endocrinol.* 6: 245–250, 1950.
33. COLE, D. F. The effects of deoxycorticosterone acetate on electrolyte distribution in the tissues of the adrenalectomized rat. *J. Endocrinol.* 6: 251–255, 1950.
34. COLLIP, J. B., D. L. THOMSON, AND G. TOBY. The effect of adrenalin on muscle glycogen in adrenalectomized, thyroidectomized and hypophysectomized rats. *J. Physiol., London* 88: 191–198, 1936.
35. CONWAY, E. J., AND D. HINGERTY. Influence of adrenalectomy on muscle constituents. *Biochem. J.* 40: 561–568, 1946.

36. COPE, O., A. B. CORKILL, E. P. MARKS, AND S. OCHOA. A study of chemical changes associated with muscular contractions in normal and adrenalectomized animals. *J. Physiol., London* 82: 305–309, 1934.
37. CORI, C. F., AND G. T. CORI. The carbohydrate metabolism of adrenalectomized rats and mice. *J. Biol. Chem.* 74: 473–494, 1927.
38. CRABBÉ, J., AND P. DEWEER. Action of aldosterone on the bladder and skin of the toad. *Nature* 202: 298–299, 1964.
39. CUSHING, H. Basophil adenomas of the pituitary body and their clinical manifestations. *Bull. Johns Hopkins Hosp.* 50: 137–195, 1932.
40. D'AGOSTINO, A. N., AND M. CHIGA. Morphologic changes in cardiac and skeletal muscle induced by corticosteroids. *Ann. NY Acad. Sci.* 138: 73–81, 1966.
41. DARROW, D. C., H. E. HARRISON, AND M. TAFFEL. Tissue electrolytes in adrenal insufficiency. *J. Biol. Chem.* 130: 487–491, 1930.
42. DAVIES, R. E. A molecular theory of muscle contraction: calcium dependent contractions with hydrogen bond formation plus ATP-dependent extensions of part of the myosin-actin cross bridges. *Nature* 199: 1068–1074, 1963.
43. DECAMPOS, F. A., W. B. CANNON, H. LUNDIN, AND T. T. WALKER. Some conditions affecting the capacity for prolonged muscular work. *Am. J. Physiol.* 87: 680–701, 1929.
44. DEDUVE, C. General properties of lysosomes. The lysosome concept. In: *Ciba Foundation Symposium on Lysosomes*, edited by A. V. S. de Reuck and M. P. Cameron. Boston: Little, Brown, 1963, p. 1–31.
45. DEDUVE, C., AND H. BEAUFAY. Tissue fractionation studies. Influence of ischaemia on the state of some bound enzymes in rat liver. *Biochem. J.* 73: 610–616, 1959.
46. DEDUVE, C., R. WATTIAUX, AND M. WIBO. Effects of fat soluble compounds on lysosomes in vitro. *Biochem. Pharmacol.* 9: 97–116, 1962.
47. DE LOECKER, W., AND F. DE WEVER. The effects of cortisol on the in vitro glycine and leucine incorporation into the proteins of the 15,000 supernatant cell fraction of skeletal muscle. *Arch. Intern. Pharmacodyn.* 183: 344–351, 1970.
48. DE LOECKER, W., E. VAN DER SCHUEREN, AND F. DE WEVER. The effects of longterm cortisol treatment on the glycine-U-^{14}C incorporation in skeletal muscle proteins of rats. *Arch. Intern. Pharmacodyn.* 183: 352–359, 1970.
49. DEUEL, N. J., L. F. HALLMAN, S. MURRAY, AND L. T. SAMUELS. Rate of absorption of glucose and of glycogen formation in normal and adrenalectomized rats. *J. Biol. Chem.* 119: 607–615, 1937.
50. DIMAURO, S., C. ANGELINI, AND C. CATANI. Enzymes of the glycogen cycle and glycolysis in various human neuromuscular disorders. *J. Neurol. Neurosurg. Psychiat.* 30: 411–415, 1967.
51. DONALDSON, H. H. Summary of data for the effects of exercise on the organ weights of the albino rat. *Am. J. Anat.* 56: 57–70, 1935.
52. DRURY, D. R. Control of blood sugar. *J. Clin. Endocrinol. Metab.* 2: 421–430, 1942.
53. DURRANT, E. P. Effect of adrenal extirpation on the activity of the albino rat. *Am. J. Physiol.* 70: 344–350, 1924.
54. EDELMAN, I. S., R. BOGOROCH, AND G. A. PORTER. On the mechanism of action of aldosterone on sodium transport: the role of protein synthesis. *Proc. Natl. Acad. Sci. US* 50: 1169–1177, 1963.
55. EDELMAN, I. S., AND G. FIMOGNARI. On the biochemical mechanism of action of aldosterone. *Recent Progr. Hormone Res.* 24: 1–3, 1968.
56. ELLIS, J. T. Degeneration and regeneration in the muscles of cortisone treated rabbits. *Am. J. Phys. Med.* 32: 240–243, 1955.
57. ELLIS, J. T. Necrosis and regeneration of skeletal muscles in cortisone-treated rabbits. *Am. J. Pathol.* 32: 993–1013, 1956.
58. ELMAN, R., AND P. ROTHMAN. Adrenal insufficiency and atrophy of the cortex following venous obstruction of the suprarenal glands. *Johns Hopkins Hosp. Bull.* 35: 54–58, 1927.
59. ENGEL, F. L. Adrenal cortex and stress in the regulation of protein metabolism. *Recent Progr. Hormone Res.* 7: 277–308, 1950.
60. FALUDI, G., J. GOTLIEF, AND J. MEYERS. Factors influencing the development of steroid-induced myopathies. *Ann. NY Acad. Sci.* 138: 62–72, 1966.
61. FERGUSON, L. A., AND I. G. WOOL. Adrenal cortical hormone and incorporation of radioactivity into nucleic acid of isolated rat diaphragm. *Proc. Soc. Exptl. Biol. Med.* 110: 529–532, 1962.
62. FIMOGNARI, G. M., O. D. FANESTIL, AND I. S. EDELMAN. Induction of RNA and protein synthesis in the action of aldosterone in the rat. *Am. J. Physiol.* 213: 954–962, 1967.
63. FLUCKIGER, E., AND F. VERZAR. Die wirkung von Aldosteron auf den Natrium, Kalium and Glykogen Stoffwechsel des isolierten Muskels. *Experientia* 10: 259–261, 1954.
64. FOSS, M. L., R. J. BARNARD, AND C. M. TIPTON. Free 11-hydroxy corticoid levels in working dogs as affected by exercise training. *Endocrinology* 89: 96–104, 1971.
65. FRENCH, I. W., AND J. F. MANERY. The effect of aldosterone on electrolytes in muscle, kidney cortex and serum. *Can. J. Biochem.* 42: 1459–1476, 1964.
66. FREYBURG, R. H., C. A. BERNSTEN, AND L. HELLMAN. Further experience with triamcinolone in treatment of patients with rheumatoid arthritis. *Arthritis Rheumat.* 1: 215–229, 1958.
67. FRITZ, I., AND R. LEVINE. Action of adrenal cortical steroids and norepinephrine on vascular responses to stress in adrenalectomized rats. *Am. J. Physiol.* 165: 457–465, 1951.
68. GANS, H. M., AND H. M. MILEY. Ergographic studies on adrenalectomized animals. *Am. J. Physiol.* 82: 1–6, 1927.
69. GAUNT, R. A., J. H. BIRNIE, AND W. J. EVERSOLE. Adrenal cortex and water metabolism. *Physiol. Rev.* 29: 281–304, 1949.
70. GOLDBERG, A. L. Protein synthesis in tonic and phasic skeletal muscle. *Nature* 217: 1219–1220, 1967.
71. GOLDBERG, A. L. Protein synthesis during work-induced growth of skeletal muscle. *J. Cell Biol.* 37: 653–658, 1968.
72. GOLDBERG, A. L. Effects of denervation and cortisone on protein catabolism in skeletal muscle. *J. Biol. Chem.* 244: 3223–3229, 1969.
73. GOLDBERG, A. L., AND H. M. GOODMAN. Relationship between growth hormone and muscular work in determining muscle size. *J. Physiol., London* 200: 655–666, 1969.
74. GOLDBERG, A. L., AND H. M. GOODMAN. Relationship between cortisone and muscle work in determining muscle size. *J. Physiol., London* 200: 667–675, 1969.
75. GOLDING, D. N., S. M. MURRAY, G. W. PEARCE, AND M. THOMPSON. Corticosteroid myopathy. *Ann. Phys. Med.* 6: 171–177, 1961.
76. GOLDSTEIN, M. S., E. R. RAMEY, I. FRITZ, AND R. LEVINE. Reversal of effects of stress in adrenalectomized animals by autonomic blocking agents. *Am. J. Physiol.* 171: 92–99, 1952.
77. GOLDSTEIN, M. S., E. R. RAMEY, AND R. LEVINE. Relation of muscular fatigue in the adrenalectomized dog to inadequate circulatory adjustment. *Am. J. Physiol.* 163: 561–565, 1950.
78. GOLDZIEHER, M. A. *The Adrenals*. New York: Macmillan, 1929.
79. GOLLNICK, P. D., R. G. SOULE, A. W. TAYLOR, C. WILLIAMS, AND C. O. IANUZZO. Exercise induced glycogenolysis and lipolysis in the rat: hormonal influence. *Am. J. Physiol.* 219: 729–733, 1970.
80. GROSSIE, J., AND C. M. SMITH. Muscle afferent activity following adrenalectomy in cats. *Am. J. Physiol.* 212: 317–323, 1967.
81. GUILLEMIN, R. Hypothalamic factors releasing pituitary hormones. *Recent Progr. Hormone Res.* 20: 89–130, 1964.
82. HALES, W. M., G. M. HASLERUD, AND D. J. INGLE. Time for

development of incapacity to work in adrenalectomized rats. *Am. J. Physiol.* 112: 65–69, 1935.
83. HARRIS, R. E., AND D. J. INGLE. The capacity for vigorous muscular activity of normal rats and rats after removal of the adrenal medulla. *Am. J. Physiol.* 130: 150–154, 1940.
84. HARROP, G. A., JR., L. J. SOFFER, W. M. NICHOLSON, AND M. STRAUSS. The effect of sodium salts in sustaining the suprarenalectomized dog. *J. Exptl. Med.* 61: 839–860, 1935.
85. HARTMAN, F. A., AND J. E. LOCKWOOD. The effect of cortin on the nervous system in adrenal insufficiency. *Proc. Soc. Exptl. Biol. Med.* 29: 141–142, 1931.
86. HARTMAN, F. A., R. H. WAITE, AND E. F. POWELL. The relation of the adrenals to fatigue. *Am. J. Physiol.* 60: 255–269, 1922.
87. HASTINGS, A. B., AND E. L. COMPERE. The effect of bilateral suprarenalectomy on certain constituents of the blood of dogs. *Proc. Soc. Exptl. Biol. Med.* 28: 376–378, 1931.
88. HENKIN, R. I., J. R. GILL, AND F. C. BARTTER. Studies on taste thresholds in normal man and patients with adrenal cortical insufficiency: the role of adrenal cortical steroids and serum sodium concentration. *J. Clin. Invest.* 42: 727–735, 1963.
89. HENNES, A. R., B. L. WAJCHENBERG, AND S. S. FAJANS. The effect of adrenal steroids on blood levels of pyruvic and alpha-ketoglutaric acid in normal subjects. *Metab. Clin. Exptl.* 6: 339–345, 1957.
90. HERMAN, M. S., AND E. R. RAMEY. Effects of hydrocortisone and epinephrine on glucose uptake by the rat diaphragm. *Endocrinology* 67: 650–656, 1960.
91. HERMAN, M. S., AND E. R. RAMEY. Epinephrine action on glucose uptake by rat diaphragm. *Am. J. Physiol.* 199: 226–228, 1960.
92. HESS, M. E., C. E. ARANSON, D. W. HOTTENSTEIN, AND J. S. KARP. Effects of adrenal cortical hormones and thyroxine on phosphorylase activity in muscle. *Endocrinology* 84: 1107–1112, 1969.
93. HOUSSAY, B. A., AND J. T. LEWIS. The relative importance to life of cortex and medulla of the adrenal glands. *Am. J. Physiol.* 64: 512–521, 1923.
94. INGLE, D. J. The time for the occurrence of cortico-adrenal hypertrophy in rats during continued work. *Am. J. Physiol.* 124: 627–630, 1938.
95. INGLE, D. J. Work performance of hypophysectomized rats treated with cortin. *Am. J. Physiol.* 122: 302–305, 1938.
96. INGLE, D. J. The work performance of adrenalectomized rats maintained on a high sodium chloride low potassium diet. *Am. J. Physiol.* 129: 278–281, 1940.
97. INGLE, D. J. Effect of two cortin-like compounds upon the body weight and work performance of adrenalectomized rats. *Endocrinology* 27: 297–304, 1940.
98. INGLE, D. J. The work performance of adrenalectomized rats treated with corticosterone and chemically related compounds. *Endocrinology* 26: 472–477, 1940.
99. INGLE, D. J. The work capacity of the rat immediately following partial adrenalectomy. *Endocrinology* 26: 478–480, 1940.
100. INGLE, D. J. The quantitative assay of adrenal cortical hormones by the muscle work test in the adrenalectomized-nephrectomized rat. *Endocrinology* 34: 191–202, 1944.
101. INGLE, D. J. Permissibility of hormone action—a review. *Acta Endocrinol.* 17: 172–186, 1954.
102. INGLE, D. J., W. M. HALES, AND G. M. HASLERUD. Influence of partial adrenalectomy on the work capacity of rats. *Am. J. Physiol.* 113: 200–204, 1935.
103. INGLE, D. J., W. M. HALES, AND G. M. HASLERUD. Work capacity in the rat after destruction of the adrenal medulla. *Am. J. Physiol.* 114: 653–656, 1936.
104. INGLE, D. J., AND R. E. HARRIS. Voluntary activity of the rat after destruction of the adrenal medulla. *Am. J. Physiol.* 114: 657–660, 1936.
105. INGLE, D. J., AND M. H. KUIZENGA. The relative potency of some adrenal cortical steroids in the muscle work test. *Endocrinology* 36: 218–226, 1945.
106. INGLE, D. J., C. H. LI, AND H. M. EVANS. The effect of pure adrenocorticotropic hormone on the work performance of hypophysectomized rats. *Endocrinology* 35: 91–95, 1944.
107. INGLE, D. J., AND J. E. NEZAMIS. The work performance of adrenalectomized rats given continuous IV infusions of glucose. *Endocrinology* 43: 261–271, 1948.
108. INGLE, D. J., M. L. PABST, AND M. H. KUIZENGA. The effect of pretreatment on the relative potency of 11-desoxycorticosterone in the muscle work test. *Endocrinology* 36: 426–430, 1945.
109. IVANYUTA, O. M. Carbohydrate-phosphorus metabolism in the skeletal muscles of adrenalectomized animals during treatment with cortisone and Vit. C. and P. *Ukr. Biokhim. Zh.* 35: 30–34, 1963.
110. JAFFE, H. L. The effects of bilateral suprarenalectomy on the life of rats. *Am. J. Physiol.* 78: 453–461, 1926.
111. JANOFF, A., G. WEISSMAN, B. W. ZWEIFACH, AND L. THOMAS. Pathogenesis of experimental shock. IV. Studies of lysosomes in normal and tolerant animals subjected to lethal trauma and endotoxemia. *J. Exptl. Med.* 116: 451–466, 1962.
112. JANOFF, A., AND B. W. ZWEIFACH. Production of inflammatory changes in microcirculation of cationic proteins extracted from lysosomes. *J. Exptl. Med.* 120: 747–765, 1964.
113. KERPPOLA, A. Inhibition of phosphorylase with cortisone and its activation with adrenaline in the rabbit. *Endocrinology* 51: 192–202, 1952.
114. KIPNIS, D. M., AND C. F. CORI. Studies of tissue permeability. III. The effect of insulin on pentose uptake of the diaphragm. *J. Biol. Chem.* 224: 681–693, 1957.
115. KIT, S., AND E. S. G. BARRON. The effect of adrenal cortical hormones on the incorporation of C^{14} into the protein of lymphatic cells. *Endocrinology* 52: 1–9, 1953.
116. KLINE, D. A procedure for the study of factors which affect the nitrogen metabolism of isolated tissues: hormonal influences. *Endocrinology* 45: 596–604, 1949.
117. KNOWLTON, A. I., AND E. N. LOEB. Depletion of carcass potassium in rats made hypersensitive with desoxycorticosterone acetate (DCA) and with cortisone. *J. Clin. Invest.* 36: 1295–1300, 1947.
118. KOSTYO, J. L. In vitro effects of adrenal steroid hormones on amino acid transport in muscle. *Endocrinology* 76: 604–613, 1965.
119. KOSTYO, J. L., AND A. F. REDMOND. Role of protein synthesis in the inhibitory action of adrenal steroid hormones on amino acid transport by muscle. *Endocrinology* 79: 531–540, 1966.
120. KOSTYO, J. L., AND J. E. SCHMIDT. Inhibitory effects of cardiac glycosides and adrenal steroids on amino acid transport. *Am. J. Physiol.* 204: 1031–1038, 1963.
121. KOVANIC, P. Lysosome breakdown following adrenalectomy in rats adapted to trauma. *Federation Proc.* 27: 355, 1968.
122. KRAHL, M. E., AND C. F. CORI. The uptake of glucose by the isolated diaphragm of normal, diabetic, and adrenalectomized rats. *J. Biol. Chem.* 170: 607–618, 1947.
123. LANDAU, B. R. Adrenal steroids and carbohydrate metabolism. In: *Vitamins and Hormones*, edited by R. S. Harris, I. G. Wool, and J. A. Loraine. New York: Acad. Press, 1965, vol. 23, p. 2–59.
124. LAPLAUD, J., AND Y. M. GARGOUIL. Potential de membrane et potentiel d'action de la fibre musculaire squelettique du Rat surrénalectomisé. *Compt. Rend. Soc. Biol.* 253: 718–723, 1961.
125. LAPLAUD, J., AND Y. M. GARGOUIL. Restauration de la repolarisation membranaire de la fibre musculaire squelettique du Rat surrénalectomisé par l'acetate de D-aldostérone et divers corticoides. *Compt. Rend. Soc. Biol.* 155: 2439–2442, 1961.
126. LAWRENCE, C. H., AND A. W. ROSE. Studies of the endocrine glands. V. The adrenals. *Endocrinology* 13: 1–39, 1929.
127. LEATHEM, J. H. Some aspects of hormone and protein

127. metabolic interrelativity. In: *Mammalian Protein Metabolism*, edited by H. N. Munro and J. H. Allison. New York: Acad. Press, 1964, vol. I, p. 343–381.
128. LEFER, A. M. Influence of corticosteroids on mechanical performance of rat papillary muscles. *Am. J. Physiol.* 214: 518–524, 1968.
129. LEONARD, S. I. The effect of hormones on phosphorylase activity in skeletal muscle. *Endocrinology* 60: 619–624, 1957.
130. LEVINE, R., B. SIMPKIN, AND W. CUNNINGHAM. Insulin sensitivity of the extrahepatic tissues of the adrenalectomized rat. *Am. J. Physiol.* 159: 111–117, 1949.
131. LEVITAN, R., AND F. J. INGELFINGER. Effect of d-aldosterone on salt and water absorption from the intact human colon. *J. Clin. Invest.* 44: 801–808, 1965.
132. LIM, V. S., AND G. W. WEBSTER. The effect of aldosterone on water and electrolyte composition of incubated rat diaphragms. *Clin. Sci.* 33: 261–270, 1967.
133. LONG, C. N. H., B. KATZIN, AND E. G. FRY. The adrenal cortex and carbohydrate metabolism. *Endocrinology* 26: 309–344, 1940.
134. LONG, C. N. H., AND O. K. SMITH. Recent studies on the adrenal cortex and carbohydrate metabolism. In: *Human Adrenal Cortex*, edited by A. R. Currie, T. Symington, and J. K. Grant. Baltimore: Williams & Wilkins, 1962, p. 268–293.
135. MANCHESTER, K. L., AND F. G. YOUNG. Hormone and protein biosynthesis in isolated rat diaphragm. *J. Endocrinol.* 18: 381–394, 1959.
136. MARINE, D., E. J. BAUMANN, AND A. CAPRA. The effect of feeding emulsions of the interrenal gland to rabbits. *Am. J. Physiol.* 72: 248–252, 1925.
137. MAUERHOFER, E. Adrenals, removal of in rats, fatigue test followed. *Z. Biol.* 74: 147–151, 1922.
138. MILNE, M. D. Biochemical and physiological changes in primary aldosteronism and in experimental potassium deficiency. In: *Human Adrenal Cortex*, edited by A. R. Currie, T. Symington, and J. K. Grant. Baltimore: Williams & Wilkins, 1962, p. 493–509.
139. MULLER, R., AND E. KUGELBERG. Myopathy in Cushing's disease. *J. Neurol. Neurosurg. Psychiat.* 22: 314–320, 1959.
140. MUNCK, A. Glucocorticoid inhibition of glucose uptake by peripheral tissues: old and new evidence, molecular mechanisms, and physiological significance. *Perspectives Biol. Med.* 14: 265–289, 1971.
141. MUNRO, H. N. General aspects of the regulation of protein metabolism by diet and hormones. In: *Mammalian Protein Metabolism*, edited by H. N. Munro and J. B. Allison. New York: Acad. Press, 1964, vol. I, p. 343–381.
142. NACHMANSOHN, D. Lactic acid formation in the muscles of adrenalectomized animals. *J. Physiol., London* 81: 36P, 1934.
143. NEUBERGER, A., AND F. F. RICHARDS. Studies of turnover in the whole animal. In: *Mammalian Protein Metabolism*, edited by H. N. Munro and J. B. Allison. New York: Acad. Press, 1964, vol. I, p. 243–297.
144. NEWSHOLME E. A., P. J. RANDLE, AND K. L. MANCHESTER. Inhibition of the phosphofructokinase reaction in perfused rat heart by respiration of ketone bodies, fatty acids and pyruvate. *Nature* 193: 270–271, 1962.
145. NOALL, M. W., T. R. RIGGS, L. M. WALKER, AND H. N. CHRISTENSEN. Endocrine control of amino acid transfer. *Science* 126: 1002–1005, 1957.
146. PELLEGRINO, C., AND C. FRANZINI. An electron microscope study of denervation atrophy in red and white skeletal muscle fibers. *J. Cell Biol.* 17: 327–349, 1963.
147. PERKHOFF, G. T., R. SILBER, F. H. TYLER, G. E. CARTWRIGHT, AND M. M. WINTROBE. Myopathy due to administration of therapeutic amounts of 17-hydroxycorticosteroids. *Am. J. Med.* 27: 891–898, 1959.
148. PETERS, R. F., M. C. RICHARDSON, M. SMALL, AND A. M. WHITE. Some biochemical effects of triamcinolone acetonide on rat liver and muscle. *Biochem. J.* 116: 349–355, 1970.
149. PORTER, G. A., R. BOGOROCH, AND I. S. EDELMAN. On the mechanism of action of aldosterone on sodium transport: the role of RNA synthesis. *Proc. Natl. Acad. Sci. US* 52: 1326–1333, 1964.
150. POWELL, R. J. Steroid and hypokalemic myopathy after corticosteroids for ulcerative colitis. *Am. J. Gastroenterol.* 52: 425–432, 1969.
151. RAMEY, E. R., AND M. S. GOLDSTEIN. The adrenal cortex and the sympathetic nervous system. *Physiol. Rev.* 37: 155–195, 1957.
152. RAMEY, E., M. S. GOLDSTEIN, AND R. LEVINE. Mechanism of muscular fatigue in adrenalectomized animals. *Am. J. Physiol.* 162: 10–16, 1950.
153. RAMEY, E., M. S. GOLDSTEIN, AND R. LEVINE. Action of norepinephrine and adrenal cortical steroids on blood pressure and work performance of adrenalectomized dogs. *Am. J. Physiol.* 165: 450–456, 1951.
154. RAMWELL, P. W., AND J. E. SHAW. Biological significance of the prostaglandins. *Recent Progr. Hormone Res.* 26: 139–173, 1970.
155. RANDLE, P. J., C. N. HALES, P. B. GARLAND, AND E. A. NEWSHOLME. The glucose fatty acid cycle: its role in insulin sensitivity and the metabolic disturbances of diabetes mellitus. *Lancet* 1: 785–789, 1963.
156. ROVETTO, M. J., AND A. M. LEFER. Electrophysiological properties of cardiac muscle in adrenal insufficiency. *Am. J. Physiol.* 218: 1015–1019, 1970.
157. RUSSELL, J. A. The relationship of the anterior pituitary and the adrenal cortex in the metabolism of carbohydrate. *Am. J. Physiol.* 128: 552–561, 1940.
158. RUSSELL, J. A. The adrenals and the hypophysis in the carbohydrate metabolism of the eviscerated rat. *Am. J. Physiol.* 140: 98–106, 1943.
159. RUSSELL, J. A., AND A. E. WILHELMI. Endocrines and muscle. In: *Structure and Function of Muscle*, edited by G. H. Bourne. New York: Acad. Press, 1960, vol. II, p. 141–198.
160. SAYERS, G. Adrenal cortex and homeostasis. *Physiol. Rev.* 30: 241–300, 1950.
161. SCHAEFFER, L. D., M. CHENOWETH, AND A. DUNN. Adrenal corticosteroid involvement in the control of phosphorylase in muscle. *Biochim. Biophys. Acta* 192: 304–309, 1969.
162. SCHWEITZER, A. The effect of adrenalectomy on the contractile power of skeletal muscle. *J. Physiol., London* 104: 21–31, 1947.
163. SECKER, J. The role of the adrenal cortex in the maintenance of the sciatic pressor reflex. *J. Physiol., London* 109: 49–52, 1949.
164. SEXTON, A. W. Isometric tension of glycerinated muscle fibers following adrenalectomy. *Am. J. Physiol.* 212: 313–316, 1967.
165. SHARP, G. W. G., AND A. LEAF. The central role of pyruvate in the stimulation of sodium transport by aldosterone. *Proc. Natl. Acad. Sci. US* 52: 1114–1121, 1964.
166. SHARP, G. W. G., AND A. LEAF. Studies in the mode of action of aldosterone. *Recent Progr. Hormone Res.* 22: 431–471, 1966.
167. SHEAHAN, M. G., AND P. J. VIGNOS, JR. Experimental corticosteroid myopathy. *Arthritis Rheumat.* 12: 491–497, 1969.
168. SIE, H. G., AND W. H. FISHMAN. Glycogen synthetase: its response to cortisol. *Science* 143: 816–817, 1964.
169. SMITH, B. Histological and histochemical changes in the muscles of rabbits given the corticosteroid triamcinolone. *Neurology* 14: 857–863, 1964.
170. SMITH, O. K., AND C. N. H. LONG. Effect of cortisol on the plasma amino nitrogen of eviscerated adrenalectomized diabetic rats. *Endocrinology* 80: 561–566, 1967.
171. SOFFER, L. J. *Diseases of the Endocrine Glands*. Philadelphia: Lea & Febiger, 1956, p. 285–286.
172. SUZUKI, T. Electron microscopic study on the effects of adrenalectomy on heart muscle. *Tohoku J. Exptl. Med.* 91: 239–253, 1967.
173. SUZUKI, T., K. OTSUKO, H. MATSUI, S. OHUKUZI, K. SAKAI,

AND Y. HARADA. Effect of muscular exercise on adrenal 17-hydroxycorticosteroid secretion in the dog. *Endocrinology* 80: 1148–1151, 1967.
174. SWINGLE, W. W. Studies on the functional significance of the suprarenal cortex. *Am. J. Physiol.* 79: 669–678, 1927.
175. SWINGLE, W. W., L. J. BRANNICK, M. OSBORN, AND D. GLENESTER. Effect of gluco- and mineralocorticoid adrenal steroids on fluid and electrolytes of fasted adrenalectomized dogs. *Proc. Soc. Exptl. Biol. Med.* 96: 446–452, 1957.
176. SWINGLE, W. W., AND A. J. EISENMAN. Studies on the functional significance of the suprarenal cortex. *Am. J. Physiol.* 79: 679–688, 1927.
177. SWINGLE, W. W., AND J. W. REMINGTON. The role of the adrenal cortex in physiological processes. *Physiol. Rev.* 24: 89–127, 1944.
178. SZENT-GYORGI, A. Free-energy relations and contraction of actomyosin. *Biol. Bull.* 96: 140–161, 1949.
179. TIPTON, C. M., P. J. STRUCK, K. M. BALDWIN, R. D. MATTHES, AND R. T. DOWELL. Response of adrenalectomized rats to chronic stress. *Endocrinology* 91: 573, 1972.
180. TROWBRIDGE, G., AND J. R. JORDON. Loss of potassium from stimulated muscles in adrenalectomized cats. *Am. J. Physiol.* 148: 222–228, 1947.
181. VELICK, S. F. The metabolism of myosin, the meromyosins, actin and tropomyosin in the rabbit. *Biochim. Biophys. Acta* 20: 228–236, 1956.
182. VOEGTLI, W. Der Einfluss des Electrolytmilieus auf Glycogenbildung und Arbeitsleustung des Isolierten Diophragmas normaler und Adrenalektomierter Tiere. *Helv. Physiol. Pharmacol. Acta* 8: 74–78, 1950.
183. WALKER, M. D., R. I. HENKIN, A. B. HARLAN, AND A. G. T. CASPER. Distribution of tritiated cortisol in blood, brain, CSF and other tissues of the cat. *Endocrinology* 88: 224–232, 1971.
184. WALKER, S. M. The response of triceps sural of normal, adrenalectomized DOCA treated and KCl treated rats to direct and indirect, single and repetitive stimulation. *Am. J. Physiol.* 149: 7–23, 1947.
185. WEISSMANN, G. Lysosomes. *New Engl. J. Med.* 273: 1084–1090, 1965.
186. WEISSMAN, G., AND L. THOMAS. Studies of lysosomes. II. The effect of cortisone on the release of acid hydrolases from a large granule fraction of rabbit liver induced by an excess of vitamin A. *J. Clin. Invest.* 42: 661–669, 1963.
187. WELLS, B. B. The influence of crystalline compounds separated from the adrenal cortex on gluconeogenesis. *Proc. Staff Meeting Mayo Clinic* 15: 294–297, 1940.
188. WHEELER, T. D., AND S. VINCENT. The question as to the relative importance to life of the cortex and medulla of the adrenal bodies. *Trans. Roy. Soc. Can. Sect. IV* 11: 125–132, 1917.
189. WICK, A. N., AND D. R. DRURY. The disposition of glucose by the extrahepatic tissues. *Ann. NY Acad. Sci.* 54: 684–692, 1951.
190. WILLIAMS, R. H. *Textbook of Endocrinology*. Philadelphia: Saunders, 1969, p. 287–379.
191. WILLIAMSON, H. E. Mechanism of the antinatriuretic action of aldosterone. *Biochem. Pharmacol.* 12: 1448–1452, 1963.
192. WINTER, C. A., AND L. FLATAKER. Work performance of trained rats as affected by cortical steroids and by adrenalectomy. *Am. J. Physiol.* 199: 863–866, 1960.
193. WINTER, C. A., AND G. C. KNOWLTON. The effect of adrenalectomy and of fasting on the functional capacity of the rat's gastrocnemius. *Am. J. Physiol.* 131: 465–469, 1940.
194. WISLOCKI, G. B., AND S. J. CROWE. Experimental observations on the adrenal and the chromaffin system. *Bull. Johns Hopkins Hosp.* 35: 187–193, 1924.
195. WOODBURY, D. M. Extrarenal effects of desoxycorticosterone, adrenocortical extract and adrenocorticotrophic hormone on plasma and tissue electrolytes in fed and fasted rats. *Am. J. Physiol.* 174: 1–19, 1953.
196. WOODBURY, D. M. Relation between the adrenal cortex and the central nervous system. *Pharmacol. Rev.* 10: 275–357, 1958.
197. WOOL, I. G. Corticosteroids and accumulation of ^{14}C labeled amino acids and histamine by isolated rat diaphragm. *Am. J. Physiol.* 199: 715–718, 1960.
198. WOOL, I. G. Accumulation of substrate by isolated rat diaphragm: a possible mechanism for the anti-inflammatory action of corticosteroids. *Nature* 186: 728, 1960.
199. WOOL, I. G., AND A. N. MOYER. Effect of actinomycin and insulin on the metabolism of isolated rat diaphragm. *Biochim. Biophys. Acta* 91: 248–256, 1964.
200. WOOL, I. G., AND E. I. WEINSHELBAUM. Incorporation of C^{14}-amino acids into protein of isolated diaphragms: role of the adrenal steroids. *Am. J. Physiol.* 197: 1089–1092, 1959.
201. WOOL, I. G., AND E. I. WEINSHELBAUM. Corticosteroids and incorporation of C^{14}-phenylalanine into protein of isolated rat diaphragm. *Am. J. Physiol.* 198: 1111–1114, 1960.
202. WOOL, I. G., AND E. I. WEINSHELBAUM. Adrenal cortical hormones and incorporation of C^{14} from amino acid precursors into muscle protein. *Am. J. Physiol.* 198: 360–362, 1960.
203. WRIGHT, E. B., AND E. J. LESTER. Effect of adrenalectomy and cortisone on peripheral nerve function. *Am. J. Physiol.* 169: 1057–1062, 1959.
204. YOUNG, D. A. Hepatic adenosine triphosphate, glucose p-phosphate, and uridine diphosphoglucose levels in fasted, adrenalectomized and control treated rats. *Arch. Biochem.* 114: 309–313, 1966.
205. ZWEMER, R. L. An experimental study of the adrenal cortex. The survival value of the adrenal cortex. *Am. J. Physiol.* 79: 641–657, 1927.
206. ZWEMER, R. L. A study of adrenal cortex morphology. *Am. J. Pathol.* 12: 107–114, 1936.

# CHAPTER 18

Corticosteroids, inflammation, and connective tissue

DAVID M. SPAIN | *Department of Pathology, Brookdale Hospital Medical Center, Brooklyn, New York*

CHAPTER CONTENTS

Inflammatory Process
General Effects and Chemical Structure of Glucocorticoid Molecules
Localization of Corticosteroids
Glucocorticoids and Vascular Permeability
Glucocorticoids and Cellular Response to Inflammation
Glucocorticoids and Lymphatic Tissue
Cortisol and the Fibroblast
Steroids and Connective Tissue
Cortisone, Lysosomes, and Inflammation
Cortisone, Platelets, and Inflammation
Conclusion

THE EFFECT of the adrenal glucocorticoid hormones on inflammation and the repair process is complex and, in most fundamental areas, still unclear. Difficulty results from the many unresolved questions concerning the pathogenesis and factors in the inflammatory process itself. Significant gaps also exist concerning knowledge of the repair process: the formation, resorption, or dissolution of reticulin, ground substance, and collagen. Glucocorticoids tend to suppress the entire inflammatory process and therefore the production of everything characteristic of it—capillary permeability, diapedesis, exudation, antibody formation, granulomatous proliferation, and the repair process. But, despite much knowledge of the many effects of corticosteroids on both cellular and metabolic levels for the different isolated, individual components of inflammation and repair, an integrated understanding of these compounds' anti-inflammatory actions is still lacking. Understanding is hindered by the marked variation in experimental models used for studying inflammation and a failure to correlate the different approaches to the problem.

INFLAMMATORY PROCESS

Inflammation is a reaction of living tissue to injury; it is comprised of a series of changes in the terminal vascular bed, in the blood, and in the connective tissue that tend to eliminate or neutralize the noxious causative agent and to repair the damaged tissue. Corticosteroids clearly act on several sites of the inflammatory process. To understand this, it is helpful to summarize the various factors thought to play a role in the acute inflammatory reaction, including the ultrastructure of the vascular wall (blood-tissue barrier). Important anatomic components of this barrier are the living endothelial cells, the intercellular junctions, the endocapillary layer, the basement membrane, collagen fibrils, elastic elements, and perivascular cells. Intercellular junctions—pathways across the blood-tissue barrier—are also involved. For a discontinuous endothelium they are remarkably simple. For continuous endothelium the pathway is more complex and less clearly understood. Three mechanisms have been postulated to explain transport along this pathway: *1*) direct passage through the endothelium without any preexisting pores or transport vesicles; *2*) transport by means of vesicles; and *3*) intercellular passage by means of pores.

The vascular phenomena basic to acute inflammation consist of changes in vessel wall tone, in rate of blood flow, and in the number and quality of formed and fluid elements of the blood. Thrombosis, hemorrhage, stasis of blood flow, and hyperemia may occur in different degrees. Crucial are the factors believed to modify the blood-tissue barrier because they alter vascular permeability and increase or decrease the exudation of formed and cellular elements.

Alterations in the rate of blood flow, increased filtration and hydrostatic pressure, and structural or functional modifications in the vascular wall account for part of the changes in vascular permeability. By ultrastructural study, two phases of increase of vascular permeability have been noted to account for much of inflammatory exudation—an immediate but transient episode of vascular leakage and a later, delayed but more permanent period of vascular leakage. These vascular leaks may result from direct injury to the vessel wall by a host of noxious agents or may be mediated chemically.

Several classes of chemical mediators have been delineated and are currently under investigation: *a*) vasoactive amines of which histamine, serotonin, epinephrine, and norepinephrine are representative; *b*) proteases and other enzymes, including the Hagamen factor, the kininogenases, plasmin, the plasma kinin system, the complement system, and the dermal permeability factors; *c*) polypeptides, including leukotaxine and related substances; *d*) polypeptides derived from known proteins, basic and acidic polypeptides, and the kinins; *e*) nucleic acids and their derivatives; and *f*) lipid-soluble acids. Increasing consideration is given to the role of the lysosomes in tissue injury and inflammation, as well as to the polymorphonuclear (PMN) leukocytes and tissue injury, as ultimately related to an increase in vascular permeability.

Cell migration as part of the exudative process, the role and function of the various cell types (granulocytes, monocytes, lymphocytes, plasma cells, and platelets), chemotaxis, and phagocytosis contribute complexity to the inflammatory process.

Special attention must be given to the mast cell because of the striking effects of the corticosteroids on these cells. The factors influencing phagocytosis, the role of complement in cell membrane stability, and the role of antibody complexes further compound the understanding since most of these elements probably interact at various levels and in time. The isolation and study of any single line of action and reaction are tedious, if not impossible—and the observations and conclusions drawn from such a study may be meaningless when related to the intact human.

The repair process, a direct extension of the inflammatory process, also involves the origin, growth, and metabolism of the fibroblast, growth stimuli, and inhibitors and the origin, fate, and chemical nature of the ground substance, collagen, and the relationship to fibrin and the fibrinolytic system (70, 71, 76).

GENERAL EFFECTS AND CHEMICAL STRUCTURE OF GLUCOCORTICOID MOLECULES

Ever since Harvey Cushing described the signs and symptoms produced in man by a basophilic adenoma of the pituitary gland, a condition associated with excessive levels of cortisol, it has been suspected that adrenal cortical steroids influence inflammation and repair. Discovery by Hench et al. (35) and Kendall (41a) of the usefulness of cortisone and ACTH on rheumatoid arthritis was the prelude to the continuing series of studies on the relationship of these steroids to inflammation and the repair process. Actually, Menckin (52) in 1942 experimentally suppressed the inflammatory process with compound E, later identified as cortisone, and Dougherty & Schneebeli (21) in 1950 demonstrated the role of cortisone in the regulation of inflammation. Spain et al. (67) inhibited wound healing and the formation of granulation tissue in mice with cortisone. Ragan et al. (59) also demonstrated some of the effects of ACTH and cortisone on connective tissue.

With the synthesis of 9α-fluoro derivatives of cortisone and hydrocortisone by Fried & Sabo (26) and with the synthesis and study of the biological activity of 1- and 6-dehydro-9α-halocorticoids by Fried et al. (25), agents more potent than the natural adrenocorticoids became available for study. It was soon learned that specific chemical groupings were responsible for the special pharmacological effects of these corticoids and that almost every portion of the cortisol molecule was important in determining biological activity.

In addition to the anti-inflammatory and granulation tissue-suppressing activity, other major effects on protein metabolism, sodium retention, potassium excretion, and hyperglycemia were noted with reduced carbohydrate tolerance. Attempts were made to alter the molecular structure to eliminate or diminish these latter effects and, at the same time, to retain the ability to suppress inflammation. Some modifications of structure have been successful in producing increases in the ratio of anti-inflammatory to sodium-retaining activity. In all compounds so far studied, however, no change in the ratio of anti-inflammatory activity to the effects on protein and carbohydrate metabolism has been noted.

Although cortisone was the first adrenal corticosteroid recognized to have anti-inflammatory activity, it is actually cortisol that is the principal anti-inflammatory adrenocortical hormone. Cortisone, to be active, must be transformed in the body to cortisol. Normally the adult adrenal gland secretes from 20 to 35 mg of cortisol per day. Such physiological quantities have little effect other than suppressing the secretion of endogenous corticosteroids. Superphysiological doses are required to produce the anti-inflammatory and other effects (47).

The structural alterations in the molecule that change absorption, protein binding, metabolic transformation rate, rate of excretion, and the ability to cross membranes can modify biological activity. The sites of alteration that increase the ratio of anti-inflammatory to sodium-retaining potency are shown in Figure 1, and some of the altered compounds are listed in Table 1.

The 4,5 double bond and the 3-ketone in ring A are essential for typical adrenocorticosteroid activity. In prednisone the introduction of a 1,2 double bond increases the effects on carbohydrate metabolism without materially changing sodium-retaining potency. The slower metabolic transformation of prednisolone, as compared to cortisol, cannot completely explain the increase in carbohydrate-regulating potency because electrolyte regulation is not increased.

The effects of 6α substitution in ring B are unpredictable. With cortisol, acute inflammatory, nitrogen-wasting, and sodium-retaining effects in man are increased. The only example of a 6α-methylated compound in wide use that has a somewhat more favorable anti-inflammatory-to-sodium-retaining ratio is 6α-methylprednisolone. All biological activities are increased by 9α-fluorination in ring B.

The presence of an oxygen function at C-11 in ring C

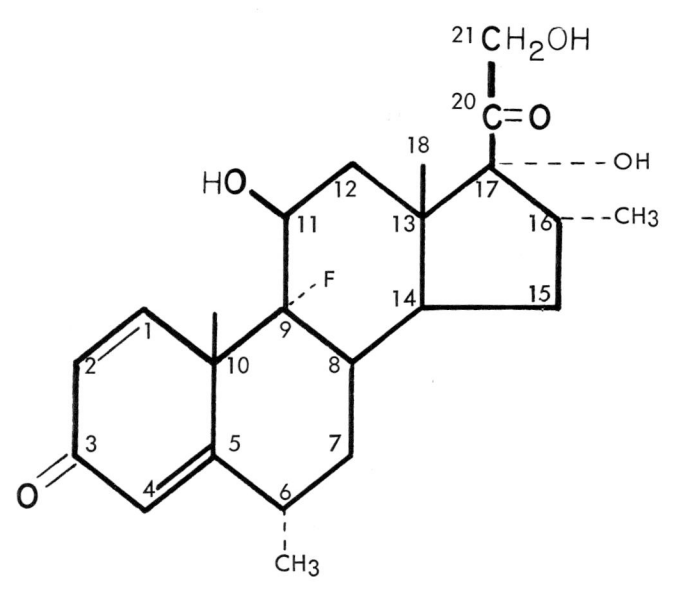

FIG. 1. Structure-activity relations of adrenocorticosteroids. *Heavier lines* indicate structure common to all anti-inflammatory steroids.

TABLE 1. *Relative Anti-inflammatory Potency and Sodium-retaining Effect of Various Therapeutic Corticoids*

Compound	Anti-inflammatory Potency	Sodium-retaining Activity
Hydrocortisone (cortisol)	1	++
Cortisone acetate	0.8	++
Prednisolone acetate (Δ^1-cortisol)	4	+
Prednisone acetate	3.5	+
Triamcinolone (9α-fluoro-16α-hydroxyprednisolone)	5	0
6α-Methylprednisolone	5	0
Paramethasone (6α-fluoro-16α-methylprednisolone)	10	0
Betamethasone (9α-fluoro-16β-methylprednisolone)	25	0
Dexamethasone (9α-fluoro-16α-methylprednisolone)	30	0
9α-Fluorohydrocortisone	15	+++++

is necessary for anti-inflammatory and carbohydrate-regulating potency but not for sodium retention. For this reason, oxidation of 11β-hydroxy compounds to 11-keto compounds significantly decreases these activities. The remaining activity may be related to metabolic transformation to the 11β-hydroxy congener.

All available anti-inflammatory steroids are 17α-hydroxy compounds produced by 16-methylation or hydroxylation in ring D. This partially modifies the activity on organic metabolism and inflammation but sharply decreases sodium retention. These 16-substituted compounds include paramethasone, dexamethasone, and triamcinolone.

The natural corticosteroids and many of the active synthetic compounds have a 21-hydroxy group. The presence of this group is essential for significant sodium-retaining potency. No glucocorticoid compound is unique in being therapeutic without eliciting some harmful effects.

LOCALIZATION OF CORTICOSTEROIDS

Corticosteroids appear to affect the inflammatory process by localizing in the inflamed or injured areas at a higher concentration than in other tissues or organs of the body. Curves plotted to show the rate of increase and decrease in the amount of ^{14}C-labeled cortisol indicate more radioactivity at the inflamed site than at any other site (18). However, measurement of radioactivity does not provide an accurate estimate of anti-inflammatory active substance because the molecule is undergoing oxidative and reductive changes that alter it into compounds with different biological activity. No specific trapping mechanism in inflamed tissue has been noted to account for the higher concentration of cortisol. The increased concentration seems rather a result of the increased blood flow and increased permeability in the early stages of the inflammatory process (18). This is nonspecific, and whether the substance involved is cortisol, trypan blue, or something else matters little (52a). Later, in inflammation resulting from differential changes in vascular permeability—part of which may have been accounted for by the cortisol itself—the situation may become reversed, that is, vascular permeability may be decreased (20).

GLUCOCORTICOIDS AND VASCULAR PERMEABILITY

As mentioned above, inflammation is a complex biological reaction characterized by an increase in vascular permeability, diapedesis, exudation, antibody formation, and granulomatous proliferation. The influence of glucocorticoids on vascular permeability is very important. Most recent findings indicate that the increase in vascular permeability may occur in the absence of venous constriction and thus support the view that a histamine type of mediation induces vascular leakage by exerting a direct effect on the endothelial cells or their junctions to cause retraction of the margins of the endothelial cells bordering large pores in the vessel wall (13). Histamine is considered one of the important mediators of vascular permeability in the inflammatory process (48, 49).

Histamine is present in most tissues and is widely distributed in most physiological fluids (71). The content of histamine in tissue is closely related to the number of mast cells present. Platelets are another important source of histamine and, with the mast cells, may constitute the major source of histamine after an injury.

Although the actual role of mast cells in the development of inflammatory reaction is not established, enough is known about the response of mast cells to various stimuli to justify some speculations about the extracellular events likely to occur as a consequence of local mast cell reactions. Within the mast cell are many biologically active substances that may affect different phases of the inflammatory process. Among these are histamine, 5-hydroxytryptamine, and various proteases (41, 79). One of the earliest observations concerning cortisol and the inflammatory process was its effect on the mast cell. Studies dating from 1950 and extending over a decade indicate that, in man and other animals, adrenal glucocorticoids will produce a diminution in the number of mast cells present at a local site of injury, as well as a change in their appearance, with the mast cells becoming vacuolated and acquiring irregular outlines. The intracellular granules that normally stain metachromatically with toluidine blue may now require an orthochromatic stain. The granules clump together to form bodies of various sizes (1, 3). Cortisol also inhibits mast cell activity in tissue cultures of embryonic skin and spleen and interferes with the uptake of $^{35}SO_4$ by mammalian mast cells. This effect of glucocorticoids on mast cells may diminish, for a period of time, the amount of histamine at the inflammatory site and thereby diminish the vascular permeability so essential to the process of inflammation. Inhibition may also take place through failure of the release of some of the other chemical mediators also present in the mast cells (41, 70, 79).

When peritoneal mast cells from previously sensitized rats are incubated in vitro with a specific antigen, histamine is liberated. Treatment of these animals with cortisol and other antirheumatic agents inhibits the antigenic histamine release from the mast cells. If the cortisol is administered toward the end of the sensitization period, it depresses the antigen-antibody reaction or enzyme release; if it is given at the beginning of the sensitization period, it inhibits antibody production (55).

The mechanics of mast cell degranulation and the process whereby cortisol inhibits degranulation are still unknown, but information about the intimate nature of the cell membrane changes occurring with degranulation are fundamental to the understanding of the release of histamine. The changes in the membrane leading to degranulation induced by the synthetic polymer amine, compound 48/80, or the changes in the membrane that inhibit degranulation, as induced by cortisol, must be a transient and reversible process since, at least with the former process, the cell does not appear to be injured (79).

Permeability factors have been isolated from tissue extracts; the appearance of some of these have been induced in rat skin and fibroblasts by various anti-inflammatory drugs, including cortisol and prednisolone. The most interesting of these is "cortisol released activating protease" obtained from rat skin. It markedly increases vascular permeability, which apparently is not related to histamine. This protease also stimulates emigration of leukocytes, digestion of dermal collagenase-ogen to free collagenase, and conversion of fibrinogen to fibrin. The ability of this cortisol-induced skin protease, as described above, plus the activation of plasminogen and the further ability to destroy bradykinin may be important in anti-inflammation. In this latter situation at least three proteases are released, one of which seems highly specific for the phenylalanine-serine bond in bradykinin (28a, 36, 71).

GLUCOCORTICOIDS AND CELLULAR RESPONSE TO INFLAMMATION

The all-important cellular response in inflammation is modified profoundly by glucocorticoids. Four cells in particular come under consideration: the polymorphonuclear leukocyte, the monocyte, the lymphocyte, and the plasma cell. The first two are most important in the nonspecific inflammatory reaction, whereas the latter two are more prominent in allergic inflammation. The more obvious end stage effects of glucocorticoids on the "inflammatory cells," whether mediated directly or indirectly, can be summarized as follows:

1. Glucocorticoids affect PMN leukocytes by depressing their stickiness, diapedesis, ameboid activity, phagocytosis, digestive power, and glycolysis, but the number of PMN leukocytes in blood increases along with their survival time (15, 27, 29, 42, 60).

2. Glucocorticoids affect monocytes by depressing mitoses, diapedesis, phagocytosis, digestive power, and granuloma formation. Intracellular parasite survival time is increased (44, 54).

3. Glucocorticoids, by their effects on lymphatic tissue and lymphocytes in particular, depress their number in the tissue and blood, and their glycolytic activity is decreased. Also active delayed hypersensitivity and the passive transfer of delayed hypersensitivity are depressed. However, donor cell activity, the transfer of delayed hypersensitivity, and lactate production seem to remain unchanged (24, 73).

4. Glucocorticoids affect plasma cells by suppressing cellular metabolism at a stage of rapid cell development so that the rate of antibody production is modified. Therefore, with primary antigenic stimuli, mitoses and antibody formation are suppressed, but with secondary antigenic stimuli, there is less effect on antibody formation and fewer mitoses are suppressed (24, 27). [For a more extensive description of the effect of glucocorticoids on inflammatory cells, see (24, 61).]

GLUCOCORTICOIDS AND LYMPHATIC TISSUE

Lymphatic tissue is involved in the inflammatory process—directly with the cells derived from lymphoid tissue present in ever increasing numbers at the site of inflammation and indirectly on the humoral level by the formation of antigen-antibody complexes. Corticoid induces the involution of lymphatic tissue and the cessation of lymphocyte mitoses. Equally significant are the metabolic processes within lymphatic tissue that are inhibited (73).

Dougherty & White (22) demonstrated that a single

treatment with adrenocortical hormone produced involution of lymphatic tissue within 3 hr. This effect persisted for about 9 hr and then diminished. Dougherty et al. (19) showed that the maximal concentration of cortisol in lymphatic tissue occurs within 15 min after administration and then diminishes. The antimitotic effect of cortisol on lymphatic tissue may be related to interference with DNA synthesis. By using adenine-8-^{14}C as a precursor, Brink-Johnsen & Dougherty (12) demonstrated that large doses of cortisol depleted nucleic acids and inhibited DNA synthesis in mouse lymphatic tissue. Stevens et al. (73), however, showed that the inhibition of DNA (in the spleen) was relatively insignificant. Nevertheless, Molomut, Spain, and Haber (52b) showed a marked reduction in spleen size in mice within 24 hr of cortisone administration. Stevens et al. (73) also noted, with leucine-1-^{14}C incorporation in the spleen, thymus, and lymph nodes, that cortisol administered for short time intervals affects protein synthesis but decreases conversion of glucose carbon into nucleic acids and protein.

Drury (23) and Ingle (39) postulated that the primary physiological effect of cortisol was to decrease glucose utilization by certain extrahepatic tissues. This would in turn lead to other metabolic changes attributed indirectly to cortisol. Cortisol may produce some of its effects by regulating genes in certain responsive cell types; Hechter & Halkerston (34) presented considerable evidence to support the contention that the mechanism of hormone action involves the regulation of gene activity, as expressed by the synthesis of specific proteins. In 1966 Goldberg & Atchley (30), by incubating DNA with cortisol obtained from human placental nuclei, observed a weakening of the intra-strand bonds of DNA. They interpreted this to mean that cortisol might activate genes by stimulating separation of the complementary strands of specific segments of DNA double helix before transcription.

Cortisol may also exert its influence by the physical disruption of the stereochemical relationships in the lamellar structures within the cell and by disturbing the spacial relationship of water structure. Based on this concept, Hechter (33) and Berendsen (4) postulated a chain reaction passing through the cell and disrupting those stereochemical relations that are essential for the operation of complex metabolic reactions, which might explain cortisol's varied effects, especially on lymphatic tissue.

CORTISOL AND THE FIBROBLAST

Cortisol produces significant morphological changes in the fibroblasts of loose connective tissue (8). Fibroblasts constitute about 90% of the cells in connective tissue and may directly or indirectly influence the function of other cells implicated in inflammation. Fibroblasts are sensitive target cells for the action of glucocorticoids (5a, 56). Many studies of the effects of cortisol on the fibroblasts have been conducted with the topical application of the steroid to experimental wounds and have been concerned with the quantity and quality of healing and scar formation. Originally, with relatively large doses of corticosteroids, the healing of experimental wounds was inhibited (59, 67, 68). Spain et al. (68) also noted, despite interference with the connective tissue repair process, no inhibition of epithelial proliferation and overgrowth occurred in these wounds, by either parenteral or topical administration of cortisone, a finding confirmed by Berliner & Nabors (8).

In other wound studies, it was found that reduction of tensile strength occurred during the substrate phase (4th day), as well as in the collagen phase (8–12th day), of wound healing (8). Tensile strength was not interfered with in the early scar maturation phase (10–12th day) (17). Corticoids may also inhibit new collagen production and promote removal of previously deposited collagen, as shown by the results of corticosteroid treatment of keloids in man (32, 43, 82).

Some of these gross effects may be mediated by the direct action of the steroid on the fibroblast. The morphological changes in the fibroblast in tissue culture treated with cortisol seem specific. These changes, consisting of a pulling in of the cytoplasmic processes, rounding up of the fibroblast, increased basophilia, and vacuolization, also occur in the intact animal. The cells may take on an epitheloid appearance. The effect is not diffusely uniform and sometimes involves groups of cells (63). The altered fibroblasts appear to resist the degenerative effects caused by inflammation that develop in the non-cortisol-treated animal.

Ultrastructural alterations in fibroblasts found in steroid-treated, 7-day wounds included dilated endoplasmic reticulum, numerous dense bodies, many intracytoplasmic filaments, and nonbanded filamentous material in the extracellular space. The plasma membrane, mitochondria, and Golgi apparatus were not altered (7). Wounds in animals with scurvy showed similar intracytoplasmic changes (62a). Among the steroids tested for suppression of fibroblast growth, fluocinolone acetonide is the most potent. It is a most active topical anti-inflammatory agent (63, 64); its potency is due to the presence of a 16,17-acetonide in the molecule.

STEROIDS AND CONNECTIVE TISSUE

Adrenal steroid hormones and connective tissue also interact on a metabolic level. With cortisol, Layton (45) inhibited the incorporation of radioactive sulfate into mucopolysaccharides of connective tissue in vitro and Bostrom et al. (11a) did the same in rats. In cartilage depleted of its matrix by papain, McCluskey & Thomas (51) noted the restoration of structure; reaccumulation of basophilic ground substance was to a large extent prevented by cortisone, cortisol, and prednisone. Mucopolysaccharide synthesis was also inhibited. Cortisone inhibited the incorporation of $^{35}SO_4$ and ^{14}C-acetate into hyaluronate and chondroitin sulfate of rat skin (65). This seems to indicate an impaired synthesis of the entire polysaccharide rather than just limited prevention of sulfate incorporation, as suggested by Bostrom et al. (11a). Bollet & Shuster (10) showed that cortisol does not inhibit the enzyme involved in the synthesis of glucosamine 6-phosphate from fructose 6-phosphate and glutamine in vitro, but intramuscular administration of cortisol does cause some decrease in the activity of this enzyme.

Cortisone also inhibits the accumulation of liberated histamine in connective tissue (31), reduces the intensity and extent of metachromatic staining of the extracellular substance (2), and depresses the hexosamine (66), which indicates a lowered total content of mucopolysaccharides.

Berliner and Dougherty (5, 6) have suggested that cortisol is metabolized by connective tissue cells. However, this aspect of glucocorticoid action in connective tissue cells, as it relates to the activity of a given steroid in lymphoid tissues, has not received any other significant experimental support; its significance therefore must be held in abeyance.

CORTISONE, LYSOSOMES, AND INFLAMMATION

The role of lysosomes in the pathogenesis of cell injury, in the autolytic phenomenon, and hence in the inflammatory process is of the utmost significance. This is especially true of the granules or lysosomes of PMN leukocytes, which contain many of the hydrolases concerned with autolysis. Lysosomes are not uniformly distributed in the cytoplasm (16). The lysosome membrane that bounds the homogeneous inner core of this organelle is impermeable to the enzymes and their substrates and prevents their mutual accessibility. At least 22 enzymes have been identified within the lysosome along with such nonenzymatic substances as chemotactic factor, cationic proteins, endogenous pyrogen, hemolysin, phagocytin, and anticoagulant, all of which are involved in the inflammatory process (53).

An injury or alteration must have occurred in the lysosomal membranes, in order for hydrolases to initiate autolysis. This is also true in the PMN leukocytes from which release of "cytases" and lysosomal hydrolases kill microorganisms, mediate late vascular leakage during the inflammatory process, and participate in the pathogenesis of the Schwartzman and Arthus phenomena (14, 37, 72).

Some bacterial endotoxins can injure lysosomal membranes and permit release of the lysosomal contents within 5 min after injection (81); however, pretreatment with hydrocortisone can prevent this release (81). Radiation, acidification, and anoxia can injure lysosomal membranes. Disintegration of lysosomes from PMN leukocytes may be enhanced as a result of an increase in glucolytic activity and the lowering of the pH that follows the onset of phagocytosis (40). Cortisone and hydrocortisone, which inhibit the rate of lysosomal rupture, may in this manner depress phagocytosis and the release of those substances mediating late venule leakage in inflammation.

More support to the theory of protective effect of cortisone on lysosomal membranes was supplied by Weissman & Dingle (80) who showed that hydrocortisone diminished the effect of ultraviolet light and thereby provoked the release of hydrolases from suspensions of rat liver lysosomes. Thomas (75) has suggested that the protective action provided by cortisone against endotoxic shock in rabbits is mediated through a steroid stabilization of lysosomal membranes.

CORTISONE, PLATELETS, AND INFLAMMATION

Platelets, or some platelet factor, are necessary for the development of immune vasculitis in rabbits receiving intradermal injection of bovine serum albumin incorporated in Freund adjuvant (50). The missing platelet factor may alter vascular permeability. Platelets contain serotonin and histamine (38), and, in rabbits, release of these substances during inflammation is associated with anaphylaxis (79a). Epinephrine, also present in platelets, can also alter vascular tone.

In rats the effect of cortisone on acute experimental inflammatory edema was investigated by tracing and measuring injected ^{131}I-albumin. The volume of edema was reduced, but tissue damage persisted (62). The inhibition of edema was related to the reduction in venule and capillary leakage. Although the role of platelets in inflammation is not entirely clear, the presence of platelets in acute experimental inflammatory edema appears also to be inhibited by cortisone (62). This suggests that platelet aggregates may enhance the inflammatory reaction via pathologically active amines, peptides, or lysosomal constituents released from them, or alternatively may help to repair the inflammatory injury.

CONCLUSION

Corticosteroids exert profound suppressive effects at almost every step of inflammation and repair—from endothelial stickiness onward—to a greater degree than do other anti-inflammatory agents. However, an integrated overall hypothesis explaining these powerful effects has not been developed.

REFERENCES

1. ASBOE-HANSEN, G. Endocrine control of connective tissue. In: *Inflammation and Diseases of Connective Tissue—a Hahneman Symposium*, edited by L. C. Mills and J. H. Moyer. Philadelphia: Saunders, 1961, p. 38–43.

3. ASBOE-HANSEN, G. Mechanism of steroid inhibition of connective tissue growth. In: *Inflammation and Diseases of Connective Tissue—a Hahneman Symposium*, edited by L. C. Mills and J. H. Moyer. Philadelphia: Saunders, 1961, p. 460-464.
4. BERENDSEN, A. J. C. Water structure in biological systems. *Federation Proc.* 25: 971-976, 1966.
5. BERLINER, D. L. Metabolism of cortisol and other steroids by connective tissue cells. In: *Inflammation and Diseases of Connective Tissues—a Hahneman Symposium*, edited by L. C. Mills and J. H. Moyer. Philadelphia: Saunders, 1961, p. 431-436.
5a. BERLINER, D. L. Biotransformation of corticosteroids as related to inflammation. *Ann. NY Acad. Sci.* 116: 1078-1083, 1964.
6. BERLINER, D. L., AND T. F. DOUGHERTY. Metabolism of cortisol by mouse connective tissue. *Federation Proc.* 17: 189, 1958.
7. BERLINER, D. L., A. J. GALLEGOS, AND G. L. SCHNEEBELI. Early morphological changes produced by anti-inflammatory steroids on tissue culture fibroblasts. *J. Invest. Dermatol.* 48: 44-49, 1967.
8. BERLINER, D. L., AND C. J. NABORS. Effects of corticosteroids on fibroblast functions. *J. Reticuloendothelial Soc.* 4: 284-313, 1967.
9. BERLINER, D. L., R. J. WILLIAMS, G. N. TAYLOR, AND C. J. NABORS. Decreased scar formation with topical corticosteroid treatment. *Surgery* 61: 619-625, 1967.
10. BOLLET, A. J., AND A. SHUSTER. Metabolism of mucopolysaccharides in connective tissue. II. Synthesis of glucosamine-6-phosphate. *J. Clin. Invest.* 39: 1114-1115, 1960.
11. BOSTROM, H., AND E. ODEBLAD. The influence of cortisone upon sulphate exchange of chondroitin sulphuric acid. *Arkiv Kemi* 6: 39, 1955.
11a. BOSTROM, H., E. ODEBLAD, AND U. FRIBERG. Qualitative and quantitative autoradiographic study on uptake of sodium sulphate in skin of adult rat. *Acta Pathol. Microbiol. Scand.* 32: 516-521, 1953.
12. BRINK-JOHNSEN, T., AND T. F. DOUGHERTY. Studies of the effect of cortisol and corticotrophin on incorporation of adenine-8-^{14}C into lymphatic tissue nucleic acids. *Acta Endocrinol.* 49: 471-477, 1965.
13. BUCKLEY, J. K., AND G. B. RYAN. Increased vascular permeability—the effect of histamine and serotonin on rat mesenteric blood vessels in vivo. *Am. J. Pathol.* 55: 329-337, 1969.
14. COCHRANE, C. G., W. O. WEIGHE, AND F. J. DIXON. The role of polymorphonuclear leukocytes in the initiation and cessation of arthus vasculitis. *J. Exptl. Med.* 110: 481-494, 1959.
15. COSTE, E., B. PIQUET, P. GONICHE, AND J. CAYLA. Cortisone, corticotropin (ACTH) acid infections. *Am. J. Med.* 52: 747, 1951.
16. DEDUVE, C., AND R. WATTIAUX. Function of lysosomes. *Ann. Rev. Physiol.* 28: 435-492, 1966.
17. DIPASQUALE, G., L. V. TRIPP, AND B. G. STINETZ. Effect of locally applied anti-inflammatory substances on rat skin wounds. *Proc. Soc. Exptl. Biol. Med.* 124: 404-407, 1967.
18. DOUGHERTY, T. F. Role of steroids in regulation of inflammation. In: *Inflammation and Diseases of Connective Tissue—a Hahneman Symposium*, edited by L. C. Mills and J. H. Moyer. Philadelphia: Saunders, 1961, p. 449-460.
19. DOUGHERTY, T. F., M. L. BERLINER, AND D. L. BERLINER. Hormonal control of lymphocyte production and destruction. In: *Progress in Hematology III*, edited by L. M. Tocantins. New York: Grune & Stratton, 1962, p. 155-169.
20. DOUGHERTY, T. F., H. E. BROWN, AND D. L. BERLINER. Metabolism of hydrocortisone during inflammation. *Endocrinology* 62: 455-460, 1959.
21. DOUGHERTY, T. F., AND G. L. SCHNEEBELI. Role of cortisone in regulation of inflammation. *Proc. Soc. Exptl. Biol. Med.* 75: 854-858, 1950.
22. DOUGHERTY, T. F., AND A. WHITE. Functional alterations in lymphoid tissue induced by adrenal cortical secretion. *Am. J. Anat.* 77: 81-110, 1945.
23. DRURY, D. R. Control of blood sugar. *J. Clin. Endocrinol. Metab.* 2: 421-430, 1942.
24. FAVOUR, C. The cellular response to inflammation and its modification by glucocorticoids. In: *Inflammation and Diseases of Connective Tissue—a Hahneman Symposium*, edited by L. C. Mills and J. H. Moyer. Philadelphia: Saunders, 1961, p. 486-501.
25. FRIED, J., K. FLOREY, G. F. SABO, J. E. HERZ, A. R. RESTIVO, A. BORMAN, AND F. M. SINGER. Synthesis and biological activity of 1 and 6 dehydro-9α-kalo corticoids. *J. Am. Chem. Soc.* 77: 4181-4182, 1955.
26. FRIED, J., AND E. F. SABO. 9α-Fluoro derivatives of cortisone and hydrocortisone. *J. Am. Chem. Soc.* 76: 1455-1456, 1954.
27. GERMUTH, F. G., G. A. NEDZEL, B. OHINGER, AND J. OYAMA. Anatomic and histological changes in rabbits with experimental hypersensitivity treated with compound E and ACTH. *Proc. Soc. Exptl. Biol. Med.* 76: 177-182, 1951.
28. GLADNER, J. A., AND J. C. HOUCK. The action of cortisol-induced enzyme preparations on bradykinin. In: *Inflammation, Biochemistry and Drug Interaction*, edited by A. Bertelli and J. C. Houck. Baltimore: Williams & Wilkins, 1961, p. 133-135.
28a. GLADNER, J. A., AND J. C. HOUCK. Cortisol released clotting enzyme. *Federation Proc.* 25: 193, 1966.
29. GLASER, R. J., J. W. BERRY, L. H. LOEB, AND W. B. WOOD, JR. Effect of cortisone in streptococcal lymphadenitis and pneumonia. *J. Lab. Clin. Med.* 38: 363-373, 1951.
30. GOLDBERG, M. L., AND W. A. ATCHLEY. The effect of hormones on DNA. *Proc. Natl. Acad. Sci. US* 55: 989-996, 1966.
31. GOTH, A., B. ALLMAN, B. MERRIT, AND J. HOLMAN. Effect of cortisone in histamine liberation induced by tiveen in the dog. *Proc. Soc. Exptl. Biol. Med.* 78: 848-852, 1951.
32. GRIFFITH, B. H. The treatment of keloids with triamcinolone acetonide. *Plastic Reconstruc. Surg.* 38: 202-208, 1966.
33. HECHTER, O. Role of water structure in the molecular organization of cell membranes. *Federation Proc.* 24: 591-601, 1965.
34. HECHTER, O., AND I. D. R. HALKERSTON. Effects of steroid hormones on gene regulation and cell metabolism. *Ann. Rev. Physiol.* 27: 133-162, 1965.
35. HENCH, P. S., E. C. KENDALL, C. H. SLOCUMB, AND H. E. POLLEY. Effect of hormone of adrenal cortex (17-hydroxy-11-dehydrocorticosterone: compound E) and of pituitary adrenocorticotropic hormone on rheumatoid arthritis. Preliminary report. *Am. J. Rheumat. Diseases* 8: 97-104, 1949.
36. HOUCK, J. C., AND V. K. SHARMA. Enzyme induction in skin and fibroblasts by anti-inflammatory drugs. In: *Inflammation, Biochemistry and Drug Interaction*, edited by A. Bertelli and J. C. Houck. Baltimore: Williams & Wilkins, 1969, p. 85-93.
37. HUMPHREY, J. H. The mechanism of the arthus reaction. I. The role of polymorphonuclear leucocytes and other factors in reversed passive arthus reactions in rabbits. *Brit. J. Exptl. Pathol.* 36: 268-282, 1955.
38. HUMPHREY, J. H., AND R. JAQUES. The histamine and serotonin content of the platelets and polymorphonuclear leucocytes of various species. *J. Physiol., London* 124: 305-310, 1954.
39. INGLE, D. J. Problems relating to the adrenal cortex. *Endocrinology* 31: 419-438, 1942.
40. KARNOVSKY, M. L. Metabolic basis of phagocytic activity. *Physiol. Rev.* 42: 143-168, 1962.
41. KELLER, R. Mast cells and inflammation. In: *Inflammation, Biochemistry and Drug Interaction*, edited by A. Bertelli and J. C. Houck. Baltimore: Williams & Wilkins, 1969, p. 234-239.
41a. KENDALL E. C. Studies related to adrenal cortex. *Federation Proc.* 9: 501-505, 1950.
42. KETCHEL, M. M., C. B. FAVOUR, AND S. H. STURGIS. In vitro action of hydrocortisone on leucocyte migration. *J. Exptl. Med.* 107: 211-218, 1958.
43. KETCHUM, L. D., J. SMITH, D. W. ROBINSON, AND F. W. MASTERS. The treatment of hypertrophic scar, keloid and scar contracture by triaminolone acetonide. *Plastic Reconstruc. Surg.* 38: 209-218, 1966.
44. KLIGMAN, A. M., G. D. BALDRIDGE, G. REBELL, AND D. M. PILLSBURY. The effect of cortisone on the pathologic responses

of guinea pigs infected cutaneously with fungii, viruses and bacteria. *J. Lab. Clin. Med.* 37: 615–620, 1951.
45. LAYTON, L. L. Effect of cortisone upon chondroitin sulfate synthesis by animal tissues. *Proc. Soc. Exptl. Biol. Med.* 76: 596–598, 1951.
46. LERNER, L. J., A. BIANCHI, A. R. TURKHEIMER, F. M. SINGER, AND A. BORMAN. Anti-inflammatory steroids: potency, duration and modification of activities. *Ann. NY Acad. Sci.* 116: 1071–1077, 1964.
47. LIDDLE, G. W., AND M. FOX. Structure-function relationships of anti-inflammatory steroids. In: *Inflammation and Diseases of Connective Tissue—a Hahneman Symposium*, edited by L. C. Mills and J. H. Moyer. Philadelphia: Saunders, 1961, p. 302–309.
48. MAJNO, G., AND M. LEVENTHAL. Pathogenesis of histamine-type vascular leakage. *Lancet* 2: 99–100, 1967.
49. MAJNO, G., AND G. E. PALADE. Studies on inflammation. I. The effect of histamine and serotonin on vascular permeability: an electron microscopic study. *J. Biophys. Biochem. Cytol.* 11: 571–605, 1961.
50. MARGARETTEN, W., AND D. G. MCKAY. The requirement for platelets in the active arthus reaction. *Am. J. Pathol.* 64: 257–270, 1971.
51. MCCLUSKEY, R. T., AND L. THOMAS. The removal of cartilage matrix in vivo by papain: prevention of recovery with cortisone, hydrocortisone and prednisolone. *Am. J. Pathol.* 35: 819–830, 1959.
52. MENKIN, V. Further studies on effect of adrenal cortex extract and of various steroids on capillary permeability. *Proc. Soc. Exptl. Biol. Med.* 51: 39–41, 1942.
52a. MENKIN, V. The anti-inflammatory problem: the effect of corticoids and ACTH (cortico tropen). In: *Inflammation and Diseases of Connective Tissue—a Hahneman Symposium*, edited by L. C. Mills and J. H. Moyer. Philadelphia: Saunders, 1961, p. 506–514.
52b. MOLOMUT, N., D. M. SPAIN, AND A. HABER. The effect of cortisone on the spleen in mice. *Proc. Soc. Exptl. Biol. Med.* 73: 416, 1950.
53. MOVAT, H. Z. The acute inflammatory reaction. In: *Inflammation, Immunity and Hypersensitivity*, edited by H. Z. Movat. New York: Harper & Row, 1971, p. 1–130.
54. NICOL, T., AND D. L. J. BILBEY. The effect of various steroids on the phagocytic activity of the reticuloendothelial system. In: *Reticuloendothelial Structure and Function*, edited by J. H. Heller. New York: Ronald Press, 1960, p. 301–320.
55. NORN, S. Influence of anti-rheumatic agents on histamine release from sensitized rat peritoneal mast cells. Mechanism of action. In: *Inflammation, Biochemistry and Drug Interaction*, edited by A. Bertelli and J. C. Houck. Baltimore: Williams & Wilkins, 1969, p. 218–220.
56. PERLMAN, D., N. A. GIUFFRE, S. A. BRINDLE, AND S. C. PAN. Cytotoxicity of steroids to mammalian cells in tissue culture. *Proc. Soc. Exptl. Biol. Med.* 111: 623–625, 1962.
57. PETERSON, R. E., C. E. PIERCE, J. B. WYNGARDEN, J. J. BUNIN, AND B. B. BRODIE. The physiologic disposition and metabolic fate of cortisone in man. *J. Clin. Invest.* 36: 1301–1312, 1957.
58. POLLEY, H. F., AND H. L. MASON. Rheumatoid arthritis—effects of certain steroids other than cortisone and of some adrenal extracts. *J. Am. Med. Assoc.* 143: 1474–1481, 1950.
59. RAGAN, C., E. L. HOWES, C. M. PLOTZ, K. MEYER, J. W. BLUNT, AND R. LATTES. The effect of ACTH and cortisone on connective tissue. *Bull. NY Acad. Med.* 26: 251–254, 1950.
60. REBUCK, J. W., AND R. C. MELLINGER. Interruption by topical cortisone of leucocyte cycles in acute inflammation in man. *Ann. NY Acad. Sci.* 56: 715–732, 1953.
61. REBUCK, J. W., R. W. SMITH, AND R. C. MELLINGER. Modification of leucocyte response in man by ACTH. In: *Inflammation and Diseases of Connective Tissue—a Hahneman Symposium*, edited by L. C. Mills and J. H. Moyer. Philadelphia: Saunders, 1961, p. 502–506.
62. REDEI, A., AND E. KELEMAN. Presence of platelets in acute experimental inflammatory edema inhibited by salicylate or cortisone. In: *Inflammation, Biochemistry and Drug Interaction*, edited by A. Bertelli and J. C. Houck. Baltimore: Williams & Wilkins, 1969, p. 247–254.
62a. ROSS, R., AND E. P. BENDITT. Wound healing and collagen formation. IV. Distortion of ribosomal patterns of fibroblasts in scurvy. *J. Cell Biol.* 22: 365–389, 1964.
63. RUHMANN, A. G., AND D. L. BERLINER. Effects of steroids on growth of mouse fibroblasts in vitro. *Endocrinology* 76: 916–927, 1965.
64. SAWYER, W. C. Treatment of resistant eczematous dermatoses with a new compound, fluocinolone acetonide. *Ann. Allergy* 20: 330–331, 1962.
65. SCHILLER, S., AND A. DORFMAN. The metabolism of mucopolysaccharides in animals: the effect of cortisone and hydrocortisone on rat skin. *Endocrinology* 60: 376–387, 1957.
66. SOBEL, H., H. A. ZUTRAUEN, AND J. MARMORSTON. Collagen and hexosamine content of skin of normal and experimentally treated rats. *Arch. Biochem.* 46: 221–231, 1953.
67. SPAIN, D. M., N. MOLOMUT, AND A. HABER. The effect of cortisone on the formation of granulation tissue in mice. *Am. J. Pathol.* 26: 710–711, 1950.
68. SPAIN, D. M., N. MOLOMUT, AND A. HABER. Biological studies on cortisone in mice. *Science* 112: 335–337, 1950.
69. SPAIN, D. M., N. MOLOMUT, AND A. HABER. The effect of cortisone on the spleen in mice. *Proc. Soc. Exptl. Biol. Med.* 73: 416, 1950.
70. SPECTOR, W. G. The acute inflammatory response. *Ann. NY Acad. Sci.* 116: 747–1084, 1964.
71. SPECTOR, W. G., AND D. A. WILLOUGHBY. *The Pharmacology of Inflammation*. London: English University Press, 1968.
72. STETSON, C. A., JR. Similarities in the mechanisms determining the arthus and Schwartzman phenomenon. *J. Exptl. Med.* 94: 347–358, 1951.
73. STEVENS, W., C. BEDKE, AND T. V. DOUGHERTY. Effect of cortisol acetate on various aspects of cellular metabolism in mouse lymphatic tissue. *J. Reticuloendothelial Soc.* 4: 254–283, 1967.
74. SWEAT, M. L., B. I. GROSSER, D. L. BERLINER, E. H. SWIM, C. J. NABORS, JR., AND T. F. DOUGHERTY. The metabolism of cortisone and progesterone by cultured uterine fibroblasts, strain U12-705. *Biochem. Biophys. Acta* 28: 591–596, 1958.
75. THOMAS, L. Physiologic and pathological alterations produced by endotoxins of gram negative bacteria. *Arch. Internal Med.* 101: 452, 1958.
76. THOMAS, L., J. W. UHR, AND L. GRANT. *International Symposium on Injury, Inflammation and Immunity*. Baltimore: Williams & Wilkins, 1964.
77. THORN, G. W., J. DALTON, J. C. LAIDLAW, F. C. GOETZ, J. F. DINGMAN, W. L. ARONS, D. H. P. STREETEN, AND B. H. MCCRACKEN. Pharmacological aspects of adrenocortical steroids and ACTH in man. *New Engl. J. Med.* 248: 232–245, 1953.
78. TOLKSDORF, S. The effect of halogenation on the biological properties of corticoids. In: *Inflammation and Diseases of Connective Tissue—a Hahneman Symposium*, edited by L. C. Mills and J. H. Moyer. Philadelphia: Saunders, 1961, p. 310–315.
79. UVNÄS, B. Mast cells and inflammation. In: *Inflammation, Biochemistry and Drug Interaction*, edited by A. Bertelli and J. C. Houck. Baltimore: Williams & Wilkins, 1969, p. 221–227.
79a. WAALKES, T. P., AND H. COBURN. Comparative effects of glycogen and histamine in the rabbit. *Proc. Soc. Exptl. Biol. Med.* 101: 122–125, 1959.
80. WEISSMAN, G., AND J. DINGLE. Release of lysosomal protease by ultraviolet irradiation and inhibition by hydrocortisone. *Exptl. Cell. Res.* 25: 207–210, 1961.
81. WEISSMAN, G., AND L. THOMAS. Studies on lysosomes. I. The effects of endotoxin, endotoxin tolerance and cortisone on the release of acid hydrolases from a granular fraction of rabbit liver. *J. Exptl. Med.* 116: 433–450, 1962.
82. WILSON, W. W. Prophylaxis against postsurgical keloids: results in 500 patients. *Southern Med. J.* 58: 751–753, 1965.

CHAPTER 19

Pathophysiology of syndromes of cortisol excess in man

RANDALL H. TRAVIS | *Department of Physiology, School of Medicine, Case Western Reserve University, Cleveland, Ohio*

CHAPTER CONTENTS

Pituitary-dependent Cortisol Excess
Extrapituitary, Extraadrenal Tumor-dependent Cortisol Excess
Adrenal Tumor-dependent Cortisol Excess
Summary

THE MOST FREQUENTLY OCCURRING adrenal disorders, exclusive of the atrophy resulting from therapeutic corticosteroid administration, are those that have in common a physiologically inappropriately elevated rate of cortisol secretion. Excessive cortisol secretion may result from *a*) inappropriate secretion of ACTH by the pituitary, *b*) ACTH production by extrapituitary, extraadrenal tumors, or *c*) excessive cortisol production by adrenal cortex tumors. These disorders have much in common but are sufficiently different etiologically, mechanistically, and in particular detail to warrant separate discusion.

PITUITARY-DEPENDENT CORTISOL EXCESS

The most common type of glucocorticoid excess (excluding iatrogenic) is the consequence of physiologically inappropriate secretion of adrenocorticotropic hormone (ACTH) by the adenohypophysis. It occurs from infancy to senility—with the peak incidence in middle life—and more frequently in females than in males (101, 153). The greater vulnerability of females has no satisfactory explanation at this time.

Cushing (33), first to describe the clinical features of hypercortisolism in 1932, attributed the syndrome to an unspecified effect of basophil adenomata of the pituitary. In 1942 Albright (3) attributed the immediate cause of the syndrome described by Cushing to increased adrenal secretion of "S hormone" (i.e., cortisol).

Increased ACTH as the cause of increased cortisol secretion in patients with cortisol excess not attributable to adrenal tumors has been well established by repeated demonstrations by bioassay and by radioimmunoassay of inappropriately high concentrations of ACTH in plasma (36, 37, 40, 101, 104, 109, 119, 138, 142, 175, 196). It is assumed that changes in plasma concentration of ACTH reflect changes in secretion rate rather than a change in rate of metabolic removal, since the little available evidence does not suggest a reduced rate of removal from plasma (123). Values of ACTH concentration in plasma tend to exceed those found in normal persons but are not invariably grossly elevated.

However, when plasma cortisol concentration and plasma ACTH concentration are simultaneously determined, plasma ACTH concentrations are manyfold higher than those found in patients with equally high cortisol concentrations in plasma that result from cortisol-secreting adrenocortical tumors (5, 101, 138) or from exogenous cortisol (196). Not only is the concentration of plasma ACTH inappropriately increased relative to plasma cortisol, but it frequently does not show the late afternoon decline observed in normal persons. Plasma cortisol also does not decline (44, 101, 142). Pituitary origin of the ACTH has been demonstrated by the fall in concentrations of plasma ACTH and plasma cortisol that follow production of destructive lesions of the pituitary by surgery or radiation (33, 136–138, 158).

In 5–10% of patients found to have pituitary-dependent hypercortisolism, there is, at the time of diagnosis, evidence for a pituitary tumor (100, 115, 135, 165). Such tumors are usually chromophobe adenomata (165).

In the 90–95% of patients in whom clinical evidence for a pituitary tumor is absent, either no morphological pathology or small basophil adenomata have been found (27, 33, 115, 153) at surgery or at autopsy. The significance of small basophil adenomata is not clear since they may occur in 3–7% of routine autopsies (29, 183) in which there is no evidence of hypercortisolism.

About 10% of patients without pituitary tumors at the time of diagnosis, who are treated by adrenalectomy, develop pituitary tumors over a period of years (29, 101,

271

138). The development of the tumor is accompanied by rising concentrations of ACTH and of melanocyte-stimulating hormone (MSH) in plasma and sometimes by recurrence of hypercortisolism from ectopic adrenal tissue or from adrenal tissue not removed at surgery (138, 175).

Both in the presence and absence of a pituitary tumor, patients with pituitary-dependent hypercortisolism exhibit reduced concentrations of ACTH in plasma and reduced secretion of cortisol when exogenous glucocorticoid is administered, although the amounts required are at least fourfold greater than the amounts required for suppression of ACTH release in normal persons (24, 100, 101, 104, 136, 138, 196). In such patients, reduction of the concentration of plasma cortisol by adrenalectomy (101, 196) or by administration of the adrenal 11β-hydroxylase inhibitor, metyrapone (138, 175), is followed by increased concentration of plasma ACTH. Normal or exaggerated increases in plasma ACTH are seen in response to insulin hypoglycemia and vasopressin infusion (36).

In responding to decreased concentration of plasma cortisol by increasing the concentration of plasma ACTH and responding to administration of glucocorticoid by decreasing the concentration of plasma ACTH, patients with pituitary-dependent hypercortisolism qualitatively, but not quantitatively, resemble normal persons. In another important way, such patients are qualitatively similar but quantitatively dissimilar to normal persons. Hellman and his colleagues (73, 193) recently concluded that in normal man cortisol is secreted episodically—about nine times per day. The greater part of the total daily cortisol secretion occurs during sleep in the early morning hours. These conclusions were based on studies in which both plasma cortisol concentration and plasma cortisol specific activity, after a pulse of isotopically labeled cortisol, were estimated at 20-min intervals throughout a day. These data permitted estimates of secretion rate during discrete intervals through the entire day. One patient with pituitary-dependent hypercortisolism, without clinical evidence of pituitary tumor, also showed a pattern of episodic secretion in which, however, episodes occurred throughout the day, occurred more frequently, and produced a pattern of cortisol concentrations in which both highs and lows were higher than in normal persons (74).

Liddle and his colleagues, who were responsible for many of the critical discoveries cited above, have interpreted the available evidence as supporting the hypothesis that the initial defect in pituitary-dependent hypercortisolism is a lesion of the hypothalamus or limbic system, which results in inappropriate overproduction of corticotropin-releasing factor (CRF) and inappropriate overproduction of ACTH, which in turn stimulates excessive secretion of cortisol with resultant structural and metabolic alterations (104). According to the hypothesis, pituitary-dependent hypercortisolism is a disorder of regulation in which the hypothalamus secretes CRF in a qualitatively normal but quantitatively abnormal manner. For a given plasma cortisol concentration, CRF secretion and ACTH release are greater than normal, which results in excessive secretion of cortisol. However, CRF and ACTH release are not suppressed to a normal extent by the increased concentration of plasma cortisol.

Not only is ACTH secretion increased in pituitary-dependent hypercortisolism, but the amount of cortisol secreted in response to a given amount of ACTH is increased (24, 25, 68, 76, 95, 106). Prolonged exposure to even small increases in ACTH increases the capacity of the adrenal cortex to secrete cortisol in normal persons (146). This phenomenon is presumably an expression of the ability of ACTH to function both as a secretagogue and as an agent promoting the development of the structural and enzymatic apparatus required for corticosteroidogenesis (89, 141).

Christy and his colleagues have described evidence suggesting the existence, in plasma of patients with pituitary-dependent hypercortisolism, of an "adrenal weight-maintaining activity," originating in the pituitary, which potentiates the activity of ACTH in maintaining the weight of the adrenal cortex in hypophysectomized rats. The physicochemical properties of this "activity" and its relationship to the biogenesis and secretion of corticosteroids are unknown (80, 170).

In addition to an adrenal effect increasing the concentration of plasma cortisol, ACTH may increase plasma cortisol by an extraadrenal effect. Kusama and colleagues (94) have reported that, in adrenalectomized human subjects, rather large quantities of ACTH increase the half-time of plasma disappearance of injected cortisol and increase the apparent volume of distribution. Compatible data were earlier reported by DeMoor et al. (35) and, in mice, by Berliner et al. (11).

The development of pituitary tumors has been attributed to prolonged, intensive stimulation by CRF. The infrequency with which pituitary tumors seem to develop in patients with adrenal insufficiency owing to destruction of the adrenal cortex has been cited in objection to this theory (158). However, it is possible that pituitary tumors do not develop in adrenal insufficiency because a degree of insufficiency that would stimulate enough CRF release to produce a tumor results in death before the tumor appears. It is also possible that a normal hypothalamus cannot produce enough CRF to induce a pituitary tumor, even with the stimulus of adrenal insufficiency, whereas the hypothalamus of the patient with pituitary-dependent hypercortisolism can, and sometimes does, produce a larger and tumorigenic amount of CRF.

Evidence at hand does not exclude the logical possibility that, rather than inappropriate secretion of CRF, there may be hypersensitivity of the adenohypophysis to normally secreted CRF. Presumably, ongoing work on the isolation and chemical characterization of CRF will allow investigation of this possibility in a definitive way.

The concentration of β-MSH in plasma is increased in pituitary-dependent hypercortisolism and tends to increase or to decrease as the concentration of plasma

ACTH increases or decreases. If the relative potency ratio of ACTH to MSH is the same in human skin as in frog skin, β-MSH is largely responsible for the hyperpigmentation of skin sometimes seen in pituitary-dependent hypercortisolism. No other activities have been ascribed to it in this disorder (1, 2). The close linkage of ACTH to β-MSH is not confined to hypercortisolism but has been observed in all situations in which simultaneous measurements have been made—glucocorticoid suppression of ACTH release, 11β-hydroxylase inhibitor administration, primary adrenal insufficiency, and ACTH-producing extrapituitary neoplasms (2).

The adrenal glands of patients with pituitary-dependent hypercortisolism are described by pathologists either as normal or as hyperplastic (27, 153). Standards for size and weight of adrenals usually employed by pathologists are derived from autopsy studies, including a substantial proportion of people dying of prolonged, severe illness, which tends to increase the size of the adrenals. Rogers & Williams (160) measured adrenal weights in endocrinologically healthy people experiencing rapid death. A mean adrenal weight of 4.5 g was found, in contrast to the normal combined weight of 12–18 g cited by pathology texts (17, 202). It is probable that the adrenals of all patients with pituitary-dependent hypercortisolism are the seat of hyperplasia, diffuse or nodular (27).

In pituitary-dependent hypercortisolism, cortisol secretion is elevated by definition and the most conspicuous and disabling manifestations of the disease are attributable to excessive cortisol action. Patients have a characteristic habitus, which includes buccal fat pads ("moon face") and supraclavicular and dorsal fat pads ("buffalo hump"). The abdomen is obese, but the extremities show little fat and much atrophy of muscles (truncal obesity) (27, 33, 101, 153, 158).

The mechanism by which this peculiar distribution of fat is brought about is unknown. In vitro experiments with rat tissues have demonstrated that glucocorticoids promote lipolysis, suppress lipogenesis, and enhance the lipolytic action of catecholamines (2, 15, 52, 81, 97, 131). The in vitro lipolytic action of ACTH and of MSH, at least in large concentrations, has been repeatedly demonstrated. However, without data concerning the net effects of insulin, ACTH, MSH, and cortisol on adipose tissues from different regions of the human body, at concentrations existing in vivo, it seems impossible to relate presently available knowledge to the state of the adipose tissue in adrenal disease in man.

Glucocorticoids have a marked stimulating effect on appetite, and fractional body fat content may increase in patients receiving such treatment (48). However, the distribution of fat in simple obesity resulting from overeating is more uniform than that described above.

Muscle atrophy and weakness, most prominent in pelvis and thighs, are characteristic findings (27, 33, 101, 130, 153). Similar changes have been reported after administration of large doses of glucocorticoids to rats (63, 64), rabbits (45, 60, 61), dogs (55), and man (41, 58, 65, 70, 113, 193). Recovery may be incomplete after excessive cortisol secretion is stopped.

Gross measurements reveal diminution in size of the muscle, and, microscopically, replacement by connective tissue and fat, diminution in fiber diameter, hyalinization, and necrosis are observed (130). Electromyographic studies reveal reduced voltage of motor units (65, 113, 130).

Numerous studies in rats have somewhat inconclusively suggested glucocorticoid enhancement of protein catabolism in muscle (63, 88, 112, 162) and have definitely demonstrated inhibition of protein anabolism (63, 88, 114, 174, 198, 199, 201). Both myofibrillar and sarcoplasmic elements are affected (63). Inhibition of anabolism may depend partly, but not entirely, on a reduced rate of amino acid penetration into cells (42, 90, 92, 174, 200, 201). The reduced rate of penetration appears to be a direct effect of the hormone, for it can be shown by addition of the hormone to the isolated tissue in vitro (90, 92).

Protein depletion is also prominent in subcutaneous connective tissue where it is manifested by thinning, friability, and pink striae—that is, discontinuities of subcutaneous tissue that allow the color of deeper tissue to be seen; they occur most frequently on the lower abdomen and are sometimes seen on shoulders, thighs, and calves (27). Easy bruisability is characteristic.

In children with pituitary-dependent cortisol excess, linear growth retardation has been frequently commented on (184, 192) and, in children treated with glucocorticoids, has been fully documented (16, 54, 145, 182). In the latter group, and presumably also in the former group, delayed skeletal maturation and osteoporosis also occur. Supporting data are available from animal experiments (9, 50, 126, 154).

These findings seem generally consistent with the known disturbances of protein metabolism and of skeletal metabolism associated with glucocorticoid excess. However, growth hormone deficiency has been suggested as an additional and specific cause by investigators who found an attenuated rise in concentration of plasma growth hormone in response to induced hypoglycemia in glucocorticoid-treated persons (57, 72, 133, 179) and in patients with pituitary-dependent cortisol excess (36, 72). Other investigators have not been able to confirm these findings. In glucocorticoid-treated subjects normal changes in concentration of plasma growth hormone have been reported in response to hypoglycemia (118, 129, 161, 164), hyperglycemia (161), and arginine infusion (133, 161). Presumably the conflicting observations concerning changes in the concentration of growth hormone in glucocorticoid-treated subjects depend on differences of experimental procedure, which are difficult to evaluate. However, it is unlikely that an absolute deficiency of growth hormone is a significant cause of growth retardation in glucocorticoid excess, for it has been the usual experience that only very large amounts of growth hormone promote growth of children (118, 128, 161, 177, 186) or rats (10, 117, 171, 177) in the presence of even modest excesses of glucocorticoids.

Osteoporosis and pathological fractures, especially of the spine (176), occur frequently in pituitary-dependent hypercortisolism. Microradiographic studies indicate both a reduced rate of bone formation and an increased rate of bone resorption (82). A possible molecular mechanism for reduced formation is suggested by the observation of reduced synthesis in vitro of protein matrix associated with reduced RNA synthesis in bone cells exposed to cortisol (150). Bone made osteoporotic by excess cortisol may remain so indefinitely, by radiologic criteria, despite return of cortisol production to normal. In children, new bone formed after treatment will be normal, whereas older, previously affected bone remains demineralized. No cause is known for failure of reconstitution of normal bone architecture after excess cortisol is no longer present (78).

The process of reducing skeletal mass in adults is possibly related to an increased incidence of cholelithiasis and nephrolithiasis in patients with glucocorticoid excess (176). The indirect evidence available suggests that appropriate secretion of parathyroid hormone and of thyrocalcitonin occurs in hypercortisolism, and regulation of the concentration of plasma calcium occurs normally (185). A direct effect of cortisol is inhibition of the action of parathyroid hormone in promoting mobilization of calcium from bone and enhancement of calcitonin action (156, 180). Apparently the effects of glucocorticoids on bone are the outcome of opposing forces: *a*) an action on protein elements tending to reduce linear growth and maturation in children and demineralization in both children and adults; and *b*) reciprocal inhibition-enhancement of the parathormone-calcitonin system, which promotes calcium retention in bones. Sustained high concentrations of glucocorticoids have net effects of demineralization and osteoporosis.

Biochemical details of the effects of glucocorticoids on metabolism of carbohydrates, proteins, and fats are described elsewhere in this volume. The most frequently observed gross metabolic findings in patients secreting excessive amounts of cortisol under the influence of the pituitary are fasting hyperglycemia and reduced glucose tolerance (27, 75, 101, 153). Additionally, there may be reduced concentrations of total inorganic phosphate in serum and increased concentration of lactate and pyruvate in serum. Tolerance to intravenously infused lactate is reduced (75). Similar observations have been made in glucocorticoid-treated rats (62, 132) in which hyperglycemia appears to be the consequence both of increased gluconeogenesis from protein (110) and also reduced extrahepatic utilization of glucose, especially by adipose tissue (15, 46, 52, 53, 111, 131, 132). Glucocorticoid impairment of glucose utilization has also been demonstrated in rodent skin (148), thymus (127, 197), and connective tissue (67).

Patients with pituitary-dependent hypercortisolism occasionally manifest hypertension, hypernatremia, metabolic alkalosis, and hypokalemia (153). This complex is characteristic of long-standing mineralocorticoid excess. However, the agent responsible has not been definitely identified. It may be cortisol, which has some ability to promote renal sodium retention and potassium loss.

Indices of aldosterone production are not usually elevated (12, 14, 23, 147, 187), consistent with the observation that continuous infusion of ACTH only transiently increases aldosterone production (13, 140, 188). The mechanism by which aldosterone secretion is caused to decline after a brief rise, during continuous ACTH infusion for several days, is not known but does not appear to depend on sodium retention or a decrease in plasma renin activity (13, 140, 188). An intraadrenal mechanism is suggested by the observation that high concentrations of ACTH inhibit in vitro production of aldosterone (84). Indices of production of both corticosterone and 11-deoxycorticosterone are usually within normal limits in patients with pituitary-dependent hypercortisolism (12, 14, 19, 20, 28, 31, 147), and consequently neither compound is responsible for the electrolyte disorder. It is surprising that production of these steroids is not increased, for experimental intravenous infusions of ACTH in man for periods up to 7 days have stimulated a sustained increase in both corticosterone and 11-deoxycorticosterone (13, 20, 28, 38, 147). Possibly the concentrations of circulating ACTH attained in these experiments were higher than those attained in pituitary-dependent cortisol excess, which, although sufficient to maintain an increased rate of cortisol, are perhaps usually insufficient to stimulate an increased rate of corticosterone and 11-deoxycorticosterone secretion.

It has been suggested that, although corticosterone and 11-deoxycorticosterone secretions appear to be regulated largely by ACTH, the renin-angiotensin system may modulate ACTH regulation of these hormones (13). That sustained ACTH stimulation of corticosterone and 11-deoxycorticosterone secretion results, in the presence of adequate sodium ion intake, in suppression of renin release, was postulated. In the presence of reduced angiotensin II, it was thought that secretion of corticosterone and 11-deoxycorticosterone would decrease, despite continuing increased concentrations of plasma ACTH.

Available evidence is strongly against this hypothesis. Infusions of angiotensin II in man do not alter indices of 11-deoxycorticosterone or corticosterone secretions (20, 147), nor does dietary sodium restriction (20, 139, 147), a potent stimulus to renin release. Also, indices of 11-deoxycorticosterone and corticosterone secretions are not elevated in a variety of clinical disorders in which ACTH release is normal but plasma renin activity is regularly increased (14, 20, 32).

Apparently, 11-deoxycorticosterone and corticosterone secretions are independent of the renin-angiotensin system in man. However, the physiology of the dog, in this respect, may be different from that of man (34, 147).

The suggestion has been offered that 18-hydroxy-11-deoxycorticosterone may be an important mineralocorticoid in man, although its role in adrenal pathophysiology remains to be assessed (83, 121, 154).

Isotopic measurements of total exchangeable potassium before and after successful treatment of cortisol excess have revealed large increases in body potassium content with improvement. Although this finding is compatible with a reduction of intracellular potassium concentration in the untreated state, a definite conclusion cannot be drawn, for improvement was associated with a grossly observable increase in muscle mass (48). Prunty et al. (155) found not only a decrease in total exchangeable potassium in untreated patients, but an increase in the ratio of exchangeable sodium to exchangeable potassium, consistent with but not conclusively proving a reduction in intracellular potassium concentration. The same result could be produced by a coincident decrease of muscle mass and increase in extracellular fluid volume, both probable events in untreated patients. The range of error in determination of values for critical quantities—extracellular fluid volume, intracellular fluid volume, and total exchangeable potassium—has prevented a conclusive demonstration of altered intracellular potassium concentration, despite even severe hypokalemia in the presence of a known tendency to renal potassium loss.

Women with pituitary-dependent hypercortisolism usually undergo some virilization: lateral recession of the scalp hairline, coarsening and increased growth of facial and body hair, acne, and clitoral enlargement (27, 33, 101, 153, 176). These changes are attributable to increased adrenal secretion of C_{19} androgens under the influence of ACTH and possibly to the increased production of androgenic metabolites of cortisol.

A small number of reports suggest a trend toward increased sexual libido in women with increased ACTH or adrenal tumors and reduced libido after surgical excision of normal adrenals (191). Indeed, it is sometimes asserted that libido in mature women is dependent on adrenal androgens. However, critical examination of the available data suggests a complex relationship in which apparently normal sexual activity may occur in the absence of adrenal androgens, and reduced libido may be experienced in the presence of excess androgens, presumably as a consequence of interplay of developmental, psychic, social, and endocrine influences.

Amenorrhea, sometimes after a period of metrorrhagia, is frequent (27). Pregnancy occurs only rarely and seems to be associated with a high rate of fetal loss (77). Infertility and amenorrhea are presumably attributable to anovulation consequent to excess adrenal steroids, rather than a primary pituitary dysfunction, for similar characteristics associated with ovarian atrophy and diminished number and maturation of ovarian follicles (79) are found in women with corticosteroid-secreting adrenal tumors (8, 43, 77, 93, 108, 149). Events of pituitary gonadotrophin secretion in hypercortisolism are largely unknown. Normal basal concentrations of plasma LH and normal increases in response to insulin hypoglycemia and to vasopressin infusion have been reported in pituitary-dependent cortisol excess and in glucocorticoid-treated women (36).

EXTRAPITUITARY, EXTRAADRENAL TUMOR-DEPENDENT CORTISOL EXCESS

Manifestations of cortisol excess concurrently with an extrapituitary, extraadrenal tumor were initially reported by Brown (21) in 1928 and subsequently reported with sufficient frequency to result in a suspicion that the association is not merely fortuitous (159). The basis of the association was demonstrated in 1962 by Meador et al. (120) who found large concentrations of ACTH-like material in plasma, and in tumors together with reduced concentrations of ACTH in the pituitary in some patients with lung tumors and cortisol excess.

An incomplete listing of organs in which ACTH-producing tumors have probably occurred includes lung and bronchi (4, 21, 22, 26, 71, 87, 99, 103, 116, 138, 155, 159, 172, 178, 181), thymus (26, 103, 125, 138, 159), pancreas (7, 69, 87, 96, 103, 120, 138, 159, 163, 189, 190), parotid (30, 99, 103, 159), liver (103), ovary (103, 143, 159), prostate (103), breast (103, 155), esophagus (103), kidney (159), thyroid (39, 159), parathyroid (157), colon (124, 159), and various peripheral neural tissues (85, 98, 103, 105, 122, 134, 169, 195).

In most of the reported cases, evidence for production and release by the tumor of a substance having adrenocorticotropic properties has been merely the coincidence of cortisol excess and the presence of the tumor. In some instances the association may have been fortuitous. However, in numerous patients, ACTH activity has been demonstrated in extracts of the tumor (30, 39, 69, 99, 103, 105, 116, 120, 122, 124, 125, 143, 152, 168, 169, 172, 181) with reduced pituitary content of ACTH (103, 105, 116, 124, 172), and there has been partial or total remission of hypercortisolism after partial or total excision of the tumor (26, 39, 69, 103, 122, 125, 134, 181, 195). This combination of observations confirms that adrenal overproduction of cortisol is attributable to adrenal stimulation by a corticotropin originating in the tumor.

Some tumors have been shown (with variable degrees of certainty) to produce not only ACTH, but also MSH (69, 96, 103, 169), gastrin (96, 103), glucagon (189), insulin (7, 189), indoles (49, 71), antidiuretic hormone (103), parathyroid hormone (103), or catecholamines (85, 98, 134, 195). Several tumors have been shown to produce more than one humoral factor in addition to ACTH. Most ACTH-producing extrapituitary tumors are highly malignant by histological and gross criteria and result in death in a few months. However, a few apparently benign ACTH-producing neoplasms have been described (26, 98, 103, 122, 124, 125, 134, 159, 195).

Evidence for the identity or near-identity of ACTH from tumors and ACTH from the pituitary consists of similarities with respect to endocrine-metabolic actions, in vivo and in vitro, chromatographic behavior, chemical or enzymatic inactivation, and immunoreactivity (103). However, MSH isolated from tumors differs from pituitary MSH both chromatographically and with respect to immunoreactivity (103, 173).

Patients with tumor-dependent cortisol excess differ from patients with pituitary-dependent cortisol excess in several important ways: men are represented in far greater numbers than women; the syndrome is rare in children; the typical adiposity and peripheral muscular atrophy of the pituitary-dependent disease is often absent; severe hypokalemic metabolic alkalosis is a characteristic rather than occasional finding; and indices of cortisol and of ACTH production tend to be greater (101). Other hormone-related features seem similar to the pituitary-dependent disease if allowance is made for the fact that the total duration of cortisol excess, before death, is characteristically only a few months.

The greater incidence in adult males than in adult females or children of either sex probably is the combined reflection of the greater incidence of malignant neoplasms of the lung in men and, perhaps, a predilection of lung tumors to produce ACTH. In the large published series, tumors of the lungs outnumber tumors of all other organs combined (4, 5, 22, 103, 105, 155, 159).

Frequent, but not invariant, absence of the moon face, buffalo hump, and truncal adiposity, despite large concentrations of plasma cortisol, has been attributed to the usually relatively brief duration of illness and to the anorexia and wasting of malignant disease. The large amounts of ACTH and other possibly lipolytic hormones released by some tumors may also be partially responsible.

The higher incidence of severe hypokalemic alkalosis in tumor-dependent cortisol excess was first noted by Bagshawe (5) and has been systematically confirmed (155). Two explanations that are not mutually exclusive have been offered. In plasma there seems to be a definite negative correlation between potassium concentration (23, 155) and cortisol concentration. Some authors believe that the generally higher concentrations of plasma cortisol found in tumor-dependent hypercortisolism are responsible for the generally more severe tendency to hypokalemic alkalosis (157). On the other hand, in contrast to the pituitary-dependent syndrome, substantial numbers of patients with tumor-dependent cortisol excess produce large quantities of corticosterone and 11-deoxycorticosterone (14, 20, 167). Perhaps greater secretion of 11-deoxycorticosterone and corticosterone occurs as a consequence of generally greater concentrations of circulating ACTH in tumor patients (101).

Patients with tumor-dependent cortisol excess respond minimally or not at all to exogenous ACTH, as measured by changes in urinary cortisol metabolites (101), consistent with the concept that the adrenal cortex is in most patients under supramaximal stimulation by corticotropin released by the tumor. Likewise, metyrapone has minimal, if any, effect on excretion of corticosteroid metabolites (101). This is the expected result if the pituitary has been suppressed for months by cortisol excess (66) and, in any case, could not substantially increase the already elevated concentrations of plasma ACTH. Exogenous glucocorticoid is expected to have no effect on tumor release of ACTH and could not reduce ACTH release by an already suppressed pituitary. Results observed in nearly all patients have been consistent with this view. Occasional apparent exceptions may have been the consequence of coincident fluctuations in the rate of release of ACTH by the tumor, independent of glucocorticoid concentration (6, 125).

ADRENAL TUMOR-DEPENDENT CORTISOL EXCESS

Both benign and malignant neoplasms of the adrenal cortex may secrete large quantities of cortisol largely or totally independent of ACTH influence. The tumors usually are unilateral but may be bilateral. Nontumorous adrenal cortex is markedly atrophic (27, 56) owing to cortisol-mediated suppression of pituitary ACTH release (101).

Carinomas are rare, may occur at any age from infancy to senility, are the most frequent cause of cortisol excess (excluding the therapeutic) in childhood, and occur overwhelmingly more frequently in females than in males (107).

Measurements of urinary steroid metabolites indicate that carcinomas may produce large quantities of a variety of corticosteroids. Excretion of large amounts of 17-ketosteroids and of dehydroepiandrosterone is usual. The excretion of large quantities of tetrahydro-11-deoxycortisol occurs frequently; this suggests that, despite secretion of excess cortisol, 11β-hydroxylation is deficient relative to the available substrate. In the presence of a relative deficiency of 11β-hydroxylase, a greater fraction of progesterone and pregnenolone is expected to be diverted to androgenic precursors of 17-ketosteroids, and indeed, severe virilization usually accompanies cortisol excess resulting from adrenal carcinoma in females (107).

Occasional patients with adrenal carcinoma experience severe fasting hypoglycemia, despite increased cortisol concentrations in body fluids and reduced tolerance to ingested glucose. It has been suggested that fasting hypoglycemia may be the consequence of greatly increased secretion of anabolic steroids (e.g., testosterone), which channels amino acids into protein synthesis and makes them unavailable for gluconeogenesis (51).

Cortisol-secreting adenomas of the adrenal cortex somewhat outnumber cortisol-secreting carcinomas; they are almost unknown in childhood and are almost entirely confined to females.

The patient's appearance and the metabolic disturbances observed are typical of cortisol excess. Cortisol concentration of plasma is increased, as is the renal excretion of cortisol metabolites. Some mild virilization reflecting increased androgen secretion may occur. However, urinary 17-ketosteroids are increased in only about one-third of patients with adenomas, in contrast with nine-tenths of patients with carcinomas (144).

Hypertension and hypokalemic alkalosis occur commonly in both benign and malignant cortisol-secreting tumors (101). This is attributable, in most instances, to secretion of excessive amounts of 11-deoxycorticosterone and corticosterone, rather than aldosterone (14, 20, 31, 147).

In patients with adrenal neoplasms, cortisol secretion usually does not increase with the administration of ACTH but may occasionally do so (59, 101, 107, 144, 166). Metyrapone has little or no influence on steroid excretion in patients with adrenal tumors, benign or malignant (101), but stimulation has been described (144, 151). Both metyrapone and exogenous ACTH may conceivably bring about a stimulation of nontumorous tissue rather than the tumor. Administration of an ordinarily pituitary-suppressing dose of a potent glucocorticoid has only rarely been reported to reduce indices of cortisol secretion (18, 59, 101, 107, 144), consistent with other evidence of marked suppression of the pituitary by tumor secretion.

SUMMARY

Three pathological syndromes associated with increased rates of cortisol secretion have been described.

1. Pituitary-dependent hypercortisolism is believed to be the consequence of an unknown defect of regulation at the hypothalamic, or higher, level resulting in an increased secretion of hypothalamic CRF and adenohypophysial ACTH. The resultant excessive cortisol secretion causes a characteristic central adiposity, hyperglycemia, protein depletion of skin and muscle, and osteoporosis. Hypokalemic alkalosis occurs only occasionally and is probably not attributable to excessive action of the mineralocorticoids, aldosterone, 11-deoxycorticosterone, or corticosterone. It may be the consequence of cortisol action or of a presently little-known or unknown mineralocorticoid.

2. Extraadrenal, extrapituitary tumor-dependent hypercortisolism is the consequence of production and release, by a usually malignant neoplasm, of a corticotropin that, by an array of chemical and biological criteria, is identical with pituitary ACTH. Characteristic metabolic manifestations of glucocorticoid excess are usually minimal, perhaps as a consequence of the usually short duration of life and the debilitation brought about by the tumor. Hypokalemic alkalosis is usual and is attributable to increased rates of secretion of corticosterone and 11-deoxycorticosterone.

3. Adrenal tumor-dependent hypercortisolism may be associated either with benign or malignant tumors. When the tumor is benign, the associated disturbances are similar to those observed in pituitary-dependent hypercortisolism, except for evidences of suppressed pituitary release of ACTH and independence of the cortisol secretion rate of ACTH. When the tumor is malignant, a deficiency of 11β-hydroxylase relative to available substrate is usual. This may at least partially account for the typical overproduction of androgens and consequent virilization of females, overwhelmingly the more frequent victims. In instances of both benign and malignant tumors, hypokalemic alkalosis occurs frequently and is attributable to high concentrations of corticosterone and 11-deoxycorticosterone in blood.

REFERENCES

1. ABE, K., W. E. NICHOLSON, G. W. LIDDLE, D. P. ISLAND, AND D. N. ORTH. Radioimmunoassay of β-MSH in human plasma and tissues. *J. Clin. Invest.* 46: 1609–1616, 1967.
2. ABE, K., W. E. NICHOLSON, G. W. LIDDLE, D. N. ORTH, AND D. P. ISLAND. Normal and abnormal regulation of β-MSH in man. *J. Clin. Invest.* 48: 1580–1585, 1967.
3. ALBRIGHT, F. Cushing's syndrome. *Harvey Lectures Ser.* 38: 123–186, 1942–1943.
4. ALLOT, E. N., AND M. O. SKELTON. Increased adrenocortical activity associated with malignant disease. *Lancet* 2: 278–283, 1960.
5. BAGSHAWE, K. D. Hyperfunction of the adrenal cortex with adrenal metastases. *Lancet* 2: 284–287, 1960.
6. BAILEY, R. E. Periodic hormonogenesis—a new phenomenon. Periodicity in function of a hormone-producing tumor in man. *J. Clin. Endocrinol. Metab.* 32: 317–327, 1971.
7. BALLS, K. F., J. T. L. NICHOLSON, H. L. GOODMAN, AND J. C. TOUCHSTONE. Functioning islet-cell carcinoma of the pancreas with Cushing's syndrome. *J. Clin. Endocrinol. Metab.* 19: 1134–1143, 1959.
8. BANK, H., R. BEER, B. LUNENFELD, E. RABAU, AND G. RUMNEY. Recurrence of adrenal carcinoma during pregnancy with delivery of a normal child. *J. Clin. Endocrinol. Metab.* 25: 359–364, 1965.
9. BECKS, H., M. E. SIMPSON, C. H. LI, AND H. M. EVANS. Effects of adrenocorticotropic hormone (ACTH) on the osseous system in normal rats. *Endocrinology* 34: 305–310 1944.
10. BECKS, H., M. E. SIMPSON, W. MARX, C. H. LI, AND H. M. EVANS. Antagonism of pituitary adrenocorticotropic hormone (ACTH) to the action of growth hormone on the osseous system of hypophysectomized rats. *Endocrinology* 34: 311–316, 1944.
11. BERLINER, D., N. KELLER, AND T. F. DOUGHERTY. Tissue retention of cortisol and metabolites induced by ACTH: an extra-adrenal effect. *Endocrinology* 68: 621–632, 1961.
12. BIGLIERI, E. G., S. HANE, P. E. SLATON, AND P. H. FORSHAM. *In vivo* and *in vitro* studies of adrenal secretions in Cushing's syndrome and primary aldosteronism. *J. Clin. Invest.* 42: 516–524, 1963.
13. BIGLIERI, E. G., M. SCHAMBELAN, AND P. E. SLATON, JR. Effect of adrenocorticotropin on desoxy-corticosterone, corticosterone and aldosterone excretion. *J. Clin. Endocrinol. Metab.* 29: 1090–1101, 1969.
14. BIGLIERI, E. G., P. E. SLATON, M. SCHAMBELAN, AND S. J. KRONFIELD. Hypermineralocorticoidism. *Am. J. Med.* 45: 170–175, 1968.
15. BLECHER, M. Serum protein-steroid hormone interactions. Effects of glucocorticoids on glucose metabolism in rat adipose isolated cells, and the influence of human plasma corticosteroid binding protein. *Endocrinology* 79: 541–546, 1966.

16. BLODGETT, F. M., L. BURGIN, D. IEZZONI, D. GRIBETZ, AND N. B. TALBOT. Effects of prolonged cortisone therapy on the status of growth, skeletal maturation, and metabolic status of children. *New Engl. J. Med.* 254: 636–641, 1956.
17. BOYD, W. *A Textbook of Pathology* (8th ed.). Philadelphia: Lea & Febiger, 1970, p. 1048.
18. BROOKS, R. V., J. DUPRE, A. N. GOGATE, I. H. MILLS, AND F. T. G. PRUNTY. Appraisal of adrenocortical hyperfunction: patients with Cushing's syndrome or "nonendocrine" tumors. *J. Clin. Endocrinol. Metab.* 23: 725–736, 1963.
19. BRORSON, I. Concentration of corticosterone and cortisol in peripheral plasma of patients with adreno-cortical hyperplasia and normal subjects. *Acta Endocrinol.* 58: 445–462, 1968.
20. BROWN, R. D., AND C. A. STROTT. Plasma deoxycorticosterone in man. *J. Clin. Endocrinol. Metab.* 32: 744–750, 1971.
21. BROWN, W. H. A case of pluriglandular syndrome: "Diabetes of bearded women." *Lancet* 2: 1022–1023, 1928.
22. CHRISTY, N. P. Adrenocorticotrophic activity in the plasma of patients with Cushing's syndrome associated with pulmonary neoplasms. *Lancet* 1: 85–86, 1961.
23. CHRISTY, N. P., AND J. H. LARAGH. Pathogenesis of hypokalemic alkalosis in Cushing's syndrome. *New Engl. J. Med.* 265: 1083–1088, 1961.
24. CHRISTY, N. P., D. LONGSON, AND J. W. JAILER. Studies in Cushing's syndrome. I. Observations on the response of plasma 17-hydroxycorticosteroid levels to corticotropin. *Am. J. Med.* 23: 910–916, 1957.
25. CHRISTY, N. P., E. Z. WALLACE, AND J. W. JAILER. The effect of intravenously-administered ACTH on plasma 17,21-dihydroxy-20-ketosteroids in normal individuals and in patients with disorders of the adrenal cortex. *J. Clin. Invest.* 34: 899–906, 1955.
26. COHEN, R. B., G. D. TOLL, AND B. CASTLEMAN. Bronchial adenomas in Cushing's syndrome: their relation to thymomas and oat cell carcinomas associated with hyperadrenocorticism. *Cancer* 13: 812–817, 1960.
27. COPE, O., AND J. W. RAKER. Cushing's disease. *New Engl. J. Med.* 253: 119–127, 1955.
28. COST, W. S. Quantitative estimation of adrenocortical hormones and their α-ketolic metabolites in urine. *Acta Endocrinol.* 42: 39–52, 1964.
29. COSTELLO, R. T. Subclinical adenoma of the pituitary gland. *Am. J. Pathol.* 12: 205–215, 1936.
30. COX, M. L., R. D. GOURLEY, AND A. E. KITABCHI. Acinic cell adenocarcinoma of the parotid with ectopic production of adrenocorticotropic hormone. *Am. J. Med.* 49: 529–533, 1970.
31. CRANE, M. G., AND J. J. HARRIS. Desoxycorticosterone secretion rates in hyperadrenocorticism. *J. Clin. Endocrinol. Metab.* 26: 1135–1143, 1966.
32. CRANE, M. G., AND J. J. HARRIS. Desoxycorticosterone secretion rates in edematous patients. *Am. J. Med. Sci.* 259: 27–31, 1970.
33. CUSHING, H. The basophil adenomas of the pituitary body and their clinical manifestations (pituitary basophilism). *Bull. Johns Hopkins Hosp.* 50: 137–195, 1932.
34. DAVIS, J. O., S. S. HOWARDS, C. I. JOHNSTON, AND T. S. WRIGHT. Deoxycorticosterone secretion in chronic experimental heart failure and during infusion of angiotensin II. *Proc. Soc. Exptl. Biol. Med.* 127: 164–168, 1968.
35. DEMOOR, P., A. HENDRIKX, AND M. HINNEKENS. Extraadrenal influence of corticotropin (ACTH) on cortisol metabolism. *J. Clin. Endocrinol. Metab.* 21: 106–109, 1961.
36. DEMURA, R., H. DEMURA, T. NANOKAWA, H. BABA, AND K. MUIRA. Responses of plasma ACTH, GH, LH and 11-hydroxycorticosteroids to various stimuli in patients with Cushing's syndrome. *J. Clin. Endocrinol. Metab.* 34: 852–859, 1972.
37. DEMURA, H., C. D. WEST, C. A. NUGENT, K. NAKAGAWA, AND F. H. TYLER. A sensitive radioimmunoassay for plasma ACTH levels. *J. Clin. Endocrinol. Metab.* 26: 1297–1302, 1966.
38. DOBAN, F. C., JR., J. C. TOUCHSTONE, AND E. M. RICHARDSON. The effect of ACTH and pathological increases in adrenocortical function on urinary alpha-ketolic steroid metabolites. *J. Clin. Invest.* 34: 485–499, 1955.
39. DONAHOWER, G. F., O. P. SCHUMACHER, AND J. B. HAZARD. Medullary carcinoma of the thyroid—a cause of Cushing's syndrome: report of two cases. *J. Clin. Endocrinol. Metab.* 28: 1199–1204, 1968.
40. DONALD, R. A. Plasma immunoreactive corticotrophin and cortisol response to insulin hypoglycemia in normal subjects and patients with pituitary disease. *J. Clin. Endocrinol. Metab.* 32: 224–231, 1971.
41. DUBOIS, E. L. Triamcinolone in the treatment of systemic lupus erythematosus. *J. Am. Med. Assoc.* 167: 1590–1599, 1958.
42. EICHHORN, J., E. SCULLY, I. D. K. HALKESTON, AND O. HECHTER. Effect of ACTH and insulin on AIB accumulation in diaphragm muscle and adrenal in vivo. *Proc. Soc. Exptl. Biol. Med.* 106: 153–157, 1961.
43. EISENSTEIN, A. B., R. KARSH, AND I. GALL. Occurrence of pregnancy in Cushing's syndrome. *J. Clin. Endocrinol. Metab.* 23: 971–974, 1963.
44. EKMAN, H., B. HOKANSSON, J. D. MCCARTHY, J. LEHMAN, AND B. SJÖGREN. Plasma 17-hydroxycorticosteroids in Cushing's syndrome. *J. Clin. Endocrinol. Metab.* 21: 684–694, 1961.
45. ELLIS, J. T. Necrosis and regeneration of skeletal muscles in cortisone-treated rabbits. *Am. J. Pathol.* 32: 993–1013, 1956.
46. ENGEL, F. L. A consideration of the roles of the adrenal cortex and stress in the regulation of protein metabolism. *Recent Progr. Hormone Res.* 6: 277–313, 1951.
47. ENGEL, F. L., AND L. KAHONA. Cushing's syndrome with malignant, corticotropin-producing tumor. *Am. J. Med.* 34: 726–734, 1963.
48. ERNEST, I. Changes in body composition after therapeutically induced remission in 12 cases of Cushing's syndrome. *Acta Endocrinol.* 54: 411–427, 1967.
49. ESCOVITZ, W. E., AND I. M. REINGOLD. Functioning malignant bronchial carcinoid with Cushing's syndrome and recurrent sinus arrest. *Ann. Internal Med.* 54: 1248–1259, 1961.
50. EVANS, H. M., M. E. SIMPSON, AND C. H. LI. Inhibiting effect of adrenocorticotropic hormone on the growth of male rats. *Endocrinology* 33: 237–238, 1943.
51. EYMONTT, M. J., G. GWINUP, F. A. KRUGER, D. E. MAYNARD, AND G. J. HAMWI. Cushing's syndrome with hypoglycemia caused by adrenocortical carcinoma. *J. Clin. Endocrinol. Metab.* 25: 46–52, 1965.
52. FAIN, J. N. Effects of dexamethasone and growth hormone on fatty acid mobilization and glucose utilization in adrenalectomized rats. *Endocrinology* 71: 633–635, 1962.
53. FAIN, J. N., R. O. SCOW, AND S. S. CHERNICK. Effects of glucocorticoids on metabolism of adipose tissue in vitro. *J. Biol. Chem.* 238: 54–58, 1963.
54. FALLIERS, C. J., L. S. TAN, J. SZENTIVANYI, J. R. JORGENSON, AND S. C. BUKANTZ. Childhood asthma and steroid therapy as influences on growth. *Am. J. Diseases Children* 104: 127–137, 1963.
55. FALUDI, G., L. C. MILLS, AND Z. W. CHAYES. Effect of steroids on muscle. *Acta Endocrinol.* 45: 68–78, 1964.
56. FORBES, A. P., AND F. ALLBRIGHT. A comparison of the 17-ketosteroid excretion in Cushing's syndrome associated with adrenal tumor and with adrenal hyperplasia. *J. Clin. Endocrinol. Metab.* 11: 926–935, 1951.
57. FRANTZ, A. G., AND M. T. RABKIN. Human growth hormone. *New Engl. J. Med.* 271: 1375–1381, 1964.
58. FREYBERG, R. H., C. A. BERNTSEN, JR., AND L. HELLMAN. Further experiences with 1,9 alpha fluoro, 16 alpha hydroxyhydrocortisone (triamcinolone) in treatment of patients with rheumatoid arthritis. *Arthritis Rheumat.* 1: 215–229, 1958.
59. GALLAGHER, T. F., A. KAPPAS, H. SPENCER, AND D. LASZLO.

Influence of invasiveness, hormones, and amphenone on steroids in adrenal cancer. *Science* 124: 487–489, 1956.
60. GERMUTH, F. G., JR., G. A. NEDZEL, B. OTTINGER, AND J. OMAYA. Anatomic and histologic changes in rabbits with experimental hypersensitivity treated with compound E and ACTH. *Proc. Soc. Exptl. Biol. Med.* 76: 177–182, 1951.
61. GLASER, G. H., AND L. STARK. Excitability in experimental myopathy. I. Measurement of refractory period; quinidine effect; cortisone myopathy. *Neurology* 8: 640–644, 1958.
62. GLENN, E. M., B. J. BOWMAN, R. B. BAYERS, AND C. E. MEYER. Hydrocortisone and some of its effects on intermediary metabolism. *Endocrinology* 68: 386–410, 1961.
63. GOLDBERG, A. L. Protein turnover in skeletal muscle. *J. Biol. Chem.* 244: 3223–3229, 1969.
64. GOLDBERG, A. L., AND H. M. GOODMAN. Relationship between cortisone and muscle work in determining muscle size. *J. Physiol., London* 200: 667–675, 1969.
65. GOLDING, D. N. Dexamethasone myopathy. *Brit. Med. J.* 2: 1129–1130, 1960.
66. GRABER, A., R. E. NEY, W. E. NICHOLSON, D. P. ISLAND, AND G. W. LIDDLE. Natural history of pituitary-adrenal recovery following long term suppression with corticosteroids. *J. Clin. Endocrinol. Metab.* 25: 11–16, 1965.
67. GRAY, J. G., W. B. PRATT, AND L. ARNOW. Effect of glucocorticoids on hexose uptake by mouse fibroblasts *in vitro*. *Biochemistry* 10: 277–284, 1971.
68. GRUMBACH, M. M., A. M. BONGIOVANNI, W. R. EBERLEIN, J. J. VAN WYK, AND L. WILKINS. Cushing's syndrome with bilateral adrenal hyperplasia: a study of the plasma 17-hydroxycorticosteroids and the response to ACTH. *Bull. Johns Hopkins Hosp.* 96: 116–125, 1955.
69. HALLWRIGHT, G. P., K. A. K. NORTH, AND J. D. REID. Pigmentation and Cushing's syndrome due to malignant tumor of the pancreas. *J. Clin. Endocrinol. Metab.* 24: 496–500, 1964.
70. HARMAN, J. B. Muscular wasting and corticosteroid therapy. *Lancet* 1: 887, 1959.
71. HARRISON, M. T., A. S. RAMSEY, D. A. D. MONTGOMERY, J. H. ROBERTSON, AND R. B. WELBOURN. Cushing's syndrome with carcinoma of bronchus and with features suggesting carcinoid tumor. *Lancet* 1: 23–25, 1957.
72. HARTOG, M., M. A. GAAFAR, AND R. FRASER. Effect of corticosteroids on serum growth hormone. *Lancet* 2: 376–378, 1964.
73. HELLMAN, L., F. NAKODA, J. CURTI, E. D. WEITZMAN, J. KREANA, H. ROFFWARG, S. ELLMAN, D. K. FUKUSHIMA, AND T. F. GALLAGHER. Cortisol is secreted episodically by normal man. *J. Clin. Endocrinol. Metab.* 30: 411–422, 1970.
74. HELLMAN, L., E. D. WEITZMAN, H. ROFFWARG, D. K. FUKUSHIMA, K. YOSHIDA, AND T. F. GALLAGHER. Cortisol is secreted episodically in Cushing's syndrome. *J. Clin. Endocrinol. Metab.* 30: 686–689, 1970.
75. HENNEMAN, D. H., AND J. P. BUNKER. The pattern of intermediary carbohydrate metabolism in Cushing's syndrome. *Am. J. Med.* 23: 34–45, 1957.
76. HINMAN, F., H. L. STEINBACH, AND P. F. FORSHAM. Preoperative differentiation between hyperplasia and tumor in Cushing's syndrome. *J. Urol.* 77: 329–338, 1957.
77. HUNT, A. B., AND W. M. MCCONAHEY. Pregnancy associated with diseases of the adrenal glands. *Am. J. Obstet. Gynecol.* 66: 970–987, 1953.
78. IANNACONE, A., J. L. GABRILOVE, S. A. BRAHMS, AND L. J. SOFFER. Osteoporosis in Cushing's syndrome. *Ann. Internal Med.* 52: 570–586, 1960.
79. IANNACONE, A., J. L. GABRILOVE, A. R. SOHVAL, AND L. J. SOFFER. The ovaries in Cushing's syndrome. *New Engl. J. Med.* 261: 775–780, 1959.
80. JAILER, J. W., D. LONGSON, AND N. P. CHRISTY. Studies in Cushing's syndrome. II. Adrenal weight-maintaining activity in the plasma of patients with Cushing's syndrome. *J. Clin. Invest.* 36: 1608–1614, 1957.
81. JEANRENAUD, B., AND A. E. RENOLD. Studies on rat adipose tissue *in vitro*. VII. Effects of adrenal cortical hormones. *J. Biol. Chem.* 235: 2217–2223, 1960.
82. JOWSEY, J., AND B. L. RIGGS. Bone formation in hypercortisonism. *Acta Endocrinol.* 63: 21–28, 1970.
83. KAGAWA, C. M., AND R. PAPPO. Renal electrolyte effects of 18-hydroxylated steroids in adrenalectomized rats. *Proc. Soc. Exptl. Biol. Med.* 109: 982–985, 1962.
84. KAPLAN, N. M., AND F. C. BARTTER. The effect of ACTH, renin, angiotensin II and various precursors on biosynthesis of aldosterone by adrenal slices. *J. Clin. Invest.* 41: 715–724, 1962.
85. KENNY, F. M., A. STAVRIDES, M. L. VOORHEES, AND R. KLEIN. Cushing's syndrome associated with an adrenal neuroblastoma. *Am. J. Diseases Children* 113: 611–615, 1967.
86. KIND, H. The role of androgenic hormones in human sexual behavior. *J. Clin. Endocrinol. Metab.* 21: 482–484, 1961.
87. KITABCHI, A. E., AND R. H. WILLIAMS. Epinephrine synthesis in Cushing's syndrome. *J. Clin. Endocrinol. Metab.* 28: 1082–1084, 1968.
88. KLINE, D. L. A procedure for the study of factors which affect the nitrogen metabolism of isolated tissues: hormonal influences. *Endocrinology* 45: 596–604, 1949.
89. KORNER, A. Ribonucleic acid and hormonal control of protein synthesis. *Progr. Biophys. Mol. Biol.* 17: 61–98, 1967.
90. KOSTYO, J. L. *In vitro* effects of adrenal steroid hormones on amino acid transport in muscle. *Endocrinology* 76: 604–613, 1965.
91. KOSTYO, J. L., AND A. F. REDMOND. Role of protein synthesis in the inhibitory action of adrenal steroid hormones on amino acid transport by muscle. *Endocrinology* 79: 531–540, 1966.
92. KOSTYO, J. L., AND J. E. SCHMIDT. Inhibitory effects of cardiac glycosides and adrenal steroids on amino acid transport. *Am. J. Physiol.* 204: 1031–1038, 1963.
93. KREINES, K., E. PERIN, AND R. SALZER. Pregnancy in Cushing's syndrome. *J. Clin. Endocrinol. Metab.* 24: 75–79, 1964.
94. KUSAMA, M., O. ABE, N. SAKAUCHI, O. TAKATONI, T. MAYAMA, R. DEMURA, AND S. KUMAOKA. Extra-adrenal action of adrenocorticotropin on cortisol metabolism. *J. Clin. Endocrinol. Metab.* 30: 778–784, 1970.
95. LAIDLAW, J. C., W. J. REDDY, D. JENKINS, N. A. HAYDAR, A. E. RENOLD, AND G. W. THORN. Advances in the diagnosis of altered states of adrenocortical function. *New Engl. J. Med.* 253: 747–753, 1955.
96. LAW, D. H., G. W. LIDDLE, H. W. SCOTT, JR., AND S. D. TAUBER. Ectopic production of multiple hormones (ACTH, MSH and gastrin) by a single malignant tumor. *New Engl. J. Med.* 273: 292–296, 1965.
97. LEBOEUF, B., A. E. RENOLD, AND G. F. CAHILL, JR. Studies on rat adipose tissue *in vitro*. IX. Further effects of cortisol on glucose metabolism. *J. Biol. Chem.* 237: 988–991, 1962.
98. LECOMPTE, P. M. Cushing's syndrome with possible pheochromocytoma. *Am. J. Pathol.* 20: 689–708, 1944.
99. LEMON, F. C., M. B. FINE, S. G. GRASSO, AND L. W. KINSELL. ACTH-like activity in a thymoma associated with gonadal dysgenesis. *J. Clin. Endocrinol. Metab.* 26: 1–5, 1966.
100. LIDDLE, G. W. Tests of pituitary-adrenal suppressibility in the diagnosis of Cushing's syndrome. *J. Clin. Endocrinol. Metab.* 20: 1539–1560, 1960.
101. LIDDLE, G. W. Cushing's syndrome. In: *The Adrenal Cortex*, edited by A. B. Eisenstein. Boston: Little, Brown, 1967, p. 523–552.
102. LIDDLE, G. W., H. L. ESTEP, J. W. KENDALL, W. C. WILLIAMS, AND A. W. TOWNES. Clinical application of a new test of pituitary reserve. *J. Clin. Endocrinol. Metab.* 19: 875–894, 1959.
103. LIDDLE, G. W., J. R. GIVENS, W. E. NICHOLSON, AND D. P. ISLAND. The ectopic ACTH syndrome. *Cancer Res.* 25: 1057–1061, 1965.
104. LIDDLE, G. W., D. ISLAND, AND C. K. MEADOR. Normal and abnormal regulation of corticotropin secretion in man. *Recent Progr. Hormone Res.* 18: 125–166, 1962.

105. LIDDLE, G. W., D. P. ISLAND, R. L. NEY, W. E. NICHOLSON, AND N. SHIMIZU. Nonpituitary neoplasms and Cushing's syndrome. *Arch. Internal Med.* 111: 471–475, 1963.
106. LINDSAY, A. E., C. J. MIGEON, C. A. NUGENT, AND H. BROWN. The diagnostic value of plasma and urinary 17-hydroxycorticosteroid determinations in Cushing's syndrome. *Am. J. Med.* 20: 15–22, 1956.
107. LIPSETT, M. B., R. HERTZ, AND G. T. ROSS. Clinical and pathophysiologic aspects of adrenocortical carcinoma. *Am. J. Med.* 35: 374–383, 1963.
108. LITOWSKY, D., AND R. V. FORD. Adrenalectomy during pregnancy. *Am. J. Obstet. Gynecol.* 83: 756–758, 1962.
109. LONDON, J., AND F. C. GREENWOOD. Homologous radioimmunoassay for plasma-levels of corticotrophin in man. *Lancet* 1: 273–276, 1968.
110. LONG, C. N. H., B. KATZIN, AND E. G. FRY. Adrenal cortex and carbohydrate metabolism. *Endocrinology* 26: 309–344, 1940.
111. LONG, C. N. H., E. G. FRY, AND M. BONNY CASTLE. The effect of cortisol on carbohydrate deposition and urea nitrogen excretion in the adrenalectomized rat. *Acta Endocrinol. Suppl.* 51: 819, 1960.
112. LOTSPEICH, W. D. Relations between insulin and pituitary hormones in amino acid metabolism. *J. Biol. Chem.* 185: 221–229, 1950.
113. MACLEAN, K., AND P. H. SHURR. Reversible amyotrophy complicating treatment with fluodrocortisone. *Lancet* 1: 701–703, 1959.
114. MANCHESTER, K. L., P. J. RANDLE, AND F. G. YOUNG. The effect of growth hormone and of cortisol on the response of isolated rat diaphragm to the stimulating effect of insulin on glucose uptake and on incorporation of amino acids into protein. *J. Endocrinol.* 18: 395–408, 1959.
115. MANNIX, H., JR., R. KARL, AND F. GLENN. Adrenalectomy for Cushing's syndrome. *Am. J. Surg.* 99: 449–457, 1960.
116. MARKS, L. J., D. L. ROSENBAUM, AND A. B. RUSSFIELD. Cushing's syndrome and corticotropin-secreting carcinoma of the lung. *Ann. Internal Med.* 58: 143–149, 1963.
117. MARX, W., M. E. SIMPSON, C. H. LI, AND H. M. EVANS. Antagonism of pituitary adrenocorticotropic hormone to growth hormone in hypophysectomized rats. *Endocrinology* 33: 102–105, 1943.
118. MATIASEVIC, D., AND H. GERSHBERG. Studies on hydroxyproline excretion and corticosteroid-induced dwarfism: treatment with human growth hormone. *Metabolism* 15: 720–729, 1966.
119. MATSUKURA, S., C. D. WEST, Y. ICHIKAWA, W. JUBIZ, G. HARADA, AND F. H. TYLER. A new phenomenon of usefulness in the radioimmunoassay of plasma adrenocorticotrophic hormone. *J. Lab. Clin. Med.* 77: 490–500, 1971.
120. MEADOR, C. K., G. W. LIDDLE, D. P. ISLAND, W. E. NICHOLSON, C. P. LUCAS, J. G. NUCKTON, AND J. A. LUETSCHER. Cause of Cushing's syndrome in patients with tumors arising from "non-endocrine" tissue. *J. Clin. Endocrinol. Metab.* 22: 693–703, 1962.
121. MELBY, J. C., S. L. DALE, AND T. E. WILSON. 18-Hydroxy-deoxy-corticosterone in human hypertension. *Circulation Res.* 28, Suppl. II: 143, 1971.
122. MELONI, C. R., J. TUCCI, J. J. CANARY, AND L. H. KYLE. Cushing's syndrome due to bilateral adrenocortical hyperplasia caused by a benign adrenal medullary tumor. *J. Clin. Endocrinol. Metab.* 26: 1192–1199, 1966.
123. MENKIN, J. W., J. E. BETHANE, R. H. DESPOINTES, AND D. H. NELSON. The rate of disappearance of ACTH activity from the blood of humans. *J. Clin. Endocrinol. Metab.* 19: 1491–1495, 1959.
124. MIURA, K., H. DEMURA, E. SATO, N. SASANO, AND N. SHIMIZU. A case of ACTH-secreting cancer of the colon. *J. Clin. Endocrinol. Metab.* 31: 591–595, 1970.
125. MIURA, K., C. SASAKI, I. KATSUSHIMA, T. OHTOMO, S. SATO, H. DEMURA, T. TORKAI, AND N. SASANO. Pituitary-adrenocortical studies in a patient with Cushing's syndrome induced by thymoma. *J. Clin. Endocrinol. Metab.* 27: 631–637, 1967.
126. MOON, H. D. Inhibition of somatic growth in castrate rats with pituitary extracts. *Proc. Soc. Exptl. Biol. Med.* 37: 34–35, 1937.
127. MORITA, Y., AND A. MUNCK. Effect of glucocorticoids *in vivo* and *in vitro* on net glucose uptake and amino acid incorporation by rat thymus cells. *Biochim. Biophys. Acta* 93: 150–157, 1964.
128. MORRIS, H. G., J. R. JORGENSEN, H. ELRICK, AND R. E. GOLDSMITH. Metabolic effects of human growth hormone in corticosteroid-treated children. *J. Clin. Invest.* 47: 436–451, 1968.
129. MORRIS, H. G., J. R. JORGENSEN, AND S. A. JENKINS. Plasma growth hormone concentration in corticosteroid treated children. *J. Clin. Invest.* 47: 427–435, 1968.
130. MULLER, R., AND E. KUGELBERG. Myopathy in Cushing's syndrome. *J. Neurol. Neurosurg. Psychiat.* 22: 314–319, 1959.
131. MUNCK, A. II. The effects *in vivo* and *in vitro* on net glucose uptake by isolated adipose tissue. *Biochim. Biophys. Acta* 57: 318–326, 1962.
132. MUNCK, A., AND S. B. KORITZ. Studies on the mode of action of glucocorticoids in rats. I. Early effects of cortisol on blood glucose and on glucose entry into muscle, liver and adipose tissue. *Biochim. Biophys. Acta* 57: 310–317, 1962.
133. NAKAGAWA, K., Y. HORIUCHI, AND K. MASHIMO. Responses of plasma growth hormone and corticosteroids to insulin and arginine with or without prior administration of dexamethasone. *J. Clin. Endocrinol. Metab.* 29: 35–40, 1969.
134. NEFF, F. C., G. TICE, G. A. WALKER, AND N. OCKERBLAD. Adrenal tumor in female infant. *J. Clin. Endocrinol. Metab.* 2: 125–127, 1942.
135. NELSON, D. H. Cushing's syndrome—pituitary or adrenal origin? *J. Chronic Diseases* 12: 499–503, 1960.
136. NELSON, D. H. Disorders of adrenal secretion in man. *Metabolism* 10: 894–901, 1961.
137. NELSON, D. H., J. W. MEAKIN, J. B. DEALY, JR., D. D. MATSON, K. EMERSON, JR., AND G. W. THORN. ACTH producing tumor of the pituitary gland. *New Engl. J. Med.* 259: 161–164, 1958.
138. NELSON, D. H., J. G. SPRUNT, AND R. B. MIMS. Plasma ACTH determinations in 58 patients before or after adrenalectomy for Cushing's syndrome. *J. Clin. Endocrinol. Metab.* 26: 722–728, 1966.
139. NEW, M. I., AND M. P. SEAMAN. Secretion rates of cortisol and aldosterone precursors in various forms of congenital adrenal hyperplasia. *J. Clin. Endocrinol. Metab.* 30: 361–371, 1970.
140. NEWTON, M. A., AND J. H. LARAGH. Effect of corticotropin on aldosterone excretion and plasma renin in normal subjects, in essential hypertension, and in primary aldosteronism. *J. Clin. Endocrinol. Metab.* 28: 1006–1013, 1968.
141. NEY, R. L., R. N. DEXTER, W. W. DAVIS, AND L. D. GARREN. A study of the mechanisms by which adrenocorticotropic hormone maintains adrenal steroidogenic responsiveness. *J. Clin. Invest.* 46: 1916–1924, 1967.
142. NEY, R. L., N. SHIMIZU, W. E. NICHOLSON, D. P. ISLAND, AND G. W. LIDDLE. Correlation of plasma ACTH concentration with adrenocortical response in normal human subjects, surgical patients, and patients with Cushing's disease. *J. Clin. Invest.* 42: 1669–1677, 1963.
143. NICHOLS, J., J. C. WARREN, AND F. A. MONTY. ACTH-like excretion from carcinoma of the ovary. *J. Am. Med. Assoc.* 182: 713–718, 1962.
144. NICHOLS, T., C. A. NUGENT, AND F. H. TYLER. Steroid laboratory tests in the diagnosis of Cushing's syndrome. *Am. J. Med.* 45: 116–128, 1968.
145. NORMAN, A. P., AND S. SANDERS. Effect of corticotrophin on skeletal maturation and linear growth. *Lancet* 1: 287–289, 1969.
146. NUGENT, C. A., K. EIK-NES, L. T. SAMUELS, AND F. H. TYLER. Changes in plasma levels of 17-hydroxycortico

steroids during the administration of adrenocorticotropin (ACTH). IV. Response to prolonged infusions of small amounts of ACTH. *J. Clin. Endocrinol. Metab.* 19: 334–343, 1959.

147. ODDIE, C. J., J. P. COGHLAN, AND B. A. SCOGGINS. Plasma deoxycorticosterone levels in man with simultaneous measurement of aldosterone, corticosterone, cortisol and 11-deoxycortisol. *J. Clin. Endocrinol. Metab.* 34: 1039–1054, 1972.

148. OVERELL, B. G., S. E. CONDON, AND V. PETROW. The effect of hormones and their analogs upon the uptake of glucose by mouse skin *in vitro*. *J. Pharm. Pharmacol.* 12: 150–153, 1959.

149. PARRA, A., AND J. CRUZ-KROHN. Intercurrent Cushing's syndrome and pregnancy. *Am. J. Med.* 40: 961–966, 1966.

150. PECK, W. A., J. BRANDT, AND I. MILLER. Hydrocortisone-induced inhibition of protein synthesis and uridine incorporation in isolated bone cells *in vitro*. *Proc. Natl. Acad. Sci. US* 57: 1599–1606, 1967.

151. PENNINGTON, L. F., R. A. KREISBERG, AND J. M. HERSHMAN. Anomalous response to metyrapone in Cushing's syndrome due to adrenocortical adenoma. *J. Clin. Endocrinol. Metab.* 30: 125–127, 1970.

152. PFOHL, R. A., AND R. P. DOE. Adrenal-pituitary studies in a patient with bronchogenic carcinoma and Cushing's syndrome. *Ann. Internal Med.* 58: 993–1002, 1963.

153. PLOTZ, C. M., A. T. KNOWLTON, AND C. RAGAN. The natural history of Cushing's syndrome. *Am. J. Med.* 13: 597–614, 1952.

154. PORTER, G. A., AND J. KINSEY. Assessment of mineralcorticoid activity of 18-hydroxy-11-deoxycorticosterone (18-OH-DOC) in the isolated toad bladder. *Endocrinology* 89: 353–357, 1971.

155. PRUNTY, F. T. G., R. V. BROOKS, J. DUPRÉ, T. M. D. GIMLETTE, J. S. M. HUTCHINSON, R. R. MCSWINEY, AND I. H. MILLS. Adrenocortical hyperfunction and potassium metabolism in patients with "nonendocrine" tumors and Cushing's syndrome. *J. Clin. Endocrinol. Metab.* 23: 737–746, 1963.

156. RAISZ, L. G., C. L. TRUMMEL, J. A. WEHER, AND H. SIMMONS. Effect of glucocorticoids on bone resorption in tissue culture. *Endocrinology* 90: 961–967, 1972.

157. RAKER, J. W., P. H. HENNEMAN, AND W. S. GRAF. Coexisting primary hyperparathyroidism and Cushing's syndrome. *J. Clin. Endocrinol. Metab.* 22: 273–280, 1962.

158. RAY, B. S. The neurosurgeon's new interest in the pituitary. *J. Neurosurg.* 17: 1–21, 1959.

159. RIGGS, B. L., JR., AND R. G. SPRAGUE. Association of Cushing's syndrome and neoplastic disease. *Arch. Internal Med.* 108: 841–849, 1961.

160. ROGERS, W. F., JR., AND R. H. WILLIAMS. Correlations of biochemical and histologic changes in the adrenal cortex. *Arch. Pathol.* 44: 126–137, 1947.

161. ROOT, A. W., A. M. BONGIOVANNI, AND W. R. EBERLEIN. Studies of the secretion and metabolic effects of human growth hormone in children with glucocorticoid-induced growth retardation. *J. Pediat.* 75: 826–832, 1969.

162. ROSE, H. G., M. C. ROBERTSON, AND T. B. SCHWARTZ. Hormonal and metabolic influences on intracellular peptidase activity. *Am. J. Physiol.* 197: 1063–1069, 1959.

163. ROSENBERG, A. A. Fulminating adrenocortical hyperfunction associated with islet-cell carcinoma of the pancreas: case report. *J. Clin. Endocrinol. Metab.* 16: 1364–1373, 1956.

164. SADEGHI-NEJAD, A., AND B. SENIOR. Adrenal function, growth, and insulin in patients treated with corticoids on alternate days. *Pediatrics* 43: 277–283, 1969.

165. SALASSA, R. M., T. P. KEARNS, J. W. KERNOHAN, R. G. SPRAGUE, AND C. S. MCCARTHY. Pituitary tumors in Cushing's syndrome. *J. Clin. Endocrinol. Metab.* 19: 1523–1539, 1959.

166. SAROFF, J., W. R. SLAUNWHITE, G. COSTA, AND A. A. SANDBERG. Steroid metabolites from cholesterol-C^{14} in a patient with adrenal cancer: effects of metopirone. *J. Clin. Endocrinol. Metab.* 23: 629–637, 1963.

167. SCHAMBELAN, M., P. E. SLATON, JR., AND E. G. BIGLIERI. Mineralocorticoid production in hyperadrenocorticism. *Am. J. Med.* 51: 299–303, 1971.

168. SCHOLZ, D. A., B. L. RIGGS, R. C. BAHN, AND G. W. LIDDLE. Adrenocortical hyperfunction associated with a corticotropin-secreting bronchogenic carcinoma: report of a case. *Proc. Staff Meeting Mayo Clinic* 38: 45–51, 1963.

169. SCHTEINGART, D. E., J. W. CONN, D. N. ORTH, T. S. HARRISON, J. E. FOX, AND J. J. BOOKSTEIN. Secretion of ACTH and β-MSH by an adrenal medullary paraganglionoma. *J. Clin. Endocrinol. Metab.* 34: 676–683, 1972.

170. SEGAL, B. M., AND N. P. CHRISTY. Potentiation of the biologic activity of ACTH by human plasma. *J. Clin. Endocrinol. Metab.* 28: 1465–1472, 1968.

171. SELYE, H. Prevention of cortisone overdosage effects with the somatotrophic hormone (STH). *Am. J. Physiol.* 171: 381–384, 1952.

172. SETHURAJAN, C., P. B. CROFT, AND M. WILKINSON. Bronchial neoplasm with endocrine, metabolic and neurological manifestations. *Neurology* 17: 1169–1173, 1967.

173. SHAPIRO, M., W. E. NICHOLSON, D. N. ORTH, W. M. MITCHELL, AND G. W. LIDDLE. Differences between ectopic MSH and pituitary MSH. *J. Clin. Endocrinol. Metab.* 33: 377–381, 1971.

174. SHIMIZU, C. S. N., AND S. A. KAPLAN. Effects of cortisone on *in vitro* incorporation of glycine into protein of rat diaphragm. *Endocrinology* 74: 709–713, 1964.

175. SHIMIZU, N., E. OGOTA, W. E. NICHOLSON, D. P. ISLAND, R. L. NEY, AND G. W. LIDDLE. Studies on the melanotropic activity of human plasma and tissues. *J. Clin. Endocrinol. Metab.* 24: 984–990, 1965.

176. SOFFER, L. J., J. EISENBERG, A. IANNACONE, AND J. L. GABRILOVE. Cushing's syndrome. *Ciba Found. Colloq. Endocrinol.* 8: 487–504, 1955.

177. SOYKA, L. F., AND J. D. CRAWFORD. Antagonism by cortisone of the linear growth induced in hypopituitary patients and hypophysectomized rats by human growth hormone. *J. Clin. Endocrinol. Metab.* 25: 469–475, 1965.

178. STEEL, K., R. D. BAERG, AND D. O. ADAMS. Cushing's syndrome in association with a carcinoid tumor of the lung. *J. Clin. Endocrinol. Metab.* 27: 1285–1289, 1967.

179. STEMPFEL, R. S., B. M. SHEIKHOLISLAM, H. E. LEBOVITZ, E. ALLEN, AND R. C. FRANKS. Pituitary growth hormone suppression with low-dosage long-acting corticoid administration. *J. Pediat.* 73: 767–773, 1968.

180. STERN, P. H. Inhibition by steroids of parathyroid hormone-induced Ca^{45} release from embryonic rat bone *in vitro*. *J. Pharmacol. Exptl. Therap.* 168: 211–217, 1969.

181. STROTT, C. A., C. A. NUGENT, AND F. N. TYLER. Cushing's syndrome caused by bronchial adenomas. *Am. J. Med.* 44: 97–104, 1968.

182. STURGE, R. A., C. BEARDWELL, M. HARTOG, D. WRIGHT, AND B. M. ANSELL. Cortisol and growth hormone secretion in relation to linear growth: patients with Still's disease on different therapeutic regimens. *Brit. Med. J.* 3: 547–551, 1970.

183. SUSMAN, W. Adenomata of the pituitary with special reference to the pituitary basophilism of Cushing. *Brit. J. Surg.* 22: 539–544, 1935.

184. TALBOT, N. B., AND E. H. SOBEL. Endocrine and other factors determining growth of children. *Advan. Pediat.* 2: 238, 1947.

185. TALMADGE, R. V., H. Z. PARK, AND J. WEBSTER. Parathyroid hormone and thyrocalcitonin function in cortisol-treated rats. *Endocrinology* 86: 1080–1084, 1970.

186. TANNER, J. M., AND R. H. WHITEHOUSE. Growth response of 26 children with short stature given growth hormone. *Brit. Med. J.* 2: 69–75, 1967.

187. TEMPLE, T. E., JR., D. J. JONES, JR., G. W. LIDDLE, AND R. N. DEXTER. Correction of hypercortisolism by o, p′ DDD without induction of aldosterone deficiency. *New Engl. J. Med.* 281: 801–805, 1969.

188. TUCCI, J. R., E. A. ESPINER, P. I. JOGGER, G. L. PAUK, AND

D. P. Lauler. ACTH stimulation of aldosterone secretion in normal subjects and in patients with chronic adrenocortical insufficiency. *J. Clin. Endocrinol. Metab.* 27: 568–575, 1967.
189. Unger, R. H., J. de V. Lochner, and A. M. Eisentraut. Identification of insulin and glucagon in a bronchogenic metastasis. *J. Clin. Endocrinol. Metab.* 24: 831–832, 1964.
190. Vance, J. E., A. E. Kitabchi, K. D. Buchanan, R. W. Stoll, D. Hollander, and F. C. Wood. Hypersecretion of insulin, glucagon and gastrin in a kindred with multiple adenomatosis. *Diabetes* 17: 299, 1968.
191. Waxenberg, S. E., M. G. Drellich, and A. M. Sutherland. The role of hormones in human behavior. I. Changes in female sexuality after adrenalectomy. *J. Clin. Endocrinol. Metab.* 19: 193–202, 1959.
192. Wegienka, L. C., and P. H. Forsham. Treatment of diseases of the adrenal cortex affecting growth and development. *Mod. Treat.* 5: 168–183, 1968.
193. Weitzman, E. D., D. Fukushima, C. Nogeire, H. Roffwarg, T. F. Gallagher, and L. Hellman. Twenty-four hour pattern of the episodic secretion of cortisol in normal subjects. *J. Clin. Endocrinol. Metab.* 33: 14–22, 1971.
194. Wells, B. B., and E. C. Kendall. The influence of corticosterone and C_{17} hydroxydehydrocorticosterone (compound E) on somatic growth. *Proc. Staff Meeting Mayo Clinic* 15: 324–332, 1940.
195. Williams, G. A., C. L. Crockett, W. W. S. Butler, III, and K. R. Crispell. The coexistence of pheochromocytoma and adrenocortical hyperplasia. *J. Clin. Endocrinol. Metab.* 20: 622, 1960.
196. Williams, W. C., D. Island, R. A. A. Oldfield, and G. W. Liddle. Blood corticotropin (ACTH) levels in Cushing's disease. *J. Clin. Endocrinol. Metab.* 21: 426–432, 1961.
197. Wira, C., and A. Munck. Specific glucocorticoid receptors in thymus cells. *J. Biol. Chem.* 245: 3436–3438, 1970.
198. Wool, I. G. Corticosteroids and accumulation of C^{14}-labelled amino acids and histamine by isolated rat diaphragm. *Am. J. Physiol.* 199: 715–718, 1960.
199. Wool, I. G., and E. I. Weichselbaum. Incorporation of C^{14}-amino acids into protein of isolated diaphragms: role of the adrenal steroids. *Am. J. Physiol.* 197: 1089–1092, 1959.
200. Wool, I. G., and E. I. Weichselbaum. Adrenal cortical hormone and incorporation of C^{14} from amino acid precursors into muscle protein. *Am. J. Physiol.* 198: 360–362, 1960.
201. Wool, I. G., and E. I. Weichselbaum. Corticosteroids and incorporation of C^{14}-phenylalanine into protein of isolated diaphragm. *Am. J. Physiol.* 198: 1111–1114, 1960.
202. Wright, G. P., and W. St. Clair Symmers. *Systemic Pathology*. New York: New American Elsevier, 1967, vol. II, p. 1080.

CHAPTER 20

Blood supply of the adrenal gland

R. E. COUPLAND | *Department of Human Morphology, University of Nottingham Medical School, Nottingham, England*

CHAPTER CONTENTS

Extraglandular Adrenal Blood Vessels
    Rat
    Rabbit
    Cat
    Dog
    Macaque
    Man
Capsular and Intracapsular Vessels
    Arteriae corticis and cortical capillaries
    Arteriae medullae and medullary capillaries
    Venous tree
    Adrenal vein
Factors Affecting Adrenal Blood Flow
Functional Significance of Regional Distribution of Blood in Adrenal Medulla

---

NOTWITHSTANDING SPORADIC STUDIES on the blood supply of the adrenal gland since the turn of the century, little progress has been made in our knowledge of the vascular pattern within the mammalian gland since the work of Flint (25). Detailed studies of the vascular architecture of glands in lower forms do not appear to have been made.

The difficulties in investigating the functional anatomy of the adrenal circulation relate to three main factors: *1*) the gland receives arterial blood from multiple branches of multiple arteries, so that in experimental animals those destined solely for adrenal tissue largely defy direct cannulation; *2*) the adrenal is a composite gland consisting of a medulla largely surrounded by a cortex; and *3*) the composite gland is under dual (i.e., hormonal and nervous) control and hence is extremely labile.

For half a century it has been known that the gland in situ under conditions of minimal stimulation (compatible with anesthesia and operative exposure) receives a blood flow of about 5 ml/min per gram (range of 4.9–7 ml/min per gram) tissue in cats (14, 57, 65). More recently, similar results have been obtained in sheep (75) in both exposed in situ glands in anesthetized animals and in conscious animals in adrenals previously transplanted to the neck.

EXTRAGLANDULAR ADRENAL BLOOD VESSELS

The details of the arterial supply to the adrenal glands differ among species and vary to some extent among individuals of the same species. However, all mammalian glands so far examined in detail are supplied by multiple branches arising from vessels that originate either directly from the aorta or from its branches arising between the point where it pierces the diaphragm and, in most cases, the level of the renal arteries.

Detailed investigations have been made on the extraglandular course of adrenal vessels in the rat, rabbit, cat, dog, macaque, and man.

Rat

In the rat (31) the main blood supply is derived from an artery that leaves the ventral aspect of the abdominal aorta rostral to the respective adrenal gland; after usually dividing into two branches it supplies the upper pole of the gland (Fig. 1). The second major source is a vessel that arises from the aorta at a more caudal level and supplies the medial aspect of the gland. Other twigs are given off inconstantly by the renal arteries. Venous drainage is by readily identifiable, single adrenal veins, which run from the left gland to the left renal vein and from the right gland to the posterior vena cava.

Rabbit

The right adrenal gland usually lies rostral to the origin of the superior mesenteric artery and is closely applied to the posterior wall of the posterior vena cava. The right adrenal vein usually opens directly into the vena cava with no free course between the gland and vessel, making experimental procedure extremely difficult in the adult without careful dissection and inevitable damage to associated blood vessels. The left adrenal presents no such problems, and its blood supply has been described in detail (31, 32).

The left adrenal gland lies anterior and anterolateral to the aorta between the origins of the superior mesenteric and renal arteries. Its main blood supply is usually derived from branches of the adrenolumbar artery. The adrenolumbar vessel normally originates from the aorta immediately rostral to the left renal artery. Branches of the adrenolumbar artery pass anterior and posterior to the gland, curve around its lateral border in a cephalic direction, and give off twigs that supply the adjacent glandular substance (Fig. 2). One posterior artery is often larger than the others and, having passed behind the adrenal supplying its posterior and upper surfaces, continues rostrally to supply the inferior surface of the diaphragm. A variable number of short branches may arise from the left renal artery and are usually distributed to the anteroinferior part of the gland. In all, the gland receives some 10 arteries, which approach from various aspects. The gland is drained by a single adrenal vein, which after a short course of 1–2 mm terminates in the left renal vein.

Cat

The blood vessels supplying the adrenal gland of the cat are more numerous than those in the rabbit and rat; vessels arise from branches of the abdominal aorta extending as far caudally as the iliolumbar arteries, as well as from the aorta itself (8). Hence renal arteries, celiac axis, and superior mesenteric, phrenic, adrenolumbar, and iliolumbar arteries may all contribute. Between 11 and 21 arteries have been observed reaching the gland and arborizing on the surface of the capsule before penetrating it (8). As in the rabbit, the gland is supplied by vessels that approach its periphery from all aspects. The venous drainage is simple and takes the form of medullary veins that open directly into the adrenolumbar veins (one on each side) as these vessels groove or tunnel through the anterior surface of the gland substance. In rare instances a left adrenal vein a few millimeters long can be traced from the gland to a less intimately related adrenolumbar vein.

Dog

The description of Flint (25) remains the classic account of the blood supply to the adrenal gland of the dog. On each side, about 21 arteries approach the gland from medial, superior, and inferior aspects and are derived from the aorta and from phrenic, renal, adrenolumbar, and, less constantly, celiac and superior mesenteric arteries (Fig. 3). Having reached the capsule, they break into fine branches that supply the parenchyma.

Two to four veins pass from each adrenal medulla to the corresponding adrenolumbar vein, and small venous channels connect the venous side of the capsular plexus to the veins accompanying the adrenal arteries and thence back to renal, phrenic, and adrenolumbar veins.

Macaque

As in lower forms, the adrenal glands receive blood from multiple branches of adjacent arteries. These form an anastomosing network adjacent to the capsule of the gland from which vessels arise to penetrate the capsule and gland substance (33). The left adrenal gland receives branches from three main vascular zones: *1)* a group of

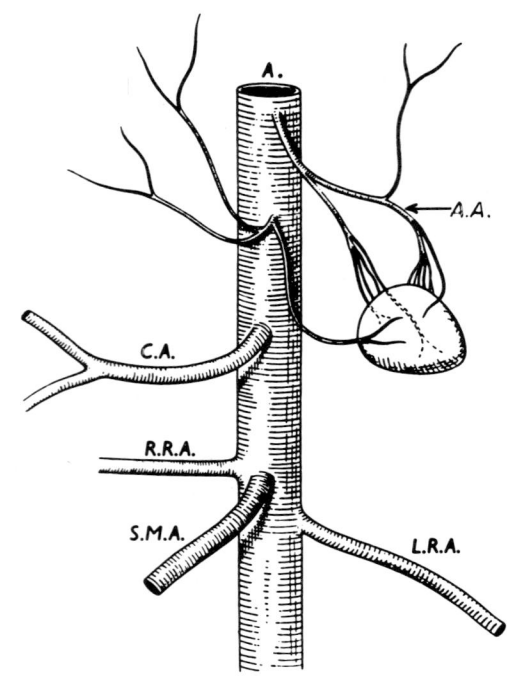

FIG. 1. Blood supply of left adrenal gland in rat. *A.*, aorta; *C.A.*, celiac artery; *R.R.A.*, right renal artery; *S.M.A.*, superior mesenteric artery; *L.R.A.*, left adrenal artery; *A.A.*, adrenal artery. [From Harrison (31).]

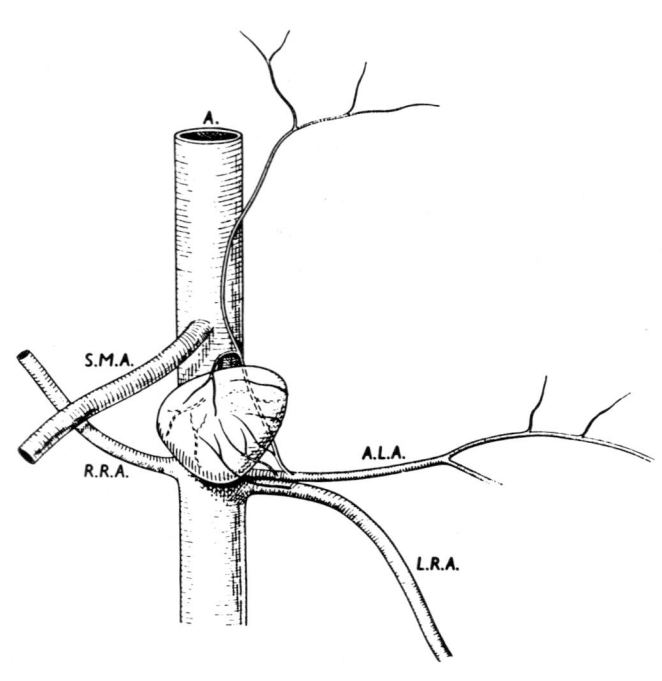

FIG. 2. Blood supply of left adrenal gland in rabbit. *A.L.A.*, adrenolumbar artery; other abbreviations as defined in Fig. 1. [From Harrrison (31).]

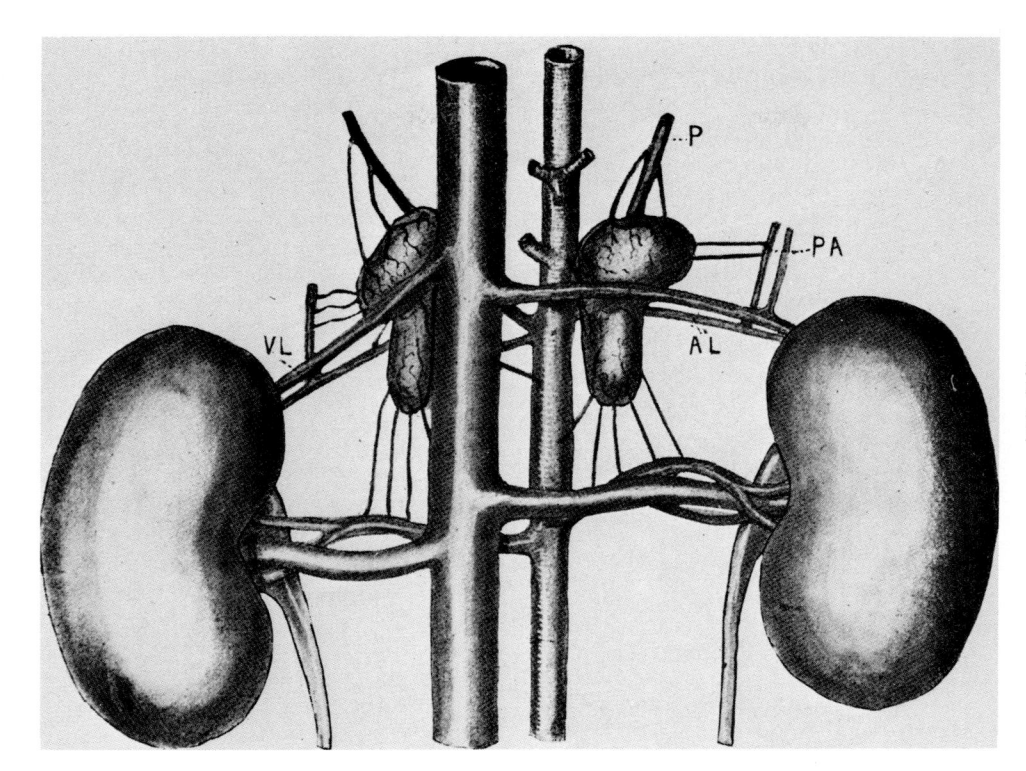

FIG. 3. Blood supply of adrenal glands in adult dog. *AL*, lumbar artery; *P*, phrenic artery; *PA*, accessory phrenic artery; *VL*, lumbar vein. [From Flint (25).]

vessels comprising the celiac axis and the adrenolumbar and inferior phrenic arteries—the latter two may and commonly do arise from the celiac artery; *2*) a middle group of two arteries that arise from the aorta; and *3*) branches from the left renal artery.

The supply to the right adrenal can be divided into vessels of superficial and deep sources (33), as viewed from the front (anterior). The superficial supply usually consists of two arteries, one arising from the aorta at the level of the right renal artery and the other from the renal artery near its origin. The former passes posteriorly to the inferior vena cava, runs rostrally, and passes medially to the gland, giving off about 15 branches; it continues as the inferior phrenic artery. The second arises near the hilus of the right kidney and sends four or five branches to the gland. The deep supply arises in the angle between the aorta and right renal artery, passes posteriorly to the inferior vena cava, and divides into 13–15 branches, which supply the medial and posterior aspects of the gland.

Adrenal veins, which are usually two in number on each side, open on the right into the inferior vena cava and on the left into the left renal vein; these have a distinct extraglandular course before reaching the major vessels.

Man

Detailed accounts of the extracapsular blood vessels of the adrenals and their variations have been published (9, 15, 26–28, 53, 54, 63), and variations in the origin and course of the adrenal and pararenal blood vessels have also been studied (1–6, 12, 22, 49, 55, 58, 59). More recently the blood supply to 200 glands has been studied by dissection of adult cadavers (27), and fetal, neonatal, and adult specimens have been examined after vascular injection of carmine latex, India ink latex, or carmine gelatin solution (53).

Nomenclature relating to the arterial blood supply of the adrenal glands commonly follows the terminology used by Gagnon (27). Thus multiple superior, middle, and inferior adrenal (suprarenal) arteries approach the upper, medial, and lower aspects of the glands as they lie in regions bounded by the inferior phrenic artery above, aorta medially, and renal artery inferiorly (Fig. 4). In general, the superior group of arteries arises from the inferior phrenic artery, the middle from the aorta, and the inferior from the renal artery. Leashes of fine adrenal vessels commonly arise from the inferior phrenic arteries and from branches of the renal arteries. Fewer and larger caliber vessels arise from the aorta and the main stem of the renal arteries and form the middle group of adrenal arteries.

The general pattern may be complicated by variations in the origins of main vessels. For example, the inferior phrenic artery may arise from the renal artery, in which case this vessel may give both middle and superior adrenal branches.

Superior adrenal arteries number 1–21 on the right and 1–23 on the left, and the average on both sides is 7.6 (27). The average number of middle adrenal arteries on both sides is 1.24 and of inferior vessels 2.75. Superior arteries do not normally branch before reaching the vicinity of the capsule, whereas the middle and inferior vessels commonly branch earlier.

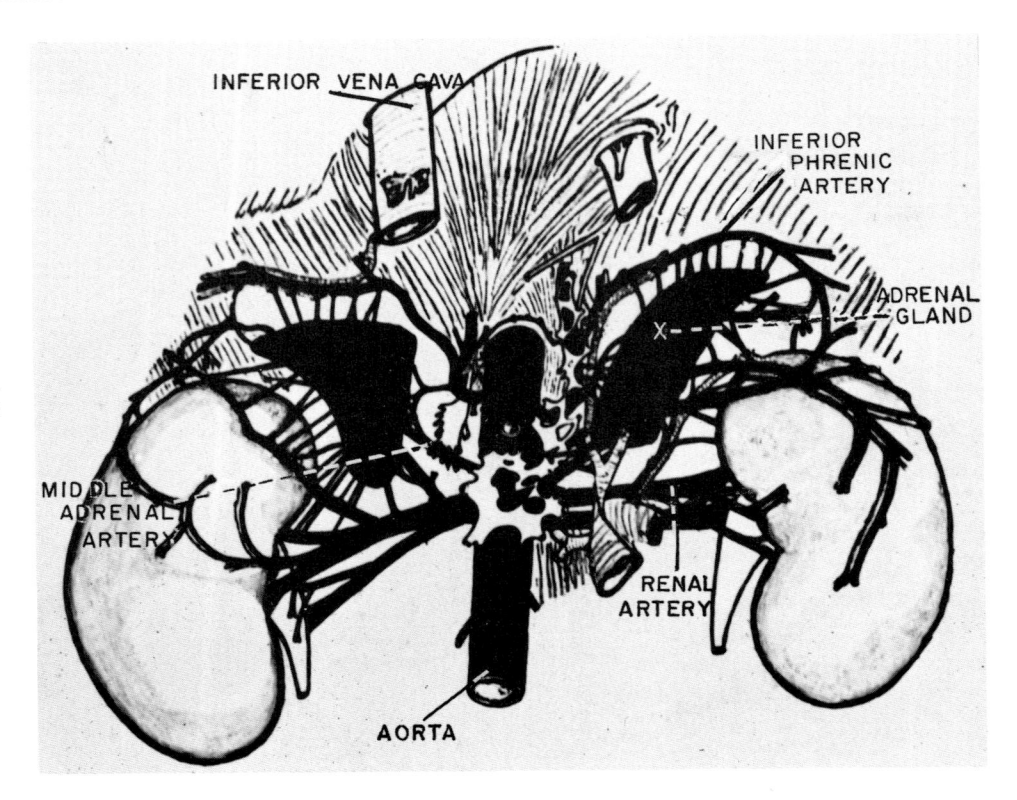

FIG. 4. Blood supply of adrenal glands in man. [After Gagnon (27).]

The main venous drainage is via the adrenal vein that emerges from the anteromedial surface of the gland to enter the renal vein on the left side and the inferior vena cava on the right. The extraglandular vein is some millimeters long on the left and virtually nonexistent on the right. The right adrenal gland is often applied directly to the posterior surface of the inferior vena cava. In addition to the drainage from the central vein into the adrenal vein, blood may also pass from surface vessels to small veins that accompany adjacent arteries—in particular, the inferior phrenics. Other veins run between the surface of the gland and tributaries of the renal veins. Anastomoses between capsular adrenal veins and branches of the hepatic portal vein have been reported (44), and in some instances the right adrenal vein or veins may join the right hepatic vein (39).

CAPSULAR AND INTRACAPSULAR VESSELS

Extracapsular arteries divide as they reach the vicinity of the gland and arborize on the surface of the capsule (Fig. 5). Anastomoses between branches of adrenal arteries either do not occur or are infrequent in the dog (25), rodent (29), and rabbit (31). In man, anastomoses, if present, may involve vessels no larger than arterioles (53). However, a complete anastomotic circle may be formed by arteries a few millimeters from the surface of the gland. Individual adrenal arteries in the dog divide five or six times on the surface of the capsule before reaching the arteriolar stage (25).

Having reached the capsule the arteries may form a capsular plexus, as in the dog (25), or penetrate the capsule to form a subcapsular plexus, as in the cat (8) and macaque (33). In the cat arteriovenous communications, as well as anastomosis between adjacent arteries, have been described on the surface of the capsule (8). In the rat a capsular plexus has been described (29), but some workers (48) refer to the plexus as being subcapsular in position. In the rabbit (31) the arteries form a capsular plexus.

The absence of anastomoses between glandular branches of the different adrenal arteries suggests that these vessels may be end arteries. Experimental evidence verifying this conclusion has been provided by ligating individual feeder vessels as they approach the gland in rabbits, rats, and cats; avascular necrosis has been demonstrated in the territory supplied by the particular branch (31). In the rabbit and cat the necrotic zone is initially confined to the zona fasciculata; in the rabbit, after some weeks the overlying zona glomerulosa is also affected. In the cat, despite the anastomotic plexus in the capsule, vascular ligation results in necrosis involving the whole thickness of the cortex in the territory of the vessel (31). The adrenal of the macaque undergoes changes similar to those of the cat after arterial ligation (33). In all species the medulla escapes damage.

From vessels lying on the surface of, or penetrating, the capsule, branches of arteriolar size arise. They are referred to as *arteriae capsulae* (25) and break into capillary nets or meshworks almost immediately.

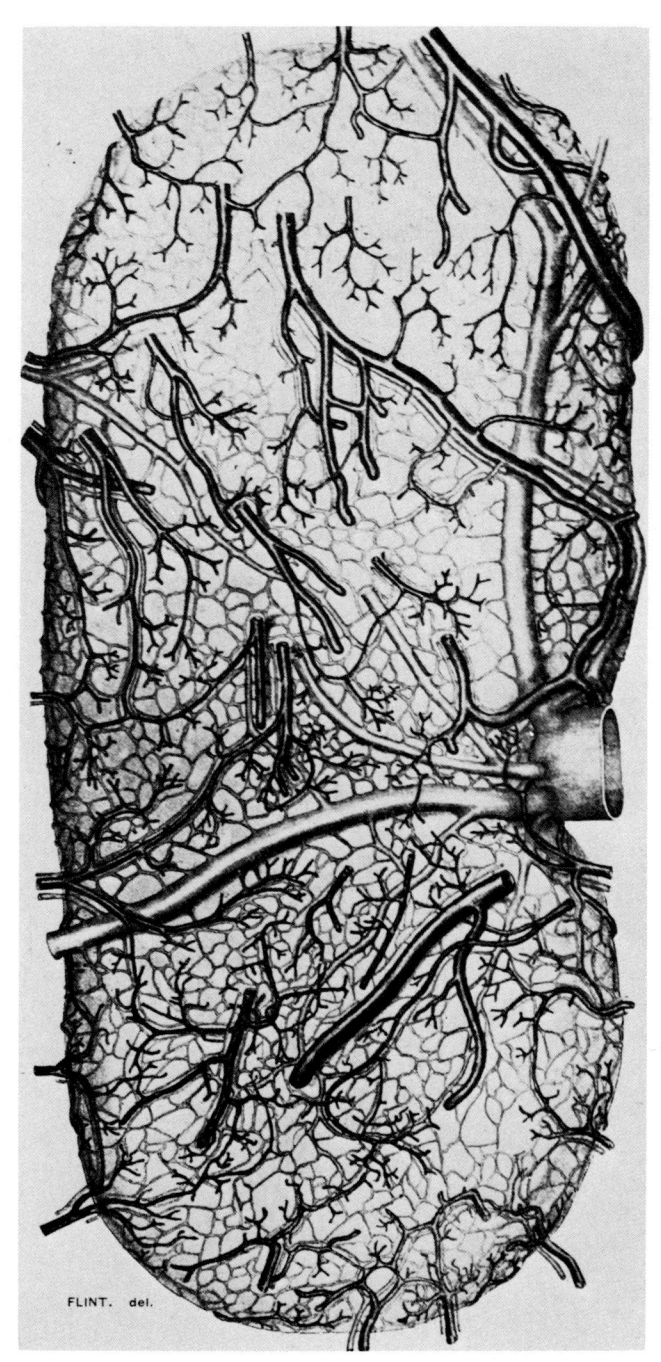

FIG. 5. Arterial (*dark*) and venous (*light*) plexuses in capsule of adrenal gland in adult dog. [From Flint (25).]

Arteriae Corticis and Cortical Capillaries

The majority of arterial branches penetrate the capsule and then either form a well-defined subcapsular plexus from which capillary vessels arise, as in the cat (8) and rat (48), or divide into capillaries that pass centrally in the septa of reticular tissue between and around cells of the zona glomerulosa (8, 25, 48) and between the cells of the zona fasciculata, anastomosing freely with each other. They continue centripetally as radially arranged channels linked by anastomotic vessels (Fig. 6).

In injected specimens a narrowing of capillary vessels was noted at the level of the outer zona fasciculata in the cat (8) and rat (48). In the zona reticularis, capillaries are wider than in outer zones and exhibit a rich intercapillary anastomosis that forms a latticework around individual cells. The essentially radial direction seen in the zona fasciculata is no longer apparent. As they approach the corticomedullary boundary, the capillaries dilate further and become first-order collecting radicles of the central adrenal vein (25, 48).

In animals such as the mouse, where the inner part of the reticular zone (X-zone of mouse) undergoes postnatal atrophy, increase in capillary density in the involutional region is marked (29). In all forms, however, increased capillary density, with rich anastomoses, occurs in the region of the zona reticularis and has indeed been referred to as a vascular dam (71–73).

Vessels intervening between arteries and veins in the adrenal gland are sometimes referred to as sinusoids (56), rather than capillaries, in consequence of their intimate association with parenchymal elements, which impart an irregular outline to their relatively large caliber, and the relative lack of supporting connective tissue.

Although the majority of vessels observed in the adrenal cortex are capillaries or sinusoids, two forms of small arteries have been identified (see Fig. 6); these are destined either to terminate in the adrenal cortex or to follow an unbranched course to the adrenal medulla where they terminate in the medullary capillary plexus. The former were designated by Flint (25) as *arteriae corticis* and supply cortical capillaries. The second group were called *arteriae medullae* (Figs. 7 and 8).

In the dog the arteriae corticis are often sixth-order branches of arteries of arteriolar size and form and end in the capillary plexus of the zona fasciculata (25). Similar vessels have been observed in the cat, rat, and mouse (8, 29, 48). In addition to these short, radially arranged, penetrating arterioles, all the more recent workers have also described looped vessels (see Fig. 8) that arise in the capsule or subcapsular region and either return to the subcapsular plexus for distribution or, after a curved course of variable length, join the capillary plexus in one of the three cortical zones.

Arteriae Medullae and Medullary Capillaries

Arteriae medullae and medullary capillaries, which were first described by Flint (25), have subsequently been seen by all workers who have followed the intraglandular arrangement of adrenal blood vessels.

The arteriae medullae pursue a radial course through the gland and are distributed exclusively to the medulla (see Figs. 6–8). In their course through the cortex, the vessels do not divide. In the dog about 50 medullary arteries occur, and they can be divided into two types, according to whether they break up into distributing

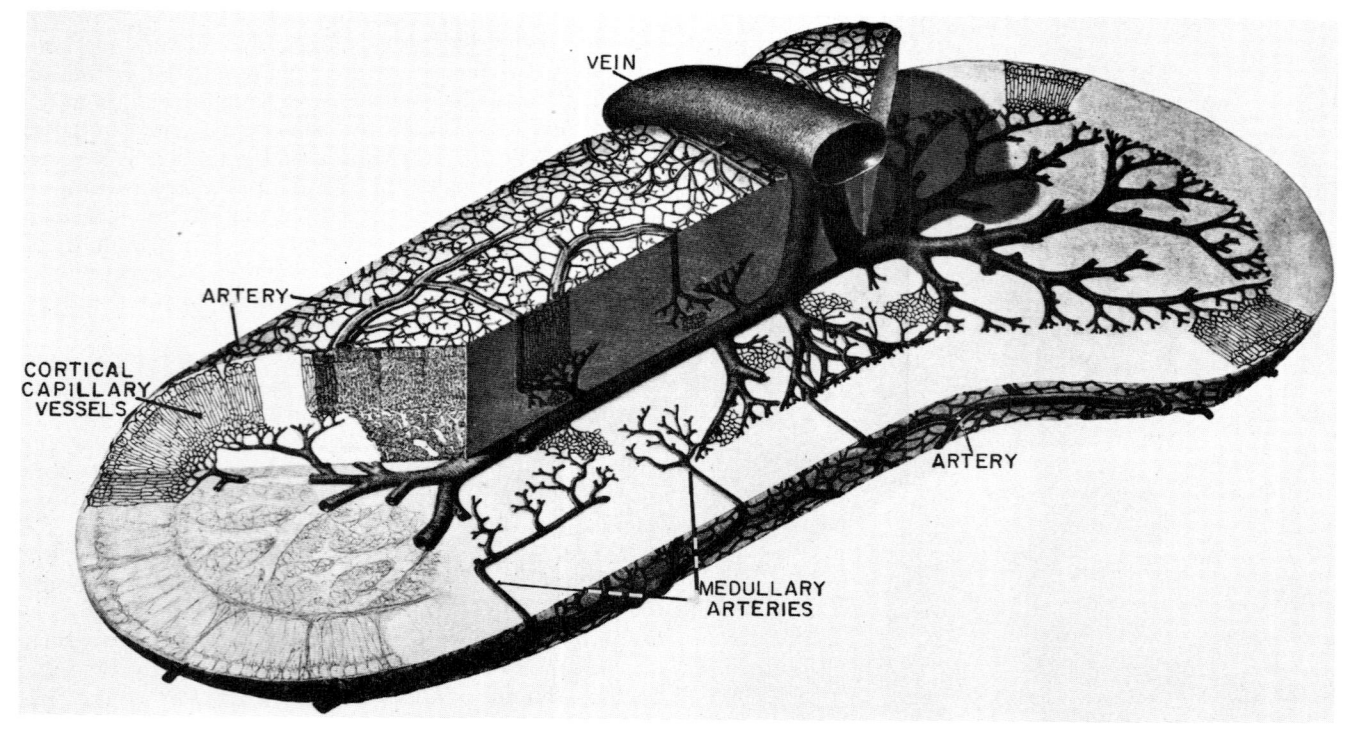

FIG. 6. Arterial blood supply and venous drainage of adrenal gland in dog. [From Flint (25).]

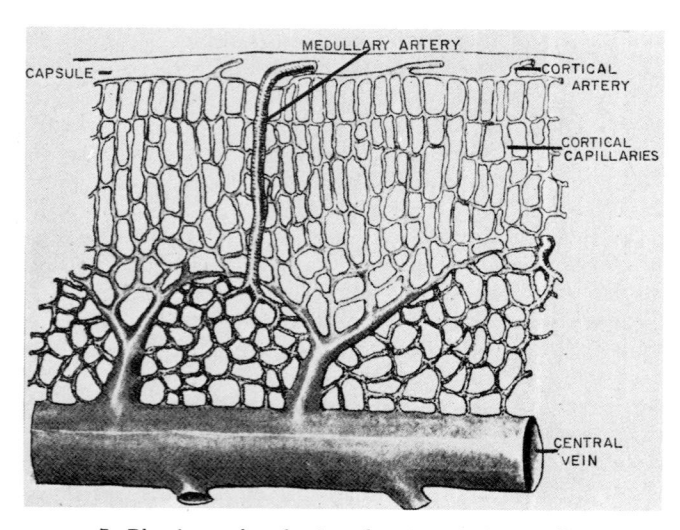

FIG. 7. Blood supply of adrenal cortex and medulla in dog. [From Flint (25).]

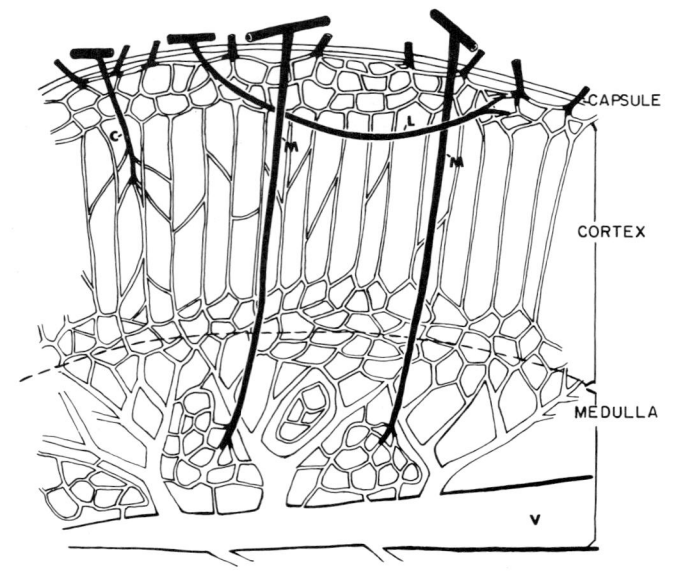

FIG. 8. Blood supply of mammalian adrenal gland. C, cortical arteries; M, medullary arteries; L, looped artery; V, central vein. [From Coupland (20).]

branches immediately or turn at the corticomedullary boundary to run for some distance parallel to the capsule before breaking into distributing branches (25). Branches of the medullary arteries ramify among cell groups that lie in the zones between the larger branches of the venous tree (8, 25, 29). In the cat, "numerous" medullary arteries were observed by Bennett & Kilham (8), and one to four medullary arteries penetrate the gland of the rat from the capsule on the opposite side to the point of emergence of the central vein (29). In the mouse a single medullary artery has been described (29), and this commonly pursues a course adjacent to the adrenal vein.

The arteriae medullae are end arteries (8, 48). They have relatively thick muscular walls in larger mammals, such as the cat (8) and ungulates (R. E. Coupland, unpublished observations).

The capillary plexus of the adrenal medulla is more

irregular and much more coarse than that of the cortex (25, 48). Capillaries run in reticular tissue between cell groups rather than between individual cells. At the corticomedullary junction, continuity between capillaries of the zona reticularis and medulla has occasionally been observed (29, 48). However, the normal direction of blood flow in these vessels has not been determined. Other capillaries drain into branches of the venous tree or form veins (venae medullae) that drain only the medullary substance and join the main trunk of the adrenal vein as it branches (25).

Venous Tree

The relatively dilated capillaries of the zona reticularis widen still further at the corticomedullary border to form the peripheral radicles of the venous tree. These first-order radicles anastomose with each other freely and unite to form bigger channels. Large channels usually do not anastomose and indeed constitute the peripheral parts of what are, in effect, terminal veins; the latter drain into the central vein (25, 29). Confluence of vessels gives rise to five orders of venous channels that terminate in the central vein [(29, 48, 54); Figs. 7 and 9].

In the mammalian adrenal medulla, chromaffin cells often exhibit polarity with respect to vascular channels, and in the cat (8) and in ungulates (19), venous and arterial capillary poles of usually columnar-shaped chromaffin cells may be identified; these cells are characteristically epinephrine-storing elements (19). Polarity of epinephrine-storing chromaffin cells relates also to innervation since nerve endings do not occur on the venous face of these cells (19, 50).

Details of the venous drainage of the adrenal gland vary among species and have been described for the dog (25), cat (8), rat (29, 48), mouse (29), and in man (26, 39, 54).

Although the majority of the blood from the gland escapes by entering the peripheral radicles of adrenal vein, other routes are available (8, 25, 26, 44, 48, 54). Thus capillaries or small veins may join the central vein as it traverses the cortical substance, surface capsular veins may anastomose with adjacent veins, and perforating veins may drain the cortical substance into capsular veins or venae comitantes of the adrenal arteries and especially into the inferior phrenic veins.

Adrenal Vein

A striking feature of the central vein of the adrenal gland is its large caliber relative to the size of the organ and the presence of longitudinal bands of smooth muscle in its wall in some species, including man, chimpanzee, hippopotamus, elephant, rhinoceros, and kangaroo (7, 11). Muscle bundles have not been described in the adrenal veins of domestic and laboratory animals.

Longitudinal muscle in the wall of the human adrenal vein was first recorded by Brunn (13). A recent study (23) of this muscle involving the reconstruction of the organ from serial sections has demonstrated a uniform and continuous layer of muscle fibers associated with the extraglandular portion of the vein; within the gland, however, it is still complete medially, but more laterally it becomes eccentric and arranged in two to four bundles. Between these bundles pass venules that drain the parenchyma. Smooth muscle can be traced as far as third- or fourth-order tributaries of the central vein in man (7, 24). Large muscle bundles, which in fixed specimens appear to protrude into the lumen of the central vein, are present in man after puberty (7).

The human adrenal vein and its medullary radicles may be divided on topographical grounds into three regions (35): *1*) the extraglandular vein extending from the appropriate gland to the inferior vena cava on the right or to the left renal vein; *2*) the central vein represented by the short, nonbranched part within the medial aspect of the gland; and *3*) the medullary veins, including all the treelike radicles that join to form the central vein.

Muscle cells can first be identified in association with the extraglandular and central vein in 20-cm fetuses and are a constant feature in 40-cm and older specimens (10, 35, 37, 41, 43, 70, 72, 73). Longitudinal muscle is already

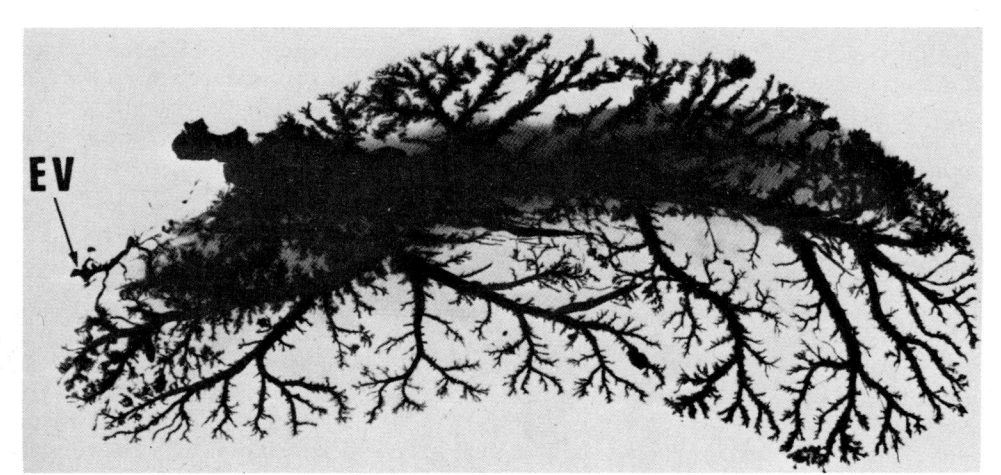

FIG. 9. Venogram of left human adrenal gland showing branches of central vein. *EV*, emissary vein. [From Dobbie & Symington (23).]

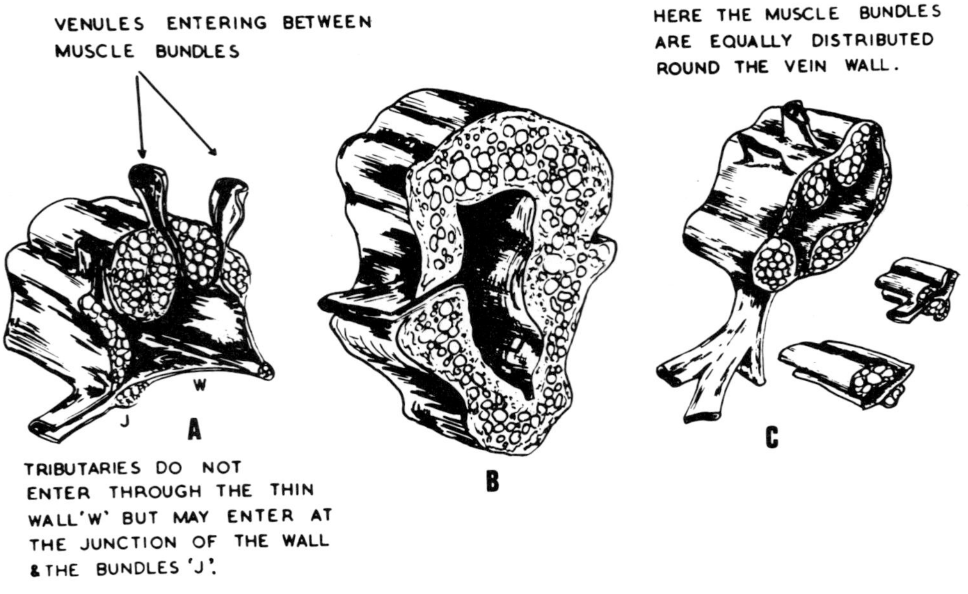

FIG. 10. Stereogram models of central vein of human adrenal gland. *A*: through body of gland; *B*: central vein external to gland; *C*: through head of gland. [From Symington (67).]

VENULES ENTERING BETWEEN MUSCLE BUNDLES

HERE THE MUSCLE BUNDLES ARE EQUALLY DISTRIBUTED ROUND THE VEIN WALL.

TRIBUTARIES DO NOT ENTER THROUGH THE THIN WALL 'W' BUT MAY ENTER AT THE JUNCTION OF THE WALL & THE BUNDLES 'J'.

well developed in the extraglandular vein during the first year of life, whereas circular fibers are rarely observed. In the adult the normal structure is an intima that contains an internal elastic layer surrounded by a medium consisting of circular smooth muscle fibers and connective tissue and an outer or adventitial layer containing longitudinal smooth muscle fibers and connective tissue. The longitudinal muscle is aggregated into thick bundles and includes a few spirally directed fibers (35). At the point of junction of the adrenal vein with the inferior vena cava or left renal vein, the longitudinal muscle coat is continuous with that of the larger vessel.

Until birth, the portion of the adrenal vein referred to as the central vein contains only a small amount of smooth muscle. Conspicuous bundles of muscle become evident during childhood; they consist of inner circular and outer longitudinal fibers, and again the latter predominate in bulk. In the adult the central and extraglandular parts of the vein have a similar appearance, the main difference being a reduction in the thickness of the muscle in the central vein, which involves both circular and longitudinal fibers (35). As the central vein is followed laterally to the medullary veins, circular fibers disappear and the longitudinal muscle becomes arranged in bundles of irregular sizes.

Heinivarra (35) considered that a subdivision of medullary veins into different types (7, 24) was irrelevant since a gradual transition in structure can be demonstrated, depending largely on size and position. Muscle, though evident in the walls of the larger veins in the neonate and even in the fetus, forms only a thin layer until the second decade of life, when longitudinally directed bundles become evident with two to four being present in the walls of the larger vessels. Some of the fibers in these bundles are longitudinal, whereas others are spiral in disposition. Smaller veins open into the larger vessels between these muscle bundles. As the venous tree is followed peripherally, muscle fibers are reduced in number and finally disappear. Dobbie & Symington (23) described an arrangement of muscle bundles in the human adrenal vein (Fig. 10) similar to that detailed by Heinivarra (35). However, they drew attention to the fact that the intraglandular portion of the adrenal vein is not surrounded by medullary tissue but that it carries with it an invaginated cuff of cortical tissue that envelops it throughout its entire length and finally merges with the cortical tissue at the tail of the gland. The main branches of the central vein are surrounded by cuffs of cortical cells, and only in the medial aspect of the gland (head region) are small venous radicles surrounded by medullary tissue (23).

Maresch (51) suggested that during contraction the longitudinal muscle bundles would encroach on the lumen and thus block it and, in addition, occlude the lumen of any small veins that joined by passing between the muscle bundles. Kutschera-Aichbergen (44) and Keil (42) suggested that, after venous occlusion, blood would travel from the interior of the gland via emissary veins to the capsule and then on to anastomotic vessels, including those associated with the hepatic portal system. Emissary veins leading to the capsular vessels have been demonstrated by vascular perfusion (23); these will be important in pathological occlusion of the central vein and should prevent total necrosis of the gland. The hypothesis of restrictive action of the musculature of the vein gained the support of many workers (7, 65, 66, 74, 79). It has been suggested that muscular contraction is induced by parasympathetic stimuli and that relaxation follows sympathetic stimulation (78). Against this possibility is the fact that only one worker (68, 69) has claimed to have definitely traced vagal fibers to the adrenal gland, whereas many others (19) have recorded their absence. Furthermore, cholinesterase-positive nerve fibers have not been observed in association with the muscle of the central vein, though as usual the smooth muscle reacts for pseudocholinesterase (18, 19).

An opposite hypothesis to the restrictive action of smooth muscle in the adrenal vein has been put forward by other workers (30, 36, 40) who suggested that contraction results in dilatation of the vein and increased blood flow. Velican (71, 73) considered that the circular muscle may have a sphincteric action on blood flow and thought that contraction of longitudinal muscle would express the contents of the medullary veins and thus inject their contents into the general circulation. Since the main medullary vein is invested in a sleeve of cortical tissue in man and veins draining cortical regions open between muscle bundles, contraction of the muscle will affect blood flow from localized cortical zones in the human gland (23). The only possible mechanical effect of contraction of the longitudinal muscle on the thin-walled venous sinuses that pass between the muscle columns is one of closure. However, where an acute angle is formed by the junction of two muscular veins, contraction will probably result in widening of the lumen at the junction and thus will assist flow (23). Since contraction of the bundles in the central vein and medullary veins in the head and body of the gland will result in encroachment of the muscle on the lumen, as well as occlusion of venous sinuses joining in this position, contraction will result in engorgement of sinuses and congestion extending back to the reticularis or even zona fasciculata. Thus the longitudinal bundles may act both as a control mechanism for medullary secretions and as sluice gates for the corticomedullary vascular dam (23).

This arrangement of the muscle bundles in the human adrenal vein suggests that blood flow through the cortex and medulla can be reduced by constriction of the normal channel of outflow. Thus, in the absence of vasoconstriction of feeding arteries, the gland will become engorged with blood as the veins become occluded, and vascular engorgement will be first evident in the medulla and zona reticularis and will gradually extend peripherally. Under these circumstances, not only may adrenocorticotropic hormone present in the blood have a better chance of reaching and affecting cells of the inner zone of the cortex (23), but back flow into capillaries fed by the arteriae medullae will result in the majority of, if not all, chromaffin cells being exposed to the high corticosteroid concentrations, which under conditions of free flow probably only affect those adjacent to the medullary venous sinuses.

FACTORS AFFECTING ADRENAL BLOOD FLOW

Because of the topographic position of the glands and the arrangement of adrenal arteries and veins, meaningful studies on the adrenal circulation are difficult to devise. To date no two workers have applied identical techniques to such studies, and variations in general methodology and temporal aspects of the studies make comparisons and attempts at conclusions regarding the effects of hormones and other chemical substances on the intrinsic circulation of the adrenal an unrewarding exercise.

Attempts were made (62) to assess adrenal blood flow by estimating the number of red blood corpuscles per cubic millimeter of cortex in glands fixed immediately after death of the animal. Using this technique the effects of blood loss, bodily exertion, sleep, psychic excitation, pain, body heating and cooling, pregnancy, gas inhalation, asphyxia, anesthetics, and subcutaneous injection of Ringer's solution, epinephrine, atropine, cocaine, acetylcholine, insulin, caffeine, pilocarpine, morphine, picrotoxin, physostigmine, nicotine, alcohol, histamine, and strychnine were measured. Clearly such a method gives no information on blood flow through the organ in part or as a whole, and an increase in number of corpuscles may result from vascular engorgement associated with decreased flow or from vasodilatation in association with increased blood flow.

This problem has also been attacked by injecting animals killed by exposure to illuminating gas with India ink and fixing the glands in formol alcohol before embedding and sectioning (29). In this work the vascular patterns present in previously normal mice of different ages were compared with those of animals that had been fed thyroid powder to induce adrenal cortical hypertrophy. Once again the size of the vascular bed rather than blood flow was recorded; the authors noted an increase in the number and diameter of cortical capillaries and dilatation of medullary veins in hypertrophied glands.

A more dynamic approach to the problems was attempted (32, 34) by injecting thorotrast into living animals and X-raying the adrenal glands in situ or X-raying frozen sections of glands after rapid removal from untreated animals and from animals previously injected intramuscularly, intraperitoneally, or intravenously with epinephrine. Blood flow through the gland was not determined, and no effect was observed on the vascular pattern up to 0.5 hr after the injection. Subsequently, increased filling of cortical vessels was observed. The delay in response was so great, however, that it was probably not due directly to epinephrine, though the workers concluded at the time that the effect presumably resulted from a vasoconstrictor action on the arteriae medullae. Similar experiments were carried out after injections of histamine, 5-hydroxytryptamine, adrenochrome, kallidin, and norepinephrine. In all cases, delayed cortical filling was observed (30–60 min after the injections), the more rapid response being observed after norepinephrine and adrenochrome. Once again the authors concluded that the main effect of the various agents was to cause constriction of arteriae medullae, which resulted in shunting of blood into cortical capillaries.

Wright (76) attempted to overcome many of the problems inherent in measurement of blood flow in the gland in situ by transplanting the left adrenal gland to the neck in sheep. He anastomosed the adrenal vessels with the carotid artery and jugular vein. Right adrenalectomy was performed before blood flow was recorded. By using these preparations a blood flow per unit mass similar to normal (14, 58) was obtained. Blood flow from the gland was estimated after infusions of various substances into the afferent vessels to the gland and into the general circulation.

The intraarterial infusion of adrenocorticotropic hormone (ACTH) at doses producing two-thirds maximal cortisol secretion had little effect on blood flow, whereas the intravenous administration of ACTH at 1-24 units/hr caused a slight but variable rise in blood flow. The results (76) were in accord with some previous work on in situ glands (38) but differed from other reports (52) in which no effect was obtained. Norepinephrine infusion into the artery at a rate of 2.4 μg/hr caused a variable reduction in blood flow, whereas angiotensin had little or no effect (76). Acetylcholine (240 μg/hr) administered by arterial infusion resulted in a 50% increase in blood flow, and 5-hydroxytryptamine administered by the same route caused a slight increase in flow. After the intraarterial infusion of bradykinin, blood flow almost doubled in some instances and always rose, and histamine had similar effects. Vasopressin caused a reduction in blood flow. The results obtained by Wright relate to blood flow from the gland and were not designed to give information about intraglandular changes in vascular pattern. Regrettably, to date no one has contributed significantly to our understanding of regional blood flow within the gland and its functional significance.

FUNCTIONAL SIGNIFICANCE OF REGIONAL DISTRIBUTION OF BLOOD IN ADRENAL MEDULLA

As indicated above, the adrenal medulla of mammals—but not, so far as is known, of lower forms—receives blood from two distinct sources: *1*) the cortical venous sinuses; *2*) the arteriae medullae. Blood passing through the sinuses connecting the cortex with the medulla comes into intimate contact with chromaffin cells that lie adjacent to the peripheral radicles of the central vein. The chromaffin cells that lie in the zones between the radicles of the adrenal veins are supplied by arterial blood through the arteriae medullae. In consequence of this arrangement, some chromaffin cells receive a primarily arterial blood supply, whereas others may be supplied primarily by cortical venous blood. This arrangement may be of importance in relation to metabolism of chromaffin cells because of relative oxygenation, P_{CO_2} of blood derived from the two sources, and the vasomotor or humoral control of the different vessels, and also by virtue of the possible effects of high concentrations of corticosteroids, which will obtain in the immediate vicinity of the cells receiving the cortical effluent. In ungulates (19) the cells lining the radicles of the venous tree are commonly epinephrine-storing elements, whereas norepinephrine-storing cells tend to occur more centrally or in zones of the medulla that lie between the major venous tributaries. Hence the arteriae medullae may be particularly concerned with supplying the norepinephrine-storing cells. This arrangement is in keeping with the findings that epinephrine-storing chromaffin cells are found in situations where high concentrations of corticosteroids are to be expected (17) and that methylation of norepinephrine is induced by exposing norepinephrine-storing cells in vitro (19–21) or in vivo (45–47, 60, 61, 77, 78) to high concentrations of corticosteroids having 11-oxy groups. Regrettably, to date, morphological and technical problems associated with the selective injection of specific vessels in the adrenal gland and the specific identifications of epinephrine- and norepinephrine-storing cells in injected material have prevented the demonstration of the regional distribution of arterial and venous blood to the two functional cell types. Hence it is still not possible to say whether the complex vascular arrangement that exists in the mammalian adrenal is directly related to and, by virtue of differing corticosteroid concentrations, responsible for epinephrine or norepinephrine synthesis and storage by the chromaffin cells of the adrenal medulla. The recent finding (R. E. Coupland and J. E. Selby, unpublished observations) that satisfactory vascular injection masses can be prepared that incorporate glutaraldehyde in sufficient concentration to allow the identification of the norepinephrine-storing cells currently suggests that a definite answer to the problem may be obtained in the relatively near future.

REFERENCES

1. ANSON, B. J., AND E. W. CAULDWELL. The anatomy of the commoner renal anomalies: ectopic and horseshoe kidneys. *J. Urol.* 36: 211–219, 1942.
2. ANSON, B. J., AND E. W. CAULDWELL. The pararenal vascular system. *Northwestern Univ. Med. School Bull.* 21: 320–328, 1947.
3. ANSON, B. J., E. W. CAULDWELL, J. W. PICK, AND L. E. BEATON. The blood supply of the kidney, suprarenal gland and associated structures. *Surg. Gynecol. Obstet.* 84: 313–320, 1947.
4. ANSON, B. J., E. W. CAULDWELL, J. W. PICK, AND L. E. BEATON. The anatomy of the pararenal system of veins with comments on the renal arteries. *J. Urol.* 60: 714–737, 1948.
5. ANSON B. J., AND L. W. RIBA. The anatomical and surgical features of ectopic kidneys. *Surg. Gynecol. Obstet.* 68: 23–44, 1939.
6. ANSON, B. J., G. A. RICHARDSON, AND W. L. MINEAR. Variations in the number and arrangements of the renal vessels: a study of the blood supply of 400 kidneys. *J. Urol.* 36: 211–219, 1936.
7. BARGMANN, W. Über den Bau der Nebennierenvenen des Menschen und der Säugetiere. *Z. Zellforsch. Mikroskop. Anat.* 17: 118–138, 1933.
8. BENNETT, H. W., AND L. KILHAM. The blood vessels of the adrenal gland of the adult cat. *Anat. Record* 77: 447–471, 1940.
9. BLEICHER, M. Les pédicules vasculaires des glandes surrénales de l'homme. *Rev. Franc. Endocrinol.* 8: 385–397, 1930.
10. BOERNER, D. Die Beziehungen der ersten Anlage der Nebenniere und iher Gefässe zueinander. *Z. Mikroskop. Anat. Forsch.* 59: 137–160, 1952.

11. BOURNE, G. H. *The Mammalian Adrenal Gland.* Oxford: Clarendon Press, 1949.
12. BOYLSTON, G. A., AND B. J. ANSON. Pelvic kidney and renal vessels in a newborn child. *J. Urol.* 40: 502–505, 1938.
13. BRUNN, A. VON. Ueber das Vorkommen organischer Muskelfasern in den Nebennieren. *Nachr. Ges. Wiss. Göttingen* 421–423, 1873. [Cited by Bargmann (7).]
14. BURTON-OPITZ, R., AND D. J. EDWARDS. The vascularity of the adrenal bodies. *Am. J. Physiol.* 43: 408–414, 1917.
15. BUSCH, W. Die arterielle Gefässversorgung der Nebennieren. *Virchows Arch. Pathol. Anat. Klin. Med.* 324: 688–699, 1954.
16. BUSCH, W. Die arterielle Gefässversorgung der Nebenniere, Zugleich ein Beitrag zur Anatomie der Nebenniere. *Z. Mikroskop. Anat. Forsch.* 6: 159–166, 1955.
17. COUPLAND, R. E. On the morphology and adrenaline-noradrenaline content of chromaffin tissue. *J. Endocrinol.* 9: 194–203, 1953.
18. COUPLAND, R. E. The distribution of cholinesterase and other enzymes in the adrenal glands of the ox and man and in a human phaeochromocytoma. In: *Cytology of Nervous Tissue. Anatomy Society of Great Britain Symposium.* London: Taylor & Francis, 1961, p. 28–32.
19. COUPLAND, R. E. *The Natural History of the Chromaffin Cell.* London: Longmans, 1965.
20. COUPLAND, R. E. Corticosterone and methylation of noradrenaline by extra-adrenal chromaffin tissue. *J. Endocrinol.* 41: 487–490, 1968.
21. COUPLAND, R. E., AND J. D. B. MACDOUGALL. Adrenaline formation in noradrenaline storing chromaffin cells *in vitro* induced by corticosterone. *J. Endocrinol.* 36: 317–324, 1966.
22. DASELER, E. H., AND B. J. ANSON. Unilateral renal agenesis: anatomical description of a specimen. *J. Urol.* 50: 155–163, 1943.
23. DOBBIE, J. W., AND T. SYMINGTON. The human adrenal gland with special reference to the vasculature. *J. Endocrinol.* 34: 479–489, 1966.
24. FERGUSON, G. The veins of the adrenal. *Am. J. Anat.* 5: 63–71, 1906.
25. FLINT, J. M. The blood vessels, angiogenesis, organogenesis, reticulum, and histology of the adrenal. *Johns Hopkins Hosp. Rep.* 153–229, 1900.
26. GAGNON, R. The venous drainage of the human adrenal gland. *Rev. Can. Biol.* 14: 350–359, 1956.
27. GAGNON, R. The arterial supply of the human adrenal gland. *Rev. Can. Biol.* 16: 421–433, 1957.
28. GÉRARD, G. Contribution à l'étude morphologique des artères des capsules surrénales chez l'homme. *J. Anat., Paris* 49: 269–303, 1913.
29. GERSH, I., AND A. GROLLMAN. The vascular pattern of the adrenal gland of the mouse and rat and its physiological response to changes in glandular activity. *Contrib. Embryol. Carnegie Inst. Wash.* 29: 113–125, 1941.
30. GROLLMANN, A. *The Adrenals.* London: Baillière, Tindall & Cox, 1963.
31. HARRISON, R. G. A comparative study of the vascularization of the adrenal gland in the rabbit, rat and cat. *J. Anat., London* 85: 12–23, 1951.
32. HARRISON, R. G. The adrenal circulation in the rabbit. *J. Endocrinol.* 15: 64–71, 1957.
33. HARRISON, R. G., AND C. W. ASLING. The anatomy and functional significance of the vascularization of the adrenal gland in the rhesus monkey (*Macaca mulatta*). *J. Anat., London* 89: 106–113, 1955.
34. HARRISON, R. G., AND M. J. HOEY. *The Adrenal Circulation.* Oxford: Blackwell, 1960.
35. HEINIVARRA, O. On the structure of the human suprarenal vein, with reference to structural changes in hypertension. *Ann. Med. Internae Fenniae* 43, Suppl. 19: 5–65, 1954.
36. HENDERSON, E. F. The longitudinal smooth muscle of the central vein of the suprarenal gland. *Anat. Record* 36: 69–78, 1927.
37. HETT, J. Ein Beitrag zu Histogenese de menschlichen Nebenniere. *Z. Mikroskop. Anat. Forsch.* 3: 179–282, 1925.
38. HOLZBAUER, M., AND M. VOGT. Corticosteroids in plasma and cells of adrenal venous blood. *J. Physiol., London* 57: 137–156, 1961.
39. JOHNSTONE, F. R. The suprarenal veins. *Am. J. Surg.* 94: 615–620, 1957.
40. KASHIWAGI, S. Funktionnelle Bedeutung der Spezifischen Struktur der Venenmuskulatur der Nebennierenmarkes und ihre Beziehung zur Adrenalinsekretion. *J. Med. Sci. Abstr. Ref. Japan J. Med. Tokyo*, 1925. [Cited by G. Velican (73).]
41. KEENE, M. F. L., AND E. E. HEWER. Observations on the development of the human suprarenal gland. *J. Anat., London* 61: 302–324, 1927.
42. KEIL, H. Note on antiquity of adreno-genital syndrome. *Bull. Hist. Med.* 23: 201–202, 1949.
43. KOHNO, S. Zur Vergleichenden Histologie und Embryologie der Nebenniere der Säuger und des Menschen. *Z. Ges. Anat. I. Z. Anat. Entwicklungs Geschichte* 77: 419–480, 1925.
44. KUTSCHERA-AICHBERGEN. Nebennierenstudien. *Frankfurter Z. Pathol.* 78: 527–628, 1922.
45. LEACH, C. S., AND H. S. LIPSCOMB. Adrenal cortical control of adrenal medullary function. *Proc. Soc. Exptl. Biol. Med.* 130: 448–451, 1966.
46. LEMPINEN, M. Extra-adrenal chromaffin tissue of the rat and the effect of cortical hormones on it. *Acta Physiol. Scand.* 62, Suppl. 231: 1–91, 1964.
47. LEMPINEN, M. Effect of hydrocortisone on histochemically demonstrable catecholamines of the para-aortic body of the rat. *Acta Physiol. Scand.* 66: 251–252, 1966.
48. LEVER, J. D. Observations on the adrenal blood vessels in the rat. *J. Anat., London* 86: 459–467, 1952.
49. LEVI, G. Le variazioni delle arterie surrenali e renali studiate col metodo statistico seriale. *Arch. Ital. Anat. Embriol.* 8: 35–71, 1909.
50. LEWIS, P. R., AND C. C. D. SHUTE. An electron and microscopic study of cholinesterase distribution in the rat adrenal medulla. *J. Microscopy* 89: 181–193, 1969.
51. MARESCH, R. Die Venenmuskulatur der menschlichen Nebennieren und ihre funktionelle Bedeutung. *Wien. Klin. Wochschr.* 34: 44–45, 1921.
52. McDONALD, I. R., AND M. REICH. Corticosteroid secretion by the autotransplanted adrenal gland of the conscious sheep. *J. Physiol., London* 147: 33–50, 1959.
53. MERKLIN, R. J. Arterial supply of the suprarenal gland. *Anat. Record* 144: 359–371, 1962.
54. MERKLIN, R. J., AND S. A. EGER. The adrenal venous system in man. *J. Intern. Colloq. Surg.* 35: 572–585, 1961.
55. MERKLIN, R. J., AND N. A. MICHELS. The variant renal and suprarenal blood supply. *J. Intern. Colloq. Surg.* 29: 41–76, 1958.
56. MINOT, C. S. On a hitherto unrecognized form of blood circulation without capillaries in the organs of vertebrata. *Proc. Boston Soc. Nat. Hist.* 29: 185–215, 1900.
57. NEUMAN, K. O. The oxygen exchange of the suprarenal gland. *J. Physiol., London* 45: 188–196, 1912.
58. PICK, J. W., AND B. J. ANSON. The inferior phrenic artery: origin and suprarenal branches. *Anat. Record* 78: 413–427, 1940.
59. PICK, J. W., AND B. J. ANSON. The renal vascular pedicle: an anatomical study of 430 body-halves. *J. Urol.* 44: 411–434, 1940.
60. POHRECKY, L., AND J. H. RUST. Studies on the cortical control of the adrenal medulla in the rat. *J. Pharmacol. exptl. Therap.* 162: 227–238, 1968.
61. ROFFI, J., AND F. MARGOLIS. Synthèse d'adrénaline dans le tissu chromaffine extra-surrénalien, chez le rat nouveau-né, sous l'effet de l'hydrocortisone ou de la corticostimuline. *Compt. Rend.* 263: 1496–1499, 1966.
62. SJÖSTRAND, T. On the principles for the distribution of the blood in the peripheral vascular system. *Skand. Arch. Physiol.* 71: 1–150, 1934.

63. Solutuchin, A. Über die Blutversorgung der Nebennieren. *Z. Anat. Entwicklungsgeschichte* 90: 288–292, 1929.
64. Spanner, R. Der Abürzungskreislauf der menschlichen Nebenniere. *Zentr. Inn. Med.* 61: 545–558, 1940.
65. Stewart, G. N. A note on some obvious consequences of the high rate of blood flow through the adrenals. *Am. J. Physiol.* 44: 92–95, 1918.
66. Stöhr, P., Jr. *Lehrbuch der Histologie und Mikroskopischen Anatomie des Menschen*. Berlin: Julius Springer, 1951.
67. Symington, T. *Functional Pathology of the Human Adrenal Gland*. Edinburgh: Livingstone, 1969.
68. Teitelbaum, H. A. The nature of the thoracic and abdominal distribution of the vagus nerves. *Anat. Record* 55: 297–317, 1933.
69. Teitelbaum, H. A. The bilateral vagus innervation of the suprarenal glands. *Bull. Med. Chir. Fac. Maryland* 19: 24, 1934.
70. Uotila, U. U. Early embryological development of fetal and permanent adrenal cortex in man. *Anat. Record* 76: 183–203, 1940.
71. Velican, C. Das Blutfördernde System der Nebenniere. *Wien. Med. Wochschr.* 9: 108, 1944.
72. Velican, C. Embryogènese de la surrénale humaine. *Arch. Anat. Microscop. Morphol. Exptl.* 36: 316–333, 1947.
73. Velican, C. Le dispositif sphinctéro-propulseur de la surrénale. *Arch. Anat. Microscop. Morphol. Exptl.* 37: 28–40, 1948.
74. Wallraff, J. *Organe mit innerer Sekretion*. München: Urban & Schwarzenberg, 1953.
75. Wiesel, J. Beitrage zur Anatomie und Entwickelung der menschlichen Nebenniere. *Arb. Anat. Inst. Wiesbaden* 19: 481–522, 1902.
76. Wright, R. D. Blood flow through the adrenal gland. *Endocrinology* 72: 418–428, 1963.
77. Wurtman, R. J. Control of epinephrine synthesis in the adrenal medulla by the adrenal cortex: hormonal specificity and dose response characteristics. *J. Endocrinol.* 79: 608–614, 1966.
78. Wurtman, R. J., and J. Axelrod. Control of enzymatic synthesis of adrenaline in the adrenal medulla by adrenal cortical steroids. *J. Biol. Chem.* 241: 2301–2305, 1966.
79. Zechwer, J. T. Possible functional significance of longitudinal muscle in adrenal veins in man. *Arch. Pathol.* 20: 9–21, 1935.

CHAPTER 21

Ultrastructure of the chromaffin cell

ODILE GRYNSZPAN-WINOGRAD | *Laboratoire de Cytologie, Université de Paris VI, Paris, France*

CHAPTER CONTENTS

General Organization of Cell
Secretory Vesicles
    Epinephrine-storing cells
    Norepinephrine-storing cells
Release of Secretory Granules
    Exocytosis profiles at free cell surface
    Exocytosis profiles at cell-to-cell apposed surface
    Presence of coated pits in granule membrane fused with plasma membrane

---

THE CHROMAFFIN CELLS, situated within the mammalian adrenal gland, are arranged in small groups and separated by numerous blood vessels, connective tissue, and nerve fibers. Nearly twenty years ago, it was recognized that, besides the organelles common to all cells, these chromaffin cells contain a characteristic structural element: vesicles with an electron-dense granule inside (14, 37, 50).

In these vesicles, catecholamines are stored with ATP, proteins, and lipids (see the chapter by Winkler and Smith in this volume of the *Handbook*). The presence of dense-cored vesicles storing secretory products are, in fact, a very frequent characteristic of glandular cells, especially of those that secrete proteins. In their general cytological organization, the chromaffin cells conform to the general features of protein-secreting cells, with the additional characteristic of being innervated as a neuron.

For the morphologist, the hamster adrenal gland has proved to be unusually favorable: as far as we know, exocytosis profiles that testify to the mechanism of release of secretory products (see the chapter by Viveros in this volume of the *Handbook*) have been observed only in this species (5, 15, 29) and occasionally in the rat (9); in this single species (the hamster) too, nerve endings of epinephrine- and norepinephrine-storing cells have been shown to be morphologically dissimilar (28).

Eränkö (20) was the first to point out that norepinephrine-storing cells are exclusively located at the periphery of the adrenal medulla just beneath the cortex in hamsters. Norepinephrine forms 20% of total adrenal catecholamines (J. Roffi, personal communication). The ultrastructure of the hamster chromaffin cell has been most extensively studied and is one of the best known (2, 5, 13, 19, 40, 51, 53). For all these reasons, the hamster chromaffin cell serves as a model in our description and in all the micrographs.

GENERAL ORGANIZATION OF CELL

Secretory vesicles are the most peripheral organelles of the chromaffin cell; although present nearly all around the cell, they are particularly numerous near the free surface of the cell, along capillaries and connective tissue (Fig. 1). Opposite the free surface, the internal part of the cell, which contains the nucleus and receives nerve terminals (Fig. 1), is rich in other organelles, such as rough endoplasmic reticulum and Golgi apparatus, which may be very close to the cell-to-cell apposed surface of the plasma membrane (Figs. 2 and 3).

In many sections, most of the rough endoplasmic reticulum is arranged in parallel arrays facing the synaptic areas (Figs. 2 and 3). Not uncommonly the cisternae and vesicles of the Golgi apparatus contain a granular material that seems to represent an early stage of the formation of the granule. Mitochondria are scattered throughout the whole cytoplasm. Single cilia have been observed attached to some chromaffin cells. Lysosome-like bodies are regularly found (Fig. 1). Microtubules are often located near the plasmalemma.

Organelles of chromaffin cells, as well as the respective capillaries and the nerve endings, are distributed so that the cell is polarized.

The free part of the plasmalemma, along capillaries and connective tissue, is covered by a basement lamina; between adjoining cells, as well as between cells and nerve terminals, there is only a small electron-lucent interspace of about 200–250 Å in width. The cell-to-cell apposed plasmalemmas possess attachment plates (Figs. 3, 4, 10, and 11*a*) at a level fairly far from the free surface. In the neighborhood of the attachment plates, the adjoining plasma membranes possess microvilli-like processes, irregularly oriented and closely interlocking when expelled granules do not lie between them. These

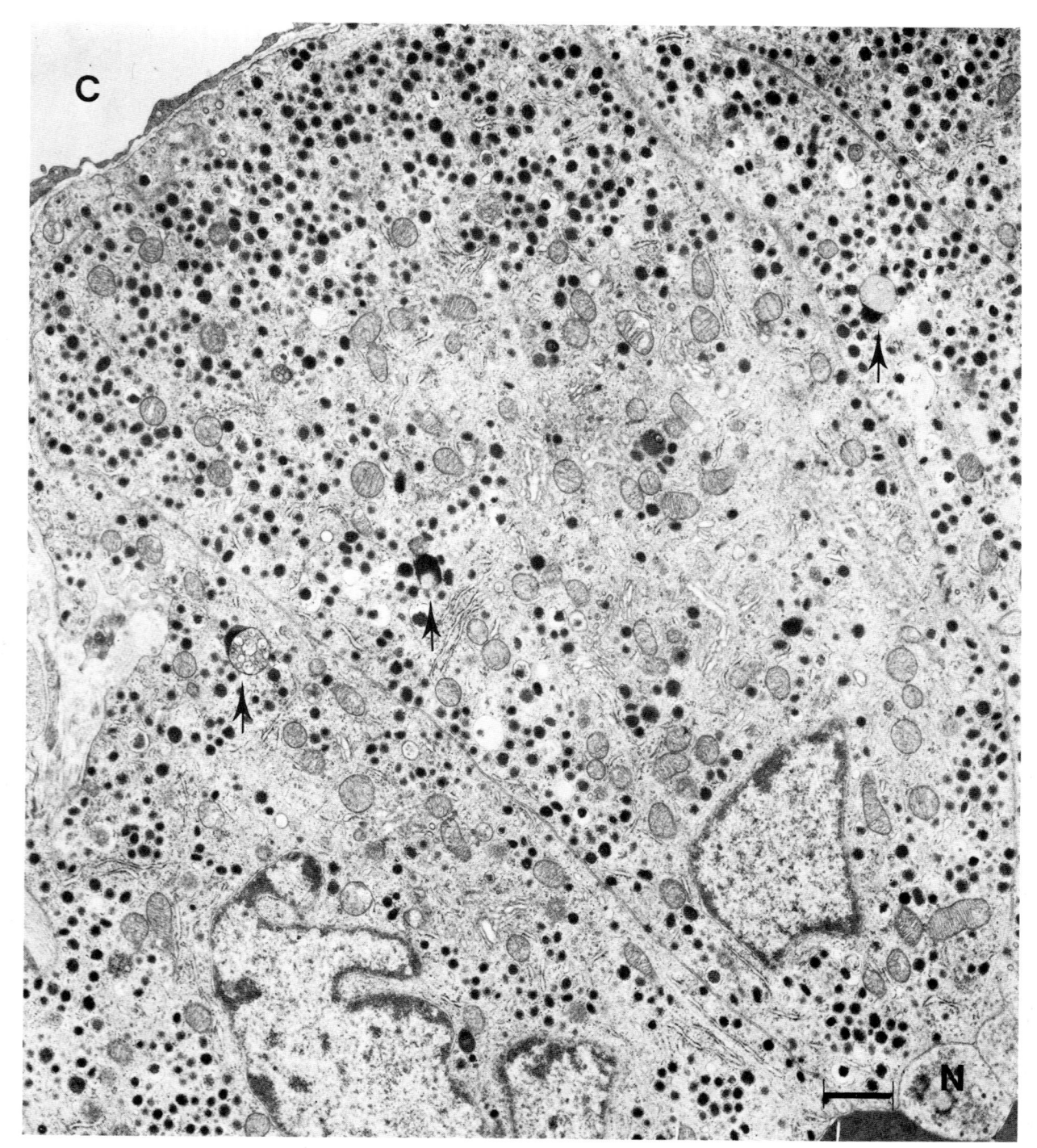

FIG. 1. Epinephrine cells. *C*, lumen of the capillary; *N*, nerve ending. Lyosome-like bodies indicated by *arrows*. Scale: 1 μm.

interdigitations (Figs. 4, 10, and 12a), which do not contain secretory granules, are not distributed regularly around the cell.

According to the observations of Coupland (9) and Elfvin (18) on the rat, the intercellular cleft may be widened between these microvilli that may be traced toward the large extracellular spaces, as if they were delimiting intercellular canaliculi. Thus the question arises if these interdigitations are concerned with the firmness of cell attachment, as it has been postulated for some types of epithelial cells (24, 36), or if they have some link with the release of secretory granules (see sub-

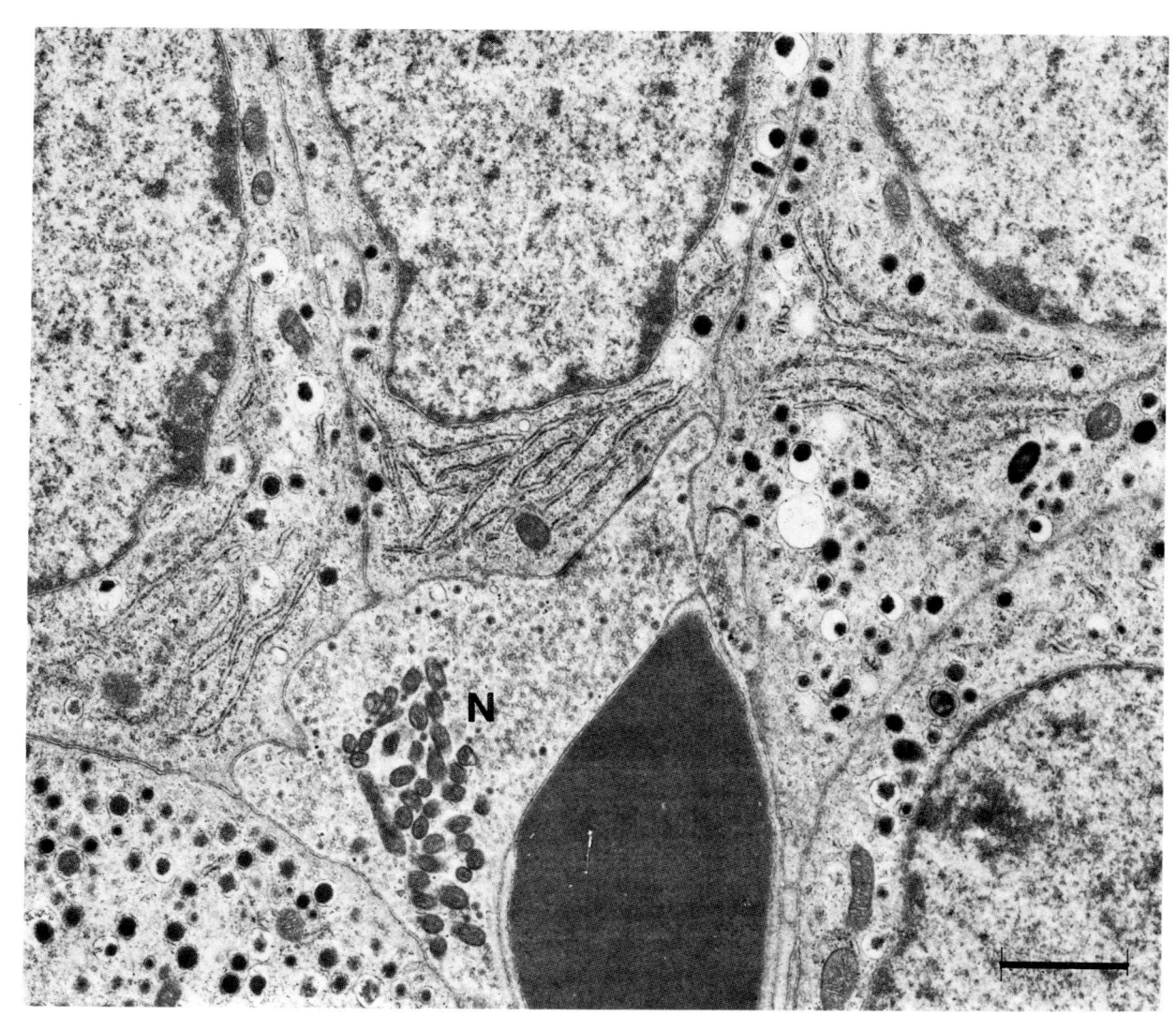

FIG. 2. Arrays of rough endoplasmic reticulum in epinephrine cells facing a voluminous nerve ending (*N*) that specifically innervates these cells. Presence of extravasated erythrocytes, which does not result from a perfusion artifact, is usual in adrenal glands, but its significance is not clearly understood. Scale: 1 μm.

section *Exocytosis Profiles at Cell-to-Cell Opposed Surface*). Because no tight junctions do occur, the basement lamina is the only morphologically visible separation between the large extracellular spaces and the intercellular cleft. Thus circulation of large molecules [see the case of peroxidase (32)] seems to be allowed all around the cell.

SECRETORY VESICLES

In material fixed in glutaraldehyde and subsequently stained with osmium tetroxide, two main types of chromaffin cells—epinephrine- and norepinephrine-storing cells (see the chapter by Coupland in this volume of the *Handbook*)—may be distinguished, in regard to their granule-containing vesicles (Fig. 5). Glutaraldehyde is an essential reagent in the procedure; with other aldehydes, such a clear-cut difference between epinephrine- and norepinephrine-storing cells cannot be obtained. However, instead of osmium tetroxide, which allows better cytological observations, other fixatives, such as potassium dichromate or permanganate, may be used.

Epinephrine-secreting cells contain granules that show only slight-to-moderate electron density; norepinephrine-secreting cells contain intensely electron-dense granules [Fig. 5; (10, 11, 48, 52)]. Epinephrine undergoes little reaction with glutaraldehyde and escapes during fixation and subsequent treatments; norepinephrine reacts with glutaraldehyde to produce an electron-dense polymer that is bound in situ. According to Coupland &

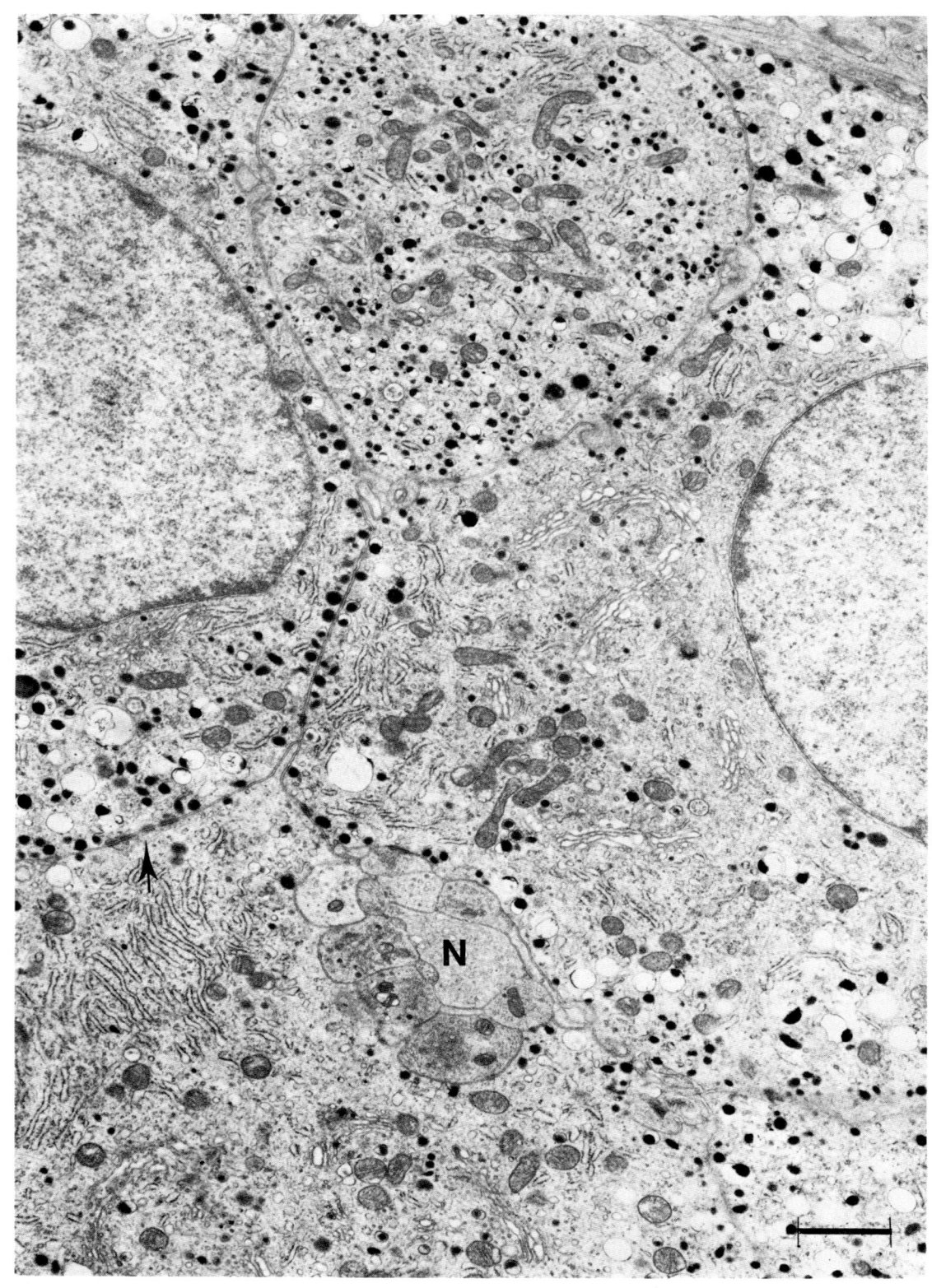

FIG. 3. Norepinephrine cells. As in epinephrine cells, the part of the cell facing the cluster of small-sized nerve endings (N) contains most of the arrays of rough endoplasmic reticulum and Golgi apparatus. Some of the attachment plates are indicated by *arrow*. Scale: 1 μm.

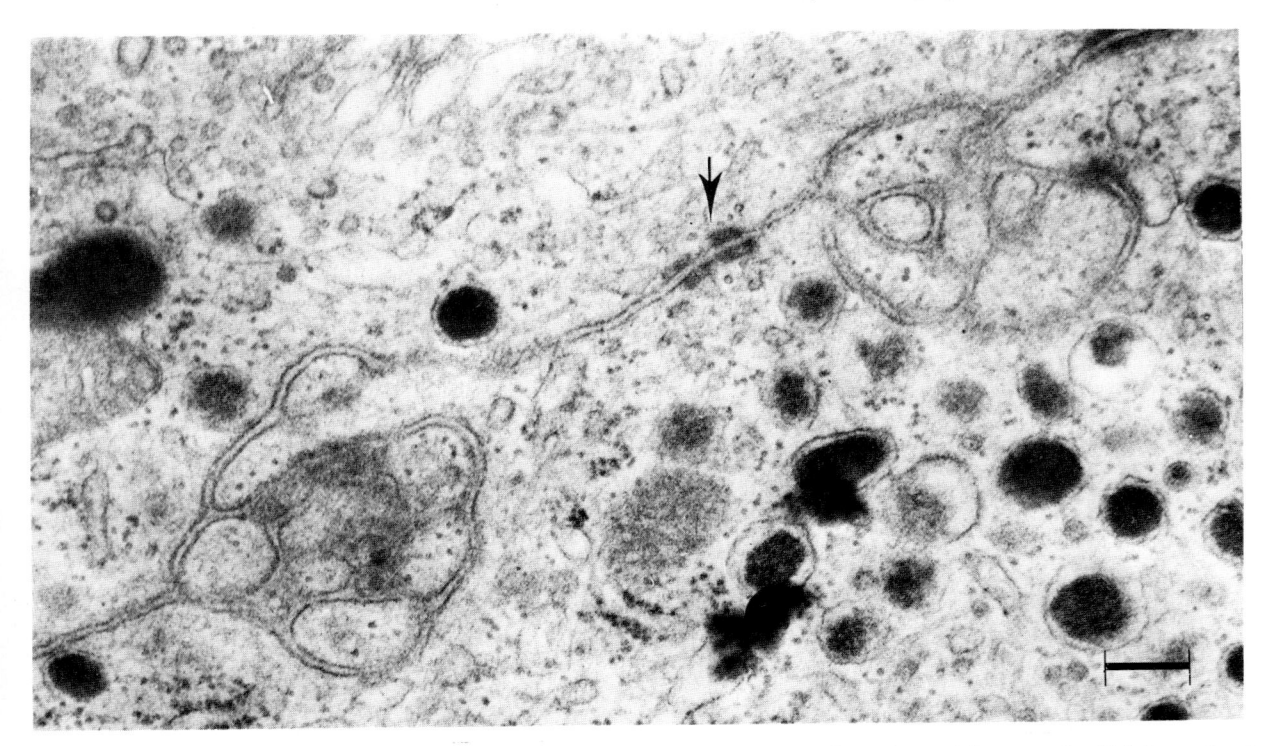

FIG. 4. Interdigitations and attachment plates (*arrows*) between 2 adjoining epinephrine cells. Scale: 0.2 μm.

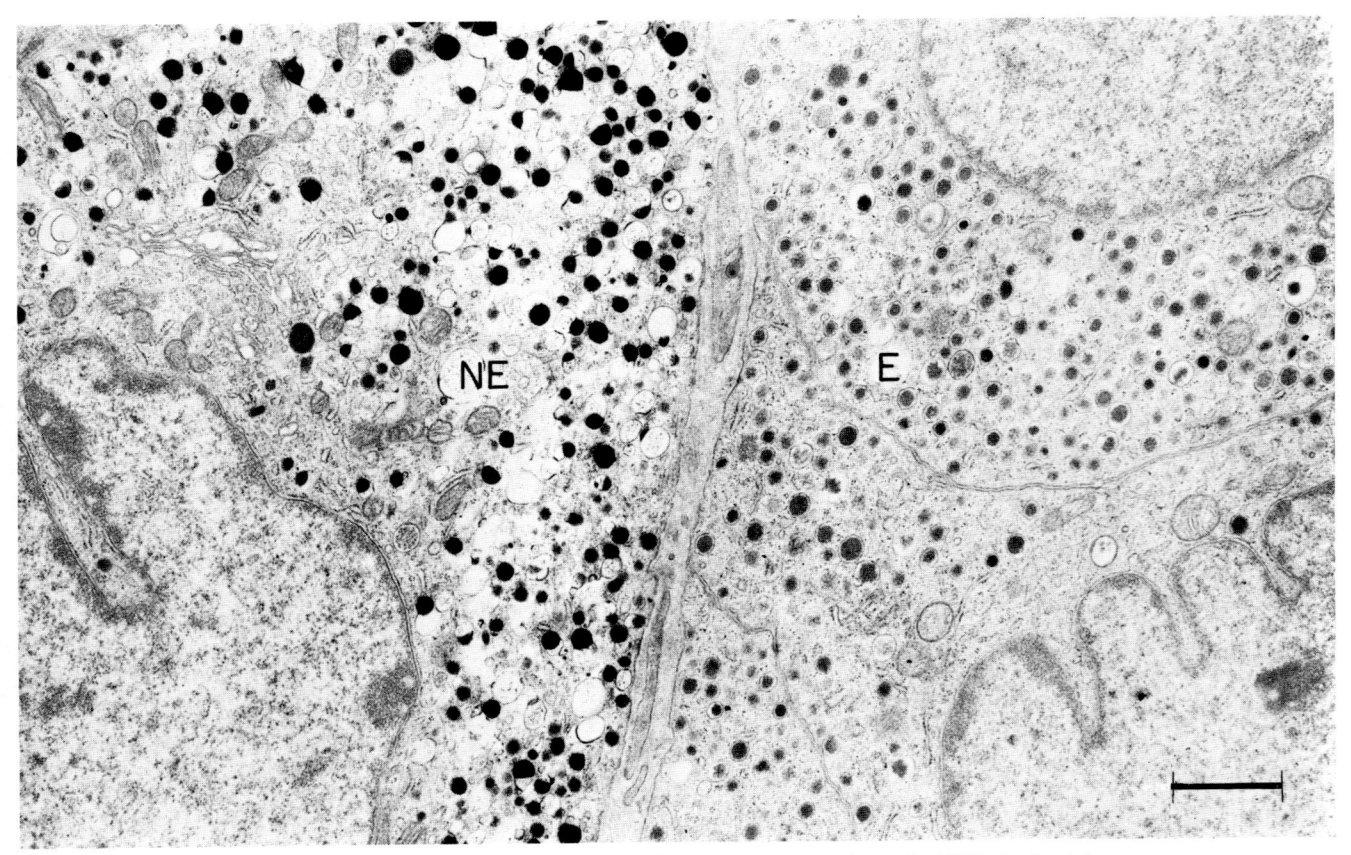

FIG. 5. Epinephrine cells (*E*) and norepinephrine cells (*NE*). Scale: 0.9 μm.

Hopwood (10) the moderate electron density of epinephrine cell granules probably results from the presence of binding substance.

Epinephrine-storing Cells

In tissue fixed in glutaraldehyde-osmium tetroxide, the shape, size, and number per cell of the granules in epinephrine cells are fairly homogeneous. A peripheral halo separates the granule from the external membrane; the most usual diameter of their sections, as observed in electron micrographs, is about 2,000 A (range 1,000–3,500 A).

The electron density and the size of the granule sections seem to depend not only on the plane of section but also on absolute values of individual granules. In the rat, D'Anzi (12) could show that the storage vesicles of the epinephrine cells are segregated into two groups, which can be differentiated on the basis of their relative electron density, size, and mass; dark granules are slightly smaller and less numerous than medium-light granules. The ratio of dark granules to medium-light granules is approximately 0.3. The significance of these two types of epinephrine-storing vesicles is unknown.

Norepinephrine-storing Cells

The granules of the norepinephrine cells are more heterogeneous than those of the epinephrine cells in their shape, size, and number per cell (Fig. 6). Nevertheless they are more electron dense than the granules of the epinephrine cells and they appear homogeneously stained in glutaraldehyde-osmium tetroxide-fixed material. In many cases, these granules are displaced toward the periphery of their vesicle; the larger the granule, the more it is displaced toward the periphery and the larger

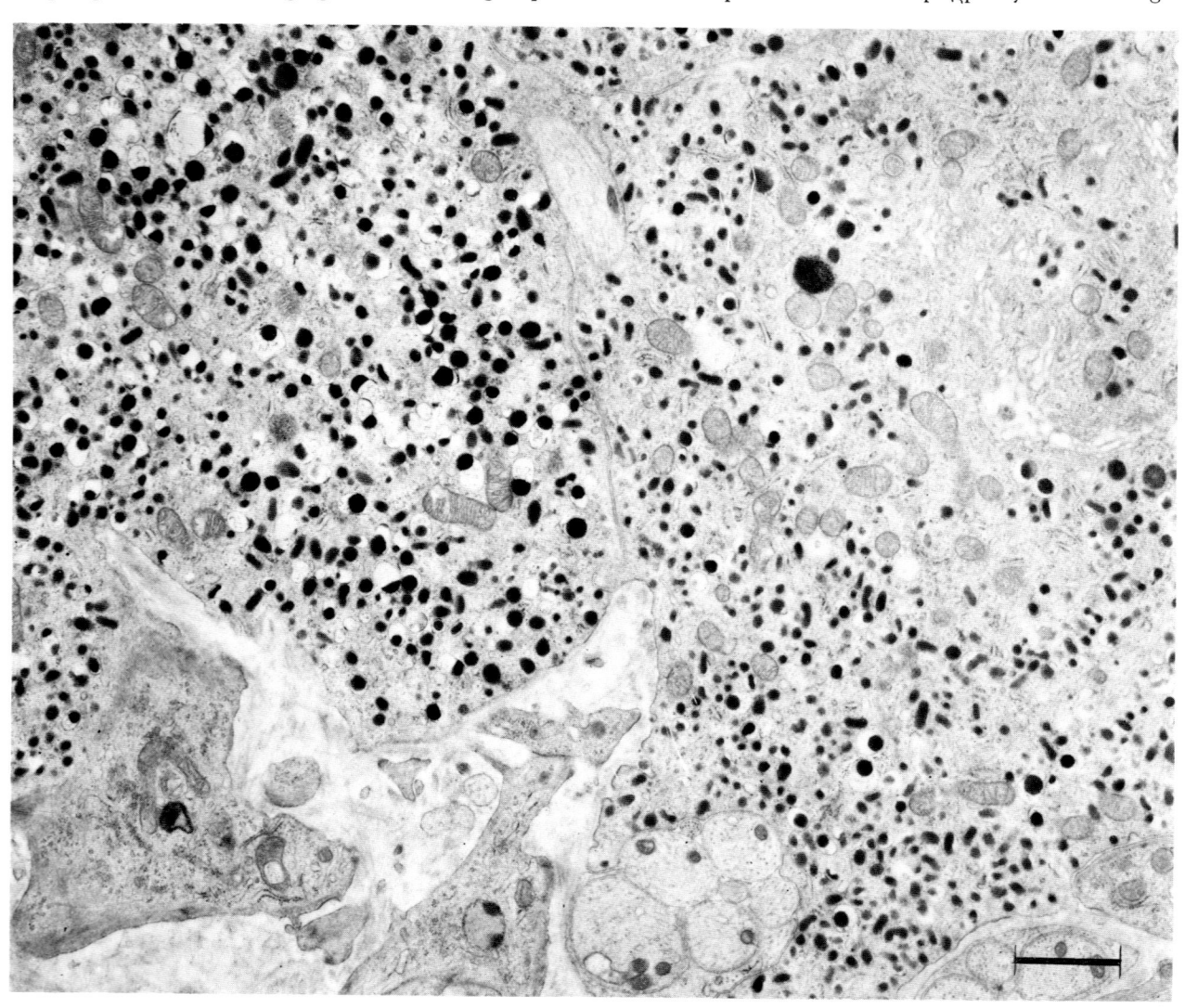

FIG. 6. Norepinephrine cells with different kinds of granules. Left cell is richer in large granules, displaced toward the periphery of their vesicle. Right cell is richer in small and flattened granules, which are less electron dense than the larger ones. Scale: 1 µm.

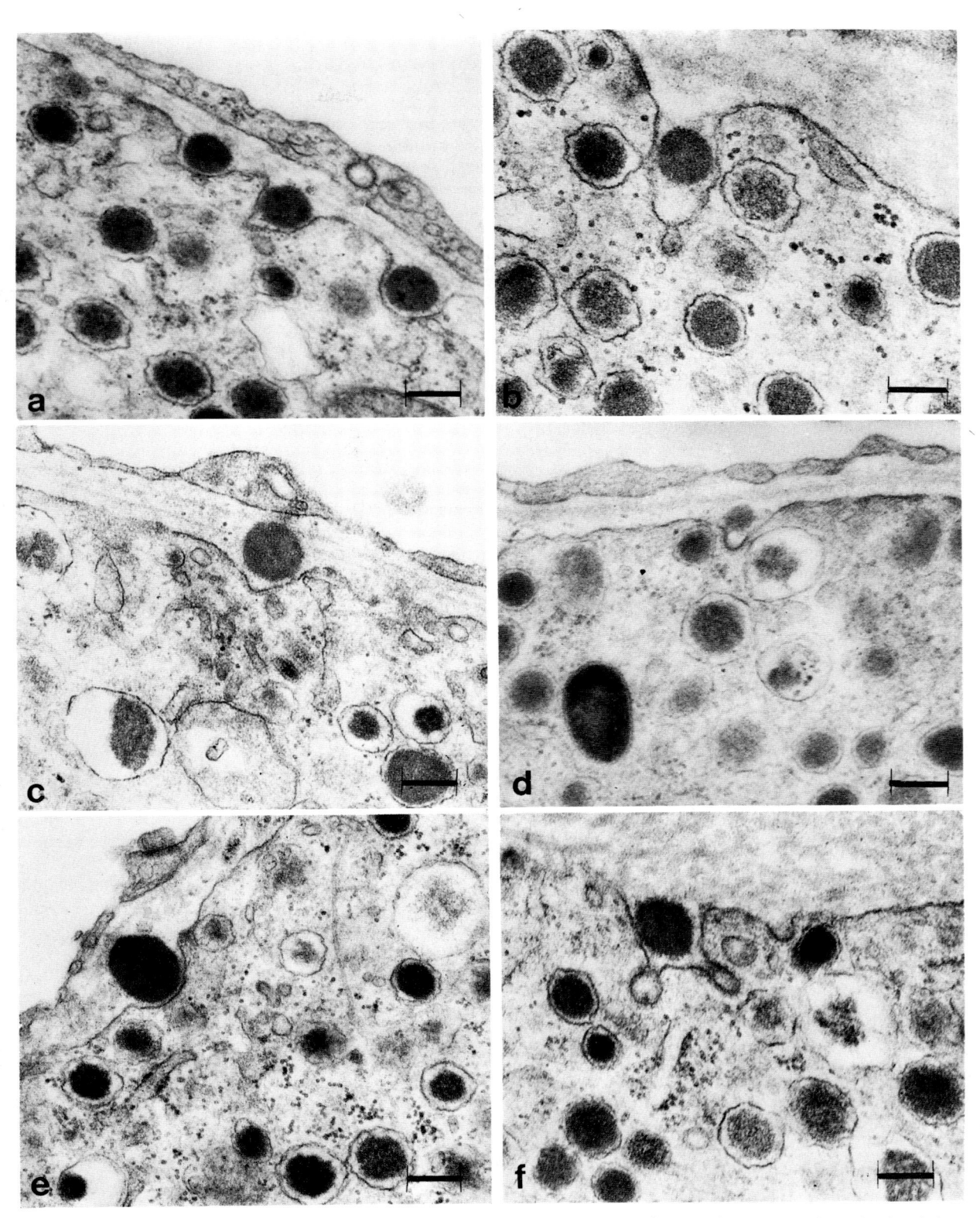

FIG. 7. Exocytosis profiles, with coated pits (*b, c, d, f*), at free surface of epinephrine cells. Expelled granules seem quite similar to intracellular granules. Scale: 0.2 μm.

is its vesicle. Coupland (9) pointed out that these displaced granules are artifacts and result from the reaction between glutaraldehyde and norepinephrine. The most usual size of these granules is the same as that of the epinephrine cells, but extreme sizes are more frequent in these cells than in the epinephrine cells. Some cells contain numerous small granules and may be even free of larger ones. The smallest granules are less electron dense than the largest ones; in the hamster the smallest granules have a typical flattened appearance (Fig. 6) and the halo between them and their membrane is very thin and sometimes inconspicuous. The significance of these small granules is not yet known. We may wonder if dopamine, known to be present in the "large crude fraction" (17, 38) is not related somehow to these granules. As Coupland (9) noticed, the small granule-containing vesicles of the Golgi zone of norepinephrine cells (as well as the granular material present inside the cisternae) have a smaller electron density and look like the epinephrine cell granules. This may represent an early stage in the formation either of granules (with only binding substance and not yet norepinephrine) or of dark and multivesicular bodies.

RELEASE OF SECRETORY GRANULES

The fact that the release of chromaffin cell secretory products involves exocytosis is accepted now on the basis of biochemical evidence (see the chapter by Viveros in this volume of the *Handbook*). Exocytosis, first described by Palade (43) in exocrine pancreas, is known to be a general mechanism for extrusion of proteins and is used by many types of exocrine and endocrine glandular cells. This release mechanism involves a fusion of the granule membrane with the plasma membrane and a fission of the fused membranes: the granule is allowed to be released directly into the extracellular medium without any prior contact with the cytoplasm of the cell.

DeRobertis and his colleagues (13, 14) were the first to suggest that the contents of the secretory granules are released into the extracellular medium after attachment of the granule membrane with the plasma membrane; nevertheless convincing micrographs showing exocytosis profiles in the adrenal medulla have been published fairly recently, and only in the hamster (5, 15, 29). In other species, observations were negative (18, 44) or extremely few in number (9).

Exotytosis profiles are seen after different kinds of fixation [osmium tetroxide, double fixation glutaraldehyde (or formol-acrolein), and osmium tetroxide] on all surfaces of the cell with some differences between the free surface and the cell-to-cell apposed surface of the plasma membrane (Figs. 7 and 13).

Exocytosis Profiles at Free Cell Surface

The free surface of the plasma membrane shows granule-containing invaginations, often omega shaped and covered by the basement lamina (Figs. 7–9). A clear space separates the granule from its membrane, now incorporated into the plasma membrane, as it does inside the cell. These profiles are quite similar to those described in other endocrine glands [i.e., adenohypophysis (8, 21, 22, 31)], A cells of endocrine pancreas (27), or neurosecretory organs (7, 41). In some neurosecretory organs, such profiles are more numerous between adjoining neurons than at the free surface (42). Although several granules may be expelled by one cell (Fig. 7a), no sequential fusions, as for zymogen granules of exocrine glands (3, 30, 33) leading to a string of connected granules, have been observed.

In the epinephrine cells, the electron density and the size of the granule sections show the same range as inside the cell (Fig. 7). No sign of evolution of the granule can be detected.

In the norepinephrine cells, the size of the granule sections also shows the same range as inside the cell, but the expelled granules are always much less electron dense (Fig. 9) and look like the epinephrine cell granules. This means (see section SECRETORY VESICLES) that as soon as the granule membrane has been ruptured norepinephrine can no longer be seen.

Exocytosis Profiles at Cell-to-Cell Apposed Surface

Enlargements of the intercellular cleft, lying near attachment plates and interdigitations or even between the interdigitations, contain an amorphous material, more electron dense than the intercellular cleft, and granules of varying size, generally smaller than the intracellular granules (Figs. 10–12); the smaller these expelled granules are, the less electron dense they are. Moreover, in the norepinephrine cells, expelled granules are less electron dense than the intracellular granules (Fig. 12).

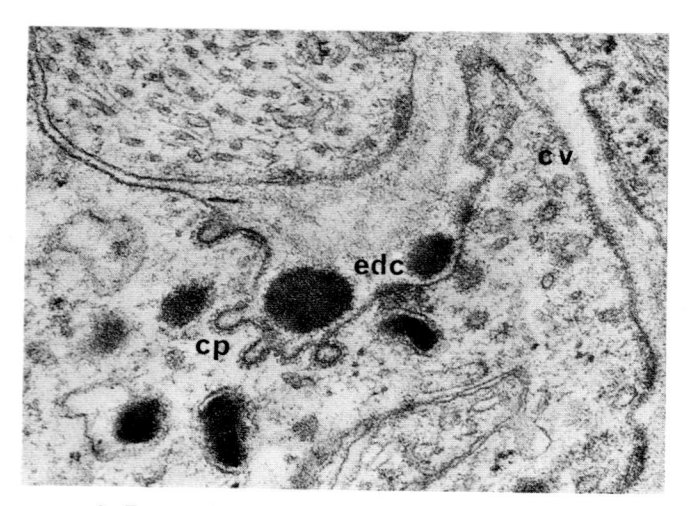

FIG. 8. Exocytosis profile with 4 coated pits (*cp*), at free surface of epinephrine cell; *cv*, coated vesicles; *edc*, extracellular dense cores. × 42,100. [From Benedeczky & Smith (5).]

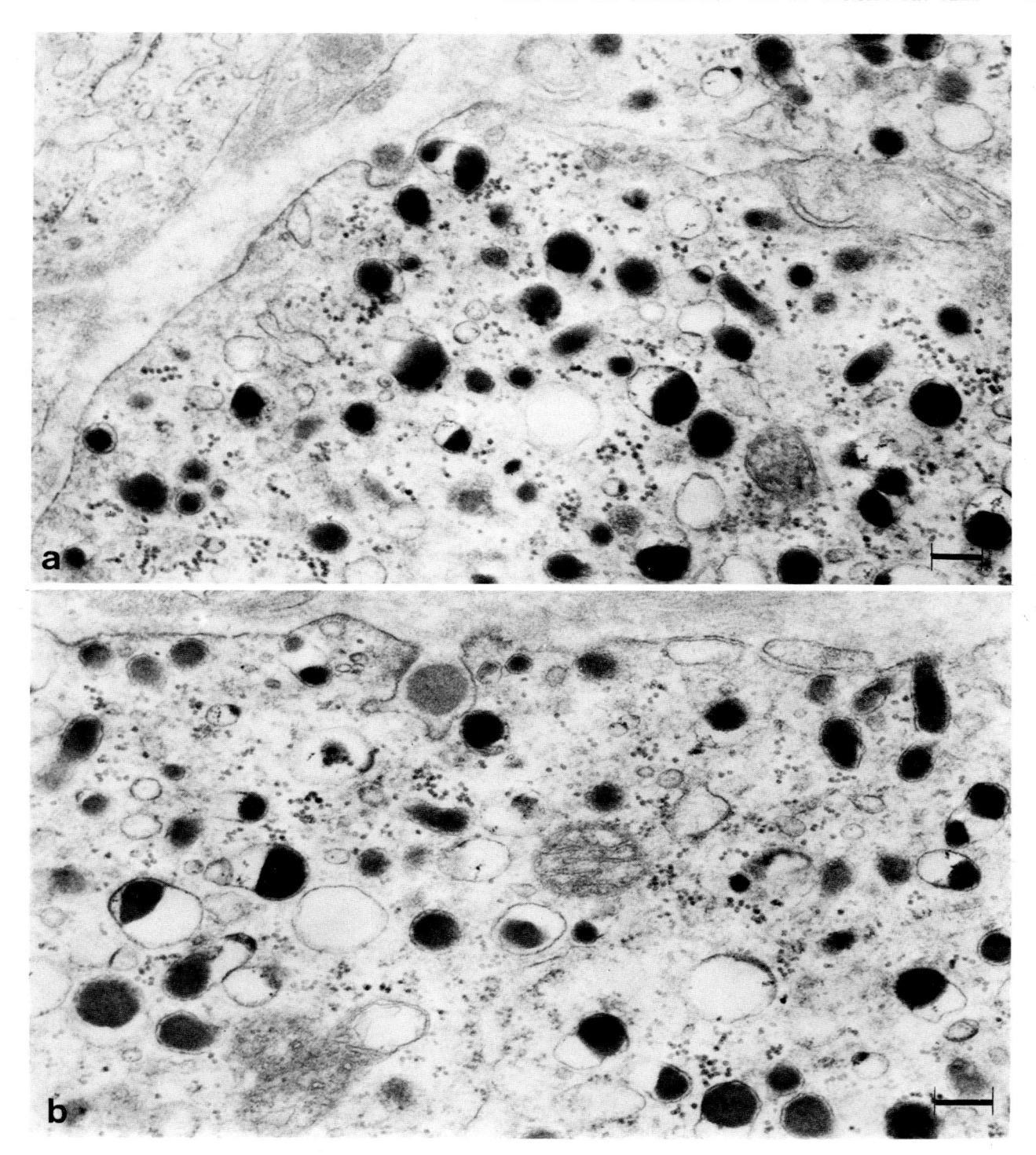

FIG. 9. Exocytosis profiles, with coated pits (*a* and *b*), at free surface of norepinephrine cells. When compared to intracellular granules of the same section, expelled granules no longer have the strong electron density that characterized norepinephrine. Scale: 0.2 μm.

Such profiles suggest a disorganization and a "dissolution" of the granule contents. Why such a disorganization of the granule contents does not seem to occur at the free surface remains obscure. Differences in the conditions of fixation (time, concentration of the fixative, washing out) of the expelled granules, according to their distance from the blood vessels by which the fixative is perfused, do not seem to account, alone, for such a dif-

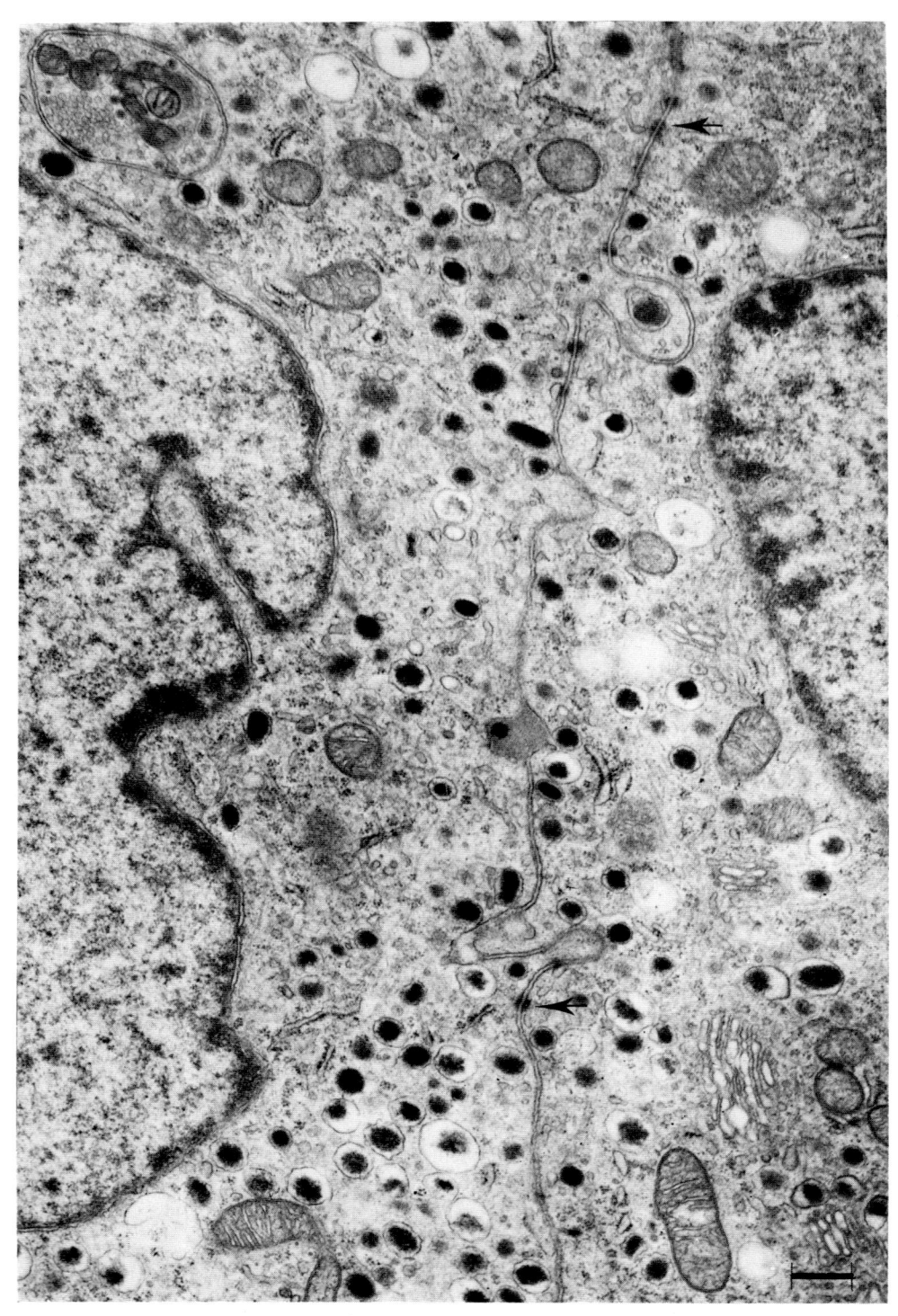

FIG. 10. Adjoining epinephrine cells showing attachment plates (*arrows*) and slightly developed interdigitations. Dilatation of intercellular cleft contains expelled granule, surrounded by moderately electron-dense material not visible elsewhere in the intercellular cleft. Scale: 0.4 μm.

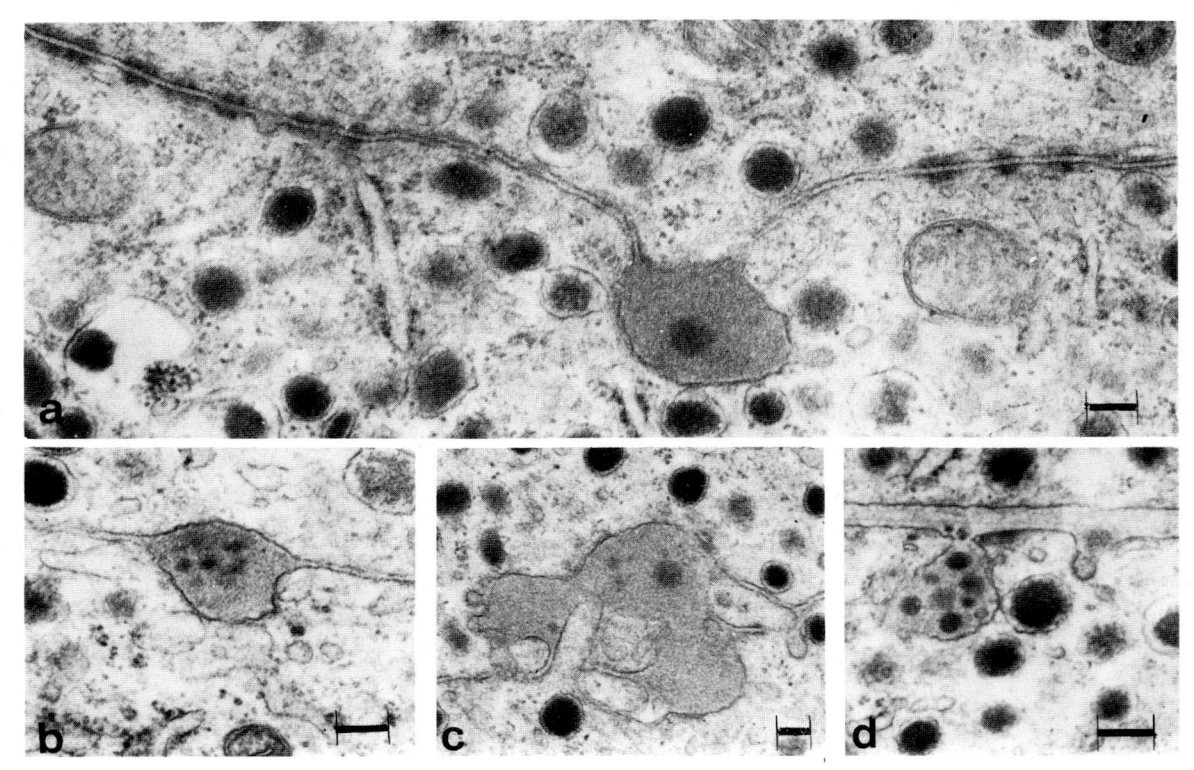

FIG. 11. Exocytosis profiles at cell-to-cell apposed surface (*a–c*) of epinephrine cells. In *d*, cells are still separated by their basal lamina. Expelled granules seem to have been disorganized into smaller and electron-lighter units and moderately electron-dense material. Scale: 0.2 μm.

ference in the exocytosis profiles. Is there a "secretion wave" from the nerve terminals to the free surface? Could it be that the earlier the granules are released, the more advanced would be their disorganization? An alternate hypothesis involves a circulation of the granules from the free surface to the intercellular cleft, where they would be disorganized. They would not cross the capillaries in any place, but only at the end of "intercellular canaliculi" (see section GENERAL ORGANIZATION OF CELL). If this were so, would all expelled granules occupy their actual release location or would some of them have not been trapped at the time of fixation? Whatever the explanation, physicochemical changes occur in the granules, in the space between the plasma membrane and the basal lamina. Beyond the basal lamina, which cannot be crossed by intact granules, granules are no longer visible.

The difference between norepinephrine, which cannot be observed extracellularly, and the other granule components (mainly chromogranins), which can be seen, is in good accordance with biochemical evidence: the release of chromogranins in perfusates lags behind that of the catecholamines (6, 35).

Presence of Coated Pits in Granule Membrane Fused with Plasma Membrane

In one-third of the observed exocytosis profile sections, the granule membrane fused with the plasma membrane showed one or more coated pits (Figs. 7–9, 11, and 12). The thickness of the section and the diameter of the coated pits being about 800–1,000 Å and the diameter of secretory vesicles about 2,500–3,000 Å, this ratio of positive observations is high enough to allow us to conclude that coated pits are always appearing in the granule membrane after its fusion-fission with the plasma membrane. The presence of coated pits in the granule membrane, after its fusion-fission with the plasma membrane, has been noticed in neurosecretory organs as well (7, 41). Morphologically similar coated pits may be found elsewhere in the plasma membrane, as in many kinds of cells [see (25)], but most of them are located in exocytosis sites and at or near interdigitations.

The presence of coated pits in the granule membrane fused with the plasma membrane is indicative of immediate changes involving fission of the granule membrane; the incorporation of the latter, after exocytosis, into the plasmalemma is not long lasting. This is in good accordance with biochemical evidence of a rapid fragmentation of the granule membrane during secretion (39, 45, 49).

In analogy to their usual destiny in other cells, these exocytosis-linked pits are probably transformed into vesicles that are retained by the cell. Are these coated pits and vesicles only devoted to the retention by the cell of the granule membranes, thus allowing the retrieval of the plasma membrane? Or do they take up some extracellular material? Indeed, in many types of cells, coated

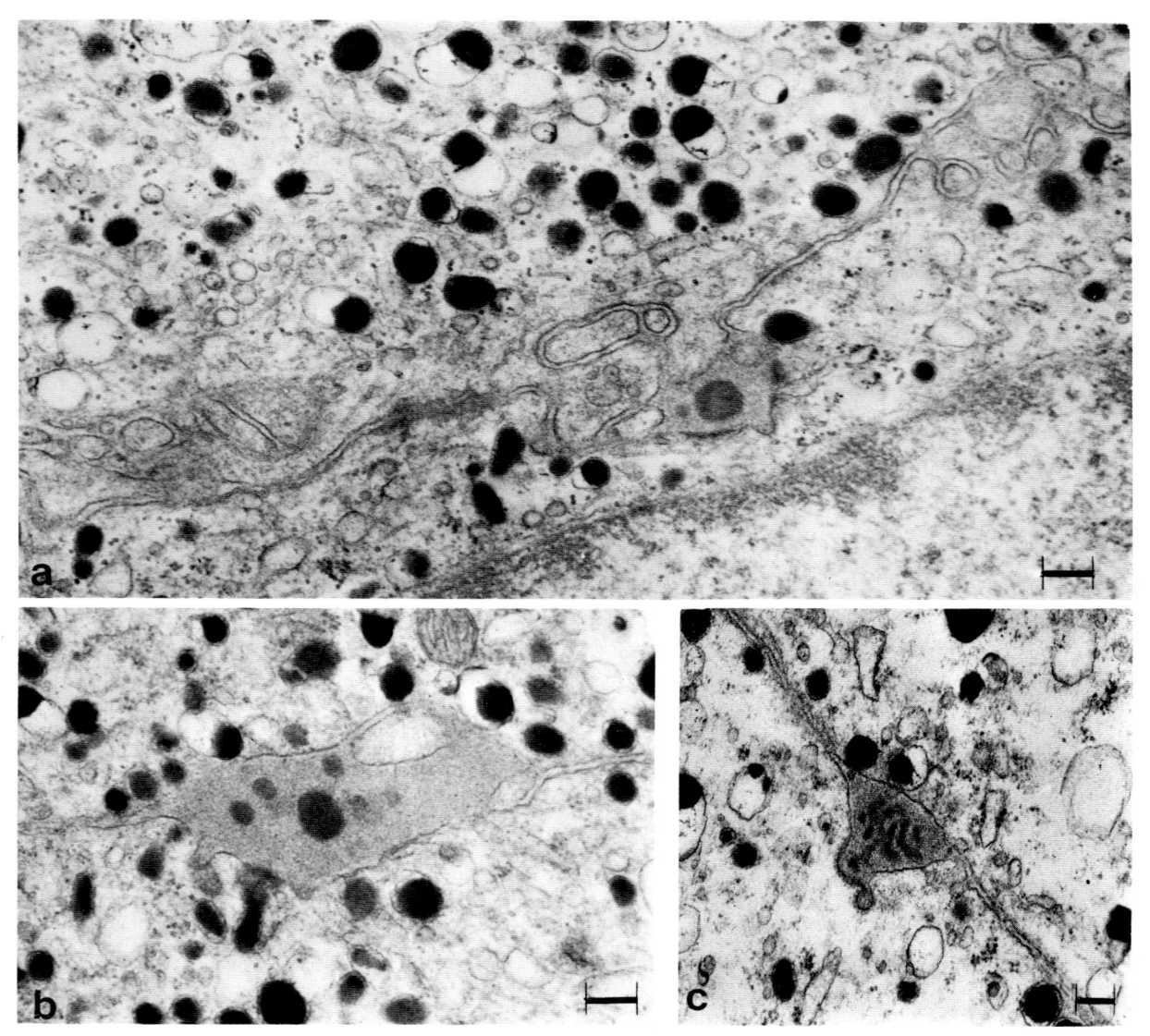

FIG. 12. Exocytosis profiles at cell-to-cell apposed surface (a-c) of norepinephrine cells. For detail, see legends to Figs. 10 and 11 for epinephrine cells, and legend to Fig. 9. Scale: 0.2 μm.

pits and vesicles are involved in extracellular protein uptake: in oocytes, yolk vesicles originate from coated pits of a larger size (4, 16, 47); in other cells, coated pits of the same size as those in the chromaffin cell take up injected proteins such as peroxidase and ferritin. After being detached from the plasma membrane as vesicles, they are believed to lose their coating and to be incorporated by lysosomes (23, 26, 46, 54). Smaller coated vesicles are regularly found in association with the Golgi apparatus; they are not involved in protein uptake, and some of them are thought to be primary lysosomes (26). Indeed, Holtzman & Dominitz (32) show that coated pits, with other tubular organelles, are involved in the uptake of peroxidase in adrenal medulla. Abrahams & Holtzman (1) observe an augmentation of pinocytosis of peroxidase after stimulation of the adrenal medulla by insulin and have concluded that a balance exists between exocytosis and endocytosis. In fact, the exact significance of the coating is not clear. Kanaseki & Kadota (34) believe that it is only a fusion-fission apparatus, without any specific link with protein uptake. Friend & Farquhar (26) postulate that it is indicative of lysosomes.

It is not known yet if the granule membrane is used again by the cell after exocytosis or is destroyed (see the chapter by Winkler and Smith in this volume of the *Handbook*). Nevertheless morphological observations allow us to conclude that, if it is used again, it is not used as a whole and intact membrane.

Although a complete morphological demonstration of exocytosis as the mechanism of release needs quantitative data comparing stimulated and nonstimulated glands, the observation of exocytosis profiles in the hamster adrenal medulla (Fig. 13) is an important first step.

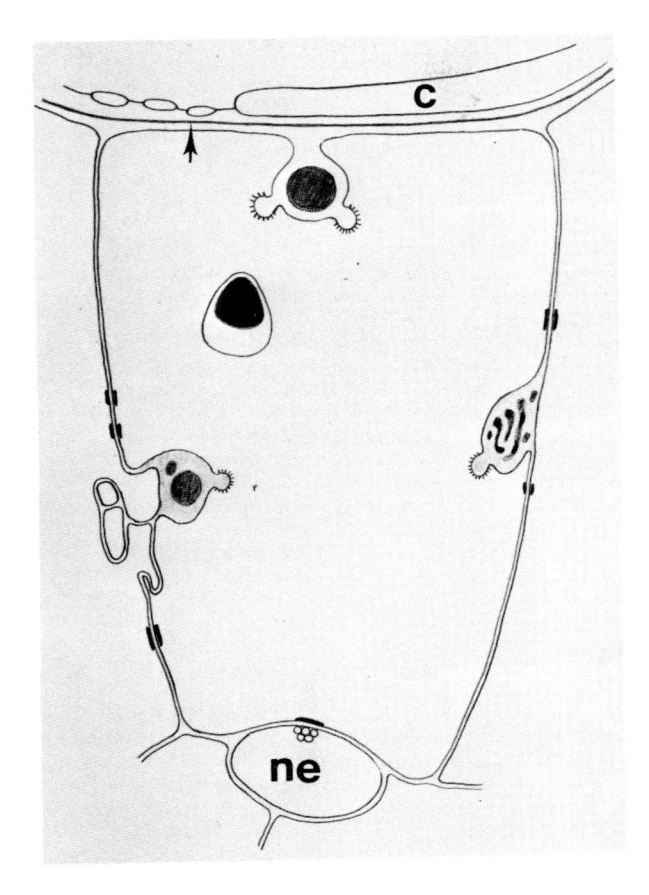

FIG. 13. Schematic representation of exocytosis profiles in chromaffin cell; c, capillary; ne, nerve ending. Coated pits appear in granule membrane after its fusion-fission with plasma membrane. Granules, expelled at free surface just beneath basal lamina (arrow), seem as compact as intracellular granules. Between adjoining plasma membranes the expelled granules appear near interdigitations and attachment plates; they are no more compact, but disorganized. Catecholamines, although kept by fixative in intracellular granules (this is true only for norepinephrine), disappear from expelled granules.

REFERENCES

1. ABRAHAMS, S. J., AND E. HOLTZMAN. Secretion and endocytosis in rat adrenal medulla cells. *Abstr. Ann. Meeting Am. Soc. Cell Biol.*, 11th, New Orleans, 1971.
2. AL-LAMI, F. Follicular arrangements in hamster adrenomedullary cells: light and electron microscopic study. *Anat. Record* 168: 161–178, 1970.
3. AMSTERDAM, A., I. OHAD, AND M. SCHRAMM. Dynamic changes in the ultrastructure of the acinar cell of the rat parotid gland during the secretory cycle. *J. Cell Biol.* 41: 753–773, 1969.
4. ANDERSON, E. Oogenesis in the cockroach, *Periplaneta americana*, with special reference to the specialization of the oolema and the fate of coated vesicles. *J. Microscopie* 8: 721–738, 1969.
5. BENEDECZKY, I., AND A. D. SMITH. Ultrastructural studies on the adrenal medulla of golden hamster: origin and fate of secretory granules. *Z. Zellforsch. Mikroskop. Anat.* 124: 367–386, 1972.
6. BLASCHKO, H., R. S. COMLINE, F. H. SCHNEIDER, M. SILVER, AND A. D. SMITH. Secretion of a chromaffin granule protein, chromogranin, from the adrenal gland after splanchnic stimulation. *Nature* 215: 58–59, 1967.
7. BUNT, A. H. Formation of coated and synaptic vesicles within neurosecretory axon terminals of the crustacean sinus gland. *J. Ultrastruct. Res.* 28: 411–421, 1969.
8. CARDELL, R. Le lobe antérieure de l'hypophyse: les cellules somatotropes et gonadotropes. In: *Structure Fine des Cellules et des Tissus*, edited by K. R. Porter and M. A. Bonneville. Paris: Ediscience, 1969, p. 71–73.
9. COUPLAND, R. E. Electron microscopic observations on the structure of the rat adrenal medulla. I. The ultrastructure and organization of chromaffin cells in the normal adrenal medulla. *J. Anat.* 99: 231–254, 1965.
10. COUPLAND, R. E., AND D. HOPWOOD. The mechanism of the differential staining reaction for adrenaline and noradrenaline-storing granules in tissues fixed in glutaraldehyde. *J. Anat.* 100: 227–243, 1966.
11. COUPLAND, R. E., A. S. PYPER, AND D. HOPWOOD. A method for differentiating between adrenaline and noradrenaline-storing cells in the light and electron microscope. *Nature* 201: 1240–1242, 1964.
12. D'ANZI, F. A. Morphological and biochemical observations on the catecholamine storing vesicles of rat adrenomedullary cells during insulin-induced hypoglycemia. *Am. J. Anat.* 125: 381–397, 1969.
13. DEROBERTIS, E., AND D. D. SABATINI. Submicroscopic analysis of the secretory process in the adrenal medulla. *Federation Proc.* 19, Suppl. 5: 70–78, 1960.
14. DEROBERTIS, E., AND A. VAZ FERREIRA. Electron microscopic study of the excretion of catechol-containing droplets in the adrenal medulla of the rabbit. *Exptl. Cell Res.* 12: 568–574, 1957.
15. DINER, O. L'expulsion des granules de la medullo-surrénale chez le hamster. *Compt. Rend.* 265: 616–619, 1967.
16. DROLLER, M. J., AND T. F. ROTH. An electron microscope study of yolk formation during oogenesis in *Lebistes reticulatus guppyi*. *J. Cell Biol.* 28: 209–232, 1966.
17. EADE, N. R. The distribution of the catecholamines in homogenates of the bovine adrenal medulla. *J. Physiol., London* 141: 183–192, 1958.
18. ELFVIN, L. G. The fine structure of the cell surface of chromaffin cells in the rat adrenal medulla. *J. Ultrastruct. Res.* 12: 263–286, 1965.
19. ELFVIN, L. G., L. E. APPELGREN, AND S. ULLBERG. High-resolution autoradiography of the adrenal medulla after injection

of tritiated dihydroxyphenylalanine(dopa). *J. Ultrastruct. Res.* 14: 277-293, 1966.
20. ERÄNKÖ, O. Distribution of fluorescing islets, adrenaline and noradrenaline in the adrenal medulla of the hamster. *Acta Endocrinol.* 18: 174-179, 1955.
21. FARQUHAR, M. C. Origin and fate of secretory granules in cells of the anterior pituitary gland. *Trans. NY Acad. Sci.* 23: 346-351, 1961.
22. FARQUHAR, M. C. Lysosome function in regulating secretion disposal of secretory granules in cells of the anterior pituitary gland. In: *Lysosomes in Biology and Pathology*, edited by J. T. Dingle and H. B. Fell. Amsterdam: North-Holland, 1969, vol. II, p. 462-482.
23. FARQUHAR, M. C., AND G. E. PALADE. Junctional complexes in various epithelia. *J. Cell Biol.* 17: 375-412, 1963.
24. FAWCETT, D. W. Physiologically significant specializations of the cell surface. *Circulation* 26: 1105-1132, 1962.
25. FAWCETT, D. W. Surface specializations of absorbing cells. *J. Histochem. Cytochem.* 13: 75-91, 1965.
26. FRIEND, D. S., AND M. G. FARQUHAR. Functions of coated vesicles during protein absorption in the rat vas deferens. *J. Cell Biol.* 35: 357-376, 1967.
27. GOMEZ-ACEBO, J., R. PARRILLA, AND J. L. R. CANDELA. Fine structure of the A and D cells of the rabbit endocrine pancreas in vivo and incubated in vitro. I. Mechanism of secretion of the A cells. *J. Cell Biol.* 36: 33-44, 1968.
28. GRYNSZPAN-WINOGRAD, O. Différences dans l'innervation des "cellules à adrénaline" et des "cellules à noradrénaline" de la medullosurrénale du hamster. *Compt. Rend.* 268: 1420-1422, 1969.
29. GRYNSZPAN-WINOGRAD, O. Morphological aspects of exocytosis in the adrenal medulla. *Phil. Trans. Roy. Soc. London Ser. B* 261: 291-292, 1971.
30. HAND, A. R. The fine structure of von Ebner's gland of the rat. *J. Cell Biol.* 44: 340-353, 1970.
31. HERLANT, M. Apport de la microscopie électronique à l'étude du lobe antérieur de l'hypophyse. In: *Cytologie de l'Adénohypophyse*, edited by J. Benoit and C. Da Lage. Paris: Centre National de la Recherche Scientifique, 1963, p. 73-90.
32. HOLTZMAN, E., AND R. DOMINITZ. Cytochemical studies of lysosomes, Golgi apparatus and endoplasmic reticulum in secretion and protein uptake by adrenal medulla cells of the rat. *J. Histochem. Cytochem.* 16: 320-336, 1968.
33. ICHIKAWA, A. Fine structural changes in response to hormonal stimulation of the perfused canine pancreas. *J. Cell Biol.* 24: 369-385, 1965.
34. KANASEKI, T., AND K. KADOTA. The "vesicle in a basket." A morphological study of the coated vesicle isolated from the nerve endings of the guinea pig brain, with special reference to the mechanism of membrane movements. *J. Cell Biol.* 42: 202-220, 1969.
35. KIRSHNER, N., AND A. G. KIRSHNER. Chromogranin A, dopamine-β-hydroxylase and secretion from the adrenal medulla. *Phil. Trans. Roy. Soc. London Ser. B* 261: 279-289, 1971.
36. KUROSUMI, K. Electron microscopic analysis of the secretion mechanism. *Intern. Rev. Cytol.* 11: 1-124, 1961.
37. LEVER, J. D. Electron microscopic observations on the normal and denervated adrenal medulla of the rat. *Endocrinology* 57: 621-635, 1955.
38. LISHAJKO, F. Occurrence and some properties of dopamine containing granules in the sheep adrenal. *Acta Physiol. Scand.* 72: 255-256, 1968.
39. MALAMED, S., A. M. POISNER, J. M. TRIFARO, AND W. W. DOUGLAS. The fate of the chromaffin granule during catecholamine release from the adrenal medulla. III. Recovery of a purified fraction of electron-translucent structures. *Biochem. Pharmacol.* 17: 241-246, 1968.
40. MICHEL-BECHET, M., G. COTTE, AND A. M. HAON. Etude ultrastructurale de la medullo-surrénale du hamster. *J. Microscopie* 2: 449-460, 1963.
41. NAGASAWA, J., W. W. DOUGLAS, AND R. A. SCHULTZ. Ultrastructural evidence of secretion by exocytosis and of "synaptic vesicle" formation in posterior pituitary glands. *Nature* 227: 407-409, 1970.
42. NORMANN, T. C. The neurosecretory system of the adult *Calliphora erythrocephala*. I. The fine structure of the corpus cardiacum with some observations on adjacent organs. *Z. Zellforsch. Mikroskop. Anat.* 67: 461-501, 1965.
43. PALADE, G. E. Functional changes in the structure of cell components. In: *Subcellular Particles*, edited by T. Hayashi. New York: Ronald Press, 1959, p. 64-80.
44. PLATTNER, H., H. WINKLER, H. HORTNAGL, AND W. PFALLER. A study of the adrenal medulla and its subcellular organelles by the freeze-etching method. *J. Ultrastruct. Res.* 28: 191-202, 1969.
45. POISNER, A. M., J. M. TRIFARO, AND W. W. DOUGLAS. The fate of chromaffin granule during catecholamine release from the adrenal medulla. II. Loss of protein and retention of lipid in subcellular fractions. *Biochem. Pharmacol.* 16: 2101-2108, 1967.
46. ROSENBLUTH, J., AND S. L. WISSIG. The distribution of exogenous ferritin in toad spinal ganglia and the mechanism of its uptake by neurons. *J. Cell Biol.* 23: 307-326, 1964.
47. ROTH, T. F., AND K. R. PORTER. Yolk protein uptake in the oocyte of the mosquito *Aedes Aegypti* L. *J. Cell Biol.* 20: 313-332, 1964.
48. TRAMEZZANI, J. H., S. CHIOCCHIO, AND G. F. WASSERMANN. A technique for light and electron microscopic identification of adrenaline and noradrenaline storing cells. *J. Histochem. Cytochem.* 12: 890-899, 1964.
49. VIVEROS, O. H., L. ARQUEROS, AND N. KIRSHNER. Mechanism of secretion from the adrenal medulla. V. Retention of storage vesicle membranes following release of adrenaline. *Mol. Pharmacol.* 6: 342-349, 1969.
50. WETZSTEIN, R. Elektronenmikroskopische Untersuchungen am Nebennierenmark von Maus, Meerschweinchen und Katze. *Z. Zellforsch. Mikroskop. Anat.* 46: 517-576, 1957.
51. WOOD, J. G. Identification of and observations on epinephrine and norepinephrine containing cells in the adrenal medulla. *Am. J. Anat.* 112: 285-304, 1963.
52. WOOD, J. G., AND R. J. BARRNETT. Histochemical demonstration of norepinephrine at a fine structural level. *J. Histochem. Cytochem.* 12: 197-209, 1964.
53. YATES, R. D., J. C. WOOD, AND D. DUNCAN. Phase and electron microscopic observations on two cell types in the adrenal medulla of the Syrian hamster. *Texas Rep. Biol. Med.* 20: 494-502, 1962.
54. ZACKS, S. I., AND A. SAITO. Uptake of exogenous horseradish peroxydase by coated vesicles in mouse neuromuscular junctions. *J. Histochem. Cytochem.* 17: 161-170, 1969.

Physiological mechanisms controlling secretory activity of adrenal medulla

G. P. LEWIS | *Department of Pharmacology, Institute of Basic Medical Sciences, Royal College of Surgeons of England, London, England*

CHAPTER CONTENTS

Peripheral Nerve Pathway
Medullary Hormones
Selective Release
Central Nerve Pathway
Functional Significance of Adrenal Discharge
Stimulation of Adrenal Discharge
    Emotional stress
    Cold, heat, and pH
    Physical stress
    Asphyxia and anoxia
    Hypotension
    Hypoglycemia
    Glucagon
    Naturally occurring substances

PERIPHERAL NERVE PATHWAY

The cholinergic nature of the preganglionic nerve to the adrenal gland, the splanchnic, was clearly shown by the classic experiments of Feldberg and his colleagues. Feldberg & Minz (54) detected a substance pharmacologically indistinguishable from acetylcholine in the venous blood from the adrenal glands during splanchnic nerve stimulation in the presence of eserine, and Feldberg et al. (56) identified the substance as acetylcholine. However, the liberation of acetylcholine from the adrenal glands during splanchnic nerve stimulation was not sufficient proof that it is the direct cause of the epinephrine discharge. In addition, the epinephrine discharge caused by splanchnic nerve stimulation itself was also greatly enhanced by eserine. They also showed that the acetylcholine receptors in the adrenals were mainly nicotinic, although they found evidence of a minor muscarinic component that could be antagonized by small doses of atropine. The presence of muscarinic transmission has recently been confirmed by Lee & Trendelenburg (98). A similar complement of receptors has been found in true sympathetic ganglion tissue (1, 89, 94, 102).

Acetylcholine is therefore the immediate physiological stimulus that causes the chromaffin cells to release their hormones, probably by acting on the outer surface of the chromaffin cells. This suggestion arose from an analogy of the junction between the preganglionic nerve ending and the chromaffin cells with the neuromuscular junction and the ganglionic synapse. At these analogous sites in the nervous system, Del Castillo & Katz (36) showed that acetylcholine applied by micropipette to the outer surface simulated the transmitter function, whereas acetylcholine applied to the inner surface did not.

Douglas & Rubin (38) examined in more detail the action of acetylcholine on the chromaffin cell of the adrenal medulla and concluded that the analogy with the neuromuscular junction and ganglionic synapse goes further. They suggested that acetylcholine evokes catecholamine secretion by promoting the inward movement of calcium across the cell membrane. This sequence of events was again analogous to that discussed by Katz (91) concerning the requirement for calcium in linking the release of chemical transmitter with the invasion of the terminal by impulses. Douglas (37) followed the concept of a "stimulus-contraction coupling" in skeletal muscle in developing the idea of a "stimulus-secretion coupling" in the adrenal medulla and other glands. The action of the transmitter acetylcholine on the cell surface is probably to increase the permeability to calcium ions. There follows an increased movement of calcium ions down an electrochemical gradient to an intracellular site, and the consequence is the release of catecholamines.

Perhaps this mechanism explains why substances that cause secretion of catecholamines from the adrenal medulla in vivo do not cause their release from isolated granules (10, 40). One might speculate that such substances exert their action via a membrane effect involving the intrusion of calcium ion. On the other hand, agents that might be expected to act via some more direct and physical means (e.g., surface active agents, pH, and certain histamine liberators) cause the release of catecholamines from isolated granules (77).

MEDULLARY HORMONES

The principal catecholamines of the adrenal medulla of mammals are epinephrine and norepinephrine, and they are usually present in amounts of 5–10 mg/g adrenal tissue.

The general pattern of change of adrenal glands throughout early life is one of a changing proportion of norepinephrine to epinephrine. During fetal and neonatal life, norepinephrine is probably the predominant catecholamine, but the proportion of epinephrine increases with age (134). The methylation of norepinephrine to epinephrine first described by Bülbring and Burn (15, 16) is intimately associated with the physiological significance of various stimuli. The sympathetic nervous system is still incompletely developed at the time of birth, and it is thus possible that the vascular tone in the fetus may be under the humoral control of norepinephrine produced by the adrenal medulla and the paraaortic bodies and that during postnatal life, as epinephrine becomes the predominant hormone, this function is gradually taken over by the nervous mechanism (30).

A similar pattern of change toward an increasing proportion of epinephrine in the adrenal medulla occurs during evolutionary development. Coupland (30) and Wright & Jones (135) have pointed out the increasing association of adrenocortical and adrenal medullary tissue throughout the vertebrates and have suggested a correlation between the proximity of cortical to medullary cells and the preponderance of epinephrine. It was implied that there was a mechanism whereby the methylation of norepinephrine might be, at least in part, controlled by adrenocortical steroids. Such a speculative functional relationship at first seems unlikely since the two tissues that make up the adrenals originate from different embryological sources and come into close juxtaposition only through a process of tissue migration. However, more recently, Wurtman & Axelrod (137) have found that glucocorticoids influence the enzymatic synthesis of epinephrine in the adrenal medulla by stimulating N-methyltransferase activity. They naturally conclude from their results that factors altering the synthesis and secretion of these corticoids may produce some of their biochemical effect as a result of changes in the availability of epinephrine. Pohorecky and Wurtman (115, 136) have also found that removal of the pituitary is followed by a gradual fall in the epinephrine content of the adrenals and that it is restored after injections of ACTH or dexamethasone.

Eränkö (44) first showed the presence of two types of cells in the adrenal medulla and later (42) showed that these cell types are related specifically to the two medullary hormones. In addition, Hillarp & Hökfelt (76) showed that all the cells of the adrenal medulla can form norepinephrine, whereas only certain specific cells are able to effect a mechanism for the methylation of norepinephrine to epinephrine and store this hormone. Whether these cells are the ones most readily available to high concentration of corticosteroids is not known. However, Eränkö (43) has shown that the islet cells containing norepinephrine are situated on the outside of the medulla nearest to the cortex. Although more epinephrine than norepinephrine appears in the adrenal venous blood on stimulation of the splanchnic nerve, even prolonged stimulation does not result in a greatly increased proportion of norepinephrine remaining in the gland (73, 80). On the other hand, nicotine, which also caused an increased proportion of epinephrine in the medullary secretion, produces a medulla containing an increased proportion of norepinephrine and depletion of epinephrine (86). This finding might mean that splanchnic nerve stimulation facilitates the methylation of norepinephrine, as suggested by Bülbring (15). However, Vogt (131) has shown that, after the adrenal glands have been chronically denervated (i.e., in complete absence of nervous stimuli), adrenal venous blood contains norepinephrine, as well as epinephrine. The composition of the secretion is determined by the degree of methylation present in the gland rather than by the type of stimulus employed.

SELECTIVE RELEASE

Recently it has become clear that there is a selective release of the two hormones and that the selectivity depends at least partly on the nature of the stimulus (17, 39, 86, 90). Hypoglycemia, like nicotine, causes a secretion rich in epinephrine and depletes the medulla of this hormone (20, 112). Brücke et al. (14) showed that carotid occlusion decreased the percentage of epinephrine in adrenal venous blood, whereas Redgate & Gellhorn (117) found that after asphyxia it was mostly epinephrine that was released. Carotid occlusion produced a medullary secretion containing a low percentage of epinephrine, whereas sciatic or brachial plexus stimulation caused a larger proportion of epinephrine in the adrenal venous blood (46).

The selective secretion of individual catecholamines might well have an important relationship to the functional significance of a particular discharge since the activities of the two hormones differ considerably. It strongly indicates that norepinephrine not only acts as the precursor of epinephrine, but functions as an independent hormone. However, Munro & Robinson (107) have shown, in human subjects with spinal lesions below T_4, a predominance of epinephrine in the plasma. The epinephrine originated in the adrenal glands since after bilateral adrenalectomy it disappeared. They concluded that norepinephrine does not normally form any considerable part of the medullary secretion in man.

CENTRAL NERVE PATHWAY

Cannon & de la Paz (23) first showed that the secretion from the adrenal medulla, together with the sympathetic nervous discharges, contributes to the signs of emotional excitement. They observed that a substance resembling epinephrine appeared in the blood during emotional behavior but disappeared after adrenalectomy. At about the same time, Elliott (41) observed that dilatation of the pupil, after removal of the superior cervical ganglion, occurs in anger when the adrenals are intact, but not during anger aroused after the glands have been excised. Cannon et al. (22) finally showed, by using the denervated heart preparation, that both emotional excitement and vigorous activity caused an increased medullary secretion manifested particularly in an increased heart rate. Furthermore, Houssay & Molinelli (84) showed the presence of a center in the brain controlling medullary secretion by observing such secretory activity on stimulation of the bulbar region, and Tournade et al. (128) not only confirmed their finding but showed that application of cocaine to the floor of the fourth ventricle reduces the secretory activity of the adrenal medulla. They suggested a state of tonic nervous activity of the adrenals that is removed by treatment with cocaine. Such a view is not consistent with that held by Cannon (21) who suggested that there is not a continuous secretion of epinephrine from the adrenal glands but that their activity is intermittent and that their real function is preparing for conditions that make particularly great requirements on the organism (e.g., during fight or flight). Meier & Bein (106) found a continuous release of norepinephrine from resting adrenal glands. However, this is not altogether neurally controlled since, even after chronic denervation, both norepinephrine and epinephrine were found in adrenal venous blood (131); although acute denervation considerably reduces the resting secretory activity, the proportion of the two catecholamines appears to remain about the same (39).

In addition to the finding that stimulation of the hypothalamus causes the release of norepinephrine from nerve endings (105), stimulation of the anterior and median region of the hypothalamus causes an increase in adrenal medullary secretion (12). Further research showed that hypothalamic stimulation increases the proportion of epinephrine in the adrenal secretion (14). Both Redgate & Gellhorn (117) and Folkow & von Euler (59) found that stimulation of different areas of the hypothalamus releases different proportions of epinephrine and norepinephrine. They concluded that the two types of adrenal cells shown by Hillarp & Hökfelt (76) to contain epinephrine and norepinephrine are innervated by separate fibers with different hypothalamic representations.

An indication that this hypothalamic center is controlled by areas of cortex was made by Kennard (92). He observed that destruction of parts of the orbital surface of the cerebral cortex of cats resulted in an increased secretion of catecholamines and suggested that this could normally exert an inhibitory influence on the sympathetic centers in the hypothalamus. Later this control was more clearly defined by Folkow and co-workers (45, 58); stimulation of certain cerebral cortical areas may enhance or inhibit secretory activity of the adrenal medulla. This cortical controlling mechanism is discriminating, since by positioning the electrode it was possible to separate the activation of fibers that are mainly responsible for a rise in blood pressure from the activation of fibers influencing pathways running to the secretory cells of the adrenal medulla. In addition, they concluded that some corticofugal fibers influencing adrenal medullary secretion seem to descend without relay stations in the hypothalamus since medullary secretion continues after destruction of the hypothalamus when certain cortical areas are stimulated.

Thus adrenal medullary secretory activity can be influenced by environmental factors that act in the central nervous system at cortical, hypothalamic, and perhaps spinal regions and by factors that stimulate or inhibit these regions reflexly.

FUNCTIONAL SIGNIFICANCE OF ADRENAL DISCHARGE

Some changes in internal or external environment of the individual stimulate certain groups of neuroeffector units, whereas others excite only the adrenal medulla. For example, exposure to moderate cold increases the activity of the sympathetic vasoconstrictor fibers in the skin vessels. A moderate fall in blood sugar levels, on the other hand, excites predominantly the cells of the adrenal medulla. Other changes, such as most types of stress, work, and emotional excitement, cause a more or less generalized increase of sympathetic activities involving both sympathetic motor nerve fibers and the adrenal medulla. These last activation patterns are referred to by Cannon (21) as "emergency reactions."

The role of the adrenal medullary hormones as activators of many physiological mechanisms in emergency situations has been recognized since the classic investigations of Cannon and his colleagues. The main biological effects of the adrenal secretion suggest such a view. The stimulating effect on the heart, the vasodilatation of skeletal muscle vessels, venoconstriction, immobilization of the gut, relaxation of bronchiolar muscle, pupillary dilatation and piloerection, and mobilization of liver glycogen and of free fatty acids, all contribute to increased efficiency of the whole organism in emergency states.

There appears to be a clear functional differentiation of the two catecholamines in that norepinephrine causes vasoconstriction, whereas epinephrine causes vasodilatation in skeletal muscle and has more important metabolic effects. Celander (27) concluded that the sympathetic vasoconstrictor nerve fibers constitute the only factor of importance eliciting constriction of the blood vessels in skeletal muscles. Epinephrine, on the other hand, is capable of producing a maximal vasodilatation at quite small concentrations. It adds an important contribution to the vasodilatation provoked by sympathetic cholinergic vasodilator fibers in skeletal muscle in helping to provide an adequate blood supply to the muscle during states of emergency (104). It has been suggested, however, that this vasodilator action of epinephrine is secondary to its metabolic action and not caused by a direct action on the vascular smooth muscle. The results of Bearn et al. (5) supported this view. They found that the increase of lactic acid production and the vasodilatation are pronounced at low doses of epinephrine but that neither effect occurs after norepinephrine administration.

In skin vessels the medullary discharge of epinephrine is overshadowed by the vasoconstriction induced by the norepinephrine liberated at sympathetic nerve endings. When norepinephrine is released from the adrenal medullary cells, the circulating catecholamine might serve to reinforce the action of the nerves.

As far as the cardiovascular system is concerned therefore the function of the adrenal medullary discharge is as a reinforcement of the motor control by the sympathetic postganglionic nerve fibers, and its role in the adjustments of the circulation does not appear to be an important one (27).

The other main function of the adrenal medulla probably involves metabolic effects (i.e., mobilization of glucose from hepatic glycogen and the breakdown into lactic acid of glycogen stored in skeletal muscles). These metabolic actions occur in tissues that are probably not under the direct control of sympathetic nerves. For example, although the hepatic blood vessels are innervated by sympathetic fibers, carbohydrate metabolism is not affected by nerve stimulation to the liver cells since the hyperglycemia observed in states of increased sympathetic activity is more or less abolished by adrenalectomy (111). However, norepinephrine has been shown to lower liver glycogen. On the other hand, the breakdown of glycogen in muscle cells is not influenced by norepinephrine (87), nor is it affected by sympathetic nerve stimulation (95); it is, however, profoundly affected by epinephrine (87).

In contrast, another metabolic effect of the autonomic sympathetic system—the mobilization of free fatty acids from adipose tissue—appears to be under the control of sympathetic nerves rather than the adrenal medulla. An increase of free fatty acids in plasma still occurs in demedullated rats subjected to cold, although the increase in plasma glucose that occurs in normal rats is suppressed. Furthermore, stimulation of the sympathetic nerves to adipose tissue, at least in certain species, results in a release of free fatty acids and glycerol into the plasma (13, 72).

STIMULATION OF ADRENAL DISCHARGE

Emotional Stress

Emotional excitement in an animal leads to a general stimulation of the sympathetic nervous system. This was first shown by Cannon & de la Paz (23) who induced emotional stress in cats by exposing them to barking dogs. In man various types of mental stress, such as anxiety and irritation, lead to an increased excretion of catecholamines. In most situations that provoke apprehension and anxiety, an increased epinephrine output has been observed, whereas norepinephrine output in general remains unchanged. Increased epinephrine excretion has been reported in connection with examinations (113), stressful working conditions (103), emotional stress (47), and psychological tests (62). In other situations usually involving excitation, norepinephrine output is increased (63, 66). In general, various investigations indicate a differential catecholamine excretion in different emotional states—passive, tense, anxious behavior tends to be associated with increased epinephrine excretion, whereas aggressive, hostile reactions are predominantly accompanied by an increased norepinephrine excretion. Bloom et al. (11), from a study in a group of paratroopers, concluded that catecholamine excretion might be related to basic personality traits. They speculate that the relatively higher correlation they found for epinephrine, as compared with norepinephrine, excretion with the various experimental conditions of their study may indicate that epinephrine secretion is a basic emergency reaction of an organism exposed to stress, whereas the norepinephrine response may be associated with complex psychophysiological relationships. In agreement with this view, Frankenhauser & Patkai (61) found a significant correlation between the performance of coding and proofreading tests carried out under distracting conditions and norepinephrine excretion but no correlation with epinephrine excretion. Frankenhauser et al. (60) suggested that secretion of catecholamines is associated with arousal, as well as emotional functions during stress. Their finding indicated that epinephrine secretion acquires an increasing importance with increasing length of the stress period, and they suggested that epinephrine secretion serves to increase arousal to counteract monotony and boredom in situations demanding sustained concentration over prolonged periods. A similar view was expressed by O'Hanlon (110). However, the view of Vogt (personal communication) is that arousal leads to the secretion of epinephrine, rather than vice versa, since there are conditions (e.g., injection of insulin) during which one can obtain a maximal secretion of epinephrine without arousal.

Emotional stress factors are usually mixed with or superimposed on physical stress factors, and the objective evaluation of such combinations is fraught with difficulties. For example, Cunningham et al. (32) have found a sustained increase in plasma and urine concentrations of norepinephrine, but no significant change in epinephrine excretion, during a stay at an altitude of 3,000–4,500 m. Becker & Kreuzer (6) in a later study tried to avoid the emotional stress factors involved in the action (i.e., the aggressive mood necessary for climbing a mountain), as well as the physical stress. They carried out experiments in low pressure chambers simulating a 3,000–4,000-m altitude. Under these conditions they found a reversed excretion pattern—an increase in epinephrine but little or no change in norepinephrine excretion. They interpreted the finding on the basis of a different type of stress.

Exposure of animals to environments with high concentrations of oxygen, particularly those accompanied by toxic symptoms, results in a pronounced sympathetic outflow (4). Shortly before and during the symptoms of oxygen toxicity, animals exhibited piloerection, elevated blood pressure, increased pulse rate, and increased blood lactic acid concentration. Cross & Houlihan (31) found that rats initially reacted to increased oxygen tensions by a depression of sympathetic nerve activity, an observation also made in man (70), but as the oxygen environment became lethal it caused a sustained sympathetic stimulation, which resulted in the release of excessive amounts of epinephrine from the adrenal medulla, as well as stimulation of sympathetic centers together with depletion of hypothalamic norepinephrine. Far from being a protective mechanism, the massive release of epinephrine augmented the pulmonary damage.

Cold, Heat, and pH

The study of the response to cold suffers also from the interference of emotional stress, and for this reason Klepping et al. (93) studied the effect of cold on adrenal medullary secretion in dogs anesthetized with pentobarbitone. They found not only a marked increase in total secretion into the adrenal vein blood, but an increase in the proportion of epinephrine. However, they had shown earlier that anesthetics themselves, particularly barbiturates, interfere with the thermoregulatory system (126). Wada et al. (133) showed that, even after adrenalectomy, exposure to cold produced a considerable increase in heart rate suggesting that sympathetic nerve activity plays an important part in the response. A similar conclusion was reached by Leduc (96) who showed a relatively smaller urinary excretion of epinephrine than of norepinephrine during exposure to cold. After adrenalectomy very little epinephrine, but still large amounts of norepinephrine, are excreted. In addition, adrenalectomized animals withstood moderate cold exposure, so long as cortical hormones were provided, which suggested that the adrenal medulla plays only a secondary role in the response to cold (see the chapter by Himms-Hagen in this volume of the *Handbook*).

Saito (119) was the first to observe that adrenal medullary secretion occurred in response to surface burns. Urinary excretion of catecholamines was found to occur after burns in man by Goodall et al. (67), but the analysis of the mechanisms of their release and of the part played by emotional stress has not been attempted.

Metabolic acidosis and alkalosis produce an increased secretion of catecholamines from the adrenal medulla. The mechanism of the increased secretion varied, however. Higashi (75) reported that metabolic acidosis acted both directly on the adrenal medullary cells and via the central nervous system when the arterial blood pH was below 6.70, but the secretion was increased only through a central nervous mechanism when the blood pH was above 6.80. In a study of alkalosis, Tamura (125) showed that adrenal secretion was increased at a blood pH above 7.76 and concluded that this was central stimulation since it was not present in splanchnicotomized dogs.

Physical Stress

Physical exercise is accompanied by an increased excretion of catecholamines in the urine (24, 71, 132). Adrenal secretion increased in dogs running on a treadmill until they were fatigued, but no such increase occurred in nonfatigued dogs (24, 71, 132). Hökfelt (79) found a decrease in the epinephrine content of the adrenal medulla after exercise in rats. Von Euler & Hellner (49) found that the relative amount of epinephrine was the same as under resting conditions and concluded that the source of the increased urinary catecholamines during exercise was both the adrenal medulla and sympathetic nerves. These authors also showed some correlation between the degree of physical exertion and catecholamine excretion and found that the most successful competitors among a group of skiers taking part in their tests were those with the highest excretion figures. This is in agreement with the finding of Munro & Robinson (108) that no increase in epinephrine levels in plasma occurred during moderate exercise in man but that in long-distance runners plasma epinephrine levels increased. However, there seems little doubt that other factors, including emotional stress, must be involved in such studies.

Asphyxia and Anoxia

Asphyxia leads to secretion of epinephrine from the adrenal glands. Houssay & Molinelli (85) found that cutting the splanchnic nerves prevented the response to anoxia and concluded that, like all responses discussed so far, the response was mediated via the splanchnic nerves. In perfusion experiments with the splanchnic nerves cut, Bülbring et al. (18) found that a period of anoxia leads to a discharge of epinephrine. This indicated therefore that the response of the adrenal glands was at least partly the result of direct stimulation of the secretory cells by local anoxia.

Asphyxia appears to represent a combination of stimuli to the central structures governing the sympathetic nervous system. Celander (27) found that in order to achieve a large secretion (e.g., 20–40% of the maximum capacity of the adrenal glands) it was necessary to prolong the asphyxia until it implied a serious threat to the organism. Von Euler & Folkow (46) also found that excitation of the adrenal medulla is a late event in the asphyxial defense response. The neurogenic adjustments always preceded and overshadowed those of the slower blood-borne catecholamines from the adrenal glands. Celander (27) has pointed to the danger of using the arterial blood pressure as an indicator of sympathetic activity and showed that during asphyxia a fall of blood pressure coincided with an increase of vasomotor nerve discharge. He suggested that the falling blood pressure was probably the result of cardiac failure and concluded that in the asphyxia defense reaction there is a predominance of sympathetic nerve activity.

Baugh et al. (3) studied anoxia induced in intact anesthetized dogs breathing 6% oxygen in nitrogen and found that many of the cardiovascular changes were prevented or moderated after acute adrenalectomy. They concluded that catecholamines released from the adrenal medulla are mainly responsible, which is in agreement with the finding of Nahas et al. (109). These authors found no change in heart rate and cardiac output in anesthetized, chronically adrenalectomized dogs during exposure to 8% oxygen in nitrogen and concluded that the adrenal medulla plays an essential role in the immediate circulatory adaptation to acute hypoxia.

Comline & Silver (28, 29) have examined the problem of asphyxia in fetal and newborn animals. During gestation the adrenal medulla appears to react directly to asphyxia, independently of the nerve supply, and the secretion consists mainly of norepinephrine. The direct response of the fetal adrenal gland to asphyxia observed in an immature sheep fetus predominates in the fetal calf throughout gestation. As the splanchnic nerve stimulation becomes effective, the direct response to asphyxia wanes. The authors suggest that the degree of development of the adrenal medulla at birth may well be related to the severity and duration of hypoxia during normal parturition, which probably varies in different species.

Hypotension

It is generally accepted that the adrenal medullary hormones do not play a significant role in the maintenance of normal blood pressure. However, there is no doubt that the glands respond to abnormally low blood pressure. In experiments in which adrenal vein blood was examined or in animals with denervated hearts, induced hypotension was accompanied by an increase in secretion of catecholamines (7, 116). In hemorrhagic hypotension also, there was an increased adrenal secretion, whereas in hypertension there was a decreased secretion (121, 127). Further it was demonstrated (119) that the secretion of catecholamines into the adrenal vein blood of unanesthetized dogs subjected to hemorrhage was proportional to the decrease in blood volume.

This response of the adrenal medulla may be partly due to anoxia brought about by a considerably reduced blood flow through the gland. Certainly reflex stimulation is a factor also since, in his classic experiments, Heymans (74) clearly demonstrated that a fall in blood pressure causes baroreceptors, located in the wall of the carotid sinus, to initiate impulses leading to the activation of the sympathetic nervous system, including increased secretion from the adrenal medulla. Kaindl & von Euler (90) demonstrated a four- to fivefold increase in total catecholamine concentration in adrenal vein blood during carotid occlusion but found that the proportions of epinephrine and norepinephrine remained unaltered. Glaviano et al. (64) observed that the high secretory rate of epinephrine was maintained over prolonged periods of low blood pressure to within minutes of complete cardiovascular and respiratory collapse. They even suggest that the released epinephrine may enter tissues and cause some of the metabolic and hemodynamic alterations found in shock.

Hypoglycemia

Hypoglycemia, such as that following an overdose of insulin, was shown to cause a secretion of catecholamines from the adrenal medulla (25). As blood glucose falls to between 110 and 70 mg/100 ml in anesthetized (or to 70–80 mg/100 ml in unanesthetized) animals, there is cardiac acceleration. If the adrenals are removed, there is no increase in heart rate, the fall in blood sugar after insulin administration occurs more rapidly, and convulsive seizures are induced sooner. The release of epinephrine appears to be a protective measure in which the catecholamine mobilizes glycogen from the liver. If this measure fails there is damage to the central nervous system that leads to convulsions.

Burn et al. (20) found that insulin depleted the medullary hormones for at least 8 hr after injection. They found an increased proportion of norepinephrine remaining in the gland, which indicated that the process of methylation was slower than that leading to accumulation of new norepinephrine. Outschoorn (112) showed that, when the blood sugar fell from 88 to 51 mg/100 ml during the first 4 hr after an injection of insulin, the adrenal medullae were depleted of epinephrine for more than 24 hr, despite the fact that the blood sugar had returned to 89 mg/100 ml 5 hr after the insulin injection.

When the sympathetic nervous system is discharging as a result of hypoglycemia, its excited state is reduced by injection of glucose. However, Dúner (39) observed that after denervation of the glands low concentration of blood sugar does not increase the medullary secretion. He went further to extend the findings of La Barre & Saric (2) in cross-circulation experiments, in showing that the local elevation of blood sugar level in the brain was accompanied by a decreased secretion of medullary hormone and that the injection of glucose into the hypothalamus caused a similar pronounced fall in secretion. More recently, Himsworth (78) showed that the hypoglycemia produced by systemic injection of 3-O-methylglucose was abolished by applying lignocaine to the hypothalamus. This finding indicated the presence of glucose-sensitive receptors in the hypothalamus, through which blood sugar level influences sympathetic nerve tone. An increase in blood sugar decreases sympathetic tone and with it the amount of glucose released into the blood. A fall in blood sugar conversely stimulates the production of glucose from the liver glycogen into the circulation.

Ikeda (88) located a similar receptor in the thoracic spinal region that is sensitive to hypoglycemia, but showed that it plays only a minor role in promoting adrenal medullary secretion and that the higher center is more essential. He found that, in dogs in which the spinal cord was transected at the level of the lowest cervical segment, the effect was still present but considerably reduced, whereas after section of the splanchnic nerves the response was almost abolished.

Glucagon

However, there might be more than one mechanism involved in the adrenal medullary response to hypoglycemia since recent findings suggest that a second pancreatic hormone, glucagon, might play some part, although the nature of its involvement is not yet clear. The increased oxygen consumption following injection of glucagon may be explained on the basis of an action on the adrenal medulla since Davidson & Salter (35) showed that the reaction was prevented by adrenalectomy. Later Scian et al. (122) showed, during infusion of glucagon into the perfused adrenal gland, a marked increase in the secretion of both epinephrine and norepinephrine. The concentration of glucagon necessary to produce this effect was just a little higher than that normally found in plasma. This action of glucagon might well explain several of its reported peripheral effects. Inhibition of the formation of muscle glycogen, decreased transfer of glucose into cells, impaired glucose tolerance, and increased lactic acid levels in plasma are all findings that could be explained in terms of known actions of epinephrine. This action of glucagon could also explain why it does not affect glucose uptake and glycogen metabolism in vitro (8).

Sarcione et al. (120) concluded that the hyperglycemic response to glucagon is the result of the combined effects of rapid hepatic glycogenolysis following activation of phosphorylase and stimulation of the release of epinephrine, which acts to depress the rate of glucose uptake by peripheral tissues. They suggest that hypoglycemia stimulates the release of glucagon, which in turn elicits the release of epinephrine. Such a mechanism could be a reinforcement of the main pathway in hypoglycemia via the hypothalamus. Von Euler et al. (50) suggested that hypoglycemia might not be the principal stimulus of epinephrine secretion since after insulin administration in man there was an increase of urinary epinephrine only after the second hour and the level was not maximal until the third hour, although the blood glucose level had already returned to normal by the end of the first hour. However, this suggestion is not consistent with the finding of Holzbauer & Vogt (83) that in dogs and man the rise in the epinephrine content of plasma starts to increase a few minutes after intravenous injection of insulin and lasts for several hours.

There seems to be little doubt that glucagon acts directly on the medullary cells. Lefebvre et al. (97) suggested that in rats part of the effect might be mediated reflexly by hypotension. In man no such fall in blood pressure concomitant with the release of medullary hormones occurred.

Naturally Occurring Substances

The release of medullary hormones as a result of the direct action of naturally occurring substances on the medullary cells themselves has been known for many years. Acetylcholine, the chemical transmitter of nerve impulses to the medullary cells, was first examined by Feldberg and associates (54, 56). Compounds related either in their chemical structure or pharmacological activity were also shown to act directly on the adrenal medulla [e.g., carbamylcholine (51), choline (57), nicotine (34, 57), pilocarpine (1, 34)]. In addition, several other naturally occurring, pharmacologically active substances, apparently unrelated to the chemical mediators, are active in stimulating directly the secretory cells of the adrenal medulla [e.g., histamine (19, 33), 5-hydroxytryptamine (118), kinins, and angiotensin (52, 53)]. Dale (33) pointed to the possible significance of the action of histamine on the adrenal medulla. He found that loss of the suprarenal glands considerably decreased the resistance of an animal to the toxic effects of histamine, and although he suggested that this might indicate the importance of the adrenal cortex, at that time still unknown, he also suggested that secretion of epinephrine by the adrenal medulla might be an important factor in the normal resistance to histamine. A similar possibility has been discussed for bradykinin (99, 114), which might well be formed in many kinds of vascular shock and is one of the most potent releasers of adrenal catecholamines. Feldberg & Lewis (52) examined the action of bradykinin and angiotensin on the cat adrenal medulla in some detail and calculated that after close-intraarterial injection the number of molecules of epinephrine released by one molecule of peptide must be at least 50 for bradykinin and several thousand for angiotensin. The release occurs with successive injections of peptide and shows a quantitative dose-response relationship. Later the same authors showed that the peptides do not act via cholinergic nerve endings because chronic denervation of the greater splanchnic nerve did not diminish their effect on the release of catecholamines (53).

Compounds that act directly on the medullary cells do not all appear to act on the same receptor. Nicotine reduces the sensitivity of the medullary cells to acetylcholine much more than that to histamine (124), and "paralyzing" doses of choline render cells insensitive to choline but only slightly reduce their sensitivity to acetylcholine or nicotine (68). Similarly, by their differential sensitivities under different conditions, bradykinin and angiotensin (53, 123) have been shown to act on receptors that differ for each peptide and from those stimulated by acetylcholine, histamine, and 5-hydroxytryptamine (102).

It seems likely that when sufficiently high concentrations of these naturally occurring substances reach the adrenal medulla, the released epinephrine will contribute to the ensuing pharmacological effects. Access of the compounds to the gland can only be via the general circulation or by some direct pathway, such as locally in an artery or lymphatic, as speculatively suggested by Feldberg & Lewis (52) for angiotensin. This would suggest that the only pathophysiological conditions in which this direct action on medullary cells may play a role would be those in which there is a high concentration of the compounds in the circulating blood, such as one might expect in shock. Some indication that this might occur comes from the experiments of Glaviano et al. (64). They found that the increased secretory activity of the adrenal medulla that occurs during hemorrhagic hypotension does not return to normal on reinfusion of the blood and restoration of the blood pressure. The increased activity during the hypotension is no doubt produced reflexly or by anoxia. However, the medullary stimulation persisting after the blood pressure has returned to normal might well be due to substances formed during hemorrhage in the animal or in the blood before reinfusion.

Perhaps the direct stimulation of adrenal medullary cells might be envisaged as another mechanism reinforcing the activated sympathetic nervous system (100) when the organism is in great peril, possibly when histamine and bradykinin are formed during shock or when angiotensin is formed during severe renal ischemia. Such a suggestion is consistent with the finding that most of these substances have been observed to stimulate other parts of the sympathetic nervous system, such as ganglia (69, 101, 129, 130) and sympathetic components of the central nervous system (9).

REFERENCES

1. AMBACHE, N. Nicotinic action of substances supposed to be purely smooth muscle stimulating; effect of $BaCl_2$ and pilocarpine on superior cervical ganglion. *J. Physiol., London* 110: 164–172, 1949.
2. BARRE, J. LA, AND R. SARIC. Sur les causes de l'augmentation postinsulinique de la teneur en adrénaline du sang veineux surrenal. *Compt. Rend. Soc. Biol.* 124: 287–289, 1937.
3. BAUGH, C. W., R. W. CORNETT, AND J. D. HATCHER. The adrenal gland and the cardiovascular changes in acute anoxia in dogs. *Circulation Res.* 7: 513–520, 1959.
4. BEAN, J. W. Effects of oxygen at increased pressure. *Physiol. Rev.* 25: 1–147, 1945.
5. BEARN, A. G., B. BILLING, AND S. SHERLOCK. The effect of adrenaline and noradrenaline on hepatic blood flow and splanchnic carbohydrate metabolism in man. *J. Physiol., London* 115: 430–441, 1951.
6. BECKER, E. J., AND F. KREUZER. Sympathoadrenal response to hypoxia. *Arch. Ges. Physiol.* 304: 1–10, 1968.
7. BEDFORD, E. A., AND H. C. JACKSON. The epinephric content of the blood in conditions of low blood pressure and "shock." *Proc. Soc. Exptl. Biol. Med.* 13: 85–87, 1916.
8. BERTHET, J. Some aspects of the glucagon problem. *Am. J. Med.* 26: 703–714, 1959.
9. BICKERTON, R. K., AND J. P. BUCKLEY. Evidence for a central mechanism in angiotensin induced hypertension. *Proc. Soc. Exptl. Biol. Med.* 106: 834–836, 1961.
10. BLASCHKO, H., P. HAGEN, AND A. D. WELCH. Observations on the intracellular granules of the adrenal medulla. *J. Physiol., London* 129: 27–49, 1955.
11. BLOOM, G., U. S. VON EULER, AND M. FRANKENHAUSER. Catecholamine excretion and personality traits in paratroop trainees. *Acta Physiol. Scand.* 58: 77–89, 1963.
12. BRAUNER, F., F. BRÜCKE, F. KAINDL, AND A. NEUMAYR. Quantitative Bestimmungen uber die Sekretion des Nebennierenmarkes bei elektrischer Hypothalamusreizung. *Arch. Intern. Pharmacodyn. Therap.* 85: 419–430, 1951.
13. BRODIE, B. B., R. P. MAICKEL, AND D. N. STERN. Autonomic nervous system and adipose tissue. In: *Handbook of Physiology. Adipose Tissue*, edited by A. E. Renold and G. F. Cahill. Washington, D.C.: Am. Physiol. Soc., 1965, sect. 5, chapt. 59, p. 583–600.
14. BRÜCKE, F., F. KAINDL, AND H. MAYER. Uber die Veranderung in der Zusammensetzung des Nebennierenmarkinkretes bei elektrischer Reizung des Hypothalamus. *Arch. Intern. Pharmacodyn. Therap.* 88: 407–412, 1952.
15. BÜLBRING, E. The methylation of noradrenaline by minced suprarenal tissue. *Brit. J. Pharmacol. Chemotherap.* 4: 234–244, 1949.
16. BÜLBRING, E., AND J. H. BURN. Liberation of noradrenaline from adrenal medulla by splanchnic stimulation. *Nature* 163: 363, 1949.
17. BÜLBRING, E., AND J. H. BURN. Liberation of noradrenaline from the suprarenal gland. *Brit. J. Pharmacol. Chemotherap.* 4: 202–208, 1949.
18. BÜLBRING, E., J. H. BURN, AND F. J. DE ELIO. The secretion of adrenaline from the perfused suprarenal gland. *J. Physiol., London* 107: 222–232, 1949.
19. BURN, J. H., AND H. H. DALE. The vaso-dilator action of histamine, and its physiological significance. *J. Physiol., London* 61: 185–214, 1926.
20. BURN, J. H., D. E. HUTCHEON, AND R. H. O. PARKER. Adrenaline and noradrenaline in the suprarenal medulla after insulin. *Brit. J. Pharmacol. Chemotherap.* 5: 417–423, 1950.
21. CANNON, W. B. Studies on the conditions of activity in endocrine organs. XXVII. Evidence that medulliadrenal secretion is not continuous. *Am. J. Physiol.* 98: 447–453, 1931.
22. CANNON, W. B., S. W. BRITTON, J. T. LEWIS, AND A. GROENEVELD. Studies on the conditions of activity in endocrine glands. XX. The influences of motion and emotion on medulliadrenal secretion. *Am. J. Physiol.* 79: 433–465, 1926.
23. CANNON, W. B., AND D. DE LA PAZ. Emotional stimulation of adrenal secretion. *Am. J. Physiol.* 28: 64–70, 1911.
24. CANNON, W. B., J. R. LINTON, AND R. R. LINTON. Conditions of activity in endocrine glands. *Am. J. Physiol.* 71: 153–162, 1924.
25. CANNON, W. B., M. A. MCIVER, AND S. W. BLISS. Studies on the conditions of activity in endocrine glands. XIII. A sympathetic and adrenal mechanism for mobilizing sugar in hypoglycemia. *Am. J. Physiol.* 69: 46–66, 1924.
26. CARLSSON, A., N-A. HILLARP, AND B. HÖKFELT. The concomitant release of adenosine triphosphate and catechol amines from the adrenal medulla. *J. Biol. Chem.* 227: 243–252, 1957.
27. CELANDER, O. The range of control exercised by the 'sympathico-adrenal system.' *Acta Physiol. Scand. Suppl.* 116: 1–32, 1954.
28. COMLINE, R. S., AND M. SILVER. The development of the adrenal medulla of the foetal and newborn calf. *J. Physiol., London* 183: 305–340, 1966.
29. COMLINE, R. S., AND M. SILVER. The release of adrenaline and noradrenaline from the adrenal glands of the foetal sheep. *J. Physiol., London* 156: 424–444, 1961.
30. COUPLAND, R. E. On the morphology and adrenaline-noradrenaline content of chromaffin tissue. *J. Endocrinol.* 9: 194–203, 1953.

31. CROSS, M. H., AND R. T. HOULIHAN. Sympathoadrenomedullary response of the rat to high oxygen exposures. *J. Appl. Physiol.* 27: 523–527, 1969.
32. CUNNINGHAM, W. L., E. J. BECKER, AND F. KREUZER. Catecholamines in plasma and urine at high altitude. *J. Appl. Physiol.* 20: 607–610, 1965.
33. DALE, H. H. Conditions which are conducive to the production of shock by histamine. *Brit. J. Exptl. Pathol.* 1: 103–114, 1920.
34. DALE, H. H., AND P. P. LAIDLAW. The significance of the suprarenal capsules in the action of certain alkaloids. *J. Physiol., London* 45: 1–26, 1912.
35. DAVIDSON, I. W. F., AND J. M. SALTER. Stimulating effect of glucagon and oxygen consumption of rats. *Federation Proc.* 17: 208, 1958.
36. DEL CASTILLO, J., AND B. KATZ. On the localization of acetylcholine receptors. *J. Physiol., London* 128: 157–181, 1955.
37. DOUGLAS, W. W. The mechanism of release of catecholamines from the adrenal medulla. *Pharmacol. Rev.* 18: 471–480, 1966.
38. DOUGLAS, W. W., AND R. P. RUBIN. The mode of action of acetylcholine on the adrenal medulla. *Biochem. Pharmacol.* 8: 20, 1961.
39. DUNER, H. The influence of the blood glucose level on the secretion of adrenaline and noradrenaline from the suprarenal. *Acta Physiol. Scand. Suppl.* 102: 481–482, 1953.
40. EADE, N. R. The release of catecholamines from isolated chromaffin granules. *Brit. J. Pharmacol. Chemotherap.* 12: 61–65, 1957.
41. ELLIOTT, T. R. The control of the suprarenal glands by the splanchnic nerves. *J. Physiol., London* 44: 374–409, 1912.
42. ERÄNKÖ, O. Distribution of adrenaline and noradrenaline in the adrenal medulla. *Nature* 175: 88–89, 1955.
43. ERÄNKÖ, O. Distribution of fluorescing islets, adrenaline and noradrenaline in the adrenal medulla of the hamster. *Acta Endocrinol.* 18: 174–179, 1955.
44. ERÄNKÖ, O. Histochemical evidence of the presence of acid-phosphatase-positive and negative cell islets in the adrenal medulla of the rat. *Nature* 168: 250–251, 1951.
45. EULER, U. S. VON, AND B. FOLKOW. The effect of stimulation of autonomic areas in the cerebral cortex upon the adrenaline and noradrenaline secretion from the adrenal gland in the cat. *Acta Physiol. Scand.* 42: 313–320, 1958.
46. EULER, U. S. VON, AND B. FOLKOW. Einfluss verschiedener afferenter Nervenreize auf die Zusammensetzung des Nebennierenmarkinkretes bei der Katze. *Arch. Exptl. Pathol. Pharmakol.* 219: 242–247, 1953.
47. EULER, U. S. VON, C. A. GEMZELL, L. LEVI, AND G. STROM. Cortical and medullary adrenal activity in emotional stress. *Acta Endocrinol.* 30: 567–573, 1959.
48. EULER, U. S. VON, AND U. HAMBERG. L-noradrenaline in the suprarenal medulla. *Nature* 163: 642–643, 1949.
49. EULER, U. S. VON, AND S. HELLNER. Excretion of noradrenaline and adrenaline in muscular work. *Acta Physiol. Scand.* 26: 183–191, 1952.
50. EULER, U. S. VON, D. IKKOS, AND R. LUFT. Adrenaline excretion during resting conditions and after insulin in adrenalectomized human subjects. *Acta Endocrinol.* 38: 441–448, 1961.
51. FELDBERG, W. Die wirkung von Lentin (carbaminoylcholinchlorid) auf die Nebennieren der Katze. *Arch. Exptl. Pathol. Pharmakol.* 168: 287–291, 1932.
52. FELDBERG, W., AND G. P. LEWIS. The action of peptides on the adrenal medulla. Release of adrenaline by bradykinin and angiotensin. *J. Physiol., London* 171: 98–108, 1964.
53. FELDBERG, W., AND G. P. LEWIS. Further studies on the effects of peptides on the suprarenal medullary of cats. *J. Physiol., London* 178: 239–251, 1965.
54. FELDBERG, W., AND B. MINZ. Das Auftreten eines Azetylcholinartigen Stoffes im Nebennierenvenenblut bei Reizung der Nervi splanchnici. *Arch. Ges. Physiol.* 233: 657–682, 1933.
55. FELDBERG, W., AND B. MINZ. Die Wirkung von Azetylcholin auf die Nebennieren. *Arch. Exptl. Pathol. Pharmakol.* 163: 66–96, 1931.
56. FELDBERG, W., B. MINZ, AND H. TSUDZIMURA. Mechanisms of nervous discharge of adrenaline. *J. Physiol., London* 81: 286–304, 1934.
57. FELDBERG, W., AND A. VERTIAINEN. Further observations on physiology and pharmacology of sympathetic ganglion. *J. Physiol., London* 83: 103–128, 1934.
58. FERGUSON, R. W., B. FOLKOW, M. G. MITTS, AND E. C. HOFF. Effect of cortical stimulation upon epinephrine activity. *J. Neurophysiol.* 20: 329–339, 1957.
59. FOLKOW, B., AND U. S. VON EULER. Selective activation of noradrenaline and adrenaline producing cells in the cat's adrenal gland by hypothalamus stimulation. *Circulation Res.* 2: 195, 1954.
60. FRANKENHAUSER, M., I. MELLIS, A. RISSLER, I. BJORKVALL, AND P. PATKAI. Catecholamine excretion as related to cognitive and emotional reaction patterns. *Psychosomat. Med.* 30: 109–120, 1968.
61. FRANKENHAUSER, M., AND P. PATKAI. Catecholamine excretion and performance during stress. *Perceptual Motor Skills* 19: 13–14, 1964.
62. FRANKENHAUSER, M., AND B. POST. Catecholamine excretion during mental work as modified by centrally acting drugs. *Acta Physiol. Scand.* 55: 74–81, 1962.
63. FRANKENHAUSER, M., K. STERKY, AND G. JARPE. Psychophysiological relations in habituation to gravitational stress. *Perceptual Motor Skills* 15: 63–72, 1962.
64. GLAVIANO, U. V., N. BASS, AND F. NYKIEL. Adrenal medullary secretion of epinephrine and norepinephrine in dogs subjected to hemorrhagic hypotension. *Circulation Res.* 8: 564–571, 1960.
65. GOLDENBERG, M., M. FABER, E. J. ALSTON, AND E. CHARGAFF. Evidence for occurrence of norepinephrine in adrenal medulla. *Science* 109: 534–535, 1949.
66. GOODALL, M. C., AND M. L. BERMAN. Urinary output of adrenaline, noradrenaline and 3-methoxy-4-hydroxymandelic acid following centrifugation and anticipation of centrifugation. *J. Clin. Invest.* 39: 1533–1538, 1960.
67. GOODALL, M. C., C. STONE, AND B. W. HAYNES. Urinary output of adrenaline and noradrenaline in severe thermal burns. *Ann. Surg.* 145: 479–487, 1957.
68. GUTMANN, P. Die Empfindlichkeit der Nebennieren von Katzen auf Cholin und Acetylcholin. *Arch. Exptl. Pathol. Pharmakol.* 166: 612–623, 1932.
69. GYERMEK, L., AND E. BINDER. Blockade of the ganglionic stimulant action of 5-hydroxytryptamine. *J. Pharmacol. Exptl. Therap.* 135: 344–348, 1962.
70. HALE, H. B., E. W. WILLIAMS, J. E. ANDERSON, AND J. P. ELLIS. Endocrine and metabolic effects of short-duration hyperoxia. *Aerospace Med.* 35: 449–451, 1964.
71. HARTMAN, F. A., R. H. WAITE, AND H. A. MCCORDOCK. The liberation of epinephrine during muscular exercise. *Am. J. Physiol.* 62: 225–241, 1922.
72. HAVEL, R. J. Autonomic nervous system and adipose tissue. In: *Handbook of Physiology. Adipose Tissue*, edited by A. E. Renold and G. F. Cahill. Washington, D.C.: Am. Physiol. Soc., 1965, sect. 5, chapt. 58, p. 575–582.
73. HERMANN, H., J. CHATONNET, AND J. VIAL. Effect of strong stimulation on the adrenal contents of adrenaline and noradrenaline, respectively. *Compt. Rend. Soc. Biol.* 146: 1318–1320, 1952.
74. HEYMANS, C. Le sinus carotidien, zone réflexogène régulatrice du tonus vagal cardiaque du tonus neurovasculaire et de l'adrenalinosecretion. *Arch. Intern. Pharmacodyn. Therap.* 35: 269–306, 1929.
75. HIGASHI, R. Effect of metabolic acidosis on adrenaline and noradrenaline secretion of the innervated and denervated adrenal gland in the dog. *Tohuku J. Exptl. Med.* 89: 77–84, 1966.
76. HILLARP, N-Å., AND B. HÖKFELT. Evidence of adrenaline

and noradrenaline in separate adrenal medullary cells. *Acta Physiol. Scand.* 30: 55–68, 1953.
77. HILLARP, N-Å., AND B. NILSON. The structure of the adrenaline and noradrenaline containing granules in the adrenal medullary cells with reference to the storage and release of the sympathomimetic amines. *Acta Physiol. Scand. Suppl.* 31: 79–107, 1954.
78. HIMSWORTH, R. L. Hypothalamic control of adrenaline secretion in response to insufficient glucose. *J. Physiol., London* 206: 411–417, 1970.
79. HÖKFELT, B. Noradrenaline and adrenaline in mammalian tissues. *Acta Physiol. Scand. Suppl.* 92: 1–134, 1951.
80. HOLLAND, W. C., AND H. J. SCHUMANN. Formation of catecholamines during splanchnic stimulation of the adrenal gland of the cat. *Brit. J. Pharmacol.* 11: 449–453, 1956.
81. HOLTZ, P., K. CREDNER, AND G. KRONEBERG. Über des sympathicomimetische pressonische Prinzip des Harns ("Urosympathin"). *Arch. Exptl. Pathol. Pharmakol.* 204: 228–243, 1947.
82. HOLTZ, P., AND H. J. SCHUMANN. Anterenol, a new adrenal cortex hormone. *Naturwiss.* 35: 159, 1948.
83. HOLZBAUER, M., AND M. VOGT. The concentration of adrenaline in the peripheral blood during insulin hypoglycaemia. *Brit. J. Pharmacol. Chemotherap.* 9: 249–252, 1954.
84. HOUSSAY, B-A., AND E-A. MOLINELLI. Secretion de l'adrenaline pourdite pas la piqûre ou l'excitation électrique du bulba. *Compt. Rend. Soc. Biol.* 91: 1045–1049, 1924.
85. HOUSSAY, B-A., AND E. A. MOLINELLI. Adrenal secretion produced by asphyxia. *Am. J. Physiol.* 76: 538–550, 1926.
86. HOUSSAY, B. A., AND C. F. RAPELA. Adrenal secretion of adrenaline and noradrenaline. *Arch. Exptl. Pathol. Pharmakol.* 219: 156–159, 1953.
87. HYNIE, S., M. WENKE, AND E. MUHLBACHOVA. Zur Charakteristik der Beeinflussung des Glycidmetabolismus durch Adrenomimetica. *Arzneimittel-Forsch.* 11: 858–861, 1961.
88. IKEDA, H. Adrenal medullary secretion in response to insulin hypoglycaemia in dogs with transection of the spinal cord. *Tohuku J. Exptl. Med.* 95: 153–168, 1968.
89. JARAMILLO, J., AND R. L. VOLLE. Nonmuscarinic stimulation and block of a sympathetic ganglion by 4-(m-chlorophenylcarbamoyloxy)-2-butynyltrimethylammonium chloride (McN-A-343). *J. Pharmacol. Exptl. Therap.* 157: 337–345, 1967.
90. KAINDL, F., AND U. S. VON EULER. Liberation of noradrenaline and adrenaline from the suprarenals of the cat during carotid occlusion. *Am. J. Physiol.* 166: 284–288, 1951.
91. KATZ, B. The transmission of impulses from nerve to muscle, and the subcellular unit of synaptic action. *Proc. Roy. Soc. London Ser. B* 155: 455–477, 1961.
92. KENNARD, M. A. Focal autonomic representation in the cortex and its relation to sham rage. *J. Neuropathol. Exptl. Neurol.* 4: 295–304, 1945.
93. KLEPPING, J., M. TANCHE, AND J. F. CIER. La sécrétion medullosurrenale dans la lutte contre le froid. *Compt. Rend. Soc. Biol.* 151: 1539–1541, 1957.
94. KONZETT, H., AND E. ROTHLIN. Die Wirkung von Erregungs- und Lähmungsmitteln der Chemorezeptoren auf ein sympathetisches Ganglion. *Wien. Klin. Wochschr.* 64: 638–639, 1952.
95. KUNTZ, A. In: *The Autonomic Nervous System* (3rd ed.), edited by J. H. Burn. London: Bailliere, Tindall, and Cox, 1946.
96. LEDUC, J. Catecholamine production and release in exposure and acclimation to cold. *Acta Physiol. Scand. Suppl.* 183: 18–38, 1961.
97. LEFEBVRE, P. J., A. M. CESSION-FOSSION, A. S. LUYCKX, J. L. LECOMTE, AND H. S. VAN CAUWENBERGE. Interrelationships glucagon-adrenergic system in experimental and clinical conditions. *Arch. Intern. Pharmacodyn. Therap.* 172: 393–404, 1968.
98. LEE, F-L., AND U. TRENDELENBURG. Muscarinic transmission of preganglionic impulses to the adrenal medulla of the cat. *J. Pharmacol. Exptl. Therap.* 158: 73–79, 1967.
99. LEWIS, G. P. The physiological and pathological functions of plasma kinins. In: *Bradykinin and Related Kinins. An International Symposium of Vaso-active Polypeptides*, edited by M. Rocha e Silva and H. A. Rothschild. Sao Paulo: Soc. Bras. Farmacol. Terap. Exptl., 1967, p. 45–51.
100. LEWIS, G. P. Peptides and the sympathetic nervous system. In: *Bradykinin and Related Kinins*, edited by F. Sicuteri, M. Rocha e Silva, and N. Black. New York: Plenum Press, 1970, p. 571–589.
101. LEWIS, G. P., AND E. REIT. The action of angiotensin and bradykinin on the superior cervical ganglion of the cat. *J. Physiol., London* 179: 538–553, 1965.
102. LEWIS, G. P., AND E. REIT. Further studies on the actions of peptides on the superior cervical ganglion and suprarenal medulla. *Brit. J. Pharmacol. Chemotherap.* 26: 444–460, 1966.
103. LEVI, L. The urinary output of adrenaline and noradrenaline during experimentally induced emotional stress in clinically different groups. *Acta Psychotherap.* 11: 218–227, 1963.
104. LINDGREN, P., AND B. UVNAS. Postulated vasodilator centre in the medulla oblongata. *Am. J. Physiol.* 176: 68–76, 1954.
105. MAGOUN, H. W., S. W. RANSON, AND A. HETHERINGTON. The liberation of adrenin and sympathin induced by stimulation of the hypothalamus. *Am. J. Physiol.* 119: 615–622, 1937.
106. MEIER, R., AND H. J. BEIN. Der Einfluss der Nebenniere auf die Kreislaufwirkung des Adrenalins. *Experientia* 4: 358, 1948.
107. MUNRO, A. F., AND R. ROBINSON. The catecholamine content of the peripheral plasma in human subjects with complete transverse lesions of the spinal cord. *J. Physiol., London* 154: 244–253, 1960.
108. MUNRO, A. F., AND R. ROBINSON. Effect of change of posture and exercise on plasma adrenaline and noradrenaline. *J. Physiol., London* 143: 20–21, 1958.
109. NAHAS, G. G., G. W. MATHER, J. D. M. WARGO, AND W. L. ADAMS. Influence of acute hypoxia on sympathectomized and adrenalectomized dogs. *Am. J. Physiol.* 177: 13–18, 1954.
110. O'HANLON, J. F. Adrenaline and noradrenaline: relation to performance in a visual vigilance task. *Science* 150: 507–509, 1965.
111. OLMSTED, J. M. D. The blood sugar after asphyxia in 'decapitate cats' and its relation to the adrenal glands. *Am. J. Physiol.* 75: 487–496, 1925.
112. OUTSCHOORN, A. S. The hormones of the adrenal medulla and their release. *Brit. J. Pharmacol. Chemotherap.* 7: 605–615, 1952.
113. PEKKARINEN, A., O. CASTREN, E. IISALO, M. KOIVUSALO, A. LAIHINEN, P. E. SIMOLA, AND B. THOMASSON. The emotional effect of matriculation examinations on the excretion of adrenaline, noradrenaline, 17-hydroxycorticosteroids into the urine and the content of 17-hydroxycorticosteroids in the plasma. In: *Biochemistry, Pharmacology and Physiology*. London: Pergamon Press, 1961, p. 117–137.
114. PIPER, P. J., H. O. J. COLLIER, AND J. R. VANE. Release of catecholamines in the guinea pig by substances involved in anaphylaxis. *Nature* 213: 838–840, 1967.
115. POHORECKY, L. A., AND R. J. WURTMAN. Adrenocortical control of epinephrine synthesis. *Pharmacol. Rev.* 23: 1–35, 1971.
116. RAPPORT, D. Studies in experimental traumatic shock. VI. The liberation of epinephrine in traumatic shock. *Am. J. Physiol.* 60: 461–475, 1922.
117. REDGATE, E. S., AND E. GELLHORN. Nature of sympathetic-adrenal discharge under conditions of excitation of control autonomic structures. *Am. J. Physiol.* 174: 475–480, 1953.
118. REID, G., AND M. RAND. Physiological actions of the partially purified serum vasoconstrictor (serotonin). *Australian J. Exptl. Biol.* 29: 401–415, 1951.
119. SAITO, S. Influence of the application of cold or heat to the dog's body upon the epinephrine output rate. *Tohuku J. Exptl. Med.* 11: 544–567, 1928.

120. Sarcione, E. J., N. Back, J. E. Sokal, B. Mehlman, and E. Knoblock. Elevation of plasma epinephrine levels produced by glucagon in vivo. *Endocrinology* 72: 523–526, 1963.
121. Satake, Y. Amount of epinephrine secreted from suprarenal glands in dogs in haemorrhage, and poisoning with quinidine, peptone, caffein, urethane and camphor. *Tohuku J. Exptl. Med.* 17: 333–344, 1931.
122. Scian, L. F., C. D. Westermann, A. S. Verdesca, and J. G. Hilton. Adrenocortical and medullary effects of glucagon. *Am. J. Physiol.* 199: 867–870, 1960.
123. Staszewska-Barczak, J., and J. R. Vane. The release of catecholamines from the adrenal medulla by peptides. *Brit. J. Pharmacol. Chemotherap.* 30: 655–667, 1967.
124. Szczygielski, J. Die adrenalinabsondernde Wirkung des Histamins und ihre Beeinflussung durch Nikotin. *Arch. Exptl. Pathol. Pharmakol.* 166: 319–332, 1932.
125. Tamura, K. Effect of metabolic alkalosis on adrenal medullary secretion in dog. *Tohuku J. Exptl. Med.* 95: 403–409, 1968.
126. Tanche, M., J. Klepping, and J. Chatonnet. Importance de l'anesthésie dans le déterminisme et l'évolution de l'hypothermie provoquée. *Compt. Rend. Soc. Biol.* 149: 1564–1567, 1955.
127. Tournade, A., and M. Chabrol. Effets des variations de la pression arterielle sur la secretion de l'adrenaline. *Compt. Rend. Soc. Biol.* 93: 934–936, 1925.
128. Tournade, A., M. Chabrol, and P. E. Wagner. Action dépressive de la cocainisation bulbaire sur l'adrénalino-sécretion et l'adrénalinemie physiologique. *Compt. Rend. Soc. Biol.* 93: 160–161, 1925.
129. Trendelenburg, U. The action of 5-hydroxytryptamine on the nictitating membrane and on the superior cervical ganglion of the cat. *Brit. J. Pharmacol. Chemotherap.* 11: 74–80, 1956.
130. Trendelenburg, U. The action of histamine and pilocarpine on the superior cervical ganglion and the adrenal glands of the cat. *Brit. J. Pharmacol. Chemotherap.* 9: 481–487, 1954.
131. Vogt, M. The secretion of the denervated adrenal medulla of the cat. *Brit. J. Pharmacol. Chemotherap.* 7: 325–330, 1952.
132. Wada, M., M. Seo, and K. Abe. Effect of muscular exercise upon the epinephrine secretion from the suprarenal gland. *Tohuku J. Exptl. Med.* 27: 65–86, 1935.
133. Wada, M., M. Seo, and K. Abe. Further studies of the influence of cold on the rate of epinephrine secretion from the suprarenal glands with simultaneous determination of the blood sugar. *Tohuku J. Exptl. Med.* 26: 381–411, 1935.
134. West, G. B., D. M. Shepherd, and R. B. Hunter. Adrenaline and noradrenaline concentrations in adrenal glands at different ages and in some diseases. *Lancet* 2: 966–969, 1951.
135. Wright, A., and I. C. Jones. Chromaffin tissue in the lizard adrenal gland. *Nature* 175: 1001–1002, 1955.
136. Wurtman, R. J. Control of epinephrine synthesis in the adrenal medulla by the adrenal cortex: hormonal specificity and dose-response characteristics. *Endocrinology* 79: 608–614, 1966.
137. Wurtman, R. J., and J. Axelrod. Control of enzymatic synthesis of adrenaline in the adrenal medulla by adrenal cortical steroids. *J. Biol. Chem.* 241: 2301–2305, 1966.

CHAPTER 23

The chromaffin granule and the storage of catecholamines

HANS WINKLER | *Institute of Pharmacology, University of Innsbruck, Innsbruck, Austria*
A. DAVID SMITH | *Department of Pharmacology, University of Oxford, Oxford, England*

CHAPTER CONTENTS

Isolation of Chromaffin Granules
    Components of large granule fraction
    Components of microsomal fraction
Composition of Chromaffin Granule
    Nucleotides
    Proteins
    Lipids
Heterogeneity of Chromaffin Granules
Mechanism of Storage of Catecholamines in Chromaffin Granule
    Permeability of chromaffin granule membrane
    Storage complex containing catecholamines
    Active uptake of catecholamines into chromaffin granule
    How is store of catecholamines maintained?
Dynamic Role of Chromaffin Granule
    Storage
    Synthesis
    Secretion
Conclusions

THREE DIFFERENT CATECHOLAMINES are found in the adrenal medulla; two of these (epinephrine and norepinephrine) occur in high concentration (1, 61, 124), and the third (dopamine) is present in only small amounts (86, 104). It is now well established that the catecholamines in this gland are stored in a specialized subcellular particle, the chromaffin granule [for reviews, see (71, 107, 122)]; the chromaffin granule is analogous to the "secretory granule" found in many other endocrine tissues (109). The subcellular fractions obtained from homogenates of adrenal medulla have been characterized in some detail, and it is now a relatively simple matter to isolate highly purified chromaffin granules on a large scale. Because of this, more is known about the composition of the chromaffin granule than about that of any other type of secretory granule, and we are now in a position where we can try to correlate our knowledge about the components of the chromaffin granule with the functions of this particle in the cell. In this chapter we concentrate on the function of the chromaffin granule as the site of storage of the secretory products of the chromaffin cell; the important role of the chromaffin granule in secretion is described in the chapter by Viveros in this volume of the *Handbook*.

ISOLATION OF CHROMAFFIN GRANULES

The first clear indication that the hormones of the adrenal medulla are stored in some kind of subcellular particle was obtained in 1953 by Blaschko & Welch (18) and by Hillarp et al. (56). These workers prepared homogenates of adrenal medullae in isosmotic sucrose solution, and first centrifuged the homogenate at low speed to remove unbroken cells and cell nuclei. When the supernatant was centrifuged at a higher speed the bulk of the catecholamines was recovered in the sediment, the so-called large granule fraction. The first electron micrographs of adrenal medulla were published by Lever (79) in 1955; he described the presence of numerous osmiophilic, membrane-limited granules in the cell that were smaller than mitochondria. It was suggested that these granules contained the hormones. Similar results were reported by Sjöstrand & Wetzstein (105) in 1956, and these authors introduced the term *chromaffin granule* for the characteristic particles of the chromaffin cell. At about the same time biochemical studies, in which the large granule fraction was further fractionated by sucrose density gradient centrifugation, also showed that the hormone-containing particles could be distinguished from mitochondria (15, 52). The morphological and biochemical approaches were correlated in 1960 by Hagen & Barrnett (41) who analyzed fractions from sucrose density gradients in the electron microscope; they found that the hormone-containing fractions were markedly enriched in osmiophilic, membrane-limited granules. It was concluded that the chromaffin granule is the site of storage of the catecholamines.

Components of Large Granule Fraction

By the use of sucrose density gradient centrifugation three different types of particle have been identified in

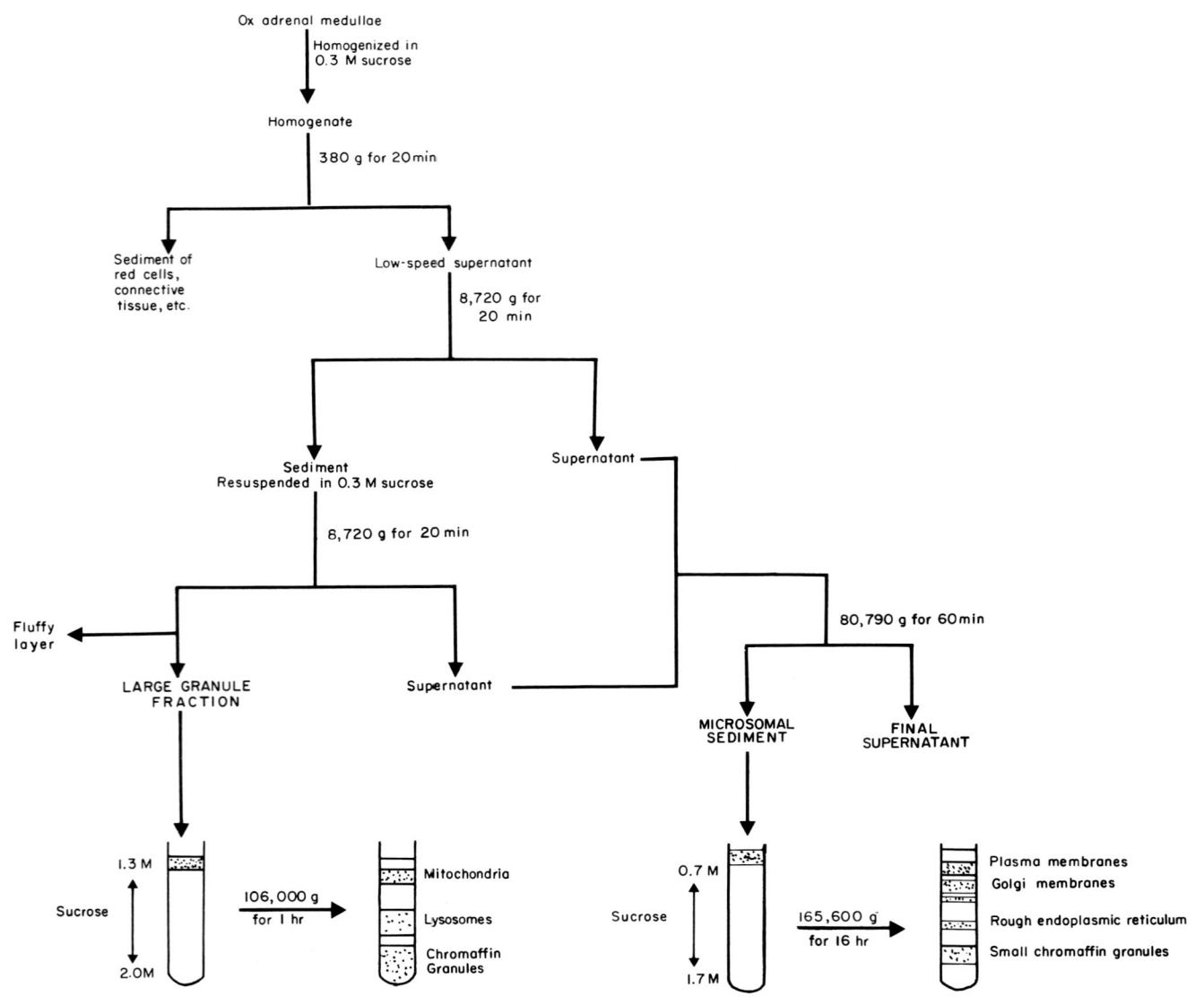

FIG. 1. Complete centrifugation scheme for obtaining subcellular fractions of chromaffin tissue. Relative centrifugal force (g) expressed in terms of average radius from center of rotation. [For full experimental details, see (4, 31, 112).]

the large granule fraction of adrenal medulla (see Fig. 1). Mitochondria remain at the top of the gradient (15) and can be separated from lysosomes, which are concentrated in the middle of the gradient at the layer of 1.6 M sucrose (112). The chromaffin granules are recovered at the bottom of the density gradient in the layers of 1.8–2.0 M sucrose. This fortuitous separation of chromaffin granules from the other components of the large granule fraction makes it easy to obtain highly purified chromaffin granules by a simplified procedure in which the resuspended large granule fraction is centrifuged on a layer of 1.6 M sucrose solution (4, 113). The chromaffin granules are obtained as a sediment. By using 1.8 M sucrose, the purity of the chromaffin granules can be further increased but at the expense of a lower yield (100a). A second modification of this method makes use of a solution containing Ficoll in deuterium oxide, which has the same density as 1.6 M sucrose but which is isosmotic (131). Other methods of preparing chromaffin granules in isosmotic solutions, such as by filtration (91), have not proved successful (131).

The fact that chromaffin granules equilibrate in layers of sucrose that are much denser than the solutions at which mitochondria equilibrate does not seem to be due to intrinsic differences between the densities of the two particles. When the large granule fraction is centrifuged on isosmotic density gradients made with silica, the chromaffin granules and mitochondria both reach about the same density ($\rho = 1.12$). However, in gradients made hyperosmotic in sucrose the chromaffin granules reach a layer of density 1.24, whereas the mitochondria remain at a layer of density 1.17 (78). The different behaviors of

TABLE 1. *Components of the Large Granule Fraction*

Particle	Component	Reference
Mitochondrion*	Monoamine oxidase	15, 76
	Succinate dehydrogenase	15
	Fumarase	112
	Cytochromes	2
	Myokinase	77
	ATPase	2
Lysosome	Acid β-glycerophosphatase	112
	Acid ribonuclease	99, 112
	Acid deoxyribonuclease	112
	Cathepsin	112
	β-Glucuronidase	112
	Arylsulfatase	112
	Phospholipase A_1	17, 115, 145
	Phospholipase A_2	17, 115, 145
Chromaffin granule†, ‡	Catecholamines	
	Adenine nucleotides	
	Chromogranins	
	Dopamine β-hydroxylase	
	Lysolecithin	

* Cholesterol:lipid phosphorus molar ratio 0.23 (14).
† Cholesterol:lipid phosphorus molar ratio 0.58 (14). ‡ See Table 3.

these two particles in hyperosmotic sucrose solutions may be due both to a more pronounced dehydration of the chromaffin granule and to a greater penetration of sucrose into the particle. When deuterium oxide is used to prepare solutions used for the density gradient, the heavy water penetrates more readily into the chromaffin granules than into mitochondria (75). This may be the reason why it is possible to separate chromaffin granules from mitochondria in a gradient made from Ficoll and heavy water (131) even though the solution is isosmotic.

The biochemical characterization of the three types of particle in the large granule fraction is well substantiated by morphological studies on the intact tissue (see the chapter by Grynszpan-Winograd in this volume of the *Handbook*). As already pointed out, the chromaffin granule was distinguished from mitochondria in the first electron-microscopic studies on the adrenal medulla. However, not until 10 years later were lysosomes, characterized by the histochemical reaction for acid phosphatase, demonstrated by electron-microscopic analysis (7, 21, 62). The histochemical method has also revealed that some chromaffin granules in the rat adrenal medulla contain a type of acid phosphatase (62). Since the biochemical studies, which showed that the bulk of the acid phosphatase is present in lysosomes, were performed on the ox adrenal medulla (112) there may be a difference between the chromaffin granules of different species. However, it has been argued that the occurrence of lead deposits in chromaffin granules is an artifact and does not represent enzyme activity (93).

Biochemical analysis of highly purified chromaffin granules has yielded much information of value in understanding the mode of storage and secretion of the secretory materials; this is discussed in detail below. Analysis of fractions enriched in mitochondria and lysosomes has provided some information about the constituents of these particles, and the data are summarized in Table 1. Of possible relevance to physiology is the wide spectrum of enzymatic activities found in lysosomes of the adrenal medulla, for it is now known that the gland responds to a stimulus by the secretion not only of the soluble contents of chromaffin granules but also of the contents of lysosomes (98, 100, 108).

Components of Microsomal Fraction

The microsomal fraction, obtained by high-speed centrifugation of the supernatant remaining after removal of the large granule fraction, is very heterogeneous. Several different components can be distinguished by sucrose density gradient centrifugation (see Fig. 1), including fragments of plasma membrane, Golgi saccules, rough endoplasmic reticulum, and small chromaffin granules (31, 32). However, the different components have not yet been purified sufficiently for chemical analysis; the composition of the total microsomal fraction has therefore been given in Table 2.

COMPOSITION OF CHROMAFFIN GRANULE

Chromaffin granules are membrane-limited organelles, and the membrane can readily be separated from the contents, so long as we make the assumption that the membrane is the only water-insoluble part of the chromaffin granule. When isolated chromaffin granules are suspended in hyposmotic buffer solution they are lysed and the content of the granules goes into solution. The membranes can be recovered from the suspension by high-speed centrifugation and can be further purified by several washing steps (141) or by density gradient centrifugation (100a). Following the pioneering work of Hillarp (54) a fairly complete analysis of the chromaffin granule has been achieved: the compositions of the content and of the membrane are listed in Table 3. It should be noted that as much as 93 % of the dry weight of chromaffin granules can be accounted for. Although it is not

TABLE 2. *Characteristic Constituents of the Microsomal Fraction**

Constituent	Reference
Acetylcholinesterase	40
5′-Nucleotidase (adenosine monophosphatase)	
Inosine diphosphatase	
Uridine diphosphatase	
Thiamine pyrophosphatase	
Adenosine triphosphatase (Ca^{2+} dependent)†	8, 32
Glucose 6-phosphatase	
Adenosine diphosphatase	
NADH cytochrome c reductase	
Cytochrome b 559	
Lysophospholipase	63b

* Cholesterol:lipid phosphorus molar ratio 0.44 (14).
† From Golgi membranes.   [Adapted from Dubois (31).]

TABLE 3. *Composition of the Bovine Adrenal Chromaffin Granule*

Constituent	Amount, % total dry wt*
Soluble content	
Catecholamines	20.5
Adenine nucleotides	15
Protein	27
Calcium	0.1
Magnesium	0.02
Membrane	
Phospholipid	17
Cholesterol	5
Protein	8
Calcium	0.06
Magnesium	0.02

* Water content of isolated chromaffin granules estimated to be 60% (72) or 68.5% (54) of wet wt. [Compiled from Borowitz et al. (19) and Hillarp (54).]

TABLE 3a. *Specific Constituents of Bovine Adrenal Chromaffin Granule*

Component	Constituent
Soluble content	Dopamine β-hydroxylase*
	Chromogranin A
Membrane	Dopamine β-hydroxylase†
	Chromomembrin B
	Cytochrome b 559
	Mg^{2+}-dependent ATPase
	Flavoprotein
	Lysolecithin

* Minor component. † Major component; formerly known as chromomembrin A.

known what makes up the remaining part of the weight, the suggestion that RNA is a major component of the particles (93) is not supported by analysis of density gradient fractions (71). One of the striking characteristics of the chromaffin granule is its high content of water-soluble substances of low molecular weight: catecholamines and adenine nucleotides comprise 35.5% of the dry weight. Obviously the chromaffin granule must not only be able to accumulate these substances very effectively, but mechanisms must also exist that prevent them from diffusing out of the particle across the membrane (see section MECHANISM OF STORAGE OF CATECHOLAMINES IN CHROMAFFIN GRANULE).

Nucleotides

The finding that chromaffin granules contain such a high concentration of catecholamines posed a problem: what acidic substance was present in the particles that could neutralize the basic amine? Hillarp & Nilson (57) realized that the presence of an acidic substance in stoichiometric amounts relative to the catecholamines would also largely account for the difference between the sum of the dry weights of the constituents (proteins, lipids, amines) known at that time and the total dry weight. Earlier suggestions that lactic acid might be present were shown to be incorrect (57), and soon Hillarp et al. (59) discovered that the acidic substance was adenosine triphosphate (ATP): the large granule fraction of ox adrenal medulla was extremely rich in this compound. It was shown that almost all the ATP was present in chromaffin granules, not in mitochondria, and it was naturally suggested that this nucleotide might be involved in the binding of the amines (12, 35). More detailed studies on purified chromaffin granules from several species (51, 60) revealed that, in addition to ATP, both ADP and AMP were present and that the total content of adenine nucleotides was sufficient to neutralize the positive charges on the molecules of catecholamines (see Table 4). Small amounts of other nucleotides (e.g., GTP) have also been found in ox adrenal chromaffin granules (29, 45).

Proteins

A characteristic feature of chromaffin granules is that the major part of their protein (77%) is water soluble after lysis by hyposmotic shock (52, 147). The water-soluble proteins have been called *chromogranins* (13) and the insoluble proteins, presumed to be components of the membrane, have been called *chromomembrins* (140). Such a distinction seems justifiable since the amino acid composition of the insoluble proteins differs markedly from that of the soluble proteins as shown in Table 5 (48, 139, 141). This does not exclude the possibility that any individual protein species might be present in both the soluble and insoluble phases, but, if it is, it will only be a minor component of one of the phases.

The bovine chromogranins have been studied in some detail (45, 73, 114, 117), and their main component is an acidic protein called chromogranin A (101), which has also been found in chromaffin granules isolated from the adrenals of horse, pig, and sheep (46, 63, 147). The chromogranins from human adrenal glands do not appear to contain a single major component, and the two main proteins that are present have a higher mobility than chromogranin A in gel electrophoresis (123). Gel electrophoresis has been particularly useful in studying the chromogranins; a typical electrophoretogram of bovine chromogranins is shown in Figure 2. Twelve different bands can be identified, although many of

TABLE 4. *Adenine Nucleotides in Adrenal Chromaffin Granules Isolated from Different Species*

Animal	Total Adenine Nucleotides, %			Ratio of Equivalents of Nucleotide Acid to Catecholamine Base
	ATP	ADP	AMP	
Fowl	60	30	7	1.01
Cat	69	22	9	0.98
Cow	87	10	3	0.98
Goat	79	16	4	1.00

Values are means calculated from the results of Hillarp & Thieme (60).

TABLE 5. *Amino Acid Composition of Chromaffin Granule Proteins*

Amino Acid Residue	Chromogranin A[b]	Dopamine β-hydroxylase[c,d]	Total chromomembrins[e]
Lys	9.4	5.8	6.1
His	2.4	3.2	2.8
Arg	8.5	6.8	7.1
Asp + Asn	8.4	9.3	9.6
Thr	2.5	6.0	4.6
Ser	6.2	6.6	7.6
Glu + Gln	26.0	13.5	15.4
Pro	8.6	5.4	5.4
Gly	3.9	4.5	4.2
Ala	5.0	4.7	5.3
Cys	0.3	1.9	0.5
Val	3.3	6.0	5.0
Met	2.2	2.1	2.9
Ile	1.0	3.9	3.7
Leu	7.3	8.6	9.9
Tyr	1.7	5.7	4.1
Phe	2.1	5.8	5.5

[a] Expressed in grams of amino acid residue per 100 g protein. [b] Data from (114). [c] Soluble. [d] Data from (64). [e] Data from (141).

some amino sugars (114) and about 3% (wt/wt) of sialic acid, mainly N-glycollyl-neuraminic acid (S. F. Bartlett, personal communication).

This unusual amino acid composition is very similar to that of the total chromogranins isolated from the adrenals of several species, including man (123). Physicochemical studies have shown that chromogranin A is not a typical globular protein: it has lower sedimentation and diffusion coefficients and a higher intrinsic viscosity than globular proteins of similar molecular weight (73, 114). The most likely explanation of the hydrodynamic properties of chromogranin A is that the conformation of the molecule approaches that of a random coil polypeptide; because the molecule carries a large excess negative charge (46 negative charges per molecule) its conformation changes according to the ionic composition of the solution (114): at low ionic strength the molecule is highly expanded but its hydrodynamic volume decreases as the ionic strength is raised. However, it can be calculated that even at an ionic strength of 0.4 the effective hydrodynamic diameter of a molecule of chromogranin A is about 120 A.

Dopamine β-hydroxylase, a characteristic constituent

them are relatively minor components. Immunochemical methods have also been used to study the occurrence and subcellular localization of chromogranin A (47, 97), although care must be taken when preparing the antiserum to check that it does not also contain antibodies to dopamine β-hydroxylase (97); this enzyme is present in trace amounts in some preparations of chromogranin A and is a highly potent antigen (39). Proteins similar to the chromogranins also occur outside the adrenal medulla. A protein cross-reacting with antibodies to chromogranin A has been found in the splenic nerve (38, 63) where it is localized in the noradrenergic vesicles (3, 30) and in the brainstem (63). Such a protein is not found in detectable amounts in several other tissues, such as liver, kidney, hypophysis, and pancreas (63).

Chromogranin A, which comprises about 40% of the chromogranins in the ox, has been purified, and several of its physical and chemical properties have been studied. It has a molecular weight of between 77,000 and 80,000 (73, 114). Claims that the molecule is composed of two identical subunits (48, 73, 117) must be treated with caution because other interpretations of the experimental results have not been excluded. The mobility of chromogranin A in gel electrophoresis under denaturing conditions is not changed by prior exposure to mercaptoethanol (63a); this makes it unlikely that subunits, if present, are bound to each other by disulfide bonds. There is excellent agreement between different laboratories about the amino acid composition of chromogranin A (see Table 5), which is characterized by a remarkably high content of glutamic acid (26% by weight), a relatively high proline content (8%), and a low content of cysteine (45, 73, 114). The protein also contains

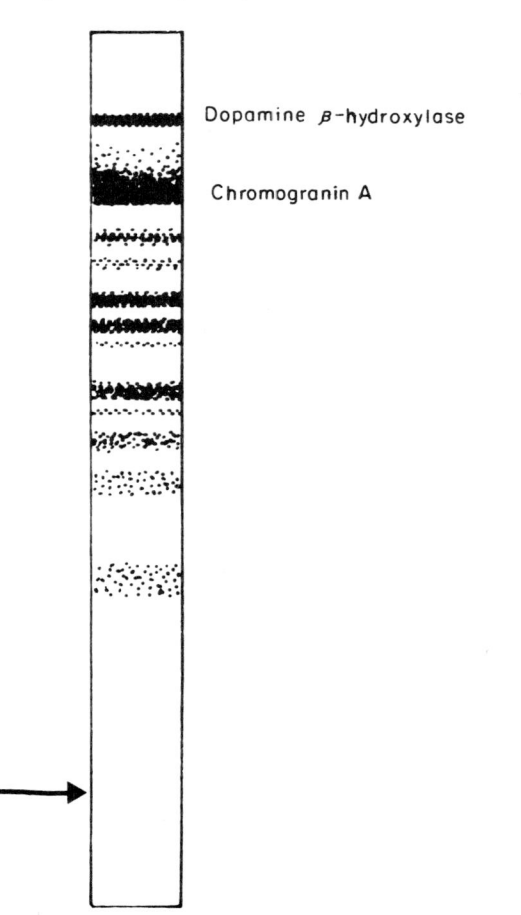

FIG. 2. Pattern of stained protein bands obtained when soluble proteins (chromogranins) of ox adrenal chromaffin granules are separated by polyacrylamide gel electrophoresis at pH 8.6. Proteins migrated from top toward anode. Arrow, position of dye marker. [For full experimental details, see (4).]

of chromaffin granules (69, 89), is the only soluble protein known to have any enzymatic activity. It is, however, only a minor component of the soluble proteins since it has been identified as the protein that gives rise to the relatively minor, slow-moving band in gel electrophoresis [see Fig. 2; (63a, 64, 111)]. The soluble dopamine β-hydroxylase has been purified, and its amino acid composition has been found to be very different from that of chromogranin A and from that of the total chromogranins (see Table 5): it contains about half as much glutamic acid by weight and is also not so rich in proline (37a, 64). Dopamine β-hydroxylase is also immunochemically distinct from chromogranin A (63a, 97), and so it seems appropriate to redefine chromogranins, in line with earlier proposals (4, 63a), as comprising chromogranin A and the other soluble proteins that are chemically and antigenically related to it. Between 50 and 80% of the total dopamine β-hydroxylase activity of chromaffin granules is recovered in the membrane fraction, depending on the species (6, 33, 136, 141): this enzyme is therefore also a component of the chromomembrins.

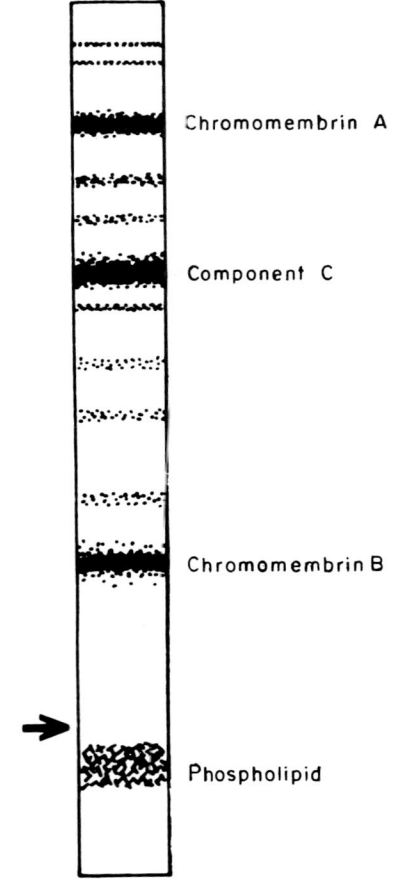

FIG. 3. Pattern of stained protein bands obtained when insoluble proteins (chromomembrins), dissolved in sodium dodecylsulfate, from ox adrenal chromaffin granules are separated by polyacrylamide gel electrophoresis at pH 6.5 in gels containing sodium dodecylsulfate. Proteins migrated from top toward anode. Arrow, position of dye marker. [For details, see (4).]

The chromomembrins, defined as those proteins remaining insoluble after hyposmotic shock (140), include dopamine β-hydroxylase, a Mg^{2+}-activated adenosine triphosphatase (2, 50, 74, 132, 141), and cytochrome b 559 (2, 36, 67, 119). Spectroscopic analysis has also indicated the presence of a flavoprotein (36). The chromomembrins are almost quantitatively solubilized when the membrane is dissolved in a solution containing sodium dodecylsulfate (141), and the proteins can then be studied by gel electrophoresis and column chromatography in the presence of the detergent. By electrophoresis, some 10–15 components can be identified, and two of these are major components that do not occur as predominant components of the membranes of mitochondrial and microsomal fractions (141). These two main components are therefore characteristic of the chromaffin granule membrane: they have been purified (66) and are called chromomembrins A and B (see Fig. 3). The amino acid compositions of the total chromomembrins (141) and of the two purified chromomembrins (66) differ from the composition of the chromogranins: the membrane proteins contain much less glutamic acid and a greater proportion of hydrophobic amino acids (see Table 5).

Chromomembrin A was first characterized by chromatography and electrophoresis of chromaffin granule membranes dissolved in sodium dodecylsulfate, but this detergent inactivates all the enzymes present in the membrane. However, when the cationic detergent cetyl pyridinium chloride is used, dopamine β-hydroxylase activity can still be measured, and this has led to the discovery that chromomembrin A is the membrane-bound form of this enzyme (64). The fact that a major protein component of the membrane is an enzyme that catalyzes the formation of norepinephrine illustrates the highly specialized nature of the chromaffin granule membrane. On the other hand, the soluble dopamine β-hydroxylase comprises only 6% of the protein in the contents of the chromaffin granule (63a). Since there is now evidence of the molecular identity of the soluble dopamine β-hydroxylase and the membrane-bound enzyme (37, 64) the earlier physicochemical studies on the enzyme purified from whole chromaffin granules, which established a molecular weight of 290,000, become easier to interpret [(68); see also the chapter by Kirshner in this volume of the *Handbook*]. It is also pertinent to ask whether molecules of dopamine β-hydroxylase can move from the soluble phase into the membrane and vice versa. The evidence so far from both biochemical (141) and physiological (135) studies suggests that this is unlikely and that, at least in the mature chromaffin granule, dopamine β-hydroxylase has a dual location, part residing within the membrane and part in the soluble contents.

It has not yet proved possible to identify chromomembrin B with any of the enzymes or electron-transfer proteins present in the chromaffin granule membrane. This protein has, however, been partially characterized: its amino acid composition is known (66), and a molecular weight of 28,500 has been estimated by gel electrophoresis (S. F. Bartlett, personal communication). Whereas dopamine β-hydroxylase is believed to be confined to the adrenal medulla and to noradrenergic nerves, where it is localized in the catecholamine-storing vesicles (110), the distribution of chromomembrin B is more widespread. By using complement fixation it has been possible to study the occurrence of a protein that cross-reacts with antiserum to bovine chromomembrin B: such antigens occur a) in adrenal chromaffin granules from several species, including man; b) in the noradrenergic vesicles of splenic nerve axons; and c) in membranes from the posterior and anterior lobes of the pituitary gland (65).

The proteins of the chromaffin granule are characterized by the distinction between the proteins of the membrane and those of the content, and by the relative lack of enzymes in this particle. The proteins of the membrane seem to be either enzymes involved in the specific functions of the particle or electron transfer proteins of unknown functions. By far the largest part of the chromogranins, the soluble proteins secreted upon stimulation of the gland (see the chapter by Viveros in this volume of the *Handbook*), is made up of an acidic glycoprotein with no known enzymatic activity. What is the significance of this protein (chromogranin A): is its main function to be found within the chromaffin granule, or is the chromaffin granule only a storehouse for this newly discovered secretory product of the adrenal medulla?

Lipids

As one would expect, the other major constituents of the chromaffin granule membrane are lipids, chiefly phospholipids and cholesterol (14, 146). Indeed the chromaffin granule membrane is relatively rich in lipids (or poor in protein) compared with other membranes: on a weight basis the protein:lipid ratio is about 0.45 (141), whereas it is greater than 1 for other membranes, with the exception of those of myelin.

The phospholipid composition of chromaffin granules (see Table 6) is quite different from those of the mitochondrial and microsomal fractions, being characterized by a high proportion of lysolecithin (14, 130, 146). It has been known for some time that the adrenal medulla is rich in lysolecithin (42), and there is now no doubt that the bulk of this phospholipid is located in the chromaffin granule (139). Analysis of the fatty acid composition of the lecithin and lysolecithin of chromaffin granules showed that the lysolecithin is the 1-acyl isomer and is probably derived from lecithin by the loss of the fatty acids in the 2 position (143). The ability of lysolecithin to cause the lysis and the fusion of biological membranes (82) has led to proposals (14, 140) that this phospholipid may be specifically located in the chromaffin granule membrane because it is required for the fusion and dissolution of membranes that occurs during the secretion of the contents of the chromaffin granule by exocytosis (see the chapter by Viveros in this volume of the *Handbook*). It would clearly be of interest to know whether lysolecithin, or the enzyme that forms it, is present in the secretory granules of other endocrine tissues since exocytosis is the likely mode of secretion from most of these cells (109).

TABLE 6. *Phospholipid Composition of Chromaffin Granules*

Species	Component	Content, % of total lipid phosphorus	Ref.
Ox	Lecithin	26.0	14
	Lysolecithin	16.8	14
	Phosphatidylethanolamine	36.1	14
	Phosphatidylserine + phosphatidylinositol	9.2	14
	Sphingomyelin	10.9	14
	Phosphatidic acid + cardiolipin	0.6	14
English	Lysolecithin	16.8	14
Austrian	Lysolecithin	16.8	146
Swiss	Lysolecithin	17.4	29a
Pig	Lysolecithin	11.3	146
Horse	Lysolecithin	7.1	146
Rat	Lysolecithin	15.4	146
Man*	Lysolecithin	11.7–23.8	16

* Pheochromocytoma.

HETEROGENEITY OF CHROMAFFIN GRANULES

The chromaffin granules in homogenates of adrenal medulla do not form a single population of particles. Apart from heterogeneity due to differences in size, four other types of heterogeneity have been identified: *1*) different particles store norepinephrine and epinephrine; *2*) two different populations of particles store epinephrine; *3*) particles contain different amounts of adenine nucleotides; and *4*) particles contain different amounts of dopamine β-hydroxylase relative to their content of catecholamines.

Morphological studies (see the chapter by Grynszpan-Winograd in this volume of the *Handbook*) have shown that norepinephrine and epinephrine are stored in separate cells. Biochemical studies have shown that the chromaffin granules from these two types of cell differ in their behavior upon density gradient centrifugation: the norepinephrine-containing particles sediment to denser regions of the gradient than the epinephrine-containing particles (34, 102). It is not known why the norepinephrine-containing granules behave differently for they contain the same proteins and phospholipids as a mixture of norepinephrine- and epinephrine-containing chromaffin granules (137). When the large granule fraction of adrenal medulla is incubated at 37 C in isotonic sucrose, the rate of release of norepinephrine into the suspending medium is biphasic: about 20% of the total norepinephrine is released very rapidly, whereas subsequently both norepinephrine and epinephrine are released slowly and at about the same rate (80, 90, 139).

TABLE 7. *Differences Between Amine Storage Pools in Bovine Adrenal Chromaffin Granules*

Characteristic	Fast-efflux Pool	Slow-efflux Pool
Catecholamine capacity	Low	High
Stability of storage complex	Low	High
Dependence on uptake activated by ATP	Low	High
Sensitivity to reserpine and to N-ethylmaleimide	Low	High
Rate of equilibration with exogenous amines	High	Low
Uptake rate of metaraminol	High	Low
Effect of structure of amine on rate of efflux	Slight	Marked

The pools were distinguished by measuring the rate of efflux of radioactive amine from isolated chromaffin granules after the particles had been loaded with the radioactive amine by incubation in vitro (106).

It is not known in which particle the rapidly released pool of norepinephrine is localized.

Another type of heterogeneity has been observed when the rate of efflux of radioactivity has been measured from chromaffin granules that had been loaded with ^{14}C-epinephrine: about 25% of the radioactivity was lost rapidly (half-life 5 min), whereas the rest was lost slowly (half-life 2–3 hr) (106, 128). Several other differences can be demonstrated between the pool with a rapid rate of efflux and the pool with a slow rate of efflux: these are listed in Table 7. It is likely, but not yet established, that each pool is present in a different population of particles (106).

The occurrence of a population of chromaffin granules containing little or no adenine nucleotides was postulated by Hillarp in 1960 (55). Hillarp found that the molar ratio of catecholamines to adenine nucleotides in chromaffin granules isolated by density gradient centrifugation of the large granules was close to 4, whereas this ratio in the large granule fraction was about 5. He suggested that up to 20% of the catecholamines in the large granule fraction might be stored in a particle that contained no adenine nucleotides and which remained in the less dense layers of a density gradient after centrifugation (55). Although there have been no subsequent studies on the distribution of all three adenine nucleotides (ATP, ADP, AMP) between density gradient fractions, some observations on the distribution of ATP (12) do support Hillarp's suggestion [for review, see (116)]. It is surprising that there has been so little work on the nucleotide-deficient chromaffin granules, for their lack of ATP is pertinent to the question of how important this nucleotide is in the binding of the catecholamines (see subsection *Storage Complex Containing Catecholamines*). It is noteworthy that the chromaffin granules isolated from some human pheochromocytomas are also deficient in ATP, and yet they contain a high concentration of catecholamines [for review, see (144)].

A third type of heterogeneity has been identified by the analysis of density gradient fractions for dopamine β-hydroxylase activity. In density gradients of the large granules from both the ox (76) and rabbit adrenals (133), the major peak of dopamine β-hydroxylase activity occurs at a slightly lower density than the peak concentration of catecholamines. This finding was discussed by Viveros et al. (133) who suggested that all chromaffin granules contain the same amount of dopamine β-hydroxylase but that their content of catecholamines varies and that it is the content of amines that largely determines the position of the particle in the density gradient. It is possible that the gland contains some chromaffin granules, perhaps newly synthesized particles (136), that contain the normal amount of dopamine β-hydroxylase but still do not have a full store of catecholamines. However, the less dense chromaffin granules might also be formed artifactually by loss of amine, but not of dopamine β-hydroxylase, during the fractionation procedure.

MECHANISM OF STORAGE OF CATECHOLAMINES IN CHROMAFFIN GRANULE

Chromaffin granules contain a very high concentration of catecholamines that corresponds to a 0.55 M solution if the amines are assumed to be present as free ions (54). How is such a high concentration achieved, and how is it maintained within the granules? Three possibilities are considered: *1*) the catecholamines may be kept inside the granules because the membrane is impermeable to them; *2*) they may be part of a macromolecular storage complex that is too large to cross the membrane; *3*) the membrane may contain an energy-dependent pump that transports catecholamines into the granules. Obviously these three mechanisms are not mutually exclusive, and it is quite possible that a combination of them accounts for the binding of the catecholamines.

Permeability of Chromaffin Granule Membrane

Isolated chromaffin granules, suspended in isosmotic sucrose solution, can be kept for several days at temperatures close to 0 C without the loss of more than small amounts of amines or ATP into the medium (35). Is this due to impermeability of the membrane to catecholamines or to the presence of a macromolecular storage complex? Experiments on the permeability of the chromaffin granule membrane to catecholamines have been carried out with suspensions of chromaffin granules at temperatures close to 0 C and at temperatures in the range of 20–37 C. Since the stability of the storage complex and the rate of active transport processes are markedly influenced by temperature (see subsection *Storage Complex Containing Catecholamines*) we must first consider the evidence for the permeability of the membrane at low temperatures. The first experiments dealing with the permeability of the membrane were reported by Carlsson & Hillarp (22) in 1958. Isolated chromaffin granules were suspended in 0.2 M epinephrine solution and left overnight at 4 C; the particles were then sedimented. The chromaffin granules now contained a higher concentration of catecholamines than before; epinephrine from the medium had passed into the granules such that the additional concentration within the granules corresponded to that in the medium. Similar results were obtained when isolated chromaffin granules were suspended in solutions containing lower concentrations (0.13–2.6 mM) of radioactively labeled catecholamines: under these conditions the concentration of radioactive amines within the granules had reached equilibrium with that in the medium already after 5 min of incubation at 4 C (72). Furthermore, when chromaffin granules that have taken up exogenous catecholamines at 4 C are resuspended in a solution not containing catecholamines, the exogenous amines rapidly diffuse out again (54, 72). These experiments show that the membrane of the chromaffin granule is permeable in both directions to catecholamines at low temperatures. However, since the endogenous catecholamines do not diffuse out of the granules at low temperature we can conclude that they must be bound in such a way that they do not rapidly equilibrate with free amines in solution inside the granule. There must therefore be a stable storage complex at low temperatures.

Membranes that are permeable to catecholamines at low temperatures probably would also be permeable at higher temperatures, and there is evidence that this is so. Large amounts of catecholamines, corresponding to 20–40% of the amines originally present in the granules, can be taken into chromaffin granules incubated in solutions (2–20 mM) of the amines at 31 C (11, 23). This type of uptake does not depend on the presence of any added cofactors, and it is probably due to passive diffusion through the membrane, just as occurs at low temperatures. However, at 31 C there is no net uptake of amines into the granules for, at this temperature, the endogenous catecholamines leak out as fast as the exogenous amines diffuse in. At 37 C the rate of loss of endogenous amines from chromaffin granules suspended in isosmotic sucrose is as high as 30% of the content per hour (53). These experiments clearly show that the chromaffin granule membrane is permeable in both directions to catecholamines at temperatures close to body temperature. They show in addition that the stability of the storage complex is much less at body temperature than at low temperatures.

We can conclude that, at temperatures ranging from 0 to 37 C, catecholamines can diffuse across the membrane of the chromaffin granule; the membrane is partly, but not necessarily freely, permeable to catecholamines. The possibility that the chromaffin granule can store a high concentration of catecholamines solely because of the impermeability of its membrane can therefore be excluded. The two remaining possibilities are that a storage complex binds the amines, or that an active transport process for catecholamines in the membrane counteracts the loss of amines from the granules and must be superimposed on the passive permeability of the membrane.

Storage Complex Containing Catecholamines

We have already pointed out that, although exogenous catecholamines can pass into chromaffin granules incubated at low temperatures, they do not mix with the endogenous store of catecholamines. Such an observation could be accounted for if the exogenous amines had entered one of the populations of chromaffin granules that normally contains only a minor part of the total store, but this seems unlikely in view of the very large amounts of catecholamines, corresponding to an additional 60% of the total store (22), that can be taken up. The stability of isolated chromaffin granules at low temperature, together with the lack of mixing of exogenous and endogenous catecholamines, argues strongly for the binding of the endogenous amines in a nondiffusible form (storage complex) at this temperature. However, at higher temperatures (31–37 C) amines taken up at low temperature (72) and those taken up at the higher temperature (128) do mix with the endogenous store of amines. The mixing is not complete, even after 5 hr (128), indicating that part of the endogenous store is still relatively nondiffusible. This partial mixing of exogenous and endogenous amines can be understood if it is assumed that at higher temperatures the hypothetical storage complex is less stable than at low temperatures and so there is a more rapid exchange between the bound, nondiffusible catecholamines in the complex and the catecholamines free in solution within the granules. Direct evidence of the lower stability of the storage complex at body temperature is the relatively rapid loss of endogenous catecholamines from isolated chromaffin granules at this temperature. Whereas very nearly all the catecholamines in chromaffin granules at low temperatures must be bound in the storage complex, it is not possible to say what proportion of the amines are bound in this way in chromaffin granules at higher temperatures. The interpretation of experiments with radioactively labeled catecholamines, which show that about 20–25% of the amines in the large granule fraction are more rapidly exchangeable at 37 C than the remainder (106, 128), is complicated by the possibility that some, if not all, of the rapidly exchangeable pool might be present in a different population of chromaffin granules (106).

We have argued that the binding of the catecholamines in isolated chromaffin granules at low temperatures is most easily accounted for if the amines are stored in a macromolecular complex and that a similar, but less stable, complex may also be present in isolated granules at body temperature. It is now necessary to look at the evidence concerning the nature and possible composition of this hypothetical storage complex. The possibility that the catecholamines are bound covalently to a macromolecule in the chromaffin granule can be excluded because the amines are freely dialyzable from the soluble extract obtained after lysis of the granules by hyposmotic shock. The binding in the complex must therefore be both noncovalent and readily reversible.

The occurrence of stoichiometric amounts of adenine nucleotides in chromaffin granules (see Table 4) naturally raises the quesion whether these participate in the formation of a complex. The fact that the negative charges on the nucleotides neutralize the positive charges on the amines is not in itself sufficient evidence that a complex is formed. Indeed it has been found that in dilute aqueous solution the interaction between molecules of epinephrine and ATP is very weak (92, 137), although it is slightly strengthened in the presence of divalent metal ions (26). A decisive discovery was made in 1969 when Berneis et al. (9) found that a very much stronger interaction occurred between amines and nucleotides in highly concentrated aqueous solutions. When amines and ATP (molar ratio 3.5:1) were present in aqueous solution in a total concentration (about 17% wt/wt) similar to that likely to occur in chromaffin granules, the average molecular weight (2,000–4,000) of solute species was greater than that of any of the individual components, indicating that aggregates containing several molecules of amines and ATP had been formed. Such aggregates were obtained when ATP was added to solutions of dopamine, norepinephrine, epinephrine, or 5-hydroxytryptamine but not with solutions of histamine or tyramine (9); the authors concluded that the formation of amine-nucleotide complexes in vitro seemed to be a common feature of those amines that are known to be stored together with ATP in storage vesicles in vivo. Further experiments gave even more striking results: when small amounts of calcium chloride were added to the solution containing catecholamines and ATP, a second liquid phase separated from the solution (10). This phase, which was denser than the original solution, contained at least 60% wt/wt of amine and ATP; it was transparent and highly viscous and was most stable at low temperatures. Measurements of the apparent average molecular weights of solutes in solutions containing norepinephrine, ATP, and divalent metal ions (Ca^{2+} or Mg^{2+}) showed that, as the temperature was lowered, aggregates of increasingly high molecular weight were formed (see Fig. 4) until, at a certain temperature, phase separation took place. The concentration of added divalent metal ions was critical: at a molar ratio of $CaCl_2$:ATP of 0.28 phase separation occurred at 6.5 C, whereas at a molar ratio of 0.72 phase separation occurred at 20 C. It can hardly be a coincidence that chromaffin granules are rich in divalent metal ions and that the molar ratio of calcium plus magnesium to ATP in the granules is in the range of 0.4–0.85 (19, 95). Furthermore the calcium in chromaffin granules at 0 C does not easily exchange with exogenous radioactive calcium ions (20), just as the endogenous catecholamines fail to exchange with exogenous amines. Aggregates of catecholamines and ATP have also been demonstrated in soluble lysates of adrenal chromaffin granules (28), which shows that the other soluble components of the particle do not inhibit the aggregation process. We can therefore conclude that the binding of catecholamines in chromaffin granules at low temperatures is due largely, if not entirely, to the formation of a second liquid phase, containing high-molecular-weight aggregates of amines, adenine nucleotides, calcium, and magnesium, that is relatively deficient in water.

An additional way in which norepinephrine can interact with adenine nucleotides has recently been discovered (84): water-insoluble complexes containing 4 moles of norepinephrine and 1 mole of ATP can be obtained in the absence of metal ions. However, epinephrine does not seem to form such complexes.

Although the properties of isolated chromaffin granules at low temperatures can now be accounted for satisfactorily, we still have to explain how the catecholamines are bound in vivo at body temperature. Is the formation of high-molecular-weight aggregates of amines, ATP, and metal ions in itself sufficient to account for the binding at body temperature? To answer this question, we must compare the behavior of isolated chromaffin granules at body temperature with what is known from in vitro studies concerning the effect of temperature on the stability of the aggregates. At low temperatures the molecular weights of the aggregates are so high that a separate phase is formed (see Fig. 4), and the catecholamines in this phase will only equilibrate very

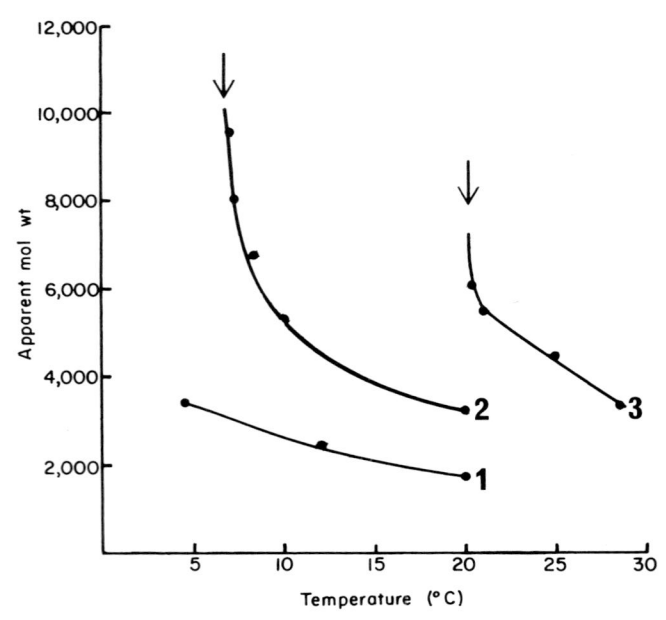

FIG. 4. Evidence for formation of high-molecular-weight aggregates in mixtures of norepinephrine and ATP (molar ratio 3.5:1) at total solute concentration of 17% wt/wt. Curves show temperature dependence of apparent molecular weight of solute species. *1*, control; *2*, calcium chloride added to give molar ratio of 0.08 relative to norepinephrine; *3*, calcium chloride added to give molar ratio of 0.24 relative to norepinephrine. *Arrows* indicate phase-separation, the lower phase containing the bulk of the solute species. [Redrawn from Berneis et al. (10).]

slowly with catecholamines in the predominantly aqueous phase. Raising the temperature causes the second phase to disappear: the aggregates are now in aqueous solution and so the catecholamines bound in the aggregates will exchange more rapidly with catecholamines free in solution. Raising the temperature still further causes the average molecular weight of the aggregates to drop (Fig. 4), and this favors the dissociation of catecholamines from the complex. (Unfortunately measurements of the average molecular weight of solute species have not yet been made in ATP and catecholamine solutions at body temperature, and so it is not even certain that high-molecular-weight aggregates exist at this temperature.) The catecholamines that have dissociated from the complex inside a chromaffin granule will diffuse out of the granule, lowering the concentration of free catecholamines inside the granule, which, in turn, will lead to further dissociation of the aggregates. If the concentration of catecholamines in the suspending medium is low enough, the complexes in the granule will dissociate completely and almost all the catecholamines will leave the chromaffin granules at temperatures above 4 C: as the temperature is raised the rate of loss of catecholamines into the medium increases and will reach a rate of about 30% of the content per hour at 37 C (53, 58). Not only are the amines lost from chromaffin granules incubated at 37 C, the ATP also diffuses out (5, 50). It seems therefore unlikely that the formation of complexes between amines and ATP is in itself sufficient to account for the binding of the amines at body temperature. Some additional factor or process must be involved in the binding in vivo that is missing from isolated chromaffin granules suspended in sucrose solution. So far we have not mentioned the possibility, originally raised by Hillarp (51), that the chromogranins might participate in the formation of a storage complex. Chromogranin A does not, in aqueous solution, bind more than small amounts of catecholamines (117), and in any case a stoichiometric binding of the catecholamines by the chromogranins is unlikely on theoretical grounds as there are about 385 molecules of catecholamine per molecule of chromogranin in the chromaffin granule (107).

A hypothetical model has nevertheless been proposed in which the catecholamines are bound to ATP, which, in turn, is bound to glutamine and asparagine side chains of chromogranin (118). An alternative idea is that the chromogranins might provide a physical environment within the chromaffin granule that helps to stabilize the aggregates formed between ATP and the catecholamines. This suggestion is made because a concentrated solution of chromogranins readily forms a gel in vitro (107, 123), and such a gel may well exist in the chromaffin granule because it contains a high concentration of chromogranins. If the aggregates of amines and ATP are present in a gel, their rate of diffusion will be considerably lower than when they are in aqueous solution. Furthermore, since the gel would be composed of negatively charged molecules of chromogranins, the diffusion of small molecules, like the catecholamines, would also be retarded [cf. the effect of hyaluronic acid on the diffusion of small molecules in a gel (85)]. We could speculate then that even at body temperature the inside of the chromaffin granule contains both an aqueous liquid phase and a gel phase and that the gel phase might stabilize the storage complex of catecholamines and ATP. Even if these speculations prove to have some foundation, we must still account for the rapid loss of catecholamines from isolated chromaffin granules compared with the stability of the store in the chromaffin granules in vivo. If it is argued that the physical properties of the contents of the chromaffin granule are alone responsible for the binding in vivo, it follows that some vital physical property must have been lost during the isolation of the chromaffin granule. This argument is difficult to test experimentally. An alternative hypothesis, more amenable to experimental verification, is that the complexes between ATP and catecholamines are stabilized in vivo by an energy-dependent process that maintains the high concentration of catecholamines and ATP within the granules. We shall now discuss the evidence for such a process.

Active Uptake of Catecholamines into Chromaffin Granule

An observation reported by Kirshner (70) in 1962 gave the first clue that the maintenance of a high concentration of catecholamines within the chromaffin granule might depend on an active (i.e., endergonic) process: he found that the addition of ATP and Mg^{2+} to a suspension of chromaffin granules in isosmotic sucrose solution at 37 C partly prevented the loss of catecholamines from the particles. Subsequent work has shown that at 31 C isolated chromaffin granules lose 22% of their catecholamines in 3 hr, but they lose only 2% in 3 hr if the suspending medium contains 5 mM ATP and 5 mM $MgCl_2$ (128). Thus, if we assume that chromaffin granules in the cell behave like those isolated and suspended in sucrose solution, the main factor that will determine the ability of chromaffin granules to maintain their store of catecholamines in vivo will be the supply of ATP.

What is the mechanism by which ATP and Mg^{2+} prevent a net loss of catecholamines from chromaffin granules? We consider four possible mechanisms: *1*) the membrane of the chromaffin granule becomes impermeable to catecholamines; *2*) the dissociation of the storage complex is inhibited; *3*) the presence of ATP causes an increased uptake of catecholamine directly into the storage complex; or *4*) the hydrolysis of ATP drives a process in the membrane that pumps those amines that have diffused out into the medium back again into the chromaffin granule, where they become bound in the storage complex.

The first and second mechanisms have been excluded by experiments involving the use of ^{14}C-labeled epinephrine, in which it was possible to determine both the rate of influx of epinephrine into the chromaffin granule

TABLE 8. *Some Properties of the Process that Actively Takes Up Catecholamines into Chromaffin Granules*

Property	Reference
Effectiveness of nucleotides	
ATP > ITP > GTP > UTP > CTP	70, 128
Effectiveness of metal ions	
Mg^{2+} = Mn^{2+} > Co^{2+}	70
Apparent K_m for ATP	
0.4 mM	70
Substrates	
Dopamine, norepinephrine, epinephrine, tyramine, 5-hydroxytryptamine	25, 76
Inhibitors	
EDTA	25, 70
N-ethylmaleimide	25, 44
Reserpine (50% inhibition at 10^{-7} M)	25, 70
Q_{10}	
2.8	70

Unless otherwise indicated, the results come from experiments with bovine chromaffin granules suspended in isosmotic sucrose solution containing ATP and Mg^{2+}.

and the rate of efflux of epinephrine out of the particle: the rate of efflux remains unchanged when ATP and Mg^{2+} are added to the medium (128), showing that the permeability of the membrane in this direction is not altered and that the storage complex can still dissociate. The prevention of the net loss of catecholamine must therefore be due to an increased uptake of catecholamine into the chromaffin granule when ATP and Mg^{2+} are present. Such an uptake process was discovered in 1962; it was shown that chromaffin granules can take up epinephrine from a dilute solution against a concentration gradient, provided that the medium contains ATP and Mg^{2+} (24, 70). Some of the properties of this uptake process are given in Table 8.

Kirshner (70) pointed out that the occurrence of an ATP-dependent uptake process in the chromaffin granule could be accounted for by two quite different hypotheses (which correspond to the third and fourth mechanisms listed above): "The binding hypothesis states that the granule membrane is freely diffusible to catecholamines and the observed uptake is a result of binding or exchange at specific sites within the granules.... The active transport hypothesis states that the catecholamines... react with some component of the granule membrane; that they are transported across the membrane and released into the interior of the granule; and that the whole is an endergonic process" (70).

In experiments designed to investigate these two possibilities, chromaffin granules are suspended in isosmotic sucrose solution containing ATP, Mg^{2+}, and ^{14}C-epinephrine at 20 C or above. After incubation the solution is cooled to 0 C and the particles are sedimented. The sediment is usually washed with cold sucrose solution before its content of radioactivity is determined. Since it is known that catecholamines can cross the membrane of the chromaffin granule by passive diffusion rather quickly at 0 C (72), only the epinephrine firmly bound inside the particle will remain after centrifugation and washing. Accordingly in these experiments one is mainly measuring the uptake of amines into the storage complex (25, 70, 81, 121, 126). This does not, however, exclude the possibility that the rate-limiting step is an active uptake across the membrane, in which case the measurement in these experiments gives a direct estimate of this uptake. In fact, most of the experimental evidence, which is summarized below, is in favor of the active transport hypothesis.

1. The uptake process is markedly temperature dependent, having a Q_{10} of 2.8 (70). This is characteristic of a chemical reaction, rather than of a binding phenomenon. If the effect of temperature is studied, with, as a control, chromaffin granules incubated with a potent inhibitor of the uptake (reserpine) to allow for the amount of epinephrine that enters by diffusion alone, a Q_{10} of 6 is found for the active process (70).

2. Chromaffin granules can take up dopamine by the ATP-dependent process, and the dopamine β-hydroxylase in the particles converts the dopamine to norepinephrine. However, when reserpine is present in the medium, not only is the uptake of dopamine prevented, but so also is its conversion to norepinephrine (70). Reserpine does not inhibit dopamine β-hydroxylase, since Kirshner found that chromaffin granules lysed by hyposmotic shock can hydroxylate dopamine in the presence of reserpine (70). The most simple explanation of these findings is that dopamine β-hydroxylase is on the inner side of the membrane, as also indicated by experiments with antiserum to the enzyme (43), and that dopamine is transported across the membrane by an ATP-dependent process.

3. The ATP-dependent uptake of epinephrine is accompanied by the hydrolysis of the ATP in the incubation medium to ADP and phosphate (70, 125), which suggests that the ATPase of chromaffin granules might be involved. This enzyme is localized exclusively in the membranous residue obtained after hyposmotic shock, and this finding, together with the fact that both the ATPase and the active uptake process are activated by magnesium ions, led Banks (2) to propose that the uptake of catecholamines is linked to the hydrolysis of ATP. Clearly the more similarities that are found between the properties of the ATPase and those of the uptake process, the more convincing is the argument that the uptake process is located in the membrane. There is, for example, a reasonable correlation between the relative rates of hydrolysis of several nucleotides by the ATPase (141), which fall in the order ATP > GTP > ITP > UTP > CTP, and the ability of these nucleotides to stimulate uptake of epinephrine (see Table 8). There is a good correlation between the ability of different halogen ions to stimulate ATP-dependent influx of ^{14}C-epinephrine and their effect on ATPase activity (127). It has also been found that both the ATPase activity (74) and the uptake of catecholamines (25, 129) are inhibited by the sulfhydryl reagent N-ethylmaleimide. Furthermore, if ATP is added to the incubation medium before the sulfhydryl reagent, the nucleotide

partly protects against both the inhibition of uptake and the inhibition of ATPase activity (44, 129). However, reserpine is a potent inhibitor of the uptake of epinephrine into chromaffin granules, giving 50% inhibition at a concentration of 10^{-7} M (70), and yet it only inhibits the ATPase by 12% at a concentration of 10^{-5} M (128). Perhaps only part of the ATPase activity is normally coupled to the transport of catecholamines. If this was so, it would account for the finding that the total ATPase activity is not activated upon the addition of epinephrine (125), although one of the criteria of a "transport" ATPase is that it is activated by the substance transported. Indeed, Taugner (125) has calculated that the activation of the ATPase activity by the addition of epinephrine would only increase the total ATPase activity by 1%, which is within the error of the method of estimation.

4. Further evidence that at least some of the ability of the chromaffin granule to take up catecholamines is a property of the membrane is the finding by Taugner (125) that membranes washed free of the soluble content can concentrate epinephrine and norepinephrine by an ATP- and Mg^{2+}-dependent process. However, although a net uptake of catecholamine was obtained, the rate of this process was only about 4% of that found with an equivalent amount of intact chromaffin granules.

Apart from one or two unsolved problems, most of the evidence described above is consistent with the active transport hypothesis, rather than with the idea that the storage complex is the site of action of ATP and Mg^{2+}. Thus we can conclude that the membrane contains the ATP-dependent uptake mechanism for catecholamines.

Chromaffin granules also possess another type of uptake system that has a high affinity for metaraminol, is only slightly stimulated by ATP, and is not inhibited by the low concentrations of reserpine that inhibit the active uptake of epinephrine (83, 106). This uptake system seems to be associated with the rapidly exchangeable pool of catecholamines (see Table 7) and may be confined to a special population of chromaffin granules. It is not known whether this uptake system is a property of the membrane or of the storage complex within the chromaffin granule.

Having reached the conclusion that the major uptake system for catecholamines is located in the membrane of the chromaffin granule, we are now able to make some sense out of the rather conflicting results in the literature concerning the permeability of the membrane to amines. Although the membrane is in fact permeable to epinephrine both at low temperatures and at body temperature, the membrane cannot be considered to be "freely" permeable (72) because it still represents a partial diffusion barrier that can be overcome by the active transport process. In other words, the transport process is superimposed upon the normal passive permeability of the membrane. The active uptake is saturated by an external catecholamine concentration of 0.5 mM (25). Accordingly, if the catecholamine concentration is raised above this level, the passive permeability of the membrane will again prevail, and indeed at these high concentrations no cofactors are needed for the uptake of catecholamines (23). At temperatures between about 20 and 37 C the active transport process is able to take up catecholamines at a rapid rate from dilute solutions, whereas passive diffusion leads to the entry of only very small amounts of amine. The amounts of amine entering by passive diffusion are not sufficient to compensate for the large amounts lost from the granules by diffusion. However, if the chromaffin granules are suspended in more concentrated solutions of catecholamines, much larger amounts of amine can enter by passive diffusion. It is obvious that the active transport process, despite its limited capacity, is going to be of much more importance in the cell because it can compensate for the spontaneous loss of catecholamines from the chromaffin granules into the cytosol.

How is Store of Catecholamines Maintained?

What are the relative contributions of the active uptake process and the storage complex to the ability of the chromaffin granule to maintain its store of catecholamine? We have attempted to illustrate the answers to this question diagrammatically in Figure 5. It is clear that both the temperature and the composition of the medium surrounding the chromaffin granules influence the relative contributions of uptake process and storage complex. At temperatures from 0 to about 20 C the storage complex of catecholamines, ATP, and divalent metal ions is fairly stable, and at these temperatures the rate of the active transport process will be very low; so the stability of the store at low temperatures reflects that of the storage complex and will be greater the lower the temperature is. At temperatures between about 20 and 37 C the aggregates of ATP, catecholamine, and metal ions are less stable, and the equilibrium

$$[(\text{catecholamine})_{3.5}(\text{metal ion})_{0.8}\, ATP]_n \rightleftharpoons$$
$$3.5n\ \text{catecholamine} + 0.8n\ \text{metal ion} + n ATP$$

will be displaced to the right as the temperature is raised. This increases the concentration of free catecholamine and ATP molecules within the chromaffin granule, and so more catecholamine passes out across the membrane by passive diffusion. Hence, if the granules are suspended in a medium that does not contain ATP and Mg^{2+}, the store will become depleted. Indeed, Hillarp (50) showed that the ATP, as well as the amines, diffuses out of the chromaffin granule under these conditions. However, if the medium contains both ATP and Mg^{2+} the active transport process will operate and the catecholamines that leave the granules will be pumped back in again. As a result of active uptake, the concentration of free catecholamine molecules in the chromaffin granule will be high and this will, by mass action, stabilize the storage complex. Accordingly the store of both catecholamine and ATP should be maintained. This is just what has been found experimentally, for the pres-

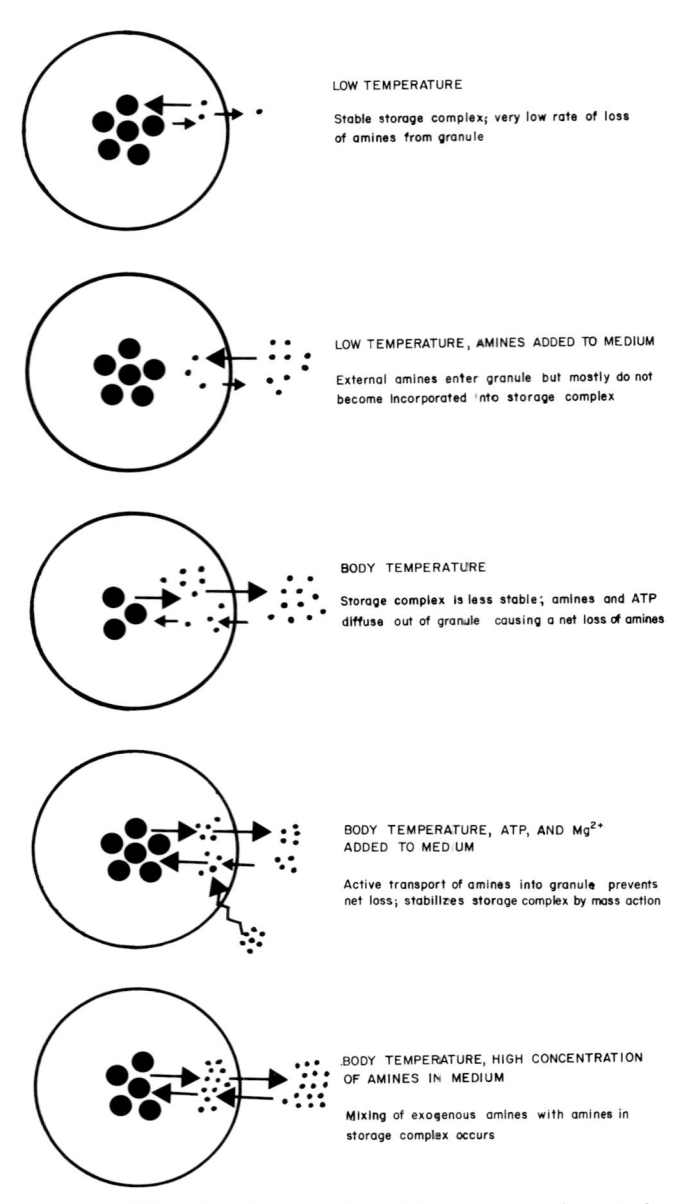

FIG. 5. Effect of environmental conditions on state of catecholamine molecules in isolated chromaffin granules. *Small black dots*, individual molecules of catecholamines or ATP; *larger black dots*, high-molecular-weight aggregates of catecholamines with ATP (i.e., the "storage complex").

ence of ATP and Mg^{2+} in the medium not only prevents the loss of catecholamines, it also prevents the loss of ATP (5). The maintenance of the store of ATP in the chromaffin granule is probably due to the mass action effect of the high concentration of free catecholamine, because only very small amounts of ATP enter the particle during incubation in vitro (5, 25, 70).

We can conclude that in vivo the storage of catecholamines within the chromaffin granule cannot be explained by one mechanism alone; on the contrary, it is the result of two processes that act together. A macromolecular complex is present inside the granule, being composed of aggregates made up of catecholamines, ATP, and divalent metal ion that are too large to pass across the membrane. This storage complex is in equilibrium with the free molecules of its components, and it is stabilized by a high concentration of catecholamine that is maintained inside the granule as a result of the uptake of amine from the medium by an endergonic process that is driven by the free energy of hydrolysis of ATP. The ATP that is hydrolyzed is present in the cytosol.

DYNAMIC ROLE OF CHROMAFFIN GRANULE

Our concept of the chromaffin granule has changed radically during the 20 years following the discovery of this particle in 1953. Whereas its function was originally believed to be that of an inert, reserve store of catecholamines, which was mobilized only when the hypothetical store in the cytosol had been released from the cell (18, 56), we now know that the chromaffin granule stores several other secretory products of the gland and that it is also directly involved in the biosynthesis and in the secretion of the catecholamines.

Storage

The role of the chromaffin granule as a store of secretory products is remarkable when we consider both the variety of substances stored (catecholamines, adenine nucleotides, chromogranins, and dopamine β-hydroxylase) and the fact that the store of secretory products comprises about 63 % of the dry weight of the chromaffin granule. We have discussed elsewhere (116) the question whether there is a significant store of catecholamines in the cytosol and concluded that there was no reason to doubt the estimate made by Hillarp (55) in 1960 that less than 10 % of the total catecholamines in the gland is normally located in the cytosol. The chromaffin granule is obviously very efficient at carrying out its role as a store of catecholamines!

Synthesis

The chromaffin granule plays a vital role in the biosynthesis of the catecholamines (see the chapter by Kirshner in this volume of the *Handbook*) because it contains the enzyme dopamine β-hydroxylase. Other parts of the cell, including the Golgi membranes (31), the empty vesicles that remain after exocytosis from chromaffin granules (see the chapter by Viveros in this volume of the *Handbook*), and possibly the cytosol (116), contain small amounts of this enzyme. However, any dopamine β-hydroxylase in the cytosol would not be functional because this part of the cell also contains potent inhibitors of the enzyme (33, 87). It is likely therefore that the conversion of dopamine to norepinephrine occurs mainly in the chromaffin granule. This conclusion is further supported by "pulse"-labeling experiments with ^{3}H-tyrosine (142) and by the finding that reserpine, which prevents the active uptake of dopamine into the chromaffin granule, inhibits the synthesis of norepinephrine in slices of adrenal medulla (138). The active uptake process in the chromaffin granule membrane is, of course, important for the biosynthesis of norepinephrine because it can concentrate the dopamine formed from 3,4-dihydroxyphenylalanine in the cytosol. If it was not for this rapid uptake of dopamine, the rate of synthesis of norepinephrine would probably be controlled by the availability (by passive diffusion) of dopamine inside the chromaffin granule.

Secretion

The physiological function of the adrenal medulla can only be fulfilled when its secretory products are released into the blood, and herein lies the ultimate role of the chromaffin granule: its function as a secretory granule that releases its entire soluble content by exocytosis [see the chapter by Viveros in this volume of the *Handbook*; (116)].

Now that we are aware of the highly efficient way in which the chromaffin cell stores and releases its secretory products, a number of new questions arise concerning the origin and fate of the chromaffin granule. Morphological studies have shown that chromaffin granules are formed in the Golgi region (see the chapter by Grynszpan-Winograd in this volume of the *Handbook*). What is the composition and what are the properties of these newly formed particles? Do they already contain catecholamines and ATP, or are these low-molecular-weight substances added later? Histochemical studies with the electron microscope have indicated that at least some of the chromaffin granules in the Golgi area of norepinephrine-containing cells already contain norepinephrine (27). However, there is other evidence showing that all the components of the chromaffin granule do not have to be brought together simultaneously. Thus, after giving insulin to animals in order to cause a reflex stimulation of the adrenal medulla, the amounts of catecholamine, ATP, and dopamine β-hydroxylase in the gland fall simultaneously because these substances are secreted, but the subsequent resynthesis of both ATP (103) and dopamine β-hydroxylase (134) occurs several hours before that of the catecholamines. So there must temporarily be a nascent chromaffin granule that contains soluble proteins and ATP but is deficient in catecholamine. Chromaffin granules rich in ATP but deficient in catecholamines also probably occur in the adrenal medullae of fetal and very young rats and rabbits (88). Independent evidence for a type of nascent chromaffin granule is provided by biochemical studies on the synthesis of chromogranins in the perfused ox adrenal gland. It appears that the chromogranins are transferred from their site of synthesis in the endoplasmic reticulum to a particle with quite different sedimentation properties from a mature chromaffin granule (142). While we can understand how the chromogranins enter the chromaffin granule, by analogy with events in other protein-secreting cells, and although we know that catecholamines can be taken up by active transport, we are still completely in the dark about the way in which large amounts of ATP are concentrated by the chromaffin granule. However, it is known that nucleotides can be rapidly transferred from their site of phosphoryla-

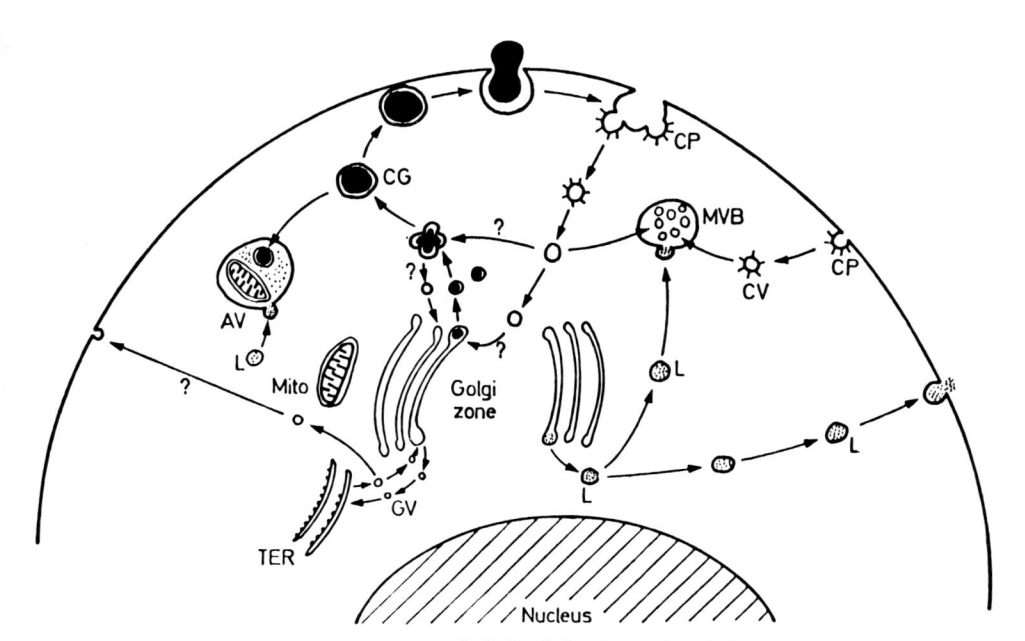

FIG. 6. Subcellular dynamics of chromaffin cell. *AV*, autophagic vacuole; *CG*, chromaffin granule; *CP*, coated pit; *CV*, coated vesicle; *GV*, Golgi vesicle; *L*, lysosome (primary); *Mito*, mitochondrion; *MVB*, multivesicular body; *TER*, transitional endoplasmic reticulum. [For detailed discussion, see (116).]

tion (in mitochondria) to the chromaffin granule (120, 142).

Another unsolved question concerns the fate of the chromaffin granule membrane after secretion of the soluble contents by exocytosis. Although morphological studies have shown that the membrane does not remain fused with the cell membrane (see the chapter by Grynzpan-Winograd in this volume of the *Handbook*) it is not known whether the membrane can be reused to envelop more secretory products, or whether it is only used once. The former pathway is, however, consistent with the finding that the rate of biosynthesis of the chromomembrins is less than that of the chromogranins in the perfused adrenal gland (142).

CONCLUSIONS

The new findings about the storage and secretory functions of the chromaffin granule show us that the function of the chromaffin cell is by no means limited to the synthesis, storage, and release of catecholamines: the chromaffin cell, like many other endocrine cells, secretes proteins. Any static pictures that we have had of the chromaffin cell as a cell organized only to make and release a low-molecular-weight hormone must therefore be discarded. The chromaffin cell shares the dynamics of all protein-secreting cells, and at the center of its organization is the chromaffin granule (see Fig. 6).

During the past 20 years we have learned a great deal about the properties of the chromaffin granule. Although this remarkable organelle will undoubtedly continue to yield us its secrets, what we already know has widened our horizons. The stage is now set for those who wish to identify the nature of the molecular interactions in the storage complex, for those who hope to unravel the intricate mechanisms involved in the dynamic pathways of the chromaffin granule within the cell, and for others who aspire to discover the functions of the proteins that are secreted from the chromaffin granules of the adrenal medulla.

REFERENCES

1. ALDRICH, T. B. A preliminary report on the active principle of the suprarenal gland. *Am. J. Physiol.* 5: 457–461, 1901.
2. BANKS, P. The adenosine-triphosphatase activity of adrenal chromaffin granules. *Biochem. J.* 95: 490–496, 1965.
3. BANKS, P., K. B. HELLE, AND D. MAYOR. Evidence for the presence of a chromogranin-like protein in bovine splenic nerve granules. *Mol. Pharmacol.* 5: 210–212, 1969.
4. BARTLETT, S. F., AND A. D. SMITH. Adrenal chromaffin granules: isolation and disassembly. In: *Methods in Enzymology*, edited by S. P. Colowick and N. O. Kaplan. New York: Acad. Press, 1974, vol. 31.
5. BAUMGARTNER, H., H. WINKLER, AND H. HÖRTNAGL. Isolated chromaffin granules maintenance of ATP content during incubation at 31°C. *European J. Pharmacol.* 22: 102–104, 1973.
6. BELPAIRE, F., AND P. LADURON. Tissue fractionation and catecholamines. I. Latency and activation properties of dopamine-β-hydroxylase in adrenal medulla. *Biochem. Pharmacol.* 17: 411–421, 1968.
7. BENEDECZKY, I. Electron histochemical localization of acid phosphatase activity in the adrenal medulla of the rat. *Nature* 214: 1243–1244, 1967.
8. BENEDECZKY, I., A. D. SMITH, AND F. DUBOIS. A cytochemical study of the calcium-activated adenosinetriphosphatase in hamster adrenal medulla: its occurrence in the Golgi region of chromaffin cells. *Histochemie* 29: 16–27, 1972.
9. BERNEIS, K. H., A. PLETSCHER, AND M. DA PRADA. Metal-dependent aggregation of biogenic amines: a hypothesis for their storage and release. *Nature* 224: 281–283, 1969.
10. BERNEIS, K. H., A. PLETSCHER, AND M. DA PRADA. Phase separation in solutions of noradrenaline and adenosine triphosphate: influence of bivalent cations and drugs. *Brit. J. Pharmacol.* 39: 382–389, 1970.
11. BERTLER, A., G. HALL, N-Å. HILLARP, AND E. ROSENGREN. Uptake of dopamine by the storage granules of the adrenal medulla *in vitro*. *Acta Physiol. Scand.* 52: 167–170, 1961.
12. BLASCHKO, H., G. V. R. BORN, A. D'IORIO, AND N. R. EADE. Observations on the distribution of catecholamines and adenosinetriphosphate in the bovine adrenal medulla. *J. Physiol., London* 133: 548–557, 1956.
13. BLASCHKO, H., R. S. COMLINE, F. H. SCHNEIDER, M. SILVER, AND A. D. SMITH. Secretion of a chromaffin granule protein, chromogranin, from the adrenal gland after splanchnic stimulation. *Nature* 215: 58–59, 1967.

14. BLASCHKO, H., H. FIREMARK, A. D. SMITH, AND H. WINKLER. Lipids of the adrenal medulla: lysolecithin, a characteristic constituent of chromaffin granules. *Biochem. J.* 104: 545–549, 1967.
15. BLASCHKO, H., J. M. HAGEN, AND P. HAGEN. Mitochondrial enzymes and chromaffin granules. *J. Physiol., London* 139: 316–322, 1957.
16. BLASCHKO, H., D. W. JERROME, A. H. T. ROBB-SMITH, A. D. SMITH, AND H. WINKLER. Biochemical and morphological studies on catecholamine storage in human phaeochromocytoma. *Clin. Sci.* 34: 453–465, 1968.
17. BLASCHKO, H., A. D. SMITH, H. WINKLER, H. VAN DEN BOSCH, AND L. L. M. VAN DEENEN. Acid phospholipase A in lysosomes of the bovine adrenal medulla. *Biochem. J.* 103: 30–32c, 1967.
18. BLASCHKO, H., AND A. D. WELCH. Localization of adrenaline in cytoplasmic particles of the bovine adrenal medulla. *Arch. Exptl. Pathol. Pharmakol.* 219: 17–22, 1953.
19. BOROWITZ, J. L. Calcium binding by subcellular fractions of bovine adrenal medulla. *Biochem. Pharmacol.* 19: 2475–2481, 1970.
20. BOROWITZ, J. L., K. FUWA, AND N. WEINER. Distribution of metals and catecholamines in bovine adrenal medulla subcellular fractions. *Nature* 205: 42–43, 1965.
21. BRADBURY, S., A. D. SMITH, AND H. WINKLER. The demonstration of lysosomes in the bovine adrenal medulla. *Experientia* 22: 142–144, 1966.
22. CARLSSON, A., AND N-Å. HILLARP. On the state of the catechol amines of the adrenal medullary granules. *Acta Physiol. Scand.* 44: 163–169, 1958.
23. CARLSSON, A., AND N-Å. HILLARP. Uptake of phenyl and indole alkylamines by the storage granules of the adrenal medulla *in vitro*. *Med. Exptl.* 5: 122–124, 1961.
24. CARLSSON, A., N-Å. HILLARP, AND B. WALDECK. A Mg^{++}-ATP dependent storage mechanism in the amine granules of the adrenal medulla. *Med. Exptl.* 6: 47–53, 1962.
25. CARLSSON, A., N-Å. HILLARP, AND B. WALDECK. Analysis of the Mg^{++}-ATP dependent storage mechanism in the amine granules of the adrenal medulla. *Acta Physiol. Scand. Suppl.* 215: 5–38, 1963.
26. COLBURN, R. W., AND J. W. MASS. Adenosine triphosphate-metal-norepinephrine ternary complexes and catecholamine binding. *Nature* 208: 37–41, 1965.

27. COUPLAND, R. E. Electron microscopic observations on the structure of the rat adrenal medulla. 1. The ultrastructure and organization of chromaffin cells in the normal adrenal medulla. *J. Anat.* 99: 231–254, 1965.
28. DA PRADA, M., K. H. BERNEIS, AND A. PLETSCHER. Storage of catecholamines in adrenal medullary granules: formation of aggregates with nucleotides. *Life Sci., Part 1* 10: 639–646, 1971.
29. DA PRADA, M., AND A. PLETSCHER. Identification of guanosine 5′-triphosphate and uridine 5-triphosphate in subcellular monoamine-storage organelles. *Biochem. J.* 119: 117–119, 1970.
29a. DA PRADA, M., A. PLETSCHER, AND J. P. TRANZER. Lipid composition of membranes of amine-storage granules. *Biochem. J.* 127: 681–683, 1972.
30. DE POTTER, W. P., A. D. SMITH, AND A. F. DE SCHAEPDRYVER. Subcellular fractionation of splenic nerve: ATP, chromogranin A and dopamine β-hydroxylase in noradrenergic vesicles. *Tissue Cell* 2: 529–546, 1970.
31. DUBOIS, F. *Membranes of the Chromaffin Cell* (B.Sc. thesis). Oxford: Univ. of Oxford, 1970.
32. DUBOIS, F., I. BENEDECZKY, AND A. D. SMITH. Membrane-bound enzymes in adrenal medulla: an adenosinetriphosphatase characteristic of the Golgi apparatus. *Biochem. J.* 122: 46–47P, 1971.
33. DUCH, D. S., O. H. VIVEROS, AND N. KIRSHNER. Endogenous inhibitor(s) in adrenal medulla of dopamine-β-hydroxylase. *Biochem. Pharmacol.* 17: 255–264, 1968.
34. EADE, N. R. The distribution of the catechol amines in homogenates of the bovine adrenal medulla. *J. Physiol., London* 141: 183–192, 1958.
35. FALCK, B., N.-Å. HILLARP, AND B. HÖGBERG. Content and intracellular distribution of adenosinetriphosphate in cow adrenal medulla. *Acta Physiol. Scand.* 36: 360–376, 1956.
36. FLATMARK, T., O. TERLAND, AND K. B. HELLE. Electron carriers of the bovine adrenal chromaffin granules. *Biochim. Biophys. Acta* 226: 9–19, 1971.
37. FOLDES, A., P. L. JEFFREY, B. N. PRESTON, AND L. AUSTIN. Dopamine β-hydroxylase of bovine adrenal medullae. A rapid purification procedure. *Biochem. J.* 126: 1209–1217, 1972.
37a. FOLDES, A., P. L. JEFFREY, B. N. PRESTON, AND L. AUSTIN. Some physical properties of bovine adrenal medullary dopamine β-hydroxylase. *J. Neurochem.* 20: 1431–1442, 1973.
38. GEFFEN, L. B., B. G. LIVETT, AND R. A. RUSH. Immunohistochemical localization of protein components of catecholamine storage vesicles. *J. Physiol., London* 204: 593–605, 1969.
39. GIBB, J. W., S. SPECTOR, AND S. UDENFRIEND. Production of antibodies to dopamine β-hydroxylase of bovine adrenal medulla. *Mol. Pharmacol.* 3: 473–478, 1967.
40. HAGEN, P. The distribution of cholinesterase in the chromaffine cell. *J. Physiol., London* 129: 50–52, 1955.
41. HAGEN, P., AND R. J. BARRNETT. The storage of amines in the chromaffin cell. In: *Adrenergic Mechanisms*, edited by J. R. Vane, G. E. W. Wolstenholme, and M. O'Connor. London: Churchill, 1960, p. 83–99.
42. HAJDU, S., H. WEISS, AND E. TITUS. The isolation of a cardiac active principle from mammalian tissue. *J. Pharmacol. Exptl. Therap.* 120: 99–113, 1957.
43. HARTMAN, B., AND S. UDENFRIEND. The application of immunological techniques to the study of enzymes regulating catecholamine synthesis and degradation. *Pharmacol. Rev.* 24: 311–330, 1972.
44. HASSELBACH, W., AND G. TAUGNER. The effect of a cross-bridging thiol reagent on the catecholamine fluxes of adrenal medulla vesicles. *Biochem. J.* 119: 265–271, 1970.
45. HELLE, K. B. Some chemical and physical properties of the soluble protein fraction of bovine adrenal chromaffin granules. *Mol. Pharmacol.* 2: 298–310, 1966.
46. HELLE, K. B. Comparative studies on the soluble protein fractions of bovine, equine, porcine and ovine adrenal chromaffin granules. *Biochem. J.* 100: 6C, 1966.
47. HELLE, K. B. Antibody formation against soluble protein from bovine adrenal chromaffin granules. *Biochim. Biophys. Acta* 117: 107–110, 1966.
48. HELLE, K. B. Biochemical studies of the chromaffin granule. 2. Properties of membrane-bound and water-soluble forms of chromogranin A and dopamine β-hydroxylase activity. *Biochim. Biophys. Acta* 245: 94–104, 1971.
49. HELLE, K. B., AND G. SERCK-HANSSEN. Chromogranin: the soluble and membrane-bound lipoprotein of the chromaffin granule. *Pharmacol. Res. Commun.* 1: 25–29, 1969.
50. HILLARP, N.-Å. Enzymic systems involving adenosinephosphates in the adrenaline and noradrenaline containing granules of the adrenal medulla. *Acta Physiol. Scand.* 42: 144–165, 1958.
51. HILLARP, N.-Å. Adenosinephosphates and inorganic phosphate in the adrenaline and noradrenaline containing granules of the adrenal medulla. *Acta Physiol. Scand.* 42: 321–332, 1958.
52. HILLARP, N.-Å. Isolation and some biochemical properties of the catecholamine granules in the cow adrenal medulla. *Acta Physiol. Scand.* 43: 82–96, 1958.
53. HILLARP, N.-Å. The release of catecholamines from the amine containing granules of the adrenal medulla. *Acta Physiol. Scand.* 43: 292–302, 1958.
54. HILLARP, N.-Å. Further observations on the state of the catecholamines stored in the adrenal medullary granules. *Acta Physiol. Scand.* 47: 271–279, 1959.
55. HILLARP, N.-Å. Different pools of catecholamines stored in the adrenal medulla. *Acta Physiol. Scand.* 50: 8–22, 1960.
56. HILLARP, N.-Å., S. LAGERSTEDT, AND B. NILSON. The isolation of a granular fraction from the suprarenal medulla, containing the sympathomimetic catecholamines. *Acta Physiol. Scand.* 29: 251–263, 1953.
57. HILLARP, N.-Å., AND B. NILSON. Some quantitative analyses of the sympathomimetic amine containing granules in the adrenal medullary cell. *Acta Physiol. Scand.* 32: 11–18, 1954.
58. HILLARP, N.-Å., AND B. NILSON. The structure of the adrenaline and noradrenaline containing granules in the adrenal medullary cells with reference to the storage and release of the sympathomimetic amines. *Acta Physiol. Scand. Suppl.* 113: 79–107, 1954.
59. HILLARP, N.-Å., B. NILSON, AND B. HÖGBERG. Adenosine triphosphate in the adrenal medulla of the cow. *Nature* 176: 1032–1033, 1955.
60. HILLARP, N.-Å., AND G. THIEME. Nucleotides in the catechol amine granules of the adrenal medulla. *Acta Physiol. Scand.* 45: 328–338, 1959.
61. HOLTZ, P., K. CREDNER, AND G. KRONEBERG. Über das sympathicomimetische pressorische Prinzip des Harns. *Arch. Exptl. Pathol. Pharmakol.* 204: 228–243, 1947.
62. HOLTZMAN, E., AND R. DOMINITZ. Cytochemical studies of lysosomes, Golgi apparatus and endoplasmic reticulum in secretion and protein uptake by adrenal medulla cells of the rat. *J. Histochem. Cytochem.* 16: 320–336, 1968.
63. HOPWOOD, D. An immunohistochemical study of the adrenal medulla of the ox. A comparison of antibodies against whole ox chromaffin granules and ox chromogranin A. *Histochemie* 13: 323–330, 1968.
63a. HÖRTNAGL, H., H. LOCHS, AND H. WINKLER. Immunological studies on the acidic chromogranins and on dopamine β-hydroxylase of bovine chromaffin granules. *J. Neurochem.* 22: 197–199, 1974.
63b. HÖRTNAGL, H., H. WINKLER, AND H. HÖRTNAGL. The subcellular distribution of lysophospholipase in bovine adrenal medulla. *European J. Biochem.* 10: 243–248, 1969.
64. HÖRTNAGL, H., H. WINKLER, AND H. LOCHS. Membrane proteins of chromaffin granules: dopamine β-hydroxylase, a major constituent. *Biochem. J.* 129: 187–195, 1972.
65. HÖRTNAGL, H., H. WINKLER, AND H. LOCHS. Immunological studies on a membrane protein (chromomembrin B) of catecholamine-storing vesicles. *J. Neurochem.* 20: 977–985, 1973.

66. HÖRTNAGL, H., H. WINKLER, J. A. L. SCHÖPF, AND W. HOHENWALLNER. Membranes of chromaffin granules, isolation and partial characterization of two proteins. *Biochem. J.* 122: 299–304, 1971.
67. ICHIKAWA, Y., AND T. YAMANO. Cytochrome 559 in the microsomes of the adrenal medulla. *Biochem. Biophys. Res. Commun.* 20: 263–268, 1965.
68. KAUFMAN, S., AND S. FRIEDMAN. Dopamine β-hydroxylase. *Pharmacol. Rev.* 17: 71–100, 1965.
69. KIRSHNER, N. Biosynthesis of adrenaline and noradrenaline. *Pharmacol. Rev.* 11: 350–357, 1959.
70. KIRSHNER, N. Uptake of catecholamines by a particulate fraction of the adrenal medulla. *J. Biol. Chem.* 237: 2311–2317, 1962.
71. KIRSHNER, N. Storage and secretion of adrenal catecholamines. *Advan. Biochem. Psychopharmacol.* 1: 71–89, 1969.
72. KIRSHNER, N., C. HOLLOWAY, AND D. L. KAMIN. Permeability of catecholamine granules. *Biochim. Biophys. Acta* 112: 532–537, 1966.
73. KIRSHNER, A. G., AND N. KIRSHNER. A specific soluble protein from the catecholamine storage vesicles of bovine adrenal medulla. 2. Physical characterization. *Biochim. Biophys. Acta* 181: 219–225, 1969.
74. KIRSHNER, N., A. G. KIRSHNER, AND D. L. KAMIN. Adenosine triphosphatase activity of adrenal medulla catecholamine granules. *Biochim. Biophys. Acta* 113: 332–335, 1966.
75. LADURON, P. *Biosynthèse, Localisation Intracellulaire et Transport des Catecholamines* (Ph.D. thesis). Louvain, Belgium: Catholic University, 1969.
76. LADURON, P., AND F. BELPAIRE. Tissue fractionation and catecholamines. 2. Intracellular distribution patterns of tyrosine hydroxylase, dopa decarboxylase, dopamine β-hydroxylase, phenylethanolamine N-methyltransferase and monoamine oxidase in adrenal medulla. *Biochem. Pharmacol.* 17: 1127–1140, 1968.
77. LAGERCRANTZ, H., B. KUYLENSTIERNA, AND L. STJÄRNE. On the origin of adenosine triphosphate in chromaffin granules. *Experientia* 26: 479–480, 1970.
78. LAGERCRANTZ, H., H. PERTOFT, AND L. STJÄRNE. Facts and artifacts in gradient centrifugation analysis of catecholamine granules. *Acta Physiol. Scand.* 78: 561–566, 1970.
79. LEVER, J. D. Electron microscopic observations on the normal and denervated adrenal medulla of the rat. *Endocrinology* 57: 621–635, 1955.
80. LISHAJKO, F. Release, re-uptake and net uptake of dopamine, noradrenaline and adrenaline in isolated sheep adrenal medullary granules. *Acta Physiol. Scand.* 76: 159–171, 1969.
81. LISHAJKO, F. Studies on catecholamine release and uptake in adrenomedullary storage granules. *Acta Physiol. Scand. Suppl.* 362, 1971.
82. LUCY, J. A. The fusion of biological membranes. *Nature* 227: 814–817, 1970.
83. LUNDBORG, P. Studies on the uptake and subcellular distribution of catecholamines and their α-methylated analogues. *Acta Physiol. Scand. Suppl.* 302, 1967.
84. MAYNERT, E. W., B. H. MOON, AND V. S. PAI. Insoluble solid complexes of norepinephrine and adenosine triphosphate. *Mol. Pharmacol.* 8: 88–94, 1972.
85. MCCABE, M. The diffusion coefficient of caffeine through agar gels containing a hyaluronic acid-protein complex. *Biochem. J.* 127: 249–253, 1972.
86. MCGOODALL, C. Studies of adrenaline and noradrenaline in mammalian heart and suprarenals. *Acta Physiol. Scand. Suppl.* 85, 1951.
87. NAGATSU, T., H. KUZUYA, AND H. HIDAKA. Inhibition of dopamine-β-hydroxylase by sulfhydryl compounds and the nature of the natural inhibitors. *Biochim. Biophys. Acta* 139: 319–327, 1967.
88. O'BRIEN, R. A., M. DA PRADA, AND A. PLETSCHER. The ontogenesis of catecholamines and adenosine-5′-triphosphate in the adrenal medulla. *Life Sci., Part 1* 11: 749–759, 1972.
89. OKA, M., K. KAJIKAWA, T. OHUCHI, H. YOSHIDA, AND R. IMAIZUMI. Distribution of dopamine-β-hydroxylase in subcellular fractions of adrenal medulla. *Life Sci.* 6: 461–465, 1967.
90. OKA, M., T. OHUCI, H. YOSHIDA, AND R. IMAIZUMI. Selective release of noradrenaline and adrenaline from isolated adrenal medullary granules. *Life Sci.* 5: 433–438, 1966.
91. OKA, M., T. OHUCHI, H. YOSHIDA, AND R. IMAIZUMI. The isolation of catecholamine storage granules from adrenal medulla by the membrane filter technique. *Life Sci.* 5: 427–432, 1966.
92. PAI, V. S., AND E. W. MAYNERT. Interactions of catecholamines with adenosine triphosphate in solutions and adrenal medullary granules. *Mol. Pharmacol.* 8: 82–87, 1972.
93. PALKAMA, A., AND L. RECHARDT. Light and electron microscopic observations on acid phosphatase activity in the adrenal medulla of the rat and mouse. *Ann. Med. Exptl. Biol. Fenniae* 48: 77–83, 1970.
94. PHILIPPU, A., AND H. J. SCHÜMANN. Effect of ribonuclease on the ribonucleic acid, adenosine-triphosphate and catecholamine content of medullary granules. *Nature* 198: 795–796, 1963.
95. PHILIPPU, A., AND H. J. SCHÜMANN. Über die Bedetung der Calcium- und Magnesiumionen für die Speicherung der Nebennierenmark-Hormone. *Arch. Exptl. Pathol. Pharmakol.* 252: 339–358, 1966.
96. RAJAN, K. S., J. M. DAVIS, AND R. W. COLBURN. Metal chelates in the storage and transport of neurotransmitters: interactions of metal ions with biogenic amines. *J. Neurochem.* 18: 345–364, 1971.
97. SAGE, H. J., W. J. SMITH, AND N. KIRSHNER. Mechanism of secretion from the adrenal medulla. 1. A microquantitative immunologic assay for bovine adrenal catecholamine storage vesicle protein and its application to studies of the secretory process. *Mol. Pharmacol.* 3: 81–89, 1967.
98. SCHNEIDER, F. H. Observations on the release of lysosomal enzymes from the isolated bovine adrenal gland. *Biochem. Pharmacol.* 17: 848–851, 1968.
99. SCHNEIDER, F. H. Lysosomal enzymes in the bovine adrenal gland. A comparison of medulla and cortex. *Biochem. Pharmacol.* 19: 819–831, 1970.
100. SCHNEIDER, F. H. Secretion from the bovine adrenal gland. Release of lysosomal enzymes. *Biochem. Pharmacol.* 19: 833–847, 1970.
100a. SCHNEIDER, F. H. Isolation of and production of antibody to cow chromaffin granule membrane. *Biochem. Pharmacol.* 21: 2627–2634, 1972.
101. SCHNEIDER, F. H., A. D. SMITH, AND H. WINKLER. Secretion from the adrenal medulla: biochemical evidence for exocytosis. *Brit. J. Pharmacol.* 31: 94–104, 1967.
102. SCHÜMANN, H. J. The distribution of adrenaline and noradrenaline in chromaffin granules of the chicken. *J. Physiol., London* 137: 318–326, 1957.
103. SCHÜMANN, H. J. Die Wirkung von Insulin und Reserpin auf den Adrenalin- und ATP-Gehalt der chromaffinen Granula des Nebennierenmarks. *Arch. Exptl. Pathol. Pharmakol.* 233: 237–249, 1958.
104. SHEPHERD, D. M., AND G. B. WEST. Hydroxytyramine in medulla of sheep, ox and cow. *J. Physiol., London* 120: 15–19, 1953.
105. SJÖSTRAND, F. S., AND R. WETZSTEIN. Elektronenmikroskopische Untersuchung der phäochromen (chromaffinen) Granula in den Markzellen der Nebenniere. *Experientia* 12: 196–199, 1956.
106. SLOTKIN, T. A., R. M. FERRIS, AND N. KIRSHNER. Compartmental analysis of amine storage in bovine adrenal medullary granules. *Mol. Pharmacol.* 7: 308–316, 1971.
107. SMITH, A. D. Biochemistry of adrenal chromaffin granules. In: *The Interaction of Drugs and Subcellular Components in Animal Cells*, edited by P. N. Campbell. London: Churchill, 1968, p. 239–292.

108. SMITH, A. D. Extracellular release of lysosomal phospholipases from the perfused adrenal gland. *Biochem. J.* 114: 72P, 1969.
109. SMITH, A. D. Storage and secretion of hormones. *Sci. Basis Med.* 74–102, 1972.
110. SMITH, A. D. Subcellular localisation of noradrenaline in sympathetic neurons. *Pharmacol. Rev.* 24: 435–457, 1972.
111. SMITH, A. D., W. P. DE POTTER, E. J. MOERMAN, AND A. F. DE SCHAEPDRYVER. Release of dopamine β-hydroxylase and chromogranin A upon stimulation of the splenic nerve. *Tissue Cell* 2: 547–568, 1970.
112. SMITH, A. D., AND H. WINKLER. The localization of lysosomal enzymes in chromaffin tissue. *J. Physiol.*, London 183: 179–188, 1966.
113. SMITH, A. D., AND H. WINKLER. A simple method for the isolation of adrenal chromaffin granules on a large scale. *Biochem. J.* 103: 480–482, 1967.
114. SMITH, A. D., AND H. WINKLER. Purification and properties of an acidic protein from chromaffin granules of bovine adrenal medulla. *Biochem. J.* 103: 483–492, 1967.
115. SMITH, A. D., AND H. WINKLER. Lysosomal phospholipases A_1 and A_2 of bovine adrenal medulla. *Biochem. J.* 108: 867–874, 1968.
116. SMITH, A. D., AND H. WINKLER. Fundamental mechanisms in the release of catecholamines. In: *Handbook of Experimental Pharmacology. Catecholamines*, edited by H. Blaschko and E. Muscholl. New York: Springer, 1972, vol. 33, p. 538–617.
117. SMITH, W. J., AND N. KIRSHNER. A specific soluble protein from the catecholamine storage vesicles of bovine adrenal medulla. 1. Purification and chemical characterization. *Mol. Pharmacol.* 3: 52–62, 1967.
118. SMYTHIES, J. R., F. ANTUN, G. YANK, AND C. YORKE. Molecular mechanisms of storage of transmitters in synaptic terminals. *Nature* 231: 185–188, 1971.
119. SPIRO, M. J., AND E. G. BALL. Studies on the respiratory enzymes of the adrenal gland. 1. The medulla. *J. Biol. Chem.* 236: 225–230, 1961.
120. STEVENS, P., R. L. ROBINSON, K. VAN DYKE, AND R. STITZEL. Studies on the synthesis and release of adenosine triphosphate-8-^{3}H in the isolated perfused cat adrenal gland. *J. Pharmacol. Exptl. Therap.* 181: 463–471, 1972.
121. STJÄRNE, L. Studies of catecholamine uptake storage and release mechanisms. *Acta Physiol. Scand. Suppl.* 228, 1964.
122. STJÄRNE, L. The synthesis, uptake and storage of catecholamines in the adrenal medulla. The effect of drugs. In: *Handbook of Experimental Pharmacology. Catecholamines*, edited by H. Blaschko and E. Muscholl. New York: Springer, 1972, vol. 33, p. 231–269.
123. STRIEDER, N., E. ZIEGLER, H. WINKLER, AND A. D. SMITH. Some properties of soluble proteins from chromaffin granules of different species. *Biochem. Pharmacol.* 17: 1553–1556, 1968.
124. TAKAMINE, J. The isolation of the active principle of the suprarenal gland. *J. Physiol.*, London 27: xxix–xxx, 1901.
125. TAUGNER, G. The membrane of catecholamine storage vesicles of adrenal medulla. Catecholamine fluxes and ATPase activity. *Arch. Pharmakol.* 270: 392–406, 1971.
126. TAUGNER, G. The effect of salts on catecholamine fluxes and adenosine triphosphatase activity in storage vesicles from the adrenal medulla. *Biochem. J.* 123: 219–225, 1971.
127. TAUGNER, G. The effects of univalent anions on catecholamine fluxes and adenosine triphosphatase activity in storage vesicles from the adrenal medulla. *Biochem. J.* 130: 969–973, 1972.
128. TAUGNER, G., AND W. HASSELBACH. Über den Mechanismus der Catecholamin-Speicherung in den "chromaffinen Granula" des Nebennierenmarks. *Arch. Pharmakol. Exptl. Pathol.* 255: 266–286, 1966.
129. TAUGNER, G., AND W. HASSELBACH. Die Bedentung der Sulfhydryl-Gruppen für den Catecholamin-Transport der Vesikel des Nebennierenmarkes. *Arch. Exptl. Pathol. Pharmakol.* 260: 58–79, 1968.
130. TRIFARÓ, J. Phospholipid metabolism and adrenal medullary activity. 1. The effect of acetylcholine on tissue uptake and incorporation of orthophosphate-^{32}P into nucleotides and phospholipids of bovine adrenal medulla. *Mol. Pharmacol.* 5: 382–393, 1969.
131. TRIFARÓ, J. M., AND J. DWORKIND. A new and simple method for isolation of adrenal chromaffin granules by means of an isotonic density gradient. *Anal. Biochem.* 34: 403–412, 1970.
132. TRIFARÓ, J. M., AND M. WARNER. Membranes of adrenal chromaffin granules. Solubilization and partial characterization of the Mg^{++}-dependent adenosine triphosphatase. *Mol. Pharmacol.* 8: 159–169, 1972.
133. VIVEROS, O. H., L. ARQUEROS, R. J. CONNETT, AND N. KIRSHNER. Mechanism of secretion from the adrenal medulla. 3. Studies of dopamine β-hydroxylase as a marker for catecholamine storage vesicle membranes in rabbit adrenal glands. *Mol. Pharmacol.* 5: 60–68, 1969.
134. VIVEROS, O. H., L. ARQUEROS, R. J. CONNETT, AND N. KIRSHNER. Mechanism of secretion from the adrenal medulla. 4. The fate of the storage vesicles following insulin and reserpine administration. *Mol. Pharmacol.* 5: 69–82, 1969.
135. VIVEROS, O. H., L. ARQUEROS, AND N. KIRSHNER. Mechanism of secretion from the adrenal medulla. 5. Retention of storage vesicle membranes following release of adrenaline. *Mol. Pharmacol.* 5: 342–349, 1969.
136. VIVEROS, O. H., L. ARQUEROS, AND N. KIRSHNER. Mechanism of secretion from the adrenal medulla. 7. Effect of insulin administration on the buoyant density, dopamine β-hydroxylase, and catecholamine content of adrenal storage vesicles. *Mol. Pharmacol.* 7: 444–454, 1971.
137. WEINER, N., AND O. JARDETZKY. A study of catecholamine nucleotide complexes by nuclear magnetic resonance spectroscopy. *Arch. Exptl. Pathol. Pharmakol.* 248: 308–318, 1964.
138. WEINER, N., AND C. O. RUTLEDGE. The actions of reserpine on the biosynthesis and storage of catecholamines. In: *Mechanisms of Release of Biogenic Amines*, edited by U. S. von Euler, S. Rosell, and B. Uvnäs. Oxford: Pergamon Press, 1966, p. 307–318.
139. WINKLER, H. Isolierung und Charakterlesierung von chromaffinen Noradrenalin-Granula aus Schweine-Nebennierenmark. *Arch. Exptl. Pathol. Pharmakol.* 263: 340–357, 1969.
140. WINKLER, H. The membrane of the chromaffin granule. *Phil. Trans. Roy. Soc. London Ser. B* 261: 293–303, 1971.
141. WINKLER, H., H. HÖRTNAGL, H. HÖRTNAGL, AND A. D. SMITH. Membranes of the adrenal medulla. Behaviour of insoluble proteins of chromaffin granules on gel electrophoresis. *Biochem. J.* 118: 303–310, 1970.
142. WINKLER, H., J. A. L. SCHÖPF, H. HÖRTNAGL, AND H. HÖRTNAGL. Bovine adrenal medulla: subcellular distribution of newly synthesised catecholamines, nucleotides and chromogranins. *Arch. Pharmakol.* 273: 43–61, 1972.
143. WINKLER, H., AND A. D. SMITH. Lipids of adrenal chromaffin granules: fatty acid composition of phospholipids, in particular lysolecithin. *Arch. Pharmakol. Exptl. Pathol.* 261: 379–388, 1968.
144. WINKLER, H., AND A. D. SMITH. Phaeochromocytoma and other catecholamine-producing tumours. In: *Handbook of Experimental Pharmacology. Catecholamines*, edited by H. Blaschko and E. Muscholl. New York: Springer, 1972, vol. 33, p. 900–933.
145. WINKLER, H., A. D. SMITH, F. DUBOIS, AND H. VAN DEN BOSCH. The positional specificity of lysosomal phospholipase A activities. *Biochem. J.* 105: 38–40c, 1967.
146. WINKLER, H., N. STRIEDER, AND E. ZIEGLER. Über Lipide, inbesondere Lysolecithin, in den chromaffinen Granula verschiedener Species. *Arch. Exptl. Pathol. Pharmakol.* 256: 407–415, 1967.
147. WINKLER, H., E. ZIEGLER, AND N. STRIEDER. Studies on the proteins from chromaffin granules of ox, horse and pig. *Nature* 211: 982–983, 1966.

CHAPTER 24

Biosynthesis of the catecholamines

N. KIRSHNER | *Department of Biochemistry, Duke University Medical Center, Durham, North Carolina*

CHAPTER CONTENTS

Biosynthetic Pathway of Norepinephrine and Epinephrine
Enzymes of Biosynthetic Pathway
   Tyrosine hydroxylase
   Dihydropteridine reductase
   Dopa decarboxylase
   Dopamine β-hydroxylase
   Phenylethanolamine *N*-methyltransferase
Regulation of Norepinephrine Synthesis
   Acute regulation in sympathetic nerves in response to stimulation
   Acute regulation in adrenal medulla in response to immediate demands
   Regulation in response to prolonged stimulation
Conclusion

THE PATHWAY for the biosynthesis of norepinephrine and epinephrine (see Fig. 1) in the adrenal medulla, as well as the pathway for the synthesis of norepinephrine in sympathetic nerves, has been known for more than a decade (7, 62, 74). More recently interest has focused on the purification and properties of each of the enzymes involved and on the mechanisms for the regulation of catecholamine synthesis. The first part of this chapter is concerned with the biochemical aspects of the individual reactions and the second part deals with the proposed mechanisms for the regulation of catecholamine synthesis.

BIOSYNTHETIC PATHWAY OF NOREPINEPHRINE AND EPINEPHRINE

Although epinephrine was one of the first hormones identified (117, 139, 143) and is a rather simple molecule, early attempts to demonstrate its formation produced conflicting and equivocal results largely because of the difficulty in detecting small amounts of newly synthesized epinephrine in the presence of large amounts of the preformed hormone (28, 64, 131, 136). With the advent of radioactive tracers and ion exchange and paper chromatography the task was greatly simplified. Because of its apparent derivation from phenylalanine or tyrosine a variety of pathways for epinephrine formation were proposed. The established sequence (Fig. 1) was first proposed by Blaschko in 1939 (6) and was based on the observations reported in 1937 and 1938 by Holtz and co-workers (61, 64) that homogenates of mammalian kidney rapidly decarboxylated 3,4-dihydroxyphenylalanine (dopa) but only very slowly decarboxylated tyrosine. Not until 1951 did Langemann (86) demonstrate that the adrenal medulla contained substantial amounts of dopa decarboxylase. Gurin & Delluva (52) were the first to demonstrate that rats formed ^{14}C- or ^{3}H-labeled epinephrine from correspondingly labeled phenylalanine. Subsequently, Udenfriend et al. (150) reported that rabbits formed ^{14}C-epinephrine from ^{14}C-tyrosine, and Udenfriend & Wyngaarden (151) found that rats utilized ^{14}C-tyrosine and ^{14}C-dopa, but not ^{14}C-tyramine or ^{14}C-phenylethylamine, in the formation of epinephrine. Leeper & Udenfriend (87) showed that rats could utilize dopamine at five to ten times the rate at which they utilized dopa for the formation of epinephrine. Rosenfeld et al. (124) found that isolated perfused calf adrenal glands readily converted DL-tyrosine-2-^{14}C to norepinephrine and that dopamine-1-^{14}C was converted to norepinephrine at a much faster rate. Only small amounts of radioactive epinephrine were formed when methionine was absent from the perfusion medium, but when methionine was present, considerable amounts of epinephrine were found. All these observations were consistent with the pathway proposed by Blaschko but did not rule out alternate sequences of reactions. One such possibility was that the side chain of dopa was hydroxylated to form dihydroxyphenylserine (dops), which would be decarboxylated to form norepinephrine (125). Injections of dops into rabbits (129) led to increased amounts of norepinephrine in the urine, and Drell et al. (29) found ^{14}C-norepinephrine in the urine of rats after injection of threo-^{14}C-dops.

Information on the sequential order of the reactions was obtained from studies in which tissue slices, homogenates, and subcellular fractions of adrenal glands were used. Demis et al. (25, 26) isolated small amounts of radioactive norepinephrine by paper chromatography from extracts of bovine adrenal homogenates incu-

FIG. 1. Pathway for synthesis of norepinephrine (*noradrenaline*) and epinephrine (*adrenaline*).

bated with ^{14}C-dopa. Hagen and Welch (53, 54) prepared dopamine-2-^{14}C from dopa-2-^{14}C by incubating the latter with a particle-free supernatant fraction prepared from homogenates of beef adrenal medulla. The dopamine-2-^{14}C was isolated by ion exchange chromatography (76) and converted to norepinephrine by incubation with a homogenate of chicken adrenal glands. Pellerin & D'Iorio (121) also demonstrated the formation of ^{14}C-dopamine and ^{14}C-norepinephrine from dopa-2-^{14}C by adrenal homogenates. Although these studies clearly showed that the adrenal medulla could form norepinephrine from dopa and dopamine, they did not rule out alternative pathways from tyrosine.

Incubation of slices of adrenal medulla with ^{14}C-labeled L-tyrosine led to the formation of ^{14}C-dopamine, ^{14}C-norepinephrine, and ^{14}C-epinephrine (50). Under identical conditions, ^{14}C-dopa was converted to ^{14}C-norepinephrine at 70–100 times the rate of conversion of tyrosine, whereas ^{14}C-tyramine did not serve as a precursor for norepinephrine. Further evidence that dopa and dopamine, but not tyramine, are metabolic intermediates was obtained by isotope dilution experiments. Addition of unlabeled dopa or dopamine to adrenal slices synthesizing norepinephrine from ^{14}C-labeled L-tyrosine greatly reduced the amounts of radioactivity incorporated into norepinephrine, whereas the addition of tyramine had no effect (50).

The subcellular localization of dopa decarboxylase in the cytosol (8) and of dopamine β-hydroxylase in the particulate fractions of cell homogenates, specifically the catecholamine storage vesicles (73), made it possible to demonstrate that dops is not an intermediate in the biogenic pathway. Aerobic incubation of ^{14}C-dopa with the particulate fraction of adrenal homogenates containing dopamine β-hydroxylase followed by anaerobic incubations with the soluble cell fraction containing dopa decarboxylase resulted in the formation of only ^{14}C-dopamine. Conversely when ^{14}C-dopa was first incubated anaerobically with the soluble cell fraction and this mixture, after boiling, was then incubated aerobically with the particulate fractions, both ^{14}C-dopamine and large amounts of ^{14}C-norepinephrine were obtained. After incubating adrenal slices with ^{14}C-tyrosine in the presence of monoamine oxidase inhibitors, Drell et al. (29) isolated radioactive dopa but could not detect any radioactive dops. These studies established the pathway from tyrosine to norepinephrine and were subsequently confirmed by studies of the substrate specificities of tyrosine hydroxylase (110), dopa decarboxylase [aromatic L-amino acid decarboxylase (92, 137)], and dopamine β-hydroxylase (20, 43, 88, 89). The final step in the formation of epinephrine, the N-methylation of norepinephrine, is catalyzed by phenylethanolamine N-methyltransferase (PNMT)—an enzyme present in the soluble cell fraction (75).

Although dopamine β-hydroxylase has a broad substrate specificity—it will hydroxylate the side chain of phenylethylamine and tyramine about equally as well as that of dopamine—the specificities of tyrosine hydroxylase, dopamine β-hydroxylase, and PNMT are such that the reaction sequence shown in Figure 1 is obligatory. For example, tyramine may be hydroxylated to *p*-hydroxyphenylethanolamine (octopamine) by dopamine β-hydroxylase, but tyramine is not N-methylated by PNMT, and neither octopamine nor its N-methylated derivative can be hydroxylated to norepinephrine or epinephrine by tyrosine hydroxylase or any other demonstrable enzyme in the adrenal gland. Alternatively dops can be decarboxylated to norepinephrine but enzymes for the formation of dops are not present in the adrenal gland; neither tyrosine nor dopa are substrates for dopamine β-hydroxylase.

ENZYMES OF BIOSYNTHETIC PATHWAY

Tyrosine Hydroxylase

The oxidation of tyrosine to dihydroxyphenylalanine is catalyzed by tyrosine hydroxylase, a mixed-function oxidase that requires molecular oxygen and a tetrahydropteridine as cosubstrate (Fig. 2). The enzyme was identified in 1964 in brain (110) and adrenal medulla (9, 111) and is of considerable importance because it may be the rate-limiting enzyme in the formation of

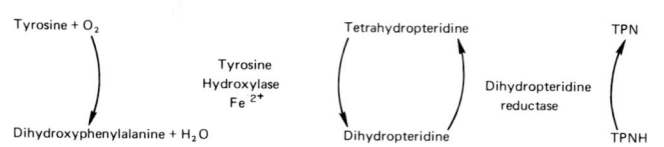

FIG. 2. Oxidation of tyrosine to dihydroxyphenylalanine.

norepinephrine (90) and subject to metabolic and genetic regulation (111, 145, 152, 154).

Studies of the subcellular distribution of tyrosine hydroxylase have produced conflicting reports. In their initial studies with bovine adrenal medulla homogenized in 0.32 M sucrose, Nagatsu et al. (111) recovered most of the enzyme activity in the particulate fraction that sedimented at 20,000 g. In similar experiments, Petrack et al. (122) recovered 90% of the activity in the particulate fraction. However, Musacchio (103) and Laduron & Belpaire (85) have shown that the distribution of enzyme between soluble and particulate fractions of adrenal medullary homogenates depends to a considerable extent on the homogenizing medium. Laduron & Belpaire (85) recovered 37–70% of the total activity in the soluble fractions and the bulk of the remainder in the nuclear fraction. Musacchio found 90% of the total activity present in bovine adrenal homogenates prepared in isotonic KCl to be in the soluble fraction after centrifugation at 100,000 g. In adrenal homogenates from rabbit, rat, and chicken, most of the activity is present in the soluble fraction (97, 102, 118, 153).

More recently, Shiman et al. (135) have suggested that tyrosine hydroxylase is present in the catecholamine storage vesicles. They claim that whole chromaffin granules do not show much activity until they have been lysed and extensively washed to remove endogenous inhibitors. However, these studies are in contradiction to those reported by Musacchio (103), Laduron & Belpaire (85), and Wurzburger & Musacchio (161). Only negligible amounts of tyrosine hydroxylase activity were associated with the storage vesicle fractions isolated by sucrose density centrifugation, even after such treatments as osmotic shock, dialysis against hypotonic buffers, and tryptic digestion. The enzyme activity found by Shiman et al. (135) undoubtedly was associated with particulate material, but it appears unlikely that the enzyme is associated with the storage vesicles. The disparate results obtained by the several groups of investigators may be explained by factors such as the property of the enzyme to form insoluble aggregates, adsorption to particulate matter or other macromolecules, the use of fresh versus frozen glands as starting material, and homogenization procedures.

Attempts to purify the native enzyme have met with only limited success (65) because of its tendency to aggregate with irreversible loss of activity (106, 161). The particulate enzyme present in homogenates of adrenal medulla can be solubilized by digestion with trypsin (122) or chymotrypsin (135). After this treatment the enzyme remains soluble and has been extensively purified by Shiman et al. (135). However, Musacchio et al. (107) have shown that the trypsin-digested enzyme has an estimated molecular weight close to 45,000, whereas the native soluble enzyme present in the 100,000-g supernatant fraction of adrenal homogenates has a molecular weight of approximately 198,000. Shiman et al. (135) estimate the molecular weight of their purified enzyme obtained after chymotryptic digestion to be about 40,000. These studies indicate that digestion with trypsin or chymotrypsin cleaves the enzyme into one or more catalytic fragments, and this treatment may alter the structural features of the protein involved in the regulation of its activity.

For maximal activity an excess of a tetrahydropteridine, or a system for reducing the quinoid form of the dihydropteridine produced during the hydroxylation of tyrosine, is required. The reducing system consists of dihydropteridine reductase and NADPH or a NADPH-generating system (135). Initial studies (111, 122) indicated that added Fe^{2+} was required for maximal activity, but Shiman et al. (135) have shown that Fe^{2+} acts to remove H_2O_2 probably generated by the nonenzymatic oxidation of the tetrahydropteridine by oxygen. Catalase or peroxidase completely obviated the requirement for Fe^{2+}.

Kinetic studies of tyrosine hydroxylase have yielded contradictory interpretations of the mechanism of the reactions. Data obtained by Ikeda et al. (65) with the partially purified native enzyme suggested that the reaction occurs sequentially—reduction of the oxidized form of the enzyme by the tetrahydropterin cofactor, dissociation of the reduced enzyme and oxidized cofactor, association of the reduced enzyme and tyrosine, and finally aerobic oxidation and release of dopa from the oxidized enzyme. To undergo a second cycle either excess reduced pteridine must be present or the oxidized pteridine must be reduced by dihydropteridine reductase and NADPH. Joh et al. (67), with a partially purified preparation obtained after tryptic digestion of the particulate enzyme, obtained data suggesting that the reaction proceeded through the formation of a quaternary complex consisting of tyrosine hydroxylase, reduced cofactor, tyrosine, and oxygen. These authors suggest that the different reaction mechanism may be due to different forms of the enzyme. The Michaelis-Menten constant (K_m) for 2-amino-4-hydroxy-6,7-dimethyltetrahydropteridine ($DMPH_4$) is 5×10^{-4} M and that for tyrosine in the presence of this cofactor has been reported to be from 1 to 10×10^{-5} M (65, 111). With the purified enzyme obtained after digestion with chymotrypsin and the natural cofactor, tetrahydrobiopterin (BH_4), Shiman et al. (135) obtained a K_m for tyrosine of 7×10^{-6} M.

Tyrosine hydroxylase exhibits a very high degree of substrate specificity toward L-tyrosine; D-tyrosine, DL-m-tyrosine, L-tryptophan, and tyramine are not hydroxylated. With either a crude (66, 135) or purified (135) preparation of the enzyme and with excess amounts of $DMPH_4$ as cofactor, phenylalanine is oxidized to tyrosine at about 5% of the rate of conversion of tyrosine to dopa. However, when BH_4 is used as cofactor with either the purified or particulate form of the enzyme, phenylalanine is converted to tyrosine at about the same rate as tyrosine is converted to dopa. Furthermore inhibition of the enzyme activity by high concentrations of tyrosine in the presence of $DMPH_4$ and a regenerating system, but not in the presence of BH_4, has been reported

(135). These observations suggest cautious interpretation of data obtained with the synthetic cofactor, as well as with modified forms of the enzyme.

The effects on tyrosine hydroxylase of a variety of analogues of tyrosine and catechol, as well as generalized enzyme inhibitors, have been studied (111, 152). Among the most potent inhibitors are 3-iodo-L-tyrosine, α-methyl-L-tyrosine, and 3-iodo-α-methyl-L-tyrosine. The catechols are weaker inhibitors and compete with $DMPH_4$. Among those tested, the most potent is 3,4-dihydroxyphenylpropylacetamide (H 22/48); in the presence of 1×10^{-4} M $DMPH_4$, 2×10^{-5} M H 22/48 causes a 50% inhibition; concentrations of 1 to 8×10^{-3} M of the other catechols were required under the same test conditions for 50% inhibition. At concentrations from 10^{-4} to 10^{-3} M, dinitrophenol, azide, p-chloromercuribenzoate, thiourea, and diethyldithiocarbamate had little effect. At 10^{-3} M, α,α'-dipyridyl was an effective inhibitor: it did not act as an iron chelator but competed with $DMPH_4$ (135).

Seven years of research on tyrosine hydroxylase has produced much information; it has also left several areas unsolved and has defined new areas where research is required. The subcellular localization of the enzyme remains controversial. Evidence is compelling that the enzyme is not localized in (149) or on the storage vesicles, although it may be closely associated with the vesicles in situ. A second unsolved point is the relation of the enzyme solubilized by proteolytic enzymes to the "native" soluble enzyme. Presently it would be rash to assume that studies utilizing the enzyme purified after proteolytic digestion can be unequivocally extrapolated to the native enzyme. Most studies on tyrosine hydroxylase have used the synthetic tetrahydropteridines as cofactors, but the studies of Shiman et al. (135) indicate important differences that may exist between these and the natural cofactor.

Dihydropteridine Reductase

Emphasis has been placed on tyrosine hydroxylase as the rate-controlling enzyme in the formation of norepinephrine (51, 90, 105, 155). However, in vivo the reaction is complex and most likely requires the participation of dihydropteridine reductase and NADPH to maintain levels of the reduced biopterin (9). All the available evidence indicates that tetrahydropteridines and dihydropteridine reductase participate in the tyrosine hydroxylase-catalyzed reaction in the same way they do in the phenylalanine hydroxylase-catalyzed reaction (9, 135). Dihydrobiopterin has been identified as the natural cofactor for phenylalanine hydroxylase (69), and this cofactor, as well as synthetic cofactors, function catalytically in both hydroxylating reactions in the presence of NADPH and dihydropteridine reductase (9, 104, 135). Lloyd & Weiner (91) have isolated dihydrobiopterin from the adrenal medulla and estimated the cofactor content of the gland to be 0.5–2.0 µg/g. Assuming that the cofactor is uniformly distributed in the cells, Musacchio (105) estimates the intracellular concentration to be 2×10^{-6} to 1×10^{-5} M, concentrations 10–50 times lower than normally used for the assay of tyrosine hydroxylase.

Kaufman (68) identified and elucidated the role of dihydropteridine reductase as a component of the phenylalanine hydroxylase system. The enzyme, isolated from sheep liver (71), utilizes NADPH to reduce the primary oxidation product, a quinoid formed from tetrahydropteridines during phenylalanine hydroxylation (70). Musacchio (104) has identified a similar enzyme in beef adrenal medulla. The enzyme requires NADPH for activity and markedly stimulates the formation of dopa from tyrosine under conditions in which the amount of tetrahydropteridine is limiting. The enzyme can reduce the quinoid form of biopterin but not biopterin itself and is not inhibited by aminopterin and methotrexate, potent inhibitors of tetrahydrofolate dehydrogenase. The enzyme has not been appreciably purified, and little information is available on its chemical and physical properties.

Musacchio (105) studied the effects of epinephrine (10^{-5} M) on the formation of dopa from tyrosine by using the complex system composed of tyrosine hydroxylase, dihydropteridine reductase, freshly prepared dimethyldihydropteridine, and a NADPH-generating system. The rate of dopa formation was a function of the amount of dihydropteridine reductase added, and at all concentrations of enzyme, 10^{-5} M epinephrine caused a 50% inhibition of dopa formation. However, in these studies it is not clear whether epinephrine was inhibiting tyrosine hydroxylase or dihydropteridine reductase. In any case the studies support the concept that feedback inhibition by norepinephrine or epinephrine may be an important regulatory mechanism (155).

Dopa Decarboxylase

Dopa decarboxylase (aromatic L-amino acid decarboxylase) was the first enzyme to be described in the norepinephrine pathway (64), even though its presence in chromaffin tissue was not demonstrated until 1952 (86). It is widely distributed in animal tissues, and except for its role in the synthesis of norepinephrine, epinephrine, and serotonin, it appears to serve no physiological function commensurate with its distribution and concentration (14, 62, 137). The enzyme exhibits a broad specificity toward aromatic amino acids (92, 137), and for this reason Lovenberg et al. (92) proposed that its name be changed to aromatic L-amino acid decarboxylase. The enzyme is most active with L-dopa as substrate; ortho- and meta-tyrosine are decarboxylated at about one-half the rate of dopa, but tyrosine itself is a very poor substrate, being decarboxylated at less than 0.5% the rate of dopa. Tryptophan, 5-hydroxytryptophan, and phenylalanine are decarboxylated at readily measurable rates, and histidine to a much lesser extent (14). For several years it was thought that dopa and 5-hydroxytryptophan were decarboxylated by separate enzymes, but evidence from several laboratories shows that the same enzyme has both activities, even though the relative rates of decarboxylation for the substrates vary from tissue to tissue (92, 137, 142). Pyridoxal phosphate is the cofactor for the reactions (71).

Most of the dopa decarboxylase activity of the adrenal medulla is readily obtained in the water-soluble fraction of homogenates, but small amounts (2–10%) are found in the storage vesicle fractions of the adrenal medulla (85), as well as in the norepinephrine-containing particles of splenic nerve homogenate (140). Because of its role in the formation of norepinephrine in sympathetic nerves, as well as in the formation of norepinephrine and epinephrine in the adrenal medulla, extensive investigations of inhibitors of the enzyme have been carried out with the aim of regulating norepinephrine synthesis in certain clinical conditions (16, 137).

Homogeneous preparations of dopa decarboxylase from bovine adrenal medulla (35) and hog kidney (14) have been reported. Fellman (35) obtained a preparation purified 20-fold from the high-speed supernatant fraction of an adrenal medulla homogenate that gave a single schlieren peak during sedimentation velocity centrifugation and a single protein peak by paper and free-flowing electrophoresis. The purified enzyme had a specific activity of 120 nmoles/min per milligram of protein. Christenson et al. (14) obtained a preparation from hog kidney that was purified 300-fold from a high-speed supernatant and had specific activity of 8,600 nmoles/min per milligram of protein. The protein was homogeneous, as indicated by sedimentation, disc gel electrophoresis, and immunologic techniques. The enzyme has a weight of 112,000 daltons and contains 0.9 mole of tightly bound pyridoxal phosphate per mole but still required the addition of pyridoxal phosphate for maximal activity. However, other data suggest that multiple forms of the enzyme may be present (14). Plots of ln c vs. r^2 for sedimentation equilibrium were linear at 4 degrees, but the plots obtained at 22 degrees were concave, and disc gel electrophoresis of the enzyme, which was homogeneous by other criteria, gave a broad band. Coulson et al. (21) obtained four peaks of dopa decarboxylase activity from the high-speed supernatant of rat liver homogenates by electrophoresis on polyacrylamide gel. Each of the bands decarboxylated both 5-hydroxytryptophan and dopa, but there appeared to be greater activity toward 5-hydroxytryptophan in the fastest-moving band and relatively greater activity toward dopa in the slowest-moving bands.

Dopamine β-hydroxylase

Dopamine β-hydroxylase is a mixed-function oxidase that catalyzes the oxidation of dopamine to norepinephrine, as shown in Figure 3 (89). Ascorbate can efficiently reduce the enzyme, but whether it is the physiological reductant is uncertain since scorbutic guinea pig hearts showed no decrease in the rate of formation of norepinephrine from tyrosine or dopamine (90). Goldstein & Joh (44) have found that $DMPH_4$ or cysteine can replace ascorbate as a cofactor for dopamine β-hydroxylase, but at equimolar concentrations they stimulate the reaction to only about one-half the extent that ascorbate does. To obtain maximal activity in vitro the presence of catalase and a dicarboxylic acid (e.g., fumarate) is required (89). Catalase protects the enzyme by decomposing hydrogen peroxide formed in the reaction mixture, and fumarate appears to increase the rate of reaction of the reduced enzyme with oxygen (45, 48); increasing the oxygen concentration can largely replace the requirement for fumarate.

Dopamine β-hydroxylase appears to be contained exclusively in the catecholamine storage vesicles (73, 85, 115), with the exception of small amounts of enzyme that may be present in vesicle membranes after vesicles release their contents and that present in newly forming vesicles (see the chapter by Viveros in this volume of the *Handbook*). The enzyme is also present in the 100,000-g supernatant prepared from glands homogenized in isotonic media, but this comes mostly from the storage vesicles disrupted during preparation. Initial studies (73, 89) suggested that all the enzyme was firmly bound to membranes of the storage vesicles, but subsequent work revealed the presence of potent endogenous inhibitors (19, 31, 89, 108, 109) in homogenates of adrenal medulla. Inactivation of the inhibitors by addition of sulfhydryl-reactive agents, such as N-ethylmaleimide (109), p-chloromercuribenzoate, Ag^+, Hg^+, or Cu^{2+}, showed the enzyme to be present in the soluble proteins obtained upon lysis of the storage vesicles in water, as well as firmly bound to storage vesicle membranes (31). The relative amounts of enzyme present in the soluble and particulate fractions of storage vesicles vary among species. In bovine and rabbit adrenal glands, about equal amounts of enzyme are found in both fractions, but in rat adrenals only about 25% is readily soluble (77).

Tissues other than the adrenal medulla also contain inhibitors of dopamine β-hydroxylase (2, 15, 19), and it seems likely that a single tissue may contain more than one inhibitor. The inhibitor from adrenal medulla has been partially purified and characterized (30). It is a sulfhydryl compound closely related to reduced glutathione but is not identical with the latter. The inhibitor from heart has also been partially characterized (15). It contains organic phosphate, carbohydrate, only trace amounts of nitrogen, and no sulfur. It is inactivated by Cu^{2+}, but unlike the inhibitor from the adrenal medulla, it is not inactivated by N-ethylmaleimide. No physiological role has been assigned to the endogenous inhibitor, or inhibitors, but in the adrenal medulla it may

$$E-(Cu^{2+})_2 + Ascorbate \rightarrow E-(Cu^+)_2 - dehydro\ ascorbate + 2H^+$$

$$E-(Cu^+)_2 + dopamine + O_2 + 2H^+ \rightarrow E-(Cu^{2+})_2 + noradrenaline + H_2O$$

Dopamine + ascorbate + O_2 → noradrenaline + dehydro ascorbate + H_2O

FIG. 3. Oxidation of dopamine to norepinephrine (*noradrenaline*) catalyzed by dopamine β-hydroxylase.

inactivate dopamine β-hydroxylase present in the membranes of the storage vesicles after secretion of their contents (see the chapter by Viveros in this volume of the *Handbook*).

The enzyme is not specific for dopamine and will oxidize a wide variety of phenylethylamines to their corresponding β-OH derivatives (20, 43, 88, 152a). Van der Schoot & Creveling (152a) have reviewed this, as well as a large body of information on inhibitors of dopamine β-hydroxylase.

Dopamine β-hydroxylase has been purified to apparent homogeneity (36, 37). It has a molecular weight of 290,000 and contains 2 moles of Cu^{2+} per mole of enzyme. The K_m for dopamine is of the order of 10^{-3} M. Studies of the partial reactions with the purified enzyme (37) and kinetic analysis (48) show the reaction to proceed sequentially. Ascorbate first reduces an approximately equivalent amount of enzyme and is oxidized to dehydroascorbate. Oxygen and substrate then react with the reduced enzyme to form the β-hydroxylated derivative, water, and the oxidized form of the enzyme. The oxygen atom incorporated into the substrate comes from molecular oxygen (76). Chemical analysis (36, 37) and electron paramagnetic resonance studies (38, 49) demonstrate that the Cu^{2+} present in the enzyme functions as the electron carrier and cycles between the monovalent and divalent forms.

Phenylethanolamine N-methyltransferase

The formation of epinephrine from norepinephrine is catalyzed by phenylethanolamine N-methyltransferase (PNMT), which transfers the S-methyl group from S-adenosylmethionine to the primary nitrogen group of norepinephrine (3, 75). In mammals PNMT is almost exclusively localized in the adrenal medulla; only very small amounts have been reported to be present in heart and brain (3, 95, 123). The enzyme is readily obtained in the water-soluble fraction of tissue homogenates (3, 75) and is generally considered to be a cytoplasmic enzyme, although approximately 10% of the total activity may be found associated with the particulate fraction of storage vesicles (44, 47). Also a cytoplasmic enzyme, S-adenosylmethionine synthetase catalyzes the formation of S-adenosylmethionine from methionine and ATP (75). Thus the adrenal medulla can efficiently use methionine as a source of methyl groups, and in fact the adrenal gland has one of the highest levels of S-adenosylmethionine of any tissue of the body (5).

Phenylethanolamine N-methyltransferase exhibits a very marked substrate specificity for a hydroxyl group on the β carbon of the side chain of phenylethylamines, but substituents on the aromatic ring have only moderate effects. Both primary and secondary phenylethanolamines can be N-methylated, but secondary amines are much poorer substrates than their corresponding primary amines (3). A low order of specificity is also displayed toward *l*- and *d*-enantiomorphs, although *l*-isomers are somewhat better substrates (3). The enzyme is inhibited by *p*-chloromercuribenzoate, has an optimal pH between 7.5 and 9 depending to some extent on the buffer used, and is not stimulated by addition of metal ions (3).

Phenylethanolamine N-methyltransferase has been purified to apparent homogeneity and has a molecular weight of 38,000 (17). Crude preparations of the enzyme are fairly stable and may be stored frozen for several months with only slight losses of activity, but the purified enzyme is quite unstable. At concentrations above 2 mg enzyme protein per milliliter, aggregation occurs with irreversible loss of activity (17). Titration with *p*-hydroxymercuribenzoate shows the presence of 8.5 moles of sulfhydryl groups per mole of enzyme; complete activity is lost upon titration of 2 moles of sulfhydryl groups per mole of enzyme. The enzyme is also markedly inhibited by concentrations of norepinephrine or epinephrine only slightly in excess of those required for maximal activity (17, 39, 40).

Kinetic studies suggest that the reaction proceeds through the formation of a ternary complex with a random order of binding in which S-adenosylmethionine is the preferred first substrate bound (17). Attempts to demonstrate the formation of a methyl enzyme as an intermediate in the reaction gave negative results (17).

The distribution of biosynthetic enzymes is such that tyrosine is oxidized to dopa and the latter decarboxylated to dopamine in the cytosol. Dopamine then enters the storage vesicles, by a mechanism that is facilitated by Mg^{2+}-ATP and inhibited by reserpine, where it is converted to norepinephrine. Norepinephrine may be stored in the vesicles, or it may be released into the cytosol where it can be methylated to epinephrine and the latter taken up and stored by the vesicles.

REGULATION OF NOREPINEPHRINE SYNTHESIS

Two different mechanisms have been proposed for regulating the rate of norepinephrine synthesis in both the adrenal medulla and sympathetic nerves: one is responsive to immediate demands for increased production, and the other is responsive to increased chronic stimulation and leads to increased total amounts of enzyme, specifically tyrosine hydroxylase. Most of the work on regulation of norepinephrine synthesis has been done on sympathetically innervated tissues, and this is briefly reviewed before proceeding with a more detailed discussion of the adrenal medulla.

Acute Regulation in Sympathetic Nerves in Response to Stimulation

The concept that tyrosine hydroxylase is the rate-limiting enzyme in norepinephrine synthesis is based on the reports by Levitt et al. (90). In isolated, perfused guinea pig hearts the amounts of norepinephrine formed from tyrosine, dopa, or dopamine increased with increasing amounts of precursor, but only with tyrosine were saturating levels of substrate achieved. Perfusion of adrenal glands or incubation of medulla slices also demonstrates that dopa and dopamine are converted to norepinephrine at much faster rates than tyrosine (50, 124). These data show that in the perfused tissue the rate-limiting step is the conversion of tyrosine to dopa but do not necessarily indicate that tyrosine hydroxylase is the rate-limiting enzyme. Levitt et al. (90) have considered the possibility that transport of tyrosine across the neuronal membrane may be a catalyzed process with a K_m comparable to that of tyrosine hydroxylase. The rate at which the dihydropteridine cofactor is reduced by dihydropteridine reductase could also be the regulator. The observation by Ikeda et al. (65) that tyrosine hydroxylase was inhibited by catechols suggested that this enzyme was subject to feedback regulation. A host of other studies (see below) have produced results consistent with the proposal that tyrosine hydroxylase is the rate-limiting and regulatory enzyme, but these studies do not completely rule out alternate possibilities.

Studies of sympathetically innervated tissues indicate that enhanced neural activity stimulates the rate of synthesis of norepinephrine. Under varying states of nervous activity the sympathetic nerves maintain their norepinephrine content at constant levels (34, 93) even though the turnover rate is increased during activity (18, 51, 116) and decreased after decentralization (58). A major role for maintaining the catecholamine stores has been attributed to the reuptake of the released amines by an amine pump localized in the neuronal membrane (55), but recent evidence suggests that de novo synthesis may also play a significant role. After administration of α-methyltyrosine, an inhibitor of tyrosine hydroxylase (138), increased neural activity causes a more rapid decline in the catecholamine levels (51). Studies of norepinephrine synthesis and release in perfused spleen (78) and heart (141) show that, during perfusion with ^{14}C-tyrosine, stimulation of the sympathetic nerves releases ^{14}C-norepinephrine with a higher specific activity than that present in the entire organ. The authors suggest that, during rapid stimulation, de novo synthesis plays a significant role in maintenance of transmitter release. The accumulation of radioactively labeled norepinephrine after administration of labeled tyrosine is increased two- to threefold as a result of nervous stimulation both in vivo (51, 116, 133, 134) and in vitro (1, 126, 157). However, the radioactive studies cannot be interpreted unequivocally as demonstrating an increased rate of norepinephrine formation for several reasons. The amount of labeled product accumulated at a single time point after the administration of a single dose of labeled precursor does not give absolute amounts of product formed. The equilibration of isotope in plasma and tissue is slow; 1 hr after the injection of a single dose of ^{14}C-tyrosine, the specific activities in heart, brain, and spleen were only one-third to one-half those in plasma (134). Stimulation may greatly increase the rate of equilibration within the neuron itself without affecting the specific activities in the parenchymal tissue. Since the nerves compose only a small portion of the total tissue, the higher specific activity in the nerves would not be detectable and would indicate only an apparent increase in the rate of norepinephrine formation. Measurement of norepinephrine accumulation during continuous perfusion of labeled precursor (134) enables estimation of minimal absolute rates of formation (assuming specific activity in the neuron is the same as in plasma) but still does not rule out the possibility that the increased accumulation observed in intact tissues compared to decentralized tissues may have been due to an increased rate of equilibration.

The increased accumulation of ^{14}C-norepinephrine after nerve stimulation has been attributed to activation of tyrosine hydroxylase by release of feedback inhibition (51, 155). It is proposed that stimulation results in the release of a chemically undetectable pool of norepinephrine that had inhibited tyrosine hydroxylase (1, 51, 157). Alternatively some other inhibitors may be released, or, as a result of nerve stimulation, a new compound that may react with a regulator site on the enzyme may be synthesized (51). Consistent with the hypothesis of end product inhibition are the reports that *a)* in the isolated vas deferens preparation, addition of norepinephrine to the bath blocks the increased formation of norepinephrine from tyrosine (1), *b)* monoamine oxidase inhibitors decrease the rate of catecholamine synthesis from tyrosine (113, 114), and *c)* nerve stimulation both in vivo and in vitro does not enhance the formation of norepinephrine from dopa (22, 133, 157). The experiments with ^{14}C-dopa may be misleading since there is essentially no endogenous pool of this compound.

Although studies of sympathetically innervated tissues indicate that neural activity stimulates the rate of norepinephrine synthesis, the intracellular distribution of biosynthetic enzyme and the cofactor requirements, including NADPH for the reduction of dihydrobiopterin and ATP for uptake of dopamine into the storage vesicles, make it extremely difficult to localize a regulatory site from in vivo studies. Little is known about dihydropteridine reductase, and this enzyme may very well be a regulatory site. Stimulation of the neuron may markedly change the levels of NADPH and ATP that would act to increase the availability of tetrahydrobiopterin and promote the uptake of dopamine into the storage vesicles. Dopa and dopamine, once formed, may be removed from the biosynthetic pathway either by leakage from the cell (56, 57) or by the action of degradative enzymes. When radioisotopic tracers are used, misleading data may be obtained because of changes in the rate of equilibration of isotope induced by stimulation, changes in the rate of delivery to the tissues resulting from altered blood flow, changes in O_2 tension, and changes in intracellular pH. The factors that regulate norepinephrine synthesis are complex, and before any conclusions can be drawn it is necessary to examine critically the experimental design and the evidence.

Acute Regulation in Adrenal Medulla in Response to Immediate Demands

A number of studies of adrenal medullary secretion suggest that rapid replacement of the secreted amine occurs during or shortly after the stimulation period. Holland & Schümann (60) electrically stimulated the splanchnic nerves of cat adrenal glands and estimated the medullary outflow of amines by comparing the blood pressure response elicited by splanchnic stimulation of the left adrenal gland to the increase in blood pressure produced by an infusion of a solution of equal parts of epinephrine and norepinephrine into the external jugular vein. The levels of amine in the right adrenal gland served as a control for the initial levels of amine in the stimulated gland. Stimulation of the left gland resulted in an estimated amine release of 584 µg/g gland into the adrenomedullary outflow but to a decrease of only 256 µg/g in the gland itself. The difference of 328 µg/g, equivalent to 38% of the amine content of the right gland, was attributed to amine synthesis during the stimulation period. The authors concluded that stimulation of the gland results in an increased rate of synthesis of norepinephrine and its methylation. In similar experiments, but with the difference that the adrenal venous blood was collected and assayed externally, Bygdeman & von Euler (12) also found that the release of amines into the blood was often considerably in excess of the loss from the gland. However, after injection of insulin or nicotine, only occasionally did release exceed losses from the gland. In another series of experiments in which the amount of epinephrine released from the medulla during insulin-induced hypoglycemia was estimated from the amount appearing in the urine, Bygdeman et al. (13) reported that depletion of the gland was accompanied by a resynthesis in 24 hr amounting to more than twice the normal content, even though at 24 hr after insulin injection the gland was markedly depleted. The concept of rapid resynthesis appears incompatible with numerous reports of other investigators that recovery of the adrenal catecholamine stores requires several days (10, 59, 150, 154) and is in direct contrast to the reports of Butterworth & Mann (11) and Eade & Wood (33). The latter two groups measured the amount of epinephrine appearing in the adrenal venous outflow after repeated injections of acetylcholine (11) or after electrical stimulation of the splanchnic nerve (33). Each group found that the amounts of epinephrine and norepinephrine in the venous outflow were quantitatively similar to the loss of amines from the stimulated glands. No evidence for rapid resynthesis of the released amines was obtained.

The differences between the observations of Holland & Schümann (60) and Bygdeman and co-workers (12, 13) and those of Butterworth & Mann (11) and Eade & Wood (33) may be due to several reasons. Eade & Wood (33) have suggested that the method of estimating the amounts of epinephrine and norepinephrine released from the adrenal medulla by comparing the blood pressure responses in the same animal to constant infusions of epinephrine and norepinephrine administered via the jugular vein may not be quantitatively valid. These authors also suggest that the pressor response observed upon stimulation of the splanchnic nerve may not be entirely due to release of epinephrine and norepinephrine. Extrapolation of the amounts of epinephrine appearing in the urine to amounts released from the adrenal gland may also not be quantitatively accurate. Another difference between the experiments is that Eade and Wood removed the control right gland before stimulating the left gland, whereas Holland and Schümann, and Bygdeman and von Euler removed the gland at the end of the experiment. Losses from the right gland during the experimental period would appear in the calculations as a decreased loss from the left gland. These conflicting reports do not allow the conclusion that during splanchnic stimulation appreciable amounts of the released amines are replaced by resynthesis.

Smith & Robinson (136) suggest that rapid resynthesis may occur in a readily secretable pool. They found that the presence of dopa or dopamine in the perfusion medium significantly retarded the declining secretory response to repeated injections of histamine. The effect of dopamine was abolished if an inhibitor of dopamine β-hydroxylase was also present in the medium. However, there were no increases in the total amounts of epinephrine and norepinephrine (perfusate plus remaining content of gland) in the presence of precursors. These observations cannot be interpreted unequivocally as evidence for increased synthesis. The observed effects may have been due to a facilitation of the response to histamine by dopa or dopamine or their metabolites. Kovacic & Robinson (79) found that after a series of 55 injections of nicotine into the perfusate from dog adrenal glands, the gland no longer responded to nicotine, but its secretory response to acetylcholine, pilocarpine, angiotensin, bradykinin, or histamine was greatly facilitated.

Other indirect evidence has also been interpreted to indicate increased rates of norepinephrine synthesis in the adrenal gland during splanchnic stimulation. Gordon et al. (51) found that 3 hr of exercise on a rotating drum caused only a moderate decrease in adrenal catecholamines, but if the animals were given α-methyltyrosine, which by itself had no effect on adrenal amine levels, before exercise a marked depletion of amines occurred. This depletion was presumed to result from failure to resynthesize the released amines. However, α-methyltyrosine inhibits tyrosine hydroxylase throughout the sympathetic nervous system and leads to lower levels of norepinephrine. In these same experiments α-methyltyrosine by itself produced in 1.5 hr a 20% decrease in heart norepinephrine, and when 1 hr of exercise was included in this period a 60% decrease occurred.

The declining levels of norepinephrine in sympathetic nerves may have resulted in lower levels of output per stimulus, which resulted in a reflexly increased rate of neuronal impulses to compensate for decreased outflow. Part or all of the decreased levels of amines in the adrenal medulla after exercise and treatment with α-methyltyrosine may have been due to an increased rate of secretion as a result of increased splanchnic stimulation rather than to an inhibition of synthesis.

Attempts to demonstrate directly an increased rate of formation of norepinephrine from tyrosine have also produced results of equivocal interpretation. Gordon et al. (51) found a two- to threefold increase in the accumulation of ^{14}C-norepinephrine formed from ^{14}C-tyrosine after 1 hr of exercise in rat adrenals, heart, brain, and spleen. If resynthesis of released amines had occurred during exercise it is surprising that there was only a two- to threefold increase in radioactively labeled amines after administration of ^{14}C-tyrosine. Since the half-life of catecholamine in rat adrenal has been reported to be 107 hr (24) very little synthesis would be expected during 1 hr in control animals, but the experiments indicate that approximately one-half the initial amines were resynthesized during the 3-hr exercise period. A possible explanation may be that most of the newly synthesized amines had been released immediately and that in the absence of de novo synthesis the endogenous stores were utilized, but this seems unlikely (see the chapter by Viveros in this volume of the *Handbook*). A more likely explanation may be that increased rates of formation of norepinephrine from tyrosine actually did occur, but they were quite small in comparison to the amount released. In the adrenal medulla, as well as in sympathetic nerves, stimulation produced no increase in the accumulation of labeled norepinephrine when ^{14}C-dopa was administered (22).

Weiner & Rutledge (158) studied slices of adrenal medulla and found that reserpine prevented the formation of dopamine and norepinephrine. The inhibition of norepinephrine formation is attributed to the blockade of dopamine uptake by the storage vesicles where it would be converted to norepinephrine. The decreased formation of dopamine is attributed to feedback inhibition of tyrosine hydroxylase by the increased concentration of cytoplasmic amines resulting from uptake blockade (65). It is interesting that tyrosine hydroxylase from human pheochromocytomas is much less sensitive to inhibition by norepinephrine than is the enzyme from the normal adrenal gland (112, 127). It has been suggested that the excessive production of catecholamines in pheochromocytomas may be due to altered sensitivity of tyrosine hydroxylase to inhibition by norepinephrine.

The evidence that stimulation of the adrenal medulla results in an immediate substantial resynthesis of norepinephrine and epinephrine is not convincing. Experiments that have compared the loss of amines from the gland to the appearance of amines in the venous outflow are in direct conflict and cannot be easily resolved. When inhibitors of tyrosine hydroxylase are used in conjunction with exercise or other types of stimuli, the possibility that the increased losses are due to a synergistic effect rather than inhibition of resynthesis has not been ruled out. The accumulation of labeled product is not a quantitative measure of synthesis and can only be used as a relative measure of synthesis provided there are no other significant changes that may affect accumulation.

Regulation in Response to Prolonged Stimulation

A variety of treatments that increase splanchnic stimulation result, within 24 to 48 hr, in marked increases in tyrosine hydroxylase activity of the adrenal gland. These treatments include sinoaortic denervation (27); insulin-induced hypoglycemia (118, 154, 156); treatment with 6-hydroxydopamine (97, 146), reserpine (99, 145, 146), phenoxybenzamine (22, 145, 146), and amphetamine (94); immobilization (84) or cold stress (144); and psychosocial stimulation (4). The increase in tyrosine hydroxylase activity also occurs in other sympathetic tissue (144, 145, 148) and appears to be a response to chronic stimulation as a mechanism for increasing steady-state levels of norepinephrine or epinephrine. The enhanced enzyme activity appears to be due to de novo protein synthesis since the rises are blocked by actinomycin D and cycloheximide (98, 118, 156).

The increase in enzyme activity in the adrenal medulla is mediated via the splanchnic innervation through the release of acetylcholine. Denervation of the gland completely abolishes the increase in tyrosine hydroxylase activity (84, 98, 118, 146, 156), but the increases can be obtained in denervated glands by repeated intravenous injections of acetylcholine into atropinized, eserinized rats (118, 120). The combination of eserine and atropine has no effect on the tyrosine hydroxylase activity of denervated glands but does cause elevation in intact glands (118, 120). Mueller et al. (101) reported that the nicotinic receptor blockers, chlorisondamine and pempidine, block the increase in tyrosine hydroxylase normally observed in superior cervical ganglia after reserpine treatment, but neither pempidine nor atropine, alone or in combination, block increases in adrenal gland activity. On the contrary, pempidine, chlorisondamine, and atropine by themselves produce increases in tyrosine hydroxylase similar to that produced by reserpine, and these effects can be blocked by transection of the splanchnic nerve. The authors suggest that the inability of the blockers to prevent the increase in adrenal tyrosine hydroxylase may be due to *a*) an incomplete blockade of the receptors, *b*) a different type of receptor, or *c*) a neurotransmitter other than acetylcholine for the adrenal medulla. The report (118) that acetylcholine can induce increases in tyrosine hydroxylase in denervated glands makes the latter possibility unlikely. Since all evidence indicates that the adrenal medulla contains only nicotinic and muscarinic receptors (see the chapter by Viveros in this volume of the *Handbook*), it is most likely that the observations (101) are explained by a lack of complete blockade.

There appears to be little relation between the increase in tyrosine hydroxylase and the degree of catecholamine depletion. Insulin-induced hypoglycemia causes an 80% depletion of the catecholamine content in 4 hr and results in a 40% increase in tyrosine hydroxylase measured 20 hr later, whereas treatment with acetylcholine and eserine produced a 20% depletion of the catecholamine content in denervated glands and a 50-60% increase in tyrosine hydroxylase (118). Mueller et al. (97, 101) found little or no decrease in the catecholamine content after treatment with 6-hydroxydopamine, atropine, and chlorisondamine but marked increases in tyrosine hydroxylase. On the other hand, Weiner & Mosimann (156) found a good correlation between the loss of catecholamines and increase in tyrosine hydroxylase in cat adrenals after insulin treatment. One might reasonably expect a relation between the degree of stimulation and the increase in tyrosine hydroxylase. The available data indicate that a series of moderate stimuli or chronic moderate stimulation is at least as effective, if not more so, than massive stimulation produced by large doses of insulin. This suggests that the stimulation threshold for maximal increases in tyrosine hydroxylase may be quite low and that secondary metabolic effects of insulin may inhibit subsequent increases in tyrosine hydroxylase.

The relation between increased levels of tyrosine hydroxylase activity and increased rates of catecholamine synthesis has not been clearly established. In earlier studies, Duner (32) and Kroneberg & Schümann (80) found that cutting the splanchnic innervation of the left adrenal gland after insulin (32) or reserpine (80) treatment resulted in a marked delay in the recovery of the depleted catecholamine stores compared to that in the intact right gland. Patrick & Kirshner (120) have confirmed these effects in rat adrenals denervated before reserpine treatment and have further shown that, if several doses of acetylcholine are administered 1 day after reserpine treatment, tyrosine hydroxylase activity increases in the denervated gland, and the denervated gland then recovers its catecholamine stores at the same time as does the intact gland. However, because of the complexity of the recovery process, it is not certain whether the accelerated recovery was due to an increased capability for norepinephrine synthesis or to an increased rate of recovery of the storage vesicles and their ability to sequester the amines. Dairman & Udenfriend (23) found two- to threefold increases in the incorporation of radioactive label into catecholamines from ^{14}C-tyrosine during a 1-hr period 24 hr after a single treatment with phenoxybenzamine and a four- to sixfold increase 24 hr after treatment with phenoxybenzamine on two successive days. At this time the tyrosine hydroxylase activity of the homogenate was twice that of controls, but 24 hr after a single dose of phenoxybenzamine no increase in tyrosine hydroxylase was observed (22, 24). Pentolinium, a ganglionic blocking agent, abolished the increased incorporation observed after a single injection of phenoxybenzamine but caused only a slight decrease in the incorporation observed after the 2-day treatment. The authors suggest that pentolinium inhibited the incorporation due only to increased neuronal stimulation and that the uninhibited, increased incorporation after two injections of phenoxybenzamine was due to the increased levels of tyrosine hydroxylase. As in other studies that employ measurement at a single time point after a single injection of ^{14}C-tyrosine, these results are ambiguous and may be equally well interpreted to indicate only an increased retention of ^{14}C-catecholamine rather than an increased rate of formation.

Reduced levels of rat adrenal tyrosine hydroxylase have been found after treatment for 4-7 days with large doses (1,000 mg/kg) of L-dopa (24). This treatment also resulted in a 70% increase in the rate of synthesis of norepinephrine and epinephrine as reflected by a reduction in the turnover half-life, but the adrenal levels of epinephrine were unchanged. The author suggests that the decreased levels of tyrosine hydroxylase indicate an attempted compensation for the increase in catecholamine synthesis resulting from bypassing the tyrosine hydroxylase reaction and that L-dopa or one of its products may inhibit the synthesis or increase the rate of degradation of the enzyme.

The levels of dopamine β-hydroxylase are also affected by increased neural stimulation (81, 82, 96, 154). Initially enzyme activities decrease because of loss of the soluble enzyme during secretion followed by recovery to normal or highly elevated levels in the next 24-48 hr. These changes have been correlated with the secretory cycle (see the chapter by Viveros in this volume of the *Handbook*), but it is believed that the increased levels of dopamine β-hydroxylase per se do not have a significant effect on the recovery of the catecholamine stores. Increased levels of phenylethanolamine N-methyltransferase after neural stimulation have been reported (147). Endocrine factors, which are discussed elsewhere in this volume, are also involved in the maintenance of activities of tyrosine hydroxylase, dopamine β-hydroxylase, and PNMT (41, 83, 100, 159, 160, 170).

The intact nerve supply exerts an effect on the normal age-dependent increases in the catecholamine stores and biosynthetic capabilities of the gland. Denervation of the gland at 23 days of age in the rat markedly slows the developmental increases in catecholamine, tyrosine hydroxylase, and dopamine β-hydroxylase content. If the animals are denervated at 8 weeks of age, the subsequent increases observed in intact glands are completely prevented (119). In the normal animal the increase in body size, as well as environmental stimuli

(4), will increase the demand for adrenal medullary secretion and lead to increased levels of tyrosine hydroxylase and dopamine β-hydroxylase.

CONCLUSION

Each of the enzymes of the biosynthetic pathway for epinephrine has been purified and partially characterized. Because of the apparent role of tyrosine hydroxylase as the rate-limiting enzyme in the pathway, it is important to obtain more definitive information on the physical and chemical properties of tyrosine hydroxylase and the manner in which it may be regulated. Further studies of dihydropteridine reductase as a possible regulatory enzyme are also indicated.

Many studies indicate that stimulation of sympathetic nerves results in an immediate increase in the rate of formation of norepinephrine from tyrosine, and this appears to be of importance in the maintenance of neurotransmitter stores. Release of feedback inhibitors of tyrosine hydroxylase has been proposed as the mechanism for regulating norepinephrine synthesis, but the putative regulatory molecule, or molecules, remains to be more firmly identified. Although acute stimulation may increase the rate of formation of catecholamines in the adrenal medulla, evidence that this results in rapid resynthesis of substantial amounts of the released amines is contradictory.

In both sympathetic nerves and adrenal medulla, prolonged or repeated stimulation results, within 24 to 48 hr, in marked increases in tyrosine hydroxylase activity. The increase in tyrosine hydroxylase activity appears to be an adaptive response of the organism for increased secretion of norepinephrine and epinephrine.

REFERENCES

1. ALOUSI, A., AND N. WEINER. The regulation of norepinephrine synthesis in sympathetic nerves: effect of nerve stimulation, cocaine, and catecholamine-releasing agents. *Proc. Natl. Acad. Sci. US* 56: 1491–1496, 1966.
2. AUSTIN, L., B. G. LIVETT, AND I. W. CHUBB. Biosynthesis of noradrenaline in sympathetic nervous tissue. *Am. Heart Assoc. Monogr.* 17: 111–117, 1967.
3. AXELROD, J. Purification and properties of phenylethanolamine-N-methyltransferase. *J. Biol. Chem.* 237: 1657–1660, 1962.
4. AXELROD, J., R. A. MUELLER, J. P. HENRY, AND P. M. STEPHENS. Changes in enzymes involved in the biosynthesis and metabolism of noradrenaline and adrenaline after psychosocial stimulation. *Nature* 225: 1059–1060, 1970.
5. BALDESSARINI, R. I., AND I. J. KOPIN. Assay of tissue levels of S-adenosylmethionine. *Anal. Biochem.* 6: 289–292, 1963.
6. BLASCHKO, H. The specific action of L-Dopa decarboxylase. *J. Physiol., London* 96: 50–51P, 1939.
7. BLASCHKO, H. The development of current concepts of catecholamine formation. *Ann. Rev. Pharmacol.* 11: 307–316, 1959.
8. BLASCHKO, H., P. HAGEN, AND A. D. WELCH. Observations on the intracellular granules of the adrenal medulla. *J. Physiol., London* 129: 27–49, 1955.
9. BRENNEMAN, A. R., AND S. KAUFMAN. The role of tetrahydropteridines in the enzymatic conversion of tyrosine to 3,4-dihydroxyphenylalanine. *Biochem. Biophys. Res. Commun.* 17: 177–183, 1964.
10. BUTTERWORTH, K. R., AND M. MANN. The adrenaline and noradrenaline content of the adrenal gland of the cat following depletion by acetylcholine. *Brit. J. Pharmacol.* 12: 415–421, 1957.
11. BUTTERWORTH, K. R., AND M. MANN. The release of adrenaline and noradrenaline from the adrenal gland of the cat by acetylcholine. *Brit. J. Pharmacol.* 12: 422–426, 1957.
12. BYGDEMAN, S., AND U. S. VON EULER. Resynthesis of catechol hormones in the cat's adrenal medulla. *Acta Physiol. Scand.* 44: 375–383, 1958.
13. BYGDEMAN, S., U. S. VON EULER, AND B. HÖKFELT. Resynthesis of adrenaline in the rabbit's adrenal medulla during insulin-induced hypoglycemia. *Acta Physiol. Scand.* 49: 21–28, 1960.
14. CHRISTENSON, J. C., W. DAIRMAN, AND S. UDENFRIEND. Preparation and properties of a homogenous aromatic L-amino acid decarboxylase from hog kidney. *Arch. Biochem. Biophys.* 141: 356–367, 1970.
15. CHUBB, I. W., B. N. PRESTON, AND L. AUSTIN. Partial characterization of a naturally occurring inhibitor of dopamine-β-hydroxylase. *Biochem. J.* 111: 243–244, 1969.
16. CLARK, W. G. Studies of inhibition of L-Dopa decarboxylase in vitro and in vivo. *Ann. Rev. Pharmacol.* 11: 330–349, 1959.
17. CONNETT, R. J., AND N. KIRSHNER. Purification and properties of bovine phenylethanolamine N-methyl transferase. *J. Biol. Chem.* 245: 329–334, 1970.
18. COSTA, E., AND N. H. NEFF. Isotopic and non-isotopic measurements of catecholamine biosynthesis. In: *Biochemistry and Pharmacology of the Basal Ganglia*, edited by E. Costa, L. Cote, and M. D. Yahr. New York: Raven Press, 1966, p. 132–150.
19. CREVELING, C. R. *Studies on Dopamine-β-Oxidase* (Doctoral thesis). Washington, D. C.: George Washington University, 1962.
20. CREVELING, C. R., J. W. DALY, B. WITKOP, AND S. UDENFRIEND. Substrates and inhibitors of dopamine-β-hydroxylase. *Biochim. Biophys. Acta* 64: 125–134, 1962.
21. COULSON, W. F., D. A. BENDER, AND J. B. JEPSON. Multiple electrophoresis peaks of rat liver decarboxylases for 3,4-dihydroxyphenylalanine and 5-hydroxytryptophan. *Biochem. J.* 115: 63–64P, 1969.
22. DAIRMAN, W., R. GORDON, S. SPECTOR, A. SJOERDSMA, AND S. UDENFRIEND. Increased synthesis of catecholamines in intact rat following administration of α-adrenergic blocking agents. *Mol. Pharmacol.* 4: 457–464, 1968.
23. DAIRMAN, W., AND S. UDENFRIEND. Increased conversion of tyrosine to catecholamines in the intact rat following elevation of tissue tyrosine hydroxylase levels by administered phenoxybenzamine. *Mol. Pharmacol.* 6: 350–356, 1970.
24. DAIRMAN, W., AND S. UDENFRIEND. Decrease in tyrosine hydroxylase and increase in norepinephrine synthesis in rats given L-Dopa. *Science* 171: 1022–1024, 1971.
25. DEMIS, A. J., H. BLASCHKO, AND A. D. WELCH. The conversion of bovine adrenal medullary homogenates. *J. Pharmacol.* 113: 14–15, 1955.
26. DEMIS, A. J., H. BLASCHKO, AND A. D. WELCH. The conversion of dihydroxyphenylalanine-2-C^{14} (DOPA) to norepinephrine by bovine adrenal medullary homogenates. *J. Pharmacol.* 117: 207–212, 1956.
27. DE QUATRO, V., R. MARONDE, T. NAGATSU, AND N. ALEXANDER. Altered norepinephrine synthesis and storage in the hypertensive buffer denervated rabbit. *Federation Proc.* 27: 240, 1968.

28. DEVINE, J. Observations on the *in vitro* synthesis of adrenaline under physiological conditions. *Biochem. J.* 34: 21–31, 1940.
29. DRELL, W., M. ESHELMAN, AND W. G. CLARK. Dihydroxyphenylserine as a precursor of arterenol. *Commun. Intern. Congr. Biochem., 1958, 4th, Abstr. 170*.
30. DUCH, D. S., AND N. KIRSHNER. Isolation and partial characterization of an endogenous inhibitor of dopamine-β-hydroxylase. *Biochim. Biophys. Acta* 236: 628–638, 1971.
31. DUCH, D. S., O. H. VIVEROS, AND N. KIRSHNER. Endogenous inhibitor(s) in adrenal medulla of dopamine-β-hydroxylase. *Biochem. Pharmacol.* 17: 255–264, 1968.
32. DUNER, H. The effect of insulin hypoglycemia on the secretion of adrenaline and noradrenaline from the suprarenal of cat. *Acta Physiol. Scand.* 32: 63–68, 1954.
33. EADE, N. R., AND C. R. WOOD. The release of adrenaline and noradrenaline from the adrenal medulla of the cat during splanchnic stimulation. *Brit. J. Pharmacol.* 13: 390–394, 1958.
34. EULER, U. S. VON, AND S. HELLNER-BJORKMAN. Effect of increased adrenergic nerve activity on the content of noradrenaline in cat organs. *Acta Physiol. Scand. Suppl.* 118: 17–20, 1955.
35. FELLMAN, J. H. Purification and properties of adrenal L-Dopa decarboxylase. *Enzymologia* 20: 366–376, 1959.
36. FRIEDMAN, S., AND S. KAUFMAN. 3,4-Dihydroxyphenylethylamine-β-hydroxylase, physical properties, copper content, and role of copper in the catalytic activity. *J. Biol. Chem.* 240: 4763–4773, 1965.
37. FRIEDMAN, S., AND S. KAUFMAN. 3,4-Dihydroxyphenylethylamine-β-hydroxylase: a copper protein. *J. Biol. Chem.* 240: 552–554PC, 1965.
38. FRIEDMAN, S., AND S. KAUFMAN. An electron paramagnetic resonance study of 3,4-dihydroxyphenylethylamine-β-hydroxylase. *J. Biol. Chem.* 241: 2256–2259, 1966.
39. FULLER, R. W., AND J. M. HUNT. Substrate specificity of phenethanolamine *N*-methyl transferase. *Biochem. Pharmacol.* 14: 1896–1897, 1965.
40. FULLER, R. W., AND J. M. HUNT. Inhibition of phenethanolamine N-methyl transferase by its product, epinephrine. *Life Sci., Part 2* 6: 1107–1112, 1967.
41. GEWIRTZ, G. P., R. KVETNANSKY, V. K. WEISE, AND I. J. KOPIN. Effect of hypophysectomy on adrenal dopamine-β-hydroxylase activity in the rat. *Mol. Pharmacol.* 7: 163–168, 1971.
42. GEWIRTZ, G. P., R. KVETNANSKY, V. K. WEISE, AND I. J. KOPIN. Effect of ACTH and dibutyryl cyclic AMP on catecholamine synthesizing enzymes in the adrenals of hypophysectomized rats. *Nature* 230: 462–464, 1971.
43. GOLDSTEIN, M., AND J. F. CONTRERA. The substate specificity of phenylamine-β-hydroxylase. *J. Biol. Chem.* 237: 1898–1902, 1962.
44. GOLDSTEIN, M., H. GANG, AND T. H. JOH. Subcellular distribution and properties of phenylethanolamine-*N*-methyl transferase. *Federation Proc.* 28: 287, 1969.
45. GOLDSTEIN, M., AND T. H. JOH. The effect of hyperbaric oxygen on dopamine-β-hydroxylase. *Biochim. Biophys. Acta* 146: 615–617, 1967.
46. GOLDSTEIN, M., AND T. H. JOH. The effect of reduced and oxidized pteridine on dopamine-β-hydroxylase activity. *Mol. Pharmacol.* 3: 396–398, 1967.
47. GOLDSTEIN, M., AND T. H. JOH. Further purification and properties of PNMT. *Federation Proc.* 29: 180, 1970.
48. GOLDSTEIN, M., T. H. JOH, AND T. Q. GARVEY, III. Kinetic studies of the enzymatic dopamine-β-hydroxylation reaction. *Biochemistry* 7: 2724–2730, 1968.
49. GOLDSTEIN, M., E. LAUBER, AND M. R. MCKEREGHAN. Studies on the purification and characterization of 3,4-dihydroxyphenylethylamine-β-hydroxylase. *J. Biol. Chem.* 240: 2066–2072, 1965.
50. GOODALL, McC., AND N. KIRSHNER. Biosynthesis of adrenaline and noradrenaline *in vitro*. *J. Biol. Chem.* 226: 213–221, 1957.
51. GORDON, R., S. SPECTOR, A. SJOERDSMA, AND S. UDENFRIEND. Increased synthesis of norepinephrine and epinephrine in the intact rat during exercise and exposure to cold. *J. Pharmacol.* 153: 440–447, 1966.
52. GURIN, S., AND A. M. DELLUVA. The biological synthesis of radioactive adrenaline from phenylalanine. *J. Biol. Chem.* 170: 545–550, 1947.
53. HAGEN, P. Biosynthesis of norepinephrine from 3,4-dihydroxyphenylethylamine (dopamine). *J. Pharmacol.* 116: 26, 1956.
54. HAGEN, P., AND A. D. WELCH. The adrenal medulla and the biosynthesis of pressor amines. *Recent Progr. Hormone Res.* 12: 27–44, 1955.
55. HEDVQUIST, P., AND L. STJÄRNE. The relative rate of recapture and *de novo* synthesis for the maintenance of neurotransmitter homeostasis in noradrenergic nerves. *Acta Physiol. Scand.* 76: 270–283, 1969.
56. HEMPEL, K., AND H. F. K. MANNL. The conversion of H³-tyrosine to H³-dopa in the adrenal glands under *in vivo* conditions. *Experientia* 22: 688–690, 1966.
57. HEMPEL, K., AND H. F. K. MANNL. Resting secretion of dopamine from the adrenal gland of the cat *in vivo*. *Experientia* 23: 919–920, 1967.
58. HERTTING, G., L. T. POTTER, AND J. AXELROD. Effect of decentralization and ganglionic blocking agents on the spontaneous release of H³-norepinephrine. *J. Pharmacol.* 136: 289–292, 1962.
59. HÖKFELT, B. Noradrenaline and adrenaline in mammalian tissues. Distribution under normal and pathological conditions with special reference to the endocrine system. *Acta Physiol. Scand. Suppl.* 92, 1951.
60. HOLLAND, W. C., AND H. J. SCHÜMANN. Formation of catecholamines during splanchnic stimulation of the adrenal gland of the cat. *Brit. J. Pharmacol.* 11: 449–453, 1956.
61. HOLTZ, P. Über Tyraminbildung im Organismus. *Arch. Exptl. Pathol. Pharmakol.* 186: 684–693, 1937.
62. HOLTZ, P. Role of L-dopa decarboxylase in the biosynthesis of catecholamines in nervous tissue and adrenal medulla. *Pharmacol. Rev.* 11: 317–329, 1959.
63. HOLTZ, P., R. HEISE, AND K. LÜDTKE. Fermentativer Abbau von *l*-dioxyphenylalanin (Dopa) durch Niere. *Arch. Exptl. Pathol. Pharmakol.* 191: 87–118, 1938.
64. HOLTZ, P., AND G. KRONENBERG. Untersuchungen über die Adrenalinbildung durch Nebennierengewebe. *Arch. Exptl. Pathol. Pharmakol.* 206: 150–163, 1949.
65. IKEDA, M., L. A. FAHIEN, AND S. UDENFRIEND. A kinetic study of bovine adrenal tyrosine hydroxylase. *J. Biol. Chem.* 241: 4452–4456, 1966.
66. IKEDA, M., M. LEVITT, AND S. UDENFRIEND. Hydroxylation of phenylalanine by purified preparations of adrenal and brain tyrosine hydroxylase. *Biochem. Biophys. Res. Commun.* 18: 482–488, 1965.
67. JOH, T. H., R. KOPET, AND M. GOLDSTEIN. A kinetic study of particulate bovine adrenal tyrosine hydroxylase. *Biochim. Biophys. Acta* 171: 378–380, 1969.
68. KAUFMAN, S. Studies on the mechanism of the enzymatic conversion of phenylalanine to tyrosine. *J. Biol. Chem.* 234: 2677–2683, 1959.
69. KAUFMAN, S. The structure of the phenylalanine hydroxylation co-factor. *Proc. Natl. Acad. Sci. US* 50: 1085–1093, 1963.
70. KAUFMAN, S. Studies on the structure of the primary oxidation product formed from tetrahydropteridines during phenylalanine hydroxylation. *J. Biol. Chem.* 239: 332–338, 1964.
71. KAUFMAN, S., W. F. BRIDGERS, F. EISENBERG, AND S. FRIEDMAN. The source of oxygen in the phenylalanine hydroxylase and dopamine-β-hydroxylase catalyzed reactions. *Biochem. Biophys. Res. Commun.* 9: 497–502, 1962.
72. KAUFMAN, S., AND B. LEVENBERG. Further studies on the

phenylalanine-hydroxylation co-factor. *J. Biol. Chem.* 234: 2683–2688, 1959.
73. KIRSHNER, N. Pathway of noradrenaline formation from Dopa. *J. Biol. Chem.* 226: 821–825, 1957.
74. KIRSHNER, N. Biosynthesis of adrenaline and noradrenaline. *Pharmacol. Rev.* 11: 350–357, 1959.
75. KIRSHNER, N., AND McC. GOODALL. The formation of adrenaline from noradrenaline. *Biochim. Biophys. Acta* 24: 658–659, 1957.
76. KIRSHNER, N., AND McC. GOODALL. Separation of adrenaline, noradrenaline and hydroxytyramine by ion exchange chromatography. *J. Biol. Chem.* 226: 207–212, 1957.
77. KIRSHNER, N., AND O. H. VIVEROS. Quantal aspects of the secretion of catecholamines and dopamine-β-hydroxylase from the adrenal medulla. In: *New Aspects of Storage and Release Mechanisms of Catecholamines*, edited by H. J. Schümann and G. Kroneberg. Berlin: Springer Verlag, 1970, p. 78–88.
78. KOPIN, I. J., G. R. BREESE, K. R. KRAUSE, AND V. K. WEISE. Selective release of newly synthesized norepinephrine from the cat spleen during sympathetic nerve activity. *J. Pharmacol.* 161: 271–278, 1968.
79. KOVACIC, B., AND R. L. ROBINSON. Facilitation of drug-induced release of adrenal catecholamines during nicotine blockade. *Federation Proc.* 27: 601, 1968.
80. KRONEBERG, G., AND H. J. SCHÜMANN. Über die Bedeutung der Innervation dur die Adrenalin-synthese im Nebennierenmark. *Experientia* 15: 234–235, 1959.
81. KVETNANSKY, R., G. P. GEWIRTZ, V. K. WEISE, AND I. J. KOPIN. Neuronal and hormonal control of elevations of adrenal tyrosine hydroxylase, dopamine-β-oxidase, and phenylethanolamine-N-methyltransferase during immobilization of rats. *Federation Proc.* 29: 277, 1970.
82. KVETNANSKY, R., G. P. GEWIRTZ, V. K. WEISE, AND I. J. KOPIN. Enhanced synthesis of adrenal dopamine-β-hydroxylase induced by repeated immobilization stress. *Mol. Pharmacol.* 7: 81–86, 1970.
83. KVETNANSKY, R., V. K. WEISE, AND I. J. KOPIN. Effect of repeated immobilization stress on rat adrenal tyrosine hydroxylase, dopamine-β-hydroxylase, and phenylethanolamine-N-methyl transferase. *Pharmacologist* 11: 274, 1969.
84. KVETNANSKY, P., V. K. WEISE, AND I. J. KOPIN. Elevation of adrenal tyrosine hydroxylase and phenylethanolamine-N-methyltransferase by repeated immobilization of rats. *Endocrinology* 87: 744–749, 1970.
85. LADURON, P., AND F. BELPAIRE. Tissue fractionation and catecholamines. II. Intracellular distribution patterns of tyrosine hydroxylase, dopa decarboxylase, dopamine-β-hydroxylase, phenylethanolamine-N-methyltransferase and monoamine oxidase in adrenal medulla. *Biochem. Pharmacol.* 17: 1127–1140, 1968.
86. LANGEMANN, H. Enzymes and their substrates in the adrenal gland of the ox. *Brit. J. Pharmacol.* 6: 318–324, 1951.
87. LEEPER, L. C., AND S. UDENFRIEND. 3,4-Dihydroxyphenylethylamine as a precursor of adrenal epinephrine in the intact rat. *Federation Proc.* 15: 298, 1956.
88. LEVIN, E. Y., AND S. KAUFMAN. Studies on the enzyme catalyzing the conversion of 3,4-dihydroxyphenylethylamine to norepinephrine. *J. Biol. Chem.* 236: 2043–2049, 1961.
89. LEVIN, E. Y., B. LEVENBERG, AND S. KAUFMAN. The enzymatic conversion of 3,4-dihydroxyphenylethylamine to norepinephrine. *J. Biol. Chem.* 235: 2080–2086, 1960.
90. LEVITT, M., S. SPECTOR, A. SJOERDSMA, AND S. UDENFRIEND. Elucidation of the rate-limiting step in norepinephrine biosynthesis in the perfused guinea-pig heart. *J. Pharmacol.* 148: 1–8, 1965.
91. LLOYD, T., AND N. WEINER. Isolation and characterization of the tyrosine hydroxylase co-factor from bovine adrenal medulla. *Pharmacologist* 12: 287, 1970.
92. LOVENBERG, W., H. WEISBACH, AND S. UDENFRIEND. Aromatic-L-amino acid decarboxylase. *J. Biol. Chem.* 237: 89–93, 1962.
93. LUCO, J. V., AND F. GONI. Synaptic fatigue and neurochemical mediators of postganglionic fibers. *J. Neurophysiol.* 11: 497–500, 1948.
94. MANDELL, A. J., AND M. MORGAN. Amphetamine-induced increase in tyrosine hydroxylase activity. *Nature* 227: 75–76, 1970.
95. McGEER, P. L., AND E. G. McGEER. Formation of adrenaline by brain tissue. *Biochem. Biophys. Res. Commun.* 17: 502–511, 1964.
96. MOLINOFF, P. B., S. BRIMIJOIN, R. WEINSHILBOUM, AND J. AXELROD. Neurally mediated increase in dopamine-β-hydroxylase activity. *Proc. Natl. Acad. Sci. US* 66: 453–458, 1970.
97. MUELLER, R. A., H. THOENEN, AND J. AXELROD. Adrenal tyrosine hydroxylase: compensatory increase in activity after chemical sympathectomy. *Science* 158: 468–469, 1969.
98. MUELLER, R. A., H. THOENEN, AND J. AXELROD. Inhibition of trans-synaptically increased tyrosine hydroxylase activity by cycloheximide and actinomycin D. *Mol. Pharmacol.* 5: 463–469, 1969.
99. MUELLER, R. A., H. THOENEN, AND J. AXELROD. Increase in tyrosine hydroxylase activity after reserpine administration. *J. Pharmacol.* 169: 74–79, 1969.
100. MUELLER, R. A., H. THOENEN, AND J. AXELROD. Effect of pituitary and ACTH on the maintenance of basal tyrosine hydroxylase activity in the rat adrenal gland. *Endocrinology* 86: 751–755, 1970.
101. MUELLER, R. A., H. THOENEN, AND J. AXELROD. Inhibition of neuronally induced tyrosine hydroxylase by nicotinic receptor blockade. *European J. Pharmacol.* 10: 51–56, 1970.
102. MUSACCHIO, J. M. Subcellular distribution of adrenal tyrosine hydroxylase. *Pharmacologist* 9: 210, 1967.
103. MUSACCHIO, J. M. Subcellular distribution of adrenal tyrosine hydroxylase. *Biochem. Pharmacol.* 17: 1470–1473, 1968.
104. MUSACCHIO, J. M. Beef adrenal medulla dihydropteridine reductase. *Biochim. Biophys. Acta* 191: 485–487, 1969.
105. MUSACCHIO, J. M. Regulation of catecholamine biosynthesis: tyrosine hydroxylase and dihydropteridine reductase. In: *Neurochemistry and Psychopharmacology of Affective Diseases of Schizophrenia*, edited by B. T. Ho. New York: Raven Press, 1971, p. 240.
106. MUSACCHIO, J. M., AND R. WURZBURGER. Aggregation of beef adrenal tyrosine hydroxylase. *Federation Proc.* 28: 159, 1969.
107. MUSACCHIO, J. M., R. J. WURZBURGER, AND G. L. D'ANGELO. Different molecular forms of bovine adrenal tyrosine hydroxylase. *Mol. Pharmacol.* 7: 136–146, 1971.
108. NAGATSU, T. Endogenous inhibitors of dopamine-β-hydroxylase. In: *Biological and Chemical Aspects of Oxygenases*, edited by K. E. Bloch and O. Hayaishi. Tokyo: Maruzen, 1966, p. 273–277.
109. NAGATSU, T., H. KUZUYA, AND H. KIDAKA. Inhibition of dopamine-β-hydroxylase by sulfhydryl compounds and the nature of the natural inhibitors. *Biochim. Biophys. Acta* 139: 319–327, 1967.
110. NAGATSU, T., M. LEVITT, AND S. UDENFRIEND. Conversion of L-tyrosine to 3,4-dihydroxyphenylalanine by cell-free preparation of brain and sympathetically innervated tissues. *Biochem. Biophys. Res. Commun.* 14: 543–549, 1964.
111. NAGATSU, T., M. LEVITT, AND S. UDENFRIEND. Tyrosine hydroxylase—the initial step in norepinephrine biosynthesis. *J. Biol. Chem.* 239: 2910–2917, 1964.
112. NAGATSU, T., T. YAMAMOTO, AND I. NAGATSU. Partial separation and properties of tyrosine hydroxylase from the human pheochromocytoma. *Biochim. Biophys. Acta* 198: 210–218, 1970.
113. NEFF, N. H., AND E. COSTA. A study of the control of catecholamine synthesis. *Federation Proc.* 25: 259, 1966.
114. NEFF, N. H., AND E. COSTA. The influence of monoamine oxidase inhibitors on catecholamine synthesis. *Life Sci.* 5: 951–959, 1966.

115. OKA, M., K. V. KAJAKAWA, I. OHUCHI, H. YOSHIDA, AND R. IMAIZAMI. Distribution of dopamine-β-hydroxylase in subcellular fractions of adrenal medulla. *Life Sci., Part 1* 6: 461–465, 1967.
116. OLEVARIO, A., AND L. STJÄRNE. Acceleration of noradrenaline turnover in the mouse heart by cold exposure. *Life Sci.* 4: 2339–2343, 1965.
117. OLIVER, G., AND E. A. SCHÄFER. On the physiological action of extracts of the suprarenal capsules. *J. Physiol., London* 16: i–ivp, 1894.
118. PATRICK, R. L., AND N. KIRSHNER. Effect of stimulation on the levels of tyrosine hydroxylase, dopamine-β-hydroxylase and catecholamines in intact and denervated rat adrenal glands. *Mol. Pharmacol.* 7: 87–96, 1971.
119. PATRICK, R. L., AND N. KIRSHNER. Effect of denervation on rat adrenal medullary tissue. *Federation Proc.* 30: 333, 1971.
120. PATRICK, R. L., AND N. KIRSHNER. Acetylcholine-induced stimulation and catecholamine recovery in denervated rat adrenals after reserpine-induced depletion. *Mol. Pharmacol.* 7: 389–396, 1971.
121. PELLERIN, J., AND A. D'IORIO. Metabolism of DL-3,4-dihydroxyphenylalanine-2-C^{14} in bovine adrenal homogenates. *Can. J. Biochem. Physiol.* 35: 151–156, 1957.
122. PETRACK, B., J. SHEPPY, AND V. FETZER. Studies on tyrosine hydroxylase from bovine adrenal medulla. *J. Biol. Chem.* 243: 743–748, 1968.
123. POHORECKY, L. A., M. ZIGMOND, H. KARTEN, AND R. J. WURTMAN. Enzymatic conversion of norepinephrine to epinephrine by the brain. *J. Pharmacol.* 165: 190–195, 1969.
124. ROSENFELD, G., L. C. LEEPER, AND S. UDENFRIEND. Biosynthesis of norepinephrine and epinephrine by the isolated perfused calf adrenal gland. *Arch. Biochem.* 74: 252–265, 1958.
125. ROSENMUND, K. W., AND H. DORNSAFT. Über oxy- und Dioxyphenylserin und die Muttersubstanz des Adrenalins. *Ber. Deut. Chem. Ges.* 52: 1734–1749, 1919.
126. ROTH, R. H., L. STJÄRNE, AND U. S. VON EULER. Acceleration of noradrenaline biosynthesis by nerve stimulation. *Life Sci.* 5: 1071–1075, 1966.
127. ROTH, R. H., L. STJÄRNE, R. J. LEVINE, AND N. J. GIARMAN. Abnormal regulation of catecholamine synthesis in pheochromocytoma. *J. Lab. Clin. Med.* 72: 397–403, 1968.
128. SCHALES, O., AND S. S. SCHALES. Dihydroxyphenylalanine decarboxylase: preparation and properties of a stable dry powder. *Arch. Biochem.* 24: 83–91, 1949.
129. SCHMITERLÖW, C. G. Formation in vivo of noradrenaline from 3,4-dihydroxyphenylserine (noradrenaline carboxylic acid). *Brit. J. Pharmacol.* 6: 127–134, 1951.
131. SCHULER, W., AND A. Z. WEIDEMANN. Über die Adrenaline synthese im Reagenzglase unter physiologischen Bedingungen. *Z. Physiol. Chem.* 233: 235–256, 1935.
132. SCHULER, W., H. BERNHARDT, AND W. REINDEL. Die Tyraminbildung aus Tyrosine mit uberlebenden Gewelschnitten und deren Beziehung zur Adrenalinsynthese. II. Mitteilung uber die Adrenalinsynthese im Reagensglase unter physiologischen Bedingungen. *Z. Physiol. Chem.* 243: 90–102, 1936.
133. SEDVALL, G. C., AND I. J. KOPIN. Acceleration of norepinephrine synthesis in vivo during sympathetic nerve stimulation. *Life Sci., Part 1* 6: 45–52, 1967.
134. SEDVALL, G. C., V. K. WEISE, AND I. J. KOPIN. The rate of norepinephrine synthesis measured in vivo during short intervals; influence of adrenergic impulse activity. *J. Pharmacol.* 159: 274–282, 1968.
135. SHIMAN, R., M. AKINO, AND S. KAUFMAN. Solubilization and partial purification of tyrosine hydroxylase from bovine adrenal medulla. *J. Biol. Chem.* 246: 1330–1340, 1970.
136. SMITH, D. J., AND R. L. ROBINSON. The dwindling secretory response of the perfused adrenal medulla of the cat to repeated injections of histamine. *J. Pharmacol.* 175: 641–648, 1970.
137. SOURKES, T. Dopa decarboxylase; substrates, coenzymes, inhibitors. *Pharmacol. Rev.* 18: 53–60, 1966.
138. SPECTOR, S., A. SJOERDSMA, AND S. UDENFRIEND. Blockade of endogenous norepinephrine synthesis by α-methyltyrosine, an inhibitor of tyrosine hydroxylase. *J. Pharmacol.* 147: 86–95, 1965.
139. STOLZ, F. Über Adrenalin und Alkyl-aminoacetobrenzcatechin. *Ber. Deut. Chem. Ges.* 37: 4149–4154, 1904.
140. STJÄRNE, L., AND F. LISHAJKO. Localization of different steps in noradrenaline synthesis to different fractions of a bovine splenic nerve homogenate. *Biochem. Pharmacol.* 16: 1719–1728, 1967.
141. STJÄRNE, L., AND A. WENNALM. Preferential secretion of newly formed noradrenaline in the perfused rabbit heart. *Acta Physiol. Scand.* 80: 428–429, 1970.
142. STREFFER, C. Eine Methode zur Bestimmung der Dekarboxylase aromatischer Aminosäuren. *Biochim. Biophys. Acta* 139: 193–195, 1967.
143. TAKAMINE, J. The blood-pressure raising principle of the suprarenal glands—a preliminary report. *Therap. Gaz.* 25: 221–224, 1901.
144. THOENEN, H. Induction of tyrosine hydroxylase in peripheral and central adrenergic neurones by cold exposure of rats. *Nature* 228: 861–862, 1970.
145. THOENEN, H., R. A. MUELLER, AND J. AXELROD. Increased tyrosine hydroxylase activity after drug-induced alteration of sympathetic transmission. *Nature* 221: 1264, 1969.
146. THOENEN, H., R. A. MUELLER, AND J. AXELROD. Trans-synaptic induction of adrenal tyrosine hydroxylase. *J. Pharmacol.* 164: 249–254, 1969.
147. THOENEN, H., R. A. MUELLER, AND J. AXELROD. Neuronally dependent induction of adrenal phenylethanolamine-N-methyltransferase. *Biochem. Pharmacol.* 19: 669–673, 1970.
148. THOENEN, H., R. A. MUELLER, AND J. AXELROD. Phase difference in the induction of tyrosine hydroxylase in cell body and nerve terminals of sympathetic neurones. *Proc. Natl. Acad. Sci. US* 65: 58–62, 1970.
149. UDENFRIEND, S. Biosynthesis and release of catecholamines. In: *Mechanisms of Release of Biogenic Amines*, edited by U. S. von Euler, S. Rosell, and B. Uvnäs. New York: Pergamon Press, 1966, p. 103–108.
150. UDENFRIEND, S., J. R. COOPER, C. T. CLARK, AND J. E. BAER. Rate of turnover of epinephrine in the adrenal medulla. *Science* 117: 663–665, 1953.
151. UDENFRIEND, S., AND J. B. WYNGAARDEN. Precursors of adrenal epinephrine and norepinephrine in vivo. *Biochim. Biophys. Acta* 20: 48–52, 1956.
152. UDENFRIEND, S., P. ZALTZMAN-NIRENBERG, AND T. NAGATSU. Inhibitors of purified beef adrenal tyrosine hydroxylase. *Biochem. Pharmacol.* 14: 835–845, 1965.
152a. VAN DER SCHOOT, J. B., AND C. R. CREVELING. Substrates and inhibitors of dopamine-β-hydroxylase. In: *Advances in Drug Research*, edited by H. J. Harper and A. B. Simmons. New York: Acad. Press, 1965, p. 47–88.
153. VIVEROS, O. H., L. ARQUEROS, R. J. CONNETT, AND N. KIRSHNER. Mechanism of secretion from the adrenal medulla. III. Studies of dopamine-β-hydroxylase as a marker for catecholamine storage vesicle membranes in rabbit adrenal glands. *Mol. Pharmacol.* 5: 60–68, 1969.
154. VIVEROS, O. H., L. ARQUEROS, R. J. CONNETT, AND N. KIRSHNER. Mechanism of secretion from the adrenal medulla. IV. The fate of the storage vesicles following insulin and reserpine administration. *Mol. Pharmacol.* 5: 69–82, 1969.
155. WEINER, N. Regulation of norepinephrine biosynthesis. *Ann. Rev. Pharmacol.* 10: 273–290, 1970.
156. WEINER, N., AND W. F. MOSIMANN. The effect of insulin on the catecholamine content and tyrosine hydroxylase activity of cat adrenal glands. *Biochem. Pharmacol.* 19: 1189–1199, 1970.

157. WEINER, N., AND M. RABADJIUA. The effect of nerve stimulation on the synthesis and metabolism of norepinephrine in the isolated guinea pig hypogastric nerve-vas deferens preparations. *J. Pharmacol.* 160: 61–71, 1968.
158. WEINER, N., AND C. O. RUTLEDGE. The actions of reserpine on the biosynthesis and storage of catecholamines. In: *Mechanisms of Release of Biogenic Amines*, edited by U. S. von Euler, S. Rosell, and B. Uvnäs. London: Pergamon Press, 1966, p. 307–318.
159. WEINSHILBOUM, R., AND J. AXELROD. Dopamine-β-hydroxylase activity in the rat after hypophysectomy. *Endocrinology* 87: 894–899, 1970.
160. WURTMAN, R. J., AND J. AXELROD. Control of enzymatic synthesis of adrenaline in the adrenal medulla by adrenal cortical slices. *J. Biol. Chem.* 241: 2301–2305, 1966.
161. WURZBURGER, R. J., AND J. M. MUSACCHIO. Subcellular distribution and aggregation of adrenal tyrosine hydroxylase. *J. Pharmacol.* 177: 155–168, 1971.

CHAPTER 25

Control of the biosynthesis of adrenal catecholamines by the adrenal medulla

NORMAN WEINER | *Department of Pharmacology, University of Colorado School of Medicine, Denver, Colorado*

CHAPTER CONTENTS

Anatomic Relationship Between Adrenal Cortex and Medulla and Synthesis of Epinephrine
Development of Adrenal Gland and Epinephrine Synthesis
Development and Catecholamine Content of Extraadrenal Chromaffin Tissue
Role of Glucocorticoids and ACTH in Epinephrine Synthesis
Regulation of Adrenal Tyrosine Hydroxylase by Adrenal Cortex
Cyclic AMP and Regulation of Adrenal Tyrosine Hydroxylase
Regulation of Adrenal Dopamine β-hydroxylase by Adrenal Cortex
Role of Ascorbic Acid in Synthesis and Catabolism of Adrenal Catecholamines
Conclusion

CATECHOLAMINE BIOSYNTHESIS in peripheral and central adrenergic neurons appears to be highly regulated. The rate of catecholamine synthesis is enhanced by acute nerve stimulation, and this enhanced rate results from increased activity of the enzyme tyrosine hydroxylase (1, 101). It appears to be mediated, at least in part, by reduced end product feedback inhibition, since exogenous norepinephrine can prevent the increased enzyme activity seen during nerve stimulation (1, 101). In the period following acute nerve stimulation, the level of activity of tyrosine hydroxylase is also increased for a short time (102). The mechanism of this effect appears to differ from that which occurs during nerve stimulation, since the increase in the activity of the enzyme is not prevented by exogenous norepinephrine. There does not seem to be any increase in the amount of the tyrosine hydroxylase enzyme, although the poststimulation increase in norepinephrine synthesis is inhibited by puromycin (102) but not by either actinomycin D or cycloheximide (89). More prolonged adrenergic nervous activity leads to enhanced levels of tyrosine hydroxylase (69, 70, 75, 90, 100) and dopamine β-hydroxylase (12, 67, 75) in both adrenergic nervous tissue and the adrenal medulla. The neurally mediated regulation of catecholamine biosynthesis has been the subject of several reviews (66, 96, 97, 99).

Catecholamine biosynthesis in the adrenal medulla is influenced by the frequency and duration of nerve impulses to the organ in a manner analogous to that in adrenergic nervous tissue. Both tyrosine hydroxylase (72, 97, 99) and phenylethanolamine *N*-methyltransferase (33, 35) are subject to end product feedback inhibition, a braking effect that would presumably be less prominent after release of catecholamines during nerve stimulation. Chronic stimulation of splanchnic nerves and chronic stimulation of the adrenal gland by pharmacological means are associated with increased levels of the enzymes tyrosine hydroxylase and dopamine β-hydroxylase (69, 70, 75, 100).

In addition to the neurally mediated factors that modify catecholamine biosynthesis in the adrenal medulla, both adrenocorticotropic hormone (ACTH) and glucocorticoids exert profound trophic effects on the adrenal medulla and on the catecholamine biosynthetic enzymes. These hormonal effects on adrenal chromaffin tissue have been intensively examined over many years, and the results of these investigations have been summarized recently (4, 5, 10, 33, 81, 113, 114). In this chapter the interrelationships between the adrenal cortex and medulla are reviewed and recent studies on the mechanisms by which ACTH and glucocorticoids affect the biosynthesis of catecholamines are emphasized. Other aspects of the regulation of catecholamine biosynthesis and the enzymology of the pertinent enzymes are discussed in the chapter by Kirshner in this volume of the *Handbook*.

ANATOMIC RELATIONSHIP BETWEEN ADRENAL CORTEX AND MEDULLA AND SYNTHESIS OF EPINEPHRINE

The variation in the anatomic relationships between the adrenal cortex and the medulla among various animal classes is considerable. This has provided a natural spectrum of variables to assess the influence of the adrenal cortex on the development and function of the adrenal medulla. Many investigators have taken advantage of the markedly different comparative anatomies of these two tissues to examine their interrelationships (18, 22, 81, 86, 111). In general, there is a correlation between the intimacy of contact of chromaffin cells of the adrenal medulla with adrenal cortical cells and the proportion of total catecholamines present in the chromaffin cells as epinephrine (22, 81). In mammals, adrenal chromaffin cells are present in the interior regions of the adrenal gland, surrounded by adrenal cortical tissue (22, 81). Shepherd & West (86) noted an overall correlation between the size of the adrenal cortex in mammals and the proportion of catecholamine present in the adrenal gland as epinephrine. In those species where the quantity of tissue in the cortex is considerably greater than that in the medulla, such as guinea pig and rabbit, the predominant catecholamine in the adrenal gland is epinephrine (104). In contrast, in cat, dog, and man, where cortical tissue constitutes a smaller fraction of the adrenal gland, a larger percentage of norepinephrine is found in the gland. In some mammalian species, such as cow, ox, horse, and sheep, the epinephrine-containing chromaffin cells predominate in the region of the adrenal medulla that is adjacent to the adrenal medullary-cortical junction. Epinephrine-containing cells in several rodent species are more variable in their distribution throughout the adrenal medulla (22, 81).

In reptiles a portion of the chromaffin tissue is attached to the surface of the adrenal gland and the remainder is present as cell clusters within the glandular tissue (9, 94, 107). In these species only norepinephrine is present in the chromaffin tissue located on the surface of the gland, whereas the chromaffin cells within the adrenal gland contain a considerable proportion of epinephrine. This is well correlated with the distribution of phenylethanolamine N-methyltransferase (PNMT), the enzyme that catalyzes the formation of epinephrine from norepinephrine. Although PNMT is present in the chromaffin tissue located on the surface of the adrenal gland, a much higher activity of this enzyme is demonstrable in the epinephrine-containing chromaffin tissue within the adrenal gland (111). Nevertheless the fact that PNMT is detectable in the extraadrenal tissue indicates that PNMT synthesis may not be absolutely dependent on glucocorticoids.

In birds chromaffin cells are distributed throughout the adrenal gland and appear to be, for the most part, in intimate contact with cortical tissue (29, 38, 104). In the chicken, for example, approximately 40–50% of the catecholamines in the adrenal gland is epinephrine (14, 86, 98). However, in other birds either epinephrine or norepinephrine may predominate. The proportion of epinephrine seems to be better correlated with the phylogeny of these animals than with the amount of adrenal cortical tissue; the later in the evolutionary scale the birds presumably appeared, the more epinephrine is present in the adrenal glands (38). The distribution of epinephrine- or norepinephrine-containing cells in the chicken adrenal medulla is not related to proximity to cortical tissue (38, 104).

In lower vertebrates, such as the dogfish, the relationship between the adrenal cortex and epinephrine synthesis is even less clear. In the dogfish, adrenal chromaffin tissue and cortical cells are completely separated (18, 87). Coupland (18) observed that the chromaffin tissue of dogfish contains very little or no epinephrine. However, Shepherd et al. (87) observed that several species of dogfish possess chromaffin tissue wherein as much as one-third of the total catecholamine content is present as epinephrine. Peyrin et al. (77) more recently reported an even greater proportion of epinephrine in chromaffin tissue of the dogfish, which is quite distal from the adrenal cortical tissue. In addition, they demonstrated that the chromaffin tissue could convert ^{14}C-norepinephrine to the N-methylated derivative.

In mammalian species the intimate relationship between the adrenal medulla and cortex is not confined to their anatomic proximity: the blood supply to the gland is also involved (see the chapter by Coupland in this volume of the *Handbook*). Multiple small adrenal arteries penetrate the substance of the adrenal cortex and ultimately supply the adrenal medulla tissue via two distinct vascular networks. The medullary arteries penetrate the substance of the adrenal cortex and enter the medulla before dividing into the capillary plexus, which supplies the latter tissue. After bathing a fraction of adrenal chromaffin cells a portion of the arterial blood enters the corticomedullary sinuses and a portion passes directly into adrenal venules and ultimately into the central vein of the adrenal gland. The second component of the vascular supply to the adrenal medulla arises from the venous drainage of the zona reticularis of the adrenal cortex. These venules enter the adrenal medulla as a portal system and, after bathing a fraction of the adrenal chromaffin cells, ultimately enter the central vein of the adrenal and thence proceed either to the adrenal lumbar vein, the renal vein, or directly into the inferior vena cava (59). Blood flow to the adrenal has been estimated to be 5 ml/g tissue per minute (22).

DEVELOPMENT OF ADRENAL GLAND AND EPINEPHRINE SYNTHESIS

The vascular arrangement of the adrenal medulla in mammals provides the means whereby secretory products of the adrenal cortex may perfuse regions of the adrenal medulla in high concentrations before entering the general circulation. Differences among species with regard to corticomedullary anatomic relationships and the general correlation between the intimacy of the anatomy of these two structures and their relative masses and the proportion of epinephrine present in chromaffin cells suggest that adrenal steroids may play a role in the biosynthesis of epinephrine. Developmental studies provide additional evidence in support of this functional relationship. Shepherd & West (86) observed that during fetal life the catecholamine content of the adrenal gland of rabbits and guinea pigs is exclusively norepinephrine. Epinephrine begins to appear in the postnatal period when adrenal cortical development is most active. Hökfelt (49) and Coupland (18, 19) observed a similar overall correlation between adrenal cortical development and the appearance of epinephrine in the adrenal gland in rat and rabbit tissue. Similar developmental relationships were noted in calf (50) and man (74, 105). In contrast, in fowl the proportions of norepinephrine and epinephrine remain fairly constant throughout life. In these animals the relative proportions of cortex and medulla in the adrenal gland also remain constant during development (86, 104). The increase of PNMT in the adrenal gland parallels the appearance of epinephrine and the overall growth of the medulla (13, 34, 86).

Roffi (82) demonstrated in rat and rabbit fetuses that the progressive increase in adrenal epinephrine and PNMT during gestation could be prevented by fetal decapitation. Injection of ACTH into the fetuses restored adrenal epinephrine and PNMT toward normal levels. Administration of cortisol either to the decapitated fetus or the mother was much less effective, although adrenal PNMT and epinephrine were elevated somewhat.

DEVELOPMENT AND CATECHOLAMINE CONTENT OF EXTRAADRENAL CHROMAFFIN TISSUE

During fetal life there is a considerable amount of extraadrenal chromaffin tissue, particularly along the major vessels and proximate to the thoracolumbar paraganglionic system (19). The catecholamine content of this extraadrenal chromaffin tissue in the newborn rabbit (19) or rat (57), for example, is largely or exclusively norepinephrine. Much of this extraadrenal chromaffin tissue involutes rapidly postnatally. The administration of glucocorticoids prevents the progressive degeneration of extraadrenal chromaffin tissue in the young rat. With large doses of glucocorticoids an actual increase in the amount of extraadrenal chromaffin tissue may be produced. In addition to maintaining or enhancing the size of this extraadrenal chromaffin tissue, glucocorticoids stimulate the appearance of epinephrine (30, 31, 56–58) and PNMT (82, 83) activity in these structures. The exact mechanism by which glucocorticoids maintain or stimulate the growth of fetal extraadrenal chromaffin tissue is not clear. It may be that these hormones either exert a generalized trophic effect on chromaffin cell tissue or stimulate the differentiation of primitive into mature chromaffin cells (10, 22, 68, 80).

ROLE OF GLUCOCORTICOIDS AND ACTH IN EPINEPHRINE SYNTHESIS

Initial experimental support for the dependence of the production of epinephrine in the adrenal medulla on cortical hormones was provided by Hökfelt (49) who observed that, after hypophysectomy, the quantity of epinephrine decreased in the adrenal gland of the rat, whereas the quantity of norepinephrine increased; the total amount of catecholamine was not changed. This effect could be reversed by administration of ACTH to the hypophysectomized animal.

Coupland & MacDougall (24) incubated preaortic chromaffin bodies of newborn rabbits in culture medium for 6 days and observed a considerable increase in the epinephrine content of the tissue in the presence of fairly high concentrations (10 μg/ml) of corticosterone. No such effect was produced when the organs were cultured in the presence of similar amounts of deoxycorticosterone (23). Coupland concluded that 11-oxysteroids were important factors in the stimulation of N-methylation of catecholamines. The amount of corticosterone employed in these studies is approximately 10 times the concentration present in rabbit or dog adrenal vein plasma and similar to the concentration present in rat adrenal venous plasma (51). Presumably the concentration of glucocorticoid bathing the adrenal chromaffin cells from the adrenal portal system could be much higher.

Pohorecky et al. (79) removed adrenal glands unilaterally from rats, dissected the tissue free of cortex, and inserted the medullae into the anterior chamber of the eye. The tissue rapidly lost its content of PNMT. Administration of large amounts of dexamethasone produced large increases in PNMT in the adrenal explant but did not affect the PNMT content of the intact adrenal gland. These results suggest that glucocorticoids are essential for the maintenance of adrenal PNMT and therefore for epinephrine formation in the adrenal medulla. However, in analogous experiments, Coupland (20, 21) assessed the proportions of norepinephrine- and epinephrine-containing cells in adrenal medullary autografts and homografts by histochemical techniques 4–6 weeks after explantation. He observed that, whereas these grafts contain relatively few adrenal cortical cells, the proportion of epinephrine- and norepinephrine-containing cells does not differ from that in the adrenal gland in situ. Coupland concluded therefore that the perfusion of the adrenal medulla by high concentrations of adrenal cortical hormones is not absolutely necessary to maintain the quantity of N-methylated amine in the chromaffin cells, although glucocorticoids may play some modulating role in this process.

Kirshner and Goodall (43, 53) demonstrated the enzymatic synthesis of epinephrine from norepinephrine in adrenal tissue and observed that the cofactor for this N-methylation was S-adenosylmethionine. The enzyme was purified and further studied by Axelrod (2) who noted its almost exclusive localization in the adrenal medulla of mammals. In hypophysectomized rats, Wurtman & Axelrod (109, 110) demonstrated a marked fall in adrenal PNMT after approximately 2–3 weeks. The effect of hypophysectomy on PNMT activity in the adrenal medulla could be reversed by administration either of ACTH or of high doses of dexamethasone. The increase in PNMT activity after dexamethasone could be inhibited by simultaneous administration of either actinomycin D or puromycin, suggesting that the increase in PNMT levels was due to enhanced synthesis of enzyme protein (110). In support of this are the recent observations of Wurtman and co-workers that labeled tyrosine incorporation into adrenal PNMT of dogs is reduced by hypophysectomy and is restored toward normal by administration of ACTH (114). The effect may not be specific, however, since profound alterations in ribosomal aggregation have been observed in adrenal tissue prepared from hypophysectomized animals. Analysis of polyribosome profiles of homogenates of rat whole adrenal prepared from both intact and hypophysectomized animals reveals a marked reduction in adrenal polyribosomes and a corresponding increase in monoribosomes in the absence of the pituitary. Similar results were obtained when high-speed supernatant fractions of adrenal medulla obtained from intact and hypophysectomized dogs were compared. The polyribosome profile obtained from adrenals of hypophysectomized animals can be restored to normal by prior treatment of the animals with either ACTH or dexamethasone (7, 114). The dependence of polyribosome stability on ACTH or glucocorticoids suggests that overall protein synthesis in adrenal tissue may be impaired in the absence of these hormones.

Although ACTH administered to hypophysectomized animals in moderate doses could restore the levels of adrenal PNMT to normal, doses of dexamethasone sufficient to provide adequate hormone replacement for most glucocorticoid-dependent metabolic functions did not elevate the levels of PNMT in the adrenal medulla. Much larger doses of dexamethasone were required for the latter effect (108). These results suggest that the levels of PNMT in the adrenal medulla are maintained by very high concentrations of glucocorticoids, which are normally secreted from the adrenal cortex into the portal vessels of the adrenal gland and reach the chromaffin cells only after minimal dilution. For other glucocorticoid-dependent functions in the body, the secretions of the adrenal cortex are diluted by blood returning from other areas of the body before reaching their target organs. Thus one would expect that glucocorticoid-dependent functions in organs other than the adrenal medulla would be considerably more sensitive to the actions of this hormone than maintenance of the levels of PNMT in the adrenal (81, 108).

It is of interest that, although ACTH or dexamethasone can elevate PNMT levels in hypophysectomized rats, treatment of rats that have intact pituitaries with large doses of these substances is not associated with an elevation of PNMT levels above normal (109, 110). However, if otherwise normal rats are implanted with a pituitary tumor, plasma corticosterone increases markedly and, after 6 weeks, adrenal epinephrine and PNMT are elevated considerably (93). Similarly, unilateral adrenalectomy is associated with a compensatory hypertrophy of the contralateral adrenal gland. After 40 days, adrenal PNMT in the remaining gland is significantly elevated, compared with that in adrenal glands of sham-operated rats of similar age (16). Thus the ability of the pituitary hormone to affect adrenal PNMT and epinephrine levels may depend on the intensity and duration of the pituitary stimulation of the adrenal cortex.

Hypophysectomy of fetal rats, by decapitation of the fetuses in utero, is associated with a marked reduction in adrenal epinephrine and PNMT at term 3–4 days later. This can be prevented by administration of ACTH or cortisol to the fetuses (64, 82). Luft & von Euler (62) observed that urinary epinephrine excretion after insulin challenge was reduced approximately 50% in women several weeks after hypophysectomy was performed as a palliative treatment for breast carcinoma. However, the posthypophysectomy patients were still able to respond with a severalfold increase in excretion of the N-methylated catecholamine. Resting levels of epinephrine and norepinephrine in urine were similar in control subjects and hypophysectomized patients. The results support the concept that glucocorticoids may play a modulating role in determining the level of PNMT in the adrenal gland, but other factors may also be important in maintaining the enzyme in chromaffin cells, perhaps including sympathetic nerve stimulation to the adrenal gland.

In the frog and other amphibians, in contrast to mammals, epinephrine is the neurotransmitter of the adrenergic postganglionic nervous system (52). In frogs PNMT activity is widely distributed in various organs, including the brain, heart, and adrenal. Hypophysectomy of these animals is not associated with a decline in the activity of the enzyme in any of these organs, nor can its activity be enhanced by glucocorticoids (112). Studies of the properties of frog PNMT indicate that it differs somewhat from the rat enzyme. For example, the frog enzyme is unstable at 47 C and has electrophoretic mobility on starch block that is different from that of the mammalian enzyme. Its pH optimum also appears to be slightly lower than that of the rat adrenal enzyme (112).

Von Euler & Ström (32) compared the catecholamine content of pheochromocytomas of the adrenal gland with that of extramedullary chromaffin cell tumors and observed that the latter tumors contained either a much lower proportion of epinephrine or no detectable epinephrine. However, some exceptions were noted by these investigators, and additional doubt was cast on this relationship by studies of Crout & Sjoerdsma (25). Pheochromocytomas not juxtaposed to the adrenal cortex, which contain high concentrations of epinephrine and presumably PNMT, also have been found by others (28, 65, 106).

Goldstein et al. (42) examined the properties of the extramedullary pheochromocytoma PNMT and observed several similarities between this enzyme and that in the frog. Both enzymes are much more affected by heat and dialysis than is the mammalian adrenal PNMT. Goldstein and co-workers (42) suggest that the extramedullary pheochromocytoma enzyme may represent the noninducible form of PNMT that is analogous to that present in the frog. However, direct evidence in support of this interesting concept, other than a few similarities in the physical properties of the enzymes, is lacking. The enzyme appears to be homogeneous in the adrenal gland of the same species, although there are isozymes of adrenal PNMT among different species (6).

Recent studies by Ciaranello et al. (17) suggest that the regulation of the levels of PNMT may differ greatly, depending on the strain of animal under study. They examined three inbred mouse strains and evaluated the effects of hypophysectomy, ACTH, dexamethasone, and neural stimulation on the levels of the adrenal enzyme. In the DBA/2J strain, PNMT levels appeared sensitive to both neural and glucocorticoid inputs. In contrast, in the C57BL/Ka strain, PNMT levels were elevated only by ACTH or cold exposure and were unaffected by dexamethasone. The cold exposure response was abolished by hypophysectomy, suggesting that only ACTH was critical in regulation of the adrenal PNMT. In a third strain, CBA/J, the predominant regulating factor appeared to be glucocorticoids and not ACTH. These strains, which appear to exhibit interesting genetic differences regarding regulation of epinephrine synthesis, may provide excellent models for dissecting out the specific mechanisms by which this enzyme may be regulated in the intact animal.

REGULATION OF ADRENAL TYROSINE
HYDROXYLASE BY ADRENAL CORTEX

The level of tyrosine hydroxylase, the enzyme that catalyzes the first step in the biosynthesis of catecholamines, also appears to be modulated by the secretions of the adrenal cortex (5). Wurtman & Axelrod (110) demonstrated that tyrosine hydroxylase activity is reduced by approximately 30% in the adrenal gland of rats 30 days after hypophysectomy. Administration of ACTH prevented the reduction of adrenal tyrosine hydroxylase activity after hypophysectomy (71). In contrast to the analogous studies of PNMT, dexamethasone given in large doses did not restore the levels of tyrosine hydroxylase to normal (71). The effect of ACTH in enhancing levels of adrenal tyrosine hydroxylase in hypophysectomized rats was similar whether the adrenal glands were innervated or not (71).

Kvetňanský and co-workers (54, 55) examined the effects of hypophysectomy, repeated immobilization stress, and adrenal denervation on the catecholamine, tyrosine hydroxylase, and PNMT levels in rat adrenal glands in order to evaluate the relative importance of neural and hormonal factors in regulating the levels of adrenal biosynthetic enzymes. They demonstrated moderate reductions in both norepinephrine and epinephrine and rather profound reductions in tyrosine hydroxylase and PNMT in adrenal glands of rats 2 weeks after hypophysectomy. In sham-operated rats, repeated immobilization stress was associated with a threefold increase in adrenal tyrosine hydroxylase activity, but only a slight elevation of adrenal PNMT. In hypophysectomized animals, tyrosine hydroxylase levels were considerably elevated after repeated immobilization stress, compared with hypophysectomized, unstressed rats, although they reached only about 20% of the levels observed in sham-operated, stressed animals. Levels of PNMT were elevated after repeated immobilization stress only in the sham-operated group. The reduction in adrenal epinephrine and norepinephrine after repetitive stress was considerably greater in the hypophysectomized rats. Administration of ACTH failed to affect either the tyrosine hydroxylase or PNMT levels of the adrenal glands of sham-operated animals. However, ACTH, but not dexamethasone, enhanced the tyrosine hydroxylase response to repeated immobilization stress in hypophysectomized rats. In the presence of either agent, PNMT levels rose after immobilization stress to the same degree as the elevations observed in sham-operated rats that were similarly stressed (55).

Denervation of one adrenal gland did not affect the levels of tyrosine hydroxylase in the denervated gland, compared with the contralateral gland, in either sham-operated or hypophysectomized rats that were not subjected to stress. Hypophysectomy was associated with a reduction in adrenal tyrosine hydroxylase in both normal and denervated glands. If these hypophysectomized animals were repeatedly stressed by immobilization, however, the level of tyrosine hydroxylase rose significantly only in the innervated gland. Administration of ACTH partially restored the tyrosine hydroxylase response of the denervated gland to repeated immobilization stress and greatly enhanced the elevation of the enzyme in the contralateral, innervated gland (54). These results confirm the importance of both nervous and hormonal factors in eliciting enhanced tyrosine hydroxylase levels in the adrenal gland. In contrast, PNMT appears to be much more importantly regulated by the hormonal factors, although nerve impulse traffic may also modulate the levels of this enzyme to some degree.

CYCLIC AMP AND REGULATION OF
ADRENAL TYROSINE HYDROXYLASE

The observation that ACTH, but not dexamethasone, administration can elevate the tyrosine hydroxylase activity in the adrenal glands of hypophysectomized rats is of interest in view of the known ability of this pituitary hormone to enhance adenylate cyclase activity in the adrenal cortex (44) and the observation that levels of tyrosine hydroxylase may be determined by levels of adenosine $3',5'$-monophosphate (cyclic AMP) in the adrenal medulla and other tissues (45, 46, 95). Waymire et al. (95) observed that dibutyryl cyclic AMP, other cyclic AMP analogues, and phosphodiesterase inhibitors all produced progressive increases in the level of tyrosine hydroxylase activity in neuroblastoma cells in culture. Similar increases in the levels of tyrosine hydroxylase activity were observed in sympathetic ganglia incubated in culture in the presence of dibutyryl cyclic AMP (63).

Gewirtz and co-workers (36) demonstrated that administration of dibutyryl cyclic AMP to rats is associated with enhanced levels of tyrosine hydroxylase in the adrenal gland. Paul et al. (76) have observed that either immobilization stress or ACTH administration is associated with increased concentrations of cyclic AMP in the adrenal gland. The increased level of cyclic AMP produced by this immobilization stress could be prevented by hypophysectomy of the rats 10 days before application of the stress. It is of interest that the change in the level of cyclic AMP after immobilization stress is confined to the adrenal cortex, even though almost 50% of the cyclic AMP content of the resting gland is in the medulla. Furthermore adrenal denervation significantly reduced the elevation in adrenal cortex cyclic AMP produced by immobilization stress but did not affect the levels of cyclic AMP in the medulla. The absence of a rise in cyclic AMP in the adrenal medulla with immobilization stress is puzzling in view of the more recent studies of Guidotti and co-workers (45, 46), who demonstrated that stimulation of the adrenal gland with carbachol is associated with a rapid but transient rise in cyclic AMP in both the adrenal medulla and cortex, followed by a rise in tyrosine hydroxylase levels 24 or more hours later. Both of these effects can be blocked by prior administration of ganglionic blocking agents. It is possible that Paul et al. (76) measured cyclic AMP levels at a time when they were no longer elevated, since the immobilization stress was for a period of 30 min and the adrenals were removed and analyzed after this period. Guidotti and co-workers (45, 46) demonstrated the peak rise in adrenal medulla cyclic AMP at 24 min, with the nucleotide levels declining after this time. However, in the latter studies, adrenal medulla cyclic AMP was still elevated at 30 min.

Adrenocorticotropic hormone is believed to stimulate adenylate cyclase activity of adrenal cortex tissue rather selectively (44). Since it is known that cyclic AMP is released from many cells intact and appears in very large concentrations in the urine (15), it is conceivable that the administration of ACTH leads to enhanced adenylate cyclase activity selectively in the adrenal cortex and that the newly formed cyclic AMP is released from cortical cells and travels to the adrenal medulla via the adrenal portal system where it enters cells in some way to induce the synthesis of tyrosine hydroxylase. Alternatively ACTH, or a substance whose production and/or secretion is stimulated by ACTH, may enter the adrenal medulla and in some manner affect the cyclic AMP system of adrenal medulla cells to elevate the intracellular levels of this cyclic nucleotide

REGULATION OF ADRENAL DOPAMINE β-HYDROXYLASE BY ADRENAL CORTEX

Dopamine β-hydroxylase levels in the adrenal gland also appear to be influenced by the adrenal cortex in a manner somewhat, although not entirely, analogous to the regulatory control of tyrosine hydroxylase (3). Weinshilboum & Axelrod (103) have observed that dopamine β-hydroxylase activity is reduced by approximately 70% in adrenal glands 3 weeks after hypophysectomy. The reduction in dopamine β-hydroxylase activity, like that of tyrosine hydroxylase, is partially reversed by administration of ACTH, but the enzyme levels in the adrenal gland are not restored by administration of large doses of glucocorticoids.

Gewirtz et al. (37) confirmed the observations that the enzyme level in the adrenal gland declines progressively for several months after hypophysectomy, although the reductions were considerably less than those observed by Weinshilboum & Axelrod (103), averaging 23 and 42% at 21 and 180 days posthypophysectomy, respectively. Daily administration of ACTH between days 8 and 14 after hypophysectomy was associated with a partial restoration of the enzyme levels in the adrenal; if ACTH was administered daily between 40 and 46 days after hypophysectomy, the enzyme levels were the same as those in adrenals of sham-operated control rats (37). Contrary to the results of Weinshilboum & Axelrod (103), Gewirtz et al. (37) were able to reverse completely the lowered adrenal dopamine β-hydroxylase levels associated with hypophysectomy by daily injection of dexamethasone between days 8 and 14 after the surgical procedure. The discrepancy may be related to the differences in the interval between hypophysectomy and glucocorticoid treatment. It is possible that the acute effects on the adrenal are related to a postsurgical stress response that can be overcome by glucocorticoids, whereas after a more prolonged period the decreased enzyme level is related to the absence of the trophic effect of ACTH on the adrenal. This latter effect, analogous to the effect on adrenal tyrosine hydroxylase, may not be reversed by glucocorticoids alone.

Gewirtz et al. (37) also examined the effects of unilateral adrenal denervation of 10 days duration and of immobilization stress on adrenal dopamine β-hydroxylase activity in sham-operated rats and in rats subjected to hypophysectomy 15 days before enzyme analysis. In the rats not subjected to immobilization stress, hypophysectomy was associated with a proportionate decline in dopamine β-hydroxylase activity in both innervated and denervated glands, although the innervated glands in both groups contained about twice as much enzyme activity as the corresponding denervated organs. Daily immobilization stress for 7 days resulted in increased levels of adrenal dopamine β-hydroxylase in both the denervated and innervated glands of sham-operated animals, although the increase was considerably greater in the innervated gland. No significant effects of immobilization stress on adrenal dopamine β-hydroxylase levels were observed in either gland in rats that had been hypophysectomized. Dopamine β-hydroxylase therefore seems to be under both neuronal and humoral control, as is tyrosine hydroxylase.

Administration of dibutyryl cyclic AMP to rats is associated with an increase in the level of dopamine β-hydroxylase activity in the adrenal gland (36). It thus appears that, by a mechanism analogous to that described for tyrosine hydroxylase, the tonic effect of ACTH on dopamine β-hydroxylase levels may be related to an effect of this hormone on adrenal cortical or adrenal medullary cyclic AMP.

ROLE OF ASCORBIC ACID IN SYNTHESIS AND CATABOLISM OF ADRENAL CATECHOLAMINES

The adrenal gland contains ascorbic acid in concentrations considerably greater than those present in most other mammalian tissues (27, 78, 84). Although the adrenal cortex contains approximately twice the concentration of ascorbic acid of the medulla, the latter is also relatively rich in this material, containing approximately 1–1.5 mg/g tissue (40, 41, 47, 78). Speculations about the role of this vitamin in adrenal medulla function have been offered for decades (78). Until recent years the most generally accepted function of ascorbic acid related to its reducing properties and its ability to stabilize catecholamines in adrenal tissue (48, 92). Although the ability of ascorbic acid to stabilize catecholamines is undisputed, the importance of this chemical interaction in vivo is not clear. In scorbutic guinea pigs, Doby & Weisinger (26) observed that adrenal medulla catecholamines were depleted. However, they also reported that blood epinephrine was elevated in these scorbutic animals, although the specificity of their assay for plasma catecholamines might be challenged. In contrast, Giroud & Martinet (39) reported that, as guinea pigs were made scorbutic, adrenal ascorbic acid levels fell progressively, but adrenal epinephrine rose to a level almost twice that of control guinea pigs.

Sayers et al. (84, 85) demonstrated that either the stress of hemorrhage or administration of ACTH was associated with a reduction in adrenal cholesterol and ascorbic acid. In man, administration of ACTH, but not of cortisone, is associated with elevated levels of ascorbic acid in plasma and enhanced ascorbic acid excretion in the urine (8). If even a proportion of this increase in plasma ascorbic acid originates from the adrenal cortex, one must presume that very high concentrations of both ascorbic acid and the glucocorticoids perfuse the adrenal medulla before entering the general circulation. Hypophysectomy is associated with a reduction in the concentration of ascorbic acid in the adrenal glands (91).

Ascorbic acid may exert a direct role in the biosynthesis of catecholamines. Tyrosine hydroxylase, generally regarded as the rate-limiting enzyme in the biosynthesis of catecholamines (72, 97), requires a reducing agent as cosubstrate (11, 72), apparently tetrahydrobiopterin (55). Ascorbic acid appears to enhance tyrosine hydroxylase activity, presumably by either maintaining the tetrahydrobiopterin in the reduced state or facilitating the conversion of dihydrobiopterin to the tetrahydro form (88). In addition to enhancing the activity of the enzyme, ascorbic acid may increase the levels of the enzyme in the adrenal gland in some as yet undefined manner. Nakashima et al. (73) have observed that adrenal tyrosine hydroxylase activity, as measured in fortified homogenates of adrenal glands, is decreased in scurvy and is restored by prior administration of ascorbic acid to the guinea pig. These workers demonstrated that this effect of ascorbic acid could be blocked by either puromycin or by actinomycin D. It is possible that the mechanism by which ACTH enhances the levels of tyrosine hydroxylase, and perhaps dopamine β-hydroxylase activity, in the adrenal medulla is mediated by its ability to enhance ascorbic acid secretion from the adrenal cortex.

Dopamine β-hydroxylase is a mixed-function oxidase that requires a reducing substance as cosubstrate. Levin & Kaufman (60) have suggested that the natural cosubstrate for this reaction is ascorbic acid. The ascorbic acid secreted during adrenal cortical stimulation may be taken up by adrenal medulla chromaffin cells and may provide the cosubstrate, which might otherwise be limiting, for the hydroxylation of dopamine to norepinephrine.

Thus factors other than glucocorticoids, which originate in the adrenal cortex, may modify the levels or activity of the catecholamine biosynthetic enzymes in the adrenal medulla. Clarification of the precise physiological role, if any, of ascorbic acid and other products of the adrenal cortex in regulating adrenal medulla catecholamine production and other aspects of catecholamine metabolism must await further research.

CONCLUSION

The investigations summarized in the preceding sections indicate the important regulatory influences that glucocorticoids and ACTH exert on several of the catecholamine biosynthetic enzymes of the adrenal medulla. The glucocorticoids appear to be important modulators of the level of the enzyme PNMT and therefore of the proportion of norepinephrine and epinephrine present in the adrenal medulla. Stress is associated with enhanced ACTH and glucocorticoid secretion, which in turn would favor epinephrine production in the adrenal medulla. Administration of the N-methylated catecholamine results in effects on target organs that might more characteristically be classified as appropriate responses to stress, as compared with the effects associated with norepinephrine infusion. Thus the adrenal medulla might be considered as one of many target organs for the adrenal cortex in which stress responses are elicited.

The levels of both tyrosine hydroxylase and dopamine β-hydroxylase appear to be more dependent on circulating ACTH levels than on glucocorticoids. More profound elevations in the levels of both enzymes in the adrenal medulla result from chronic increases in nervous impulses to the gland. The quantitative interrelationships between ACTH and nerve stimulation as determinants of the levels of these two enzymes remain to be clarified. Genetic factors are also important in the expression of these effects. Systematic analyses of other factors, including age, sex, season, and various types of stress inputs, have not been conducted. It is likely that many, if not all, of these inputs will modulate the relative importance of neural and hormonal factors in this system.

Finally the molecular basis for actions of the humoral and neural factors responsible for regulating the catecholamine biosynthetic enzymes of the adrenal medulla has not been clarified. Cyclic AMP may be involved in this process, but other factors, such as ascorbic acid, may also be implicated. It is not yet clear whether increased synthesis and release of cyclic AMP from the adrenal cortex is an intermediate step in the ACTH-induced elevation of the levels of tyrosine hydroxylase and dopamine β-hydroxylase of the adrenal medulla. It is likely that many other substances that have not yet been identified are released from the adrenal cortex during ACTH stimulation and that some of these factors (e.g., ascorbic acid) may mediate effects on catecholamine synthesis in the adrenal medulla.

REFERENCES

1. ALOUSI, A., AND N. WEINER. The regulation of norepinephrine synthesis in sympathetic nerves. Effect of nerve stimulation, cocaine and catecholamine releasing agents. *Proc. Natl. Acad. Sci. US* 56: 1491–1496, 1966.
2. AXELROD, J. Purification and properties of phenylethanolamine-N-methyl transferase. *J. Biol. Chem.* 237: 1657–1660, 1962.
3. AXELROD, J. Dopamine-β-hydroxylase: regulation of its synthesis and release from nerve terminals. *Pharmacol. Rev.* 24: 233–243, 1972.
4. AXELROD, J. Neural and hormonal control of catecholamine synthesis. *Res. Publ. Assoc. Res. Nervous Mental Disease* 50: 229–240, 1972.
5. AXELROD, J., R. A. MUELLER, AND H. THOENEN. Neuronal and hormonal control of tyrosine hydroxylase and phenylethanolamine N-methyltransferase activity. In: *Bayer Symposium II. New Aspects of Storage and Release Mechanisms of Catecholamines*, edited by H. J. Schümann and G. Kroneberg. New York: Springer Verlag, 1970, p. 212–219.
6. AXELROD, J., AND E. S. VESELL. Heterogeneity of N- and O-methyltransferases. *Mol. Pharmacol.* 6: 78–84, 1970.
7. BALIGA, B. S., L. A. POHORECKY, H. N. MUNRO, AND R. J. WURTMAN. Control of adrenal medullary protein synthesis by corticosteroids. *Biochim. Biophys. Acta* 299: 337–343, 1973.
8. BECK, J. C., J. S. L. BROWNE, AND K. R. MACKENZIE. The effect of adrenocorticotrophic hormone and cortisone on the metabolism of ascorbic acid. In: *Proceedings of the Second Clinical ACTH Conference. Research*, edited by J. R. Mote. New York: Blakiston, 1951, vol. 1, p. 355–366.
9. BISCARDI, A. M., AND G. F. WASSERMANN. Release of catecholamines from adrenalinogenic and noradrenalinogenic tissue by the action of nicotine "in vitro." *Arch. Intern. Pharmacodyn. Therap.* 159: 424–433, 1966.
10. BLASCHKO, H. Catecholamine biosynthesis. *Brit. Med. Bull.* 29: 105–109, 1973.
11. BRENNEMAN, A. R., AND S. KAUFMAN. The role of tetrahydropteridines in the enzymatic conversion of tyrosine to 3,4-dihydroxyphenylalanine. *Biochem. Biophys. Res. Commun.* 17: 177–183, 1964.
12. BRIMIJOIN, S., AND P. B. MOLINOFF. Effects of 6-hydroxydopamine on the activity of tyrosine hydroxylase and dopamine-β-hydroxylase in sympathetic ganglia of the rat. *J. Pharmacol. Exptl. Therap.* 178: 417–425, 1971.
13. BRUNDIN, T. Catecholamines in adrenals from fetal rabbits. *Acta Physiol. Scand.* 63: 509–510, 1965.
14. BURACK, W. R., N. WEINER, AND P. B. HAGEN. The effect of reserpine on the catecholamine and adenine nucleotide content of chicken adrenals. *J. Pharmacol. Exptl. Therap.* 130: 245–250, 1960.
15. BUTCHER, R. W., AND E. W. SUTHERLAND. Adenosine 3',5'-phosphate in biological materials. I. Purification and properties of cyclic 3',5-nucleotide phosphodiesterase and use of this enzyme to characterize adenosine 3',5'-phosphate in human urine. *J. Biol. Chem.* 237: 1244–1250, 1962.
16. CIARANELLO, R. D., J. D. BARCHAS, AND J. VERNIKOS-DANELLIS. Compensatory hypertrophy and phenylethanolamine N-methyltransferase (PNMT) activity in the rat adrenal. *Life Sci.* 8: 401–407, 1969.
17. CIARANELLO, R. D., J. N. DORNBUSCH, AND J. D. BARCHAS. Regulation of adrenal phenylethanolamine N-methyltransferase activity in three inbred mouse strains. *Mol. Pharmacol.* 8: 511–520, 1972.
18. COUPLAND, R. E. On the morphology and adrenaline-noradrenaline content of chromaffin tissue. *J. Endocrinol.* 9: 194–203, 1953.
19. COUPLAND, R. E. The development and fate of the abdominal chromaffin tissue in the rabbit. *J. Anat.* 90: 527–537, 1956.
20. COUPLAND, R. E. The effects of insulin, reserpine and choline 2:6-xylylether bromide on the adrenal medulla and on medullary autografts in the rat. *J. Endocrinol.* 17: 191–196, 1958.
21. COUPLAND, R. E. Synthesis and storage of pressor amines in adrenal medullary grafts. *J. Endocrinol.* 18: 162–164, 1959.
22. COUPLAND, R. E. *The Natural History of the Chromaffin Cell.* London: Longmans, Green, 1965.
23. COUPLAND, R. E. Corticosterone and methylation of noradrenaline by extra-adrenal chromaffin tissue. *J. Endocrinol.* 41: 487–490, 1968.
24. COUPLAND, R. E., AND J. D. B. MACDOUGALL. Adrenaline formation in noradrenaline-storing chromaffin cells in vitro induced by corticosterone. *J. Endocrinol.* 36: 317–324, 1966.
25. CROUT, J. R., AND A. SJOERDSMA. Turnover and metabolism of catecholamines in patients with pheochromocytoma. *J. Clin. Invest.* 43: 94–102, 1964.
26. DOBY, T., AND I. WEISINGER. Veränderungen des Adrenalingehaltes des Blutes und der Nebennieren während des Skorbuts normaler bzw. schilddrüsenloser Meerschweinchen. *Z. Physiol. Chem.* 255: 259–266, 1938.
27. DURY, A. The correlation of the circulating polymorphonuclear leucocytes (neutrophiles) with the adrenal ascorbic acid in the rat. *Endocrinology* 43: 336–348, 1948.
28. ENGELMAN, K., AND W. G. HAMMOND. Adrenaline production by an intrathoracic phaeochromocytoma. *Lancet* 1: 609–611, 1968.
29. ERÄNKÖ, O. Distribution of adrenaline and noradrenaline in the hen adrenal gland. *Nature* 179: 417–418, 1957.
30. ERÄNKÖ, O., M. LEMPINEN, AND L. RÄISÄNEN. Adrenaline and noradrenaline in the organ of Zuckerkandl and adrenals of newborn rats treated with hydrocortisone. *Acta Physiol. Scand.* 66: 253–254, 1966.
31. ERÄNKÖ, O., M. LEMPINEN, AND L. RÄISÄNEN. Effect of hydrocortisone administration in utero on the adrenaline and noradrenaline content of extra-adrenal chromaffin tissue in the rat. *Acta Physiol. Scand.* 69: 255–256, 1967.
32. EULER, U. S. V., AND G. STRÖM. Present status of diagnosis and treatment of pheochromocytoma. *Circulation* 15: 5–13, 1957.
33. FULLER, R. W. Control of epinephrine synthesis and secretion. *Federation Proc.* 32: 1772–1781, 1973.

34. FULLER, R. W., AND J. M. HUNT. Activity of phenethanolamine N-methyl transferase in the adrenal glands of foetal and neonatal rats. *Nature* 214: 190, 1967.
35. FULLER, R. W., AND J. M. HUNT. Inhibition of phenylethanolamine N-methyl transferase by its product, epinephrine. *Life Sci.* 6: 1107–1112, 1967.
36. GEWIRTZ, G. P., R. KVETŇANSKÝ, V. K. WEISE, AND I. J. KOPIN. Effect of ACTH and dibutyryl cyclic AMP on catecholamine synthesizing enzymes in the adrenals of hypophysectomized rats. *Nature* 230: 462–464, 1971.
37. GEWIRTZ, G. P., R. KVETŇANSKÝ, V. K. WEISE, AND I. J. KOPIN. Effect of hypophysectomy on adrenal dopamine-β-hydroxylase activity in the rat. *Mol. Pharmacol.* 7: 163–168, 1971.
38. GHOSH, A. A comparative study of the histochemistry of the avian adrenals. *Gen. Comp. Endocrinol. Suppl.* 1: 75–80, 1962.
39. GIROUD, A., AND M. MARTINET. Augmentation de l'adrenalinogénese au cours de la carence C. *Bull. Soc. Chim. Biol.* 23: 456–458, 1941.
40. GIROUD, A., AND N. SANTA. Variations sexuelles du cortex et de la médullosurrénale. Variations ponderalés et taux de l'acide ascorbique. *Compt. Rend. Soc. Biol.* 133: 420–421, 1940.
41. GLICK, D., AND G. R. BISKIND. The histochemistry of the adrenal gland. I. The quantitative distribution of vitamin C. *J. Biol. Chem.* 110: 1–7, 1935.
42. GOLDSTEIN, M., H. GANG, AND T. H. JOH. Subcellular distribution and properties of phenylethanolamine-N-methyl transferase (PNMT). *Federation Proc.* 28: 287, 1969.
43. GOODALL, McC., AND N. KIRSHNER. Biosynthesis of adrenaline and noradrenaline in vitro. *J. Biol. Chem.* 226: 213–221, 1957.
44. GRAHAME-SMITH, D. C., R. W. BUTCHER, R. L. NEY, AND E. W. SUTHERLAND. Adenosine 3′,5′-monophosphate as the intracellular mediator of the action of adrenocorticotropic hormone on the adrenal cortex. *J. Biol. Chem.* 242: 5535–5541, 1967.
45. GUIDOTTI, A., AND E. COSTA. Involvement of adenosine 3′,5′-monophosphate in the activation of tyrosine hydroxylase elicited by drugs. *Science* 179: 902–904, 1973.
46. GUIDOTTI, A., B. ZIVKOVIC, R. PFEIFFER, AND E. COSTA. Involvement of 3′,5′-cyclic adenosine monophosphate in the increase of tyrosine hydroxylase elicited by cold exposure. *Arch. Pharmacol.* 278: 195–206, 1973.
47. HARRIS, L. J., AND S. N. RAY. Vitamin C in the suprarenal medulla. *Biochem. J.* 27: 2006–2010, 1933.
48. HEARD, R. D. H., AND A. D. WELCH. The perfusion of the adrenal gland with reference to the mechanism of adrenaline stabilization. *Biochem. J.* 29: 998–1008, 1935.
49. HÖKFELT, B. Noradrenaline and adrenaline in mammalian tissues. *Acta Physiol. Scand. Suppl.* 92: 1–134, 1952.
50. HOLTON, P. High concentration of noradrenaline in calves' suprarenals. *Nature* 167: 858–859, 1951.
51. HOLZBAUER, M., AND M. VOGT. Corticosteroids in plasma and cells of adrenal venous blood. *J. Physiol., London* 157: 137–156, 1961.
52. HOLZBAUER, M., AND D. F. SHARMAN. The distribution of catecholamines in vertebrates. In: *Catecholamines*, edited by H. Blaschko and E. Muscholl. Berlin: Springer Verlag, 1972, p. 110–185.
53. KIRSHNER, N., AND McC. GOODALL. The formation of adrenaline from noradrenaline. *Biochim. Biophys. Acta* 24: 658–659, 1957.
54. KVETŇANSKÝ, R., G. P. GEWIRTZ, V. K. WEISE, AND I. J. KOPIN. Effect of hypophysectomy on immobilization-induced elevation of tyrosine hydroxylase and phenylethanolamine-N-methyl transferase in the rat adrenal. *Endocrinology* 87: 1323–1329, 1970.
55. KVETŇANSKÝ, R., V. K. WEISE, AND I. J. KOPIN. Elevation of adrenal tyrosine hydroxylase and phenylethanolamine-N-methyl transferase by repeated immobilization of rats. *Endocrinology* 87: 744–749, 1970.
56. LEMPINEN, M. Effect of cortisone on extra-adrenal chromaffin tissue of the rat. *Nature* 199: 74–75, 1963.
57. LEMPINEN, M. Extra-adrenal chromaffin tissue of the rat and the effect of cortical hormones on it. *Acta Physiol. Scand. Suppl.* 231: 1–91, 1964.
58. LEMPINEN, M. Effect of hydrocortisone on histochemically demonstrable catecholamines of the para-aortic body of the rat. *Acta Physiol. Scand.* 66: 251–252, 1966.
59. LEVER, J. D. Observations on the adrenal blood vessels in the rat. *J. Anat.* 86: 459–467, 1952.
60. LEVIN, E. Y., AND S. KAUFMAN. Studies on the enzyme catalyzing the conversion of 3,4-dihydroxyphenylethylamine to norepinephrine. *J. Biol. Chem.* 236: 2043–2049, 1961.
61. LLOYD, T., AND N. WEINER. Isolation and characterization of a tyrosine hydroxylase cofactor from bovine adrenal medulla. *Mol. Pharmacol.* 7: 568–580, 1971.
62. LUFT, R., AND U. S. VON EULER. Effect of insulin hypoglycemia on urinary excretion of adrenaline and noradrenaline in man after hypophysectomy. *J. Clin. Endocrinol. Metab.* 16: 1017–1025, 1956.
63. MACKAY, A. V. P., AND L. L. IVERSEN. Increased tyrosine hydroxylase activity of sympathetic ganglia cultured in the presence of dibutyryl cyclic AMP. *Brain Res.* 48: 424–426, 1972.
64. MARGOLIS, F. L., J. ROFFI, AND A. JOST. Norepinephrine methylation in fetal rat adrenals. *Science* 154: 275–276, 1966.
65. MIĆIĆ, R., M. KIĆIĆ, AND S. ADANJA. Phaeochromocytoma of urinary bladder. *Acta Endocrinol.* 39: 1–12, 1962.
66. MOLINOFF, P. B., AND J. AXELROD. Biochemistry of catecholamines. *Ann. Rev. Biochem.* 40: 465–500, 1971.
67. MOLINOFF, P. B., W. S. BRIMIJOIN, R. WEINSHILBOUM, AND J. AXELROD. Neurally mediated increases in dopamine-β-hydroxylase activity. *Proc. Natl. Acad. Sci. US* 66: 453–458, 1970.
68. MOSCONA, A. A., AND R. PIDDINGTON. Enzyme induction by corticosteroids in embryonic cells: steroid structure and inductive effect. *Science* 158: 496–497, 1967.
69. MUELLER, R. A., H. THOENEN, AND J. AXELROD. Increase in tyrosine hydroxylase activity after reserpine administration. *J. Pharmacol. Exptl. Therap.* 169: 74–79, 1969.
70. MUELLER, R. A., H. THOENEN, AND J. AXELROD. Adrenal tyrosine hydroxylase: compensatory increase in activity after chemical sympathectomy. *Science* 163: 468–469, 1969.
71. MUELLER, R. A., H. THOENEN, AND J. AXELROD. Effect of pituitary and ACTH on the maintenance of basal tyrosine hydroxylase activity in the rat adrenal gland. *Endocrinology* 86: 751–755, 1970.
72. NAGATSU, T., M. LEVITT, AND S. UDENFRIEND. Tyrosine hydroxylase. The initial step in norepinephrine biosynthesis. *J. Biol. Chem.* 239: 2910–2917, 1964.
73. NAKASHIMA, Y., R. SUZUE, H. SANADA, AND S. KAWADA. Effect of ascorbic acid on tyrosine hydroxylase activity in vivo. *Arch. Biochem. Biophys.* 152: 515–520, 1972.
74. NIEMINEVA, K., AND A. PEKKARINEN, Determination of adrenalin and noradrenalin in the human foetal adrenals and aortic bodies. *Nature* 171: 436–437, 1953.
75. PATRICK, R. L., AND N. KIRSHNER. Effect of stimulation on the levels of tyrosine hydroxylase, dopamine-β-hydroxylase and catecholamines in intact and denervated rat adrenal glands. *Mol. Pharmacol.* 7: 87–96, 1971.
76. PAUL, M. I., R. KVETŇANSKÝ, H. CRAMER, S. SILBERGELD, AND I. J. KOPIN. Immobilization stress induced changes in adrenocortical and medullary cyclic AMP content in the rat. *Endocrinology* 88: 338–344, 1971.
77. PEYRIN, L., J. F. CIER, AND G. PERES. La méthylation de la noradrénaline et les interrelations corticomedullaires chez la Roussette. *Ann. Endocrinol.* 30: 1–38, 1969.
78. PIRANI, C. L. Review: relation of vitamin C to adrenocortical function and stress phenomena. *Metabolism* 1: 197–222, 1952.
79. POHORECKY, L. A., R. S. PIEZZI, AND R. J. WURTMAN. Steroid induction of phenylethanolamine-N-methyl transferase in adrenomedullary explants: independence of adrenal innervation. *Endocrinology* 86: 1466–1468, 1970.

80. POHORECKY, L. A., AND R. J. WURTMAN. Induction of epinephrine-forming enzyme by glucocorticoids: steroid hydroxylation and inductive effect. *Nature* 219: 392–394, 1968.
81. POHORECKY, L. A., AND R. J. WURTMAN. Adrenocortical control of epinephrine synthesis. *Pharmacol. Rev.* 23: 1–35, 1971.
82. ROFFI, J. Influence des corticosurrénales sur la synthèse d'adrénaline chez le foetus et le nouveau-né de rat et de lapin. *J. Physiol., Paris* 60: 455–494, 1968.
83. ROFFI, J., AND F. MARGOLIS. Synthèse d'adrénaline dans le tissu chromaffine extra-surrénalien, chez le rat nouveau-né sous l'effet de l'hydrocortisone ou de la corticostimuline. *Compt. Rend.* 263: 1496–1499, 1966.
84. SAYERS, G., M. A. SAYERS, T. Y. LIANG, AND C. N. H. LONG. The cholesterol and ascorbic acid content of the adrenal, liver, brain and plasma following hemorrhage. *Endocrinology* 37: 96–110, 1945.
85. SAYERS, G., M. A. SAYERS, T. LIANG, AND C. N. H. LONG. The effect of pituitary adrenotrophic hormone on the cholesterol and ascorbic acid content of the adrenal of the rat and the guinea pig. *Endocrinology* 38: 1–9, 1946.
86. SHEPHERD, D. M., AND G. B. WEST. Noradrenaline and the suprarenal medulla. *Brit. J. Pharmacol.* 6: 665–674, 1951.
87. SHEPHERD, D. M., G. B. WEST, AND V. ERSPAMER. Chromaffin bodies of various species of dogfish. *Nature* 172: 509, 1953.
88. STONE, K. J., AND B. H. TOWNSLEY. The effect of L-ascorbate on catecholamine biosynthesis. *Biochem. J.* 131: 611–613, 1973.
89. THOA, N. B., D. G. JOHNSON, I. J. KOPIN, AND N. WEINER. Acceleration of catecholamine formation in the guinea-pig vas deferens following hypogastric nerve stimulation: roles of tyrosine hydroxylase and new protein synthesis. *J. Pharmacol. Exptl. Therap.* 178: 442–449, 1971.
90. THOENEN, H., R. A. MUELLER, AND J. AXELROD. Trans-synaptic induction of adrenal tyrosine hydroxylase. *J. Pharmacol. Exptl. Therap.* 169: 249–254, 1969.
91. TYSLOWITZ, R. Effect of hypophysectomy on the concentration of ascorbic acid in the adrenals of the rat. *Endocrinology* 32: 103–108, 1943.
92. VERLY, A. Oxydation de l'adrénaline et de la vitamine C. Actions réciproques. *Arch. Intern. Physiol.* 56: 1–24, 1948.
93. VERNIKOS-DANELLIS, J., R. CIARANELLO, AND J. BARCHAS. Adrenal epinephrine and phenylethanolamine N-methyl transferase (PNMT) activity in the rat bearing a transplantable pituitary tumor. *Endocrinology* 83: 1357–1358, 1968.
94. WASSERMANN, G., AND J. H. TRAMEZZANI. Separate distribution of adrenaline- and noradrenaline-secreting cells in the adrenal of snakes. *Gen. Comp. Endocrinol.* 3: 480–489, 1963.
95. WAYMIRE, J. C., N. WEINER, AND K. N. PRASAD. Regulation of tyrosine hydroxylase activity in cultured mouse neuroblastoma cells: elevation induced by analogs of adenosine 3′,5′-cyclic monophosphate. *Proc. Natl. Acad. Sci. US* 69: 2241–2245, 1972.
96. WEINER, N. The regulation of adrenergic neurotransmitter metabolism. In: *Progress in Endocrinology. Proceedings of the Third International Congress of Endocrinology.* Amsterdam: Excerpta Medica Foundation, 1969, p. 294–301. (Intern. Congr. Ser. 184.)
97. WEINER, N. Regulation of norepinephrine biosynthesis. *Ann. Rev. Pharmacol.* 10: 273–290, 1970.
98. WEINER, N., W. R. BURACK, AND P. B. HAGEN. The effect of insulin on the catecholamine and adenine nucleotide content of chicken adrenals. *J. Pharmacol. Exptl. Therap.* 130: 251–255, 1960.
99. WEINER, N., G. CLOUTIER, R. BJUR, AND R. I. PFEFFER. Modification of norepinephrine synthesis in intact tissue by drugs and during short-term adrenergic nerve stimulation. *Pharmacol. Rev.* 24: 203–221, 1972.
100. WEINER, N., AND W. F. MOSIMANN. The effect of insulin on the catecholamine content of cat adrenal glands. *Biochem. Pharmacol.* 19: 1189–1199, 1970.
101. WEINER, N., AND M. RABADJIJA. The effect of nerve stimulation on the synthesis and metabolism of norepinephrine in the isolated guinea-pig hypogastric nerve-vas deferens preparation. *J. Pharmacol. Exptl. Therap.* 160: 61–71, 1968.
102. WEINER, N., AND M. RABADJIJA. The regulation of norepinephrine synthesis. Effect of puromycin on the accelerated synthesis of norepinephrine associated with nerve stimulation. *J. Pharmacol. Exptl. Therap.* 164: 103–114, 1968.
103. WEINSHILBOUM, R. M., AND J. AXELROD. Dopamine-β-hydroxylase activity in the rat after hypophysectomy. *Endocrinology* 87: 894–899, 1970.
104. WEST, G. B. The comparative pharmacology of the suprarenal medulla. *Quart. Rev. Biol.* 30: 116–137, 1955.
105. WEST, G. B., D. M. SHEPHERD, AND R. B. HUNTER. Adrenaline and noradrenaline concentrations in adrenal glands at different ages and in some diseases. *Lancet* 2: 966–969, 1951.
106. WINKLER, H., AND A. D. SMITH. Phaeochromocytoma and other catecholamine producing tumors. In: *Catecholamines*, edited by H. Blaschko and E. Muscholl. Berlin: Springer Verlag, 1972, p. 900–933.
107. WRIGHT, A., AND I. CHESTER JONES. Chromaffin tissue in the lizard adrenal gland. *Nature* 175: 1001–1002, 1955.
108. WURTMAN, R. J. Control of epinephrine synthesis in the adrenal medulla by the adrenal cortex: hormonal specificity and dose-response characteristics. *Endocrinology* 79: 608–614, 1966.
109. WURTMAN, R. J., AND J. AXELROD. Adrenaline synthesis: control by the pituitary gland and adrenal glucocorticoids. *Science* 150: 1464–1465, 1965.
110. WURTMAN, R. J., AND J. AXELROD. Control of enzymatic synthesis of adrenaline in the adrenal medulla by adrenal cortical steroids. *J. Biol. Chem.* 241: 2301–2305, 1966.
111. WURTMAN, R. J., J. AXELROD, AND J. TRAMEZZANI. Distribution of the adrenaline-forming enzyme in the adrenal gland of a snake, *Xeondon merremii*. *Nature* 215: 879–880, 1967.
112. WURTMAN, R. J., J. AXELROD, E. S. VESELL, AND G. T. ROSS. Species difference in inducibility of phenylethanolamine-N-methyl transferase. *Endocrinology* 82: 584–590, 1968.
113. WURTMAN, R. J., AND L. A. POHORECKY. Adrenocortical control of epinephrine synthesis in health and disease. *Advan. Metab. Disorders* 5: 53–76, 1971.
114. WURTMAN, R. J., L. A. POHORECKY, AND B. S. BALIGA. Adrenocortical control of the biosynthesis of epinephrine and proteins in the adrenal medulla. *Pharmacol. Rev.* 24: 411–426, 1972.

CHAPTER 26

Secretomotor control of adrenal medullary secretion: synaptic, membrane, and ionic events in stimulus-secretion coupling

W. W. DOUGLAS | *Department of Pharmacology, Yale University School of Medicine, New Haven, Connecticut*

CHAPTER CONTENTS

Historical Background
Responses to Stimulation of Splanchnic Nerves
  Spatial recruitment, overlap, and convergence
  Frequency-response relations
  Splanchnic-adrenal fatigue
  Preferential secretion of epinephrine and norepinephrine
Basal Secretion, Denervation, and Supersensitivity
Cholinergic Nature of Secretomotor Fibers
Acetylcholine Receptors
  Nicotinic and muscarinic receptors
  Preferential secretion of epinephrine and norepinephrine
Cholinesterase and Cholinesterase Inhibitors
Secretagogues Other than Acetylcholine
Intracellular Recording with Microelectrodes
  Resting transmembrane potentials
  Depolarization in response to acetylcholine
  Inward sodium and calcium currents
  Electrical properties of chromaffin cells
Ions and Secretion
  Calcium is essential and sufficient for responses to acetylcholine
  Potassium stimulates and also requires calcium
  Calcium itself is a secretagogue
  Strontium and barium are calcium substitutes and stimulants
  Magnesium inhibits responses to acetylcholine, potassium, calcium, strontium, and barium
  Sodium lack and potentiation of basal and evoked secretion
  Potassium lack and potentiation of basal and evoked secretion
  Stimulant effects of ouabain
  Prolonged sodium deprivation inhibits
Role of Depolarization
Termination of Secretory Responses and Calcium Inactivation
Membrane and Ionic Events: a Summing-up
Parallels with Excitation-Contraction Coupling
Chromaffin Cell as Model System

SYNAPTIC AND CELLULAR EVENTS controlling secretion of adrenal medullary hormones—*secretion* here meaning release or discharge of secretory product—are considered in this chapter. Such usage, although frowned on by some morphologists and others who would retain for secretion its older meaning of elaboration and sequestration of secretory product, is customary in physiology and gaining in popularity in biology as the older sense of the word is being supplanted by the terms *synthesis* and *storage*. Discussion is restricted to the influence of the secretomotor nerves on the medullary chromaffin cells and the problem of *stimulus-secretion coupling*, which has been defined as "embracing all the events occurring in the cell exposed to its immediate stimulus (in this instance the synaptic transmitter, acetylcholine, released by the secretomotor nerves) that lead, finally, to the appearance of the characteristic secretory product (here the catecholamines) in the extracellular environment" (45). Since morphological and biochemical aspects of stimulus-secretion coupling are treated in detail in other chapters (see the chapters by Grynszpan-Winograd and Viveros, respectively, in this volume of the *Handbook*) they are touched on here only to the extent required for a coherent account; the main emphasis is given to membrane and ionic events. It will be recognized, however, that this separate consideration of phenomena constituting part of an ill-defined sequence is somewhat arbitrary, and the present chapter is certainly intended to be read in conjunction with the other two mentioned above.

HISTORICAL BACKGROUND

Studies on the adrenal medulla have had prominent and germinal influences on the development of a variety of physiological concepts, not only within the field of endocrinology but in those of chemical transmission and secretion in general, including secretion by such disparate entities as exocrine cells and neurons. This is readily understandable, for the adrenal gland is an exceptionally favorable test object. It is anatomically obvious, accessible, and provided with a comparatively simple vasculature that allows perfusion and quantitative recovery of venous effluent. It possesses well-defined secretomotor nerves liberating a known, simple, available, chemical substance, acetylcholine (ACh); and the cholinergic synapses between nerves and chromaffin cells are vulnerable to alkaloids, such as nicotine and physostigmine, which have long been studied by pharmacologists and which, along with many other drugs, provide valuable tools for analyzing synaptic function. Moreover, the medullary hormones, the catecholamines, have such potent, rapid, and reproducible cardiovascular actions that the crudest experiments with watery extracts reveal their presence and but little skill is required for their bioassay—and still less for their detection and measurement by sensitive fluorometric procedures.

The anatomic discreteness of the adrenal glands allowed their recognition by the ancients, and their association with the sympathetic nervous system, although less venerable, was well known more than a century ago. Despite this, the function of these glands, including the medulla with which we are presently concerned, eluded discovery right up to the end of the 19th century when many more subtle physiological mechanisms had long since been unraveled (158). By 1895, however, Oliver & Schäfer (138) had witnessed the remarkable effects of adrenal extracts on heart and blood vessels and made the essential point that "it appears established that like the thyroid gland, the suprarenal capsules are to be regarded, although ductless, as strictly secreting glands." Shortly thereafter the Polish physiologist Czybulski (31) detected the cardiovascular principle in adrenal venous blood. It remained only to account for the old anatomic observation of the close relation between suprarenal capsules and the sympathetic nervous system and the fact that sympathetic nerves could be traced to the medullary region. In retrospect, it is puzzling that this proved so difficult, for secretomotor control of exocrine glands had been demonstrated by Ludwig some 50 years earlier, had been studied by Bernard and many others, and was familiar to physiologists at the end of the 19th century (1); moreover the effects of stimulating the splanchnic nerves were, within a few years—in the 1920s—considered sufficiently striking to be included in a much-used student laboratory manual (118). In any event, both Oliver & Schäfer (138) and Biedl (11), a dominant figure in the study of glands of "inner secretion" (endocrinology, as we now call it), failed to find any response to splanchnic stimulation. It is interesting to speculate on the degree to which prejudice against the notion of innervation of an endocrine gland contributed to their negative results. By 1898, however, Dreyer (69), in his work at Johns Hopkins, had confirmed Czybulski's discovery and succeeded in demonstrating an increase in the amount of cardiovascular principle (catecholamine) in the adrenal venous blood on electrical stimulation of the splanchnic nerves. Triumphantly he wrote that his analysis furnished "the first demonstration of the actual existence of nerves for controlling internal secretion." Although greeted at first with some skepticism, his results were elegantly corroborated a decade later by Tscheboksaroff (179) and by Elliott (72), the latter writing:

From the variety of methods and rapidity with which adrenaline loss can be induced through the splanchnic nerves it appears probable that suprarenal glands are played upon by the splanchnic nerves in the emotional and vasomotor reflexes with almost as delicate and ever-changing an adjustment as are the muscles of the peripheral tissues connected with the sympathetic nerves.

Thus was the adrenal medulla established as an innervated endocrine organ. For long it was regarded as something of an oddity because endocrine glands generally seemed not to be innervated. But time has proved the medullary pattern more prophetic than bizarre: the important influence of the central nervous system over a host of endocrine cells, particularly those of the anterior pituitary, is a commonplace today, and many endocrine cells formerly believed without innervation do in fact receive a nervous supply. Clearly today's subdiscipline of neuroendocrinology has its roots in adrenal medullary physiology.

In 1913 Elliott (73) made a further critical contribution by pointing out that adrenal chromaffin cells develop from the same anlage as sympathetic ganglion cells and, like the latter, are innervated by first-order, 'preganglionic,' sympathetic fibers. Elliott's placement of inverted commas around preganglionic indicates his recognition of the inappropriateness of applying this term to fibers innervating chromaffin cells, but no alternative has been proposed.

RESPONSES TO STIMULATION OF SPLANCHNIC NERVES

The secretomotor sympathetic (preganglionic) fibers innervating the adrenal chromaffin cells run mainly in the ipsilateral splanchnic nerves—greater, lesser, and least (122, 164, 189). In the cat, Marley & Prout (125) found that stimulation of the greater splanchnic evoked an output of catecholamines about twice that resulting from stimulation of the remaining splanchnic nerves together, and a similar pattern is evident in dogs (122, 164). In addition, some secretomotor innervation is provided by small leashes of sympathetic fibers running separately from the more visible aggregates constituting the splanchnic nerves proper (189), and, in the cat at least, there appears to be a minute contribution from the contralateral sympathetic chain (123).

In most experiments only the greater splanchnic nerves have been stimulated. Nevertheless responses are striking, and catecholamine output can often be raised more than 100-fold above the basal level with electrical pulses of optimal duration, intensity, and frequency. The response, as judged by the concentration of catecholamines in the adrenal venous effluent, begins within a second or two of stimulation and reaches a maximum value shortly thereafter and well within the first minute of stimulation (59). At its height the rate of secretion in the cat, when measured over a period of about 10 sec, often exceeds 20 μg/min, and a rate of several micrograms per minute may be sustained for many minutes thereafter.

CHAPTER 26: STIMULUS-SECRETION COUPLING

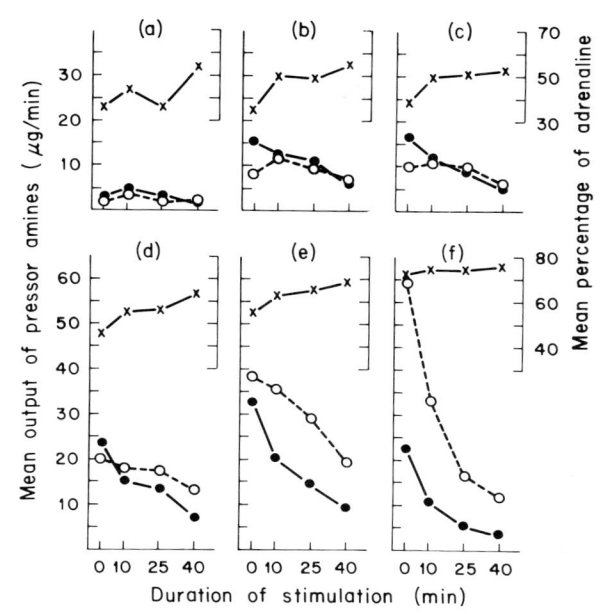

FIG. 1. Output of pressor amines from bovine adrenal glands during prolonged electrical stimulation of splanchnic nerves at various ages. ●, norepinephrine (noradrenaline); ○, epinephrine (adrenaline); ×, % epinephrine (adrenaline). Calves a) less than 1 week, b) 2–3 weeks, c) 4–5 weeks, d) 7–11 weeks, e) 15–30 weeks; and cows f) 2–3 years. Records show how responsiveness develops from newborn to adult, tendency for output of both amines to wane during prolonged stimulation, and effect of such stimulation on proportions of two amines in effluent. [From Silver (167).]

During such prolonged stimulation the gland is releasing approximately 1% of its content each minute. Although the rate falls progressively with time (Fig. 1), stimulation for an hour or so commonly reduces the gland's amine content to about half the initial value (21, 71).

Maturation of the splanchnic-adrenal synapse occurs at different periods in different species. In the sheep the system is functional well before birth (26), whereas in the calf (27, 167) splanchnic stimulation has relatively little effect at birth—despite the presence of large amounts of catecholamines in the adrenal—and elicits powerful secretory responses only some weeks later (see Fig. 1).

Spatial Recruitment, Overlap, and Convergence

Experiments on the cat (125) have demonstrated spatial recruitment of the secretory response upon stimulation of the various splanchnic nerves or stimulation of the greater splanchnic with increasingly strong stimuli; moreover catecholamine output in response to stimulation of the first and second splanchnic nerves has been greater than the sum of the responses to stimulation of the nerves separately. There is thus no sign of occlusion; rather, the result indicates the presence of a subliminal fringe and overlap of innervation. This overlap is also evident from experiments showing that, after partial chronic degeneration, secretory responses to stimulation of remaining nerve fibers are enhanced (125, 168). Histological studies by Hillarp (98) show that a single splanchnic neuron innervates clusters of chromaffin cells and that individual cells may receive innervation from several neurons.

Frequency-Response Relations

The rate of catecholamine output increases with the frequency of splanchnic stimulation over a wide range. The most effective frequency, when measured over periods lasting a minute or more, varies with the species and experimental conditions but lies in the range 15–40 Hz (123, 124, 131, 139, 155, 167, 173). At higher frequencies the secretory response falls off for reasons undetermined (123, 167, 173).

When electrical stimulation is restricted to periods sufficiently brief to avoid the problem of fatigue (see subsection *Splanchnic-Adrenal Fatigue*), catecholamine output per test period increases with the number of shocks applied to the nerves. In addition, the catecholamine output per shock increases with increasing stimulus frequency (109, 123–125, 173). Possibly this effect (Fig. 2) results from increased acetylcholine (ACh) output per impulse (101) or from accumulation of ACh as release outstrips destruction (173). Alternatively the explanation could reside at the level of the chromaffin cells: depolarizing synaptic potentials (48) may sum, there may be an accumulation of free intracellular calcium as influx outpaces inactivation (see subsection *Splanchnic-Adrenal Fatigue*), or again some recapture of catecholamines may occur at low frequencies of stimulation (109, 125).

Splanchnic-Adrenal Fatigue

In his early work Elliott (72) noted that medullary secretion wanes during sustained splanchnic stimulation even when the total catecholamine content of the gland is little reduced and when nicotine still evokes vigorous responses. Such fatigue (see Fig. 1) has been noted many times (19, 71, 124, 167). It is countered to some extent by cholinesterase inhibition and might therefore reflect diminishing ACh output from the splanchnic nerve terminals (124). Here again, however, it is likely that

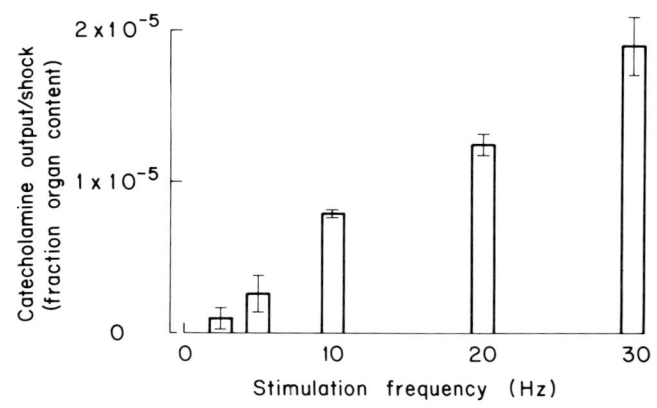

FIG. 2. Catecholamine output per supramaximal shock to greater splanchnic nerve in cat increases with increasing frequency of stimulation. [From Stjärne (173).]

much of the effect is postsynaptic, since chromaffin cells stimulated directly with ACh or potassium (see Fig. 11) also yield quite rapidly waning responses (62, 64).

Preferential Secretion of Epinephrine and Norepinephrine

The presence of epinephrine- and norepinephrine-containing cells in adrenal glands of various species has been discussed in previous chapters, and evidence that different reflex stimuli can release the two amines in different proportions has been presented (see the chapter by Lewis in this volume of the *Handbook*). Clearly there exist secretomotor fibers innervating one or other of the two cell types, preferentially if not selectively. Attempts to demonstrate preferential innervation by stimulating the splanchnic nerves with pulses of different intensities and frequencies or by stimulating during partial nerve block (131) have met with little success. But this is understandable. There is no reason to suppose the electrical properties of the different secretomotor fibers should be distinct. In the dog the ratio of epinephrine to norepinephrine discharged increases at higher frequencies of stimulation (131, 155), but in cats (124) and calves (167) this occurs rarely or not at all. Prolonged stimulation of cat adrenals sometimes (19, 124), but not always (121, 125, 139), shifts the ratio in favor of norepinephrine, and Bülbring & Burn (19) suggested that cells normally secreting epinephrine may release the precursor norepinephrine as methylation lags behind secretion. This explanation now seems unsatisfactory since even after prolonged stimulation much of the original catecholamine content is still present and the rate of synthesis, moreover, is very low (21, 71). On first view the discovery that some dopamine escapes from cat (96, 97, 145) and sheep (119) adrenals might be considered support for the precursor hypothesis. However, dopamine escapes even during "basal" secretion, and the percentage, which is small, does not increase with stimulation. For these and other reasons, dopamine in the adrenal effluent has been considered an end product, or adrenal hormone, in its own right and not merely a precursor. Furthermore, in contradistinction to the cat adrenal, the calf adrenal (167) tends to discharge an increasing percentage of epinephrine during prolonged stimulation (see Fig. 1). It therefore seems simplest, at present, to suppose the changes in the proportions of the amines observed with varying parameters of stimulation reflect differences in synaptic behavior and susceptibility to fatigue of the different neuroeffector populations.

BASAL SECRETION, DENERVATION, AND SUPERSENSITIVITY

In animals provided with catheters chronically implanted in the adrenal veins, a continuous basal output of catecholamines is evident in the absence of any overt stimulus, such as pain, emotion, or hypoglycemia, and in the presence or absence of anesthesia. This basal secretion is reduced when the splanchnic nerves are sectioned acutely and is thus partly due to ongoing secretomotor discharge from the central nervous system (CNS) (164). The small residual secretion is resistant to cholinergic blocking drugs (57, 61, 124) and cannot therefore be attributed to leakage of ACh from the cholinergic terminals (101, 103). Moreover basal secretion is demonstrable after chronic denervation (70, 122, 124, 155, 164, 181). Vogt (181), for example, found that pairs of cat adrenals chronically denervated released about 50 ng catecholamine per minute, a rate roughly 0.1–1% that attainable by maximal repetitive electrical stimulation of the splanchnic nerves. According to Marley & Prout (125), a single cat adrenal releases only about 5–10 ng catecholamine in response to a single maximal shock applied to the greater splanchnic nerve. Clearly then, adrenal chromaffin cells possess considerable spontaneous secretory activity. In this respect they resemble their developmental homologues, ordinary neurons, whose spontaneous secretion reveals itself in the familiar miniature potentials that may be recorded postsynaptically (101, 103).

Adrenal medullary cells maintain their typical histological appearance after chronic denervation and transplantation (29, 75), but, like many other cells, they then exhibit the phenomenon of supersensitivity. Thus, when part of the splanchnic supply to the gland is severed and allowed to degenerate, the secretory response to stimulation of the remaining nerves is enhanced (123, 168).

CHOLINERGIC NATURE OF SECRETOMOTOR FIBERS

The experiments by Feldberg and associates (81–84) are classics in the development of the theory of chemical transmission. Here, in the medulla, they obtained the first evidence for chemical transmission of nerve impulses at a site other than the peripheral autonomic neuroeffector junctions. Moreover their demonstration of the cholinergic nature of nerves, already recognized to be homologous with preganglionic fibers elsewhere in the sympathetic system, provided a spur for the classic work by Feldberg & Gaddum (79) on sympathetic ganglia, which in turn yielded the first clear evidence of nerve-to-nerve communication by chemical means. The development of this exciting story—yet another illustration of the heuristic value of adrenal medullary studies—is presented in a monograph by Minz (130), which also catalogues the evidence for the cholinergic nature of the splanchnic nerves. This evidence follows the now familiar pattern: *a*) ACh is present in the adrenal medulla; *b*) ACh appears in the adrenal venous effluent during splanchnic stimulation, provided cholinesterase is inhibited; *c*) ACh evokes medullary secretion when injected close arterially into adrenals either normally innervated, acutely denervated, or chronically denervated; *d*) secretion in response to splanchnic stimulation or ACh injection is potentiated by cholinesterase-inhibiting drugs; and *e*) drugs, such as nicotine or hexamethonium, that inhibit responses to ACh also inhibit responses to splanchnic stimulation.

The splanchnic secretomotor fibers innervating the chromaffin cells thus conform to the general pattern of cholinergic first-order efferent axons found throughout the sympathetic outflow and studied in great detail at the sympathetic ganglion (15). That adrenal and ganglionic synapses show similar pharmacological behavior is not surprising in view of their common ancestry [(124); see subsection *Nicotinic and Muscarinic Receptors*].

ACETYLCHOLINE RECEPTORS

Splanchnic nerve endings make synaptic-like contacts with chromaffin cells, and clearly the ACh they release gains immediate access to these cells. The question now to be considered is how exposure to ACh causes the chromaffin cells to secrete.

The elegant microiontophoretic studies of Del Castillo & Katz (36) have shown that ACh exerts its typical effect at the endplate region of skeletal muscle when applied to the outside of the plasma membrane but not to the inside. For this and other reasons, including the fact that ACh and many of its antagonists are polar substances that would not be expected to traverse membranes readily, it is generally held that ACh receptors at various sites, regardless of their function, are located on the outer surface of the cell. However, despite widespread interest and intense study, little is yet known of the molecular nature of any ACh receptor. The general view is that the receptor molecule is a protein, but neither this protein nor its reactive moieties have been identified, nor is it clear whether a single ACh molecule or several are required to activate a receptor or how activation is transduced into the membrane response characteristic of the particular cell (132, 137, 154). On the other hand, a fairly clear picture is emerging of the consequences of acetylcholine's interaction with membranes. In every instance examined, including neurons (the cells that on developmental grounds are most likely to behave as chromaffin cells), the response is an increase in the permeability of the plasma membrane to one or more of the species of inorganic ions most abundant in the cell and its environment—commonly the cations Na^+, K^+, and Ca^{2+}, but sometimes anions, such as Cl^-. In some instances the permeability increase may be selective for a particular ion (e.g., potassium in the heart); in others, including neurons and motor endplates, it is rather unspecific and involves several ion species (91). Evidence to be presented in later sections indicates that ACh receptors on the chromaffin cell are also located on the membrane and that their activation involves an increase in permeability to Na^+ and Ca^{2+}.

Nicotinic and Muscarinic Receptors

In his classic pharmacological studies on the cardiovascular actions of ACh, Dale (32) demonstrated that, after muscarine-like actions are blocked by atropine, ACh has readily demonstrable nicotine-like stimulant effects on sympathetic ganglia and adrenal medulla. Later he classified the action of ACh on medullary chromaffin cells as of the "nicotine" type (33). The "nicotine receptors" of the chromaffin cells closely resemble those of the developmentally homologous sympathetic ganglion cells: they are stimulated and blocked by the same classes of cholinomimetic and cholinergic blocking drugs, of which tetramethylammonium and hexamethonium are the respective archetypes, and are distinguished from nicotine receptors of motor endplates by refractoriness to compounds such as decamethonium (124, 183).

Although there is no doubt that acetylcholine's action as a secretagogue at the adrenal medulla is predominantly nicotinic, Dale's classification has tended to delay general awareness of the existence in chromaffin cells of ACh receptors of the muscarinic sort. The fact that drugs are commonly screened for medullary stimulant action on atropinized animals is witness to this. Yet, paradoxically, evidence for the existence of muscarine receptors on chromaffin cells is about as old as that for nicotine receptors. Thus pilocarpine, a classic muscarine-like alkaloid, was shown to evoke adrenal medullary secretion in 1912 (34), the same year that Cannon et al. (22) demonstrated unequivocally the direct medullary response to nicotine; in their paper of 1934 Feldberg et al. (84) demonstrated that muscarine itself evoked medullary secretion by an action typical of that alkaloid in its sensitivity to the blocking effect of atropine. Their findings have been confirmed and extended to other muscarine-like drugs in cats (57, 115, 162) and dogs (104–106). Both muscarinic and nicotinic receptors are clearly present on the chromaffin cells themselves, although not necessarily on the same cells, for both nicotine- and muscarine-like drugs elicit responses from isolated chromaffin cells (48). The lack of consideration afforded the muscarinic receptors is attributable to their relatively minor importance in the normal animal, as evidenced by the persistence of vigorous responses after full atropinization and the powerful blocking effects of antinicotinic drugs, such as hexamethonium. Indeed, in the ox (A. D. Smith, unpublished observations), muscarine-like drugs are quite ineffective. Nevertheless it is interesting that muscarine-like drugs have been used clinically in provocative tests for adrenal medullary tumors—pheochromocytoma (113).

Preferential Secretion of Epinephrine and Norepinephrine

Nicotine and pilocarpine release epinephrine and norepinephrine in different proportions from adrenal glands of cats. The former releases relatively large amounts of norepinephrine, and the ratio of amines released by ACh shifts in favor of epinephrine after atropinization (57, 129, 162). Such a differential effect has not been found in dogs (104, 105), but in rats treated chronically with nicotine, Eränkö (74) found a selective hyperplasia of the norepinephrine-containing cell islets. The functional significance attached to the differential responses is obscure.

CHOLINESTERASE AND CHOLINESTERASE INHIBITORS

Although diffusion of ACh from the site of its release offers a theoretical mechanism for terminating the action of the splanchnic neurons, there is abundant cholinesterase activity on splanchnic terminals, chromaffin cells, and interstitial cells (30, 117, 141), and it is clear that enzymatic destruction of the transmitter is important since cholinesterase inhibitors, such as physostigmine, increase the output of catecholamines in response to splanchnic stimulation. Such drugs also augment catecholamine output after splanchnicotomy, which indicates that, provided hydrolysis is slowed, ACh spontaneously released from the splanchnic terminals may be sufficient to elicit secretion (122). Increased secretion of catecholamines is one of the common consequences of systemic poisoning with cholinesterase inhibitors (100).

SECRETAGOGUES OTHER THAN ACETYLCHOLINE

Medullary secretion can be evoked by several autacoids besides ACh: the amines, histamine and 5-hydroxytryptamine (147, 171); and the polypeptides, bradykinin and angiotensin (80, 147, 157, 172). The effects have been observed in a variety of species but vary in intensity with experimental condition [cf. (28, 182)]. The drugs continue to exert their effect after cholinergic block and have been shown, in isolated chromaffin cells, to act directly on the plasma membrane (48). It is uncertain, however, whether any of these substances in physiological conditions—or even pathophysiological conditions, such as anaphylaxis—achieves in the blood a concentration comparable to that found effective in the pharmacological studies, and medullary stimulation by these drugs might be dismissed as of little functional significance. The phenomenon is mentioned here mainly because it speaks in a language, as yet not understood, of the organization of the chromaffin cell membrane and offers a possible insight into the essential events involved in eliciting secretion. The uniqueness of ACh and its physiological specificity as a medullary secretagogue reside then mainly in the anatomic arrangement of cholinergic innervation, which assures its delivery to the chromaffin cells in high concentration.

For a more comprehensive listing of adrenal medullary stimulants the reader is referred to other reviews (160, 164). It is noteworthy that asphyxia is a direct stimulus to fetal adrenal chromaffin cells before splanchnic maturation (26).

INTRACELLULAR RECORDING WITH MICROELECTRODES

Recording of transmembrane potential with glass microelectrodes has long been established as a valuable means of analyzing function at various neuroeffector junctions, but application of the method to the adrenal medulla has not proved easy: the cells are loosely suspended in a spongelike matrix surrounded by a substantial layer of cortical cells and are difficult to record

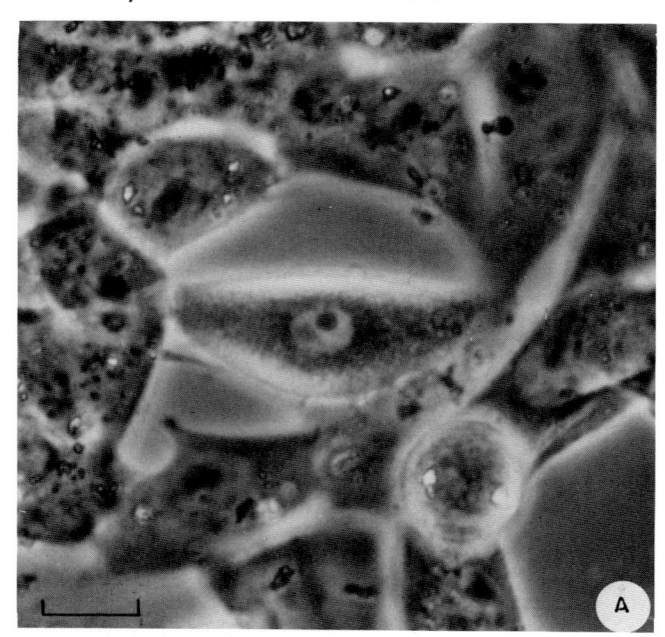

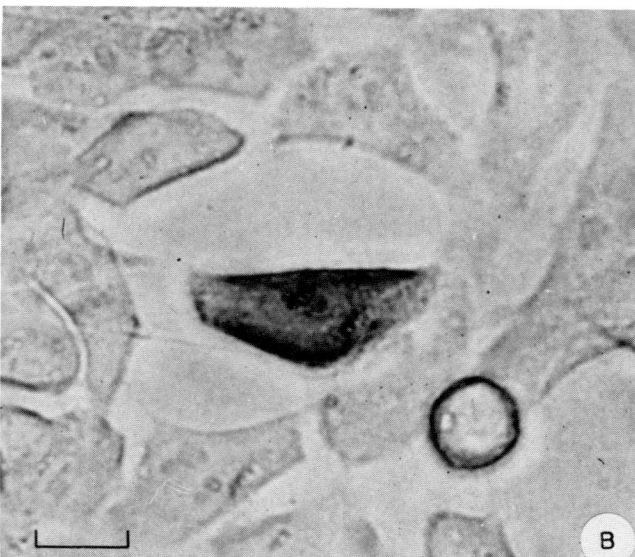

FIG. 3. Isolated chromaffin cell, maintained in tissue culture conditions, of the sort used in in vitro studies of effects of acetylcholine. *A*: phase contrast view. Chromaffin cell is spindle shaped and lies in the *center* of the field; it is surrounded by hamster lung cells of the feeder culture. *B*: same group of cells viewed under bright field after staining with Zenker's fluid. Identity of cell is confirmed by chromaffin reaction. *Horizontal bar* represents 10 μ. [From Douglas et al. (48).]

from; moreover they are mingled with various other cells, including stray ganglion cells, from which they must be distinguished.

Resting Transmembrane Potentials

To overcome these technical difficulties Douglas et al. (48) disaggregated gerbil adrenal medullae, maintained the isolated cells under favorable tissue culture conditions, and impaled positively identified chromaffin cells under direct visual control (Figs. 3 and 4). They observed resting potentials of 25–30 mv (see Figs. 6–8). Comparable values have been obtained from populations of cells, presumably chromaffin cells, in the medullary regions (Fig. 5) of adrenal glands from other species (78, 126). When compared with nerves, resting potential is relatively low and the curve relating this potential to $[K^+]_o$ relatively flat (Fig. 6). This probably reflects a relatively high permeability of chromaffin cells to sodium: the chromaffin cells hyperpolarize (see Fig. 8) when $[Na^+]_o$ is lowered (49).

Depolarization in Response to Acetylcholine

By recording the mean membrane potential from populations of isolated chromaffin cells before, during,

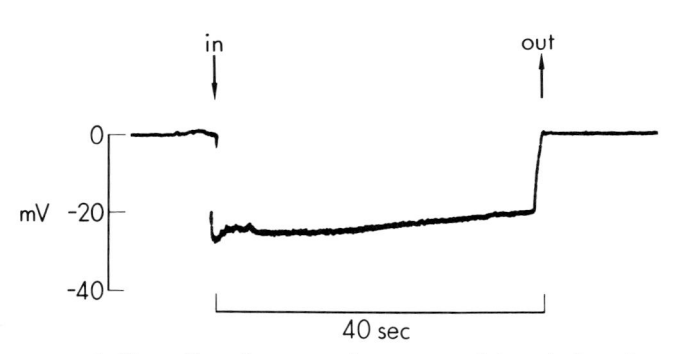

FIG. 4. Recording of transmembrane potential made from isolated gerbil adrenal chromaffin cell in vitro, such as that illustrated in Fig. 3. Electrode inserted at *first arrow* and withdrawn at *second arrow*. [From Douglas et al. (48).]

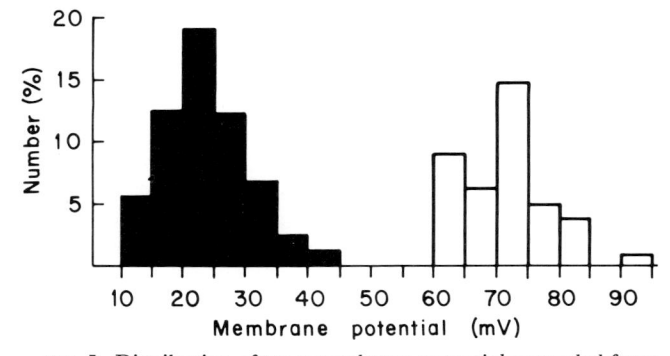

FIG. 5. Distribution of transmembrane potentials recorded from medullary (*filled columns*) and cortical (*open columns*) regions of rats' adrenal glands in vivo. Frequency of resting membrane potentials in 287 cells is depicted. [From Fawcett (78).]

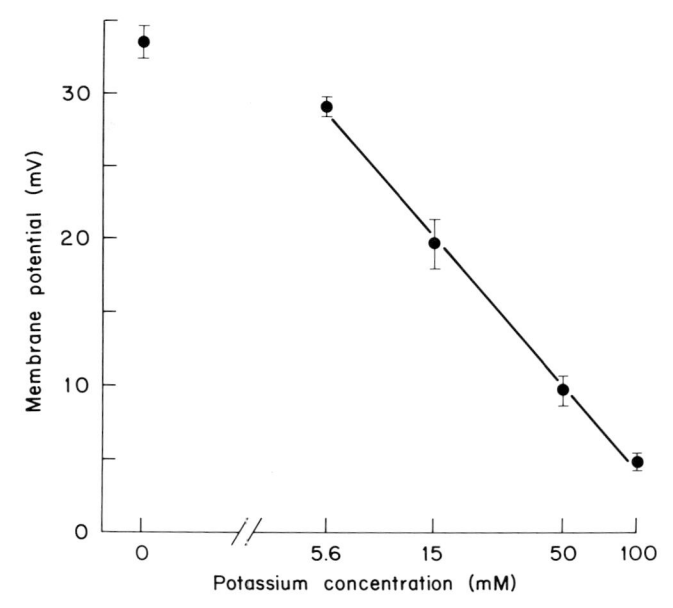

FIG. 6. Relation between potassium concentration of the medium and membrane potential of gerbil chromaffin cells in vitro. [From Douglas et al. (49).]

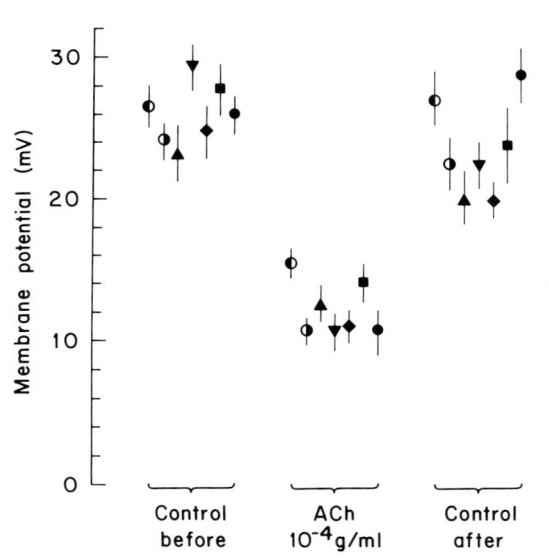

FIG. 7. Depolarizing effect of acetylcholine (*ACh*) on adrenal chromaffin cells. The 7 different symbols represent results of 7 experiments, each carried out on a different population of isolated gerbil chromaffin cells. *Points* show mean membrane potential (±SE) recorded from the population before, during, and after exposure to ACh. [From Douglas et al. (48).]

and after exposure to ACh, it was discovered that ACh depolarizes the cells (48). The effect was detectable with ACh in concentrations of about 3×10^{-6} g/ml and grew with increasing concentration. With 10^{-4} g/ml ACh, transmembrane potential was less than half the resting value (Fig. 7). In a few experiments, acetylcholine was delivered by micropipette close to chromaffin cells during recording of potentials and the depolarizing responses were observed to develop rapidly (102).

Inward Sodium and Calcium Currents

The finding that ACh-induced depolarization varies with log $[Na^+]_o$ and also with log $[Ca^{2+}]_o$ over a wide range (Figs. 8 and 9) indicates that the response is due largely to inward currents of both these cations, with Na being quantitatively more important (49). Although conductance measurements have yet to be made, these currents probably result from a primary action of ACh which increases permeability of the plasmalemma to allow these ions to run passively down their electrochemical gradient. The effect of ACh on the chromaffin cell, which involves both sodium and calcium, apparently conforms to a rather general pattern found at excitatory junctions—nervous synapses and neuromuscular junctions (91)—and contrasts, for example, with its effect on the specialized tissue of the heart involving selective increase in permeability to potassium and hyperpolarization. Although the important task of defining the detailed behavior of the adrenal synapse in vivo remains, the inference from the above is obvious: that acetylcholine's effect as a secretagogue is probably referable to this membrane action.

Electrical Properties of Chromaffin Cells

Initial results have indicated that resting membrane conductance in chromaffin cells is much higher than in neurons and that no spike generation occurs when depolarizing pulses are passed directly across the membrane through intracellular electrodes (102). Many years ago, Cannon & Rosenblueth (23) found that electric current passed through chronically denervated adrenal glands failed to elicit catecholamine secretion. The difficulty of depolarizing small cells suspended in a mass of short-circuiting material with such field stimulation is obvious, and possible loss of electrical excitability as a consequence of chronic denervation has to be considered. Nevertheless the result is in harmony with the findings on the isolated chromaffin cells and suggestive of electrical inexcitability. A more rigorous study of normal chromaffin cells in situ is obviously needed, but from results described below, it is already evident that medullary secretion can be evoked in the absence of sodium, the most common spike-generating ion.

IONS AND SECRETION

Some years before the demonstration of the effect of ACh on membrane potential and ionic fluxes in the chromaffin cell, Douglas & Rubin (61, 63) explored the possibility that such effects might underlie acetylcholine's ability to evoke medullary secretion. Their approach was to examine the influence of the ionic environment on spontaneous and ACh-evoked secretion, and for this they used cats' adrenal glands perfused with a variety of artificial media. Their experiments revealed the unique importance of calcium and led them to suggest that influx of calcium might be the central event in what they termed "stimulus-secretion coupling." The finding that stimulation increases ^{45}Ca uptake in the adrenal medulla [(52, 53); see also (161)], although less definitive than the later demonstration of inward calcium current already described, buttressed the idea, as did a number of other observations. A survey of the evidence follows.

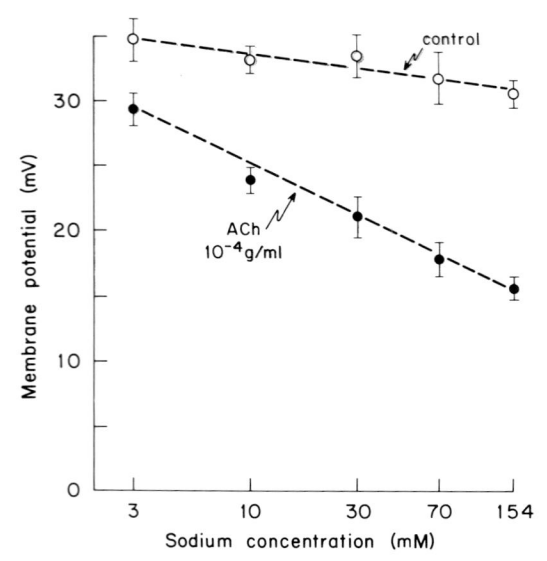

FIG. 8. Relation between sodium concentration of the medium, "resting" potential (○), and depolarization in response to acetylcholine (●) in gerbil chromaffin cells in vitro. Note that as $[Na]_o$ is lowered the cells hyperpolarize slightly and the depolarizing response to acetylcholine (ACh) diminishes. [From Douglas et al. (49).]

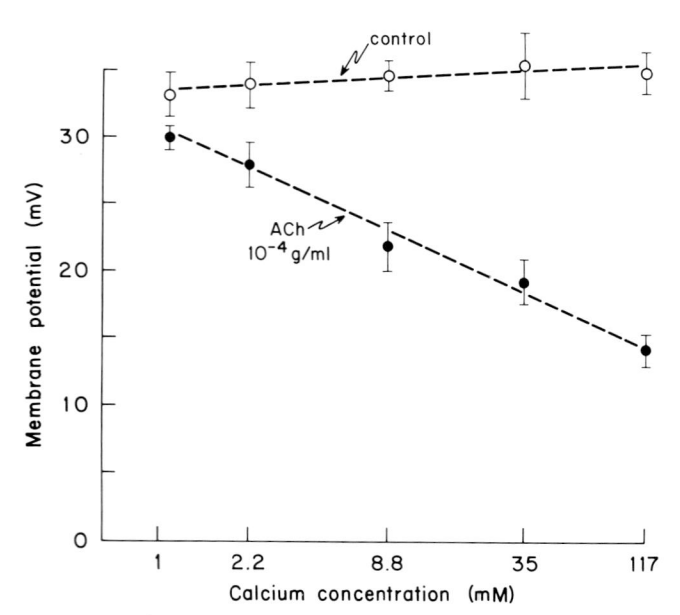

FIG. 9. Relation between calcium concentration of the medium, "resting" potential (○), and depolarization in response to acetylcholine (●) in gerbil chromaffin cells in vitro. Experiments were carried out in absence of sodium, tonicity being maintained by sucrose. Note that, as $[Ca]_o$ is increased, cells hyperpolarize slightly and depolarizing response to acetylcholine (ACh) increases. [From Douglas et al. (49).]

Calcium is Essential and Sufficient for Responses to Acetylcholine

Although inward sodium current is the major factor in the electrophysiology of the adrenal medulla, secretory responses to ACh can be elicited long after sodium has been removed from the perfusing medium and replaced, for example, by sucrose. Clearly sodium influx is not needed for stimulus-secretion coupling. Likewise the other ions commonly present in the extracellular environment—K^+, Mg^{2+}, and Cl^-—can be dispensed with. Acetylcholine will, in fact, elicit secretion during adrenal perfusion with a medium consisting simply of isosmotic sucrose and calcium together with the impermeant anion, SO_4^{2-}. If calcium is omitted from this, or from any conventional perfusion medium, however, ACh rapidly loses its effectiveness (Fig. 10). Clearly then, calcium is not only necessary but sufficient for acetylcholine's action as a secretagogue (61, 63).

Furthermore the output of catecholamines in response to ACh is directly correlated with the concentration of calcium in the medium over a wide range. This may be shown by perfusing glands alternately with media containing different amounts of calcium and testing the response to ACh during each perfusion period (61) or by perfusing continuously with an ACh-containing medium and varying the calcium concentration (63). The latter method allows an especially vivid illustration of the control exerted by $[Ca^{2+}]_o$ (Fig. 11). Figure 11 illustrates that elevation of $[Ca^{2+}]_o$ in the absence of the secretagogue, ACh, is without effect (see also Fig. 12). It will be recalled that inward calcium current, upon exposure to ACh, also increases as $[Ca^{2+}]_o$ is raised [(49); see Fig. 9].

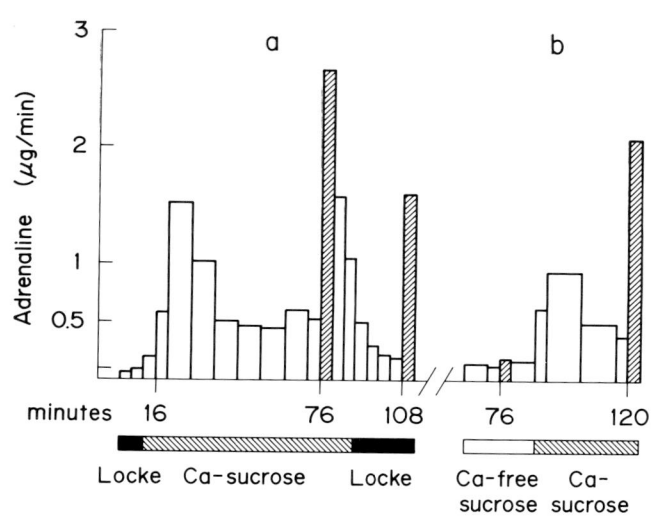

FIG. 10. Stimulant effect of acetylcholine on adrenal secretion during perfusion with isosmotic sucrose (free of Na or K) and its dependence on calcium. Acetylcholine was infused during the period shown by *hatching* in *vertical columns*. *a*: Response in Ca-containing sucrose is followed by control response in Locke's solution (*Locke*). *b*: Response is preceded by response in Ca-free sucrose. Note also increase in "resting" output of catecholamines in sucrose medium and its dependence on Ca. [From Douglas & Rubin (63).]

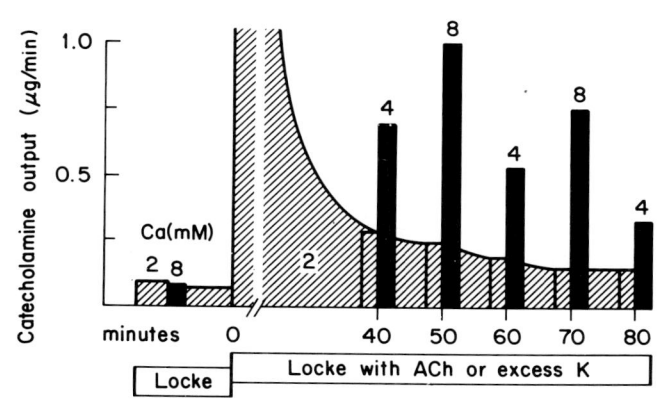

FIG. 11. Schematic portrayal of experiments contrasting the effects, on catecholamine secretion from perfused adrenal glands of cats, of elevating extracellular calcium concentration before and during exposure to the secretagogues, acetylcholine (*ACh*) and excess potassium. During perfusion with the control medium, Locke's solution (*Locke*), elevation of $[Ca]_o$ has little effect on spontaneous output of catecholamines. After introduction of acetylcholine (10^{-5} g/ml) or potassium (50 mM), secretion promptly increases to 10 or more μg/min. Thereafter secretion diminishes with time, as indicated by *cross-hatched area*, despite the continued presence of the secretagogue, but during this period elevations in $[Ca]_o$ are now accompanied by corresponding increases in catecholamine output. [Adapted from Douglas & Rubin (63).]

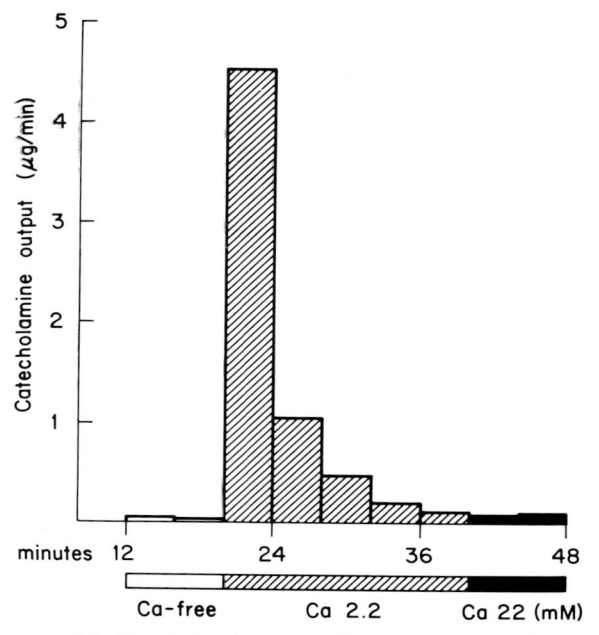

FIG. 12. Catecholamine output from a cat's adrenal gland perfused first for 20 min with Ca-free "Locke's solution," then with Locke's solution containing 2.2 mM Ca, and finally with a "high-Ca Locke's solution" containing 22 mM Ca. *Time scale* indicates minutes from beginning Ca-free perfusion. Note that after Ca-deprivation the reintroduction of Ca, in the conventional concentration (2.2 mM), causes intense secretion but that 10-fold elevation of $[Ca]_o$ during perfusion with the conventional Ca-containing medium does not. [Adapted from Douglas & Rubin (63).]

Besides ACh, numerous medullary secretagogues of widely different chemical structure have now been shown to require calcium. These include nicotine (62, 110) and the nicotine-like drugs, lobeline, tetraethylammonium, DMPP (dimethyl-4-phenylpiperazinium), and tetramethylammonium (62); muscarine and the muscarine-like drugs, pilocarpine and methacholine (147); carbachol, a drug possessing both muscarinic and nicotinic activity (5); histamine, 5-hydroxytryptamine, angiotensin, and bradykinin (147); and various other drugs (160). Most, and perhaps all, of these substances act on membrane receptors. Examples of each of the classes cited have been shown to depolarize chromaffin cells (49). One possibility is that calcium deprivation interferes with drug-receptor binding (142), but the diversity of substances affected argues against this, and the evidence of an alternative role for calcium (see subsection *Calcium Itself Is a Secretagogue*) renders such speculation unnecessary. The explanation clearly does not apply to the substance of most physiological interest, ACh, whose depolarizing action persists in Ca-free media (49).

Potassium Stimulates and Also Requires Calcium

In the expectation that ACh might depolarize chromaffin cells, Douglas & Rubin (61) tested the effect, in perfusion experiments, of increasing $[K^+]_o$ 10-fold from the conventional 5.6 mM to 56 mM. This, they found, stimulated catecholamine output no less intensely than ACh. The response to excess K proved resistant to cholinergic blocking agents, hexamethonium and atropine [(61); W. W. Douglas and R. P. Rubin, unpublished observations], and thus seemed to involve the chromaffin cells directly. Vogt's demonstration (181) that potassium injections stimulate chronically denervated adrenal glands pointed in the same direction, and both the suspected site and mechanism were confirmed when elevation of $[K^+]_o$ was shown to depolarize isolated chromaffin cells, presumably by reducing the ratio $[K^+]_i:[K^+]_o$ (49). Depolarization seems the most probable explanation of potassium's stimulant effect. There are no grounds for suspecting the existence of membrane receptors for K comparable to those for ACh and other drugs, and the action of K can scarcely be intracellular since the K concentration there is higher than the extracellular concentrations eliciting secretion. Moreover, both Rb^+ and Cs^+, which are known for their K^+-like depolarizing action on other tissues, behave like K^+ on the adrenal medulla (170). Depolarization, as is well known, accounts for the stimulating effect of excess K on nerves and muscles where it increases membrane permeability to Na and Ca just as does the passage of depolarizing current (3, 166). Such considerations, and the obvious importance of calcium for medullary responses to ACh and the other secretagogues, led to the view that excess K stimulates medullary secretion by promoting influx of calcium ions (61). Support for this interpretation came from the following observations: excess K, like ACh and the other secretagogues discussed, fails to evoke secretion when Ca is omitted from the extracellular environment, and the magnitude of the secretory response to K increases with increasing $[Ca^{2+}]_o$ over a wide range (61, 63); excess K increases Ca uptake in the medulla (52), and when this is blocked by local anesthetics, secretion also is blocked (161); and finally (see Fig. 11) chromaffin cells exposed to a maintained depolarizing concentration of potassium secrete catecholamines at a rate paralleling closely experimental fluctuations in $[Ca^{2+}]_o$ (63). The simplest explanation is that K-induced depolarization increases the permeability of the chromaffin cell membrane and allows Ca ions to run into the cell down their electrochemical gradient (61). What is particularly striking is that chromaffin cells exposed to excess K behave like those exposed to ACh: in both instances the secretory apparatus becomes responsive to extracellular calcium. It will be recalled that in the absence of these secretagogues even quite substantial increases in $[Ca^{2+}]_o$ have little or no effect on catecholamine secretion (see Figs. 11 and 12).

Calcium Itself Is a Secretagogue

During the course of their perfusion studies, Douglas & Rubin (61) observed a remarkable phenomenon (Fig. 12) strongly reinforcing their view that calcium acts as a mediator or coupling agent linking stimulus to secretory response. When adrenals were perfused with Ca-free Locke's solution for about 15 min (during which time output of catecholamines fell to very low levels), the reintroduction of calcium, in the conventional concentration (2 mM), was itself sufficient to induce medullary secretion of an intensity comparable with the maximum attainable with ACh or nerve stimulation. The response, which passed after several minutes, could be repeated many times in a single preparation and stood in vivid contrast to the inefficacy of introducing calcium, even in large amount, during perfusion with normal Ca-containing media. It was thus clear that calcium, in the concentration normally present in the extracellular environment, is itself sufficient to induce secretion and that its ability to act as a secretagogue can be unmasked simply by depriving the chromaffin cell of calcium for a brief period.

This important result was interpreted along the lines illustrated schematically in Figure 13 (41–43, 61). It is supposed that the chromaffin cell membrane, like that of other cells (133), requires calcium for the maintenance of its normal properties, including relative impermeability to calcium; that in the absence of calcium, membrane permeability increases, an assumption borne out by the demonstration that removal of calcium causes a loss of potassium from the adrenal (W. W. Douglas and A. M. Poisner, unpublished observations) and depolarization of the chromaffin cells (49); that calcium introduced in such conditions readily traverses the unduly permeable membrane; that calcium on entering the cell sets the secretory mechanism in motion; and that the secretory response ceases when the cell membrane has

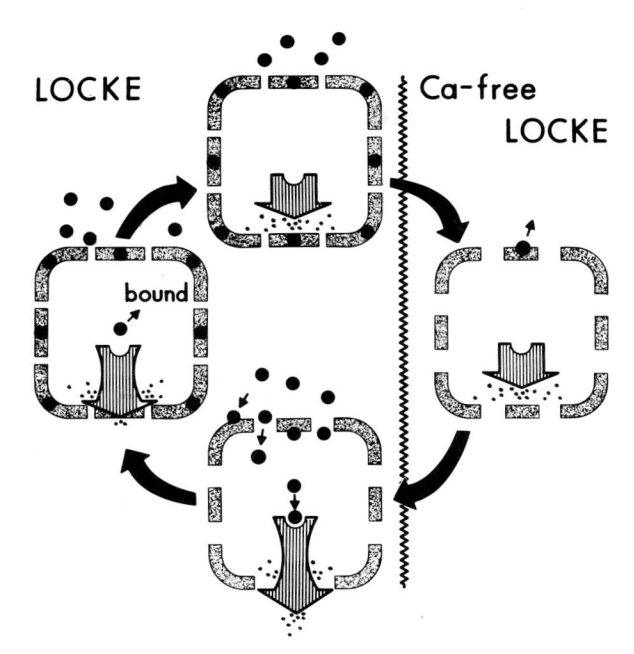

FIG. 13. Schematic portrayal of events thought to underlie stimulant effect of Ca after perfusion with a Ca-free medium (41, 62). Calcium in cell membrane and extracellular environment is represented by *closed circles*. The Ca-deprived cell loses Ca from its membrane, which then becomes permeable to that ion. On reintroducing Ca, some penetrates the leaky membrane and activates the secretory process here represented by the *arrow*. Stimulant effect ceases when membrane reacquires its complement of Ca and becomes relatively impermeable to that ion, and as free Ca inside the cell is bound and extruded. LOCKE, Locke's solution. [From Douglas (42).]

reacquired its normal complement of calcium and relative impermeability to that ion and when the calcium that has entered the cell is inactivated by binding and extrusion (see section TERMINATION OF SECRETORY RESPONSES AND CALCIUM INACTIVATION). The crucial point is the discovery that calcium itself, in the absence of ACh or any other secretagogue, can evoke intense secretory activity.

Strontium and Barium Are Calcium Substitutes and Stimulants

The effects of the alkaline earths on the saline-perfused adrenal have been studied in some detail (64, 65).

Strontium behaves much like calcium: it has little tendency to increase secretion when added to the usual Ca-containing perfusion medium, but its addition potentiates responses to ACh or K. Strontium substitutes for calcium in sustaining secretory responses to ACh or K and, like Ca, will itself evoke intense secretion when introduced into glands perfused for some time with Ca-free media.

Barium is in some respects similar to Sr and Ca but in others remarkably different. Like Sr, it can substitute for Ca and sustain responses to ACh or K, provided it is present in relatively low concentration, and, like both Ca and Sr, it stimulates secretion intensely when introduced to Ca-deprived glands. In contrast to Ca and Sr, however, it stimulates strongly when added in quite small amounts (about 2 mM) during perfusion with conventional Ca-containing medium. Barium is, in fact, a potent secretagogue, just as it is a potent and familiar spasmogen of smooth muscle.

The secretory responses to Ba or Sr that may be elicited from Ca-deprived preparations can be obtained after prolonged calcium deprivation and exposure to ethylenediaminetetraacetate (EDTA). Moreover successive responses to these ions decline no more rapidly than do those obtained in comparable experiments involving intermittent introduction of calcium. Nor does brief perfusion with calcium arrest the progressive decline in the responses to Ba or Sr. For these various reasons it has been suggested that Sr and Ba act directly on the normally Ca-sensitive apparatus and thereby induce secretion and do not owe their effect to displacement of bound calcium. If this interpretation is correct, the efficacy of these related alkaline earths provides a clue to the biochemical nature of the calcium receptor (64). The medullary stimulant effect of Ba has yet to be fully explained. Barium has a larger ion and hydrated ion radius than Ca or Sr (90, 134) and would not be expected to penetrate the cell membrane more easily. It has, however, been observed to depolarize chromaffin cells and may itself carry inward depolarizing current (49); it may facilitate its own entry, and that of extracellular Ca, by displacing plasmalemmal Ca (65).

Magnesium Inhibits Responses to Acetylcholine, Potassium, Calcium, Strontium, and Barium

Magnesium has no stimulant effect on medullary secretion whether tested on normal or Ca-deprived glands (63–65). Moreover the presence or absence of the usual complement of Mg (about 1 mM) has little influence on the acute secretory response to ACh or K. However, concentrations of Mg above 5 mM or so inhibit responses to these stimuli. This inhibition increases with increasing Mg concentration and can be overcome by raising $[Ca^{2+}]_o$ (63). Simply on the general grounds of the prevalent antagonism between calcium and magnesium in various biological processes, this inhibition by magnesium could be considered yet another link in the chain of evidence implicating calcium in stimulus-secretion coupling. However, it is not necessary to rely on such general inference: the antagonism can be shown directly. As noted above, it is possible to induce medullary secretion by introducing Ca to Ca-deprived glands, and Mg given at the same time inhibits this Ca effect (63). The site of magnesium's inhibitory action is uncertain. Possibly it interferes with Ca influx, perhaps by competing for a common carrier or "pore"; there has long been evidence that Mg inhibits resting influx of Ca into squid axon (99), and more recently it has been found to depress the depolarization-dependent Ca influx into squid axon (3). But an additional or alternative mechanism must be considered, namely that Mg antagonizes Ca at the intracellular site where Ca induces secretion (63). In the Ca-deprived cell the introduction of Mg, in contrast to the other alkaline earths, does not initiate secretion but inhibits the secretory stimulant effect of Ca simultaneously introduced. Yet the ionic radius of Mg is smaller, and it would be expected to penetrate more readily than the other alkaline earths. The possibility of an intracellular Mg-Ca antagonism has also been raised by observations on the posterior pituitary where the inhibitory effect of Mg on Ca influx is much less striking than its inhibitory effect on release of posterior pituitary hormones (56).

Sodium Lack and Potentiation of Basal and Evoked Secretion

Experiments on adrenals perfused alternately with conventional media rich in Na and media containing little or no Na (Na being replaced with sucrose) have revealed that responses to ACh or K not only persist in Na-deficient media but are potentiated (Fig. 14); that Na-deficient media themselves cause an increase in the basal output of catecholamines; and that both effects are Ca dependent (61, 63). Since analogous phenomena had earlier been observed in muscles—low $[Na^+]_o$ potentiating stimulus-evoked contraction or itself inducing contraction—and these muscle responses appeared to be due to increased Ca influx and accumulation, it was argued that the effects on medullary secretion might be similarly explained. In addition, it was suggested that lowering $[Na^+]_o$ might be expected to result in hyperpolarization—an expectation borne out by subsequent intracellular recordings from chromaffin cells (48)—and that hyperpolarization facilitates both the Ca-dependent release of neurohumors and the Ca-dependent contraction of muscles, possibly by increasing the electrical gradient contributing to inward Ca movement and increasing the amount of membrane-bound Ca mobilized by stimulation (61, 63). The subsequent discovery that evoked secretion of neurohypophysial hormones (55) and secretion of neurohumors (12, 107) are similarly potentiated by lowering $[Na^+]_o$, together with kinetic studies of the phenomenon (152), harmonize with the view that Ca and Na compete at a common site in the release process and indicate that the release mechanism is partly inactivated by the high Na concentration of the normal ionic environment.

An additional factor to be considered here is the recently discovered mechanism of Na-Ca exchange across nerve and other membranes (2, 156), which apparently utilizes the energy of the normally steep electrochemical gradient for Na across the membrane (outside to inside) to eject intracellular Ca and seems to be important for the maintenance of free intracellular Ca at the extremely low levels (2, 108) characteristic of cytoplasm. In this mechanism, Na and Ca compete not only extracellularly for influx but intracellularly for efflux, with the result that lowering $[Na^+]_o$ not only increases influx of Ca^{2+} but diminishes Ca^{2+} extrusion, both effects favoring accumulation of intracellular Ca^{2+}. Banks and his colleagues (8, 9) have proposed that this may account for both the increased basal and evoked secretion elicited by Na deprivation.

Potassium Lack and Potentiation of Basal and Evoked Secretion

Omission of K during adrenal perfusion raises the basal secretion of catecholamines (9) and potentiates responses to ACh (61, 63) or carbachol (9). Here again analogy with muscle has suggested that the explanation may reside in increased Ca influx possibly linked to hyperpolarization (49, 61, 63). Alternatively, or additionally, it may lie in interference with the Na-Ca exchange mechanism (8). Since this Na-Ca exchange is driven by the electrochemical gradient for Na across the plasmalemma it ultimately depends on the maintenance of this gradient through active extrusion of Na by plasmalemmal Na-K ATPase, the familiar "sodium pump." Removal of extracellular K will inhibit the sodium pump, allow Na to accumulate intracellularly, diminish the Na gradient, increase the intracellular concentration of Na that competes with Ca for extrusion, and thereby favor intracellular accumulation of Ca^{2+}. Support for this interpretation comes from studies of the effects of ouabain described below (7).

Stimulant Effects of Ouabain

Ouabain is one of a group of cardiac glycosides long known to potentiate muscle contraction and, in high concentration, to induce contraction. As long ago as 1918 Loewi (120) emphasized that their effects on the heart closely resemble those elicited by raising $[Ca^{2+}]_o$

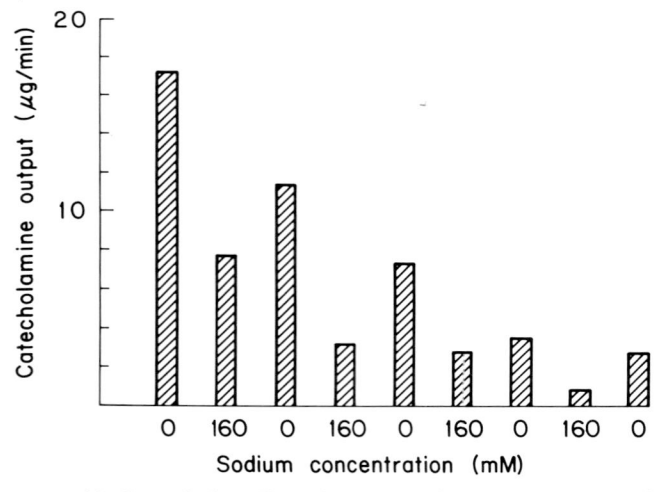

FIG. 14. Potentiating effect of sodium omission. A cat's adrenal gland was perfused for alternate periods of 14 min with Locke's solution containing 160 mM Na (*160*) or Na-free Locke's solution (*0*). Acetylcholine (10^{-5} g/ml) was introduced during the last 2 min of each perfusion period. Output of catecholamines on successive tests is depicted by *vertical columns*. [From Douglas & Rubin (63).]

and suggested that the glycosides sensitize the heart to Ca. The pivotal function of Ca in excitation-contraction coupling has now become a commonplace, but analysis of the effects of the glycosides has revealed no direct effect on Ca but, on the contrary, a highly specific and characteristic inhibitory effect on Na-K ATPase. The discovery of the Na-Ca exchange mechanism has offered a solution to the dilemma because, as just described, inhibition of the sodium pump will indirectly favor Ca influx and impede Ca efflux (156). Once again there is a parallel between contraction and secretion, for while the interaction between Na, Ca, and ouabain was being explored on various muscles, ouabain was found to potentiate secretion of chemical transmitters (13, 14), insulin (94, 95), and medullary catecholamines [(7, 8); Fig. 15], and in each instance the effect has been attributed to increased $[Na^+]_i$, which favors a rise in $[Ca^{2+}]_i$. Ouabain itself, in sufficiently high concentration, elicits secretion, but the extent to which the Na-Ca exchange mechanism is responsible here is unclear. As $[Na^+]_i$ increases, $[K^+]_i$ will fall, and the resulting depolarization will itself stimulate.

When considered together, the evidence from K-deprived or ouabain-exposed glands certainly suggests that a rise in $[Na^+]_i$ favors secretion. The behavior of the Na-Ca exchange mechanism, which in such circumstances would be expected to allow Ca accumulation within the cell, provides a plausible explanation of the secretory stimulant effects. A rise in the background level of intracellular free Ca would, on this hypothesis, suffice to augment spontaneous secretory activity and would also lead to higher levels of free Ca being reached during the phasic Ca entry occurring on exposure to K or ACh. Moreover, according to the Na-Ca exchange hypothesis, elevated $[Na^+]_i$ will impede extrusion of Ca that enters during stimulation. There is also the interesting possibility that elevated $[Na^+]_i$ may facilitate phasic entry of Ca (see subsection *Prolonged Sodium Deprivation Inhibits*).

Prolonged Sodium Deprivation Inhibits

In adrenal glands perfused with solutions where sucrose replaces most or all of the Na, successive secretory responses to ACh diminish more rapidly than usual (9, 63). About 90 min may elapse before responses are profoundly depressed, but failure is hastened when Na is replaced with Li or choline, substitutions known to facilitate the loss of Na_i (8, 9). These observations, coupled with the indications (see subsection *Stimulant Effects of Ouabain*) that elevated $[Na^+]_i$ potentiates secretion, have prompted Banks and his colleagues (8, 9) to suggest that influx of Ca into the chromaffin cell during stimulation is regulated by intracellular Na. A similar possibility had been raised with regard to release of transmitters from neurons (13, 14). However, medullary responses to stimulation may be sustained in Na-free media simply by increasing $[Ca^{2+}]_o$, which suggests that Na_i is facilitatory, rather than mandatory, for Ca entry (8). In the absence of any direct evidence that intra-

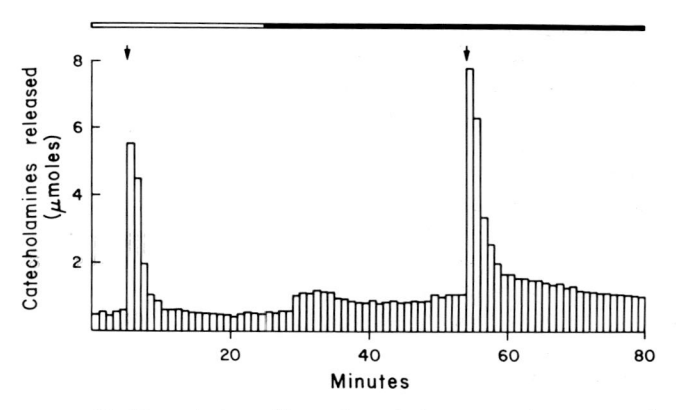

FIG. 15. Potentiating effect of ouabain on spontaneous and stimulated release of catecholamines by perfused bovine adrenal gland. Gland was perfused with Tyrode's solution for 30 min before beginning of experiment. *Open bar* indicates perfusion with Tyrode's solution; *filled bar* indicates perfusion with Tyrode's solution containing 0.1 mM ouabain. Stimulation (*arrows*) was with carbamylcholine (0.5 ml, 10 mM injected into perfusion stream). [From Banks (7).]

cellular sodium contributes to phasic Ca influx (2), other explanations should be considered for the ultimate failure of medullary secretion during Na-free perfusion. For example, it is conceivable that low $[Na^+]_i$ might facilitate Ca binding and inactivation (see section TERMINATION OF SECRETORY RESPONSES AND CALCIUM INACTIVATION), or perhaps Na is involved in the secretory process set in motion by Ca.

It is quite apparent that the actions of the alkaline earths and alkali metals on medullary secretion are complex and their interactions still more so. And to compound the difficulty of interpretation there is the central uncertainty over the site and intimate molecular mechanism of calcium's action in evoking secretion. Clearly speculation here, and in the literature, is outstripping the evidence.

ROLE OF DEPOLARIZATION

Depolarization of the chromaffin is clearly insufficient, by itself, to evoke catecholamine secretion.
1. No secretion accompanies the depolarizing effects of ACh or excess K when Ca is absent (61, 63).
2. Chromaffin cells deprived of Ca for sufficiently long periods depolarize (49), but their output of catecholamines falls (61, 63).
3. Excess Mg inhibits secretion to ACh or K but does not prevent depolarization (49, 61, 63).
4. Depolarization unaccompanied by secretion can be obtained in the presence of the local anesthetic, tetracaine, in concentrations that preferentially block inward Ca movement (47, 161).

Clearly then, depolarization can be dissociated from secretion by a variety of maneuvers preventing Ca influx.
The question whether Ca influx, by itself, is sufficient to evoke secretion, or is effective only when the cell

membrane is depolarized, is not so easily answered. From the curve relating $[Na^+]_o$ to resting potential and ACh-induced depolarization (see Fig. 8) and other evidence (49), it is evident that low $[Na^+]_o$ hyperpolarizes and that during a superimposed ACh-induced depolarization the membrane potential may fall little or not at all below the normal resting value observed in conventional Na-rich environments. Yet low $[Na^+]_o$ increases basal and ACh-stimulated secretion. Increased basal secretion seems thus to occur as resting potential is rising, and the potentiation of evoked secretion apparently takes place in the face of weakened depolarizing responses. If the arguments presented earlier are correct and lowering $[Na^+]_o$ increases basal secretion by causing free Ca to accumulate intracellularly, then the obvious conclusion is that Ca can indeed induce secretion without depolarization. The potentiated responses to ACh could be interpreted along the same lines, but the situation is more complex. Some depolarization is still taking place; moreover this depolarization, as well as the Ca influx and secretion, witnesses the fact that the basic action of ACh on the membrane is still present and that the secretory response is clearly occurring against a background of an altered plasmalemma (45). It must be borne in mind that ion fluxes and potential changes are merely secondary manifestations of ACh-induced plasmalemmal properties. What is, however, evident from the experiments is that secretion in response to ACh is not directly correlated with the drug's depolarizing effect. Further testimony to this lies in the finding that ACh can stimulate catecholamine efflux from glands already completely depolarized by media with a high K concentration [(63); see Fig. 16]. Since comparable behavior has been noted in smooth muscle and ACh has been demonstrated to increase membrane conductance at motor endplates exposed to excess K it has been suggested that ACh may have an effect in increasing membrane permeability additive with that of excess K and further that it may be able to mobilize or displace Ca more effectively than excess K (42, 63). Whatever the explanation, ACh can clearly evoke secretion independently of its membrane depolarizing actions.

TERMINATION OF SECRETORY RESPONSES AND CALCIUM INACTIVATION

The abundance of cholinesterase in and around the medullary synapses will assure prompt hydrolysis of ACh liberated by the splanchnic nerves and dissipation of the immediate stimulus to the chromaffin cells *pari passu* with cessation of splanchnic discharge. Membrane permeability and potential can both be expected to recover rapidly. On the calcium hypothesis of stimulus-secretion coupling (45, 61), the free intracellular Ca assumed to mediate the secretory response must somehow be inactivated. On general grounds, and more immediately by analogy once more with muscle contraction, it was initially supposed (41, 61) that this free Ca is reduced to nonstimulant levels by two mechanisms: *1*) binding to cellular components, and *2*) extrusion across the plasmalemma. The importance of Ca extrusion and the involvement of the Na-Ca exchange mechanism have been treated in preceding sections and need no further comment. The possibility of Ca inactivation by binding, such as occurs in muscle (184), has been explored in several studies (18, 92, 148). Poisner & Hava (148) have obtained a microsomal fraction from the adrenal medulla that accumulates Ca through an ATP-dependent process similar in its properties to that of sarcoplasmic reticulum. The structures giving rise to this fraction are unidentified, but thiocyanate, which depresses calcium accumulation by the fraction, also potentiates catecholamine output from perfused glands. Since mitochondria avidly accumulate Ca and perhaps contribute to Ca inactivation in muscle (24, 25, 116), they too could participate in truncating secretory responses. It must, however, be emphasized that, although the electrophysiological evidence (see Fig. 9) demonstrates unequivocally that Ca ions carry inward current across the chromaffin cell membrane exposed to ACh, it does not follow that the level of free Ca thereby rises throughout the cytoplasm: the Ca may move no further than the inner surface of the membrane (45). Furthermore membranes carry net negative charges (arising mainly from ionized carboxyl and phosphate groups of protein and phospholipid) and have a high affinity for cations, and Ca^{2+} in particular. The inner surface of the plasmalemma might therefore be of importance in dissi-

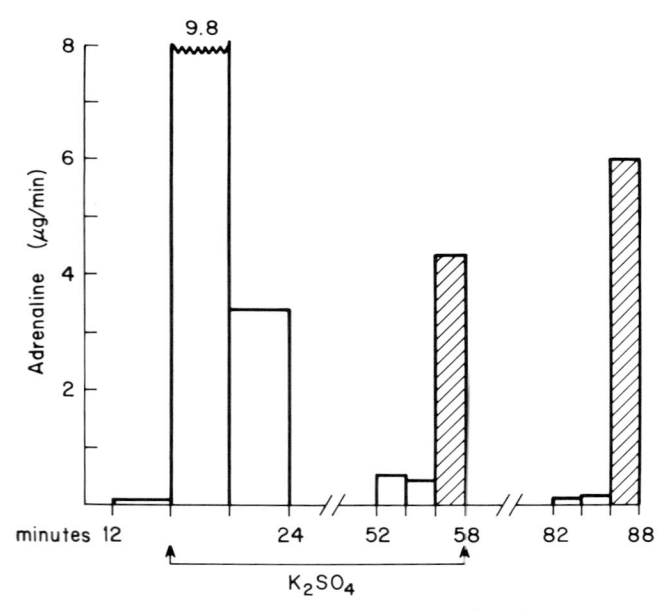

FIG. 16. Stimulant effect of acetylcholine (ACh) on catecholamine output from cat's adrenal gland perfused with "Locke's solution" containing 126 mM K_2SO_4 to depolarize chromaffin cells. Acetylcholine (10^{-4} g/ml) was introduced during last 2 min of perfusion with this medium and evoked response indicated by *hatched vertical column*. Perfusion was then switched back to Locke's solution and response to ACh again tested. [From Douglas & Rubin (63).]

pating local elevations in free Ca, its "buffering" capacity perhaps being restored by the Na-Ca exchange mechanism.

MEMBRANE AND IONIC EVENTS: A SUMMING-UP

It is evident from the preceding account that a great variety of findings can now be marshalled in support of the hypothesis that ACh evokes medullary secretion by causing Ca ions to penetrate the adrenal medullary cells and the conception that Ca is a mediator in stimulus-secretion coupling (Fig. 17).

A satisfying feature of this scheme is that it holds the mechanism of action of ACh as a secretagogue to be essentially similar to its action as a synaptic transmitter at other sites in the body where it excites or inhibits at nervous or neuroeffector synapses, namely an action on the plasma membrane whereby permeability to commonly occurring ions is increased. But there are clearly many unanswered questions. The nature of the ACh receptors and how their activation increases membrane permeability are no clearer here than at other sites of cholinergic transmission. Much also remains to be learned of the detailed behavior of the medullary synapse, something not possible in isolated chromaffin cells whatever their other advantages; furthermore it may well prove that extracellular Na has a more important role under normal conditions than is evident when excess K or injected ACh are used to stimulate: if the action of synaptically delivered ACh is highly localized—as seems not unlikely from the anatomic evidence and the abundance of cholinesterase—then inward Na current at the immediate postsynaptic site may be of importance in achieving electrotonic depolarization adequate to induce optimal Ca influx over the entire cell surface (49). Secretion is not limited to synaptic regions (see the chapter by Grynszpan-Winograd in this volume of the *Handbook*). Moreover, although the demonstration of inward Ca current shows that Ca traverses the cell membrane, there is no evidence on the degree of cytoplasmic penetration achieved or the critical site where Ca acts. Nor has the locus of antagonistic effect of Na and Mg been clearly established: both ions may interfere with Ca influx, but there are also hints of an action at the level of the "Ca receptor" whose activation promotes secretion (49, 56, 64). It is also not yet certain whether this Ca receptor accepts Ba and Sr or whether these ions act by displacing bound Ca. And, finally doubt still exists whether Ca delivered to its critical site is itself sufficient to activate secretion or does so effectively only in conjunction with a plasmalemmal modification. If the latter is true, then the "modification" must be something that can be induced not only by ACh but by a spectrum of stimulant drugs and ions, such as K and Ba, or indeed by Ca deprivation.

From all this it is quite evident that, although more is perhaps known of stimulus-secretion coupling in the chromaffin cell than in any other cell, an enormous amount remains to be learned, and those of us who delight in experiment would scarcely wish it otherwise.

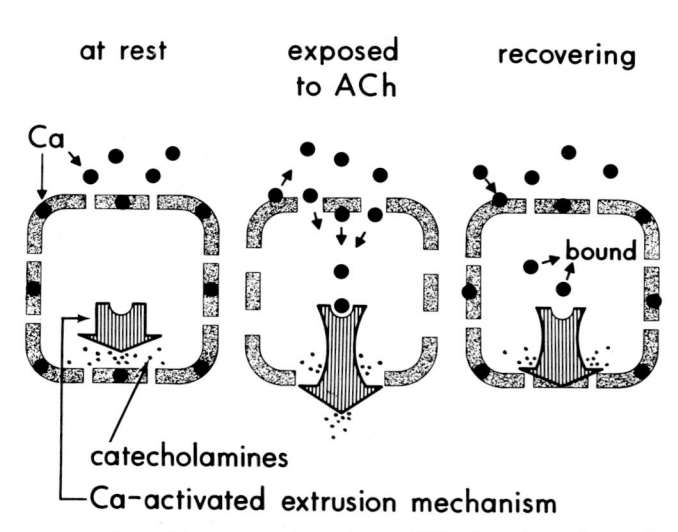

FIG. 17. Calcium-entry hypothesis (62) of action of acetylcholine (*ACh*) on chromaffin cell based on the arguments schematized in Fig. 13 and other evidence described in text. Acetylcholine induces increased permeability of cell membrane (possibly by "decalcifying" it as depicted here) and thereby allows Ca ions to enter and activate secretion (exocytosis). When ACh is withdrawn the membrane recovers its relative impermeability to Ca^{2+}, excess Ca^{2+} within cell is bound and extruded, and secretion ceases. [From Douglas (42).]

One thing is, however, clear: namely, that the secretory process dependent on Ca is what De Duve (35) has termed exocytosis. When the importance of Ca in medullary secretion first became evident a great variety of schemes had been proposed for catecholamine secretion [see (44, 45)], and the suggestion that Ca had to do with the phenomenon now known as exocytosis (61, 63) rested on slender electron-microscopic evidence (38, 39) and the always precarious argument by analogy with other systems—Ca was, at about the same time, found essential for protein secretion in exocrine glands (54) where morphological evidence for exocytosis (140) was much more convincing. At the present time, however, this interpretation is much better founded. The use of appropriate species has yielded a rich harvest of unequivocal electron-microscopic images of exocytosis (10, 40, 93, 135). Moreover, as a result of the introduction (42, 59) and vigorous development [see (112) and the chapter by Viveros in this volume of the *Handbook*] of the method of defining medullary secretion by analyzing the adrenal effluent for various cellular constituents, there is now the necessary qualitative and quantitative chemical evidence to establish exocytosis beyond a doubt as the principal and probably only significant mechanism of catecholamine extrusion (see the chapter by Viveros in this volume of the *Handbook*).

Although calcium's function is clearly concerned with exocytosis, this function is scarcely better defined today than when the unique importance of the ion first became apparent and when the vague suggestion was made that it might induce exocytosis—or "pinocytosis in reverse," as it was then called—by somehow altering the physicochemical state of the cytoplasm and the interacting granule and plasma membranes (61, 63). This does not imply a paucity of conjecture. On the contrary, there have been a variety of proposals—for example, that Ca either annuls net negative and mutually repulsive surface charges on granule and plasmalemma (6, 8, 127, 143) and thus allows approximation, cationic bridging, and interaction (but this, at best, is an incomplete scheme because Mg, which might be expected to behave similarly, is ineffective), or activates an enzyme possibly involved in membrane fusion and fission, such as a phospholipase or nucleotidase (see section PARALLELS WITH EXCITATION-CONTRACTION COUPLING), or does both (46). These and other ideas are considered more fully in the chapter by Viveros in this volume of the *Handbook*. Here, however, it is appropriate to devote some discussion to one particular line of conjecture that is a direct outgrowth of the pattern of ionic influences on medullary secretion with which the present chapter has mainly been concerned.

PARALLELS WITH EXCITATION-CONTRACTION COUPLING

It has doubtless become apparent that there are remarkable similarities in the influences of the inorganic ions on medullary secretion and muscular contraction. Indeed, it was awareness of this parallelism that prompted coining of the term "stimulus-secretion coupling" (61), which is clearly patterned after Sandow's (163) term "excitation-contraction coupling."

The choice of "stimulus," rather than "excitation," was a deliberate one based on two considerations. First, in the secretory context the stimulus (in this instance, acetylcholine) was definable, whereas excitation was not. It will be recalled that when Sandow (163) devised his term he was dealing with striated muscle where excitation could be fairly satisfactorily defined as the propagated electrical disturbance, the action potential, arising secondarily to synaptic activation. Clearly the situation in the chromaffin cell is quite different, and no such simple definition is possible. The evidence is that the chromaffin cells are electrically inexcitable (do not generate impulses), and there is no correspondingly clear set of phenomena mediating synaptic activation and functional response: drug-receptor interaction and the accompanying membrane phenomena (chemical, ionic, and electrical) are, as we have seen, as yet inextricably interwoven. Second, "excitation," in Sandow's usage, is a state clearly secondary to, and indeed spatially separated from, the initiating synaptic events and thus does not include phenomena that, for secretion, it was felt desirable and even essential to embrace. *Stimulus-secretion coupling* is thus a relatively broad term encompassing all events following exposure of the cell to its secretagogue—including any state that might conceivably be considered as excitation—and resulting in the appearance of secretory product in the extracellular environment (45).

The parallel behavior is evident from the following list of statements, each of which applies not only to adrenal medullary secretion but also to muscle contraction of one type or another. The works cited after each statement document the secretory phenomena and include references to the corresponding findings in muscles.

1. Calcium is necessary for the response (61).
2. The response varies with $[Ca^{2+}]_o$ over a wide range (61, 63).
3. Calcium itself stimulates when the membrane barrier is removed (61).
4. Acetylcholine depolarizes and so too does excess K (48, 49).
5. The stimulant effect of ACh can be mimicked by depolarizing concentrations of K (49, 61).
6. Local anesthetics block responses and Ca influx to ACh or K (47, 161).
7. Stimulation by ACh or K causes inward Ca flux (52, 53).
8. Acetylcholine can still evoke responses from the completely depolarized preparation (63).
9. Strontium substitutes for Ca, but various other divalent ions do not (64).
10. Barium stimulates, and this effect does not require Ca_o^{2+} (65).
11. Magnesium has little effect at physiological concentrations but inhibits responses to ACh, K, and Ba (61, 63, 64).
12. Reduction in $[Na^+]_o$ or $[K^+]_o$ potentiates evoked responses and increases basal responses (8, 61, 63).
13. Ouabain potentiates evoked responses and induces spontaneous responses (7, 8).
14. Chloride ion can be replaced with SO_4^{2-} (63).
15. Responses are energy dependent and blocked by metabolic inhibitors (111, 159).

It is possible that this remarkable parallelism is simply a consequence of common involvement of Ca in two disparate processes and merely reflects the similarity of factors controlling transmembrane Ca fluxes and intracellular levels of free Ca. However, the parallel behavior has led to the hypothesis that a common process is involved in contraction and secretion (64) and has prompted the suggestion that efforts to define the mechanism of calcium's action in secretion could benefit from knowledge of calcium's action in contraction and its role within the broader unitary framework of stimulus-response coupling (42). Attempts to explain calcium's role in secretion in terms of events involved in contraction have taken a variety of forms. Poisner & Trifaró (149) suggested that the processes of membrane fusion and rupture underlying exocytosis may involve a reaction reminiscent of molecular events in contraction in which Ca facilitates a splitting of plasmalemmal ATP by ATPase activity of the chromaffin granules [see also (143, 150, 177, 178); see the chapter by Viveros in this volume of the *Handbook*]. Another possibility suggested by the work of Lacy and his colleagues on insulin secretion (114) is that microtubules or similar entities participate in some contraction-like process, inducing exocytosis. The inhibitory effects of colchicine and some related drugs on medullary secretion have been considered to support this scheme (144), but analysis suggests that colchicine acts at some stage earlier in stimulus-secretion coupling than exocytosis—possibly at the level of the ACh receptor or associated membrane phenomena—for the drug has little effect on K-evoked secretion (66, 176). Cytochalasin B, a substance exerting a spectrum of pharmacological effects in which microfilaments have been implicated (186), also inhibits medullary secretion (67). However, this effect of cytochalasin may well involve a mechanism quite unrelated to microfilaments (68). Despite these uncertainties, a contractile basis for secretion by exocytosis remains an intriguing prospect, and it is still "conceivable that nature uses similar devices at the molecular level to effect these two seemingly disparate responses, contraction and secretion" (45). The appeal of the unitary hypothesis should not, however, obscure the possibility that the Ca-sensitive mechanism in secretion is quite different. For example, although the evidence is confusing, there are hints that exocytosis may involve activation of phospholipase activity or at least lysolecithin, which is normally present in the chromaffin granule membrane (16, 17, 60, 153, 174, 175, 187, 188).

CHROMAFFIN CELL AS MODEL SYSTEM

It remains to place the results and conclusions from the chromaffin cell within the broader context of secretion in general. In a lecture delivered in 1967 (45), it was argued that the chromaffin cell provides a useful model system, that the pattern of stimulus-secretion coupling evident there probably applies to many other secretory cells, that the essence of stimulation in each instance is the promotion of Ca entry, and that calcium's function is always to activate exocytosis. At the time, it was possible to document the need for Ca in secretion in cells from each of the classic categories—exocrine, endocrine, and neuroendocrine—as well as various other cells with secretory function, such as ordinary neurons, leukocytes, and mast cells. Exocytosis was by then clearly established as the mode of secretion in the chromaffin cell (see the chapter by Viveros in this volume of the *Handbook*). Evidence for its operation in other cells was less compelling and in many instances fragmentary or nonexistent, but it was already abundantly clear from electron microscopy that secretory products in most cells, including neurons, were packaged in rather similar membrane-limited granules differing essentially only in size, and the exocytosis concept (35, 140) offered a neat, if not generally accepted, mechanism for their extrusion. Moreover, economy of hypothesis required the common requirement for Ca to be attributed to some mechanism shared by the diverse cells, and exocytosis, which involves essentially only the plasmalemma and the membranous wrappings of the secretory material, offered the only obvious possibility: it seemed reasonable to suppose this mechanism involves similar reactions in different cells and operates independently of the nature of the secretory product. Now several years later, the list of cells that can with confidence be considered to secrete by exocytosis has expanded greatly (76), and Ca seems to be a universal requirement (160). Furthermore the behavior of certain endocrine glands, such as the anterior pituitary and islets of Langerhans, follows in surprising detail the pattern established for the chromaffin cells. For example, responses to the physiological secretagogues (hypophysiotropic hormones, and glucose, respectively) are mimicked by simple elevation of $[K^+]_o$ and vary with $[Ca^{2+}]_o$; moreover, Ba is stimulant, and Mg inhibits (20, 88, 94, 95, 127, 128, 160, 165). Still closer to the chromaffin cells in their secretory behavior toward ions and drugs are neurons and neurohypophysial fibers. This, coupled with their similar developmental origins, has made it particularly attractive to suppose that these possess the same secretory mechanism as the chromaffin cell and that similar chemical approaches to defining secretion would be helpful (42, 44–46). One of the most exciting recent developments has been the accumulation of such chemical, as well as morphological, evidence pointing to the operation of comparable Ca-activated exocytosis in nerves (85–87, 89, 101, 169, 185) and neurohypophysial terminals (46, 50, 51, 77, 180).

The chromaffin cell seems then to have established its worth as a model possessing the essential quality: predictive value. The obverse of this coin should not, however, be ignored. As the basic similarities between the chromaffin cell and other cells exporting packaged materials become increasingly evident, it follows that many lessons learned from these other systems may be expected to apply to the chromaffin cell. The field of secretion stands to benefit as much as any other from the comparative approach.

REFERENCES

1. Babkin, B. P. *Secretory Mechanisms of the Digestive Glands.* New York: Harper, 1944.
2. Baker, P. F. Sodium-calcium exchange across the nerve cell membrane. In: *Calcium and Cellular Function,* edited by A. W. Cuthbert. New York: St. Martin's, 1970, p. 96–109.
3. Baker, P. F., A. L. Hodgkin, and E. B. Ridgway. Depolarization and calcium entry in squid giant axons. *J. Physiol., London* 218: 709–755, 1971.
4. Baker, P. F., H. Meves, and E. B. Ridgway. Phasic entry of calcium in response to depolarization of giant axons of *Loligo. J. Physiol., London* 216: 70–71P, 1971.
5. Banks, P. Effects of stimulation by carbachol on the metabo-

lism of the bovine adrenal medulla. *Biochem. J.* 97: 555–560, 1965.
6. BANKS, P. An interaction between chromaffin granules and calcium ions. *Biochem. J.* 101: 18–20c, 1966.
7. BANKS, P. The effect of ouabain on the secretion of catecholamines and on the intracellular concentration of potassium. *J. Physiol., London* 193: 631–637, 1967.
8. BANKS, P. Involvement of calcium in the secretion of catecholamines. In: *Calcium and Cellular Function*, edited by A. W. Cuthbert. New York: St. Martin's, 1970, p. 148–162.
9. BANKS, P., R. BIGGINS, R. BISHOP, B. CHRISTIAN, AND N. CURRIE. Sodium ions and the secretion of catecholamines. *J. Physiol., London* 200: 797–805, 1969.
10. BENEDECZKY, I., AND A. D. SMITH. Ultrastructural studies on the adrenal medulla of golden hamster: origin and fate of secretory granules. *Z. Zellforsch. Mikroskop. Anat.* 124: 367–386, 1972.
11. BIEDL, A. Beiträge Zur Physiologie der Nebeniere: die Innervation der Nebennieren. *Arch. Ges. Physiol.* 67: 443–483, 1897.
12. BIRKS, R. I., AND M. W. COHEN. Effects of sodium on transmitter release from frog motor nerve terminals. In: *Muscle*, edited by W. M. Paul, E. E. Daniel, C. M. Kay, and G. Monckton. New York: Pergamon Press, 1965, p. 403–420.
13. BIRKS, R. I., AND M. W. COHEN. The action of sodium pump inhibitors on neuromuscular transmission. *Proc. Roy. Soc. London, Ser. B* 170: 381–399, 1968.
14. BIRKS, R. I., AND M. W. COHEN. The influence of internal sodium on the behaviour of motor nerve endings. *Proc. Roy. Soc. London Ser. B* 170: 401–421, 1968.
15. BIRKS, R. I., AND F. C. MACINTOSH. Acetylcholine metabolism of a sympathetic ganglion. *Can. J. Biochem. Physiol.* 39: 787–827, 1961.
16. BLASCHKO, H., H. FIREMARK, A. D. SMITH, AND H. WINKLER. Phospholipids and cholesterol in particulate fractions of adrenal medulla. *Biochem. J.* 98: 24P, 1966.
17. BLASCHKO, H., H. FIREMARK, A. D. SMITH, AND H. WINKLER. Lipids of the adrenal medulla: lysolecithin, a characteristic constituent of chromaffin granules. *Biochem. J.* 104: 545–549, 1967.
18. BOROWITZ, J. L. Effect of acetylcholine on the subcellular distribution of ^{45}Ca in bovine adrenal medulla. *Biochem. Pharmacol.* 18: 715–723, 1969.
19. BÜLBRING, E., AND J. H. BURN. Liberation of noradrenaline from the suprarenal gland. *Brit. J. Pharmacol. Chemotherap.* 4: 202–208, 1949.
20. BURGUS, R., AND R. GUILLEMIN. Hypothalamic releasing factors. *Ann. Rev. Biochem.* 39: 499–526, 1970.
21. BUTTERWORTH, K. R., AND M. MANN. A quantitative comparison of the sympathomimetic amine content of the left and right adrenal glands of the cat. *J. Physiol., London* 136: 294–299, 1957.
22. CANNON, W. B., J. C. AUB, AND C. A. L. BINGER. A note on the effect of nicotine injection on the adrenal medulla. *J. Pharmacol. Exptl. Therap.* 3: 379–385, 1912.
23. CANNON, W. B., AND A. ROSENBLUETH. Excitabilité électrique de la surrénale dénervée. *Compt. Rend. Soc. Biol.* 124: 1262–1264, 1937.
24. CARAFOLI, E., P. PATRIARCA, AND C. S. ROSSI. A comparative study of the role of mitochondria and the sarcoplasmic reticulum in the uptake and release of Ca^{++} by the rat diaphragm. *J. Cellular Physiol.* 74: 17–30, 1969.
25. CARAFOLI, E., AND C. S. ROSSI. Calcium transport in mitochondria. In: *Advances in Cytopharmacology*, edited by F. Clementi and B. Cecarelli. New York: Raven Press, 1971, vol. 1, p. 209–227.
26. COMLINE, R. S., I. A. SILVER, AND M. SILVER. Factors responsible for the stimulation of the adrenal medulla during asphyxia in the foetal lamb. *J. Physiol., London* 178: 211–238, 1965.
27. COMLINE, R. S., AND M. SILVER. The development of the adrenal medulla of the foetal and new-born calf. *J. Physiol., London* 183: 305–340, 1966.
28. COMLINE, R. S., M. SILVER, AND D. G. SINCLAIR. The effects of bradykinin, angiotensin and acetylcholine on the bovine adrenal medulla. *J. Physiol., London* 196: 339–350, 1968.
29. COUPLAND, R. E. The effects of insulin, reserpine and choline 2:6-xylylether bromide on the adrenal medulla and on medullary autografts in the rat. *J. Endocrinol.* 17: 191–196, 1958.
30. COUPLAND, R. E. *The Natural History of the Chromaffin Cell.* London: Longmans, Green, 1965, p. 1–279.
31. CZYBULSKI, N. [Quoted in Dreyer (69).]
32. DALE, H. H. The action of certain esters and ethers of choline and their relation to muscarine. *J. Pharmacol. Exptl. Therap.* 6: 147–190, 1914.
33. DALE, H. H. Acetylcholine as a transmitter of the effects of nerve impulses. In: *Adventures in Physiology*. London: Pergamon Press, 1953, p. 611–635.
34. DALE, H. H., AND P. O. LAIDLAW. The significance of the suprarenal capsules in the action of certain alkaloids. *J. Physiol., London* 45: 1–26, 1912.
35. DE DUVE, C. Endocytosis. In: *Lysosomes*, edited by A. V. S. DeReuck and M. P. Cameron. London: Churchill, 1963, p. 126.
36. DEL CASTILLO, J., AND B. KATZ. On the localization of acetylcholine receptors. *J. Physiol., London* 128: 157–181, 1955.
37. DE POTTER, W. P., A. F. DE SCHAEPDRYVER, E. J. MOERMAN AND A. D. SMITH. Evidence for the release of vesicle-proteins together with noradrenaline upon stimulation of the splenic nerve. *J. Physiol., London* 204: 102–104P, 1969.
38. DEROBERTIS, E. D. P., AND D. D. SABATINI. Submicroscopic analysis of the secretory process in the adrenal medulla. *Federation Proc.* 19: 70–78, 1960.
39. DEROBERTIS, E. D. P., AND A. VAZ FERREIRA. Electron microscope study of the excretion of catechol-containing droplets in the adrenal medulla. *Exptl. Cell Res.* 12: 568–574, 1957.
40. DINER, O. L'expulsion des granules de la médullosurrénale chez le hamster. *Compt. Rend.* 265: 616–619, 1967.
41. DOUGLAS, W. W. Acetylcholine as a secretagogue: calcium-dependent links in "stimulus-secretion coupling" at the adrenal medulla and submaxillary gland. In: *Pharmacology of Cholinergic and Adrenergic Transmission.* London: Pergamon Press, 1965, vol. 3, p. 95–111.
42. DOUGLAS, W. W. Calcium dependent links in stimulus-secretion coupling in the adrenal medulla and neurohypophysis. In: *Mechanisms of Release of Biogenic Amines*, edited by U. S. von Euler, S. Rosell, and B. Uvnäs. London: Pergamon Press, 1966, p. 267–290.
43. DOUGLAS, W. W. The mechanism of release of catecholamines from the adrenal medulla. *Pharmacol. Rev.* 18: 471–480, 1966.
44. DOUGLAS, W. W. Stimulus-secretion coupling in the adrenal medulla and the neurohypophysis: cellular mechanisms of release of catecholamines and posterior pituitary hormones. In: *Neurosecretion*, edited by F. Stutinsky. Berlin: Springer, 1967, p. 178–190.
45. DOUGLAS, W. W. Stimulus-secretion coupling: the concept and clues from chromaffin and other cells. (The First Gaddum Memorial Lecture). *Brit. J. Pharmacol.* 34: 451–474, 1968.
46. DOUGLAS, W. W. How do neurones secrete peptides? Exocytosis and its consequences, including synaptic vesicle formation, in the hypothalamoneurohypophyseal system. *Progr. Brain Res.* 39: 21–38, 1973.
47. DOUGLAS, W. W., AND T. KANNO. The effect of amethocaine on acetylcholine-induced depolarization and catecholamine secretion in the adrenal chromaffin cell. *Brit. J. Pharmacol. Chemotherap.* 30: 612–619, 1967.
48. DOUGLAS, W. W., T. KANNO, AND S. R. SAMPSON. Effects of acetylcholine and other medullary secretagogues and antagonists on the membrane potential of adrenal chromaffin

cells: an analysis employing techniques of tissue culture. *J. Physiol., London* 188: 107–120, 1967.
49. DOUGLAS, W. W., T. KANNO, AND S. R. SAMPSON. Influence of the ionic environment on the membrane potential of adrenal chromaffin cells and on the depolarizing effect of acetylcholine. *J. Physiol., London* 191: 107–121, 1967.
50. DOUGLAS, W. W., AND J. NAGASAWA. Membrane vesiculation at sites of exocytosis in the neurohypophysis, adenohypophysis and adrenal medulla: a device for membrane conservation. *J. Physiol., London* 218: 94–95P, 1971.
51. DOUGLAS, W. W., J. NAGASAWA, AND R. A. SCHULZ. Electronmicroscopic studies on the mechanism of secretion of posterior pituitary hormones and significance of microvesicles ("synaptic" vesicles): evidence of secretion by exocytosis and formation of microvesicles as a by-product of this process. *Mem. Soc. Endocrinol.* 19: 353–378, 1971.
52. DOUGLAS, W. W., AND A. M. POISNER. Stimulation of uptake of calcium-45 in the adrenal gland by acetylcholine. *Nature* 192: 1299, 1961.
53. DOUGLAS, W. W., AND A. M. POISNER. On the mode of action of acetylcholine in evoking adrenal medullary secretion: increased uptake of calcium during the secretory response. *J. Physiol., London* 162: 385–392, 1962.
54. DOUGLAS, W. W., AND A. M. POISNER. The influence of calcium on the secretory response of the submaxillary gland to acetylcholine or to noradrenaline. *J. Physiol., London* 165: 528–541, 1963.
55. DOUGLAS, W. W., AND A. M. POISNER. Stimulus-secretion coupling in a neurosecretory organ: the role of calcium in the release of vasopressin from the neurohypophysis. *J. Physiol., London* 172: 1–18, 1964.
56. DOUGLAS, W. W., AND A. M. POISNER. Calcium movement in the neurohypophysis of the rat and its relation to the release of vasopressin. *J. Physiol., London* 172: 19–30, 1964.
57. DOUGLAS, W. W., AND A. M. POISNER. Preferential release of adrenaline from the adrenal medulla by muscarine and pilocarpine. *Nature* 208: 1102–1103, 1965.
58. DOUGLAS, W. W., AND A. M. POISNER. Evidence that the secreting adrenal chromaffin cell releases catecholamines directly from ATP-rich granules. *J. Physiol., London* 183: 236–248, 1966.
59. DOUGLAS, W. W., A. M. POISNER, AND R. P. RUBIN. Efflux of adenine nucleotides from perfused adrenal glands exposed to nicotine and other chromaffin cell stimulants. *J. Physiol., London* 179: 130–137, 1965.
60. DOUGLAS, W. W., A. M. POISNER, AND J. M. TRIFARÓ. Lysolecithin and other phospholipids in the adrenal medulla of various species. *Life Sci.* 5: 809–815, 1966.
61. DOUGLAS, W. W., AND R. P. RUBIN. The role of calcium in the secretory response of the adrenal medulla to acetylcholine. *J. Physiol., London* 159: 40–57, 1961.
62. DOUGLAS, W. W., AND R. P. RUBIN. Mechanism of nicotinic action at the adrenal medulla: calcium as a link in stimulus-secretion coupling. *Nature* 192: 1087–1089, 1961.
63. DOUGLAS, W. W., AND R. P. RUBIN. The mechanism of catecholamine release from the adrenal medulla and the role of calcium in stimulus-secretion coupling. *J. Physiol., London* 167: 288–310, 1963.
64. DOUGLAS, W. W., AND R. P. RUBIN. The effects of alkaline earths and other divalent cations on adrenal medullary secretion. *J. Physiol., London* 175: 231–241, 1964.
65. DOUGLAS, W. W., AND R. P. RUBIN. Stimulant action of barium on the adrenal medulla. *Nature* 203: 305–307, 1964.
66. DOUGLAS, W. W., AND M. SORIMACHI. Colchicine inhibits adrenal medullary secretion evoked by acetylcholine without affecting that to potassium. *Brit. J. Pharmacol.* 45: 129–132, 1972.
67. DOUGLAS, W. W., AND M. SORIMACHI. Effects of cytochalasin B and colchicine on secretion of posterior pituitary and adrenal medullary hormones. *Brit. J. Pharmacol.* 45: 143–144P, 1972.
68. DOUGLAS, W. W., AND Y. UEDA. Mast cell secretion (histamine release) induced by 48-80: calcium-dependent exocytosis inhibited strongly by cytochalasin only when glycolysis is rate-limiting. *J. Physiol., London* 234: 97–98P, 1973.
69. DREYER, G. P. On secretory nerves to the suprarenal capsules. *Am. J. Physiol.* 2: 203–219, 1898.
70. DUNER, H. The influence of the blood glucose level on the secretion of adrenaline and noradrenaline from the suprarenal. *Acta Physiol. Scand. Suppl.* 28: 102, 1953.
71. EADE, N. R., AND D. R. WOOD. The release of adrenaline and noradrenaline from the adrenal medulla of the cat during splanchnic stimulation. *Brit. J. Pharmacol. Chemotherap.* 13: 390–394, 1958.
72. ELLIOTT, T. R. The control of the suprarenal glands by the splanchnic nerves. *J. Physiol., London* 44: 374–409, 1912.
73. ELLIOTT, T. R. The innervation of the adrenal glands. *J. Physiol., London* 46: 285–290, 1913.
74. ERÄNKÖ, O. Nodular hyperplasia and increase of noradrenaline content in the adrenal medulla of nicotine-treated rats. *Acta Pathol. Microbiol. Scand.* 36: 210–218, 1955.
75. ERÄNKÖ, O. Adrenaline and noradrenaline in adrenal autografts. *Nature* 178: 603, 1956.
76. FAWCETT, D. W., J. A. LONG, AND A. L. JONES. The ultrastructure of endocrine glands. *Recent Progr. Hormone Res.* 25: 315–368, 1969.
77. FAWCETT, C. P., A. E. POWELL, AND H. SACHS. Biosynthesis and release of neurophysin. *Endocrinology* 83: 1299–1310, 1968.
78. FAWCETT, P. R. W. An electrophysiological study of the rat adrenal gland *in vivo. J. Neurol. Sci.* 8: 381–383, 1969.
79. FELDBERG, W., AND J. H. GADDUM. The chemical transmitter at synapses in a sympathetic ganglion. *J. Physiol., London* 81: 305–319, 1934.
80. FELDBERG, W., AND G. P. LEWIS. Further studies on the effects of peptides on the suprarenal medulla of cats. *J. Physiol., London* 178: 239–251, 1965.
81. FELDBERG, W., AND B. MINZ. Die Wirkung von Acetylcholin auf die Nebennieren. *Arch. Exptl. Pathol.* 163: 66–96, 1931.
82. FELDBERG, W., AND B. MINZ. Die blutdrucksteigernde Wirkung des Acetylcholins an Katzen nach Entfernen der Nebennieren. *Arch. Exptl. Pathol.* 165: 261–290, 1932.
83. FELDBERG, W., AND B. MINZ. Das Auftreten eines acetylcholinartigen Stoffes im Nebennierenvenenblut bei Reizung der Nervi splanchnici. *Arch. Ges. Physiol.* 233: 657–682, 1934.
84. FELDBERG, W., B. MINZ, AND H. TSUDZIMURA. The mechanism of the nervous discharge of adrenaline. *J. Physiol., London* 81: 286–304, 1934.
85. FILLENZ, M. Fine structure of noradrenaline storage vesicles in nerve terminals of the rat vas deferens. *Phil. Trans. Roy. Soc. London Ser. B* 261: 319–323, 1971.
86. GEFFEN, L. B., AND B. G. LIVETT. Synaptic vesicles in sympathetic neurones. *Physiol. Rev.* 51: 98–157, 1971.
87. GEFFEN, L. B., B. G. LIVETT, AND R. A. RUSH. Immunohistochemical localization of chromogranins in sheep sympathetic neurones and their release by nerve impulses. In: *New Aspects of Storage and Release Mechanism of Catecholamines*, edited by H. J. Schümann and G. Kroneberg. Berlin: Springer, 1970, p. 58–72.
88. GESCHWIND, I. I. Mechanisms of release of anterior pituitary hormones: studies *in vitro. Mem. Soc. Endocrinol.* 19: 221–229, 1971.
89. GEWIRTZ, G. P., AND I. J. KOPIN. Release of dopamine β-hydroxylase with norepinephrine during cat splenic nerve stimulation. *Nature* 227: 406–407, 1970.
90. GILLARD, R. D. The simple chemistry of calcium and its relevance to biological systems. In: *Calcium and Cellular Function*, edited by A. W. Cuthbert. New York: St. Martin's, 1970, p. 3–9.
91. GINSBORG, B. L. Ion movements in junctional transmission. *Pharmacol. Rev.* 19: 289–316, 1967.
92. GOZ, B. Properties of a microsomal adenosine triphosphatase from the adrenal medulla. *Biochem. Pharmacol.* 16: 593–596, 1967.

93. GRYNSZPAN-WINOGRAD, O. Morphological aspects of exocytosis in the adrenal medulla. *Phil. Trans. Roy. Soc. London Ser. B* 261: 291–292, 1971.
94. HALES, C. N., AND R. D. G. MILNER. The role of sodium and potassium in insulin secretion from rabbit pancreas. *J. Physiol., London* 194: 725–743, 1968.
95. HALES, C. N., AND R. D. G. MILNER. Cations and the secretion of insulin from rabbit pancreas in vitro. *J. Physiol., London* 199: 177–187, 1968.
96. HEMPEL, K., AND H. F. K. MÄNNL. Resting secretion of dopamine from the adrenal glands of the cat in vivo. *Experientia* 23: 919–920, 1967.
97. HEMPEL, K., AND H. F. K. MÄNNL. Quantitative Analyse der Catecholamin-Biosynthese des Nebennierenmarks in vivo und Ruhesekretion neugebildeter Amine unter besonderer Berücksichtigung des Dopamins. *Arch. Exptl. Pathol. Pharmakol.* 264: 363–388, 1969.
98. HILLARP, N-Å. Structure of the synapse and the peripheral innervation apparatus of the autonomic nervous system. *Acta Anat.* 2, Suppl. 4: 1–153, 1946.
99. HODGKIN, A. L., AND R. D. KEYNES. Movements of labelled calcium in squid giant axons. *J. Physiol., London* 138: 253–281, 1957.
100. HOLMSTEDT, B. Pharmacology of organophosphorus cholinesterase inhibitors. *Pharmacol. Rev.* 11: 567–688, 1959.
101. HUBBARD, J. I. Mechanism of transmitter release. *Progr. Biophys. Mol. Biol.* 21: 33–124, 1970.
102. KANNO, T., AND W. W. DOUGLAS. Effect of rapid application of acetylcholine or depolarizing current on transmembrane potentials of adrenal chromaffin cells. *Proc. Can. Federation Biol. Soc.* 10: 39, 1967.
103. KATZ, B. *The Release of Neural Transmitter Substances* (The Sherrington Lectures x). Springfield, Ill.: Thomas, 1969, p. 1–60.
104. KAYAALP, S. O., AND R. J. MCISAAC. In vivo release of catecholamines from the adrenal medulla by selective activation of cholinergic receptors. *Arch. Intern. Pharmacodyn. Therap.* 176: 168–175, 1968.
105. KAYAALP, S. O., AND R. J. MCISAAC. Muscarinic component of splanchnic-adrenal transmission in the dog. *Brit. J. Pharmacol.* 36: 286–293, 1969.
106. KAYAALP, S. O., AND R. K. TÜRKER. Evidence for muscarinic receptors in the adrenal medulla of the dog. *Brit. J. Pharmacol.* 35: 265–270, 1969.
107. KELLY, J. S. Antagonism between Na^- and Ca^{2+} at the neuromuscular junction. *Nature* 205: 296–297, 1965.
108. KEYNES, R. D., AND P. R. LEWIS. The intracellular calcium contents of some invertebrate nerve fibres. *J. Physiol., London* 134: 399–407, 1956.
109. KIRKEPEKAR, S. M., AND P. CERVONI. Effect of cocaine, phenoxybenzamine and phentolamine on the catecholamine output from spleen and adrenal medulla. *J. Pharmacol. Exptl. Therap.* 142: 59–70, 1963.
110. KIRSHNER, N., H. J. SAGE, AND W. J. SMITH. Mechanism of secretion from the adrenal medulla. 2. Release of catecholamines and storage vesicle protein in response to chemical stimulation. *Mol. Pharmacol.* 3: 254–265, 1967.
111. KIRSHNER, N., AND W. J. SMITH. Metabolic requirements for secretion from the adrenal medulla. *Life Sci., Part 1* 8: 799–803, 1969.
112. KIRSHNER, N., AND O. H. VIVEROS. Quantal aspects of the secretion of catecholamines and dopamine-β-hydroxylase from the adrenal medulla. In: *New Aspects of Storage and Release Mechanisms of Catecholamines*, edited by H. J. Schümann and H. G. Kroneberg. Berlin: Springer, 1970, p. 78–88.
113. KOELLE, G. B. Parasympathomimetic agents. In: *The Pharmacological Basis of Therapeutics* (4th ed.), edited by L. S. Goodman and A. Gilman. New York: Macmillan, 1970, p. 466–477.
114. LACY, P. E., S. L. HOWELL, D. A. YOUNG, AND C. J. FINK. New hypothesis of insulin secretion. *Nature* 219: 1177–1179, 1968.
115. LEE, F. L., AND U. TRENDELENBURG. Muscarinic transmission of preganglionic impulses to the adrenal medulla of the cat. *J. Pharmacol. Exptl. Therap.* 158: 73–79, 1967.
116. LEHNINGER, A. L. Mitochondria and calcium ion transport. *Biochem. J.* 119: 129–138, 1970.
117. LEWIS, P. R., AND C. C. D. SHUTE. An electron-microscopic study of cholinesterase distribution in the rat adrenal medulla. *J. Microscopy* 89: 181–193, 1969.
118. LIDDELL, E. G. T., AND C. SHERRINGTON. *Mammalian Physiology*. Oxford: Clarendon, 1923.
119. LISHAJKO, F. Dopamine secretion from the isolated perfused sheep adrenal. *Acta Physiol. Scand.* 79: 405–410, 1970.
120. LOEWI, O. Über den Zusammenhang Zwischen Digitalis— und Kalziumwirkung. *Arch. Exptl. Pathol. Pharmakol.* 83: 366–380, 1918.
121. LUND, A. Release of adrenaline and noradrenaline from the adrenal gland. *Acta Pharmacol. Toxicol.* 7: 309–320, 1951.
122. MALMEJAC, J. Activity of the adrenal medulla and its regulation. *Physiol. Rev.* 44: 186–218, 1964.
123. MARLEY, E. The adrenergic system and sympathomimetic amines. *Advan. Pharmacol.* 3: 168–266, 1964.
124. MARLEY, E., AND W. D. M. PATON. The output of sympathetic amines from the cat's adrenal gland in response to splanchnic nerve activity. *J. Physiol., London* 155: 1–27, 1961.
125. MARLEY, E., AND G. I. PROUT. Physiology and pharmacology of the splanchnic adrenal medullary junction. *J. Physiol., London* 180: 483–513, 1965.
126. MATTHEWS, E. K. Membrane potential measurement in cells of the adrenal gland. *J. Physiol., London* 189: 139–148, 1967.
127. MATTHEWS, E. K. Calcium and hormone release. In: *Calcium and Cellular Function*, edited by A. W. Cuthbert. New York: St. Martin's, 1970, p. 163–182.
128. MCCANN, S. D., AND J. C. PORTER. Hypothalamic pituitary stimulating and inhibiting hormones. *Physiol. Rev.* 49: 240–284, 1969.
129. MIELE, E. The nicotinic stimulation of the cat adrenal medulla. *Arch. Intern. Pharmacodyn. Therap.* 179: 343–351, 1969.
130. MINZ, B. *The Role of Humoral Agents in Nervous Activity*. Springfield, Ill. Thomas, 1955.
131. MIRKIN, B. L. Factors influencing the selective secretion of adrenal medullary hormones. *J. Pharmacol. Exptl. Therap.* 132: 218–225, 1961.
132. *Molecular Properties of Drug Receptors* (Ciba Foundation Symposium), edited by R. Porter and M. O'Connor. London: Churchill, 1970.
133. MORRILL, G. E., H. R. KABACK, AND E. ROBBINS. Effect of calcium on intracellular sodium and potassium concentrations in plant and animal cells. *Nature* 204: 641–642, 1964.
134. MULLINS, L. T. The macromolecular properties of excitable membranes. *Ann. NY Acad. Sci.* 94: 390–404, 1961.
135. NAGASAWA, J., AND W. W. DOUGLAS. Thorium dioxide uptake into adrenal medullary cells and the problem of recapture of granule membrane following exocytosis. *Brain Res.* 37: 141–145, 1972.
136. NASTUK, W. L., AND C. LIU. Muscle postjunctional membrane: change in chemosensitivity produced by calcium. *Science* 154: 266–267, 1966.
137. O'BRIEN, R. D., M. E. ELDEFRAWI, AND A. T. ELDEFRAWI. Isolation of acetylcholine receptors. *Ann. Rev. Pharmacol.* 12: 19–34, 1972.
138. OLIVER, G., AND E. A. SCHÄFER. The physiological effects of extracts of suprarenal capsules. *J. Physiol., London* 18: 230–276, 1895.
139. OUTSCHOORN, A. S. The hormones of the adrenal medulla and their release. *Brit. J. Pharmacol. Chemotherap.* 7: 605–615, 1952.
140. PALADE, G. E. Functional changes in the structure of cell components. In: *Subcellular Particles*, edited by T. Hayashi. New York: Ronald Press, 1959, p. 64–83.
141. PALKAMA, A. Demonstration of adrenomedullary catechol-

amines and cholinesterases at electron microscopic level in the same tissue section. *Ann. Med. Exptl. Fenn.* 45: 295-306, 1967.
142. PATON, W. D. M., AND A. M. ROTHSCHILD. The effect of varying calcium concentration on the kinetic constants of hyoscine and mepyramine antagonism. *Brit. J. Pharmacol. Chemotherap.* 24: 432-436, 1965.
143. POISNER, A. M. Release of transmitters from storage: a contractile model. In: *Biochemistry of Simple Neuronal Models*, edited by E. Costa and E. Giacobini. New York: Raven Press, 1970, p. 95-108.
144. POISNER, A. M., AND J. BERNSTEIN. A possible role of microtubules in catecholamine release from the adrenal medulla: effect of colchicine, vinca alkaloids and deuterium oxide. *J. Pharmacol. Exptl. Therap.* 177: 102-108, 1971.
145. POISNER, A. M., AND W. W. DOUGLAS. The release of dopamine on stimulation of the adrenal medulla. *Pharmacologist* 7: 168, 1965.
146. POISNER, A. M., AND W. W. DOUGLAS. Preferential release of adrenaline from the adrenal medulla by muscarine and pilocarpine. *Nature* 208: 1102-1103, 1965.
147. POISNER, A. M., AND W. W. DOUGLAS. The need for calcium in adrenomedullary secretion evoked by biogenic amines, polypeptides, and muscarinic agents. *Proc. Soc. Exptl. Biol. Med.* 123: 62-64, 1966.
148. POISNER, A. M., AND M. HAVA. The role of adenosine triphosphate and adenosine triphosphatase in the release of catecholamines from the adrenal medulla. IV. Adenosine triphosphate-activated uptake of calcium by microsomes and mitochondria. *Mol. Pharmacol.* 6: 407-415, 1970.
149. POISNER, A. M., AND J. M. TRIFARÓ. The role of ATP and ATPase in the release of catecholamines from the adrenal medulla. 1. ATP-evoked release of catecholamines, ATP, and protein from isolated chromaffin granules. *Mol. Pharmacol.* 3: 561-571, 1967.
150. POISNER, A. M., AND J. M. TRIFARÓ. The role of adenosine triphosphate and adenosine triphosphatase in the release of catecholamines from the adrenal medulla. 3. Similarities between the effects of adenosine-triphosphate on chromaffin granules and on mitochondria. *Mol. Pharmacol.* 5: 294-299, 1969.
151. POTTER, L. T. Role of intraneuronal vesicles in the synthesis, storage and release of noradrenaline. *Circulation Res.* 21, Suppl. 3: 13-24, 1967.
152. RAHAMIMOFF, R. Role of calcium ions in neuromuscular transmission. In: *Calcium and Cellular Function*, edited by A. W. Cuthbert. New York: St. Martin's, 1970, p. 131-147.
153. RAMWELL, P. W., J. E. SHAW, W. W. DOUGLAS, AND A. M. POISNER. Efflux of prostaglandin from adrenal glands stimulated with acetylcholine. *Nature* 210: 273-274, 1966.
154. RANG, H. P. Drug receptors and their function. *Nature* 231: 91-96, 1971.
155. RAPELA, C. E. Differential secretion of adrenaline and noradrenaline. *Acta Physiol. Latinoam.* 6: 1-14, 1956.
156. REITER, M. Cardioactive steroids with special reference to calcium. In: *Calcium and Cellular Function*, edited by A. W. Cuthbert. New York: St. Martin's, 1970, p. 270-279.
157. ROBINSON, R. L. Stimulation of the catecholamine output of the isolated, perfused adrenal gland of the dog by angiotensin and bradykinin. *J. Pharmacol. Exptl. Therap.* 156: 252-257, 1967.
158. ROLLESTON, H. D. The suprarenal bodies. *Brit. Med. J.* 1: 629-633, 645-748, 1895.
159. RUBIN, R. P. The metabolic requirements for catecholamine release from the adrenal medulla. *J. Physiol., London* 202: 197-209, 1969.
160. RUBIN, R. P. The role of calcium in the release of neurotransmitter substances and hormones. *Pharmacol. Rev.* 22: 389-428, 1970.
161. RUBIN, R. P., M. B. FEINSTEIN, S. D. JAANUS, AND M. PAIMRE. Inhibition of catecholamine secretion and calcium exchange in perfused cat adrenal glands by tetracaine and magnesium. *J. Pharmacol. Exptl. Therap.* 155: 463-471, 1967.
162. RUBIN, R. P., AND E. MIELE. A study of the differential secretion of epinephrine and norepinephrine from the perfused cat adrenal gland. *J. Pharmacol. Exptl. Therap.* 164: 115-121, 1968.
163. SANDOW, A. Excitation-contraction coupling in muscular response. *Yale J. Biol. Med.* 25: 176-201, 1952.
164. SATAKE, Y. *Secretion of Adrenaline and Sympathin*. Tokyo: Nangando, 1955.
165. SCHOFIELD, J. G., AND E. N. COLE. Behaviour of systems releasing growth hormone *in vitro*. *Mem. Soc. Endocrinol.* 19: 185-201, 1971.
166. SHANES, A. M. Electrochemical aspects in excitable cells. *Pharmacol. Rev.* 10: 59-273, 1958.
167. SILVER, M. The output of adrenaline and noradrenaline from the adrenal medulla of the calf. *J. Physiol., London* 152: 14-29, 1960.
168. SIMEONE, F. A. Sensitization of the adrenal gland by partial denervation. *Am. J. Physiol.* 122: 186-190, 1938.
169. SMITH, A. D., W. P. DE POTTER, E. H. MOERMAN, AND A. F. DE SCHAEPDRYVER. Release of dopamine β-hydroxylase and chromogranin A upon stimulation of the splenic nerve. *Tissue Cell* 2: 547-568, 1970.
170. SORIMACHI, M. Effects of alkali metal and other monovalent ions on the adrenomedullary secretion. *European J. Pharmacol.* 3: 235-241, 1968.
171. STASZEWSKA-BARCZAK, J., AND J. R. VANE. The release of catecholamines from the adrenal medulla by histamine. *Brit. J. Pharmacol. Chemotherap.* 25: 728-742, 1965.
172. STASZEWSKA-BARCZAK, J., AND J. R. VANE. The release of catecholamines from the adrenal medulla by peptides. *Brit. J. Pharmacol. Chemotherap.* 30: 655-667, 1967.
173. STJÄRNE, L. Quantal or graded secretion of adrenal medullary hormone and sympathetic transmitter. In: *New Aspects of Storage and Release Mechanisms of Catecholamines*, edited by H. J. Schümann and G. Kroneberg. New York: Springer, 1970, p. 112-127.
174. TRIFARÓ, J. Phospholipid metabolism and adrenal medullary activity. 1. The effect of acetylcholine on tissue uptake and incorporation of orthophosphate-^{32}P into nucleotides and phospholipids of bovine adrenal medulla. *Mol. Pharmacol.* 5: 382-393, 1969.
175. TRIFARÓ, J. The effect of Ca^{2+} omission on the secretion of catecholamines and the incorporation of orthophosphate-^{32}P into nucleotides and phospholipids of bovine adrenal medulla during acetylcholine stimulation. *Mol. Pharmacol.* 5: 420-431, 1969.
176. TRIFARÓ, J. M., B. COLLIER, A. LASTOWECKA, AND D. STERN. Inhibition by colchicine and by vinblastine of acetylcholine-induced catecholamine release from the adrenal gland: an anticholinergic action, not an effect on microtubules. *Mol. Pharmacol.* 8: 264-267, 1972.
177. TRIFARÓ, J. M., AND J. DWORKIND. Phosphorylation of membrane components of adrenal chromaffin granules by adenosine triphosphate. *Mol. Pharmacol.* 7: 52-65, 1971.
178. TRIFARÓ, J. M., AND A. M. POISNER. The role of ATP and ATPase in the release of catecholamines from the adrenal medulla. 2. ATP-evoked fall in optical density of isolated chromaffin granules. *Mol. Pharmacol.* 3: 572-580, 1967.
179. TSCHEBOKSAROFF, M. Über sekretorische Nerven der Nebennieren. *Arch. Ges. Physiol.* 137: 59-122, 1911.
180. UTTENTHAL, L. O., B. G. LIVETT, AND D. B. HOPE. Release of neurophysin together with vasopressin by a Ca^{2+}-dependent mechanism. *Phil. Trans. Roy. Soc. London Ser. B* 261: 379-380, 1971.
181. VOGT, M. The secretion of the denervated adrenal medulla of the cat. *Brit. J. Pharmacol. Chemotherap.* 7: 325-330, 1952.
182. VOGT, M. Release of medullary amines from the isolated perfused adrenal gland of the dog. *Brit. J. Pharmacol. Chemotherap.* 24: 561-565, 1965.

183. VOLLE, R. L., AND G. B. KOELLE. Ganglionic stimulating and blocking agents. In: *The Pharmacological Basis of Therapeutics* (4th ed.), edited by L. S. Goodman and A. Gilman. New York: Macmillan, 1970, p. 585-600.
184. WEBER, A., R. HERZ, AND I. REISS. Study of the kinetics of calcium transport by isolated fragmented sarcoplasmic reticulum. *Biochem. Z.* 345: 329-369, 1966.
185. WEINSHILBOUM, R. M., N. B. THOA, D. G. JOHNSON, I. J. KOPIN, AND J. AXELROD. Proportional release of norepinephrine and dopamine-β-hydroxylase from sympathetic nerves. *Science* 174: 1349-1351, 1971.
186. WESSELS, N. K., B. S. SPOONER, J. F. ASH, M. P. BRADLEY, M. A. LUDUENA, E. L. TAYLOR, J. R. WREN, AND K. M. YAMADA. Microfilaments in cellular and developmental processes. *Science* 171: 135-143, 1971.
187. WINKLER, H. The membrane of the chromaffin granule. *Phil. Trans. Roy. Soc. London Ser. B* 261: 293-303, 1971.
188. WINKLER, H., N. STRIEDER, AND E. ZIEGLER. Über Lipide, insbesondere Lysolecithin, in den chromaffinen Granula verschiedener Species. *Arch. Pharmakol. Exptl. Pathol.* 256: 407-415, 1967.
189. YOUNG, J. Z. Partial degeneration of the nerve supply of the adrenal. A study in autonomic innervation. *J. Anat.* 73: 540-550, 1939.

CHAPTER 27

Mechanism of secretion of catecholamines from adrenal medulla

OSVALDO HUMBERTO VIVEROS | *Departamento de Neurobiología, Instituto de Ciencias Biológicas, Universidad Católica de Chile, Santiago, Chile*

CHAPTER CONTENTS

Subcellular Origin of Adrenomedullary Secretion
    Apocrine or holocrine secretion
    Secretion by increased permeability of plasma membrane to catecholamines
    Catecholamine secretion by increased amine outflow from storage vesicle into cytoplasm
    Direct extrusion of catecholamine storage vesicle content into extracellular space
    Fate of storage vesicle membrane
    Quantal secretion from adrenal medulla
    Release of newly synthesized catecholamines from adrenal gland
Excitation-Secretion Coupling
    Factors that may determine amount of material secreted in response to stimulus
    Chromaffin cell motility
    Electrophysiology of adrenomedullary cell in relation to secretion
    Ionic requirements for secretion
    Adrenal chromaffin cell energy metabolism in relation to secretion
    Effects of drugs on secretion
    Relevance of catecholamine release from isolated storage vesicles to study of adrenal chromaffin cell secretion
    Mechanism of membrane fusion
    Some general hypotheses for excitation-secretion coupling
    Adaptability of excitation-secretion mechanism of adrenomedullary cell to homeostatic demands

SECRETION has been defined in *Webster's Third New International Dictionary* as

    1a: The act or process of segregating, elaborating, and releasing some material that is either specialized to perform some function in the organism (as saliva) or is isolated for excretion from the body (as urine); b: a product of such secretion formed in the animal or plant body (as the cellulose wall of a plant cell or the pancreatic juice of an animal); *sometimes:* any such product that performs a specific useful function in the organism—distinguished from excretion.

Several other definitions have also been proposed (55, 62, 107, 156, 158, 175, 292); some of these have limited the

Cited unpublished work from this laboratory has been supported by CONICYT Grant 39-70 and Catholic University Research Fund Grant 37/72.

use of the term secretion to what Webster's Dictionary calls "release," as mentioned above (7, 62). This last phase of the secretory process has also been called "extrusion" (156, 175). Both *release* and *extrusion* are also frequently used to refer to any increase in the concentration of secretory products outside a secretory cell, including that caused by noxious agents that alter the integrity of the cell.

In this chapter, *secretion* includes only the events occurring in a secretory cell, such as a specific response to a physiological stimulus or to any other stimulus that can activate any step of the normal pathway that necessarily leads to the appearance of the characteristic secretory product in the extracellular space. The increase in extracellular catecholamines by any other mechanism, or when in doubt, is called *release*. When referring to the whole complex cell function of elaborating, segregating, transporting, storing, and secreting a secretory product, the term *secretory process* or *secretory function* is preferred.

Jacobj (152) in 1892 showed that electrical stimulation of the dog's great splanchnic nerve or direct stimulation of the adrenal gland reduced the amplitude of contraction of the gut and thus provided the first evidence on how the adrenal gland could be made to secrete biologically active substances. Demonstration of pressor activity of adrenal medulla extracts by Oliver & Schäfer (226) was soon followed by the finding of increased pressor activity on the adrenal venous blood of the dog during splanchnic nerve stimulation (80). Feldberg and co-workers (100, 101) showed that acetylcholine was the physiological stimulus for secretion and found both nicotinic and muscarinic receptors in the medullary cells. Houssay & Molinelli (145) in 1928 had already shown that Ca^{2+} was necessary in inducing secretion from the adrenal gland, but not until the extensive studies of Douglas and co-workers (62) from 1961 on was attention called to Ca^{2+} as a universal, necessary step in stimulus-secretion coupling. The demonstration by Blaschko & Welch (27) and Hillarp et al. (138) that catecholamines are stored in high concentrations with ATP and soluble proteins within membrane-bound, electron-dense granules (27, 47, 120, 138)—hereinafter called the chromaffin vesicle—and the large amount of information on the biochemistry of the chromaffin cell and its organelles (164, 277) have made possible a precise definition of the most important subcellular elements that participate in the secretory mechanism, even though all the steps involved in stimulus-secretion coupling at the molecular level in this and other cells have not yet been sorted out.

SUBCELLULAR ORIGIN OF ADRENOMEDULLARY SECRETION

In order to discover how the catecholamines are transferred from their storage sites to the extracellular space in response to a stimulus, the immediate intracellular source of the secreted amines and the minimum number of intracellular elements that interact to obtain this transfer must first be determined.

Many early workers using the light microscope tried to determine the subcellular structures that stored the catecholamines and the changes that occurred during the secretory cycle (7, 18). Cramer (49, 50) fixed the adrenomedullary cells by exposure to osmic acid vapors. When he induced strong, acute, reflex splanchnic stimulation in rats by the injection of beta-tetrahydronaphthylamine, ether anesthesia, CO_2 breathing, or exposure to low temperature for a short period of time, the chromaffin cells showed marked reduction of their typical cytoplasmic osmiophilic granulations, and these were observed in large numbers in adjacent subendothelial spaces and capillaries. Cramer concluded that there was "clear evidence that the osmiophilic adrenaline granule would leave the cell to pass into the blood vessels during stimulation leaving a laked cell" (50). Vincent (300) and Hion (142) observed a decrease in the chromaffin reaction in the adrenal medulla after neurogenic secretion induced by exercising rats in the cold or until exhaustion. A similar finding was reported by Hillarp (129) after secretion induced by insulin, beta-tetrahydronaphthylamine, and cold exposure. The chromaffin reaction, which stains all catecholamine-containing cells, and the iodate reaction and formol calcium-induced fluorescence, which is selective for norepinephrine cells, have been frequently used as semiquantitative assays for selective secretion of one or the other of the amines by different forms of reflexly induced secretion (1, 90, 136, 214) or drug-induced depletion (118).

A view different from Cramer's proposal was adopted by Bennett (18) and Hillarp et al. (137). Bennett, in a detailed study of the adrenal medulla of the cat, described "secretory granules," 0.5–4 μ in diameter, that showed chromaffin, silver, and osmium reactions but were also stained bright red by acid fuchsin and by the Altman-Kull method for mitochondria. Stimulation of the splanchnic nerve for 1 min resulted in an increase in the chromaffin reaction, an increase in the proportion of cells showing "secretory droplets," an increase in the number and size of the secretory droplets throughout the gland, and an increased amount of chromaffin and acid fuchsin-positive material in the venous vessels. Hillarp et al. (137) induced catecholamine secretion in rats by beta-tetrahydronaphthylamine or insulin hypoglycemia until catecholamine depletion was complete as judged by the disappearance of the chromaffin and ammoniacal silver reactions. Small pieces of medulla or isolated cells were mechanically obtained from the contralateral unfixed gland for vital observation under the phase and darkfield microscopes. Cells from both control and depleted adrenals showed highly refractive granular structures, less than 1 μ in diameter, that could be isolated after homogenization and differential centrifugation in a fraction containing most of the catecholamines (138) and 80% of the total succinic dehydrogenase and were intensely stained with Janus green (137). They concluded that catecholamine depletion "does not change the number, size or general appearance of the specific catecholamine granules." Both of these groups concluded that secretion occurred with conservation of the catecholamine "storage granules" within the chromaffin cell.

Not until the first electron-microscopic observations of the adrenal medulla (57, 185, 276, 311) did it become clear that the catecholamine storage structures were definitely different from mitochondria and that the large majority of the chromaffin granules or vesicles were well below the resolving power of the light microscope (47, 185). What had been observed represented either the larger of the electron microscopically visible chromaffin vesicles or aggregates of granules (47). In some instances the observed structures were in all probability mitochondria (18, 137).

Subsequent ultrastructural and biochemical work has given rise to numerous hypotheses on the immediate origin of the secreted catecholamines.

Apocrine or Holocrine Secretion

Graumann (116) reported a follicular arrangement of the adrenomedullary cells of the golden hamster. Many of these follicles contained a periodic acid-Schiff-reactive material, which appeared to originate by degeneration of the apical portion of the chromaffin cell. Franzen (106) made similar observations and proposed that, in the adrenal gland of the golden hamster, secretion products are extruded by merocrine secretion at the basal portion of the cell, whereas holocrine secretion occurs into the lumen of the follicle. All these observations have been made on the unstimulated gland, and it is not known whether the rate of degeneration is increased by stimulation, what fraction of the output of the gland originates by holocrine or apocrine secretion, or whether the observed changes represent normal or pathologic turnover of the cells in the gland and are not at all related to the secretory function. More recent studies show no increased secretion of cytoplasmic enzymes (168, 169, 229, 268, 302, 304) or catecholamine storage vesicle membrane components (168, 169, 268, 298, 302, 304) on stimulation of the adrenal medulla of the cow, rabbit, and rat. This evidence does not support holocrine or apocrine secretion by the chromaffin cell in these species. Similar studies of secretion should be performed on golden hamster adrenal medulla to establish whether apocrine or holocrine processes are involved in secretion of catecholamines.

Secretion by Increased Permeability of Plasma Membrane to Catecholamines

Blaschko & Welch (27) in 1953, after finding "that the adrenaline content of the adrenal medullary cell is divided between the cytoplasmic sap which contains less than 30% of the total activity and the particulate fraction" expressed that

> the question of the equilibrium between adrenaline in the particulate fraction and the cytoplasmic sap is closely bound up with that of the mechanism of release. According to current ideas, the liberation of acetylcholine from the splanchnic nerve results in an increased permeability of the membrane of the secretory cell. This would lead to a loss of adrenaline present in the cytoplasmic sap.... Two possibilities have to be considered with regards to how the adrenaline content of the sap is maintained: either the granule allows adrenaline to pass into the cell sap, be it by diffusion or active transport, or the granule disintegrates and thus gives off its adrenaline to the cell sap.

Hillarp (135) proposed a dynamic equilibrium between a free cytoplasmic pool and a bound intergranular pool of amines in the chromaffin cell. The stimulus would produce a short transient increase in plasma membrane permeability, which would allow the catecholamines to escape to the extracellular space. Hillarp (135) also proposed that the free cytoplasmic catecholamine pool might control catecholamine synthesis by feedback inhibition. A similar view for secretion from the adrenal medulla was held by von Euler (95, 96).

A somewhat more elaborate proposal was made by Maas & Colburn (193). The stimulus would activate both the plasma membrane and the vesicle membrane ATPases, and the former would split the ATP from hypothetical ATP-metal-phospholipid complexes at the plasma membrane, which would increase its micellar conformation and hence its permeability to hydrophilic solutes, including catecholamines. The vesicle membrane ATPase would remove the ATP from an ATP-catecholamine-metal-phospholipid complex and thus make it more lipid soluble and permit it to diffuse out through the otherwise impermeable vesicle membrane into the cytoplasm. A variation of the cytoplasmic hypothesis has been proposed by several authors for the release of catecholamines from sympathetic nerves (3, 94, 97, 121, 289). The impulse would directly release a very small pool of norepinephrine bound to releasing sites on the plasma membrane. The sites on the plasma membrane would then be rapidly refilled directly from the storage sites by resynthesis or reuptake of the released amine (94, 97, 289) or from the cytoplasmic pool, which in turn would be in equilibrium with the vesicle storage pool (3, 121).

Burack & Draskóczy (35) argued against an extragranular origin for the secreted catecholamines since the specific activity of the catecholamines in the venous effluent of the adrenal gland of rats that had received ^{3}H-dopa for 3 days before the experiment was identical with the specific activity of the medullary amines. More direct evidence against the plasma membrane sites or the cytoplasm as the immediate origin of the secreted catecholamines comes from the finding that, during secretion, all the soluble content of the storage vesicle, including large-size proteins, is extruded into the extracellular space (16, 74, 168, 169, 268, 302, 304) with no release of enzymes presumed to be free in the cytoplasm (168, 169, 229, 268, 302, 304).

Catecholamine Secretion by Increased Amine Outflow from Storage Vesicle into Cytoplasm

Blaschko's and Welch's second proposal (27) on the origin of the catecholamines secreted after intracytoplasmic "disintegration" of the granule soon gained many supporters. Hillarp and co-workers (137) found no morphological changes in chromaffin cells immediately after secretion and concluded that there was a fast transport of the amines from the granules through the cytoplasm into the extracellular space. This hypothesis was strengthened when Carlsson and associates (42, 43) showed, after inducing reflex secretion by morphine or insulin administration to cats, rats, and sheep, a 70% depletion of the amines, acid-labile phosphate, and adenine nucleotide in the large granular fraction of an isotonic homogenate, with no increase in ADP, AMP, adenosine, or inorganic phosphate in the granular fraction and no increase in any of these substances and/or catecholamines in the supernatant. In the large granular fraction prepared from rat and sheep medulla, there was a 12 and 25% decrease, respectively, in the protein content. From these studies the authors concluded that there was no secretion of the whole granular contents since they had expected a 35–40% decrease in the total granular proteins. Philippu and Schümann (230, 271, 272) found that the addition of Ca^{2+} to an isotonic sucrose suspension of the large granule fraction of bovine adrenal medulla increased the spontaneous release of catecholamines, ATP, Ca^{2+}, and Mg^{2+}, as measured by their decreased content in the pellet at the end of the incubation period; however, there was no decrease in the protein content. They concluded that the action of the acetylcholine secreted at the splanchnic-adrenomedullary junction is mediated through an increased Ca^{2+} entry, and this cation increases the permeability of the storage vesicle membrane or disrupts the storage complex, which releases the catecholamines that diffuse to the exterior of the cell.

This hypothesis was also supported by morphological studies with the electron microscope. Wetzstein (311) and Yates (323), after inducing secretion by insulin hypoglycemia in the mouse and Syrian hamster, have distinguished three groups of cells

> cells of group 1 had granules comparable to those of control tissue, group 2 showed granules with a reduction in density and size of the central core, while the cells of group 3 were

devoid of granules. The findings indicate that catecholamine loss is accompanied by changes in granule ultrastructure, catecholamines can be released from the adrenomedullary cells without complete granule destruction.

De Robertis & Vaz Ferreira (57) reported in their experiments with splanchnic nerve stimulation that "more seldom one may find droplets (chromaffin granules) that seem to undergo loss of catechol content while in the interior of the cytoplasm...." Similar observations have been made after 1–3 days of reserpine treatment in the hamster (322). Smitten (286) described progressive loss of electron density without membrane rupture of the chromaffin granules in rats that develop mild hypoglycemic symptoms after insulin injection. After intense convulsive shock the chromaffin granules adopted irregular forms, with membrane protrusions and final fragmentation into many small electron-dense droplets distributed throughout the cytoplasm, which appeared completely filled with small vesicles 30–70 mμ in diameter, either empty or with only a dense core. Smitten concluded that whether secretion occurred by dissolution of the granular content or by fragmentation of the intracytoplasmic granules depended on the intensity of the stimulus (286). Lever & Findlay (186) have reported that granules with large discontinuities or openings on their membrane are found in the unstimulated adrenomedullary cells of the guinea pig. These perforated granules are randomly distributed in the cytoplasm and are not preferentially seen close to the plasma membrane. They have made similar findings on the β cells of the pancreas of the rabbit and guinea pig and propose that secretion proceeds by intracytoplasmic release of the granular content through these openings.

The same biochemical evidence that argues against secretion originating in an increased plasma membrane permeability to catecholamines also makes the hypothesis that secretion originates in intracytoplasmic release of catecholamines no longer tenable. Additional evidence against intracytoplasmic discharge of catecholamines is provided in subsequent sections of this chapter.

Direct Extrusion of Catecholamine Storage Vesicle Content into Extracellular Space

De Robertis & Vaz Ferreira (57) were the first to give experimental evidence and to suggest that the storage vesicle might discharge its content directly into the interstitium with no loss of cytoplasmic material by close apposition or fusion of vesicle and plasma membrane and with a localized increase in permeability or actual rupture of the fused membrane. This mechanism of cell secretion has lately been proposed for practically every cell that segregates its products for export within a membranous envelope (62, 175). De Robertis and co-workers (55–57) have described the changes induced in the chromaffin cell of the rabbit adrenal medulla when the splanchnic nerve is stimulated supramaximally at 40–100 pulses/sec.

There is an apparent increase in the size of the droplets with diminution of electron density and a conspicuous attachment of many of them to the cell membrane. The process of attachment can be observed also in normal glands but is less frequent.... This process, in its highest degree, leads to the complete excretion of catechols leaving only the membrane (57).

Several authors have also found storage vesicles close to, or attached to, the inner surface of the cell membrane in unstimulated (46, 47, 58, 84, 186, 232) and stimulated adrenal glands (115, 286, 323). Coupland (46, 47), in the unstimulated rat adrenal, and Graf (115), in the reserpine-treated mouse adrenal, have shown "caveolae" (indentations on the plasma membrane), which may represent fusions of plasma and vesicle membranes after secretion has occurred. Only recently, Diner (58), by glutaraldehyde perfusion of the unstimulated medulla of the hamster, obtained clear-cut images of invaginations of the free external surface of the plasma membrane, each of which contains the dense core of a chromaffin granule and which in all probability has its origin in the fusion and opening of vesicle and plasma membranes. These exocytotic figures were not found where the plasma membrane of one chromaffin cell was facing another, although the frequency of simple contact between vesicle and plasma membrane was the same all over the periphery of the cell. However, several authors have claimed that secretion occurs throughout the periphery of the chromaffin cell (18, 84, 185).

Unfortunately there are very few quantitative observations on the frequency of vesicle membrane and plasma membrane contacts, of plasma membrane invaginations, and of exocytotic figures in control and stimulated adrenal glands. Yates reported no significant increase in vesicle and plasma membrane contacts in the chromaffin cell when Syrian hamsters treated with insulin (323) or reserpine (322) were compared to control animals. Smitten (286) occasionally saw vesicle and plasma membrane fusions in the rat adrenomedullary cells after insulin hypoglycemia. D'Anzi (51) made a thorough statistical investigation of the number, diameters, and association with the plasma membrane of the storage vesicles of epinephrine- and norepinephrine-containing cells in the rat at several time intervals after insulin administration. He found no changes in the norepinephrine-containing cells and no change in storage vesicle diameter of epinephrine-containing cells, but a drastic reduction in the number of vesicles—from 7.3 ± 0.2 vesicle profiles per square micron immediately after subcutaneous injection of insulin to 0.4 vesicle profiles per square micron 3 hr later. At this time the epinephrine content of the gland had fallen to about one-fifth the initial values. The cytoplasm displayed an abundance of smooth-surfaced membranes and small vesicles having a semi-electron-opaque content. In none of the experimental groups examined was an increase in the number of associations between storage vesicle membrane and plasmalemma observed. Lever (185), in the first electron-microscopic observation of the adrenal medulla, had also reported that the only obvious change in the catecholamine storage vesicles of rats exposed to 3–5 C for 2 hr just before killing was the disappearance of most of the electron-dense vesicles from many cells, whereas a few always retained their normal granular appearance.

Another way in which the storage vesicle could directly secrete its content into the extracellular space could be by the export of the whole vesicle out of the cell followed by its disruption. This possibility was also originally proposed by Blaschko & Welch (27) as a result of the pressor effect observed when the large granular fraction obtained from an adrenal medulla homogenate was resuspended in isotonic media and intravenously administered. The pressor effect was much smaller than that caused by injection of the same amount of material previously lysed by resuspension in water. These results led the authors to suggest that part of the pressor material stored in the granules was immediately active. On the same grounds, and since the storage vesicles were thought to be contained within the endoplasmic cisterna which was supposed to be continuous with the extracellular space, this hypothesis was also subscribed to by Hagen & Barrnett (120). Gori (113) obtained electron micrographs showing numerous intact storage granules traversing the plasma membrane and maintaining their structure in the subendothelial space and capillary lumen of the adrenal gland of the dwarf mouse. Elfvin (84) has also reported electron-dense particles, 300–700 A in diameter, in the intercellular and free surfaces of the chromaffin cell of the rat. Grillo (119) has recently proposed such a mechanism for the secretion of dense core and clear synaptic vesicles from the nerve terminals in the rat atria. Lever (185) and Coupland (46, 47) have deliberately sought storage vesicles or material resembling dense cores in the subendothelial space and capillary lumen but have not observed these particles or their contents.

The electron-microscopic evidence is contradictory and suggests both exocytosis and storage vesicle expulsion as possible mechanisms for secretion from the adrenal gland. There is obvious need of further quantitative experiments and, as discussed later in this chapter, better and faster methods of fixation to preserve what may be the morphological basis of secretion.

If the storage vesicle was to secrete its content directly into the extracellular space, all the soluble components of this vesicle, or their metabolites, should appear in the venous effluent of the gland (unless part of the secreted products were taken up or retained by the tissue). Simultaneously the gland should show a decreased content, unless the rate of resynthesis is high enough to immediately replace the losses. Vesicle membrane constituents should also be detected in the extracellular space if the whole vesicle is exported during secretion. Substances free in the chromaffin cell cytoplasm, or characteristic of other cell organelles, should be retained within the cell. Such an approach has been successfully applied to the studies of secretion from the polymorphonuclear leukocyte (318, 321), the posterior hypophysis (98, 261), the exocrine pancreas (6), and the rat mast cell (88, 154, 155), as well as the adrenal medulla. An extensive knowledge of the chemistry of the different cell compartments of the chromaffin cell is required to establish what substances may be characteristic of each one and be suitable as endogenous tracers [(164, 166, 277); Table 1].

The chemical analysis of the adrenal medulla of different species by Hillarp and co-workers (131, 134, 140) showed that the catecholamine storage vesicles were extremely rich in adenine nucleotides and soluble protein (4.5 and 9.2% of the wet wt, respectively, for bovine adrenal storage vesicles). Carlsson and associates (42, 43) subsequently showed that strong stimulation of the adrenal gland in various species was followed by a large

TABLE 1. *Endogenous Tracers of Subcellular Compartments in Adrenomedullary Cell*

Compartment	Tracer	References
Plasmalemma	Adenyl cyclase	176
	Na K ATPase	N. Kirshner, unpublished observations
Cytoplasm	Lactic dehydrogenase	268
	Tyrosine hydroxylase	162, 180
	Phenylethanolamine N-methyltransferase	162, 165, 180
	Dihydroxyphenylalanine decarboxylase	180
Chromaffin vesicle		
Soluble	Catecholamines	25, 27, 138, 139
	ATP	42, 74, 131, 140, 141
	Total chromogranins	16, 135, 162, 169, 262, 268, 277, 278
	Chromogranin A	135, 161, 162, 168, 262, 268, 277, 278
	Dopamine β-hydroxylase	82, 162, 172, 180, 301, 304
Particulate	Cholesterol	24, 168, 268, 298, 315
	Total phospholipids	24, 168, 268, 298, 315
	Lysolecithin	24, 268, 315
	Dopamine β-hydroxylase	82, 162, 163, 172, 180, 301, 304
Mitochondria	Monoamine oxidase	180
	Succinic dehydrogenase	176
	Fumarase	280
	Cytochrome oxidase	180
Lysosome	Acid ribonuclease	176, 180, 263, 266, 280
	Acid deoxyribonuclease	263, 266, 280
	Acid phosphatase	176, 280
	β-Glucuronidase	180, 263, 266
	Phospholipases A₁ and A₂	26, 282
Microsome	Glucose 6-phosphatase	18
	RNA	176

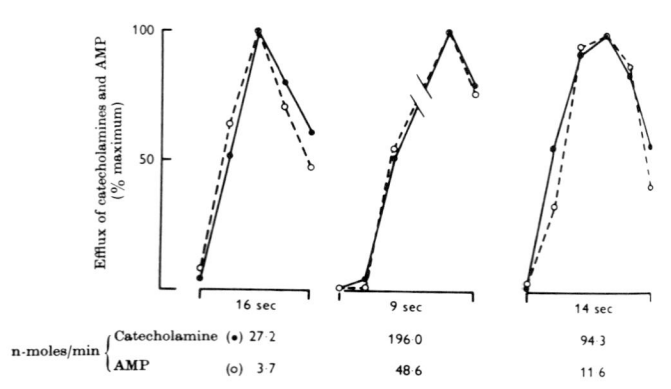

FIG. 1. Parallel time courses of efflux of catecholamines and AMP in 3 adrenal glands stimulated for 16, 9, and 14 sec through their splanchnic nerves. Each pair of curves was constructed by measuring catecholamines and AMP in successive drops emerging from the venous cannula after beginning stimulation and by expressing results as percentage of maximal value in each experiment. *Figures* below each graph represent absolute value of this maximum (1 drop was lost in the middle experiment). [From Douglas & Poisner (72).]

decrease in the catechol and adenine nucleotide content of the large granular fraction. Similar findings were reported after insulin administration to chickens by Schümann (269, 270) and Weiner et al. (308). Stjärne (288) studied the fate of the storage vesicle adenine nucleotide during secretion. He perfused cattle adrenal glands with Tyrode's solution and gave repeated injections of acetylcholine. Although he could not find ATP, ADP, or AMP in the pooled perfusate at the end of the experiment, he found two major peaks on cation exchange chromatograms, one of which was identified as hypoxanthine. Only very small corresponding peaks were obtained when the adrenomedullary extract was chromatographed, which suggested that this material had its origin in the ATP that had disappeared from the gland during perfusion. Douglas, Poisner, and Rubin (71, 74) were first to make a quantitative study of the release of adenine nucleotides and to suggest that their results, as well as the previous information, could be better explained if secretion was assumed to occur by what Douglas called "facilitated diffusion by membrane fusion." He proposed that fusion of the plasma and vesicle membranes resulted in an increased permeability to catecholamines and adenine nucleotides, but not to the intravesicular protein (61). This explanation was preferred over exocytosis with membrane disruption to account for the very small increase in effluent protein found on stimulation of the perfused adrenal gland (71). When catecholamine secretion was induced in the perfused cat adrenal by acetylcholine, nicotine, carbachol, high potassium concentration, reintroduction of calcium into a gland previously perfused in calcium-free media (71, 74), or splanchnic nerve stimulation (71, 72), there was a large increase in the AMP content of the venous effluent; only small amounts of ADP and ATP were found. The molar ratio of catecholamines to total adenine nucleotides was approximately 4, very close to the ratio for the isolated storage vesicles of the cat adrenal found by Hillarp & Thieme (141). Both catecholamines and nucleotides showed a strictly parallel rise and fall during continued splanchnic stimulation even when each drop of the venous effluent was analyzed [(72); Fig. 1]. The constancy of the ratio is also maintained at different times during continuous acetylcholine exposure, despite the progressive fall in the rate of secretion. The ratio of catecholamines to adenine nucleotides is also approximately 4 on the residual secretion induced by nerve stimulation during perfusion of the gland with hexamethonium plus atropine. The difference in the adenosine nucleotide composition between the effluent, where 96% of the nucleotides is AMP (72), and the storage vesicles, where 69% is ATP (141), was explained on the basis that exogenous ATP was 94–99% hydrolyzed in one passage through the gland (73). If adrenal phosphatases are inhibited by perfusion with calcium- and magnesium-free media plus EDTA and secretion is elicited by introduction of barium in the Locke's solution, the hydrolysis of ATP is greatly reduced and the molar ratio of catecholamines to ATP varies from $1,924 \pm 721$ in normal Locke's solution to 11.1 ± 1.4 in calcium- and magnesium-free Locke's solution. The ratio of catecholamines to total adenine nucleotides in this last group was 4.7 ± 0.3, and partial inhibition of adenosine phosphatases did not impair the stimulating effect of barium (73). Similar observations have been made after stimulation of cat adrenals with amphetamines and other phenylethylamines (259) and after stimulation of bovine adrenals with carbachol (10). In the latter case the adenine nucleotides were further degraded largely to xanthine, hypoxanthine, and AMP; ^{32}P-labeled ATP metabolites are released from carbachol-stimulated adrenals of cats that have received ^{32}P-labeled orthophosphate daily for 5–7 days before the experiment (125, 291). Since adenine nucleotide permeability through cell membranes is severely restricted, the constancy of the catecholamine-to-nucleotide ratio suggested that both substances might originate from the storage vesicle and leave the cell by a common mechanism. Although the data on the simultaneous release of catecholamines and adenine nucleotides established that the storage vesicles are the source of the secreted compounds, these observations did not distinguish whether secretion occurred by exocytosis, "facilitated diffusion by membrane fusion," extrusion of the whole vesicle, or even intracytoplasmic release with a carrier system for catecholamines and ATP.

Conclusive evidence has been obtained for direct secretion from the intravesicular to the extracellular space (16, 168, 169, 262, 264, 265, 268, 302–306). Hillarp (132) showed that 77% of the total protein of the catecholamine storage vesicles isolated from cow adrenals was readily solubilized upon lysis of the vesicles in water. Smith et al. (285) solved the crude storage vesicle protein by gel filtration and found a major fraction that accounted for 35% of the total soluble protein and had a molecular weight close to 40,000 by sedimentation equilibrium and sedimentation diffusion analysis. Further studies (126, 181, 279, 281, 284) showed that this major peak has a molecular weight close to 80,000 and hydrodynamic radius of 62 A, is very rich in acidic amino acids, and dissociates into two identical chains in 6 M guanidine hydrochloride plus 0.1 M mercaptoethanol. The earlier reported molecular weight of 40,000 was probably caused by separation of the subunits before the measurements were made. Smith & Winkler (281) analyzed the total soluble storage vesicle protein by starch gel electrophoresis and found eight bands, which were given the generic name of chromogranins (23); the major protein has been called chromogranin A. Duch et al. (81, 82) found that the endogenous inhibitors of dopamine β-hydroxylase (4, 81, 82, 216, 217) could be completely inhibited by Cu^{2+} and other sulfhydryl-reactive reagents, which led them to discover that dopamine β-hydroxylase is not only a vesicle membrane-bound enzyme (162, 187, 301) but that it is also normally present in the water-soluble fraction of the vesicles (82, 301, 303, 304). Laduron & Belpaire (180) found a similar subcellular distribution of dopamine β-hydroxylase. Other characteristic features of the chromaffin vesicle are a high calcium content, most of which becomes soluble on lysis with water (29, 32, 231), and a high cholesterol-to-phospholipid ratio (24) and high lysolecithin content (315, 316) of the membrane fraction. Cytochrome b-559 (8, 148) and a Mg^{2+}- or Ca^{2+}-dependent adenosine triphosphatase (8, 130, 167) have been described in the water-insoluble residue of purified catecholamine storage vesicles. Winkler et al. (313) have recently found 15 protein bands on polyacrylamide gel electrophoresis of the water-insoluble residue dissolved in phenolacetic acid urea; one of the major bands from the vesicle membranes seems to be absent in microsomal or mitochondrial membranes and in the water lysate of the storage vesicles and may prove to be a useful marker in studying the fate of the vesicle membrane during the secretory cycle.

Banks & Helle (16) confirmed the report of Douglas & Poisner (71) that there are only relatively small increases in the amounts of protein in the perfusates of adrenal glands stimulated with carbachol. Banks & Helle (16) reported a mean 32.2 ± 7.5-fold increase in catecholamine content and a 1.65 ± 0.25-fold increase in protein content in the efflux of four different bovine adrenal glands during the stimulation period. However, the ratio of the increase in catecholamines (μmoles) in the perfusate during stimulation to the corresponding increase in proteins (mg) was 7.6 ± 1.74, which is reasonably close to the value of 9.8 reported by Smith for the ratio of catecholamines to soluble protein in the purified catecholamine storage vesicles from bovine adrenal glands (277). More important was that the protein present in the perfusate during the stimulation period, when combined with an antiserum prepared against the soluble protein of the chromaffin granule, produced a precipitate. No precipitation was obtained with the protein derived from the control period perfusates. Banks and

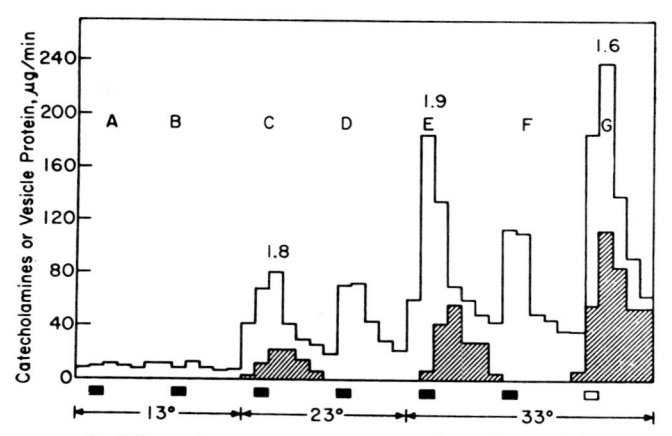

FIG. 2. Effect of temperature on secretion of catecholamines and vesicle protein. Each *bar* represents a 2-min sample. Between temperature changes, gland was perfused for 30 min with the warmer solution. Temperature of gland was monitored with thermistor needle probe inserted into cortex. Catecholamines, *open bars*; vesicle protein, *shaded bars*; stimulation period with acetylcholine, *solid horizontal bars*; stimulation period with nicotine, *horizontal open bar*. Numbers above bars are net catecholamine: vesicle protein ratios. [From Kirshner et al. (169).]

Helle concluded that secretion from the adrenal medulla was accompanied by the release of soluble protein from the chromaffin granules (16).

Kirshner and co-workers (168, 169, 262), with purified antichromogranin A sera, identified the vesicle protein in effluents from both control and stimulated bovine adrenal glands by immunoelectrophoresis and by quantitative microcomplement fixation. Furthermore they found that the storage vesicle protein was released in the same amount relative to catecholamines as that found in the intact gland when acetylcholine, nicotine, or Ba^{2+} was used as the stimulating agent. The secretion of both the specific protein and the catecholamines by acetylcholine and nicotine was Ca^{2+} dependent and was increased to the same extent by increasing the perfusion temperature from 13 to 23 C and then to 33 C (Fig. 2). Perfusion with diisopropylfluorophosphate enhanced the effect of acetylcholine in stimulating the release of catecholamines and vesicle protein, probably because of inhibition of acetylcholinesterase, whereas cocaine at 5×10^{-5} g/ml inhibited the secretion of catecholamines and protein. In none of these experiments was it possible to demonstrate in the effluent of the stimulated glands the presence of the cytoplasmic enzyme, phenylethanolamine N-methyltransferase (mol wt 38,000) even when the perfusates had been concentrated 10-fold. In these experiments it was usually found that the peak increase in protein secretion after pharmacological stimulation would lag 1 min behind the peak increase in catecholamines; this is probably explained by the lower rate of diffusion of the protein through the interstitial spaces or across the endothelial lining of the capillaries. The vesicle protein must be able to permeate the capillary wall since it has also been found in the venous effluent of the in situ, blood-perfused adrenal gland of the anesthetized calf stimulated through the splanchnic nerve (23). Very little protein seems to leave the gland through the lymphatic system in vivo since the ratio of catecholamines to chromogranin A in the venous effluent during stimulation was equal to or below the ratio found in the isolated granules (23). This might be related to the presence of fenestrae in the capillary endothelium of the adrenal gland (85).

Sage et al. (262) also showed that the distribution of specific antigenic protein closely paralleled the distribution of catecholamines after centrifugation of the large granule fraction through a sucrose density gradient and found that 55% of the total chromogranin A in the adrenal gland homogenate was stored in the catecholamine storage vesicle. The ratio of catecholamines (μg) to specific vesicle protein (μg) in the large granular fraction was 1.6 and in the perfusates from the stimulation period 1.7 (169). The ratios of catecholamines to specific protein in the other fractions obtained by differential centrifugation of the adrenal medulla homogenate were not significantly different from the former ratios, which further indicates that chromogranin A and catecholamines have a common distribution in the intact cell. The large proportion of the total specific protein in the large granular fraction, the distribution of the protein in the sucrose density gradient, and the fact that phenylethanolamine N-methyltransferase did not appear in the extracellular fluid during stimulation, even though the vesicle protein has a larger hydrodynamic radius than the enzyme, are consistent with a secretory process in which the vesicle contents are discharged directly to the exterior of the cell (169).

Kirshner and co-workers (168), based on their detailed studies on chromogranin A secretion, reported that, of the total increase in protein content of the adrenal effluent during stimulation, only 20–40% could be accounted for by the increase in chromogranin A. These results were soon confirmed by Schneider et al. (268) and extended to the other seven protein fractions that could be resolved by gel electrophoresis of the soluble vesicle proteins. In these experiments the isolated perfused bovine adrenal glands were stimulated with carbachol. Chromogranin A, as determined by complement fixation, comprised 48.2 ± 20.4% of the increase in total protein, which is essentially the same as the proportion of chromogranin A to total soluble protein in the lysate of purified chromaffin vesicles (47.6 ± 17.8%). Starch gel electrophoresis of the effluent and lysate protein indicated that 43 and 41%, respectively, of total protein is chromogranin A. The ratio of the net increase in catecholamines (μmole) to net increase in chromogranin A in the adrenal effluent during stimulation was 11.9 ± 5.0, whereas the ratio in the storage vesicle lysate was 10.1 ± 3.9. In the control adrenal effluent only one major protein component appeared to have a mobility corresponding to serum albumin. This band did not increase during stimulation of the gland and was not present in the lysate of the chromaffin granules. Starch gel electrophoresis of the protein obtained from the perfusates collected during stimulation indicated eight bands that closely corresponded to those of the soluble proteins from the storage vesicle lysate. The amino acid composition of the total protein found in the perfusate during stimulation minus the composition of the effluent protein during the control period was almost identical with that of chromogranins and different from that of the protein obtained from control perfusates. Schneider et al. (268) did not find any increased release of lactate dehydrogenase (effective hydrodynamic radius approximately 37 A, mol wt 140,000) or lysolecithin during stimulation. There was a small increment in phospholipids, cholesterol, and fatty acids, but the corresponding ratio of the net increase of lipid to net increase in catecholamines in the effluent was very much lower than the corresponding ratios in the total chromaffin granules. On the basis of these data, they concluded that the entire soluble contents of chromaffin granules are secreted by exocytosis from the adrenal medulla upon stimulation (268). Later work by Schneider (265) with polyacrylamide gel electrophoresis has shown the presence of at least two other distinct bands in the effluent protein obtained during carbachol stimulation of the cortex-free adrenal medulla that are not present in the chromaffin granule lysate. Furthermore, Schneider has shown that adrenal medulla lysosomal enzymes are secreted from the adrenal gland in response to many of the agents that induce catecholamine secretion; this response is Ca^{2+} dependent and blocked by the same agents that block catecholamine secretion (263–266).

Duch et al. (81, 82) and Viveros and co-workers (301–303) found that dopamine β-hydroxylase (mol wt 290,000) activity was distributed within the storage vesicle in a fixed proportion of bound to water-soluble enzyme, which varied with animal species, and so provides a simple marker for study of the fate of the storage vesicle content and membrane during the secretory and recovery period. Acetylcholine or nicotine stimulation of the perfused adrenal gland increased the outflow of catecholamines and soluble enzyme in the same proportion. Perfusion with Ca^{2+}-free Locke's solution produced a parallel decrease in the stimulated secretion of both substances. There was no measurable phenylethanolamine N-methyltransferase or tyrosine hydroxylase (cytoplasmic enzyme, mol wt 150,000) in the perfusates during the stimulation or the control periods (303, 304).

Most of the earlier biochemical evidence for exocytosis had been obtained by pharmacological stimulation of the isolated adrenal gland perfused with salt solutions. Only Douglas & Poisner (72) had determined adenine nucleotides during splanchnic stimulation of the in situ Locke-perfused adrenal gland of the anesthetized cat, and Blaschko and co-workers (23) had found increased chromogranin A in the adrenal venous blood during stimulation of the splanchnic nerve in the anesthetized calf. Viveros and associates (172, 302, 303, 305, 306) obtained biochemical evidence for exocytosis in vivo by inducing reflex stimulation of the adrenal gland of unanesthetized animals. Their basic assumption was that, if the rate of secretion of cell components by neurogenic stimu-

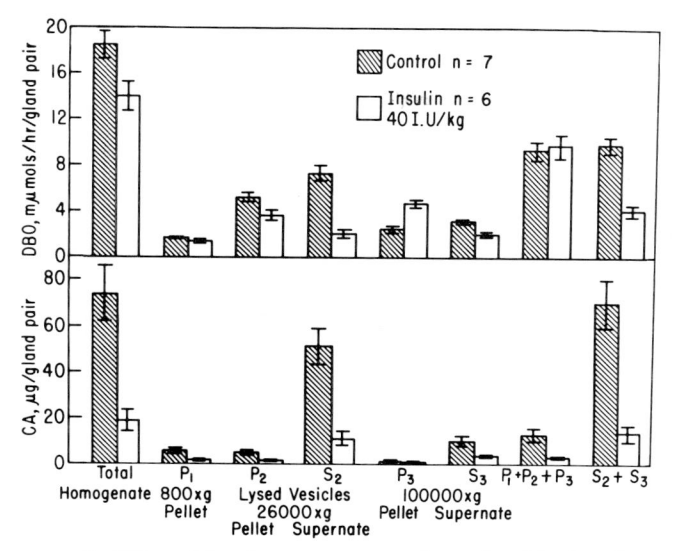

FIG. 3. Effect of insulin treatment on dopamine β-hydroxylase (*DBO*) and catecholamine (*CA*) content and distribution in rabbit adrenals. Glands from control and insulin-treated animals were subjected to differential centrifugation. Note decrease of DBO in the P₂ fraction of insulin-treated animals and compensatory increase in the P₃ fraction. Insulin-treated animals were killed 4 hr after receiving 40 IU/kg insulin iv. [From Kirshner & Viveros (172).]

lation is faster than the rate of resynthesis of these components, secretion should result in a decrease of the endogenous tracers of the different subcellular pools that participate in the secretory process. A second assumption is that the normal rate of destruction of these components is also low relative to the rate of secretion and is not increased during short periods of stimulation. Reflex adrenomedullary stimulation was elicited by insulin-induced hypoglycemia maintained for a period of 3 or 4 hr. Rabbits were selected as experimental animals since their adrenal glands primarily contain epinephrine, which is specifically secreted as part of the homeostatic response to hypoglycemia. When the animals were killed during the secretion period (Fig. 3) there was a large decrease in the catecholamine content of the gland, a smaller but significant decrease in total dopamine β-hydroxylase, and no change in the content of tyrosine hydroxylase or phenylethanolamine *N*-methyltransferase (302, 303). Most of the decrease in amines and dopamine β-hydroxylase could be accounted for by the corresponding losses from the soluble fraction of the catecholamine storage vesicles (172, 306). There was no significant recovery of the amine content and dopamine β-hydroxylase activity of the gland during the first 21 hr after the last dose of insulin [(302, 306); O. H. Viveros, L. Arqueros, and N. Kirshner, unpublished observations], which suggested that resynthesis was not a complicating factor. Depletion of dopamine β-hydroxylase was a result of secretion and not merely a consequence of amine depletion since relatively low doses of reserpine (or after blockade of the splanchnic-adrenomedullary junction by chlorisondamine, high doses of reserpine) did result in large decreases in adrenal catecholamine content but no decrease in dopamine β-hydroxylase levels (302, 306). If high doses of reserpine were given without preventing the effect of increased splanchnic discharge on the adrenal medulla, the catecholamines were depleted at a much faster rate, and a simultaneous decrease in dopamine β-hydroxylase content resembled the effect of insulin. These results confirm the theory that catecholamines are secreted from the adrenal gland by direct continuity of the intravesicular space and the extracellular space in response to neurogenic stimulation in a conscious animal. The smaller decrease in total dopamine β-hydroxylase compared to the decrease in catecholamines indicated that part of the enzyme present in the storage vesicle was not leaving the gland together with the secreted amines and suggested that the vesicle membrane might not be extruded. Similar findings have been recently reported after insulin-induced hypoglycemia (229) and immobilization stress in rats (176).

We now know that the early experiments in which insulin was found to produce a parallel decrease in catecholamine and adenine nucleotide of the large granular fraction (42, 43) or in purified storage vesicles (269, 270, 308) can be better explained by exocytosis than by intracytoplasmic release of the vesicle content. We also know that Carlsson and co-workers (42, 43) could not expect to find more than a 25% decrease of the total protein in the large granular fraction after 70% depletion of catecholamines since this fraction still contained 80% of the mitochondria originally present in the gland homogenate (137, 138) and probably even more of the lysosomes. Schümann (270) had also reported no change in the protein content of the large granular fraction after giving insulin to chickens; nevertheless his data show a significant decrease of protein in the "dense granule" fraction after centrifugation of the large granules in a sucrose density gradient.

Fate of Storage Vesicle Membrane

Bennett (19) in 1956 proposed the concept of membrane flow. Transport of ions and other molecules or particles into and out of, or within, the cell could result from the formation or synthesis of membranes in one region of the cell where they would vesiculate and flow to another region of the cell to discharge their content; elimination of the membrane could occur by intracellular digestion or extracellular extrusion. Palade (228) pointed out that in secretory cells the movement of vesicles should be bidirectional with a centrifugal limb from the Golgi region to the plasmalemma and a centripetal limb of empty vesicles moving back to the Golgi to be reused.

Several reports suggested that the vesicle membranes were retained within the adrenal gland after secretion. Schneider et al. (268) found only a small increase in cholesterol, phospholipids, and fatty acids and no increase in lysolecithin in the effluent of the perfused bovine adrenal gland during carbachol stimulation. Trifaró et al. (298) did not find any significant increase in phospholipids or cholesterol in the effluent of the in vitro perfused bovine adrenal gland stimulated with acetylcholine. In a similar experiment, Poisner et al. (246) repeated the acetylcholine stimulation 20 times; in the large granular fraction of the stimulated glands the catecholamine content was 59.4 ± 4.7% and the protein content 71.2 ± 5.0% of the corresponding values in the unstimulated gland, but there was no significant change in the phospholipid or cholesterol content of this fraction. If the large granular fraction was further resolved by centrifugation through a discontinuous sucrose density gradient, the decrease of catecholamines and protein was largest in the interphase between 1.8 and 2.25 M sucrose. This fraction, compared to the same fraction from an unstimulated gland, was significantly depleted of phospholipid (58.4 ± 6.1%) and cholesterol (46.5 ± 9.8%). There was no significant increase in the phospholipid or cholesterol of any other fraction along the gradient. Malamed et al. (194) subsequently showed that, after repeated stimulation of the perfused adrenal gland of the cat with acetylcholine followed by isolation of a granular fraction by filtration of the homogenate through progressively smaller millipore filters up to 0.45-μ diameter, it was possible to obtain a fraction rich in electron-translucent vesicles, most of which had diameters smaller than the electron-dense core vesicles isolated by the same procedure from unstimulated adrenals. The authors concluded from these series of experiments that the membrane of the vesicle was retained within the chromaffin cell and that it probably did not stay attached to the plasma membrane for a long period of time since there was no decrease of lipids in the total large granular fraction. They also suggested that the small electron-lucent vesicles observed with the electron microscope could result from artifactual fragmentation of the vesicles that had already released their content and become more fragile or alternatively could result from intracellular fragmentation after secretion. Another possible explanation for these results could be that the whole storage vesicle was secreted into the subendothelial space followed by disruption of the membrane, which might not be able to traverse the capillary wall (246).

All these studies, though suggestive, have suffered from several limitations. Total phospholipids, cholesterol, fatty acids, and individual phospholipids like lysolecithin are constituents of membranes from all organelles within the cell (277). Changes in their distribution within a certain subcellular fraction will be masked by dilution. In addition, these substances are too nonspecific to show displacement of the vesicle membrane from one subcellular fraction to another as a result of secretion or during the process of recovery. All smooth-surface membranes have the same appearance in the electron microscope. Consequently it is not possible to follow the fate of the vesicle membrane, after it loses its characteristic electron-opaque content, with any degree of certainty with currently available morphological techniques. Finally experiments with isolated perfused glands limit the time of the experimental study to acute immediate changes in the empty vesicle membranes and do not allow a study of the recovery phase of the secretory cycle.

More definitive information on the fate of the storage vesicle membrane during and after secretion has been obtained by Viveros and associates (172, 302, 303, 305, 306) using membrane-bound dopamine β-hydroxylase as a specific marker of the storage vesicle membrane after reflexly induced secretion, which permitted them to follow the fate of the membrane for prolonged periods of time. After 3 or 4 hr of insulin-induced secretion [Fig. 3; (172, 305)] there was a 78% decrease in the catecholamine content of the gland but only a 25% decrease in total dopamine β-hydroxylase. The bulk of the decrease of amines (71.3 ± 13.8%) and enzyme (81.6 ± 21.9%) comes from the soluble fraction of the storage vesicle. The total quantity of membrane-bound enzyme within the gland does not change during secretion, but there is a 37% decrease in the amount of membrane-bound enzyme that sediments in the large granular fraction and a corresponding increase in the enzyme content of the microsomal fraction. When vesicle membranes were prepared by lysing the large granular fraction in distilled water, they would still sediment at 26,000 g × 20 min. When this fraction was centrifuged to equilibrium through a sucrose density gradient, there was only one peak of dopamine β-hydroxylase activity corresponding to a specific gravity of 1.12 g/cm^3. The enzyme recovered in the microsomal fraction after the vesicles had secreted their contents had the same buoyant density. The decrease in the sedimentation rate of the membranes of the storage vesicle after secretion should then result from a decrease in their size (172, 305). Several recent morphological reports show the formation of microvesicles shortly after secretion in different cells: neurosecretory axons of the blow fly (219); axons of the posterior hypophysis of the hamster (215); and parotid acinar cells of the rat (2). It has been proposed that these microvesicles originate from fragmentation of the membranes of the empty secretory vesicles after extrusion of their content. Also consistent with this hypothesis are the results of Malamed et al. (194) and the observations of Diner (58). She (58) observed an increased frequency of micropinocytotic figures over portions of the external membrane of the chromaffin cell that seem to originate from the vesicle membrane after fusion and release of their contents. Smith (278) has proposed a similar microvesiculation to occur at the varicosities of noradrenergic axons where the small, dense and clear vesicles would originate from fragmentation of the large, dense core vesicles after secretion of their content by exocytosis. These small vesicles should still be able to synthesize, store, and release norepinephrine.

Whole granule extrusion with microvesiculation in the extracellular space and retention of the microvesicles within the interstitium for four or more hours without being removed by the lymphatic system seems highly unlikely. Morphological observations made after secretion and reported by D'Anzi (51) show, 4 hr after insulin administration, a 90% decrease in the number of dense core granules and a 63% depletion of the epinephrine content of the gland but do not show an abnormal amount of electron-translucent microvesicles in the subendothelial space.

The direct association of vesicle membrane and plasma membrane is probably very short-lived since there was no increase of dopamine β-hydroxylase in the 800-g pellet, which contains the bulk of adenyl cyclase activity [(163); R. L. Patrick and N. Kirshner, unpublished observations], an enzyme currently believed to be closely associated with plasma membranes. The fragility or short duration of the membrane fusion may underlie the difficulties in showing exocytotic figures in the adrenomedullary cells.

Viveros et al. (302) have studied the amine incorporation and storage capacity of the storage vesicles that sediment with the large granular fraction after insulin-induced secretion. After 3 hr of insulin hypoglycemia the catecholamine content of the large granular fraction was 42.0 ± 2.2% of controls, and the ^{14}C-epinephrine incorporation capacity of this fraction was 55.0 ± 3.3% of controls. Although in these experiments only the total dopamine β-hydroxylase in the large granular fraction was measured, it is possible to calculate that over 95% of the vesicle membranes were sedimenting in this fraction. In another group of experiments where particle-bound and soluble enzyme was measured [(172); O. H. Viveros, L. Arqueros, and N. Kirshner, unpublished observations], it was found that only half of the vesicles that had emptied their contents would fragment enough not to sediment at 26,000 g × 20 min. This means that in the former experiments not all the decrease in ^{14}C-epinephrine incorporation capacity can be attributed to a reduction in the number of vesicles (filled and empty) present in the large granular fraction. It can be calculated that, if the empty or partially empty storage vesicles of this fraction had a normal incorporation capacity, the uptake of ^{14}C-epinephrine after secretion should have been between 71 and 95% of controls. Furthermore after 4 hr of insulin hypoglycemia there is a 2.5-fold increase in the microsomal-bound dopamine β-hydroxylase but a 50% decrease in the amine content of this fraction [see Fig. 3; (172)]. From this evidence it is highly unlikely that the catecholamine storage vesicles of the adrenal medulla are functionally active after secreting their content. Nevertheless more direct evidence on the incorporation and storage capacity of the microsomal microvesicles in vitro and on the synthetic and secretory function of the gland after neurogenically induced depletion is necessary.

Viveros, Arqueros, and Kirshner (unpublished observations) have examined the subcellular distribution of adrenal amines and dopamine β-hydroxylase between 20 and 144 hr after stopping a 4-hr period of neurogenic stimulation in the rabbit. After 20 hr of recovery, there is a small increase (103 units) in the amount of particulate enzyme that sediments in the large granular fraction. At the same time there is a very significant decrease (257 units) in the amount of microsomal-bound enzyme, which returns to normal levels. The mean value for the total enzyme in the gland decreases by 148 units (not significant), despite a 10% increase in the mean catecholamine content. When the large granular fraction is further resolved in a sucrose density gradient, the amount of enzyme bound to empty-vesicle membranes decreased significantly after 20 hr of recovery, whereas the enzyme in the filled-vesicle fraction increased by only half the amount lost from the empty-vesicle membranes. From these data, it can be calculated that at least 70–85% of the empty-vesicle membranes are not directly reutilized for the formation of new vesicles. Nothing is yet known of the mechanisms of membrane digestion. As in other cells, presumably the empty membranes are engulfed by lysosomes.

Quantal Secretion from Adrenal Medulla

Spontaneous, as well as depolarization-induced, secretion of neurotransmitters at chemical synapses probably is the result of the release of integral multiples of a multimolecular package or quantum of transmitter of approximately the same size (53, 158, 202). Del Castillo & Katz (53) proposed that these quanta are preformed within the axon terminal before release takes place and may correspond to the synaptic vesicles. Folkow and co-workers (104, 105) and Stjärne and associates (289, 290) have argued against the proposal that the total content of the noradrenergic synaptic vesicle is the subcellular unit of quantal release. They have calculated that only 3–10% of the content of a single vesicle would be released from each varicosity on maximal stimulation of the outflow to a sympathetically innervated organ.

Until recently it was not possible to establish if secretion from other cells was quantal because of the limitations in the analytical methods, which are not yet sensitive enough to measure secretion from one individual cell or from a portion of its membrane, as can be done at chemical synapses. Biochemical studies on the adrenal medulla have given evidence consistent with the idea that secretion occurs by an all-or-none release of the contents of the vesicles. Viveros and co-workers (172, 305) have demonstrated that storage vesicle membranes equilibrate at a substantially lower density than intact vesicles obtained from normal animals when centrifuged through a sucrose gradient. Unlysed, partially depleted vesicles obtained from reserpine-treated rabbits equilibrate at an intermediate position. In this latter case, the partially depleted vesicles retain all the dopamine β-hydroxylase, both soluble and particulate, which results in a large increase in the ratio of enzyme to catecholamines. If each vesicle secretes through a cycle of partial extrusions of its soluble content, the ratio of dopamine β-hydroxylase to amines should also increase since a fixed amount of enzyme is firmly bound to the vesicle membrane (50% of the total enzyme in storage vesicles from normal rabbits). Partial secretion from each vesicle during exocytosis should also result in an increase in the enzyme-to-catecholamine ratio in the vesicles (Fig. 4). On the other hand, if secretion occurs by extrusion of the

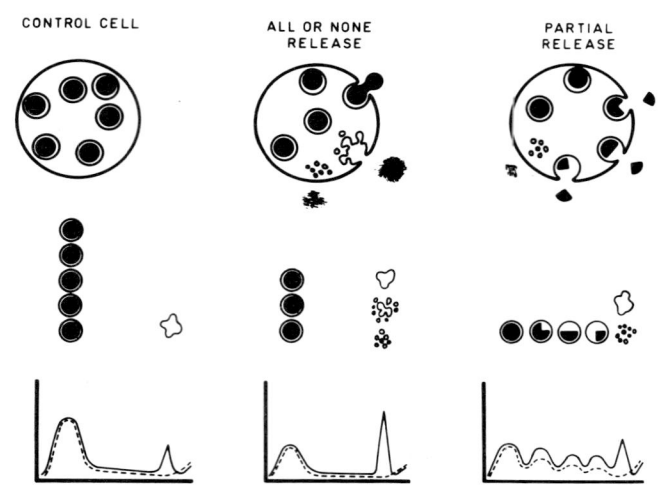

FIG. 4. Diagrammatic representation of all-or-none and partial release. *Upper row*: hypothetical distribution of filled, partially empty, and empty storage vesicles within adrenomedullary cell. *Middle row*: vesicles after homogenization; notice that some vesicles have been disrupted as the result of mechanical stress. *Lower row*: dopamine β-hydroxylase (——) and catecholamines (----) after isopycnic centrifugation of large granular fraction through a linear sucrose density gradient; denser region of gradient is to *right-hand side* of each graph. Although amine secretion by all-or-none release of soluble content from each vesicle only decreases dense vesicle peak with a corresponding increase in empty vesicle fraction (lighter dopamine β-hydroxylase peak), partial release induces appearance of new enzyme and amine peaks of lesser buoyancy with an enzyme-to-amine ratio that continuously increases as vesicles become more depleted and lighter. Number of new peaks should be a function of amount of soluble material released each time a vesicle fuses with the plasma membrane; relative size of each peak will be determined by probability of filled, empty, and partially empty vesicles to participate in secretion and by magnitude of depletion of chromaffin cell.

total content of the storage vesicle, the remaining vesicles should have the same buoyant density and dopamine β-hydroxylase-to-catecholamine ratio as those of control animals, and at the same time one should expect an increase in the particulate enzyme present in the empty vesicle membranes that equilibrate at the lower density. When the large granule fraction obtained from rabbits that had been under insulin hypoglycemia for 3 hr was centrifuged through sucrose density gradients, there was only one peak of filled vesicles, which was reduced in size but had the same equilibrium density and dopamine β-hydroxylase-to-catecholamine ratio as the vesicles from control animals. As discussed earlier, there also was an increase in empty vesicle membranes. These results indicate that neurogenic stimulation resulted in all-or-none discharge of the total content of those vesicles that participated in the response (172, 305). Thus the secretion from the adrenomedullary cell is quantal.

Each storage vesicle is a multimolecular package of catecholamines, ATP, soluble proteins, and ions. It has been calculated that the mean catecholamine content on each adrenal chromaffin vesicle is 2.4×10^6 molecules in the cat (172) and 8×10^6 molecules in the chicken (34).

Kirshner & Viveros (172) have calculated that only one quantum per cell would be secreted if every cell innervated by the first splanchnic nerve in the cat would respond equally to a maximal stimulus applied to the nerve trunk. Even if these calculations were off by a factor of 10, the "quantal content" of the secretory response by the chromaffin cell to a stimulus seems to be made up of much larger but fewer packets than the quantal content of the excitatory postsynaptic potential at the neuromuscular junction, where several hundred quanta are simultaneously released per impulse (56, 201), or at the giant synapse of the squid stellate ganglion, where 10^4 or more units are simultaneously released (212). Confirmation of the quantal nature and determination of the quantal content of the adrenomedullary secretion require development of sensitive methods to measure secretion from individual cells.

Release of Newly Synthesized Catecholamines from Adrenal Gland

The biochemical evidence discussed in the preceding sections indicates that the direct origin of the secreted catecholamines from the adrenal medulla is the storage vesicle and that secretion occurs by direct communication of the intravesicular and extracellular spaces by a pore large enough to permit the outflow of other soluble vesicle components as large as dopamine β-hydroxylase (290,000 mol wt, 75 A hydrodynamic radius). This type of secretion probably corresponds to the exocytosis seen in the electron microscope.

The evidence also indicates that secretion from each vesicle is all or none and that the empty vesicle membranes rapidly flow back into the cytoplasm by micropinocytosis to be digested at a later time. These empty vesicles do not incorporate amines from the media and are probably not functional since it takes several days for vesicles to regain their normal catecholamine content and to recover the ATP-Mg^{2+}-dependent catecholamine incorporation capacity [(302); O. H. Viveros, L. Arqueros, and N. Kirshner, unpublished observations]. Catecholamine and protein secretion in the isolated gland is known to proceed for several hours in the complete absence of catecholamine or protein precursors in the perfusion media, as well as in the presence of protein synthesis inhibitors (17, 176, 229). These data and the biochemical evidence for exocytosis indicate that secretion occurs from the pool of already stored amines. Any newly synthesized amines that are secreted may originate from replacement of those amines that leak from mature storage vesicles or may be secreted from newly formed vesicles that have acquired their amine content from new synthesis.

Several early reports suggest rapid resynthesis of amines, during and shortly after stimulation (38, 39, 144); however, in these studies the amine release and resynthesis rates have been measured by very indirect methods. More direct methods have failed to show an increased rate of synthesis or secretion of newly formed amines during stimulation (37, 83). In the following discussion of the mechanisms that may couple excitation of the cell to secretion, we assume that this chain of events is directed to the secretion of the substances contained only within storage vesicles. Nevertheless we should keep in mind that most of the experiments in which secretion of amines and other subcellular components into the extracellular space have been determined were done in vitro with no supply of precursors for synthesis of catecholamines or other adrenal cell components. The in vivo experiments, where only the changes in content and distribution of different materials in the gland at the end of the secretory period were measured, are based on the assumption that no important resynthesis of exportable materials occurs during the secretory period and so the possibility cannot be discarded that a small part of the secreted material comes from a newly made pool that is never stored and, as a consequence, does not change the amine to other tracer ratios in the subcellular compartments of the chromaffin cell.

EXCITATION-SECRETION COUPLING

The term *stimulus-secretion coupling* was coined by Douglas & Rubin (75) and has been defined by Douglas (62) to "embrace all the events occurring in the cell exposed to its immediate stimulus that leads, finally, to the appearance of the characteristic secretory product in the extracellular environment." In this review an attempt is made to define more precisely this term, including all the events occurring in the chromaffin cell, as a specific response to its physiological stimulus, or any other stimulus that can activate any step of the normal pathway, which necessarily leads to the appearance of all the soluble components of the storage vesicle in the extracellular space. Despite the very large number of substances and conditions that have been found to stimulate, block, or be necessary for the release of catecholamines, and, despite the large number of hypotheses that partly cover some of these effects, we are left with few solid facts, and these cannot yet be included in one general hypothesis susceptible to experimental confirmation. The reader is referred to the chapter by Douglas in this volume of the *Handbook* for detailed analysis of the interaction of the stimulating agent with the receptor site, of the electrophysiological changes that follow this interaction, and of the ionic dependence of secretion. The author only briefly reviews this subject in order to point to some of the proposals that need to be more fully documented. The general plan followed in this section is to discuss first some general factors that determine the secretory response to a stimulus when the experimenter is studying the excitation-secretion coupling of a large population of cells. Then there is a brief review of some of the basic cell functions (e.g., protoplasmic movement, electrophysiology, ionic requirements, energy metabolism in the chromaffin cell) that might be related to secretion induced by nerve stimulation, by its transmitter acetylcholine, or by cholinomimetic substances. The effects of other drugs that stimulate or modify catecholamine secretion are then described, and a discussion of the relevance of in vitro release to cell secretion follows. Finally some of the current hypotheses for excitation-secretion coupling are discussed.

Factors That May Determine Amount of Material Secreted in Response to Stimulus

To study the link between a well-defined stimulus applied to the isolated adrenal medulla and the resulting secretion, it is necessary to establish quantitatively the stimulus-response relationship that can be affected by a number of experimental variables, as well as by the past history of the gland in situ.

Although the threshold response and maximal rates of secretion, as well as the shape of the dose-response curve of an isolated gland, may in part result from its past history (e.g., total number of vesicles per cell, vesicle content, changes in the amount of catecholamines and of amine synthesizing enzymes), the reproducibility of the stimulus-response curve should not significantly be affected by such processes since they are long-lasting and slowly developing effects.

The changes in the size of the response to a preset stimulus that occurs during an acute experiment are usually associated with decreased response of each cell to the stimulus (tachyphylaxis), which is later discussed in detail, or variation in the spontaneous release of catecholamines and in the number of responding cells.

Variation in the number of responding cells frequently can arise from spontaneous changes in the homogeneity of the perfusion during the experiment and sometimes can result from the vasoactive properties of the agent tested or other variations in the composition of the perfusing media. Changes in the spontaneous release are extremely important when measurements are made in the in situ gland and result from reflex splanchnic activity and probably from endocrine homeostatic mechanisms; this increase may result in an apparent decrease in responsiveness as the spontaneous rate approaches the maximal rate of secretion. The causes for the in vivo changes have been already discussed by Malmejac (196). Destruction of cells by surgical trauma, inadequate perfusion rates, or badly perfused areas of medulla resulting in progressive cell deterioration will give high basal secretion, which will vary in time. Even perfectly healthy cells, acutely or chronically denervated, have a low basal output of catecholamines (307), which appears to be only partially Ca^{2+} dependent (75, 169, 307) and varies greatly with the composition of the perfusion media. No information is available on the origin of this remnant amine release, which could represent leakage of amines through the plasmalemma or the spontaneous secretion of a few quanta, similar to the appearance of miniature postsynaptic potentials at chemical synapses.

Chromaffin Cell Motility

Observations on cytoplasmic movements in secretory cells are extremely few, despite the early observations by Gladstone & van Heyningen (112) and the detailed study of Woodin and co-workers (318, 319, 321) on the drastic changes induced by the secretory stimulus in the polymorphonuclear leukocyte. Stimulation of polymorphonuclear leukocytes with a specific secretory agent results in cytoplasmic solation and conversion of the normal orderly streaming of the secretory granules, and other cell organelles, into Brownian motion. The granules that come in contact with the inner surface of the plasma membrane adhere, and granular enzymes simultaneously appear in the extracellular fluid. In the absence of Ca^{2+} in the suspension medium, the same phenomenon will be observed, with the exception that the granules bounce against the plasma membrane and no secretion occurs (319). Cytoplasmic gel-to-sol transformations and the involvement of a motile system in excitation-secretion coupling have been also postulated to explain the effect of drugs that interact with microtubules in several secretory cells (179, 188, 195, 317), including the adrenal chromaffin cell (236–238). Isolated normal adrenal chromaffin cells, as well as pheochromocytoma cells in tissue culture, have been described by Costero et al. (45) to undergo rhythmic movements of alternating retraction and expansion, recorded with time lapse cinematography through a phase contrast microscope. Chévez and Costero (personal communication) have also observed cyclosis (sometimes interrupted by brief periods of random movement) of the cytoplasmic organelles of cultured normal adrenal medulla cells. Unfortunately no observations have been made in the presence of stimulating agents. A frequent observation made by morphologists is the vacuolar appearance of the cytoplasm and ill-defined fixation of cytoplasm and organelles in stimulated chromaffin cells compared to control cells (18, 50). Coupland (47) has called attention to this phenomenon by stating, "In stimulated glands fixation becomes a still more difficult problem since stimulated cells are even more friable and more easily damaged by manipulation than normal ones." Although the causes of this "friability" have not been established and may be multiple, they might in part be a consequence of changes in the physical state of the cytoplasm as a result of stimulation. Although most of the storage vesicles are below the resolution of the light microscope, changes in the movement of larger organelles and measurements of refractive index and cytoplasmic viscosity of resting and stimulated chromaffin cells may cast some light on the early events of excitation-secretion coupling.

Electrophysiology of Adrenomedullary Cell in Relation to Secretion

Because of technical difficulties, there are very few observations on the electrophysiology of the adrenomedullary cell. Matthews (204, 205) has recorded low intracellular resting potentials of bisected adrenals superfused with Kreb's-Henseleit solutions from rats, rabbits, and kittens. In this experimental condition the resting membrane potentials range from -20.4 ± 0.57 mv in the rat to -31.7 ± 1.3 mv in the cat and are extremely insensitive to changes in external K^+ concentration. Douglas and associates (63–66, 157) have also found low resting potentials in the isolated chromaffin cells of the adrenal of the gerbil that had been kept for 6–10 hr in a feeder tissue culture. These cells have a resting potential in the control media of -32.8 ± 0.2 mv and show a linear inverse relation to the external concentration of Na^+ and K^+ in the extracellular fluid. The extracellular concentration of Ca^{2+} does not affect the membrane potential except when it is absent from the extracellular fluid, in which case a substantial depolarization occurs.

The complete replacement of Cl^- by SO_4^{2-} does not modify the resting potential. Increasing concentrations of Ba^{2+} and Mg^{2+} have been reported to depolarize the chromaffin cell in the presence or absence of Na^+ in the extracellular fluid (66). Whether these effects could also be seen in the absence of Ca^{2+} has not been reported.

Early reports have demonstrated the release of catecholamines by direct electrical stimulation of the adrenal gland (41, 80, 128, 200). However, this was probably the result of intraglandular stimulation of the splanchnic nerve endings or cellular damage by excessive current intensity since this release could not be repeated by using field stimulation in the perfused bovine adrenal gland where the cholinergic synapse was blocked by hexamethonium and atropine (O. Viveros, unpublished observations), nor were action potentials set up when the membrane of an isolated cell was rapidly depolarized by passing current across it (157).

There are no reports of direct recording of the intracellular potential during splanchnic nerve stimulation. In the isolated cells from the gerbil, acetylcholine (3×10^{-6} to 10^{-3} g/ml) produces a dose-dependent depolarization (65). This is approximately the same range of concentrations that will cause from threshold to maximal stimulation of secretion in perfused adrenal glands of other species. The depolarizing effect of acetylcholine falls linearly with the log of the external concentration of Na^+ and, in Na^+-free medium, increases linearly with the log of extracellular Ca^{2+} concentration. Acetylcholine will also depolarize the chromaffin cell in the presence of Na^+ and complete absence of Ca^{2+} (66). Acetylcholine-induced depolarization is not modified by replacing Cl^- with SO_4^{2-} in the extracellular fluid or by the addition of Mg^{2+} in concentrations as great as 20.0 mM. Douglas and co-workers (63, 66) concluded that acetylcholine depolarizes the chromaffin cell by increasing the conductance to both Na^+ and Ca^{2+}.

In the presence of hexamethonium the depolarizing effect of acetylcholine is significantly reduced, and in the presence of hexamethonium and atropine it is completely abolished. These drugs do not block the depolarizing effect of K^+ or other secretagogues (65). The depolarizing effect of acetylcholine or K⁺ in balanced salt media or in Ca²⁺-free media is not significantly modified by amethocaine. This drug completely blocks depolarization when acetylcholine is added in a medium where Ca²⁺ is the only extracellular cation (63). These data suggest that hexamethonium and atropine block the effects of acetylcholine at the receptor level (65), whereas amethocaine selectively blocks the increase in Ca²⁺ conductance (63). The depolarization obtained by equimolar replacement of Na⁺ by K⁺ in the extracellular fluid is not affected by the presence or absence of normal concentrations of Ca²⁺ (2.2 mM) (66). There are no studies of the contribution of Ca²⁺ current, if any, during the depolarization induced by increasing the extracellular concentration of K⁺.

Nicotine, pilocarpine, histamine, 5-hydroxytryptamine, angiotensin, and bradykinin, at concentrations similar to those that induce catecholamine secretion in isolated adrenal glands, also depolarized the gerbil chromaffin cell (65). The depolarizing effects of nicotine and pilocarpine were completely antagonized by hexamethonium and atropine, respectively. Hexamethonium plus atropine did not significantly modify the depolarizing effects of histamine and angiotensin.

In summary, depolarization is not in itself a sufficient stimulus to induce secretion from the chromaffin cell since acetylcholine, K⁺, and other stimulants depolarize the cell in the absence of Ca²⁺, which, as discussed later, is required for secretion (62, 75). Amethocaine blocks acetylcholine secretion, and in a sucrose medium in which Ca²⁺ is the only cation, it also blocks depolarization but does not significantly modify depolarization in Na⁺-containing media (63). Increased Mg²⁺ concentration in the extracellular fluid blocks secretion, and by itself induces depolarization, but does not block acetylcholine-induced depolarization. The effectiveness of acetylcholine as a secretagogue is increased immediately after removal of Na⁺ from the perfusion medium (13, 77), despite the fact that low Na⁺ concentration hyperpolarizes the adrenal chromaffin cell; under these conditions, acetylcholine reduces the increased resting potential to very much the same value as that of the normal resting potential (66). Douglas et al. (66) proposed that

> depolarization in response to acetylcholine may be no more than the electrical sign of increased permeability to ions such as sodium and calcium, and is not, in itself, a key event in stimulus-secretion coupling. The evidence is held to favor the view that movement of calcium into the chromaffin cells on exposure to acetylcholine is responsible for evoking secretion.

In other secretory cells, such as the adrenocortical cells, the physiological stimulus for secretion does not depolarize the cell to any measurable extent and depolarization and secretion can be completely uncoupled (207, 208). However, in chemical synapses, secretion of neurotransmitter and depolarization in the presence of Ca²⁺ seem to be tightly coupled, probably because the increase in Ca²⁺ permeability of the axonal membrane is a function of depolarization (158, 160). Since in the chromaffin cell it has not been possible to obtain secretion under conditions that do not cause depolarization (all stimulants studied will more or less depolarize the cells in conditions in which they induce secretion), Douglas (62) has stated

> although it is possible that calcium entry is sufficient in itself to evoke secretion, it must be borne in mind that in no instance have we succeeded in evoking secretion without there being some change in the chemistry of the plasma membrane as revealed by movement of ions or change in potential. None of our evidence tells whether calcium would be effective in the absence of this unidentified change in membrane chemistry.

In this respect it should be kept in mind that acetylcholine has other effects on the chromaffin cell, such as the increase in phospholipid turnover (143, 294) that occurs in Ca²⁺-free media (295). It has not been established if, for this and other actions of acetylcholine on the chromaffin cell (e.g., increase in the synthesis of catecholamine synthesizing enzymes), the second messenger results from changes in ion conductance or if it is coupled through other metabolic pathways. We do not know whether the secretory stimulus or depolarization may, simultaneously with the increase in Ca²⁺ conductance, activate some other parallel Ca²⁺-independent system, which may also be an absolute requirement for secretion similar to the Ca²⁺-independent changes in cytoplasmic movements seen in polymorphonuclear leukocytes (321). The importance of depolarization in the coupling mechanism will probably not be fully established until more sophisticated electrophysiological techniques are available that may permit measurements of secretory activity induced by acetylcholine or other secretagogues while the chromaffin cell potential is held constant at some preset value.

Ionic Requirements for Secretion

Houssay & Molinelli (145) observed in 1928 that the pressor effect obtained upon splanchnic stimulation in the dog disappeared after intravenous injections of sodium citrate or oxalate and was recovered by calcium chloride injection. These effects were interpreted as an impairment of adrenomedullary secretion by calcium removal and not as an effect at the adrenergic receptor site. Since then it has repeatedly been shown that calcium is an absolute requirement for excitation of a secretory cell to secrete its export product into the extracellular fluid. The requirement for Ca²⁺ and other ions in secretion from the adrenal gland and other secretory cells has been thoroughly documented in several recent reviews (13, 61, 62, 158, 206, 247, 250, 255, 275, 292, 321). A brief survey of the pertinent experimental evidence is necessary for the discussion of the several hypotheses that have been proposed to explain the role of different ions in stimulus-secretion coupling.

The isolated or in vivo adrenal gland will maintain a low resting output of catecholamines and respond to acetylcholine and several other stimulants for several hours if perfused with a balanced salt solution. When all ions except Ca²⁺ are replaced by sucrose, there is an initial increase in the base-line output of amines that soon returns to control levels; acetylcholine retains the ability to evoke secretion of catecholamines, which is lost in sucrose Ca^{2+}-free media or in any other isotonic media free of calcium (75, 77). Other secretagogues are also ineffective in Ca^{2+}-free media (76, 287).

Reintroduction of normal concentrations of Ca^{2+} into a Ca^{2+}-free medium will transiently increase the output of catecholamines, although sudden increases of Ca^{2+} above normal levels in the perfusion media does not evoke secretion. The effectiveness of acetylcholine as a secretagogue improves as a function of the concentration of Ca^{2+} in the medium. Increased Mg^{2+} concentration will prevent the effect of Ca^{2+} reintroduction into a Ca^{2+}-free medium and competitively antagonize the effects of increasing concentrations of Ca^{2+} on the response to acetylcholine (75, 77); Ba^{2+} and Sr^{2+} will induce secretion if introduced in the absence of Ca^{2+}, and Ba^{2+} will also act as a secretagogue at normal Ca^{2+} concentrations; Ba^{2+}, Sr^{2+}, and to a lesser degree Mn^{2+} will sustain acetylcholine- or K^+-induced secretion in the absence of Ca^{2+}. This effect is not shared by Mg^{2+}, Co^{2+}, Ni^{2+}, or Zn^{2+} (78, 79).

Prolonged perfusions with Ca^{2+}-containing, Na^+-free media made isosmotic by replacement with Li^+ or choline will decrease and eventually completely block the secretory response to acetylcholine or increased K^+ (13–15). The complete absence of K^+ or the presence of ouabain in the media will increase the basal rate of amine release, as well as the stimulation by acetylcholine or by Ca^{2+} reintroduction (12, 13). As already mentioned, replacing Na^+ with K^+ in an otherwise normal medium will induce secretion, which is proportional to the log of the extracellular ion concentration. This effect is also shared by Rb^+, Cs^+, and NH_4^+. These effects are not blocked by hexamethonium or atropine but are blocked by excess of Mg^{2+} or lack of Ca^{2+} (287).

Banks and co-workers (12–15) have suggested that not the extracellular, but the intracellular, concentration of Na^+ is important in stimulus-secretion coupling. Ouabain or K^+-free media may exert their effects by impairing the K^+-dependent sodium pump and thereby increasing the intracellular sodium concentration since they do not potentiate secretion in Na^+-free media. The slow development of blockade of secretion in Na^+-free media may result from intracellular Na^+ depletion. The intracellular Na^+ should not directly affect secretion but could modulate the action of calcium by controlling Ca^{2+} entry into the secretory cell (13).

Borowitz (30) determined the subcellular distribution of ^{45}Ca retained in the perfused bovine adrenal gland after loading it with the tracer for a total of 7 min followed by a 53-min washout period. He found that all the organelles contained several times more ^{45}Ca per milligram of protein than the cell supernatant. The largest concentration of ^{45}Ca for both control and acetylcholine-stimulated glands was found in a mixed mitochondrial-lysosomal fraction, which contained 8 and 10 times more counts per milligram of protein, respectively, than the corresponding supernatants. The chromaffin granules obtained from glands that had been loaded with ^{45}Ca in the presence of acetylcholine showed a proportionally larger increase in ^{45}Ca retention compared to the other organelles. No net increase in total calcium was found in these experiments. Borowitz has also shown that ^{45}Ca added just before homogenizing the gland in 0.3 M sucrose (30) or to mitochondrial and chromaffin granule fragments (29) will result in a concentration of the tracer in all subcellular fractions as compared to the $100{,}000 \times g$ supernatant. The binding of ^{45}Ca was reduced by 150 mM sodium chloride (29). Banks (8) and Goz (114) have described in the bovine adrenal medulla a microsomal Ca^{2+}-activated adenosine triphosphatase that is inhibited by 100 mM sodium chloride (114). Poisner and Hava (237, 242) have reported an ATP-dependent binding of calcium by microsomal and mitochondrial fractions of adrenal medulla prepared by millipore filtration but failed to find inhibition of ^{45}Ca uptake into microsomes by Na^+ (242). An alternative explanation for the effects of intracellular Na^+ on secretion is that sodium may increase Ca^{2+} concentration at the coupling site by interfering with a Ca^{2+}-inactivating mechanism, perhaps with Ca^{2+} binding into one of the above-mentioned organelles.

Despite the central importance of Ca^{2+} in stimulus-secretion coupling, few efforts have been made to define its locus of action in chromaffin and other secretory cells. Miledi & Slater (213) could not obtain secretion of neurotransmitter from the giant synapse of the squid in a Ca^{2+}-free medium when Ca^{2+} was locally applied by microiontophoresis at a "synaptic spot" immediately inside the presynaptic axon in the presence or absence of impulse invasion of the terminal; when the Ca^{2+} pipette was at the same spot, but outside the axon, release of as little as 10^{-14} to 10^{-13} moles of Ca^{2+} per second was enough to maintain the secretory capacity of the presynaptic spike. Katz and Miledi (158, 159) further showed in the tetrodotoxin-treated neuromuscular junction of the frog in Ca^{2+}-free media that this ion must be present during the depolarization for secretion to occur; if the local release of calcium was delayed so it would reach the membrane during the synaptic delay, there was no secretion of transmitter. These authors have proposed (158, 159, 213) that depolarization opens a gate or provides a carrier to calcium ions, which allows Ca^{2+} to move through a very steep concentration gradient toward the inside of the axon membrane and thus reach the critical sites of the release reaction; very few molecules of Ca^{2+} should be necessary to activate this process and the releasing sites must be at the membrane or in very close continuity to the membrane, because of the short time that is available for Ca^{2+} diffusion, and should be accessible only from the outside of the axon.

On the other hand, in the polymorphonuclear leukocyte, where Ca^{2+} has also been proposed to react with some critical site at the plasma membrane (321), the stimulus seems to be able to start the excitation-secretion sequence in the absence of calcium ions. These initial reaction(s) must still be active for some time after removal of the stimulus, since secretion can proceed by late introduction of Ca^{2+} into the surrounding fluid. The early Ca^{2+}-independent events in stimulus-secretion coupling in the leukocyte consists in transformation of cytoplasmic streaming into Brownian movement and swelling of the secretory granules (319, 321).

Since reintroduction of Ca^{2+} into a Ca^{2+}-free medium in perfused adrenal gland stimulates secretion, it is not possible to determine whether any priming of the chromaffin cell by the stimulus in the absence of this ion occurs. Nevertheless there have been several reports, based on studies with the electron microscope, of generalized chromaffin granule swelling with changes in the density and disposition of the electron-dense core shortly after stimulation of the adrenal medulla (47, 55, 57). These changes are similar to occurrences in the leukocyte, but these studies have not been repeated in the absence of calcium.

Douglas & Poisner (67, 68) exposed perfused cat adrenal glands to Locke's solution containing 0.5–1.0 $\mu c/ml$ ^{45}Ca for 10 min and subsequently washed the glands by further perfusion with Locke's solution for 100 min. At all times, 2.2 mM $CaCl_2$ was present in the perfusing fluids. At the end of the experiment, the medullae were dissected from the cortices and ^{45}Ca determined in both tissues, as well as in the effluent collected during the 100 min of washout. In all experiments one gland from each animal was stimulated by introducing acetylcholine for 2 min into the ^{45}Ca-Locke's solution. Control glands retained ^{45}Ca equivalent to 264 ± 69 pmoles/mg dry wt. The stimulated glands retained ^{45}Ca equivalent to 732 ± 142 pmoles/mg dry wt. The increased retention of ^{45}Ca in the stimulated gland was assumed to be the result of increased calcium uptake during the 2-min exposure to acetylcholine. From the amount retained in the gland at the end of the washout period and the time of exposure to ^{45}Ca, the authors calculated that a minimal value for the rate of uptake of calcium into the resting adrenomedullary cells was 0.50 ± 0.7 pmole/mg dry wt per second and for the stimulated cells 4.3 ± 0.8 pmoles/mg dry wt per second. Stimulation of the gland with 56 mM KCl produced a similar increase in ^{45}Ca retention (67). Since 100 min of perfusion with Locke's solution after loading the gland with ^{45}Ca also washes out part of the ^{45}Ca initially present in the intracellular space, a value closer to reality could be obtained by extrapolation of the last exponential of the washout curve back to zero time. Retention of ^{45}Ca determined by extrapolation was 15 times higher for the whole gland than the values obtained after 100 min of washout, and the rates of uptake should be corrected in this proportion (68), the assumption being that the washout rates for cortex and medulla are similar (washout was done in whole glands). The authors concluded "that these findings support the suggestion that acetylcholine evokes catecholamine secretion from the medulla by promoting the uptake of calcium" (68).

Rubin et al. (256) did similar experiments in the cat adrenal gland. In all the experiments, ^{45}Ca (in Locke's solution containing 2 mM ^{42}Ca) was perfused for 5 min, in the presence of 2.2×10^{-4} M acetylcholine, followed by a 60-min washout with Ca^{2+}-free Locke's solution. The effluent was collected at 5-min intervals, and the radioactivity remaining in the whole gland at the end of the washout and in the effluents was measured. The ^{45}Ca washout curves in these glands have at least three exponentials with half-lives of 1.5, 6.5, and 27.5 min, respectively. The last value was presumed to represent ^{45}Ca efflux from cellular sites, whereas the first two values were presumed to be of extracellular origin. Extrapolation of the slowest washout curve to zero time indicated that $19.1 \pm 0.8\%$ of the total ^{45}Ca initially present in the gland (at the start of the washout period) was in the intracellular space; when this value was divided by the time of exposure of the gland to ^{45}Ca, a rate for the cellular uptake of calcium of 7.3–10.7 pmoles/mg dry wt per second (whole gland) was obtained. When tetracaine (amethocaine), at a concentration that caused 90% inhibition of the secretory response of the adrenal gland to acetylcholine, was also included in the Locke's solution during the loading period, the half-lives of the washout curves were not significantly different from half-lives of the washout curves of glands not treated with tetracaine, but the extrapolated zero time uptake of ^{45}Ca was reduced by 50%. The authors concluded that tetracaine inhibits secretion by interfering with Ca^{2+} entry into the medullary chromaffin cell (256).

Borowitz (30) has determined the ^{45}Ca retention in the medulla of perfused bovine adrenal glands when loaded for 7 min followed by a 53-min washout period with normal Locke's solution. When 100 $\mu g/ml$ of acetylcholine was included in the ^{45}Ca-Locke's solution during the loading period, the increase in the retained calcium was proportional to the percent of the total catecholamine store released during stimulation with acetylcholine. There was no net increase in calcium content in the stimulated adrenal medulla or in any of its organelles compared to unstimulated glands. The ^{45}Ca accumulated in all subcellular organelles and the percent increase in chromaffin vesicles was slightly but significantly higher than in other fractions. Borowitz (30) concluded that his data supported the hypothesis that calcium may act at an intracellular site to initiate the release process and that the exchange of calcium in chromaffin granules with calcium in the environment increases during stimulation of the adrenal medulla with acetylcholine; ^{45}Ca has also been shown to accumulate in a vesicular fraction after stimulation of the polymorphonuclear leukocyte (321) and in the cat salivary glands (36). In the latter experiments (36, 321), the data have been interpreted to suggest the accumulation of ^{45}Ca in vesicles that are empty as a result of secretion or because they may be newly formed. This would not appear to be the case in the adrenal medulla since empty vesicles no longer sediment with the purified vesicle fraction (172, 305). Borowitz (31) suggests that the increased uptake of ^{45}Ca into the storage vesicles is due to an increased synthesis of catecholamines and that Ca^{2+} is part of the storage complex. An alternate hypothesis might be that stimulation may somehow induce some form of activation of the storage complex, as has been proposed for the in vitro effects of ATP and Mg by Ferris et al. (103) and result in the increased Ca^{2+} exchange (30), as well as in morphological swelling and changes in electron opacity and granularity of the storage vesicle core (47, 55, 57).

The data that have been reported on ^{45}Ca retention in control and drug-treated adrenals is difficult to interpret. The calcium uptake rates during the ^{45}Ca-loading period, calculated from the data of Douglas & Poisner (68), are 7.5 ± 0.11 pmoles/mg dry wt per second for the resting gland and 64.5 ± 1.2 pmoles/mg dry wt per second for the stimulated gland when the necessary correction is made for the zero time washout. By using the values reported by Borowitz et al. (32) of 25 μmoles of Ca^{2+} per gram protein for the adrenal medulla, a value of 70% for the water content of the adrenal gland, and uptake rates reported by Douglas & Poisner (63), it is possible to calculate a half-life for the intracellular calcium pool of the resting medulla of 9.2 min and of 1.0 min for the stimulated gland. These rates appear to be extremely high and are many times higher than the rates that can be obtained by using the slope of the last exponential decline in their typical washout curve. Similar results are obtained by using the data of Rubin et al. (256).

Because of the short times used for ^{45}Ca loading, the differences found by calculating the uptake rates in the same experiment by the two different methods could readily result if it takes a few minutes for ^{45}Ca to distribute equally throughout the extracellular compartments. That no equilibrium in the extracellular space was obtained in this experiment is further suggested by the very large proportion of the total ^{45}Ca, which washes out at the faster rate, present in the gland at the end of the loading period. The representative curve reported by Douglas & Poisner (68) shows that approximately 1% of the total ^{45}Ca in the gland at zero washout time is in the slow "intracellular" pool, 19% is in the intermediate pool, and 80% is in the fast pool. The mean washout curves of 14 glands loaded with ^{45}Ca in the presence of acetylcholine reported by Rubin et al. (256) showed approximately 19% of the total ^{45}Ca in the slow pool, 6% in the intermediate pool, and 75% in the fast pool. The first and second exponentials on a washout curve are supposed to represent the decline of the tracer as it washes out of the intravascular and interstitial compartment. The shape of the washout curves suggests that, at the time acetylcholine was given and when washout commenced, most of the tracer still was in the intravascular compartment and the ability of the cell to take up ^{45}Ca was greatly determined by diffusion at the capillary-interstitial barrier. A slight change in the capillary surface area-permeability product should result in large changes in the apparent uptake rates by the chromaffin cell. In the author's experience, introduction of acetylcholine into the solution perfusing a dog, sheep, or bovine adrenal gland rarely results in measurable changes in perfusion pressure but almost always results in increased amounts of hemoglobin in the gland effluent, even after 60 min of washout before the first stimulation. Successive stimulations have similar effects, although reduced amounts of protein appear in the perfusates. These observations indicate that acetylcholine results in redistribution of the blood flow through the gland, opening vessels that otherwise are closed, and this effect probably is not at the arterioles since it does not decrease perfusion pressure.

As a consequence it is impossible to decide if the increase in ^{45}Ca retention in adrenal glands reported in the literature is due to an effect of acetylcholine on the medullary cells, to an increase in the capillary exchange area in the gland, or to a combination of both phenomena.

Rubin et al. (256) have studied ^{45}Ca exchange in the adrenal medulla by loading the gland with ^{45}Ca, washing out the extracellular space for 60 min when the third exponential phase of ^{45}Ca decline has started, reintroducing Ca^{2+} into the Ca^{2+}-free medium, and measuring the excess of ^{45}Ca released by this procedure in the presence and absence of other ions and drugs. Introduction of 3×10^{-4} M tetracaine or 5×10^{-3} M Mg^{2+} 20 min before reintroduction of 2 mM Ca^{2+} resulted in a 64% and 51% reduction, respectively, in ^{45}Ca "exchange." However, as Borowitz (30, 31) has shown, after 60 min of washout most, if not all, of the ^{45}Ca is bound to subcellular organelles, including the catecholamine storage vesicles. These vesicles release their calcium into the media when disrupted and should also secrete ^{45}Ca by exocytosis. Arqueros, Figueroa, Martínez, and Viveros (unpublished observations) have shown that acetylcholine or K^+ will also induce ^{45}Ca outflow when the washout is with Locke's solution containing 2.2 mM calcium. Furthermore catecholamine and ^{45}Ca outflow is blocked in a parallel fashion by different secretion blockers, even by those that have been postulated to act at a later step than that proposed for Ca^{2+} in stimulation-secretion coupling (103, 243). During acetylcholine or K^+ perfusion, Ca^{2+}-free media will also block the outflow of ^{45}Ca and catecholamines, whereas Ba^{2+} will still be active both as a catecholamine and ^{45}Ca secretagogue. All the stimulants tried released ^{45}Ca and catecholamines in the same proportion with the exception of ^{42}Ca reintroduction, which released proportionally more ^{45}Ca. It is difficult to assess the relation of this extra calcium release to the secretory process.

The author of this review is not trying to imply from the previous discussion that it is not necessary for calcium to enter the cell to activate the coupling mechanism, or to imply that acetylcholine does not increase calcium uptake or that ^{45}Ca washout curves from the adrenal gland are useless. On the contrary, although there are other methods to use in studying ion fluxes, ^{45}Ca washout curves may give very important information if they are done with different ^{45}Ca-loading times and at different concentrations of calcium ions in the loading and washout media and if simultaneous measurements of the extracellular compartments are included. Nevertheless methods that measure small transient changes in Ca^{2+} efflux, which may not result in increased bound calcium, are also necessary in studying this very important function. One of these methods has already been used by Douglas and co-workers (63, 66) who measured the changes in membrane potential induced by acetylcholine when Ca^{2+} was the only permeant ion in the extracellular fluid. This is indisputable evidence that acetylcholine can increase calcium conductance. Despite the difficulties of this method, it could provide a very large amount of valuable knowledge on the correlation between Ca^{2+} movement and secretion.

At the moment, whether Ca^{2+} must enter the chromaffin cell to permit excitation-secretion coupling and how much calcium is necessary for this action are questions with no direct answers. Douglas & Poisner (70) have made some kinetic studies in vitro on ^{45}Ca retention by the neurohypophysis of the rat and have compared them to similar experiments where secretion of vasopressin was measured (60, 69). They found that ^{45}Ca retention at the end of the washout period was a linear function of the external concentration of CaCl$_2$ in the loading media (0.44–8.8 mM) in the presence of either 5.6 or 56 mM KCl; ^{45}Ca retention was close to five times greater in the high-K$^+$ than in the normal-K$^+$ media, even in 8.8 mM Ca^{2+} when secretion is largely inhibited; MgCl$_2$ (10 or 20 mM), which greatly reduces K$^+$-stimulated vasopressin secretion, only blocked by 15 and 30%, respectively, the K$^+$-stimulated ^{45}Ca-retention; Na$^+$-free media, which activate vasopressin release, did not modify K$^+$-induced ^{45}Ca retention by the neurohypophysis. Perfusion without Ca^{2+} conditions a secretory response to reintroduction of Ca^{2+} into the perfusion fluid (13, 75, 77) supposedly because decalcifying the membrane should make it more permeable to Ca^{2+} and allow it to flow into the cell and reach its active site. Arqueros, Martinez, and Viveros (unpublished observations) have found a significant decrease in ^{45}Ca retention in the cortex-free, perfused bovine adrenal gland when Ca^{2+} is omitted during the preloading period, followed by a ^{45}Ca-loading period in Locke's solution with 2.2 mM Ca^{2+} and a washout period in Ca^{2+}-free Locke's solution, which is exactly the reverse of what was expected. The lack of increase in ^{45}Ca retention could be explained if the amount of calcium necessary to activate the secretory mechanism is so small that it cannot be shown by the washout-retention method [the same is suggested by Douglas and Poisner's experiments in the neurohypophysis (70)], or if the calcium necessary for secretion acts at the plasmalemma and does not penetrate into the cytoplasm, or if the active site is intracellular but the calcium that acts on it is not retained but goes back into the extracellular pool. Miledi & Slater (213) have also shown that minimal amounts of calcium are necessary to induce neurotransmitter secretion, and van Breemen & McNaughton (299) have recently demonstrated that, of the total "intracellular" increase in ^{45}Ca influx induced in vascular smooth muscle by high K$^+$ measured by the usual washout methods, only about 5% seems to be really intracellular and this is the Ca^{2+} necessary to activate the contractile system.

Adrenal Chromaffin Cell Energy Metabolism in Relation to Secretion

Banks (9) found a 50% increase in oxygen consumption in strips of bovine adrenal medulla when carbachol was added to the Tyrode's solution, but the carbachol-induced secretory response to the perfused gland was not modified by anoxia. Kirshner and co-workers found that the rate of catecholamine and chromogranin A secretion induced by acetylcholine was temperature dependent (Fig. 2), with a Q$_{10}$ of 2–3 (168), and that acetylcholine-, nicotine-, or Ba^{2+}-stimulated secretion could be completely prevented by combination of one oxidative phosphorylation blocker (CN$^-$, oligomycin, antimycin) with an inhibitor of glycolysis (iodoacetate) (170, 171). Blockade of either metabolic pathway alone did not modify secretion.

Rubin (253, 254) confirmed these experiments and further showed that anoxia plus glucose-free media depressed secretion induced by high concentrations of acetylcholine and that glucose-free media plus CN$^-$ blocked the response to calcium reintroduction into a Ca^{2+}-free, high-K$^+$ Locke's solution. No decrease or a very small decrease in the glycogen content of the medulla was found even after repeated stimulation of secretion in a control medium, but there was a 60–70% decrease if stimulation was done in a medium equilibrated with nitrogen. Glucose deprivation plus anoxia caused an increase in the spontaneous catecholamine output, which was Ca^{2+} dependent. Cyanide potentiated the secretory response to calcium reintroduction in the presence of glucose, but the response was gradually blocked in the absence of glucose. After metabolic blockade, perfusion of the gland with ATP, creatine phosphate, phosphoenolpyruvate, or 3′,5′-AMP did not provide an energy source for the response to calcium reintroduction. Rubin (253) has proposed "that an interaction between calcium and high energy nucleotides is a step in the sequence of events leading to the extrusion of catecholamines."

Because of the large number of cell functions that depend on ATP, it has not been determined if energy is directly required for some step, or steps, in excitation-secretion coupling or if it is needed to maintain some general function, such as normal cell membrane excitability or cytoplasmic motility.

Effects of Drugs on Secretion

Such a large number of substances depress or increase the outflow of catecholamines from the adrenal gland that this topic deserves an extensive review on its own; only a few selected examples are cited here.

The definition of secretion stated in the introduction to this chapter limits the substances that can be called secretagogues to those that activate "any of the steps of the normal excitation-secretion pathway that necessarily leads to the appearance of the secretory product in the extracellular space." Since these steps are far from being established, we have empirically defined a secretagogue by its capacity to induce the last step in excitation-secretion coupling—exocytosis. Stimulation of cholinergic receptors, reduction of membrane potential, and calcium or energy dependency for secretion provide important suggestive evidence on how certain drugs may act but are not sufficient criteria, at least at the present time, to serve as indicators of distinct steps in the secretory process. Only biochemical evidence—the simultaneous release of catecholamines and other substances contained within the storage vesicles—provides unequivocal evidence of secretion.

Very few drugs have been tested for their capacity to produce exocytosis. The biochemical test distinguishes at least three different types of catecholamine-releasing agents. First, lytic agents, in addition to the increasing outflow of soluble storage-vesicle components, release large amounts of cytoplasmic proteins such as lactate dehydrogenase. Ethylenediamine at pH 11.4 (264) and Triton X-100 (266, 267) have been shown to belong to this group. Snake and bee venom, as well as lysolecithin-induced release may result from lytic activity (99). A second type of releasing agent selectively releases catecholamines; Schneider (267) has found that exposure of the perfused bovine adrenal medulla to acetaldehyde (≥ 1.0 mM) caused a dose-related secretion of catecholamines and adenine nucleotides but no significant release of chromogranins or lactate dehydrogenase. The ratio of catecholamines to adenine nucleotides was twice that found upon stimulation with carbachol. Catecholamine secretion was not prevented by hexamethonium, tetracaine, Ca^{2+}-free media, or decreasing the temperature of the perfusion fluid to 23 C. Schneider (267) has proposed that this specific release of amines might result by altering the properties of the vesicle membrane or from direct interference of acetaldehyde with the amine storage complex either by forming a Schiff base with the primary amine group of norepinephrine or by interaction with the soluble proteins in chromaffin granules. A third type of releasing agent is the adrenomedullary secretagogue; exocytosis has been well established for acetylcholine, nicotine (168, 169, 304), carbachol (264, 265, 268), and barium (169). Stimulation of amine release by high K^+ concentrations and by Ca^{2+} reintroduction probably is the result of exocytosis since the ratio of adenine nucleotides to catecholamines in the effluent is close to the ratio inside the storage vesicle (74); the only criterion missing is that these procedures have not been shown to increase outflow of cytoplasmic components.

Phenylethylamine seems to act on the bovine adrenal medulla through a combination of selective amine release and secretion. Schneider (264) has shown that under normal circumstances phenylethylamine will increase the outflow of both catecholamines and vesicle protein but that the ratio of catecholamines to proteins is higher than for carbachol or for the isolated vesicles. In Ca^{2+}-free media the catecholamine response of phenylethylamine was reduced by two-thirds but release of chromogranins was completely blocked. There may be a species difference in the mechanisms by which sympathomimetic amines cause release. Rubin & Jaanus (257, 259) have found that perfusion in a Ca^{2+}-free medium, or with 5 mM Mg^{2+}, or with hexamethonium blocks the catecholamine-releasing effect of amphetamine, phenylethylamine, phenylpropylamine, and tyramine in the cat adrenal gland. On the other hand, Philippu & Schümann (230, 231) and Oka et al. (220) have found no, or only a weak, depression of the effects of phenylethylamine and tyramine on the bovine adrenal medulla in Ca^{2+}-free media.

Since nicotine and pilocarpine depolarize the chromaffin cell (65) and since the catecholamine-releasing effect of nicotinic (tetramethylammonium, lobeline, dimethylphenylpiperazinium) and muscarinic drugs (muscarine, pilocarpine, methacholine) is calcium dependent (76, 239) the release of catecholamines by these drugs most probably results from exocytosis. Similar evidence is available for serotonin and histamine (65, 239), and these may be classified tentatively as secretagogues.

Rasmussen (250) has proposed a general hypothesis of cell secretion in which the stimulus promotes Ca^{2+} uptake and simultaneously increases the production of $3',5'$-AMP, which in turn may regulate intracellular Ca^{2+} inactivation and mobilization and may also activate a kinase system that is involved in the transport of the storage vesicles to the releasing sites. When cyclic AMP and its dibutyryl derivative were perfused through the adrenal gland, they were completely ineffective in releasing catecholamines (163). Aminophylline, an inhibitor of cyclic AMP phosphodiesterase, evokes release of catecholamines only at concentrations of 5×10^{-3} M or above (163). There are no reports on the release of other vesicular and cytoplasmic components by aminophylline, nor are there measurements of intracellular cyclic AMP in the adrenal gland after administration of this drug or any other known secretagogue.

Angiotensin and bradykinin have been reported to depolarize the chromaffin cell of the gerbil (65) and induce Ca^{2+}-dependent secretion in the cat adrenal medulla (239). On the other hand, Robinson, with prolonged perfusion with Ca^{2+}-free media (251), has found, at most, only a 50% reduction of the increase in catecholamine output evoked by these peptides in the adrenal gland of the dog.

Large doses of Segontin and reserpine induce amine release from the adrenal gland, which is not calcium dependent (220, 231). The data do not enable one to differentiate between lysis and selective release of catecholamines and other vesicle components. Two drugs that are used as histamine-releasing agents, compounds 48/80 and 1935 L, also increase the outflow of catecholamines in the perfused adrenal of the rat; their effects are not modified by hexamethonium or promethazine (181). Arginine infusion, which is known to induce insulin, growth hormone, and glucagon release, will double the rate of amine release into the adrenal vein during a 30-min infusion period, and after removal of arginine there is further increase in the release during the following 30 min (149). It is not possible to establish the mechanism of action of these drugs with the information available.

Studies of the mechanism of action of inhibitors of catecholamine secretion, especially of those agents that seem to work at some step after the interaction of the secretagogue and its corresponding receptor sites, are of great importance for the understanding of the steps involved in excitation-secretion coupling. Of this group, Mg^{2+} stands in its own right for its universal capacity to inhibit Ca^{2+}-dependent secretion. The acetylcholine-induced depolarization of the chromaffin cell is not affected by Mg^{2+} (0.0–20.0 mM) either in normal or Ca^{2+}-free media (66), despite the fact that Mg^{2+} within the concentrations tested will completely block the secretory effect of acetylcholine, of high K^+ concentration, or of Ca^{2+} reintroduction (77, 78). The inhibitory effects of Mg^{2+} are competitively antagonized by increasing the concentration of Ca^{2+} in the extracellular fluid. Douglas & Rubin (77) have proposed that Mg^{2+} might be competitively blocking a Ca^{2+} "channel" in the plasma membrane and impeding the access of Ca^{2+} to its active site. Nevertheless Mg^{2+} by itself will depolarize the chromaffin cell membrane, which suggests that it permeates the chromaffin cell membrane with relative ease (66). Depolarization-induced ^{45}Ca uptake into the posterior lobe of the hypophysis is not significantly modified even in the presence of very high concentrations of Mg^{2+} (70). It is then more probable that Mg^{2+} competes with Ca^{2+} (and Ba^{2+} or Sr^{2+}) at the excitation-secretion coupling active site, while being incapable by itself of activating the site. These sites are probably only a small proportion of the total sites with which Ca^{2+} can interact. Unfortunately there are no reports of the effects of acetylcholine on membrane potentials when Mg^{2+} or Mg^{2+} plus Ca^{2+} are the only extracellular cations, nor are there radiotracer studies on the transmembrane fluxes of Mg^{2+} in the resting and stimulated chromaffin cell. The studies on the blockade of ^{45}Ca "exchange" by Mg^{2+} are difficult to interpret (256).

Local anesthetics inhibit catecholamine secretion from the adrenal at relatively low concentrations. Amethocaine, which selectively blocks Ca^{2+} conductance (63), and other local anesthetics will produce a dose-dependent block of the secretory response to acetylcholine and to Ca^{2+} reintroduction in a high-K^+ medium, which can be antagonized by increasing the acetylcholine or the Ca^{2+} concentration (150, 211, 256, 260). Although some of these agents will block acetylcholine-induced release at concentrations 100 times lower than what is needed to block secretion by Ca^{2+} reintroduction, others will give similar dose-response curves for both agonists. Rubin and co-workers (213, 260) have concluded that, whereas some local anesthetics will exclusively block Ca^{2+} movement during secretion, those that structurally resemble acetylcholine will block first at the cholinergic receptor and only later interfere with the movement of Ca^{2+}. Guanethidine similarly blocks adrenomedullary secretion (151). Although it has been proposed that propranolol blocks secretion by interfering with Ca^{2+} movement, since the dose-response curves for inhibition of Ca^{2+}- and acetylcholine-induced secretion are identical, this blockade is not reversed by increasing the concentration of Ca^{2+} used as a stimulant (150). Since there are no electrophysiological or ^{45}Ca uptake studies after treatment with these drugs, with the exception of amethocaine, it is not clear if all of them produce a general block of Ca^{2+} conductance or if some of them might compete directly at the Ca^{2+} active site or even interfere at a later step along the excitation-secretion pathway. In this respect, the noncompetitive inhibition exerted by propranolol seems extremely interesting and may provide a more specific way to determine the site of action of calcium.

Another group of substances that show a widespread capacity to block secretion are the microtubule-disrupting agents, colchicine, colcemide, vinblastine, vincristine, podophylotoxin, and griseofulvin. One or several of these drugs have been shown to block secretion of lysosomal enzymes (196, 248) and histamine (188) from leukocytes, insulin from the pancreas (179), and ^{131}I from previously labeled thyroid gland slices (218, 317). Williams & Wolff (317) found that colchicine binds to a soluble 6S protein from bovine thyroid gland. Poisner & Bernstein (238) have recently reported that colchicine, vinblastine, and vincristine inhibit acetylcholine- and nicotine-induced secretion of catecholamines from the perfused bovine adrenal gland. Small numbers of microtubular structures with no apparent special orientation within the cell have been observed under the electron microscope in the adrenomedullary cells (46, 47). Rasmussen (250) has proposed the existence of a microtubule-microfilament cytoskeleton radially arranged in the secretory cells that would be activated as a consequence of the secretory stimulus and move the secretory vesicles toward the cell surface. Whittaker (312) and Lacy et al. (179) have proposed a direct connection between storage vesicles and the external membrane through a microtubular system, the lumen of which would become enlarged in the presence of Ca^{2+} (312). Since such an elaborate cytoskeleton has not been observed, an alternative explanation could be that microtubule-disrupting drugs impair the general motile function of the cell by stopping organelle movement within a gelled cytoplasm, by impeding Brownian motion, by displacing the filled vesicles toward the plasma membrane, and by removing the empty vesicles from the attachment sites. Experiments on the inhibition of leukocyte degranulation by N-ethylmaleimide suggests this last mechanism of action (321).

Winkler et al. (314) and Plattner et al. (232) did not find microtubules in their beautiful study of the ultrastructure of the adrenal medulla of the cat by the freeze-etching method. They also reported that in their preparations large numbers of granules seemed to be aligned and probably in very close contact with the plasma membrane since frontal views of plasma membrane exposed by the fracture planes were seen "bulging" in several places as if the vesicles lay close below it (232). On the basis of this evidence, they proposed that the stimulus, or the influx of calcium, did not induce the attachment of the vesicles to the plasma membrane but merely caused the granule to discharge its content (232, 314). In chemically fixed glands, by far the largest proportion of the plasma membrane is free from direct contact with chromaffin granules, and although this could be an artifact of fixation, the large number of attached vesicles seen by the freeze-etching method may also be artifactual as a result of the high osmolarity of the antifreezing medium (approximately 10 times plasma osmolarity).

Gardier et al. (108) showed that N,N-diisopropyl-N'-isoamyl-N'-diethylaminoethylurea (P-286) blocked the pressor response to an intravenous injection of acetylcholine or to splanchnic nerve stimulation in the anesthetized dog, whereas there was no apparent ganglionic blockade; P-286 has also been shown to block acetylcholine (103)-, neostigmine-, and dimethyl-phenylpiperazinium-induced secretion but only partially to reduce the effect of tyramine in the perfused bovine adrenal gland (109). Segontin (103, 248) and N-ethylmaleimide (103) are also potent blockers of adrenomedullary secretion; these compounds are referred to later in relation to the in vitro release of catecholamines from storage vesicles.

Hedqvist (124) has shown that prostaglandins PGE_1 and PGE_2 markedly and reversibly inhibit the responses to sympathetic nerve stimulation and cause a reduction in the amount of catecholamines secreted. This effect can be reversed by increasing extracellular calcium concentration, and Hedqvist has proposed that prostaglandins might inhibit calcium influx. Ramwell et al. (249) reported increased efflux of prostaglandin from the perfused cat adrenal stimulated with acetylcholine; later, Shaw & Ramwell (274) found that only acetylcholine increased the release of prostaglandins from the perfused adrenal gland of the cow or rat, whereas nicotine or Ca^{2+} reintroduction did not have this effect. Miele (210) has recently observed that PGE_1 and $PGF_{1\alpha}$ do not modify catecholamine secretion from the adrenal gland that has been evoked by several different agents and thereby concluded that prostaglandins are not involved in modulating excitation-secretion coupling in the adrenal medulla.

Finally, when analyzing the mechanism of action of inhibitors of secretion, we should deal with the observation of decreased rate of secretion observed on frequent or repeated exposure of the gland to the same agonist (direct tachyphylaxis) (77, 174, 183, 283, 287) or when a different secretagogue is introduced after prolonged exposure to a previous stimulating agent (crossed tachyphylaxis) (174, 183, 258). A similar decline is also found during stimulation of the splanchnic nerve at a constant frequency, even though the content of medullary amines may not be significantly depleted (86, 87).

Smith & Robinson (283) injected histamine, at 10-min intervals and in doses that varied from just above threshold to maximal effects, into the inflow cannula perfusing isolated cat adrenal glands. By about the fifth injection, the response to each of these doses had fallen to about one-third of the corresponding initial response, and little further drop occurred as the injections were continued. Dopa or dopamine, but not tyrosine, significantly retarded the rate of decline of the secretory response to 1 μg of histamine (which initially gave a response approximately 20% of maximal), and this effect was partially blocked by diethyldithiocarbamate, which was supposedly acting as a dopamine β-hydroxylase inhibitor. The authors suggested that the "dwindling" response of the perfused adrenal to histamine was the result of depletion of a "readily secretable" pool of catecholamines whose maintenance would largely depend on the synthesis of the amines and to a lesser extent on the movement of the storage vesicles to the periphery. The maintenance of a nearly steady rate of secretion after the fast decline in the response and the recovery of the response after a period of rest possibly resulted from this mobilization (283). Smith & Robinson (283) took the important precaution of removing the contralateral gland to determine total initial content of catecholamines before perfusing and stimulating the other gland. When the total amount of catecholamines in the venous effluent of the perfused gland was added to the amount remaining in the gland at the end of the experiment, the resulting value exactly matched the initial catecholamine content as determined in the contralateral gland, both for the glands that received either histamine alone and for those that received histamine plus dopamine (283). This experiment shows that in neither condition was there a measurable increase in amine synthesis; furthermore, whereas the mean decrease in catecholamine content in the histamine-stimulated gland was 18.8% of the total initial content, the mean amount secreted by the gland that received histamine plus dopamine was 28.6%. These data are more easily explained if dopamine improves mobilization or some other of the steps in excitation-secretion coupling.

There are various other data in the literature that tend to disprove that tachyphylaxis results from depletion of some "easily releasable pool." Kovacic & Robinson (174) injected 500 μg nicotine at 100-sec intervals 55 times into the inflow perfusing adrenals of dogs. Such a schedule initiates catecholamine secretion at a very fast rate, which rapidly starts declining exponentially so that at 75 min secretion is still about twice the prestimulation level. When nicotinic-type drugs (e.g., dimethylphenylpiperazinium, tetramethylammonium) were injected immediately after the 55th injection of nicotine, they increased secretion only by 5–20% of the amount released by these drugs before the repeated nicotine treatment. On the other hand, there was a large potentiation to the response of acetylcholine, high K^+, pilocarpine, histamine, angiotensin, and bradykinin compared to the corresponding responses before the repeated injections of nicotine. Lee & Trendelenburg (183) reported similar findings in the adrenal of the cat in situ. Rubin & Jaanus (258) found that the perfused adrenal gland of the cat rapidly developed direct and crossed tachyphylaxis after repeated injections of tyramine, phenylethylamine, d-amphetamine, and acetylcholine, which was not the result of a depleted pool since the initial maximal response to any of the agonists could be attained by increasing the amount injected. Furthermore the response to acetylcholine could be completely recovered by increasing the concentration of Ca^{2+} in the perfusion media. Increased concentrations of Ca^{2+} would also improve but not completely recover the response to amphetamine and not modify the response to tyramine or phenylethylamine. In the experiments referred to above the total amounts of catecholamines secreted or the amounts left in the gland at the end of the experiment were not given. Douglas & Rubin (77) have included experiments in which one cat adrenal gland was constantly perfused with Locke's solution containing 10^{-5} g/ml acetylcholine and two others perfused with high K^+ (56 mM and 126 mM, respectively). In all three experiments the introduction of the secretagogue greatly increased the rate of secretion, which declined exponentially; after 30 min the rates were still 10–20 times higher than the control rates. During this whole period, the cumulative amount of catecholamines released was close to 94 µg for the acetylcholine-stimulated glands and 80 and 177 µg for the K^+-stimulated glands [the catecholamine content of one cat adrenal gland is approximately 300 µg (199)]. At this time the calcium concentration in the first two glands was increased from 2.2 to 8.8 mM, and there was an immediate four- to fivefold rise in the rate of secretion; the third gland perfused with isosmotic KCl received acetylcholine (10^{-4} g/ml), which increased the secretory rate nearly 10 times. All these data suggest that the development of tachyphylaxis by the adrenomedullary chromaffin cell to a certain secretagogue (and related compounds) may partly result from the turning on of some inactivation system particular to that specific secretagogue, whereas the main common pathway for excitation-secretion coupling and other incoming branches, as well as the accessibility to the catecholamine pool, are left unaltered or are even improved.

We can express other factors that may determine the rate of response to a stimulus as a function of the total number of releasing sites, the total number of filled and empty vesicles, and the probability for filled and for empty vesicles to react with the releasing sites. The probability of reaction between vesicles and releasing sites should be determined by *a*) the time a vesicle must remain attached before it extrudes its content and is removed, which in turn will depend on the efficiency of some hypothetical removal system, *b*) the rate of mobilization of filled vesicles toward the releasing sites (which could be active or passive), *c*) the distance between the position of the vesicle at the time of the stimulus and the releasing sites at the plasma membrane, and *d*) affinity constants of the filled and the empty vesicles for the releasing sites. The system just described assumes that the releasing sites are only at the free plasma membrane and that they are blocked while a vesicle remains attached to the membrane.

Ultrastructural evidence from the stimulated salivary cells (2) and exocrine pancreas (147) shows that filled vesicles may also extrude their contents through previously attached empty vesicles, which suggests that increased numbers of empty vesicles may not interfere with secretion. In theory the stimulus could modify the number of releasing sites or the affinity constant, which could also be a complex function of the concentration of Ca^{2+} and other ions in the media surrounding the releasing sites. A different hypothesis concerned with the probability of interaction of the storage vesicles with the releasing sites is discussed below.

The decline in secretory activity during prolonged splanchnic nerve stimulation is further complicated by factors that determine the secretion of acetylcholine at the nerve terminal. Marley and co-workers (199, 200) have given evidence that most of the decline in catecholamine secretion during splanchnic stimulation results from preganglionic "fatigue."

Since secretion is the culmination of a complex series of events, it should be obvious that a declining secretion rate in response to continued stimulation does not necessarily mean that this effect is due to various pools of more or less easily releasable amines.

Relevance of Catecholamine Release from Isolated Storage Vesicles to Study of Adrenal Chromaffin Cell Secretion

Since Blaschko & Welch (27) and Hillarp et al. (138) reported that adrenal catecholamines were stored at high concentrations within particles, there have been many studies on the effects of secretagogues, ions, and secretion blockers on the spontaneous release of amines from these storage particles in vitro. Very soon after their initial study of the amine storage particles, Blaschko and co-workers (25) reported that acetylcholine was ineffective in increasing the spontaneous rate of amine release from the vesicles suspended in isotonic sucrose at 37 C. This observation has been confirmed many times in sucrose (230, 273) or in different media containing salts (117), including calcium ions (117, 230). It is now quite evident that the action of acetylcholine is not directly at the storage site but is mediated by activating a receptor, probably at the plasma membrane.

The studies on the releasing capacity of calcium in vitro are conflicting: Hillarp (133) did not find any changes in the spontaneous release of amines from isolated bovine medullary granules at 37 C in a sucrose-histidine or a KCl-histidine medium on addition of 1.0 mM $CaCl_2$. Philippu and Schümann (230, 231, 271, 272) found that calcium concentrations of 2.5, 5.0, and 10 mM would increase the spontaneous rate of release of catecholamines in a sucrose medium at 37 C by 40, 100, and 140%, respectively. Other vesicle components, such as ATP, Ca^{2+}, and Mg^{2+}, were also released into the media in a proportion similar to that within the storage vesicle. The Ca^{2+}-induced release was not temperature dependent: catecholamines were released in as great a quantity at 37 C as at 0 C (231). Oka et al. (222) reported a similar release by Ca^{2+} from a bovine storage vesicle preparation purified by millipore filtration and suspended in NaCl-Tris buffer, but Greenberg & Kolen (117) reported that this effect was only seen in NaCl-

Tris buffer, whereas inhibition of release was found when Ca^{2+} (2.5×10^{-3} to 25 mM) was added to rat adrenomedullary vesicles suspended in KCl-Tris or in KCl-phosphate buffer.

Lishajko (191, 192) has recently reported a significant increase in the release of all soluble components from bovine adrenomedullary granules suspended in 130 mM phosphate buffer when calcium ions are added at concentrations of 3 mM or more. This effect is temperature and time dependent, and the effective concentration of Ca^{2+} is reduced 10-fold if RNA is added to the medium. Lishajko found that the releasing effect of Ca^{2+} occurred only in phosphate buffers; no Ca^{2+} effect was observed in unbuffered sucrose, NaCl, or KCl. The effectiveness of the release by Ca^{2+} seems to be proportional to the amount of calcium phosphate precipitate that is formed and can be reproduced by the addition of freshly formed calcium phosphate to the storage vesicle suspension. This effect is blocked by the addition of Mg^{2+} or ATP; Ba^{2+}, Sr^{2+}, and Mg^{2+} cannot substitute for Ca^{2+} as a releasing agent. Lishajko (191, 192) has proposed that this effect might result from the formation of a calcium phosphate complex within the vesicle membrane and in vivo it may serve to bridge the vesicle and plasma membrane and thereby promote their fusion and the extrusion of the vesicle content. Although this is an attractive hypothesis, it loses much of its weight by the lack of effect of Ba^{2+} and Sr^{2+} in vitro.

Another possible explanation for the coupling effect of calcium is based on the ability of this ion to reduce the surface potential of natural and artificial membranes (198). Banks (11) found that chromaffin granules suspended in a medium containing 270 mM sucrose plus 150 mM KCl migrated toward the anode, but when 2 mM $CaCl_2$ was added to the medium, electrophoretic mobility was reduced by 60% and completely stopped at 5 mM Ca^{2+}. When Banks observed his preparation under the phase contrast microscope, he found that the particles would clump together on addition of Ca^{2+}; at 5 mM Ca^{2+} there were no more free individual granules. These clumps have not been observed under the electron microscope, and the extent of attachment and fusion of the storage vesicle membranes or fusion of the vesicles themselves remains to be established. Since Banks found that magnesium ions had the same effect as calcium, he proposed that for exocytosis to occur the "granules should first become attached to the inner surface of the cell membrane, and this should be followed by a re-arrangement of the lipoproteins in both membranes so that the content of the granules can be extruded." He further suggested that this last step could result from "calcium holding the granule and cell membranes in close juxtaposition and can also act as a cofactor for an enzyme, such as phospholipase, involved in re-organizing the membrane structure. The enzyme could confer specificity for divalent cations in the secretory response" (11). The inner surface of the cell membrane also seems to have a negative charge (209), which would normally prevent the vesicles from coming in close apposition to the releasing sites, and consequently an increased concentration of divalent cations may greatly increase the probability of secretion by decreasing the surface potential in one or both membranes.

Among the most exciting observations of the last 2 years in the study of biogenic amines are those based on the experiments by Berneis and associates (20, 21, 233) on the formation in vitro of macromolecular aggregates of amines, ATP, and Ca^{2+} or Mg^{2+} when they are mixed in the concentrations known to occur in the storage organelles in vivo. The size and the stability of these complexes are critically dependent on the proportion of divalent cation to amines in the mixture; at concentrations much above or below the concentrations of Ca^{2+} or Mg^{2+} found inside the storage vesicles the system will become unstable at room temperature. The authors have proposed that such a critical dependence on the concentration of cation in the media may explain the dual effect of these ions on uptake and release of amines. Because the concentration of calcium and magnesium within the catecholamine storage vesicle (32) is well above the concentration in the extracellular fluid, and at least for Ca^{2+} several orders of magnitude higher than in the cytoplasm (22), it is difficult to visualize extrusion of catecholamines resulting from an increased influx of calcium into the chromaffin cell during depolarization. On the other hand, the lower Ca^{2+} concentration in the extracellular fluid as compared to the vesicle content might determine a very fast dissociation of the storage complex as soon as there is free communication between the intravesicular and interstitial space. Such a sudden disruption of the complex should greatly increase the intravesicular osmotic pressure, and as a result, water should move through the vesicle membrane into the intravesicular space and flush the content out into the interstitium. Much further work is needed in this area before we can fully understand the relation of this "storage complex" studied in vitro and the mechanism of incorporation, storage, and release of amines from vesicles in vivo.

Another system that has generated much interest in recent years is the release in vitro of catecholamines from isolated storage vesicles by addition of ATP and Mg^{2+} to the suspension media. This system was originally described by Oka and co-workers (221, 223) who found that the release rate of catecholamines from bovine chromaffin vesicles suspended in isotonic NaCl or KCl was doubled or tripled upon addition of ATP and Mg^{2+} to the media. This effect was time and temperature dependent; Mg^{2+} could not be replaced by Ca^{2+}, and ADP gave only a small fraction of the effect of ATP. The effect was not present when ATP or Mg^{2+} alone was added to the salt medium or when ATP plus Mg^{2+} was added to vesicles suspended in sucrose. When the optical density (OD) of this suspension was measured at 520 mμ, as an indication of structural changes of the vesicles (173), there was a time-dependent decrease in OD, which suggested that the vesicles were increasing in volume. The authors suggested that this change in OD was related to the activity of the vesicle membrane ATPase and in some undetermined way led to the release of catecholamines (223). Poisner and Trifaró (235, 243–245, 297) showed that ATP and Mg^{2+} also induce release of endogenous ATP and protein from the vesicle suspension, that hydrolysis of ATP occurs at the same time as release of catecholamines, and that inhibitors of the vesicle membrane ATPase will also inhibit catecholamine release (243) and the fall in OD at 540 mμ (297). Trifaró & Dworkind (296) have recently shown that the membrane of the storage vesicles becomes phosphorylated by ATP in the same experimental conditions that sustain ATP-Mg^{2+}-dependent release. Poisner & Trifaró (243) proposed that upon stimulation Ca^{2+} and ATP previously bound to the plasma membrane would become free in the cytoplasm and extracellular Ca^{2+} would enter the cell; Ca^{2+} would link anionic groups in the plasma membrane to those in the membrane of chromaffin granules. The vesicle membrane ATPase can simultaneously act on the released ATP, and this interaction results in some conformational change in the vesicle membrane, which breaks a hypothetical bond between these membranes and a catecholamine-ATP-protein complex. This permits the egress of these substances at the area of increased permeability (243). The authors do not clearly state the origin of the increase in plasma membrane permeability, but they imply that it is the result of displacement of bound calcium by depolarization and ATP breakdown by the vesicle ATPase. On the basis of the similarities between release of catecholamines in vitro and mitochondrial contraction (245) and of excitation-secretion coupling and excitation-contraction coupling, these authors have suggested that the granule membrane ATPase may function as a mechanochemical transducer (243) to produce "an active ejection of transmitter" (237). Although there might be some kind of contractile system in the vesicle membrane that requires ATP and Mg^{2+}, this is not substantiated by the available evidence. The light scattering measurements done on vesicle suspensions always show an increase in the amount of scattered light, and a corresponding decrease in OD (190, 223, 245, 297), on addition of ATP plus Mg^{2+}, which is exactly the opposite of what is expected if the vesicle contracts. Trifaró & Poisner (297) did not see any changes in OD when ATP and Mg^{2+} were added to vesicles previously lysed in water [the addition of ATP to intact or disrupted mitochondria still produces a decrease in light scattering (184)]. Increases in light scattering produced by a suspension of chromaffin vesicles is seen with every agent that will lyse the storage vesicle (hypo-osmotic media, a variety of detergents, phospholipase A), as had been shown by Hillarp & Nilson (139) in 1954.

The ATP-Mg^{2+}-induced release in vitro might be a more complex expression of storage vesicle function than initially envisioned. Lishajko has shown that ATP-Mg^{2+}-stimulated release does not occur in isotonic potassium phosphate or sodium acetate media, unless chloride ions are present at concentrations greater than 50 mM (189). Ferris, Viveros, and Kirshner (unpublished observations) have found that of 10 different organic and inorganic anions only Cl^-, Br^-, and I^- will support ATP-Mg^{2+}-dependent release in vitro.

The only evidence that such a system may be one of the steps in excitation-secretion coupling comes from the observations by Ferris et al. (102, 103) that N-ethylmaleimide, N,N-diisopropyl-N'-isoamyl-N'-diethylaminoethylurea (P-286), and prenylamine blocked, at very similar concentrations, both ATP-Mg^{2+}-induced release in vitro and the effect of a maximal concentration of acetylcholine in the perfused bovine adrenal gland. These last two drugs had no effect on vesicle membrane ATPase. Inhibitors of glycolysis or oxidative phosphorylation, by themselves or in combination, or propranolol, at concentrations known to block catecholamine secretion, did not modify ATPase activity or ATP-Mg^{2+}-induced release in vitro. Soluble dopamine β-hydroxylase was released by ATP and Mg^{2+} in the same proportion as catecholamines, and the ratio of enzyme to catecholamines in the medium was identical with the ratio inside the vesicles.

Because the same conditions that stimulate and block ATP-Mg^{2+} release in a chloride medium stimulate and inhibit catecholamine incorporation in nonchloride, as well as in chloride, media, Ferris et al. (103) proposed that both release and incorporation of catecholamines might result if ATP, through a reaction requiring Mg^{2+}, would "activate" the vesicle storage complex. The activated complex could exchange or incorporate amines but could also become disrupted if some other factor, like Cl^-, Br^-, or I^-, were present in the media. The intravesicular osmolarity should increase and result in a subsequent influx of water leading to lysis of the vesicles or distension of the vesicle surface to the extent of becoming permeable to protein. In the intact gland, the disruption of the complex and the influx of water after the vesicles have become attached to the plasma membrane may be an important physiological mechanism for the extrusion of the vesicle contents to the exterior of the cell (103).

The more important argument against the involvement of such a system in excitation-secretion coupling is the rather high concentration of chloride required for release in vitro, whereas prolonged perfusion with a chloride-free medium does not inhibit catecholamine secretion from the perfused gland (75, 77). In later work, Ferris, Viveros, and Kirshner (unpublished observations) have found that a fraction from the postmicrosomal supernatant of the adrenal medulla greatly potentiates ATP-Mg^{2+}-induced release in chloride media and maintains high rates of stimulated release even in media completely free of chloride ions; furthermore they have also obtained evidence, by the use of sucrose density gradient centifugation, that release in vitro from each vesicle is all or none, as seems to be the case with secretion (172, 305).

A similar ATP-Mg^{2+}-dependent release in vitro has been found in parotid and pancreas zymogen granules (324, 351), posterior pituitary granules (240), and cholinergic synaptic vesicles (203). The Mg^{2+} concentration in the cytoplasm of the adrenomedullary cell seems to be close to 5 mM (32); even if a large proportion was bound such that the concentration of free Mg^{2+} would be similar to that found in red cells (0.1–0.25 mM) (252), this should be close to the optimal concentration, found in vitro, for the ATP-Mg^{2+}-stimulated release (243). There are no data available on the concentration of free ATP in the cytoplasm of the chromaffin cell, but rather large amounts of ATP are apparently associated with plasma membranes (33, 40). Also Cecchi et al. (44) have shown that several glycolytic enzymes are firmly bound to a plasma membrane fraction of squid retinal nerves and that incubation of the membranes with ADP or GDP and orthophosphate resulted in ATP synthesis. Even if ATP concentration in the cytoplasm is high, the low concentration of intracellular chloride should prevent intracytoplasmic ATP-Mg^{2+}-stimulated release from occurring while providing the energy necessary to incorporate the amines into the storage complex. If stimulation would in some way increase the concentration of the postmicrosomal supernatant factor at or near the plasma membrane, the intravesicular dissociation of the storage complex may start. This should result in increased intravesicular pressure and, to a certain extent, in increased volume. As a consequence of the increased pressure and increased diameter, the membrane tension should increase (Laplace's law). From studies of the effects of hypoosmotic solutions on the integrity of vesicles (139), it is known that the normal tension at the vesicle membrane should be very close to the maximum stress it can hold without breaking or becoming extremely permeable. If now the vesicle membrane, as the result of the action of calcium or from some other factor, becomes fused with the plasma membrane, the radius of curvature of the fused area will be between the radius of curvature of a normal vesicle (approximately 100 mμ) and the radius of curvature of the cell membrane (10 μ for a sphere, several times more for the free subendothelial surface of the cell). The tension on this common membrane will also be a function of both intravesicular and intracellular pressure. The vesicle membrane should preferentially break through the area of fusion. As discussed later, the factors that promote fusion of the membrane should also decrease the resistance to stress of such a membrane.

Another alternative explanation for the ATP-Mg^{2+}-induced release in vitro, and presumably in vivo, would be that these substances do act at the membrane of the vesicle in such a way that adhesion and fusion of the vesicles are promoted. The vesicles would progressively increase in size, and the increased radius of curvature at constant pressure will result in progressively increasing vesicle membrane tension until it finally bursts. The normal tension in any vesicle may be so close to breaking the membrane that just the extra tension added by the fusion with the plasma membrane might be enough to open a continuity to the extracellular space.

Mechanism of Membrane Fusion

Fusion of cellular membranes (plasma membrane and membranes from cell organelles) is an absolute requisite not only for the secretory function of the cell, but for lysosomal function and plasma membrane replacement and growth; also cell fusion is a common result of viral infection. It is certainly striking how few experiments have been published on membrane fusion in general, none of them on the fusion of the membranes of secretory vesicles.

Probably the best studied form of membrane fusion is the fusion of the plasma membrane of neighboring cells by certain types of viruses resulting in the production of multinucleated syncytia (122). The active part of the virus seems to be a protein of the viral envelope (122), and both energy production (225) and calcium ions (224) are necessary for fusion to proceed. The first obvious changes during fusion are clumping of the cells together and the appearance of small cytoplasmic bridges between apposed cells; the bridges increase in number and size with time. Electron microscopy has not resolved the precise structural basis of fusion (122).

Blioch et al. (28) studied the adhesion between artificial phospholipid membranes in aqueous solutions in the presence of different concentrations of various ions. The phospholipids were extracted from brain, and a heptane-phospholipid solution was placed over the ends of two small tubes to form a black or a colored membrane (a few hundred A thick). By applying gentle pressure from the inside of the tubes the lipid films bulged and came into contact with each other. After some time, there was a sudden change in the shape of the contact area and adhesion was assumed to have occurred. The authors mention that in some instances the transverse membrane broke and a continuous phospholipid membrane tube was formed, but only the "times of adhesion" were reported. Times of adhesion were reduced from infinite time to 16 $\pm$ 2 sec and 32 $\pm$ 4 sec for colored and black membranes, respectively, by substituting 100 mM KCl for distilled water. Calcium chloride and magnesium chloride reduced the adhesion times for colored films to 2.7 $\pm$ 0.3 and 6.9 $\pm$ 0.7 sec. These times were further reduced by trivalent and tetravalent cations, whereas anions were ineffective. There was no attempt to characterize the "adhesion" of the membranes by electron microscopy or by trying to reform the individual membranes by washing the ions out and by chelation. The authors proposed that the adhesion between synaptic vesicles and the membrane at the nerve ending may arise by a similar mechanism and further postulated that there should be a specific mechanism to reduce the normal intracellular concentration of Mg^{2+} (which should be high enough to induce membrane adhesion in the resting terminal) in the region between the axonal membrane and synaptic vesicles (28). Ionic bridging between chromaffin vesicle and plasma membranes as the specific effect of Ca^{2+} in secretion has also been proposed (243).

Calcium, as well as other divalent cations, is necessary in maintaining adhesion of neighboring cells (111, 198) by decreasing electrostatic repulsion or by establishing ionic bridges between adjacent membranes, but the cells maintain their individualities and the plasma membranes do not fuse. It is then evident that simple membrane bridging or reduction of the surface potential by calcium may contribute, but is not sufficient for cellular membranes to fuse. Furthermore these actions are not specific for calcium, but all divalent cations have similar effects (110, 198).

Dingle (59) has proposed, on the basis of the action of foam stabilizing and antifoaming agents, that the fusion of lipoprotein membranes might be related to a high surface tension and displacement of the external protein monolayer. Howell & Lucy (146) have proposed that fusion should result from increased proportion of phospholipid molecules in the micellar configuration. In any case the membrane will be unstable, and these authors have suggested that anything that will decrease the stability of the plasma and vesicle membrane, such as relative high proportion of short-chain fatty acids, incorporation of *cis*-isomers, presence of polar group in the hydrocarbon chain, presence of wedge-shaped molecules, such as lysolecithin, or any other change that decreases the molecular packing, should result in an increased fusion ability (59, 146). Howell & Lucy (146) have treated chicken red blood cells with lysolecithin for 30 sec at 37 C, followed by glutaraldehyde fixation. Many cells lyse as a result of the treatment, and red cell ghosts are seen sticking together when observed under the phase contrast microscope. With the electron microscope, some of the ghosts are seen fused together to form a multinucleated syncytium. The earliest morphological change reported is the formation of small cytoplasmic bridges. This report, as well as those on cell fusion by viruses, suggests that the time the interposed membrane takes to open after one membrane comes in contact and fuses with the other must be extremely short. A study at earlier times in such a system may provide valuable evidence on the initial stages of fusion. Lysolecithin-induced fusion apparently does not require calcium ions in the medium (146).

The membranes of the adrenomedullary storage vesicle are unusually rich in a lysolecithin (24, 315, 316), which may originate by the action of a phospholipase A_2 on the lecithin of the vesicle membrane (315). Acid hydrolases in the chromaffin cell are stored in lysosomal particles that can be separated from storage vesicles (266, 280, 282) and contain phospholipase A_1 and A_2 (26, 282). Blaschko et al. (24) and Banks (11) have proposed that the influx of Ca^{2+} might activate these phospholipases, and Schneider (263, 266) has found increased release of lysosomal enzymes from the adrenal medulla under all conditions that increase catecholamine secretion (by exocytosis). Feldberg (99) found that lysolecithin and bee and cobra venom, which are rich in phospholipases, increased the release of catecholamines from the cat adrenal gland with no apparent lysis of the chromaffin cells when histologically studied.

On the other hand, Winkler et al. (316) and Trifaró (294) have not found increased amounts of lysolecithin in the storage vesicle fraction obtained from stimulated adrenal glands. However, in the measurements of the amount of lysolecithin after stimulation, the expected increase should be in the fractions where the plasma membrane (low-speed sediment) and the empty vesicle membranes are distributed (microsomal pellet and 1.12 specific gravity in sucrose density gradients).

Other proposals on the mechanism by which calcium can make the plasma membrane unstable at the site of contact with the vesicle membrane have been advanced. Woodin & Weineke (320, 321) suggested that stimulation will increase the calcium concentration at the membrane releasing sites and promote adhesion of the vesicles. Once adhesion is established, Ca^{2+} is removed by formation of calcium phosphate as a result of the activity of the granule-membrane ATPase; the decrease in plasma membrane-bound Ca^{2+} and ATP should make the membranes unstable or at least more permeable. Douglas (62) proposed that the removal of ATP bound to the plasma membrane by the Ca^{2+}-dependent ATPase of the attached chromaffin vesicle may lead to membrane fusion and to the release of the content of the granule. This hypothesis, although very attractive because of its inherent simplicity, does not easily account for the specificity for calcium ions and inhibitory actions of Mg^{2+} since the vesicle membrane enzyme is activated more by Mg^{2+} than by Ca^{2+} (8, 167, 313).

Some General Hypotheses for Excitation-Secretion Coupling

Up to now, we have discussed some of the hypothetical steps that may form part of the excitation-secretion pathway; we now refer to some of the hypotheses in which the mechanism of secretion is considered in a more general fashion.

Del Castillo and Katz (53, 158) have proposed a model for release of transmitter substances in which the rate of collision between vesicular and axonal membrane is very high at all times but release occurs only in the statistically improbable event of two reactive molecules or specific sites, one on each membrane, meeting and starting off a reaction that causes the vesicle and plasma membranes to burst open. Excitation will permit Ca^{2+} to move into the membrane and temporarily increase by a large factor the number of reactive sites so the statistical probability of release is increased, and for the same total number of collisions a much larger fraction becomes successful.

Matthews has recently published a most interesting

paper (206) applying quantitative kinetic terms to the electrostatic theory of vesicle-plasma membrane interaction previously proposed by Banks (11) and Blioch et al. (28). Matthews (206) has calculated that the most probable minimal time it will take a 200-mµ vesicle to reach the plasma membrane by Brownian motion through a cytoplasm of 0.06 poise viscosity and a distance of 5 µ is 33 sec, but it will take only 0.13 msec if the vesicle was 10 mµ from the periphery. He also calculated that, if the vesicle membrane had similar surface charges of equal sign and about -25 mv, the mean kinetic energy of such a vesicle in Brownian movement would be too low to overcome the electrostatic repulsion and make contact with the plasma membrane. Nevertheless it should be expected that the largest vesicles within the population would occasionally acquire enough kinetic energy to break the barrier. The author has proposed that this may account for the quantal or basal release of transmitter.

Matthews (206) proposed that, in the unstimulated secretory cell with a resting transmembrane potential of -20 to -70 mv developed across a membrane of 200 A, the electric field should be large enough to maintain dipole orientation and ionization of macromolecular fixed charges. At this time free calcium in cytoplasm is low. Depolarization of the cell by the stimulus will make the electric field collapse, and Ca^{2+} previously bound inside the membrane may become available at the inner surface together with more Ca^{2+} entering the cell. Divalent cations are very effective in decreasing the membrane surface potential, and the potential energy barrier to granule-cell membrane interaction should disappear. When a granule closely approaches the plasma membrane (e.g., 5 A), adhesion may be aided by cross-linking of cell and granule membranes resulting from ion triplet formation; desolvation may occur and stabilize the adhesion and thereby encourage fusion (206).

In these two hypotheses the secretion rate is mainly determined by the increased number of releasing sites at the membrane, the difference being that in the hypothesis of del Castillo & Katz (53) the idea of specific releasing sites is implied, whereas in the hypothesis advanced by Matthews (206) the attachment site could be any negatively charged group or area of the plasma membrane. On the other hand, Woodin & Weineke (321), from their observations on the rarity with which they found exocytotic figures on the plasma membrane of the stimulated polymorphonuclear leukocyte and from other evidence, have concluded that the total number of releasing sites is very low and that fusion occurs only at the site of the potassium pump of the cell membrane. This releasing site still needs calcium to become active and supposedly binds the ion as a result of stimulation. In their concept the increased probability of release seems to be mainly a function of the noncalcium-dependent gel-to-sol transformation of the cytoplasm, which allows the granules to collide by Brownian motion against the plasma membrane.

On the basis of current information, it is obvious that hypotheses in which only changes in the number of releasing sites are considered the main effect of excitation cannot easily explain the early events induced in the leukocyte by stimulation, nor can they account for the effects of microtubular disrupting agents. On the other hand, it is difficult to envision how the polymorphonuclear leukocyte may have only a few releasing sites and become completely degranulated within a minute (321). An alternative explanation for the absence of exocytotic figures is that the duration of such a fusion may be extremely short-lived and labile.

I would like to propose as a working hypothesis that secretion from the adrenal medulla may be determined by several necessary steps, probably not all of which are in causal or temporal sequence but may be independent and perhaps coexistent.

The normal excitation-secretion pathway may be organized as follows (Fig. 5).

1. Interaction of the secretagogue with any of the many adrenomedullary receptors (e.g., nicotinic, muscarinic), or direct depolarization, alters the conformation of the membrane such that there is an increase in conductance to sodium, calcium, and possibly other ions.

2. The increased membrane conductance to some ion other than calcium or other changes at the membrane result in cytoplasmic solvation. As a consequence orderly movement of the cytoplasm and organelles stops and Brownian movement of the particles through a medium of decreased viscosity starts. Random movement will direct some of the storage vesicles toward the plasmalemma.

3. The surface potentials of the plasma membrane and peripheral vesicles are reduced or abolished by the increase in calcium concentration in this area. As a result both membranes come into direct contact with one another. This contact may be stabilized by a Ca^{2+} bridge linking the two negatively charged surfaces.

4. Additionally the Ca^{2+} may react with a specific site or sites on the plasma membrane, and thus an increase in the probability of fusion of the internal layer of the plasma membrane to the external layer of the vesicle membrane results. In this reaction Ba^{2+} and Sr^{2+}, but not Mg^{2+}, may substitute for Ca^{2+}. The hypothetical site for activation of membrane fusion could be some specific molecular component of the membrane that, directly on binding to calcium, results in structural changes in the membrane, or Ca^{2+} could activate an enzyme system that may have such an effect (phospholipases, *cis-trans*-isomerases, an actomyosin system that on contraction may expose the lipid phase of the membrane). The resulting area of fusion becomes a weak point in the vesicle membrane because of the local increase in tension that results from the larger radius of curvature and the additive effects of vesicle and cell internal pressures.

5. The catecholamine storage complex starts to dissociate by an increase in the concentration of ATP,

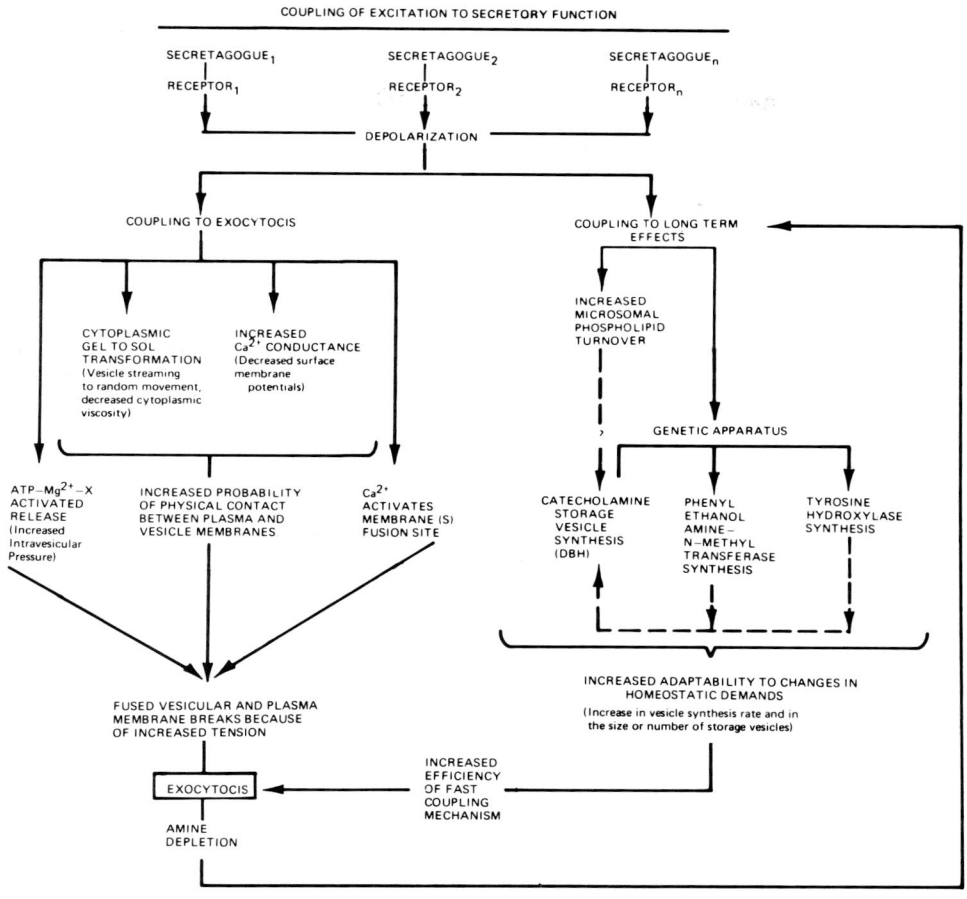

FIG. 5. Excitation-secretion pathway. *DBH*, dopamine β-hydroxylase.

Mg^{2+}, or the X factor, which is replaced by Cl^- in vitro, in the medium surrounding the vesicle. This activation of the storage complex, as a result of stimulation, may affect all vesicles in the cell or more probably is localized to its periphery. The activation of this step may result from a true increase in concentration of some of the required factors, or activation may occur because the vesicle moves into close proximity with the cell membrane where these factors may normally exist in high concentration. As a consequence the pressure inside the vesicle increases and the vesicle membrane becomes more unstable. The increased intravesicular pressure will then result in the opening of the fused area into the extracellular space. The complete and rapid dissociation of the storage complex, when exposed to the composition of the interstitial fluid, may help flush out the vesicle content.

In this scheme, after Step 1 is activated, the subsequent steps could proceed simultaneously and independently of each other. Step 3 may be not relevant or of only minor importance, depending on the values for the surface potentials of the plasma and vesicle membrane within the cell, which in turn should depend on the free concentration of Mg^{2+}. This concentration is enough to completely neutralize the negative charge of the storage vesicle in vitro (11) and also probably enough to bind most of the negative groups on the inner side of the plasma membrane (209). If this were the case, adherence between vesicles and plasma membrane could be prevented by the region of cytoplasmic gel near the plasmalemma and by cytoplasmic movements (55, 153).

Inhibition of any one of these individual steps should result in blockade of the secretory response to stimulation. The independence of the obligatory reactions after activation of the first suggests that one or more steps may be blocked without affecting the others. Step 1 is blocked by the corresponding receptor blocking drugs, Step 2 may be the site blocked by microtubule disrupting agents, Steps 3 and 4 by blockers of calcium conductance, like amethocaine, and Step 5 by inhibitors of the $ATP-Mg^{2+}-Cl^-$-dependent release in vitro. On the other hand, inhibition of metabolism may block every one of the five steps.

These five obligatory steps for secretion may be modified by a variety of other factors, such as the inactivation system that seems to be turned on each time a particular receptor is activated and may result in tachyphylaxis, or the mechanism by which increased intracellular sodium may potentiate secretion.

There is nothing novel in the hypothetical scheme here presented. On the contrary, it is merely an attempt to summarize our knowledge and, where there is no knowledge, to include some of the current ideas on excitation-secretion coupling. The scarcity of experimental facts on adrenomedullary secretion (as in most secretory cells) and the profusion of plausible hypotheses have required extrapolation from other systems and the author's own prejudiced interpretations, although he knows full well that the same data could be fitted to many different schemes.

Adaptability of Excitation-Secretion Mechanism of Adrenomedullary Cell to Homeostatic Demands

Since in all probability the empty catecholamine vesicles cannot be immediately reused to accumulate, store, and secrete catecholamines, the adrenomedullary cell should have a maximal capacity to respond to increased splanchnic stimulation related to the number of vesicles that a well-rested cell can store. Once complete depletion is attained, the rate of secretion would be totally dependent on the rate at which a new vesicle is made and is able to fuse with the plasma membrane. The turnover time for the catecholamines in the adrenals of different species is between 3 days and a week (127). A relatively mild, chronic stimulus, such as exposure to cold, may persistently increase adrenal amine output by two- to sevenfold (182) and would result in complete depletion of the gland in a few days if replenishment of vesicles and catecholamine stores did not occur.

Viveros and co-workers (302, 303) showed that, between 24 and 48 hr after neurogenic stimulation, the adrenal tyrosine hydroxylase levels are significantly increased and maintained for several days; the initial decrease in dopamine β-hydroxylase is followed within days by increases to levels significantly higher than the controls. Reserpine treatment is also followed by a large increase in dopamine β-hydroxylase levels, and the authors proposed that this increase probably was the result of making a whole new population of vesicles to replace those damaged by reserpine. De Quattro et al. (54) also showed increased levels of tyrosine hydroxylase after chronically increasing the rate of splanchnic discharge as a result of sinoaortic denervation. Early observations had shown that chronic adrenomedullary stimulation results in a significant increase in the volume of the adrenal medulla and in its amine content (89, 91–93, 195, 234), as well as in the histochemical reaction for acid and alkaline phosphatase (1, 89, 93, 214). The capacity of the adrenal medulla to regulate the functional levels of the amine synthesizing machinery has been confirmed by several authors (5, 123, 176–178, 229, 234, 309, 310). Since the rate of mitosis in the adult adrenal medulla is extremely low (197), the evidence presented by Viveros and associates (301, 302) suggests that the increase in catecholamine content results from an increased amine storage capacity of each vesicle or from a larger number of vesicles per cell.

If the vesicles from chronically stimulated glands contain larger than normal amounts of amines and protein and the probability of release of each granule is unchanged, a stimulus of equal intensity should induce a greater secretion of the hormone from the chronically stimulated gland than from the control gland; a larger number of vesicles of normal content should also result in increased secretion, provided the probability of release is kept constant. Since the efficiency of excitation-secretion coupling has not been measured in such a gland and compared to that in glands from normal animals or to chronically denervated glands nothing can be said of the effects of chronic adrenomedullary activity on the probability of release, which in itself may be changed by chronic hyperfunction; at any rate the chronically stimulated gland seems to be better fitted to respond for longer periods of time and probably also at a faster rate to increased homeostatic demands (177).

The chromaffin cell has repeatedly proven to be an excellent model of the physiology of the noradrenergic system, as well as of other secretory cells, including chemical synapses. If the adrenal chromaffin cell can "learn" to improve its response by chronic stimulation resulting in a larger number or size of secreted quanta, a similar mechanism that may function in other endocrine cells may be strongly suggested. Such a mechanism may be the basis for the increased density of synaptic vesicles in the rod terminals of the outer plexiform layer of the retina and in the neuropile of the lateral geniculate nucleus of light-reared rats (48) and may also be the explanation for the "functional opening of a synapse" as a consequence of increased activity through that nervous pathway.

The author is indebted to the Fulbright-Hays Program for a travel grant during the preparation of the manuscript and to Dr. Norman Kirshner for his continuous kindness and encouragement.

REFERENCES

1. Allen, J. M. The influence of cold, inanition and insulin shock upon the histochemistry of the adrenal medulla of the mouse. *J. Histochem. Cytochem.* 4: 341–346, 1956.
2. Amsterdam, A., I. Ohad, and M. Schramm. Dynamic changes in the ultrastructure of the acinar cell of the rat parotid gland during the secretory cycle. *J. Cell Biol.* 41: 753–773, 1969.
3. Anden, N. E., A. Carlsson, and T. Häggendal. Adrenergic mechanisms. *Ann. Rev. Pharmacol.* 9: 119–134, 1969.
4. Austin, L., B. G. Livett, and I. W. Chubb. Biosynthesis of noradrenaline in sympathetic nervous tissue. *Circulation Res.* 21, Suppl. 3: 111–117, 1967.
5. Axelrod, J., R. A. Mueller, and H. Thoenen. Neuronal and hormonal control of tyrosine hydroxylase and phenylethanolamine N-methyltransferase activity. In: *New Aspects of Storage and Release Mechanisms of Catecholamines*, edited by H. J. Schümann and G. Kroneberg. Berlin: Springer Verlag, 1970, p. 212–219.
6. Babkin, B. P. *Secretory Mechanism of Digestive Glands.* New York: Hoeber, 1950.
7. Bachmann, R. Die Niebenniere. In: *Handbuch der Mikro-*

skopischen Anatomie des Menschen, edited by W. von Möllendorf and W. Bargman. Berlin: Springer Verlag, 1954, vol. VI, part 5, p. 1–952.
8. BANKS, P. The adenosine triphosphatase activity of adrenal chromaffin granules. *Biochem. J.* 95: 490–496, 1965.
9. BANKS, P. Effects of stimulation by carbachol in the metabolism of the bovine adrenal medulla. *Biochem. J.* 97: 555–560, 1965.
10. BANKS, P. The release of adenosine triphosphate catabolites during the secretion of catecholamines by bovine adrenal medulla. *Biochem. J.* 101: 536–541, 1966.
11. BANKS, P. An interaction between chromaffin granules and calcium ions. *Biochem. J.* 101: 18–20c, 1966.
12. BANKS, P. The effect of ouabain on the secretion of catecholamines and on the intracellular concentration of potassium. *J. Physiol., London* 193: 631–637, 1967.
13. BANKS, P. Involvement of calcium in the secretion of catecholamines. In: *Calcium and Cellular Function*, edited by A. W. Cuthbert. New York: St. Martin's, 1970, p. 148–162.
14. BANKS, P., R. BIGGINS, R. BISHOP, B. CHRISTIAN, AND N. CURRIE. Sodium ions and the secretion of catecholamines. *J. Physiol., London* 200: 797–805, 1969.
15. BANKS, P., R. BIGGINS, R. BISHOP, B. CHRISTIAN, AND N. CURRIE. Monovalent cations and the secretion of catecholamines. *J. Physiol., London* 201: 47–48P, 1969.
16. BANKS, P., AND K. HELLE. The release of protein from the stimulated adrenal medulla. *Biochem. J.* 97: 40–41c, 1965.
17. BAUDUIN, H., J. REUSE, AND J. E. DUMONT. Non-dependence of secretion on protein synthesis. *Life Sci., Part 2* 6: 1723–1731, 1967.
18. BENNETT, H. S. Cytological manifestations of secretion in the adrenal medulla of the cat. *Am. J. Anat.* 69: 333–381, 1941.
19. BENNETT, H. S. The concept of membrane flow and membrane vesiculation as mechanism of active transport and ion pumping. *J. Biophys. Biochem. Cytol. Suppl.* 2: 99–103, 1956.
20. BERNEIS, K. H., M. DAPRADA, AND A. PLETSCHER. Metal dependent aggregation of biogenic amines: a hypothesis of their storage and release. *Nature* 224: 281–283, 1969.
21. BERNEIS, K. H., A. PLETSCHER, AND M. DA PRADA. Phase separation in solution of noradrenaline and adenosine triphosphate: influence of bivalent cations and drugs. *Brit. J. Pharmacol.* 39: 382–389, 1970.
22. BIANCHI, C. P. *Cell Calcium*. London: Butterworths, 1968.
23. BLASCHKO, H., R. S. COMLINE, F. H. SCHNEIDER, M. SILVER, AND A. D. SMITH. Secretion of a chromaffin granule protein, chromogranin, from the adrenal gland after splanchnic stimulation. *Nature* 215: 58–59, 1967.
24. BLASCHKO, H., H. FIREMARK, A. D. SMITH, AND H. WINKLER. Phospholipids and cholesterol in particulate fractions of adrenal medulla. *Biochem. J.* 98: 24P, 1966.
25. BLASCHKO, H., P. HAGEN, AND A. D. WELCH. Observations on the intracellular granules of adrenal medulla. *J. Physiol., London* 129: 27–49, 1955.
26. BLASCHKO, H., A. D. SMITH, H. WINKLER, H. VAN DEN BOSCH, AND L. L. M. VAN DEENEN. Acid phospholipase A in lysosomes of the bovine adrenal medulla. *Biochem. J.* 103: 30–32c, 1967.
27. BLASCHKO, H., AND A. D. WELCH. Localization of adrenaline in cytoplasmatic particles of the bovine adrenal medulla. *Arch. Exptl. Pathol. Pharmakol.* 219: 17–22, 1953.
28. BLIOCH, Z. L., I. M. GLAGOLEVA, E. A. LIBERMAN, AND V. A. NENASHEV. A study of the mechanism of quantal transmitter release at a chemical synapse. *J. Physiol., London* 199: 11–35, 1968.
29. BOROWITZ, J. L. Calcium binding by subcellular fractions of bovine adrenal medulla. *J. Cell Physiol.* 69: 305–310, 1967.
30. BOROWITZ, J. L. Effect of acetylcholine on the subcellular distribution of Ca^{45} in bovine adrenal medulla. *Biochem. Pharmacol.* 18: 715–723, 1969.
31. BOROWITZ, J. L. Catecholamine binding complex in bovine adrenal medulla. Possible involvement of calcium. *Biochem. Pharmacol.* 19: 2475–2481, 1970.
32. BOROWITZ, J. L., K. FUWA, AND N. WEINER. Distribution of metals and catecholamines in bovine adrenal medulla subfractions. *Nature* 205: 42–43, 1965.
33. BOYD, I. A., AND T. FORRESTER. The release of adenosine triphosphate from frog skeletal muscle in vitro. *J. Physiol., London* 199: 115–135, 1968.
34. BURACK, W. R., E. AVERY, P. R. DRASKÓCZY, AND N. WEINER. The number of catecholamine storage granules in the adrenal medulla. In: *Technical Documentary Report No. 62–119*. USAF School of Aerospace Medicine, Aerospace Medical Division (AFSC), Brooks Air Force Base, Texas, 1962, p. 1–4.
35. BURACK, W. R., AND P. R. DRASKÓCZY. The mode of secretion of catecholamines from the adrenal medulla. *J. Pharmacol. Exptl. Therap.* 138: 165–169, 1962.
36. BURFORD, H. J., AND J. B. GILL. Calcium and secretion in normal and supersensitive submaxillary glands of the cat. *Biochem. Pharmacol.* 17: 1881–1892, 1968.
37. BUTTERWORTH, K. R., AND M. MANN. The release of adrenaline and noradrenaline from the adrenal gland of the cat by acetylcholine. *Brit. J. Pharmacol.* 12: 422–426, 1957.
38. BYGDEMAN, S., AND U. S. VON EULER. Resynthesis of catechol hormones in the cat's adrenal medulla. *Acta Physiol. Scand.* 44: 375–383, 1958.
39. BYGDEMAN, S., U. S. VON EULER, AND B. HÖKFELT. Resynthesis of adrenaline in the rabbit's adrenal medulla during insulin-induced hypoglycemia. *Acta Physiol. Scand.* 49: 21–28, 1960.
40. CALLEJA, G. B., AND G. T. REYNOLDS. Experimental demonstration of ATP on the muscle cell surface. *Rev. Can. Biol.* 29: 395–398, 1970.
41. CANNON, W. B., AND A. ROSENBLUETH. L'excitabilité électrique de la surrénale dénervée. *Compt. Rend. Soc. Biol.* 124: 1262–1264, 1937.
42. CARLSSON, A., AND N-Å. HILLARP. Release of adenosine triphosphate along with adrenaline and noradrenaline following stimulation of the adrenal medulla. *Acta Physiol. Scand.* 37: 235–239, 1956.
43. CARLSSON, A., N-Å. HILLARP, AND B. HÖKFELT. The concomitant release of adenosine triphosphate and catecholamines from the adrenal medulla. *J. Biol. Chem.* 227: 243–252, 1957.
44. CECCHI, X., M. CANESSA-FISCHER, A. MATURANA, AND S. FISCHER. The molecular organization of nerve membranes. II. Glycolytic enzymes and ATP synthesis by plasma membranes of squid retinal axons. *Arch. Biochem. Biophys.* 145: 240–247, 1971.
45. COSTERO, I., A. CHÉVEZ, L. PERALTA, E. MONROY, AND F. RAMÓN. Rhythmic cellular movements in tissue culture of pheochromocytoma and adrenal medulla. *Texas Rep. Biol. Med.* 23, Suppl. 1: 213–220, 1965.
46. COUPLAND, R. E. Electron microscopic observations on the structure of the rat adrenal medulla. I. The ultrastructure and organization of chromaffin cells in the normal adrenal medulla. *J. Anat.* 99: 231–254, 1965.
47. COUPLAND, R. E. *The Natural History of the Chromaffin Cell*. London: Longmans, Green, 1965.
48. CRAGG, B. G. Are there structural alterations in synapses related to functioning. *Proc. Roy. Soc. London Ser. B* 171: 319–323, 1968.
49. CRAMER, W. Further observations on the thyroid-adrenal apparatus. A histochemical method for the demonstration of the adrenaline granules in the suprarenal gland. *J. Physiol., London* 52: viii–x, 1918.
50. CRAMER, W. *Fever, Heat Regulation, Climate and Thyroid-Adrenal Apparatus*. London: Longmans, Green, 1928.
51. D'ANZI, F. A. Morphological and biochemical observations on the catecholamine storing vesicles of rat adrenomedullary cells during insulin induced hypoglycemia. *Am. J. Anat.* 125: 381–397, 1969.
52. DEL CASTILLO, J., AND B. KATZ. Quantal components of the end plate potential. *J. Physiol., London* 124: 560–573, 1954.
53. DEL CASTILLO, J., AND B. KATZ. La base "quantale" de la

transmission neuro-musculaire. In: *Microphysiologie Comparée des Elémentes Excitables.* Paris: Colloq. Intern. CNRS, 1957, vol. 67, p. 245–258.
54. DE QUATTRO, V., R. MARONDE, T. NAGATSU, AND N. ALEXANDER. Altered norepinephrine synthesis and storage in the hypertensive buffer denervated rabbit (Abstract). *Federation Proc.* 27: 240, 1968.
55. DE ROBERTIS, E. D. P., W. W. NOWINSKI, AND F. A. SAEZ. *Cell Biology.* Philadelphia: Saunders, 1965.
56. DE ROBERTIS, E. D. P., AND D. D. SABATINI. Submicroscopic analysis of the secretory process in the adrenal medulla. *Federation Proc.* 19, Suppl. 5: 70–78, 1960.
57. DE ROBERTIS, E., AND A. VAZ FERREIRA. Electron microscopic study of the excretion of catechol-containing droplets in the adrenal medulla. *Exptl. Cell Res.* 12: 568–574, 1957.
58. DINER, O. L'expulsion des granules de la médullo-surrénale chez le hamster. *Compt. Rend.* 265: 616–619, 1967.
59. DINGLE, J. T. Vacuoles, vesicles and lysosomes. *Brit. Med. Bull.* 24: 141–145, 1968.
60. DOUGLAS, W. W. A possible mechanism of neurosecretion: release of vasopressin by depolarization and its dependence on calcium. *Nature* 197: 81–82, 1963.
61. DOUGLAS, W. W. Calcium-dependent links in stimulus-secretion coupling in the adrenal medulla and neurohypophysis. In: *Mechanism of Release of Biogenic Amines,* edited by U. S. von Euler, S. Rosell, and B. Uvnäs. Oxford: Pergamon Press, 1966, p. 267–289.
62. DOUGLAS, W. W. Stimulus-secretion coupling: the concept and clues from chromaffin and other cells. *Brit. J. Pharmacol.* 34: 451–474, 1968.
63. DOUGLAS, W. W., AND T. KANNO. The effect of amethocaine on acetylcholine-induced depolarization and catecholamine secretion in the adrenal chromaffin cell. *Brit. J. Pharmacol.* 30: 612–619, 1967.
64. DOUGLAS, W. W., T. KANNO, AND S. R. SAMPSON. Intracellular recording from adrenal chromaffin cells: effects of acetylcholine, hexamethonium and potassium on membrane potentials. *J. Physiol., London* 186: 125–126P, 1966.
65. DOUGLAS, W. W., T. KANNO, AND S. R. SAMPSON. Effects of acetylcholine and other medullary secretagogues and antagonists on the membrane potential of adrenal chromaffin cells: an analysis employing techniques of tissue culture. *J. Physiol., London* 188: 107–120, 1967.
66. DOUGLAS, W. W., T. KANNO, AND S. R. SAMPSON. Influence of the ionic environment on the membrane potential of adrenal chromaffin cells and on the depolarizing effects of acetylcholine. *J. Physiol., London* 191: 107–121, 1967.
67. DOUGLAS, W. W., AND A. M. POISNER. Stimulation of uptake of Ca^{45} in the adrenal gland by acetylcholine. *Nature* 192: 1299, 1961.
68. DOUGLAS, W. W., AND A. M. POISNER. On the mode of action of acetylcholine in evoking adrenal medullary secretion: increased uptake of calcium during the secretory response. *J. Physiol., London* 162: 385–392, 1962.
69. DOUGLAS, W. W., AND A. M. POISNER. Stimulus-secretion coupling in a neurosecretory organ: the role of calcium in the release of vasopressin from the neurohypophysis. *J. Physiol., London* 172: 1–18, 1964.
70. DOUGLAS, W. W., AND A. M. POISNER. Calcium movement in the neurohypophysis of the rat and its relation to the release of vasopressin. *J. Physiol., London* 172: 19–30, 1964.
71. DOUGLAS, W. W., AND A. M. POISNER. Efflux of adenine nucleotides and their derivatives and of protein from adrenal glands during stimulation of the splanchnic nerve or exposure to acetylcholine (Abstract). *Proc. Intern. Congr. Physiol. Sciences, 23rd, Tokyo, 1965,* p. 484.
72. DOUGLAS, W. W., AND A. M. POISNER. Evidence that the secreting adrenal chromaffin cell releases catecholamines directly from ATP-rich granules. *J. Physiol., London* 183: 236–248, 1966.
73. DOUGLAS, W. W., AND A. M. POISNER. On the relation between ATP splitting and secretion in the adrenal chromaffin cell: extrusion of ATP (unhydrolysed) during release of catecholamines. *J. Physiol., London* 183: 249–256, 1966.
74. DOUGLAS, W. W., A. M. POISNER, AND R. P. RUBIN. Efflux of adenine nucleotides from perfused adrenal glands exposed to nicotine and other chromaffin cell stimulants. *J. Physiol., London* 179: 130–137, 1965.
75. DOUGLAS, W. W., AND R. P. RUBIN. The role of calcium in the secretory response of the adrenal medulla to acetylcholine. *J. Physiol., London* 159: 40–57, 1961.
76. DOUGLAS, W. W., AND R. P. RUBIN. Mechanism of nicotinic action at the adrenal medulla: calcium as a link in stimulus-secretion coupling. *Nature* 192: 1087–1089, 1961.
77. DOUGLAS, W. W., AND R. P. RUBIN. The mechanism of catecholamine release from the adrenal medulla and the role of calcium in stimulus-secretion coupling. *J. Physiol., London* 167: 288–310, 1963.
78. DOUGLAS, W. W., AND R. P. RUBIN. The effects of alkaline earths and other divalent cations on adrenal medullary secretion. *J. Physiol., London* 175: 231–241, 1964.
79. DOUGLAS, W. W., AND R. P. RUBIN. Stimulant action of barium on the adrenal medulla. *Nature* 203: 305–307, 1964.
80. DREYER, G. P. On secretory nerves to the suprarenal capsules. *Am. J. Physiol.* 2: 203–219, 1899.
81. DUCH, D. S., O. H. VIVEROS, AND N. KIRSHNER. Endogenous inhibitors of dopamine-β-hydroxylase (Abstract). *Federation Proc.* 27: 837, 1968.
82. DUCH, D. S., O. H. VIVEROS, AND N. KIRSHNER. Endogenous inhibitors in adrenal medulla of dopamine-β-hydroxylase. *Biochem. Pharmacol.* 17: 255–264, 1968.
83. EADE, N. R., AND D. R. WOOD. The release of adrenaline and noradrenaline from the adrenal medulla of the cat during sphanchnic stimulation. *Brit. J. Pharmacol.* 13: 390–394, 1958.
84. ELFVIN, L-G. The fine structure of the cell surface of chromaffin cells in the rat adrenal medulla. *J. Ultrastruct. Res.* 12: 263–286, 1965.
85. ELFVIN, L-G. The ultrastructure of the capillary fenestrae in the adrenal medulla of the rat. *J. Ultrastruct. Res.* 12: 687–704, 1965.
86. ELLIOT, T. R. The control of the suprarenal glands by the splanchnic nerves. *J. Physiol., London* 44: 374–409, 1912.
87. ELLIOT, T. R. The innervation of the adrenal glands. *J. Physiol., London* 46: 285–290, 1913.
88. ELLIS, H. V., A. R. JOHNSON, AND N. C. MORAN. Selective release of histamine from rat mast cells by several drugs. *J. Pharmacol. Exptl. Therap.* 175: 627–631, 1970.
89. ERÄNKÖ, O. Nodular hyperplasia and increase of noradrenaline content in the adrenal medulla of nicotine treated rats. *Acta Pathol. Microbiol. Scand.* 36: 210–218, 1955.
90. ERÄNKÖ, O., AND M. HÄRKÖNEN. Distribution and concentration of adrenaline and noradrenaline in the adrenal medulla of the rat following depletion induced by muscular work. *Acta Physiol. Scand.* 51: 247–253, 1961.
91. ERÄNKÖ, O., AND M. HÄRKÖNEN. Long term effects of muscular work on the adrenal medulla of the mouse. *Endocrinology* 69: 186–187, 1961.
92. ERÄNKÖ, O., V. HOPSU, AND L. RAÏSÄNEN. Effect of prolonged administration of nicotine on the medullary volume and the distribution of noradrenaline in the adrenals of the rat, the mouse, and the guinea pig. *Endocrinology* 65: 293–297, 1959.
93. ERÄNKÖ, O., V. HOPSU, AND L. RAÏSÄNEN. Changes induced by prolonged administration of nicotine in the distribution of cholinesterases and acid phosphatase in the adrenal medulla of the rat. *J. Neurochem.* 4: 332–337, 1959.
94. EULER, U. S. VON. Catecholamines in nerve and organ granules. In: *Mechanisms of Release of Biogenic Amines,* edited by U. S. von Euler, S. Rosell, and B. Uvnäs. Oxford: Pergamon Press, 1966, p. 211–222.
95. EULER, U. S. VON. Adrenal medullary secretion and its neural control. In: *Neuroendocrinology,* edited by L. Martini

and W. F. Ganong. New York: Acad. Press, 1967, vol. II, p. 283-333.
96. EULER, U. S. VON. Some aspects of the mechanisms involved in adrenergic neurotransmission. *Perspect. Biol. Med.* 12: 79-94, 1968.
97. EULER, U. S. VON. Effect of some metabolic factors and drugs in uptake and release of catecholamines in vitro and in vivo. In: *New Aspects of Storage and Release Mechanisms of Catecholamines*, edited by H. J. Schümann and G. Kroneberg. Berlin: Springer Verlag, 1970, p. 144-158.
98. FAWCETT, C. P., A. E. POWELL, AND H. SACHS. Biosynthesis and release of neurophysin. *Endocrinology* 83: 1299-1310, 1968.
99. FELDBERG, W. The action of bee venom, cobra venom and lysolecithin on the adrenal medulla. *J. Physiol., London* 99: 104-118, 1940.
100. FELDBERG, W., AND B. MINZ. Das Auftreten eines acetylcholinartigen Stoffes im Nebennierenvenenblut bei Reizung der Nervi splanchnici. *Arch. Ges. Physiol.* 233: 657-682, 1934.
101. FELDBERG, W., B. MINZ, AND H. TSUDZIMURA. The mechanism of the nervous discharge of adrenaline. *J. Physiol., London* 81: 286-304, 1934.
102. FERRIS, R. M., O. H. VIVEROS, L. ARQUEROS, AND N. KIRSHNER. Effects of drugs on adenosine triphosphate-magnesium stimulated uptake and release of catecholamines in isolated adrenal storage vesicles (Abstract). *Federation Proc.* 28: 287, 1969.
103. FERRIS, R. M., O. H. VIVEROS, AND N. KIRSHNER. Effects of various agents on the Mg^{2+}-ATP stimulated incorporation and release of catecholamines by isolated bovine adrenomedullary storage vesicles and on secretion from the adrenal medulla. *Biochem. Pharmacol.* 19: 505-514, 1970.
104. FOLKOW, B., AND J. HÄGGENDAL. Some aspects of the quantal release of the adrenergic transmitter. In: *New Aspects of Storage and Release Mechanisms of Catecholamines*, edited by H. J. Schümann and G. Kroneberg. Berlin: Springer Verlag, 1970, p. 91-97.
105. FOLKOW, B., J. HÄGGENDAL, AND B. LISANDER. Extent of release and elimination of noradrenaline at peripheral adrenergic nerve terminals. *Acta Physiol. Scand. Suppl.* 307: 1-38, 1967.
106. FRANZEN, D. Beiträge zur Morphologie und Chemohistologie des Nebennierenmarks des Goldhamsters (Mesocricetus auratus). *Anat. Anz.* 115: 35-58, 1964.
107. GABE, M., AND L. ARVY. Gland cells. In: *The Cell*, edited by J. Brachet and A. E. Mirsky. New York: Acad. Press, 1961, vol. 5, part 2, p. 1-88.
108. GARDIER, R. W., B. E. ABREU, A. B. RICHARDS, AND H. C. HERRLICH. Specific blockade of the adrenal medulla. *J. Pharmacol. Exptl. Therap.* 130: 340-345, 1960.
109. GARRETT, J., W. E. OSSWALD, E. RODRIGUES-PEREIRA, AND S. GUIMĀRAES. Catecholamine release from the isolated perfused adrenal. *Arch. Exptl. Pathol. Pharmakol.* 250: 325-336, 1965.
110. GILLARD, R. D. The simple chemistry of calcium and its relevance to biological systems. In: *Calcium and Cellular Function*, edited by A. W. Cuthbert. New York: St. Martin's, 1970, p. 3-9.
111. GINGELL, D., D. R. GARROD, AND J. F. PALMER. Divalent cations and cell adhesion. In: *Calcium and Cellular Function*, edited by A. W. Cuthbert. New York: St. Martin's, 1970, p. 59-64.
112. GLADSTONE, G. P., AND W. E. VAN HEYNINGEN. Staphylococcal leucocidins. *Brit. J. Exptl. Pathol.* 38: 123-137, 1957.
113. GORI, Z. M. Electron microscopic study on the excretion of the catechol-containing droplets across the cell membranes and capillary walls (Abstract). In: *Third European Regional Conference on Electron Microscopy*. Prague: Publishing House of the Czechoslovak Academy of Sciences, 1964, p. 493-494.
114. GOZ, B. Properties of a microsomal adenosine triphosphatase from the adrenal medulla. *Biochem. Pharmacol.* 16: 593-596, 1967.

115. GRAF, J. Zur Strukturbindung und Secretion der Catecholamine. Histochemische und pharmakologische Untersuchimgen mit dem Electromikroskop. *Arch. Intern. Pharmacodyn.* 159: 170-184, 1966.
116. GRAUMANN, W. Beobachtungen über Bildung und Sekretion perjodatreaktiver Stoffe im Nebennierenmark des Goldhamsters. *Z. Anat. Entwicklungsgesch.* 119: 415-430, 1956.
117. GREENBERG, R., AND C. A. KOLEN. Effects of acetylcholine and calcium ions on the spontaneous release of epinephrine from catecholamine granules. *Proc. Soc. Exptl. Biol. Med.* 121: 1179-1184, 1966.
118. GREENBERG, R., AND J. E. P. TORNAN. Effects of drugs on the histologically visualized catecholamines of the adrenal medulla of the rat. *Arch. Intern. Pharmacodyn.* 159: 87-108, 1966.
119. GRILLO, M. Extracellular synaptic vesicles in the mouse heart. *J. Cell Biol.* 47: 547-553, 1970.
120. HAGEN, P., AND R. J. BARRNETT. The storage of amines in the chromaffin cell. In: *Adrenergic Mechanisms*, edited by R. J. Vane, G. E. W. Wolstenholme, and M. O'Connor. London: Churchill, 1960, p. 83-99.
121. HÄGGENDAL, J. Some further aspects on the release of the adrenergic transmitter. In: *New Aspects of Storage and Release Mechanisms of Catecholamines*, edited by H. J. Schümann and G. Kroneberg. Berlin: Springer Verlag, 1970, p. 100-109.
122. HARRIS, H. *Cell Fusion*. Oxford: Clarendon Press, 1970.
123. HARTMAN, B. K., P. B. MOLINOFF, AND S. UDENFRIEND. Increased rate of synthesis of dopamine beta hydroxylase (DBH) in adrenals of reserpinized rats (Abstract). *Pharmacologist* 12: 286, 1970.
124. HEDQVIST, P. Studies on the effects of prostaglandins E_1 and E_2 on the sympathetic neuromuscular transmission in some animal tissues. *Acta Physiol. Scand. Suppl.* 345: 1-40, 1970.
125. HEDQVIST, P., H. LAGERCRANTZ, AND L. STJÄRNE. Adenine nucleotides and catecholamine mobilization in adrenal medulla and in sympathetic nerves. *Acta Physiol. Scand.* 74: 40-41A, 1968.
126. HELLE, K. Some chemical and physical properties of the soluble protein fraction of bovine adrenal chromaffin granules. *Mol. Pharmacol.* 2: 298-310, 1966.
127. HEMPEL, K., AND H. F. K. MÄNNL. Quantitative Analyse der Catecholamin-Biosynthese des Nebennierenmarks in Vivo und Ruhesekretion neugebildeter Amine unter besonnonderer Berücksichtigung des Dopamins. *Arch. Exptl. Pathol. Pharmakol.* 264: 363-388, 1969.
128. HERMANN, H., F. JOURDAN, G. MORIN, AND J. VIAL. Adrénalinosécrétion par excitation directe de la glande surrénde énervée chez le chien. *Compt. Rend. Soc. Biol.* 122: 579-582, 1936.
129. HILLARP, N.-Å. Structure of the synapse and the peripheral innervation apparatus of the autonomic nervous system. *Acta Anat. Suppl.* IV: 1-153, 1946.
130. HILLARP, N.-Å. Enzymic systems involving adenosinephosphatases in the adrenaline and noradrenaline containing granules of the adrenal medulla. *Acta Physiol. Scand.* 42: 144-165, 1958.
131. HILLARP, N.-Å. Adenosinephosphates and inorganic phosphate in the adrenaline and noradrenaline containing granules of the adrenal medulla. *Acta Physiol. Scand.* 42: 321-332, 1958.
132. HILLARP, N.-Å. Isolation and some biochemical properties of the catecholamine granules in the cow adrenal medulla. *Acta Physiol. Scand.* 43: 82-96, 1958.
133. HILLARP, N.-Å. The release of catecholamines from the amine containing granules of the adrenal medulla. *Acta Physiol. Scand.* 43: 292-302, 1958.
134. HILLARP, N.-Å. Further observations on the state of the catecholamines stored in the adrenal medullary granules. *Acta Physiol. Scand.* 47: 271-279, 1959.
135. HILLARP, N.-Å. Catecholamines: mechanisms of storage and release. *Acta Endocrinol.* 50, Suppl. 1: 181-185, 1960.
136. HILLARP, N.-Å., AND B. HÖKFELT. Cytological demonstration

of noradrenaline in the suprarenal medulla under conditions of varied secretory activity. *Endocrinology* 55: 255–260, 1954.

137. HILLARP, N.-Å., B. HÖKFELT, AND B. NILSON. The cytology of the adrenal medullary cells with special reference to the storage and secretion of the sympathomimetic amines. *Acta Anat.* 21: 155–167, 1954.

138. HILLARP, N.-Å., S. LAGERSTEDT, AND B. NILSON. The isolation of a granular fraction from the suprarenal medulla, containing the sympathomimetic catecholamines. *Acta Physiol. Scand.* 29: 251–263, 1953.

139. HILLARP, N.-Å., AND B. NILSON. The structure of the adrenaline and noradrenaline containing granules in the adrenal medullary cells with reference to the storage and release of the sympathomimetic amines. *Acta Physiol. Scand. Suppl.* 113: 79–107, 1954.

140. HILLARP, N.-Å., B. NILSON, AND B. HÖGBERG. Adenosine triphosphate in the adrenal medulla of the cow. *Nature* 176: 1032–1033, 1955.

141. HILLARP, N.-Å., AND G. THIEME. Nucleotides in the catecholamine granules of the adrenal medulla. *Acta Physiol. Scand.* 45: 328–338, 1959.

142. HION, V. Zur Histologie der Nebennieren bei Erschöpften tieren. *Folia Neuropathol. Estoniana* 7: 178–189, 1927.

143. HOKIN, M. R., B. G. BENFEY, AND L. E. HOKIN. Phospholipids and adrenaline secretion in guinea pig adrenal medulla. *J. Biol. Chem.* 233: 814–817, 1958.

144. HOLLAND, W. C., AND H. J. SCHÜMANN. Formation of catecholamines during splanchnic stimulation of the adrenal gland of the cat. *Brit. J. Pharmacol.* 11: 449–453, 1956.

145. HOUSSAY, B. A., AND E. A. MOLINELLI. Excitabilité des fibres adrenalinosecretoires der nerf grand splanchnique. Fréquences, seuil et optimum des stimulus. Role de l'ion calcium. *Compt. Rend. Soc. Biol.* 99: 172–174, 1928.

146. HOWELL, J. I., AND J. A. LUCY. Cell fusion induced by lysolecithin. *FEBS* 4: 147–150, 1969.

147. ICHIKAWA, A. Fine structural changes in response to hormonal stimulation of the perfused canine pancreas. *J. Cell Biol.* 24: 369–385, 1965.

148. ICHIKAWA, Y., AND T. YAMANO. Cytochrome 559 in the microsomes of the adrenal medulla. *Biochem. Biophys. Res. Commun.* 20: 263–268, 1965.

149. IMMS, F. J., D. R. LONDON, AND R. L. B. NEAME. The secretion of catecholamines from the adrenal gland following arginine infusion in the rat. *J. Physiol., London* 200: 55–56P, 1969.

150. JAANUS, S. D., E. MIELE, AND R. P. RUBIN. The analysis of the inhibitory effect of local anaesthetics and propranolol on adrenomedullary secretion evoked by calcium or acetylcholine. *Brit. J. Pharmacol.* 31: 319–330, 1967.

151. JAANUS, S. D., E. MIELE, AND R. P. RUBIN. The action of guanethidine on the adrenal medulla of the cat. *Brit. J. Pharmacol.* 33: 560–569, 1968.

152. JACOBJ, C. Beiträge zur physiologischen und pharmakologischen Kenntniss der Darmbewegungen mit besonderorer Berückschtigung der Beziehung der Nebenniere zu Denselben. *Arch. Exptl. Pathol. Pharmakol.* 29: 171–211, 1892.

153. JAHN, T. L., AND E. C. BOVEE. Protoplasmatic movements within cells. *Physiol. Rev.* 49: 793–862, 1969.

154. JOHNSON, A. R., AND N. C. MORAN. Selective release of histamine from rat mast cells by compound 48/80 and antigen. *Am. J. Physiol.* 216: 453–459, 1969.

155. JOHNSON, A. R., AND N. C. MORAN. The selective release of histamine from rat mast cells. In: *Cellular and Humoral Mechanisms in Anaphylaxis and Allergy*, edited by H. Z. Movat. Basel: Karger, 1969, p. 122–128.

156. JUNQUEIRA, L. C. U., AND G. C. HIRSCH. Cell secretion: a study of pancreas and salivary glands. In: *International Review of Cytology*, edited by G. H. Bourne and J. F. Danielli. New York: Acad. Press, 1956, vol. v, p. 323–354.

157. KANNO, T., AND W. W. DOUGLAS. Effect of rapid application of acetylcholine or depolarizing current on trans-membrane potentials of adrenal chromaffin cells (Abstract). *Proc. Can. Federation Biol. Soc.* 10: 39, 1969.

158. KATZ, B. *The Release of Neural Transmitter Substances*. Liverpool: Liverpool Univ. Press, 1969.

159. KATZ, B., AND R. MILEDI. The timing of calcium action during neuromuscular transmission. *J. Physiol., London* 189: 535–544, 1967.

160. KATZ, B., AND R. MILEDI. A study of synaptic transmission in the absence of nerve impulses. *J. Physiol., London* 192: 407–436, 1967.

161. KIRSHNER, A. G., AND N. KIRSHNER. A specific soluble protein from the catecholamine storage vesicles of bovine adrenal medulla. II. Physical characterization. *Biochim. Biophys. Acta* 181: 219–225, 1969.

162. KIRSHNER, N. Pathway of noradrenaline formation from Dopa. *J. Biol. Chem.* 226: 821–825, 1957.

163. KIRSHNER, N. Storage and secretion of adrenal catecholamines. In: *Advances in Biochemical Psychopharmacology*, edited by E. Costa and P. Greengard. New York: Raven Press, 1969, vol. 1, p. 71–89.

164. KIRSHNER, N. The adrenal medulla. In: *The Structure and Function of Nervous Tissue*, edited by G. H. Bourne. New York: Acad. Press, 1972, vol. 5, p. 163–204.

165. KIRSHNER, N., AND McC. GOODALL. The formation of adrenaline from noradrenaline. *Biochim. Biophys. Acta* 24: 658–659, 1957.

166. KIRSHNER, N., AND A. G. KIRSHNER. Chromogranin A, dopamine-β-hydroxylase and secretion from the adrenal medulla. *Phil. Trans. Roy. Soc. London Ser. B* 261: 279–289, 1971.

167. KIRSHNER, N., A. G. KIRSHNER, AND D. L. KAMIN. Adenosine triphosphatase activity of adrenal medulla catecholamine granules. *Biochim. Biophys. Acta* 113: 332–335, 1966.

168. KIRSHNER, N., H. J. SAGE, W. J. SMITH, AND A. G. KIRSHNER. Release of catecholamines and specific protein from adrenal glands. *Science* 154: 529–531, 1966.

169. KIRSHNER, N., H. J. SAGE, AND W. J. SMITH. Mechanism of secretion from the adrenal medulla. II. Release of catecholamines and storage vesicle protein in response to chemical stimulation. *Mol. Pharmacol.* 3: 254–265, 1967.

170. KIRSHNER, N., AND W. J. SMITH. Metabolic requirements for secretion from the adrenal medulla (Abstract). *Science* 154: 422, 1966.

171. KIRSHNER, N., AND W. J. SMITH. Metabolic requirements for secretion from the adrenal medulla. *Life Sci., Part 1* 8: 799–803, 1969.

172. KIRSHNER, N., AND O. H. VIVEROS. Quantal aspects of the secretion of catecholamines and dopamine-β-hydroxylase from the adrenal medulla. In: *New Aspects of Storage and Release Mechanisms of Catecholamines (Bayer-Symposium II)*, edited by H. J. Schümann and G. Kroneberg. Berlin: Springer Verlag, 1970, p. 78–88.

173. KOCH, A. L. Some calculations on the turbidity of mitochondria and bacteria. *Biochim. Biophys. Acta* 51: 429–441, 1961.

174. KOVACIC, V., AND R. L. ROBINSON. Drug-induced secretion of catecholamines by the perfused adrenal gland of the dog during nicotine blockade. *J. Pharmacol. Exptl. Therap.* 175: 178–182, 1970.

175. KUROSUMI, K. Electron microscopic analysis of the secretion mechanism. In: *International Review of Cytology*, edited by G. H. Bourne and J. F. Danielli. New York: Acad. Press, 1961, vol. 11, p. 1–124.

176. KVETŇANSKÝ, R. V., G. P. GEWIRTZ, V. K. WIESE, AND I. J. KOPIN. Enhanced synthesis of adrenal dopamine-β-hydroxylase induced by repeated immobilization in rats. *Mol. Pharmacol.* 7: 81–86, 1971.

177. KVETŇANSKÝ, R., AND L. MIKULAJ. Adrenal and urinary catecholamines in rats during adaptation to repeated immobilization stress. *Endocrinology* 87: 738–743, 1970.

178. KVETŇANSKÝ, R., AND L. MIKULAJ. Elevation of adrenal

tyrosine hydroxylase and phenylethanolamine-N-methyl transferase by repeated immobilization stress. *Endocrinology* 87: 744–749, 1970.
179. LACY, P. E., S. L. HOWELL, D. A. YOUNG, AND J. C. FINK. New hypothesis of insulin secretion. *Nature* 219: 1177–1179, 1968.
180. LADURON, P., AND F. BELPAIRE. Tissue fractionation and catecholamines. II. Intracellular distribution patterns of tyrosine hydroxylase, dopa-decarboxylase, dopamine-β-hydroxylase, phenylethylamine-N-methyltransferase and monoamine oxydase in adrenal medulla. *Biochem. Pharmacol.* 17: 1127–1140, 1968.
181. LECOMTE, J., AND A. CESSION-FOSSION. Action stimulante de deux histamino-libérateurs sur la medullosurrénale du rat. *Compt. Rend. Soc. Biol.* 159: 2282–2283, 1965.
182. LEDUC, J. Catecholamine production and release in exposure and acclimation to cold. *Acta Physiol. Scand. Suppl.* 183: 1–101, 1961.
183. LEE, F. L., AND U. TRENDELENBURG. Muscarinic transmission of preganglionic impulses to the adrenal medulla of the cat. *J. Pharmacol. Exptl. Therap.* 158: 73–79, 1967.
184. LEHNINGER, A. L. Water uptake and extrusion by mitochondria in relation to oxidative phosphorylation. *Physiol. Rev.* 42: 467–517, 1962.
185. LEVER, J. D. Electron microscopic observations on the normal and denervated adrenal medulla of the rat. *Endocrinology* 57: 621–635, 1955.
186. LEVER, J. D., AND J. A. FINDLAY. Similar structural bases for the storage and release of secretory material in adrenomedullary and β-pancreatic cells. *Histochemie* 74: 317–324, 1966.
187. LEVIN, E. Y., B. LEVENBERG, AND S. KAUFMAN. The enzymatic conversion of 3,4-dihydroxy-phenylethylamine to norepinephrine. *J. Biol. Chem.* 235: 2080–2086, 1960.
188. LEVY, D. A., AND J. A. CARLTON. Influence of temperature on the inhibition by colchicine of allergic histamine release. *Proc. Soc. Exptl. Biol. Med.* 130: 1333–1336, 1969.
189. LISHAJKO, F. Influence of chloride ions and ATP-Mg^{++} on the release of catecholamines from isolated adrenal medullary granules. *Acta Physiol. Scand.* 75: 255–256, 1969.
190. LISHAJKO, F. Osmotic factors determining the release of catecholamines from isolated chromaffin cell granules. *Acta Physiol. Scand.* 79: 64–75, 1970.
191. LISHAJKO, F. Releasing effect of calcium and phosphate on catecholamines, ATP, and protein from chromaffin cell granules. *Acta Physiol. Scand.* 79: 575–584, 1970.
192. LISHAJKO, F. Effect of calcium phosphate and RNA on the release of catecholamines, ATP and protein from isolated medullary granules. *Life Sci., Part 1* 9: 695–699, 1970.
193. MAAS, J. W., AND R. W. COLBURN. Coordination chemistry and membrane function with particular reference to the synapse and catecholamine transport. *Nature* 208: 41–46, 1965.
194. MALAMED, S., A. M. POISNER, J. M. TRIFARÓ, AND W. W. DOUGLAS. The fate of the chromaffin granule during catecholamine release from the adrenal medulla. III. Recovery of a purified fraction of electron-translucent structures. *Biochem. Pharmacol.* 17: 241–246, 1968.
195. MALAWISTA, S. E., AND K. G. BENSCH. Human polymorphonuclear leucocytes: demonstration of microtubules and effect of colchicine. *Science* 156: 521–522, 1967.
196. MALMEJAC, J. Activity of the adrenal medulla and its regulation. *Physiol. Rev.* 44: 186–218, 1964.
197. MALVALDI, G., P. MERCACCI, AND M. P. VIOLA-MAGNI. Mitosis in adrenal medullary cells. *Experientia* 24: 475–476, 1968.
198. MANERY, J. F. Effects of Ca ions in membranes. *Federation Proc.* 25: 1804–1810, 1966.
199. MARLEY, E., AND W. D. M. PATON. The output of sympathetic amines from the cat's adrenal gland in response to splanchnic nerve activity. *J. Physiol., London* 155: 1–27, 1961.

200. MARLEY, E., AND G. I. PROUT. Physiology and pharmacology of the splanchnic adrenal medullary junction. *J. Physiol., London* 180: 483–513, 1965.
201. MARTIN, A. R. A further study of the statistical composition of the end plate potential. *J. Physiol., London* 130: 114–122, 1955.
202. MARTIN, A. R. Quantal nature of synaptic transmission. *Physiol. Rev.* 46: 51–66, 1966.
203. MATSUDA, T., F. HATA, AND H. YOSHIDA. Stimulatory effect of Na$^+$ and ATP on the release of acetylcholine from synaptic vesicles. *Biochim. Biophys. Acta* 150: 739–741, 1968.
204. MATTHEWS, E. K. Membrane potential measurement in cells of the adrenal gland and the effects of potassium. *J. Physiol., London* 184: 22–23P, 1966.
205. MATTHEWS, E. K. Membrane potential measurement in cells of the adrenal gland. *J. Physiol., London* 189: 139–148, 1967.
206. MATTHEWS, E. K. Calcium and hormone release. In: *Calcium and Cellular Function*, edited by A. W. Cuthbert. New York: St. Martin's, 1970, p. 163–182.
207. MATTHEWS, E. K., AND M. SAFFRAN. Steroid production and membrane potential measurement in cells of the adrenal cortex. *J. Physiol., London* 189: 149–161, 1967.
208. MATTHEWS, E. K., AND M. SAFFRAN. Effect of ACTH on the electrical properties of adrenocortical cells. *Nature* 219: 1369–1370, 1968.
209. MEVES, H. Experiments on internally perfused squid giant axons. *Ann. NY Acad. Sci.* 137: 807–817, 1966.
210. MIELE, E. Lack of effect of prostaglandin E$_1$ and F$_{1\alpha}$ on adrenomedullary catecholamine secretion evoked by various agents. In: *Prostaglandins, Peptides and Amines*, edited by P. Mantegazza and E. W. Horton. London: Acad. Press, 1969, p. 85–93.
211. MIELE, E., AND R. P. RUBIN. Further evidence for the dual action of local anaesthetics on the adrenal medulla. *J. Pharmacol. Exptl. Therap.* 161: 296–301, 1968.
212. MILEDI, R. Spontaneous synaptic potentials and quantal release of transmitter in the stellate ganglion of the squid. *J. Physiol., London* 192: 379–406, 1967.
213. MILEDI, R., AND C. R. SLATER. The action of calcium on neuronal synapses in the squid. *J. Physiol., London* 184: 473–498, 1966.
214. MIRAGLIA, T. Histochemical studies on the adrenal medullary cells of the marmoset (Callithrix jacchus). *J. Histochem. Cytochem.* 13: 595–598, 1965.
215. NAGASAWA, J., W. W. DOUGLAS, AND R. A. SCHULZ. Ultrastructural evidence for secretion by exocytosis and of "synaptic vesicle" formation in posterior pituitary glands. *Nature* 227: 407–409, 1970.
216. NAGATSU, T. Endogenous inhibitors of dopamine-β-hydroxylase. In: *Biological and Chemical Aspects of Oxygenases*, edited by K. E. Block and O. Hayaishi. Tokyo: Maruzen, 1966, p. 273–277.
217. NAGATSU, T., H. KUSUYA, AND H. KIKADA. Inhibition of dopamine-β-hydroxylase by sulfhydryl compounds and the nature of the natural inhibitors. *Biochim. Biophys. Acta* 139: 319–327, 1967.
218. NÈVE, P., C. WILLEMS, AND J. E. DUMONT. Involvement of the microtubule-microfilament system in thyroid secretion. *Exptl. Cell Res.* 63: 457–460, 1970.
219. NORMANN, T. C. Experimentally induced exocytosis of neurosecretory granules. *Exptl. Cell Res.* 55: 285–287, 1969.
220. OKA, M., T. OHUCHI, H. YOSHIDA, AND R. IMAIZUMI. The importance of calcium in the release of catecholamines from the adrenal medulla. *Japan. J. Pharmacol.* 15: 348–365, 1965.
221. OKA, M., T. OHUCHI, H. YOSHIDA, AND R. IMAIZUMI. Effect of adenosine triphosphate and magnesium on the release of catecholamines from adrenal medullary granules. *Biochim. Biophys. Acta* 97: 170–171, 1965.
222. OKA, M., T. OHUCHI, H. YOSHIDA, AND R. IMAIZUMI. Selec-

tive release of noradrenaline and adrenaline from isolated adrenal medullary particles. *Life Sci.* 5: 433-438, 1966.
223. OKA, M., T. OHUCHI, H. YOSHIDA, AND R. IMAIZUMI. Stimulatory effect of adenosine triphosphate and magnesium on the release of catecholamines from adrenal medullary granules. *Japan. J. Pharmacol.* 17: 199-207, 1967.
224. OKADA, Y., AND F. MURAYAMA. Requirement of calcium ions for the cell fusion reaction of animal cells by HVJ. *Exptl. Cell Res.* 44: 527-551, 1966.
225. OKADA, Y., F. MURAYAMA, AND K. YAMADA. Requirement of energy for the cell fusion reaction of Ehrlich ascites tumor cells by HVJ. *Virology* 28: 115-130, 1968.
226. OLIVER, G., AND E. A. SCHÄFER. On the physiological action of extracts of the suprarenal capsules. *J. Physiol., London* 16: i-ivp, 1894.
227. OZAKI, M., Y. SUZUKI, Y. YAMORI, AND K. OKAMOTO. Adrenal catecholamine content in the spontaneously hypertensive rat. *Japan. Circulation J.* 32: 1367-1372, 1968.
228. PALADE, G. E. Functional changes in the structure of cell components. In: *Subcellular Particles*, edited by T. Hayashi. New York: Ronald Press, 1959, p. 64-80.
229. PATRICK, R. L., AND N. KIRSHNER. Effect of stimulation on the levels of tyrosine hydroxylase, dopamine-β-hydroxylase, and catecholamines in intact and denervated rat adrenal glands. *Mol. Pharmacol.* 7: 87-96, 1971.
230. PHILIPPU, A., AND H. J. SCHÜMANN. Der Einfluss von Calcium auf die Brenzakatechinaminfreitsetzung. *Experientia* 18: 138-140, 1962.
231. PHILIPPU, A., AND H. J. SCHÜMANN. Über die Bedeutung der Calcium und Magnesium für die Speicherung der Nebennierenmark-Hormone. *Arch. Exptl. Pathol. Pharmakol.* 252: 339-358, 1966.
232. PLATTNER, H., H. WINKLER, H. HÖRTNAGL, AND W. FALLER. A study of the adrenal medulla and its subcellular organelles by the freeze-etching method. *J. Ultrastruct. Res.* 28: 191-202, 1969.
233. PLETSCHER, A., K. H. BERNEIS, AND M. DA PRADA. A biophysical model for the storage and release of biogenic monoamines at the level of the storage organelles. In: *Biochemistry of Simple Neuronal Models*, edited by E. Costa and E. Giacobini. New York: Raven Press, 1970, p. 205-211.
234. POHORECKY, L., AND J. H. RUST. Studies on the cortical control of the adrenal medulla in the rat. *J. Pharmacol. Exptl. Therap.* 162: 227-238, 1968.
235. POISNER, A. M. Inhibition of ATP-induced effects on chromaffin granules (Abstract). *Federation Proc.* 28: 287, 1969.
236. POISNER, A. M. Actomyosin-like protein from the adrenal medulla (Abstract). *Federation Proc.* 29: 545, 1970.
237. POISNER, A. M. Release of transmitters from storage: a contractile model. In: *Biochemistry of Simple Neuronal Models*, edited by E. Costa and E. Giacobini. New York: Raven Press, 1970, p. 95-108.
238. POISNER, A. M., AND J. BERNSTEIN. A possible role of microtubules in catecholamine release from the adrenal medulla: effect of colchicine, vinca alkaloids, and Deuterium oxide. *J. Pharmacol. Exptl. Therap.* 177: 102-108, 1971.
239. POISNER, A. M., AND W. W. DOUGLAS. The need for calcium in adrenomedullary secretion evoked by biogenic amines, polypeptides, and muscarinic agents. *Proc. Soc. Exptl. Biol. Med.* 123: 62-64, 1966.
240. POISNER, A. M., AND W. W. DOUGLAS. A possible mechanism of release of posterior pituitary hormones involving adenosine triphosphate and an adenosine triphosphatase in the neurosecretory granules. *Mol. Pharmacol.* 4: 531-540, 1968.
241. POISNER, A. M., W. W. DOUGLAS, AND R. POISNER. ATP and ATPase in zymogen granules from bovine pancreas (Abstract). *Pharmacologist* 10: 199, 1968.
242. POISNER, A. M., AND M. HAVA. The role of adenosine triphosphate and adenosine triphosphatase in the release of catecholamines from the adrenal medulla. IV. Adenosine triphosphate-activated uptake of calcium by microsomes and mitochondria. *Mol. Pharmacol.* 6: 407-415, 1970.

243. POISNER, A. M., AND J. M. TRIFARÓ. The role of ATP and ATPase in the release of catecholamines from the adrenal medulla. I. ATP-evoked release of catecholamines, ATP, and protein from isolated chromaffin granules. *Mol. Pharmacol.* 3: 561-571, 1967.
244. POISNER, A. M., AND J. M. TRIFARÓ. Release of catecholamines from isolated adrenal chromaffin granules by endogenous ATP. *Mol. Pharmacol.* 4: 196-199, 1968.
245. POISNER, A. M., AND J. M. TRIFARÓ. The role of adenosine triphosphate and adenosine triphosphatase in the release of catecholamines from the adrenal medulla. III. Similarities between the effects of adenosine triphosphate on chromaffin granules and on mitochondria. *Mol. Pharmacol.* 5: 294-299, 1969.
246. POISNER, A. M., J. M. TRIFARÓ, AND W. W. DOUGLAS. The fate of the chromaffin granule during catecholamine release from the adrenal medulla. II. Loss of protein and retention of lipid in subcellular fractions. *Biochem. Pharmacol.* 16: 2101-2108, 1967.
247. RAHAMIMOFF, R. Role of calcium ions on neuromuscular transmission. In: *Calcium and Cellular Function*, edited by A. W. Cuthbert. New York: St. Martin's, 1970, p. 131-147.
248. RAJAN, K. T. Lysosomes and gout. *Nature* 210: 959-960, 1966.
249. RAMWELL, P. W., J. E. SHAW, W. W. DOUGLAS, AND A. M. POISNER. Efflux of prostaglandin from adrenal glands stimulated with acetylcholine. *Nature* 210: 273-274, 1966.
250. RASMUSSEN, H. Cell communication, calcium ions, and cyclic adenosine monophosphate. *Science* 170: 404-412, 1970.
251. ROBINSON, R. L. Stimulation of the catecholamine output of the isolated perfused adrenal gland of the dog by angiotensin and bradykinin. *J. Pharmacol. Exptl. Therap.* 156: 252-257, 1967.
252. ROSE, I. A. The state of magnesium in cells as estimated from the adenylate kinase equilibrium. *Proc. Natl. Acad. Sci. US* 61: 1079-1086, 1968.
253. RUBIN, R. P. The metabolic requirements for catecholamine release from the adrenal medulla. *J. Physiol., London* 202: 197-209, 1969.
254. RUBIN, R. P. The role of energy metabolism in calcium evoked secretion from the adrenal medulla. *J. Physiol., London* 206: 181-192, 1970.
255. RUBIN, R. P. The role of calcium in the release of neurotransmitter substances and hormones. *Pharmacol. Rev.* 22: 389-428, 1970.
256. RUBIN, R. P., M. B. FEINSTEIN, S. D. JAANUS, AND M. PAIMRE. Inhibition of catecholamine secretion and calcium exchange in perfused cat adrenal glands by tetracaine and magnesium. *J. Pharmacol. Exptl. Therap.* 155: 463-471, 1967.
257. RUBIN, R. P., AND S. D. JAANUS. A study of the release of catecholamines from the adrenal medulla by indirectly acting sympathomimetic amines. *Arch. Exptl. Pathol. Pharmakol.* 254: 125-137, 1966.
258. RUBIN, R. P., AND S. D. JAANUS. Tachyphylaxis to the stimulant actions of the indirectly acting sympathomimetic amines and acetylcholine on the adrenal medulla. *Arch. Exptl. Pathol. Pharmakol.* 256: 464-475, 1967.
259. RUBIN, R. P., AND S. D. JAANUS. The release of nucleotide from the adrenal medulla by indirectly acting sympathomimetic amines. *Biochem. Pharmacol.* 16: 1007-1012, 1967.
260. RUBIN, R. P., AND E. MIELE. The relation between the chemical structure of local anaesthetics and inhibition of calcium evoked secretion from the adrenal medulla. *Arch. Exptl. Pathol. Pharmakol.* 260: 298-308, 1968.
261. SACHS, H. Neurosecretion. In: *Handbook of Neurochemistry*, edited by A. Lajtha. New York: Plenum Press, 1970, vol. IV, p. 373-428.
262. SAGE, H. J., W. J. SMITH, AND N. KIRSHNER. Mechanism of secretion from the adrenal medulla. I. A microquantitative immunologic assay for bovine adrenal catecholamine storage vesicle protein and its application to studies of the secretory process. *Mol. Pharmacol.* 3: 81-89, 1967.

263. SCHNEIDER, F. H. Observations on the release of lysosomal enzymes from the isolated bovine adrenal gland. *Biochem. Pharmacol.* 17: 845–851, 1968.
264. SCHNEIDER, F. H. Drug induced release of catecholamines, soluble protein and chromogranin A from the isolated bovine adrenal gland. *Biochem. Pharmacol.* 18: 101–107, 1969.
265. SCHNEIDER, F. H. Secretion from the cortex-free bovine adrenal medulla. *Brit. J. Pharmacol.* 37: 371–379, 1969.
266. SCHNEIDER, F. H. Secretion from the bovine adrenal gland. Release of lysosomal enzymes. *Biochem. Pharmacol.* 19: 833–847, 1970.
267. SCHNEIDER, F. H. Acetaldehyde-induced catecholamine secretion from the cow adrenal medulla. *J. Pharmacol. Exptl. Therap.* 177: 109–118, 1971.
268. SCHNEIDER, F. H., A. D. SMITH, AND H. WINKLER. Secretion from the adrenal medulla: biochemical evidence for exocytosis. *Brit. J. Pharmacol.* 31: 94–104, 1967.
269. SCHÜMANN, H. J. The distribution of adrenaline and noradrenaline in chromaffin granules from the chicken. *J. Physiol., London* 137: 318–326, 1957.
270. SCHÜMANN, H. J. Die Wirkung von Insulin und Reserpin auf den Adrenalin und ATP-Gehalt der chromaffinen Granula des Nebennierenmarks. *Arch. Exptl. Pathol. Pharmakol.* 233: 237–249, 1958.
271. SCHÜMANN, H. J. Medullary particles. *Pharmacol. Rev.* 18: 433–438, 1966.
272. SCHÜMANN, H. J., AND A. PHILIPPU. Zum Mechanismus der durch Calcium und Magnesium verursachten Freisetzung der Nebennierenmarkhormone. *Arch. Exptl. Pathol. Pharmakol.* 244: 466–476, 1963.
273. SCHÜMANN, H. J., AND E. WEIGMANN. Über den Angriffspunkt der indirekten Wirkung sympathicomimetischer Amine. *Arch. Exptl. Pathol. Pharmakol.* 240: 275–284, 1960.
274. SHAW, J. E., AND P. W. RAMWELL. Prostaglandin release from the adrenal gland. In: *Prostaglandins*, edited by S. Bergstrom and B. Samuelson. Stockholm: Almqvist & Wiksell, 1967, p. 291–299.
275. SIMPSON, L. L. The role of calcium in neurohumoral and neurohormonal extrusion processes. *J. Pharm. Pharmacol.* 20: 889–910, 1968.
276. SJÖSTRAND, F. S., AND R. WETZSTEIN. Electronenmikroskopische Untersuchung der phäochromen (chromaffinen) Granula in den Markzellen der Nebenniere. *Experientia* 12: 196–199, 1956.
277. SMITH, A. D. Biochemistry of adrenal chromaffin granules. In: *The Interaction of Drugs and Subcellular Components on Animal Cells*, edited by P. N. Campbell. London: Churchill, 1968, p. 239–292.
278. SMITH, A. D. Proteins of vesicles from sympathetic axons: chemistry, immunoreactivity, and release upon stimulation. *Neurosci. Res. Program Bull.* 8: 377–385, 1970.
279. SMITH, A. D., AND H. WINKLER. Studies of soluble protein from adrenal chromaffin granules. *Biochem. J.* 95: 42P, 1965.
280. SMITH, A. D., AND H. WINKLER. The localization of lysosomal enzymes in chromaffin tissue. *J. Physiol., London* 183: 179–188, 1966.
281. SMITH, A. D., AND H. WINKLER. Purification and properties of an acidic protein from chromaffin granules of bovine adrenal medulla. *Biochem. J.* 103: 483–492, 1967.
282. SMITH, A. D., AND H. WINKLER. Lysosomal phospholipases A_1 and A_2 of bovine adrenal medulla. *Biochem. J.* 108: 867–874, 1968.
283. SMITH, D. J., AND R. L. ROBINSON. The dwindling secretory response of the perfused adrenal medulla of the cat to repeated injections of tyramine. *J. Pharmacol. Exptl. Therap.* 175: 641–648, 1970.
284. SMITH, W. J., AND N. KIRSHNER. A specific soluble protein from the catecholamine storage vesicles of bovine adrenal medulla. Purification and chemical characterization. *Mol. Pharmacol.* 3: 52–62, 1967.
285. SMITH, W. J., A. KIRSHNER, AND N. KIRSHNER. Soluble proteins of the chromaffin granules on the adrenal medulla (Abstract). *Federation Proc.* 23: 350, 1964.
286. SMITTEN, N. A. Cytological and ultrastructural pattern of the secretory activity of adrenomedullary cells. *Arch. Anat. Microscop. Morphol. Exptl.* 54: 145–162, 1965.
287. SORIMACHI, M. Effects of alkali metal and other monovalent ions on the adrenomedullary secretion. *European J. Pharmacol.* 3: 235–241, 1968.
288. STJÄRNE, L. Studies of catecholamine uptake, storage and release mechanisms. *Acta Physiol. Scand. Suppl.* 228: 1–97, 1964.
289. STJÄRNE, L. Quantal or graded secretion of adrenal medullary hormone and sympathetic neurotransmitter. In: *New Aspects of Storage and Release Mechanisms of Catecholamines*, edited by H. J. Schümann and G. Kroneberg. Berlin: Springer Verlag, 1970, p. 112–127.
290. STJÄRNE, L., P. HEDQVIST, AND S. BYGDEMAN. Neurotransmitter quantum released from sympathetic nerves in cat's skeletal muscle. *Life Sci., Part 1* 8: 189–196, 1969.
291. STJÄRNE, L., P. HEDQVIST, AND H. LAGERCRANTZ. Catecholamines and adenine nucleotide material in effluent from stimulated adrenal medulla and spleen. A study of the exocytosis hypothesis for hormone secretion and neurotransmitter release. *Biochem. Pharmacol.* 19: 1147–1158, 1970.
292. STOMORKEN, H. The release reaction of secretion. *Scand. J. Haemotol. Suppl.* 9: 1–24, 1969.
293. THIENES, C. H. Chronic nicotine poisoning. *Ann. NY Acad. Sci.* 90: 239–248, 1960.
294. TRIFARÓ, J. M. Phospholipid metabolism and adrenal medullary activity. I. The effect of acetylcholine on tissue uptake and incorporation of orthophosphate-P^{32} into nucleotides and phospholipids of bovine adrenal medulla. *Mol. Pharmacol.* 5: 382–393, 1969.
295. TRIFARÓ, J. M. The effect of Ca^{2+} omission on the secretion of catecholamines and the incorporation of orthophosphate-P^{32} into nucleotides and phospholipids of bovine adrenal medulla during acetylcholine stimulation. *Mol. Pharmacol.* 5: 420–431, 1969.
296. TRIFARÓ, J. M., AND J. DWORKIND. Phosphorylation of membrane components of adrenal chromaffin granules by adenosine triphosphate. *Mol. Pharmacol.* 7: 52–65, 1971.
297. TRIFARÓ, J. M., AND A. M. POISNER. The role of ATP and ATPase in the release of catecholamines from the adrenal medulla. II. ATP-evoked fall in optical density of isolated chromaffin granules. *Mol. Pharmacol.* 3: 527–580, 1967.
298. TRIFARÓ, J. M., A. M. POISNER, AND W. W. DOUGLAS. The fate of the chromaffin granule during catecholamine release from the adrenal medulla. I. Unchanged efflux of phospholipid and cholesterol. *Biochem. Pharmacol.* 16: 2095–2100, 1967.
299. VAN BREEMEN, C., AND E. McNAUGHTON. The separation of cell membrane calcium transport from extracellular calcium exchange in vascular smooth muscle. *Biochem. Biophys. Res. Commun.* 39: 567–574, 1970.
300. VINCENT, S. The effects of fatigue and temperature on the adrenal bodies of the rat. *Quart. J. Exptl. Physiol.* 15: 319–326, 1925.
301. VIVEROS, O. H., L. ARQUEROS, R. J. CONNETT, AND N. KIRSHNER. Mechanism of secretion from the adrenal medulla. II. Studies of dopamine-β-hydroxylase as a marker for catecholamine storage vesicle membranes in rabbit adrenal glands. *Mol. Pharmacol.* 5: 60–68, 1969.
302. VIVEROS, O. H., L. ARQUEROS, R. J. CONNETT, AND N. KIRSHNER. Mechanism of secretion from the adrenal medulla. IV. The fate of the storage vesicles following insulin and reserpine administration. *Mol. Pharmacol.* 5: 69–82, 1969.
303. VIVEROS, O. H., L. ARQUEROS, AND N. KIRSHNER. Mechanism of secretion from the adrenal medulla. The fate of the catecholamine storage vesicles (Abstract). *Federation Proc.* 27: 601, 1968.
304. VIVEROS, O. H., L. ARQUEROS, AND N. KIRSHNER. Release of catecholamines and dopamine-β-oxidase from the adrenal medulla. *Life Sci., Part 1* 7: 609–618, 1968.

305. VIVEROS, O. H., L. ARQUEROS, AND N. KIRSHNER. Quantal secretion from adrenal medulla: all or none release of storage content. *Science* 165: 911–913, 1969.
306. VIVEROS, O. H., L. ARQUEROS, AND N. KIRSHNER. Mechanism of secretion from the adrenal medulla. v. Retention of storage vesicle membranes following release of adrenaline. *Mol. Pharmacol.* 5: 342–349, 1969.
307. VOGT, M. The secretion of the denervated adrenal medulla of the cat. *Brit. J. Pharmacol.* 7: 325–330, 1952.
308. WEINER, N., W. R. BURACK, AND P. B. HAGEN. The effect of insulin on the catecholamines and adenine nucleotides of adrenal glands. *J. Pharmacol. Exptl. Therap.* 130: 251–255, 1960.
309. WEINER, N., AND W. F. MOSIMANN. The effect of insulin on the catecholamine content and tyrosine hydroxylase activity of cat adrenal glands. *Biochem. Pharmacol.* 19: 1189–1199, 1970.
310. WEINSHILBOUM, R., AND J. AXELROD. Dopamine-β-hydroxylase activity in the rat after hypophysectomy. *Endocrinology* 87: 894–899, 1970.
311. WETZSTEIN, R. Electronenmikroskopische Untersuchungen am Nebennierenmark von Maus, Meerschweinchen und Katz. *Histochemie* 46: 517–576, 1957.
312. WHITTAKER, V. P. Structure and function of animal-cell membranes. *Brit. Med. Bull.* 24: 101–106, 1968.
313. WINKLER, H., H. HÖRTNAGL, H. HÖRTNAGL, AND A. D. SMITH. Membranes of the adrenal medulla. Behaviour of insoluble proteins of chromaffin granules on gel electrophoresis. *Biochem. J.* 118: 303–310, 1970.
314. WINKLER, H., H. PLATTNER, H. HÖRTNAGL, AND W. PFALLER. Zum Secretionsmechanismus der Katecholamine: eine Untersuchung des Nebennierenmarks mit der Gefrierätztechnik. *Arch. Exptl. Pathol. Pharmakol.* 264: 324–325, 1969.
315. WINKLER, H., AND A. D. SMITH. Lipids of adrenal chromaffin granules: fatty acid composition of phospholipids, in particular lysolecithin. *Arch. Exptl. Pathol. Pharmakol.* 261: 379–388, 1968.
316. WINKLER, H., N. STRIEDER, AND E. ZIEGLER. Uber Lipide, insbesondere Lysolecithin, in den chromaffinen Granula verschiedener Species. *Arch. Exptl. Pathol. Pharmakol.* 256: 407–415, 1967.
317. WILLIAMS, J. A., AND J. WOLFF. Possible role of microtubules in thyroid secretion. *Proc. Natl. Acad. Sci. US* 67: 1901–1908, 1970.
318. WOODIN, A. M. The passage of proteins and particles across the surface of cells. In: *The Structure and Function of the Membranes and Surfaces of Cells*, edited by D. J. Bell and J. K. Grant. Cambridge: Cambridge Univ. Press, 1963, p. 126–139.
319. WOODIN, A. M., J. E. FRENCH, AND V. T. MARCHESI. Morphological changes associated with the extrusion of protein induced in the polymorphonuclear leucocyte by staphylococcal leucocidin. *Biochem. J.* 87: 567–571, 1963.
320. WOODIN, A. M., AND A. A. WEINEKE. The participation of calcium, adenosine triphosphate and adenosine triphosphatase in the extrusion of granule proteins from the polymorphonuclear leucocyte. *Biochem. J.* 90: 498–509, 1964.
321. WOODIN, A. M., AND A. A. WIENEKE. Site of protein secretion and calcium accumulation in the polymorphonuclear leucocyte treated with leucocidin. In: *Calcium and Cellular Function*, edited by A. W. Cuthbert. New York: St. Martin's, 1970, p. 183–197.
322. YATES, R. D. A light and electron microscopic study correlating the chromaffin reaction and granule ultrastructure in the adrenal medulla of the Syrian hamster. *Anat. Record* 142: 237–250, 1964.
323. YATES, R. D. Fine structural alterations of adreno-medullary cells of the Syrian hamster following intraperitoneal injections of insulin. *Texas Rep. Biol. Med.* 22: 756–763, 1964.
324. YOSHIDA, H., N. MIKI, H. ISHIDA, AND I. YAMAMOTO. Release of amylase from zymogen granules by ATP and a low concentration of Ca^{2+}. *Biochim. Biophys. Acta* 158: 489–490, 1968.

CHAPTER 28

Catecholamines in blood

B. A. CALLINGHAM | *Department of Pharmacology, University of Cambridge, Cambridge, United Kingdom*

CHAPTER CONTENTS

Assay Methods
Concentrations of Catecholamines in Peripheral Plasma
  Epinephrine and norepinephrine contents of normal human plasma
  Epinephrine and norepinephrine contents of blood plasma of experimental animals
Dopamine in Blood
Plasma Concentrations after Catecholamine Administration
Factors Causing Change in Plasma Catecholamines
  Hypoglycemia
  Hypoxia
  Hypercapnia and acidemia
  Hemorrhage and hypotension
  Temperature changes
  Muscular work
  Mental activity and emotional stress
  Plasma catecholamines in disease
Drugs and Plasma Catecholamines
  Nicotine
  Anesthetics
Catecholamines in Adrenal Venous Blood
  Resting secretion
  Stimulated release of adrenal medullary amines
    Electrical stimulation
    Cholinergic drugs
    Hypoglycemia
    Hypoxia
    Hypotension
    Histamine
    Polypeptides and other substances
Overflow of Norepinephrine from Sympathetically Innervated Organs

---

SINCE THE TURN OF THE CENTURY, many workers have been intrigued by the possibility that the active principles of the adrenal medulla could be found circulating freely in the blood. This has naturally led to a vast number of chemical and biological assay methods designed to detect and measure the minute amounts that in fact occur. It has become clear in the last 20 years or so that many of these techniques have yielded values that we now know are far too high. As assays have improved, the apparent amounts of the catecholamines in the blood have fallen steadily. The currently available methods are sufficiently reliable to indicate that tiny amounts of epinephrine and norepinephrine can be found in the blood of man and other animals. The errors involved and the variation between individuals still make it very difficult to give precise values. Most are accompanied by huge standard errors. Quite recently a third catecholamine, dopamine, has also been found in the blood in surprisingly large and variable amounts.

ASSAY METHODS

The first chemical methods of assay were colorimetric, the earliest apparently being that of Battelli (3) in 1902 who attempted to estimate epinephrine in blood. These proved to be neither sensitive nor specific enough, and early biological methods were, on the whole, equally unsatisfactory. The presence of other pressor and depressor substances invalidated most of the results. Not until 1935 did Page (136) report pressor activity in normal blood that was due to an active principle soluble in water and organic solvents. Von Euler & Sjöstrand (44) subsequently found pressor activity in alcoholic extracts of human blood and plasma and in their dialysates. Again contamination with depressor substances prevented any accurate identification of the pressor agent. Improved techniques of both extraction and estimation were required. Currently alumina is commonly employed as a means of extracting the catechol constituents from blood plasma. Ion-exchange resins are also widely employed, especially where extraction of the basic metabolites is required. Catecholamines are also isolated by paper chromatography, particularly when followed by bioassay.

Until recently the only chemical methods of assay that stood any chance of estimating the normal amounts of the blood catecholamines involved fluorimetry. The amines, after separation from other blood constituents, are converted into derivatives possessing characteristic fluorescence spectra that can be detected and assayed at high sensitivity and specificity. Two basic methods are available, both of which have been modified in many ways by many experimenters, each of whom claims particular advantages for his own method not shared by any other. This multiplicity of techniques reflects the great difficulties that confront the unwary. In consequence these methods are described and their attendant problems discussed in many reviews (12, 69, 162).

One method, usually referred to as the *trihydroxyindole* (THI) *method*, involves the oxidation of the catecholamine to its corresponding chrome compound followed by rearrangement to the highly fluorescent lutine in the presence of strong alkali and an antioxidant. Coupled with reliable extraction procedures, this technique has provided most of the presently acceptable evidence. The other method in which the catecholamine is oxidized and coupled with ethylenediamine to yield a fluorescent derivative appears to be more sensitive than the THI method but is also much less specific. Many results obtained with this ethylenediamine (EDA) method were in error because of this lack of specificity in the assay combined with inadequate extraction techniques. Although this problem has been resolved to a large degree by improvements in the extraction of the catecholamines, the method is no longer used. Values determined by this method for the circulating amounts of epinephrine and norepinephrine in the peripheral blood plasma under resting conditions have therefore largely been excluded from this chapter. However, comparative results obtained by the EDA method may be valuable and are included when appropriate. The EDA method is sensitive and reliable after the catecholamines, converted to stable acetylated derivatives, have been separated by paper chromatography (92).

Radiochemical methods that appear to be both sensitive and able to provide an accurate estimate of the errors involved in their use are now available. One such method can detect as little as 0.25 ng of either epinephrine or norepinephrine (38).

The most successful bioassay for catecholamines in blood has proved to be the rat blood pressure method. Sensitivity of a very high order has been achieved by the use of drugs such as cocaine and imipramine to prevent the inactivation of the injected catecholamines by uptake into the sympathetic neurons (65), or by pronethalol to convert the biphasic response to epinephrine into a larger, purely pressor one (177). Many other methods involving isolated tissues have been employed, often with great success. These methods have been exploited by Vane and his colleagues (176) for the detection of the catecholamines circulating in the blood of man and other animals. In their technique the blood is taken from the animal and superfused directly over selected tissues, such as a strip of rat stomach and hen rectal caecum arranged in series. The blood is then returned to the experimental animal, but not to the human volunteer.

CONCENTRATIONS OF CATECHOLAMINES IN PERIPHERAL PLASMA

The amounts of circulating catecholamines are almost always expressed in terms of the content in the blood plasma. The amines are relatively stable in frozen plasma and can be stored in this form before assay, but the influence of the red cells appears to be unpredictable (12). A recent study has confirmed that the preparation of the plasma sample can be a major source of error (18). However, the amine content of whole blood is usually reported when the blood is directly assayed without any preparation or where the content is estimated from such effects as rises in the blood pressure or contractions of the nictitating membrane induced by catecholamines released in the same animal by some experimental procedure.

Many factors influence the values obtained for the concentrations of the catecholamines in the peripheral blood plasma. First, the amount present at any one time represents the balance of the amounts released, on the one hand, and the amounts removed by uptake and by catabolism and excretion, on the other. Second, the actual source of the catecholamines varies. It is safe to assume that the norepinephrine originates from two major sources: the adrenal medulla and the postganglionic sympathetic nerve endings. In contrast, epinephrine originates almost exclusively from the adrenal medulla. The contribution of the extramedullary chromaffin tissues is difficult to assess. The relative proportions of the catecholamines may vary widely depending on the particular vessel from which the blood sample is taken. Differences can be expected between the contents of blood from the brachial vein and the renal vein, for example. The overflow from the different sympathetically innervated organs will vary from time to time and influence the content of locally obtained samples. The ability of the tissues to take up the amines that enter them is also of importance. This is highlighted by the observation of Ferreira & Vane (49) that, although epinephrine in the blood can pass through the lungs unscathed, 30% of the norepinephrine is taken up. This organ could have an important influence on the relative proportions of amines, particularly when they originate from the adrenal medulla.

Epinephrine and Norepinephrine Contents of Normal Human Plasma

Because the sensitivity of the presently available methods is such that comparatively large volumes (12–20 ml or more) of blood are required to obtain a reasonably reliable estimate of its catecholamine content[1], most information has been derived from estimations of samples taken from normal human subjects under resting conditions. Particularly in experimental animals but also in man, there is some difficulty in defining exactly what represents resting conditions. Even in man the stress of the collection procedure may be sufficient to raise the amount of the circulating catecholamines. This can be overcome by allowing the subject to rest for at least 30 min after insertion of a catheter into a blood vessel (20). In a study of the effects of the insertion of the catheter on the blood pressure, heart rate, and plasma norepineph-

---

[1] Recently a method has been reported that requires only 0.75 ml or less of plasma (136a).

rine levels in volunteers, Klensch (87) showed that it was not sufficient to wait until the heart rate had returned to normal after venipuncture before taking the blood sample. Although the heart rate and blood pressure had returned to normal within 10 min, plasma norepinephrine was still higher than in samples taken several minutes later. Samples obtained by venipuncture have been shown to yield consistently higher plasma epinephrine values than those obtained through an indwelling catheter (18).

Some of the available estimates of the epinephrine and norepinephrine levels in the plasma of normal human subjects are given in Table 1. These values have been selected because sufficient data in each case have been obtained to compensate for the major sources of error in the method. The amounts of epinephrine estimated are extremely small and at the limit of the sensitivity of the method. Many of the values represent the mean of a large number of estimations varying from zero to the maximum. Moreover one author, with a very sophisticated THI method, failed to find any at all (67).

In Table 2 the epinephrine and norepinephrine concentrations obtained for the plasma of male and female subjects by the use of a radioactive double isotope assay technique are summarized.

There is sufficient evidence to suggest that the venous plasma of normal human subjects contains about 0.05 ng/ml of epinephrine and about 0.3 ng/ml of norepinephrine. However, these values represent a very subjective and approximate estimate. They only include free catecholamines circulating in the blood and do not take into account conjugated amine. Häggendal (68) showed that normal human plasma contained conjugated norepinephrine in concentrations of two to three times those of the free amine. In 10 healthy subjects he found 0.7 ng/ml of conjugated norepinephrine, compared with 0.3 ng/ml of free norepinephrine, but was unable to detect any free or conjugated epinephrine.

Although differences in plasma catecholamine contents between male and female subjects have been reported from time to time [e.g., by Hochuli (78) with the EDA method] the present evidence indicates that they are only slight if they occur at all; certainly they are not statistically significant. In fact many investigators employ volunteers of both sexes in their experiments.

In man, the concentration of the catecholamines in the circulating blood is influenced to some extent by the age of the subject, the concentration increasing with age (Tables 3 and 3a). A similar relationship appears to hold with respect to the mean arterial blood pressure. The changes are relatively small and are only likely to be seen in studies involving large numbers of observations. With small numbers the differences may be lost in the errors of the assay technique. It perhaps should be added that the THI method used in this study was rigorously controlled to limit the errors involved as much as possible.

Significant differences have been found in the catecholamine content of blood samples drawn from various regions of the body. Vendsalu (178) demonstrated that

TABLE 1. *Concentration of Epinephrine and Norepinephrine in Blood Plasma of Normal Subjects*[a]

| Plasma Concentrations, ng/ml[b] |||| Percentage Recovery || Ref. |
| Epinephrine || Norepinephrine || Epi-nephrine | Norepi-nephrine | |
Arterial	Venous	Arterial	Venous			
0.01 ±0.10[c]	0.01 ±0.07[c]	0.20 ±0.12[c]	0.34 ±0.15[c]	78	83	146
	0.06 ±0.05[c]		0.30 ±0.07[c]	70–90[d]	70–90[d]	21
0.23 ±0.02[c]	0.07 ±0.01[c]	0.31 ±0.02[c]	0.40 ±0.02[c]	80.2 ±13.1	83.0 ±11.4	178
	0[c]		0.30 ±0.11[e]	73 ±29	71 ±16	67
	0.08 ±0.05[c]		0.17 ±0.05[c]	91.8 ±3[f]		135
	0.04 ±0.04[c]		0.24 ±0.09[c]	79 ±9	72.4 ±9	63
			0.29 ±0.11[e,g]	72–92		179

[a] Determined with THI method. [b] Value expressed ±SD. [c] Value not corrected for percentage recovery. [d] Range given is 1 mean deviation. [e] Value corrected for percentage recovery. [f] Norepinephrine recovery not significantly different from epinephrine. [g] Determined with automated THI method; total plasma catecholamines expressed as norepinephrine.

TABLE 2. *Concentration of Epinephrine and Norepinephrine in Plasma of Normal, Resting Subjects**

| Sex | Number of Subjects | Plasma Concentration, ng/ml ||||
| | | Epinephrine || Norepinephrine ||
		Mean ± SD	Range	Mean ± SD	Range
Male	12	0.06±0.04	0–0.11	0.20±0.08	0.10–0.31
Female	10	0.04±0.03	0–0.10	0.21±0.09	0.10–0.37
Total	22	0.05±0.03	0–0.11	0.20±0.08	0.10–0.37

* Determined by double isotope assay. [Adapted from Engelman & Portnoy (38).]

the lowest amounts were obtained from the hepatic vein and the highest from the vena cava and left renal vein because of blood coming from the adrenal medulla. Häggendal (68) also found very low concentrations of amines in the hepatic vein. Lammerant & de Herdt (90) simultaneously withdrew blood samples from four vessels in dogs with an artificial pneumothorax 120–180 min after administration of the anesthetic. Lowest concentrations of total catecholamine were found in the pulmonary vein (0.81 ng/ml) and the highest in the pulmonary artery (about 2.24 ng/ml). This difference may be due to the uptake of norepinephrine by the lung tissue (49). Blood in the aortic arch contained 1.11 ng/ml.

Differences between arterial and venous contents of the catecholamines in human subjects are apparent (see above) and have been investigated by some workers.

TABLE 3. *Comparison of Mean Resting Blood Pressure and Venous Plasma Norepinephrine in Man*

Mean Blood Pressure, mmHg	Number of Subjects*	Plasma NE, ng/ml†,‡	Heart Rate§
90–104	36	0.248	68.7
105–109	21	0.314	72.5
110–114	43	0.309	71.6
115–119	46	0.307	70.6
120–124	26	0.342	75.7
125–129	23	0.352	70.8
130–139	26	0.393	78.1
140–149	17	0.353	86.1

NE, norepinephrine.   * Total 238.   † Values not corrected for percentage recovery during extraction and assay procedure.   ‡ Mean 0.328.   § Mean 73.2.   [Adapted from Klensch (87).]

TABLE 3a. *Comparison of Age and Venous Plasma Norepinephrine in Man*

Age	Number of Subjects	Plasma NE, ng/ml	Mean Systolic BP, mmHg	Mean Heart Rate
20–29	21	0.266	112	71.6
30–39	4	0.266	113	71.3
40–49	28	0.273	118	72.3
50–59	33	0.280	116	67.0
60–68	9	0.350	124	67.2

NE, norepinephrine; BP, blood pressure. [Adapted from Klensch (87).]

Weil-Malherbe & Bone (186), by using the EDA method, found that in six subjects the epinephrine content in arterial plasma was greater than that in venous plasma but that the norepinephrine content in arterial plasma was lower in three of the subjects and higher in the other three. Higher norepinephrine contents in the arterial plasma have been shown by others (54, 146). Vendsalu (178) obtained a highly significant difference (0.09 ± 0.02 ng/ml) between the brachial artery and anticubital vein contents. The opposite appears to be the case for epinephrine, the arterial content exceeding the venous. Again, Vendsalu found a highly significant difference (0.16 ± 0.02 ng/ml) between arterial and venous epinephrine contents.

Although the resting levels are very low and subject to considerable error, it may be concluded that the positive arteriovenous difference in the case of epinephrine is due to uptake of the amine originating from the adrenal medulla by the tissues of the body. The higher venous concentration of norepinephrine represents overflow of the sympathetic neurotransmitter (41). The fact that small amounts of the catecholamines can be detected in the resting supine subject would indicate a basal release from the adrenal medulla and sympathetic neurons sufficient for a small fraction to escape the uptake processes that confront it.

Epinephrine and Norepinephrine Contents of Blood Plasma of Experimental Animals

Table 4 summarizes some values for epinephrine and norepinephrine in blood obtained, as far as one can judge, under conditions that minimize the stress experienced by the animal; these conditions are very difficult to define, and the values reported are almost certainly influenced by them, as well as being subject to the errors described above. In addition, quite large volumes of blood are required for successful estimation of the catecholamines.

DOPAMINE IN BLOOD

Street & Roberts (169) have found variable amounts of dopamine in the peripheral blood of cats anesthetized with chloralose. In one group of six animals, dopamine concentration was 4.75 ± 2.15 ng/ml, compared with 1.15 ± 0.17 and 1.66 ± 0.44 ng/ml for norepinephrine and epinephrine, respectively. Dopamine concentration varied widely from animal to animal, from 0.69 to 14.46 ng/ml. Kelly et al. (85) found much lower concentrations in conscious sheep and goats (0.1–0.4 ng/ml).

A resting secretion of dopamine from the adrenal glands of anesthetized cats has been demonstrated by assay of the adrenal venous blood of animals pretreated with ^{3}H-tyrosine. With this approach, Hempel & Männl (73, 74) have shown that up to 50% of the catecholamine in the adrenal venous effluent could be dopamine. They calculated that a single cat adrenal gland under their conditions released 10 ng/kg per min of ^{3}H-dopamine. However, they were unable to obtain any secretion of labeled dopamine in the rabbit, since its conversion to norepinephrine was complete.

TABLE 4. *Concentration of Epinephrine and Norepinephrine in Blood Plasma of Various Animals*

Species	Epinephrine	Norepinephrine	Reference
Rat[a]	1.83	1.01	29
Rat[b]	10.80	5.20	1
Rat[c,d]			60
Male	1.38 ± 0.15	0.73 ± 0.16	
Estrous	2.75 ± 0.39	0.44 ± 0.05	
Diestrous	1.98 ± 0.13	1.14 ± 0.24	
Metestrous	2.17 ± 0.56	1.08 ± 0.25	
Pregnant	2.33 ± 0.10	0.26 ± 0.13	
Dog	0.41	1.05	1
Dog[e]	0.10	0.18	118
Dog[e]	0.45	0.44	165
Sheep	0.27	0.52	1
Calf[f]	0.76 ± 0.02	1.00 ± 0.33	110
Carp[f]	0.15 ± 0.03	1.6 ± 0.3	112

Plasma Concentration, ng/ml.   [a] Serum content.   [b] Animals probably stressed by collection procedures.   [c] Animals anesthetized with pentobarbitone.   [d] Values expressed ± SE.   [e] Animals anesthetized with thiopentone.   [f] Values expressed ± SD.

PLASMA CONCENTRATIONS AFTER CATECHOLAMINE ADMINISTRATION

The catecholamines released into the circulation do not last for long. Their existence can only be maintained by the continuous release of fresh amines from the adrenal medulla or by overflow from the postganglionic sympathetic neurons. The half-life of the catecholamines in the peripheral blood has been calculated to be less than 20 sec (49), which is of the same order as the circulation time in the cat or dog (164). Uptake into neuronal and nonneuronal tissues is of great importance (see the chapter by Iversen in this volume of the *Handbook*).

The disappearance of injected catecholamines is also extremely rapid, even when huge nonphysiological doses are used. Concentrations of both epinephrine and norepinephrine in plasma fell to normal levels in dogs and rabbits within 5 to 10 min after injections of 50–100 μg/kg, norepinephrine returning more rapidly than epinephrine (104, 140). Recovery times of about 1–3 min have been reported by others (122, 185). The use of radioactively labeled catecholamines has enabled lower doses to be used. Initial loss from the circulation is very rapid; for example, after the intravenous injection of 25 μg/kg of ^{3}H-norepinephrine into cats, there was an initial fall to 35 ng/ml in 2 min after which the rate of disappearance slowed such that at 120 min the plasma content was 2.7 ng/ml (23). This residual concentration presumably represents the slow release of labeled amine from the sites of uptake (2).

Even after intravenous infusions of epinephrine and norepinephrine that raise the plasma concentrations to several times their normal values, the recovery is rapid. Reports indicate that during the infusion of the catecholamines the concentrations measured in the peripheral plasma rise to a plateau level, which persists until the infusion ceases (21, 185). Infusions of epinephrine and norepinephrine into human subjects at rates varying between 10 and 30 μg/min produced plateau levels after about 5–10 min of 3 ng/ml of epinephrine and 5 ng/ml of norepinephrine (22). A plateau of the level in plasma has also been shown to occur after lower rates of infusion (178). In normal subjects, 0.07 μg/kg per min of epinephrine produced a plasma concentration of 0.05 ng/ml, and 0.08 μg/kg per min of norepinephrine produced a concentration of 1.5–2.0 ng/ml between 7.5 and 10 min after commencing the infusion.

Infusion of dl-^{3}H-norepinephrine at a rate of 0.05 μg/kg per min into five normal subjects for 1 hr led to peak concentrations in plasma immediately before the end of the infusion (56). The concentration fell rapidly to 33% of the peak value within 10 min of ceasing the infusion. Subsequently the loss was much more gradual, the radioactivity reaching background levels in about 24–30 hr. These results agreed closely with those found in the cat (2, 187). Infusion of epinephrine into pregnant women yields results identical to those obtained in non-pregnant women and in other animals (191), the plasma epinephrine concentrations returning to normal within 10 min. However, it seems that most of the methods used to measure unlabeled catecholamines after infusion are unable to detect the small amounts of the infused amines that are subsequently released from the tissues, or alternatively the material that is released replaces some of the endogenous catecholamines circulating in the blood. In assays of labeled amines small amounts can be detected for up to several hours after injection or infusion. With the THI method, Häggendal & Svedmyr (70) showed that, after an infusion of 0.1 μg/kg per min of epinephrine into five normal subjects, the plasma concentration reached a peak of 0.7 ng/ml from a normally undetectable level 20 min after beginning the infusion. This value fell even though the infusion was continued for another 10 min. However, the plasma concentration was nearly 0.2 ng/ml 30 min after stopping the infusion and 0.1 ng/ml 1 hr later. It seems probable that they were able to detect the overflow of amine taken up during the infusion since there was no detectable endogenous plasma epinephrine to interfere. Tissue uptake is reflected in the arteriovenous difference in plasma concentrations of the amines after infusion (144). Very high infusion concentrations of 10 μg/kg per min of epinephrine for about 80 min produced an arterial concentration of 201 ng/ml, compared with a venous concentration of 70 ng/ml.

There are some reports that increases in the plasma concentration of one amine occur when the other is infused (52, 95). Conversely a fall in the norepinephrine concentration was found during the infusion of small amounts of epinephrine into pregnant women (191). However, when the infusion concentration of epinephrine was raised, the fall in norepinephrine became an increase. Nevertheless the weight of evidence is against such an interrelationship. Neither Vendsalu (178) nor Manger et al. (107), who used the EDA method, observed such changes. Similarly no alteration in the plasma concentration of norepinephrine was seen during the infusion of epinephrine into normal or hyperthyroid patients (70). If the infusion leads to a rise in blood pressure, secretion from the adrenal gland may be reduced (106, 156). It is reasonable to suspect the validity of the assay result when the concentration of one amine is much greater than that of the other (53).

FACTORS CAUSING CHANGE IN PLASMA CATECHOLAMINES

Many factors have been found to influence the responses of the sympathetic nervous system and the release of hormones from the adrenal medulla. Much emphasis has been placed on the effects of stress since Cannon (13) first defined the part that these hormones play in what he described as the "fight or flight" reaction to stressful situations. He demonstrated the presence of the medullary hormone in the blood from the adrenal glands of cats exposed to barking dogs. With his assay technique, none could be found in the adrenal venous blood of cats not stressed in this way. Most of the subsequent evidence is based on experiments employing conditions that often severely stress the animal or human volunteer, since it is then possible to estimate the secretory response they produce. However, changes in the plasma catecholamines can reasonably be expected in the normal maintenance of homeostasis. The relative importance of the adrenal medulla and the postganglionic nerve endings as the source of these amines depends largely on the nature of the particular stimulus employed.

Hypoglycemia

Houssay et al. (80) and Cannon et al. (15) first showed that insulin hypoglycemia caused an increased secretion of catecholamines from the adrenal gland. Dunér (34) measured the epinephrine and norepinephrine content of the adrenal venous blood of the cat. He found that the injection of insulin was followed by a fall in the blood sugar that was maximal after about 35 min, at which time epinephrine output from the gland increased to over 10 times the resting value. This was accompanied by a much smaller rise in norepinephrine output. As the blood sugar returned to normal the amine secretion declined. Similar results have been obtained in man and other animals. Holzbauer & Vogt (79) showed, by using bioassay, that injections of insulin in the dog increased the amount of epinephrine in the peripheral venous plasma from control values of 0.08–0.24 ng/ml to 0.25–6.4 ng/ml. In the human subject the plasma epinephrine level rose from 0.06 ng/ml to 1.8 ng/ml, whereas the blood sugar fell from 121 to 55 mg/100 ml 45 min after the injection of insulin. The plasma norepinephrine concentration always remained below the sensitivity of the assay techniques. The raised epinephrine concentration in the blood associated with insulin hypoglycemia fell sharply when glucose was administered (116). Later workers, with refined THI methods of assay, have also found rises in the plasma concentrations of epinephrine without any change in the norepinephrine content in the peripheral blood (178). Häggendal (68) gave 0.1 unit/kg of insulin to human subjects and found after 30 min an increase in the epinephrine content of plasma withdrawn from the brachial vein from 0 to 0.5 ng/ml, together with the appearance of traces of conjugated epinephrine. No change was seen in the norepinephrine content. The amounts of free amines in hepatic vein plasma were very low both before and after insulin injection.

The denervated adrenal gland is insensitive to the action of insulin (25), and it has been suggested that regions in the hypothalamus might be responsible for controlling the rate of secretion of adrenal catecholamines when the blood sugar was abnormally high (33). In the sheep a comparison of the effects of insulin on the secretion of epinephrine and norepinephrine into the adrenal venous blood of anesthetized intact, decerebrate, and spinal animals indicates that neurons situated in the brainstem caudal to the hypothalamus are capable of stimulating the adrenal medulla in hypoglycemia (28). In the intact sheep anesthetized with sodium pentobarbitone, insulin increased the output of epinephrine in the venous drainage from the left adrenal gland from 5 to 83.2 ng/kg per min for epinephrine and from 2.7 to 14.2 ng/kg per min for norepinephrine. It seems that when the catecholamine content of adrenal venous blood is measured, there is an increase in norepinephrine as well as epinephrine, although on a much lower scale, an effect not seen when blood is taken from vessels some distance away. This rise in norepinephrine output does not appear to have any important function since only epinephrine can protect the animal against the effects of insulin (23). The possibility remains that the rise is an artifact caused by the use of differential assays that are known to be suspect when one amine is present in excess over the other (53).

Hypoxia

In 1911 Cannon & Hoskins (14) showed that acute hypoxia caused increased adrenal medullary output in the experimental animal. The amount of catecholamine in the blood plasma is correlated with the degree of reduction in the oxygen tension (103). In the anesthetized dog, anoxia produced by exposure to pure nitrogen for 2 min caused an increase in the total amine content in the pulmonary arterial plasma from 2.2 to 128 ng/ml and in the pulmonary venous plasma from 0.81 to 41 ng/ml. Asphyxia by occluding the trachea of the anesthetized cat may selectively increase the secretion of epinephrine (90). However, no change in plasma amines was reported when human subjects breathed a gas mixture containing 10% oxygen for 15 min (50).

Comline and his colleagues (24–26) have measured the output of epinephrine and norepinephrine in the adrenal venous effluent in fetal, newborn, and adult sheep and cattle. In the fetal calf, for example, between 180 days gestation and term, asphyxia by exposure of the mother to reduced oxygen tension or by clamping the umbilical cord induced the release of adrenal hormone, which in the fetal animal is predominantly norepinephrine. The action of the stimulus was directly on the adrenal cells because the response was unaffected by denervation of the glands. As the animal developed, this direct effect became less important and disappeared completely by 24 hr after birth when the splanchnic nerves became the exclusive means whereby asphyxia induced the release of adrenal amines. The splanchnic nerves, however, did not become maximally effective until 2–3 weeks after birth. In the carp, asphyxia raised the epinephrine content of the peripheral plasma from 0.15 to a maximum of 0.73 ng/ml and the norepinephrine from 1.6 to 3.6 ng/ml (112).

Changes in the circulating amounts of catecholamines have been reported in human subjects under conditions of prolonged hypoxia. Cunningham et al. (30) found an increase in the total blood amines, measured as norepinephrine, in a group involved in a mountaineering expedition as they climbed from sea level. Before the climb, which took a period of weeks, the mean plasma content was about 0.8 ng/ml, whereas at an altitude of 4,560 m it reached 1.6 ng/ml. On their return to sea level the plasma content fell to 0.5 ng/ml, a value lower than that found during the stressful weeks of training and preparation before the climb. However, only slight and insignificant rises in plasma epinephrine content have been noted in subjects born at over 3,200 m and living for over a year at an altitude of 4,600 m, where the resting oxygen saturation of the arterial blood was 82%. No changes were observed in subjects previously living at sea level if their blood was examined 36 hr after bringing them up to the same height (124). It has been suggested that guinea pigs and rats, at least, can adapt to prolonged hypoxia (168). Exposure of these animals to a gas mixture of 7.5% oxygen in nitrogen significantly decreased the catecholamine content of their adrenal glands at periods of up to 12 hr. On further exposure the adrenal content returned to normal levels because of an increase in the rate of synthesis.

On the other hand, exposure to increased oxygen tensions may lead to a rise in the circulating catecholamines (29). Rats subjected to lethal pressures of oxygen (e.g., 4,500 mmHg), which caused convulsions, had serum contents of 2.15 and 7.89 ng/ml of norepinephrine and epinephrine, respectively, compared with control values of 1.01 and 1.83 ng/ml, respectively. Serum epinephrine was significantly increased at lower oxygen tensions where the norepinephrine was either unchanged or lowered. Below the minimum lethal pressure of 690 mmHg of oxygen, no changes were seen in the serum content of either amine.

Hypercapnia and Acidemia

Increases in the carbon dioxide concentration of blood, both with and without attendant hypoxia, provide an extremely potent stimulus for the release of catecholamines (119, 172). The increase in concentration of plasma epinephrine resulting from hemorrhage is greatly reduced if the concomitant acidosis is prevented (31). A decrease in blood pH and apnea without hypoxia caused a rise in the catecholamines in dog plasma (129–131). There was no increase in amine concentration if the blood pH was maintained during the rise in P_{CO_2} by Tris buffer. The increase, caused by release of that amine from the adrenal medulla, is largely in the epinephrine content of the blood. It has been suggested that the epinephrine release is only seen when the blood pH falls below 6.8 (125, 172), but Nahas et al. (131) have detected increases in circulating epinephrine levels at arterial pH of 6.9–7.1 and arterial P_{CO_2} between 96 and 103 mmHg. Assay of adrenal venous blood has indicated an increase in output from the gland, made up largely of epinephrine, in hypercapnic acidosis with a pH of 6.93 and a P_{CO_2} of 127 mmHg (17).

Nahas and his colleagues (115, 132) have studied the ef-

TABLE 5. *Influence of pH and P_{CO_2} on Catecholamine Output of Dog Adrenal Gland Perfused with Blood*

Perfusion Fluid				Total Catecholamine Output, ng/gland per min
Blood	pH	P_{CO_2}, mmHg	HCO₃, mEq/liter	
Control	7.41	32	20.5	70
+ 10% CO₂	6.84*	176*	29.6*	532*
+ Lactic acid				
31 mM	7.02*	49.2*	11.2*	98
46 mM	6.86*	29*	6.3*	237*

* Value significantly different from control. [Adapted from Nahas et al. (132).]

fects of acidemia on the dog adrenal gland perfused with blood in situ. They measured both epinephrine and norepinephrine but expressed their results in terms of total amine. At a normal pH the output of amine averaged 70 ng/gland per min. This was increased by 100% after the pH of the perfusing blood was reduced to between 6.96 and 7.10 (see Table 5). These authors confirm the suggestion first proposed by Morris & Millar (125) that in the dog hypercapnic acidosis can directly stimulate adrenal medullary secretion. Morris and Millar measured peripheral blood plasma in anesthetized intubated dogs breathing various mixtures of carbon dioxide in oxygen. In animals pretreated with a ganglion blocking drug and in which adrenal denervation had been done, no release of amines occurred at a pH of 7.02 but a release amounting to about 30% of that of normal animals was seen at a pH of 6.71. The differences in the results reported by these two groups of workers (115, 125, 132) may be due to the inherent higher sensitivity of the assay of adrenal venous effluent.

It seems likely that the H⁺ concentration is responsible for the direct stimulation of the adrenal medulla, since at a pH of 6.81 the same increase in output was produced with a P_{CO_2} of 34 mmHg as with a P_{CO_2} of 150 mmHg (132). The situation is different in the fetal lamb, where changes in P_{CO_2}, pH, and lactic acid levels during asphyxia appeared to have little effect on the catecholamine output from the gland (24).

Hemorrhage and Hypotension

Gross hemorrhage leading to falls in blood pressure results in rises in the contents of epinephrine and norepinephrine in plasma (61, 117). Millar & Benfey (117) measured epinephrine and norepinephrine in the peripheral plasma of anesthetized dogs and found that the falls in blood pressure increased the circulating amines to 49 ng/ml and 27 ng/ml, respectively. That a proportion of the norepinephrine rise was due to overflow from the adrenergic neurons was shown in adrenalectomized dogs (118). In these animals a fall in the blood pressure to a level of 52 mmHg caused an increase in the plasma norepinephrine from 0.19 to 0.57 ng/ml without any effect on the residual epinephrine. This rise was significantly enhanced after treatment with phenoxybenzamine. The increased amounts of amines that occur after hemorrhage fall again when the blood loss is compensated (184).

Darby & Watts (31) found that a fall in blood pressure of anesthetized dogs to 40 mmHg produced by hemorrhage increased the circulating epinephrine in a way that closely paralleled the onset of uncompensated acidosis. If this were corrected by intravenous tromethamine or sodium bicarbonate, the rise was greatly reduced. After 15 min of hypotension, in control animals the epinephrine in the peripheral plasma had risen from a control value of 1.0 ng/ml to 8.0 ng/ml; after 60 min it rose to 23 ng/ml. However, after 60 min of hypotension in animals treated with tromethamine, the plasma epinephrine content was only 3.0 ng/ml.

Rises in plasma epinephrine, but not in norepinephrine, have been reported in dogs during endotoxin shock (147, 165).

Temperature Changes

Norepinephrine has been implicated in the acclimatization to a cold environment, during which its urinary excretion is raised (94). Rats given norepinephrine survive longer than untreated animals when exposed to a temperature of −20 C.

Small but significant rises in plasma norepinephrine, but not epinephrine, were observed in male volunteers who allowed a shower of water at 0–2.5 C to fall on their chests (84). It was suggested that the intense vasomotor responses, such as large increases in cardiac output, pulse rate, and pulse pressure, were caused by the sympathetic innervation to the heart and blood vessels rather than by discharge from the adrenal medulla, which led to an increase in norepinephrine alone when measured by the EDA method.

An increase in the excretion of catecholamines has been seen in men exposed to hot climates (72). The greatest increases coincided with the maximum temperatures or the maximum amounts of solar radiation. However, seasonal variations in the excretion of catecholamines have been found in two widely differing climates (48, 81). Epinephrine excretion is increased in the winter to about double that in summer, whereas norepinephrine excretion is unaffected.

Increases in the temperature of anesthetized dogs cause an elevation in both the plasma catecholamines and histamine (171). The total catecholamine rose to two to three times the control level of 3.6 ng/ml when the temperature of the animals reached 39.5–40 C. Maximum plasma concentrations (7.6–35.8 ng/ml) were reached at temperatures of 40.5–41 C. These concentrations tended to fall when the animal collapsed.

Muscular Work

Muscular work or exercise has many times been shown to increase the concentrations of the catecholamines in plasma. Usually it is the norepinephrine that is first affected, rises in epinephrine concentration becoming detectable only if the activity is severe, for example, running a quarter mile or more (126). Klensch (88) found a rise in venous plasma norepinephrine, from 0.2 to 0.42 ng/ml, when subjects exercised on the bicycle ergometer at a rate of 100 watts for 10 min. Very similar results are found when urinary catecholamines are measured (36, 41). Plasma norepinephrine rose to four and six times the resting level without change in epinephrine levels in two normal men performing muscular work at rates of 600 and 900 kg/min (68). The plasma concentration of conjugated norepinephrine rose by 50%. However, the urinary contents of both free and conjugated dopamine are unaltered during the severe muscular work involved in a hard military cross-country race lasting for 2.5 hr (71). Under these conditions the excretion of epinephrine and norepinephrine increased.

Mild stimuli, such as postural changes, modify the plasma and urinary contents of norepinephrine. A rise in the plasma content of this amine is seen when subjects are tilted from the horizontal to the vertical or some intermediate plane (77, 126), whereas little or no alteration in plasma epinephrine is observed. This change in epinephrine is reflected in urinary output (170). On the other hand, total body immersion for 6 hr reduced the urinary excretion of norepinephrine by about 40% (58).

Disease may modify the subject's response to exercise. Exercise, which in the normal subject did not increase plasma catecholamine levels, did so in patients suffering from angina pectoris (55). Braunwald and his colleagues (7, 20) found that patients with heart disease in the absence of congestive failure responded to moderate exercise in the same way as normal subjects: both groups showed slight rises in plasma norepinephrine. However, when congestive failure was present the resting level of norepinephrine tended to be above the normal range, and after exercise the increase was considerably greater. There were no consistent changes in any of the groups. These authors (7, 20) subjected their control group of normal subjects to severe exercise to obtain an increase in plasma norepinephrine that amounted to rather more than twice the normal level.

Mental Activity and Emotional Stress

Changes in the concentration of plasma catecholamines are associated with changes in mental activity, especially when the subject is confronted with a stressful situation. An increase in the epinephrine content of plasma on waking has been detected by the EDA method (150), and studies of urinary catecholamines have indicated that the excretion of both epinephrine and norepinephrine is reduced during sleep (36, 83).

It seems that conditions involving increased mental or emotional activity usually produce an increase in both plasma and urinary epinephrine. If physical work or unpleasant stimulation is superimposed, there is an accompanying increase in norepinephrine. Muscular work unaccompanied by mental stress causes increases in norepinephrine level only (134).

Increased excretion of epinephrine occurs in human subjects in situations that provoke fear, for example, traveling by air before a parachute descent (6), viewing a frightening film (98), and undergoing a psychiatric interview (37). In rhesus monkeys with indwelling catheters in the vena cava, increases in norepinephrine alone occurred when the animals were exposed to unpleasant but familar stimuli. Epinephrine was increased, with or without norepinephrine increase, when there was a threat of something unpleasant, but its occurrence was unpredictable or the animal was uncertain how to respond (111).

Anxiety produced in more subtle ways can markedly increase the levels of catecholamines (134); for example, attempting to proofread in a fairly noisy environment (99) and conversion from a regular salary to a piece-work system of payment (97) have been found to be highly effective. Even the mild stresses experienced in one's normal employment may be sufficient to produce catecholamine levels as high as can be found in pheochromocytoma (100).

An important correlation between the maintenance of vigilance and circulating epinephrine was first demonstrated by O'Hanlon (133). He showed, with the EDA method, that in subjects performing a simple visual task their highest efficiency was associated with a raised epinephrine content in plasma. As this content declined, so did their performance. These observations were subsequently confirmed and extended by a further study in which he employed the THI method for the assay of the plasma catecholamines (134).

Plasma Catecholamines in Disease

Raised concentrations of plasma catecholamines have been reported for a variety of diseases, such as pheochromocytoma, severe eclampsia, myocardial infarction, and Raynaud's disease (52), but in phenylketonuria the amine levels may be lower than normal.

Tumors of the sympathetic tissues, both in the adrenal gland and in other parts of the body, often release large amounts of catecholamines into the circulating blood. The relative amounts of the different amines and the varying quantities in the blood withdrawn from different vessels provide a valuable means of identifying and locating the tumor (64, 75, 178). Frequently the release of catecholamines from the tumor is intermittent, which leads to paroxysmal hypertension. In one such situation, the concentration of norepinephrine in plasma rose from 5.6 to 98 ng/ml during an attack, but 5 min later it fell sharply to 13.2 ng/ml (57). In general the contents of catecholamines in plasma vary greatly between individuals but are almost always much higher than normal, with norepinephrine being the predominant amine, particularly when the tumor is extramedullary. Manipulation of the tumor at surgery can lead to a very great increase in the circulating catecholamines, as can the

TABLE 6. *Plasma Catecholamines in Myocardial Infarction*

Clinical Group[a]	Mortality	Mean Systolic BP, mmHg	Plasma Catecholamines, ng/ml[b, c]	
			Epinephrine	Norepinephrine
A[e]	7 of 9	64	0.27 ± 0.10^d	4.1 ± 0.6^d
B[f]	2 of 8	86	0.12 ± 0.06^d	1.5 ± 0.42^d
C[g]	1 of 8	124	0.09 ± 0.04	0.61 ± 0.22^d
D[h]			0.08 ± 0.04	0.29 ± 0.06

BP, blood pressure. [a] Twenty-five male patients with myocardial infarction. [b] Measured on admission to intensive care. [c] Value ±SD. [d] Value significantly different from clinical group D. [e] Clinical shock. [f] Abnormal blood pressure, central venous pressure, and heart rate. [g] Normal blood pressure, central venous pressure, and heart rate. [h] Control group without myocardial infarction. [Adapted from Griffiths & Leung (62).]

use of an anesthetic such as ether. Under halothane anesthesia a reduced loss of amines into the circulation during operation and handling of the tumor has been reported (39).

In rheumatic and valvular heart disease not complicated by either congestive failure or angina pectoris, the concentrations of plasma epinephrine and norepinephrine lie within normal limits both before and after exercise (20). In congestive failure, not only is the resting level often slightly raised, but there is a much greater increase on exercise than occurs in normal subjects. The plasma catecholamines are increased in myocardial infarction both in man and experimental animals (55, 157). Significant rises in norepinephrine to 0.6 ng/ml from a control value of 0.28 ng/ml in the absence of any rise in epinephrine have been seen in a group of male patients with a recent history of myocardial infarction (113). However, although Griffiths & Leung (62) confirmed the preferential release of norepinephrine, they found a small but significant increase in epinephrine; the greatest increase in circulating amines was observed in those patients with the highest subsequent mortality (Table 6). The authors claim that the amount of circulating catecholamines provides a useful guide to the prognosis of patients with myocardial infarction.

Large rises in the circulating amines have been seen in patients suffering from Raynaud's disease (139). Values of 25 and 22 ng/ml of epinephrine and norepinephrine, respectively, were seen, compared with undetectable levels in normal subjects. Further increases, up to 46 and 98 ng/ml, respectively, occurred when the patients' limbs were cooled.

DRUGS AND PLASMA CATECHOLAMINES

Drugs may alter the amounts of the catecholamines in the circulation in several ways. For example, the drug may interact directly with the chromaffin cells to liberate catecholamines, either by exocytosis or by displacement of their amine stores. This action may be exerted at the adrenal medulla or on the adrenergic neurons, or both.

Conversely the drug may prevent the release of the catecholamines. A further possibility could be the inhibition of the normal pathways of catecholamine inactivation, which would be expected to lead to an increase in the plasma amines. Cocaine, an inhibitor of uptake$_1$ [i.e., an inhibitor of norepinephrine and epinephrine uptake into adrenergic neurons (see the chapter by Iversen in this volume of the *Handbook*)] provides an example of this last mode of action. Trendelenburg (174) injected 25 µg of norepinephrine into anesthetized cats and took blood plasma samples 1, 2, and 3 min later. In control experiments the plasma content of norepinephrine fell from 74.5 ng/ml at 1 min to 15.2 at 3 min. With administration of 5 mg/kg of cocaine, the plasma norepinephrine reached 144.2 ng/ml at 1 min and fell more slowly to 56.0 at 3 min. Similar effects are seen with the uptake$_2$ inhibitor [i.e., extraneuronal uptake (see the chapter by Iversen in this volume of the *Handbook*)], phenoxybenzamine, which has been reported to cause a rise in plasma norepinephrine in the cat (188). If in the anesthetized dog the blood pressure is maintained, there is no change in the concentration of plasma epinephrine or norepinephrine (118). If, however, the blood pressure is allowed to fall, the resulting rise in concentration of plasma amines is greatly potentiated by phenoxybenzamine. Before administration of the drug, the plasma contents were 0.10 and 0.18 ng/ml of epinephrine and norepinephrine, respectively; 180 min after 20 mg/kg of phenoxybenzamine was administered the plasma contents reached 23 ng/ml of epinephrine and 8.7 ng/ml of norepinephrine.

Many drugs cause a release of catecholamines from the chromaffin cells. However, reserpine, a drug that depletes almost all the body stores of amines by an effect on vesicle storage, usually produces little rise in the plasma catecholamines. In the rabbit, however, injections of 1–2.3 mg/kg of this drug led to rises in the plasma epinephrine of between 2 and 22 times (127). Norepinephrine values were not significantly changed.

Nicotine

It is well known that acetylcholine and other drugs that stimulate nicotinic receptors will cause the release of catecholamines. Carbachol, for example, has been shown to increase the catecholamine concentrations in plasma of cats (4). A dose of 0.2 mg/kg of carbachol after atropine caused increases in the total plasma catecholamines from control values of less than 1 ng/ml to 12.9, 19.2, and 46.5 ng/ml in three cats. After adrenalectomy, smaller rises were still seen, but now norepinephrine was predominant.

Nicotine itself, when given to the experimental animal or when administered in tobacco smoke to the human subject, results in increases in the plasma amines. In a dose of 0.2 mg/kg injected into the aorta of the deeply anesthetized dog, nicotine led to a rise in the total catecholamines in the peripheral plasma from a control value of 2.4 ± 0.2 ng/ml to 40.7 ± 15.3 ng/ml (189). There appeared to be a selective effect on epinephrine. Potassium chloride given by this route also caused a rise in the plasma amines. Epinephrine rose from 1.4 to 60 ng/ml, and norepinephrine from 2.0 to 11.5 ng/ml. Smoking a cigarette was found to increase the plasma norepinephrine concentration by 26 % (88). If the subject undertook moderate exercise the increase was 110 %. The plasma epinephrine content was altered only if the exercise continued for double the usual time. Nonesterified fatty acids (NEFA) in plasma rose to 60 % above normal after smoking a cigarette. Increases in the excretion of catecholamines and in plasma NEFA have been measured after both cigar and cigarette smoking (86). However, the rises are not as great after cigar smoking, possibly because of variations in the amount of nicotine absorbed as a result of the amount of smoke inhaled.

Anesthetics

Elliott (35) in 1912 showed that ether, chloroform, and urethane all depleted the adrenal glands of their catecholamine content. Since that time there have been many reports of rises in the plasma amines during surgical anesthesia. These rises may be further modified by other factors, such as acidemia, hypoxia, and changes in body temperature. Drug treatment may also have some influence.

Diethyl ether readily increases the concentration of plasma catecholamines. In rats the arterial plasma content of epinephrine, measured biologically, rose to 1–6 ng/ml after a short exposure to ether (180). The content was reduced to less than 0.5 ng/ml if the animals had been subjected to adrenal demedullation before the experiment.

In dogs and rabbits where the plasma epinephrine content was about 1 ng/ml during ether anesthesia, concomitant respiratory failure increased it to about 16 ng/ml and to 75 ng/ml in cardiovascular collapse (183). Use of the EDA method has shown that large rises in concentration of epinephrine and norepinephrine in plasma occur in dogs under deep surgical anesthesia produced by diethyl ether, divinyl ether, and chloroform (152). The plasma amines were not significantly altered by thiopentone. When ether was given to animals already anesthetized with thiopentone, the concentration of plasma catecholamines rose considerably but fell to about normal by 30 min after withdrawal of the ether. Millar & Morris (121) showed that ether caused highly significant increases in the concentration of plasma norepinephrine in man and dogs. Rises in the epinephrine content were also found, but they were more marked in the dog than in man. There was still a rise in the concentration of plasma norepinephrine in adrenalectomized dogs, which indicated some extramedullary action of the anesthetic. This rise was enhanced in the presence of hypercapnia. A relationship has been suggested, in human subjects, between the concentration of ether in the inspired gas and the plasma content of catecholamines (5). Exposure of the subject to 5, 10, and 15 % ether caused increases of norepinephrine concentration in the plasma from a control value of 0.16 ng/ml to 0.19, 0.67, and 1.52 ng/ml, respectively. Cyclopropane anesthesia also leads to a release of catecholamines, but halothane does not (121). Although no change in the plasma amines was seen in uncomplicated anesthesia, significant rises occurred if hypercapnia were allowed to develop. Methoxyfluorane behaved in a similar manner (120). Trichloroethylene superimposed on nitrous oxide and oxygen anesthesia also caused no significant increase in the plasma amines (175).

Barbiturates do not raise the concentration of plasma amines to any extent (33, 122, 152) and are probably the most satisfactory anesthetics for experiments involving the measurement of plasma catecholamines. However, they may depress the sensitivity of sympathetic tissue to releasing agents (189). In dogs, thiopentone, unlike ether and cyclopropane, causes no change in the myocardial content of catecholamines (101). Phenobarbitone and pentobarbitone both cause an initial loss of amine from the heart, but the content is restored even though the anesthesia is maintained (166). Halothane may also depress the release of catecholamines into the plasma; thus it has been recommended as a suitable anesthetic in the removal of chromaffin cell tumors (39).

Urethane has long been known to induce the release of catecholamines. Satake (160) found an increase in the plasma catecholamine content of dogs after injections of urethane. More recently, Spriggs (166) has shown that urethane anesthesia in the rat causes an increase in the cardiac stores of epinephrine by uptake of this amine from the circulation after its release from the adrenal medulla.

CATECHOLAMINES IN ADRENAL VENOUS BLOOD

Resting Secretion

There have been many attempts to determine the output of the adrenal gland under resting conditions. In most cases this has involved cannulation of the adrenal vein in anesthetized animals. Consequently the values obtained are many and varied and are usually influenced by the almost insurmountable difficulties encountered in the collection of blood samples in this manner (40, 105). Since the glands are so sensitive to stress, the surgery involved can easily increase the rate of catecholamine output. The cannulation of the adrenal vein can stimulate the glands to increase their output, by the loss of blood and by depriving the animal of the secretion of one gland. Even if there is no fall in blood pressure on cannulation, the output can triple (105), and as the experiment progresses, the adrenal output may rise severalfold (59, 82, 105). Great care must be exercised in the selection of a suitable anesthetic, and acidemia and hypercapnia must be prevented at all costs. The use of indwelling cannulae in the conscious animal may produce the most reliable values.

The evidence indicates that there is always some release of catecholamines into the adrenal vein, even after denervation. It is impossible completely to prevent this adrenal secretion by infusion of epinephrine into the experimental animal (106, 156), although the secretion from the gland is reduced when the blood pressure is artificially raised and increased when the blood pressure falls (173). A basal secretion rate of about 15 ng/kg per min was observed in conscious dogs with adrenal glands transplanted into the neck (182).

Recently, Sapira & Bron (158) have estimated the catecholamine content of the adrenal venous blood of conscious human subjects. Blood samples were obtained by inserting a catheter into the left adrenal vein of 13 patients undergoing angiography. These authors found an extremely wide variation in the resting rate of epinephrine secretion both between patients and within the same individual. In general, much smaller amounts of norepinephrine than epinephrine were released, and 60% of the samples contained no norepinephrine at all. No correlation could be seen between the simultaneous epinephrine and norepinephrine contents of the adrenal venous blood. The mean resting rate of epinephrine secretion from one human adrenal gland was calculated to be 272 ng/min. However, the values ranged from 52 to 644 ng/min. In four anesthetized patients, total epinephrine output between 230 and 610 ng/min has been reported (145). Ether anesthesia in man produced adrenal vein contents of 50–200 ng/ml of epinephrine and 7–16 ng/ml of norepinephrine (161). The output of the human adrenal medulla has been calculated indirectly from the rate of infusion of epinephrine needed to maintain a given concentration in the peripheral plasma. Values of 8 ng/kg per min (178) and 10 ng/kg per min (22) have been found by this approach; they compare very well with the figure of 8.7 ng/kg per min obtained by direct measurement (158).

A wide variation in resting output from the gland is often seen in the experimental animal because of the changing conditions of the experiment, together with the possibility that the release of the amines is intermittent (158). In Table 7 some values for this resting secretion are summarized.

Stimulated Release of Adrenal Medullary Amines

The adrenal medulla can be induced to release its hormones in a variety of ways. Reflex release as a result of baroreceptor stimulation is one example. Naturally occurring substances and the neurotransmitter, acetylcholine, may directly stimulate the chromaffin cells to release their amine store. These substances, together with synthetic drugs, can be administered to the experimental animal. Appropriate brain regions and splanchnic nerves can be stimulated electrically. Some of these methods have already been mentioned in this chapter, but reference is made to them again where they have been shown to increase the catecholamine content of the adrenal venous blood.

TABLE 7. *Resting Secretion of Epinephrine and Norepinephrine from One Adrenal Gland*

Species	Adrenal Output, ng/kg per min		Ref.
	Epinephrine	Norepinephrine	
Man*	8.7		158
Pig*	10.9		159
Cat†	30	70	89
	6.2 (0.8–11.0)	37 (26–75)	34
	10–120	6–67	59
Dog†	40 (0.9–205)	14 (0.8–64)	155
Dog†			105
Newborn	86	105	
75-Day-old	120	15	
Adult	183	34	
Calf†,‡			163
Birth to 1 week	22	25	
2–5 weeks	176	94	
8–30 weeks	130	40	
Sheep†	5	2.7	28

* Catheter sample from conscious subject. † Adrenal vein sample from anesthetized subject. ‡ Splanchnic nerves cut 15–30 min before sampling.

ELECTRICAL STIMULATION. Preferential release of either amine from the adrenal gland has been reported in response to stimulation of certain areas in the hypothalamus (9, 51, 148) and amygdala (64, 149). For example, stimulation of the anterior hypothalamus may cause a preferential release of norepinephrine, whereas epinephrine is associated with stimulation of the regions adjacent to the mammillary bodies (148).

Bülbring & Burn (10) showed that stimulation of the splanchnic nerve in the spinal cat (i.e., a cat with spinal cord transected in the neck and the brain destroyed) caused the release of both epinephrine and norepinephrine from the adrenal gland. The output rises to a maximum at an optimum stimulation rate of 30–60 Hz (108, 109). Supramaximal stimulation of the splanchnic nerve with 10 shocks at 1 Hz caused the release of 5–10 ng of amine per shock (109). Stimulation at the optimal rate for either 200 or 256 shocks produced 3–5 ng per shock. If the stimulation were continued for 10 min the adrenal secretion fell to less than 0.5 ng and finally declined to background levels.

There have been several reports that the relative proportions of the two amines released into the adrenal vein depend on the frequency of stimulation (143). In cats anesthetized with dial-urethane the amount of total catecholamine released from the gland rose from about 10 ng/kg per min at 1 Hz to 18 ng/kg per min at 10 Hz, together with a rise in the proportion of epinephrine from 27 to 60% (89). However, this change is not seen in the calf, for example (163); in the dog the frequency range required is nonphysiological (123).

CHOLINERGIC DRUGS. Although the main action of acetylcholine in releasing catecholamines from the adrenal chromaffin cells is mediated through nicotinic receptors, muscarinic receptors may also be involved (47). The muscarinic receptors have been implicated in the neuronal release of adrenal catecholamines (96). Douglas & Poisner (32) showed that, in the cat, stimulation of these muscarinic receptors with muscarine or pilocarpine caused a preferential release of epinephrine into the venous effluent from the gland. Nicotine, on the other hand, in low concentrations may lead to a preferential loss of norepinephrine (157). This is also seen with dimethylphenylpiperazinium iodide (DMPP) (114). However, the evidence is at present not at all clear concerning the possibility that the muscarinic receptors are associated with the epinephrine-containing cells [(143); see the chapter by Douglas in this volume of the *Handbook*]. It has been pointed out that most of the results were obtained from adrenal glands perfused with Locke's solution at pH 7 and not with blood (143). This procedure has been shown to cause some damage to the adrenal cells together with a selective loss of epinephrine (132).

HYPOGLYCEMIA. Insulin-induced hypoglycemia leads to the preferential increase in epinephrine output from the adrenal medulla as a result of stimulation of centers in the brainstem or hypothalamus. In the sheep the output from the left adrenal gland rose from control values of 5.0 and 2.7 ng/kg per min of epinephrine and norepinephrine, respectively, to 83.2 and 14.2 ng/kg per min, respectively, after insulin was administered (28). The increased output began between 30 min and 1 hr after the injection and continued for several hours. In the dog, where the resting output of epinephrine was 7.5 ng/kg per min, insulin induced a rise to a peak value of 31.9 ng/kg per min (190).

The hyperglycemic compound, diazoxide, has been shown to induce the release of both adrenal and extramedullary catecholamines (102). The effect on the adrenal is at least partially direct and independent of the hypotension that the drug produces. Cross-perfusion experiments indicated that a dose of 2.0 mg/kg increased the adrenal output from about 110 and 10 ng/min of epinephrine and norepinephrine, respectively, in the control period to about 620 and 110 ng/min, respectively, in a group of five dogs.

HYPOXIA. Hypoxia and asphyxia are powerful stimuli causing the release of adrenal medullary hormones in experimental animals. In the cat, for example, the output can reach 1 μg/kg per min (42) or even higher (19). The dog responds in a similar manner (105). In the newborn animal the epinephrine output rose from 86 to 680 ng/kg per min and the norepinephrine from 105 to 420 ng/kg per min. In the older dog the corresponding rises were from 120 to 866 and from 16 to 468 ng/kg per min, respectively. Splanchnic denervation greatly reduces or abolishes the response to asphyxia (25). In the fetal lamb, severe hypoxia produced by ligature of the umbilical cord led to increases in adrenal output (24). At 115 days gestation the secretion of norepinephrine reached 900 ng/min from a resting level of about 40 ng/min by a direct effect of the stimulus on the gland. This effect of asphyxia could be mimicked by the intraarterial injection of sodium cyanide, which in doses of 2–5 mg caused an immediate increase in the adrenal output from a resting level of 50 and 90 ng/min for epinephrine and norepinephrine, respectively, to 240 and 770 ng/min, respectively. At about 140 days gestation the adrenal gland became much more sensitive to small falls in P_{O_2} because of the influence of the now functional splanchnic nerve. In the calf the adrenal response to asphyxia is mediated through the direct component until birth (26). Rapid changes in the sensitivity of the gland occur in the first 24 hr after birth. At first it is hypersensitive because the direct and neuronal components act together, but the sensitivity falls again and does not return to the level in the newborn until 2–3 weeks later. At this time the effect of asphyxia is mediated almost entirely through the splanchnic nerve.

HYPOTENSION. The increase in secretion of adrenal catecholamines in hypotension and the decrease in hypertension are mediated through reflex control from the carotid sinus (76). The carotid occlusion reflex invoked by clamping the carotid arteries usually leads to increase in the adrenal output. For example, Kaindl & von Euler (82) found an increase in the rate of adrenal secretion of total catecholamines from a control level of 73 ng/kg per min to 230 ng/kg per min without change in the relative proportions of the two amines. This effect was only seen in animals in which the vagus nerves had been cut.

Many investigators have reported that the adrenal amine secretion steadily increased during the course of an experiment involving an anesthetized animal (59, 105). Increases of about four to five times the initial secretion have been observed probably because of attempts by the animal to maintain its blood pressure (82).

Both acidemia and hypercapnia are effective stimulants of adrenal medullary release. In the fetal lamb, however, both at 115 and 140 days gestation, hypercapnia had only a very slight effect on the adrenal gland, and it did not potentiate the responses to asphyxia (24). Intraarterial lactic acid, in doses of between 4 and 10 mg, caused a significant increase in norepinephrine output from a control level of 90 ± 31 ng/min to 170 ± 19 ng/min in the fetus at 115 days gestation. In conscious pigs with indwelling catheters collecting the venous blood from the left adrenal gland, loss of 30% of the blood volume in 30 min increased the catecholamine output from a control value of 10.9 to 133 ng/kg per min, but only after the blood loss had stopped. The same loss of blood spread over 90 min was without any measurable effect (159).

HISTAMINE. Burn & Dale (11) first showed that adrenalectomy abolished the secondary rise in blood pressure that followed the injection of histamine in the cat. Direct measurement of the epinephrine and norepinephrine contents of the adrenal venous blood of anesthetized dogs indicated a release of both amines after very large intravenous doses of histamine or the production of anaphylaxis (155). Doses of histamine ranging from 0.5 to 10 mg were required to induce an increase of medullary output, which in some instances amounted to about 50–60 times the resting level. However, not all reports indicate that histamine releases catecholamines. For example, the injection of 40 μg/kg of histamine into the aorta of anesthetized dogs did not alter the total plasma catecholamines from the control value of 5.2 ± 2.8 ng/ml (189).

Staszewska-Barczak & Vane (167) measured the catecholamine content in blood of both cats and dogs by the blood-bathed organ technique after intravenous and intraarterial injections of histamine. Doses of 10–20 μg resulted in a secretion consisting almost entirely of epinephrine. Adrenalectomy and treatment with antihistamines prevented this release in both species. In the cat epinephrine release was unaffected by section of the spinal cord, but in the dog it was reduced. The authors conclude that, in the dog at least, three mechanisms are involved in the release of adrenal medullary hormones by histamine: stimulation of chemo- or baroreceptors, stimulation of the nerve endings in the adrenal medulla, and a direct effect on the chromaffin cells caused by histamine in high concentrations.

POLYPEPTIDES AND OTHER SUBSTANCES. In the cat, Feldberg & Lewis (45, 46) have shown that bradykinin and angiotensin are powerful stimulants of adrenal medullary release. Injection of these compounds into the stump of the celiac artery of cats eviscerated by removal of stomach, spleen, and intestines caused a discharge of catecholamines from the gland that could be measured on the denervated nictitating membrane and blood pressure of the same animal. It was estimated that each molecule of bradykinin could release about 50 molecules of catecholamine, and angiotensin several thousands. Under these conditions, vasopressin, oxytocin, and substance P were ineffective. Neither denervation nor treatment with hexamethonium reduced the potency of the releasing agents. Angiotensin, injected intravenously in the adrenalectomized cat, still produced a small effect. Since no direct action could be seen it was concluded that it could exert some action on extramedullary stores of catecholamines. Bradykinin and angiotensin, as well as histamine, SRS-A, and the injection of antigen into sensitized animals, cause the release of epinephrine into the circulation of the guinea pig (27, 141, 142). This release is prevented by adrenalectomy.

The ability of these agents to release catecholamines seems to depend on the species of animal studied. In the calf, for instance, intraarterial injection of bradykinin or angiotensin raised the adrenal medullary output to only just above the control value (27). In the same animals, acetylcholine or splanchnic stimulation increased the output by between 10- and 100-fold. The release of the catecholamines in response to these polypeptides in the dog adrenal gland is seen in the isolated organ perfused with Locke's solution (154, 181) and also in the anesthetized animal (137). After adrenalectomy the initial rise in plasma catecholamines was as large as that found in the intact animal, but it soon fell to the resting level, even though the angiotensin infusion continued. Recently angiotensin I has been found to possess a direct effect on the adrenal medulla not dependent on its conversion to angiotensin II (138).

OVERFLOW OF NOREPINEPHRINE FROM SYMPATHETICALLY INNERVATED ORGANS

Cannon & Uridil (16) stimulated the sympathetic nerves to the cat's liver and found, by detecting its effects on the denervated heart of the same animal, that the transmitter substance overflowed into the circulation. However, the resting levels of catecholamines in the circulation from all sources are very low, and the contribution of the adrenal glands is difficult to assess. Nearly all the epinephrine disappears after adrenalectomy, but the norepinephrine remains about the same. Price (145) found that, in human subjects, adrenalectomy reduced the plasma epinephrine content from 0.25 to 0.02 ng/ml, whereas the norepinephrine content showed an insignificant rise from 1.1 to 1.2 ng/ml. These changes are closely reflected in the urinary excretion of the amines (143). The lack of effect on the plasma norepinephrine may be due to either an insignificant output of this amine from the adrenal medulla in the normal animal or to a compensatory rise in the contribution from the other organs when this source is lost.

A great deal of information has accumulated from experiments in which the output from individual organs has been estimated by sampling the amine content of their venous effluent. In the isolated blood-perfused spleen, stimulation of the splenic nerves does not give rise to measurable amounts of norepinephrine until the rate of stimulation exceeds 10 Hz (8). The overflow from the organ for each stimulus steadily rises to a maximum of about 0.8 ng at around 30 Hz. The output is unaffected by the simultaneous inhibition of both monoamine oxidase and catechol-O-methyltransferase but is potentiated by phenoxybenzamine. At low rates of stimulation this amounted to a fivefold increase, but by 30 Hz it was only just significant. In the saline-perfused spleen in the presence of both cocaine and phenoxybenzamine, a norepinephrine overflow of 43.2 ± 7.4 ng/min could be detected at a stimulation rate of 0.5 Hz (66). At a stimulation rate of 1 Hz, the output was three times as great.

Maximal release of norepinephrine occurred at 2 Hz, where it reached 5.5 ng per stimulus.

Estimation of the catecholamine content of the various vessels supplying and leaving the heart indicates that this organ can release norepinephrine into the circulation. The direct release of this amine into the left chambers of the heart has been suggested to occur in acute coronary occlusion in the dog; the amine content of the pulmonary venous and aortic arch blood plasma was increased from control values of 0.19 and 0.5 ng/ml to 0.75 and 2.25 ng/ml, respectively (40).

The perfused inferior mesenteric ganglion of the dog releases epinephrine and norepinephrine (128). The resting output, originating from the chromaffin cells of the paraganglia, varied widely between preparations when they were perfused with a modified Locke's solution. Outputs in the range of 0.7–40 ng/min and 0.7–25 ng/min of norepinephrine and epinephrine, respectively, were found. The very high values were probably due to the presence of small amounts of the organ of Zuckerkandl. Stimulation of the inferior splanchnic nerves did not change the resting release of catecholamines. The output doubled, however, after stimulation of the ascending mesenteric nerves. Both acetylcholine and DMPP increased the output by between 6 and 100 times. Drugs that stimulated muscarinic receptors were almost without effect, whereas bradykinin had only weak action and angiotensin inhibited release.

The plasma catecholamines originate in almost all parts of the body by virtue of the sympathetic innervation to the various organs and to the vascular smooth muscle. They are also released from the chromaffin cells of the adrenal medulla and possibly from the scattered paraganglion tissue. The relative importance of these various sites of amine release depends on the nature of the stimulus. In some situations, the adrenal gland alone is involved, but in others an integrated response of the whole sympathetic system results. At present it is only with some difficulty that the contribution of the adrenal medulla can be discovered, usually by finding the effect of adrenalectomy on the plasma catecholamine response to the particular stress. Application of catheterization techniques, together with improved assay methods in which only a fraction of the volume of blood needed in the present methods is used, should provide the way to determine the behavior of the different sympathetically innervated organs both in the response of the animal to stress and in the maintenance of homeostasis.

REFERENCES

1. ANTON, A. H., AND D. F. SAYRE. A study of the factors affecting the aluminum oxide-trihydroxyindole procedure for the analysis of catecholamines. *J. Pharmacol. Exptl. Therap.* 138: 360–375, 1962.
2. AXELROD, J., H. WEIL-MALHERBE, AND R. TOMCHICK. The physiological disposition of ³H epinephrine and its metabolite metanephrine., *J. Pharmacol. Exptl. Therap.* 127: 251–256, 1959.
3. BATTELLI, M. F. Dosage colorimetrique de la substance active des capsules surrénales. *Compt. Rend. Soc. Biol.* 54: 571–573, 1902.
4. BERTLER, Å., A. CARLSSON, M. LINDQVIST, AND T. MAGNUSSON. On the catecholamine levels in blood plasma after stimulation of the sympathoadrenal system. *Experientia* 14: 184–185, 1958.
5. BLACK, G. W., L. MCARDLE, H. MCCULLOUGH, AND V. K.

N. UNNI. Circulating catecholamines and some cardiovascular, respiratory, metabolic and pupillary responses during diethyl ether anaesthesia. *Anaesthesia* 24: 168–179, 1969.
6. BLOOM, G., U. S. VON EULER, AND M. FRANKENHAEUSER. Catecholamine excretion and personality traits in paratroop trainees. *Acta Physiol. Scand.* 58: 77–89, 1963.
7. BRAUNWALD, E., C. A. CHIDSEY, D. C. HARRISON, T. E. GAFFNEY, AND R. L. KAHLER. Studies on the function of the adrenergic nerve endings in the heart. *Circulation* 28: 958–969, 1963.
8. BROWN, L. The release and fate of the transmitter liberated by adrenergic nerves. *Proc. Roy. Soc. London Ser. B* 162: 1–19, 1965.
9. BRÜCKE, F., F. KAINDL, AND H. MAYER. Über die Veränderung in der Zusammensetzung des Nebennierenmarkinkretes bei elektrischer Reizung des Hypothalamus. *Arch. Intern. Pharmacodyn. Therap.* 88: 407–412, 1952.
10. BÜLBRING, E., AND J. H. BURN. Liberation of noradrenaline from the suprarenal gland. *Brit. J. Pharmacol. Chemotherap.* 4: 202–208, 1949.
11. BURN, J. H., AND H. H. DALE. The vasodilator action of histamine and its physiological significance. *J. Physiol., London* 61: 185–214, 1926.
12. CALLINGHAM, B. A. The catecholamines. Adrenaline; noradrenaline. In: *Hormones in Blood* (2nd ed.), edited by C. H. Gray and A. L. Bacharach. London: Acad. Press, 1967, p. 519–599.
13. CANNON, W. B. *Bodily Changes in Pain, Hunger, Fear and Rage.* New York: Appleton, 1929.
14. CANNON, W. B., AND R. G. HOSKINS. The effects of asphyxia, hypernoea and sensory stimulation on adrenal secretion. *Am. J. Physiol.* 29: 274–279, 1911.
15. CANNON, W. B., M. A. MCIVER, AND S. W. BLISS. Studies on the conditions of activity in endocrine glands. XIII. A sympathetic and adrenal mechanism for mobilizing sugar in hypoglycemia. *Am. J. Physiol.* 69: 46–66, 1924.
16. CANNON, W. B., AND J. E. URIDIL. Studies on the conditions of activity in endocrine glands. VIII. Some effects on the denervated heart of stimulating the nerves of the liver. *Am. J. Physiol.* 58: 353–364, 1921.
17. CANTU, R. C., G. G. NAHAS, AND W. M. MANGER. Effect of hypercapnic acidosis and of hypoxia on adrenal catecholamine output of the spinal dog. *Proc. Soc. Exptl. Biol. Med.* 122: 434–437, 1966.
18. CARRUTHERS, M., P. TAGGART, N. CONWAY, D. BATES, AND W. SOMERVILLE. Validity of plasma-catecholamine estimations. *Lancet* 2: 62–67, 1970.
19. CELANDER, O. The range of control exercised by the 'sympathetico-adrenal system.' *Acta Physiol. Scand. Suppl.* 116: 1–132, 1954.
20. CHIDSEY, C. A., D. C. HARRISON, AND E. BRAUNWALD. Augmentation of the plasma nor-epinephrine response to exercise in patients with congestive heart failure. *New Engl. J. Med.* 267: 650–654, 1962.
21. COHEN, G., AND M. GOLDENBERG. The simultaneous fluorimetric determination of adrenaline and noradrenaline in plasma. II. Peripheral venous plasma concentrations in normal subjects and in patients with pheochromocytoma. *J. Neurochem.* 2: 71–80, 1957.
22. COHEN, G., B. HOLLAND, J. SHA, AND M. GOLDENBERG. Plasma concentration of epinephrine and norepinephrine during intravenous infusions in man. *J. Clin. Invest.* 38: 1935–1941, 1959.
23. COMLINE, R. S., AND A. V. EDWARDS. The effects of insulin on the new born calf. *J. Physiol., London* 198: 383–404, 1968.
24. COMLINE, R. S., I. A. SILVER, AND M. SILVER. Factors responsible for the stimulation of the adrenal medulla during asphyxia in the foetal lamb. *J. Physiol., London* 178: 211–238, 1965.
25. COMLINE, R. S., AND M. SILVER. The release of adrenaline and noradrenaline from the adrenal glands of the foetal sheep. *J. Physiol., London* 156: 424–444, 1961.
26. COMLINE, R. S., AND M. SILVER. The development of the adrenal medulla of the foetal and new born calf. *J. Physiol., London* 183: 305–340, 1966.
27. COMLINE, R. S., M. SILVER, AND D. G. SINCLAIR. The effects of bradykinin, angiotensin and acetylcholine on the bovine adrenal medulla. *J. Physiol., London* 196: 339–350, 1968.
28. CRONE, C. The secretion of adrenal medullary hormones during hypoglycaemia in intact, decerebrate and spinal sheep. *Acta Physiol. Scand.* 63: 213–224, 1965.
29. CROSS, M. H., AND R. T. HOULIHAN. Sympathoadrenalmedullary response of the rat to high oxygen exposures. *J. Appl. Physiol.* 27: 523–527, 1969.
30. CUNNINGHAM, W. L., E. J. BECKER, AND F. KREUZER. Catecholamines in plasma and urine at high altitudes. *J. Appl. Physiol.* 20: 607–610, 1965.
31. DARBY, T. D., AND D. T. WATTS. Acidosis and blood epinephrine levels in hemorrhagic hypotension. *Am. J. Physiol.* 206: 1281–1284, 1964.
32. DOUGLAS, W. W., AND A. M. POISNER. Preferential release of adrenaline from the adrenal medulla by muscarine and pilocarpine. *Nature* 208: 1102–1103, 1965.
33. DUNÉR, H. The influence of the blood glucose level on the secretion of adrenaline and noradrenaline from the suprarenal. *Acta Physiol. Scand. Suppl.* 102: 1–77, 1953.
34. DUNÉR, H. The effect of insulin hypoglycaemia on the secretion of adrenaline and noradrenaline from the suprarenal of the cat. *Acta Physiol. Scand.* 32: 63–68, 1954.
35. ELLIOTT, T. R. The control of the suprarenal glands by the splanchnic nerves. *J. Physiol., London* 44: 374–409, 1912.
36. ELMADJIAN, F. Epinephrine, norepinephrine and aldosterone: release and excretion. In: *Man's Dependence on the Earthly Atmosphere*, edited by K. E. Schaefer. New York: Macmillan, 1962, p. 100–116.
37. ELMADJIAN, F., J. M. HOPE, AND E. T. LAMSON. Excretion of epinephrine and norepinephrine in various emotional states. *J. Clin. Endocrinol. Metab.* 17: 608–620, 1957.
38. ENGELMAN, K., AND B. PORTNOY. A sensitive double-isotope derivative assay for norepinephrine and epinephrine. *Circulation Res.* 26: 53–57, 1970.
39. ETSTEN, B. E., AND S. SHIMOSATO. Halothane anesthesia and catecholamine levels in a patient with pheochromocytoma. *Anesthesiology* 26: 688–691, 1965.
40. EULER, U. S. VON. *Noradrenaline*. Springfield, Ill.: Thomas, 1956.
41. EULER, U. S. VON. The catecholamines. Adrenaline; noradrenaline. In: *Hormones in Blood* (1st ed.), edited by C. H. Gray and A. L. Bacharach. London: Acad. Press, 1961, p. 515–582.
42. EULER, U. S. VON, AND B. FOLKOW. Einfluss verschiedener afferenter Nervenreize auf die Zusammensetzung des Nebennierenmarkinkretes bei der Katze. *Arch. Exptl. Pathol. Pharmakol.* 219: 242–247, 1953.
43. EULER, U. S. VON, C. FRANKSSON, AND J. HELLSTRÖM. Adrenaline and noradrenaline output in urine after unilateral and bilateral adrenalectomy in man. *Acta Physiol. Scand.* 31: 1–5, 1954.
44. EULER, U. S. VON, AND T. SJÖSTRAND. Pressor activity in blood and plasma from normal subjects and patients with essential hypertension. *Acta Med. Scand.* 119: 1–17, 1944.
45. FELDBERG, W., AND G. P. LEWIS. The action of peptides on the adrenal medulla. Release of adrenaline by bradykinin and angiotensin. *J. Physiol., London* 171: 98–108, 1964.
46. FELDBERG, W., AND G. P. LEWIS. Further studies on the effects of peptides on the suprarenal medulla of cats. *J. Physiol., London* 178: 239–251, 1965.
47. FELDBERG, W., B. MINZ, AND H. TSUDZIMURA. The mechanism of the nervous discharge of adrenaline. *J. Physiol., London* 81: 286–304, 1934.
48. FELLER, R. P., AND H. B. HALE. Human urinary catecholamines in relation to climate. *J. Appl. Physiol.* 19: 37–39, 1964.
49. FERREIRA, S. H., AND J. R. VANE. Half-lives of peptides and amines in the circulation. *Nature* 215: 1237–1240, 1967.

50. FLOHR, H., H. KLENSCH, R. FELIX, AND P. GEISLER. Plasmakatecholaminkonzentrationen in akuter Hypoxie. Fluorimetrische Messungen im arteriellen und mischvenösen menslichen Blut. *Arch. Ges. Physiol.* 290: 225–230, 1966.
51. FOLKOW, B., AND U. S. VON EULER. Selective activation of noradrenaline and adrenaline producing cells in the cat's adrenal gland by hypothalamic stimulation. *Circulation Res.* 2: 191–195, 1954.
52. FRANZEN, F., AND K. EYSELL. Biologically active amines found in man. Oxford: Pergamon Press, 1969.
53. GADDUM, J. H. Bioassay procedures. *Pharmacol. Rev.* 11: 241–249, 1959.
54. GARCÍA, U. H., AND J. M. WALLACE. Acción de la actividad física y de la infusión intravenosa de epinefrina y nor-epinefrina sobre los niveles plasmáticos de ambas aminas en sujetos normales (Abstract). *Intern. Congr. Physiol. Sci., 21st, Buenos Aires, 1959*, p. 102–103.
55. GAZES, P. C., J. A. RICHARDSON, AND E. F. WOODS. Plasma catecholamine concentration in myocardial infarction and angina pectoris. *Circulation* 19: 657–661, 1959.
56. GITLOW, S., M. MENDLOWITZ, E. KRUK, S. WILK, R. WOLF, AND N. NAFTCHI. Norepinephrine metabolism in essential hypertension. *J. Clin. Invest.* 42: 934–935, 1963.
57. GOLDFIEN, A., M. S. ZILELI, R. H. DESPOINTES, AND J. E. BETHUNE. The effect of hypoglycemia on the adrenal secretion of epinephrine and norepinephrine in the dog. *Endocrinology* 62: 749–757, 1958.
58. GOODALL, McC., M. McCALLY, AND D. F. GRAVELINE. Urinary adrenaline and noradrenaline response to a simulated weightless state. *Am. J. Physiol.* 206: 431–436, 1964.
59. GRANT, R., P. LINDGREN, A. ROSEN, AND B. UVNÄS. The release of catechols from the adrenal medulla on activation of the sympathetic vasodilator nerves to the skeletal muscles in the cat by hypothalamic stimulation. *Acta Physiol. Scand.* 43: 135–154, 1958.
60. GREEN, R. D., III, AND J. W. MILLER. Catecholamine concentrations: changes in plasma of rats during estrous cycle and pregnancy. *Science* 151: 825–826, 1966.
61. GREEVER, C. J., AND D. T. WATTS. Epinephrine levels in peripheral blood during irreversible hemorrhagic shock in dogs. *Circulation Res.* 7: 192–195, 1959.
62. GRIFFITHS, J., AND F. LEUNG. The sequential estimation of plasma catecholamines and whole blood histamine in myocardial infarction. *Am. Heart J.* 82: 171–179, 1971.
63. GRIFFITHS, J. C., F. Y. T. LEUNG, AND T. J. MCDONALD. Fluorimetric determination of plasma catecholamines: normal human epinephrine and norepinephrine levels. *Clin. Chim. Acta* 30: 395–405, 1970.
64. GRIM, C. E., J. F. GLENN, J. O. WYNN, J. CAULIE GUNNELLS, JR., AND N. C. DURHAM. Bilateral pheochromocytoma. The application of a plasma catecholamine bioassay for tumor localization. *Am. Heart J.* 74: 809–815, 1967.
65. GUNNE, L-M., AND D. J. REIS. Changes in brain catecholamines associated with electrical stimulation of amygdaloid nucleus. *Life Sci.* 2: 804–809, 1963.
66. HAEFELY, W., A. HÜRLIMANN, AND H. THOENEN. Relation between the rate of stimulation and the quantity of noradrenaline liberated from sympathetic nerve endings in the isolated perfused spleen of the cat. *J. Physiol., London* 181: 48–58, 1965.
67. HÄGGENDAL, J. An improved method for fluorimetric determination of small amounts of adrenaline and noradrenaline in plasma and tissues. *Acta Physiol. Scand.* 59: 242–254, 1963.
68. HÄGGENDAL, J. The presence of conjugated adrenaline and noradrenaline in human blood plasma. *Acta Physiol. Scand.* 59: 255–260, 1963.
69. HÄGGENDAL, J. Newer developments in catecholamine assay. *Pharmacol. Rev.* 18: 325–329, 1966.
70. HÄGGENDAL, J., AND N. SVEDMYR. The effect of triiodothyronine treatment on the catecholamine content of the blood during infusion of adrenaline in man. *Acta Physiol. Scand.* 66: 103–105, 1966.
71. HÄGGENDAL, J., AND B. WERDINIUS. Dopamine in human urine during muscular work. *Acta Physiol. Scand.* 66: 223–225, 1966.
72. HALE, H. B., E. W. WILLIAMS, AND J. P. ELLIS, JR. Catecholamine excretion during heat deacclimatization. *J. Appl. Physiol.* 18: 1206–1208, 1963.
73. HEMPEL, K., AND H. F. K. MÄNNL. Resting secretion of dopamine from the adrenal glands of the cat in vivo. *Experientia* 23: 919–920, 1967.
74. HEMPEL, K., AND H. F. K. MÄNNL. Dopamin, ein neuer Bestandteil des Nebennieren—Inkrets. *Arch. Exptl. Pathol. Pharmakol.* 263: 222, 1969.
75. HERMANN, H., AND R. MORNEX. *Human Tumours Secreting Catecholamines.* Oxford: Pergamon Press, 1964.
76. HEYMANS, C. Le sinus carotidien, zone réflexogène regulatrice du tonus vagal cardiaque du tonus neurovasculaire et de l'adrénalosécrétion. *Arch. Intern. Pharmacodyn. Therap.* 35: 269–306, 1928.
77. HICKLER, R. B., J. T. HAMLIN, III, AND R. E. WELLS, JR. Plasma norepinephrine response to tilting in essential hypertension. *Circulation* 20: 422–426, 1959.
78. HOCHULI, E. Adrenalin—und Noradrenalinbestimmungen in Blutplasma in der Schwangerschaft, unter der Geburt und bei Schwangerschaftstoxikose. *Geburtsh. Frauenheilk.* 20: 835–842, 1960.
79. HOLZBAUER, M., AND M. VOGT. The concentration of adrenaline in the peripheral blood during insulin hypoglycaemia. *Brit. J. Pharmacol. Chemotherap.* 9: 249–252, 1954.
80. HOUSSAY, B. A., J. T. LEWIS, AND E. A. MOLINELLI. Rôle de la sécrétion d'adrénaline pendant l'hypoglycémie produit par l'insuline. *Compt. Rend. Soc. Biol.* 91: 1011–1013, 1924.
81. JOHANSSON, G., M. FRANKENHAEUSER, AND W. W. LAMBERT. *Seasonal Variations in Catecholamine Output.* Report No. 269. Stockholm: Psychology Laboratory, University of Stockholm, 1968.
82. KAINDL, K., AND U. S. VON EULER. Liberation of nor-adrenaline and adrenaline from the suprarenals of the cat during carotid occlusion. *Am. J. Physiol.* 166: 284–288, 1951.
83. KÄRKI, N. T. The urinary excretion of noradrenaline and adrenaline in different age groups; its diurnal variations and the effect of muscular work on it. *Acta Physiol. Scand. Suppl.* 132: 1–96, 1956.
84. KEATINGE, W. R., M. B. McILROY, AND A. GOLDFIEN. Cardiovascular responses to ice-cold showers. *J. Appl. Physiol.* 19: 1145–1150, 1964.
85. KELLY, M., D. F. SHARMAN, AND P. TEGERDINE. Dopamine in the blood of the ruminant. *J. Physiol., London* 210: 130P, 1970.
86. KERSHBAUM, A., S. BELLET, J. JIMENEZ, AND L. J. FEINBERG. Differences in effects of cigar and cigarette smoking on free fatty acid mobilization and catecholamine excretion. *J. Am. Med. Assoc.* 195: 1095–1098, 1966.
87. KLENSCH, H. Der basale Noradrenalinspiegel im peripheren venösen Blut des Menschen. *Arch. Ges. Physiol.* 290: 218–224, 1966.
88. KLENSCH, H. Blut-Katecholamine und—Fettsäuren beim Stress durch Rauchen und durch körperliche Arbeit. *Z. Kreislaufforsch.* 55: 1035–1044, 1966.
89. KLEVANS, L. R., AND G. L. GEBBER. Comparison of differential secretion of adrenal catecholamines by splanchnic nerve stimulation and cholinergic agents. *J. Pharmacol. Exptl. Therap.* 172: 69–76, 1970.
90. LAMMERANT, J., AND P. DE HERDT. Catecholamine plasma levels in the pulmonary artery, the pulmonary vein and the arterial tree of open-chest dogs during ambient air breathing and during acute anoxia. *Arch. Intern. Physiol.* 73: 81–96, 1965.
91. LAMMERANT, J., P. DE HERDT, AND C. DE SCHRYVER. Direct release of myocardial catecholamines into the left heart chambers: the enhancing effect of acute coronary occlusion. *Arch. Intern. Pharmacodyn. Therap.* 163: 219–226, 1966.
92. LAVERTY, R., AND D. F. SHARMAN. The estimation of small quantities of 3,4-dihydroxyphenylethylamine in tissues. *Brit. J. Pharmacol. Chemotherap.* 24: 538–548, 1965.

93. LEBLANC, J., AND M. POULIOT. Importance of noradrenaline in cold adaption. *Am. J. Physiol.* 207: 853–856, 1964.
94. LEDUC, J. Catecholamine production and release in exposure and acclimatization to cold. *Acta Physiol. Scand. Suppl.* 183: 1–100, 1961.
95. LEDUC, J., R. DUBREUIL, AND A. D'IORIO. Distribution of adrenaline and noradrenaline in the normal and hyperthyroid rat following adrenaline administration. *Can. J. Biochem. Physiol.* 33: 283–288, 1955.
96. LEE, F-L., AND U. TRENDELENBURG. Muscarinic transmission of preganglionic impulses to the adrenal medulla of the cat. *J. Pharmacol. Exptl. Therap.* 158: 73–79, 1967.
97. LEVI, L. The stress of everyday work as reflected in productiveness, subjective feelings and urinary output of adrenaline and noradrenaline under salaried and piecework conditions. *J. Psychosomat. Res.* 8: 199–202, 1964.
98. LEVI, L. The urinary output of adrenaline and noradrenaline during pleasant and unpleasant emotional states. *Psychosomat. Med.* 27: 80–85, 1965.
99. LEVI, L. Life stress and urinary excretion of adrenaline and noradrenaline. In: *Prevention of Ischemic Heart Disease*, edited by W. Raab. Springfield, Ill.: Thomas, 1966, p. 85–95.
100. LEVI, L. Stressors, stress tolerance, emotions and performance in relation to catecholamine excretion. In: *Emotional Stress*, edited by L. Levi. New York: Elsevier, 1967, p. 192–200.
101. LI, T-H., L. H. LAASBERG, AND B. E. ETSTEN. Effects of anesthetics on myocardial catecholamines. *Anesthesiology* 25: 641–649, 1964.
102. LOUBATIÈRES, A., M. M. MARIANI, AND R. ALRIC. The action of diazoxide on insulin secretion, medullo-adrenal secretion, and the liberation of catecholamines. *Ann. NY Acad. Sci.* 150: 226–241, 1968.
103. LUDEMANN, H. H., M. G. FILBERT, AND M. CORNBLATH. Application of a fluorometric method for adrenaline-like substances in peripheral plasma. *J. Appl. Physiol.* 8: 59–66, 1955.
104. LUND, A. Elimination of adrenaline and noradrenaline from the organism. *Acta Pharmacol. Toxicol.* 7: 297–308, 1951.
105. MALMEJAC, J. Activity of the adrenal medulla and its regulation. *Physiol. Rev.* 44: 186–218, 1964.
106. MALMEJAC, J., G. NEVERRE, M. BIANCHI, AND H. BOITEAU. Limites entre lesquelles se situe la sécrétion médullo-surrénale physiologique. *Compt. Rend. Soc. Biol.* 150: 1944–1947, 1956.
107. MANGER, W. M., K. G. WAKIM, AND J. L. BOLLMAN. *Chemical Quantitation of Epinephrine and Norepinephrine in Plasma.* Springfield, Ill.: Thomas, 1959.
108. MARLEY, E., AND W. D. M. PATON. The output of sympathetic amines from the cat's adrenal gland in response to splanchnic nerve activity. *J. Physiol., London* 155: 1–27, 1961.
109. MARLEY, E., AND G. I. PROUT. Physiology and pharmacology of the splanchnic-adrenal medullary junction. *J. Physiol., London* 180: 483–513, 1965.
110. MARTIN, L. E., AND C. HARRISON. An automated method for the determination of noradrenaline and adrenaline in tissues and biological fluids. *Anal. Biochem.* 23: 529–545, 1968.
111. MASON, J. W., G. MANGAN, JR., J. V. BRADY, D. CONRAD, AND D. McK. RIOCH. Concurrent plasma epinephrine, norepinephrine and 17-hydroxycorticosteroid levels during conditioned emotional disturbance in monkeys. *Psychosomat. Med.* 23: 344–353, 1961.
112. MAZEAUD, M. Influence de divers facteurs sur l'adrénalinémie et la noradrénalinémie de la carpe. *Compt. Rend. Soc. Biol.* 158: 2018–2021, 1964.
113. McDONALD, L., C. BAKER, C. BRAY, A. McDONALD, AND N. RESTIEAUX. Plasma-catecholamines after cardiac infarction. *Lancet* 2: 1021–1023, 1969.
114. MIELE, E. The nicotinic stimulation of the cat adrenal medulla. *Arch. Intern. Pharmacodyn. Therap.* 179: 343–351, 1969.
115. MILHAUD, A., W. M. MANGER, AND G. G. NAHAS. Action direct de l'acidémie sur la médullosurrénale isolée et perfusée du chien *in vitro*. *Compt. Rend. Soc. Biol.* 161: 1294–1302, 1967.
116. MILLAR, R. A. The fluorimetric estimation of epinephrine in peripheral venous plasma during insulin hypoglycemia. *J. Pharmacol. Exptl. Therap.* 118: 435–445, 1956.
117. MILLAR, R. A., AND B. G. BENFEY. The fluorimetric estimation of adrenaline and noradrenaline during haemorrhagic hypotension. *Brit. J. Anaesthesia* 30: 158–165, 1958.
118. MILLAR, R. A., E. B. KEENER, AND B. G. BENFEY. Plasma adrenaline and noradrenaline after phenoxybenzamine administration, and during haemorrhagic hypotension in normal and adrenalectomized dogs. *Brit. J. Pharmacol. Chemotherap.* 14: 9–13, 1959.
119. MILLAR, R. A., AND M. E. MORRIS. Apneic oxygenation in adrenalectomized dogs. *Anesthesiology* 22: 433–439, 1961.
120. MILLAR, R. A., AND M. E. MORRIS. A study of methoxyflurane anaesthesia. *Can. Anaesthetists Soc. J.* 8: 210–215, 1961.
121. MILLAR, R. A., AND M. E. MORRIS. Sympatho-adrenal responses during general anaesthesia in the dog and man. *Can. Anaesthetists Soc. J.* 8: 356–386, 1961.
122. MILLER, J. W., AND H. W. ELLIOTT. Plasma sympathin concentrations of dogs. *Proc. Soc. Exptl. Biol. Med.* 87: 487–488, 1954.
123. MIRKIN, B. L. Factors influencing the selective secretion of adrenal medullary hormones. *J. Pharmacol. Exptl. Therap.* 132: 218–225, 1961.
124. MONCLOA, F., M. GÓMEZ, AND A. HURTADO. Plasma catecholamines at high altitudes. *J. Appl. Physiol.* 20: 1329–1331, 1965.
125. MORRIS, M. E., AND R. A. MILLAR. Blood pH/plasma catecholamine relationships: respiratory acidosis. *Brit. J. Anaesthesia* 34: 672–681, 1962.
126. MUNRO, A. F., AND R. ROBINSON. The catecholamine content of the peripheral plasma in human subjects with complete transverse lesions of the spinal cord. *J. Physiol., London* 154: 244–253, 1960.
127. MUSCHOLL, E., AND M. VOGT. The concentration of adrenaline in the plasma of rabbits treated with reserpine. *Brit. J. Pharmacol. Chemotherap.* 12: 532–535, 1957.
128. MUSCHOLL, E., AND M. VOGT. Secretory responses of extramedullary chromaffin tissue. *Brit. J. Pharmacol. Chemotherap.* 22: 193–203, 1964.
129. NAHAS, G. G. Influence du tamponnement du gaz carbonique sur les catécholamines du sang au cours de l'hypercapnie. *Compt. Rend.* 248: 294–297, 1959.
130. NAHAS, G. G., E. C. JORDAN, AND J. C. LIGOU. Effects of a "CO_2 buffer" on hypercapnia of apneic oxygenation. *Am. J. Physiol.* 197: 1308–1316, 1959.
131. NAHAS, G. G., J. C. LIGOU, AND B. MEHLMAN. Effects of pH changes on O_2 uptake and plasma catecholamine levels in the dog. *Am. J. Physiol.* 198: 60–66, 1960.
132. NAHAS, G. G., D. ZAGURY, A. MILHAUD, W. M. MANGER, AND G. D. PAPPAS. Acidemia and catecholamine output of the isolated canine adrenal gland. *Am. J. Physiol.* 213: 1186–1192, 1967.
133. O'HANLON, J. F., JR. Adrenaline and noradrenaline: relation to performance in a visual vigilance task. *Science* 150: 507–509, 1965.
134. O'HANLON, J. F., JR. *Vigilance, the Plasma Catecholamines and Related Biochemical and Physiological Variables.* Technical Report 787-2. Goleta, Calif.: Human Factors Research, Inc., 1970.
135. O'HANLON, J. F., JR., H. C. CAMPUZANO, AND S. M. HORVATH. A fluorometric assay for subnanogram concentrations of adrenaline and noradrenaline in plasma. *Anal. Biochem.* 34: 568–581, 1970.
136. PAGE, I. H. Pressor substances from the body fluids of man in health and disease. *J. Exptl. Med.* 61: 67–96, 1935.
136a. PASSON, P. G., AND J. D. PEULER. A simplified radiometric assay for plasma norepinephrine and epinephrine. *Anal. Biochem.* 51: 618–631, 1973.
137. PEACH, M. J., AND G. D. FORD. The actions of angiotensin II on canine myocardial and plasma catecholamines. *J. Pharmacol. Exptl. Therap.* 162: 92–100, 1968.
138. PEACH, M. J., F. MERLIN BUMPUS, AND P. A. KHAIRALLAH.

Release of adrenal catecholamines by angiotensin I. *J. Pharmacol. Exptl. Therap.* 176: 366–376, 1971.
139. PEACOCK, J. H. Peripheral venous blood concentrations of epinephrine and norepinephrine in primary Raynaud's disease. *Circulation Res.* 7: 821–827, 1959.
140. PEKKARINEN, A. Studies on the chemical determination, occurrence and metabolism of adrenaline in the animal organism. *Acta Physiol. Scand. Suppl.* 54: 1–111, 1948.
141. PIPER, P. J., H. O. J. COLLIER, AND J. R. VANE. Release of catecholamines in the guinea-pig by substances involved in anaphylaxis. *Nature* 213: 838–840, 1967.
142. PIPER, P. J., AND J. R. VANE. The assay of catecholamines released into the circulation of the guinea-pig by angiotensin. *J. Physiol., London* 188: 20–21p, 1967.
143. POHORECKY, L. A., AND R. J. WURTMAN. Adrenocortical control of epinephrine synthesis. *Pharmacol. Rev.* 23: 1–35, 1971.
144. POOLE, T. R., AND D. T. WATTS. Peripheral blood epinephrine levels in dogs during intravenous infusion. *Am. J. Physiol.* 196: 145–148, 1959.
145. PRICE, H. L. Circulating adrenaline and noradrenaline during diethyl ether anaesthesia in man. *Clin. Sci.* 16: 377–387, 1957.
146. PRICE, H. L., AND M. L. PRICE. The chemical estimation of epinephrine and norepinephrine in human and canine plasma. II. A critique of the trihydroxyindole method. *J. Lab. Clin. Med.* 50: 769–777, 1957.
147. REDDIN, J. L., B. STARZECKI, AND W. W. SPINK. Comparative hemodynamic and humoral response of puppies and adult dogs to endotoxin. *Am. J. Physiol.* 210: 540–544, 1966.
148. REDGATE, E. S., AND E. GELLHORN. Nature of sympatheticoadrenal discharge under conditions of excitation of central autonomic structures. *Am. J. Physiol.* 174: 475–480, 1953.
149. REIS, D. J., AND L-M. GUNNE. Brain catecholamines. Relation to the defense reaction evoked by amygdaloid stimulation in cat. *Science* 149: 450–451, 1965.
150. RENTON, G. H., AND H. WEIL-MALHERBE. Adrenaline and noradrenaline in human plasma during natural sleep. *J. Physiol., London* 131: 170–175, 1956.
151. RICHARDSON, J. A., E. F. WOODS, AND E. E. BEGWELL. Circulating epinephrine and norepinephrine in coronary occlusion. *Am. J. Cardiol.* 5: 613–618, 1960.
152. RICHARDSON, J. A., E. F. WOODS, AND A. K. RICHARDSON. Plasma concentrations of epinephrine and norepinephrine during anesthesia. *J. Pharmacol. Exptl. Therap.* 119: 378–384, 1957.
153. RITZEL, G., W. A. HUNZINGER, AND H. STAUB. Über des Verhalten der optischen Isomeren von Adrenalin im Blut. *Experientia* 14: 205–207, 1958.
154. ROBINSON, R. L. Stimulation of the catecholamine output of the isolated perfused adrenal gland of the dog by angiotensin and bradykinin. *J. Pharmacol. Exptl. Therap.* 156: 252–257, 1967.
155. ROBINSON, R. L., AND K. E. JOCHIM. Histamine and anaphylaxis on adrenal medullary secretion in dogs. *Am. J. Physiol.* 199: 429–432, 1960.
156. ROBINSON, R. L., AND D. T. WATTS. Inhibition of adrenal secretion of epinephrine during infusion of catecholamines. *Am. J. Physiol.* 203: 713–716, 1962.
157. RUBIN, R. P., AND E. MIELE. A study of the differential secretion of epinephrine and norepinephrine from the perfused cat adrenal gland. *J. Pharmacol. Exptl. Therap.* 164: 115–121, 1968.
158. SAPIRA, J. D., AND K. BRON. Human epinephrine secretion. Direct measurement of the secretion of epinephrine from the human adrenal medulla. *J. Clin. Endocrinol. Metab.* 33: 436–447, 1971.
159. SAPIRA, J. D., L. C. CAREY, AND R. A. CURTIN. The effect of hemorrhage on the adrenal epinephrine secretory rate in swine. *Clin. Res.* 19: 52, 1971.
160. SATAKÉ, Y. The amount of epinephrine secreted from the suprarenal glands in dogs in hemorrhage, and poisoning with guanidine, peptone, caffeine, urethane, camphor, etc. *Tohoku J. Exptl. Med.* 17: 333–344, 1931.

161. SERÓR, J., R. STOPPA, PLANE, AND BIANCHI. De l'hyperépinéphrie dans la maladie de Buerger. Quelques dosages hormonaux. *Mem. Acad. Chir.* 84: 586–591, 1958.
162. SHARMAN, D. F. Methods of determination of catecholamines and their metabolites. In: *Methods in Neurochemistry*, edited by R. Fried. New York: Dekker, 1971, vol. 1, p. 83–127.
163. SILVER, M. The output of adrenaline and noradrenaline from the adrenal medulla of the calf. *J. Physiol., London* 152: 14–29, 1960.
164. SPECTOR, W. S. *Handbook of Biological Data.* Philadelphia: Saunders, 1956.
165. SPINK, W. W., J. REDDIN, S. J. ZAK, M. PETERSON, B. STARZEKI, AND E. SELJESKOG. Correlation of plasma catecholamine levels with hemodynamic changes in canine endotoxin shock. *J. Clin. Invest.* 45: 78–85, 1966.
166. SPRIGGS, T. L. B. The effects of anaesthesia induced by urethane or phenobarbitone upon the distribution of peripheral catecholamines in the rat. *Brit. J. Pharmacol. Chemotherap.* 24: 752–758, 1965.
167. STASZEWSKA-BARCZAK, J., AND J. R. VANE. The release of catecholamines from the adrenal medulla by histamine. *Brit. J. Pharmacol. Chemotherap.* 25: 728–742, 1965.
168. STEINSLAND, O. S., S. S. PASSO, AND G. G. NAHAS. Biphasic effect of hypoxia on adrenal catecholamine content. *Am. J. Physiol.* 218: 995–998, 1970.
169. STREET, D. M., AND D. J. ROBERTS. The presence of dopamine in cat spleen and blood. *J. Pharm. Pharmacol.* 21: 199–201, 1969.
170. SUNDIN, T. The effect of body posture on the urinary excretion of adrenaline and noradrenaline. *Acta Med. Scand.* 161, Suppl. 336: 1–59, 1958.
171. SYMBAS, P. N., M. JELLINEK, T. COOPER, AND C. HANLON. Effect of hypothermia on plasma catecholamines and histamine. *Arch. Intern. Pharmacodyn. Therap.* 50: 132–136, 1964.
172. TENNEY, S. M. Sympatho-adrenal stimulation by carbon dioxide and the inhibitory effect of carbonic acid on epinephrine response. *Am. J. Physiol.* 187: 341–346, 1956.
173. TOURNADE, A., AND M. CHABROL. Effets des variations de la pression artérielle sur la sécrétion de l'adrenaline. *Compt. Rend. Soc. Biol.* 93: 934–936, 1925.
174. TRENDELENBURG, U. The supersensitivity caused by cocaine. *J. Pharmacol. Exptl. Therap.* 125: 55–65, 1959.
175. UNNI, V. K. N., L. McARDLE, AND G. W. BLACK. Sympathoadrenal, respiratory and metabolic changes during trichloroethylene anaesthesia. *Brit. J. Anaesthesia* 42: 429–433, 1970.
176. VANE, J. R. The release and fate of vaso-active hormones in the circulation. *Brit. J. Pharmacol.* 35: 209–242, 1969.
177. VANOV, S., AND M. VOGT. Catecholamine-containing structures in the hypogastric nerves of the dog. *J. Physiol., London* 168: 939–944, 1963.
178. VENDSALU, A. Studies on the adrenaline and noradrenaline in human plasma. *Acta Physiol. Scand. Suppl.* 173: 1–123, 1960.
179. VIKTORA, J. K., A. BAUKAL, AND F. W. WOLFF. New automated fluorimetric methods for estimation of small amounts of adrenaline and noradrenaline. *Anal. Biochem.* 23: 513–528, 1968.
180. VOGT, M. Plasma adrenaline and release of ACTH in normal and demedullated rats. *J. Physiol., London* 118: 588–594, 1952.
181. VOGT, M. Release of medullary amines from the isolated perfused adrenal gland of the dog. *Brit. J. Pharmacol. Chemotherap.* 24: 561–565, 1965.
182. WADA, M., M. SEO, AND K. ABE. Effects of muscular exercise upon the epinephrine secretion from the suprarenal gland. *Tohoku J. Exptl. Med.* 27: 65–86, 1935.
183. WATTS, D. T. Epinephrine in the circulating blood during ether anesthesia. *J. Pharmacol. Exptl. Therap.* 114: 203–210, 1955.
184. WATTS, D. T., AND A. D. BRAGG. Blood epinephrine levels

during spontaneous reinfusion of blood in hemorrhagic shock in dogs. *J. Pharmacol. Exptl. Therap.* 122: 81–82A, 1958.
185. WATTS, D. T., AND T. R. POOLE. Peripheral blood epinephrine levels following intravenous administration of the materials. *Federation Proc.* 16: 344, 1957.
186. WEIL-MALHERBE, H., AND A. D. BONE. On the occurrence of adrenaline and noradrenaline in blood. *Biochem. J.* 58: 132–141, 1954.
187. WHITBY, L. G., J. AXELROD, AND H. WEIL-MALHERBE. The fate of ^{3}H-norepinephrine in animals. *J. Pharmacol. Exptl. Therap.* 132: 193–201, 1961.
188. WILLEY, G. L. Effect of antisympathomimetic drugs on the plasma concentrations of catecholamines. *Brit. J. Pharmacol. Chemotherap.* 19: 365–374, 1962.
189. WOODS, E. F., J. A. RICHARDSON, A. K. RICHARDSON, AND R. F. BOZEMAN, JR. Plasma concentrations of epinephrine and arterenol following the actions of various agents on the adrenals. *J. Pharmacol. Exptl. Therap.* 116: 351–355, 1956.
190. WURTMAN, R. J., A. CASPAR, L. A. POHORECKY, AND F. C. BARTTER. Impaired secretion of epinephrine in response to insulin among hypophysectomized dogs. *Proc. Natl. Acad. Sci. US* 61: 522–528, 1968.
191. ZUSPAN, F. P., G. H. NELSON, AND R. P. AHLQUIST. Epinephrine infusions in normal and toxemic pregnancies. *Am. J. Obstet. Gynecol.* 92: 1102–1106, 1965.

CHAPTER 29

Adrenergic receptors

NEIL C. MORAN | *Department of Pharmacology, Division of Basic Health Sciences, Emory University, Atlanta, Georgia*

CHAPTER CONTENTS

Development of Concept of Receptors
    Definition of receptor
    Attempts to define adrenergic receptors chemically
    Operational concept of receptor
    Classification of receptors
Development of Classification for Adrenergic Receptors
Adrenergic Receptors That Subserve Metabolic Responses
    Carbohydrate metabolism
    Lipid metabolism
    Calorigenesis
Cardiovascular System
    Heart
    Blood vessels
        Veins
        Coronary arteries
        Pulmonary vessels
Nonvascular Smooth Muscle
    Gastrointestinal
    Spleen
    Nictitating membrane
    Iris
    Uterus
    Respiratory tract
Skeletal Muscle
Central Nervous System
Miscellaneous Systems
    Melanophore responses
    Skin gland secretions
    Other effects
Role of Adrenergic Receptors in Sympathoadrenal Responses
Conclusions

DEVELOPMENT OF CONCEPT OF RECEPTORS

The concept of cellular receptors for drugs and neurohumoral transmitters is derived from two sources: Paul Ehrlich's theory of sites with which drugs selectively react to alter cellular function, and Langley's (90) suggestion that a specific "receptive substance" mediates the actions of neurohumors or related drugs. Several facts about epinephrine helped shape these early views of receptors. Oliver & Schäfer (128) first demonstrated the physiological and hyperglycemic actions of extracts of the adrenal gland. Lewandowsky (96) found that sympathetically denervated organs retained their responsiveness to epinephrine. Elliott (45, 46) demonstrated that extracts of the adrenal gland produced responses in animals similar to those obtained with stimulation of the sympathetic nerves, a similarity that led Barger & Dale (7) to propose the term *sympathomimetic* to describe chemical agents whose actions mimicked the effects of sympathetic nerve stimulation. Dale (35) recognized that epinephrine and nerve stimulation produce both excitatory and inhibitory responses in various organs and that derivatives of ergot blocked primarily excitatory effects of sympathetic stimuli.

The first rigorous and quantitative appraisal of receptors was that of A. J. Clark (33) who concluded, "... the more accurate quantitative data can be interpreted as the expression of a chemical reaction between the drug and specific receptors, which latter [i.e., receptors] in a large number of cases appear to be situated on the cell surface." Many reviews have appeared since Clark's work, the most recent and comprehensive being that of Waud (158) to which the reader is referred for a complete and detailed evaluation of the quantitative aspects of receptor theory and for references to previous evaluations.

This chapter is concerned with adrenergic receptors[1], those specific sites of cells that respond to adrenergic stimuli (i.e., norepinephrine released from adrenergic nerve endings; norepinephrine or epinephrine released into the blood from the adrenal medulla; drugs related chemically to these catecholamines). The primary emphasis is on classification of receptors. However, other aspects of receptor evaluation in general are discussed.

[1] The terminology for receptors is not uniform. Ahlquist first classified "adrenotropic" receptors, but recently he has used the more commonly employed term, "adrenergic receptor." The term "adrenoceptor" is used in some writing and apparently is standard in the *British Journal of Pharmacology*. It can be argued that the suffix, -ergic, with its connotation of work is inappropriate in that the "work" is done by the effector cells and not by the receptors. However, this strict definition would require abandonment of the term "adrenergic neuron" in that the neuron does not perform the work. I prefer to retain the common form adrenergic receptor in this chapter in the sense that adrenergic neurons and adrenergic receptors mediate the final effect of norepinephrine. Furthermore I prefer to use alpha and beta as modifiers of adrenergic rather than of receptor (e.g., alpha adrenergic receptor rather than adrenergic alpha receptor).

Definition of Receptor

Underlying several views of receptors is the assumption of a highly specific, molecular interaction between a drug, a hormone, or a neurohumor, on the one hand, and a specific component of a cell, on the other hand, and that this interaction alters the function of the cell.

Schueler (146) defined a receptor as

In general a pattern *R* of forces of diverse origin forming a part of some biological system and having roughly the same dimensions as a certain pattern *M* of forces presented by the drug molecule such that between patterns *M* and *R* a relationship of complementarity for interaction exists.

This definition centers on a pattern of forces as part of a structural "mosaic of any tissue component...without involving one...in the consideration of these entities in a holistic sense."

Although he did not define a receptor concisely, Clark (33) concluded that many types of actions of drugs and hormones could be explained only on the basis of reactions with specific receptors. He stated that the receptor theory could account for such diverse factors in drug action as *a*) the "extraordinary specificity of the actions of drugs" whereby slight changes in chemical constitution can markedly alter the biological action, *b*) the phenomenon of drug antagonism, and *c*) the fact that different tissues vary in their pattern of response to a given drug, suggesting that receptors in various tissues vary slightly in their patterns.

Various types of bonds can be involved in drug-receptor interactions, from covalent bonds with high energy to noncovalent (dipole) bonds of low energy and low specificity (e.g., van der Waals forces). It is probable that weak, noncovalent bonds are more important in the specificity of drug-receptor interactions. The three-dimensional structures of drugs and hormones and of receptor molecules are of great importance in terms of complementarity. Furthermore, although individual dipole-induced bonds are weak and require close approximation between the two molecules (van der Waals forces diminish with the seventh power of the intermolecular distance), a constellation of appropriately oriented groups on each molecule can amplify the attracting forces. Furthermore the fact that drugs and neurohumors, particularly catecholamines, appear not to be chemically modified as a result of the interaction with the receptors and the fact that many drug effects are readily reversible suggest simple molecular attractions, rather than high-energy chemical reactions, for most actions of drugs and neurohumors.

The concept of receptors is based on several established facts about many drugs and hormones.

1. There is a high degree of specificity. This is seen in terms of chemical structure and in terms of the exceedingly small number of molecules of many drugs that is required to elicit effects. The structure of the drug or hormone is important in terms of molecular size, the number and arrangement of the atoms, and the three-dimensional configuration. Seemingly minor differences in configuration, such as that between the stereoisomers, D(−)-norepinephrine and L(+)-norepinephrine, can be the basis of marked quantitative differences in biological activity.

2. Concentration-response curves (i.e., the quantitative relation between the concentration of the drug and the degree of biological response) are similar to adsorption isotherms, enzyme-substrate reaction curves, and drug-protein binding curves. These similarities suggest that the concentration-effect curve is a representation of the molecular interaction between molecules of drug or hormone and receptor molecules.

3. Interaction of receptor and drug or hormone (agonists) results in a biological response, such as contraction of smooth muscle (i.e., agonist-receptor interaction can be conceived of as an initiating or "triggering" reaction).

4. Selective antagonism is most readily explained by blockade or occlusion of receptors.

5. Complete reversibility of effect, very rapid with most agonists and slow with competitive antagonists, suggests that a specific receptor is reversibly binding the drug.

Attempts to Define Adrenergic Receptors Chemically

Two lines of attack on chemical definition of adrenergic receptors have so far yielded little fundamental insight into their actual nature. One is an attempt to define adrenergic receptors as theoretical depictions of the three-dimensional surface of the receptor and possible reactive sites on the basis of the three-dimensional structure of agonist and antagonist molecules and their reactive groups. Belleau (11) and Bloom & Goldman (21) have speculated on the nature of adrenergic receptors in these terms. However, this approach has been of limited value because it has not led to definitive experimental tests of the hypotheses. As with other methods of analysis of receptors, much of the emphasis is on the interaction of the agonist and the receptor with little consideration of the steps subsequent to the agonist-receptor interaction.

The second method is isolation of the receptor itself. Important steps have been made in this direction, but particularly in terms of the cholinergic receptor (106). Lefkowitz and associates (91, 91a, 91b) have reported the isolation of a protein fraction from the dog heart that they assert has the properties of the beta adrenergic receptor. Their conclusion is based on comparison of binding affinities of sympathomimetic amines and adrenergic blocking drugs with the biological actions of these drugs on the heart. However, they did not demonstrate a difference in binding constants for the two enantiomorphs of norepinephrine. They also found a low binding affinity for propranolol, a very active antagonist of beta receptor-mediated function in the intact heart. Cuatracasas (personal communication), however, has concluded that this protein represents binding sites specific for catechol and not specific for beta adrenergic agonists or antagonists. Cuatracasas also could show no difference between D(−)-norepinephrine and L(+)-norepinephrine in terms of binding constants. He thinks that this protein has so many catechol binding sites that they obscure the detection of the much smaller number of possible stereospecific catecholamine binding sites. At this time there is no clear evidence for the isolation and characterization of the beta receptor. However, work such as that of Lefkowitz and associates and Cuatracasas points the way toward the ultimate isolation of the receptor.

Operational Concept of Receptor

Despite the extensive literature on receptors, most knowledge comes from experiments in which a tissue, such as an intestinal strip, is exposed to an agonist, either alone or in the presence of an antagonist, and a response, such as contraction, is measured. Only a few facts are known, namely, the chemical structures of the agonist and antagonist, their concentrations in the organ bath (and presumably therefore their concentrations at the receptors), the complex nature of the tissue, and finally the degree of response, such as that determined by the movement of a pen or lever. The reaction can be depicted as

$$\text{agonist} + \text{tissue} \rightarrow \text{effect}$$

Little is known about the events between addition of the drug to the bath and the ensuing response. However, if the assumption is valid that there are several steps between the site of action of the drug and the cellular machinery that mediates the final response, we can postulate a multi-step, sequential reaction that is initiated at the receptor as follows:

$$A + R \rightarrow AR \rightarrow a \rightarrow b \rightarrow c \rightarrow n \rightarrow \text{effect}$$

The reaction between agonist (A) and receptor (R) can be considered the triggering reaction.

In the absence of knowledge of the receptor itself and of the intermediate steps, the receptor can be operationally defined as all the steps from the true receptor to the effect (109), that is

$$A + \underbrace{[R \rightarrow AR \rightarrow a \rightarrow b \rightarrow c \rightarrow n]}_{\text{operational receptor}} \rightarrow \text{effect}$$

As knowledge of individual steps is acquired, the operationally defined receptor can be contracted accordingly. Thus, if steps c to final effect are elucidated and it is clear that A does not have an effect at any of those steps, then the operationally defined receptor becomes

$$A + [R \rightarrow AR \rightarrow a \rightarrow b] \rightarrow c \rightarrow n \rightarrow \text{effect}$$

Finally, when all the steps are known and the receptor itself is isolated and identified, the operational receptor becomes identical with the true receptor, as

$$A + [R] \rightarrow AR \rightarrow a \rightarrow b \rightarrow c \rightarrow n \rightarrow \text{effect}$$

Thus the operationally defined receptor is the most proximal step, or steps, of a multi-step, sequential reaction. Where detailed steps are not known, the receptor is then defined as the entire sequence.

Where several types of responses to a single agonist can be measured in a given system, one must distinguish between a single type and two or more different subtypes of receptors. The single receptor type with two types of effects can be expressed schematically

$$A + R \rightarrow AR \begin{array}{c} \nearrow a_1 \rightarrow b_1 \rightarrow c_1 \rightarrow n_1 \rightarrow \text{effect}_1 \\ \searrow a_2 \rightarrow b_2 \rightarrow c_2 \rightarrow n_2 \rightarrow \text{effect}_2 \end{array}$$

Variations on this theme can be visualized with different branch points and with more than two different effects. Multiple types of receptors that react to a single type of agonist produce multiple effects

$$A + R_1 \rightarrow AR_1 \rightarrow a_1 \rightarrow b_1 \rightarrow c_1 \rightarrow n_1 \rightarrow \text{effect}_1$$
$$A + R_2 \rightarrow AR_2 \rightarrow a_2 \rightarrow b_2 \rightarrow c_2 \rightarrow n_2 \rightarrow \text{effect}_2$$

Certain criteria must be established to classify receptors in terms of a single receptor type with multiple responses or multiple receptor types with either a single effect or multiple effects. First, the specificity of agonists must be established and the order of potency in an homologous series of agonists for one effect must be similar to that for a second effect if a single receptor type is claimed. Different orders of potency point to different receptor types whether the effects are qualitatively the same (as in two types of smooth muscle) or are different. Second, selectivity of antagonism should be established. Although selective blockade is a powerful method for receptor classification, it is often not practical because antagonists for a given type of effect may not exist or several antagonists may be known, but their specificity may be in doubt. However, if an antagonist is available it must block all types of effects elicited by a single agonist if they all are to be ascribed to a single receptor type. If an antagonist blocks only one of two or more effects, multiple receptors must be postulated or one must consider the possibility that the antagonist does not block any of the putative receptors.

Some of the problems involved in the use of antagonists are readily seen in schematic presentations of reaction sequences and the operational receptor concept. If the postulated reaction is a single receptor type with a single effect and if nothing is known about the discrete steps distal to the receptor, the site of blockade of an antagonist must be broadly designated by the operational definition of the receptor, that is

$$A + \underbrace{[R \rightarrow AR \rightarrow a \rightarrow b \rightarrow c \rightarrow n]}_{\text{site of blockade = operational receptor}} \rightarrow \text{effect}$$

even though the site of blockade is undoubtedly more discrete and specific. Furthermore, if two compounds, perhaps of considerably different chemical structure, antagonize the effect, it is hazardous to assume that they both act at the true receptor (i.e., at a single site), even though they both would have to be considered to block the receptor as it is defined in an operational sense. Thus one can depict two blocking agents, B_1 and B_2, in the following scheme

$$A + \boxed{R} \rightarrow AR \rightarrow a \rightarrow b \rightarrow \boxed{c} \rightarrow n \rightarrow \text{effect}$$

$$\underbrace{\text{"real" site}}_{\text{of } B_1} \quad \underbrace{\text{"real" site}}_{\text{of } B_2}$$

$$\underbrace{\qquad\qquad\qquad\qquad\qquad}_{\text{operationally defined site of action of } B_1 \text{ and } B_2}$$

Lack of knowledge of the intermediate steps in reaction sequences can lead to the false assumption that two effects are mediated through two different receptor types if a single blocking agent antagonizes only one of the two effects. Thus

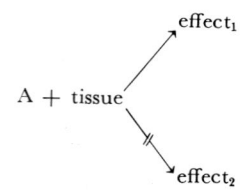

$$A + \text{tissue} \begin{array}{c} \nearrow \text{effect}_1 \\ \searrow \!\!\!\!\!/\!\!\!\!\! \text{effect}_2 \end{array}$$

That is, the use of antagonism by B_2 alone would suggest classification of two receptors, when in fact the site of action of B_2 might be at a distal locus in one of two divergent sequences. Thus

$$A + R \rightarrow AR \begin{array}{c} \nearrow a_1 \rightarrow b_1 \rightarrow c_1 \rightarrow n_1 \rightarrow \text{effect}_1 \\ \searrow a_2 \rightarrow b_2 \rightarrow \boxed{c_2} \rightarrow n_2 \rightarrow \text{effect}_2 \end{array}$$

$$\underbrace{\qquad\qquad}_{\text{actual site of } B_2 \text{ action}}$$

In this instance, the use of orders of potency as the main criterion would be the most useful method in showing that only one receptor type is involved and that therefore the antagonist probably does not act at the receptor.

The use of selective blockade in establishing the validity of the conclusion of two receptor types is schematically depicted as

$$A + R_1 + B_1 \xrightarrow{/\!\!/} \text{effect}_1 \quad A + R_1 + B_2 \rightarrow \text{effect}$$
$$A + R_2 + B_2 \xrightarrow{/\!\!/} \text{effect}_2 \quad A + R_2 + B_1 \rightarrow \text{effect}_2$$

The pattern of two or more receptors in a single tissue in which sequential reactions converge on a common type of effect can be expressed as

$$\begin{array}{c} A + R_1 \rightarrow AR_1 \rightarrow a_1 \rightarrow b_1 \rightarrow c_1 \searrow \\ \qquad\qquad\qquad\qquad\qquad\qquad\quad n \rightarrow \text{effect} \\ A + R_2 \rightarrow AR_2 \rightarrow a_2 \rightarrow b_2 \rightarrow c_2 \nearrow \end{array}$$

Differing orders of potency would help to dissociate the receptor types, as would selective blockade. The use of blockade alone, however, could lead to the erroneous classification of a single receptor type if an antagonist acted to block the effect, not at a receptor, but at distal sites in both reaction sequences or at a single site beyond convergence of the two sequences.

Classification of Receptors

With wider acceptance of the concept of receptors for drugs, neurohumors, and hormones, the classification of receptors has been more thoroughly and extensively evaluated. Ahlquist's (3) proposal in 1948 of two types of adrenergic receptors and the subsequent validation of his classification by the discovery of beta adrenergic blocking drugs have strongly influenced efforts toward refined classification and identification of drug receptors in general.

Classification of adrenergic receptors into subtypes requires assumptions as outlined above: *a*) the order of potency of a homologous series of compounds (e.g., phenylethylamines) will be the same in all systems if the receptor type is the same; and *b*) selective blockade will help define separate receptor types (Table 1). In both of these approaches to receptor classification it is assumed that accessibility of both agonists and antagonists to receptor sites is a negligible factor; that is, there would not be great differences in diffusibility through tissue barriers among a group of closely related chemical compounds.

Furchgott (58) has emphasized the importance of proper experimental conditions for evaluating receptors. Among these are the elimination of indirect effects of drugs (e.g., induced release of catecholamines) and antagonism of all processes, other than passive diffusion, that effectively remove the agonists from the area of the receptor. In the case of adrenergic agonists, uptake of norepinephrine and, to a lesser extent, of epinephrine by adrenergic nerves is the most active removal process and can be antagonized by cocaine, imipramine, and other drugs.

DEVELOPMENT OF CLASSIFICATION
FOR ADRENERGIC RECEPTORS

The problem of resolution of the fact that adrenergic stimuli could produce opposite types of responses (i.e., excitatory and inhibitory) has attracted attention for over half a century. When Dale (35) observed that ergot derivatives antagonized only certain actions of epinephrine, he concluded that ergot has a "paralytic action on motor elements of that myotrophic structure or substance which is excited by adrenaline and by impulses in fibres of the true sympathetic system; the inhibitor elements on the same being relatively or absolutely unaffected."

Although there had been early proposals of adrenergic receptors, by the mid 1930s the most widely accepted explanation of the dual responses to adrenergic stimuli was that of Cannon & Rosenblueth (30) that two substances, sympathin E (excitatory) and sympathin I

TABLE 1. *General Classification of Adrenergic Receptors*

Basis of Classification	Receptor Types			
	Alpha	Beta₁	Beta₂	Dopamine
Potency of agonists	NE ≥ E > D > I	I > E ≥ NE > D	I > E ≫ NE > D	D ≫ EN
Selective blockade				
Alpha antagonists (e.g., POB, PHEN, ERG)	Block	No block	No block	No block
Beta antagonists				
General (e.g., DCI, PROP)	No block	Block	Block	No block
Beta₁ type (e.g., PRAC)	No block	Block	Weak block	No block
Beta₂ type (e.g., BUTOX)	No block	Weak block	Block	No block
Dopamine antagonists (e.g., HAL)	No block	No block	No block	Weak block

NE, norepinephrine; E, epinephrine; I, isoproterenol; D, dopamine; POB, phenoxybenzamine; PHEN, phentolamine; ERG, ergot alkaloids; DCI, dichloroisoproterenol; PROP, propranolol; PRAC, practolol; BUTOX, butoxamine; HAL, haloperidol; EN, epinine.

(inhibitory), mediated the effects through a single receptor type[2].

The work of von Euler (51, 52) led to the wide acceptance of the concept of a single adrenergic neurohumoral mediator (i.e., norepinephrine). Because it is difficult to explain the varying effects of sympathetic nervous system activity on the basis of a single mediator and also because the adrenergic blocking drugs known before 1950 have a restricted range of blockade (121) (i.e., they are all like the ergot alkaloids in that they do not antagonize either the excitatory responses of the heart or most inhibitory responses of other tissues), Ahlquist (3) proposed two types of receptors, which he noncommittally called alpha and beta adrenotropic receptors.

Ahlquist approached receptor classification by comparing the orders of potency of several closely related agonists on several types of physiological systems. He used six sympathomimetic amines with the following characteristics: *a*) they produced effects in the same dose range as epinephrine; *b*) at equivalent doses they had similar durations of action; *c*) they had identical actions on the myocardium; and *d*) none produced tachyphylaxis. Their relative potencies were compared on a variety of physiological systems, both in vivo and in vitro.

Five of Ahlquist's compounds were racemic mixtures; all are catecholamines, and all have a hydroxyl group at the β position on the side chain. There are three variations of structure on the nitrogen: *1*) R-NH₂ = norepinephrine; *2*) R-NHCH₃ = epinephrine; and *3*) R-NHC₃H₇ = isoproterenol (isopropylnorepinephrine), where R represents the following structure.

[2] It is difficult to find a consistent and precise definition of the term *sympathin* in the work of Cannon and his colleagues. On the one hand, Cannon seemed to consider sympathin E and sympathin I as mediators per se, but in other contexts he alluded to the sympathins being formed as a result of the reaction of the mediator and a receptive substance. Whether Cannon had finally refined his definition of sympathin to one or the other of the connotations is not relevant today. He obviously was not satisfied with the "one mediator-one receptor" concept.

$$HO\text{-}C_6H_3(OH)\text{-}CHOH\text{-}CH_2\text{-}$$

Two compounds were derived from epinephrine and norepinephrine by the addition of a methyl group to the α carbon of the side chain. A sixth compound was the levo isomer of epinephrine.

Ahlquist found D(−)-epinephrine to be the most potent and DL(+,−)-isoproterenol the least potent agent on a variety of "excitatory" responses, such as vasoconstriction. However, the order of potency was different for the excitatory responses of the heart— isoproterenol was most potent and DL(+,−)-norepinephrine least potent. Furthermore, in assessing the inhibitory response of intestinal relaxation, he found the order of potency to be identical to that of the excitatory responses, except for that of the heart. Finally, the potency order for inhibitory responses of the uterus and blood vessels (vasodilatation) was identical with that on the heart. Thus Ahlquist concluded that there must be two types of adrenergic receptors, but they could not be classified simply as inhibitory and excitatory. Instead, he arbitrarily designated two receptor types based on the two main orders of potency of the agonists. Thus those receptors that subserve responses on which D(−)-epinephrine was the most potent were designated *alpha* and those on which isoproterenol was most potent as *beta* receptors. He stated, "Although there are two kinds of adrenotropic receptors they cannot be classified simply as excitatory or inhibitory since each kind of receptor may have either action depending on where it is found."

It is unfortunate that Ahlquist did not use compounds of the same stereochemical configuration. Both alpha and beta receptors "recognize" the D(−) forms of phenylethanolamines "better" than the L(+) forms. Furthermore two of Ahlquist's compounds were α-methyl derivatives of epinephrine and norepinephrine in which the additional center of asymmetry provides compounds with four stereoisomers instead of two. It is interesting to speculate that Ahlquist might not have described two adrenergic receptors if D(−)-isoproterenol were less active than it actually is. If it were of the same potency or only slightly more potent than D(−)-epinephrine, the racemic mixture of isoproterenol would have been less potent than D(−)-epinephrine, and Ahlquist would have found D(−)-epinephrine to be the most potent compound in all his test systems. There would therefore have been little justification for classifying two types of adrenergic receptors. The potency of D(−)-isoproterenol, however, is so much greater than that of D(−)-epinephrine on "beta" systems that its priority was assured even when diluted with the L(+) form of the compound. Had Ahlquist used D(−)-norepinephrine instead of DL(+, −)-norepinephrine he probably would have found it equal to or of greater potency than D(−)-epinephrine on the "excitatory" response he classified alpha. An interesting critical appraisal of the usage of ratios of activities of isomers in receptor analysis can be found in the work of Patil and colleagues (132).

Ahlquist's proposed classification of adrenergic receptors went largely unnoticed for 10 years except for an alternative classification by Lands (86) of "differentiated" and "undifferentiated" receptors. The acceptance of this classification was due to the discovery by Slater and Powell (135, 151) in 1957 of a new type of adrenergic blocking agent, dichloroisoproterenol (DCI). Dichloroisoproterenol antagonized many responses to sympathomimetic drugs that the conventional adrenergic blocking drugs did not, and conversely it did not block the effects that the conventional blocking drugs did. Powell & Slater (135) found only a nonspecific depression of the isolated frog heart by DCI and concluded that, although the stimulant effect of epinephrine was reduced, the specificity of this antagonism "remains in doubt" because of the direct depressant effect of the blocking compound itself. They did not mention Ahlquist's classification of adrenergic receptors but rather stated that the drug "was combining with certain 'adrenergic inhibitory sites' without itself causing much physiological effect and yet was competing for these sites with physiologically active amines."

Knowledge of the actions of DCI was soon expanded to include the fact that it competitively and selectively blocks the effects of sympathomimetic drugs and of sympathetic nerve stimulation on the heart (41, 56, 115). Moran & Perkins (115) proposed that DCI blocks those adrenergic receptors Ahlquist had designated as beta, that DCI be termed a "beta adrenergic blocking drug," and that the older adrenergic antagonists, such as ergot alkaloids, the beta haloalkylamines, and phentolamine, be called "alpha adrenergic blocking drugs." Thus the discovery of DCI and its characterization as an antagonist of beta adrenergic receptors helped establish the validity of Ahlquist's classification of adrenergic receptors.

Soon after the discovery of DCI, other beta adrenergic blocking drugs were introduced. The first and most notable were pronethalol and propranolol (18, 19).

One inconsistency in Ahlquist's classification has been the fact that norepinephrine is a potent activator of cardiac beta receptors but not of smooth muscle beta adrenergic receptors. This discrepancy led Lands and co-workers (87) to propose two separate subtypes of beta receptors, namely beta$_1$ and beta$_2$. Other lines of evidence obtained from new drugs, both antagonists and agonists, have lent support to this proposed subclassification.

The development of the concepts of alpha and beta adrenergic receptors has been reviewed elsewhere (110–113). The current status of the classification of these receptors is summarized in Table 2, which is a representation of the author's view of the most reasonable classification at this time.

ADRENERGIC RECEPTORS THAT SUBSERVE METABOLIC RESPONSES

The literature on metabolic effects of sympathomimetic amines is extensive, dating back to early observations of the hyperglycemic and calorigenic actions of epinephrine. Since the discovery of cyclic AMP as the "second messenger" in the mediation of the glycogenolytic effect of epinephrine (154) and the discovery of beta adrenergic blocking drugs, the volume of literature has increased in frightening proportions. Fortunately, much of the work of the past decade has been admirably condensed in several reviews and proceedings of symposia (47–49, 71, 73, 142). Consequently this section merely summarizes and highlights the material found in these reviews and in selected papers. Robison and associates have provided a particularly valuable review of the metabolic effects of catecholamines with reference to receptors and cyclic AMP [(142); see also the chapter by Williamson in this volume of the *Handbook*].

Much of the work on metabolic actions of catecholamines was not designed to assess receptor types. Many studies dealt with only a single adrenergic agonist (e.g., epinephrine), instead of a series of agonists, to allow evaluation of orders of potency. Blocking drugs, when used, have often been used indiscriminately so that assessment of selectivity of blockade is not possible. Many investigators have been oriented primarily toward mechanisms of action and not toward classification of receptors. Furthermore metabolic and biochemical studies often require more experimental procedures and may be more complex and less exact than corresponding physiological systems. For example, a smooth muscle system in vitro enables an investigator to evaluate a wide range of concentrations of several agonists with and without antagonists in a relatively short period of time on one sample of tissue. This is difficult to do in experiments that require removal of samples of blood or tissue for chemical analysis.

Two major conclusions can now be drawn on the basis of a large body of experimental evidence.

1. The activation of beta adrenergic receptors is associated with increased production of cyclic AMP through increased activity of adenylate cyclase, although it is not established that all beta adrenergic responses are mediated by cyclic AMP. On the other hand, glucagon, which produces some metabolic effects similar to those of catecholamines, also increases the content of cyclic AMP through stimulation of adenylate cyclase but not via beta adrenergic receptors.

2. Adrenergic responses mediated via alpha receptors are not associated with activation of adenylate cyclase. On the contrary, it has been suggested that alpha receptor activation is associated with decreased production of cyclic AMP.

There are three major metabolic effects of catecholamines: *1)* glycogenolysis; *2)* lipolysis; and *3)* calorigenesis, all of which are clearly secondary to activation of beta adrenergic receptors. Glycogenolysis and lipolysis can be linked directly to the influence of cyclic AMP, but the calorigenic action is not so directly related to elevated cyclic AMP content in tissue.

Carbohydrate Metabolism

Glycogenolysis represents a clear example of a multistep sequential reaction in which the adrenergic receptor is the most proximal part of the sequence. The present understanding of the main sequence in adrenergically induced hepatic glycogenolysis is depicted in Figure 1. This scheme shows neither the concomitant changes in activity of glycogen synthetase that results from increased cyclic AMP nor the enhanced gluconeogenesis.

Adrenergic and glucagon receptors are readily distinguished by the use of selective beta adrenergic blockade. That is, propranolol antagonizes the effects of catecholamines but not of glucagon. Furthermore neither catecholamine nor glucagon acts at steps distal to the receptor-adenylate cyclase system. Thus the operational definition places adrenergic and glucagon receptors proximal to the production of cyclic AMP. However, this definition does not distinguish between receptors as integral parts of the enzyme or as separate entities albeit coupled to the enzyme.

Unequivocal classification of the adrenergic receptor that subserves glycogenolysis in the liver has been hindered by two problems: *1)* both alpha and beta adrenergic blocking drugs have been reported to antagonize adrenergically induced hyperglycemia; and *2)* differences in the responses of various species have been notable, especially the relative lack of potency of isoproterenol in the rat compared with other species.

Although, as stated above, neither catecholamine nor glucagon has important effects on the distal parts of the reaction sequence leading to glycogenolysis, it is not so certain that the actions of antagonist drugs are limited to the receptors. Blocking drugs frequently have effects

TABLE 2. *Classification of Adrenergic Receptors in Selected Tissues*

Tissue	Receptor
Heart	
Increased contractility	Beta$_1$
Increased pacemaker frequency	Beta$_1$
Increased conduction velocity	Beta$_1$
Blood vessels	
Arterial constriction	Alpha
Arterial dilatation	Beta$_2$ in skeletal muscle and perhaps in heart; dopamine in kidney and mesentery
Venoconstriction	Beta$_2$
Bronchioles	
Dilatation	Beta$_2$
Gastrointestinal tract	
Decreased motility	Alpha possibly at neuronal site; beta in smooth muscle
Contraction (sphincters)	Alpha and beta
Uterus	
Relaxation	Beta, influenced by estrous state and pregnancy
Contraction	Alpha
Spleen	
Contraction	Alpha
Relaxation	Beta
Nictitating membrane	
Contraction	Alpha
Relaxation	Beta
Iris	
Radial muscle, contraction	Alpha
Skin	
Erector pilae contraction	Alpha
Skin darkening, amphibians and reptiles	Beta
Skin lightening, amphibians and reptiles	Alpha
Secretion of skin glands, toads	Alpha
Exocrine glands	
Pancreatic secretion	Alpha
Salivary secretion, with amylase	Beta
Sweat	Alpha
Inhibition of milk ejection	Possibly beta
Skeletal muscle	
Fast muscle, augmented contraction	Beta
Slow muscle, decreased contraction	Beta
Extraocular, induced contraction	Alpha
Neuromuscular transmission, enhanced	Alpha
Central nervous system	
Consummatory behavior	
Thirst	Beta
Water satiety	Alpha
Hunger	Alpha
Satiety	Beta
Metabolism	
Glycogenolysis	Beta
Lipolysis	Beta
Calorigenesis	Beta
Insulin secretion inhibition	Alpha

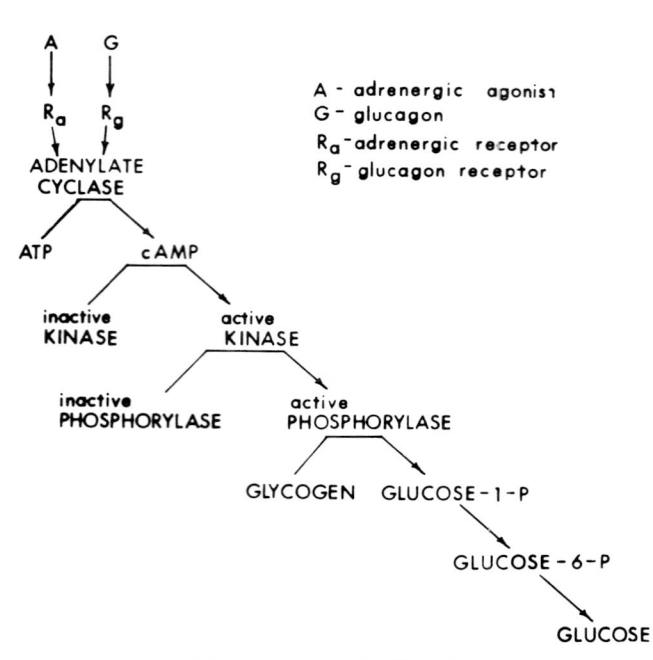

FIG. 1. Sequential reactions in the liver in hyperglycemia induced by an adrenergic agonist or by glucagon. The scheme is based on the assumption of discrete receptors for adrenergic agonists and for glucagon, neither of which are directly part of the adenylate cyclase enzyme. This scheme does not include the contribution of gluconeogenesis in the elaboration of glucose. *cAMP*, cyclic AMP.

other than the selective receptor antagonism for which they are most noted. For example, propranolol is a potent local anesthetic drug, and therefore some effects (e.g., cardiac antiarrhythmic) of propranolol must be interpreted in the light of the possibility that the local anesthetic action, and not the blockade of the beta adrenergic receptor, is responsible.

In the early studies of adenylate cyclase, Sutherland and his colleagues (117) noted that ergotamine, as well as DCI, antagonized the epinephrine-induced production of cyclic AMP in broken cell preparations of liver and cardiac muscle. The experiments of Northrup and Parks (126, 127) suggest that dihydroergotamine acts at a more distal site than does DCI. In both intact animals (127) and in isolated perfused livers (126), hepatic production of glucose in response to epinephrine and cyclic AMP was inhibited by dihydroergotamine, whereas DCI inhibited only the effect of epinephrine.

It seems reasonable to conclude that inhibition of glycogenolysis by alpha blocking drugs represents nonspecific antagonism and does not warrant identifying metabolic receptors as alpha nor does it warrant refusal to classify them as beta.

The rat has posed a particular problem to classification of metabolic adrenergic receptors because it has seemed so resistant to the effects of isoproterenol. Hornbrook (75) reviewed previous work and found that isoproterenol was less active than epinephrine and norepinephrine in elevating blood sugar and in augmenting activation of liver phosphorylase in rats, whereas the three amines were equiactive in augmenting cyclic AMP formation in the isolated perfused rat liver. In contrast, isoproterenol in the dog is more potent than the other two amines in terms of producing hyperglycemia, activating liver phosphorylase, and augmenting cyclic AMP formation. Recent work by Newton & Hornbrook (120) shows that the order of potency of the three catecholamines in increasing the activity of adenylate cyclase in rat liver homogenates is isoproterenol > epinephrine > norepinephrine. Also propranolol produced complete inhibition of the effects of isoproterenol at 10^{-5} M and greater than 80% blockade at 10^{-6} M. Ergotamine and phenoxybenzamine, in contrast, produced no more than 50% blockade of isoproterenol at 10^{-4} M. Thus it is clear that the adrenergic receptor for hepatic glycogenolysis in the rat is of the beta type.

Newton and Hornbrook observed a unique aspect of the action of isoproterenol in the rat. By utilizing anesthetized rats in which samples of the liver were excised for assay of phosphorylase, they found that isoproterenol was nearly inactive when given subcutaneously, although epinephrine increased phosphorylase activity when given by this route. In contrast, isoproterenol was more potent than epinephrine and norepinephrine when infused intravenously. Subcutaneous administration of a large dose of isoproterenol antagonized the effect of intravenously infused isoproterenol. These results suggest that previous reports of inactivity of isoproterenol as a hyperglycemic agent in the rat might reflect this autoinhibitory action of the amine when given subcutaneously. Newton and Hornbrook found no obvious explanation for the autoinhibitory effect.

Catecholamines inhibit release of insulin from the pancreas, presumably via alpha adrenergic receptors; that is, phentolamine and ergotamine antagonize the inhibitory actions both in vitro and in vivo (142). In contrast, isoproterenol, particularly in the presence of phentolamine, increases release of insulin, an effect that is antagonized by propranolol and mediated by a beta adrenergic receptor. It is likely that the dominant effect physiologically is the alpha receptor-mediated inhibition of insulin release, an effect that would add to the elevated blood glucose brought about through augmented glycogenolysis.

Lipid Metabolism

Adrenergically induced lipolysis can be antagonized in vitro by both beta and alpha adrenergic blocking drugs. However, the blocking effects of alpha antagonists are nonspecific. Sympathetic nerve stimulation and intraarterial infusions of norepinephrine in dogs release both glycerol and free fatty acids from subcutaneous (55) and omental fat (6). The effects of both nerve stimulation and norepinephrine infusion are selectively antagonized by the beta blocking drugs. It seems clear therefore that both in vitro and in vivo the adrenergic receptor for lipolysis has the characteristics of a beta adrenergic receptor, although subclassification is not established (142). Adrenergically induced lipolysis appears to be mediated via a lipase that is activated by cyclic AMP. Whether a kinase is intermediate between cyclic AMP and lipase is not clear (142).

Calorigenesis

The calorigenic effect of catecholamines has been known for many years. The increase in heat production elicited by exposure to cold is similar to that produced by administration of sympathomimetic amines in that both types are antagonized by beta adrenergic blocking drugs. The mechanism of the calorigenic response is not known. Attempts to reproduce it by the use of dibutyryl cyclic AMP have not been successful. Robison et al. (142) suggest that several factors combine to augment oxygen consumption; these include the heightened oxidative metabolism of brown fat stimulated by norepinephrine, the hyperlacticacidemia that occurs secondary to muscle glycogenolysis, hyperglycemia, elevated free fatty acids in the plasma, and the calorigenic process of formation and metabolism of cyclic AMP itself (see the chapter by Himms-Hagen in this volume of the *Handbook*).

CARDIOVASCULAR SYSTEM

Adrenergic receptors in the cardiovascular system can be classified as: alpha receptors, which subserve all vasoconstriction, whether in arteries or veins; and beta receptors, which subserve active adrenergic vasodilatation and all cardiac responses to adrenergic stimuli. Until the past few years this classification fitted most of the facts derived from experimental data. However, detailed analysis of the actions of adrenergic agonists and antagonists on various parts of the circulatory system and of various cardiovascular modalities yields a less clear picture of adrenergic receptors.

1. Division of beta receptors into two subtypes, beta$_1$ for the heart and beta$_2$ for active adrenergic vasodilatation, has been proposed (87).

2. The concept that cardiac adrenergic receptors are only beta has been challenged by the proposal that alpha receptors coexist with beta receptors in the heart (67, 68).

3. Vasodilator responses to dopamine in certain vascular beds have been proposed to be subserved by specific "dopamine" receptors (62).

Heart

Classification of cardiac adrenergic receptors has been approached most extensively and rigorously in terms of heart rate and, particularly, contractile force. Other modalities, such as membrane action potentials, intracardiac conduction, ion fluxes, and metabolic processes, have been studied in less detail, and therefore the conclusions regarding receptor types are not as well founded.

Ahlquist (3) found the order of potency of six sympathomimetic amines as cardiac stimulants and vasodilators to be the same (i.e., isoproterenol was the most potent cardiac stimulant and vasodilator). He therefore put cardiac adrenergic receptors in the beta class. Confirmation of this classification came with the discovery of the blocking actions of DCI on the heart. Moran & Perkins (115) found isoproterenol to be more potent than either norepinephrine or epinephrine on rate and contractility in dog heart in situ and in rabbit heart in vitro. They then found that DCI selectively antagonized adrenergic stimuli in both dog and rabbit heart. In the dog the cardiac responses to intravenous injections of epinephrine, norepinephrine, isoproterenol, and ephedrine and to electrical stimulation of the cardiac sympathetic nerves were blocked by DCI, whereas the inotropic effects of digoxin, calcium chloride, and theophylline were not altered. The positive chronotropic effects of theophylline were not blocked by doses of DCI that antagonized the chronotropic effects of adrenergic stimuli. Subsequently other authors reported similar results with DCI (41, 56) and with other new beta adrenergic blocking drugs, such as pronethalol (19) and propranolol (18).

Identification of the cardiac adrenergic receptors in terms of selectivity of blockade was reassessed several years after the discovery of DCI because of previous reports that alpha adrenergic blocking drugs antagonized adrenergically induced changes in rate and force. Two groups of investigators (116, 122) simultaneously showed that alpha adrenergic blocking drugs did not antagonize the effects of adrenergic stimuli on myocardial contractility and on pacemaker rate, in both isolated heart tissue and dog heart in situ. Apparent antagonism by alpha adrenergic blocking drugs was due to nonspecific effects of the blocking drugs.

There have been recent challenges of the concept that the cardiac receptors are all beta. Alpha receptors in the heart have been suggested in addition to beta receptors. Govier et al. (68) evaluated the effects of agonists and antagonists on the functional refractory period of rabbit atria and concluded that beta receptors mediated decreased refractory period and that alpha receptors mediated increased refractory period. However, complete dose-response curves of agonists were not evaluated, and selectivity of blockade was not fully established for either pronethalol or phenoxybenzamine. Subsequently, Govier (67) reported evidence favoring the view that alpha receptors, as well as beta receptors, subserve the positive inotropic effect of adrenergic stimuli in isolated guinea pig atria. Similar results were obtained by Benfey & Varma (12) on contractility and functional refractory period of rabbit atria. In contrast, Yoo & Lee (168) were unable to show any evidence of alpha receptors in spontaneously beating rabbit atria, and Krell & Patil (85) found none for rate in the guinea pig heart. The proposal that alpha receptors exist in mammalian heart muscle requires confirmation.

All beta adrenergic receptors in the mammalian heart are of a common type based on orders of potency and selective blockade. That is, the sinoatrial node receptors are not different in functional pattern from those in atrial or ventricular muscle (20, 25). In addition, the responses elicited by sympathetic nerve stimulation are selectively antagonized by beta adrenergic blocking drugs (112, 115).

Several lines of evidence suggest that the beta receptors of the heart represent a subtype of beta receptor. Lands et al. (87) have proposed labeling beta receptors as beta$_1$ and beta$_2$, the former for the heart and the latter for smooth muscle and perhaps metabolic effects. The fact that norepinephrine is more potent as a cardiac stimulant than as a vasodilator and bronchodilator, for example, has placed the cardiac adrenergic receptors in a slightly different category from the receptors of smooth muscle that subserve inhibitory responses or relaxation. Several new drugs have emphasized these differences. First, beta adrenergic blocking compounds that have minor substitutions on the side chain have marked differences in blocking activity at different sites. The addition of a methyl group on the α carbon of DCI and closely related amines reduced cardiac adrenergic blocking potency 15-fold without altering the potency for antagonizing vasodilatation responses (95, 109). Subsequently, practolol, a new beta adrenergic blocking drug of the propranolol class, was found to be more selective as a cardiac beta blocker than as an antagonist of smooth muscle relaxation (43). Finally, a new agonist, salbutamol, has been developed; it appears to have much greater activity on beta receptors of smooth muscle than on those of the heart (26). Thus evidence from studies on orders of potency of agonists and from studies on new beta adrenergic blocking drugs supports the proposal by Lands and colleagues to classify two types of beta receptors: beta$_1$ for the heart and beta$_2$ for smooth muscle.

The metabolic responses to adrenergic stimuli were discussed in greater detail in a previous section. At this point, however, it is relevant to discuss cardiac adrenergic receptors in the context of metabolic systems in the heart. Although adrenergic stimuli augment consumption of oxygen and uptake and utilization of glucose, lactate, and fatty acids, it is in the area of glycogenolysis that most detailed work has been done; such studies provide a picture of the relation of metabolic systems to adrenergic receptors.

For many years catecholamines have been known to increase breakdown of glycogen in the heart. Hess & Haugaard (72) related the activation of cardiac phosphorylase by sympathomimetic amines to the augmentation of contractility. Mayer & Moran (105) demonstrated the selective blockade by DCI of the augmentation of contractility and activation of phosphorylase in the dog heart in situ. They proposed that the glycogenolytic action of adrenergic stimuli be classified as mediated by beta receptors.

Subsequent work has clearly shown that the antecedent events (i.e., the stimulation of the adenylate cyclase system) are related to beta receptors. Several recent reviews have provided detailed evaluation of the evidence (50, 103, 104, 142). All available evidence indicates that activation of beta adrenergic receptors in mammalian myocardium results in increased content of cyclic AMP and in augmented activity of enzymes distal to adenylate cyclase in the glycogenolytic pathway (i.e., phosphorylase kinase and phosphorylase). Furthermore adrenergic stimuli augment activation of glycogen synthetase (163). These responses are correlated with the inotropic response to adrenergic stimuli, in that there are comparable orders of potency and all responses are selectively blocked by beta adrenergic blocking drugs, are potentiated by methylxanthines that inhibit phosphodiesterase, and are dissociable from comparable responses induced by glucagon (i.e., augmented contractility, elevated cyclic AMP, activation of phosphorylase and of synthetase) by means of selective blockade of the adrenergically induced effects of beta antagonists.

Although both glycogenolysis and contractile activity are increased through activation of beta adrenergic receptors in the mammalian heart, it is not clear whether both are mediated beyond the receptor by cyclic AMP (see the chapter by Williamson in this volume of the *Handbook*). A unitary view favors cyclic AMP as a second messenger for both effects, although through divergent pathways. Evidence for this view comes from the demonstration by Robison et al. (141) that the peak response of tissue cyclic AMP after infusion of epinephrine into the isolated perfused rat heart occurred 15 sec earlier than the peak response of contractile force. Both the rise in concentration of cyclic AMP in tissue and the contractile force response were blocked by pronethalol. Neither cyclic AMP nor several of its derivatives injected into the perfusion fluid elicited responses on contractile force. Namm & Mayer (118) found increases in cardiac contractile force in dogs in response to epinephrine with no change in cyclic AMP. However, there were augmented activities of phosphorylase b kinase and phosphorylase. Namm & Mayer (118) concluded that their method for taking samples of myocardium would result in destruction of the newly formed cyclic AMP during the biopsy but that cyclic AMP was probably responsible for the augmented contractile force. Also consistent with the hypothesis is the work of Skelton et al. (150) who showed that dibutyryl cyclic AMP (a derivative of cyclic AMP that is thought to enter cells more readily than cyclic AMP and to be more resistant to phosphodiesterase) augments contractile force of cat papillary muscle; cyclic AMP itself was inactive. The effect of dibutyryl cyclic AMP was not antagonized by propranolol in concentrations that blocked the effects of epinephrine.

In contrast, Kjekhus et al. (82) found evidence that cyclic AMP does not mediate the positive inotropic effect of catecholamines. In perfused, isolated guinea pig hearts, addition of dimethylsulfoxide (DMSO) to the perfusion fluid to facilitate entry of cyclic AMP augmented the effect of added cyclic AMP on phosphorylase. Addition of cyclic AMP, with or without DMSO, did not increase contractile force. Addition of epinephrine or isoproterenol produced both chronotropic and inotropic responses in DMSO-treated hearts with changes equivalent to those in normally perfused hearts. These authors conclude that the positive inotropic effect of catecholamines is not mediated by a direct action of cyclic AMP on the contractile apparatus. They suggest instead that the hypothesis of Rasmussen & Tenenhouse (138) is feasible; that is, catecholamine-induced activation of adenylate cyclase results in conversion of membrane-bound ATP to cyclic AMP via adenylate cyclase with a consequent release of calcium from the calcium-membrane-ATP complex. Thus catecholamines may increase contractile force as a consequence of the secondary release of calcium as cyclic AMP is formed from ATP. There has been no evidence that the putative alpha receptors in the heart mediate any metabolic response to adrenergic stimuli.

In summary, although a great deal of evidence supports the view that the adenylate cyclase system is identical to, or in close association with, the cardiac beta adrenergic receptor and that cyclic AMP is a common second messenger in the mediation of the effects of adrenergic stimuli, there are enough contradictory data at this time to warrant a circumspect attitude toward the hypothesis. Figure 2 depicts two possible schemes in which adrenergic and glucagon receptors might be coupled to the contractile system.

Functional modalities of the heart other than contractility have not been studied rigorously in terms of classification of adrenergic receptors. Dale recognized that ergot did not block the positive chronotropic effect of epinephrine, and Ahlquist classified the adrenergic receptors subserving heart rate as beta. The discovery of DCI clearly established the beta category. The electrical manifestation of sinoatrial node pacemaker function has been studied less consistently. West et al. (162) appear to be the first to have shown that D(−)-epinephrine increases the slope of the prepotential (diastolic depolarization; phase 4 depolarization) of the sinoatrial node pacemaker cells. Little work has been done on sinoatrial pacemakers with adrenergic blocking drugs. Strauss et al. (153) showed that sotalol, a beta adrenergic blocking drug without local anesthetic activity, produced a surmountable type of antagonism of isoproterenol when the spontaneous rate of isolated sinoatrial node preparations of the rabbit, recorded either with intracellular microelectrodes or surface bipolar electrodes, was used as an index. Although transmembrane potentials were recorded, the effects of isoproterenol and sotalol on phase 4 potential slopes were not reported.

Davis & Temte (38) found that epinephrine increased phase 4 depolarization of isolated Purkinje fibers of the dog and that propranolol in low concentration blocked the effect. No analysis of orders of potency of agonist was made, nor was an alpha adrenergic blocking agent tested. Giotti et al. (61) observed both beta- and alpha-mediated effects in isolated Purkinje fibers of the sheep. Iso-

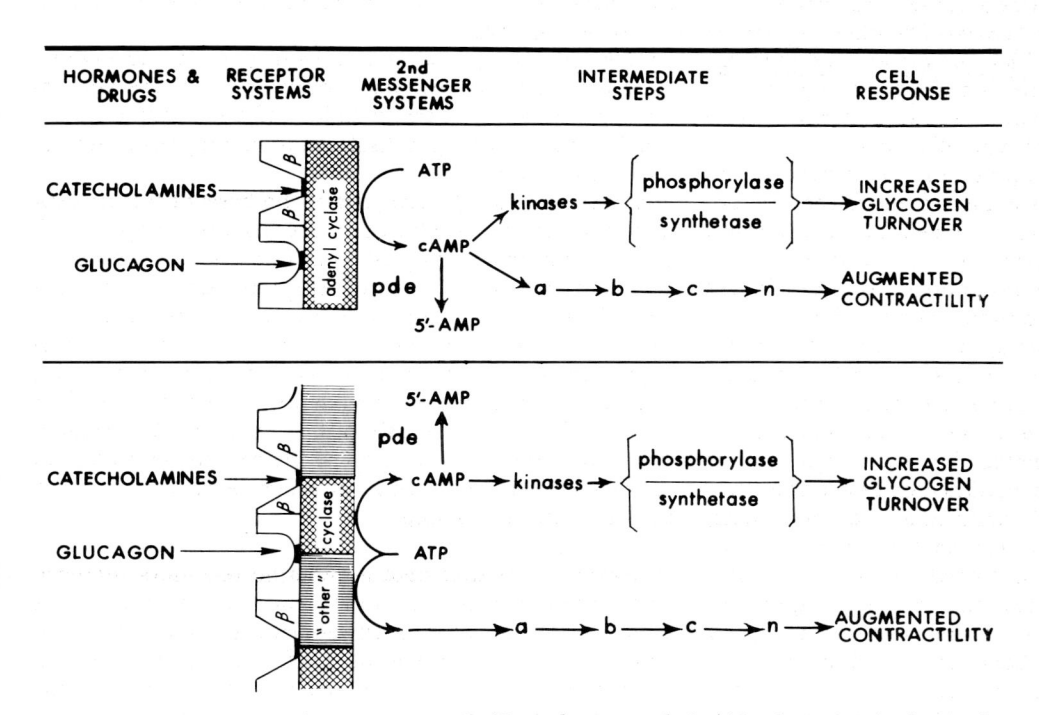

FIG. 2. Two alternate relationships between the beta adrenergic receptor and the adenylate cyclase system in the heart. *Upper* scheme is based on unitary hypothesis of Sutherland and colleagues that all beta adrenergic responses of the heart are mediated by cyclic AMP as a second messenger. In the *lower* scheme, it is assumed that the positive inotropic effect of adrenergic agonists may not be mediated by cyclic AMP. *Pde*, phosphodiesterase.

proterenol, norepinephrine, and epinephrine all increased the slope of phase 4 depolarization and the frequency of spontaneous generation of action potentials in the fibers, isoproterenol being more potent than the other two amines. Propranolol blocked this effect. In the presence of propranolol, norepinephrine decreased phase 4 depolarization, and in some preparations not treated with propranolol, norepinephrine decreased the slope of phase 4 and this action was blocked by phentolamine. These data were the basis for the authors' conclusion that there are both alpha and beta receptors in sheep Purkinje tissue.

Pappano (129) found that isoproterenol, norepinephrine, and epinephrine increased duration of the plateau phase without altering the total duration of the action potential of isolated, electrically stimulated atria of guinea pigs. Propranolol blocked this effect. Epinephrine was found to prolong the duration of the action potential, an effect not blocked by propranolol but antagonized by phentolamine and dihydroergotamine. Rahn & Reuter (136) found that epinephrine (5×10^{-7} g/ml) increased the resting membrane potential and shortened the duration of the action potential of guinea pig atria. Pretreatment with a beta adrenergic blocking drug reversed these effects of epinephrine. No alpha adrenergic blocking drug was used.

Atrioventricular conduction is augmented by adrenergic stimuli (36, 74, 157). Berkowitz et al. (15) showed that propranolol in both animals and man prolongs atrioventricular conduction, an effect they attribute to beta adrenergic blockade, although they did not evaluate the quinidine-like effect of the drug. Kabella & Mendez (79) found that, in dogs in which sinoatrial node function was excluded by crushing the node and thereby leaving the atrioventricular (AV) node as the dominant pacemaker, the increase in heart rate elicited by adrenergic stimuli was blocked by propranolol. Furthermore the adrenergically induced shortening of the refractory period of the AV node was antagonized by propranolol. Whitsit & Lucchesi (165) also observed prolongation of AV functional refractory period in dogs, but they did not test the effects of a sympathomimetic drug. However, on the basis of the higher potency of dl-propranolol compared with d-propranolol (which has little beta receptor-blocking action) they concluded that the effect of the prolongation was primarily due to receptor blockade.

Cardiac arrhythmias elicited by adrenergic agents are now generally held to be mediated by beta adrenergic receptors. The genesis of ventricular ectopic beats, either single or multiple, and ventricular fibrillation that can occur with large doses of "cardiotonic" sympathomimetic amines are complex and involve augmented automaticity of pacemakers in the ventricular system (probably in the Purkinje fibers) and simultaneous suppression of sinoatrial (SA) node pacemakers as a result of augmented reflex vagal activity. Shortly after the discovery of DCI, several workers demonstrated its ability to antagonize adrenergically induced ventricular arrhythmias in animals (42, 60, 107, 114). It was then noted that DCI and some related beta adrenergic blocking drugs have local anesthetic properties (108). Dextro isomers of pronethalol and propranolol have antiarrhythmic effects but are weak beta adrenergic blocking compounds (99). It is obvious that certain types of experimental and clinical arrhythmias are mediated by beta receptors, but it should not be concluded that all arrhythmias blocked by beta adrenergic blocking drugs are of adrenergic origin.

Blood Vessels

Adrenergic receptors in blood vessels generally fall in the category of alpha for mediation of vasoconstriction and beta for vasodilatation. Where this general rule does not appear to be valid, it is probable that rigorous, careful evaluations have not been accomplished. According to this general rule, all blood vessels, both arteries and veins, that are innervated by the sympathetic nervous system appear to respond to nerve activity by vasoconstriction through alpha receptors. In contrast, there is serious question about the innervation of blood vessels in terms of nerve-mediated active vasodilatation, as opposed to passive vasodilatation as a result of withdrawal of sympathetic vasoconstrictor activity. Furthermore, present evidence favors the view that beta adrenergic receptors in blood vessels are primarily located in the arteries of skeletal muscles. That is, studies based on the use of isoproterenol as a beta vasodilating agent indicate that isoproterenol is more potent in skeletal muscle than in other tissues and that the magnitude of the vasodilator response is greater.

The classification of two types of vascular adrenergic receptors goes back to Dale's discovery that the antagonism of the vasoconstrictor effect of epinephrine in the dog by extracts of ergot disclosed a vasodepressor action. The dual actions of epinephrine (i.e., vasoconstriction and vasodilatation) were part of the basis of the concept of two types of neurohumoral mediators—sympathin E and sympathin I. Ahlquist's classification of adrenergic receptors categorized those receptors subserving vasoconstriction as alpha and those subserving vasodilatation as beta. Ahlquist designated beta vasodilatation primarily in the skeletal muscles and the coronary vessels and, to a slight extent, in mesenteric vessels. Powell & Slater (135) then established the fact that DCI blocked the vasodepressor effect of epinephrine and isoproterenol in the cat and the vasodilator effect of isoproterenol in the hind limb of the dog.

Although one can demonstrate by the use of injections of isoproterenol that beta adrenergic receptors subserve vasodilatation, especially in skeletal muscle, it has been difficult to demonstrate a nerve-mediated beta adrenergic vasodilatation. Viveros et al. (156) have used a refined technique of perfusion of a gracilis muscle of the dog and have obtained evidence for neurogenically mediated vasodilatation. Furthermore they have found vasodilatation in response to small doses of norepinephrine, in contrast to previous investigators who have observed vasodilatation in the hind limb only with large doses of this amine. Because both sympathetic nerve stimulation and norepinephrine cause vasoconstriction, Viveros and co-workers used an alpha adrenergic blocking drug. Because of the sympathetic-cholinergic vasodilator system in dogs, they used atropine. When both of these blocking drugs were used, nerve stimulation (both motor nerve to the muscle and lumbar sympathetic nerve) and intraarterial injections of norepinephrine produced vasodilator responses that were blocked by propranolol. This work suggests a close relation between adrenergic nerve endings and beta receptors in muscle blood vessels. The high potency of norepinephrine detected by Viveros and associates casts doubt on the validity of the classification by Lands et al. (87) of vasodilator adrenergic receptors as beta$_2$. The work of Viveros et al. (156) requires validation before one can fully accept the view that beta adrenergically mediated vasodilatation can be nerve mediated.

Dopamine, the catecholamine precursor of norepinephrine, has been found to dilate blood vessels in the renal and mesenteric beds through a receptor distinct from the beta receptor (62). There is no evidence that this is a neurogenically mediated effect, nor is there any evidence that dopamine receptors have a physiological role in modulating visceral blood flow.

VEINS. Most reports now show that veins are primarily populated by alpha adrenergic receptors subserving contraction. Coupar (35) found human saphenous vein strips in vitro to have this pattern. He found D(−)-epinephrine to be most potent and D(−)-isoproterenol to be least potent as stimulants of contraction. Alpha adrenergic blocking drugs antagonized the contractile effects of both norepinephrine and isoproterenol, whereas propranolol did not. Only variable and small relaxant responses to isoproterenol were obtained. Similar results were found in strips of rabbit vena cava.

Some reports suggested that a major aspect of venoconstriction is mediated by beta receptors (44, 80). The conclusions of these reports are open to criticism, however. Eckstein & Hamilton (44) administered isoproterenol to human subjects by vein, and the venoconstriction that followed might have been a reflex response to the fall in blood pressure. Kaiser et al. (80) assessed changes in venous capacitance by measuring displacement of blood from the hind part of the dogs into or from a reservoir. The changes in reservoir volume can be accounted for by changes in arterial, as well as venous, capacitance and relaxation of hepatic venous sphincters.

Abboud et al. (1) found small, consistent venodilator responses to isoproterenol in the foreleg of dogs. This effect of isoproterenol had the characteristics of a beta receptor-mediated action on the basis of selective blockade. They used the technique of estimating segmental resistance, which consists of constant flow perfusion of the limb with measurement of pressures in large and small arteries and veins.

Intraarterial injection of isoproterenol reduces vascular resistance without venous constriction (1, 147). Zsoter (169) measured distensibility of a single vein and found no effect of low doses of isoproterenol on superficial veins of man or femoral and jugular veins of the dog. Large doses of isoproterenol were not used.

Thus there is no good evidence that venoconstriction is mediated by beta receptors. Rather, adrenergically induced venoconstriction appears to be entirely alpha.

CORONARY ARTERIES. Most evidence supports the concept that adrenergic vasoconstriction mechanisms exist in coronary vessels and are subserved by alpha receptors. Adrenergic coronary vasodilatation is presumably mediated by beta receptors. However, because of the unique characteristics of the coronary circulation, it is difficult to determine the function of these receptors in physiological adjustments of blood flow. It is difficult to separate changes in coronary resistance caused by active vasodilatation and vasoconstriction from changes secondary to alterations in ventricular wall tension, contraction of myocardium, and metabolism of the heart muscle.

Klocke et al. (83) evaluated alpha and beta receptors in the coronary circulation of the dog heart in situ. They compared responses to isoproterenol in the heart arrested by the intravenous infusion of potassium chloride (to eliminate the influence of alterations of heart rate and myocardial contractile force on coronary blood flow) with those in the regularly beating heart. They found that increased flow occurred with intraarterial injections of isoproterenol, and in the potassium-arrested heart the response was independent of metabolism or decreased myocardial oxygenation. The responses were blocked by pronethalol. However, alpha blocking agents were not evaluated, nor were other vasodilating agonists used. They concluded that the coronary vessels are supplied with a mechanism for adrenergically induced vasodilatation, but its significance is uncertain.

Zuberbuhler & Bohr (170) found that isolated strips of small coronary arteries (250–500 μ) from dogs had a predominance of beta receptors, as judged by the relaxation produced by catecholamines and antagonism of this response by pronethalol. Large coronary arteries have a predominance of alpha receptors, as judged by adrenergically induced, contractile responses that are blocked by phenoxybenzamine. Norepinephrine was more potent than epinephrine as a relaxant but less potent as a constrictor; the concentrations of norepinephrine were less than the normal concentration of the material in the blood.

Increased coronary vascular resistance in response to beta adrenergic blocking drugs has been attributed to the antagonism of neurogenic beta vasodilatation that unmasks alpha vasoconstriction. Whitsitt & Lucchesi (164), however, concluded that this increased coronary vascular resistance, seen with beta blocking drugs, is due largely to the decreased heart rate and the secondary decreased requirement of the myocardium for energy and the nonspecific reduction in myocardial contractility. Since increased coronary arterial resistance follows administration of propranolol in dogs pretreated with reserpine, Whitsitt & Lucchesi (164) concluded that the increased coronary resistance in normal dogs after administration of propranolol is not due to unmasking alpha constrictor activity.

Pitt et al. (133) have found evidence for both alpha and beta receptors in coronary vessels of the unanesthetized dog. Intravenous injections of isoproterenol and epinephrine led to increased coronary blood flow in dogs with heart rates held constant by electrical stimulation. These changes occurred with only slight changes in cardiac output. Intracoronary artery injections of isoproterenol caused an immediate increase in coronary flow before changes in heart rate or contractile activity occurred. Propranolol blocked the early increase in coronary flow caused by both intravenous and intraarterial injections of the amines. Coronary vasoconstriction occurred after intravenous phenylephrine and intraarterial norepinephrine in some animals. Phenoxybenzamine appeared to block the constrictor effect of norepinephrine.

Broadley (27) outlined four components of coronary vascular response to catecholamines in isolated, perfused guinea pig hearts: *1*) an initial phase of vasoconstriction mediated by alpha adrenergic receptors; *2*) a secondary constriction resulting from extravascular compression during the augmented myocardial contraction; *3*) a prolonged dilatation probably caused by increased cardiac metabolism; and *4*) a direct vasodilatation mediated by beta$_2$ receptors. The latter effect is largely obscured by the metabolically mediated dilatation. Broadley concluded that the major effect of catecholamines is an increase in myocardial blood flow as a result of the augmented metabolism. Similarly, Parratt & Wadsworth (130) concluded that in dogs the markedly augmented blood flow that results from administration of isoproterenol is due to augmented metabolism, with a small component due to active vasodilatation via beta$_2$ adrenergic receptors in the coronary vessels.

A number of workers has described a rapidly developing and transient coronary vasoconstriction during stellate ganglion stimulation in unanesthetized animals (69) and in anesthetized dogs (16). Feigl (53, 54) has sought an answer to the possibility that there is a sympathetic cholinergic vasodilator system in the heart, as in canine skeletal muscle. He was not able to show this with hypothalamic stimulation, even when the stimulation caused vasodilatation in skeletal muscles. Feigl (53) showed that stimulation of the stellate ganglion increases coronary flow, an effect converted to a decrease by propranolol. Similarly stimulation of the hypothalamus in the area that increases skeletal muscle blood flow augments coronary flow and increases heart rate. The cardiac effects, but not the skeletal muscle vasodilatation, were blocked by propranolol. These experiments do not rule out the possibility of a beta receptor-mediated coronary vasodilatation in response to augmented sympathetic nerve activity to the heart. Thus it is clear that coronary vasoconstriction can result from sympathetic nerve stimulation, but it is not clear whether there is a nerve-mediated vasodilatation separate from the vasodilatation that is secondary to the augmented cardiac metabolism. The possible role of sympathetically induced coronary vasoconstriction is obscure. Possibly it is involved in redistribution of myocardial blood flow during heightened myocardial activity (10).

Adam et al. (2) measured coronary blood flow in anesthetized dogs and evaluated the responses to cardiac sympathetic nerve stimulation and to intravenously administered norepinephrine before and after treatment with practolol, the agent that selectively blocks beta$_1$ receptors. The augmented coronary flow induced by these two forms of adrenergic stimulation was converted to a vasoconstrictor effect by practolol. However, the vasodilator effect of epinephrine and isoproterenol was only slightly reduced in magnitude. Practolol blocked the tachycardia and the augmented rate of change of isovolumic intraventricular pressure (dP/dt) that is produced by all forms of beta adrenergic stimuli. Phentolamine in the presence of practolol blocked the increased coronary resistance produced by nerve stimulation and by norepinephrine. Ross & Jorgensen (143) obtained similar results.

PULMONARY VESSELS. Evaluation of receptors in pulmonary blood vessels is difficult. In the intact animal changes in pulmonary blood flow and resistance are in large measure due to changes in cardiac output because of the low resistance and high capacitance of the pulmonary vascular circuit. Furthermore changes in bronchiolar resistance influence pulmonary blood flow secondary to the changes in alveolar pressures.

Epinephrine and norepinephrine constrict vessels of the perfused, isolated lung, and this action is blocked by alpha adrenergic blocking drugs. Castro de la Mata et al. (31) have evaluated the effects of adrenergic agonists and antagonists on the perfused, in situ lung of the dog. They found a pattern of vasoconstriction in response to epinephrine, norepinephrine, and postganglionic sympathetic nerve stimulation. Because this response was not blocked by DCI but was blocked by tolazoline, an alpha adrenergic antagonist, these authors concluded that the effect was alpha receptor mediated. The vasodilator effect of isoproterenol in this preparation was blocked by DCI. They concluded that the pulmonary vessels have beta adrenergic receptors that subserve vasodilatation. However, it is not possible with this preparation to clearly separate direct vascular effects from effects secondary to actions on the heart. Although the lobe of the lung was perfused from a pump by-passing the right heart, the drainage was directly into the left atrium. Thus alterations in left atrial and left ventricular contractility can affect pulmonary resistance. Isoproterenol not only reduced the perfusion pressure but also reduced left atrial pressure. This effect could be due to vasodilatation directly or to the secondary effect of cardiac stimulation with reduction of left atrial pressure. Since both of these effects are mediated by beta receptors, blockade by DCI would not distinguish between pulmonary vessels and heart. The use of one of the new selective agents would help in this type of assessment; that is, practolol as a cardiac (beta₁) antagonist would prevent isoproterenol-induced myocardial stimulation with minimal blockade of vascular receptors. Furthermore the beta₂-type agonist, such as salbutamol, should dilate pulmonary vessels without cardiac stimulation if the pulmonary vessels have beta₂ receptors.

Ingram et al. (78) have also found pulmonary vascular responses to sympathetic nerve stimulation in the dog lung perfused but isolated in situ to be alpha adrenergically mediated vasoconstriction, based on antagonism of the changes by phenoxybenzamine and no blockade by propranolol. Intraarterial injections of norepinephrine also produced alpha adrenergically mediated vasoconstriction. However, they interpreted the effects of nerve stimulation to be on large pulmonary vessels, based on reduced compliance and no change in peripheral resistance. The effects of injected norepinephrine were interpreted to be on small arteries as well because of the rise the drug produced in peripheral resistance.

Thus adrenergic stimulation, both by means of injected drugs and by nerve stimulation, causes pulmonary vasoconstriction via alpha adrenergic receptors. The question of the existence of beta receptor-mediated vasodilatation cannot be answered on the basis of current data.

NONVASCULAR SMOOTH MUSCLE

Gastrointestinal

Dale (35) observed that the inhibitory effect of epinephrine and of splanchnic nerve stimulation on the intestine was not blocked by ergot, whereas excitatory responses of intestinal sphincter muscle were blocked. Interpreted in terms of current receptor classification, Dale's work suggests that the relaxant effect of adrenergic stimuli is subserved by beta receptors. However, Ahlquist originally classified intestinal relaxation as an alpha adrenergic function, and subsequently Ahlquist & Levy (4) concluded that adrenergically induced relaxation of the ileum of the dog in situ is subserved by both alpha and beta receptors. The effect of phenylephrine was blocked by an alpha adrenergic blocking agent but not by DCI, the effect of isoproterenol was blocked by DCI and not by the alpha antagonist, and the effects of epinephrine were only partially blocked by either type of blocking agent alone but completely by the combination of alpha and beta antagonists. Subsequent work by other investigators (57, 100, 139, 144) has confirmed the observation of Ahlquist and Levy.

In an attempt to explain two classes of receptors, both of which subserve the same type of response, Van Rossum & Mujić (144) and Reddy & Moran (139) proposed that alpha adrenergically induced intestinal relaxation is due to hyperpolarization and inhibition of nerve impulse formation secondary to activation of receptors located on the cell surface of motor neurons in the myenteric plexuses. Beta adrenergically induced relaxation is due to changes in smooth muscle contractility secondary to activation of receptors located directly in the smooth muscle. Histochemical studies provided a basis for this hypothesis in that Norberg (125) and others have shown that adrenergic neurons in the small intestine of the guinea pig terminate primarily in apposition with intramural ganglion cells, with very few terminating at smooth muscle cells. Furthermore, Lum et al. (100) found that damage to neuronal elements of the gut induced by cold storage diminished the alpha-mediated part of relaxation but had little effect on the beta part.

Bowman & Hall (22) challenged the concept of localization of alpha receptors on intramural neurons; they favored the view that both alpha and beta receptors are part of smooth muscle cells—*alpha* receptors on the cell surface and the beta receptors within the cell. On the other hand, Kosterlitz et al. (84) argue that the most likely site of alpha adrenergic receptors in small intestine is on neuronal elements and that beta receptors are a part of smooth muscle cells.

Bartlet & Hassan (8) have evaluated the adrenergic receptors in the chick rectum and the guinea pig colon. They concluded that the guinea pig colon has both alpha and beta receptors but that the rectum of the chick has a predominance of beta receptors. Adrenergically induced contractions of the sphincter of Odi (choledochoduodenal junction) of the cat appears to be mediated by alpha receptors and relaxation by beta receptors (98). In contrast, Reddy & Moran (139) found that pyloric and ileocolic sphincter areas of the rabbit contracted in response to epinephrine, norepinephrine, and methoxamine—responses that were blocked by phentolamine but not by DCI. Isoproterenol caused relaxation of these sphincters in low concentrations and contraction in high concentrations. Both responses to isoproterenol were blocked by DCI and not by phentolamine. They concluded that sphincters contain both alpha and beta receptors, both subserving contraction.

Several investigators have observed contractile responses to sympathomimetic amines in nonsphincter intestinal preparations—in the rat colon pretreated with pronethalol (140), in the guinea pig stomach (5, 70), and in the guinea pig colon pretreated with a beta blocking drug (59). Phentolamine partially blocked the contractions of the guinea pig colon induced by the sympathomimetic amines, which suggested that alpha receptors subserve contraction (59).

Cyclic AMP has been implicated in the relaxant effect of catecholamines on intestine. Bueding et al. (28) found a correlation between relaxation and increase in cyclic AMP in guinea pig intestinal muscle in response to epinephrine. Wilkenfeld & Levy (166) found that theophylline and diazoxide, inhibitors of phosphodiesterase, potentiated the inhibitory effect of isoproterenol on isolated rabbit ileum and that imidazole, a compound that enhances the activity of phosphodiesterase, inhibited the effect of isoproterenol. Neither the inhibitors nor the enhancer of phosphodiesterase altered the relaxant effect of phenylephrine. These authors concluded that the data are compatible with the view that cylic AMP mediates the beta receptor route of intestinal relaxation but not the alpha receptor route.

Catecholamines reduce or abolish spontaneous spike discharge and hyperpolarization of the intestinal smooth muscle membranes (29). Davis (39) proposed that the reduction of spike discharge is due to stimulation of beta receptors and the hyperpolarization to stimulation of alpha receptors. Davis' studies were conducted with beta blocking drugs which have some agonistic action, and his conclusions were based on the use of these drugs as agonists. Depolarization of the metabolically depressed taenia coli is attributed to stimulation of alpha receptors.

Weisbrodt et al. (160) concluded that both alpha and beta receptors subserve relaxation in guinea pig taenia coli induced to contract by 35 mM KCl. Beta adrenergically induced relaxation was not accompanied by changes in membrane potential of spike activity, whereas the alpha receptor-mediated effect was associated with reduction of spike activity. Aminophylline relaxed the KCl-contracted taenia coli independently of alpha and beta adrenergic receptors. In 90 mM KCl the gut strips underwent marked depolarization with abolition of spike activity, and in this condition no alpha receptor component of relaxation could be detected.

Spleen

Bickerton (17) carefully evaluated adrenergic receptor types in isolated strips of cat spleen. All the characteristics, such as order of potency of catecholamines, selective blockade, and receptor protection, supported the conclusion that the receptors subserving contraction are alpha. Bickerton also concluded that DCI and isoproterenol act also on alpha receptors "either directly or indirectly." Furthermore he found evidence that beta receptors subserve relaxation. Subsequently, Ignarro & Titus (77) evaluated the receptors in mouse spleen and concluded that both alpha and beta adrenergic receptors are in the mouse spleen subserving contraction and relaxation, respectively.

Nictitating Membrane

The smooth muscle of the nictitating membrane contracts in response to postganglionic sympathetic nerve stimulation and to blood-borne epinephrine and norepinephrine. These responses are blocked by alpha adrenergic blocking drugs (121). Ahlquist (3) classified the adrenergic receptors in the nictitating membrane of the cat as solely alpha, but adrenergic stimuli also elicit relaxation of the membrane, the characteristics of which (order of potency of agonists and selective blockade) indicate a beta receptor function (152).

Pluchino & Trendelenburg (134) utilized the nictitating membrane of the cat in evaluating the relation of alpha and beta adrenergic receptors to denervation and decentralization supersensitivity. They concluded that one type of denervation supersensitivity is restricted to those amines taken up by normal adrenergic nerve endings, whereas decentralization supersensitivity is of a qualitatively different type and is localized to postsynaptic sites. Furthermore it was postulated that decentralization supersensitivity is restricted to those agents that have excitatory actions; that is, there is not supersensitivity to beta relaxant effect on the membrane.

Langer & Trendelenburg (89) came to the interesting conclusion that decentralization produces postsynaptic changes such that the alpha adrenergic blocking drug, phenoxybenzamine, became less effective as an antagonist of adrenergically induced contraction of the cat nictitating membrane. The decrease in effectiveness developed in a time course similar to that of the development of decentralization supersensitivity and was related to the postsynaptic changes that accompany decentralization. They speculate that the changes consist either of an increase in receptor population or an improvement in the link between activation of the receptor and contraction of the smooth muscle. They were unable to distinguish between these two possibilities.

Iris

Ahlquist (3) classified the adrenergic receptors in the cat iris as solely alpha. This conclusion was reached later by Bennet et al. (13) on the basis of responses to intraocular injections of agonists in the rabbit. They concluded that the rabbit iris dilator has only alpha receptors but that isoproterenol is an effective agonist on this receptor. The vasculature of the iris of the rabbit appeared to have both alpha and beta receptors subserving vasoconstriction and vasodilation, respectively.

The usual responses to alpha adrenergic blockade are miosis, enophthalmos, ptosis, and, in animals, relaxation of the nictitating membrane. Beta adrenergic blocking drugs do not have these effects even in large doses. The blocking effects of ergot on the cat pupil were first recognized by Dale and were later demonstrated for Dibenamine by Nickerson & Goodman (123).

Patil (131) studied isolated strips of cattle iris sphincter and concluded that this muscle has mainly beta adrenergic receptors that subserve relaxation. He concluded that slight excitatory alpha adrenergic effects could be demonstrated. An unusual feature of his work is low degree of effectiveness of propranolol as a beta adrenergic antagonist compared with the high effectiveness of sotatol. In other tissues, such as the heart, propranolol is the more potent beta blocker.

Uterus

Adrenergic receptors of uterine muscle are difficult to classify, inasmuch as the responses of the uterus vary widely depending on the species of animal, the stage of the estrous cycle, and whether the uterus is from a pregnant or nonpregnant animal. Generally all adrenergically induced inhibitory responses of the uterus are mediated by beta receptors, and all adrenergically induced contractile responses are mediated by alpha receptors. Dale (35) noted that the relaxant effects of epinephrine on the uterus were not antagonized by ergot. Nickerson & Goodman (123) then showed that Dibenamine blocks the epinephrine-induced contraction of the nonpregnant rabbit uterus and even reverses the effect, but it has no effect on the relaxant action of epinephrine on the nonpregnant cat uterus. Nickerson & Hollenberg (124) have pointed out that a number of alpha adrenergic blocking drugs stimulate the uteri of various species and under a variety of conditions but that this effect is unrelated to alpha adrenergic blockade.

Ahlquist (3) originally classified the uterus as having both alpha and beta adrenergic receptors, the alpha receptor subserving contraction and the beta relaxation. Rudzik & Miller (145) proposed that both alpha and beta receptors subserve relaxation, but this concept was disputed by Levy & Tozzi (94) who presented evidence that inhibitory responses to adrenergic stimuli were activated only by beta receptors.

The uteri of various species respond differently from one another, particularly in reference to the state of estrus (119). Human uterus at term relaxes in response to isoproterenol, and the effect is antagonized by propranolol. It is concluded that the adrenergic receptor subserving uterine relaxation in the human female at term is a beta receptor (101).

Tsai & Fleming (155) studied the effects of adrenergic agents on uteri isolated from cats in various hormonal states. By using selective blockade and orders of potencies of norepinephrine, epinephrine, and isoproterenol, they found that the uterus of the virgin cat is relaxed via beta receptors and that the uterus under the influence of progesterone contracts via alpha receptors. Estrogen treatment appears to create a more variable situation. These authors suggest that hormonal states cause a shift in the balance of alpha to beta receptors.

Respiratory Tract

Adrenergically induced relaxation of bronchiolar and tracheal smooth muscle appears to be entirely subserved by beta$_2$-type receptors. Ahlquist did not study tracheobronchial muscle in his first classification of adrenergic receptors. However, he did classify bronchial receptors as beta on the basis of the work of Lands et al. (88) in which isoproterenol was found to be a more potent bronchodilator than epinephrine. Powell & Slater (135) showed that DCI prevented isoproterenol-induced relaxation of the isolated tracheal chain of the guinea pig, an observation that supported Ahlquist's classification. Castro de la Mata et al. (31) then showed the same phenomenon in the dog and also described a slight bronchoconstriction in response to epinephrine, norepinephrine, and postganglionic sympathetic nerve stimulation. This bronchoconstriction is blocked by tolazoline, an alpha adrenergic antagonist. There are no thorough studies of the receptors in tracheobronchial smooth muscle.

Indirect evidence based on the observation that propranolol increases airway resistance in some patients with bronchial asthma suggests that the beta receptors are innervated and that there is a certain degree of "normal" sympathetic bronchiolar dilatation. However, it is possible that propranolol might increase airway resistance by means other than bronchiolar beta adrenergic receptor blockade, such as reflexly or centrally induced parasympathetic bronchoconstriction or increased pulmonary vascular pressure because of cardiac depression.

The most potent of the common sympathomimetic amines as bronchodilators is isoproterenol (several less commonly used drugs are more potent). Norepinephrine appears to have little bronchodilating activity in animal or man. It should be pointed out that a similar statement has been made often for norepinephrine with regard to vasodilatation in skeletal muscle until the recent work of Viveros et al. (156) in which norepinephrine was shown to be a potent vasodilator when injected intra-arterially into the gracilis muscle of the dog. One must consider the possibility that bronchiolar beta receptors are innervated and that norepinephrine is a potent activator of these receptors, but so far these possibilities have not been adequately tested.

Several new drugs have selective agonist action on bronchiolar beta receptors, in contrast to their weak action on the heart; among these, salbutamol is the most widely studied (26). Its structure protects it from oxidation by monoamine oxidase, from O-methylation by catechol-O-methyltransferase, and from uptake by adrenergic neurons. Consequently it produces a long-lasting bronchodilatation that is blocked by propranolol. The discovery of salbutamol helps validate the classification of beta adrenergic receptors into two subtypes, beta$_1$ and beta$_2$.

SKELETAL MUSCLE

Oliver & Schäfer (128) first observed the augmented contractions of indirectly stimulated gastrocnemius muscle in the dog by injections of extracts of the adrenal gland. Not until many years later was it found that catecholamines have both direct and indirect effects on skeletal muscle and that the responses of slow-contracting muscles differ from those of fast-contracting muscles.

Three recent reviews have provided excellent evaluations of the effects of adrenergic stimuli on skeletal muscle and analyses of the types of adrenergic receptors (23, 24, 137). Consequently this section merely summarizes the conclusions of these authors. The reader is referred to the reviews for details and specific references (see also the chapter by Tomita in this volume of the *Handbook*).

Sympathomimetic amines produce direct but opposite effects on fast-contracting and slow-contracting mammalian muscles. However, the responses of both types of muscle are mediated by beta adrenergic receptors. Fast-contracting muscles respond to sympathomimetic amines by augmented twitch tension, increased total duration of contraction, and slightly slowed rate of rise of tension. The prolonged twitch results in increased fusion during tetanic contractions. Catecholamine treatment causes a greater increase in peak tension of incomplete tetanus than of single twitches. However, the tension of complete tetanus is not altered. These effects are independent of innervation and circulatory changes. Based on order of potency of catecholamines and on selective blockade, one can conclude that the adrenergic receptor is of the beta type.

Slow-contracting skeletal muscles respond to adrenergic stimuli in an opposite manner (i.e., decreased twitch tension, shortening of the duration of the contraction, decreased fusion of incomplete tetani, and diminished tension of incomplete tetani). Tension developed with full tetanus is not altered. The order of potency of agonists and selective blockade places the adrenergic receptor type as beta.

The effect on mammalian fast-contracting muscles is thought to result from prolongation of the active state and that in slow-contracting muscles from a shortening of the active state.

Both types of muscles show the same type of change in membrane activity, namely, increased demarcation potential resulting from hyperpolarization of the membrane. The analysis of receptor types shows these membrane responses to be mediated via beta receptors.

Other types of muscles show different types of responses. The extraocular muscles of the cat can be induced to contract by addition of catecholamines or stimulation of the superior cervical ganglion. The response of this muscle is mediated via alpha adrenergic receptors. Amphibian and avian muscles do not respond to catecholamines with changes in tension. However, both show increased demarcation potentials mediated by beta adrenergic receptors. Chronically denervated mammalian skeletal muscle responds to adrenergic stimuli via beta receptors with increased fibrillatory frequency, increased tone, and increased demarcation potential.

Both slow- and fast-contracting mammalian skeletal muscle and muscle of amphibians and birds are also affected by adrenergic stimuli indirectly. Catecholamines exert an initial facilitatory effect on neuromuscular transmission, presumably by enhancing liberation of acetylcholine from prejunctional nerve terminals. The effect is mediated through alpha adrenergic receptors. In addition, there is a slight, later postjunctional inhibitory action on the muscle, probably hyperpolarization of the membrane, via a beta adrenergic receptor.

Human skeletal muscle is not so clearly separated into fast and slow types, but rather each muscle is made up of varying amounts of slow and fast components. However, the direct effects of the catecholamines on human muscle contraction are related to beta receptors. Neuromuscular transmission is augmented by an alpha receptor-mediated effect of catecholamines. The tremors and the weakness felt in back muscles during infusions of epinephrine and by patients with pheochromocytomas may be related to the decreased fusion of the slower components in postural muscles with incomplete tetanus.

The antifatigue action of adrenergic stimuli in mammalian fast-contracting muscles is primarily the alpha receptor-mediated prejunctional effect. Postjunctional beta receptor-mediated effects play a small role in fatigued fast muscle of mammals but none in fatigued slow muscle or amphibian muscle. In the latter two types only the prejunctional effects are important in defatiguing action.

It is probable that only the direct action on slow-contracting muscles has physiological significance, inasmuch as the effective doses of epinephrine for the fast-contracting muscles are higher than can occur after adrenal medullary secretion (see the chapter by Tomita in this volume of the *Handbook*).

CENTRAL NERVOUS SYSTEM

Although there is little question that adrenergic neurons exist in mammalian brain, the characteristics of central adrenergic receptors are vague. The complexity of the central nervous system, the problems of limiting delivery of drugs to restricted areas of the brain, the difficulty in separating central from peripheral actions when drugs are administered systemically, and the lack of certainty about adrenergic systems as such in the central nervous system all contribute to the sparse literature on central adrenergic receptors. Finally, where attempts at classification of central adrenergic receptors have been made, rigorous adherence to criteria for classification has been lacking.

The most interesting and well-defined work on adrenergic receptors in the central nervous system is that on "consummatory behavior." From the work of two different groups (63, 92, 93) has emerged the concept that the hypothalamus of rats has systems involved in the regulation of water and food intake. A beta adrenergic thirst system in the lateral hypothalamus is opposed by an alpha adrenergic water-satiety system in the ventromedial hypothalamus. A beta adrenergic food-satiety system in the lateral hypothalamus is opposed by an alpha adrenergic hunger center in the ventromedial hypothalamus. The evidence for this concept is reasonable, although not rigorous. The strong evidence is that derived from injections of adrenergic agonists and antagonists directly into the hypothalamus. However, there has been no attempt to classify these receptors on the basis of orders of potency of agonists, and the data on selective blockade are erratic. The physiological role of these adrenergic systems and their relations with other systems are not clear. For example, if the adrenergic component of the hunger control system alone were of physiological importance, treatment of an animal with a beta adrenergic blocking drug should increase hunger and lead to increased weight. Even though no published evidence suggests such an effect, it seems likely that significant weight gain would have been observed in animals and human beings with chronic administration of propranolol. Either these adrenergic systems play little role, or the experimental alterations of water and food intake by adrenergic blocking drugs is spurious, or other systems, such as cholinergic and others, dominate.

Marley & Stephenson (102) have tentatively concluded that the behavioral effects of catecholamines infused into the brains of young chickens are due to stimulation of alpha adrenergic receptors. When norepinephrine, isoproterenol, and α-methylnorepinephrine were infused into the hypothalamic regions of chicks, behavioral sleep accompanied by hypothermia, hypotension, and lowered oxygen consumption was produced. Electrocortical sleep activity was observed but was not closely correlated with behavioral sleep. The sleep activity was antagonized by prior treatment of the animals with phenoxybenzamine but not with propranolol. The hypothermic effects were attributed to beta receptor mediation or to a receptor with both alpha and beta characteristics since both phenoxybenzamine and phentolamine blocked this action. The authors (102) discuss the possibility that the blockade might be nonselective.

MISCELLANEOUS SYSTEMS

Melanophore Responses

Melanin granules in the melanophores of vertebrates can be controlled by hormonal and pharmacological substances. Dispersion of the granules into the dendritic processes of melanophores in amphibians and reptiles causes darkening of the skin. Aggregation of the granules causes lightening. Catecholamines cause both types of responses, the darkening response being due to stimulation of beta adrenergic receptors and the lightening response resulting from alpha adrenergic receptor activation. Differentiation of these receptor types has been accomplished by evaluation of orders of potency of adrenergic agonists and by selective blockade (64, 65). Furthermore adrenergically induced melanin granule dispersion is mediated separately from that caused by melanophore-stimulating hormone (66). Whereas all amphibians and reptiles appear to have beta receptors, some seem to lack alpha receptors in the melanophores (65). Goldman and Hadley have found indirect evidence suggesting that cyclic AMP is involved as a second messenger in the darkening response to adrenergic stimuli in toad (65) and lizard (66) skin.

Skin Gland Secretions

Benson & Hadley (14) have evaluated the secretion from the granular (serous or poison) glands of *Rana pipiens* and *Xenopus laevis*. By using the criteria of order of potency of four catecholamines and selective blockade, they concluded that adrenergically activated secretion of these glands is entirely mediated through alpha receptors. It is believed that the secretion is induced by the contraction of smooth muscles around the glands. Watlington (159) has suggested that the secretion of the mucous glands of anurans may be regulated by beta adrenergic receptors.

Other Effects

The rate of flow of juice from an isolated pancreas of the rabbit was found to be influenced by adrenergic agents in a pattern suggesting alpha receptor mediation (76). Norepinephrine and isoproterenol reduced flow rate, norepinephrine being 100 times more potent than isoproterenol, and the effect of the two catecholamines was blocked by phenoxybenzamine and not by propranolol. Hubel (76) critically examined the possibilities of the site of action and concluded that the alpha receptors are part of secretory cells and that adrenergic effects on the pancreatic duct and blood vessels could not account for this effect in vitro.

Norepinephrine antagonizes the effect of antidiuretic hormone on urine flow in rats, an effect completely blocked by phenoxybenzamine but not by propranolol (97). This alpha receptor-mediated action of norepinephrine appears to be independent of vascular effects of the amine.

Catecholamines and sympathetic nerve stimulation are known to inhibit oxytoxin-stimulated milk ejection from mammary glands. Chan (32) studied the inhibitory effect of a series of sympathomimetic amines in rabbits and found the order of potency to be isoproterenol > epinephrine > norepinephrine. Administration of either phenoxybenzamine alone or phenoxybenzamine plus pronethalol failed to antagonize the inhibitory action of these amines. Chan concluded that the amines inhibit oxytocin-induced milk ejection by acting directly on mammary tissue independently of their effects on blood flow to the mammary glands. They also concluded that the effect of epinephrine is not mediated by either alpha or beta receptors. However, the order of potency of the amines suggests a beta function. Adrenergic blockade was probably not adequately evaluated. It seems unreasonable to categorically conclude that beta receptors are not involved.

Catecholamines have a unique effect on salivary glands in stimulating the flow of saliva and the secretion of amylase and potassium. The amylase secretion is attributed to a beta receptor-mediated effect on the basis of selective blockade by beta adrenergic blocking drugs (9, 81), whereas the potassium secretion is related to an alpha-mediated effect (9). Isoproterenol also causes increased salivary gland weight and augmented synthesis of DNA in salivary glands. Since the effect is inhibited by propranolol, it is probably mediated by a beta receptor (142).

Potassium flux in most systems is considered an alpha

receptor-mediated response to adrenergic stimuli. The alpha-mediated fluxes are related to altered membrane permeability and appear not to be associated with the other metabolic actions of adrenergic stimuli. In contrast, the potassium efflux from the liver is a beta receptor-mediated function but is slower in time course. The relation of catecholamine action on movements of other ions to the type of adrenergic receptors involved is not clear. Daniel et al. (37) have reviewed the relation of ionic fluxes to adrenergic receptors.

Adrenergic stimulation increases synthesis of melatonin in pineal glands (167). Weiss & Costa (161) have shown that pineal gland adenylate cyclase is increased only by catecholamine sympathomimetic amines and not by other hormones. Furthermore the effect is selectively blocked by beta adrenergic blocking drugs. Since dibutyryl cyclic AMP can increase the synthesis of melatonin in pineal glands (148), the augmented synthesis induced by adrenergic stimuli might be mediated via cyclic AMP.

ROLE OF ADRENERGIC RECEPTORS IN SYMPATHOADRENAL RESPONSES

The adrenergic receptors are the first step in the mediation of cellular responses to catecholamines, whether the latter are released from sympathetic nerve terminals or the adrenal medulla or are of exogenous origin. The sympathoadrenal system is both a nervous system and an endocrine system, in contrast to the parasympathetic system, which is strictly a nervous system. Therefore one must consider the effects of blood-borne mediators, as well as the effects of mediators released from nerves, in assessing the adrenergic responses of an organism to exercise and to emotional states, such as anxiety, fear, and anger.

Epinephrine is a potent activator of both alpha and beta$_1$ and beta$_2$ adrenergic receptor-effector systems. In contrast, norepinephrine is a more selective activator of alpha and beta$_1$ receptors than it is of beta$_2$ receptors. Epinephrine is at least as potent as norepinephrine on alpha and beta$_1$ receptors and considerably more potent than norepinephrine on beta$_2$ receptors. In most adult mammals, epinephrine is the major hormone of the adrenal medulla; that is, it comprises more than 75% of the adrenal catecholamine content in species such as rabbit, guinea pig, cow, and man (51). Furthermore the adrenal gland output in response to stress in animals, such as the adult dog, is nearly entirely epinephrine (101a). Thus in most adult mammals, epinephrine is the major adrenal medullary hormone and is also more able to elicit a generalized response than is norepinephrine; that is, it is capable of effective activation of all adrenergic receptors that are accessible from the bloodstream. Norepinephrine, on the other hand, in most mammals seems to be less a hormone than a neurohumoral mediator with influence restricted to alpha and beta$_1$ receptors.

From a functional standpoint, it is not clear why, in many animal species in which epinephrine is the major adrenal catecholamine in adults, norepinephrine is the primary adrenal medullary hormone in neonatal and young animals. Nor is it clear why, functionally, adult mammals, such as cats, have a high proportion of adrenal catecholamines as norepinephrine (51). Goodall (66a) classified animals on the basis of the epinephrine content in their adrenal glands, which suggested that aggressive animals (i.e., the hunters), such as the cat, have a relatively high proportion of norepinephrine in the adrenals (approximately 50%), whereas nonaggressive animals (i.e., the hunted), such as the rabbit, zebra, and baboon, have very high epinephrine contents (the baboon, for example, having 100% epinephrine). Von Euler (51) has commented that the high proportion of norepinephrine in feline animals "may be associated with their peculiar kinds of activity which is typically one of sudden attacks. Under such circumstances a quick release of a vasoconstrictor may be desirable from the point of view of blood pressure homeostasis." It is difficult to see how release of norepinephrine into the bloodstream would cause a prompter vasoconstriction than would neurally released norepinephrine. The speed of nerve conduction is so rapid that the vasoconstrictor influence of sympathetic nerve activation to the blood vessels would be faster than the influence of catecholamines released from the adrenal into the bloodstream by the period of at least one circulation time. Furthermore, according to the tabulation published by von Euler (51), the whale has the highest content of adrenal medullary norepinephrine of any mammalian species listed. The whale is not considered to be an aggressive animal that attacks suddenly.

It is reasonable to conclude that the relative content of catecholamines in the adrenal medulla has no well-defined relation to the mode of life of the animal; that is, aggressivity versus passivity or sedentary versus active behavior. However, it is also obvious that we have little knowledge on which to base a definition of such relationships. More information is needed about the patterns of distribution of adrenergic receptor types in many species of animals and the relative output of norepinephrine and epinephrine from the adrenal glands in response to various types of stress.

During exercise the sympathoadrenal system is mobilized, and the responses are mediated by alpha and beta receptors, as shown in Figure 3. Some of these responses, such as vasoconstriction and cardiac augmentation, are clearly mediated by neurally released norepinephrine, as well as by circulating catecholamines. The direct relation of other adrenergic responses to neurally released norepinephrine is not as clear. It is possible that blood-borne catecholamines are more important in activating receptors for certain metabolic effects, such as hepatic glycogenolysis, than is neurally released norepinephrine. However, lipolytic responses in dogs are clearly induced by neurally released norepinephrine (6, 54). In all neurally induced activation of

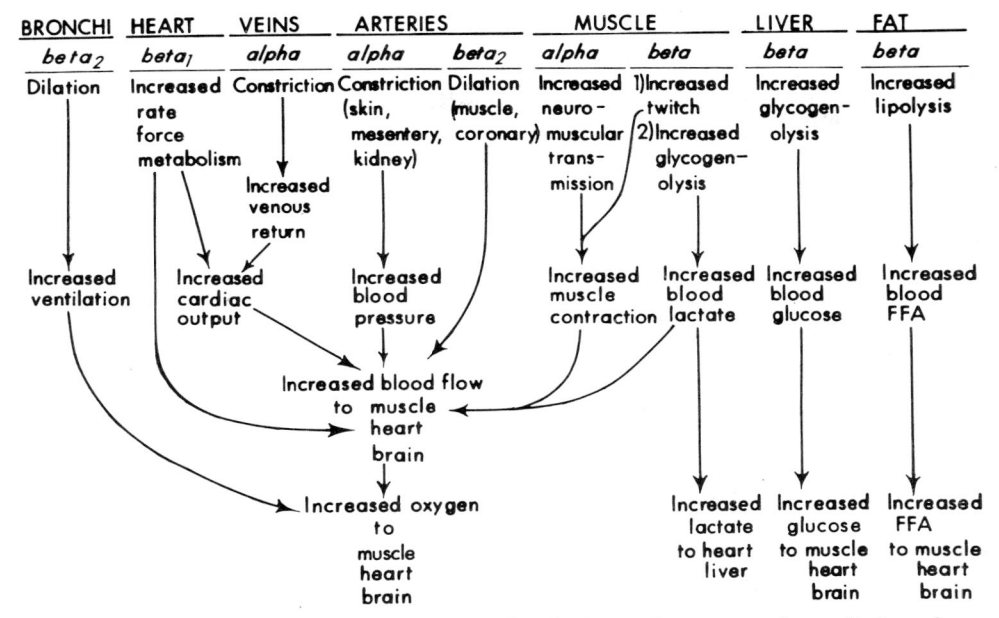

BRONCHI	HEART	VEINS	ARTERIES		MUSCLE		LIVER	FAT
beta$_2$	beta$_1$	alpha	alpha	beta$_2$	alpha	beta	beta	beta
Dilation	Increased rate force metabolism	Constriction	Constriction (skin, mesentery, kidney)	Dilation (muscle, coronary)	Increased neuromuscular transmission	1) Increased twitch 2) Increased glycogenolysis	Increased glycogenolysis	Increased lipolysis

FIG. 3. Role of adrenergic receptors in mediation of sympathoadrenal responses to exercise. Beta adrenergic receptors are subdivided into beta$_1$ and beta$_2$ types only where evidence is definitive. Otherwise, the general classification of beta is used. Some responses, such as vasoconstriction and cardiac augmentation, are mediated by neuronally released norepinephrine, as well as by blood-borne catecholamines. In other responses the role of neuronally released norepinephrine is not certain. *FFA*, free fatty acids.

adrenergic receptors, secondary activation can also occur in response to blood-borne catecholamines.

The importance of the adrenal medulla as a part of the sympathoadrenal system is seen in the experiments of Donald et al. (40) on trained racing greyhounds. They found that complete denervation of the heart by autotransplantation did not adversely affect the ability of the dogs to run a measured course and to respond with augmented heart rate. The tachycardia in dogs with denervated hearts was slow in onset after the beginning of the run, and the recovery of heart rate to normal was slower than in normal dogs. In the absence of cardiac nerves, cardio-acceleration in response to exercise was clearly caused by catecholamines released from the adrenal medulla. Administration of propranolol to normal dogs did not seriously impair running performance and only slightly reduced the exercise tachycardia. However, in dogs with denervated hearts treated with propranolol, there was no exercise tachycardia, and the dogs collapsed at the end of the run. Thus the neural response of the heart to exercise is fast and is a sum of augmented sympathetic nerve activity and withdrawal of vagus nerve activity, the net effect being higher concentrations of norepinephrine at the sinoatrial node cell beta receptors and lower concentrations of acetylcholine at the cholinergic receptors with resultant tachycardia. The cardiac response to adrenal medullary catecholamines is slower in onset and offset than to neurally released norepinephrine. However, the adrenal catecholamines will sustain the cardiac part of the physical performance. The absence of both neural and hormonal adrenergic responses is detrimental to sustained physical exercise.

CONCLUSIONS

Adrenergic receptors are divided into two main classes, alpha and beta. Alpha receptors are most likely located on cell surfaces in order to mediate rapid excitatory responses, such as smooth muscle contraction, and rapid inhibitory responses, such as hyperpolarization of neuronal membranes and inhibition of glandular secretion. Alpha receptor-mediated responses have been postulated to be a result of decreased cellular cyclic AMP. The evidence for this postulate is, however, not strong enough to warrant acceptance at this time.

Beta adrenergic receptors can be subdivided into beta$_1$ and beta$_2$ types, but the subclassification is not yet rigorously established for all types of beta adrenergic responses. Beta$_1$ adrenergic receptors mediate cardiac responses, and beta$_2$ receptors appear to mediate smooth muscle relaxation. It is not certain whether beta adrenergically mediated metabolic responses are beta$_1$ or beta$_2$. In most cells, increased beta adrenergic activity is associated with augmented activity of adenylate cyclase and increased production of cyclic AMP. Glycogenolytic and lipolytic responses to adrenergic stimuli are clearly mediated by cyclic AMP. However, it is not established whether other responses, such as increased heart rate and force, are mediated by the cyclic nucleotide.

Sutherland and his colleagues have proposed an

attractive unitary hypothesis; they suggest that responses of cells to adrenergic stimuli are mediated by increases and decreases in intracellular cyclic AMP, beta receptors increasing cyclic AMP and alpha receptors diminishing cyclic AMP. The adrenergic receptors have not been identified as part of the adenylate cyclase system, although the beta adrenergic receptor would appear to be closely coupled to it. If alpha receptors play a part in modulating intracellular cyclic AMP, it is probable that they also are closely coupled to the enzyme system.

ADDENDUM

Two important books have been published in 1972 and 1973. *Catecholamines* (1A), a detailed and comprehensive addition to the literature, deals with the entire scope of catecholamines from their synthesis to their effects. Furchgott's chapter (4A) on the classification of adrenergic receptors lays particular stress on receptor theory as derived from kinetic analyses of drug interactions. However, his conclusions regarding classification of adrenergic receptors are similar to those presented in the present chapter. Trendelenburg (9A), in a chapter on classification of sympathomimetic amines, provides interesting information on adrenergic receptors from the standpoint of structure-activity relationships of agonists. *Frontiers in Catecholamine Research* (10A) provides a comprehensive view of many aspects of current research in catecholamines, but the treatment of adrenergic receptors is less systematic and analytical than that in *Catecholamines*.

The initial optimism about isolation of beta adrenergic receptors has been dispelled by several papers. Molinoff (7A) has presented a thorough and critical assessment of the criteria required to validate a catecholamine binding material as a receptor. Lefkowitz (6A) in a reappraisal of his work has presented a more circumspect analysis of the attempts at isolation of the putative beta adrenergic receptor [cf. (91, 91a, 91b)]. Most importantly, Cuatracasas and colleagues (2A) have published a careful study of binding of ^{3}H-norepinephrine to subcellular particles and to intact cells and conclude that the fraction of dog heart Lefkowitz isolated as the beta adrenergic receptor is probably a specific catechol binding material and not specific for catecholamines. They could find no evidence of stereospecific binding of norepinephrine. Certain compounds that have the catechol moiety but no nitrogen (inactive as sympathomimetic drugs) inhibited ^{3}H-norepinephrine binding, and other compounds that lack a catechol moiety but are active sympathomimetic drugs failed to inhibit binding of tritiated norepinephrine. Cuatracasas and co-workers concluded that the previously reported binding of ^{3}H-norepinephrine to subcellular fractions is probably related to a process totally separate from binding to the true receptors, but shares with the receptors only the recognition of the catechol moiety. They suggest that true receptors are probably sparse and that detection of the receptors will require radioactively labeled catecholamines of much higher specific activity than are presently available.

Several groups of investigators have adduced evidence to support the hypothesis that alpha adrenergic receptors on adrenergic nerve terminals are involved in the modulation of the release of norepinephrine (3A, 5A, 8A). Alpha adrenergic agonists inhibit the release of norepinephrine from adrenergic neurons, and alpha adrenergic blocking agents enhance transmitter release. Beta adrenergic agonists and antagonists appear to have no significant effect on transmitter release. Thus, regardless of the type of receptor on effector cells innervated by adrenergic nerves, the release of norepinephrine from adrenergic nerve endings might be modulated by a feedback mechanism via prejunctional alpha adrenergic receptors in a variety of tissues, including heart, spleen, nictitating membrane, and brain. [See REFERENCES, p. 472.]

REFERENCES

1. ABBOUD, F. M., J. W. ECKSTEIN, AND B. G. ZIMMERMAN. Venous and arterial responses to stimulation of beta adrenergic receptors. *Am. J. Physiol.* 209: 383-389, 1965.
2. ADAM, K. R., S. BOYLESS, AND P. C. SCHOLFIELD. Cardio-selective β-adrenoceptor blockade and the coronary circulation. *Brit. J. Pharmacol.* 40: 534-536, 1970.
3. AHLQUIST, R. P. A study of the adrenotropic receptors. *Am. J. Physiol.* 153: 586-600, 1948.
4. AHLQUIST, R. P., AND B. LEVY. Adrenergic receptive mechanism of canine ileum. *J. Pharmacol. Exptl. Therap.* 127: 146-149, 1959.
5. BAILEY, D. M. Some effects of sympathomimetic amines on isolated smooth muscle preparation from the stomach of the guinea pig. *Brit. J. Pharmacol.* 34: 204P, 1968.
6. BALLARD, K., AND S. ROSELL. Adrenergic neurohumoral influences on circulation and lipolysis in canine omental adipose tissue. *Circulation Res.* 28: 389-396, 1971.
7. BARGER, G., AND H. H. DALE. Chemical structure and sympathomimetic actions of amines. *J. Physiol., London* 41: 19-59, 1910.
8. BARTLET, A. L., AND T. HASSAN. Adrenoceptors of the chick rectum. *Brit. J. Pharmacol.* 39: 817-821, 1970.
9. BATZRI, S., Z. SELINGER, AND M. SCHRAMM. Potassium ion release and enzyme secretion: adrenergic regulation by α- and β-receptors. *Science* 174: 1029-1031, 1971.
10. BECKER, L. C., N. J. FORTUIN, AND B. PITT. Effect of ischemia and antianginal drugs on the distribution of radioactive microspheres in the canine left ventricle. *Circulation Res.* 28: 263-269, 1971.
11. BELLEAU, B. Stereochemistry of adrenergic receptors: newer concepts on the molecular mechanism of action of catecholamines and antiadrenergic drugs at the receptor level. *Ann. NY Acad. Sci.* 139: 580-605, 1967.
12. BENFEY, B. G., AND D. R. VARMA. Interactions of sympathomimetic drugs, propranolol and phentolamine on atrial refractory period and contractility. *Brit. J. Pharmacol.* 30: 603-611, 1967.
13. BENNET, D. R., D. A. REINKE, E. ALPER, T. BAUM, AND H. VASQUEZ-LEON. The action of intraocularly administered adrenergic drugs on the iris. *J. Pharmacol. Exptl. Therap.* 134: 190-198, 1961.
14. BENSON, B. J., AND M. E. HADLEY. In vitro characterization of adrenergic receptors controlling skin gland secretion in two anurans *Rana pipiens* and *Xenopus laevis*. *Comp. Biochem. Physiol.* 30: 856-864, 1969.
15. BERKOWITZ, W. D., A. L. WIT, S. H. LAU, C. STEINER, AND A. N. DAMATO. The effects of propranolol on cardiac conduction. *Circulation* 40: 855-862, 1969.
16. BERNE, R. M., H. DEGEEST, AND M. N. LEVY. Influence of the cardiac nerves on coronary resistance. *Am. J. Physiol.* 208: 763-769, 1965.
17. BICKERTON, R. K. The response of isolated strips of cat spleen to sympathomimetic drugs and their antagonists. *J. Pharmacol. Exptl. Therap.* 142: 99-110, 1963.
18. BLACK, J. W., A. F. CROWTHER, R. G. SHANKS, L. H. SMITH, AND A. C. DORNHORST. New adrenergic beta-receptor antagonist. *Lancet* 1: 1080-1081, 1964.
19. BLACK, J. W., AND J. S. STEPHENSON. Pharmacology of a new adrenergic beta-receptor blocking compound (nethalide). *Lancet* 2: 311-314, 1962.
20. BLINKS, J. R. Evaluation of the cardiac effects of several β-adrenergic blocking agents. *Ann. NY Acad. Sci.* 139: 673-685, 1967.
21. BLOOM, B. M., AND I. M. GOLDMAN. The nature of catecholamine-adenine mononucleotide interactions in adrenergic mechanisms. *Advan. Drug Res.* 3: 121-169, 1966.

22. BOWMAN, W. C., AND M. T. HALL. Inhibition of rabbit intestine by α- and β-adrenoceptors. *Brit. J. Pharmacol.* 38: 399-415, 1970.
23. BOWMAN, W. C., AND M. W. NOTT. Actions of sympathomimetic amines and their antagonists on skeletal muscle. *Pharmacol. Rev.* 21: 27-72, 1969.
24. BOWMAN, W. C., AND C. RAPER. Adrenotropic receptors in skeletal muscle. *Ann. NY Acad. Sci.* 139: 741-753, 1967.
25. BRISTOW, M., AND R. D. GREEN. A quantitative study of beta-adrenergic receptors in rabbit atria. *European J. Pharmacol.* 12: 120-123, 1970.
26. BRITTAIN, R. T. A comparison of the pharmacology of salbutamol with that of isoprenaline, orciprenaline and trimetoquinol. *Postgrad. Med. J. Suppl.* 47: 11-16, 1971.
27. BROADLEY, K. J. An analysis of the coronary vascular responses to catecholamines, using a modified Langendorff heart preparation. *Brit. J. Pharmacol.* 40: 617-629, 1970.
28. BUEDING, E., R. W. BUTCHER, J. HAWKINS, A. R. TIMMS, AND E. W. SUTHERLAND. Effects of epinephrine on adenosine 3',5'-monophosphate and hexose phosphates in intestinal smooth muscle. *Biochem. Biophys. Acta* 115: 173-178, 1966.
29. BÜLBRING, E. Biophysical changes produced by adrenaline and noradrenaline. In: *Ciba Foundation Symposium on Adrenergic Mechanisms*, edited by J. R. Vane, G. E. W. Wolstenholme, and M. O'Connor. Boston: Little, Brown, 1960, p. 275-287.
30. CANNON, W. B., AND A. ROSENBLUETH. *Autonomic Neuroeffector Systems.* New York: Macmillan, 1937.
31. CASTRO DE LA MATA, R., M. PENNA, AND D. M. AVIADO. Reversal of sympathomimetic bronchodilatation by dichloroisoproterenol. *J. Pharmacol. Exptl. Therap.* 135: 197-203, 1962.
32. CHAN, W. Y. Mechanism of epinephrine inhibition of the milk ejecting response to oxytocin. *J. Pharmacol. Exptl. Therap.* 147: 48-53, 1965.
33. CLARK, A. J. *General Pharmacology. Heffters Handbuch der Experimentellen Pharmakologie.* Berlin: Springer, 1937, vol. 4, p. 216.
34. COUPAR, J. M. The effect of isoprenaline on adrenoceptors in human saphenous vein. *Brit. J. Pharmacol.* 39: 465-475, 1970.
35. DALE, H. H. On some physiological actions of ergot. *J. Physiol., London* 34: 163-206, 1906.
36. DAMATO, A. N., S. H. LAU, R. H. HELFANT, E. STEIN, W. D. BERKOWITZ, AND S. I. COHEN. Study of atrioventricular conduction in man using electrode catheter recordings of His bundle activity. *Circulation* 39: 287-296, 1969.
37. DANIEL, E. E., D. M. PATON, G. S. TAYLOR, AND B. J. HODGSON. Adrenergic receptors for catecholamine effects on tissue electrolytes. *Federation Proc.* 29: 1410-1425, 1970.
38. DAVIS, L. D., AND J. V. TEMTE. Effects of propranolol on the transmembrane potentials of ventricular muscle and Purkinje fibers of the dog. *Circulation Res.* 22: 661-677, 1968.
39. DAVIS, W. G. The effects of beta adrenoceptor blocking agents on the membrane potential and spike generation in the smooth muscle of the guinea-pig taenia coli. *Brit. J. Pharmacol.* 38: 12-19, 1970.
40. DONALD, D. E., D. A. FERGUSON, AND S. E. MILBURN. Effect of beta-adrenergic receptor blockade on racing performance of greyhounds with normal and with denervated hearts. *Circulation Res.* 22: 127-134, 1968.
41. DRESEL, P. E. Blockade of some cardiac actions of adrenaline by dichloroisoproterenol. *Can. J. Biochem. Physiol.* 38: 375-381, 1960.
42. DRESEL, P. E., K. L. MACCANNELL, AND M. NICKERSON. Cardiac arrhythmias induced by minimal doses of epinephrine in cyclopropane-anesthetized dogs. *Circulation Res.* 8: 948-955, 1960.
43. DUNLOP, D., AND R. G. SHANKS. Selective blockade of adrenoceptive beta receptors in the heart. *Brit. J. Pharmacol.* 32: 201-218, 1968.
44. ECKSTEIN, J. W., AND W. K. HAMILTON. Effects of isoproterenol on peripheral venous tone and transmural right atrial pressure in man. *J. Clin. Invest.* 38: 342-346, 1959.
45. ELLIOTT, T. R. On the action of adrenaline. *J. Physiol., London* 31: 20-22, 1904.
46. ELLIOTT, T. R. Action of adrenaline. *J. Physiol., London* 32: 401-467, 1905.
47. ELLIS, S. The effects of sympathomimetic amines and adrenergic blocking agents on metabolism. In: *Physiological Pharmacology*, edited by W. S. Root and I. G. Hoffman. New York: Acad. Press, 1967, vol. 4, p. 179-241.
48. ELLIS, S. Symposium on adrenergic receptors mediating metabolic responses. *Federation Proc.* 29: 1350-1428, 1969.
49. ELLIS, S., B. L. KENNEDY, A. J. EUSEBI, AND N. H. VINCENT. Autonomic control of metabolism. *Ann. NY Acad. Sci.* 139: 826-832, 1967.
50. EPSTEIN, S. E., G. S. LEVEY, AND C. L. SKELTON. Adenyl cyclase and cyclic AMP. Biochemical links in the regulation of myocardial contractility. *Circulation* 43: 437-450, 1971.
51. EULER, U. S. VON. *Noradrenaline: Chemistry, Physiology, Pharmacology and Clinical Aspects.* Springfield, Ill.: Thomas, 1956.
52. EULER, U. S. VON. Adrenergic neurotransmitter functions. *Science* 173: 202-206, 1971.
53. FEIGL, E. O. Sympathetic control of coronary circulation. *Circulation Res.* 20: 262-271, 1967.
54. FEIGL, E. O. Carotid sinus reflex control of coronary blood flow. *Circulation Res.* 23: 223-237, 1968.
55. FREDHOLM, B., AND S. ROSELL. Effects of adrenergic blocking agents on lipid mobilization from canine subcutaneous adipose tissue after sympathetic nerve stimulation. *J. Pharmacol. Exptl. Therap.* 159: 1-7, 1968.
56. FURCHGOTT, R. F. The receptors for epinephrine and norepinephrine (adrenergic receptors). *Pharmacol. Rev.* 11: 429-441, 1960.
57. FURCHGOTT, R. F. Receptors for sympathomimetic amines. In: *Ciba Foundation Symposium on Adrenergic Mechanisms*, edited by J. R. Vane, G. E. W. Wolstenholme, and M. O'Connor. Boston: Little, Brown, 1960, p. 246-252.
58. FURCHGOTT, R. F. The pharmacological differentiation of adrenergic receptors. *Ann. NY Acad. Sci.* 139: 553-570, 1967.
59. GAGNON, D. J., AND S. BELISLE. Stimulatory effects of catecholamines on the isolated rat colon after beta-adrenergic blockade with oxprenolol and propranolol. *European J. Pharmacol.* 12: 303-309, 1970.
60. GILBERT, J. L., G. LANGE, AND C. McC. BROOKS. Influence of sympathomimetic pressor drugs on arrhythmias caused by multiple stimuli. *Circulation Res.* 7: 417-423, 1959.
61. GIOTTI, A., F. LEDDA, AND P. F. MANNAIONI. Electrophysiological effects of alpha- and beta-receptor agonists and antagonists on Purkinje fibres of sheep heart. *Brit. J. Pharmacol.* 695-696P, 1968.
62. GOLDBERG, L. I. Cardiovascular and renal actions of dopamine: potential clinical applications. *Pharmacol. Rev.* 24: 1-29, 1972.
63. GOLDMAN, H. W., D. LEHR, AND E. FRIEDMAN. Antagonistic effects of alpha and beta-adrenergically coded hypothalamic neurones on consummatory behavior in the rat. *Nature* 231: 453-455, 1971.
64. GOLDMAN, J. M., AND M. E. HADLEY. *In vitro* demonstration of adrenergic receptors controlling melanophore responses of the lizard, *Anolis carolinensis*. *J. Pharmacol. Exptl. Therap.* 166: 1-7, 1969.
65. GOLDMAN, J. M., AND M. E. HADLEY. The *beta* adrenergic receptor and cyclic 3',5'-adenosine monophosphate: possible roles in the regulation of melanophore responses of the spadefoot toad, *Scaphiopus couchi*. *Gen. Comp. Endocrinol.* 13: 151-163, 1969.
66. GOLDMAN, J. M., AND M. E. HADLEY. Evidence for separate receptors for melanophore stimulating hormone and cate-

cholamine regulation of cyclic AMP in the control of melanophore responses. *Brit. J. Pharmacol.* 39: 160–166, 1970.
66a. GOODALL, McC. Studies of adrenaline and noradrenaline in mammalian heart and suprarenals. *Acta Physiol. Scand. Suppl.* 24: 85, 1951.
67. GOVIER, W. C. Myocardial *alpha* receptors and their role in the production of a positive inotropic effect by sympathomimetic agents. *J. Pharmacol. Exptl. Therap.* 159: 82–90, 1968.
68. GOVIER, W. C., N. C. MUSAL, P. WHITTINGTON, AND A. BROOM. Myocardial *alpha* and *beta* adrenergic receptors as demonstrated by atrial functional refractory-period changes. *J. Pharmacol. Exptl. Therap.* 154: 255–263, 1966.
69. GRANATA, L., R. A. OLSSON, A. HUVOS, AND D. E. GREGG. Coronary inflow and oxygen usage following cardiac sympathetic nerve stimulation in unanesthetized dogs. *Circulation Res.* 16: 114–120, 1965.
70. GUIMARAES, S. Alpha excitatory, alpha inhibitory and beta inhibitory adrenergic receptors in the guinea pig stomach. *Arch. Intern. Pharmacodyn.* 170: 188–201, 1969.
71. HAGEN, J. H., AND J. P. HAGEN. Action of adrenalin and noradrenalin on metabolic systems. In: *Actions of Hormones on Molecular Processes*, edited by G. Litwack and D. Kitchevsky. New York: Wiley, 1964, p. 268–319.
72. HESS, M. E., AND N. HAUGAARD. The effect of epinephrine and aminophylline on the phosphorylase activity of perfused contracting heart muscle. *J. Pharmacol. Exptl. Therap.* 122: 169–175, 1958.
73. HIMMS-HAGEN, J. Sympathetic regulation of metabolism. *Pharmacol. Rev.* 19: 367–461, 1967.
74. HOFFMAN, B. F., AND P. F. BRANEFIELD. *Electrophysiology of the Heart.* New York: McGraw-Hill, 1960, p. 207.
75. HORNBROOK, K. R. Adrenergic receptors for metabolic responses in the liver. *Federation Proc.* 29: 1381–1385, 1970.
76. HUBEL, K. A. Response of rabbit pancreas in vitro to adrenergic agonists and antagonists. *Am. J. Physiol.* 219: 1590–1594, 1970.
77. IGNARRO, L. J., AND E. TITUS. The presence of antagonistically acting *alpha* and *beta* adrenergic receptors in the mouse spleen. *J. Pharmacol. Exptl. Therap.* 160: 72–80, 1968.
78. INGRAM, R. H., J. P. SZIDON, R. SKALAK, AND A. P. FISHMAN. Effects of sympathetic nerve stimulation on the pulmonary arterial tree of the isolated lobe perfused in situ. *Circulation Res.* 22: 801–815, 1968.
79. KABELLA, E., AND R. MENDEZ. Action of propranolol on the atrioventricular node and on its response to adrenaline and isoprenaline. *Brit. J. Pharmacol.* 26: 473–481, 1966.
80. KAISER, G. A., J. ROSS, JR., AND E. BRAUNWALD. Alpha and beta adrenergic receptor mechanisms in the systemic venous bed. *J. Pharmacol. Exptl. Therap.* 144: 156–162, 1964.
81. KATZ, R. L., AND I. D. MANDEL. Action and interaction of alpha and beta adrenergic blockers on parotid and submaxillary secretions in man. *Proc. Soc. Exptl. Biol. Med.* 128: 1140–1145, 1968.
82. KJEKHUS, J. K., P. D. HENRY, AND B. E. SOBEL. Activation of phosphorylase by cyclic AMP without augmentation of contractility in the perfused guinea pig heart. *Circulation Res.* 29: 468–478, 1971.
83. KLOCKE, F. J., G. A. KAISER, J. ROSS, JR., AND E. BRAUNWALD. An intrinsic adrenergic vasodilator mechanism in the coronary vascular bed of the dog. *Circulation Res.* 16: 376–382, 1965.
84. KOSTERLITZ, H. W., R. J. LYDON, AND A. J. WATT. The effects of adrenaline, noradrenaline and isoprenaline on inhibitory α- and β-adrenoceptors in the longitudinal muscle of the guinea-pig ileum. *Brit. J. Pharmacol.* 30: 398–413, 1970.
85. KRELL, R. D., AND P. N. PATIL. Combinations of *alpha* and *beta* adrenergic blockers in isolated guinea pig atria. *J. Pharmacol. Exptl. Therap.* 170: 263–271, 1969.

86. LANDS, A. M. Sympathetic receptor action. *Am. J. Physiol.* 169: 11–21, 1952.
87. LANDS, A. M., A. ARNOLD, J. P. MCAULIFF, F. P. LUDUENA, AND R. G. BROWN, JR. Differentiation of receptor systems activated by sympathomimetic amines. *Nature* 214: 597–598, 1967.
88. LANDS, A. M., V. L. NASH, H. M. MCCARTHY, H. R. GRANGER, AND B. L. DERTINGER. The pharmacology of N-alkyl homologues of epinephrine. *J. Pharmacol. Exptl. Therap.* 90: 110–119, 1947.
89. LANGER, S. Z., AND U. TRENDELENBURG. Decrease in effectiveness of phenoxybenzamine after chronic denervation and chronic decentralization of the nictitating membrane of the pithed cat. *J. Pharmacol. Exptl. Therap.* 163: 290–299, 1968.
90. LANGLEY, J. N. Observations on the physiological actions of extracts of the supra-renal bodies. *J. Physiol., London* 27: 237–413, 1901.
91. LEFKOWITZ, R. J., AND E. HABER. A fraction of the ventricular myocardium that has the specificity of the cardiac beta-adrenergic receptor. *Proc. Natl. Acad. Sci. US* 68: 1773–1777, 1971.
91a. LEFKOWITZ, R. J., E. HABER, AND D. O'HARA. Identification of the cardiac beta-adrenergic receptor protein: solubilization and purification by affinity chromatography. *Proc. Natl. Acad. Sci. US* 69: 2828–2832, 1972.
91b. LEFKOWITZ, R. J., G. W. G. SHARP, AND E. HABER. Specific binding of β-adrenergic catecholamines to a subcellular fraction from cardiac muscle. *J. Biol. Chem.* 248: 342–349, 1973.
92. LEIBOWITZ, S. F. Reciprocal hunger-regulating circuits involving alpha- and beta-adrenergic receptors located, respectively, in the ventromedial and lateral hypothalamus. *Proc. Natl. Acad. Sci. US* 67: 1063–1070, 1970.
93. LEIBOWITZ, S. F. Hypothalamic alpha- and beta-adrenergic systems regulate both thirst and hunger in the rat. *Proc. Natl. Acad. Sci. US* 68: 332–334, 1971.
94. LEVY, B., AND S. TOZZI. The adrenergic receptive mechanism of the rat uterus. *J. Pharmacol.* 142: 178–184, 1963.
95. LEVY, B., AND B. E. WILKENFELD. An analysis of selective beta receptor blockade. *European J. Pharmacol.* 5: 227–234, 1969.
96. LEWANDOWSKY, M. Wirkung des Nebennierenextrakts auf die glatten Muskeln der Haut. *Z. Physiol.* 14: 433, 1900.
97. LIBERMAN, B., L. A. KLEIN, AND C. R. KLEEMAN. Effect of adrenergic blocking agents on the vasopressin inhibiting action of norepinephrine. *Proc. Soc. Exptl. Biol. Med.* 133: 131–134, 1970.
98. LIEDBERG, G., AND C. G. A. PERSSON. Adrenoceptors in the cat choledochoduodenal junction studied in situ. *Brit. J. Pharmacol.* 39: 619–626, 1970.
99. LUCCHESI, B. R., L. S. WHITSITT, AND T. IWAMI. Effect of propranolol and its dextro-isomer on experimentally induced arrhythmia. In: *Cardiovascular Beta Adrenergic Responses*, edited by A. A. Kattus, G. Ross, and V. Hall. Berkeley: Univ. of California Press, 1970, p. 21–43.
100. LUM, B. K. B., M. H. KERMANI, AND R. D. HEILMAN. Intestinal relaxation produced by sympathomimetic amines in the isolated rabbit jejunum: selective inhibition by adrenergic blocking agents and by cold storage. *J. Pharmacol. Exptl. Therap.* 154: 463–471, 1966.
101. MAHON, W. A., D. W. J. REID, AND R. A. DAY. The in vivo effects of *beta* adrenergic stimulation and blockade of the human uterus at term. *J. Pharmacol. Exptl. Therap.* 156: 178–185, 1967.
101a. MALMEJAC, J. Activity of the adrenal medulla and its regulation. *Physiol. Rev.* 44: 186–218, 1964.
102. MARLEY, E., AND J. D. STEPHENSON. Effects of catecholamines infused into the brain of young chickens. *Brit. J. Pharmacol.* 40: 639–658, 1970.
103. MAYER, S. E. Adrenergic receptors for metabolic receptors in the heart. *Federation Proc.* 29: 1367–1372, 1970.

104. MAYER, S. E. Adenyl cyclase as a component of the adrenergic receptor. In: *Ciba Foundation Symposium on Molecular Properties of Drug Receptors*, edited by R. Porter and M. O'Connor. London: Churchill, 1970, p. 43–56.
105. MAYER, S. E., AND N. C. MORAN. Relation between pharmacologic agumentation of cardiac contractile force and the activation of myocardial glycogen phosphorylase. *J. Pharmacol. Exptl. Therap.* 129: 271–281, 1960.
106. MILEDI, R., P. MOLINOFF, AND L. T. POTTER. Isolation of the cholinergic receptor protein of *Torpedo* electric tissue. *Nature* 229: 554–557, 1971.
107. MOORE, J. I., AND H. H. SWAIN. Sensitization to ventricular fibrillation. I. Sensitization by a substituted propiophenone, U-0882. *J. Pharmacol. Exptl. Therap.* 128: 243–252, 1960.
108. MORALES-AUGILERÁ, A., AND E. M. VAUGHAN WILLIAMS. The effects on cardiac muscle of β-receptor antagonists in relation to their activity as local anesthetics. *Brit. J. Pharmacol.* 24: 332–338, 1965.
109. MORAN, N. C. Pharmacological characterization of adrenergic receptors. *Pharmacol. Rev.* 18: 503–512, 1966.
110. MORAN, N. C. (editor). New adrenergic blocking drugs: their pharmacological, biochemical and clinical actions. *Ann. NY Acad. Sci.* 139: 541–1009, 1967.
111. MORAN, N. C. Aims of the conference. Conference on new adrenergic blocking drugs: their pharmacological, biochemical and clinical actions. *Ann. NY Acad. Sci.* 139: 545–548, 1967.
112. MORAN, N. C. The development of beta adrenergic blocking drugs: a retrospective and prospective evaluation. *Ann. NY Acad. Sci.* 139: 649–660, 1967.
113. MORAN, N. C. Beta adrenergic blockade. An historical review and evaluation. In: *Cardiovascular Beta Adrenergic Responses*, edited by A. A. Kattus, G. Ross, and V. Hall. Berkeley: Univ. of California Press, 1970, p. 1–20.
114. MORAN, N. C., J. I. MOORE, A. K. HOLCOMB, AND G. MUSHET. Antagonism of adrenergically induced cardiac arrhythmias by dichloroisoproterenol. *J. Pharmacol. Exptl. Therap.* 136: 327–335, 1962.
115. MORAN, N. C., AND M. E. PERKINS. Adrenergic blockade of the mammalian heart by a dichloro analogue of isoproterenol. *J. Pharmacol. Exptl. Therap.* 124: 223–237, 1958.
116. MORAN, N. C., AND M. E. PERKINS. An evaluation of adrenergic blockade of the mammalian heart. *J. Pharmacol. Exptl. Therap.* 131: 192–201, 1961.
117. MURAD, F., Y-M. CHI, T. W. RALL, AND E. W. SUTHERLAND. Adenyl cyclase. III. The effect of catecholamines and cholinesters on the formation of adenosine $3',5'$-phosphate by preparations from cardiac muscle and liver. *J. Biol. Chem.* 237: 1233–1238, 1962.
118. NAMM, D. H., AND S. E. MAYER. Effects of epinephrine on cyclic $3',5'$-AMP, phosphorylase kinase, and phosphorylase. *Mol. Pharmacol.* 4: 61–69, 1968.
119. NASMYTH, P. A. The effect of adrenergic agents on smooth muscle other than those of the vascular system. In: *Physiological Pharmacology*, edited by W. S. Root and F. G. Hoffman. New York: Acad. Press, 1967, vol. 4, p. 129–178.
120. NEWTON, N. E., AND K. R. HORNBROOK. Effects of adrenergic agents on carbohydrate metabolism of rat liver: activities of adenyl cyclase and glycogen phosphorylase. *J. Pharmacol. Exptl. Therap.* 181: 479–488, 1972.
121. NICKERSON, M. The pharmacology of adrenergic blockade. *Pharmacol. Rev.* 1: 27–101, 1949.
122. NICKERSON, M., AND G. C-M. CHAN. Blockade of responses of isolated myocardium to epinephrine. *J. Pharmacol. Exptl. Therap.* 133: 186–191, 1961.
123. NICKERSON, M., AND L. S. GOODMAN. Pharmacological properties of a new adrenergic blocking agent: N,N-dibenzyl β-chloroethylamine (Dibenamine) *J. Pharmacol. Exptl. Therap.* 89: 167–185, 1947.
124. NICKERSON, M., AND N. K. HOLLENBERG. Blockade of α-adrenergic receptors. In: *Physiological Pharmacology*, edited by W. S. Root and F. G. Hoffman. New York: Acad. Press, 1967, vol. 4, p. 243–305.
125. NORBERG, K. A. Adrenergic innervation of the intestinal wall studied by fluorescence microscopy. *Intern. J. Neuropharmacol.* 3: 379–382, 1964.
126. NORTHRUP, G. Effects of adrenergic blocking agents on epinephrine and $3',5'$-AMP-induced responses in the perfused rat liver. *J. Pharmacol. Exptl. Therap.* 159: 22–28, 1968.
127. NORTHRUP, G., AND R. E. PARKS, JR. The effects of adrenergic blocking agents and theophylline on $3',5'$-AMP-induced hyperglycemia. *J. Pharmacol. Exptl. Therap.* 145: 87–91, 1964.
128. OLIVER, G., AND E. A. SCHÄFER. Physiological effects of the suprarenal capsules. *J. Physiol., London* 18: 230–276, 1895.
129. PAPPANO, A. J. Propranolol-insensitive effects of epinephrine on action potential repolarization in electrically driven atria of the guinea pig. *J. Pharmacol. Exptl. Therap.* 177: 85–95, 1971.
130. PARRATT, J. R., AND R. M. WADSWORTH. The effect of "selective" β-adrenoceptor blocking drugs on the myocardial circulation. *Brit. J. Pharmacol.* 39: 296–308, 1970.
131. PATIL, P. N. Adrenergic receptors of the bovine iris sphincter. *J. Pharmacol. Exptl. Therap.* 166: 199–307, 1969.
132. PATIL, P. N., D. G. PATEL, AND R. D. KRELL. Steric aspects of adrenergic drugs. XV. Use of isomeric activity ratio as a criterion to differentiate adrenergic receptors. *J. Pharmacol. Exptl. Therap.* 176: 622–633, 1971.
133. PITT, B., E. C. ELLIOT, AND D. E. GREGG. Adrenergic receceptor activity in the coronary arteries of the unanesthetized dog. *Circulation Res.* 21: 75–84, 1967.
134. PLUCHINO, S., AND U. TRENDELENBURG. The influence of denervation and of decentralization on the *alpha* and *beta* effects of isoproterenol on nictitating membrane of the pithed cat. *J. Pharmacol. Exptl. Therap.* 163: 257–265, 1968.
135. POWELL, C. E., AND I. H. SLATER. Blocking of inhibitory adrenergic receptors by a dichloro analog of isoproterenol. *J. Pharmacol. Exptl. Therap.* 122: 480–488, 1967.
136. RAHN, K. H., AND H. REUTER. Die Wirkung von β-Receptoren blockierenden Substanzen auf die durch Adrenalin gesteigerte ^{42}K-Abgabe des Meerschweinchenvorhofs. *Arch. Exptl. Pathol. Pharmakol.* 253: 484–494, 1966.
137. RAPER, C. Receptors for catecholamines in skeletal muscle. A comparison with cardiac muscle and autonomic ganglia. *Circulation Res.* 21, Suppl. III: 147–155, 1967.
138. RASMUSSEN, H., AND A. TENENHOUSE. Cyclic adenosine monophosphate, Ca^{++} and membranes. *Proc. Natl. Acad. Sci. US* 59: 1364–1370, 1968.
139. REDDY, V., AND N. C. MORAN. An evaluation of the adrenergic receptor types in isolated segments of the small intestine of the rabbit. *Arch. Intern. Pharmacodyn.* 176: 326–336, 1968.
140. REGOLI, D., AND J. R. VANE. A sensitive method for the assay of angiotensin. *Brit. J. Pharmacol.* 23: 351–359, 1964.
141. ROBISON, G. A., R. W. BUTCHER, I. ØYE, H. E. MORGAN, AND E. W. SUTHERLAND. The effect of epinephrine on adenosine $3',5'$-phosphate levels in the isolated perfused rat heart. *Mol. Pharmacol.* 1: 168–177, 1965.
142. ROBISON, G. A., R. W. BUTCHER, AND E. W. SUTHERLAND. *Cyclic AMP*. New York: Acad. Press, 1971, chapt. 6.
143. ROSS, G., AND C. R. JORGENSEN. Effects of a cardio-selective beta-adrenergic blocking agent on the heart and coronary circulation. *Cardiovascular Res.* 4: 148–153, 1970.
144. ROSSUM, J. M. VAN, AND M. MUJIĆ. Classification of sympathomimetic drugs on the rabbit intestine. *Arch. Intern. Pharmacodyn.* 155: 418–431, 1965.
145. RUDZIK, A. D., AND J. W. MILLER. The mechanism of uterine inhibitory action of relaxin-containing ovarian extracts. *J. Pharmacol. Exptl. Therap.* 138: 82–87, 1962.
146. SCHUELER, F. W. *Chemobiodynamics and Drug Design*. New York: McGraw-Hill, 1960, p. 139.
147. SHARPEY-SCHAFER, E. P., AND J. GINSBURG. Humoral agents

and venous tone. Effects of catecholamines, 5-hydroxytryptamine, histamine and nitrites. *Lancet* 2: 1337–1340, 1962.
148. SHEIN, H. M., AND R. J. WURTMAN. Cyclic adenosine monophosphate: stimulation of melatonin and serotonin syntheses in cultured rat pineals. *Science* 166: 519–520, 1969.
149. SIEGEL, J. H., J. P. GILMORE, AND S. J. SARNOFF. Myocardial extraction and production of catecholamines. *Circulation Res.* 9: 1336–1350, 1961.
150. SKELTON, C. L., G. S. LEVEY, AND S. E. EPSTEIN. Positive inotropic effects of dibutyryl cyclic adenosine 3′,5′-monophosphate. *Circulation Res.* 26: 35–43, 1970.
151. SLATER, I. H., AND C. E. POWELL. Blockade of adrenergic inhibitory receptor sites by 1-(3′,4′,-dichlorophenyl)-2-isopropylaminoethanol hydrochloride. *Federation Proc.* 16: 336, 1957.
152. SMITH, C. B. Relaxation of the nictitating membrane of the spinal cat by sympathomimetic amines. *J. Pharmacol. Exptl. Therap.* 142: 163–170, 1963.
153. STRAUSS, H. C., J. T. BIGGER, JR., AND B. F. HOFFMAN. Electrophysiological and beta-receptor blocking effects of MJ 1999 on dog and rabbit cardiac tissue. *Circulation Res.* 26: 661–678, 1970.
154. SUTHERLAND, E. W. An introduction. In: *Cyclic AMP*, by G. A. Robison, R. W. Butcher, and E. W. Sutherland. New York: Acad. Press, 1971, p. 1–16.
155. TSAI, T. H., AND W. W. FLEMING. The adrenotropic receptors of the cat uterus. *J. Pharmacol. Exptl. Therap.* 143: 268–272, 1964.
156. VIVEROS, O. H., D. G. GARLIC, AND E. M. RENKIN. Sympathetic beta adrenergic vasodilatation in skeletal muscle of the dog. *Am. J. Physiol.* 215: 1218–1225, 1968.
157. WALLACE, A. G., AND S. J. SARNOFF. Effects of cardiac sympathetic nerve stimulation on conduction in the heart. *Circulation Res.* 14: 86–92, 1964.
158. WAUD, D. R. Pharmacological receptors. *Pharmacol. Rev.* 20: 49–88, 1968.
159. WATLINGTON, C. O. Effect of adrenergic stimulation on ion transport across skin of living frogs. *Comp. Biochem. Physiol.* 24: 965–974, 1968.
160. WEISBRODT, N. W., C. C. HUG, JR., AND P. BASS. Separation of the effects of *alpha* and *beta* adrenergic receptor stimulation on taenia coli. *J. Pharmacol. Exptl. Therap.* 170: 272–280, 1970.
161. WEISS, B., AND E. COSTA. Selective stimulation of adenyl cyclase of rat pineal gland by pharmacologically active catecholamines. *J. Pharmacol. Exptl. Therap.* 161: 310–319, 1968.
162. WEST, T. C., G. FALK, AND P. CERVONI. Drug alteration of transmembrane potentials in atrial pacemaker cells. *J. Pharmacol. Exptl. Therap.* 117: 245–252, 1956.
163. WILLIAMS, B. J., AND S. E. MAYER. Hormonal effects on glycogen metabolism in the rat heart *in situ*. *Mol. Pharmacol.* 2: 454–464, 1966.
164. WHITSITT, L. S., AND B. R. LUCCHESI. Effect of propranolol and its stereoisomers upon coronary vascular resistance. *Circulation Res.* 21: 305–317, 1967.
165. WHITSITT, L. S., AND B. R. LUCCHESI. Effects of beta-receptor blockade and glucagon on the atrioventricular conduction transmission system in the dog. *Circulation Res.* 23: 585–595, 1968.
166. WILKENFELD, B. E., AND B. LEVY. The effects of theophylline, diazoxide and imidazole on isoproterenol-induced inhibition of the rabbit ileum. *J. Pharmacol. Exptl. Therap.* 169: 61–67, 1969.
167. WURTMAN, R. J., J. AXELROD, AND D. E. KELLY. *The Pineal*. New York: Acad. Press, 1968.
168. YOO, C. S., AND W. C. LEE. Blockade of the cardiac actions of phenylephrine by bretylium or cocaine. *J. Pharmacol. Exptl. Therap.* 172: 274–281, 1970.
169. ZSOTER, T. The effect of aminophylline and isoproterenol on venous distensibility. *Can. J. Physiol. Pharmacol.* 46: 225–228, 1968.
170. ZUBERBUHLER, R. C., AND D. F. BOHR. Responses of coronary smooth muscle to catecholamines. *Circulation Res.* 16: 431–440, 1965.

REFERENCES IN ADDENDUM

1A. BLASCHKO, H., AND E. MUSCHOLL (editors). *Catecholamines. Handbook of Experimental Pharmacology*. Berlin: Springer, 1972, vol. 33.
2A. CUATRACASAS, P., G. P. E. TELL, V. SICA, I. PARIKH, AND K-J. CHANG. Noradrenaline binding and the search for catecholamine receptors. *Nature* 247: 92–97, 1974.
3A. FARNEBO, L-O., AND B. HAMBERGER. Catecholamine release and receptors in brain slices. In: *Frontiers in Catecholamine Research*, edited by E. Usdin and S. Snyder. New York: Pergamon Press, 1973, p. 589–593.
4A. FURCHGOTT, R. F. The classification of adrenoceptors (adrenergic receptors). An evaluation from the standpoint of receptor theory. In: *Catecholamines. Handbook of Experimental Pharmacology*, edited by H. Blaschko and E. Muscholl. Berlin: Springer, 1972, vol. 33, p. 283–335.
5A. LANGER, S. Z. The regulation of transmitter release elicited by nerve stimulation through a presynaptic feedback mechanism. In: *Frontiers in Catecholamine Research*, edited by E. Usdin and Snyder. New York: Pergamon Press, 1973, p. 543–549.
6A. LEFKOWITZ, R. J. Toward isolation of a β-adrenergic binding protein. In: *Frontiers in Catecholamine Research*, edited by E. Usdin and S. Snyder. New York: Pergamon Press, 1973, p. 361–368.
7A. MOLINOFF, P. Methods of approach for the isolation of β-adrenergic receptors. In: *Frontiers in Catecholamine Research*, edited by E. Usdin and S. Snyder. New York: Pergamon Press, 1973, p. 357–360.
8A. STARKE, K. Regulation of catecholamine release: α-receptor mediated feedback control in peripheral and central neurones. In: *Frontiers in Catecholamine Research*, edited by E. Usdin and S. Snyder. New York: Pergamon Press, 1973, p. 561–565.
9A. TRENDELENBURG, U. Classification of sympathomimetic amines. In: *Catecholamines. Handbook of Experimental Pharmacology*, edited by H. Blaschko and E. Muscholl. Berlin: Springer, 1972, vol. 33, p. 336–362.
10A. USDIN, E., AND S. SNYDER (editors). *Frontiers in Catecholamine Research*. New York: Pergamon Press, 1973.

CHAPTER 30

Catecholamines and the cardiovascular system

ERIC NEIL | *Middlesex Hospital Medical School, London, England*

CHAPTER CONTENTS

Relative Importance of Cardiovascular Effects of Circulating
    Catecholamines and of Sympathetic Innervation
Regional Vascular Beds
    Muscle vessels
    Cutaneous vessels
    Cerebral vessels
    Renal vessels
    Splanchnic and hepatic vessels
    Coronary vessels
    Pulmonary vessels
    Veins
Catecholamines and Cardiac Function
    Catecholamines and heart rate—electrophysiological studies
    Conduction velocity
    Inotropic effects of catecholamines
        Isolated papillary muscle preparation
        Heart-lung preparation
    Myocardial oxygen usage

FLOW THROUGH THE CAPILLARIES—the prime function of the circulation—is governed by Ohm's law:

$$\text{flow} = \frac{\text{potential energy}}{\text{resistance}}$$

Poiseuille (128) showed that the resistance to the flow of fluid through a tube was determined by the fourth power of the tube radius (r), by the length of the tube (L), and by the viscosity (η) of the fluid:

$$\text{Resistance} \propto \frac{\eta L}{r^4}$$

The main determinant of resistance is the radius of the arterioles. Arteriolar caliber is tonically reduced by sympathetic vasoconstrictor discharge and is increased by the local action of metabolites derived from tissue activity.

In the circulation, flow is provided by cardiac output, which in turn presupposes a satisfactory venous return to prime the cardiac pump. The thin-walled veins contain 65–70% of the blood volume, and modifications of the transmural pressure caused by postural influences would have a profound effect on venous capacity and therefore venous return if it were not for appropriate variations in the venoconstrictor impulse activity of the sympathetic nerves that supply the veins.

Cardiac output per minute is the product of the heart rate and the stroke volume, and each of these factors is increased by sympathetic activity. Heart rate is also influenced by vagal discharge, which reduces it.

Sympathetic impulse activity and cardiac vagal discharge are both reflexly modified by a negative feedback system. Stretch receptors in the aortic arch and the carotid sinus signal the mean stretch and the pulsatile stretch of the arterial system (22, 39). If the arterial pressure rises, increased sino-aortic afferent activity reflexly inhibits cardiac and vasoconstrictor sympathetic discharge and reflexly increases cardiac vagal impulse activity. As a result the rise in blood pressure is minimized. Conversely a fall in blood pressure sets in chain reflex adjustments that tend to prevent this fall from being unduly large (53, 71–73, 91).

Most of these facts were understood by the time Oliver and Schäfer performed their first experiment in 1893, but how the sympathetic nerves exerted their effects on the heart and blood vessels was not.

It is in some ways ironic that their pioneer experiments on the humoral influence of the adrenal medulla on the cardiovascular system have served to demonstrate the importance of the sympathetic innervation of the heart and vasculature compared with the influence of circulating medullary hormones on these structures. Their evidence that adrenal medullary extracts could cause such striking cardiovascular effects led to an intensive study of the chemical nature of the active principle. It took 50 years to prove that one of the active principles—norepinephrine—secreted by the adrenal medulla was itself secreted by the postganglionic nerve endings of the cardiovascular sympathetic nerves.

Few experiments can have given such dramatic results as that first one performed by Oliver and Schäfer in Autumn 1893. Only the classic demonstration, by Bayliss & Starling (13), of pancreatic secretion induced by humoral means could be said to have rivaled it.

Hill (76) in 1895 refers to Oliver's ingenious instrument, the arteriometer, which Oliver himself (120) described in a book written in the same year. The arteriometer, which measured the diameter of an artery, and the hemodynamometer, which measured the blood pressure, were employed by Oliver in 1894 to observe the effect of an extract of the suprarenal gland administered to his own child; the extract decreased the size of the radial artery and raised the blood pressure. According to Schäfer (136), this particular observation was never published. However, Oliver came from Harrogate to London in Autumn 1893 to meet Schäfer (they had both been pupils of the great teacher, William Sharpey) and to persuade him to test the efficacy of suprarenal extract in raising the blood pressure in an experimental animal. The results were striking enough—the hypertension evoked sufficed to drive the mercury clean out of the Ludwig manometer—to lead to their classic joint investigation, published in full in 1895 (122).

They studied the cardiovascular changes induced by suprarenal extracts administered intravenously to the dog and other mammals. Additionally, Oliver (121) examined the effect of the extracts on the rate of flow of Ringer's solution through the denervated arterial system of the frog.

The huge rise of arterial blood pressure that followed the injection of the extract was ascribed to arteriolar contraction because *a)* it occurred "even when concomitant vagus action caused a great diminution in the rate and force of the heart's beats," *b)* it caused "almost complete cessation of the flow of circulating fluid through the arterioles (of the frog)," and *c)* it usually caused "contraction of isolated organs" (enclosed by a plethysmograph) (136).

The effect of extracts on the isolated perfused frog ventricle was to accelerate the rhythm and to increase the strength of contraction. Effects on the mammalian heart in the intact circulation depended on whether or not the vagi were intact. With intact vagi the extract provoked inhibition of atrial contraction, but with the vagi cut there resulted only augmentation and acceleration of the atria and ventricles. This they attributed to a direct effect of the extract on the heart.

Further experiments proved that the active principle was contained only in the medulla and that extracts made from glands of patients suffering from Addison's disease were ineffective in causing cardiovascular effects when injected into dogs.

The active principle of the suprarenal medulla was purified by Abel & Crawford (2) in 1897 and isolated by Takamine (152) in 1901, who called it adrenaline (now epinephrine). It was the first of the natural hormones to be isolated and the first to be synthesized—in 1904 by Stolz (147, 148).

The striking similarity between the responses to stimulation of the sympathetic nervous system and the effects of epinephrine in the organism had already been noted by Lewandowsky (100) and by Langley (98), and further work by Elliott (41, 42) led him to suggest that the transmitter substance liberated by the sympathetic nerve endings was epinephrine.

Barger & Dale (12) and Cannon & Uridil (26) noted differences between the effects of sympathetic stimulation and those of epinephrine and thus doubted that epinephrine was the transmitter. Loewi (104) showed that stimulation of the cardiac sympathetic nerves in the frog caused the liberation of a sympathicomimetic substance, which he later identified as epinephrine (105, 106). This perpetuated the idea that epinephrine was the sympathetic transmitter—which it is in the frog heart, but not in mammalian species. Although Bacq (7) suggested that norepinephrine was the sympathetic transmitter, not until 1946, when von Euler (46) showed that the extracts of various organs and of sympathetic nerves contained a sympathomimetic substance with chemical properties and biological effects similar to those of norepinephrine, was any direct evidence obtained that the primary sympathetic transmitter was norepinephrine. Peart (125) showed that splenic sympathetic nerve stimulation caused the release of large amounts of norepinephrine, together with small quantities of epinephrine.

Meanwhile the influence of the pregangionic splanchnic nerves on the secretion of the adrenal glands had been documented. The first good evidence naturally had to await the demonstration of Oliver and Shäfer that the adrenal medulla released a pressor hormone. In 1899 Dreyer (36) pointed out that the venous effluent from a suprarenal gland exerted a greater pressor effect when injected into another animal if the effluent was collected during splanchnic stimulation of the gland than if it was sampled from the resting gland. Elliott (42) confirmed and considerably extended these studies by assaying the effects of suprarenal extracts on the blood pressure of pithed cats. He showed that the two glands contained similar amounts of "active pressor substance" and that ether, chloroform, and urethane anesthesia depleted this material. Fright (induced in cats by morphine or by β-tetrahydronaphthylamine) or afferent stimulation of the sciatic nerve exhausted the glandular content of epinephrine only if the splanchnic nerve supply was intact; section of the relevant splanchnic nerve prevented exhaustion of the gland. Faradic stimulation of the splanchnic nerve itself caused depletion of its content of the pressor substance, which made possible the correct identification of the dual hump of arterial blood pressure caused by such stimulation as being due to a combination of splanchnic vasoconstriction followed by an outpouring of the suprarenal medullary hormone.

In 1911 Cannon and co-workers (24, 25) found that emotion and asphyxia provoked an increase of adrenal medullary discharge, and the introduction of the denervated heart by Cannon provided a very sensitive method of assaying adrenal discharge.

Space does not permit discussion of the controversy, which lasted for years, about whether there is a resting secretion of adrenal medullary hormone, or hormones [see (83, 108)]. The modern viewpoint differs little from the conclusions reached by Hoskins in 1922 and by McDowall in 1938 that the resting secretion of the catecholamine, or catecholamines, is unimportant.

Moreover, Hoskins also wrote that "the medulla apparently serves merely to reinforce the sympathetic system in times of stress," which is likewise the view today.

Holtz et al. (81) showed for the first time that the suprarenal medulla contained norepinephrine, as well as epinephrine, and this was quickly confirmed by Holtz & Schümann (82) and von Euler & Hamberg (48), among others. Hökfelt provided details of the distribution of norepinephrine and epinephrine in mammalian tissues (79). Eränkö (44) found that treatment with formaldehyde solution caused fluorescence of adrenal medullary cells containing much norepinephrine and little epinephrine and nonfluorescence of cells containing epinephrine and not much norepinephrine. Hillarp & Hökfelt (77) showed and Eränkö (45) confirmed that norepinephrine was easily oxidized by potassium iodate to give insoluble pigments and that this reaction could be used to identify the norepinephrine-producing cells in the adrenal medulla. Falck & Torp (51) confirmed the great sensitivity of the formaldehyde vapor technique. The physiological role of the circulating catecholamines in influencing cardiovascular activity could be seriously assessed only when methods became available for their accurate determination in body fluids and tissues. The development of such methodology [for reviews, see (47, 49, 79, 85, 135)] has at last allowed a proper appraisal of the relative importance of the contribution of adrenal medullary secretions of catecholamine to cardiovascular regulation compared with that of the sympathetic postganglionic release of norepinephrine at strategic sites of the circulatory system.

One problem that puzzled the earlier investigators was the transience of action of the catecholamines when injected into the bloodstream. It was first considered that destruction by tissue enzymes was mainly, if not entirely, responsible for catecholamine inactivation. More recently, with the advent of the use of radioactively labeled compounds, it has become clear that tissue uptake, notably by postganglionic noradrenergic nerve endings, is of greater importance in removing the catecholamines from the circulation. The evidence for this statement has been admirably marshaled by Iverson [(85, 86); see the chapter by Iversen in this volume of the *Handbook*]. The hypersensitivity of sympathetically denervated structures to circulating catecholamine can thus be satisfactorily explained. Similarly it has been demonstrated that cocaine, long known to potentiate the action of epinephrine and norepinephrine, blocks the uptake of these compounds by the postganglionic nerve endings by competing with them for a common uptake site.

RELATIVE IMPORTANCE OF CARDIOVASCULAR EFFECTS OF CIRCULATING CATECHOLAMINES AND OF SYMPATHETIC INNERVATION

Celander (27) was the first to compare quantitatively the cardiovascular effects of circulating catecholamines with the effects of sympathetic innervation. He compared the effects of stimulating the local sympathetic nerve supply of the blood flow through various regional circuits (skin, muscle, kidney, and spleen) perfused at constant pressure with the effects induced by the intravenous infusion of either epinephrine or norepinephrine.

Skin and renal vessels and vessels of the spleen were far more responsive to the effects of stimulation of their local sympathetic nerve supply than to those of the catecholamines administered either by the intravenous or by the intraarterial route (Fig. 1).

The vessels of skeletal muscle showed only constriction in response to their regional sympathetic stimulation or to the infusion of norepinephrine. However, epinephrine induced vasodilatation when the infusion rate was less than 4 μg/kg·min and provoked only a mild constriction at higher rates of infusion (Fig. 2).

In further experiments, Celander stimulated the splanchnic nerve to one adrenal gland at rates that reached the highest frequency likely to be seen in physiological circumstances—10 pulses/sec (53). The adrenal medullary secretion of catecholamines thereby provoked caused a rise in blood pressure (the cats were spinalized) and a contraction of the nictitating membrane. These responses were recorded, and the rate of liberation of catecholamine they represented was assayed by comparing it with those induced by known rates of catecholamine infusion.

From such experiments, Celander concluded that the maximum secretion rate provoked by splanchnic nerve stimulation did not exceed 5 μg/kg·min. He argued, probably correctly, that even the strongest reflex activation of medullary secretion seen in physiological condi-

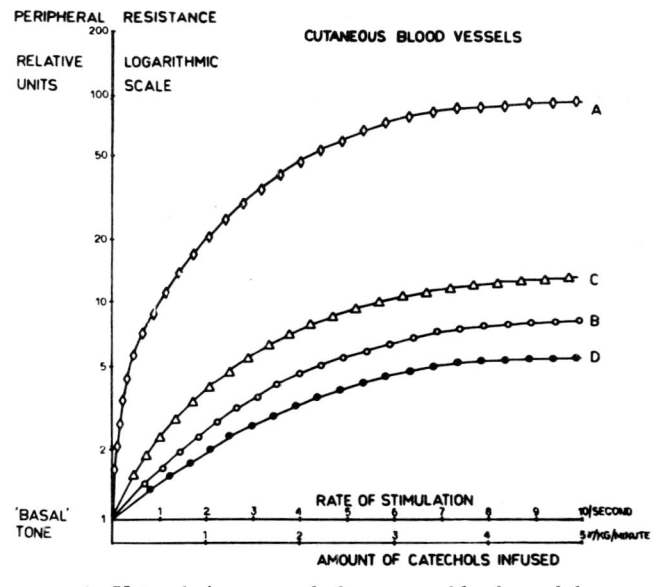

FIG. 1. *Upper abscissa*: control of cutaneous blood vessels by sympathetic constrictor nerve fibers (*A*) and by both adrenal medullae (*B*). *Lower abscissa*: effects of *l*-epinephrine (*C*) and *l*-norepinephrine (*D*) on control of cutaneous blood vessels. [From Celander (27).]

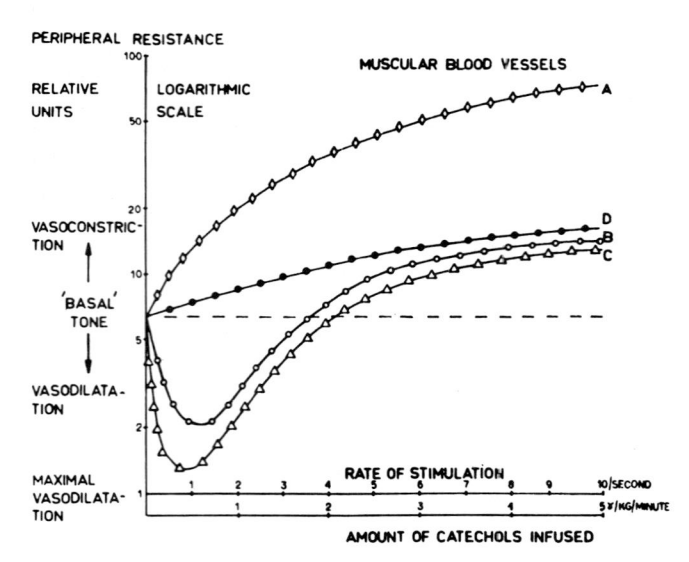

FIG. 2. *Upper abscissa*: control of muscular blood vessels by sympathetic constrictor nerve fibers (*A*) and by both adrenal medullae (*B*). *Lower abscissa*: effects of *l*-epinephrine (*C*) and *l*-norepinephrine (*D*) on control of muscular blood vessels. Note marked "*basal*" tone normally exhibited by sympathetically decentralized muscular blood vessels. [From Celander (27).]

tions was not as high as this, but in all his comparisons between the effects of local stimulation of the sympathetic nerves supplying a regional vascular bed and those of catecholamines, he used the response obtained by infusing them at a rate of 5 µg/kg·min.

His conclusions were clear. Either in resting conditions or in those associated with maximal rates of medullary secretion, the vascular effects of reflex activation of adrenal catecholamine liberation were trivial in comparison with those evoked by increased sympathetic impulse traffic in the vasomotor nerves.

Folkow et al. (55) and Ljung (102, 103) have estimated the local concentration of norepinephrine to be of the order of 1 µg/ml in the neuromuscular junctional gap at vasoconstrictor nerve endings in the smooth muscle wall of the arterioles. They calculated that the maximal plasma concentration of catecholamines occurring in intense reflex activation of adrenal medullary secretion could not exceed 50 ng/ml. As Mellander & Johansson (113) point out, the sympathetic nerve endings have a fairly restricted distribution in the muscle layer of the media of the arterioles and venules, so that circulating catecholamines are likely to reach a much greater number of muscle cells in the media. Nevertheless the order of concentration locally achieved by the effects of sympathetic stimulation should far exceed that resulting from the diffusion of blood-borne catecholamines, and this is in keeping with Mellander's results.

The muscle vessels alone exhibit a response to moderate increases in the plasma epinephrine concentration that differs qualitatively from that induced by sympathetic stimulation. In most adult animals the adrenal medulla secretes both epinephrine and norepinephrine, and the proportions of the two amines do not seem to vary much in any one species when the secretion rate is increased from its low resting level to maximal levels seen in asphyxia or to more moderate levels, as provoked, for example, by carotid occlusion (89).

However, in the adult rabbit the medullary secretion is almost solely epinephrine (79, 109, 138), and Korner and his colleagues (28, 93, 94, 157) have shown that anoxia provokes changes in the muscle circulation that depend on whether or not the animal is adrenalectomized. After adrenalectomy, anoxia provokes vasoconstriction of the muscle vascular bed, whereas the intact rabbit demonstrates muscle hyperemia during anoxia. The adrenal medullary secretion in arterial hypoxia contributes to the subsequent splanchnic vasoconstriction (60, 109). In summary, the cardiovascular effects of an increase in the circulating catecholamine concentration are less important than those of increased impulse activity in the cardiovascular sympathetic nerves, which probably always occurs concomitantly. This must be borne in mind when considering the ensuing pages in which the features of the response of the various regional vascular circuits and of the heart to the catecholamines are presented in more detail.

It might seem more logical to consider the effects of the catecholamines on cardiac activity first, since the heart provides the energy for the circulation. However, so much work has been devoted to the effects of the medullary hormones on the muscle vascular bed—much of it performed quantitatively on unanesthetized man—that we consider this first; details of the responses of the other regional circulations are discussed before the influence of epinephrine and norepinephrine on cardiac rate and force are considered.

REGIONAL VASCULAR BEDS

Muscle Vessels

The local direct action of epinephrine on the blood vessels of muscle has been demonstrated by infusion into the brachial or femoral artery in man (Fig. 3). Forearm or calf blood flow was measured by venous occlusion plethysmography [see (11) for references]. In doses from 0.001 to 1 µg/min for the human forearm and 1 to 8 µg/min for the calf, given for 5–10 min, the initial effect is a transient vasodilatation to a peak flow of two to five times the resting value during the first 1–2 min of the infusion. This quickly subsides, and the flow falls to near the resting level. When infusion is terminated, flow may rise for a subsequent 3 min before returning to normal (96, 162). The use of epinephrine antagonists has demonstrated that the flow pattern during infusion represents a balance between a constrictor action and a vasodilator effect. Thus preliminary treatment with chlorpromazine or phenoxybenzamine, which blocks the constrictor effects but not the vasodilator influence of epinephrine, causes the response to infusion of epinephrine to become purely dilator. Conversely pronethalol given intraarterially abolishes all dilator responses to epinephrine in the muscle vessels, and epinephrine infusion provokes vasoconstriction, which subsides within 2 min of stopping the infusion (162).

The balance of opposing constrictor and dilator actions of epinephrine on muscle blood vessels has been explained in two ways.

    1. Ahlquist in 1948 (3) postulated separate constrictor (α) receptors and dilator (2) receptors in the vessel wall—a concept that has been elaborated by others (65). Since vasoconstriction alone prevails when doses greater than 1 μg/min are given, whereas small doses result in dilatation, it can be presumed that the β receptors have a lower threshold to epinephrine. The "after-dilatation" seen on cessation of intraarterial epinephrine infusion can be attributed to a rapid wearing off of the α response, whereas the β response continues a little longer. It is possible that the evanescent effect of the α receptor response may be due to epinephrine uptake by the sympathetic noradrenergic vasoconstrictor terminals, which presumably innervate the α receptors themselves but not the β receptors. Phenoxybenzamine and chlorpromazine block the α receptors, and epinephrine infusion then causes only β receptor excitation and vasodilatation. Pronethalol blocks β receptors, and epinephrine thereupon induces pure vasoconstriction. It is not known whether the α and β receptors are to be found on the same smooth muscle fiber or whether separate fibers exist, one exhibiting α-type response and the other the β receptor characteristics. The dilator receptors in skin vessels must be of a different nature from those in muscle, since even the administration of α-blocking drugs causes no vasodilator response of skin vessels to intraarterial infusion of epinephrine (162). Nevertheless dilator receptors must exist in skin vessels, for histamine, acetylcholine, bradykinin, and adenosine triphosphate cause cutaneous dilatation (66). Moreover muscle blood vessels themselves must also contain further receptors—christened γ receptors by Green & Kepchar (65)—which mediate the dilator effects of acetylcholine, either infused or delivered naturally by the sympathetic cholinergic vasodilator fiber nerve endings.

    2. Lundholm (107) claimed that the muscle vasodilatation induced by epinephrine was due to the release of lactic acid from the muscles. It is indisputable that lactic acid concentration may rise in the venous blood when epinephrine levels are increased, but this lacticacidemia is not thought to cause the muscle vessel vasodilatation (92). De la Lande & Whelan (96) were unable to provoke muscle vasodilatation by infusing either sodium lactate or lactic acid solutions buffered to pH values as low as 3.3. Lactic acid given simultaneously with epinephrine infusions had no dilator effect. The doses were sufficient to raise the lactate level to a value far in excess of that seen during epinephrine infusion. Whelan & de la Lande (162) quote Shanks' finding that the dilator response to epinephrine is blocked by dichloroisopropyl norepinephrine, which does not prevent the rise in lactic acid output from the muscles. Barcroft &

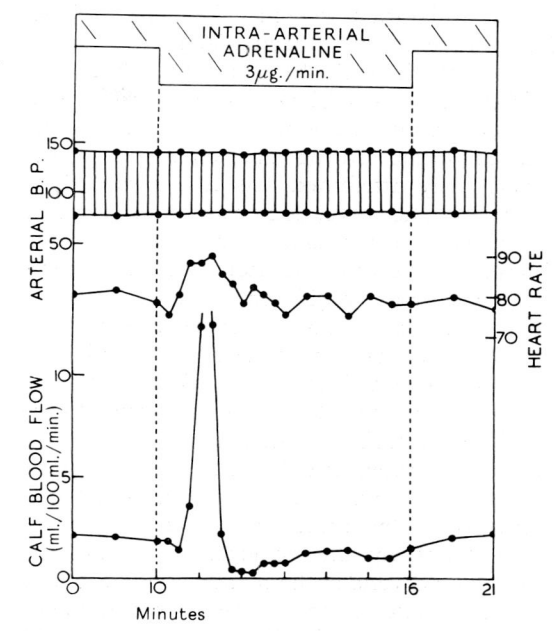

FIG. 3. Intraarterial infusion of epinephrine (*ADRENALINE*) causes transient vasodilatation in calf. Vasodilatation is due to direct local action of epinephrine in skeletal muscle blood vessels. *B.P.*, blood pressure. [From Allen et al. (6).]

McArdle (unpublished observations) found a normal response of the forearm vessels to intravenous epinephrine in a patient whose muscles contained no phosphorylase and concluded that the vasodilator response could not be due to the action of epinephrine on carbohydrate metabolism in muscle.

The pattern of blood flow and of venous oxygen saturation changes during epinephrine infusions might be due to the opening of thoroughfare channels and the diversion of the blood into nonmetabolic conduits. Rosell & Uvnäs (130) have shown that the sympathetic vasodilator nerves act in this manner in animals, but evidence of such action is lacking in man.

In experiments with animals, Mellander (112) showed that the skeletal muscle resistance vessels responded to epinephrine infusion by dilating when the dose given was 0.3–0.5 μg/kg·min. In such responses the use of "isovolumetric" hind limb revealed that the dilatation was confined to the precapillary resistance vessels, the postcapillary venules showing only constriction. The consequent reduction of total flow resistance led to a reduced precapillary-to-postcapillary resistance ratio, which caused an increase of P_{cap} (mean capillary pressure) with increased filtration of fluid into the interstitium and a rise in limb volume. Such results are compatible with a localization of β receptors predominantly in the precapillary resistance vessels.

When epinephrine is given by continuous intravenous infusion in man in doses of 5–30 μg/min, again there is a transient marked vasodilatation of the forearm for 1–2 min, but with continued infusion the flow settles to a level about double that of the resting value. On stopping infusion no after-dilatation is seen (6). Duff & Swan (38) found that subjects sympathectomized some months previously, although showing the transient initial vasodilatation of forearm muscle blood vessels in response to intravenous epinephrine infusion, did not manifest the sustained vasodilatation during the remainder of the infusion period; they attributed this to a sympathetic reflex. Whelan (161), however, demonstrated that simple blocking of the nerves to the forearm by local anesthesia did not abolish the sustained dilator response to epinephrine infusion. He considered that intravenous epinephrine caused the release of some intermediate vasodilator substance (as yet unidentified) and suggested that this accounted for the difference in the patterns of forearm muscle blood vessel response to intravenous and intraarterial infusion. Whelan & de la Lande (162) have pointed out that an increased sensitivity of the chronically sympathectomized muscle blood vessels to epinephrine (resulting from failure of uptake of the catecholamine by the nonexistent sympathetic nerve endings) would render them more susceptible to the α receptor constrictor action of the infused epinephrine and would thus mask the "secondary" sustained vasodilatation.

Peripheral actions of norepinephrine in man were first investigated by Barcroft & Konzett (9); the amine was shown to be invariably vasoconstrictor to muscle blood vessels when given intraarterially. However, when it was administered intravenously, Barcroft et al. (10) sometimes found that flow either remained unchanged or actually increased. This occasional dilator response was absent in sympathectomized subjects or in subjects in whom the regional nerves had been blocked by local anesthesia. Barcroft and co-workers concluded that the vasodilatation was central in origin—it resulted from an inhibition of the vasomotor center caused by an increased sino-aortic baroreceptor discharge resulting from the systemic hypertension provoked by the drug infusion.

The dilatation thus provoked in the forearm by intravenous infusion of norepinephrine was prevented by the adrenergic blocking agent, phenoxybenzamine, which blocks the α receptor constrictor response to intraarterial infusions of norepinephrine, and hence in turn prevents the systemic hypertension that reflexly provokes the dilatation seen on intravenous infusion.

Cutaneous Vessels

Both epinephrine and norepinephrine evoke constriction of resistance and capacitance vessels and an increase in the precapillary-to-postcapillary resistance ratio (11, 66, 112). In man the intravenous infusion of 20 μg/min of either epinephrine or norepinephrine causes a striking fall in the blood flow through the hand during the period of infusion. In the case of norepinephrine infusion, the blood flow regains normal values quickly, but after an intravenous infusion of epinephrine, blood flow not only regains itself quickly but reaches a higher value than that registered during the preinfusion "control" period (11, 151). This hyperemia shown by blood flow in the hand is not seen in the sympathectomized limb (37), nor does it occur after intrabrachial arterial infusion of epinephrine (151); it is presumably caused by an inhibition of sympathetic vasoconstrictor discharge. However, as Barcroft and Swan have argued, this is not likely to be a medullary depressor reflex of sympathetic vasomotor activity because it often coincides with a period of systemic arterial hypotension. They concluded that the after-dilatation following intravenous infusion of epinephrine was due to a direct depression of vasoconstrictor discharge by an action of epinephrine on the transmission of sympathetic impulses in the regional sympathetic ganglia (11).

Iontophoresis of epinephrine has been used to suppress the skin circulation (40). Such therapy prevents the normal responses of the forearm skin vessels to body heating.

Cutaneous arteriovenous anastomoses constrict particularly strongly in response to the catecholamines. This is not due to a greater shortening of the smooth muscle elements in their walls but is attributable to the high wall-to-lumen ratio in these arteriovenous shunt vessels.

Cerebral Vessels

The deep cerebral vascular circuit is featured by a relative paucity of terminal arterioles and precapillary sphincters compared with that such as is displayed by other systemic regional vascular beds (129). The terminal arterioles and precapillary sphincters are grouped as resistance vessels (56) and in other vascular beds receive a dense innervation by sympathetic noradrenergic fibers. The cerebral vascular circuit, however, demonstrates a relatively sparse sympathetic innervation, and it is generally agreed that cerebral vascular resistance is mainly determined by local chemical factors, of which the most important is the hydrogen ion concentration of the cerebral interstitial fluid (56, 129).

Norepinephrine, given intravenously in doses sufficient to provoke systemic hypertension, reduces deep cerebral blood flow but does not alter cerebral oxygen usage. Epinephrine, however, increases cerebral oxygen usage, and the increased cerebral blood flow that occurs during an intravenous infusion of epinephrine is probably attributable to the increased concentration of metabolites and hydrogen ion concentration acting locally on the cerebral arterioles (90). In experiments on isolated 4-mm lengths of the middle cerebral artery of the cat, Nielsen & Owman (117) found epinephrine to be a more effective constrictor than norepinephrine, although norepinephrine exerted its action more promptly. Hence the cerebral vasodilatation seen during intravenous infusion of epinephrine is indeed probably due to the metabolic effects of the drug.

Renal Vessels

Both epinephrine and norepinephrine cause renal vasoconstriction, and direct flow measurements made in the dog (144) show them to be almost equally effective in this respect when given intraarterially in doses of 5 µg. In each case the greatest degree of resistance change is seen in the afferent arterioles (137). Celander (27) measured renal venous outflow directly in the cat and was unable to find a consistent decrease in flow in response to either catecholamine even when they were infused in amounts up to 1 µg/kg·min. Such a dosage is very large compared with the amounts of catecholamine that can be maximally secreted from the adrenal medullae. Celander reported that 5–8 µg/kg·min of catecholamine infused intravenously was required to lower renal blood flow to 50% of its control value. Electrical stimulation of the renal sympathetic nerves produced a much greater degree of vasoconstriction.

In the autonomic response to hemorrhage, adrenal medullary secretion plays a relatively minor role (94, 95) compared with that of the sympathetic discharge.

Splanchnic and Hepatic Vessels

In the perfused liver, both epinephrine and norepinephrine exert a vasoconstrictor action at all dosage levels.

In man, Bradley (19) found that the intramuscular injection of 1 mg epinephrine increased hepatic flow. Beam et al. (14) showed that an intravenous infusion of epinephrine of 0.1 µg/kg·min increased liver blood flow but almost doubled splanchnic oxygen usage. Norepinephrine, which exerted only a minor effect on splanchnic oxygen usage, reduced hepatic blood flow.

The intestinal vessels are constricted by epinephrine or norepinephrine when infused intravenously (69), but the peak vasoconstriction is transient and vascular resistance returns toward the control level during the perfusion (8, 35). This "autoregulatory escape" also features the response of the intestinal vessels to sympathetic vasoconstrictor fiber stimulation and at least in part seems to be due to a redistribution of blood flow from mucosal to submucosal vessels (113).

Korner and his colleagues (157) have demonstrated that adrenal medullary secretion plays an important role in accentuating the rise in portal vascular resistance caused by hypoxia in the rabbit.

Coronary Vessels

Epinephrine and norepinephrine can cause an increase in coronary blood flow (15), but this has been attributed by many workers to the stimulation of myocardial cells that leak vasodilator metabolites rather than to a direct effect on the coronary arteries (67, 68, 126, 127). However, β adrenergic receptor activity, as manifested by coronary relaxation, has been demonstrated in isolated strips of the coronary arteries immersed in solutions containing catecholamines (17, 164). Similarly catecholamines have been shown to cause vasodilatation in the coronary vessels of the nonbeating heart (33). After blockade of β receptors, coronary vasoconstriction has been documented in thoracotomized animals. Pitt et al.

(127) studied the effect of intravenous and intracoronary injections of epinephrine and norepinephrine on coronary flow in unanesthetized dogs. Intracoronary norepinephrine administration increased mean coronary blood flow by about 50% before heart rate or aortic pressure changes. After β receptor blockade, epinephrine decreased coronary flow. They concluded that there are α receptors in the coronary vessels and that the effects of either epinephrine or norepinephrine may depend on the relative proportions of α and β adrenergic receptors.

Pulmonary Vessels

Daly & Hebb (32) have reviewed the effects of catecholamines on the pulmonary vascular circuit critically. In some species (e.g., the dog), under certain circumstances, epinephrine and norepinephrine can cause dilatation, but usually both are constrictor. The rat, guinea pig, rabbit, and cat show mainly or purely vasoconstrictor responses to epinephrine and norepinephrine.

That sympathetic nervous stimulation causes vasoconstriction in the pulmonary vascular circuit of the dog was unequivocally demonstrated by Daly in 1958 (32). These neurogenic effects on pulmonary flow resistance are usually fairly weak; even maximal sympathetic stimulation seldom increases the resistance more than by about 30%. However, sympathetic vasoconstriction may be important in reducing pulmonary capacity and thereby expelling substantial fractions of the pulmonary blood reservoir to the left heart. This may be the really significant response of the pulmonary circuit either to sympathetic discharge or to circulating catecholamines.

It has hitherto been inferred that the effects of sympathetic stimulation or those of catecholamine infusion on pulmonary vascular resistance (PVR) are solely due to constriction of the arteries, arterioles, and veins of the pulmonary circuit. Lately, however, some additional and perhaps important effects of catecholamines have been reported.

Hemorrhagic systemic arterial hypertension causes a marked rise in PVR. Bø & Hognestad (18) have investigated the role of the catecholamines liberated from the adrenal medullae in contributing to this increase in PVR that occurs after blood loss. The normal blood catecholamine concentration of 1 µg/liter rises to 20–100 µg/liter during hemorrhagic hypotension (131) mainly because of the outpouring of adrenal catecholamines. Bleeding induces a rise of PVR, which is much greater when the adrenal glands are innervated than when the nerves supplying the glands are cut. Hemorrhagic hypotension normally causes a fall in the number of circulating thrombocytes, but this thrombocytopenia is much less marked if bleeding is carried out after adrenal denervation. Mustard & Packham (115) showed that the infusion of catecholamines induces the aggregation of thrombocytes; the aggregates liberate vasoconstrictor substances. In keeping with these results, Bø and Hognestad found that the infusion of catecholamines into animals subjected to adrenal denervation and bleeding not only caused a rise of pulmonary vascular resistance but simultaneously induced a fall in their thrombocyte count. The mechanism whereby increased blood catecholamine concentrations induce thrombocytic aggregation is not believed to be direct (153). However, Bø & Hognestad (18) have also demonstrated that the pulmonary vascular resistance does not rise much when thrombocytopenic animals are bled, which indicates that thrombocytic aggregation is responsible, if indirectly, for the striking increase of pulmonary resistance.

Veins

The earlier references to the influence of epinephrine on venous tone and capacity are reviewed by Franklin (59).

Epinephrine and norepinephrine constrict the veins of the systemic and pulmonary circuits (4, 5, 47, 113). Again the effect of the circulating catecholamines seems subservient to that of the sympathetic discharge to these structures. Nevertheless their contribution to the reduction in capacity of the vascular bed, which aids in the maintenance of venous return to the heart, should not be ignored. Mellander (112) showed that the administration of epinephrine in such amounts as to elicit pronounced dilatation in the muscle often caused constriction of the venules and veins. Mellander & Johansson (113) have suggested that the β receptors are localized predominantly in the precapillary resistance vessels, whereas the α receptors are distributed to both the precapillary and postcapillary sections of the muscle vascular bed.

Few electrophysiological studies of the smooth muscle of veins have been made, except on the longitudinal muscle of mammalian portal and anterior mesenteric veins. Circular smooth muscle in the anterior mesenteric veins rarely shows spontaneous electrical activity, unlike that of longitudinal muscle, which usually does (87, 88, 143, 149). Spontaneous electrical activity of the longitudinal muscle of the portal vein is increased by norepinephrine and epinephrine (80). Each catecholamine in high concentration depolarizes the isolated rat portal vein and converts the bursts of action potentials, which decline in amplitude as the depolarization develops. Johansson et al. (87), who recorded these observations of norepinephrine, were uncertain whether the reduction in amplitude of the action potentials represented asynchrony of electrical activity or a depolarization of such degree that an action potential could not develop. By using intracellular recording, Funaki and Bohr (61, 62) found that epinephrine did cause progressive depolarization to a degree that was incompatible with the development of an action potential.

CATECHOLAMINES AND CARDIAC FUNCTION

Both epinephrine and norepinephrine directly exert positive chronotropic, inotropic, and dromotropic effects on the heart. Östlund (123) obtained marked positive chronotropic and inotropic responses when either the isolated squid heart or the isolated rat heart was perfused with solutions containing either catecholamine in a concentration of 0.01 µg/ml.

Catecholamines and Heart Rate— Electrophysiological Studies

Single fibers of spontaneously beating cultures of embryonic chick heart can be impaled by microelectrodes, and the action potentials they develop are similar to those manifest by cells in the adult sinoatrial node (163). In cultures of cardiac tissue from young embryos, typical pacemaker potentials can be recorded in many single fibers of either the atrium or the ventricle, but in cultures of cardiac tissue obtained from older embryos, ventricular fibers and most of the atrial fibers lose this pacemaker activity.

When single cardiac cells of the ventricle of the adult heart are impaled, the resting membrane potential is about 85–90 mv (inside negative to outside). The fibers are not themselves spontaneously active but can be excited electrically, whereupon there is a rapid depolarization of the membrane and the transmembrane potential quickly changes from −90 mv to about +20 mv. This fulminant depolarization constitutes the upstroke of the action potential and is similar in cardiac fibers of either atrium or ventricle. Repolarization in atrial fibers occurs at a fairly constant speed, but in ventricular fibers, after an initial sharp fall of transmembrane potential from +20 to near 0 mv, the transmembrane potential is maintained at approximately 0 mv for 150–200 msec before the final repolarization occurs fairly abruptly [Fig. 4; (23, 31, 34, 78, 159, 160)]. During diastole the transmembrane resting potential remains

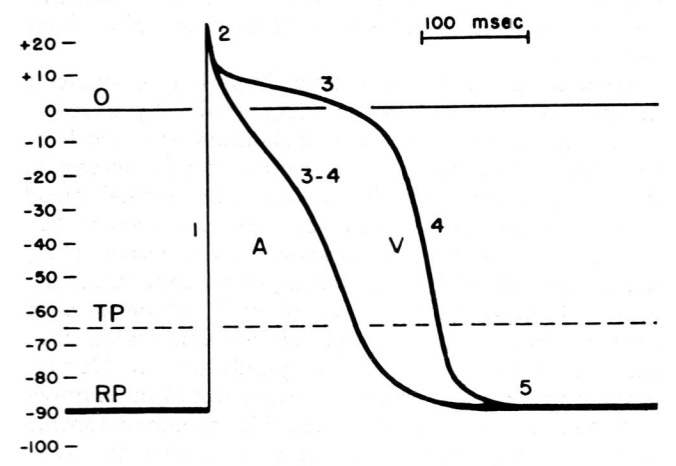

FIG. 4. Schematic representation of transmembrane potentials of atrial (*A*) and ventricular (*V*) muscle. *O*, line of zero potential; *TP*, threshold potential; *RP*, resting potential. *Numbers* refer to different phases of action potential: *1*, depolarization; *2*, reversal; *3*, plateau; *4*, repolarization; *5*, steady level of resting potential. [From Hoffman (78a).]

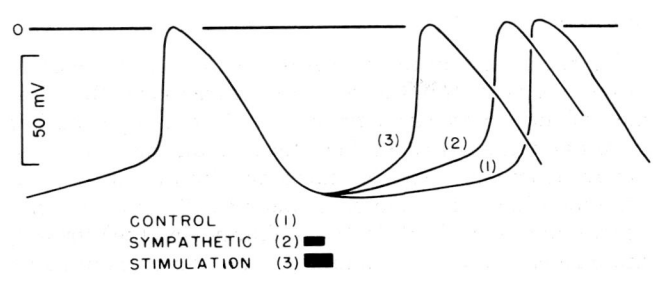

FIG. 5. Schematic representation of transmembrane potentials recorded from sinoatrial pacemaker fiber during sympathetic stimulation. Area of *dark bars* indicates relative strength of stimulation. [From Hoffman (78a).]

unchanged until the arrival of a propagated excitation wave.

Excitation occurs as a result of a shift in the membrane potential from the resting level toward zero level. If the membrane potential is reduced to a critical level (−55 mv), the threshold potential depolarization becomes regenerative and the action potential "takes off."

Cells of the sinoatrial node, certain atrial cells, and cells in the His-Purkinje tissue exhibit automaticity. Some of these show spontaneous phase 5 depolarization (Fig. 5) of a degree sufficient to reach the threshold potential, which propagates and excites neighboring cells; the cell initiating such an action potential is termed a *pacemaker*. Other automatic cells demonstrate latent pacemaker activity characterized by a slow depolarization in phase 5, which is, however, inadequate of itself to reach the critical threshold value required to initiate an action potential (84, 118, 154).

The true pacemaker cells are found in the sinoatrial node. Three major variables influence the rate of beat of the pacemaker cells: *1*) the magnitude of the resting potential achieved after completion of repolarization; *2*) the slope of the pacemaker potential; and *3*) the level of the threshold potential.

The resting potential of sinoatrial node cells is lower than that of neighboring atrial cells, and the slope of their pacemaker potential is higher. It is for such reasons that sinoatrial node activity determines the rate of the heart.

The direct electrophysiological observation of the effects of sympathetic stimulation on the natural pacemaker has been possible only on the sinus venosus of the frog heart (84, 154). Sympathetic stimulation increases the slope of the pacemaker potential and accelerates the beat rate. The application of epinephrine or norepinephrine to the sinoatrial node of the rabbit heart produces similar results.

The application of catecholamine through a micropipette to a latent pacemaker area (i.e., a cell or group of cells that do show pacemaker potentials, albeit of a smaller slope than that of the sinoatrial node fibers) often results in a shift of the pacemaker to the site of application. The addition of epinephrine to the fluid bathing excised Purkinje cells increases their rate of beat and likewise increases the slope of their pacemaker potentials (124, 154). Such observations account for the incidence of extrasystoles after intravenous injections of catecholamines. These are especially prone to occur in the intact animal after the intravenous injection of epinephrine or norepinephrine in amounts that provoke systemic hypertension and reflex vagal inhibition of the sinoatrial node; this nodal inhibition favors the development of heterotopic pacemakers.

The effect of catecholamines on the slope of the pacemaker potential and on the rate of spontaneous rhythm has been investigated thoroughly during the last 20 years. Catecholamines do not greatly influence the resting conductance or the sodium conductance involved in generating the action potential (155). Noble, Trautwein, and their colleagues have used voltage clamp techniques to study the changes in time- and voltage-dependent current that underlie the pacemaker potential in Purkinje fibers (70, 118, 119). The most important time-dependent change in the pacemaker potential is a decrease in the potassium current (i_{K_2}) after repolarization at the end of the action potential (119, 158). This reduction in i_{K_2} allows the inward background currents to cause progressive depolarization of the membrane (Fig. 6) until the threshold membrane potential is reached, from which the action potential fulminantly develops. Hauswirth et al. (70) showed that epinephrine accelerates this rate of decay of the potassium current and that pronethalol, which blocks β receptors, abolishes this effect of epinephrine.

Vagal excitation (or acetylcholine) causes hyperpolarization of the pacemaker cells and reduces or abolishes the slope of the pacemaker potential. These

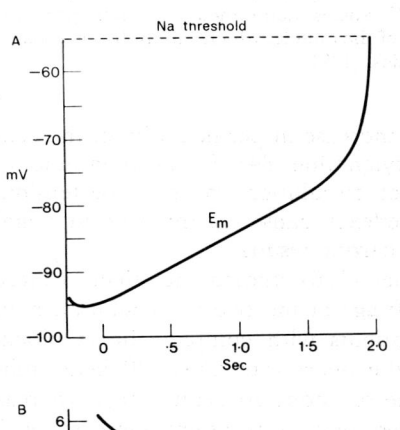

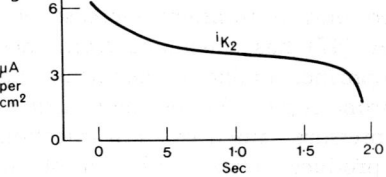

FIG. 6. *A*: variation in membrane potential (E_m) during pacemaker activity. [Adapted from Vassalle (158).] *B*: changes in potassium current (i_{K_2}) calculated from voltage clamp results. [Adapted from Noble & Tsien (119).]

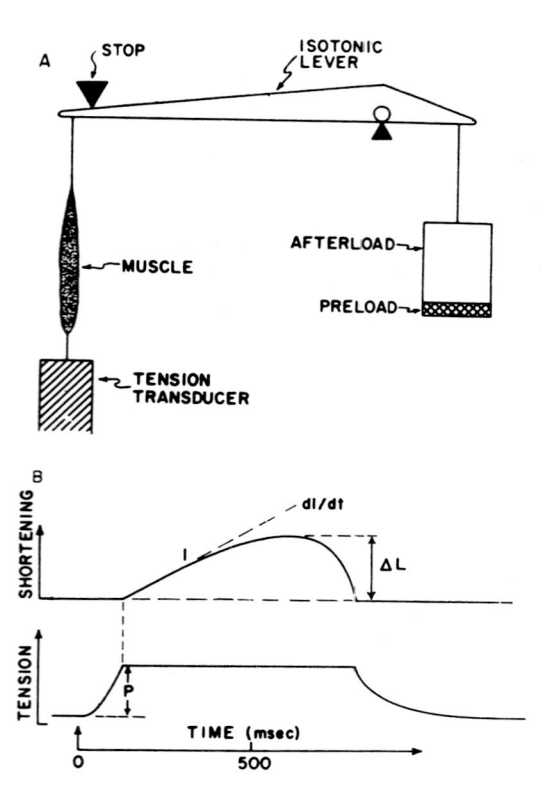

FIG. 7. Afterloaded isotonic contraction. *A*: schematic diagram of apparatus. Cat papillary muscle is attached below to *tension transducer*. Free upper end of muscle is connected to *isotonic lever*. Initial length of muscle is established by small *preload*. A *stop*, which keeps initial length of muscle constant before onset of contraction, is then set. Loads added to preload are only encountered by muscle with onset of contraction. *B*: recording of force (*tension*) and *shortening* for an afterloaded contraction. With stimulation, force development begins. When force (*P*) equals load, shortening begins at a maximal rate (*dl/dt* or *V*) and is maintained for a short period of time. Δ*L*, net shortening of the muscle, which equals distance load is moved. [From Sonnenblick (139).]

effects are due to an increase in permeability of the cells to K^+ caused by acetylcholine (84). If catecholamine infusion into the intact circulation causes hypertension, then baroreceptor reflexes cause an increase in vagal discharge and bradycardia results.

Nathanson & Miller (116) studied the effect of large intravenous doses (30 µg) of the two catecholamines on the heart rate of patients with complete heart block. Epinephrine raised the heart rate about 30 beats/min (from a control value of about 40 beats/min), whereas norepinephrine caused only a transient increase of 5 beats/min. Von Euler (47) has concluded from these results that norepinephrine, unlike epinephrine, has only a slight direct chronotropic effect on the ventricles. However, the rise of pressure caused by both injections was such as might produce reflex inhibition of the sympathetic fibers supplying the ventricular pacemaker cells, and norepinephrine caused a greater increase of systolic and pulse pressure in this experiment.

Conduction Velocity

Epinephrine slightly increases the conduction velocity in the dog heart and shortens the ventricular QRS complex of the electrocardiogram (21). Norepinephrine has a similar but slightly weaker effect. Transmission in the atrioventricular node is markedly improved with a corresponding reduction of as much as 40 % in the atrioventricular delay (110, 150). As Trautwein (154) stresses, the effects of the catecholamines and sympathomimetic agents on conduction velocity do not explain the arrhythmias they may produce. Such arrhythmias are essentially due to the enhanced tendency of the fibers of the conduction system to produce spontaneous excitation.

Inotropic Effects of Catecholamines

ISOLATED PAPILLARY MUSCLE PREPARATION. The slim, cylindrical shape of the isolated cardiac papillary muscle allows its use in experiments conducted in the muscle bath, where its contractile performance in response to a single electrical stimulation can be studied (1, 140, 141). Both isometric and isotonic contractions can be analyzed.

The initial length of the muscle is established by a small preload and fixed by the micrometer stop above the lever (Fig. 7). Thereafter additional loads added to the preload can have no effect on the resting muscle length but are encountered by the muscle only as it contracts. Such additional loads are termed *afterload*. Obviously the total load during muscle contraction is equal to the preload plus the afterload. Adjustment of the lever system allows isometric recording. The tension developed during isometric contraction is increased (up to a point) by increasing the resting length of the muscle before stimulation (Fig. 8). This of course is a demonstration of the Frank-Starling principle—that the force of contraction developed is proportional to the "end-diastolic" length of the fibers. When norepinephrine or epinephrine is added to the muscle bath (0.05 µg/ml),

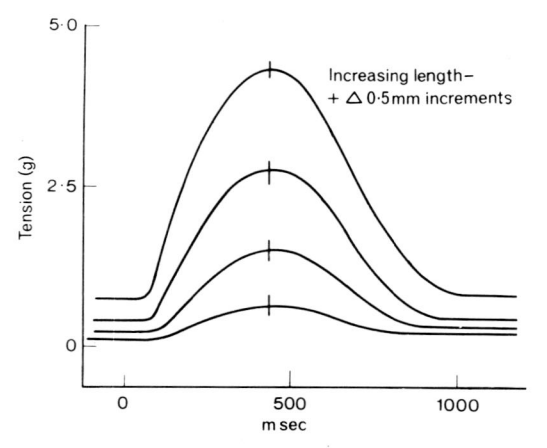

FIG. 8. Four superimposed isometric muscle twitches obtained from cat papillary muscle. From below upward, 4 twitches were obtained at initial lengths of 8.5, 9.0, 9.5, and 10.0 mm. [From Sonnenblick (139).]

velocity of contraction (Fig. 11). This increase in the maximal velocity of contraction of the muscle indicates that the catecholamines accelerate the rate-determining processes of the contractile mechanism of cardiac muscle.

Sonnenblick (140) has expanded these studies in his investigation of the active state in cardiac papillary muscle by using a modified quick-release method. His results bear out the earlier conclusions of Abbott & Mommaerts (1) and others (20, 97) that there is some delay in the development of the active state but that this can be abbreviated by the catecholamines. Norepinephrine accelerates the onset of the active state, increases its

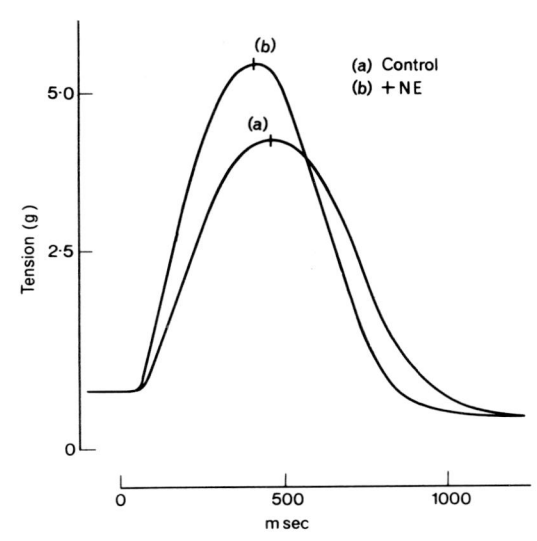

FIG. 9. Two isometric muscle twitches obtained at same initial length; a, control twitch; b, twitch obtained when norepinephrine (NE) was added to bathing solution to a concentration of 0.5 µg/ml. [From Sonnenblick (139).]

however, the contraction provoked at any given resting length occurs more briskly, develops a higher tension, and subsides more quickly (Fig. 9). This is designated a positive inotropic effect and must be clearly differentiated from the change in performance caused by altering the initial length of the muscle.

The results of isometric recordings are difficult to analyze satisfactorily because of the structural arrangement of the cardiac muscle fibers. These comprise a contractile element in series with an elastic element. The active state developed by the contractile element causes changes in the elastic elements. Hence isotonic recording is necessary in studying the force-velocity relations of cardiac muscle accurately and thus to investigate the influence of catecholamines on such performance. In isotonic recording, when the muscle is stimulated, its contractile elements begin to shorten, and thereby the series elastic elements are stretched and external force is developed. Once the force generated equals the load, the afterload is lifted and force thereafter remains constant. While the afterload is being moved, the series elastic elements are of constant length and muscle shortening is recorded as the shortening of the contractile elements only.

The force-velocity relation can be studied either at different resting lengths or at any one muscle length, with and without the addition of catecholamines to the muscle bath. In Figure 10 the force-velocity relation of the muscle is illustrated at two initial lengths. It will be noted that, although the force the muscle develops is increased by increasing its initial length, the maximal velocity it can achieve (with negligible load) is not. However, when norepinephrine is added the muscle can develop not only a greater force but also a greater

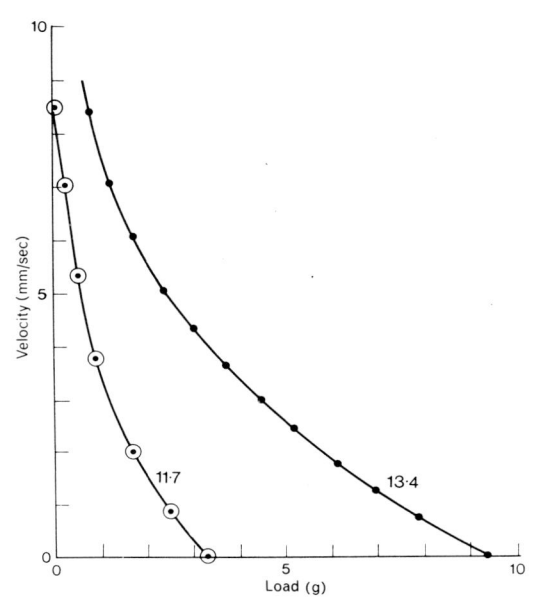

FIG. 10. Force-velocity curves for papillary cardiac muscle. Initial muscle lengths were 11.7 and 13.4 mm. Note that when initial length is greater, muscle develops a greater P_0 (maximal force) but not a greater V_{max}. [From Sonnenblick (139).]

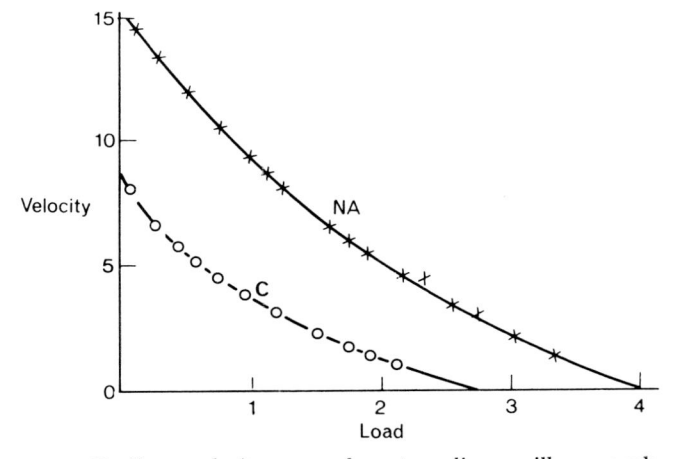

FIG. 11. Force-velocity curves for cat cardiac papillary muscle (velocity in mm/sec, load in g). C, control; NA, after addition of norepinephrine (0.05 µg/ml) to muscle bath. Norepinephrine increases both P_0 and V_{max} (positive inotropic action). [From Sonnenblick (139).]

maximum intensity, shortens its duration, and accelerates its rate of decline.

This delay in the onset of the activation state is worth noting. Hill (75) suggested that the diffusion of an activating substance from a superficial site along a skeletal muscle 100 μ in diameter would not be rapid enough to explain the rapidity of activation. More recently, evidence has accumulated that the sarcoplasmic reticulum releases calcium in the immediate vicinity of each sarcomere and that Ca^{2+} diffuses only a short distance to induce contraction. The sarcoplasmic reticulum is much more sparse in cardiac than in skeletal muscle, but the cardiac fiber has a diameter of only 5–10 μ, so it is not unlikely that activation follows release of some activating substance, such as Ca^{2+}, from the superficial site (99). Entman et al. (43) have claimed that the positive inotropic effects of epinephrine may result from an increase in the sarcotubular calcium pool, which induces activation of an adenylate cyclase localized to the sarcoplasmic reticulum; the increased adenylate cyclase concentration itself activated by epinephrine causes the production of cyclic 3',5'-AMP. The increased concentration of cyclic AMP augments myocardial contractility (110).

HEART-LUNG PREPARATION. The fundamental relation between the initial length of skeletal muscle and its force of contraction was described by Fick (52) in 1882 and by Blix (16) in 1895. Frank (58) in 1895 extended these results to cardiac muscle, and Starling in the Linacre Lecture of 1915 summarized his results on the performance of the dog heart-lung preparation (145). Starling stated

The law of the heart is therefore the same as that of skeletal muscle, namely that the mechanical energy set free on passage from the resting to the contracted state depends on the area of "chemically active surfaces", i.e. on the length of the muscle fibre.

In the same lecture, Starling stated

If a man starts to run his muscular movements pump more blood into the heart. As a result the heart is over filled. Its volume, both in systole and diastole, enlarge progressively until by the lengthening of the muscle fibres so much more active surfaces are brought into play within the fibres that the energy of the contraction becomes sufficient to drive on into the aorta during each systole the largely increased volume of blood entering the heart from the veins during diastole.

Such a statement by itself does not take into account the influence of the cardiac sympathetic nerves or that of circulating catecholamines. However, in a lecture given in 1920, Starling (146) indicated that the effect of such agents might well serve to offset the increase of end-diastolic volume so that the cardiac dilatation "becomes imperceptible in the intact animal and is not revealed, for instance, by any radiographic study of the heart during exercise."

Sarnoff and his colleagues (134) showed that catecholamines or cardiac sympathetic stimulation strikingly increased the external work of the paced heart developed from any given left ventricular end-diastolic pressure (Fig. 12). A family of so-called ventricular function curves can be obtained in this manner.

Linden (101) has demonstrated that the maximal rate of development of pressure during the isometric phase of left ventricular contraction (dP/dt_{max}) is considerably increased either by the infusion of catecholamines or by stimulation of the cardiac sympathetic fibers.

Covell et al. (30) have carried out force-velocity studies on the intact heart and have shown that the force-velocity relation is more sensitive than is the ventricular function curve in revealing the positive inotropic effects of catecholamines or of other agents. The force-velocity relations of the ventricle are not afterload dependent and provide information regarding both speed and force in the myocardium—two factors that may not be altered to the same extent, or even in the same direction.

The most direct application of the force-velocity relation in the intact heart is with the single isovolumic beat (secured by inflating a balloon in the aortic root during diastole to prevent ventricular ejection during the following beat). During isovolumic systole, fiber shortening must be zero, so the velocity of contraction of the con-

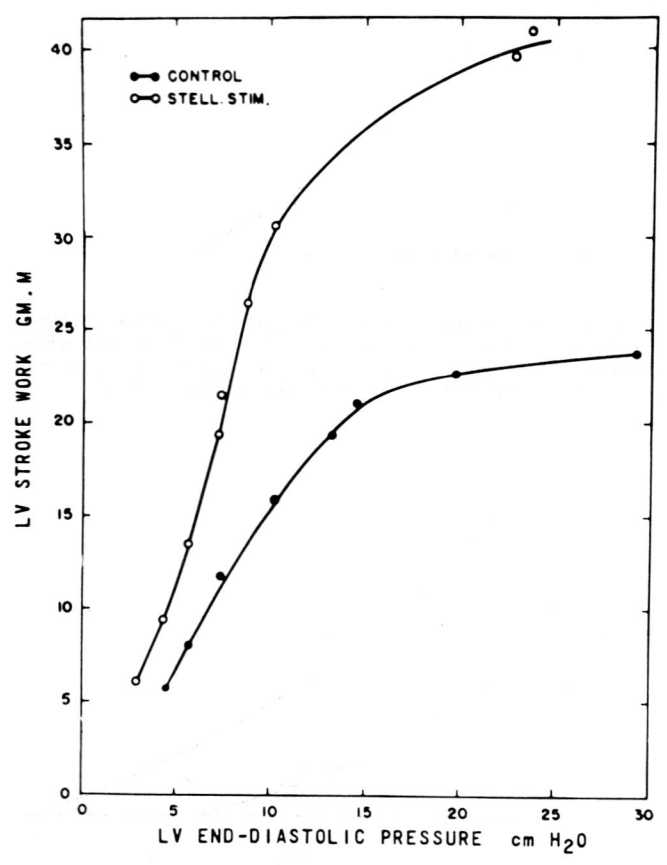

FIG. 12. Relation between left ventricular (*LV*) stroke work (in gram meters, *GM.M*) and end-diastolic pressure in ventricle before (*closed circles*) and during (*open circles*) stimulation of left stellate ganglion (*STELL. STIM.*), freed except for nerves to the heart. Both vagi sectioned in neck. Constant heart rate of 171 beats/min throughout. [From Sarnoff & Mitchell (134).]

tractile element (V_{CE}) must be offset by the velocity of lengthening of the series elastic element (V_{SE}). The series elastic element is an exponential spring, hence its velocity of lengthening is the rate of tension development (dT/dt) divided by its modulus of elasticity (dT/dl), which is a measurement of stiffness (141). As dT/dl is linearly related to the tension or stress

$$dT/dl = kT + C$$

where k and C are constants

$$V_{SE} = \frac{dT/dt}{kT + C}$$

$$T = \frac{PR_i^2}{R_o^2 - R_i^2}$$

where R_i and R_o are the internal and external radii of the ventricle and P is the intraventricular pressure.

In the isovolumic phase of contraction

$$\frac{dT/dt}{kT + C} = \frac{dP/dt}{kP + C} = V_{SE} = V_{CE}$$

Studies of this nature have revealed that, in the intact heart, increasing preload causes an increase in maximal tension developed during contraction but does not increase the maximal speed of contraction. The infusion of catecholamines increases both the maximal tension and the maximal speed of contraction.

The Hill equation (74) for skeletal muscle states

$$(P + a)V = (P_0 - P)b$$

where a equals the heat release associated with shortening and P equals the load. When P equals zero, V is maximal (V_{max}). The ratio a/P_0 in cardiac muscle is constant so V_{max} varies directly with b, which is the rate constant for the energy flux from the contractile elements as a function of the load. Thus V_{max} is proportional to the rate of turnover of the force-generating process. As the catecholamines increase V_{max}, one might expect that they should increase myocardial oxygen usage, $M\dot{V}O_2$.

Myocardial Oxygen Usage

Sonnenblick et al. (142) list the most important determinants of $M\dot{V}O_2$ as: *a*) intramyocardial tension (stress), which depends on intraventricular pressure, volume, and myocardial mass (132)

$$T = \frac{PR_i^2}{R_o^2 - R_i^2}$$

b) heart rate, which determines the cumulative tension developed; *c*) the contractile state characterized by V_{max}; *d*) the energy associated with shortening against load (i.e., the external work of the heart); and *e*) the resting metabolism of the heart.

The equation

$$T = \frac{PR_i^2}{R_o^2 - R_i^2}$$

indicates that the endocardiac pressure is a measure of the tension if the initial volume of the heart is not altered, as noted in 1915 by Evans & Matsuoka (50).

Evans and Matsuoka concluded that the major determinant of $M\dot{V}O_2$ was the aortic pressure. Sarnoff et al. (133) found a good correlation between $M\dot{V}O_2$ and the tension-time index—the total area under the ventricular pressure pulse multiplied by the number of beats per minute—which gives the time that tension is maintained. Monroe & French (114), however, showed that the release of pressure in an isovolumetrically contracting ventricle, midway through the course of systole, reduced $M\dot{V}O_2$ by only 10%. They concluded that the development of tension, rather than its maintenance, was the main determinant of $M\dot{V}O_2$. Gregg (67) found little correlation between integrated pressure and $M\dot{V}O_2$ during exercise or during cardiac sympathetic nerve stimulation. Sonnenblick et al. (142) showed that catecholamine infusions, calcium infusions, and paired electrical stimulation of the ventricle, alone or in concert, strikingly increased $M\dot{V}O_2$ and the velocity of myocardial fiber shortening but always lowered the tension-time index. They proposed that the velocity of myocardial contraction was the main determinant of $M\dot{V}O_2$. Previously, Sarnoff et al. (133) had found that catecholamines did not increase $M\dot{V}O_2$, despite their undoubted efficacy in promoting increased contractility. Graham et al. (64) have resolved the problem by showing that the effect of norepinephrine on $M\dot{V}O_2$ depends on its two influences—that of reducing the end-diastolic volume and that of its positive inotropic action. The decrease in ventricular volume leads to a decrease in intramyocardial tension required to develop intraventricular pressure and hence tends to reduce $M\dot{V}O_2$. The positive inotropic action of the catecholamine (i.e., its effect on contractility) increases $M\dot{V}O_2$. The net result of these two opposing effects is an increase of contractility with little or no change in $M\dot{V}O_2$.

Thus any positive inotropic agent (e.g., acetylstrophanthidin) given in heart failure with ventricular dilatation reduces $M\dot{V}O_2$ by decreasing heart size, despite the increase of that fraction of the oxygen usage required by the augmented contractility. When the same drug is administered to a normal individual, the increased $M\dot{V}O_2$ caused by increased contractility usually offsets the decrease of oxygen usage caused by the reduction in the end-diastolic volume.

The mammalian heart contains a large amount of norepinephrine, which corresponds to its postganglionic sympathetic nerve supply. In the common laboratory animals the norepinephrine content is 1–2 µg/g heart (79). The frog heart contains only epinephrine and, as first proved by Loewi (105, 106), epinephrine is the chemical transmitter of the sympathetic nerve endings in this species. Goodall (63) showed that denervation of the mammalian heart depleted its norepinephrine content, which was regained as the sympathetic nerve supply regenerated.

Chidsey & Braunwald (29) found that the norepinephrine content of human atria was about 1.8 µg/g, by using material removed at cardiac operation from patients who had no history of heart failure. Atrial tissue from patients who manifested some degree of heart failure contained much lower concentrations of norepinephrine; about 15% of these patients had atrial norepinephrine concentrations less than 10% of the average normal values. In studies of heart failure produced in dogs, tricuspid insufficiency and pulmonary stenosis induced artificially led to right ventricular failure and a right ventricular content of norepinephrine that was grossly reduced compared with normal values. In a discussion of the evidence, Chidsey & Braunwald (29) concluded that the depletion of norepinephrine content of the heart in studies of man and dog was consonant with a diminution of the number of noradrenergic nerve endings in the failing heart. As they point out, the normal heart has the Frank-Starling mechanism and the positive inotropic effect of the catecholamines to aid its performance in conditions of increased circulatory activity. Failure of the heart reduces stroke work at any given diastolic volume, and as a consequence, the heart tends to enlarge. If the sympathetic nerves are functionally active, however, this tendency to dilatation can be combated by increased cardiac sympathetic activity. Once the sympathetic influence wanes in magnitude and efficacy, cardiac function has no extrinsic support.

REFERENCES

1. ABBOTT, B. C., AND W. F. H. M. MOMMAERTS. A study of inotropic mechanisms in the papillary muscle preparation. *J. Gen. Physiol.* 42: 533–551, 1959.
2. ABEL, J. J., AND A. C. CRAWFORD. On the blood pressure raising constituent of the suprarenal capsule. *Johns Hopkins Hosp. Bull.* 8: 151–157, 1897.
3. AHLQUIST, R. P. A study of the adrenotropic receptors. *Am. J. Physiol.* 153: 586–600, 1948.
4. ALEXANDER, R. S. The influence of constrictor drugs on the distensibility of the splanchnic venous system. *Circulation Res.* 2: 140–147, 1954.
5. ALEXANDER, R. S. The peripheral venous system. In: *Handbook of Physiology. Circulation*, edited by W. F. Hamilton and P. Dow. Washington, D.C.: Am. Physiol. Soc., 1963, sect. 2, vol. II, p. 1075–1098.
6. ALLEN, W. J., H. BARCROFT, AND O. G. EDHOLM. The action of adrenaline on the blood vessels in human skeletal muscle. *J. Physiol., London* 105: 255–267, 1946.
7. BACQ, Z. M. Recherches sur la physiologie du systeme nerveux autonome, et particulièrement du sympathique, d'après la théorie neurohumorale. *Ann. Physiol.* 10: 467–528, 1934.
8. BAKER, R., AND D. MENDEL. Some observations on "autoregulatory escape" in cat intestine. *J. Physiol., London* 190: 229–240, 1967.
9. BARCROFT, H., P. GASKELL, J. T. SHEPHERD, AND R. F. WHELAN. The effect of noradrenaline infusions on the blood flow through the human forearm. *J. Physiol., London* 123: 443–450, 1954.
10. BARCROFT, H., AND H. KONZETT. On the actions of noradrenaline, adrenaline and isopropylnoradrenaline on the arterial blood pressure, heart rate and muscle blood flow in man. *J. Physiol., London* 110: 194–204, 1949.
11. BARCROFT, H., AND H. J. C. SWAN. *Sympathetic Control of Human Blood Vessels*. London: Arnold, 1953, p. 1–165.
12. BARGER, G., AND H. H. DALE. Chemical structure and the sympathomimetic actions of amines. *J. Physiol., London* 41: 19–59, 1910.
13. BAYLISS, W. M., AND E. H. STARLING. The mechanism of pancreatic secretion. *J. Physiol., London* 28: 325–353, 1902.
14. BEARN, A. G., B. BILLING, AND S. SHERLOCK. The effect of adrenaline and noradrenaline on hepatic blood flow and splanchnic carbohydrate metabolism. *J. Physiol., London* 115: 430–441, 1951.
15. BERNE, R. Regulation of coronary blood flow. *Physiol. Rev.* 44: 1–64, 1964.
16. BLIX, M. Die Länge und die Spannung des Muskels. *Skand. Arch. Physiol.* 5: 173–207, 1895.
17. BØ, G., AND J. HOGNESTAD. The role of the adrenal medulla in post hemorrhagic pulmonary hypertension. *Acta Physiol. Scand.* 83: 124–132, 1971.
18. BOHR, D. R. Adrenergic receptors in coronary arteries. *Ann. NY Acad. Sci.* 139: 799–807, 1967.
19. BRADLEY, S. E. The hepatic circulation. In: *Handbook of Physiology. Circulation*, edited by W. H. Hamilton and P. Dow. Washington, D.C.: Am. Physiol. Soc., 1963, sect. 2, vol. II, p. 1387–1438.
20. BRADY, A. J. Active state in cardiac muscle. *Physiol. Rev.* 48: 570–600, 1968.
21. BRENDEL, W., H. GLADEWITZ, F. HILDEBRANDT, AND W. TRAUTWEIN. Elektrophysiologische Untersuchungen am Hertz-Lungen-Präparet nach Starling. *Cardiologia* 18: 345–359, 1951.
22. BRONK, D. W., AND G. STELLA. Afferent impulses in carotid sinus nerve. I. The relation of the discharge from single end organs to arterial blood pressure. *J. Cell. Comp. Physiol.* 1: 113–130, 1932.
23. BROOKS, C. MCC., B. F. HOFMAN, E. E. SUCKLING, AND O. ORIAS. *Excitability of the Heart*. New York: Grune & Stratton, 1955.
24. CANNON, W. B., AND R. G. HOSKINS. The effects of asphyxia, hyperpnoea and sensory stimulation on adrenal secretion. *Am. J. Physiol.* 29: 274–279, 1911.
25. CANNON, W. B., AND D. DE LA PAZ. Emotional stimulation of adrenal secretion. *Am. J. Physiol.* 28: 64–70, 1911.
26. CANNON, W. B., AND J. E. URIDIL. Studies on the conditions of activity in endocrine glands. VIII. Some effects on the denervated heart of stimulating the nerves of the liver. *Am. J. Physiol.* 58: 353–364, 1921.
27. CELANDER, O. The range of control exercised by the sympathico-adrenal system. *Acta Physiol. Scand. Suppl.* 116: 1–132, 1954.
28. CHALMERS, J. P., P. I. KORNER, AND S. W. WHITE. The control of the circulation in skeletal muscle during hypoxia in the rabbit. *J. Physiol., London* 184: 698–716, 1966.
29. CHIDSEY, C. A., AND E. BRAUNWALD. Sympathetic activity and neurotransmitter depletion in congestive heart failure. *Pharmacol. Rev.* 18: 685–700, 1966.
30. COVELL, J. W., J. ROSS, JR., E. H. SONNENBLICK, AND E. BRAUNWALD. Comparison of the force-velocity relation and the ventricular function curve as measures of the contractile state of the intact heart. *Circulation Res.* 19: 364–372, 1966.
31. CRANEFIELD, P. F., AND B. F. HOFFMAN. Electrophysiology of single cardiac cells. *Physiol. Rev.* 38: 41–76, 1958.
32. DALY, I. DE B., AND C. O. HEBB. *Pulmonary and Bronchial Vascular Systems*. London: Arnold, 1966, p. 1–432.
33. DOUTHEIL, U. Wirkung von Brenzcatechinaminen auf die

Coronardurchblutung an asystolischen Hundeherzen. *Arch. Ges. Physiol.* 287: 111–123, 1966.
34. DRAPER, M. H., AND S. WEIDMANN. Cardiac resting and action potentials recorded with an intracellular electrode. *J. Physiol., London* 115: 75–94, 1951.
35. DRESEL, P., AND L. WALLENTIN. Effects of sympathetic vasoconstrictor fibres, noradrenaline and vasopressin on the intestinal vascular resistance during constant blood flow or blood pressure. *Acta Physiol. Scand.* 66: 427–436, 1966.
36. DREYER, G. P. Secretory nerve to the suprarenal capsules. *Am. J. Physiol.* 2: 203–219, 1899.
37. DUFF, R. S. Effect of adrenaline and noradrenaline on blood vessels of the hand before and after sympathectomy. *J. Physiol., London* 129: 53–64, 1955.
38. DUFF, R. S., AND H. J. C. SWAN. Further observations on the effect of adrenaline on the blood flow through skeletal muscle. *J. Physiol., London* 114: 41–55, 1951.
39. EAD, H. W., J. H. GREEN, AND E. NEIL. A comparison of the effects of pulsatile and nonpulsatile blood flow through the carotid sinus on the reflexogenic activity of the sinus baroreceptors in the cat. *J. Physiol., London* 118: 509–519, 1952.
40. EDHOLM, O. G., R. H. FOX, AND R. K. MCPHERSON. Effect of body heating on the circulation in skin and muscle. *J. Physiol., London* 134: 612–619, 1956.
41. ELLIOTT, T. R. The action of adrenaline. *J. Physiol., London* 32: 401–467, 1905.
42. ELLIOTT, T. R. The control of the adrenal glands by the splanchnic nerves. *J. Physiol., London* 44: 374–409, 1912.
43. ENTMAN, M. L., G. S. LEVEY, AND S. E. EPSTEIN. Mechanism of action of epinephrine and glucagon on the canine heart. *Circulation Res.* 25: 429–438, 1969.
44. ERÄNKÖ, O. On the histochemistry of the adrenal medulla of the rat with special reference to acid phosphatase. *Acta Anat.* 16, Suppl. 17, 1952.
45. ERÄNKÖ, O. The histochemical demonstration of noradrenaline in the adrenal medulla of rats and mice. *J. Histochem. Cytochem.* 4: 11–13, 1956.
46. EULER, U. S. VON. A specific sympathomimetic ergone in adrenergic nerve fibres (sympathin) and its relation to adrenaline and noradrenaline. *Acta Physiol. Scand.* 12: 73–97, 1946.
47. EULER, U. S. VON. Noradrenaline, chemistry, physiology, pharmacology and clinical aspects. Springfield, Ill.: Thomas, 1956.
48. EULER, U. S. VON, AND U. HAMBERG. L-Noradrenaline in the suprarenal medulla. *Nature* 163: 642–643, 1949.
49. EULER, U. S. VON, AND F. LISHAWKO. Improved technique for the fluorometric determination of catecholamines. *Acta Physiol. Scand.* 51: 348–361, 1961.
50. EVANS, C. L., AND Y. MATSUOKA. The effect of various mechanical conditions on the gaseous metabolism and efficiency of the mammalian heart. *J. Physiol., London* 49: 378–405, 1915.
51. FALCK, B., AND A. TORP. A fluorescence method for histochemical demonstration of noradrenaline in the adrenal medulla. *Med. Exptl.* 5: 429–432, 1961.
52. FICK, A. *Mechanische Arbeit und Wärmeentwicklung beider Muskelthätigkeit.* Leipzig: Brockhaus, 1882.
53. FOLKOW, B. Impulse frequency in sympathetic vasomotor fibres correlated to the release and elimination of the transmitter. *Acta Physiol. Scand.* 25: 49–76, 1952.
54. FOLKOW, B., AND U. S. VON EULER. Selective activation of noradrenaline and adrenaline producing cells in the suprarenal gland of the cat by hypothalamic stimulation. *Circulation Res.* 2: 191–195, 1954.
55. FOLKOW, B., J. HAGGENDAL, AND B. LISSANDER. Extent of release and elimination of noradrenaline at peripheral adrenergic nerve terminals. *Acta Physiol. Scand. Suppl.* 307: 1–38, 1967.
56. FOLKOW, B., AND E. NEIL. *Circulation.* Oxford: Oxford Univ. Press, 1971.
57. FOLKOW, B., AND R. SIVERTSSON. Aspects of the difference in vascular "reactivity" between cutaneous resistance vessels and A-V anastomoses. *Angiologica* 1: 338–345, 1964.

58. FRANK, O. Zur Dynamik der Herzmuskels. *Z. Biol.* 32: 370–447, 1895.
59. FRANKLIN, K. J. *A Monograph on Veins.* Springfield, Ill.: Thomas, 1937, p. 1–410.
60. FUKUDA, T., AND T. KOBAYASHI. On the relation of chemoreceptor stimulation to epinephrine secretion in anoxaemia. *Japan. J. Physiol.* 11: 467–475, 1961.
61. FUNAKI, S. Spontaneous spike-discharges of vascular smooth muscle. *Nature* 191: 1102–1103, 1961.
62. FUNAKI, S., AND D. F. BOHR. Electrical and mechanical activity of isolated vascular smooth muscle of the rat. *Nature* 203: 192–194, 1964.
63. GOODALL, McC. Studies of adrenaline and noradrenaline in mammalian heart and suprarenals. *Acta Physiol. Scand. Suppl.* 85, 1951.
64. GRAHAM, T. P., J. W. COVELL, E. H. SONNENBLICK, J. ROSS, JR., AND E. BRAUNWALD. Control of myocardial oxygen consumption: relative influence of contractile state and tension development. *J. Clin. Invest.* 47: 375–385, 1968.
65. GREEN, H. D., AND J. H. KEPCHAR. Control of peripheral vascular resistance in major systemic vascular beds. *Physiol. Rev.* 39: 617–686, 1959.
66. GREENFIELD, A. D. M. The circulation through the skin. In: *Handbook of Physiology. Circulation,* edited by W. F. Hamilton and P. Dow. Washington, D.C.: Am. Physiol. Soc., 1963, sect. 2, vol. II, p. 1325–1351.
67. GREGG, D. E. Physiology of the coronary circulation. *Circulation* 27: 1128–1137, 1963.
68. GREGG, D. E. The coronary circulation in the unanaesthetised dog. In: *Coronary Circulation and Energetics of the Myocardium,* edited by G. Marchetti and B. Taccardi. Basel: Karger, 1967, p. 54–63.
69. GRIM, E. The flow of blood in the mesenteric vessels. In: *Handbook of Physiology. Circulation,* edited by W. F. Hamilton and P. Dow. Washington, D.C.: Am. Physiol. Soc., 1963, sect. 2, vol. II, p. 1439–1457.
70. HAUSWIRTH, O., D. NOBLE, AND R. W. TSIEN. Adrenaline: mechanism of action on the pacemaker potential in cardiac Purkinje fibres. *Science* 162: 916–917, 1968.
71. HERING, H. E. *Die Karotissinus Reflex auf Herz und Gefässe.* Leipzig: Steinkopff, 1927.
72. HEYMANS, C. *Le Sinus Carotidien et les Autres Zones Vasosensibles Réflexogènes.* London: Lewis, 1929.
73. HEYMANS, C., AND E. NEIL. *Reflexogenic Areas of the Cardiovascular System.* London: Churchill, 1958.
74. HILL, A. V. The heat of shortening and the dynamic constants of muscle. *Proc. Roy. Soc. London Ser. B* 126: 136–195, 1938.
75. HILL, A. V. On the time required for diffusion and its relation to processes in muscle. *Proc. Roy. Soc. London Ser. B* 135: 446–453, 1948.
76. HILL, L. The influence of the force of gravity on the circulation of the blood. *J. Physiol., London* 18: 15–53, 1895.
77. HILLARP, N-Ä., AND B. HÖKFELT. Evidence of adrenaline and noradrenaline in separate adrenal medullary cells. *Acta Physiol. Scand.* 30: 55–68, 1953.
78. HOFFMAN, B. F., AND D. H. SINGER. Appraisal of the effects of catecholamines on cardiac electrical activity. *Ann. NY Acad. Sci.* 139: 914–939, 1967.
78a. HOFFMAN, B. F. Origin of the heart beat. In: *Cardiovascular Functions,* edited by A. A. Luisada. New York: McGraw-Hill, 1962.
79. HÖKFELT, B. Noradrenaline and adrenaline in mammalian tissues. *Acta Physiol. Scand. Suppl.* 92: 1–134, 1951.
80. HOLMAN, M. E., C. B. KASBY, AND M. B. SUTHERS. Some properties of the smooth muscle of rabbit portal vein. *J. Physiol., London* 196: 111–132, 1968.
81. HOLTZ, P., K. KREDNER, AND G. KRONEBERG. Über das sympathico mimetische pressorische Prinzip des Harns ("Urosympathin"). *Arch. Exptl. Pathol. Pharmakol.* 204: 228–243, 1947.
82. HOLTZ, P., AND H-J. SCHÜMANN. Arterenol ein neues Hormon des Nebennierenmarks. *Naturwissenschaften* 5: 159, 1948.

83. HOSKINS, F. G. The relation of the adrenals to the circulation. *Physiol. Rev.* 2: 343–360, 1922.
84. HUTTER, O. F., AND W. TRAUTWEIN. Vagal and sympathetic effects on the pacemaker fibres in the sinus venosus of the heart. *J. Gen. Physiol.* 39: 715–733, 1956.
85. IVERSEN, L. L. The inhibition of noradrenaline uptake by drugs. *Advan. Drug Res.* 2: 5–23, 1965.
86. IVERSEN, L. L. *The Uptake and Storage of Noradrenaline in Sympathetic Nerves*. London: Cambridge, 1967, p. 1–253.
87. JOHANSSON, B., O. JONSSON, J. AXELSSON, AND B. WAHLSTRÖM. Electrical and mechanical characteristics of vascular smooth muscle response to norepinephrine and isoproterenol. *Circulation Res.* 619–633, 1967.
88. JOHANSSON, B., AND B. LJUNG. Sympathetic control of rhythmically active vascular smooth muscle as studied by a nerve-muscle preparation of portal vein. *Acta Physiol. Scand.* 70: 299–311, 1967.
89. KAINDL, F., AND U. S. VON EULER. Liberation of noradrenaline and adrenaline from the suprarenals of the cat during carotid occlusion. *Am. J. Physiol.* 166: 284–288, 1951.
90. KING, B. D., L. SOKOLOFF, AND R. L. WECHSLER. The effects of L-epinephrine and L-norepinephrine upon cerebral circulation and metabolism in man. *J. Clin. Invest.* 31: 373–379, 1952.
91. KOCH, E. *Die Reflektorische Selbsteuerung des Kreislaufes*. Leipzig: Steinkopff, 1931, p. 1–234.
92. KONTOS, H. A., D. W. RICHARDSON, AND J. L. PATTERSON. Relationship between the metabolic and vasodilator effects of epinephrine in human forearm muscle. *Circulation Res.* 21: 679–689, 1967.
93. KORNER, P. I. Integrative neural cardiovascular control. *Physiol. Rev.* 51: 312–367, 1971.
94. KORNER, P., J. P. CHALMERS, AND S. W. WHITE. Some mechanisms of reflex control of the circulation by the sympathoadrenal system. *Circulation Res.* 20, Suppl. III: 157–170, 1967.
95. KORNER, P. I., G. S. STOKES, S. W. WHITE, AND J. P. CHALMERS. Role of the autonomic nervous system in the renal vasoconstriction response to hemorrhage in the rabbit. *Circulation Res.* 20: 676–685, 1967.
96. LANDE, I. S. DE LA, AND R. F. WHELAN. The effect of antagonists on the response of the forearm vessels to adrenaline. *J. Physiol., London* 148: 548–553, 1959.
97. LANGER, G. A. Ion fluxes in cardiac excitation and contraction and their relation to myocardial contractility. *Physiol. Rev.* 48: 708–757, 1968.
98. LANGLEY, J. N. Observations on the physiological actions of extracts of the suprarenal bodies. *J. Physiol., London* 27: 237–256, 1901.
99. LEE, K. S. Role of cardiac sarcoplasmic reticulum in excitation-contraction coupling. In: *Factors Influencing Myocardial Contractility*, edited by R. D. Tanz, F. Kavaler, and J. Roberts. New York: Acad. Press, 1967, p. 363.
100. LEWANDOWSKY, M. Wirkung des Nebennierenextrakts auf die glatten Muskeln der Haut. *Z. Physiol.* 14: 433, 1900.
101. LINDEN, R. J. The heart-ventricular function. *Anaesthesia* 23: 566–584, 1968.
102. LJUNG, B. Use of partial α-receptor blockade for estimation of transmitter concentration at vasoconstrictor nerve endings. *Acta Physiol. Scand.* 73: 6–7A, 1968.
103. LJUNG, B. Local transmitter concentrations in vascular smooth muscle during vasoconstrictor activity. *Acta Physiol. Scand.* 77: 212–223, 1969.
104. LOEWI, O. Über humorale Ubertragbarkeit der Herznervenwirkung. *Arch. Ges. Physiol.* 189: 239–242, 1921.
105. LOEWI, O. Quantitative und qualitative Untersuchungen über den Sympathicusstoff. *Arch. Ges. Physiol.* 237: 504–514, 1936.
106. LOEWI, O. Über den Adrenalingehalt des Säugerherzens. *Arch. Intern. Pharmacodyn.* 57: 139–140, 1937.
107. LUNDHOLM, L. The mechanism of the vasodilator effect of adrenaline. *Acta Physiol. Scand. Suppl.* 133: 1–156, 1956.
108. MALMEJAC, J. Activity of the adrenal medulla and its regulation. *Physiol. Rev.* 44: 186–218, 1964.
109. MATSUDA, K., T. HOSHI, AND S. KAMEYAMA. Action of acetylcholine and adrenaline upon the membrane potential of the atrio-ventricular node (Tawara). *Tohoku J. Exptl. Med.* 68: 16, 1958.
110. MAYER, S. E., B. J. WILLIAMS, AND J. M. SMITH. Adrenergic mechanisms in cardiac glycogen metabolism. *Ann. NY Acad. Sci.* 139: 686–702, 1967.
111. MCDOWALL, R. J. S. *The Control of the Circulation of the Blood*. London: Longmans, Green, 1938, p. 1–619.
112. MELLANDER, S. Comparative studies on the adrenergic neurohumoral control of resistance and capacitance blood vessels in the cat. *Acta Physiol. Scand. Suppl.* 176: 1–86, 1960.
113. MELLANDER, S., AND B. JOHANSSON. Control of resistance, exchange and capacitance functions in the peripheral circulation. *Pharmacol. Rev.* 20: 117–196, 1968.
114. MONROE, R. G., AND G. N. FRENCH. Left ventricular pressure-volume relationships and myocardial oxygen consumption in the isolated heart. *Circulation Res.* 9: 362–374, 1961.
115. MUSTARD, J. F., AND M. A. PACKHAM. Factors influencing platelet function: adhesion, release and aggregation. *Pharmacol. Rev.* 22: 97–187, 1970.
116. NATHANSON, N. H., AND H. MILLER. The action of norepinephrine and of epinephrine on the ventricular rate of heart block. *Am. Heart J.* 40: 374–381, 1950.
117. NIELSEN, K. C., AND C. OWMAN. Contractile response and amine receptor mechanisms in isolated middle cerebral artery of the cat. *Brain Res.* 27: 33–42, 1971.
118. NOBLE, D. Application of Hodgkin-Huxley equations to excitable tissues. *Physiol. Rev.* 46: 1–50, 1966.
119. NOBLE, D., AND R. W. TSIEN. The kinetics and rectifier properties of the slow potassium current in cardiac Purkinje fibres. *J. Physiol., London* 195: 185–214, 1968.
120. OLIVER, G. *Pulse Gauging*. London: Lewis, 1895.
121. OLIVER, G. The action of animal extracts on the peripheral vessels. *J. Physiol., London* 21: 22–23P, 1897.
122. OLIVER, G., AND E. A. SCHÄFER. The physiological effects of extracts of the suprarenal capsules. *J. Physiol., London* 18: 230–276, 1895.
123. ÖSTLUND, E. The distribution of catecholamines in lower animals and their effect on the heart. *Acta Physiol. Scand. Suppl.* 112, 1954.
124. OTSUKA, M. Die Wirkung von Adrenaline auf Purkinje fasem von Säugetierherzen. *Arch. Ges. Physiol.* 266: 512–517, 1968.
125. PEART, W. S. The nature of splenic sympathin. *J. Physiol., London* 108: 491–501, 1949.
126. PITT, B. Sympathetic control of the coronary circulation in the unanaesthetized dog. In: *Coronary Circulation and Energetics of the Myocardium*, edited by G. Marchetti and B. Taccardi. Basel: Karger, 1967, p. 89–95.
127. PITT, B., E. C. ELLIOT, AND D. E. GREGG. Haemodynamic effects of catecholamines on the coronary circulation in the unanaesthetized dog. *Federation Proc.* 25: 401, 1966.
128. POISEUILLE, J. L. M. Recherches expérimentales sur le mouvement des liquides dans les tubes de très petits diamètres. *Mém. Savant Etrangers* 9: 433–544, 1846.
129. PURVES, M. J. *The Physiology of the Cerebral Circulation*. London: Cambridge, 1972.
130. ROSELL, S., AND B. UVNÄS. Vasomotor activity and oxygen uptake in skeletal muscles of the anaesthetized cat. *Acta Physiol. Scand.* 54: 209–222, 1962.
131. ROSENBERG, J. C., R. C. LILLEHEI, J. LONGERBEAM, AND B. ZIMMERMANN. Studies on hemorrhagic shock and endotoxin shock in relation to vasomotor changes and circulating epinephrine, norepinephrine and serotonin. *Ann. Surg.* 154: 611–627, 1961.
132. SANDLER, H., AND H. T. DODGE. Left ventricular tension and stress in man. *Circulation Res.* 13: 91–102, 1963.
133. SARNOFF, S. J., E. BRAUNWALD, G. H. WELCH, JR., R. B. CASE, W. N. STAINSBY, AND R. MACRUZ. Haemodynamic de-

terminants of oxygen consumption of the heart with special reference to the Tension-Time Index. *Am. J. Physiol.* 192: 148–156, 1958.
134. SARNOFF, S. J., AND J. H. MITCHELL. The control of the function of the heart. In: *Handbook of Physiology. Circulation*, edited by W. F. Hamilton and P. Dow. Washington, D.C.: Am. Physiol. Soc., 1962, sect. 2, vol. I, p. 489–532.
135. SCHAEPDRYVER, A. F. DE. *On the Secretion, Distribution and Excretion of Adrenaline and Noradrenaline.* Bruges: St. Catherine Press, 1959.
136. SCHÄFER, E. A. The Oliver Sharpey Lectures on the present condition of our knowledge regarding the functions of the suprarenal capsules. *Brit. Med. J.* May 30 and June 6: 1–10, 1908.
137. SELKURT, E. The renal circulation. In: *Handbook of Physiology. Circulation*, edited by W. F. Hamilton and P. Dow. Washington, D.C.: Am. Physiol. Soc., 1963, sect. 2, vol. II, p. 1457–1516.
138. SHEPHERD, D. M., AND G. B. WEST. Noradrenaline and accessory chromaffin tissue. *Nature* 170: 42–43, 1952.
139. SONNENBLICK, E. H. Force-velocity relations in mammalian heart muscle. *Am. J. Physiol.* 202: 931–939, 1962.
140. SONNENBLICK, E. H. Active state in heart muscle. Its delayed onset and modification by inotropic agents. *J. Gen. Physiol.* 50: 661–676, 1967.
141. SONNENBLICK, E. H., W. W. PARMLEY, AND C. W. PARMLEY. The contractile state of the heart as expressed by force-velocity relations. *Am. J. Cardiol.* 23: 488–503, 1969.
142. SONNENBLICK, E. H., J. ROSS, JR., AND E. BRAUNWALD. Oxygen consumption of the heart. New concepts of its multifactorial determination. *Am. J. Cardiol.* 22: 328–336, 1969.
143. SPEDEN, R. C. Excitation of vascular smooth muscle. In: *Smooth Muscle*, edited by E. Bulbring, A. F. Brading, A. W. Jones, and T. Tomita. London: Arnold, 1970, p. 558–588.
144. SPENCER, M. P., A. B. DENISON, AND H. D. GREEN. The direct renal vascular effects of epinephrine and norepinephrine before and after adrenergic blockade. *Circulation Res.* 2: 537–540, 1954.
145. STARLING, E. H. *The Linacre Lecture on the Law of the Heart.* London: Longmans, Green, 1918.
146. STARLING, E. H. On the circulatory changes associated with exercise. *J. Roy. Army Med. Corps* 34: 258–275, 1920.
147. STOLZ, F. Über Adrenalin und Alkylaminoacetobrenzcatechin. *Ber. Deut. Chem.* 37: 4149–4154, 1904.
148. STOLZ, F. Synthese der wirksamen Substanz der Nebennieren-Synthetisches Suprarenin. *Chem. Z.* 2: 981–982, 1906.
149. SUTTER, M. C. The pharmacology of isolated veins. *Brit. J. Pharmacol. Chemotherap.* 24: 742–751, 1965.
150. SWAIN, H. H., AND C. L. WEIDNER. A study of substances which alter intraventricular conduction in the isolated dog heart. *J. Pharmacol.* 120: 137–148, 1957.
151. SWAN, H. J. C. Observations on a central dilator action of adrenaline in man. *J. Physiol., London* 112: 426–437, 1951.
152. TAKAMINE, J. The isolation of the active principle of the suprarenal gland. *J. Physiol., London* 27: 29–30, 1901.
153. THOMAS, D. P. The role of platelet catecholamines in the aggregation of platelets by collagen and thrombin. *Exptl. Biol. Med.* 3: 129–134, 1968.
154. TRAUTWEIN, W. Generation and conduction of impulses in the heart as affected by drugs. *Pharmacol. Rev.* 15: 277–330, 1963.
155. TRAUTWEIN, W., AND R. F. SCHMIDT. Zur Membranwirkung des Adrenalin an der Herzmuskelfaser. *Arch. Ges. Physiol.* 271: 715–725, 1960.
156. UCHIDA, E., D. F. BOHR, AND S. W. HOOBLER. A method for studying isolated rsistance vessels from rabbit mesentery and brain and their response to drugs. *Circulation Res.* 21: 525–536, 1967.
157. UTHER, J. B., S. N. HUNYOR, J. SHAW, AND P. I. KORNER. Bulbar and suprabulbar control of the cardiovascular autonomic effects during arterial hypoxia in the rabbit. *Circulation Res.* 26: 491–506, 1970.
158. VASSALLE, M. An analysis of cardiac pacemaker potential by means of "voltgage clamp" technique. *Am. J. Physiol.* 210: 1335–1341, 1966.
159. VAUGHAN WILLIAMS, E. M. The action of beta-receptor blocking agents on cardiac muscle. In: *Symposium on the Coronary Circulation and Energetics of the Myocardiuum*, edited by B. Marchetti and B. Taccardi. Basel: Karger, p. 118–124, 1967.
160. WEIDMANN, S. Cardiac electrophysiology in the light of recent morphological findings. *Harvey Lectures Ser.* 61: 1–16, 1967.
161. WHELAN, R. F. Vasodilatation in human skeletal muscles during adrenaline infusions. *J. Physiol., London* 118: 575–587, 1952.
162. WHELAN, R. F., AND I. S. DE LA LANDE. Action of adrenaline on limb blood vessels. *Brit. Med. Bull.* 19: 125–131, 1963.
163. WOLLENBERGER, A. Rhythmic and arrhythmic contractile activity of single myocardial cells cultured in vitro. *Circulation Res.* 14, Suppl. 2: 184–201, 1964.
164. ZUBERBUHLER, R. C., AND D. F. BOHR. Responses of coronary smooth muscle to catecholamines. *Circulation Res.* 16: 431–440, 1965.

Reflex respiratory effects of circulating catecholamines

N. JOELS | Department of Physiology, The Medical College of St. Bartholomew's Hospital, London, England

CHAPTER CONTENTS

Epinephrine-induced Apnea
   Acute anemia of respiratory center
   Direct depression of respiratory center
   Increased blood supply to respiratory center
   Reflex inhibition of respiration
Epinephrine- and Norepinephrine-induced Hyperpnea
   Central effects of epinephrine and norepinephrine
   Metabolic effects of catecholamines
   Effects of catecholamines on arterial chemoreceptors
   Mechanism of chemoreceptor stimulation by catecholamines
Effects of Catecholamines on Respiratory Reflexes
Physiological Significance of Respiratory Stimulation by Catecholamines
Catecholamine Secretion and Chemoreceptor Stimulation of Respiration at Birth
Summary and Conclusions

IN THEIR CLASSIC STUDY of the physiological effects of extracts of the adrenal glands published in 1895, Oliver & Schäfer (86) found that intravenous injection of such extracts depressed respiration in anesthetized dogs and rabbits. This finding was soon confirmed in rabbits, as well as in cats and dogs, by many other workers (3, 13, 61, 65, 67, 95, 101); Langley (65), in particular, noted that the injections sometimes caused complete cessation of breathing.

However, Nice et al. (85) pointed out that the doses of epinephrine administered in previous studies were exceedingly large and reported that injections of epinephrine into the jugular vein of cats and dogs in the more modest doses of 3 and 6 µg, respectively, led to an increased depth of respiration and a small fall in blood pressure; with larger doses there was respiratory depression and a rise in blood pressure similar to that observed by Oliver & Schäfer (86). Small doses of epinephrine have been shown also to cause respiratory stimulation in anesthetized animals of other species, including rabbit (84), horse, and mule (1), and in experiments on conscious human subjects, hyperpnea has been invariably the response to epinephrine (11, 12, 26, 27, 41, 104).

Whelan & Young (104) found that infusion of norepinephrine similarly led to hyperpnea in man, though norepinephrine was less effective than epinephrine in this respect. The occurrence of norepinephrine-induced hyperpnea in human subjects has since been confirmed many times (4, 28–30, 68). Stimulation of respiration by norepinephrine has also been demonstrated in the anesthetized and conscious rabbit (109) and in the anesthetized cat (60).

Thus moderate doses of epinephrine and norepinephrine have been shown repeatedly to stimulate respiration in both man and other animals. Before considering the mechanisms that may bring about this stimulation, however, it is convenient first to discuss the inhibition of respiration, epinephrine-induced apnea ("adrenaline apnoea"), which can be produced by larger amounts of catecholamine.

EPINEPHRINE-INDUCED APNEA

Oliver and Schäfer used extracts of adrenal gland in water, alcohol, and glycerine in which the quantities of epinephrine itself were of course unknown. However, some of the doses that produced respiratory depression or apnea in other studies are listed in Table 1.

A number of explanations were proposed to account for the inhibition of respiration by epinephrine. These included *a*) acute anemia of the respiratory center caused by constriction of the medullary vessels, *b*) a direct depressant action of the drug on the respiratory center, *c*) washing-out of a respiratory stimulant from the center by an increased medullary blood flow, and *d*) reflex depression resulting from the raised arterial pressure.

Acute Anemia of Respiratory Center

Roberts (93) concluded that epinephrine-induced apnea was of central origin and due to acute anoxia of

TABLE 1. *Doses of Epinephrine Producing Respiratory Depression or Apnea*

Species	Dose*, μg	Ref.
Dog	100	93
	20	84
	1,000	105
	400–500	51
	10–40	49
	300	47
	50–200	74
Cat and dog	100–1,000	96
	50–100	98
Cat	1,000	14
	2.5–15	84
	20	76
	100–200	108
	250	51
Rabbit and cat	100	77

* Injected intravenously.

the respiratory center resulting from cerebral vasoconstriction, since it still occurred after vagotomy or when a blood pressure compensator was used to prevent the accompanying hypertension. Mellanby & Huggett (77) at the time agreed with this theory; in addition, they showed that apnea did not occur after the vasoconstrictor action of epinephrine had been blocked with ergotoxine, a finding confirmed by McDowall (76). However, this view became untenable when cerebral venous outflow was shown to increase during epinephrine-induced apnea (63) or when epinephrine was added to the blood perfusing the brain (96).

Direct Depression of Respiratory Center

Direct depression of the respiratory center, first suggested by Szymonowicz (101), was a widely held explanation for epinephrine-induced apnea (13, 14, 63, 76, 84, 85). Huggett & Mellanby (56), who previously suggested that epinephrine-induced apnea was due to medullary anemia (77), now also supported the theory of a specific depression of the respiratory center since they subsequently showed that epinephrine had no effect on the activity of other medullary centers, such as the cardio-inhibitory, vasomotor, and swallowing centers. However, a direct depressant effect of epinephrine on the respiratory center is not consistent with the observations that, when epinephrine is injected into the carotid or vertebral arteries, the respiratory inhibition is of relatively slow onset (93) and the depression is less than that produced by intravenous injection of the same dose of the drug (97). Even stronger evidence against the idea that epinephrine-induced apnea is due to direct depression of the respiratory center was provided by Schmidt (97) who showed that, if the cerebral vessels were perfused at constant blood flow, the addition of epinephrine to the perfusate failed to alter breathing, and by Heymans & Heymans (49) who performed cross-circulation experiments in which the head of a dog was supplied with blood from a donor dog. Injection of epinephrine into the arterial inflow to this isolated head never depressed its respiratory movements.

Increased Blood Supply to Respiratory Center

As has been noted above, epinephrine-induced apnea is associated with an increase, rather than a decrease, in cerebral blood flow (63, 96), and it was proposed that the increased blood supply led to respiratory depression by reducing the concentration of a chemical stimulant in the cells of the respiratory center. This view was largely abandoned with the discovery of the reflex contribution to the production of the apnea.

Reflex Inhibition of Respiration

Because many workers showed that epinephrine would produce respiratory depression after vagotomy (13, 77, 85, 93, 96, 105) and that nasal movements are reduced by epinephrine even when the spinal cord has been divided in the cervical region, the intervention of afferent nervous stimuli in epinephrine-induced apnea was completely discounted. However, in 1926 Heymans & Heymans (49) reported experiments in which the isolated head of one dog, connected with its trunk only by the vagus nerves, was perfused by a donor dog. It has already been mentioned that injection of epinephrine into the circulation perfusing such an isolated head did not reduce respiratory movements of the head. On the other hand, if epinephrine was injected into the trunk of the recipient animal, there was a profound depression of respiratory movements in the head (Fig. 1). That this depression was not due to a specific effect of epinephrine,

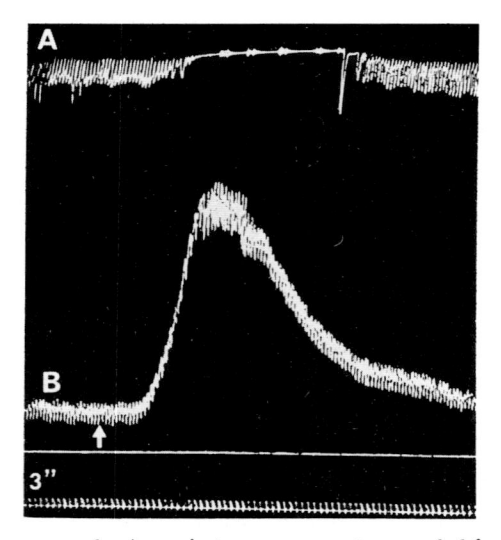

FIG. 1. *A*: respiratory movements, recorded from larynx, of isolated head of a dog (the "recipient") perfused with blood from donor animal. *B*: blood pressure in trunk of recipient dog that was connected to the head solely by vagus nerves. Time marker: 3-sec intervals. At *arrow*, intravenous injection of 40 μg epinephrine into trunk of recipient. Note hypertension in trunk and apnea of isolated head. [From Heymans & Heymans (49).]

but resulted from stimulation of the aortic arch baroreceptors by the hypertension it produced, was confirmed by the production of similar respiratory depression when blood pressure was raised by injecting 250 ml of Tyrode's solution into the isolated trunk and by the absence of any effect of epinephrine when pressure in the trunk was prevented from rising by a blood pressure compensator.

These experiments showed that epinephrine-induced apnea could be engendered by a reflex mechanism with its afferent pathway in the vagus. Nevertheless, in the intact animal, epinephrine-induced apnea still occurs after vagotomy, and this phenomenon needed explanation before a wholly reflex origin for epinephrine-induced apnea could be generally accepted. The explanation was afforded by Heymans & Bouckaert (47) who showed that an increase or decrease in pressure within the isolated perfused carotid sinuses of a dog would decrease or increase, respectively, the breathing and that after section of both sinus and depressor nerves intravenous injection of previously effective doses of epinephrine did not produce any appreciable reduction in respiratory rate or amplitude. These findings were confirmed for the cat by Wright (108), who demonstrated that the apnea produced in this species by epinephrine after vagotomy was similarly abolished by cutting the sinus nerves (Fig. 2) and, contrary to Roberts (93) but in agreement with Heymans & Heymans (49), that the apnea could be prevented if a blood pressure compensator was used (Fig. 3). Thereafter general acceptance was given to the view that epinephrine-induced apnea is a reflex response to stimulation of carotid sinus and aortic arch baroreceptors by the rise in arterial pressure, and this would also account for the parallelism, noted by McDowall (76), between the apnea and the slowing of the heart induced by epinephrine, since both would be dependent on afferent impulses from the same sources. Nevertheless some authors still claimed that epinephrine exerted an additional depressant effect on the respiratory center. Thus Schmidt (98) reported that, though section of the sinus and aortic nerves abolished

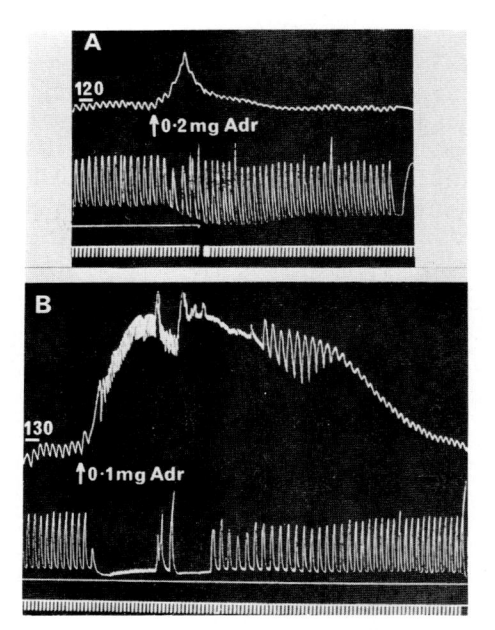

FIG. 3. Cat anesthetized with chloralose and with vagi intact. *Upper trace*, arterial pressure; *middle trace*, respiration; and *bottom trace*, time in 2-sec intervals. A: with compensator, injection of 200 μg epinephrine (*Adr*) causes only a small rise in blood pressure and little change in breathing. B: without compensator, injection of 100 μg epinephrine (*Adr*) causes marked hypertension and apnea. [From Wright (108).]

epinephrine-induced apnea in nearly every case, there were instances in which this was not so. These discrepancies were explained by Marri & Hauss (74). They showed that epinephrine failed to produce apnea after sinus and aortic nerve section when the animals were in good condition, but that, if blood pressure was lowered by bleeding or if respiration was depressed by morphine, epinephrine continued to inhibit the breathing even after the nerves were cut (74). Presumably in these situations the respiratory center would have been exposed to an abnormally high tension of CO_2; this would have been significantly reduced by the increased cerebral blood flow resulting from the hypertension produced by epinephrine injection. Similar considerations may apply to more recent experiments (51) in which epinephrine depressed respiration after the vagus and glossopharyngeal nerve roots had been cut in animals with the brainstem transected in the rostral portion of the medulla. Though no values for blood pressure were given, it is likely to have been reduced as a result of the extensive intracranial surgery, and because both carotid arteries were tied cerebral blood flow before injection of epinephrine would have been impaired further. Moreover the extent to which respiration can be considered normal in such a preparation is also debatable.

EPINEPHRINE- AND NOREPINEPHRINE-INDUCED HYPERPNEA

Stimulation of respiration by both epinephrine and norepinephrine has been described many times in con-

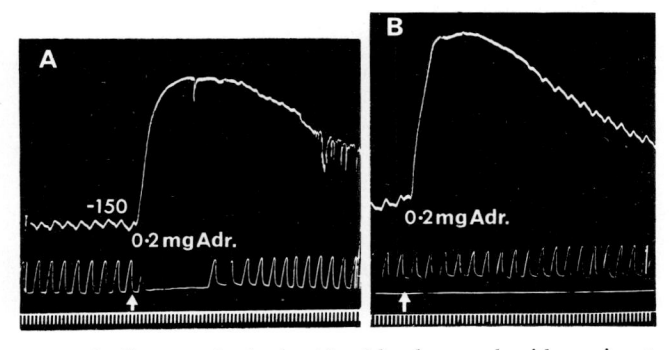

FIG. 2. Cat anesthetized with chloralose and with vagi cut. *Upper trace*, arterial blood pressure; *middle trace*, respiratory movements; *bottom trace*, time in 2-sec intervals. A: intravenous injection of 200 μg epinephrine (*Adr.*) at arrow leads to hypertension and apnea. B: after denervation of both sinuses, intravenous injection of 200 μg epinephrine (*Adr.*) at arrow produces hypertension but no apnea. [From Wright (108).]

scious human subjects; Tables 2 and 3 list some of these reports, together with the doses administered and an indication of the increases in ventilation that resulted. Many of these authors drew attention to the fact that the increased pulmonary ventilation resulted primarily from a greater tidal volume with only a minimal increase in respiratory rate. In anesthetized animals, hyperpnea can also be induced by moderate doses of epinephrine, as was first demonstrated in cats and dogs by Nice et al. (85) and subsequently confirmed both in these and other species (Table 2). Norepinephrine has similarly been shown to induce hyperpnea in animals (Table 3).

Various explanations have been proposed for this stimulation of breathing. Principal among these are a) that the hyperpnea is due to a central action of the catecholamines, b) that it results from their metabolic effects, and c) that it is a reflex response to increased activity of the arterial chemoreceptors in the carotid and aortic bodies. These possibilities, which are not necessarily mutually exclusive, are now considered in turn.

Central Effects of Epinephrine and Norepinephrine

Changes in neuronal activity caused by the direct action of catecholamines are reviewed elsewhere in this volume [see the chapter by Vogt in this volume of the Handbook; (72, 94)], but the drugs might also produce effects within the central nervous system indirectly through changes in cerebral blood flow. The literature on the effects of epinephrine on the cerebral vasculature is confusing but has been summarized by Sokoloff (100). In animals, epinephrine appears to slightly constrict the cerebral vessels, but this weak action is outweighed by the passive dilatation produced by the accompanying rise in systemic blood pressure (107) or by the chemical vasodilator effects of the increased cerebral metabolism that occurs with pressor doses of epinephrine (62). Thus, if blood pressure is unchanged, cerebral blood flow is also unchanged or slightly reduced; if blood pressure is increased, cerebral blood flow follows it passively. In man, there is no evidence for a constrictor effect of epinephrine on cerebral vessels, and nonpressor doses given by intramuscular injection probably have little effect on cerebral blood flow or metabolism (99), though intravenous administration has been reported to cause cerebral vasodilatation and increased blood flow (44). Pressor doses, however, increase cerebral blood flow proportionately to the rise in systemic arterial pressure, with cerebral vascular resistance remaining unchanged (44, 62). By contrast there is general agreement that in man intravenous infusions of pressor doses of norepinephrine constrict the cerebral vessels, the rise in cerebral vascular resistance being greater than the rise in mean arterial pressure so that there is a moderate reduction in blood flow to the brain (62, 80). During these studies falls in arterial CO_2 content on catecholamine administration were noted with norepinephrine (62, 99), but only one of these groups (62) found a similar fall with epinephrine as well. The changes in CO_2 were attributed to hyperventilation though ventilation did not appear to have been measured.

The ability of epinephrine and norepinephrine to alter the activity of the brain either directly or through modification of cerebral blood supply does not mean, however, that this is the mechanism producing the increase in respiration. Nice et al. (85) suggested that epinephrine-induced hyperpnea was the result of central stimulation since the hyperpnea persisted after cutting the vagi. However, it should be remembered that this hypothesis was advanced before the discovery of the part played in respiratory regulation by the peripheral arterial chemoreceptors in the carotid bodies. Central stimulation by epinephrine was also proposed as the cause of the hyperpnea when the drug was added to the fluid perfusing the vascularly isolated brain (16), but the results of these experiments were very variable in that, whereas respiration was stimulated in some tests, in others it was un-

TABLE 2. *Dose of Epinephrine Used to Produce Hyperpnea*

Species*	Dose	Increase in Respiratory Minute Volume, %	Ref.
Conscious man	1–1.5 mg, sc (1,000–1,500 μg)	34–63	41
	0.5 ml 1:1,000, im (500 μg)	4–45	102
	0.5–1.0 mg, sc (500–1,000 μg)	30–68	12
	0.5 ml 1:1,000, sc (500 μg)	23	69
	0.025–0.1 μg/kg·min		26
	0.5 ml 1:1,000, sc (500 μg)		27
	10–20 μg/min, iv	13–153	104
	20 μg/min, iv		15
	10 μg/min, iv or ia		20
	0.15 μg/kg·min	40	68
Horse and mule	5–10 μg/kg		1
Unanesthetized dog	0.0006–0.0025 mg/kg·min, iv (0.6–2.5 μg/kg·min)	20–75	11
Dog	0.6 ml 1:100,000, iv (6 μg)		85
	0.5 ml 1:10,000, iv (50 μg)		57
	0.5 ml 1:100,000, iv (5 μg)		84
Cat	0.3 ml 1:100,000, iv (3 μg)		85
	0.5–3.0 ml 1:200,000, iv (2.5–15 μg)		84
	1.0 μg/kg·min, iv	22	46
	0.8 μg/kg·min, iv	14	60

Sc, subcutaneous; im, intramuscular; ia, intraarterial; iv, intravenous. * Anesthetized, unless otherwise indicated.

TABLE 3. *Dose of Norepinephrine Used to Produce Hyperpnea*

Species	Dose[a,b]	Increase in Respiratory Minute Volume, %	Ref.
Man[c]	7–15		92
	10–20	39–70	104
	10	20–50	4
	5–10		30
	8–15		29
Cat[d]	0.8 μg/kg·min	8	60

[a] Intravenously injected. [b] Values expressed in μg/min, unless otherwise noted. [c] Conscious. [d] Anesthetized.

changed or even depressed. From experiments in which doses of epinephrine, large enough normally to produce apnea, stimulated breathing if a blood pressure compensator was used to prevent the rise in pressure and consequent increased stimulation of the carotid sinus and aortic arch baroreceptors, Wright (108) also concluded that epinephrine could stimulate respiration by a central action. However, as will be discussed subsequently, there must have been considerable stimulation of the carotid and aortic body chemoreceptors under these circumstances.

More recently, Coles et al. (20) attempted to determine whether the stimulant action of epinephrine and norepinephrine on respiration in man is the result of a direct action on the respiratory or any other center in the brain. In patients undergoing cerebral angiography for diagnostic purposes, epinephrine or norepinephrine was infused at 1–2 μg/min into one carotid or vertebral artery. In no instance was respiration altered, though the cerebral vessels were well outlined by the injection of contrast medium through the same needle. Only when the dose infused was raised to 10 μg/min was there an increase in respiration, but this dose was sufficient to stimulate breathing when injected intravenously. In a similar investigation on anesthetized cats and rabbits, Young (109) found that injection into the vertebral artery of 0.12–0.25 μg epinephrine, which increased minute volume when injected intravenously, either had no effect on respiration or led to an increase in ventilation smaller than that produced by intravenous injection of the same dose.

Thus there is little evidence that the action of catecholamines on the central nervous system, exerted either directly or through alterations in its blood supply, is primarily responsible for the respiratory stimulation when these drugs are injected or infused. On the other hand, whether such actions contribute to effects mediated by other mechanisms has yet to be determined.

Metabolic Effects of Catecholamines

Epinephrine stimulates metabolism and thereby produces a rise in heat production with increased oxygen consumption, increased carbon dioxide production, and generally a rise in the respiratory quotient. In many accounts of the stimulation of respiration by epinephrine, these effects on metabolism were also observed and thought to be responsible for the hyperpnea both in conscious man (12, 41, 102) and in the unanesthetized dog (11). However, epinephrine stimulates lactic acid production, as well as oxidative metabolism, and in experiments during which blood lactic acid levels were measured while epinephrine was infused intravenously at approximately 2–5 μg/min (26) or injected subcutaneously in a dose of 0.5 mg (27) the increase in respiration was attributed to the accompanying rise in blood lactate concentration. A more precise correlation of the respiratory effects of epinephrine with its various metabolic actions was attempted by Griffith et al. (46). Anesthetized cats were infused with various concentrations of the drug. The lowest rate of infusion to definitely increase pulmonary ventilation was 1 μg/kg·min, though the blood sugar level was increased with infusion at only half this rate. Oxygen consumption possibly increased also at this lower rate of infusion, but appreciable increases in O_2 consumption only occurred with infusions of 1 μg/kg·min or more. This was also the threshold for elevation of the blood lactic acid level.

However, a number of studies in the 1950s suggested that the stimulating action of epinephrine in man is to a large extent independent of the accompanying increases in oxygen consumption and lactic acid production. Whelan & Young (104) infused human subjects with 10–20 μg/min of epinephrine or norepinephrine for periods of 10 min. The pattern of response was similar with both catecholamines. During the first 5 min of the infusion respiration increased and alveolar CO_2% fell, presumably as a result of the increased minute volume; but during the second half of the infusion, ventilation, and to a lesser extent alveolar CO_2%, tended toward their original values (Fig. 4). A fall in alveolar CO_2 during epinephrine-induced hyperpnea had also been observed by Lyman et al. (69). This fall would seem to have been the cause of the decline in ventilation during the second 5 min of the infusion period, since Barcroft et al. (4) subsequently showed that, if 2–5% CO_2 was added to the inspired air of subjects receiving an infusion of norepinephrine, the increase in respiratory minute volume was sustained over the whole of a 15-min infusion with only a very small fall in alveolar P_{CO_2} accompanying the hyperpnea (Fig. 5).

The fall in alveolar P_{CO_2} (69, 104) suggests that in-

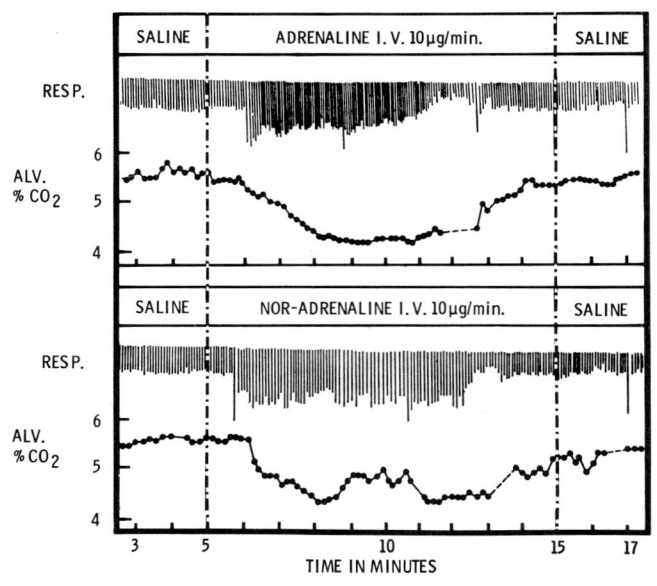

FIG. 4. Stethograph records of alveolar (*ALV.*) air CO_2% during intravenous (*I.V.*) infusions of epinephrine (*ADRENALINE*) and norepinephrine (*NOR-ADRENALINE*), at rate of 10 μg/min for 10 min. *RESP.*, respiration. [Redrawn from Whelan & Young (104).]

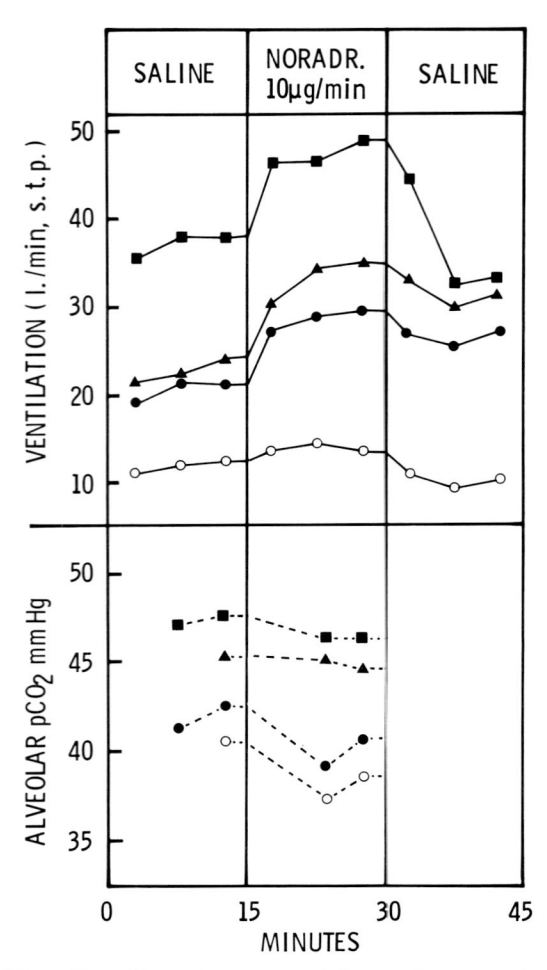

FIG. 5. Effect of breathing mixtures containing varying amounts of CO$_2$ on respiratory response to infusion of norepinephrine (*NORADR*); results obtained in one subject. ○, 2% CO$_2$; ●, 4% CO$_2$; ▲, 4.5% CO$_2$; ■, 5% CO$_2$. S.t.p., standard temperature and pressure. [Redrawn from Barcroft et al. (4).]

that their findings also excluded lactic acid accumulation as a cause of catecholamine-induced hyperpnea since the onset of the increased rate and depth of breathing occurred only 1–1.5 min after the commencement of the infusion and the respiratory changes were at their peak shortly afterward, whereas measurements of lactic acid concentration during infusion of similar amounts of epinephrine (5) showed that the blood lactate was not significantly raised until 10 min after beginning the infusion and moreover that norepinephrine had negligible effects on lactic acid concentration. That the stimulating action of epinephrine on respiration is not initiated by the release of acid metabolites into the bloodstream was also indicated by the observation (15) that a rise in plasma pH of 0.03–0.10 unit and a fall in plasma CO$_2$ tension of 3–8 mmHg accompanied the increased breathing during infusion of 20 μg/min epinephrine. There was no fall in CO$_2$ combining power until the second 5-min period of the infusion, when the peak of the hyperventilation was over and the pH and P$_{CO_2}$ were returning to their normal values (Fig. 6).

Some of the conclusions just discussed were challenged subsequently by Lundholm & Svedmyr (68). In contrast to Bradley et al. (15), Lundholm and Svedmyr reported that plasma pH fell and P$_{CO_2}$ rose with the onset of epinephrine infusion (Fig. 7), so that the increase they measured in CO$_2$ elimination must have been due to an increase in CO$_2$ production. They dismissed the contrary findings (15) of a rise in pH and a fall in P$_{CO_2}$ on the grounds that Bradley and his associates carried out their analyses on samples that had been stored as whole blood in ice, a procedure that, according to Lundholm and Svedmyr, in itself leads to a lowering of plasma P$_{CO_2}$ and a rise in pH. In their own experiments the plasma was separated before storage, but on repeating the experiments with samples stored as whole blood in a manner similar to that of Bradley and co-workers, they

creased metabolic CO$_2$ production cannot be a major factor in epinephrine hyperpnea. This is consistent with the finding by Reale et al. (92) that norepinephrine, like epinephrine, increased the rate and depth of respiration but produced no consistent change in oxygen consumption, whereas epinephrine infused in the same dosage (7–15 μg/min) increased oxygen uptake by about 10%. Whelan & Young (104) also compared the effects of epinephrine and norepinephrine on oxygen uptake with their effects on breathing. They found the average increase in minute volume with norepinephrine to be at least 75% of that during infusion of the same dose of epinephrine. On the other hand, oxygen consumption increased during epinephrine infusion by an average of over 30%, but the changes with norepinephrine were negligible. Thus, as these authors point out, the rise in oxygen uptake produced by epinephrine can neither be attributed to the increased activity of the respiratory muscles nor can it be responsible for much of the stimulation of respiration. Whelan & Young (104) suggested

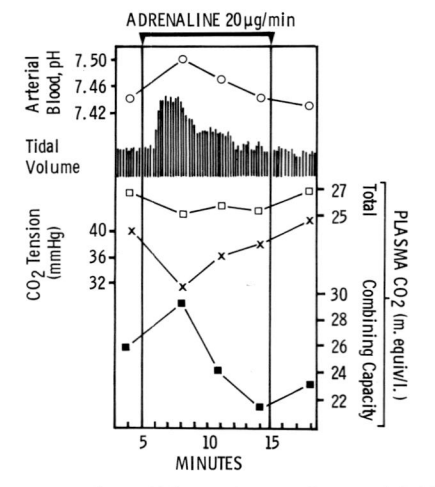

FIG. 6. Acid-base changes in arterial blood during infusion of L-epinephrine (*ADRENALINE*), 20 μg/min for 10 min. During infusion, respiratory rate rose from its resting value of 13 breaths per min to 21 breaths per min at the height of respiratory stimulation. [Redrawn from Bradley et al. (15).]

were able to reproduce the latters' (15) results. Although changes in the composition of the stored blood samples might account for the finding by Bradley and his colleagues of a lowered plasma P_{CO_2} and raised plasma pH during epinephrine infusion, this would not explain the reduced end-tidal P_{CO_2} values noted by Whelan & Young (see Fig. 4). However, Lundholm & Svedmyr (68) drew attention to the finding by Matell (75) of a difference between the end-tidal P_{CO_2} and the P_{CO_2} of the arterial blood during exercise and suggested that a similar lack of correlation between end-tidal and arterial P_{CO_2} might occur during epinephrine infusion.

With norepinephrine infusion, Lundholm & Svedmyr (68) found ventilation to increase by about 40%, a rise similar to that produced by epinephrine infusion, but there was now an initial increase in plasma pH and fall in P_{CO_2}, even though the plasma had been separated before storage (Fig. 8). In confirmation of results obtained by Bearn et al. (5), lactic acid concentration, which rose appreciably with epinephrine infusion, increased only slightly with norepinephrine infusion.

Thus Lundholm & Svedmyr (68) concluded that the increased ventilation induced by epinephrine infusion could be explained, at least in part, by increased CO_2 production. From measurements of the changes in CO_2 elimination, oxygen uptake, and plasma bicarbonate concentration, they calculated that about half of this increased CO_2 production derived from increased oxygen consumption and the remainder from increased acidity in the tissues. On the other hand, the effect of norepinephrine on breathing could not be similarly accounted for, since the initial phase of respiratory stimulation was associated with a reduction of the plasma P_{CO_2} and an increase in the plasma pH, which appeared to indicate that the increase in CO_2 elimination resulted from the washing-out of CO_2 and not from increased CO_2 production. Although their experiments provided no information concerning the mechanism responsible for the initial stimulating effect of norepinephrine on respiration, Lundholm & Svedmyr (68) suggested that

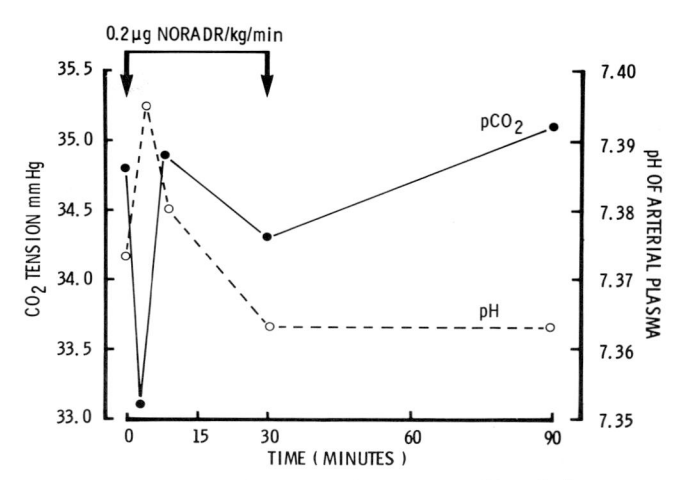

FIG. 8. Effect of infusing norpinephrine (*NORADR*) on pH (*open circles, dashed line*) and P_{CO_2} (*closed circles, solid line*) in plasma from arterial blood. [Redrawn from Lundholm & Svedmyr (68).]

norepinephrine might influence breathing by stimulating the arterial chemoreceptors and that part of the effect of epinephrine might be expressed in this way also.

Effects of Catecholamines on Arterial Chemoreceptors

In the course of experiments examining the effects of intravenous norepinephrine infusions on the respiratory responses of unanesthetized human subjects to the inhalation of various gas mixtures, Cunningham et al. (29) showed that such infusions specifically increased the sensitivity to hypoxia and predicted that in the absence of hypoxia norepinephrine would be without effect on the respiration. This conclusion was confirmed shortly afterward by Cunningham et al. (30) who found that, whereas at normal and low alveolar oxygen tensions a change in the infusion from saline to norepinephrine, or vice versa, was followed by a substantial increase or decrease, respectively, in ventilation, at high alveolar P_{O_2} levels of approximately 650 mmHg such changes had no consistent effect. Lundholm & Svedmyr (68) also noted that the stimulant action of norepinephrine in conscious man was abolished when the subject breathed pure oxygen, while Joels & White (60) found that in the anesthetized cat the inhalation of oxygen abolished the increase in ventilation normally produced by epinephrine infusion, as well as that resulting from norepinephrine infusion (Fig. 9).

The link between the level of alveolar P_{O_2} and the production of respiratory stimulation by catecholamines suggested that the arterial chemoreceptors of the carotid and aortic bodies, which in response to a reduction of arterial P_{O_2} initiate a vigorous discharge of afferent nerve impulses (9, 35, 37, 53, 106) and reflexly increase ventilation (25, 48, 50), might contribute to respiratory stimulation by catecholamines.

This possibility was investigated by Joels & White (60) who observed the effects of epinephrine and norepinephrine infusions on the ventilation of cats breathing

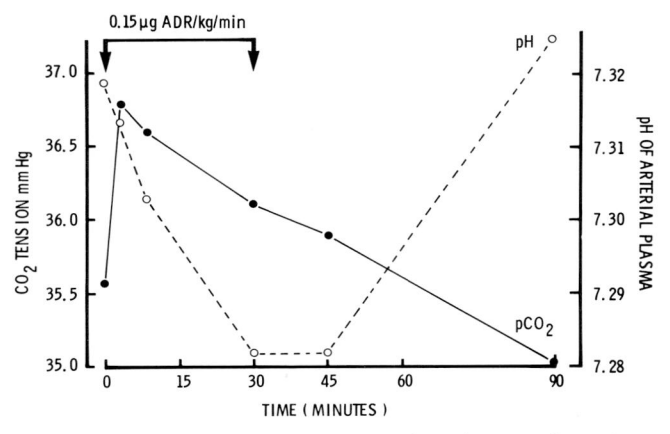

FIG. 7. Effect of infusing epinephrine (*ADR*) on pH (*open circles, dashed line*) and P_{CO_2} (*closed circles, solid line*) in plasma from arterial blood. Plasma was separated before storage. [Redrawn from Lundholm & Svedmyr (68).]

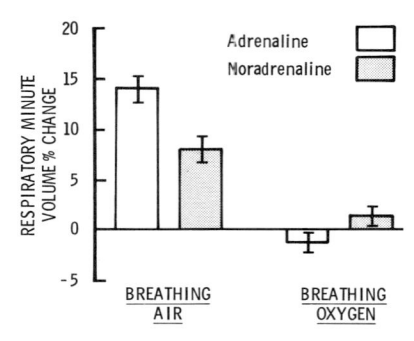

FIG. 9. Effects of catecholamine infusion on ventilation of cats breathing room air and on that of cats breathing 100% O_2. During room air breathing, average dose of both epinephrine (*Adrenaline*) and norepinephrine (*Noradrenaline*) was 0.8 µg/kg·min. While breathing 100% O_2, average dose of epinephrine was 0.8 µg/kg·min and that of norepinephrine was 1.1 µg/kg·min. *Vertical bars* represent ±1 SEM. [From Joels & White (60).]

room air before and after denervation of the carotid and aortic bodies by section of the carotid sinus and aortic nerves. Cutting these nerves also interrupts the afferent fibers from the baroreceptors of the carotid sinus and aortic arch, which in turn leads to a rise in systemic pressure. Since the blood flow through the carotid bodies, and presumably the aortic bodies, is dependent on the level of arterial pressure (31, 90) and since the discharge from the arterial chemoreceptors can be altered by changes in blood flow (43, 64, 65), changes in blood pressure following sinus and aortic nerve section were minimized by the use of a compensator. Measurements of ventilation made during the fifth minute of catecholamine infusion, when both blood pressure and respiration had attained a steady state, showed that, whereas infusion of epinephrine or norepinephrine at 1.5–2.0 µg/kg·min increased ventilation by an average of 7% when the sinus and aortic nerves were intact, after the nerves were cut such infusions had no effect on breathing (Fig. 10). The importance of the arterial chemoreceptors for respiratory stimulation by catecholamines was further demonstrated by experiments in which epinephrine and norepinephrine were administered by close-arterial infusion to the region of one carotid bifurcation, so as to gain immediate access to one carotid body. Though the dose (0.1–0.2 µg/kg·min) was only one-tenth that given by intravenous infusion in the preceding studies, the increase in ventilation (10–11%) was possibly greater. Moreover, after the dividing of the corresponding sinus nerve, the catecholamines were ineffective in these smaller doses, even though the innervation of both aortic bodies and the contralateral carotid body remained intact [Fig. 11; (60)]. Similarly, Byck (17) has reported that injections of norepinephrine into the carotid artery evoked reflex stimulation of respiration in anesthetized dogs, and Anichkov & Belen'kii (2) cite experiments by Kuznetsov and Belen'kii, both of whom found that perfusion of the isolated carotid sinus with 10^{-5} to 10^{-6} epinephrine induced a modest increase in respiration in decerebrate cats. On the other hand,

reference has already been made to the observation (20) that intracarotid infusion of 1–2 µg/min of epinephrine or norepinephrine failed to increase ventilation in conscious human subjects. However, because the observations were made in the course of cerebral angiography these patients were probably breathing 100% O_2, which could account for the lack of stimulation. Young (109) also noted that intracarotid injections of epinephrine and norepinephrine in cats did not alter the ventilation. In Young's experiments, however, the injections were made into the common carotid artery rostral to an occluding arterial clip and, as Lee et al. (66) pointed out, under these circumstances the chemoreceptors, stimulated by stagnant hypoxia, might already have been discharging heavily.

Additional evidence indicating participation of the carotid body chemoreceptors in the ventilatory response to catecholamines was obtained by Joels & White (60) from records of the action potential discharge of chemoreceptor fibers in the sinus nerve. The discharge was increased by epinephrine and norepinephrine, whether

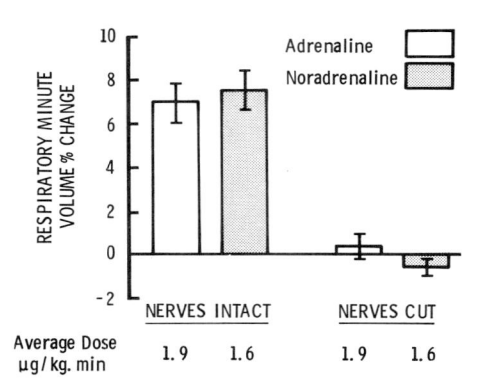

FIG. 10. Effect of carotid sinus and aortic nerve section on respiratory response to intravenous infusion of epinephrine (*Adrenaline*) and norepinephrine (*Noradrenaline*). *Vertical bars* represent ±1 SEM. [From Joels & White (60).]

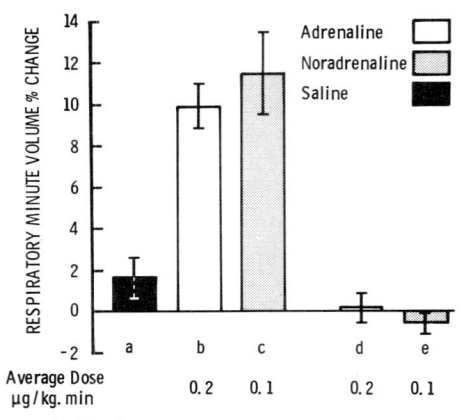

FIG. 11. Changes in ventilation produced by intracarotid infusion of catecholamines. *a–c*: carotid sinus nerve intact. *d* and *e*: after section of carotid sinus nerve on side of infusion. [From Joels & White (60).]

these drugs were infused intravenously or, in lesser dosage, close arterially (Fig. 12).

These findings strongly suggest that the stimulation of ventilation during the early minutes of catecholamine infusion is largely reflex in origin and initiated from the carotid and aortic body chemoreceptors. This could account for the fall in P_{CO_2} observed at this stage by Bradley et al. (15) with epinephrine infusion and by Whelan & Young (104) and Lundholm & Svedmyr (68) with norepinephrine infusion. However, since the infusions were relatively brief, no more than 5–8 min in duration, this conclusion does not exclude the possibility that increased metabolic CO_2 production and the formation of lactic acid may play an important role in stimulating respiration when catecholamines are administered for more prolonged periods. In this connection, attention has already been drawn to studies (5) in which there was no significant rise in lactic acid concentration before the tenth minute of epinephrine infusion. Lundholm & Svedmyr (68) found only a small increase of lactate level by the eighth minute of infusion, but the rise did not reach its peak until the end of the 30-min infusion period.

Nevertheless the work of Joels & White (60) indicates that epinephrine may be enhancing the respiratory response even during the early minutes of epinephrine infusion by an effect additional to its action on the chemoreceptors. When the percentage increases in chemoreceptor discharge during infusions of epinephrine and norepinephrine were compared with the corresponding percentage increases in ventilation, it was found that, for a similar increase in chemoreceptor discharge, hyperpnea was greater during infusion of epinephrine. Since in these experiments epinephrine failed to stimulate respiration after chemoreceptor denervation it was suggested that this additional effect of epinephrine might be a facilitation of the central response to the increased chemoreceptor discharge.

Mechanism of Chemoreceptor Stimulation by Catecholamines

Landgren & Neil (64) drew attention to the sensitivity of the arterial chemoreceptors to a reduction in local blood flow, as illustrated by the intense chemoreceptor activity evoked by the stagnant hypoxia of hemorrhagic hypotension. The suggestion that chemoreceptor stimulation by catecholamines could also be due to a reduced blood flow may appear inconsistent with the observations of Daly et al. (31) who found that the intravenous injection of 10–25 µg epinephrine increased the flow through the carotid body of the cat. However, injection of this amount of epinephrine produces a marked rise in systemic pressure that in the experiments of Daly and his associates must have been sufficient to outweigh any local vasoconstrictor action at the carotid body. In some unpublished experiments of their series in which a compensator was used to prevent the rise in systemic pressure, carotid body blood flow was reduced after epinephrine injection (M. de Burgh Daly, personal communication). Neil & Joels (81) showed that, when the glomus was

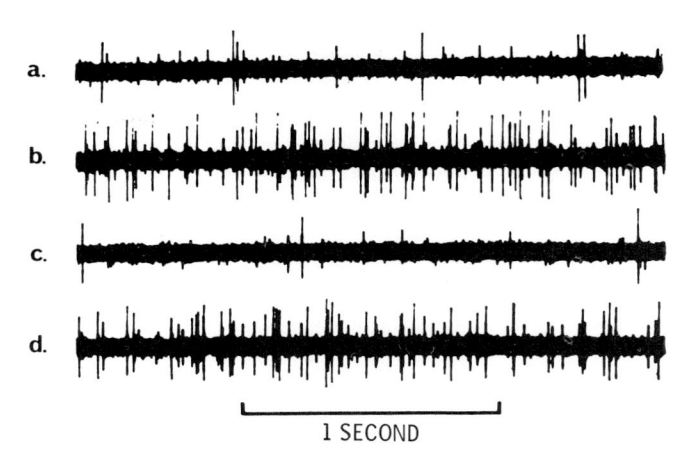

FIG. 12. Cat anesthetized with chloralose. Effect of intraarterial infusion of epinephrine and norepinephrine through cannula in left lingual artery on discharge in a few-fiber filament of left carotid sinus nerve; a: immediately before infusion; b: 2 min after commencing infusion of epinephrine (0.25 µg/kg·min); c: 2 min after ceasing infusion; and d: 2 min after commencing infusion of norepinephrine (0.13 µg/kg·min). Blood pressure remained at 120 mmHg throughout. [From Joels & White (60).]

perfused at a constant pressure, the addition of norepinephrine to the perfusate led to an increase in chemoreceptor discharge, presumably through an increase in vascular resistance and a consequent reduction in flow. Lee et al. (66) used a different approach to the same problem: they recorded aortic chemoreceptor discharge during hypoxia and compared the effects on this discharge of raising the blood pressure either by an intravenous injection of catecholamine or by tightening a snare around the abdominal aorta. Though raising the pressure by either means reduced the hypoxic discharge, the activity at any given level of arterial pressure was greater when epinephrine or norepinephrine was used to vary the blood pressure.

Blood flow in the carotid body can also be varied by changes in sympathetic activity. The blood vessels of the glomus are richly innervated by postganglionic fibers from the superior cervical ganglion. Daly et al. (31) found that stimulation of the peripheral cut end of the cervical sympathetic nerve reduced blood flow through the carotid body by 55%, and similar changes were found on sympathetic stimulation by Purves (91). Floyd & Neil (39) noted that the discharge in the postganglionic sympathetic fibers was greater in hypoxia or hemorrhage, situations in which chemoreceptor activity is also intensified. Correspondingly, electrical stimulation of the postganglionic sympathetic fibers increased chemoreceptor activity (38, 39). Nevertheless any increase in the activity of the sympathetic supply to the chemoreceptors that may occur during catecholamine infusion cannot be essential for the stimulation of ventilation or the enhanced chemoreceptor discharge since both are seen in animals in which the cervical sympathetic nerves have been divided (60).

There is a second nervous pathway that can be influenced by catecholamines and through which the sensitivity of the chemoreceptors may be altered. Both the sinus nerves and the aortic nerves contain efferent, as well as afferent, fibers, and it has recently been shown that the activity in these efferent fibers increases after intravenous injection of epinephrine (10, 83). In parallel studies (82) these efferent fibers were excited by electrical stimulation of the distal ends of the cut sinus and aortic nerves; this led to a depression of chemoreceptor discharge. Though stimulation of the sinus nerve efferents usually increased carotid body blood flow as well, the responses of carotid body blood flow and reduced chemoreceptor activity were not temporally related. Moreover close-arterial injection of atropine abolished the effect of efferent stimulation on blood flow, but the effect on chemoreceptor discharge persisted. It therefore seems improbable that the increased carotid body blood flow on efferent stimulation was responsible for the depression of chemoreceptor activity.

A reduction in chemoreceptor activity brought about by an increased efferent discharge in the sinus and aortic nerves after injection of epinephrine would of course oppose the previously described stimulant effect of this drug on the arterial chemoreceptors. However, the doses used in these studies of efferent activity were high, at least 20 µg in a single injection, and fall into the range of dosages (see Table 1) in which epinephrine induces apnea in response to baroreceptor stimulation by the resultant hypertension. Whether epinephrine affects the activity in efferent fibers of the sinus and aortic nerves when given in the much smaller doses associated with hyperpnea remains unknown.

In addition to these effects of catecholamines on the blood vessels of the carotid and aortic bodies and on their efferent nerve supply, a more direct excitatory action on the chemoreceptors has also been envisaged. The cells of the carotid body contain large quantities of catecholamines (19, 110), and this has led to the suggestion that catecholamines may act as a "transmitter" in this situation, being discharged from the chemoreceptor cells to excite the neighboring chemoreceptor afferent nerve terminals. This hypothesis cannot be tested by experiments in which the carotid body is perfused through its own vasculature because the vasoconstrictor effects of the catecholamines cannot then be excluded. However, in studies on the superfused carotid body suspended in a stream of oxygenated saline, Biscoe (6) obtained stimulation with epinephrine and norepinephrine, though a high concentration of the drugs (10^{-5} g/ml) was required. But in later, more extensive studies (36, 110) the authors were unable to excite the superfused carotid body with catecholamines. Moreover, Zapata et al. (110) also found that after cats had been treated with reserpine, which greatly reduced the carotid body content of epinephrine and norepinephrine, reflex respiratory responses to hypoxia were unaffected, an observation arguing against a transmitter function for catecholamines at this site. Thus the reduction in local blood flow produced by these amines remains the most likely cause for chemoreceptor stimulation by these drugs.

EFFECTS OF CATECHOLAMINES
ON RESPIRATORY REFLEXES

The effects of norepinephrine on the changes in pulmonary ventilation produced by alterations in alveolar P_{O_2} and P_{CO_2} have been investigated in man (29, 30). In these experiments the composition of the inspired air could be adjusted to maintain any desired levels of alveolar P_{O_2} and P_{CO_2}, despite changes in ventilation. The findings revealed that norepinephrine increases the sensitivity to hypoxia, and to hypercapnia as well, provided the oxygen tension is not elevated. When mixtures containing high tensions of oxygen were inspired, however, norepinephrine infusion failed to modify the ventilation. These results in unanesthetized man are paralleled by findings in the anesthetized cat (60). Both epinephrine and norepinephrine infusions increased the respiration while the animals were breathing room air, low-oxygen mixtures, or 5% CO_2 in air but failed to increase the respiration while the animals breathed pure oxygen or 5% CO_2 in oxygen.

The stimulant action of catecholamines in these circumstances seems once again to originate largely at the arterial chemoreceptors. Hypoxia stimulates the chemoreceptors, and mention has been made of the observation in cats ventilated with low-oxygen mixtures that at comparable levels of arterial pressure the discharge from the aortic chemoreceptors was greater during catecholamine infusions (66). A rise in P_{CO_2} will also stimulate the chemoreceptors (9, 35, 37, 54, 58, 106), and considerable evidence suggests that hypoxia and hypercapnia in combination exert a more than additive effect (37, 53, 59, 81, 87). It seems likely that catecholamine infusion increases the sensitivity to CO_2 indirectly by intensifying the hypoxic response and thus magnifying the interaction of hypoxia and hypercapnia, rather than directly by acting on the CO_2 response. The arguments are beyond the scope of this review, but the interested reader should consult Torrance (103).

PHYSIOLOGICAL SIGNIFICANCE OF RESPIRATORY
STIMULATION BY CATECHOLAMINES

Though many investigators have shown that respiration can be increased by the injection or infusion of relatively small doses of catecholamines, the physiological importance of this observation depends on whether or not the adrenal medulla is capable of secreting the hormones in comparable amounts.

Several measurements have been made of catecholamine output from the left adrenal gland during stimulation of its nerve supply by collecting and subsequently assaying the venous effluent from the gland. Celander (18) found in the cat that up to 5 µg/kg·min could be released by splanchnic nerve stimulation, though in other studies on the cat slightly smaller values have been reported [2 μg/kg·min (52); 50 μg over 50 min of stimulation (34); 38 μg over 10 min of stimulation (73)].

Catecholamine secretion from the adrenal medulla can also be provoked by electrical stimulation of the hypothalamus. Folkow & von Euler (40) found that this led to a secretion of 1–2.5 μg/kg·min, and even when only low or moderate intensities of hypothalamic stimulation were used, an average catecholamine output of 0.7 μg/kg·min was obtained, the maximum output in these circumstances being 1.6 μg/kg·min (45). These rates of catecholamine secretion in response to stimulation of the splanchnic nerve or the hypothalamus in the anesthetized cat are at least as great and generally much larger than the rates of infusion (0.8–1.0 μg/kg·min) used to produce hyperpnea in the cat (46, 60). Moreover the values obtained during stimulation of the splanchnic nerve or the hypothalamus in these experiments represent output from the left adrenal gland only. Doubtless the combined production by both glands would be correspondingly greater.

Nevertheless, though electrical stimulation of the hypothalamus or splanchnic nerve can elicit the production of catecholamines in amounts that have been shown to increase pulmonary ventilation, any suggestion that catecholamines may contribute to the stimulation of respiration in physiological circumstances depends on the demonstration that sufficient hormone can be liberated by more natural stimuli. Asphyxia is one of the most potent of such stimuli. Houssay & Molinelli (55) found an epinephrine output of about 2 μg/kg·min during asphyxia in the dog, and a similar rate of secretion (mean 1.3 μg/kg·min; maximum 2–2.5 μg/kg·min) was reported by Celander (18) in the cat. More recently, Malmejac (70) observed an output of 0.7 μg/kg·min in dogs subjected to asphyxia, and after 10 min of asphyxia, Millar (78) found the plasma level of epinephrine to have risen from 1.05 to 18.3 μg/liter and of norepinephrine from 0.99 to 11.4 μg/liter. Comparable quantities of catecholamines appear to be released during hemorrhage. Galviano et al. (42) removed 20–25% of the blood volume in dogs, and both they and Malmejac (70), in similar bleeding experiments, recorded catecholamine outputs from one adrenal gland of up to 1 μg/kg·min. Manger et al. (71) measured plasma levels of catecholamines in dogs and found that removing one-third of the blood volume increased the epinephrine content from 1.0 to 7.8 μg/liter and the norepinephrine content from 2.5 to 3.6 μg/liter. In a similar investigation Millar & Benfey (79) noted that, after a hemorrhage of 48 ml/kg, plasma epinephrine and norepinephrine rose from control levels of less than 0.5 μg/liter to 15.8 and 6.0 μg/liter, respectively.

Thus there seems little doubt that catecholamines may enter the bloodstream as a result of severe physiological stresses in amounts sufficient to stimulate respiration. However, further investigation is needed to determine whether this secretion of catecholamines contributes significantly to the overall respiratory stimulus in situations such as asphyxia or hemorrhage, or whether its effects are far outweighed by the respiratory responses to the associated changes in blood gases and alterations in cardiac output and blood pressure.

CATECHOLAMINE SECRETION AND CHEMORECEPTOR STIMULATION OF RESPIRATION AT BIRTH

In the fetal lamb the cardiovascular response to hypoxia is unaffected by cutting the carotid sinus nerves but abolished by vagotomy or aortic nerve section, which suggests that in fetal life only the aortic chemoreceptors are responsive to hypoxia (32). Nevertheless the carotid bodies must be potentially active since the intracarotid injection of cyanide, which provides a more powerful stimulus to the chemoreceptors than does hypoxia, induces a cardiovascular response that disappears after the sinus nerves are cut (33).

In newborn lambs the carotid body chemoreceptors have been shown to respond to changes in arterial P_{O_2}. Minute ventilation was increased by hypoxia (89) and was reduced during inspiration of 100% O_2, but these changes no longer occurred after carotid body denervation. Chemoreceptor impulse traffic in the sinus nerve was similarly increased by hypoxia and reduced by 100% O_2 (8). The cause of this increase in sensitivity of the carotid chemoreceptors that takes place at about the time of parturition is not fully established, but one major contributing factor may be an alteration in the volume or distribution of carotid body blood flow resulting from an increase in sympathetic activity. Thus, in an investigation (7) in which clamping the umbilical cord of the fetal lamb delivered 1–2 days before term led to an increase in carotid chemoreceptor activity and the taking of a breath, the increase in chemoreceptor discharge was preceded by a large rise in the discharge recorded from postganglionic cervical sympathetic nerve fibers.

An elevated concentration of circulating catecholamines would also enhance chemoreceptor responsiveness by its effect on carotid body blood flow, and the fetal adrenal medulla has been shown to be capable, at the time of parturition, of producing large amounts of catecholamines in response to asphyxia. In the fetal lamb mean outputs from one gland of 0.5 μg/kg·min (22), with peak values of 1.0 μg/kg·min (21), have been measured. A similar catecholamine production of 0.5–1.0 μg/kg·min during asphyxia at or near term has been reported in the fetal calf (23) and fetal foal (24). The fetal calf and foal are of particular interest since in these species the sympathetic innervation of the adrenal medulla is poorly developed at the time of birth and catecholamine secretion results largely from a direct effect of hypoxia on the gland (23, 24). Whether or not a similar immaturity of the sympathetic nerve supply to other organs exists at this time is unknown, but the studies on the fetal lamb discussed above suggest that, if in the calf and foal the sympathetic supply to the carotid bodies was also relatively undeveloped, the release of catecholamines from the adrenal medulla during asphyxia at parturition might assume correspondingly greater importance in the initiation of breathing.

SUMMARY AND CONCLUSIONS

Early observations indicated that the injection of epinephrine depressed breathing or even led to a temporary respiratory arrest, epinephrine-induced apnea ("adrenaline apnea"). Subsequently, when more modest doses were used, both epinephrine and norepinephrine were found to increase respiration in unanesthetized human subjects, as well as in anesthetized animals.

The apnea following larger doses of epinephrine is reflex in origin: it is due to an increased discharge from the carotid sinus and aortic arch baroreceptors that results from the rise in arterial pressure produced by the epinephrine. Thus epinephrine-induced apnea does not occur if the carotid sinus and aortic nerves have been cut or if a compensator is used to prevent a rise in the blood pressure.

Increases in respiration have been reported when epinephrine and norepinephrine were infused intravenously in doses of about 0.8 µg/kg·min in anesthetized animals and 0.2 µg/kg·min in conscious man. It seems unlikely that any central effect of the catecholamines, either a direct effect on respiratory neurons or an indirect effect exerted through alterations in cerebral blood flow, is responsible for the hyperpnea. Recent studies suggest that the hyperpnea resulting from epinephrine infusion may result in part from the metabolic effects of epinephrine leading to increased CO_2 production and lowered arterial pH resulting from the formation of lactic acid, though this does not explain the similar increase in ventilation produced by norepinephrine.

The arterial chemoreceptors appear to be of major importance for the production of catecholamine hyperpnea, particularly during the first minutes. This is suggested by the failure of catecholamine infusion to increase respiration in subjects breathing 100% O_2 and is further supported by a similar failure of catecholamine infusion to stimulate breathing in animals in which the chemoreceptors of the carotid and aortic bodies have been denervated by carotid sinus and aortic nerve section. In addition, these doses of epinephrine and norepinephrine evoke an increased discharge in chemoreceptor fibers of the sinus nerve. The most likely cause for this chemoreceptor stimulation by catecholamines is a reduction in local blood flow caused by the vasoconstrictor action of these drugs.

There is still little direct evidence to indicate whether respiratory stimulation by catecholamines is of physiological importance. However, catecholamines can be released from the adrenal medulla by stimulation of the hypothalamus or the splanchnic nerve in quantities exceeding those needed to increase breathing when infused intravenously. Comparable amounts can be released by physiological stresses, such as asphyxia and hemorrhage.

Catecholamine secretion may participate in the initiation of breathing at birth. The carotid bodies are relatively insensitive in the fetus but become sensitive to hypoxia at parturition. Increased sympathetic activity appears to contribute to this increased sensitivity, but it has also been shown that in the full-term fetus asphyxia leads to an active secretion of catecholamines by the adrenal medulla, and this may be an additional factor increasing the responsiveness of the chemoreceptors.

REFERENCES

1. AMOROSO, E. C., F. R. BELL, A. S. KING, AND H. ROSENBERG. Carotid nerve reflexes and effects of adrenaline in the horse and mule. *J. Physiol., London* 109: 29p, 1949.
2. ANICHKOV, S. V., AND M. L. BELEN'KII. *Pharmacology of the Carotid Body Chemoreceptors.* Oxford: Pergamon Press, 1963, p. 126.
3. BADANO, F. Azione del succo di capsule surrenali sul sistema cardiovascolare e sulla respirazione. *Clin. Med. Ital.* 37: 375–386, 1898.
4. BARCROFT, H., V. BASNAYAKE, O. CELANDER, A. F. COBBOLD, D. J. C. CUNNINGHAM, M. G. M. JUKES, AND I. M. YOUNG. The effect of carbon dioxide on the respiratory response to noradrenaline in man. *J. Physiol., London* 137: 365–373, 1957.
5. BEARN, A. G., B. BILLING, AND S. SHERLOCK. The effect of adrenaline and noradrenaline on hepatic blood flow and splanchnic carbohydrate metabolism in man. *J. Physiol., London* 115: 430–441, 1951.
6. BISCOE, T. J. Some effects of drugs on the isolated superfused carotid body. *Nature* 208: 294–295, 1965.
7. BISCOE, T. J., AND M. J. PURVES. Cervical sympathetic and chemoreceptor activity before and after the first breath of the new-born lamb. *J. Physiol., London* 181: 70–71p, 1965.
8. BISCOE, T. J., AND M. J. PURVES. Carotid body chemoreceptor activity in the new-born lamb. *J. Physiol., London* 190: 443–454, 1967.
9. BISCOE, T. J., M. J. PURVES, AND S. R. SAMPSON. The frequency of nerve impulses in single carotid body chemoreceptor afferent fibres recorded *in vivo* with intact circulation. *J. Physiol., London* 208: 121–131, 1970.
10. BISCOE, T. J., AND S. R. SAMPSON. Rhythmical and nonrhythmical spontaneous activity recorded from the central cut end of the sinus nerve. *J. Physiol., London* 196: 327–338, 1968.
11. BOOTHBY, W. M., AND I. SANDIFORD. The calorigenic action of adrenalin chlorid. *Am. J. Physiol.* 66: 93–123, 1923.
12. BORNSTEIN, A. Über Adrenalinglykämie. *Biochem. Z.* 114: 157–164, 1921.
13. BORUTTAU, H. Erfahrungen über die Nebennieren. *Arch. Ges. Physiol.* 78: 97–128, 1899.
14. BOUCKAERT, J. Contribution à l'étude de l'influence de l'adrénaline sur la respiration. *Arch. Néerl. Physiol.* 7: 285–291, 1922.
15. BRADLEY, R. D., P. GASKELL, W. W. HOLLAND, G. DE J. LEE, AND I. M. YOUNG. The acid-base changes in arterial blood during adrenaline hyperpnea in man. *J. Physiol., London* 124: 213–218, 1954.

16. BROWN, E. D. Observations on the effect of epinephrine on the medullary centres. *J. Pharmacol. Exptl. Therap.* 8: 195–203, 1916.
17. BYCK, R. Carotid chemoreceptor stimulation by nicotine and some sympathomimetic amines. *Federation Proc.* 16: 287, 1957.
18. CELANDER, O. The range of control exercised by the sympathico-adrenal system. *Acta Physiol. Scand. Suppl.* 116: 102–106, 1954.
19. CHIOCCHIO, S. R., A. M. BISCARDI, AND J. H. TRAMEZZANI. Catecholamines in the carotid body of the cat. *Nature* 212: 834–835, 1966.
20. COLES, D. R., F. DUFF, W. H. T. SHEPHERD, AND R. F. WHELAN. The effect on respiration of infusions of adrenaline and noradrenaline into the carotid and vertebral arteries in man. *Brit. J. Pharmacol. Chemotherap.* 11: 346–350, 1956.
21. COMLINE, R. S., I. A. SILVER, AND M. SILVER. Factors responsible for the stimulation of the adrenal medulla during asphyxia in the foetal lamb. *J. Physiol., London* 178: 211–238, 1965.
22. COMLINE, R. S., AND M. SILVER. The release of adrenaline and noradrenaline from the adrenal glands of the foetal sheep. *J. Physiol., London* 156: 424–444, 1961.
23. COMLINE, R. S., AND M. SILVER. The development of the adrenal medulla of the foetal and new-born calf. *J. Physiol., London* 183: 305–340, 1966.
24. COMLINE, R. S., AND M. SILVER. Catecholamine secretion by the adrenal medulla of the foetal and new-born foal. *J. Physiol., London* 126: 659–682, 1971.
25. COMROE, J. H., AND C. F. SCHMIDT. The part played by reflexes from the carotid body in the chemical regulation of respiration in the dog. *Am. J. Physiol.* 121: 75–97, 1938.
26. CORI, C. F., AND K. W. BUCHWALD. Effect of continuous intravenous injection of epinephrine on the carbohydrate metabolism, basal metabolism and vascular system of normal man. *Am. J. Physiol.* 95: 71–78, 1930.
27. COURTICE, F. C., C. G. DOUGLAS, AND J. G. PRIESTLEY. Carbohydrate metabolism and muscular exercise. *Proc. Roy. Soc. London, Ser. B* 127: 41–64, 1939.
28. CUNNINGHAM, D. J. C., E. N. HEY, AND B. B. LLOYD. The effect of intravenous infusion of noradrenaline on the respiratory response to carbon dioxide in man. *Quart. J. Exptl. Physiol.* 43: 394–399, 1958.
29. CUNNINGHAM, D. J. C., E. N. HEY, J. M. PATRICK, AND B. B. LLOYD. The effect of noradrenaline infusion on the relation between pulmonary ventilation and the alveolar P_{O_2} and P_{CO_2} in man. *Ann. NY Acad. Sci.* 109: 756–771, 1963.
30. CUNNINGHAM, D. J. C., B. B. LLOYD, AND J. M. PATRICK. The respiratory effect of infused noradrenaline at raised partial pressures of oxygen in man. *J. Physiol., London* 165: 45–46p, 1963.
31. DALY, M. DE BURGH, C. J. LAMBERTSEN, AND A. SCHWEITZER. Observations on the volume of blood flow and oxygen utilization of the carotid body in the cat. *J. Physiol., London* 125: 67–89, 1954.
32. DAWES, G. S., S. L. B. DUNCAN, B. V. LEWIS, C. L. MERLET, J. B. OWEN-THOMAS, AND J. T. REEVES. Hypoxaemia and aortic chemoreceptor function in foetal lambs. *J. Physiol., London* 201: 105–116, 1969.
33. DAWES, G. S., S. L. B. DUNCAN, B. V. LEWIS, C. L. MERLET, J. B. OWEN-THOMAS, AND J. T. REEVES. Cyanide stimulation of the systemic arterial chemoreceptors in foetal lambs. *J. Physiol., London* 201: 117–128, 1969.
34. EADE, N. R., AND D. R. WOOD. The release of adrenaline and noradrenaline from the adrenal medulla of the cat during splanchnic stimulation. *Brit. J. Pharmacol. Chemotherap.* 13: 390–394, 1958.
35. EULER, U. S. VON, G. LILJESTRAND, AND Y. ZOTTERMAN. The excitation mechanism of the chemoreceptors of the carotid body. *Skand. Arch. Physiol.* 83: 132–152, 1939.
36. EYZAGUIRRE, C., AND H. KOYANO. Effects of some pharmacological agents on chemoreceptor discharges. *J. Physiol., London* 178: 410–437, 1965.
37. EYZAGUIRRE, C., AND J. LEWIN. Chemoreceptor activity of the carotid body of the cat. *J. Physiol., London* 159: 222–237, 1961.
38. EYZAGUIRRE, C., AND J. LEWIN. The effect of sympathetic stimulation on carotid nerve activity. *J. Physiol., London* 159: 251–267, 1961.
39. FLOYD, W. F., AND E. NEIL. The influence of the sympathetic innervation of the carotid bifurcation on chemoreceptor and baroreceptor activity in the cat. *Arch. Intern. Pharmacodyn. Thérap.* 91: 230–239, 1952.
40. FOLKOW, B., AND U. S. VON EULER. Selective activation of noradrenaline and adrenaline producing cells in the cat's adrenal gland by hypothalamic stimulation. *Circulation Res.* 2: 191–195, 1954.
41. FUCHS, D., AND N. ROTH. Untersuchungen über die Wirkung des Adrenalins auf den respiratorischen Stoffwechsel. *Z. Exptl. Pathol. Therap.* 10: 187–190, 1912.
42. GALVIANO, V. V., N. BASS, AND F. NYKIEL. Adrenal medullary secretion of epinephrine and norepinephrine in dogs subjected to hemorrhagic hypotension. *Circulation Res.* 8: 564–571, 1960.
43. GERNANDT, B., G. LILJESTRAND, AND Y. ZOTTERMAN. Adrenaline apnea. *Acta Physiol. Scand.* 9: 367–377, 1945.
44. GIBBS, F. A., E. L. GIBBS, AND W. G. LENNOX. The cerebral blood flow in man as influenced by adrenalin, caffein, amyl nitrite and histamine. *Am. Heart J.* 10: 916–924, 1935.
45. GRANT, R., P. LINDGREN, A. ROSEN, AND B. UVNÄS. The release of catechols from the adrenal medulla on activation of the sympathetic vasodilator nerves to the skeletal muscles in the cat by hypothalamic stimulation. *Acta Physiol. Scand.* 43: 135–154, 1958.
46. GRIFFITH, F. R., F. E. EMERY, AND J. E. LOCKWOOD. Effect of adrenalin on pulmonary ventilation: proportionality with dose. *Am. J. Physiol.* 129: 155–164, 1940.
47. HEYMANS, C., AND J. J. BOUCKAERT. Sinus caroticus and respiratory reflexes. I. Cerebral blood flow and respiration. Adrenaline apnoea. *J. Physiol., London* 69: 254–266, 1930.
48. HEYMANS, C., J. J. BOUCKAERT, AND L. DAUTREBANDE. Sinus carotidien et réflexes respiratoires. II. Influences respiratoires réflexes de l'acidose, de l'alcalose, de l'anhydride carbonique, de l'ion hydrogène et de l'anoxemie. Sinus carotidiens et échanges respiratoires dans les poumons et au dela des poumons. *Arch. Intern. Pharmacodyn. Thérap.* 39: 400–448, 1930.
49. HEYMANS, J. F., AND C. HEYMANS. Recherches physiologiques et pharmacodynamiques sur la tête isolée du chien. *Arch Intern. Pharmacodyn. Thérap.* 32: 9–41, 1926.
50. HEYMANS, J. F., AND C. HEYMANS. Sur les modifications directes et sur la régulation réflexe de l'activité du centre respiratoire de la tête isolée du chien. *Arch. Intern. Pharmacodyn. Thérap.* 33: 273–370, 1927.
51. HOFF, H. H., C. G. BRECKENRIDGE, AND J. E. CUNNINGHAM. Adrenaline apnea in the medullary animal. *Am. J. Physiol.* 160: 485–489, 1950.
52. HOLLAND, W. C., AND H. J. SCHÜMANN. Formation of catechol amines during splanchnic nerve stimulation of the adrenal gland of the cat. *Brit. J. Pharmacol. Chemotherap.* 11: 449–453, 1956.
53. HORNBEIN, T. F., Z. J. GRIFFO, AND A. ROOS. Quantitation of chemoreceptor activity: interrelation of hypoxia and hypercapnia. *J. Neurophysiol.* 24: 561–568, 1961.
54. HORNBEIN, T. F., AND A. ROOS. Specificity of H ion concentration as a carotid chemoreceptor stimulant. *J. Appl. Physiol.* 18: 580–584, 1963.
55. HOUSSAY, B. A., AND E. A. MOLINELLI. Adrenal secretion produced by asphyxia. *Am. J. Physiol.* 76: 538–550, 1926.
56. HUGGETT, A. ST. G., AND J. MELLANBY. The action of adrenalin on the central nervous system. *J. Physiol., London* 59: 387–394, 1924.
57. JACKSON, D. E. An experimental investigation of certain

phenomena relating to the action of drugs on the rate of oxygen consumption in the animal body. *J. Lab. Clin. Med.* 2: 145–158, 1916.
58. JOELS, N., AND E. NEIL. Chemoreceptor impulse activity evoked by perfusion of the glomus at various P_{CO_2} and pH values. *J. Physiol., London* 154: 7P, 1960.
59. JOELS, N., AND E. NEIL. The influence of anoxia and hypercapnia, separately and in combination, on chemoreceptor impulse discharge. *J. Physiol., London* 155: 45–46P, 1961.
60. JOELS, N., AND H. WHITE. The contribution of the arterial chemoreceptors to the stimulation of respiration by adrenaline and noradrenaline in the cat. *J. Physiol., London* 197: 1–23, 1968.
61. KAHN, R. H. Beobachtungen über die Wirkung des Nebennierenextractes. *Arch. Anat. Physiol., Physiol. Abt.* 522–537, 1903.
62. KING, B. D., L. SOKOLOFF, AND R. L. WECHSLER. The effects of l-epinephrine and l-nor-epinephrine upon cerebral circulation and metabolism in man. *J. Clin. Invest.* 31: 273–279, 1952.
63. KUNO, Y. On the effect of adrenaline on the respiratory centre. *J. Physiol., London* 60: 148–154, 1925.
64. LANDGREN, S., AND E. NEIL. Chemoreceptor impulse activity following haemorrhage. *Acta Physiol. Scand.* 23: 158–167, 1951.
65. LANGLEY, J. N. Observations on the physiological action of extracts of the suprarenal bodies. *J. Physiol., London* 27: 237–256, 1901.
66. LEE, K. D., R. A. MAYOU, AND R. W. TORRANCE. The effect of blood pressure upon chemoreceptor discharge to hypoxia, and the modification of this effect by the sympathetic-adrenal system. *Quart. J. Exptl. Physiol.* 49: 171–183, 1964.
67. LOEWI, O., AND H. MEYER. Über die Wirkung synthetischer, dem Adrenalin verwandter Stoffe. *Arch. Exptl. Pathol. Pharmakol.* 53: 213–226, 1905.
68. LUNDHOLM, L., AND N. SVEDMYR. Studies on the stimulating effects of adrenaline and noradrenaline on respiration in man. *Acta Physiol. Scand.* 67: 65–75, 1966.
69. LYMAN, R. S., E. NICHOLLS, AND W. S. MCCANN. The respiratory exchange and blood sugar curves of normal and diabetic subjects after epinephrin and insulin. *J. Pharmacol. Exptl. Therap.* 21: 343–356, 1923.
70. MALMEJAC, J. Activity of the adrenal medulla and its regulation. *Physiol. Rev.* 44: 186–218, 1964.
71. MANGER, W. M., J. L. BOLLMAN, F. T. MAHER, AND J. BERKSON. Plasma concentration of epinephrine and nor-epinephrine in hemorrhagic and anaphylactic shock. *Am. J. Physiol.* 190: 310–316, 1957.
72. MARLEY, E. Behavioural and electrophysiological effects of catecholamines. *Pharmacol. Rev.* 18: 753–768, 1966.
73. MARLEY, E., AND W. D. M. PATON. The output of sympathetic amines from the cat's adrenal gland in response to splanchnic nerve activity. *J. Physiol., London* 155: 1–27, 1961.
74. MARRI, R., AND W. HAUSS. Au sujet de l'influence de l'adrénaline sur la respiration. *Arch. Intern. Pharmacodyn. Thérap.* 63: 469–480, 1939.
75. MATELL, G. Time-courses of changes in ventilation and arterial gas tensions in man induced by moderate exercise. *Acta Physiol. Scand. Suppl.* 206: 1–53, 1963.
76. MCDOWALL, R. J. S. The effects of adrenaline on respiration. *Quart. J. Exptl. Physiol.* 18: 325–332, 1928.
77. MELLANBY, J., AND A. ST. G. HUGGETT. The adrenalin and vagal types of apnea. *J. Physiol., London* 57: 395–404, 1923.
78. MILLAR, R. A. Plasma adrenaline and noradrenaline during diffusion respiration. *J. Physiol., London* 150: 79–90, 1960.
79. MILLAR, R. A., AND B. G. BENFEY. The fluorometric estimation of adrenaline and noradrenaline during haemorrhagic hypotension. *Brit. J. Anaesthesiol.* 30: 158–165, 1958.
80. MOYER, J. H., G. MORRIS, AND H. SNYDER. A comparison of the cerebral hemodynamic responses to aramine and nor-epinephrine in the normotensive and the hypotensive subject. *Circulation* 10: 265–270, 1954.

81. NEIL, E., AND N. JOELS. The carotid glomus sensory mechanism. In: *The Regulation of Human Respiration*, edited by D. J. C. Cunningham and B. B. Lloyd. Oxford: Blackwell Sci. Publ., 1963, p. 163–171.
82. NEIL, E., AND R. G. O'REGAN. The effects of electrical stimulation of the distal end of the cut sinus and aortic nerves on peripheral arterial chemoreceptor activity in the cat. *J. Physiol., London* 215: 15–32, 1971.
83. NEIL, E., AND R. G. O'REGAN. Efferent and afferent activity recorded from few-fibre preparations of otherwise intact sinus and aortic nerves. *J. Physiol., London* 215: 33–47, 1971.
84. NICE, L. B., AND A. J. NEILL. The action of adrenaline on respiration. *Am. J. Physiol.* 73: 661–664, 1925.
85. NICE, L. B., J. L. ROCK, AND R. O. COURTRIGHT. The influence of adrenalin on respiration. *Am. J. Physiol.* 34: 326–331, 1914.
86. OLIVER, G., AND E. A. SCHÄFER. The physiological effects of extracts of the suprarenal capsules. *J. Physiol., London* 18: 230–276, 1895.
87. OTEY, E. S., AND T. BERNTHAL. Interaction of hypoxia and hypercapnia at the carotid bodies in chemoreflex stimulation of breathing. *Federation Proc.* 19: 373, 1960.
88. PURVES, M. J. Respiratory and circulatory effects of breathing 100% O_2 in the new-born lamb before and after denervation of the carotid chemoreceptors. *J. Physiol., London* 185: 42–59, 1966.
89. PURVES, M. J. The effects of hypoxia in the new-born lamb before and after denervation of the carotid chemoreceptors. *J. Physiol., London* 185: 60–77, 1966.
90. PURVES, M. J. The effect of hypoxia, hypercapnia and hypotension upon carotid body blood flow and oxygen consumption in the cat. *J. Physiol., London* 209: 395–416, 1970.
91. PURVES, M. J. The role of the cervical sympathetic nerve in the regulation of oxygen consumption of the carotid body of the cat. *J. Physiol., London* 209: 417–431, 1970.
92. REALE, A., A. KAPPERT, C. SKOGLUND, AND G. C. SUTTON. The effect of l-nor-adrenaline on the oxygen consumption of human beings. *Acta Physiol. Scand.* 20: 153–159, 1950.
93. ROBERTS, F. The effect of adrenaline upon respiration. *J. Physiol., London* 55: 346–353, 1921.
94. SALMOIRAGHI, G. C. Central adrenergic synapses. *Pharmacol. Rev.* 18: 717–726, 1966.
95. SALVIOLI, I., AND P. PEZZOLINI. Sur le différent mode d'agir des extracts medullaire et cortical des capsules surrénales. *Arch. Ital. Biol.* 37: 380–382, 1902.
96. SCHMIDT, C. F. The influence of cerebral blood-flow on respiration. I. The respiratory responses to changes in cerebral blood-flow. *Am. J. Physiol.* 84: 202–222, 1928.
97. SCHMIDT, C. F. The action of adrenalin on the respiratory center, with remarks upon the treatment of severe respiratory depression. *J. Pharmacol. Exptl. Therap.* 35: 297–311, 1929.
98. SCHMIDT, C. F. Carotid sinus reflexes to the respiratory center. II. Attempt at evaluation. *Am. J. Physiol.* 102: 119–137, 1932.
99. SENSENBACH, W., L. MADISON, AND L. OCHS. A comparison of the effects of l-nor-epinephrine, synthetic l-epinephrine, and U.S.P. epinephrine upon cerebral blood flow and metabolism in man. *J. Clin. Invest.* 32: 226–232, 1953.
100. SOKOLOFF, L. The action of drugs on the cerebral circulation. *Pharmacol. Rev.* 11: 1–85, 1959.
101. SZYMONOWICZ, L. Die Function der Nebenniere. *Arch. Ges. Physiol.* 64: 97–164, 1896.
102. TOMPKINS, E. H., C. C. STURGIS, AND J. T. WEARN. Studies on epinephrine. II. The effects of epinephrin on the basal metabolism in soldiers with "irritable heart," in hyperthyroidism and in normal men. *Arch. Intern. Med.* 24: 269–283, 1919.
103. TORRANCE, R. W. Prolegomena. In: *The Wates Foundation Symposium on Arterial Chemoreceptors*, edited by R. W. Torrance. Oxford: Blackwell Sci. Publ., 1968, p. 1–40.

104. WHELAN, R. F., AND I. M. YOUNG. The effect of adrenaline and noradrenaline infusions on respiration in man. *Brit. J. Pharmacol. Chemotherap.* 8: 98–102, 1953.
105. WHITEHEAD, R. W., AND D. C. ELLIOTT. Electrocardiographic studies of the action of alpha lobelin and epinephrin on the mammalian heart. *J. Pharmacol. Exptl. Therap.* 31: 145–176, 1927.
106. WITZLEB, E. W. The excitation of chemoreceptors by arterial hypoxia and hypercapnia. In: *The Regulation of Human Respiration*, edited by D. J. C. Cunningham and B. B. Lloyd. Oxford: Blackwell Sci. Publ., 1963, p. 173–182.
107. WOLFF, H. G. The cerebral circulation. *Physiol. Rev.* 16: 545–596, 1936.
108. WRIGHT, S. Action of adrenaline and related substances on respiration. *J. Physiol., London* 69: 493–499, 1930.
109. YOUNG, I. M. Some observations on the mechanism of adrenaline hyperpnoea. *J. Physiol., London* 137: 374–395, 1957.
110. ZAPATA, P., A. HESS, E. L. BLISS, AND C. EYZAGUIRRE. Chemical, electron microscopic and physiological observations on the role of catecholamines in the carotid body. *Brain Res.* 14: 473–496, 1969.

CHAPTER 32

Action of catecholamines on bronchial smooth muscle

J. G. WIDDICOMBE | *Department of Physiology, St. George's Hospital Medical School, Tooting, London, England*

CHAPTER CONTENTS

Innervation of Bronchial Muscle
Methods of Study of Catecholamine Action
  In vitro
  In vivo
    Direct
    Indirect
Actions of Exogenous Catecholamines
  β-Adrenoceptor stimulant drugs
  α-Adrenoceptor stimulant drugs
Lung Tissue Catecholamines
Actions of Blood-borne Catecholamines
Sympathetic Nervous Transmitters
Conclusions

BECAUSE BRONCHIAL SMOOTH MUSCLE is a tissue readily subjected to in vitro experiments and because of the importance of such work in the therapy of lung diseases, such as asthma, its pharmacology has been extensively studied for over 60 years. Thus literature on the action of exogenous catecholamines on airway smooth muscle is extensive [for reviews, see (1, 12, 13, 21, 48, 59, 70, 71, 74)]. To a certain extent these studies can be correlated with what is known about the innervation of the airways, and their relevance to possible endogenous catecholamine action is usually obvious. However, three major parts of the whole picture are drawn only sketchily.

1. The nature of the transmitter between sympathetic nerves and airway smooth muscle has not been established.

2. The relative importance of sympathetic, as compared with parasympathetic, nerves is uncertain, and their interactions have been little studied.

3. Study of the possible action of blood-borne catecholamines on airway smooth muscle has been largely neglected for experimental animals and almost entirely ignored for man.

Furthermore the investigation of catecholamine action is complicated because use of exogenous drugs emphasizes many species differences and also differences between various parts of the airways (e.g., trachea, bronchi, bronchioles). The extensive use of catecholamines in the treatment of asthma has led to many pharmacological studies, but quantitative application of these results to normal airways is clearly unreliable.

INNERVATION OF BRONCHIAL MUSCLE

Tracheobronchial smooth muscle is innervated by both the parasympathetic and the sympathetic nervous systems. Parasympathetic fibers are located in the vagus nerves; they are constrictor in function, and acetylcholine is the chemical transmitter. Postganglionic sympathetic fibers arise in the thoracic sympathetic trunk and utilize catecholamines as transmitters; the stellate ganglion sends fibers by the cervical sympathetic nerve and the recurrent laryngeal nerve to the trachea, and by the ansa subclavia and the cardio-pulmonary branches from the upper 1–4 sympathetic ganglia to the lungs. The sympathetic fibers mingle with those of the vagus and its branches to form common afferent and efferent nerve bundles to the lungs and the respiratory tract. This general description of the innervation of the lungs has been frequently reviewed (21, 48, 70, 71, 74) and seems to apply to all mammalian species studied.

There have been many studies of both the anatomy and histology of the pulmonary nerves. However, the histological studies have tended to concentrate on afferent end organs and fibers or on parasympathetic (cholinergic) efferent fibers and their ganglion cells. Sympathetic (adrenergic) efferent postganglionic fibers have been less frequently studied, although recently the fluorescence method of Hillarp and Falck has been applied, but mainly with emphasis on the innervation of blood vessels in the lung (21). The method has revealed catecholamine-containing inclusions in nerves in the bronchial muscle of cat (19), rat (75), dog, and guinea pig (30). The fact that they are found throughout the muscle of the entire bronchial tree down to respiratory bronchioles may indicate that airways of all sizes have a sympathetic adrenergic innervation but does not indicate if such innervation is more potent in one part of the respiratory tract than in another. The chemical nature of the catecholamine displayed by the fluorescence method has not been established.

The dominant nervous control of airway smooth muscle, both in the sense of tonic and of reflexly induced activity, is parasympathetic, cholinergic, and constrictor (70, 71). Atropine increases airway caliber in unanesthetized man and in anesthetized experimental mammals, as judged both by changes in airway resistance to flow and by measurement of anatomic dead space, and blocks reflexly induced bronchoconstrictions in both types of subjects.

The physiological role of sympathetic catecholamine-mediated control is probably slight, at least in healthy lungs. In pathological situations, which are beyond the scope of this review, it is possible that sympathetic nerves to airway muscle play a larger part. The evidence on the physiological role of the sympathetic nerves is mainly indirect, and careful experiments testing the action of sympathetic nerves are few. The best and recent study by Nadel and his colleagues (8) showed that supramaximal stimulation (60 Hz) of the sympathetic nerves to the dog's lung increased the diameter of the airways from bronchi to 0.5-mm bronchioles. The response was absent when there was no vagal bronchoconstrictor tone or when constrictor tone was strong, and the dilator influence never completely inhibited vagal constriction. Both vagal and sympathetic actions were homolateral.

METHODS OF STUDY OF CATECHOLAMINE ACTION

In Vitro

Preparations of airway tissues suspended in organ baths can show the quantitative action of drugs and other chemicals on airway smooth muscle and on the intrinsic innervation of the smooth muscle. Among the methods most frequently used is that in which tracheal or bronchial rings or chains are made to move an isotonic lever. Although these methods can provide little information about endogenous hormonal or chemical actions or establish the nature of nerve transmitters, they are valuable for two reasons: *1*) they test whether a drug is acting locally on the neuromuscular apparatus of the airways rather than reflexly, by an action on the central nervous system or by the release of chemical mediators somewhere other than in the airway smooth muscle; and *2*) they allow the direct observation and assay of drug actions and interactions. Such in vitro preparations can be made from most vertebrate species of appropriate body size, including man.

In Vivo

DIRECT. Direct in vivo methods are essential in studying the role of the extrinsic innervation of airway smooth muscle and in establishing whether chemicals and drugs have an action in a physiological situation. The two variables influenced by airway smooth muscle contraction and most readily measured are the resistance to airflow in the respiratory tract and the geometric dimensions of the airways.

The only convenient method of measuring "total" airways resistance is with the body plethysmograph (18, 27), which gives a value for resistance to flow from alveoli to external atmosphere (including laryngeal and upper airway resistance). Although this method is usually applied to cooperating humans, methods based on similar principles have been applied to experimental mammals (57). An approximation of airways resistance can be obtained by assessing "total lung resistance to flow," from the pressure-volume-flow relations of the entire lung (24, 33, 52, 56), or by the "interruptor" technique (10). The derived values include not only airways resistance, but also the viscous resistance to flow of the lung tissues, which is about 20% of the total and therefore probably does not constitute a major error. Bouhuys and his colleagues (23, 26) have recently developed methods for the measurement of total lung resistance in small experimental animals, and their technique shows great promise in the study of airway pharmacology.

Airway geometry can be assessed in several ways. Anatomic dead space can be measured by using foreign or physiological gases and indicates the total volume of the airways, including upper airways, up to the point at which alveolar and respiratory tract gases become mixed (18). Radiographic methods indicate linear dimensions of the airways; they have the advantage of being "direct," but values are usually only applicable to localized regions and, with an exception, to the larger airways (40, 70). The exception is the use of tantalum dust as a radio-opaque medium; this allows accurate measurement of airway diameter down to 0.5 mm and has been successfully applied to man and experimental animals (54). A useful experimental method is the measurement of volume changes in the cervical trachea isolated in situ and in vivo; this preparation provides a direct assessment of tracheal caliber and easy access to blood supply and to sympathetic and parasympathetic nerves (33, 56, 72). However, it should not be assumed that pharmacological results obtained with it will be the same for the intrapulmonary bronchi and bronchioles. The method has so far only been applied to dog and cat, although there is no reason to suppose that smaller mammals will prove intractable.

INDIRECT. Methods based on changes in lung compliance (the volume-pressure relation) cannot be reliably interpreted in terms of bronchial smooth muscle activity, unless it can be unequivocally established that the compliance change is due to alterations in airway smooth muscle contraction (70). Compliance is also affected by changes in surfactant and in the pulmonary vascular bed and by collapse of the lungs. The extensive use of the method of Konzett & Rössler (44) by pharmacologists reflects its convenience and its sensitivity as an index of compliance rather than its reliability as a technique for assessing bronchial caliber or smooth muscle tone (49, 70). Methods such as measurement of fast expired volume (FEV) and peak flow rate (PFR) have been frequently used in man. They give values influenced by bronchial caliber and smooth muscle tone and are of considerable clinical value and convenience, but they provide no data meaningful in terms of airway geometry and are greatly influenced by factors other than airway smooth muscle contraction (18). Histology of the airways, in particular by rapid-freezing techniques (55), can give valuable but nonquantitative information. The recent measurements of frequency-dependent compliance point to a potentially valuable research method for determining the resistance of the bronchioles and smaller airways, but its general application and assessment have not yet taken place (73).

In summary, the actions of drugs, such as catecholamines, on airway smooth muscle may be indicated or determined by in vitro or indirect in vivo methods, but the relation of such experiments to the physiological situation can only be established by more direct measurements of airways resistance or caliber in vivo. Both types of analysis are complementary and essential for an adequate interpretation of airway physiology and pharmacology.

ACTIONS OF EXOGENOUS CATECHOLAMINES

β-Adrenoceptor Stimulant Drugs

Catecholamines that act on β receptors relax the airway smooth muscle. This has been known since 1912 when Dixon & Ransom (25) and Trendelenburg (68) showed that adrenal extracts could cause bronchodilatation, if there was pre-existing smooth muscle tone. Isoproterenol was shown by Konzett (42, 43) in 1940 to be about 10 times more active than epinephrine, and, until the last few years, isoproterenol has been the drug of choice in the treatment of asthma. (There are probably thousands of references to the use of this and similar β receptor stimulant drugs, especially in relation to clinical and pharmacological studies. For 1971 alone an incomplete survey of journals from Western Europe and North America estimated 250 references. Hereafter only a few key and/or recent papers and reviews are cited.) Isoproterenol relaxes isolated tracheobronchial preparations of most mammalian species and prevents the action of drugs, such as acetylcholine and histamine, that cause contraction (21, 70). In intact healthy man, isoproterenol, given as an aerosol or intravenously, increases anatomic dead space by 25–40% and decreases airways resistance by 30–50% (70); its action in patients with bronchoconstriction can be considerably greater. Although there may be some quantitative species differences, and even differences between trachea and bronchi (35, 50), the overwhelming consensus of the literature is that drugs acting on β receptors inhibit the tone and prevent the contraction of airway smooth muscle and that the potency order of the most relevant drugs is isoproterenol > epinephrine > norepinephrine > phenylephrine. (Potency ratios vary greatly in different species and experiments but in general they are of the order 500:50:5:1, respectively.) These relaxant and blocking responses are prevented by β receptor blocking agents, such as dichloroisoproterenol and propranolol (1, 21, 70).

In 1967 Lands and co-workers (45) introduced the concept of two types of β receptors: β_1 receptors, which, for example, mediate the inotropic and chronotropic actions of adrenergic nerves on the heart; and β_2 receptors, which mediate the actions of catecholamines on peripheral vascular beds and on bronchial smooth muscle.

Several drugs that are potent relaxors of airway smooth muscle but have little action on the heart are now in clinical use; these include salbutamol, terbutaline, and isoethamine (1, 4, 6, 7, 20, 38). Although the clinical importance of these drugs is clearly great, the extent to which they indicate pharmacological receptor mechanisms is less clear. Many studies have shown that these drugs have actions quantitatively different from those of isoproterenol or epinephrine on cardiac, as compared with bronchial, muscle, but there is some inconsistency in the actions of the drugs on different tissue preparations and on different species, which probably makes the classification of β receptors into β_1 and β_2 types an oversimplification (32, 38). There is a therapeutic convenience in labeling a bronchodilator drug a "β_2 stimulant," but the research telling us how its mode of action differs from a cardiac "β_1 stimulant" does not seem to have been done.

α-Adrenoceptor Stimulant Drugs

A number of publications now report that α receptor stimulant catecholamines and drugs can, in the presence of β receptor antagonists, cause contraction of isolated airway smooth muscle from both man and other species [e.g., (9, 34, 63, 64)]. It must be emphasized that these contractions in response to stimulation only occur when β receptors are blocked and that even powerful α receptor stimulants, such as phenylephrine and norepinephrine, almost invariably cause airway smooth muscle relaxation in the absence of β blocking drugs (1, 9, 59). Other publications indicate that α receptors mediating contraction are absent, sparse, or weak (31, 34, 51). Conversely drugs that block α receptors can potentiate the action of catecholamines that stimulate β receptors and thereby relax airway smooth muscle, but the careful and extensive study of Foster (31) indicates that the underlying mechanism is complex and not a simple α receptor block.

Some of the in vitro studies can be criticized because the doses of drugs used were very high or because the involvement of cholinergic contractile mechanisms was not always ruled out.

In vivo studies in animals have also given contradictory results (8, 22). In man α receptor stimulants can cause bronchoconstriction in the presence of β blocking drugs, but some investigations have shown that the constriction is prevented (36, 47) or reduced (41, 63) by atropine, which suggests that the α receptor stimulants are acting via vagal cholinergic pathways.

It is difficult to summarize the confused and contradictory literature on airway α receptors. It is possible tentatively to conclude that a) in appropriate circumstances α receptor stimulant drugs can cause contraction of tracheobronchial smooth muscle; b) the concentrations of agonists and antagonists are often greatly in excess of those applied in other studies; c) their mode of action may be not only on α or β receptors but may involve other biological processes, such as cholinergic mechanisms; d) the in vitro experiments cannot be cited as positive support for an α receptor-mediated contractile mechanism with a physiological role in the intact animal. The whole problem may have a clinical application: it has been suggested that the hypersensitivity of bronchial smooth muscle in asthmatics is associated with, or even due to, an increase in potency of an α receptor-mediated contractile mechanism (67), since β blocking drugs can aggravate asthma (17, 51, 60).

LUNG TISSUE CATECHOLAMINES

Although the lung tissue content of catecholamines and related enzymes has been studied, interpretation of these studies is hampered by a fundamental problem: there are at least three adrenergic motor systems in the lungs (i.e., to pulmonary circulation, to bronchial circulation, and to airway smooth muscle), and the methods do not allow their differentiation. In particular, sympathetic supply to the pulmonary vascular bed is abundant, and the transmitter is probably norepinephrine (21). Studies on tracheal muscle might be informative. Therefore the following summary is brief, since it applies to total adrenergic innervation and not necessarily to bronchial smooth muscle innervation.

Over 90% of the total extractable catecholamine in mammalian lung is dopamine (28, 62). In early work using relatively insensitive methods (61) no measurable dopa decarboxylase, which would convert dopa to dopamine, was found in the lungs and it was considered possible that the dopamine reaches the lungs from the circulating blood (5). By contrast, the sympathetic nerves to pulmonary vessels contain roughly equal amounts of dopamine and norepinephrine (29). Tyramine, in concentrations high relative to those for other tissues, has been described in cat lungs (65).

The conversion pathway for lung dopamine to norepinephrine and epinephrine is not established, but rabbit lung can catalyze the formation of epinine from dopamine, and epinine could be converted to epinephrine by dopamine β-oxidase (2).

Axelrod (3) has shown that the lungs can take up relatively large quantities of blood-borne norepinephrine, whereas epinephrine was taken up at a far slower rate. The importance of the lungs as tissue absorbents of many blood-borne hormones has recently been emphasized (69), but the exact sites of uptake have not been determined.

With regard to the breakdown of catecholamines in the lungs, the tissue contains both catechol-O-methyltransferase and monoamine oxidase, the latter in concentrations only exceeded by the liver and kidney (37).

ACTIONS OF BLOOD-BORNE CATECHOLAMINES

Since in the absence of β blocking drugs catecholamines, such as epinephrine and norepinephrine, relax airway smooth muscle in vitro, it is possible that release of these hormones from the adrenal medulla in vivo might have a similar action via the bloodstream. This possibility seems to have been studied mainly in the guinea pig, in which adrenal medullary hormones are released in anaphylaxis (58, 66). The rate of output of epinephrine into the blood recorded in this condition (0.02–1 μg/min) is sufficient to lessen drug-induced bronchoconstrictions in the guinea pig (14). Collier and his co-workers (15, 16) have shown that β receptor blockade intensifies the bronchoconstriction in anaphylaxis in guinea pigs. This could be brought about by a local action on bronchial smooth muscle, which would change either the effect of catecholamine transmitters released in the lungs or the effect of blood-borne catecholamines released from the adrenal medulla. The observation that adrenalectomy also potentiates the bronchoconstriction resulting from anaphylaxis favors the latter explanation (39). In cats, too, Colebatch (11) has shown that adrenalectomy augments the bronchoconstriction caused by intravenous administration of histamine, presumably by preventing the action of blood-borne catecholamines.

The action on bronchial muscle of catecholamines released from the adrenal medulla of man does not seem to have been studied. The fact that parenterally administered epinephrine is a recognized and effective therapy for anaphylactic bronchoconstrictions shows that blood-borne catecholamines are able to relax airway muscle but does not indicate that those released from the adrenal medulla do so as well.

SYMPATHETIC NERVOUS TRANSMITTERS

Information on the nature of the transmitter at the postganglionic sympathetic nerve endings to bronchial smooth muscle has been sought in two types of experiments. In both the thoracic sympathetic nerves to the lungs are stimulated electrically; however, in one instance the transmitter is assayed in the effluent fluid of perfused lung, and in the other bronchomuscular contraction is estimated and the effects of various blocking drugs are studied.

When the sympathetic nerves are stimulated electrically a chemical is released into pulmonary venous blood of perfused cat lungs. Chromatographic and pharmacological tests originally showed this substance to have properties similar to those of isoproterenol but not to epinephrine or norepinephrine (46). No norepinephrine was detected, although it is the transmitter at sympathetic endings to the pulmonary vascular bed (21). The conclusion that isoproterenol might be the sympathetic transmitter is made less tenable because no appreciable amount of isoproterenol can be extracted from either the thoracic sympathetic nerve trunks (53) or lung tissue (46a). Experiments with tracheal muscle might be helpful since they would eliminate the complication due to release of transmitters from the pulmonary vasculature.

The use of pharmacological blocking agents during sympathetic nerve stimulation has been applied on several occasions, although the parasympathetic (cholinergic) nerves have been studied far more extensively by this approach. The experiments support the evidence based on use of exogenous catecholamines that the sympathetic transmitter that relaxes the muscle acts on β receptors, but these experiments give little definite information about its nature (apart from the teleological argument that the order of effectiveness would be isoproterenol > epinephrine > norepinephrine). Thus β receptor blocking drugs, such as dichloroisoproterenol, block the bronchodilation caused by sympathetic nervous stimulation in the presence of smooth muscle tone (1, 59). Whether the transmitter has an action also on the hypothetical α receptors, and would therefore tend to cause constriction or lessen dilation, is more uncertain, although this has been claimed (22). However, the careful experiments of Nadel and co-workers (8), who used "direct" radiographic methods of measuring bronchial and bronchiolar tone in dogs with nervously induced bronchoconstrictions, provide convincing evidence that in these conditions transmitter release does not have an α receptor action. A priori it seems unlikely that norepinephrine is the transmitter, since this is primarily an α receptor stimulant; in the absence of good indications that isoproterenol is involved, epinephrine must be the strongest candidate for the transmitter, in which case it must be concluded that α receptor constrictor mechanisms are insignificant in physiological conditions. Pharmacologically and clinically these mechanisms could be of greater importance.

CONCLUSIONS

This review should make it clear that we are ignorant of many of the basic facts about catecholamine action on bronchial smooth muscle. Although it is certain that the main pharmacological mechanism involves a β receptor relaxation, we are uncertain as to the nature of the adrenergic transmitter and whether blood-borne catecholamines have a significant action. Controversy clouds the problems of the nature of the β receptors (or, perhaps, β_2 receptors) and whether α receptors (constrictor) exist or are of physiological significance. Some of the experiments designed to study these problems should not be difficult to perform.

REFERENCES

1. Aviado, D. M. *Sympathomimetic Drugs*. Springfield, Ill.: Thomas, 1970.
2. Axelrod, J. Enzymic formation of adrenaline and other catechols from monophenols. *Science* 140: 499–500, 1963.
3. Axelrod, J., L. G. Whitby, G. Hertting, and I. L. Kopin. Studies on the metabolism of catecholamines. *Circulation Res.* 9: 715–719, 1961.
4. Bergman, J., H. Persson, and K. Wetterlin. Two new groups of selective stimulants of adrenergic β-receptors. *Experientia* 25: 899–901, 1969.
5. Blaschko, H. The development of current concepts of catecholamine formation. *Pharmacol. Rev.* 11: 307–316, 1959.
6. Brittain, R. T. A comparison of the pharmacology of salbutamol with that of isoprenaline, orciprenaline and trimetoquinol. *Postgrad. Med. J. Suppl.* 47: 11–16, 1971.
7. Brittain, R. T., D. C. Jack, and A. C. Ritchie. Recent β-adrenoreceptor stimulants. *Advan. Drug Res.* 5: 197–253, 1970.
8. Cabezas, G. A., P. D. Graf, and J. A. Nadel. Sympathetic versus parasympathetic nervous regulation of airways in dogs. *J. Appl. Physiol.* 31: 651–655, 1971.
9. Chahl, L. A., and S. R. O'Donnell. Actions of phenylephrine on β-adrenoreceptors. *Brit. J. Pharmacol.* 37: 41–51, 1969.
10. Clements, J. A., J. T. Sharp, R. P. Johnson, and J. O. Elam. Estimation of pulmonary resistance by repetitive interruption of airflow. *J. Appl. Physiol.* 38: 1262–1270, 1959.
11. Colebatch, H. J. H. The humoral regulation of alveolar ducts. In: *Airway Dynamics, Physiology and Pharmacology*, edited by A. Bouhuys. Springfield, Ill.: Thomas, 1970, p. 169–189.
12. Collier, H. O. J. Humoral factors in bronchoconstriction. In: *Scientific Basis of Medicine. Annual Reviews*. London: Athlone Press, 1968, p. 308–355.
13. Collier, H. O. J. Endogenous bronchoactive substances and their antagonism. *Advan. Drug Res.* 5: 95–107, 1970.
14. Collier, H. O. J., J. A. Holgate, M. Schachter, and P. G. Shorley. The bronchoconstrictor action of bradykinin in the guinea-pig. *Brit. J. Pharmacol.* 15: 290–297, 1960.
15. Collier, H. O. J., and G. W. L. James. Humoral factors affecting pulmonary inflation during acute anaphylaxis in the guinea-pig in vivo. *Brit. J. Pharmacol.* 30: 283–301, 1967.
16. Collier, H. O. J., and G. W. L. James. Humoral factors in airway function, with particular reference to anaphylaxis in the guinea-pig. In: *Airway Dynamics, Physiology and Pharmacology*, edited by A. Bouhuys. Springfield, Ill.: Thomas, 1970, p. 239–252.
17. Connolly, C. K., and J. C. Batten. Comparison of the effect of alprenolol and propranolol on specific airway conductance in asthmatic patients. *Brit. Med. J.* ii: 515–516, 1970.
18. Cotes, J. E. *Lung Function* (2nd ed.). Oxford: Blackwell, 1968.
19. Dahlström, A., K. Fuxe, T. Hökfelt, and K-A. Norberg. Adrenergic innervation of the bronchial muscle in the cat. *Acta Physiol. Scand.* 66: 507–508, 1966.
20. Daly, I. de B., and C. Hebb. *Pulmonary and Bronchial Vascular Systems*. London: Arnold, 1966.

21. DALY, M. J., J. B. FARMER, AND G. P. LEVY. Comparison of the bronchodilator and cardiovascular actions of salbutamol, isoprenaline and orciprenaline. *Brit. J. Pharmacol.* 43: 624–638, 1971.
22. DE LA MATA, C. R., M. PENNA, AND D. M. AVIADO. Reversal of sympathetic bronchodilation by dichloroisoproterenol. *J. Pharmacol. Exptl. Therap.* 135: 197–203, 1962.
23. DENNIS, M. W., AND J. S. DOUGLAS. Control of bronchomotor tone in spontaneously breathing unanaesthetised guinea-pigs. In: *Airway Dynamics, Physiology and Pharmacology*, edited by A. Bouhuys. Springfield, Ill.: Thomas, 1970, p. 253–262.
24. DIAMOND, L. Utilization of changes in pulmonary resistance for the evaluation of bronchodilator drugs. *Arch. Intern. Pharmacodyn.* 168: 239–250, 1967.
25. DIXON, W. E., AND F. RANSOM. Bronchodilator nerves. *J. Physiol., London* 45: 413–428, 1912.
26. DOUGLAS, J. S., M. W. DENNIS, P. RIDGWAY, AND A. BOUHUYS. Airway dilation and constriction in spontaneously breathing guinea-pigs. *J. Pharmacol. Exptl. Therap.* 180: 98–109, 1972.
27. DUBOIS, A. B., S. Y. BOTELHO, AND J. H. COMROE. A new method for measuring airway resistance in man using a body plethysmograph: values in normal subjects and in patients with respiratory disease. *J. Clin. Invest.* 35: 327–335, 1956.
28. EULER, U. S. VON, AND F. LISHAJKO. Dopamine in mammalian lung and spleen. *Acta Physiol. Pharmacol. Neérl.* 6: 295–303, 1957.
29. EULER, U. S. VON, AND F. LISHAJKO. Catecholamines in the vascular wall. *Acta Physiol. Scand.* 42: 333–341, 1958.
30. FILLENZ, M., AND R. I. WOODS. Sensory innervation of the airways. In: *Breathing: Hering-Breuer Centenary Symposium*, edited by R. Porter. London: Churchill, 1970, p. 101–107.
31. FOSTER, R. W. The nature of the adrenergic receptors of the trachea of the guinea-pig. *J. Pharm. Pharmacol.* 18: 1–12, 1966.
32. FURCHGOTT, R. F. Pharmacological characteristics of adrenergic receptors. *Federation Proc.* 29: 1352–1361, 1970.
33. GREEN, M., AND J. G. WIDDICOMBE. The effects of ventilation of dogs with different gas mixtures on airway calibre and lung mechanics. *J. Physiol., London* 186: 363–381, 1966.
34. GUIRGIS, H. M., AND R. S. MCNEILL. The nature of the adrenergic receptors in isolated human bronchi. *Thorax* 24: 613–615, 1969.
35. HAWKINS, D. F., AND W. D. M. PATON. Responses of isolated bronchial muscle to ganglionically active drugs. *J. Physiol., London* 144: 193–219, 1958.
36. HERXHEIMER, H., AND I. LANGER. Untersuchungen über die bronchokonstriktorische Wirkung des β-Rezeptorblockers Propranolol bei Meerschweinchen und Patienten mit Asthma bronchiale. *Klin. Wochschr.* 45: 1149–1153, 1967.
37. IISALO, E. Enzyme action on noradrenaline and adrenaline. *Acta Pharmacol. Toxicol.* 19, Suppl. 1: 1–90, 1962.
38. JACK, D. An introduction to salbutamol and other modern β-adrenoreceptor stimulants. *Postgrad. Med. J. Suppl.* 47: 8–11, 1971.
39. JAMES, G. W. L. The use of the in vivo trachea preparation of the guinea-pig to assess drug action on the lung. *J. Pharm. Pharmacol.* 21: 379–386, 1900.
40. KILBURN, K. H. Dimensional responses of bronchi in apneic dogs to airway pressure, gases and drugs. *J. Appl. Physiol.* 15: 229–234, 1960.
41. KOCK, M. A. DE. Mechanism of bronchial obstruction in man. In: *Bronchitis III*, edited by N. G. M. Orie and R. van der Lende. Assen: Thomas, 1970, p. 300–311.
42. KONZETT, H. Neue broncholytische hochwirksame Körper der Adrenalinreihe. *Arch. Exptl. Pathol. Pharmakol.* 197: 27–40, 1940.
43. KONZETT, H. Zur Pharmakologie neuer adrenalinverwandter Körper. *Arch. Exptl. Pathol. Pharmakol.* 197: 41–56, 1940.
44. KONZETT, H., AND R. RÖSSLER. Versuchsanordnung zu Untersuchungen an der Bronchialmuskulatur. *Arch. Exptl. Pathol. Pharmakol.* 195: 71–74, 1940.
45. LANDS, A. M., A. ARNOLD, J. P. MCAULIFF, F. P. LUDUENA, AND T. G. BROWN. Differentiation of receptor systems activated by sympathomimetic amines. *Nature* 214: 597–598, 1967.
46. LOCKETT, M. F. The transmitter released by stimulation of bronchial sympathetic nerves. *Brit. J. Pharmacol.* 12: 86–96, 1957.
46a. LOCKETT, M. F. [Cited by Daly & Hebb (20).]
47. MACDONALD, A. G., C. G. INGRAM, AND R. S. MCNEILL. The effect of propranolol on airway resistance. *Brit. J. Anaesthesiol.* 39: 919–926, 1967.
48. MACKLIN, C. C. The musculature of the bronchi and lungs. *Physiol. Rev.* 9: 1–60, 1929.
49. MARCELLE, R. Limits of indirect methods for evaluating bronchomotor reactions in guinea-pigs. *Arch. Intern. Pharmacodyn.* 183: 406–409, 1970.
50. MCDOUGAL, M. D., AND G. B. WEST. The action of drugs on isolated mammalian smooth muscle. *Brit. J. Pharmacol.* 8: 26–29, 1953.
51. MCNEILL, R. S. The effect of β-antagonists on the bronchi. *Postgrad. Med. J. Suppl.* 47: 14–16, 1971.
52. MEAD, J., AND J. L. WHITTENBERGER. Physical properties of human lungs measured during spontaneous respiration. *J. Appl. Physiol.* 5: 779–796, 1953.
53. MUSCHOLL, E., AND M. VOGT. The action of reserpine on the peripheral sympathetic system. *J. Physiol., London* 141: 132–155, 1958.
54. NADEL, J. A., G. A. CABEZAS, AND J. H. M. AUSTIN. In vivo roentgenographic examination of parasympathetic innervation of small airways. Use of tantalum and a fine spot x-ray tube. *Invest. Radiol.* 6: 9–17, 1971.
55. NADEL, J. A., H. J. P. COLEBATCH, AND C. R. OLSEN. Location and mechanism of airway constriction after barium sulfate microembolism. *J. Appl. Physiol.* 19: 387–394, 1964.
56. NADEL, J. A., AND J. G. WIDDICOMBE. Effect of changes in blood gas tensions and carotid sinus pressure on tracheal volume and total lung resistance to airflow. *J. Physiol., London* 163: 13–33, 1962.
57. PALECEK, F. Measurement of ventilatory mechanics in the rat. *J. Appl. Physiol.* 27: 149–156, 1969.
58. PIPER, P. P., H. O. J. COLLIER, AND J. R. VANE. Release of catecholamines in the guinea-pig by substances involved in anaphylaxis. *Nature* 213: 838–840, 1967.
59. PRUSS, T. P., AND D. M. AVIADO. Drugs for the therapy of pulmonary disorders. *Ann. Rep. Med. Chem.* 55–62, 1969.
60. RICHARDSON, P. S., AND G. M. STERLING. Effects of β-adrenergic receptor blockade on airway conductance and lung volume in normal and asthmatic subjects. *Brit. J. Med.* ii: 143–147, 1969.
61. SCHÜMANN, H. J. Über den Hydroxytyramin- und Noradrenalingehalt der Lunge. *Arch. Exptl. Pathol. Pharmakol.* 234: 282–290, 1958.
62. SCHÜMANN, H. J. Formation of adrenergic transmitters. In: *Adrenergic Mechanisms*, edited by J. R. Vane, G. E. W. Wolstenholme, and M. O'Connor. London: Churchill, 1960, p. 6–16.
63. SIMONSSON, B. G., R. ANDERSSON, N. P. BERGH, B. E. SKOOGH, AND N. SVEDMYR. In vivo and in vitro studies of pharmacological effects on different receptors regulating bronchial tone in man. In: *Bronchitis III*, edited by N. G. M. Orie and R. van der Lende. Assen: Thomas, 1970, p. 334–342.
64. SIRO-BRIGIANI, G. Pharmacologic reactivity of tracheobronchial muscle of ten species of animals. *Arch. Ital. Sci. Farmacol.* 15: 214–231, 1965.
65. SPECTOR, S., K. MELMON, W. LOVENBERG, AND A. SJOERDSMA. The presence and distribution of tyramine in mammalian tissue. *J. Pharmacol. Exptl. Therap.* 140: 229–235, 1963.
66. STASZEWSKA-BARCZAK, J., AND J. R. VANE. The release of catecholamines from the adrenal medulla. *Brit. J. Pharmacol.* 25: 728–742, 1965.
67. SZENTIVANYI, A. The β-adrenergic theory of the atopic abnormality in bronchial asthma. *J. Allergy* 42: 203–232, 1968.
68. TRENDELENBURG, P. Physiologische und pharmakologische Untersuchungen an der isolierten Bronchialmuskulatur. *Arch. Exptl. Pathol. Pharmakol.* 69: 79–107, 1912.

69. VANE, J. R. The release and assay of hormones in the circulation. In: *Scientific Basis of Medicine. Annual Reviews.* London: Athlone Press, 1968, p. 336–359.
70. WIDDICOMBE, J. G. Regulation of tracheobronchial smooth muscle. *Physiol. Rev.* 43: 1–37, 1963.
71. WIDDICOMBE, J. G. The regulation of bronchial calibre. In: *Recent Advances in Respiratory Physiology*, edited by C. G. Caro. London: Arnold, 1966, p. 48–82.
72. WIDDICOMBE, J. G., AND J. A. NADEL. Reflex effects of lung inflation on tracheal volume. *J. Appl. Physiol.* 18: 681–686, 1963.
73. WOOLCOCK, A. J., N. J. VINCENT, AND P. T. MACKLEM. Frequency dependence of compliance as test for obstruction in small airways. *J. Clin. Invest.* 48: 1097–1106, 1969.
74. WYSS, O. A. M. La motilité de la paroi bronchique. *Bronches* 2: 101–151, 1952.
75. ZUSSMAN, W. V. Fluorescent localization of catecholamine stores in the rat lung. *Anat. Rev.* 156: 19–29, 1966.

CHAPTER 33

Role of circulating catecholamines in the gastrointestinal tract

J. B. FURNESS
G. BURNSTOCK | *Department of Zoology, University of Melbourne, Parkville, Victoria, Australia*

CHAPTER CONTENTS

Effects of Catecholamines on Gastrointestinal Motility
    General considerations: nonsphincter muscle
    Sphincter muscle
    Muscularis mucosae
    Receptor sites
    Summary
Effects of Catecholamines on Gastrointestinal Vasculature
    General observations
    Dilator effects
    Local reactions
    Duration of action
    Summary
Effects of Catecholamines on Gastrointestinal Secretion
    Gastric acid secretion
    Mucous secretion
Effects of Catecholamines on Gastrointestinal Absorption
Conditions Leading to Increased Levels of Circulating
    Catecholamines and Their Effects on the Gut
    Shock
    Intense Emotion
    Exercise
    Pheochromocytoma
    Summary
Possible Involvement of Catecholamines in Ulceration
Adrenergic Nerves as Source of Circulating Catecholamines
Relative Roles of Circulating and Locally Released
    Catecholamines
Plasma Levels of Catecholamines and the Sensitivity of
    Gastrointestinal Structures
    Summary
Conclusions

CIRCULATING CATECHOLAMINES are only part of a system of nervous and hormonal mechanisms that regulate the functions of the gut. None of these is adequately understood on its own, and the nuances of their interplay are complex. Gastrointestinal function is influenced by catecholamines released locally from sympathetic nerves, as well as by those released into the circulation. Moreover, conditions leading to increased discharge of catecholamines into the circulation also activate sympathetic nerves. The roles of adrenergic nerves in the gastrointestinal tract are considered in a recent review article (133).

Catecholamines affect, directly or indirectly, almost every aspect of gastrointestinal function. They have been shown to influence motility, blood flow, secretion, absorption, and the activity of enteric neurons. These functions are interdependent, and the apparent simplicity of determining the mode of action of catecholamines is deceptive. Among the wealth of data available, are many seemingly conflicting observations, as well as considerable agreement. It is also clear that serious doubt can be placed on several accepted "textbook" generalizations. For example, the common statement that sphincter muscle is contracted by catecholamines overlooks a great deal of contrary evidence. In addition, the view that catecholamines act simply to constrict the splanchnic vasculature does not take into account the redistribution of blood flow in the gut wall or the autoregulatory escape observed during continued exposure to catecholamines.

This chapter may be divided into two parts. The first part deals with the sites and nature of the actions of catecholamines on the gastrointestinal tract. In the first two sections of this part, the results of studies of the actions of catecholamines on gastrointestinal motility and on the distribution and flow of blood in the gastrointestinal tract are collated and analyzed. These sections are followed by short summaries so that, if the reader desires, the thesis presented in the review can be followed without referring to the extensive data collected under these headings. On the other hand, details of the original investigations are provided for those who require them. In the second part, conditions that alter the levels of circulating catecholamines are examined and their effects on gastrointestinal function are discussed. The results of these and other studies are used as a basis for

---

This work was supported by the National Heart Foundation of Australia, the Australian Research Grants Committee, the National Health and Medical Research Council, and the John Halliday Fellowship of the Life Insurance Medical Research Fund of Australia and New Zealand.

analysis of the physiological role of blood-borne catecholamines. A synthesis of the authors' views on the role of circulating catecholamines is presented at the end of the chapter.

Several problems related to this subject have not been considered. For example, there is no discussion of extra-adrenal chromaffin tissue, which may contribute to the catecholamines entering the circulation. In addition, epinephrine and norepinephrine are assumed to be the only catecholamines secreted that could significantly influence the gastrointestinal tract. Information about the distribution and chemistry of chromaffin tissue can be obtained from Coupland's monograph (35). This chapter is confined to research on mammals.

EFFECTS OF CATECHOLAMINES ON
GASTROINTESTINAL MOTILITY

General Considerations: Nonsphincter Muscle

The clearest and the earliest observed effects of catecholamines on the gut were their powerful actions in inhibiting the movement and reducing the tone of the intestine. The original recognition that the secretions of the adrenal glands inhibited gastrointestinal motility was in 1892 by Jacobj (181) who observed that stimulation of the nerves to the suprarenals or direct stimulation of the glands after all nervous connections had been severed brought the movements of the intestine to a complete standstill. The work of Jacobj and of Oliver & Schäfer (255) inspired a great deal of research on the actions of extracts of the adrenals. In the next few years several authors confirmed the potency of adrenal extracts in inhibiting gut movements (38, 210, 256, 257). The active component of the glands, shown by Moore (243) to be confined to the medulla, was isolated and identified soon thereafter (5, 314). Subsequently the sensitivity of gut muscle to the pure extract, epinephrine, was investigated. Magnus (227) found that the longitudinal muscle of isolated segments of the small intestine of the cat was relaxed by 5×10^{-9} g/ml of epinephrine. Relaxation of rabbit small intestine by 2×10^{-10} g/ml epinephrine was observed by Hoskins (173). This great sensitivity to epinephrine led Cannon & de la Paz (65) to use isolated segments of the cat's intestine as assay organs for estimating the catecholamine content of the adrenal effluent.

Contraction of nonsphincter parts of the intestines of most mammals is inhibited by catecholamines. In some animals, small regions have been shown to contract, although the general response of the intestine is relaxation (89, 295). In contrast, epinephrine appears to cause contraction of most parts of the gut of the horse (6, 50, 315).

Generalization concerning the action of catecholamines on the movement of gastric muscle is difficult, in that differences between species and between areas of the stomach are considerable. For example, the stomachs of ruminants, even within the one species, are in some cases contracted and in others relaxed by catecholamines (323). There is unanimity that the stomach of the cat is relaxed by catecholamines (45, 46, 87, 230, 261, 308, 327). Inhibition in response to catecholamines has also been observed in mouse and rat stomach (44, 129, 261). Although the overall reaction of the guinea pig stomach is relaxation (151, 152), in some areas or under special conditions, contraction has been observed (154, 308). The stomach of the dog can be either contracted or relaxed by catecholamines, the response depending largely on the initial tone (46, 207, 235, 244, 245, 247, 308, 317). Muren (245) has made the interesting observation that inhibitory responses are most frequently observed when excitatory vagal influences on the stomach are prominent but that, under conditions of reduced vagal influence, even a stomach highly contracted by carbachol is sometimes further contracted by epinephrine or norepinephrine. The usual response of the musculature of the rabbit stomach to catecholamines is contraction, although relaxation may also be observed (44, 129, 207, 308). The contractions of the human stomach were augmented by epinephrine in the work of Loeper & Verpy (223), although inhibition was observed in the single specimen studied by Smith (308). Danielopulu & Carniol (91) reported that low concentrations of epinephrine were excitatory and high concentrations inhibitory to the human stomach, but their records do not substantiate this. With the injection of a low concentration, a slight inhibition is shown in their record, and the augmenter effect is not observed until about 5 min after injection, when little of the injected epinephrine would be remaining in the gastric circulation. With a high concentration, their record shows an immediate inhibition of stomach movements and a return beyond the original level of activity after about 5 min. Anderson & Morris (12) found inhibition of the human stomach by epinephrine, except that a slight and inconsistent increase in gastric movements was sometimes observed with very low doses. By direct observation through a fistula, Wolf & Wolff (344) noted relaxation of the human gastric musculature caused by epinephrine. Graham (148) observed relaxation of the human stomach with a threshold dose of 5×10^{-9} g/ml. This result was confirmed by Bennett & Whitney (32). More recently, Haffner et al. (158) have found that epinephrine sometimes contracts and in other cases relaxes isolated strips from the human stomach.

Sphincter Muscle

Both Elliott (104, 105) and Dale (87) observed that catecholamines had an excitatory action on the smooth muscle of the sphincters of the gastrointestinal tract. Elliott's (105) generalization that the movement of mammalian gastrointestinal muscle is inhibited by catecholamines except in the regions of the sphincters, where it is contracted, has been retained even by authors of recent review articles (211, 348). A large volume of contradictory evidence concerning, particularly, the responses of sphincters and of the stomach suggests that this generalization should be reevaluated.

Langley (210) noted that the cardiac sphincter of the rabbit was relaxed by epinephrine. Although Smith (308) found epinephrine inactive on this muscle, Langley's observation has since been confirmed (44, 49, 345). In contrast, epinephrine contracts this sphincter in dog (21, 22, 308), cat (75, 308, 327), opossum (72), and in man (21, 22).

In the literature there is disagreement concerning the actions of catecholamines on the pyloric sphincter in rat, dog, rabbit, cat, and man. It is now clear that both excitatory and inhibitory receptors for catecholamines mediate effects on the pyloric muscle of these species. Nakanishi (246) reported contraction of the sphincter by epinephrine in the rat, whereas Armitage & Dean (15) could only find relaxation. In the dog, Winkelstein & Aschner (342) reported contraction, but Thomas & Wheelon (320) observed relaxation, as have later investigators (21, 46, 88). In a later publication, Thomas (317) reported that epinephrine occasionally contracted the pyloric sphincter of the dog. Most investigators agree that the pyloric sphincter of the rabbit contracts in response to epinephrine (105, 274, 308, 318), but Brown & McSwiney (44) state that epinephrine has an inhibitory action on the rabbit pylorus. Smith (308) found contraction of the pyloric sphincter in the cat, but this could not be confirmed by Thomas (318). Brown et al. (46) reported inhibition of the cat pyloric sphincter by epinephrine. In man, Loeper & Verpy (223) found that epinephrine hastened the evacuation of the stomach, a phenomenon that could result from a relaxation of the pyloric sphincter. Shipley & Blackfan (304) subsequently observed relaxation of the human fetal pylorus in response to epinephrine. However, Smith (308) observed contraction of the sphincter in the one preparation he examined. The results of other studies make it clear that an inhibitory action of catecholamines on the human pyloric sphincter is dominant (21, 22, 32, 158, 316). It should be noted that about one-third of the pyloric strips examined by Haffner et al. (158) were contracted by epinephrine, which indicates that responses in vitro are mediated through both excitatory and inhibitory receptors.

The ileocolic sphincter in cats, dogs, and rabbits is contracted by catecholamines (21, 87, 105, 138, 168, 206, 274, 307). In contrast, relaxation of the human ileocolic sphincter was reported by White et al. (340) and by Buirge (52) who observed the movements of the exposed human ileocolic junction directly and also used intraluminal balloons to record movements. More recently, low doses of epinephrine have been reported to increase sphincter tone, and high doses to cause relaxation (221). Gazet & Jarrett (138) found that epinephrine caused contraction of the human ileocolic sphincter in vitro. They suggested that, because of the narrow sphincter area in man, balloon methods may be principally recording the relaxation of adjacent nonsphincter areas of gut. Bass et al. (21) also noted contraction of the human ileocolic sphincter.

Contraction of the internal anal sphincter of most mammals seems to be induced by epinephrine, an exception being that of the rabbit (210). Although the internal anal sphincters of the cat and of man are usually contracted by catecholamines, relaxation may also occur (196, 260).

We believe it would be wise if Elliott's frequently quoted generalization that catecholamines cause contraction of the gastrointestinal sphincters were treated cautiously. There is no sphincter for which exceptional observations cannot be found, and in the pylorus (even though there is some argument as to its status as a sphincter) relaxation is observed more often than is contraction. The available evidence suggests that all sphincters contain receptors for catecholamines through which either excitation or inhibition can be mediated. Further work must be carried out before the sites and roles of receptors in sphincter areas can be evaluated.

Muscularis Mucosae

Few experimenters have examined the responses of the muscularis mucosae to catecholamines; in the majority of cases excitatory responses have been observed. Thorell (322) observed that epinephrine caused contraction of the muscularis mucosae in the dog and rabbit stomachs. In the pig the muscularis mucosae of the cardia relaxed in response to epinephrine, but in other parts of the stomach it contracted. In the cat, most areas of the mucosal muscle were relaxed, but in the region of the cardia it was contracted by epinephrine. Thorell found that the muscularis mucosae of the body of the human stomach was contracted by epinephrine, but Walder (332) noted contraction near the greater curvature and relaxation in the region of the lesser curvature. Walder always observed relaxation in response to norepinephrine. In the rabbit epinephrine contracts the muscularis mucosae of the small intestine (156), and in the dog it contracts the muscularis mucosae of the small intestine and mid-colon (199). Primary relaxation of the muscularis mucosae in the dog was never observed in any experiment where epinephrine was the only drug added (199). The threshold concentration was between 5×10^{-7} and 5×10^{-8} g/ml. Epinephrine depolarizes and causes an increase in the frequency of action potentials in the muscularis mucosae of the pig esophagus (55). Catecholamines also induce contraction in the smooth muscle that extends into the villi (137, 198, 199).

Receptor Sites

The inhibition of intestinal movements by catecholamines results from actions at several sites and through several receptor mechanisms (Fig. 1). Based on the work of Ahlquist (3), receptors for adrenergic agonists have been classified α and β, according to their order of responsiveness to a series of sympathomimetic amines. Selective antagonists for the two receptor types have

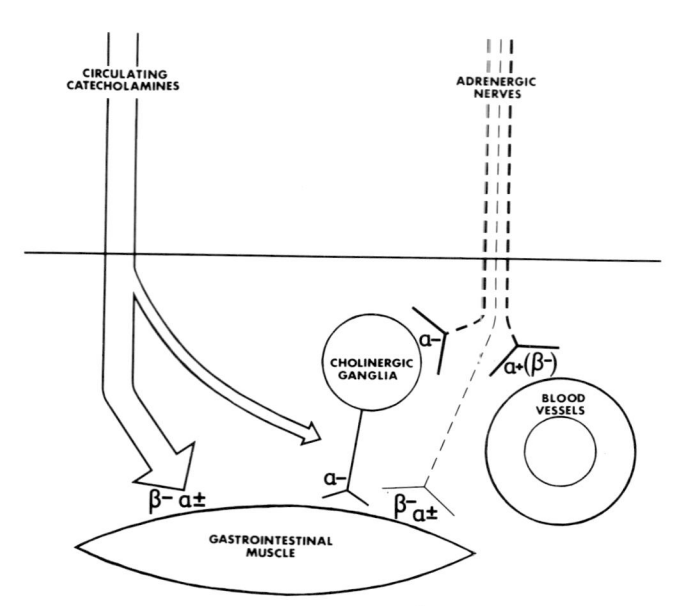

FIG. 1. Diagrammatic representation of arrangement of adrenergic receptors in gastrointestinal tract and of their major modes of activation. Positions of α and β receptors and the types of effect they mediate, either excitatory (+) or inhibitory (−), are indicated. This diagram is a deliberate simplification to which exceptions are known; the text should be consulted for a more detailed analysis.

been introduced and used to differentiate between them. It was soon apparent that the identification by Ahlquist of intestinal adrenoceptors as being of the α type could not be maintained (128, 209). Ahlquist & Levy (4) then discovered that a combination of α and β blocking agents could effectively antagonize the actions of epinephrine and norepinephrine on the canine ileum. Their conclusion that the gut contains both α and β receptors is now widely accepted (211, 295).

Intestinal motility is inhibited by the action of catecholamines in reducing the release of acetylcholine from nerve fibers in the gut wall and by their direct action on the muscle cells (see Fig. 1). It may be broadly stated that the activation of α adrenergic receptors inhibits the excitatory neural elements of the enteric plexuses of the gut and that β receptors are involved only in direct inhibitory actions of epinephrine or norepinephrine on the smooth muscle. However, catecholamines may also act directly on the muscle via α receptors; the α receptors on the muscle can subserve either excitation or inhibition.

The work of Jacobj (181) is the first to suggest that catecholamines may indirectly inhibit the motility of the gut by acting on excitatory nerves; Jacobj considered that sympathoadrenal discharge blocked the excitatory influence of the vagus by a mechanism separate from the direct action on the musculature. This view was again advanced by McDougal & West (232) and Kosterlitz & Robinson (203); the former authors proposed an α adrenergic inhibition of transmission from excitatory nerves to the muscle of the guinea pig ileum. This conclusion was supported by Chiu & Lee (71), Beleslin & Varagić (31) and Lee & Tseng (212), who examined the effects of catecholamines on the peristaltic reflex, and by the work of Muren (245) cited in the subsection *General Considerations: Nonsphincter Muscle*. Kosterlitz & Watt (204) showed that inhibitory actions of catecholamines on nerve-mediated contractions of the guinea pig ileum involved an interaction with both α and β receptors but that only β receptors were involved in inhibiting the direct action of acetylcholine on the muscle. These experiments were performed after ganglion blockade, so it can be assumed that catecholamines, acting through α receptors, inhibit the release of acetylcholine from neurons in the gut wall. Similar results have also been obtained by Oberdorf & Kroneberg (252). Moreover direct measurement of acetylcholine release from the gut reveals an adrenergic inhibition of the release of transmitter from the cholinergic fibers innervating the smooth muscle (27, 202, 262, 296, 313, 329). These experiments suggest that adrenoceptors located on cholinergic axons inhibit acetylcholine release. Experiments on the inhibition of cholinergic excitation of gastric and intestinal muscle by adrenergic nerves indicate that similar receptors are also located on the cell bodies of the cholinergic neurons (133, 189). The observation that α inhibitory effects can be selectively reduced by cold storage of the rabbit jejunum or duodenum further suggests that they are associated with intestinal nerves (224, 225, 290). Moreover, in the taenia coli of the guinea pig, where α, as well as β, receptors are found on the muscle cells, cold storage does not block the inhibition mediated through either α or β receptors (303a). A very interesting exception to the inhibitory action of catecholamines on cholinergic neurons has been found by Christensen & Daniel (73) who showed that norepinephrine, acting through α receptors, contracts the longitudinal muscle of the feline esophagus. This contraction is antagonized by atropine and potentiated by physostigmine. Continued exposure to hemicholinium also reduces the contraction, which can be restored by choline after the hemicholinium is washed from the tissue. These results suggest that catecholamines act on cholinergic nerves in this part of the gut to promote rather than inhibit the release of acetylcholine.

The adrenergic inhibition of the release of acetylcholine in the gastrointestinal tract seems to be mediated entirely through α receptors, whereas β receptors subserve direct inhibition of the muscle of nearly all parts of the gut. At least two exceptions to the latter statement are known. Reddy (274) has found that isoproterenol contracts the muscle of the pyloric and ileocecal sphincters in the rabbit and that dichloroisoproterenol blocks this contraction. Excitation, also mediated through β receptors, has been found in the circular muscle of the duodenal bulb of the dog (88). There have been far too few studies of the receptor types of intestinal circular muscle to claim that this is exceptional. However, Ahlquist & Levy (4) found β inhibitory receptors in the circular muscle of the dog ileum. Harry (161) found a predominance of α inhibitory receptors in the circular muscle of the guinea pig ileum but little to suggest the presence of β receptors either inhibiting or exciting the muscle.

The actions of catecholamines on the smooth muscle of the gut involve changes in cell metabolism and in ionic movements. A discussion of the cellular basis for the action of catecholamines is beyond the scope of this review; the subject is dealt with in several recent articles (13, 14, 42, 51, 53a, 90, 133, 190, 205).

Several additional mechanisms for the action of catecholamines on gastrointestinal motility have been only partly investigated. A widespread nonadrenergic inhibitory innervation of the gut has been found in mammals (55a–57, 134). Adrenergic effects on these nerves were examined by Jansson & Martinson (189) who found that the activation of adrenergic fibers to the cat stomach did not modify the relaxation mediated by nonadrenergic inhibitory fibers. Nonadrenergic, noncholinergic excitatory fibers can also affect gut muscle (10, 11, 132, 134), but the influence catecholamines may have on these nerves in not known. The possibility of adrenergic effects on afferent nerves has not been evaluated. It is known that motility may be influenced by changes in blood flow, and because catecholamines affect the gastrointestinal vasculature (see section EFFECTS OF CATECHOLAMINES ON GASTROINTESTINAL VASCULATURE), an indirect effect on motility could be anticipated; such an indirect action of catecholamines on motility is unlikely to be significant (133).

Summary

Epinephrine and norepinephrine inhibit the movements of most nonsphincter parts of the muscularis externa of the mammalian intestine. However, at least in one species, the horse, catecholamines appear to cause contraction of all parts of the intestine. Catecholamines also inhibit contraction of gastric muscle, but in most species excitation can also be observed, and in the dog and rabbit excitation appears to be dominant.

The action of catecholamines on sphincter muscle has been incompletely analyzed. Although the effects in particular cases have been described, no theory to predict whether excitation or inhibition should be expected in any novel situation can be reasonably proposed. The muscularis mucosae of the gastrointestinal tract usually contracts when exposed to catecholamines.

Catecholamines affect gastrointestinal motility by direct interaction with receptors on the muscle cells and also by interference with the release of acetylcholine from axons innervating the musculature (see Fig. 1). Both α and β receptors are found on the muscle. The β receptors almost always mediate inhibition, but α receptors can be either inhibitory or excitatory. Where catecholamines cause contraction of the gut, this is generally an α receptor action. Interference with the release of acetylcholine is mediated through α receptors in all situations so far examined. With only one exception, epinephrine and norephinephrine have been shown to inhibit acetylcholine release.

EFFECTS OF CATECHOLAMINES ON
GASTROINTESTINAL VASCULATURE

General Observations

In their work on the effects of extracts of the suprarenals, Oliver & Schäfer (255) state, "The great rise in blood pressure which invariably follows the injection of the extract is due very largely to the contraction of the arterioles of the splanchnic area." Since then, a great deal of observation has demonstrated that the vessels of the gastrointestinal tract are constricted by epinephrine and norepinephrine. Brodie & Dixon (41) found that the venous outflow from the isolated intestine, perfused at constant pressure, was diminished by epinephrine. Similar decreases in blood flow were noted by subsequent investigators (58, 75, 119, 200, 297). Increased resistance of the intestinal vasculature to flow of blood was noted by Binit et al. (35), Deal & Green (92), and Selkurt et al. (298). Other authors have used various plethysmographic devices to record decreases in intestinal volume in response to epinephrine infusion (53, 74, 144, 346). MacLean et al. (231) obtained a similar result by recording intestinal weight changes. Blanching of the intestinal mucosa has been noted in response to either local or systemic application of catecholamines (100, 127, 305, 344). Grayson & Swan (150) have associated a decrease in bowel temperature caused by catecholamines with a decrease in blood flow.

It is unlikely that circulating catecholamines have any direct influence on the flow of lymph; epinephrine and norepinephrine have small effects, only in high concentrations, on lymph flow (37, 267). However, sympathetic nerves act on the larger lymph vessels, which are adrenergically innervated (116, 131, 289).

The results of most investigations indicate that catecholamines act to decrease the flow of blood through the stomach and intestines and also to decrease the volume of blood that can be held in this part of the vasculature. Three points should be noted: *1*) the overall decrease in blood flow and blood volume does not necessarily indicate a decrease in blood supply to all parts of the intestinal wall, in fact, redistribution of the circulation may take place and thereby increase flow in some areas; *2*) as well as having receptors for catecholamines that mediate constriction of the splanchnic vasculature, the vessels also contain receptive mechanisms for dilatation that can be revealed in some circumstances; *3*) the maximum constrictor effect of catecholamines on the gastrointestinal arteries is not maintained.

Dilator Effects

Dilatation of intestinal blood vessels was noted by Ogawa (254) with low concentrations of epinephrine (2×10^{-8} g/ml), but constriction was observed if the concentration was increased. Similar results were obtained by Bülbring & Burn (53), but Clark (76) found that constriction was caused by the lowest effective dose of epinephrine. Experiments with ergotamine and other adrenergic blocking drugs show that, as would be interpreted today, intestinal blood vessels contain α excitatory and β inhibitory adrenoceptors (53, 75, 153), the β receptors being more easily activated by low concentrations of agonists. Other authors have observed partial dilatation after the initial constricting action of catecholamines (see subsection *Duration of Action*).

Local Reactions

There have been numerous studies on isolated parts of the splanchnic circulation, those on the mesenteric vessels being reasonably simple to interpret, but the results of those on intrinsic vessels still are not sufficiently clear-cut for the redistribution of blood flow to be understood. Campbell (60) initially showed that epinephrine contracts the muscle of isolated mesenteric arteries. This has been confirmed by several authors (228, 233, 281, 310).

Changes in the caliber of the vessels draining the gastrointestinal tract, the mesenteric and portal veins, influence the volume of blood in the splanchnic region. Where the reactions of these vessels to catecholamines have been directly examined, a constrictor action has been found [(60, 82, 97, 102, 123, 155, 171, 191); see also (124)]. It is clear that constriction of the mesenteric veins always occurs if no other drug is added, but it must be remembered that weak dilatation can be observed after blockade of α receptors (123, 171, 191).

The different layers of the gut wall (muscularis externa, submucosa, mucosa) are supplied by parallel vascular circuits that arise from the mesenteric arteries. The layers have individual vascular patterns and nutritional requirements, which are reflected in the relative blood flows through the layers at rest; the flow through the mucosa is about four times that through the muscle (94, 193a). The important question is whether these relative flows are changed by catecholamines, and particularly whether there is a diversion of flow from the mucosa, which could weaken its resistance to ulceration (see section POSSIBLE INVOLVEMENT OF CATECHOLAMINES IN ULCERATION). In the dog, norepinephrine causes a slight decrease in total gastric blood flow associated with a diminished mucosal and an augmented muscle blood flow, that is, a diversion of blood away from the mucosa (95). The response to epinephrine depends on the activity of the gastric mucosa; in the nonsecreting stomach, where blood flow is low, epinephrine causes an increase (95), but when blood flow and secretion are stimulated by gastrin, epinephrine decreases mucosal blood flow (185). Comparable studies on the human stomach are not available, although visual observations indicate that epinephrine restricts mucosal blood flow (127, 344). Observation of the passage of microspheres of various sizes through the gastric vasculature suggests that epinephrine causes a preferential flow through wide arteriovenous connections (265). The increase in overall resistance of the gastrointestinal vasculature in response to catecholamines is not maintained (see subsection *Duration of Action*), but the restriction of blood flow through the canine gastric mucosa persisted throughout infusions of norepinephrine (0.5 µg/kg per min) lasting 90 min (86). In the intestine of the cat, restriction of mucosal blood flow during adrenergic nerve stimulation is maintained even when the overall increase in resistance has waned (120).

Duration of Action

In 1930 Clark (75) showed that the decrease in intestinal volume and in venous outflow caused by epinephrine was not sustained and soon gave way to vasodilatation. This phenomenon, also seen after sympathetic stimulation, has been called *autoregulatory escape*. Autoregulatory escape in the intestinal vasculature following the constrictor action of catecholamines has been confirmed by many authors [e.g. (99, 144, 153, 231, 284, 297, 346)]. Autoregulatory escape is not confined to constrictions caused by catecholamines; it occurs with a variety of unrelated agents, such as angiotensin, prostaglandin $F_{2\alpha}$, and vasopressin (165a, 303). There is some evidence that the activation of β adrenoceptors can contribute to the escape phenomenon during norepinephrine infusions (284), but it is clear that a shift in dominance from α to β receptors can only explain part of the autoregulatory escape from the constrictor action of catecholamines (165a, 278, 300). The various experiments cited have shown that catecholamines restrict blood flow through the intestine only during the first 1 or 2 min of infusion. From the studies of Folkow et al. (120) it seems that, even in the escape phase of continued sympathetic stimulation, there is a sustained suppression of blood flow through the mucosa and a marked increase in submucosal flow. This suggests that the activity of adrenergic nerves might facilitate blood flow through arteriovenous shunts, although histochemical studies do not reveal a specialized adrenergic innervation of shunt vessels (131). Further investigation indicates that shunting during autoregulatory escape is through nutritional vessels, not "true" shunts that would bypass the capillary bed (98). Dresel et al. (98) suggest that blood flow diversion from the mucosa during continued sympathetic activity may suppress secretory and absorptive activity and so decrease the nutritional demands of the intestine. Although autoregulatory escape occurs in the intestine, the larger veins (capacitance vessels) maintain their constriction in response to catecholamines (77, 236, 253). The sustained constriction may be important in the redistribution of blood during sympathoadrenal discharge. The splanchnic circulation contains about 20% of the total blood volume, 70% of this 20% in the veins (40). Stimulation of adrenergic vasoconstrictor fibers has been shown to divert 30–40% of the splanchnic blood volume to other parts of the circulation.

Summary

The overall effect of catecholamines is initially to reduce blood flow through the stomach and intestine and to reduce substantially the blood volume of the splanchnic vasculature. There is evidence to suggest that blood flow is diverted away from the mucosa, partially by preferential shunting in the submucosa. The initial constriction is followed after a few minutes by an autoregulatory escape. However, even during this secondary dilatation, the mucosa remains ischemic. In addition, the constriction of the large mesenteric and portal veins seems to persist, and so the splanchnic blood volume remains reduced.

EFFECTS OF CATECHOLAMINES ON
GASTROINTESTINAL SECRETION

Gastric Acid Secretion

Several studies in the early decades of this century revealed an increase in gastric acid secretion in response to epinephrine (220, 223, 285, 351). In these studies the basal secretion was inevitably low, and the effects of anesthesia and operative conditions were not assessed. (This criticism also applies to much of the later work.) Other observers at this time noted a decrease in secretion (7, 167, 242), a result that has been substantiated by more recent studies (121, 160, 185, 222, 250, 266, 287, 321, 344). It has been noted often that gastric blood flow and secretion change together, either both increasing or both decreasing. It is difficult to demonstrate a causal relationship (183), although several authors have proposed that catecholamine-induced changes in secretion are secondary to changes in mucosal blood flow (121, 321). It must be appreciated that any change in mucosal blood flow derives from a summation of several effects of catecholamines. Constriction of the arterial inflow and particularly of mucosal arterioles would tend to decrease flow, whereas the general rise in arterial pressure acts to force more blood into the mucosal circulation. Thompson & Vane (321) have found that, in the rare cases in which blood flow is increased by catecholamines, secretion is also increased, but that the general occurrence is a decrease in both. Jacobson (184) measured changes in the ratio of blood flow to secretory rate and found that norepinephrine decreased but that prostaglandin E increased this ratio. Jacobson reasoned that, in the case of norepinephrine, the change in secretion was subservient to the change in blood flow. Some results have been interpreted to indicate that part of the inhibition of gastric secretion by catecholamines is independent of vascular effects (23, 160, 266). In conclusion, it may be stated that, although their effects are small (78, 169), catecholamines generally act to inhibit gastric acid secretion, principally as a result of reducing mucosal blood flow.

Mucous Secretion

The arguments outlined above apply also to the action of catecholamines on the secretion of mucus, in which a decrease, in some cases allied to inhibition of mucosal blood flow, has been observed (242, 250, 280, 344). Reports of increases in mucous secretion are, however, quite common. Langley (210) found that large doses of epinephrine increased the secretion of mucus from the esophagus of the cat. Similar increases have been found in the stomachs of cats (26) and dogs (17) and in the duodenums of dogs (162). The mucoid secretion of the antrum of the dog's stomach has been reported to be unaffected by epinephrine (237). According to Hartiola & Toivonen (162), the secretion of the mucous glands of the duodenum is relatively independent of blood flow. It is apparent from most investigations that catecholamines do not have a strong influence on mucous production. Changes arise from alteration of mucosal perfusion and possibly also from direct stimulation of secretion.

EFFECTS OF CATECHOLAMINES ON
GASTROINTESTINAL ABSORPTION

There is no evidence to suggest that catecholamines have other than an indirect effect on absorption. Evidently absorption must have some dependence on blood flow, and any agent that alters blood flow will also tend to influence absorption. This was recognized in 1896 by Reid (275) who noted that, when blood flow was reduced by stimulation of the mesenteric nerves or by clamping of vessels to the gut, absorption was also reduced. Several other investigators have confirmed a dependence of absorption on blood flow (157, 192, 302). Cori & Cori (84) found that epinephrine reduced the absorption of glucose in the rat. However, Friedman & Byers (126) found that neither epinephrine nor norepinephrine had an appreciable effect on cholesterol, phospholipid, or triglyceride absorption. In contrast, Winne (343) found a decreased absorptive capacity during a norepinephrine-induced decrease in blood flow. Although the action of catecholamines on absorption is probably only through alteration of blood flow, Schanker et al. (294) and Varro et al. (326) have concluded that blood flow plays only a minor role in limiting absorption. From the literature cited above, it is apparent that extreme depression of blood flow (as occurs during mechanical occlusion of the mesenteric arteries) inhibits absorption but that absorption is largely independent of smaller changes in blood flow. Only exceptionally or when their action is sustained, would circulating catecholamines be expected to influence the uptake of intestinal contents.

CONDITIONS LEADING TO INCREASED LEVELS OF CIRCULATING CATECHOLAMINES AND THEIR EFFECTS ON THE GUT

Secretion from the adrenal medulla is elicited by a variety of circumstances. In this section the effects of shock, intense emotion, exercise, and pheochromocytoma are reviewed. Catecholamines are also released by anoxia, lowered body temperature, and several other conditions (85, 163), but in most of these instances effects on the gut are not well understood. For example, both cold and anoxia affect the movements of the isolated gut (113, 132, 201, 231). In addition, drugs, such as nicotine, that release medullary catecholamines can also relax gastrointestinal muscle through other mechanisms (9, 56, 142, 227).

Shock

Increased levels of circulating catecholamines are found in cases of acute hypotension arising in anaphylactic, hemorrhagic, bacterial, or other conditions of shock. In 1916 Bedford & Jackson (29) reported that experimental shock increased the output of epinephrine from the suprarenal bodies [see also (28)]. Shock induced by handling of the intestine, by hemorrhage, or by occlusion of the vena cava increased the potency of plasma samples from the dog adrenal vein in causing relaxation of the isolated rabbit intestine. Exclusion of the adrenals by ligation completely abolished this effect. This result was confirmed in traumatic (269) and hemorrhagic shock (324). Shock induced by peptone poisoning markedly increased catecholamine secretion into the circulation, assay indicating increases between 5 and 30 times in one group and between 12 and 200 times in a second group of dogs (335). In anaphylactic shock a 20- to 30-fold increase in secretion of catecholamines was found (293a).

More recent work with chemical, as well as biological, assay has confirmed the elevation of plasma catecholamines during shock and shown that both epinephrine and norepinephrine are released in significant amounts (143, 226, 240, 282, 333, 334, 336). The increase in circulating catecholamines is paralleled by an increase in the activity of the sympathetic nervous system. There can be little doubt that the increased sympathoadrenal activity in shock is a damaging factor in the gut: the released catecholamines constrict the peripheral blood vessels and thus heighten the ischemia of visceral organs. In the gut, restriction of blood flow is greatest in the mucosa (270). The severe stress on the mucosa has been extensively documented; vascular congestion, bleeding into the lumen of the intestine, mucosal ulceration, and ischemic necrosis have been reported in various types of shock (36, 108, 115, 125, 217, 241, 331, 335). Mucosal damage and rupture of blood vessels occurs in epidemic hemorrhagic fever (176). Therapy involving the use of α blocking agents may alleviate conditions of shock (147, 218, 259, 276, 301, 341) and thus enhance the effectiveness of other procedures[1]. Freeman et al. (125) reported that sympathetic denervation, including the denervation of the adrenal glands, prevented the development of shock in hemorrhaged dogs and also prevented the necrosis of the intestinal mucosa that normally results from substantial hemorrhage. Prior sympathetic denervation of the intestine, without denervation of the adrenals, also increases the survival rate of animals in shock, which suggests that the local release of norepinephrine is of importance in intensifying the effects of shock (114). However, the large increase in circulating catecholamines must affect the blood flow through the intestine and probably contributes to mucosal damage. If hypotension is not so severe as to cause shock, catecholamines may contribute to a beneficial redistribution of blood away from the splanchnic vessels and to the heart and central nervous system. It has been shown that the reduction in splanchnic blood volume in hemorrhage is proportionally much greater than is the reduction in total blood volume, which suggests that such a redistribution does occur (277).

McNeill et al. (234) have recently cast doubt on the commonly held belief that adrenergic mechanisms are responsible for intestinal vasoconstriction in hemorrhage. These authors measured superior mesenteric artery blood flow and pressure in cats and found that phenoxybenzamine or adrenalectomy plus sympathectomy were ineffective in relieving the vasoconstriction. However, removal of the kidneys and hypophysis was effective, which suggests that angiotensin and vasopressin contribute to intestinal vasoconstriction in acute hypotension. It should be noted that the hemorrhage was insufficient to cause shock and the anesthetic used (pentobarbital) is known to inhibit transmission through sympathetic ganglia (113a) and to depress supraspinal autonomic reflexes (293). Therefore the experiments do not exclude the contribution of locally released or circulating catecholamines to intestinal vasoconstriction in hemorrhagic shock.

Active absorption of glucose was inhibited in cases of shock (83, 145, 157), but passive absorption was not affected (157). In other experiments acute hemorrhage did not influence chloride or glucose absorption (213, 216). Inhibition of absorption appears to be associated

---

[1] Chien (70) has pointed out that pretreatment with α blocking agents reduces the volume of blood that has to be removed to achieve the same degree of hypotension observed in control animals, if constant pressure conditions are maintained. This lessens the value of such experiments in determining the importance of therapy with blockade of α receptors. This criticism does not apply to studies where the bleeding was the same in both experimental and control animals (276).

with sustained shock. It is likely that the restriction of mucosal blood flow does not immediately influence absorption but that after a sustained period of anoxia the ability of the mucosa to take up substances from the intestinal contents is impaired.

The effects of hemorrhage on gastrointestinal motility in dogs have been investigated by several workers. Decreases in tone and in spontaneous movement of the duodenum (159), ileum (330), and colon (214, 215) have been observed. Some disagreement with these results has been brought forward by Necheles et al. (248) who found that hemorrhage increased colonic motility, although it caused depression in the upper gastrointestinal tract. In the ileum an increase in the transit time of a charcoal-acacia meal was found, which the authors described as highly significant (215), although they had previously interpreted similar data as showing no significant difference between bled and control animals (214). Hamilton et al. (159) found that adrenalectomy abolished the inhibition of the canine duodenum in response to hemorrhage. Another experiment relevant to this problem was performed by Youmans et al. (349) who found that hypotension induced by acetylcholine caused the inhibition of denervated intestinal fistulas and that bilateral adrenalectomy substantially reduced the inhibition.

Intense Emotion

Changes in the levels of circulating catecholamines and alteration in gastrointestinal function have been associated with the strong emotions of the defense reaction, variously described as fear, rage, apprehension, excitement, or a combination of these. Manifestations of the relation between gastrointestinal and emotional changes are discussed in detail by Alvarez (8).

In 1898 Cannon (61) used an X-ray technique to examine the movements of the stomach of the cat. He found that when the cat entered into a struggle to be loose or showed signs of fright or rage the regular gastric movements suddenly stopped. The whole stomach, including the pylorus, relaxed, and movement returned only when the cat was calmed. Bickel & Sasaki (34) showed that excitement in a dog inhibited secretion from the stomach. The dog, even though it was very hungry and took food, exhibited very little gastric secretion after fury induced by the presence of a cat. Cannon (62) recognized that these and other observations paralleled the effects of the activation of sympathetic nerves and that the inhibition of stomach movement was reduced by section of the splanchnic nerves. In an investigation of the possible involvement of the adrenals in the emotional effects on stomach and intestinal movements (65), blood taken from the vena cava central to the adrenal vein relaxed an isolated strip of gut if the donor cat had been excited. This effect was not observed if the adrenals were removed or if the blood was taken from a quiet animal. Further implication that circulating factors are involved in this reaction comes from experiments in which the movements of denervated intestinal fistulas were inhibited by fright (347). Increase in circulating catecholamines in conditions of excitement or other strong emotion was confirmed by several authors (64, 106, 195, 291, 292).

The involvement of emotion in the control of the mucosal circulation was examined by Drury et al. (100). They observed rapid and extreme pallor of the mucosa of the colon when a dog was alarmed. The reaction was still observed after adrenalectomy, but the removal of most of the sympathetic nerves delayed the onset of pallor and rendered the pallor less marked. Although the vessels of the gastrointestinal tract are constricted when an animal is frightened, the systemic blood pressure and heart rate are increased at the same time and a decrease in mesenteric arterial blood flow is not necessarily observed (288). Recent studies have confirmed that fright may reduce blood flow to the gastrointestinal tract (286, 287). The features of the defense reaction can also be elicited by stimulation of the hypothalamic defense area (2, 103). The changes observed include release of catecholamines into the bloodstream and constriction of intestinal vessels (2, 77, 149). The nausea associated with these emotions in human beings is well known and sometimes may lead to vomiting (8).

Exercise

Apparently the first indication that exercise increases the secretion of the adrenal medulla comes from the work of Battelli & Boatta (24) in 1902. They used a colorimetric method to determine the catecholamine content of the adrenals of normal dogs and of dogs made to run until exhausted and found that adrenal amine content could be reduced to as little as one-third by this treatment. A number of studies using bioassay techniques have subsequently documented the secretion of catecholamines associated with exercise (66, 164, 165). Von Euler & Hellner (112) studied urinary catecholamines after muscular exertion in humans and found both epinephrine and norepinephrine levels increased. They interpreted the results as indicating an increased activity of adrenergic nerves combined with an augmented adrenal secretion. Increase in the secretion of both catecholamines was also found by Kärki (194). In extreme cases, the rate of epinephrine accumulation in the urine increased 25 times and that of norepinephrine 35 times. Gasser & Meek (136), Hartman et al. (165), and Itikawa (179) showed that exclusion of the adrenals reduced sympathomimetic effects of muscular exertion.

The contractions and tone of the dog's stomach are reduced by exercise; the greater the exertion of the animal the greater is the inhibition (67). When the exercise is vigorous, the period of inhibition outlasts the exercise. Carlson (67) found that running also inhibited the movements of the human stomach and, as in dogs, the inhibition was proportional to the exertion involved. Dickson & Wilson (96) examined the movements of the human stomach at rest and immediately after "violent exercise"

—a sprint of 400 yards. Such exercise invariably inhibited gastric movements. Some authors proposed that exercise should result in constriction of splanchnic vessels even without direct evidence (18, 172). Earlier than this, in 1907, Weber reported that anticipation of exercise in hypnotized patients led to a decrease in the volume of the abdominal viscera. More direct evidence of constriction of intestinal vessels during exercise was obtained by Barcroft & Florey (20) who observed color changes in the mucosa of sections of exteriorized colon. They considered that the pallor induced by exercise was partly due to excitement of the dogs. Herrick et al. (166) subsequently used the thermostromuhr method to estimate superior mesenteric artery flow in the dog and found that, in most cases, blood flow to the intestine increased during exercise. However, they assumed that there was constriction of the splanchnic vasculature but that the increase in systemic blood pressure overcame the increased resistance of the intestinal vessels. This hypothesis is supported by the work of Rushmer et al. (288) who found that exercise had only a small decremental effect on blood flow in the superior mesenteric artery of the dog. Although the average flow per unit time was not significantly altered, the flow per pulse was diminished, which suggested increased resistance to flow in the intestinal vasculature. More recently, a decrease of 20% in the flow of blood to the gut of dogs during exercise has been reported (54).

Pheochromocytoma

Although earlier reports suggested that excessive release of catecholamines in cases of tumors of chromaffin tissue gave rise to the symptoms of pheochromocytoma, Beer et al. (30) in 1937 were the first to give a clear documentation. By using the denervated artery of the rabbit ear to assay pressor substances in the patient's blood, they found that, after a hypertensive attack, a blood sample would constrict the assay artery and that this constriction was blocked by ergotamine. After removal of the adrenal tumor both the symptoms and the pressor activity of the blood disappeared. Later studies, in which both biological and chemical assays were used, confirmed the increase in the secretion of catecholamines in pheochromocytoma (107, 110, 146).

The case reports for patients with chromaffin tumors indicate that effects on the gastrointestinal tract are prominent. Of 18 case histories reviewed by Howard & Barker (175), 15 patients suffered attacks of nausea associated with vomiting. In later reviews 42 of 100 patients examined were nauseous (319), and in infantile pheochromocytoma 46 of 95 children suffered nausea and vomiting (312). Mucosal ulceration and hemorrhage into the lumen of the gut have been reported in several cases of pheochromocytoma (47, 81, 122, 139, 175, 239, 279, 299, 309); abdominal pain is also a general symptom of pheochromocytoma. The appearance of patients during a pheochromocytomic attack is very similar to the fight-or-flight appearance associated with the defense reaction (236).

Summary

The gastrointestinal changes associated with elevations of circulating catecholamines are remarkably similar, despite differences in the primary causes. Shock, the defense reaction, and exercise are all associated with constriction of the vessels of the gut. Although this has not been directly observed during pheochromocytomic attacks, it is likely to occur. Other changes that parallel the actions of catecholamines, such as gastric and intestinal relaxation and inhibition of absorption and secretion, have also been observed. The nausea frequently encountered during emotional crises or in pheochromocytoma may be associated with distension of the relaxed stomach wall.

POSSIBLE INVOLVEMENT OF CATECHOLAMINES IN ULCERATION

Gastric ulceration occurs when the digestive powers of the gastric juices overcome the resistance of the mucosa. Therefore any factor that tends to weaken the mucosa will facilitate the formation of ulcers, and several authors have suggested that mucosal ischemia may be such a factor (19, 178, 258, 306). Similar conditions can probably precipitate ulceration of the esophagus, small intestine, and colon. The severe and sustained ischemia caused by catecholamines would provide the conditions for development of ulcers. In fact, in conditions like shock and pheochromocytoma, petechiae and vascular congestion of the mucosa occur, and the stress is sometimes sufficiently severe to cause ulceration and bleeding into the lumen of the gut (36, 47, 108, 115, 122, 125, 175, 217, 239, 241, 279, 299, 309, 331, 335). Examination of the gastric and intestinal mucosa in man and other animals after exposure to shock reveals extensive and severe ulceration (125, 263, 264, 338). Sympathectomy, which included adrenal denervation, prevented the mucosal damage that normally accompanies severe hemorrhage in dogs (125). De Busscher (93) and Illingworth (178) suggest that an important element in creating the mucosal conditions conducive to ulceration is the opening of submucosal arteriovenous anastomoses, which permit a diversion of blood from the mucosa. As outlined above, catecholamines cause a preferential flow of blood through shunt vessels in the gut wall. Large doses of epinephrine (16–17 μg/kg per min) can cause hemorrhagic necrosis of the intestinal mucosa of dogs (219). Brown et al. (48) found localized areas of necrosis and mucosal hemorrhage after they subjected dogs to a series of infusions of *l*-norepinephrine (2.8 μg/kg per min) over a period of several days. A similar rate of catecholamine release could be expected under conditions of extreme stress.

In situations in which there is hypersecretion of catecholamines, mucosal damage is sometimes severe, and catecholamine infusion causes similar effects. Thus catecholamines released in pheochromocytoma and in stressful situations contribute to mucosal damage.

ADRENERGIC NERVES AS SOURCE OF CIRCULATING CATECHOLAMINES

The possibility that postganglionic sympathetic nerves, as well as chromaffin tissue, contribute to the catecholamines in the circulation was investigated by Cannon & Britton (64) and Newton et al. (249). It was found that excitement still caused a slow acceleration of the denervated heart in cats in which the adrenals had been demedullated, the extraadrenal chromaffin tissue in the kidney region had been removed, and the abdominal sympathetic chains had been extirpated. When the remaining (thoracic) sympathetic chains were removed, the acceleration was no longer observed. These results were confirmed in several investigations [see (63, 283)].

Clear evidence for an extraadrenal, blood-borne action of catecholamines on the intestine was provided by Youmans & Meek (350) who examined the reflex relaxation of Thiry or Thiry-Vella fistulas of the jejunum. When the rectum of the dog was irritated, there was a marked inhibition of the movements of the fistulas. This inhibition was not affected by vagotomy or by demedullation of the adrenal glands; however, it was abolished if the splanchnic nerves were sectioned and the lumbar sympathetic chains removed. If the fistula, but not the rest of the intestine, was denervated by interrupting the nerves accompanying its pedicle, reflex inhibition of the muscle of the fistula was still observed, although it appeared after a greater delay. This inhibition was observed after demedullation of the adrenal glands. It is likely that norepinephrine was released in sufficient quantity at the nerve endings of the innervated part of the intestine to enter the bloodstream and relax the denervated fistula. Reflex release of catecholamines from extraadrenal chromaffin tissue could also contribute to the effect. It should be noted that the denervated segments had greater than normal sensitivity to epinephrine.

The possibility that an overflow of norepinephrine from vasoconstrictor fibers could cause intestinal inhibition has been discussed by Celander (69) and Kock (200). They consider that stimulation at "physiological" impulse frequencies in the splanchnic nerves (up to 8-10 impulses/sec), or reflexes involving the central nervous system do not exert any direct control over intestinal motility, but that artificial stimulation of splanchnic or paravascular nerves at greater frequencies can release sufficient transmitter from vascular endings to inhibit gastrointestinal motility. More recent work suggests that adrenergic nerve endings in the enteric plexuses are likely to be the principal source of norepinephrine that diffuses to the muscle during aphysiological stimuli (133). That substantial overflow of catecholamines into the bloodstream is abnormal is supported by Brown et al. (43) who were unable to detect any overflow from the small intestine of the cat even at stimulation frequencies up to 50/sec, although their bioassay technique would be expected to detect less than 5 μg/liter. Only when binding of norepinephrine in the tissue was blocked was overflow demonstrable. With a radiometric method, Boullin et al. (39) found that tritium-labeled catecholamines could be detected in the effluent of the isolated cat colon even without stimulation of adrenergic nerves.

It is concluded that norepinephrine released from adrenergic nerves does enter the bloodstream in small amounts, but in comparison with the adrenal glands, adrenergic nerves are not an important source of circulating amines.

RELATIVE ROLES OF CIRCULATING AND LOCALLY RELEASED CATECHOLAMINES

An extensive study of the relative roles of circulating and locally released catecholamines has been made by Kock (200) who examined blood flow and motility in the jejunum of anesthetized cats. Kock investigated reflex intestinal inhibition and vasoconstriction caused by carotid occlusion, graded hemorrhage, afferent nerve stimulation, and intestinal distension. He found that the inhibition of intestinal motility caused by carotid occlusion, hemorrhage, or afferent stimulation was slow in onset (involving a 15-sec or greater delay) and that it was abolished by exclusion of the adrenals. Constriction of the intestinal vessels was insensitive to removal of the adrenals but was blocked by interruption of the sympathetic vasomotor nerves. The intestino-intestinal inhibitory reflex involved an immediate intestinal relaxation that was abolished by section of the sympathetic nerves but not by adrenal exclusion [see (133)]. Kock concluded that the delayed intestinal inhibition caused by central reflexes was mediated by circulating catecholamines but that intestinal vasoconstriction was in response to increased vasomotor nerve activity. He also pointed out that epinephrine significantly reduced intestinal motility at concentrations too low to have measurable vascular effects.

The conclusion that direct effects of circulating catecholamines are more important than direct effects of adrenergic nerves in the central reflex relaxation of gastrointestinal muscle and that adrenergic vasomotor fibers are more important than circulating catecholamines for vascular effects is confirmed in several of the studies previously cited. In shock the intense vasoconstriction of intestinal vessels can be greatly reduced by sympathetic denervation (114), and yet then inhibition of intestinal movement is abolished by adrenalectomy (159). During reflex activation of the sympathoadrenal system in the defense reaction, the intestinal vasoconstriction is insensitive to adrenalectomy but can be abolished by sympathetic denervation (100). The roles of local and circulating catecholamines in the intestinal inhibition during the defense reaction apparently have not been directly compared. However, Jansson et al. (188) examined effects of stimulation of the hypothalamic defense area in adrenalectomized cats. They found that the sympathetic discharge inhibited transmission from cholinergic nerves to the gastric muscle, but they could find little evidence of a direct inhibition of the stomach by catecholamines released from adrenergic nerves. On the other hand, activation of the defense reaction causes a significant secretion of catecholamines from the adrenal glands (64, 65, 106, 195, 292). The experiments of Youmans et al. (349) suggest that the inhibition of the intestine during hypotension in the dog is principally produced by circulating factors. These authors found that, after hypotension induced by acetylcholine, extrinsically denervated intestinal fistulas were more markedly inhibited than were innervated fistulas. Bilateral removal of the adrenal medullae delayed and reduced the intestinal inhibition. Youmans et al. (349) considered that the residual response was due to an overflow from adrenergic vasomotor fibers into the circulation. Recent work (109) suggests that release of medullary catecholamines contributes to the intestino-intestinal inhibitory reflex; the reflex initiated by stimulation of afferent mesenteric nerves was reduced by bilateral adrenalectomy or by transection of the splanchnic nerves. No response was observed in reserpine-treated animals.

The distribution of adrenergic nerve endings in the intestine gives some indication of the relative roles of locally released and circulating catecholamines. Not until the fluorescence histochemical method for adrenergic nerves became available could their distribution in the gastrointestinal tract be meaningfully examined [see (133)]. With this method, Norberg (251) and Jacobowitz (182) found that very few adrenergic nerve fibers innervate the intestinal musculature but that the ganglia of the myenteric plexuses are richly supplied with adrenergic endings. The dense adrenergic innervation of the myenteric ganglia has been confirmed in several investigations (25, 130, 133, 134a, 271). Adrenergic fibers, although sparsely distributed, can be found in the nonsphincter muscle of the gut, especially in the circular muscle and in taeniae of the longitudinal coat (1, 25, 33, 130, 133, 134a, 135, 141, 170, 182, 251, 272). The adrenergic innervation of intestinal blood vessels has only recently been examined in detail (131). The arteries and arterioles supplying the gastrointestinal tract are all heavily innervated; innervation of the veins within the gut wall is very sparse (131). However, the large mesenteric veins taking blood from the intestine and the hepatic portal veins are heavily innervated. The arrangement of adrenergic fibers confirms that locally released norepinephrine affects intestinal motility indirectly by acting on the intramural ganglia and that there is a direct effect on the intestinal vasculature from adrenergic vasomotor endings [see (133)].

There is convincing evidence that adrenergic nerves to the cat stomach only influence motility by their action on cholinergic neurons of the enteric ganglia under physiological conditions. In such studies the authors have been concerned to use only "physiological" rates of stimulation [i.e., less than 8–10 impulses/sec (68, 69, 117, 133)] or to activate adrenergic fibers reflexly[2]. Jansson &

[2] Although these studies indicate that adrenergic nerves have little direct effect on gastric muscle in vivo, some studies have

Martinson (189) found that the activation of an intestino-gastric reflex did not affect the basal myogenic tone of the stomach. However, if vagal cholinergic fibers were stimulated, the reflex excitation of the sympathetic nerves did inhibit the contractions. In contrast, the gastric contraction caused by exogenous acetylcholine was unaffected by the reflex impulses in adrenergic nerves to the stomach. Direct stimulation of the adrenergic supply to the stomach produced prompt inhibition at low frequencies of stimulation only when vagal excitatory fibers were active. In contrast, only delayed and sluggish inhibition was observed in atropine-treated animals. These results were confirmed in chronically vagotomized cats, which develop cholinergic contractile waves in the gastric musculature (187), in the case of responses elicited by stimulation of the hypothalamic defense area (188) and of somatic afferents (186). Similar conclusions have been made for the jejunum and colon of the cat (177, 197). Jansson (186) distinguished a short latency (4–5 sec) inhibition of cholinergic excitation in the stomach and a long latency (18–25 sec) inhibition in the absence of cholinergic tone. He suggested that the first response was due to the activation of the efferent adrenergic nerves to the stomach and that the latter was caused by secretion of catecholamines from the adrenal medulla.

Circulating catecholamines might also be expected to act on the intrinsic ganglia, because epinephrine has been shown to inhibit the emptying phase of the peristaltic reflex at a lower concentration than was required to antagonize the preparatory contraction of the longitudinal muscle (203). A concentration of 12.5 µg/liter was sufficient to cause inhibition of the emptying phase, but 50 µg/liter was required to reduce the longitudinal contraction. However, the excitatory effect of exogenous acetylcholine was not inhibited by even 150 µg/liter of epinephrine. This result seems to be in conflict with the studies outlined above, which suggest that the intramural ganglia are less sensitive than is the muscle to the actions of catecholamines. The results of Kosterlitz & Robinson (203) could be due to a direct action of catecholamines on the circular muscle, which reduces the emptying phase even though no reduction in longitudinal muscle response was seen, perhaps because the longitudinal muscle was stimulated supramaximally.

PLASMA LEVELS OF CATECHOLAMINES AND SENSITIVITY OF GASTROINTESTINAL STRUCTURES

Two measures of the secretion of catecholamines are useful in assessing possible effects on the gut. Catecholamine concentrations in plasma may be compared with the concentrations that influence isolated segments of the gastrointestinal tract. Unfortunately concentrations in

demonstrated direct adrenergic actions on the gut in vitro with low frequencies of stimulation; inhibition after blockade of muscarinic receptors has been reported at frequencies of stimulation of adrenergic fibers as low as 1 or 2 per second [(56, 59, 140); see also (133)].

plasma have usually been estimated from blood samples in peripheral veins or in places remote from the gastrointestinal tract. However, it is probable that peripheral arterial concentrations in other areas are similar to those reaching the gut, and availability of reliable data allows estimation of expected arterial levels from known venous concentrations of catecholamines. In the other method, rates of secretion from the adrenals are compared with rates of infusion (with the adrenals excluded) necessary to affect the gut.

A detailed study of the concentrations of epinephrine and norepinephrine in human arterial and venous plasma has been made by Vendsalu (328). He found arterial levels of slightly less than 0.3 µg/liter epinephrine and about 0.35 µg/liter norepinephrine. However, the veins (excluding the vena cava anterior to the adrenal veins) contained significantly lower concentrations of epinephrine and slightly higher concentrations of norepinephrine. In the upper part of the inferior vena cava, epinephrine levels were significantly higher than in the arteries, but norepinephrine levels were about the same. There was almost no difference in norepinephrine concentrations in the inferior vena cava anterior and posterior to the adrenal inflow.

These results indicate that, in man, the adrenals continually release low levels of epinephrine but very little norepinephrine. Most of the epinephrine loss in passing from the inferior vena cava into the arterial circulation is probably due to dilution with venous blood from other sources, although the heart does extract catecholamines from the blood (16, 268, 339). It appears that some epinephrine is lost in passing through the capillary bed but at rest this is largely compensated by norepinephrine, which is swept into the circulation from the discharge of adrenergic nerves. Other investigations have given similar results, except that estimations of norepinephrine by the ethylenediamine method are apparently too high because of some interfering substance in the blood (79, 325). Rather higher arterial plasma concentrations, about 2 µg/liter, have been found in dogs (208, 325).

The resting secretion of catecholamines has been measured in both cats and dogs by analyzing the outflow from one adrenal gland; the catecholamine outflow is usually between 0.01 and 0.15 µg/kg body wt per minute (101, 118, 174, 193, 234). In cats about 70–80% of the resting outflow is norepinephrine, but in dogs epinephrine accounts for about 85–90%. In man, basal secretion has been calculated as 0.01 and 0.04 µg/kg per minute for epinephrine and norepinephrine, respectively (80). This apparent preponderance of norepinephrine in the effluent is in conflict with the results of Vendsalu (328).

Infusions of catecholamines at rates of up to 0.2 µg/kg per minute into a peripheral vein (with the adrenals excluded) could be expected to mimic the resting secretion. By utilizing Vendsalu's (328) comparison of caval vein epinephrine concentration (anterior to the adrenal veins) and arterial epinephrine concentration, it is reasonable to suppose that intraarterial infusion should be at about half the venous rate to be equivalent for the area supplied by the artery used for infusion.

Celander (68) has estimated the output of adrenal catecholamines in the cat in response to asphyxia and to stimulation of the splanchnic nerves. The intestines, omentum, and spleen were removed to avoid a contribution from adrenergic nerves in these organs, and the right adrenal gland was excluded. The denervated nictitating membrane or the blood pressure responses of a spinal animal were used to assay the catecholamines released. Control doses of amines were given by intravenous injection. The physiological output can be calculated by doubling the assay amount, the two adrenals being considered equivalent. From these results the maximum rate of secretion of catecholamines that could be expected physiologically would be 5 µg/kg per minute (assuming that stimulation at frequencies above 8–10 impulses/sec is aphysiological). Celander found the maximum secretory rate during asphyxia to be 2–2.5 µg/kg per minute, with the average rate being 1–1.3 µg/kg per minute. In dogs peripheral arterial levels of catecholamines can increase to 74 µg/liter in acute anoxia (208). Carotid occlusion produces a far less impressive increase in adrenal output, to about 0.4–0.5 µg/kg per minute (111, 193); the authors' values, calculated for a single adrenal, have been doubled to give an estimate of total output. However, hypothalamic stimulation results in almost maximal adrenal output, 4–5 µg/kg per minute (118). Catecholamine levels of plasma in various cases of shock have been estimated in dogs (240, 273, 282, 311). Concentrations of epinephrine of about 20–40 µg/liter and of norepinephrine of about 7–20 µg/liter have been found in the inferior vena cava in endotoxin or hemorrhagic shock (282). Epinephrine levels of up to 82 µg/liter were found. Arterial concentrations of 7–50 µg/liter (epinephrine) and 1–27 µg/liter (norepinephrine) and peripheral venous concentrations of 5–12 µg/liter (epinephrine) and 5–22 µg/liter (norepinephrine) have been reported (240, 273, 311).

The basal level of secretion of catecholamines appears to be close to the threshold for direct effects on gastrointestinal muscle. Minimal inhibitory effects of epinephrine are seen at 0.2–5 µg/liter (173, 232). More recent studies indicate that minimal effective concentrations for both norepinephrine and epinephrine are in this range (128, 148). Kock (200) found that the intravenous infusion of as little as 0.08 µg/kg per minute of l-epinephrine base caused inhibition of the jejunum of the cat. The intestine was three to five times less sensitive to norepinephrine. Average minimal concentrations causing intestinal inhibition were 0.13 and 0.64 µg/kg per minute for l-epinephrine and l-norepinephrine, respectively. Kock found that maximal intestinal inhibition could be obtained with an infusion of 1–1.2 µg/kg per minute of l-epinephrine. Even a slight rise in the secretion of catecholamines into the circulation can therefore be expected to affect gastrointestinal motility, and maximal effects can readily be obtained with submaximal stimulation of secretion. However, 2.4 µg/kg per minute was required to reduce intestinal blood flow by 30%. Altura (7a) has shown that precapillary sphincters in the rat mesentery are significantly constricted by concentrations of epinephrine (0.01–0.1 µg/liter) and norepinephrine (0.1–1 µg/liter) which could be expected in the blood under resting conditions. Fluorescence histochemical studies show that these vessels are not adrenergically innervated (J. B. Furness, unpublished observations). The longer, innervated arterioles were on average 500–1,000 times less sensitive than the precapillary sphincters, so only at peak rates of secretion would circulating catecholamines be expected to constrict these vessels. Muscular venules were even less sensitive and are unlikely to be affected by circulating catecholamines. Kewenter (197) observed nearly maximal intestinal inhibition with 0.3 µg/kg per minute, a dose of norepinephrine that had almost no effect on intestinal blood flow. Relaxation of the cat stomach in response to l-epinephrine (0.5–1.2 µg/kg per min) was shown by Martinson (230). A depression of gastric mucosal blood flow and secretion has been shown by Jacobson et al. (185) with an infusion of 1 µg/kg per minute of epinephrine base into a peripheral vein. In these experiments, background secretion and blood flow were elevated by histamine.

Summary

Any increase in the levels of circulating catecholamines will relax gastrointestinal muscle, and maximal effects can be expected with moderate increases. The gastrointestinal vasculature is less sensitive to catecholamines, but levels of catecholamines attained physiologically do affect the gastrointestinal arterioles; in fact, constriction can be great enough to inhibit gastric secretion.

CONCLUSIONS

Some general conclusions can be drawn concerning the manner in which catecholamines affect the gastrointestinal tract. These involve revision of some widely accepted views and also lead to a more precise description of the sites and mechanisms of catecholamine action on the gut.

Motility and muscular tone are decreased by catecholamines in most areas of the gut. However, in the stomach, although inhibition is the usual response in most species, excitation is often observed and is sometimes the dominant response.

The generalization that the muscle of the gastrointestinal sphincters is always contracted by catecholamines is no longer tenable. Cardiac, ileocolic, and anal sphincters are in most cases contracted, but the pyloric sphincter is more often relaxed. Available evidence suggests that all sphincters contain receptors for catecholamines, which can mediate either excitation or inhibition. The relative importance of these receptor types remains to be determined.

The sites of catecholamine action on the gastrointestinal tract are summarized in Figure 1. Catecholamines inhibit the movements of the gut both directly and by an antagonism of the release of acetylcholine. As far as is known, the inhibition of transmission from cholinergic neurons is in all cases mediated through α receptors. These α receptors are present both on the cell bodies and at the terminals of the cholinergic neurons. Receptors of the β type are located on the muscle and are almost invariably inhibitory. However, the activation of α receptors on the muscle may in some places contract but in others relax the gut. Excitation of the gut in response to catecholamines, where it occurs, is nearly always mediated by α receptors on the muscle. The basal concentrations of catecholamines in the blood are close to the threshold for relaxation of nonsphincter gastrointestinal muscle, so that any increased adrenal discharge will inhibit gastrointestinal movement. On the other hand, there is only a sparse adrenergic innervation of the nonsphincter muscle, and the reflex activation of the sympathetic nerves to the intestine or their stimulation at physiological frequencies has little direct inhibitory effect on the musculature. Thus circulating catecholamines are of greater importance than is locally released norepinephrine in mediating direct effects on the nonsphincter muscle. In contrast, catecholamines released from adrenergic nerves are principally involved in the inhibition of the contractions of the gut caused by cholinergic nerves and in actions on sphincter muscle (133).

Catecholamines cause an initial constriction of intestinal arteries that is replaced within a few minutes by dilatation of some vessels. This results in an initial decrease in flow followed by a sustained increase. However, the mucosa of the gastrointestinal tract remains ischemic, even during the secondary phase. Under conditions of stress, the ischemia of the mucosa can be sufficiently intense to cause lasting damage and to contribute to ulceration. The gastrointestinal capacitance vessels maintain their constriction during continued exposure to catecholamines, and thereby diversion of blood volume from the splanchnic vasculature to the general circulation is sustained. During sympathoadrenal discharge, effects on the intestinal vasculature are principally mediated by the adrenergic nerves, but catecholamines released from the adrenals reach sufficient concentration in the plasma to act directly on the intestinal arteries. Effects on the capacitance vessels are mediated almost entirely by adrenergic nerves.

Secretory and absorptive processes of the gastrointestinal tract are largely insensitive to the direct actions of catecholamines. Both secretion and absorption tend to be reduced by catecholamines, principally as a result of reduced blood flow through the mucosa.

We gratefully acknowledge the helpful criticism of Drs. Graeme Campbell, Marcello Costa, Marion McCulloch, and David Storey.

REFERENCES

1. ÅBERG, G., AND O. ERÄNKÖ. Localization of noradrenaline and acetylcholinesterase in the taenia of the guinea-pig caecum. *Acta Physiol. Scand.* 69: 383–384, 1967.
2. ABRAHAMS, V. C., S. M. HILTON, AND A. ZBROZYNA. Active muscle vasodilatation produced by stimulation of the brain stem: its significance in the defence reaction. *J. Physiol., London* 154: 491–513, 1960.
3. AHLQUIST, R. P. A study of the adrenotropic receptors. *Am. J. Physiol.* 153: 586–600, 1948.
4. AHLQUIST, R. P., AND B. LEVY. Adrenergic receptive mechanism of canine ileum. *J. Pharmacol. Exptl. Therap.* 127: 146–149, 1959.
5. ALDRICH, T. B. A preliminary report on the active principle of the suprarenal gland. *Am. J. Physiol.* 5: 457–461, 1901.
6. ALEXANDER, F. The action of some humoral agents on the horse intestine. *Quart. J. Exptl. Physiol.* 35: 11–24, 1949.
7. ALPERN, D. Zur Frage der Beziehung der inneren zur Äusseren Sekretion. *Biochem. Z.* 136: 551–563, 1923.
7a. ALTURA, B. M. Chemical and humoral regulation of blood flow through the precapillary sphincter. *Microvascular Res.* 3: 361–384, 1971.
8. ALVAREZ, W. C. *Nervousness, Indigestion and Pain.* New York: Hoeber, 1943.
9. AMBACHE, N. Unmasking, after cholinergic paralysis by botulinum toxin, of a reversed action of nicotine on the mammalian intestine, revealing the probable presence of local inhibitory ganglion cells in the enteric plexuses. *Brit. J. Pharmacol.* 6: 51–67, 1951.
10. AMBACHE, N., AND M. A. FREEMAN. Atropine resistant longitudinal muscle spasms due to excitation of non-cholinergic neurones in Auerbach's plexus. *J. Physiol., London* 199: 705–728, 1968.
11. AMBACHE, N., J. VERNEY, AND M. A. ZAR. Evidence for the release of two atropine-resistant spasmogens from Auerbach's plexus. *J. Physiol., London* 207: 761–782, 1970.
12. ANDERSON, W. F., AND N. MORRIS. The effects of atropine, prostigmin, adrenaline and calcium on the movements of the fasting human stomach. *J. Pharmacol. Exptl. Therap.* 77: 258–265, 1943.
13. ANDERSSON, R., AND E. MOHME-LUNDHOLM. Studies on the relaxing actions mediated by stimulation of adrenergic α- and β- receptors in taenia coli of the rabbit and guinea-pig. *Acta Physiol. Scand.* 77: 372–384, 1969.
14. ANDERSSON, R., AND E. MOHME-LUNDHOLM. Metabolic actions in intestinal smooth muscle associated with relaxation mediated by adrenergic α- and β-receptors. *Acta Physiol. Scand.* 79: 244–261, 1970.
15. ARMITAGE, A. K., AND A. C. B. DEAN. The effects of pressure and pharmacologically active substances on gastric peristalsis in a transmurally stimulated rat stomach-duodenum preparation. *J. Physiol., London* 182: 42–56, 1966.
16. AXELROD, J., H. WEIL-MALHERBE, AND R. TOMCHICK. The physiological disposition of H^3-epinephrine and its metabolite metanephrine. *J. Pharmacol. Exptl. Therap.* 127: 251–256, 1959.
17. BABKIN, B. P. *Secretory Mechanism of the Digestive Glands* (2nd ed.). New York: Hoeber, 1950.
18. BAINBRIDGE, F. A. *The Physiology of Muscular Exercise* (2nd ed.). London: Longmans, 1923.
19. BARBORKA, C. J., AND E. C. TEXTER. *Peptic Ulcer.* Boston: Little, Brown, 1955.
20. BARCROFT, J., AND H. FLOREY. The effects of exercise on the vascular conditions in the spleen and the colon. *J. Physiol., London* 68: 181–189, 1929.
21. BASS, D. D., T. J. USTACH, T. HAMBRECHT, AND M. M. SCHUSTER. In-vitro pharmacologic differentiation of sphincteric and nonsphincteric muscle. *Clin. Res.* 16: 527, 1968.
22. BASS, D. D., T. J. USTACH, AND M. M. SCHUSTER. In vitro pharmacologic differentiation of sphincters and non-sphincteric muscle. *Johns Hopkins Med. J.* 127: 185–191, 1970.
23. BASS, P., AND M. A. PATTERSON. Gastric secretory responses to drugs affecting adrenergic mechanisms in rats. *J. Pharmacol. Exptl. Therap.* 156: 142–149, 1967.
24. BATTELLI, F., AND G. B. BOATTA. Influence de la fatigue sur la quantité d'adrénaline existant dans les capsules surrénales. *Compt. Rend. Soc. Biol.* 54: 1203–1205, 1902.
25. BAUMGARTEN, H. G. Über die Verteilung von Catecholaminen im Darm des Menschen. *Z. Zellforsch. Mikroskop. Anat.* 83: 133–146, 1967.
26. BAXTER, S. G. Sympathetic secretory innervation of the gastric mucosa. *Am. J. Digest. Diseases* 1: 36–39, 1934.
27. BEANI, L., C. BIANCHI, AND A. CREMA. The effect of catecholamines and sympathetic stimulation on the release of acetylcholine from the guinea-pig colon. *Brit. J. Pharmacol.* 36: 1–17, 1969.
28. BEDFORD, E. A. The epinephric content of the blood in conditions of low blood pressure and shock. *Am. J. Physiol.* 43: 235–257, 1917.
29. BEDFORD, E. A., AND H. C. JACKSON. The epinephric content of the blood in conditions of low blood pressure and shock. *Proc. Soc. Exptl. Biol. Med.* 13: 85–87, 1916.
30. BEER, E., F. H. KING, AND M. PRINZMETAL. Pheochromocytoma with demonstration of pressor (adrenaline) substance in the blood preoperatively during hypertensive crises. *Ann. Surg.* 106: 85–91, 1937.
31. BELESLIN, D., AND V. VARAGIĆ. The effect of catecholamines and anticholinesterases on the peristaltic reflex of the isolated guinea-pig ileum. *Arch. Intern. Pharmacodyn.* 148: 123–134, 1964.
32. BENNETT, A., AND B. WHITNEY. A pharmacological investigation of human isolated stomach. *Brit. J. Pharmacol.* 27: 286–298, 1966.
33. BENNETT, M. R., AND D. C. ROGERS. A study of the innervation of the taenia coli. *J. Cell Biol.* 33: 573–596, 1967.
34. BICKEL, A., AND K. SASAKI. Experimentelle Untersuchungen über den Einfluss von Affekten auf die Magensaft Sekretion. *Deut. Med. Wochschr.* 31: 1829–1831, 1905.
35. BINIT, L., M. BURSTEIN, AND D. COULLAUD. Sur les réactions vasomotrices au niveau de l'intestin grêle. *Compt. Rend. Soc. Biol.* 148: 1954–1958, 1954.
36. BLALOCK, A. Shock: further studies with particular reference to the effects of haemorrhage. *Arch. Surg.* 29: 837–857, 1934.
37. BLOMSTRAND, R., C. FRANKSSON, AND B. WERNER. *The Transport of Lymph in Man.* Uppsala: Appelbergs Boktryckeri, 1965.
38. BORUTTAU, H. Erfahrungen über die Nebennieren. *Arch. Ges. Physiol.* 78: 97–128, 1899.
39. BOULLIN, D. J., E. COSTA, AND B. B. BRODIE. Evidence that blockade of adrenergic receptors causes overflow of norepinephrine in cat's colon after nerve stimulation. *J. Pharmacol. Exptl. Therap.* 157: 125–134, 1967.
40. BRADLEY, S. E. The hepatic circulation. In: *Handbook of Physiology. Circulation,* edited by W. F. Hamilton and P. Dow. Washington, D.C.: Am. Physiol. Soc., 1963, sect. 2, vol. II, p. 1387–1438.
41. BRODIE, T. G., AND W. E. DIXON. Contributions to the physiology of the lungs. II. On the innervation in the pulmonary blood vessels and some observations on the action of suprarenal extract. *J. Physiol., London* 30: 476–502, 1904.
42. BRODY, T. M., AND J. H. MCNEILL. Adrenergic receptors for metabolic responses in skeletal and smooth muscles. *Federation Proc.* 29: 1375–1378, 1970.
43. BROWN, G. L., B. N. DAVIES, AND J. S. GILLESPIE. The release of chemical transmitter from the sympathetic nerves of the intestine of the cat. *J. Physiol., London* 143: 41–54, 1958.
44. BROWN, G. L., AND B. A. MCSWINEY. Reaction to drugs of strips of the rabbit's gastric musculature. *J. Physiol., London* 61: 261–267, 1926.

45. Brown, G. L., and B. A. McSwiney. The movements and reaction to drugs of strips of the gastric musculature of the cat and dog. *Quart. J. Exptl. Physiol.* 16: 9–39, 1926.
46. Brown, G. L., B. A. McSwiney, and W. J. Wadge. The sympathetic innervation of the stomach. I. The effect on the stomach of stimulation of the thoracic sympathetic trunk. *J. Physiol., London* 70: 253–260, 1930.
47. Brown, R. B., and M. Borowsky. Further observation on intestinal lesions associated with pheochromocytoma. *Ann. Surg.* 151: 683–692, 1960.
48. Brown, R. B., B. H. Rice, and J. E. Szakas. Intestinal bleeding and perforation complicating treatment with vasoconstrictors. *Ann. Surg.* 150: 790–798, 1959.
49. Brücke, F., and G. Spring. Über die Wirkung sympathicotroper Stoffe auf den Schliessmuskel der Kardia. *Arch. Exptl. Pathol. Pharmakol.* 245: 374–382, 1963.
50. Brunaud, M., and C. Labouche. L'adrénaline, agent contracturant des fibres longitudinals du duodenum du cheval. *Compt. Rend. Soc. Biol.* 141: 167–169, 1947.
51. Bueding, E., and E. Bülbring. Relationship between energy metabolism of intestinal smooth muscle and the physiological actions of epinephrine. *Ann. NY Acad. Sci.* 139: 758–761, 1967.
52. Buirge, R. E. Experimental observations on the human ileocaecal valve. *Surgery* 16: 356–369, 1944.
53. Bülbring, E., and J. H. Burn. Sympathetic vasodilatation in skin and intestine of the dog. *J. Physiol., London* 87: 254–274, 1936.
53a. Bülbring, E., and H. Kuriyama. The action of catecholamines on guinea-pig taenia coli. *Phil. Trans. Roy. Soc. London Ser. B* 265: 115–121, 1973.
54. Burns, G. P., and W. G. Schenk. Effects of digestion and exercise on intestinal blood flow and cardiac output. An experimental study in the conscious dog. *Arch. Surg.* 98: 790–794, 1969.
55. Burnstock, G. Membrane potential changes associated with stimulation of smooth muscle by adrenaline. *Nature* 186: 727–728, 1960.
55a. Burnstock, G. Purinergic nerves. *Pharmacol. Rev.* 24: 509–581, 1972.
56. Burnstock, G., G. Campbell, and M. J. Rand. The inhibitory innervation of the taenia of the guinea-pig caecum. *J. Physiol., London* 182: 504–526, 1966.
57. Burnstock, G., G. Campbell, D. Stachell, and A. Smythe. Evidence that adenosine triphosphate or a related nucleotide is the transmitter substance released by non-adrenergic inhibitory nerves in the gut. *Brit. J. Pharmacol.* 40: 668–688, 1970.
58. Burton-Opitz, R. The vascularity of the liver. VI. The influence of the greater splanchnic nerves on venous inflow. *Quart. J. Exptl. Physiol.* 5: 189–196, 1912.
59. Campbell, G. The inhibitory nerve fibres in the vagal supply to the guinea-pig stomach. *J. Physiol., London* 185: 600–612, 1966.
60. Campbell, J. A. The effects of certain animal extracts upon the blood vessels. *Quart. J. Exptl. Physiol.* 4: 1–17, 1911.
61. Cannon, W. B. The movements of the stomach studied by means of röntgen rays. *Am. J. Physiol.* 1: 359–382, 1898.
62. Cannon, W. B. The influence of emotional states on the functions of the alimentary canal. *Am. J. Med. Sci.* 137: 480–487, 1909.
63. Cannon, W. B., and Z. M. Bacq. Studies on the conditions of activity in endocrine organs. XXVI. A hormone produced by sympathetic action on smooth muscle. *Am. J. Physiol.* 96: 392–412, 1931.
64. Cannon, W. B., and S. W. Britton. Studies on the conditions of activity in endocrine glands. XX. The influence of motion and emotion on medulliadrenal secretion. *Am. J. Physiol.* 79: 433–465, 1927.
65. Cannon, W. B., and D. de la Paz. Emotional stimulation of adrenal secretion. *Am. J. Physiol.* 28: 64–70, 1911.
66. Cannon, W. B., J. R. Linton, and R. R. Linton. Conditions of activity in endocrine glands. XIV. The effects of muscle metabolites on adrenal secretion. *Am. J. Physiol.* 71: 153–162, 1924.
67. Carlson, A. J. *The Control of Hunger in Health and Disease.* Chicago: Univ. of Chicago Press, 1916.
68. Celander, O. The range of control exercised by the sympathicoadrenal system. *Acta Physiol. Scand. Suppl.* 116: 1–132, 1954.
69. Celander, O. Are there any centrally controlled sympathetic inhibitory fibres to the musculature of the intestine? *Acta Physiol. Scand.* 47: 299–309, 1959.
70. Chien, S. Role of the sympathetic nervous system in hemorrhage. *Physiol. Rev.* 47: 214–288, 1967.
71. Chiu, C. Y., and C. Y. Lee. The effects of some adrenergic blocking agents on the inhibition of peristalsis caused by sympathomimetic amines. *J. Formosan Med. Assoc.* 60: 1128, 1961.
72. Christensen, J. Pharmacologic identification of the lower oesophageal sphincter. *J. Clin. Invest.* 49: 681–691, 1970.
73. Christensen, J., and E. E. Daniel. Electric and motor effects of autonomic drugs on the longitudinal oesophageal smooth muscle. *Am. J. Physiol.* 211: 387–394, 1966.
74. Clark, C. G., and J. R. Vane. The cardiac sphincter in the cat. *Gut* 2: 252–262, 1961.
75. Clark, G. A. The selective vaso-constrictor action of adrenaline. *J. Physiol., London* 69: 171–184, 1930.
76. Clark, G. A. The vaso-dilator action of adrenaline. *J. Physiol., London* 80: 429–440, 1934.
77. Cobbold, A., B. Folkow, O. Lundgren, and I. Wallentin. Blood flow, capillary filtration coefficients and regional blood volume responses in the intestine of the cat during stimulation of the hypothalamic defence area. *Acta Physiol. Scand.* 61: 467–475, 1964.
78. Code, C. F. The inhibition of gastric secretion. *Pharmacol. Rev.* 3: 59–106, 1951.
79. Cohen, G., and M. Goldenberg. The simultaneous fluorimetric determination of adrenaline and noradrenaline in plasma. II. Peripheral venous plasma concentrations in normal subjects and in patients with pheochromocytoma. *J. Neurochem.* 2: 71–80, 1957.
80. Cohen, G., B. Holland, J. Sha, and M. Goldenberg. Plasma concentrations of epinephrine and norepinephrine during intravenous infusions in man. *J. Clin. Invest.* 38: 1935–1941, 1959.
81. Cone, T. E., M. S. Allen, and H. A. Pearson. Pheochromocytoma in children: report of three familial cases in two unrelated families. *Pediatrics* 19: 44–56, 1957.
82. Connet, H. Effect of adrenaline on venous blood pressure. *Am. J. Physiol.* 54: 96–121, 1920.
83. Cordier, D., and M. Touze. Troubles de l'absorption intestinale du glucose au cours du choc traumatique. *Compt. Rend. Soc. Biol.* 142: 91–93, 1948.
84. Cori, C. F., and G. T. Cori. The mechanism of epinephrine action. 3. The influence of epinephrine on the utilization of absorbed glucose. *J. Biol. Chem.* 79: 343–355, 1928.
85. Coupland, R. E. *The Natural History of the Chromaffin Cell.* London: Longmans, 1965.
86. Cowley, D. J., and C. F. Code. Effects of secretory inhibitors on mucosal blood flow in nonsecreting stomach of conscious dogs. *Am. J. Physiol.* 218: 270–274, 1970.
87. Dale, H. H. On some physiological actions of ergot. *J. Physiol., London* 34: 163–206, 1906.
88. Daniel, E. E. Electrical and contractile responses of the pyloric region to adrenergic and cholinergic drugs. *Can. J. Physiol. Pharmacol.* 44: 951–979, 1966.
89. Daniel, E. E. Pharmacology of the gastrointestinal tract. In: *Handbook of Physiology. Alimentary Canal*, edited by C. F. Code. Washington, D.C.: Am. Physiol. Soc., 1968, sect. 6, vol. IV, p. 2267–2324.
90. Daniel, E. E., D. M. Paton, G. S. Taylor, and B. J. Hodgson. Adrenergic receptors for catecholamine effects on tissue electrolytes. *Federation Proc.* 29: 1410–1425, 1970.
91. Danielopulu, D., and A. Carniol. Action de l'adrénaline

sur l'estomac de l'homme. Voie intraveineuse et voie gastrique. *Compt. Rend. Soc. Biol.* 97: 716-718, 1922.
92. Deal, C. P., and H. D. Green. Comparison of change in mesenteric resistance following splanchnic nerve stimulation with responses to epinephrine and norepinephrine. *Circulation Res.* 4: 38-44, 1956.
93. De Busscher, G. Étude morphologique et considérations physiologiques sur la vascularisation de l'estomac. *Acta Gastroenterol. Belgica* 11: 333-351, 1948.
94. Delany, J. P., and E. Grim. Canine gastric blood flow and its distribution. *Am. J. Physiol.* 207: 1195-1201, 1964.
95. Delany, J. P., and E. Grim. Experimentally induced variations in canine gastric blood flow and its distribution. *Am. J. Physiol.* 208: 353-358, 1965.
96. Dickson, W. H., and M. J. Wilson. The control of the motility of the human stomach by drugs and other means. *J. Pharmacol. Exptl. Therap.* 24: 33-51, 1924.
97. Donegan, J. F. The physiology of the veins. *J. Physiol., London* 55: 226-245, 1921.
98. Dresel, P., B. Folkow, and I. Wallentin. Rubidium[86] clearance during neurogenic redistribution of intestinal blood flow. *Acta Physiol. Scand.* 67: 173-184, 1966.
99. Dresel, P., and I. Wallentin. Effects of sympathetic vasoconstrictor fibres, noradrenaline and vasopressin on the intestinal vascular resistance during constant blood flow or blood pressure. *Acta Physiol. Scand.* 66: 427-436, 1966.
100. Drury, A. N., H. Florey, and M. E. Florey. The vascular reactions of the colonic mucosa of the dog to fright. *J. Physiol., London* 68: 173-180, 1929.
101. Dunér, H. The influence of the blood glucose level on the secretion of adrenaline and noradrenaline from the suprarenal. *Acta Physiol. Scand. Suppl.* 102: 1-77, 1953.
102. Edmunds, C. W. Some vasomotor reactions of the liver, with special reference to the presence of vasomotor nerves to the portal vein. *J. Pharmacol. Exptl. Therap.* 6: 569-590, 1915.
103. Eliasson, S., B. Folkow, P. Lindgren, and B. Uvnäs. Activation of sympathetic vasodilator nerves to the skeletal muscles in the cat by hypothalamic stimulation. *Acta Physiol. Scand.* 23: 333-351, 1951.
104. Elliott, T. R. On the innervation of the ileo-colic sphincter. *J. Physiol., London* 31: 157-168, 1904.
105. Elliott, T. R. The action of adrenaline. *J. Physiol., London* 32: 401-467, 1905.
106. Elliott, T. R. The control of the suprarenal glands by the splanchnic nerves. *J. Physiol., London* 44: 374-409, 1912.
107. Engel, A., and U. S. von Euler. Diagnostic value of increased urinary output of noradrenaline and adrenaline in pheochromocytoma. *Lancet* 2: 387, 1950.
108. Erlanger, J., and H. S. Gasser. Studies in secondary traumatic shock. II. Shock due to mechanical limitation of blood flow. *Am. J. Physiol.* 49: 151-173, 1919.
109. Esaki, A. Pharmacological study on the intestinal inhibitory and depressor reflexes caused by afferent mesenteric nerve stimulation. *Fukuoka Acta Med.* 60: 221-234, 1969.
110. Euler, U. S. von. Increased urinary excretion of noradrenaline and adrenaline in cases of pheochromocytoma. *Ann. Surg.* 134: 929-933, 1951.
111. Euler, U. S. von, and B. Folkow. Einfluss verschiedener afferenter Nervenreize auf die Zusammensetzung des Nebennierenmarkinkretes bei der Katze. *Arch. Exptl. Pathol. Pharmakol.* 219: 242-247, 1953.
112. Euler, U. S. von, and S. Hellner. Excretion of noradrenaline and adrenaline in muscular work. *Acta Physiol. Scand.* 26: 183-191, 1952.
113. Evans, C. L. The physiology of plain muscle. *Physiol. Rev.* 6: 358-398, 1926.
113a. Exley, K. A. Depression of autonomic ganglia by barbiturates. *Brit. J. Pharmacol.* 9: 170-181, 1954.
114. Fine, J. Shock and peripheral circulatory insufficiency. In: *Handbook of Physiology. Circulation*, edited by W. F. Hamilton. Washington, D.C.: Am. Physiol. Soc., 1965, sect. 2, vol. III, p. 2037-2069.

115. Fine, J., E. D. Frank, H. A. Ravin, S. H. Rutenberg, and F. B. Schweinburg. Bacterial factor in traumatic shock. *New Engl. J. Med.* 260: 214-220, 1959.
116. Florey, H. Observations on the contractility of lacteals. II. *J. Physiol., London* 63: 1-18, 1927.
117. Folkow, B. Impulse frequency in sympathetic vasomotor fibres correlated to the release and elimination of the transmitter. *Acta Physiol. Scand.* 25: 49-76, 1952.
118. Folkow, B., and U. S. von Euler. Selective activation of noradrenaline and adrenaline producing cells in the cat's adrenal gland by hypothalamic stimulation. *Circulation Res.* 2: 191-195, 1954.
119. Folkow, B., J. Frost, and B. Uvnäs. Action of adrenaline, noradrenaline and some other sympathomimetic drugs on the muscular, cutaneous and splanchnic vessels of the cat. *Acta Physiol. Scand.* 15: 412-420, 1948.
120. Folkow, B., D. H. Lewis, D. Lundgren, S. Mellander, and I. Wallentin. The effect of the sympathetic vasoconstrictor fibres on the distribution of capillary blood flow in the intestine. *Acta Physiol. Scand.* 61: 458-466, 1964.
121. Forrest, A. P. M., and C. F. Code. Effect of postganglionic sympathectomy on canine gastric secretion. *Am. J. Physiol.* 177: 425-429, 1954.
122. Fougar, F. R. Essential and paroxysmal hypertension: contrasted by case reports. *Am. J. Pathol.* 15: 741-764, 1939.
123. Franklin, K. J. The pharmacology of the isolated vein ring. *J. Pharmacol. Exptl. Therap.* 26: 215-225, 1925.
124. Franklin, K. J. *A Monograph on Veins*. London: Thomas, 1937.
125. Freeman, N. E., S. A. Shaffer, A. E. Schecter, and H. E. Holling. The effect of total sympathectomy on the occurrence of shock from hemorrhage. *J. Clin. Invest.* 17: 359-368, 1938.
126. Friedman, M., and S. O. Byers. Effects of epinephrine and norepinephrine on lipid metabolism of the rat. *Am. J. Physiol.* 199: 995-999, 1960.
127. Friedman, M. H. F., and W. J. Snape. Color changes in the mucosa of the colon in children as affected by food and psychic stimuli. *Federation Proc.* 5: 30, 1946.
128. Furchgott, R. F. The receptors for epinephrine and norepinephrine (adrenergic receptors). *Pharmacol. Rev.* 11: 429-442, 1959.
129. Furchgott, R. F. The pharmacological differentiation of adrenergic receptors. *Ann. NY Acad. Sci.* 139: 553-570, 1967.
130. Furness, J. B. The origin and distribution of adrenergic nerve fibres in the guinea-pig colon. *Histochemie* 21: 295-306, 1970.
131. Furness, J. B. The adrenergic innervation of the vessels supplying and draining the gastrointestinal tract. *Z. Zellforsch. Mikroskop. Anat.* 113: 67-82, 1971.
132. Furness, J. B. Secondary excitation of intestinal smooth muscle. *Brit. J. Pharmacol.* 41: 213-226, 1971.
133. Furness, J. B., and M. Costa. The adrenergic innervation of the gastrointestinal tract. *Ergeb. Physiol.* 69: 1-54, 1974.
134. Furness, J. B., and M. Costa. The nervous release and the action of substances which affect intestinal muscle through neither adrenoreceptors nor cholinoreceptors. *Phil. Trans. Roy. Soc. London Ser. B* 265: 123-133, 1973.
134a. Gabella, G., and M. Costa. Le fibre adrenergiche nel canale alimentare. *G. Accad. Med. Torino* 130: 1-12, 1967.
135. Gabella, G., and M. Costa. Adrenergic innervation of the intestinal smooth musculature. *Experientia* 25: 395-396, 1969.
136. Gasser, H. S., and W. J. Meek. A study of the mechanisms by which muscular exercise produces acceleration of the heart. *Am. J. Physiol.* 34: 48-71, 1914.
137. Gáti, T., G. Ludány, and A. Sántha. Über die Wirkung der Phenothiazine auf die Darmzottenbewegung. *Arch. Intern. Pharmacodyn.* 113: 390-399, 1958.
138. Gazet, J. C., and R. J. Jarrett. The ileocoecocolic sphincter. Studies *in vitro* in man, monkey, cat and dog. *Brit. J. Surg.* 51: 368-370, 1964.
139. Gendel, B. R., and M. Ende. Pheochromocytoma: a report

of an unusual case with gastrointestinal bleeding. *Gastroenterology* 19: 344–348, 1951.
140. GILLESPIE, J. S. Electrical response of mammalian smooth muscle to stimulation of the extrinsic sympathetic and parasympathetic nerves. *Physiologist* 3: 65, 1960.
141. GILLESPIE, J. S. Electrical activity in the colon. In: *Handbook of Physiology. Alimentary Canal*, edited by C. F. Code and W. Heidel. Washington, D.C.: Am. Physiol. Soc., 1968, sect. 6, vol. IV, p. 2093–2120.
142. GILLESPIE, J. S., AND B. R. MACKENNA. The inhibitory action of nicotine on the rabbit colon. *J. Physiol., London* 152: 191–205, 1960.
143. GLAVIANO, V. V., N. BASS, AND F. NYKIEL. Adrenal medullary secretion of epinephrine and norepinephrine in dogs subjected to hemorrhagic hypotension. *Circulation Res.* 8: 564–571, 1960.
144. GOETZ, R. H. The control of the blood flow through the intestine as studied by the effect of adrenaline. *Quart. J. Exptl. Physiol.* 29: 321–332, 1939.
145. GOLDBERG, M., AND J. FINE. Traumatic shock. XI. Intestinal absorption in hemorrhagic shock. *J. Clin. Invest.* 24: 445–450, 1945.
146. GOLDENBERG, M. Adrenal medullary function. *Am. J. Med.* 10: 627–641, 1951.
147. GOURZIS, J. T., M. W. HOLLENBERG, AND M. NICKERSON. Involvement of adrenergic factors in the effects of bacterial endotoxin. *J. Exptl. Med.* 114: 593–604, 1961.
148. GRAHAM, J. D. P. The effect of drugs on the motility of isolated strips of human stomach muscle. *J. Pharm. Pharmacol.* 1: 95–102, 1949.
149. GRANT, R., P. LINDGREN, A. ROSEN, AND B. ÜVNAS. The release of catechols from the adrenal medulla on activation of the sympathetic vasodilator nerves to the skeletal muscles in the cat by hypothalamic stimulation. *Acta Physiol. Scand.* 43: 135–154, 1958.
150. GRAYSON, J., AND H. J. C. SWAN. Action of adrenaline, noradrenaline and dihydroergocornine on the colonic circulation. *Lancet* 1: 488–490, 1950.
151. GREEFF, K., AND P. HOLTZ. Untersuchungen am isolierten Vagus—Magenpräparat. *Arch. Exptl. Pathol. Pharmakol.* 227: 427–435, 1955.
152. GREEFF, K., H. KASPERAT, AND W. OSSWALD. Paradoxe Wirkung elektrischen Vagusreizung am isolierten Magen und Herzvorhofpräparat. *Arch. Exptl. Pathol. Pharmakol.* 243: 528–545, 1962.
153. GREEN, H. D., C. P. DEAL, S. BARDHANABAEDYA, AND A. B. DENISON. The effects of adrenergic substances and ischaemia on the blood flow and peripheral resistance of the canine mesenteric vascular bed before and during adrenergic blockade. *J. Pharmacol. Exptl. Therap.* 113: 115–123, 1955.
154. GUIMARÃES, S. Alpha excitatory, alpha inhibitory and beta inhibitory adrenergic receptors in the guinea-pig stomach. *Arch. Intern. Pharmacodyn.* 179: 188–201, 1969.
155. GUNN, J. A., AND F. B. CHEVASSE. The action of adrenin on veins. *Proc. Roy. Soc. London Ser. B* 86: 192–197, 1913.
156. GUNN, J. A., AND S. W. F. UNDERHILL. Experiments on the surviving mammalian intestine. *Quart. J. Exptl. Physiol.* 8: 275–296, 1915.
157. GUTHRIE, J. E., AND J. H. QUASTEL. Absorption of sugars and amino acids from isolated surviving intestine after experimental shock. *Arch. Biochem. Biophys.* 62: 485–496, 1956.
158. HAFFNER, J. F. W., I. LIAVAG, AND J. SETEKLIEV. Excitatory adrenergic receptors in the human stomach and pylorus. *Scand. J. Gastroenterol.* 4: 145–150, 1969.
159. HAMILTON, A. S., D. A. COLLINS, AND M. J. OPPENHEIMER. Effects of blood pressure on intestinal motility. *Federation Proc.* 3: 17, 1944.
160. HARRIES, E. H. L. The effect of noradrenaline on the gastric secretory response to histamine in the dog. *J. Physiol., London* 133: 498–505, 1956.
161. HARRY, J. The site of action of sympathomimetic amines on the circular muscle strip from the guinea-pig isolated ileum. *J. Pharm. Pharmacol.* 16: 332–336, 1964.
162. HARTIOLA, K. J. V., AND T. TOIVONEN. Studies on the effect of adrenaline and noradrenaline on the duodenal secretion in dog. *Acta Physiol. Scand.* 31: 125–130, 1954.
163. HARTMAN, F. A., AND K. A. BROWNELL. *The Adrenal Gland*. Philadelphia: Lea and Febiger, 1949.
164. HARTMAN, F. A., R. H. WAITE, AND H. P. MCCORDOCK. The liberation of epinephrine during muscular exercise. *Am. J. Physiol.* 62: 225–241, 1922.
165. HARTMAN, F. A., R. H. WAITE, AND E. F. POWELL. The relation of the adrenals to fatigue. *Am. J. Physiol.* 60: 255–269, 1922.
165a. HENRICH, H., AND J. LUTZ. Das vasculäre Escape—Phänomen am Intestinalkreislauf und seine Auslösung durch unterschiedliche vasoconstriktorische Substanzen. *Arch. Ges. Physiol.* 329: 82–94, 1971.
166. HERRICK, J. F., J. H. GRINDLAY, E. J. BALDES, AND F. C. MANN. Effect of exercise on the blood flow in the superior mesenteric, renal and common ileac arteries. *Am. J. Physiol.* 128: 338–344, 1940.
167. HESS, W. R., AND R. GRUNDLACH. Der Einfluss des Adrenalins auf die Sekretion des Magensaftes. *Arch. Ges. Physiol.* 185: 122–136, 1920.
168. HINRICHSEN, J., AND A. C. IVY. Studies on the ileo-cecal sphincter of the dog. *Am. J. Physiol.* 96: 494–507, 1931.
169. HIRSCHOWITZ, B. I. The control of pepsinogen secretion. *Ann. NY Acad. Sci.* 140: 709–723, 1967.
170. HOLLANDS, B. C. S., AND S. VANOV. Localization of catecholamines in visceral organs and ganglia of the rat, guinea-pig and rabbit. *Brit. J. Pharmacol.* 25: 307–316, 1965.
171. HOLMAN, M. E., C. B. KASBY, M. B. SUTHERS, AND J. A. F. WILSON. Some properties of the smooth muscle of rabbit portal vein. *J. Physiol., London* 196: 111–132, 1968.
172. HOOKER, D. R. The effect of exercise on the venous blood pressure. *Am. J. Physiol.* 28: 235–248, 1911.
173. HOSKINS, R. G. A consideration of some biologic tests for epinephrine. *J. Pharmacol. Exptl. Therap.* 3: 93–99, 1911.
174. HOUSSAY, B. A., AND C. E. RAPELA. Adrenal secretion of adrenaline and noradrenaline. *Arch. Exptl. Pathol. Pharmakol.* 219: 156–159, 1953.
175. HOWARD, J. E., AND W. H. BARKER. Paroxysmal hypertension and other clinical manifestations associated with benign chromaffin cell tumors (phaeochromocytomata). *Bull. Johns Hopkins Hosp.* 61: 371–410, 1937.
176. HULLINGHORST, R. L., AND A. STEER. Pathology of epidemic hemorrhagic fever. *Ann. Internal Med.* 38: 77–101, 1953.
177. HULTÉN, L. Extrinsic nervous control of colonic motility and blood flow: an experimental study in the cat. *Acta Physiol. Scand. Suppl.* 335: 1–116, 1969.
178. ILLINGWORTH, L. F. W. *Peptic Ulcer*. London: Livingstone, 1953.
179. ITIKAWA, K. The paradoxical pupil reaction in cats, before and after interfering with the suprarenal medulla. *Tohoku J. Exptl. Med.* 28: 1–25, 1936.
181. JACOBJ, C. Beiträge zur physiologischen und pharmakologischen Kenntniss der Darmbewegungen mit besonderer Berücksichtigung der Beziehung der Nebenniere zur Denselben. *Arch. Exptl. Pathol. Pharmakol.* 29: 171–211, 1892.
182. JACOBOWITZ, D. Histochemical studies of the autonomic innervation of the gut. *J. Pharmacol. Exptl. Therap.* 149: 358–364, 1965.
183. JACOBSON, E. D. Secretion and blood flow in the gastrointestinal tract. In: *Handbook of Physiology. Circulation*, edited by C. F. Code. Washington, D. C.: Am. Physiol. Soc., 1967, sect. 6, vol. II, p. 1043–1062.
184. JACOBSON, E. D. Comparison of prostaglandin E_1 and norepinephrine on the gastric mucosal circulation. *Proc. Soc. Exptl. Biol. Med.* 133: 516–519, 1970.
185. JACOBSON, E. D., R. H. LINFORD, AND M. I. GROSSMAN. Gastric secretion in relation to mucosal blood flow studied by a clearance technique. *J. Clin. Invest.* 45: 1–13, 1966.

186. JANSSON, G. Effect of reflexes of somatic afferents on the adrenergic outflow to the stomach in the cat. *Acta Physiol. Scand.* 77: 17–22, 1969.
187. JANSSON, G., AND B. LISANDER. On adrenergic influence on gastric motility in chronically vagotomized cat. *Acta Physiol. Scand.* 76: 463–471, 1969.
188. JANSSON, G., B. LISANDER, AND J. MARTINSON. Hypothalamic control of adrenergic outflow to the stomach in the cat. *Acta Physiol. Scand.* 75: 176–186, 1969.
189. JANSSON, G., AND J. MARTINSON. Studies on the ganglionic site of action of sympathetic outflow to the stomach. *Acta Physiol. Scand.* 68: 184–192, 1966.
190. JENKINSON, D. H., AND I. K. M. MORTON. Adrenergic blocking drugs as tools in the study of the actions of catecholamines on the smooth muscle membrane. *Ann. NY Acad. Sci.* 139: 762–771, 1967.
191. JOHANSSON, B., AND B. LJUNG. Sympathetic control of rhythmically active vascular smooth muscle as studied by a nerve-muscle preparation of portal vein. *Acta Physiol. Scand.* 70: 299–311, 1967.
192. JOSKE, R. A., M. H. SHAMMAA, AND G. D. DRUMMEY. Intestinal malabsorption following temporary occlusion of the superior mesenteric artery. *Am. J. Med.* 25: 449–455, 1958.
193. KAINDL, F., AND U. S. VON EULER. Liberation of noradrenaline and adrenaline from the suprarenals of the cat during carotid stimulation. *Am. J. Physiol.* 166: 284–288, 1951.
193a. KAMPP, M., AND O. LUNDGREN. Blood flow and flow distribution in the small intestine of the cat as analysed by the Kr^{85} wash-out technique. *Acta Physiol. Scand.* 72: 282–297, 1968.
194. KÄRKI, N. T. The urinary excretion of noradrenaline and adrenaline in different age groups, its diurnal variation and the effect of muscular work on it. *Acta Physiol. Scand. Suppl.* 132: 1–96, 1956.
195. KELLAWAY, C. H. The hyperglycaemia of asphyxia and the part played therein by the suprarenals. *J. Physiol., London* 53: 211–235, 1919.
196. KERREMANS, R., AND F. PENNINCKX. A study *in vitro* of adrenergic receptors in the rectum and in the internal anal sphincter of the cat. *Gut* 11: 709–714, 1970.
197. KEWENTER, J. The vagal control of the jejunal and ileal motility and blood flow. *Acta Physiol. Scand. Suppl.* 251: 1–68, 1965.
198. KING, C. E., AND L. ARNOLD. The activities of the intestinal mucosal motor mechanism. *Am. J. Physiol.* 59: 97–121, 1922.
199. KING, C. E., AND M. H. ROBINSON. The nervous mechanism of the muscularis mucosae. *Am. J. Physiol.* 143: 325–355, 1945.
200. KOCK, N. An experimental analysis of mechanisms engaged in reflex inhibition of intestinal motility. *Acta Physiol. Scand. Suppl.* 164: 1–54, 1959.
201. KOSTERLITZ, H. W., AND G. M. LEES. Pharmacological analysis of intrinsic intestinal reflexes. *Pharmacol. Rev.* 16: 301–339, 1964.
202. KOSTERLITZ, H. W., AND R. J. LYDON. The action of choline, adrenaline and phenoxybenzamine on the innervated longitudinal muscle strip of the guinea-pig ileum. *Brit. J. Pharmacol.* 32: 442p, 1968.
203. KOSTERLITZ, H. W., AND J. A. ROBINSON. Inhibition of the peristaltic reflex of the isolated guinea-pig ileum. *J. Physiol., London* 136: 249–262, 1957.
204. KOSTERLITZ, H. W., AND A. J. WATT. Adrenergic receptors in the guinea-pig ileum. *J. Physiol., London* 177: 11p, 1965.
205. KURIYAMA, H. Effects of ions and drugs on the electrical activity of smooth muscle. In: *Smooth Muscle*, edited by E. Bülbring, A. Brading, A. Jones, and T. Tomita. London: Arnold, 1970, p. 366–395.
206. KURODA, M. Observations of the effects of drugs on the ileo-colic sphincter. *J. Pharmacol. Exptl. Therap.* 9: 187–195, 1916.
207. KURODA, S. Pharmakodynamische Studien zur Frage der Magenmotilität. *Z. Ges. Exptl. Med.* 39: 341–354, 1924.
208. LAMMERANT, J., AND P. DE HERDT. Catecholamines plasma levels in the pulmonary artery, the pulmonary vein and the arterial tree of open-chest dogs during acute anoxia. *Arch. Intern. Physiol. Biochim.* 73: 81–96, 1965.
209. LANDS, A. M. Sympathetic receptor action. *Am. J. Physiol.* 169: 11–21, 1952.
210. LANGLEY, J. N. Observations on the physiological action of extracts of the supra-renal bodies. *J. Physiol., London* 27: 237–256, 1901.
211. LEE, C. Y. Adrenergic receptors in the intestine. In: *Smooth Muscle*, edited by E. Bülbring, A. F. Brading, A. W. Jones, and T. Tomita. London: Arnold, 1970, p. 549–557.
212. LEE, C. Y., AND L. F. TSENG. A further study on the adrenergic inhibition of the peristaltic reflex of the gut. *Abstr. Intern. Cong. Pharmacol.*, 3rd, Sao Paulo, Brazil, *1966*, p. 117.
213. LIERE, E. J. VAN, D. W. NORTHRUP, AND C. K. SLEETH. The effect of acute hemorrhage on absorption in the small intestine. *Am. J. Physiol.* 124: 102–105, 1938.
214. LIERE, E. J. VAN, D. W. NORTHUP, AND J. C. STICKNEY. The effect of anemic anoxia on peristalsis of the small and large intestine of the dog. *Federation Proc.* 3: 50, 1944.
215. LIERE, E. J. VAN, D. W. NORTHUP, AND J. C. STICKNEY. The effects of anemic anoxia on the motility of the small and large intestine. *Am. J. Physiol.* 142: 260–264, 1944.
216. LIERE, E. J. VAN, D. W. NORTHUP, AND J. C. STICKNEY. The null effect of hemorrhage on intestinal absorption of chloride in the presence of sulphate. *Proc. Soc. Exptl. Biol. Med.* 66: 260–262, 1947.
217. LILLEHEI, C. W., J. L. DIXON, AND O. H. WANGENSTEEN. Relation of anemia and hemorrhagic shock to experimental ulcer production. *Proc. Soc. Exptl. Biol. Med.* 68: 125–128, 1948.
218. LILLEHEI, R. C., J. R. LONGERBEAM, J. H. BLOCH, AND W. G. MANAX. The nature of irreversible shock: experimental and clinical observations. *Ann. Surg.* 160: 682–708, 1964.
219. LILLEHEI, R. C., J. K. LONGERBEAM, AND J. C. ROSENBERG. The nature of irreversible shock: its relationship to intestinal changes. In: *Shock: Pathogenesis and Therapy*, edited by K. D. Bock. Berlin: Springer, 1962, p. 106–129.
220. LIM, R. K. S. The question of a gastric hormone. *Quart. J. Exptl. Physiol.* 13: 79–103, 1922.
221. LIOTTA, D., V. ZUPPONE, AND A. H. GIFFONIELLO. Extudios sobre la motilidad y la farmacologia del esfinter ileocecal y del ileon terminal el hombre. *Prensa Med. Arg.* 44: 3093–3096, 1957.
222. LIPPMANN, W. Reduction of gastric acid secretion and ulcer formation by 3,3-dimethyl-1-(3-methylamino-propyl)-1-phenylpthalon (LU3-010); an inhibition of noradrenaline uptake. *J. Pharm. Pharmacol.* 22: 568–573, 1970.
223. LOEPER, M., AND G. VERPY. L'action de l'adrénaline sur le tractus digestif. *Compt. Rend. Soc. Biol.* 80: 703–705, 1917.
224. LUM, B. K. B., R. D. HEILMAN, AND M. A. GAUNT. Selective loss of responsiveness to alpha adrenergic receptor stimulation after cold storage of the rabbit intestine. *European J. Pharmacol.* 1: 109–113, 1967.
225. LUM, B. K. B., M. H. KERMANI, AND R. D. HEILMAN. Intestinal relaxation produced by sympathomimetic amines in the isolated rabbit jejunum; selective inhibition by adrenergic blocking agents and by cold storage. *J. Pharmacol. Exptl. Therap.* 154: 463–471, 1966.
226. LUND, A. Release of adrenaline and noradrenaline from the suprarenal gland. *Acta Pharmacol. Toxicol.* 7: 309–320, 1951.
227. MAGNUS, R. Versuche am überlebenden Dünndarm. 5. Mitteilung. Wirkungsweise und Angriffspunkt einiger Gifte am Katzendarm. *Arch. Ges. Physiol.* 108: 1–71, 1905.
228. MALIK, K. U., AND G. M. LING. Modification by acetylcholine of the response of rat mesenteric arteries to sympathetic stimulation. *Circulation Res.* 25: 1–10, 1969.
229. MALMEJAC, J. Sur la nature de la sécrétion médullo-surrénale. Discussion sur des théories dualiste et uniciste. *Bull. Acad. Roy. Med. Belg.* 23: 50–70, 1958.
230. MARTINSON, J. Vagal relaxation of the stomach. Experi-

mental re-investigation of the concept of the transmission mechanism. *Acta Physiol. Scand.* 64: 453–462, 1965.
231. MacLean, L., E. Brackney, and M. Visscher. Effects of epinephrine, norepinephrine and histamine on canine intestine and liver weight continuously recorded in vivo. *J. Appl. Physiol.* 9: 237–240, 1956.
232. McDougal, M. D., and G. B. West. The inhibition of the peristaltic reflex by sympathomimetic amines. *Brit. J. Pharmacol.* 9: 131–137, 1954.
233. McGregor, D. D. The effect of sympathetic nerve stimulation on vasoconstriction responses in perfused mesenteric blood vessels of the rat. *J. Physiol., London* 177: 21–30, 1965.
234. McNeill, J. R., R. D. Stark, and C. V. Greenway. Intestinal vasoconstriction after hemorrhage: roles of vasopressin and angiotensin. *Am. J. Physiol.* 219: 1342–1347, 1970.
235. McSwiney, B. A., and G. L. Brown. Reversal of the action of adrenaline. *J. Physiol., London* 62: 52–64, 1926.
236. Mellander, S., and B. Johansson. Control of resistance, exchange, and capacitance functions in the peripheral circulation. *Pharmacol. Rev.* 20: 117–196, 1968.
237. Menguy, R., and A. E. Thompson. Regulation of the secretion of mucous from the gastric antrum. *Ann. NY Acad. Sci.* 140: 797–803, 1967.
238. Meyers, M. A. *Diseases of the Adrenal Glands.* Springfield, Ill.: Thomas, 1963.
239. Miles, R. H. Pheochromocytoma—interesting experiences with three cases. *Ann. Surg.* 149: 925–935, 1959.
240. Millar, R. A., and B. G. Benfey. The fluorimetric estimation of adrenaline and noradrenaline during haemorrhagic hypotension. *Brit. J. Anaesthesia* 30: 158–165, 1958.
241. Ming, S. C., and R. Leviton. Acute hemorrhagic necrosis of the gastrointestinal tract. *New Engl. J. Med.* 263: 59–65, 1960.
242. Moll, H., and E. R. Flint. The depressive influence of the sympathetic nerves on gastric acidity. *Brit. J. Surg.* 16: 283–307, 1928.
243. Moore, B. On the chemical nature of a physiological active substance occurring in the suprarenal gland. *J. Physiol., London* 17: 14–17, 1895.
244. Muren, A. Gastric motor responses to adrenaline and noradrenaline after treatment with a parasympathicolytic agent. *Acta Physiol. Scand.* 39: 188–194, 1957.
245. Muren, A. Influence of the vagal innervation on gastric motor responses to adrenaline and noradrenaline. *Acta Physiol. Scand.* 39: 195–202, 1957.
246. Nakanishi, M. The innervation of the pyloric sphincter in the cat. *J. Physiol., London* 58: 480–484, 1924.
247. Nakazato, Y., K. Saito, and A. Ohga. Gastric motor and inhibitor response to stimulation of the sympathetic nerve in the dog. *Japan. J. Pharmacol.* 20: 131–141, 1970.
248. Necheles, H., L. Walker, and W. Olson. A gradient of gastrointestinal motility following hemorrhage. *Federation Proc.* 5: 75–76, 1946.
249. Newton, H. F., R. L. Zwemer, and W. B. Cannon. The mystery of emotional acceleration of the denervated heart after the exclusion of known humoral accelerators. *Am. J. Physiol.* 96: 377–391, 1931.
250. Nicoloff, D. M., E. T. Peter, N. H. Stone, and O. H. Wangensteen. Effect of catecholamines on gastric secretion and blood flow. *Ann. Surg.* 159: 32–36, 1964.
251. Norberg, K-Å. Adrenergic innervation of the intestinal wall studied by fluorescence microscopy. *Intern. J. Neuropharmacol.* 3: 379–382, 1964.
252. Oberdorf, A., and G. Kroneberg. Alpha- und beta-sympathicomimetische Wirkung am elektrischgereizten isolierten Meerschweinchenileum. *Arch. Exptl. Pathol. Pharmakol.* 267: 195–207, 1970.
253. Öberg, B. Effects of cardiovascular reflexes on net capillary fluid transfer. *Acta Physiol. Scand. Suppl.* 229: 1–98, 1964.
254. Ogawa, S. Beiträge zur Gefässwirkung des Adrenalins. *Arch. Exptl. Pathol. Pharmakol.* 67: 89–110, 1912.
255. Oliver, G., and E. A. Schäfer. The physiological action of extract of the suprarenal capsules. *J. Physiol., London* 18: 230–276, 1895.
256. Ott, I. The peristaltic action of the intestine. Action of certain agents upon it. New function of the spleen. *Med. Bull. Philadelphia* 19: 376–381, 1897.
257. Pal, J. Über Beziehungen zwischen Circulation, Motilität und Tonus des Darmes. *Wien. Med. Presse.* 44: 2017–2026, 1901.
258. Palmer, E. D., and D. P. Buchanan. On the ischemic basis of peptic ulcer. 1. Historical definition of present status. *Ann. Internal Med.* 38: 1187–1205, 1953.
259. Palmerio, C., A. Nabor, R. Minton, and J. Fine. Limitations of antiadrenergic therapy for refractory traumatic shock. *Proc. Soc. Exptl. Biol. Med.* 124: 623–627, 1967.
260. Parks, A. G., D. J. Fishlock, J. D. H. Cameron, and H. May. Preliminary investigation of the pharmacology of the human internal anal sphincter. *Gut* 10: 674–677, 1969.
261. Paton, W. D. M., and J. R. Vane. An analysis of the responses of the isolated stomach to electrical stimulation and to drugs. *J. Physiol., London* 165: 10–46, 1963.
262. Paton, W. D. M., and E. S. Vizi. The inhibitory action of noradrenaline and adrenaline on acetylcholine output by guinea-pig ileum longitudinal muscle strip. *Brit. J. Pharmacol.* 35: 10–28, 1969.
263. Penner, A., and A. I. Bernheim. Acute postoperative esophageal, gastric and duodenal ulcerations: a further study of the pathologic changes in shock. *Arch. Pathol.* 28: 129–140, 1939.
264. Penner, A., and L. J. Druckerman. Enterocolitis as a postoperative complication and its significance. *Gastroenterology* 11: 478–487, 1948.
265. Peters, R., and N. Womack. Hemodynamics of gastric secretion. *Ann. Surg.* 148: 537–550, 1958.
266. Pradhan, S. N., and H. W. Wingate. Effects of some adrenergic blocking agents on gastric secretion in dogs. *Arch. Intern. Pharmacodyn.* 162: 303–310, 1966.
267. Pullinger, B. D., and H. W. Florey. Some observations on the structure and functions of lymphatics: their behavior in local oedma. *Brit. J. Exptl. Pathol.* 16: 49–61, 1935.
268. Raab, W., and W. Gigee. Specific avidity of the heart muscle to absorb and store epinephrine and norepinephrine. *Circulation Res.* 3: 553–558, 1955.
269. Rapport, D. Studies in experimental traumatic shock. VI. The liberation of epinephrine in traumatic shock. *Am. J. Physiol.* 60: 461–475, 1922.
270. Rayner, R. P., L. D. MacLean, and E. Grim. Intestinal tissue blood flow in shock due to endotoxin. *Circulation Res.* 8: 1212–1217, 1960.
271. Read, J. B., and G. Burnstock. Comparative histochemical studies of adrenergic nerves in the enteric plexuses of vertebrate large intestine. *Comp. Biochem. Physiol.* 27: 505–517, 1968.
272. Read, J. B., and G. Burnstock. Adrenergic innervation of the gut musculature in vertebrates. *Histochemie* 17: 263–272, 1969.
273. Reddin, J. L., B. Starzecki, and W. W. Spink. Comparative hemodynamic and humoral responses of puppies and adult dogs to endotoxin. *Am. J. Physiol.* 210: 540–544, 1966.
274. Reddy, V. *A Pharmacological Analysis of Adrenergic Receptors in the Isolated Small Intestine of the Rabbit* (M.Sc. thesis). Atlanta, Ga.: Emory University, 1960.
275. Reid, E. W. The influence of the mesenteric nerves on intestinal absorption. *J. Physiol., London* 20: 298–309, 1896.
276. Remington, J. W., W. F. Hamilton, G. H. Boyd, W. F. Hamilton, Jr., and M. M. Caddell. Role of vasoconstriction in the response of the dog to hemorrhage. *Am. J. Physiol.* 161: 116–124, 1950.
277. Reynell, P. C., P. A. Marks, C. Chidsey, and S. E. Bradley. Changes in splanchnic blood volume and splanchnic blood flow in dogs after haemorrhage. *Clin. Sci.* 14: 407–419, 1955.

278. RICHARDSON, D. R., AND P. C. JOHNSON. Changes in mesenteric capillary flow during norepinephrine infusion. *Am. J. Physiol.* 219: 1317–1323, 1970.

279. ROACH, P. J. Gastrointestinal bleeding in pheochromocytoma and following the administration of norepinephrine (Arterenol). *Arch. Internal Med.* 104: 175–177, 1959.

280. ROGERS, J., J. M. RAKE, AND E. ABLAHADAIN. The stimulation and inhibition of gastric secretion which follows the subcutaneous administration of certain organ extracts. *Am. J. Physiol.* 48: 79–92, 1919.

281. ROGERS, L. A., R. A. ATKINSON, AND J. P. LONG. Responses of isolated perfused arteries to catecholamines and nerve stimulation. *Am. J. Physiol.* 209: 376–382, 1965.

282. ROSENBERG, J. C., J. K. LILLEHEI, J. K. LONGERBEAM, AND B. ZIMMERMANN. Studies on hemorrhagic and endotoxin shock in relation to vasomotor changes and endogenous circulating epinephrine, norepinephrine and serotonin. *Ann. Surg.* 154: 611–627, 1961.

283. ROSENBLUETH, A. *The Transmission of Nerve Impulses at Neuroeffector Junctions and Peripheral Synapses.* New York: Wiley, 1950.

284. ROSS, G. Effects of catecholamines on splanchnic blood flow before and after beta adrenergic blockade. In: *Cardiovascular Beta Adrenergic Responses*, edited by A. A. Kattus, G. Ross, and V. E. Hall. Berkeley: Univ. of California Press, 1970.

285. ROTHSCHILD, F. Die klinische Bedeutung der fraktionierten Magenausheberung unter besonderer Berücksichtigung der Gesamtchloride und der Neutralchloride. *Arch. Verdauungskrankheiten* 35: 286–310, 1925.

286. RUDICK, J., W. G. GUNTHEROTH, AND L. M. NYHUS. Recent observations on gastric blood flow and acid secretion. In: *Gastric Secretion: Mechanisms and Control*, edited by T. K. Shnitka, J. A. L. Gilbert, and R. C. Harrison. Oxford: Pergamon Press, 1967, p. 53–69.

287. RUDICK, J., L. S. SEMB, W. G. GUNTHEROTH, G. L. MULLINS, H. N. HARKINS, AND L. M. NYHUS. Gastric blood flow and acid secretion in the conscious dog under various physiological and pharmacological stimuli. *Surgery* 58: 47–56, 1965.

288. RUSHMER, R. F., D. L. FRANKLIN, R. L. VON CITTERS, AND O. A. SMITH. Changes in peripheral blood flow distribution in healthy dogs. *Circulation Res.* 9: 675–687, 1961.

289. RUSZNYAK, I., M. FOLDI, AND G. SZABO. *Lymphatics and Lymph Circulation. Physiology and Pathology* (2nd ed.). Oxford: Pergamon Press, 1967.

290. SALIMI, M., R. Z. KERMANI, B. DJAHANSOUZ, AND S. H. GOLSHAN. Impairment of alpha receptor activity induced by cold storage in the isolated rabbit duodenum. *Pharmacology* 4: 341–346, 1970.

291. SATAKE, Y., M. SUGAWARA, AND M. WATANABE. A method for collecting the blood from the suprarenal gland. *Tohoku J. Exptl. Med.* 8: 501–534, 1927.

292. SATAKE, Y., M. WATANABE, AND T. SUGAWARA. Effect of fastening and of sensory stimulation upon the rate of epinephrine output from the suprarenal gland in dogs. The fourth report. *Tohoku J. Exptl. Med.* 9: 1–40, 1927.

293. SATO, A., N. TSUSHIMA, AND B. FUJIMORI. Reflex potentials of lumbar sympathetic trunk with sciatic nerve stimulation in cats. *Japan. J. Physiol.* 15: 532–539, 1965.

293a. SATO, H., M. OHGURI, AND M. WADA. Epinephrine discharge, blood sugar and blood pressure in anaphylactic shock of dogs, non-anaesthetized, non-fastened. *Tohoku J. Exptl. Med.* 28: 504–519, 1935.

294. SCHANKER, L. S., P. A. SHORE, B. B. BRODIE, AND C. A. M. HOGBEN. Absorption of drugs from the stomach. 1. The rat. *J. Pharmacol. Exptl. Therap.* 120: 528–540, 1957.

295. SCHATZMANN, H. J. Action of acetylcholine and epinephrine on intestinal smooth muscle. In: *Handbook of Physiology. Alimentary Canal*, edited by C. F. Code. Washington, D. C.: Am. Physiol. Soc., 1968, sect. 6, vol. IV, p. 2173–2191.

296. SCHAUMANN, W. Zusammenhänge zwischen der Wirkung der Analgetika und Sympathicomimetic auf den Meerschweinchen-Dünndarm. *Arch. Exptl. Pathol. Pharmakol.* 233: 112–124, 1958.

297. SCHWIEGK, H. Untersuchungen uber die Leberdurchblutung und den Pfortaderkreislauf. *Arch. Exptl. Pathol. Pharmakol.* 168: 693–714, 1932.

298. SELKURT, E., M. SCIBETTA, AND T. CULL. Hemodynamics of intestinal circulation. *Circulation Res.* 6: 92–99, 1958.

299. SELYE, H. *Textbook of Endocrinology.* Montreal: Acta Endocrinologica, Inc., 1949.

300. SHANBOUR, L. L., AND E. D. JACOBSON. Autoregulatory escape in the gut. *Gastroenterology* 60: 145–148, 1971.

301. SHAPIRO, P., B. BRONSTHER, E. D. FRANK, AND J. FINE. Host resistance to hemorrhagic shock. XI. Role of deficient flow through intestine in development of irreversibility. *Proc. Soc. Exptl. Biol. Med.* 97: 372–376, 1958.

302. SHAW, R. S., AND E. P. MAYNARD. Acute and chronic thrombosis of mesenteric arteries associated with malabsorption. *New Engl. J. Med.* 258: 874–878, 1958.

303. SHEHADEH, Z., W. E. PRICE, AND E. D. JACOBSON. Effects of vasoactive agents on intestinal blood flow and motility in the dog. *Am. J. Physiol.* 216: 386–392, 1969.

303a. SHIBATA, S., K. HATTORI, AND D. TIMMERMAN. Effect of cold storage on the response of guinea-pig taenia coli to certain catecholamines and other agents. *European J. Pharmacol.* 11: 321–331, 1970.

304. SHIPLEY, P. G., AND K. D. BLACKFAN. The pharmacological action of adrenaline on the sphincter pylori of the foetus. *Bull. Johns Hopkins Hosp.* 33: 159–162, 1922.

305. SHOSKES, M. Responses of colonic muscle to local application of drugs. *Gastroenterology* 10: 305–309, 1948.

306. SIRCUS, W. The aetiology of peptic ulcer. In: *Peptic Ulceration*, edited by C. Wells and J. Kyle. Edinburgh: Livingstone, 1960, p. 11–36.

307. SMETS, W. La contraction de la valvule iléo-caecale. *Compt. Rend. Soc. Biol.* 122: 793–795, 1936.

308. SMITH, M. I. The action of the autonomic drugs on the surviving stomach. A study of the innervation of the stomach. *Am. J. Physiol.* 96: 232–243, 1918.

309. SPATT, S. D., AND D. M. GRAYZEL. Pheochromocytoma of the adrenal medulla, a clinicopathological study of five cases. *Am. J. Med. Sci.* 216: 39–50, 1948.

310. SPEDEN, R. N. Excitation of vascular smooth muscle. In: *Smooth Muscle*, edited by E. Bulbring, A. Brading, A. Jones, AND T. Tomita. London: Arnold, 1970, p. 558–588.

311. SPINK, W. W., J. L. REDDIN, S. J. ZAK, M. PETERSON, B. STARZECKI, AND E. SELJESKOG. Correlation of plasma catecholamine levels with hemodynamic changes in canine endotoxin shock. *J. Clin. Invest.* 45: 78–85, 1966.

312. STACKPOLE, R. H., M. M. MELICOW, AND A. C. USON. Pheochromocytoma in children. *J. Pediat.* 63: 315–330, 1963.

313. TACCA, M. DEL, G. SOLDANI, M. SELLI, AND A. CREMA. Action of catecholamines on release of acetylcholine from human taenia coli. *European J. Pharmacol.* 9: 80–84, 1970.

314. TAKAMINE, J. Adrenaline, the active principle of the suprarenal glands and its mode of preparation. *Am. J. Pharmacol.* 73: 523–531, 1901.

315. TANAKA, U., AND Y. OHKUHO. Pharmacological studies on the autonomic nerves of the small intestine of the horse. 1. Sympathetic innervation of the small intestine. *Japan. J. Vet. Sci.* 2: 321–339, 1940.

316. TEZNER, O., AND M. TUROLT, Studien über die Wirkung der Verschiebung der K- und Ca-Ionen auf den überlebenden menschlichen Magen. *Z. Ges. Exptl. Med.* 24: 1–10, 1921.

317. THOMAS, J. E. The action of adrenaline on the pyloric sphincter. *Proc. Soc. Exptl. Biol. Med.* 23: 748–750, 1926.

318. THOMAS, J. E. A further study of the nervous control of the pyloric sphincter. *Am. J. Physiol.* 88: 498–518, 1929.

319. THOMAS, J. E., E. D. ROOKE, AND W. F. KVALE. The neurologist's experience with pheochromocytoma. A review of one hundred cases. *J. Am. Med. Assoc.* 197: 754–758, 1966.

320. THOMAS, J. E., AND H. WHEELON. The nervous control of the pyloric sphincter. *J. Lab. Clin. Med.* 7: 375–391, 1922.
321. THOMPSON, J. E., AND J. R. VANE. Gastric secretion induced by histamine and its relationship to the rate of blood flow. *J. Physiol., London* 121: 433–444, 1953.
322. THORELL, G. Untersuchungen über die Bewegungen und Innervationsverhält nisse der Muscularis mucosae des Magens. *Skand. Arch. Physiol.* 50: 205–282, 1927.
323. TITCHEN, D. A. Nervous control of motility of the forestomach of ruminants. In: *Handbook of Physiology. Alimentary Canal*, edited by C. F. Code. Washington, D.C.: Am. Physiol. Soc., 1968, sect. 6, vol. v, p. 2705–2724.
324. TOURNADE, A., AND M. CHABROL. Effects des variations de la pression artérièlle sur la sécrétion de l'adrénaline. *Compt. Rend. Soc. Biol.* 93: 934–936, 1925.
325. VALK, A. DE T., AND H. L. PRICE. The chemical estimation of epinephrine and norepinephrine in human and canine plasma. I. A critique of the ethylenediamine condensation method. *J. Clin. Invest.* 35: 837–841, 1956.
326. VARRO, V., G. BLAHO, L. CSERNAY, I. JUNG, AND F. SZARVAS. Effect of decreased local circulation on the absorptive capacity of a small intestine loop in the dog. *Am. J. Digest. Diseases* 10: 170–177, 1965.
327. VEACH, H. O. Studies on the innervation of smooth muscle. III. Splanchnic effects on the lower end of the oesophagus and stomach of the cat. *J. Physiol., London* 60: 457–478, 1925.
328. VENDSALU, A. Studies on adrenaline and noradrenaline in human plasma. *Acta Physiol. Scand. Suppl.* 173: 1–123, 1960.
329. VIZI, E. S. The inhibitory action of noradrenaline and adrenaline on release of acetylcholine from guinea-pig ileum longitudinal strips. *Arch. Exptl. Pathol. Pharmakol.* 259: 199–200, 1968.
330. WAKIM, K. G., AND J. W. MASON. The influence of hemorrhage and of depletion of plasma proteins on intestinal activity. *Gastroenterology* 4: 92–101, 1945.
331. WALCOTT, W. W. Blood volume in experimental hemorrhagic shock. *Am. J. Physiol.* 143: 247–253, 1945.
332. WALDER, D. N. The muscularis mucosae of the human stomach. *J. Physiol., London.* 120: 365–372, 1953.
333. WALKER, W. F., M. S. ZILELI, F. W. RUETTER, W. C. SCHOEMAKER, D. FRIEND, AND F. D. MOORE. Adrenal medullary secretion in hemorrhagic shock. *Am. J. Physiol.* 197: 773–780, 1959.
334. WALTON, R. P., J. A. RICHARDSON, R. P. WALTON, AND W. L. THOMPSON. Sympathetic influences during hemorrhagic hypotension. *Am. J. Physiol.* 197: 223–230, 1959.
335. WATANABE, M. Simultaneous determination of the blood sugar content and epinephrine output from the suprarenal gland in the non-anaesthetized, non-fastened dog during peptone poisoning. *Tohoku J. Exptl. Med.* 9: 412–453, 1927.
336. WATTS, D. T. Arterial blood epinephrine levels during hemorrhagic hypotension in dogs. *Am. J. Physiol.* 184: 271–274, 1956.
337. WEBER, E. Über die Ursache der Blutverschiebung im Körper bei verschiedenen psychischen Zuständen. *Arch. Physiol.* 293–348, 1907.
338. WEIL, M. H. Morphologic changes in dogs following the production of shock with endotoxin and their comparison to the morphologic changes occurring during shock associated with bacteremia in patients. *J. Clin. Invest.* 37: 940–941, 1958.
339. WHITBY, L. G., J. AXELROD, AND H. WEIL-MALHERBE. The fate of H^3-norepinephrine in animals. *J. Pharmacol. Exptl. Therap.* 132: 193–201, 1961.
340. WHITE, H. L., W. R. RAINEY, B. MONAGHAN, AND A. S. HARRIS. Observation on the nervous control of the ileocaecal sphincter and on intestinal movements in an unanaesthetized human subject. *Am. J. Physiol.* 108: 449–457, 1934.
341. WIGGERS, H. G., R. G. INGRAHAM, F. ROEMHILD, AND H. GOLDBERG. Vasoconstriction and the development of irreversible hemorrhagic shock. *Am. J. Physiol.* 153: 511–520, 1948.
342. WINKELSTEIN, A., AND P. W. ASCHNER. The pressure factors in the biliary-duct system of the dog. *Am. J. Med. Sci.* 168: 812–819, 1924.
343. WINNE, D. Der Einfluss einiger Pharmaka auf die Darmdurchblutung und die Resorption tritiummarkierten Wassers aus dem Dünndarm der Ratte. *Arch. Exptl. Pathol. Pharmakol.* 254: 199–224, 1966.
344. WOLF, S. G., AND H. G. WOLFF. *Human Gastric Function: An Experimental Study of a Man and His Stomach.* New York: Oxford, 1943.
345. WOLNER, E., AND F. BRÜCKE. Über Tyraminresistente adrenergische Mechanismen in der Kardia des Kaninchens. *Arch. Exptl. Pathol. Pharmakol.* 254: 91–100, 1966.
346. WOODS, G., V. NELSON, AND E. NELSON. The effect of small amounts of ergotamine on the circulatory response to epinephrine. *J. Pharmacol. Exptl. Therap.* 45: 403–418, 1932.
347. YOUMANS, W. B. *Nervous and Neurohumoral Regulation of Intestinal Motility.* New York: Interscience, 1949.
348. YOUMANS, W. B. Innervations of the gastrointestinal tract. In: *Handbook of Physiology. Alimentary Canal*, edited by C. F. Code. Washington, D.C.: Am. Physiol. Soc., 1968, sect. 6, vol. IV, p. 1655–1633.
349. YOUMANS, W. B., K. W. AUMANN, H. F. HANEY, AND F. WYNIA. Reflex cardiac acceleration and liberation of sympathomimetic substances in unanaesthetized dogs during acetylcholine hypotension. *Am. J. Physiol.* 128: 467–474, 1940.
350. YOUMANS, W. B., AND W. J. MEEK. Reflex and humoral gastro-intestinal inhibition in unanaesthetized dogs during rectal stimulation. *Am. J. Physiol.* 120: 750–756, 1937.
351. YUKAWA, G. Klinisch—experimentelle Untersuchungen der Adrenalin—Wirkung auf die Magendrüsen. *Arch. Verdauungskrankheiten* 14: 166–185, 1908.

CHAPTER 34

Action of catecholamines on skeletal muscle

T. TOMITA | *Department of Physiology, Faculty of Medicine, Kyushu University, Fukuoka, Japan*

CHAPTER CONTENTS

Direct Action of Catecholamines on Muscle Fiber
    Effects of catecholamines in normal ionic environment
        Fast muscles
        Slow muscles
    Effects of catecholamines in different external potassium
        concentrations
        Excess potassium
        Low potassium
    Adrenoreceptors
    Effects of ouabain and temperature on catecholamine action
        Ouabain
        Low temperature
    Electrical changes
    Mechanism of action on muscle fiber
Action of Catecholamines on Neuromuscular Transmission
    Facilitatory action
    Inhibitory action
    Effects on end-plate potential
    Effects on miniature end-plate potential
    Mechanism of increase of transmitter release
Conclusions

THE ACTIONS OF SYMPATHOMIMETIC amines on skeletal muscles are complicated because they vary with condition of the muscle, type of muscle, and species. Furthermore the amines influence both the muscle fibers themselves and the neuromuscular junction.

Since many reviews concerning classic mechanical (9, 14, 22, 36) and biochemical (25, 27, 38, 81) studies are available, this review is confined mainly to recent biophysical findings in mammalian muscles.

DIRECT ACTION OF CATECHOLAMINES ON MUSCLE FIBER

Effects of Catecholamines in Normal Ionic Environment

Mammalian skeletal muscles have been classified as fast or slow muscle on the basis of their speed of contraction. Fast or twitch muscles, such as tibialis anterior and extensor digitorum longus, contract rapidly—they reach the peak tension in 30 msec or less in an isometric twitch. They require high frequencies of stimulation before complete tetanic fusion of twitches occurs. These muscles are functionally phasic, flexor-type muscles that contract only occasionally. On the other hand, slow muscles, such as soleus, tend to be tonic in nature and function in the maintenance of posture. In contrast to twitch muscles, tonic muscles have much slower contraction times—they reach the peak of an isometric twitch in 40 msec or more and may be tetanized at lower frequencies.

Fast and slow muscles differ not only in their contractile and functional properties but also in the activity of the various enzymes they contain (3, 21, 30, 79). Fast muscles have highly active myosin adenosine triphosphatase (ATPase), high capacity to utilize glycogen, low rate of lipid metabolism, low rate of oxidative metabolism, and low content of myoglobin. The reverse is true for slow muscles. Thus the activities of the enzymes involved in anaerobic glycolysis are higher in fast muscles than in slow muscles, whereas the activities of enzymes involved in aerobic pathways are higher in slow muscles. Histochemical studies of muscle fibers have shown that fast muscles contain predominantly fibers that stain intensely for phosphorylase but poorly for succinic dehydrogenase and other oxidative enzymes.

FAST MUSCLES. Epinephrine and other sympathomimetic amines increase the maximum twitch tension of unfatigued, fast-contracting skeletal muscles in various species when the stimulation is applied directly after complete curarization or after chronic denervation (7, 15, 34, 35, 73). In normal nonfatigued muscles the same changes are observed when the muscles are stimulated through their nerves (17). The maximum increase in twitch tension is 15–16% in the tibialis anterior of the cat in situ (15, 35). However, the maximum tetanic tension is not increased (15) or may be depressed (35).

In Figure 1A the typical response of a fast-contracting muscle, tibialis anterior of the rabbit, in situ to epinephrine is shown. When twitch tension is increased by injection of catecholamines, the peak is usually delayed, the duration is prolonged, and the rate of relaxation is slightly decreased without change in the rising phase. Therefore incomplete tetanic contractions are increased both in tension and fusion by epinephrine, as shown in

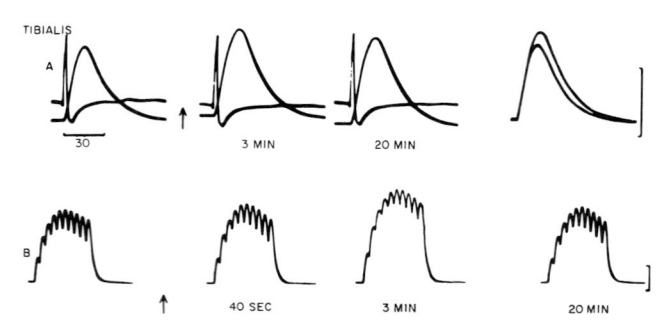

FIG. 1. Effects of epinephrine on fast-contracting muscles. *A*: tibialis anterior of rabbit anesthetized with urethane. Maximal twitches and gross muscle action potentials elicited by motor nerve stimulation every 10 sec. First record is control response. Epinephrine (10 μg/kg) injected intravenously at *arrow*. Subsequent contractions were recorded at the time after injection shown. Last record shows first 2 twitches superimposed. *B*: tibialis anterior of cat anesthetized with chloralose. Incomplete tetani (40 pulses/sec for 0.25 sec). Epinephrine (8 μg/kg) given intravenously at *arrow*. Note that epinephrine augments contractions, with little change in action potentials. Time calibrations in msec. Tension calibration on *right* equivalent to 0.5 kg. [Adapted from Bowman & Raper (14).]

the records of Figure 1*B* taken from the tibialis anterior of the cat in situ. These effects are produced in the fast-contracting tibialis anterior, gastrocnemius, and extensor digitorum longus muscle of cats, dogs, rabbits, guinea pigs, and rats (14) and in the isolated diaphragm preparation of the rat (35).

In most experiments on the rat diaphragm stimulated either through its nerve or directly after curarization, the time from stimulus to peak tension is delayed after epinephrine application by 3–20%, usually with a concomitant increase in tension. However, in some experiments the time to peak is prolonged without change in tension (35). These effects have also been observed in the guinea pig extensor digitorum longus with isoproterenol (N. Tashiro and T. Tomita, unpublished observations). In this muscle the time course of twitch tension differs depending on stimulus duration. The time from the beginning of the twitch to peak tension (i.e., peak tension time) is about 20 msec at 30 C, when the stimulus duration is less than 2 msec. However, the peak tension time is about 35 msec with a maximal 20-msec pulse, although the magnitude of tension is more than three times as great as the maximum tension obtained with a maximal 2-msec pulse. There is little difference in the isoproterenol effects between responses evoked by a 2-msec and by a 20-msec pulse.

The delay of the time to peak tension is not due to a reduction of the propagation velocity along the muscle fiber, since the delay of the time to peak is nearly the same whether the muscle is stimulated indirectly through its nerve or directly by simultaneous stimulation at many places along the muscle (35).

In the guinea pig diaphragm, effects of isoproterenol are weak and variable. The rate of relaxation is sometimes increased, rather than decreased, as in the rat diaphragm, with little change in the maximum tension, particularly when the twitch is evoked by short current pulses (less than 2 msec). These responses of the guinea pig diaphragm may be related to the fact that this is not a typical fast muscle. The time course of twitch is slower than that of the rat diaphragm, which is histochemically classified as a red muscle (2), although two other fiber types, white and intermediate, can also be identified on the basis of myosin ATPase activities (84).

Goffart & Ritchie (35) and Jurna et al. (48) concluded that epinephrine and isoproterenol increase the maximum twitch tension by prolonging the active state in the tibialis anterior muscle of the cat and in the isolated diaphragm muscle of the rat.

SLOW MUSCLES. In the slow-contracting muscles (e.g., soleus muscle of cats, rabbits, guinea pigs, and rats; crureus muscle of cats; plantaris muscle of dogs) it has been reported that twitch tension, evoked through the muscle's nerve or by direct stimulation of the muscle with 0.5–1-msec pulses, is reduced and that the rate of relaxation is increased by epinephrine and by isoproterenol (11, 14, 15, 47). In Figure 2*A* the characteristic response of the cat soleus in situ to epinephrine is illustrated. The maximum decrease in twitch tension is 20% in the soleus muscle of the cat in situ (15). This may be caused by shortening of the active state of the muscle (8, 47, 48). Incomplete tetanic contractions of slow-contracting muscles are reduced by catecholamines both in tension and in fusion (Fig. 2*B*). The same effect is produced in the slow motor units present in human muscles (68). Decreased fusion caused by catecholamines may be responsible for the tremor produced by these drugs.

When the effects of isoproterenol were examined in the guinea pig soleus after complete curarization, the responses differed depending on the stimulus parameters. The peak tension time is about 40 msec with a 2-msec

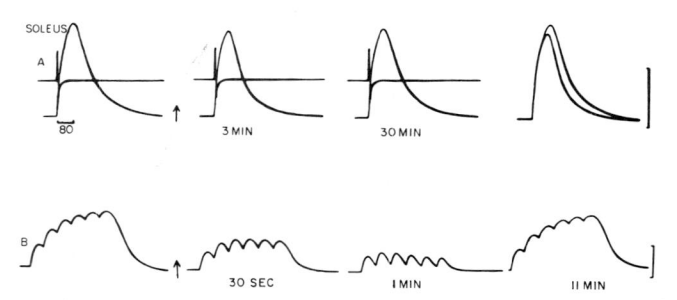

FIG. 2. Effects of epinephrine on soleus of cat anesthetized with chloralose. *A*: maximal twitches and gross muscle action potentials elicited by motor nerve stimulation every 10 sec. First record is control response. Epinephrine (1 μg/kg) injected intravenously at *arrow*. Subsequent responses recorded at the time after injection shown. Last record shows first 2 twitches superimposed. *B*: incomplete tetani (6 pulses/sec for 1 sec). Epinephrine (2 μg/kg) given intravenously at *arrow*. Note depression of contractions by epinephrine, with little change in action potentials. Time calibration in msec. Tension calibration on *right* equivalent to 0.5 kg. [Adapted from Bowman & Raper (14).]

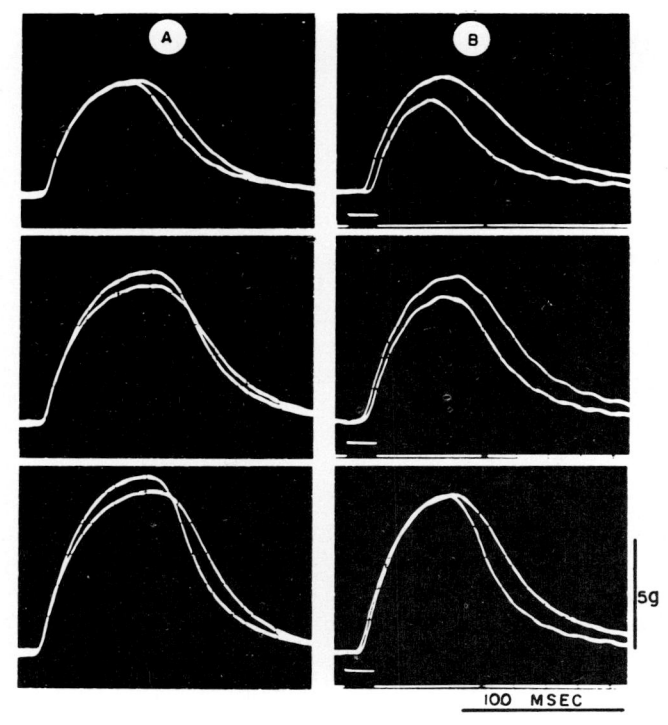

FIG. 3. Isolated guinea pig soleus in presence of d-tubocurarine (5×10^{-6} g/ml). Two different preparations (A and B) at 35 C stimulated directly with 20-msec pulse of 3 different intensities. Each frame shows superimposed traces of isometric twitches (3 twitches at 10-sec interval) before and 5 min after isoproterenol (10^{-6} g/ml). Isoproterenol shortened twitch duration with changes in twitch size.

pulse and 55–60 msec with a 20-msec pulse at 35 C. The maximum tension evoked by a 20-msec pulse is only twice that caused by a 2-msec pulse, the increase being less in the soleus than in the extensor digitorum longus. Twitches are usually reduced by isoproterenol when the stimulus intensity is weak or the pulse duration is less than 2 msec. However, they are usually potentiated by isoproterenol when the intensity is near the maximum and the pulse duration is more than 5 msec, as shown in Figure 3. The duration of the twitch is, however, always shortened mainly because of the acceleration of relaxation. Isoproterenol does not necessarily increase the rate of relaxation but in some conditions causes the relaxation to begin earlier.

In the guinea pig soleus, in contrast to the fast-contracting muscles, a change in the resting tension is often produced by isoproterenol. This is particularly clear after the first application. The tension change is diphasic with a transient decrease followed by a gradual prolonged increase.

It is known that at birth all limb muscles in mammals are slow-contracting, and differentiation into fast and slow types occurs during the first few weeks after birth (19). Despite the uniformly slow contraction, the effects of epinephrine in the kitten are the same as those in the adult cat. Thus in the tibialis anterior and flexor digitorum longus of the young kitten, the tension and the times to peak tension and to half-relaxation are increased by the catecholamines. The effects of epinephrine on the soleus muscle of young kittens are variable and weak.

Buller et al. (20) have shown that, when a nerve from a phasic motoneuron of a cat has been transplanted to innervate a slow muscle, the mechanical properties are transferred so that it becomes a fast muscle even in the adult. The soleus muscles cross-innervated with the nerve that formerly innervated the flexor digitorum longus resemble a true phasic muscle in contraction and in response to catecholamines. The twitch tension is now increased by epinephrine, as in a fast muscle, but its speed of relaxation is still increased, as in the normal soleus (9, 11).

Effects of Catecholamines in Different External Potassium Concentrations

EXCESS POTASSIUM. In the isolated diaphragm of the rat, potentiation of the contraction by catecholamines is much more clearly demonstrated when the contractions are first depressed by increasing the external K concentration to 10–12 mM (12, 37, 56, 63).

When the external K is increased from 4.6–5.9 to 10–13 mM, twitch tension is gradually increased, whether stimulation is applied through the nerve or directly to the muscle. This increase is associated with a prolongation of the contraction time by 3–18% (35). This potentiation is, however, only transient and is followed by depression (12, 37).

In the extensor digitorum longus and the diaphragm of the guinea pig, it is necessary to increase the external K concentration to 15–18 mM in order to demonstrate clearly the depression of twitch tension after an initial potentiation. The potentiation of twitch tension by excess K is observed only when a short pulse of less than 2 msec or a weak pulse of more than 10 msec is used.

The magnitude of the potentiation of twitch tension by isoproterenol in the K-depressed extensor digitorum longus and diaphragm of the guinea pig greatly varies from one preparation to another. In some preparations no effect can be observed; the reason for this failure is not clear.

In the guinea pig soleus, potentiation of the twitch by isoproterenol is always clearly demonstrated after the tension is depressed in Krebs solution containing 11 mM K. A recovery of the tension is observed even when it has been nearly completely depressed by excess K (Fig. 4). When short, stimulating pulses (less than 2 msec) are used, isoproterenol depresses the twitch tension in the normal K concentration, as described above. However, after the twitch tension has been reduced in the K-excess solution, isoproterenol always potentiates the twitch evoked by the same stimulus and a suppression of twitch tension is never observed. The time course of twitch is not appreciably changed during the potentiation of twitch by isoproterenol. When the K concentration is increased

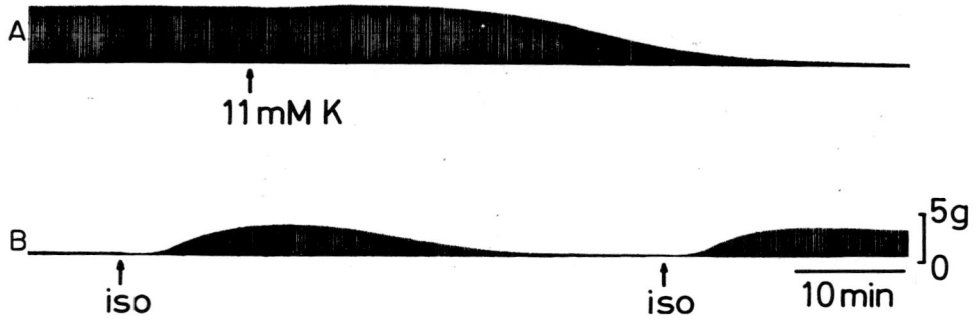

FIG. 4. Effects of isoproterenol (10^{-6} g/ml) on isometric twitches of isolated guinea pig soleus at 35 C in Krebs solution containing excess K and d-tubocurarine (5×10^{-6} g/ml). Direct stimulation with 20-msec pulse at 10-sec interval throughout. Isoproterenol (*iso*) was administered into organ bath through which the bathing solution flowed continuously. Note recovery of twitch in presence of isoproterenol.

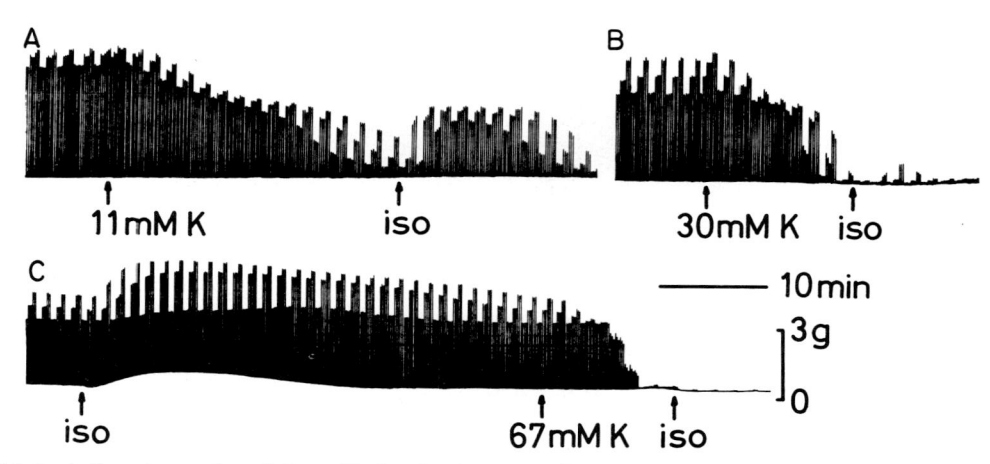

FIG. 5. Effects of isoproterenol (10^{-6} g/ml) on isometric twitches of isolated guinea pig soleus at 35 C in Krebs solution containing increasing concentrations of K ions. Effect in 11 mM K (*A*). Note reduction at 30 mM K (*B*) or abolition at 67 mM K (*C*) of isoproterenol (*iso*) effect. Typical effect of isoproterenol in normal Krebs solution is shown in *C*. Three stimuli (20-msec pulse) with 3 different intensities given at 10-sec intervals throughout.

further to more than 30 mM, the effects of isoproterenol become weak or disappear, as shown in Figure 5.

LOW POTASSIUM. The guinea pig extensor digitorum longus and diaphragm are rather insensitive to low K (0.6 mM) solution. However, in K-free Krebs solution, twitch tension gradually decreases and the effects of isoproterenol are reduced. In the rat diaphragm stimulated through its nerve, prolonged immersion in K-free Tyrode's solution reverses the effect of isoproterenol to a depression of the twitch tension (33). However, in the guinea pig extensor digitorum longus, no reversal of the effect is observed.

In the guinea pig soleus, the twitch tension is increased and prolonged by reducing the external K concentration to 0.6 mM or to zero. Isoproterenol depresses the twitch tension evoked either by 2-msec or 20-msec pulse and accelerates the relaxation, when given after the twitch has been augmented by low concentration of K. Thus, in a solution low in K, the effects of isoproterenol on tension are reversed, although the acceleration of relaxation remains the same. This reduction of tension by isoproterenol is less when the stimulus strength is near maximum and the tension is not depressed below the level observed at the normal K concentration. The effect of isoproterenol on the twitch tension is abolished after prolonged immersion (150 min) in K-free solution.

Adrenoreceptors

In direct effects on the contractions of both fast- and slow-contracting skeletal muscles, *l*-isoproterenol is about twice as potent as *l*-epinephrine, whereas *l*-norepinephrine is weaker than *l*-epinephrine (12, 14, 15, 63). Since a relatively high concentration is necessary to influence the contraction of fast muscles, the effect of norepinephrine and epinephrine on these muscles does not seem to have any physiological significance. Slow-contracting muscles are much more sensitive to epinephrine than fast-contracting muscles. Therefore it has been suggested that an action of epinephrine on slow-contracting, postural muscles may be an explanation for

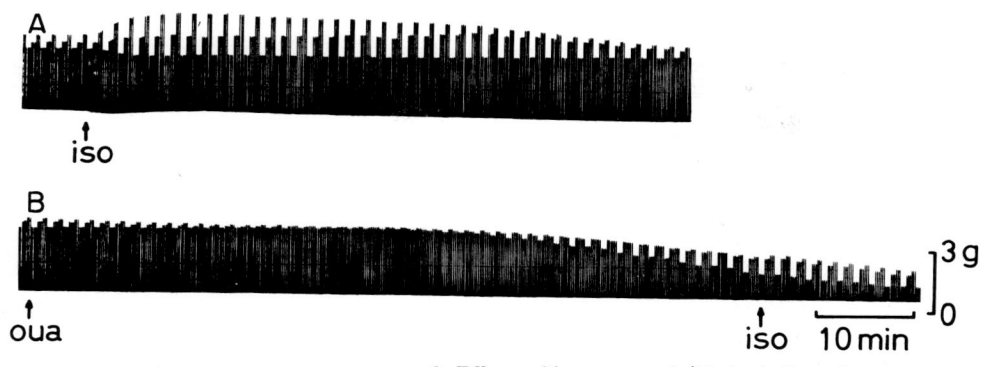

FIG. 6. Effects of isoproterenol (10^{-6} g/ml) on isometric twitches of isolated guinea pig soleus at 35 C in normal Krebs solution (A) and in presence of 2×10^{-6} g/ml ouabain (B). Isoproterenol (*iso*) was given 80 min after ouabain-containing solution (*oua*) had started to flow (B). Stimulations with 20-msec pulses at 10-sec intervals and with 3 different intensities. All solutions contained d-tubocurarine (5×10^{-6} g/ml).

the feeling of weakness in the limbs experienced as a result of fright or during epinephrine infusions (15).

The effects of catecholamines are not affected by α receptor blocking agents, such as Dibenamine, phenoxybenzamine, or phentolamine, but are suppressed by β receptor blocking agents, such as dichloroisoproterenol, pronethalol, propranolol, or isopropylmethoxamine. In the K-depressed muscles the relative potencies of catecholamines and the action of blocking agents are the same. From these results, it is concluded that the direct action of catecholamines on the muscle fiber is mediated by β receptors (8, 9).

Recently, it has been proposed that there are two types of β receptor, $β_1$ and $β_2$, and that the effects on muscle contractions are mediated via $β_2$ receptors (10, 63). The ability of various sympathomimetic compounds to increase the twitches of the K-depressed rat diaphragm is correlated with their ability to dilate the guinea pig bronchioles and to inhibit contraction of the rat uterus, but not with their ability to stimulate the rabbit heart or to relax the rabbit intestine.

Effects of Ouabain and Temperature on Catecholamine Action

OUABAIN. Effects of ouabain ($1-5 \times 10^{-6}$ g/ml) on the twitch tension of the guinea pig extensor digitorum longus and soleus are similar to those of excess (11 mM) K, but the effects appear much more slowly. There is a slight potentiation of the twitch before depression occurs, particularly when the stimulus is weak. When isoproterenol (10^{-6} g/ml) is applied after the depression by ouabain, a weak but clear potentiation is observed in the extensor digitorum longus, whereas little effect is produced in the soleus (Fig. 6), in contrast to the augmentation of twitch tension after treatment with excess K.

The strong potentiating effect of isoproterenol on the twitch of the soleus observed in the presence of excess K is also greatly suppressed by ouabain ($2-5 \times 10^{-6}$ g/ml), when it is added to the solution with a high K concentration, as shown in Figure 7.

LOW TEMPERATURE. In both the tibialis anterior and soleus muscle of the cat and rabbit, the twitch tension is reduced by a fall in temperature from 36 to about 30 C. Effects of epinephrine on the tension and time course of the twitches in these muscles at about 30 C are similar to those at 36 C (8).

The twitch tension of the guinea pig extensor digitorum longus evoked directly by 2-msec pulse is increased and slowed when the temperature is lowered from 32 to 20 C, as shown in Figure 8A. The effect of isoproterenol at 20 C is essentially the same as at 32 C (see Fig. 8B, C), although it appears slowly at the lower temperature.

In the guinea pig soleus, lowering the temperature from 35 to 20 C reduces the twitch (see Fig. 8D). When stimulation is submaximal, there is an initial small potentiation of twitch tension during cooling. As the temperature is lowered, the effects of isoproterenol on the soleus appear more gradually, are prolonged, and become weaker. At 20 C, isoproterenol has little effect on the twitch size (Fig. 9) but still accelerates the falling phase (see Fig. 8F).

The effects of lowering temperature on the isoproterenol action on the K-depressed soleus of the guinea pig are similar. In these preparations the potentiating effects of isoproterenol are still produced at 18 C, but they appear very gradually and the degree of potentiation is much smaller than that at 35 C (Fig. 10). Cooling reversibly increases the resting tension in the excess K solution, and this is partially antagonized by isoproterenol.

When the temperature is raised after an isoproterenol application, a large potentiation of twitch occurs both in normal K (see Fig. 9) and in excess K solution (see Fig. 10A and C). Although there is a potentiation in response to an increase in temperature itself, the pretreatment with isoproterenol strongly augments this process, even after isoproterenol has been completely washed out from the organ bath. This potentiation is reduced by ouabain applied simultaneously with isoproterenol (see Fig. 10B). When the preparation is

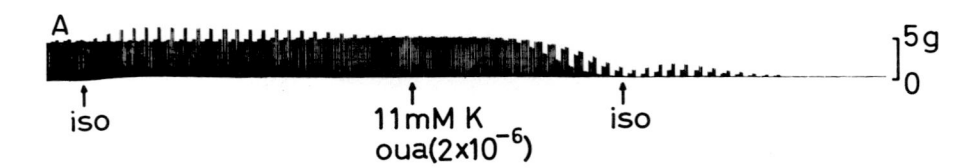

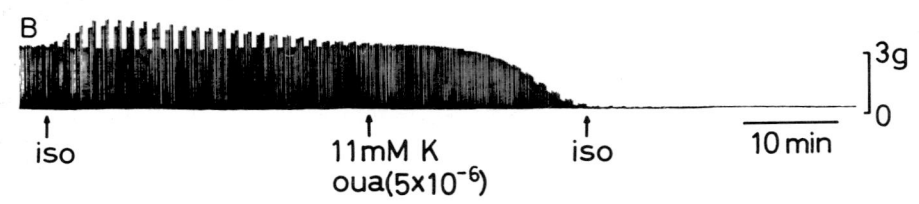

FIG. 7. Effects of isoproterenol (10^{-6} g/ml) on isometric twitches of isolated guinea pig soleus at 35 C in presence of 11 mM K and ouabain (*oua*). Krebs solution containing 11 mM K and ouabain (2×10^{-6} g/ml in *A*; 5×10^{-6} g/ml in *B*) started to flow at *arrow*, and isoproterenol (*iso*) given when twitch was suppressed. Stimulations with 20-msec pulses of 3 different intensities at 10-sec intervals throughout. All solutions contained *d*-tubocurarine (5×10^{-6} g/ml).

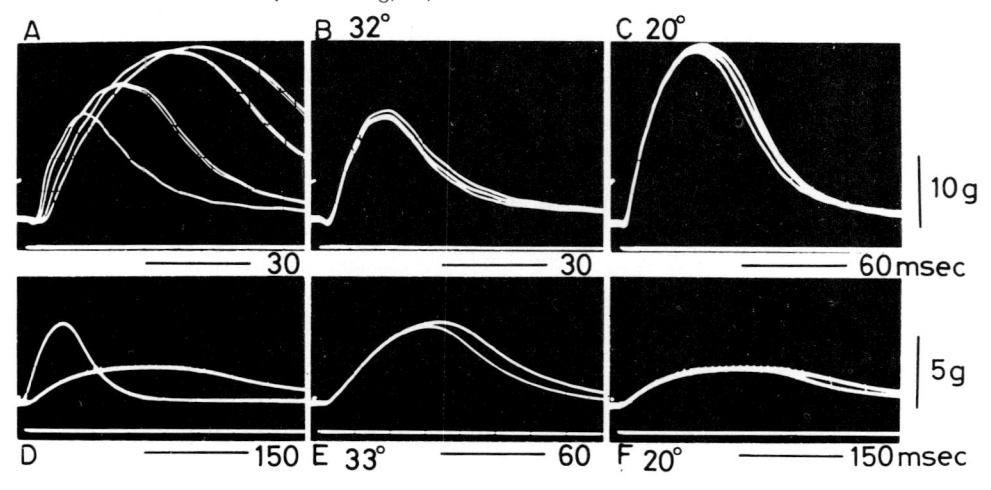

FIG. 8. Effects of temperature on isolated guinea pig extensor digitorum longus (*A–C*) and soleus (*D–F*). Maximal isometric twitches elicited by direct stimulation (2-msec pulses every 10 sec) in Krebs solution containing *d*-tubocurarine (5×10^{-6} g/ml). *A*: superimposed records showing increase and slowing of twitches by lowering temperature (3 responses at 32, 28, 24, and 20 C). *B*: 3 twitches were recorded before and 3 and 5 min after isoproterenol at 32 C. *C*: similar to *B*, but 10 and 15 min after isoproterenol at 20 C. Note that isoproterenol potentiated twitches in extensor, and also note slower sweep speed in *C*. *D*: superimposed records showing decrease and slowing of twitches in soleus by lowering temperature from 33 to 20 C. *E*: 3 twitches recorded before and 5 min after isoproterenol at 33 C. *F*: similar to *E*, but 15 min after isoproterenol at 20 C. Note that isoproterenol reduced and shortened twitch at 33 C, but at 20 C it accelerated falling phase without effect on twitch size. Also note faster sweep speed in *E*.

treated with ouabain (5×10^{-6} g/ml) for more than 30 min before isoproterenol application, the potentiation of twitches caused by warming is greatly suppressed. Relaxation caused by warming is not affected by ouabain.

Electrical Changes

Investigations of catecholamine action on the electrical properties of the muscle membrane are rather limited, compared to mechanical properties. Catecholamines increase the demarcation (injury) potential of the fast-contracting tibialis anterior of the cat in situ (13, 18). As with the effects on twitch tension, isoproterenol is slightly more potent and norepinephrine slightly less potent than epinephrine in hyperpolarizing the membrane.

An increase in demarcation potential is also produced by the catecholamines in the slow-contracting soleus of the cat (13), although the mechanical responses to the amines differ from those observed in the tibialis anterior. With intracellular microelectrodes, Krnjević &

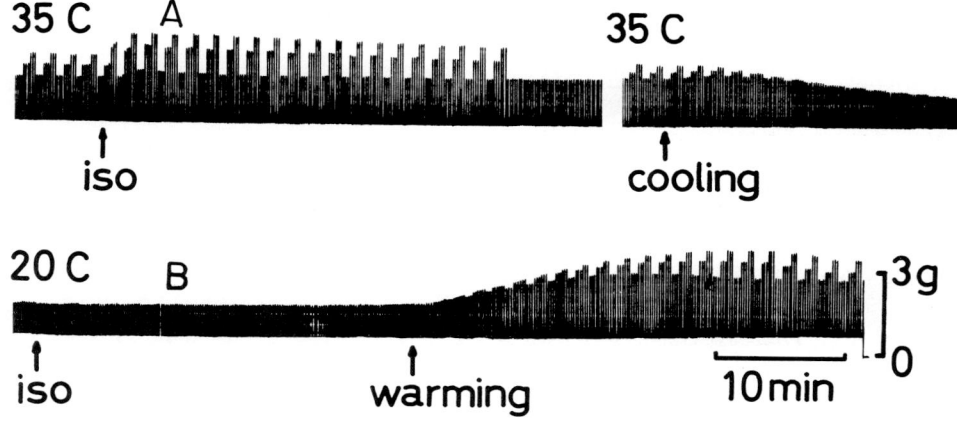

FIG. 9. Effect of isoproterenol on isometric twitch tension in isolated guinea pig soleus at different temperatures (35 and 20 C). Krebs solution contained d-tubocurarine (5×10^{-6} g/ml). A 20-msec pulse was given at 10-sec intervals with 3 different intensities. A: isoproterenol (iso) effects at 35 C, and effects of cooling to 20 C. B: isoproterenol effect at 20 C, and effects of warming to 35 C. Note little effect of isoproterenol at 20 C.

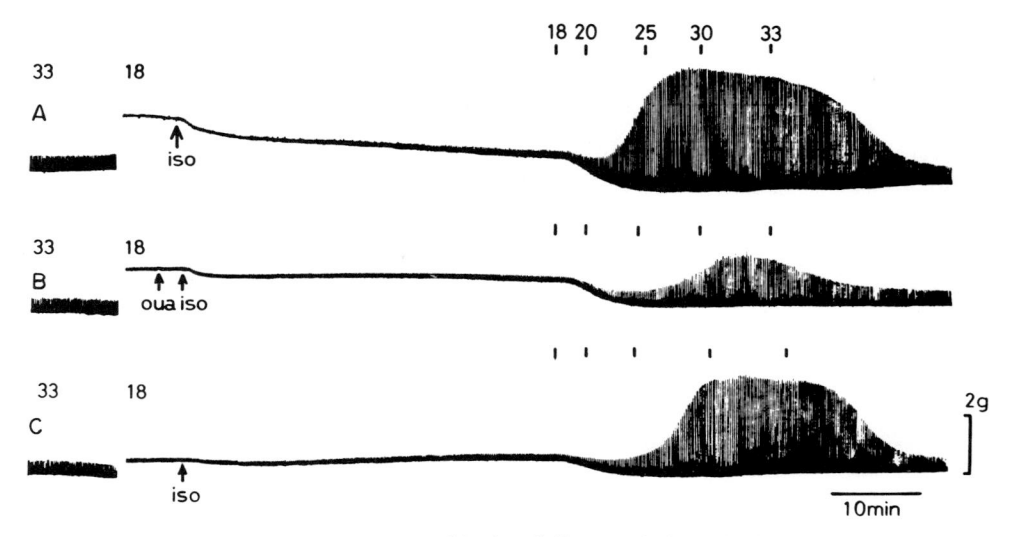

FIG. 10. A and C: potentiation of twitches by warming from 18 to 33 C after pretreatment with isoproterenol (10^{-6} g/ml). B: suppression of potentiation by simultaneous application of ouabain (2×10^{-6} g/ml). Krebs solution contained 11 mM K and tubocurarine (5×10^{-6} g/ml). Constant stimulation with 5-msec pulses at 10-sec intervals throughout. Interval between records in each trace is 30 min, during which temperature was lowered to 18 C and contracture developed. Oua, ouabain; iso, isoproterenol.

Miledi (58) were unable to find any significant change in the resting potential in response to epinephrine (2–5×10^{-6} g/ml) in the isolated rat diaphragm at room temperature (about 22 C). These negative results are in agreement with the observations on frog muscle made by Hutter & Loewenstein (45), although epinephrine has no direct effect on the contraction in this preparation, in contrast to the mammalian muscles.

On the other hand, Kuba (60) found that, at 32–34 C, the muscle membrane in the rat diaphragm is hyperpolarized by 3–4 mv by both epinephrine and isoproterenol at a concentration of 5×10^{-6} g/ml or more. The hyperpolarization caused by epinephrine is increased when the external K concentration is reduced, but blocked when Na is replaced with tris-(hydroxymethyl) amino methane. A concomitant increase in input resistance of the muscle membrane occurs during hyperpolarization. The changes in membrane potential and resistance are blocked by a β blocking agent, pronethalol, but not by an α blocking agent, phentolamine. In fish red muscle, Hidaka & Kuriyama (39) also observed hyperpolarization and an increase in membrane resistance as a result of treatment with epinephrine.

In the guinea pig, isoproterenol (10^{-6} g/ml) hyperpolarizes the muscle membrane from 66–71 mv to 73–78 mv in the soleus at 33 C, whereas little change is observed in the extensor digitorum longus (82). Hyperpolarization observed in the soleus by isoproterenol is abolished in K-free solution, at low temperature (18 C), and by treatment with ouabain (2×10^{-6} g/ml), which suggests an involvement of the Na-K pump in this process.

Isoproterenol relaxes the spontaneous tone and also the acetylcholine contracture of avian slow fibers (chicken anterior latissimus dorsi and pigeon latissimus dorsi). This effect is mediated through β adrenergic receptors, since it is blocked by pronethalol but not by Dibenamine. When isoproterenol (2×10^{-7} g/ml) produces relaxation in Krebs solution containing 5.9 mM K, depolarization is small but significant (2.7 mv). In Krebs solution containing 1 mM K, isoproterenol produces hyperpolarization by about 9 mv. This hyperpolarizing effect observed in 1 mM K solution is blocked by replacement of Na with Li and by treatment with ouabain (10^{-4} M). From these results, Somlyo & Somlyo (80) have suggested that isoproterenol stimulates the Na pump. The different effects on the membrane potential in 5.9 and 1 mM K solutions may be explained by assuming that the K-to-Na coupling ratio varies with the external K concentration.

Epinephrine increases the demarcation potential by 7–17% in the domestic fowl gastrocnemius (78). However, in this preparation, no effect of epinephrine is observed on the twitches when directly stimulated after complete curarization.

In the denervated soleus muscle of rat that has been rendered Na rich by soaking in a cold, K-free Krebs solution, isoproterenol depolarizes the membrane by about 5 mv during the recovery process in the Krebs solution containing 10 mM K at 37 C (24).

Mechanism of Action on Muscle Fiber

Understanding of the mechanism of catecholamine action on contraction is incomplete. Electrophysiological investigations are clarifying some important factors involved in the action of catecholamines. A possible difference between the excitation-contraction coupling in the slow muscle and that in the fast muscle should be thoroughly investigated, because this may underlie some differences in effects of catecholamines. There are many biochemical observations, but the correlation of these findings with muscle function is still a matter of speculation.

Epinephrine and other sympathomimetic amines stimulate glycogenolysis in skeletal muscles (23, 27, 57, 76). Epinephrine activates adenyl cyclase, which catalyzes the conversion of ATP to the cyclic nucleotide, 3',5'-AMP. Phosphorylase *b* kinase, activated by the cyclic AMP, converts inactive phosphorylase *b* to active phosphorylase *a* [(41, 42); see also the chapter by Himms-Hagen in this volume of the *Handbook*]. Phosphorylase *a* catalyzes the breakdown of glycogen with the production of hexose phosphates (4). The glucose 6-phosphate is subsequently catabolized through the Embden-Meyerhof pathway with the production of lactic acid.

These metabolic activations by catecholamines may affect some process in the muscle contraction. If the speed of contraction is determined by myosin ATPase, as suggested by Bárány (3), catecholamines may affect the twitch by modifying the reaction between the myosin ATPase and ATP probably because of an increase in ATP supply. It is also possible, however, that Ca released from the sarcoplasmic reticulum determines the process of contraction. Then catecholamines may exert their effect on the process of Ca release or reuptake.

As in the potentiating effect on the twitch, the effect of catecholamines on muscle glycogenolysis is mediated through β receptors (29, 55, 70, 72), more precisely β_2 receptors (63). The relative potencies of catecholamines in increasing the twitches correlate with their relative potencies in stimulating glycogenolysis (29).

Epinephrine can potentiate twitches in the K-depressed rat diaphragm even in the presence of the glycolytic inhibitor, iodoacetate, or under anaerobic conditions (12, 27, 28). Therefore the action of epinephrine on the twitch is probably independent of the Embden-Meyerhof pathway or oxidative phosphorylation.

Formation of cyclic 3',5'-AMP or an increase in hexose-phosphate level, or both, may be related to the action of epinephrine on muscle contractility (9). Thus, in fast-contracting muscles, cyclic 3',5'-AMP may facilitate the release of Ca from the sarcoplasmic reticulum or may suppress the reuptake of Ca and thereby increase the concentrations of intracellular free Ca. The adenyl cyclase, which synthesizes cyclic 3',5'-AMP, is localized in fractions containing the calcium-accumulating granules derived from the sarcoplasmic reticulum (77). Cyclic 3',5'-AMP may also increase the sensitivity of actomyosin to Ca ions, as suggested by Uchida & Mommaerts (83). On the other hand, in slow-contracting muscles, cyclic AMP may potentiate the process of reuptake of Ca ions by the sarcoplasmic reticulum and thereby increase the rate of decay of the active state.

In the guinea pig soleus, a slow-contracting muscle, it is possible to demonstrate the potentiation of twitch tension by isoproterenol when a strong and long stimulating current pulse is used and also when the twitch has been previously suppressed by excess K. It is therefore tempting to speculate that catecholamines facilitate the release of Ca in both fast- and slow-contracting muscles. The decrease of twitch tensions evoked by nerve stimulation or by direct stimulation with short or weak pulses in the soleus muscle could partly result from a reduction in numbers of active fibers caused by an increase in threshold resulting from the hyperpolarization of the muscle membrane.

Since the effects of isoproterenol on twitch size in the guinea pig soleus are blocked by removal of external K ion, by ouabain, and by lowering the temperature, it is possible that the action, at least in this muscle, is mediated by a potentiation of the active ion transport system (i.e., the Na-K pump). The Na-K pump may affect the contraction not only by changing the membrane potential, but also by modifying the distribution of intracellular Ca, as observed in squid giant axon (1). An in-

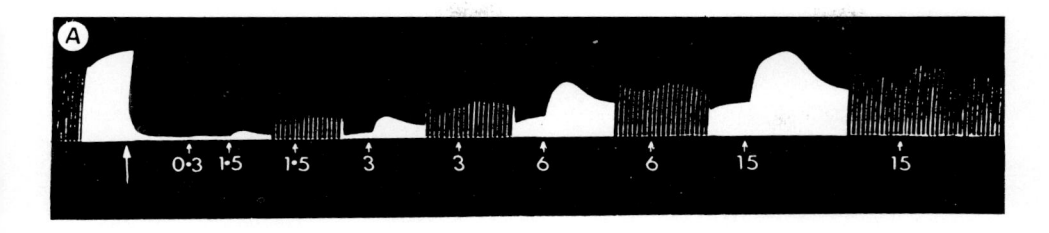

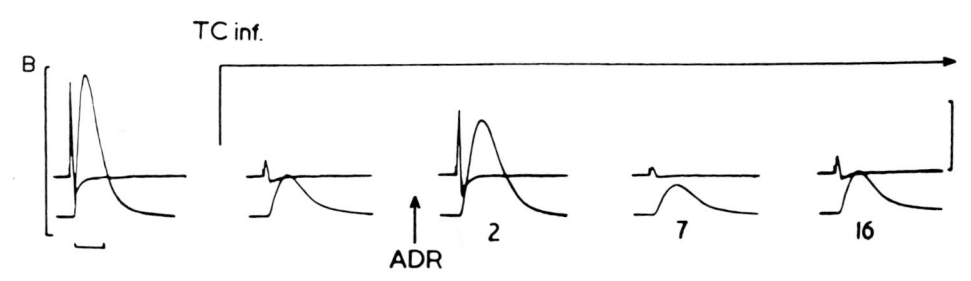

FIG. 11. Maximal twitches of tibialis anterior of cat anesthetized with chloralose and pentobarbitone sodium. *A*: stimulation of motor nerve once every 10 sec, or for alternate periods, once every second (50-μsec pulse). At *larger arrow* tubocurarine (0.25 mg/kg) was injected intravenously. *Numbers* below *small arrows* indicate doses of epinephrine (μg/kg) injected intravenously. *B*: twitches and gross muscle action potentials. At *TC inf*. tubocurarine infusion (0.58 mg/kg per hr) was started. At *arrow* epinephrine (*ADR*) was injected intravenously (10 μg/kg). Responses are shown at 2, 7, and 16 min after epinephrine injection. Note that changes in twitch tension are accompanied by corresponding changes in amplitude of gross action potentials. Tension on *left*, 1 kg; time *below*, 30 msec; action potential on *right*, 20 mv. [Adapted from Bowman & Raper (13).]

crease in the resting potential may be a predominant factor in the recovery of the twitch in the K-depressed muscle, as suggested by Bowman and co-workers (9, 12). Activation of the Na-K pump by catecholamines is also suggested from studies on the resting potential in the rat diaphragm (24), the guinea pig soleus (82), and the avian muscle (80). However, a change in resting potential does not seem to be the only factor influencing contraction, since there is no close relation between changes in membrane potential and contraction caused by catecholamines (9, 80).

ACTION OF CATECHOLAMINES ON
NEUROMUSCULAR TRANSMISSION

Facilitatory Action

The effects of catecholamines on the contractions of noncurarized, nonfatigued muscles are mainly due to actions on the muscle fibers themselves. However, in a partially curarized muscle the facilitatory action on neuromuscular transmission is the more important factor in increasing twitch tension. Examples of the anticurare effect of epinephrine observed in a tibialis anterior of an anesthetized cat are shown in Figure 11. The potentiation of twitch is more pronounced at the higher stimulation frequency. The contraction is increased as a result of recruitment of muscle fibers previously blocked by tubocurarine (see Fig. 11*B*), and the fast and slow muscles have the same sensitivity to this facilitatory action of the amines (13).

The catecholamines are believed to exert their effect by enhancing the release of acetylcholine by the nerve impulse. Epinephrine may also relieve presynaptic failure of conduction in a rapidly stimulated preparation (58). Other phenolic compounds, including phenol and catechol, also have facilitatory effects similar to those of catecholamines in fish (59), frog (71, 75), and cat (7).

Norepinephrine and epinephrine are much stronger than isoproterenol in facilitating neuromuscular transmission. In contrast to the direct action on the muscle fibers, the effect on the neuromuscular junction is abolished by the α receptor blocking drugs but is unaffected by the β receptor blocking drugs (8, 13, 14, 65).

Epinephrine and norepinephrine augment the potentiating effects of neostigmine, succinylcholine, and decamethonium; this is chiefly the result of increased repetitive firing of the muscle fibers and is blocked by the previous intravenous injection of the α receptor blocking drugs, Dibenamine, phenoxybenzamine, and phentolamine (13, 14). The repetitive firing produced in the motor nerve by anticholinesterases is also augmented by epinephrine (6).

According to Breckenridge et al. (16), epinephrine and theophylline potentiate the twitch of the cat gastrocnemius in situ evoked by sciatic nerve stimulation, when an anticholinesterase, neostigmine, is also present. The combined injection of epinephrine, neostigmine, and theophylline caused a striking potentiation of the contraction. This potentiation is blocked by propranolol, and it is not observed when the muscle is stimulated directly after complete curarization. Bowman & Nott

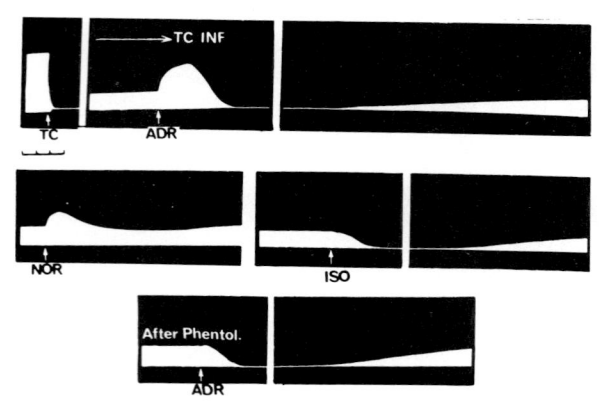

FIG. 12. Maximal twitches of tibialis anterior of cat anesthetized with chloralose and pentobarbitone sodium. At *TC* a single intravenous injection of tubocurarine (0.3 mg/kg) was given. During recovery from this dose, intravenous infusion (0.58 mg/kg per hr) of tubocurarine (*TC INF*) was started. At *ADR*, *NOR*, and *ISO*, 10 μg/kg of epinephrine, norepinephrine, and isoproterenol, respectively, were injected intravenously. Second response to epinephrine was recorded after intravenous injection of 2 mg/kg phentolamine (*Phentol*). Gaps in responses to epinephrine and isoproterenol each correspond to 10 min. Time calibration in minutes. [From Bowman & Raper (13).]

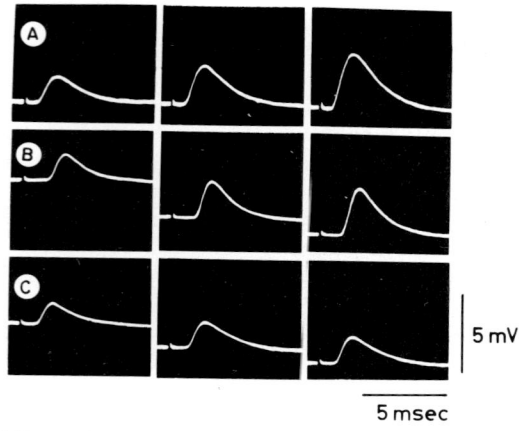

FIG. 13. Effects of catecholamines on end-plate potentials in solution containing *d*-tubocurarine (1×10^{-6} g/ml). *A*: norepinephrine (1×10^{-6} g/ml); *B*: epinephrine (1×10^{-6} g/ml); and *C*: isoproterenol (1×10^{-6} g/ml) in 3 different preparations. First record, control; second, 5 min; and third, 10 min after application of drugs taken from same end-plate. [Adapted from Kuba (60).]

(9) have suggested that this effect of propranolol is not due to a β adrenergic blocking action but to its local anesthetic action.

Inhibitory Action

Epinephrine is known to enhance the block of neuromuscular transmission caused by tubocurarine after the initial facilitatory action, as shown in Figure 12. After an intravenous injection of phentolamine, effects of epinephrine become similar to those of isoproterenol, which produces only suppression of transmission without the initial potentiation. Isoproterenol is the most potent, epinephrine slightly less, and norepinephrine the least active in enhancing tubocurarine paralysis, and the effect is abolished by the β receptor blocking drugs (13).

The inhibitory action of catecholamines is observed in situ in fast muscles: tibialis anterior and gastrocnemius of the cat (13) and flexor digitorum longus of the rabbit (26, 74); and in slow muscle: soleus of the cat (13); and also in the avian gastrocnemius muscle (78). The inhibitory effect is only observed clearly when rapid stimulation of more than 1 cycle/sec is used.

The inhibitory action of the amines on neuromuscular transmission has not been observed when the unfatigued, isolated phrenic nerve-diaphragm preparation was used (17, 58), except as described in one report by Montagu (73). This suggests that the action in the intact animal may result from changes in blood flow or in the plasma K concentration (17, 58). However, since blood pressure and flow recordings show responses different from those of muscle contractions it is concluded that the effects on the transmission are not a consequence of vascular change caused by catecholamines (13, 74, 78).

Catecholamines increase the demarcation potential in tibialis anterior and soleus muscles of the cat, and the time course of the potential change corresponds to that of the augmentation of the neuromuscular block by the amines. Hyperpolarization of the muscle membrane produced by catecholamines is supposed to be the mechanism for an increase in the tubocurarine block. The hyperpolarization increases the threshold so that the number of active muscle fibers would be reduced when the transmission is partially suppressed (13).

Effects on End-plate Potential

Norepinephrine increases the amplitude of the end-plate potential (EPP) without affecting the postjunctional properties [fish red muscle (39), frog skeletal muscle (46), rat diaphragm (58, 60)]. Figure 13 shows examples of effects of catecholamines on the EPPs in the rat diaphragm evoked by phrenic nerve stimulation in the presence of tubocurarine (1×10^{-6} g/ml).

Epinephrine may increase the resting membrane potential and the membrane resistance of the muscle fiber, in addition to its presynaptic actions, which are the same as those of norepinephrine [fish red muscle (39), rat diaphragm (60)]. Isoproterenol acts only on the postjunctional membrane to enhance the membrane resistance and increase the membrane potential [rat diaphragm (60)]. These effects on the muscle membrane also lead to an increase in the EPP.

The potentiating action of norepinephrine on the amplitude of the EPP is blocked by an α blocking agent, such as phentolamine, but not by a β blocking agent, such as pronethalol [fish (39), frog (46), rat (60)]. This finding concurs with the idea that the adrenergic α receptors are present in the motor nerve ending to increase transmitter release, whereas the β receptors are present in the muscle fibers (9, 14).

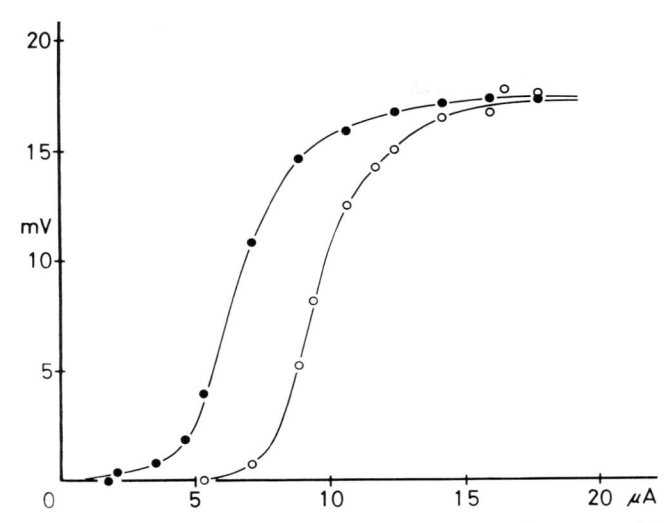

FIG. 14. Relation between amplitude of end-plate potential (*ordinate*) and current intensity (*abscissa*) in presence (●) and absence (○) of norepinephrine (5×10^{-6} g/ml). [From Kuba & Tomita (62).]

End-plate currents and action currents of the nerve terminal can be recorded with an extracellular glass electrode placed at the end-plate region. These recordings in the rat diaphragm indicate that both norepinephrine and epinephrine increase the end-plate current, whereas isoproterenol has no effect (60). Augmentation of the end-plate current is abolished by phentolamine, but not by pronethalol.

In the rat diaphragm the acetylcholine (ACh) potential produced by iontophoretically applied ACh is not affected by norepinephrine. Kuba (60) has reported that epinephrine and isoproterenol potentiate the amplitude of the ACh potentials, in contrast to the finding of Krnjević & Miledi (58). However, this potentiation is probably not due to an increase in the sensitivity of end-plate to ACh, but to the increase in the membrane potential and resistance. It has also been reported that norepinephrine increases the depolarization in frog muscle caused by adding ACh to the bathing solution (45) and that epinephrine enhances the ACh potential evoked iontophoretically in fish muscle (39).

When a brief depolarizing pulse of strong intensity is applied to the nerve terminal through an external electrode in the presence of tetrodotoxin and prostigmine, an EPP can be produced (50–52, 61). Figure 14 shows the relation between the current intensity and the amplitude of the EPP in a solution with and without norepinephrine. Norepinephrine simply shifts the EPP-current intensity relation toward a weaker current intensity, without changing the slope of the relation or the maximum amplitude of the EPPs.

Effects on Miniature End-plate Potential

Norepinephrine and epinephrine increase the frequency of the miniature end-plate potentials (MEPPs), whereas isoproterenol has little effect (46, 58). Epinephrine and isoproterenol, but not norepinephrine, increase the amplitude of MEPPs. Examples of norepinephrine effects on MEPP are shown in Figure 15.

The frequency of MEPPs can be increased by depolarizing the nerve terminal with a locally applied steady current. The generation of a spike in the terminal is suppressed with tetrodotoxin, which has no effect on the MEPPs. The increase in the frequency is nearly exponential, with a linear increase in depolarizing current intensity. Figure 16 shows this relation with and without norepinephrine. The curve showing the relation between MEPP frequency and current intensity is shifted in parallel along the frequency axis (abscissa) toward weaker intensity, without change in the slope (62).

The frequency of MEPPs is higher with higher external Ca concentration, $[Ca]_o$, between 0.01 and 7.5 mM at constant $[Na]_o$ (136 mM) and $[Mg]_o$ (1 mM). The increase in MEPP frequency with increasing $[Ca]_o$ is potentiated in the presence of norepinephrine, as shown in Figure 17. In other words, the effects of norepinephrine on spontaneous release of ACh are potentiated by an increase in the external Ca concentration.

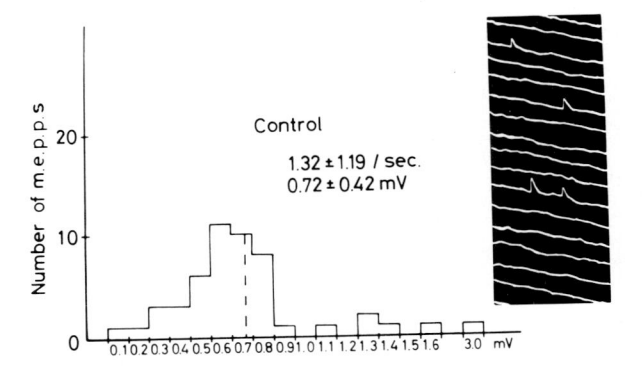

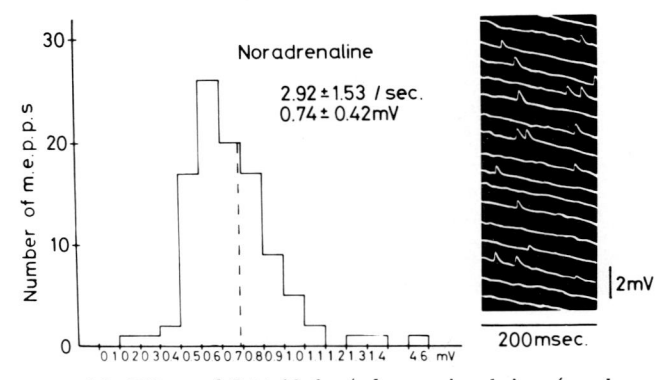

FIG. 15. Effects of 5×10^{-6} g/ml norepinephrine (*noradrenaline*) on amplitude and numbers of miniature end-plate potentials (*m.e.p.p.s*) recorded in normal Krebs solution during a 40-sec period. *Right*: sample records of miniature end-plate potentials. *Left*: histograms of miniature end-plate potentials. Results obtained 5 min after norepinephrine application. *Dashed lines* indicate mean amplitude of miniature end-plate potentials ($\pm$ SD) on *abscissa*, which was unchanged. Increase in frequency from 1.32 to 2.92 pulses/sec is significant ($P < 0.001$). [From Kuba (60).]

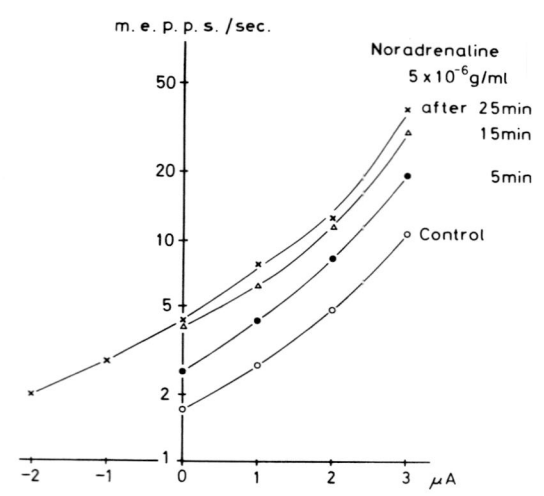

FIG. 16. Relation between miniature end-plate potential frequency and current intensity used for nerve terminal depolarization in presence of tetrodotoxin (1×10^{-7} g/ml) and prostigmine (2×10^{-7} g/ml). Frequency of miniature end-plate potentials is plotted as *ordinate* on logarithmic scale; current intensity is plotted as *abscissa*. ○: control; ●, △, and ×: 5, 15, and 25 min, respectively, after application of 5×10^{-6} g/ml norepinephrine (*noradrenaline*). [From Kuba & Tomita (62).]

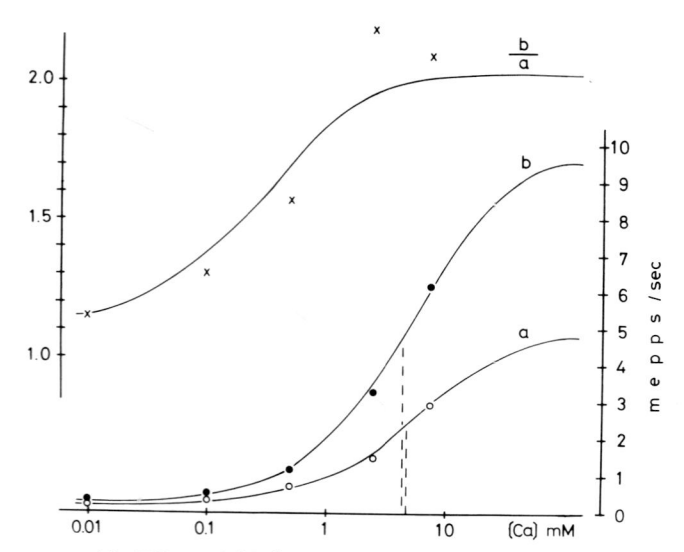

FIG. 17. Effect of $[Ca]_o$ on norepinephrine action. *Abscissa*: $[Ca]_o$ on logarithmic scale. ○: frequencies of miniature end-plate potentials (*m e p p s*) in control solution; ●: frequencies in presence of norepinephrine (5×10^{-6} g/ml). ×: ratios between frequencies in presence and absence of norepinephrine at each $[Ca]_o$; they refer to ordinate on *left*. Curves (*a*, control; *b*, norepinephrine) are theoretically obtained from Equation 2 (see text). Upper curve ($\frac{b}{a}$) indicates ratio between curves *b* and *a*. Vertical dashed lines correspond to values of dissociation constants (K) in Equation 2 in presence or absence of norepinephrine. Note no change in dissociation constant by norepinephrine. [From Kuba & Tomita (62).]

In the presence of 0.01 mM Ca, the increase in EPP frequency by norepinephrine is only 1.15 times the control value, whereas in 2.5 and 7.5 mM $[Ca]_o$ the increases in EPP frequency are 2.18 and 2.08 times the control value, respectively.

When $[Na]_o$ is reduced to 76 mM or to 56 mM in Krebs solution containing 0.5 mM $[Ca]_o$ and 1.2 mM $[Mg]_o$, the frequency of MEPPs is increased. The increase in the frequency of EPPs by norepinephrine is also enhanced as the $[Na]_o$ is reduced. When Ca and Na concentrations are both changed, the action of norepinephrine becomes stronger when the ratio of $[Ca]_o$ to $[Na]_o^2$ is larger. This is expected if Ca and Na ions compete for anionic sites and the amount of Ca bound with these sites controls the action of norepinephrine. Magnesium ions (6 mM) reduce the MEPP frequency and slightly suppress the norepinephrine action.

Mechanism of Increase of Transmitter Release

The process of transmitter release from the nerve terminal may be divided into the following steps, according to the recent studies on the neuromuscular junction of the frog and rat and on the giant synapse of the squid (43, 44, 49, 51–53): *a*) depolarization of the nerve terminal membrane; *b*) Ca entry into the nerve terminal resulting from an increase in the Ca conductance; *c*) binding of Ca with the critical site, X, of the release reaction; and *d*) an increase in probability of acetylcholine release by the Ca-receptor complex, CaX. The last step (*d*) probably includes several more processes in which vesicles in the terminal fuse with the internal surface of the nerve membrane and by which the transmitter in the vesicle is released.

The presynaptic actions of norepinephrine and epinephrine are unlikely to result from a change in the resting potential of the nerve ending. If the increase in release of transmitter by norepinephrine were due to hyperpolarization of the nerve terminal, it would be difficult to explain the increase in the frequency of MEPP since this is generally associated with depolarization of the nerve terminal (64). Another reason for assuming that there is no effect on the membrane potential of the nerve ending is the observation that catecholamines have no effect on the action current of the nerve ending in the rat diaphragm (60). The input resistance of the terminal membrane probably also remains unchanged in the presence of norepinephrine, since the slope of MEPP-current intensity relation is not modified. Thus norepinephrine does not seem to have any detectable effect on the electrical properties of the nerve membrane.

Maeno & Edwards (66) have studied the relation between the mean quantal content of the EPP and the frequency of stimulation (0.3–10 cycles/sec) in the frog sartorius muscle treated with excess (8–18 mM) Mg ions. The logarithm of the mean quantal content is proportional to the frequency of stimulation. They have explained this facilitation by an increase in the amount of ACh quanta readily available for release, through activation of the process that mobilizes ACh from the stored form. The mean quantal content of the

EPP is expressed as the product of the probability of the release of a quantum and the amount of available transmitter.

Acetylcholine release caused by a nerve impulse may be modified either through a change in the probability of quantum release or through a change in the transmitter mobilization. The mechanism of drug action on ACh release may be analyzed based on changes in the relation between the mean quantal content and the frequency of stimulation. Epinephrine and external Ca ions alter the release probability and do not affect the transmitter mobilization process [(66); T. Maeno, personal communication].

According to the model proposed by Hubbard et al. (43), acetylcholine release takes place as follows

$$[Ca] + [X] \underset{}{\overset{K}{\rightleftarrows}} [CaX] \quad \downarrow k_0 \quad \downarrow k_1 \quad (1)$$
$$\text{release} \quad \text{release}$$

where k_0, k_1, and K are rate constants and dissociation constant, respectively, in each process shown in Equation 1. With some assumptions, the frequency of MEPP can be expressed by Equation 2 (43, 44)

$$f = \frac{F\left(k_0 \frac{K}{[Ca]} + k_1\right)}{k_1\left(\frac{K}{[Ca]} + 1\right)} \quad (2)$$

where F is the frequency when all receptors are combined with Ca. The frequency (f_0) independent of $[Ca]_o$ is found to be 0.25 pulse/sec in the rat diaphragm (62). When $[Ca]_o$ is close to zero, Equation 2 is reduced to

$$f_0 = F\frac{k_0}{k_1} = 0.25 \text{ pulse/sec} \quad (3)$$

The values for F and K can be determined by using Equations 2 and 3 to obtain a theoretical curve fitting the observed frequency with different Ca concentrations. In the absence of norepinephrine, F is estimated to be 4.75 pulses/sec, which is similar to the value of 4.94 pulses/sec reported by Hubbard et al. (43). The value for K is 4.55 mM. The ratio of the rate constant of Ca-dependent release to that of Ca-independent release, k_1/k_0, is 19. The constants in the presence of norepinephrine (5 × 10⁻⁶ g/ml) are 9.5 pulses/sec for F, 4.47 mM for K, and 33 for k_1/k_0. The theoretical curves in Figure 17 are based on Equation 2 and use these values; they are in fairly good agreement with the experimental results. From these analyses, it may be assumed that norepinephrine does not change the dissociation constant (K) of the reaction between Ca and X, but increases both the maximum frequency (F) and the ratio (k_1/k_0) of the rate constant of X and CaX in the release process.

In normal solution

$$F = k_1 \cdot X_t = 4.75 \text{ pulses/sec}$$

where X_t is the total receptors, and

$$f_0 = (k_0/k_1)F = 0.25 \text{ pulse/sec}$$

In the presence of norepinephrine they are 9.50 and 0.29 pulses/sec, respectively. Thus, if $[X_t]$ remains constant, k_0 is slightly increased (15%) and k_1 is doubled by norepinephrine. Therefore it may be concluded that norepinephrine does not affect Ca binding, with the site X acting for release, but that it acts on the last step responsible for release of ACh after Ca has combined with the active site to increase the probability of transmitter release. The effects of Mg and Na ions may be explained by assuming a competition between these ions and Ca ions for the site X, as suggested by many investigators (5, 32, 54).

The effect of catecholamines is potentiated when the probability of ACh release is first augmented by changing external Ca and Na concentrations or by depolarizing the nerve terminal with current. Modification of catecholamine action by alteration in the external ionic composition and in the membrane potential suggests that the amines act on the membrane rather than the internal structure. However, it is possible that the amines modify the metabolism inside the nerve terminal and that this leads to a change in the membrane property increasing the release probability.

CONCLUSIONS

Catecholamines influence the contraction of skeletal muscles by acting directly on muscle fibers, as well as indirectly on neuromuscular transmission. The direct effects on the muscle fibers are blocked by the β receptor blocking drugs. Isoproterenol is about twice as potent as epinephrine, whereas norepinephrine is less potent (14). Both in fast- and slow-contracting muscles, twitch tension is increased by isoproterenol, if direct stimulation is applied with pulses of longer than 3 msec and of supramaximal intensities. This potentiation appears to be related to activation of the Na-K pump. When short pulses of less than 3 msec are used, a reduction of twitch tension is observed in the slow-contracting muscles. This may be partly due to hyperpolarization of the membrane caused by isoproterenol. The falling phase of the contraction of fast-contracting muscles is prolonged by isoproterenol, whereas that of slow-contracting muscles is shortened.

Neuromuscular transmission, which has been partially suppressed by curare, is facilitated by epinephrine and norepinephrine but is scarcely affected by isoproterenol; these actions of the catecholamines are abolished by the α receptor blocking drugs. The same facilitatory effects on transmission are observed in both fast- and slow-contracting muscles. Norepinephrine augments the end-plate potential by raising the probability of release of transmitter quanta. However, in the normal noncurarized muscle the effects of epinephrine on contractions are mainly the result of its direct action on the muscle fibers.

The fast-contracting muscles are much less sensitive to epinephrine than the slow-contracting muscles. The minimal effective intravenous doses of epinephrine necessary to increase the tension of the tibialis anterior muscle are between 3 and 10 µg/kg (15). Since a rapid intravenous injection of 1 µg epinephrine in an average-sized cat probably corresponds to a concentration that is reached by the maximum physiological output from the suprarenal medulla in extreme stress (31), the effects of epinephrine on the fast-contracting skeletal muscles seem to have little physiological significance.

On the other hand, the minimal effective intravenous doses of epinephrine necessary to affect the slow-contracting muscles are between 0.06 and 0.5 µg/kg (15), which result in concentrations of circulating epinephrine that are within the physiological range. Thus, during emergency states, the tension of the slow-contracting muscles may be decreased and a degree of fusion in incomplete tetanic contractions may be decreased by the circulating epinephrine. The concentration of epinephrine released from the suprarenal medulla in response to hypoxia is sufficient to produce a detectable effect on the soleus in the cat (9, 14). The action of epinephrine on slow-contracting muscles may be the cause of the well-known feeling of weakness and enhancement of tremor in the limbs experienced during fright or during infusion of epinephrine in man (67, 68), although it is possible that sensitization of the stretch reflex by epinephrine partially contributes to the increase in tremor (40, 69).

I thank Professor E. Bülbring and Dr. Allan W. Jones for help in preparation of this manuscript.

REFERENCES

1. BAKER, P. F., M. P. BLAUSTEIN, A. L. HODGKIN, AND R. A. STEINHARDT. The influence of calcium on sodium efflux in squid axons. *J. Physiol., London* 200: 431–458, 1969.
2. BÄR, U., AND M. C. BLANCHAER. Glycogen and CO_2 production from glucose and lactate by red and white skeletal muscle. *Am. J. Physiol.* 209: 905–909, 1965.
3. BÁRÁNY, M. ATPase activity of myosin correlated with speed of muscle shortening. *J. Gen. Physiol.* 50: 197–218, 1967.
4. BELFORD, J., AND M. R. FEINLEIB. Effect of stimulation and catecholamines on glucose-6-phosphate content of intact skeletal muscle. *Biochem. Pharmacol.* 13: 125–127, 1964.
5. BIRKS, R. I., P. G. R. BURSTYN, AND O. R. FIRTH. The form of sodium-calcium competition at the frog myoneural junction. *J. Gen. Physiol.* 52: 887–907, 1968.
6. BLABER, L. C., AND W. C. BOWMAN. The effects of some drugs on the repetitive discharges produced in nerve and muscle by anticholinesterases. *Intern. J. Neuropharmacol.* 2: 1–16, 1963.
7. BLABER, L. C., AND J. P. GALLAGHER. The facilitatory effects of catechol and phenol at the neuromuscular junction of the cat. *Neuropharmacology* 10: 153–159, 1971.
8. BOWMAN, W. C., A. A. J. GOLDBERG, AND C. RAPER. A comparison between the effects of a tetanus and the effects of sympathomimetic amines on fast- and slow-contracting mammalian muscles. *Brit. J. Pharmacol.* 19: 464–484, 1962.
9. BOWMAN, W. C., AND M. W. NOTT. Actions of sympathomimetic amines and their antagonists on skeletal muscle. *Pharmacol. Rev.* 21: 27–72, 1969.
10. BOWMAN, W. C., AND M. W. NOTT. Actions of some sympathomimetic bronchodilator and beta-adrenoceptor blocking drugs on contractions of the cat soleus muscle. *Brit. J. Pharmacol.* 38: 37–49, 1970.
11. BOWMAN, W. C., AND C. RAPER. Adrenaline and slow-contracting skeletal muscles. *Nature* 193: 41–43, 1962.
12. BOWMAN, W. C., AND C. RAPER. The effects of adrenaline and other drugs affecting carbohydrate metabolism on contractions of the rat diaphragm. *Brit. J. Pharmacol.* 23: 184–200, 1964.
13. BOWMAN, W. C., AND C. RAPER. Effects of sympathomimetic amines on neuromuscular transmission. *Brit. J. Pharmacol.* 27: 313–331, 1966.
14. BOWMAN, W. C., AND C. RAPER. Adrenotropic receptors in skeletal muscle. *Ann. NY Acad. Sci.* 139: 741–753, 1967.
15. BOWMAN, W. C., AND E. ZAIMIS. The effects of adrenaline, noradrenaline and isoprenaline on skeletal muscle contractions in the cat. *J. Physiol., London* 144: 92–107, 1958.
16. BRECKENRIDGE, B. MCL., J. H. BURN, AND F. M. MATSCHINSKY. Theophylline, epinephrine, and neostigmine facilitation on neuromuscular transmission. *Proc. Natl. Acad. Sci. US* 57: 1893–1897, 1967.
17. BROWN, G. L., E. BÜLBRING, AND B. D. BURNS. The action of adrenaline on mammalian skeletal muscle. *J. Physiol., London* 107: 115–128, 1948.
18. BROWN, G. L., M. GOFFART, AND M. VIANNA DIAS. The effects of adrenaline and of sympathetic stimulation on the demarcation potential of mammalian skeletal muscle. *J. Physiol., London* 111: 184–194, 1950.
19. BULLER, A. J., J. C. ECCLES, AND R. M. ECCLES. Differentiation of fast and slow muscles in the cat hind limb. *J. Physiol., London* 150: 399–416, 1960.
20. BULLER, A. J., J. C. ECCLES, AND R. M. ECCLES. Interactions between motoneurones and muscle in respect of the characteristic speeds of their responses. *J. Physiol., London* 150: 417–439, 1960.
21. BULLER, A. J., W. F. H. M. MOMMAERTS, AND K. SERAYDARIAN. Enzymic properties of myosin in fast and slow twitch muscles of the cat following cross-innervation. *J. Physiol., London* 205: 581–597, 1969.
22. BURN, J. H. The relation of adrenaline to acetylcholine in the nervous system. *Physiol. Rev.* 25: 377–394, 1945.
23. CORI, C. F. Mammalian carbohydrate metabolism. *Physiol. Rev.* 11: 143–275, 1931.
24. DOCKRY, M., R. P. KERNAN, AND A. TANGNEY. Active transport of sodium and potassium in mammalian skeletal muscle and its modification by nerve and by cholinergic and adrenergic agents. *J. Physiol., London* 186: 187–200, 1966.
25. DRUMMOND, G. I. Microenvironment and enzyme function: control of energy metabolism during muscle work. *Am. Zoologist* 11: 83–97, 1971.
26. DYBING, F. The effects of noradrenaline and isoprenaline (isopropylnoradrenaline) on neuromuscular transmission during partial curarization. *Acta Pharmacol. Toxicol.* 10: 364–370, 1954.
27. ELLIS, S. Relation of biochemical effects of epinephrine to its muscular effects. *Pharmacol. Rev.* 11: 469–479, 1959.
28. ELLIS, S., AND S. B. BECKETT. The action of epinephrine on the anaerobic or the iodoacetate-treated rat's diaphragm. *J. Pharmacol.* 112: 202–209, 1954.

29. Ellis, S., A. H. Davis, and H. L. Anderson. Effects of epinephrine and related amines on contraction and glycogenolysis of the rat's diaphragm. *J. Pharmacol.* 115: 120–125, 1955.
30. Eversole, L. R., and S. M. Standish. Histochemical demonstration of muscle fiber types. *J. Histochem. Cytochem.* 18: 591–594, 1970.
31. Folkow, B. Nervous control of the blood vessels. *Physiol. Rev.* 35: 629–663, 1955.
32. Gage, P. W., and D. M. J. Quastel. Competition between sodium and calcium ions in transmitter release at mammalian neuromuscular junctions. *J. Physiol., London* 185: 95–123, 1966.
33. Goffart, M. Inversion d'action de l'adrénaline sur le muscle strié et taux du K^+ musculaire. *Compt. Rend. Soc. Biol.* 141: 1278–1279, 1947.
34. Goffart, M. Recherches relatives a l'action de l'adrénaline sur le muscle strié de mammifère. I. Potentiation par l'adrénaline de la contraction maximale du muscle non fatigué. *Arch. Intern. Physiol.* 60: 318–366, 1952.
35. Goffart, M., and J. M. Ritchie. The effect of adrenaline on the contraction of mammalian skeletal muscle. *J. Physiol., London* 116: 357–371, 1952.
36. Gruber, C. M. The significance of epinephrine in muscle activity. *Endocrinology* 3: 145–153, 1919.
37. Hajdu, I., and R. J. S. McDowell. Some actions of calcium and potassium in the rat diaphragm. *J. Physiol., London* 108: 10p, 1949.
38. Haugaard, N., and M. E. Hess. Actions of autonomic drugs on phosphorylase activity and function. *Pharmacol. Rev.* 17: 27–69, 1965.
39. Hidaka, T., and H. Kuriyama. Effects of catecholamines on the cholinergic neuromuscular transmission in fish red muscle. *J. Physiol., London* 201: 61–71, 1969.
40. Hodgson, H. J. F., C. D. Marsden, and J. C. Meadows. The effect of adrenaline on the response to muscle vibration in man. *J. Physiol., London* 202: 98–99p, 1969.
41. Hornbrook, K. R., and T. M. Brody. The effect of catecholamines on muscle glycogen and phosphorylase activity. *J. Pharmacol.* 140: 295–307, 1963.
42. Hornbrook, K. R., and T. M. Brody. Phosphorylase activity in rat liver and skeletal muscle after catecholamines. *Biochem. Pharmacol.* 12: 1407–1415, 1963.
43. Hubbard, J. I., S. F. Jones, and E. M. Landau. On the mechanism by which calcium and magnesium affect the spontaneous release of transmitter from mammalian motor nerve terminals. *J. Physiol., London* 194: 355–380, 1968.
44. Hubbard, J. I., S. F. Jones, and E. M. Landau. On the mechanism by which calcium and magnesium affect the release of transmitter by nerve impulses. *J. Physiol., London* 196: 75–86, 1968.
45. Hutter, O. F., and W. R. Loewenstein. Nature of neuromuscular facilitation by sympathetic stimulation in the frog. *J. Physiol., London* 130: 559–571, 1955.
46. Jenkinson, D. H., B. A. Stamenović, and B. D. L. Whitaker. The effect of noradrenaline on the end-plate potential in twitch fibres of the frog. *J. Physiol., London* 195: 743–754, 1968.
47. Jurna, I., and W. Rummel. Die Wirkung von Adrenalin und Noradrenalin auf die Spannungsentwicklung von Soleus und Tibialis anterior der Katze. *Arch. Ges. Physiol.* 275: 137–151, 1962.
48. Jurna, I., W. Rummel, and H. Schäfer. Die abfallende Phase des aktiven Zustandes des Tibialis anterior, Gastrocnemius und Soleus der Katze und ihre Beeinflussung durch Dehnung und Sympathicomimetica. *Arch. Ges. Physiol.* 277: 513–522, 1963.
49. Katz, B. The Croonian Lecture. The transmission of impulses from nerve to muscle, and the subcellular unit of synaptic action. *Proc. Roy. Soc. London Ser. B* 155: 455–477, 1962.
50. Katz, B., and R. Miledi. Release of acetylcholine from a nerve terminal by electric pulses of variable strength and duration. *Nature* 207: 1097–1098, 1965.
51. Katz, B., and R. Miledi. Tetrodotoxin and neuromuscular transmission. *Proc. Roy. Soc. London Ser. B* 167: 8–22, 1967.
52. Katz, B., and R. Miledi. The release of acetylcholine from nerve endings by graded electric pulses. *Proc. Roy. Soc. London Ser. B* 167: 23–38, 1967.
53. Katz, B., and R. Miledi A study of synaptic transmission in the absence of nerve impulses. *J. Physiol., London* 192: 407–436, 1967.
54. Kelly, J. S. Antagonism between Na^+ and Ca^{2+} at the neuromuscular junction. *Nature* 205: 296–297, 1965.
55. Kennedy, B. L., and S. Ellis. Interactions of sympathomimetic amines and adrenergic blocking agents at receptor sites mediating glycogenolysis. *Federation Proc.* 22: 449, 1963.
56. Knox, J. A. C., R. J. S. McDowall, and K. A. Montagu. The action of adrenaline on the rat diaphragm. *J. Physiol., London* 112: 36–37p, 1951.
57. Krebs, E. G., R. J. DeLange, R. G. Kemp, and W. D. Riley. Activation of skeletal muscle phosphorylase. *Pharmacol. Rev.* 18: 163–171, 1966.
58. Krnjević, K., and R. Miledi. Some effects produced by adrenaline upon neuromuscular propagation in rats. *J. Physiol., London* 141: 291–304, 1958.
59. Kuba, K. The action of phenol on neuromuscular transmission in the red muscle of fish. *Japan. J. Physiol.* 19: 762–774, 1969.
60. Kuba, K. Effects of catecholamines on the neuromuscular junction in the rat diaphragm. *J. Physiol., London* 211: 551–570, 1970.
61. Kuba, K., and T. Tomita. Effect of prostigmine on the time course of the end-plate potential in the rat diaphragm. *J. Physiol., London* 213: 533–544, 1971.
62. Kuba, K., and T. Tomita. Noradrenaline action on nerve terminal in the rat diaphragm. *J. Physiol., London* 217: 19–31, 1971.
63. Lands, A. M., F. P. Luduena, and H. J. Buzzo. Differentiation of receptors responsive to isoproterenol. *Life Sci.* 6: 2241–2249, 1967.
64. Liley, A. W. The effects of presynaptic polarization on the spontaneous activity at the mammalian neuromuscular junction. *J. Physiol., London* 134: 427–443, 1956.
65. Maddock, W. O., V. M. Rankin, and W. B. Youmans. Prevention of the anti-curare action of epinephrine by dibenamine. *Proc. Soc. Exptl. Biol. Med.* 67: 151–153, 1948.
66. Maeno, T., and C. Edwards. Neuromuscular facilitation with low-frequency stimulation and effects of some drugs. *J. Neurophysiol.* 32: 785–792, 1969.
67. Marsden, C. D., T. H. Foley, D. A. L. Owen, and R. G. McAllister. Peripheral β-adrenergic receptors concerned with tremor. *Clin. Sci.* 33: 53–65, 1967.
68. Marsden, C. D., and J. C. Meadows. The effect of adrenaline on the contraction of human muscle. *J. Physiol., London* 207: 429–448, 1970.
69. Marsden, C. D., J. C. Meadows, G. W. Lange, and R. S. Watson. Effect of deafferentation on human physiological tremor. *Lancet* 2: 700–702, 1967.
70. Mayer, S. E., N. C. Moran, and J. Fain. The effect of adrenergic blocking agents on some metabolic actions of catecholamines. *J. Pharmacol.* 134: 18–27, 1961.
71. Mogey, G. A., and P. A. Young. The antagonism of curarizing activity by phenolic substances. *Brit. J. Pharmacol.* 4: 359–365, 1949.
72. Mohme-Lundholm, E., and N. Svedmyr. Influence of nethalide on the phosphorylase activating effects of adrenaline and isoprenaline in experiments on isolated rat diaphragm. *Acta Physiol. Scand.* 61: 192–194, 1964.
73. Montagu, K. A. On the mechanism of action of adrenaline in skeletal nerve-muscle. *J. Physiol., London* 128: 619–628, 1955.
74. Naess, K., and T. Sirnes. A synergistic effect of adrenaline and d-tubocurarine on the neuromuscular transmission. *Acta Physiol. Scand.* 29: 293–306, 1953.

75. Otsuka, M., and Y. Nonomura. The action of phenolic substances on motor nerve endings. *J. Pharmacol.* 140: 41–45, 1963.
76. Posner, J. B., R. Stern, and E. G. Krebs. Effects of electrical stimulation and epinephrine on muscle phosphorylase, phosphorylase *b* kinase, and adenosine-3',5'-phosphate. *J. Biol. Chem.* 240: 982–985, 1965.
77. Rabinowitz, M., L. Desalles, J. Meisler, and L. Lorand. Distribution of adenyl-cyclase activity in rabbit skeletal muscle fractions. *Biochim. Biophys. Acta* 97: 29–36, 1965.
78. Raper, C., and W. C. Bowman. Effects of catecholamines on the gastrocnemius muscle of the domestic fowl. *European J. Pharmacol.* 4: 309–316, 1968.
79. Romanul, F. C. A. Enzymes in muscle. I. Histochemical studies of enzymes in individual muscle fibers. *Arch. Neurol.* 11: 355–368, 1964.
80. Somlyo, A. P., and A. V. Somlyo. Pharmacology of excitation-contraction coupling in vascular smooth muscle and in avian slow muscle. *Federation Proc.* 28: 1634–1642, 1969.
81. Sutherland, E. W., and T. W. Rall. The relation of adenosine-3',5'-phosphate and phosphorylase to the actions of catecholamines and other hormones. *Pharmacol. Rev.* 12: 265–299, 1960.
82. Tashiro, N. Effects of isoproterenol on contractions of directly stimulated fast and slow skeletal muscles of the guinea-pig. *Brit. J. Pharmacol.* 48: 121–131, 1973.
83. Uchida, K., and W. F. H. M. Mommaerts. Modification of the contractile response of actomyosin by cyclic adenosine-3',5'-phosphate. *Biochem. Biophys. Res. Commun.* 10: 1–3, 1963.
84. Zolovick, A. J., R. L. Norman, and M. R. Fedde. Membrane constants of muscle fibers of rat diaphragm. *Am. J. Physiol.* 219: 654–657, 1970.

CHAPTER 35

Catecholamines in relation to the eye

M. L. SEARS | *Department of Ophthalmology and Visual Science, Yale University School of Medicine, New Haven, Connecticut*

CHAPTER CONTENTS

Adrenergic Pathways to Eye and Ocular Structures
Metabolism, Uptake, Storage, and Release of Ocular
　　Catecholamines
Denervation
Degeneration Release
Tissue Function
　Adnexa
　　Orbits and lids
　　Nictitans
　　Extrinsic muscles
　　Lacrimal gland
　Eye
　　Blood flow
　　Intraocular pressure
　　Cornea and lens
　　Intrinsic muscle
　　Vitreous
Adrenergics and Ocular Pigment
　Relation of mydriasis to iris pigmentation
　Pigment in nuclear portion of crystalline lens
Retina
Adrenal Medulla

INFORMATION ABOUT THE MECHANISM of catecholamine synthesis, storage, release, transport, and degradation and about the distribution and organization of nerve fibers within the autonomic ground plexus has led to a better understanding of the physiology of adrenergic nerves. Some of this information has come from experiments done in the richly innervated iris [(100, 147, 150, 204, 290, 293, 294); Fig. 1]. The dense innervation of the iris and the ease with which the pupil can be studied probably account for the steady interest in the reactivity of the iris as a pharmacological tool, behavioral indicator, and signpost to disease (280). Recent demonstrations of direct adrenergic effects on eye pressure (18, 54, 279, 375, 380) have stimulated interest in other aspects of the physiology of catecholamines in the eye.

Eyelid retraction; protrusion of the nictitating membrane (nictitans); trophic influences on the epithelia of the cornea, lens, and pigment cell layers; reflex pupillary dilation; negative (distance) accommodation; supranuclear control of miosis and ciliary tonus in sleep; tonic vergences of the eyes; regulatory influences over ocular blood flow and intraocular pressure; and a possible modulating effect on intraretinal transmission of neural impulses are among the ocular functions ascribed to catecholamines. The influence of the adrenal medullary secretion on these parameters is discussed in detail at the end of this chapter.

ADRENERGIC PATHWAYS TO EYE AND OCULAR STRUCTURES

The adrenergic innervation to the mammalian eye is derived from the sympathetic division of the autonomic nervous system (252). Fibers of the sympathetic division pass from the upper end of the midbrain, down ventral to the posterior commissure, and divide soon after into two bundles. One of these bundles lies in the lateral aspect of the midbrain and descends in the reticular formation of the pons and medulla. The other descends in the medial longitudinal fasciculus. The fibers from the medulla continue downward in the anterolateral column of the cervical region and synapse with the preganglionic cell bodies located in the intermediolateral cell column of the 12th thoracic and upper third or fourth lumbar segments of the spinal cord. The axons of these cells, largely myelinated fibers, traverse the ventral root to form the white communicating rami of the thoracic and lumbar nerves and thus reach the trunk ganglia of the sympathetic chain. On entering the trunk ganglia, these fibers may synapse within a nest of ganglion cells, pass up or down the sympathetic trunk to synapse with ganglion cells at a higher or lower level, or pass through the trunk ganglia and out to one of the collateral or intermediary sympathetic ganglia.

Fibers to the eye are carried to the sympathetic trunk from the cord in the white rami of the upper two thoracic and lower cervical nerves (393). They ascend to synapse mainly with cells in the superior cervical ganglion. The experiments of Langley (268a) provide evidence that the preganglionic fibers involved in sympathetic innervation of the eye arise in the upper thoracic segment of the spinal cord. He demonstrated that stimulation of the ventral roots of the upper three thoracic nerves, but not those of the lower cervical or fourth thoracic nerve, regularly elicited pupillary dilation. Thus preganglionic fibers ruling the innervation

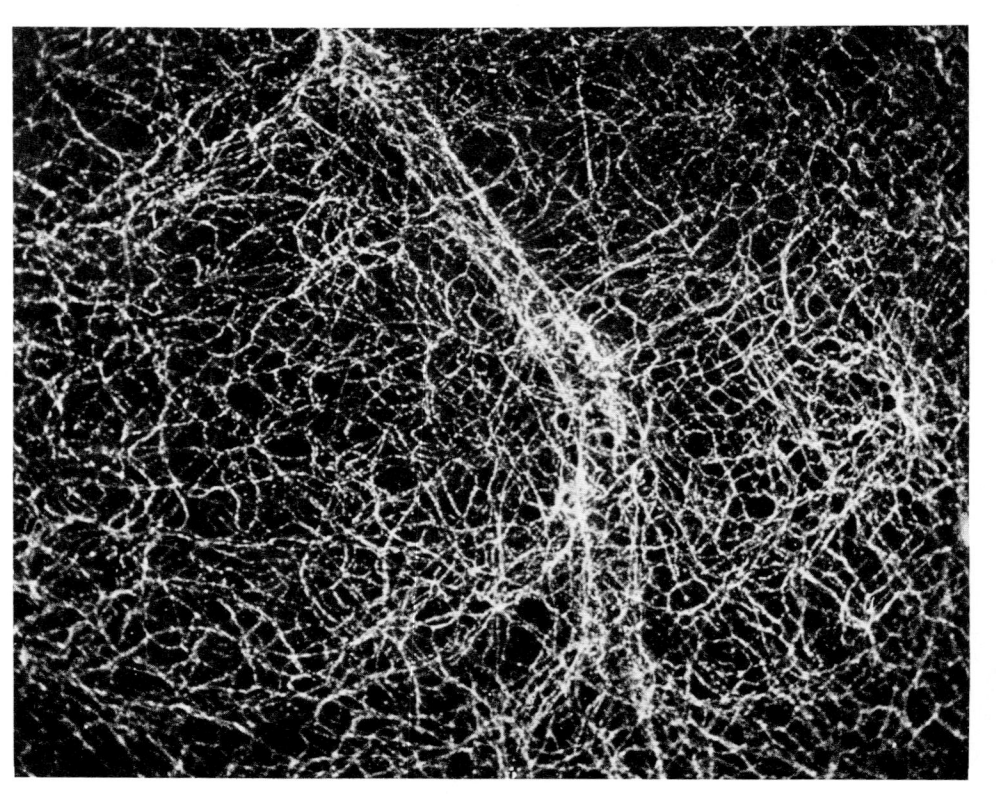

FIG. 1. Fluorescence photomicrograph of stretch preparations from dilator muscle of rat iris. Preparations were dried at room temperature for 5–20 min and treated with formaldehyde gas (from paraformaldehyde) at 80 C for 1 hr. In addition to fluorescent nerve fibers in muscle, a vascular plexus is clearly visible. [From Falck (150).]

of the dilator muscle of the iris leave the spinal cord in the upper three thoracic nerves. The second thoracic nerve constitutes the bulk of those preganglionic fibers to the iris, whereas the nictitans is subserved by the third.

Branches of the sympathetic trunk are composed of postsynaptic, predominantly unmyelinated fibers. Those innervating the eye are derived almost exclusively from the ipsilateral superior cervical sympathetic ganglion (252, 280, 393). The experiments in which Langley used nicotine supported the belief that this ganglion is the chief source of postganglionic fibers to the eye. This compound has a special property of blocking the synaptic transmission of impulses conducted from the center to the peripheral ganglion. Thus electrical stimulation of fibers proximal to the block, or at the synapse at the superior cervical ganglion, is without effect on the eye, whereas electrical stimulation of the ganglion itself or fibers distal to it yields a response. Histofluorescence studies done in the iris after ipsilateral superior cervical ganglionectomy confirm Langley's original observations (141).

The distribution of postganglionic fibers to the eye may vary (393). From the superior cervical ganglion some fibers run upward, along with a few fibers from the middle or inferior cervical ganglion, or both, and enter into the formation of plexuses about the internal and external carotid arteries. Further distribution to the eye is made through the Gasserian ganglion to the nasal branch of the ophthalmic division of the trigeminal nerve. The long ciliary nerves arising from this branch carry the noradrenergic fibers into the eye through the sclera into the suprachoroidal space, where a plexus is formed from which fibers proceed to the dilator muscle of the iris. Other postganglionic fibers run to plexuses along the internal carotid artery. The cavernous plexus is the nearest to the eye. It has fibers that pass without synapse through the ciliary ganglion to enter the globe with the short ciliary nerves. In the cat, at least, and probably in man as well, postganglionic fibers leaving the superior cervical ganglion via the superior carotid nerve pass between the tympanic plates of the auditory bulla and the inferior surface of the petrous bone. Some of these fibers appear within the middle ear (26). Others course between the petrous bone and the tympanic plates of the bulla, then pass between the articulation of the petrous portion of the temporal and sphenoid bones to join the under surface of the Gasserian ganglion before reaching the orbit with the first division of the fifth nerve (393).

Another circuitous cephalad route for postganglionic fibers is from the stellate ganglion to the vertebral artery (393). A plexus here is apparently continuous with a plexus around the basilar and internal carotid vessels. It is doubtful that fibers from this route gain access to the eye. Other possible variations in innervational distribution include the presence of accessory ganglia within the cranial vault or orbit itself. There is considerable skepticism (280) about the existence of accessory sympathetic ganglia to the eye originally described by the early anatomists. It has been recently demonstrated, however, that small ganglia or aggregates of sympathetic ganglion cells may be seen partially or completely embedded in ventral spinal roots, usually at the site of origin of white communicating rami, particularly in the first and second thoracic segments (252) and in cervical segments of dogs (447). The possibility has not been ruled out that some postganglionic fibers from such ganglia reach the sympathetic trunk through white communicating rami for distribution to the brachial plexus. A similar arrangement may exist for fiber distribution to the eye. These cells probably failed to reach the primordia of the sympathetic trunk ganglia. The link between these cells and distal organs need not traverse the sympathetic trunk. Such pathways would not be interrupted by extirpation of the trunk ganglia (317). However, after unilateral superior cervical ganglionectomy, the permanence of miosis, the lack of demonstrable histofluorescence in samples of iris preparations from rats, rabbits, and cats taken from the eye months or even years after surgical denervation (141), and the ipsilateral failure of uptake and binding by the iris of exogenously administered norepinephrine (353) argue in favor of the exclusiveness of the superior cervical ganglion as the source of postganglionic fibers to the eye. There are observations supporting an opposing argument.

1. Species or strain differences may account for inconsistencies in the above observations [e.g., innervation in man and dog may be different from that in rabbits (447)].
2. Concentrations of catecholamines below 10 µg/g may not be resolved by histofluorescence in tissue sections as thin as 5–10 µ (326) and could be missed without serial examination of sections of iris.
3. An ipsilateral effector response to nicotine (which requires intact innervation to produce an adrenergic response) in some unilaterally ganglionectomized rabbits and cats (13) may be evidence that some sympathetic function remains. This would support the idea that either cross innervation or aberrant ganglia (287) supply some postganglionic fibers to the eye.
4. Hypotony lasting several days has been induced by the topical application of epinephrine to one eye of several patients who had undergone bilateral stellate ganglionectomy (M. L. Sears, unpublished observations). This response was far more exaggerated than that seen in patients with unilateral Horner's syndrome similarly tested [see section DENERVATION; (373)].

The final puzzle is the similar augmented mydriasis and aqueous outflow in bilaterally versus unilaterally ganglionectomized rabbits after intracamerally administered norepinephrine (Fig. 2). These effects of denervation might imply the existence of cephalad ganglia (287), as well as a cross innervation in some

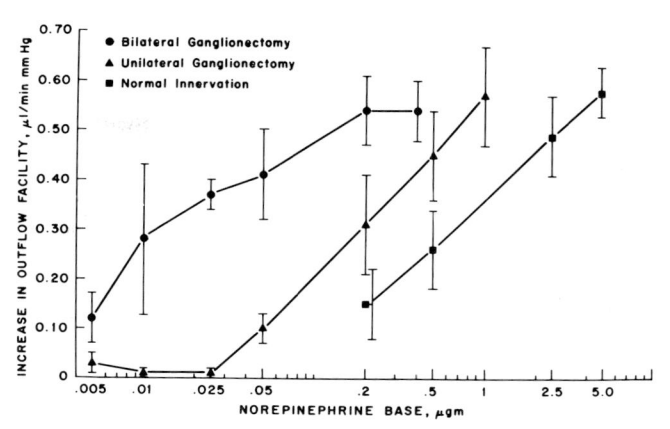

FIG. 2. Increase in outflow of aqueous humor in rabbit eye after intracamerally administered norepinephrine. Response in normal animal compared with response after unilateral and bilateral cervical ganglionectomy.

species. It is possible, however, that this latter effect of bilateral ganglionectomy is mediated by some neurohumoral path other than from the pineal or other sympathetically innervated central nervous system structures. In conclusion, most evidence favors an ipsilateral innervation to the eye derived exclusively from the superior cervical ganglion.

METABOLISM, UPTAKE, STORAGE, AND RELEASE OF OCULAR CATECHOLAMINES

The prominent ground plexus of adrenergic nerves within the uvea (iris, ciliary body, choroid) of the eye is responsible for a very high content of the adrenergic neurotransmitter, norepinephrine, in tissue. Yet, despite this dense innervation and high concentration of norepinephrine in these tissues, the watery fluids of the eye are virtually devoid of the neurohumor [(129, 376); Fig. 3]. These observations appear even more striking when one considers that the pupil is continuously moving. An enormous capacity and efficiency for inactivation of physiological amounts of the catecholamine are present. A study relating the mode of inactivation of norepinephrine in the eye directly to the termination of a physiological event, such as pupillary dilation, has not yet been done. Unless contrary evidence is presented, it must be assumed that the termination mechanism is directly related to the efficiency of reuptake and binding of released catecholamine into the nerve terminal. Recent evidence suggests that enzymatic degradation may play more of a role in the termination of a physiological event than has been allowed in recent years (175, 230, 231). In the eye, however, the high rate of blood flow (51) through the uvea and the absence of degradative enzymes in the aqueous humor (438) suggest that the circulatory removal in the uvea and reuptake and binding of norepinephrine by the iris play the prominent roles in regulating pupillary dilation. After denervation, despite no change in catechol-O-methyltransferase (COMT) levels (438)

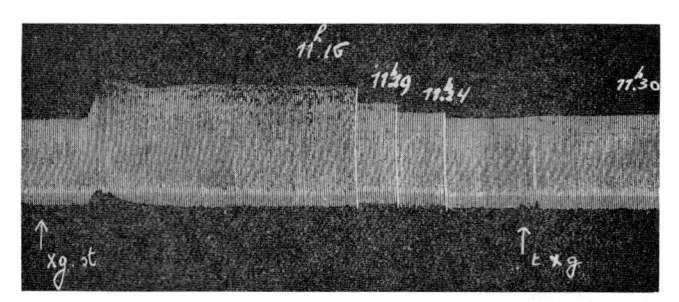

FIG. 3. Influence of aqueous humor, removed from rabbit immediately after prolonged stimulation of cervical sympathetic, on isolated heart of *Bufo calamita*. [From Bacq (15).]

and only moderate changes in monoamine oxidase (MAO) levels (438) in the ocular tissues, there is a prolonged persistence of norepinephrine in the aqueous humor (376). These findings further support the primacy of reuptake as the mode of inactivation. Finally enhancement of ocular adrenergic activities by inhibiton of COMT or MAO, or both, has not been conclusively demonstrated, although admittedly inhibitors of COMT are not well suited to the eye and MAO inhibitors have on occasion given rise to prolonged (455) but not augmented responses. In these latter instances, however, the range and potency of the intrinsic activity of the MAO inhibitors have not been evaluated. [The histochemistry, pharmacology, and toxicology of ocular MAOs and their inhibitors have received a great deal of attention (225, 242, 246, 284, 309, 318, 335, 348, 405, 438, 455).]

Experimental evidence for this uptake process of norepinephrine by the eye tissues could be reflected by *a*) an increase over endogenous levels after an injection of norepinephrine, *b*) uptake of a label (14, 112), or *c*) under certain conditions, an arteriovenous difference in the concentration of norepinephrine in the blood perfusing the uvea. Evidence of *a* comes mainly from qualitative studies showing an increase in histofluorescence of the iris after intracamerally and topically administered norepinephrine (290), and of *b* from studies on the isolated iris (192, 201, 220, 290, 293) and from in vivo studies comparing both irises of animals injected intravenously with labeled norepinephrine at intervals after unilateral ganglionectomy (243, 376). Experiments of the third type have not been done. Values obtained from uptake studies done in the iris must be corrected for a relatively large intercellular space (228) and a small extraneuronal compartment (228, 353). The location of the uptake process is primarily axonal (202); after denervation, irises exposed to low or ordinary amounts of norepinephrine take up less than 5% of the amount taken up by the normally innervated iris (220, 228). Mast cells, a potential locus, although plentiful in the posterior uvea, are scarce in the iris (275, 388). Extraneuronal uptake is thus negligible under ordinary circumstances. At high concentrations of norepinephrine a secondary uptake process occurs. Now the barrier to diffusion appears to break down so that a loose tissue binding occurs. Accumulation of the catecholamine takes place within the iris, but only to a small extent by comparison with cardiac tissue (219, 220).

The membrane pump thus is the dominant and most important mechanism for the initial uptake of norepinephrine. The properties of the interaction between the carrier in the membrane and norepinephrine and the transport phenomena indicate that the process requires energy and that it obeys saturation kinetics. The process is saturable in vitro at a norepinephrine concentration of 0.15 μg/ml (228). The half-maximum constant for l-norepinephrine uptake is 1.4–1.7×11^{-6} M (220, 228), compared with a value of 2.7×10^{-7} M for the heart (219). Stereospecificity is not as easily demonstrated in the iris as in cardiac tissue (220); D and L forms of both epinephrine and norepinephrine are equipotent inhibitors of ^{3}H-norepinephrine uptake (220). Isoprenaline is not taken up (100). Uptake of injected norepinephrine can increase the content of norepinephrine in the tissues of the heart and salivary glands two- to threefold (398). Accumulation studies indicate somewhat less of an increase in tissue content in the guinea pig iris (228, 374). This finding implies that under steady-state conditions a large capacity for uptake is present and reflects the continuous tonic activity of the adrenergic fibers.

It is the granule mechanism that is important for the storage capacity of the nervous terminals and for the intraneuronal retention of norepinephrine. Under varying physiological circumstances, the norepinephrine content of sympathetic tissue does not change. This remarkable constancy of content is related to the conservation mechanism (i.e., reuptake of the neurohumor across the neuronal membrane and then rebinding within the storage vesicles). Even under stress when adrenergic activity is considerably increased, changes of levels in tissue are not markedly altered. With enhanced nervous activity, synthesis of norepinephrine is increased both in vivo (176) and in vitro (357). With reduced levels of activity, axonal norepinephrine inhibits its own synthesis. Both of these observations support the idea of a feedback regulation of end products of biosynthesis. In this connection, note that electrical stimulation of the cervical sympathetic trunk does not markedly change the fluorescence seen in iris terminals (104). The absence of visible change is not a certain reflection of qualitative changes in axonal levels of norepinephrine, especially at higher concentrations (227). On the other hand, it is difficult to demonstrate the transmitter in the aqueous humor without the help of blockade of reuptake (129). This finding would suggest that inactivation by reuptake, along with the augmented synthesis associated with nervous activity (197), preserves the constancy of the neuronal norepinephrine.

Identification of the specific pool responsible for release has not been made. Evidence does indicate that the intracellular pool represented by the granules of the iris terminals may be the site susceptible to release by nervous stimulation and tyramine administration (152). Until specific sites of release are identified the feedback mechanisms also remain elusive.

The presence of pools of different sizes impairs the study of the turnover of norepinephrine. Although studies of turnover rates may reveal how the sympathetic nervous system adapts to different levels of activity, the presence of pools of various sizes makes interpretation difficult (66, 73). The influence of heterogenous pools on the determination of synthesis rates of norepinephrine is considerable. Pools located deep within the nerve should turn over slowly as compared with those located close to the synaptic region. Further, the influence of each pool upon turnover values depends on its susceptibility to release. Large pools indicate slow turnover. In the ordinary physiology of the adrenergic nerve it may be the small labile pool that is the important one. Within these limitations, tissues may be grouped according to the turnover time of the norepinephrine they contain. For example, the turnover time for peripheral tissues (i.e., iris, heart, salivary gland) is 8-15 hr (66, 128, 374). The norepinephrine of cervical ganglia has a short turnover, only 2 hr (66). This difference between the cell body and peripheral axon may only reflect a difference in binding capacity. It is not necessary to postulate a migration of vesicles from the ganglia to the nerve terminals in the iris to maintain constancy of their norepinephrine content. After reserpine administration the reappearance of norepinephrine in the cell body before its appearance in the terminal may merely indicate the more rapid turnover of norepinephrine in the former. The half-life of the storage vesicle is much longer than the turnover rate of norepinephrine. Also the enzymes and substrates necessary for synthesis in peripheral tissues, like the iris, are present. Therefore, as norepinephrine leaks or is discharged, the vesicles probably maintain a constant norepinephrine content (107) by local synthesis, as well as by reuptake (176, 197, 357).

DENERVATION

In man a lesion of the cervical sympathetic nerve was first described in a wounded soldier.

> The pupil of the right eye is very small, that of the left eye unusually large. There is a slight, but very distinct ptosis of the right eye and its outer angle appears as though it were dropped a little lower than the inner angle. The ball of the right eye looks smaller than that of the left. . . . The conjunctiva of the right eye is somewhat redder than that of the left . . . the right eye . . . is . . . myopic . . . face distinctly flushed on the right side only and pale on the left.

These clinical signs were recorded and attributed to an ipsilateral lesion of the cervical sympathetic nerve in 1864 by Keen, Morehouse, and Mitchell (232a, 238), the latter a neurologist and former student of Claude Bernard (41, 42). Later, in 1869 Horner completed the clinical characterization of the lesion (216). Horner's syndrome, as it is called today, includes all these features: miosis, ptosis, enophthalmos, narrowing of the palpebral fissure, and dilation of the conjunctival vessels. Anhidrosis and rise in temperature of the affected side of the face will occur if the lesion is below the bifurcation of the carotid. (The sympathetic fibers for sweat leave at the bifurcation to travel with the facial nerve.) Transient decrease in eye pressure (92, 216, 399) and an increase in amplitude of accommodation occur. Heterochromia, cataract, and facial hemiatrophy are associated less frequently (174, 347).

Three developments have generated recent interest in sympathetic denervation of the eye.

1. Denervation is of use in controlling observations made with histofluorescence microscopy, in helping to show details of the iridic adrenergic ground plexus (290, 291, 295), and in observing the exciting changes taking place during embryogenesis of reinnervating adrenergic nerves (293).

2. Direct- and indirect-acting amines have been shown to differ from each other in their effect on innervated and denervated tissue (156-158). These differences permit the use of various amines in the topographic localization of a lesion in the sympathetic system.

3. The outflow resistance of a sympathetically denervated eye decreases strikingly upon the exogenous administration of alpha-active adrenergic compounds (379). When this denervation supersensitivity of the outflow channels became known (131, 380), a clinical search began for adrenergic potentiators capable of producing a fall in intraocular pressure in patients with glaucoma (elevated resistance to outflow of aqueous humor).

The idea that the resistance to outflow of aqueous humor could be lowered in response to norepinephrine after sympathetic denervation of the eye evolved from experiments in which the influence of the sympathetic nervous system on eye pressure was explored. At about the turn of the century a number of clinical observations had indicated that shortly after cervical sympathectomy, possibly ganglionectomy, a drop in ipsilateral intraocular pressure ensued (226). (The extensive dissection of the neck required in a superior cervical ganglionectomy in man makes it unlikely that the operation described was anything more than either removal of the stellate ganglion, or perhaps the middle cervical ganglion.) Subsequent trials, however, showed that intraocular pressure was more labile after cervical sympathectomy (3, 276) and that intraocular pressure was not permanently reduced to any significant degree (282, 350). A series of laboratory investigations then developed (178, 179, 319, 363). Stimulation of the cervical sympathetic nerves caused an apparent increase in the drainage of aqueous fluid into the aqueous veins of the rabbit (187). Effects on intraocular pressure after cervical sympathetic stimulation appeared inconsistent

(223). The transient volumetric changes that occurred were hard to separate from effects on inflow and outflow, determinants of the equilibrium level of intraocular pressure. The same held true for stellate ganglion blockage of the sympathetic input to the eye (303). Beginning in 1955 the effect of surgical denervation on the factors determining the steady-state level of eye pressure was reinvestigated in detail. Twenty-four hours after superior cervical ganglionectomy in rabbits a decrease in eye pressure occurred (279), but the fall in pressure did not occur after preganglionic section of the cervical sympathetic chain (266). An increase in the outflow of aqueous humor accounted for the fall in intraocular pressure that did occur after ganglionectomy (267, 375). Sears & Bárány (375) hypothesized that the decrease in the resistance to outflow of aqueous humor resulted from the release of norepinephrine from the degenerating sympathetic nerve terminals of the iris into the anterior chamber where the neurohumor acted on a receptor in the outflow channels. The outflow channels (trabecular area) are ordinarily perfused only by aqueous humor and not by the blood circulation. Therefore direct access to the area is via the aqueous humor. The transient nature of the ganglionectomy effect (18)—its persistence after death, but its disappearance 30 min later (23)—supported the idea that the responsible agent was released into the anterior chamber and then was either metabolized or washed away. The persistence of the resistance reduction in the dead eye, as well as the failure of carotid ligation to block the effect (353), proved its independence of circulatory changes and of variations in intraocular pressure [see (102, 199) for contrary views].

The analysis of the relation between the ganglionectomy effect on outflow resistance and the release of norepinephrine from degenerating nerve endings provides evidence for the presence of an alpha adrenergic receptor for outflow. The decrease in resistance after ganglionectomy is *a*) largely prevented by prior elimination of norepinephrine stores with reserpine (18) and α-methyl-*m*-tyrosine (353) and completely prevented with α-methyltyrosine (353); *b*) blocked by the prior administration of phentolamine (18, 198), Dibenamine (375), and dibenzyline (353); *c*) preceded by a decrease in the endogenous catecholamine content of the iris [(377); Fig. 4]; *d*) related directly to the appearance of norepinephrine in the perfusate (aqueous humor of the anterior chamber) [(376); Fig. 5]; and *e*) duplicated by substances causing release of norepinephrine, such as reserpine [(353); Fig. 6], and by a close-intracameral injection of norepinephrine [(379, 380); see Fig. 2].

The site of the adrenergic receptor has not been identified. It most likely has a "trabecular locus" situated in or near the endothelial lining of the channels of outflow in the iridocorneal (chamber) angle (380). These cells appear similar to, and contain organelles found in, other cells that respond to adrenergic compounds (79). In the rabbit, stimulation results from alpha-active (131, 379, 380) and beta-active (180) substances but not from their precursors or metabolites (380). Although the spaces of Fontana appear to be the only regions in the rabbit chamber angle containing an adrenergic innervation (133), the trabecular area is nonetheless responsive to norepinephrine and furthermore takes up and binds norepinephrine perfused through the anterior chamber (46).

Innervation of the chamber angle has long been the object of investigation. Early work with silver staining depicted nerve fibers in the trabecular area, some of which were found to make turns around the pillars of the trabeculae (64). Since 1954 many workers have claimed an innervation for the meshwork or inner wall, or both, of the canal of Schlemm (84, 154, 213, 214). With electron microscopy the search for nerves is difficult, but several were found in the human eye, mainly in the inner trabecular area. In two human eyes, nerves were found running along the inner wall of the canal; Schwann sheaths abutted directly against the endothelial lining. Myelinated and unmyelinated nerves were seen terminating in the meshwork, and in one instance a small bundle of unmyelinated nerves was seen in a peninsula of connective tissue in the lumen of the canal (L. Feeney, personal communication). Histofluorescence studies have indicated that most of these nerves are not adrenergic (135), except in the guinea pig, where an abundance of adrenergic terminals is seen with both histofluorescence technique (133) and electron microscopy (Fig. 7). In the latter instance the criteria for the presence of adrenergic nerve terminals have been satisfied (188). On occasion these adrenergic terminals have been seen in the uveal trabeculum of the human eye (Fig. 8).

The nervous innervation of the iridocorneal angle has not yet been systematically studied with specific staining and denervation techniques along with analysis of fine structure. Several questions must be answered.

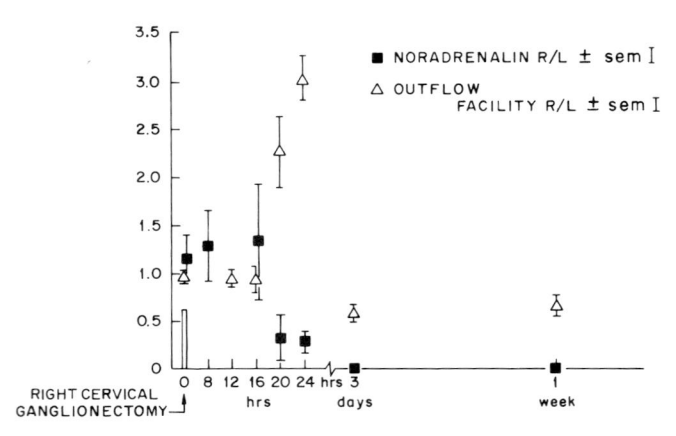

FIG. 4. Outflow facility and iridic norepinephrine (*noradrenalin*) after unilateral cervical ganglionectomy. Progressive disappearance of endogenous iridic norepinephrine correlated with increase in outflow facility. Ratio of denervated to normally innervated iris (R/L) ± SEM plotted on ordinate. [From Sears et al. (377).]

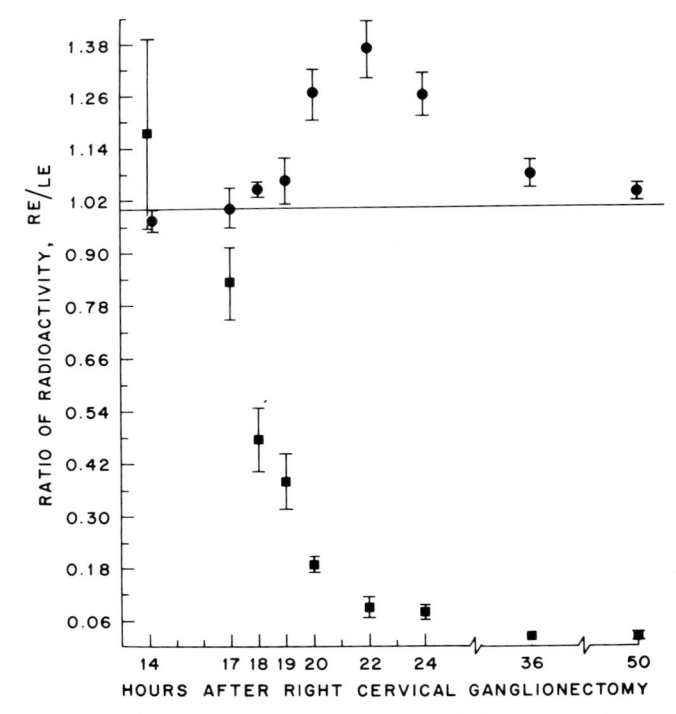

FIG. 5. Retention (■) and appearance (●) of tritiated norepinephrine by iris and ciliary processes of rabbits after unilateral cervical ganglionectomy. ^{3}H-norepinephrine, 5 μg/kg (170 nc/kg), was injected intravenously, and 2 hr later tissues were removed at intervals after ganglionectomy indicated on abscissa. Results were plotted on ordinate as ratio (counts/min of tritium) of denervated to normally innervated iris (*RE/LE*). Each experimental point represents mean ± SEM of at least 6 animals. [From Sears & Gillis (376).]

Do the nerves pass through the trabecular region on their way to the cornea, or are there real terminals? Evidence has been presented to indicate the latter (325, 427). If so, do these terminals serve the endothelium of the canal of Schlemm, the trabeculae, or the forward prolongation of ciliary muscle? In this regard, it is interesting to consider the anatomy of the region in more detail. In lower forms the scleral spur is poorly developed. Smooth muscle cells are often found in the guinea pig and rabbit. This uveal mesh, especially in the guinea pig, has numerous adrenergic terminals (133, 325). Terminals are found in the uveal mesh in man, but there is little evidence for them near or anterior to the well-developed scleral spur, in the corneoscleral meshwork. Finally, if the corneoscleral trabecula is the tendon for the meridional ciliary muscle (254), innervation would not be expected there. What innervation is found would then be presumably related only to muscle cells in the uvea (i.e., anterior portions of the ciliary muscle, especially the longitudinal part).

The singular or isolated response of the outflow channels to adrenergic agents is difficult to demonstrate by other than an intracameral route. Topical, intravitreal, or systemic administration gives small and/or varied effects. This observation suggests that, under ordinary circumstances, norepinephrine released into the anterior chamber is efficiently inactivated by the mechanism of reuptake and binding by the iridic adrenergic nerves. Thus a trabecular effect on outflow resistance from even low doses of norepinephrine delivered into a denervated eye by intracameral injection is assured. As little as 10 ng norepinephrine base, corresponding to 2.5×10^{-7} M, in the anterior chamber is active (380). In the normally innervated eye, however, at least 1×10^{-5} M is required to produce any decrease in resistance. Thus, whereas outflow channels are responsive to intracamerally administered norepinephrine, the response is greatly limited by the presence of a normal innervation, even when the eye is treated with large amounts of exogenous norepinephrine. Analogous conclusions can be drawn from experiments on the effects of cervical sympathetic nerve stimulation on intraocular pressure (83). The efficient reuptake mechanism prevents the depletion of iridic stores and thwarts the detection of neurohumor in the anterior chamber in most instances. On the other hand, if the animal is first treated with cocaine, detectable quantities of the neurohumor are present in the aqueous humor (15, 123, 129, 283, 336). The physiological counterpart of these observations is found in the changes of outflow resistance after stimulation of the cervical sympathetic nerve. Although some trend toward a decrease can be seen, pretreatment with cocaine elicits a distinct reduction in the resistance to aqueous outflow (330).

The special effect of superior cervical sympathetic ganglionectomy on eye pressure (degeneration release) was useful in establishing the presence of an adrenergic influence on aqueous outflow. When it was further found that supersensitivity denervation (131, 379, 380) ensued and could be duplicated in human Horner's syndrome (373), a search for compounds that might mimic or produce denervation was undertaken. The first such study employed topical administration of guanethidine followed by topical administration of

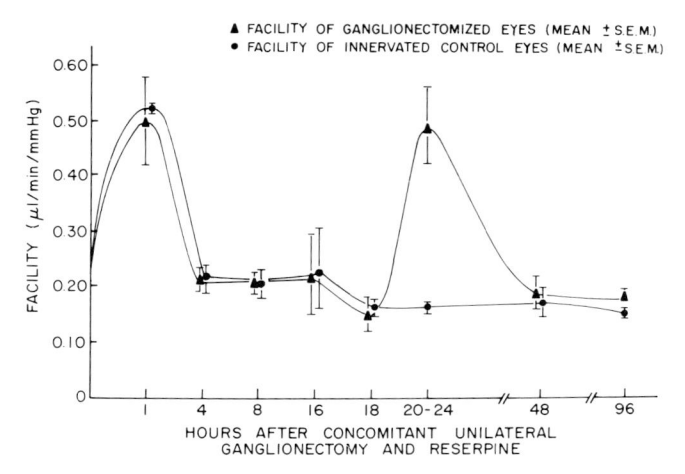

FIG. 6. Effect on outflow facility of intravenously administered reserpine compared with that of unilateral cervical ganglionectomy. Release of norepinephrine into anterior chamber with each method produces 2.5-fold increases in outflow. [From Rosser & Sears (353).]

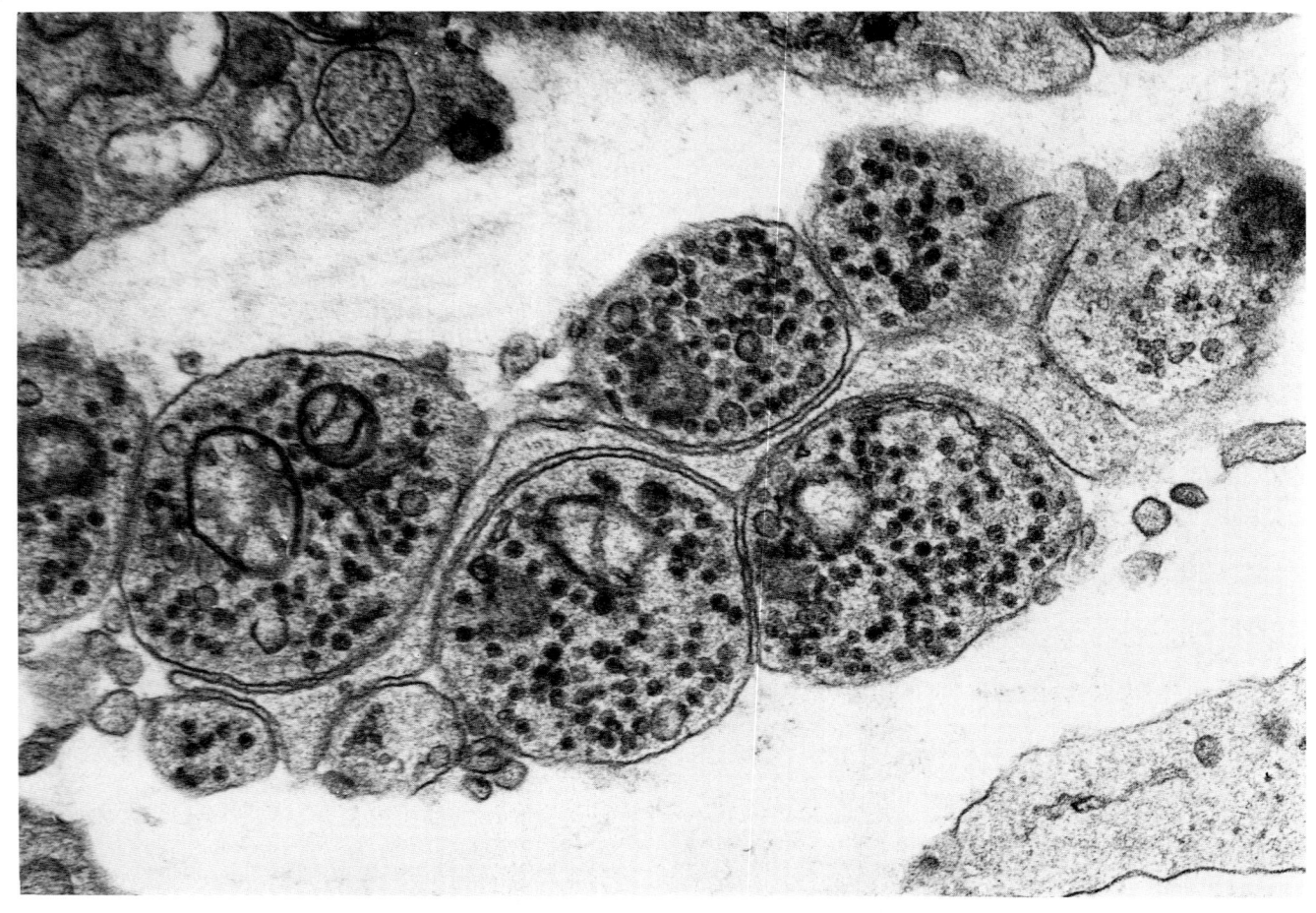

FIG. 7. Nerve bundle within uveal meshwork of chamber angle of eye of guinea pig. Numerous dense core vesicles, naked neurites, and (swollen) mitochondria are seen. Trabecular tissue at *left top*. Permanganate fixation. × 23,400. (From S. Nishida and M. Sears, unpublished observations.)

epinephrine (232). This combination caused a reduction in eye pressure, but the effect could be elicited for only 1 week. A search for other compounds, such as cocaine analogues, that can affect axonal reuptake and binding has continued. These compounds (e.g., protriptylene) have been used, together with a subsequent dose of epinephrine, with very limited success (264). The degeneration of adrenergic nervous terminals seen with 6-hydroxydopamine (240) has prompted its trial (212). Whether any nontoxic, chemical supersensitivity denervation of ocular adrenergic receptors can satisfactorily be achieved and then become a significant modality in the treatment of glaucoma patients (195, 442) remains unanswered. To date, in the human eye the most dramatic supersensitivity denervation effects on eye pressure have been observed in patients with acquired Horner's syndrome (373) where, with incomplete denervation, the magnitude of the effect of topical epinephrine is inversely related to the duration of the lesion and its closeness to the eye. In complete postganglionic lesions (268), the augmented response is elicited at a maximum value indefinitely.

DEGENERATION RELEASE

Hours after superior cervical ganglionectomy, transmitter from degenerating sympathetic fibers causes not only a decreased resistance to outflow of aqueous humor in the rabbit eye (16–20 hr), but also provokes the onset of these phenomena: mydriasis at 16 hr in rabbits and other animals (25, 377); decrease in mitoses of corneal epithelium at 12–16 hr in rabbits and rats [Fig. 9; (167, 304)]; contraction of the nictitans at 18 hr in cats (261); constriction of the ear vessels at 20 hr in rabbits (25); exophthalmos and retraction of the lids at 13–15 hr in rats (285); and secretion from salivary glands in cats (91, 145). These effects are transient.

The transient "ganglionectomy effect" (18) on outflow resistance is caused by release of stored transmitter from degenerating adrenergic terminals (18, 375) within the iris (353). Transient glandular secretion was also described (91, 145), and later the degeneration contraction of the denervated nictitans was reported (261). These phenomena were expected to occur because shortly after denervation the nerve endings in

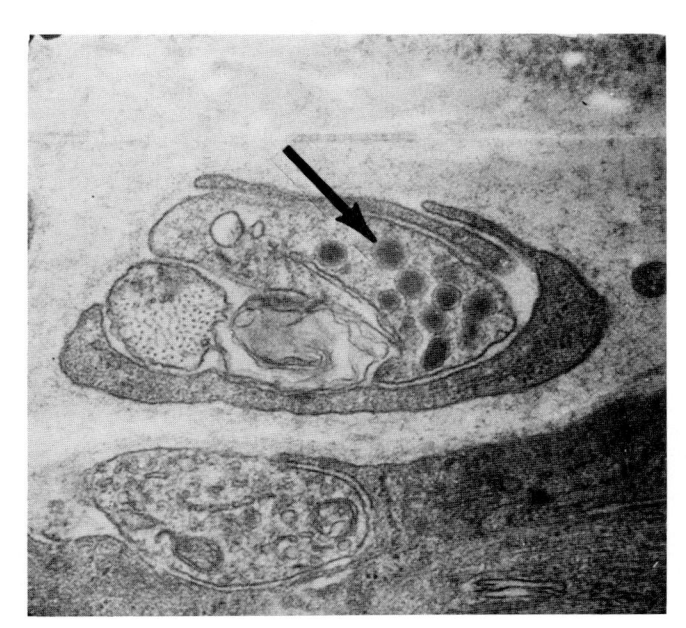

FIG. 8. Dense core vesicles (*arrow*) in terminal region of noradrenergic axon of trabeculum of human eye. Neurofibrils are seen at *left*, cut in cross section. Axon is exposed to aqueous humor and is partly covered by cytoplasm of Schwann cell, which is hard to distinguish from cytoplasm of trabecular endothelium. Glutaraldehyde fixation. × 43,100. (From Y. Shiose, unpublished observations.)

sympathetically innervated organs lose their transmitter content (34, 129, 237, 293, 377, 441).

> The variability of the intervals between axotomy and degeneration release of transmitter is not only due to the interval required for "the message of the missing cell body" to reach the terminals but comprises a time which is different for terminals in different organs (412).

In the case of the reduction in aqueous outflow resistance, the correlation between loss of transmitter from tissue and the appearance of the neurohumor in a place that probably affects the appropriate receptor has been studied in detail in the rabbit (25, 353, 376, 377, 410–412). Similar studies have been made with nictitans (261, 262, 430). After superior cervical ganglionectomy, mydriasis and the decrease in resistance to aqueous outflow commencing, respectively, between 14.5 and 16 hr and between 16 and 20 hr can probably be accounted for by the release of norepinephrine resulting from degeneration. The total depletion of norepinephrine stores completely eliminates the drop in resistance (353). Doses of adrenergic blocking agents reaching the anterior chamber in adequate concentration also abolish the effect. The time lag between onset and peak effects can be explained (see Fig. 10) by a progressive degeneration of binding sites. The terminals will trap the transmitter until they themselves deteriorate. In fact, the early phase of mydriasis begins when uptake and binding by the iris begin to fail. So that animals could be followed over a long period of time after ganglionectomy, the changes in eye pressure may be measured by tonometry. Therefore recording pressure changes and outflow with direct manometry and perfusion techniques is eliminated. The pressure measurement, however, includes the resistance component and other factors as well. The lowering in resistance will begin a little earlier than the change in pressure (see Fig. 10) and coincide even more closely with the early mydriasis. As the uptake of amines by the axonal amine pump diminishes (243, 293, 376, 390), the sensitivity to the transmitter release may increase progressively during degeneration contraction (262) and cause a striking response.

A second wave of mydriasis and a curious hyperemia during the later phases of degeneration release occur, however (412). Whether a two-step depletion of catecholamine stores seen in some denervation experiments (293) could explain the two waves of mydriasis is not known. Persistence of norepinephrine within the anterior chamber (see Fig. 5) may help prolong, but not delay, mydriasis. However, both the delayed mydriasis and hyperemia are resistant to antiadrenergic agents (412). The technique of bretylium delay has been used to analyze these phenomena (25). The effects of intrinsic differences among different terminals [(25); e.g., ear vessels vs. iris vessels vs. dilator muscle of the iris] and differences in the distribution and affinity of bretylium for normal terminals and for those that degenerate at different rates are factors that complicate the analysis (285). In the instance of iridic hyperemia, a substance other than norepinephrine is probably formed

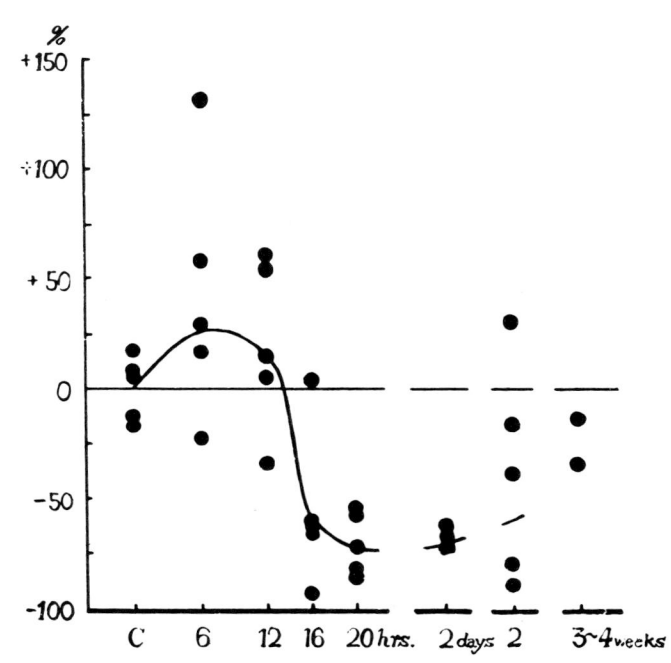

FIG. 9. Mitotic rates after sympathetic denervation. Ordinate, mitotic increase and decrease (%); abscissa, intervals after denervation; C, control; *solid line*, time course of average rate. Conspicuous decrease of mitotic rate takes place after lag period of 16 hr. [From Mishima (304).]

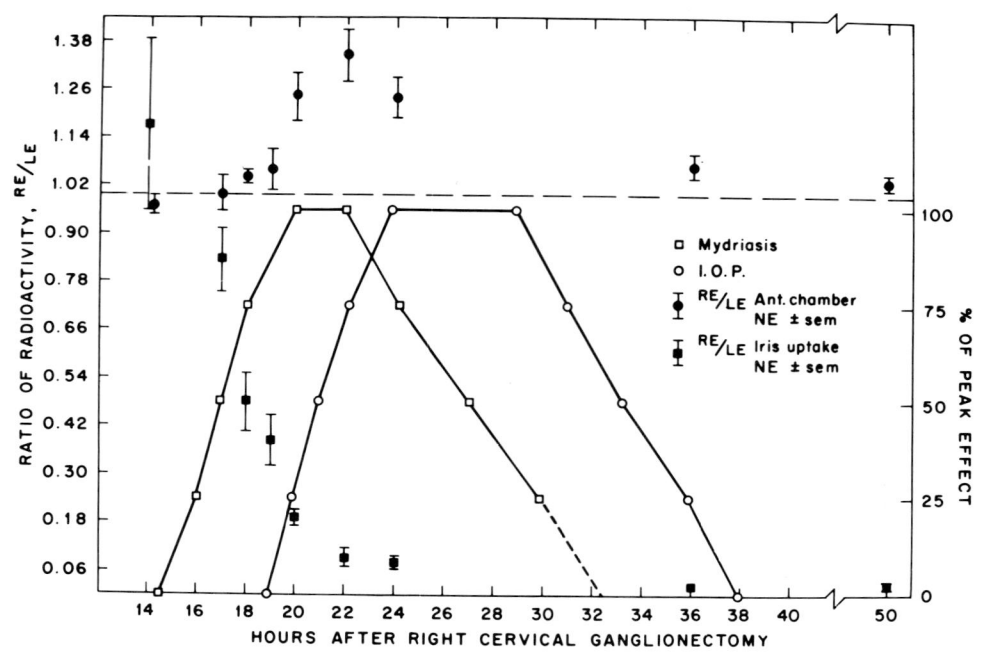

FIG. 10. Relation between progressive disappearance of binding capacity of norepinephrine (*NE*) by iris, appearance of norepinephrine in anterior chamber (*Ant. chamber*), and effect of degeneration release of norepinephrine on mydriasis and intraocular pressure (*I.O.P.*). Values plotted as % peak effect of increase in pupillary diameter and tonometric decrease in intraocular pressure, and as ratio of radioactivity, denervated to control, right eye to left eye (*RE/LE*), as in Fig. 5. (See text for discussion.) Degeneration mydriasis begins as binding sites in iris deteriorate. Reduction in intraocular pressure corresponds to appearance of norepinephrine in anterior chamber—compare values at 50% of peak effect. [Adapted from Sears & Gillis (376) and Bárány & Treister (24a).]

and/or liberated when sympathetic nervous system terminals degenerate (319a). Pretreatment of the ganglionectomized animal with either indomethacin or acetylsalicylic acid (aspirin), known prostaglandin synthetase inhibitors, prevents the hyperemia. This suggests that release of one or more of the prostaglandins causes the degeneration hyperemia. Furthermore the release of prostaglandins is dependent on the presence or release of norepinephrine because pretreatment with an inhibitor of norepinephrine biosynthesis, α-methyltyrosine, also prevents the hyperemia. Interactions between the adrenergic system and prostaglandins have been well studied for other systems (197a).

TISSUE FUNCTION

Adnexa

ORBITS AND LIDS. In mammals, bundles of smooth muscle fibers are unevenly distributed in at least three places within the periorbital tissue. In certain places they are concentrated to form the orbital muscle of Müller. In the orbital cavity of rodents, this muscle is a well-developed orbital membrane covering the bony floor and lateral wall. The muscle may act as a protruder and is different from the striated retractor bulbi supplied by the sixth nerve. The latter retracts the globe and supports it when the head is dependent, as in feeding.

Smooth muscle fibers, also called the muscles of Müller, are present in the lids. They originate among the fibers of the levator palpebrae superioris (upper lid) and from the prolongation of the inferior rectus (lower lid), and insert into the proximal margins of the tarsal plates of the lids. Posterior to the Gasserian ganglion, adrenergic filaments from the carotid plexus pass to branches of the third nerve to innervate the superior and inferior palpebral smooth muscles. These fibers widen the palpebral fissure. The width of the fissure may reflect the psychic state of the subject, but it also depends on the combined tone of the levator palpebrae superioris and the sympathetically innervated Müller muscles.

Apart from the ptosis of Horner's syndrome, the chief clinical interest in adrenergic function of lid structure lies in the retraction often observed in patients with thyrotoxicosis and in the ptosis in subjects with myxedema (273). The fact that both the upper and lower lids are involved supports the opinion that the Müller muscles are primarily concerned. In the thyrotoxicosis, although there is no mydriasis, the presence of high adrenergic tone is indicated by the fact that the lid retraction can be reduced by reserpine (81) or guanethidine (171). The local use of adrenergic blocking agents in therapy of the stare and retraction came from the idea that lid retraction may be mediated by the sympathetic nervous system and, conversely, from the observation that ptosis occurred after the topical use of guanethidine. After the beneficial effect of this drug was reported (82, 171, 391), additional studies employing alpha and beta blockade were done (103). Although it is clear that depletion or prevention of release of norepinephrine will relieve lid retraction, the action of the alpha and beta blocking agents on the lid is not completely explained. These compounds are irritating after topical application. Furthermore beta blocking agents have a local anesthetic action (224, 387); however, they have abolished lid retraction in some patients. This observation, taken together with the lack of mydriasis (an alpha-dominated function) in the thyrotoxic patient and the ameliorating effect of beta blockade on many of the signs of thyroid toxicity (81), suggests that lid retraction may be mediated by a beta receptor. Support to this idea is given by the observation that triiodothyronine causes a decrease in eye pressure that was prevented by pretreatment with propranolol (193), a beta blocking agent. Phentolamine also had a blocking effect, but it was small.

It is difficult to explain an apparent enhanced sensitivity to catecholamines in the thyrotoxic patient. The effect of thyroid feeding on COMT and MAO activity is not significant. There is no difference in the concentration of catecholamines and their metabolites in plasma and urine of normal and hyperthyroid dogs or in the plasma and urine of normal and hyperthyroid patients. It is unlikely that thyroid hormones act via an increase in concentration of free catecholamines. After infusion into normal and thyroxine-pretreated rats, catecholamine uptake into the various tissues was very similar in the two groups. Studies in man also indicate that thyroid hormones do not reduce the uptake of circulating catecholamines. There is presently no explanation for the action of triiodothyronine; it may sensitize the receptor to catecholamines or act directly on either alpha or beta receptors.

NICTITANS. The nictitans may be thought of as a soft contact lens that protects the cornea and eye from noxious influences but also provides the eye with an accessory, transparent refractive device when its optical power becomes altered, as in underwater diving.

For the most part the membrane is passive in its movements. It is forced out across the cornea by the propulsive action of a pyramidal-shaped muscle, the retractor bulbi, as it pulls the eyeball inward. The stimulus for this movement may be more than a localized corneal provocation, but a generalized (autonomic) sympathetic effect as well (2). The return of the membrane is largely passive but may be helped by the action of the orbital muscle of Müller. Muscle fibers of the nictitans among placentals are vestigial, but in the frog two distinct muscular mechanisms move the nictitans (396). The membrane folds inside the thickness of the lower lid and forms an N-shaped structure in cross section. The third nerve innervates the lower lid while the sixth nerve innervates the depressor membrane nictitans.

In the bird, both mechanisms are present with a separate lower lid and nictitans.

In the cat, stimulation of thoracic segments, $D_1 \rightarrow D_4$ and sometimes D_5, causes active retraction of the nictitans. Reflex protrusion is elicited via the afferents of the fifth nerve and efferents of the sixth nerve (351). In rodents, often the retractor bulbi attached to the posterior surface of the sclera is intimately wound around the tendon of the nictitans. Therefore the membrane is drawn over the cornea with retractor action. In some mammals both innervations are present, but the sixth nerve mechanism has no connection with the plica or the lid.

The muscular part of the nictitans has been of most interest to the physiologist in studies of sympathetic fiber thresholds (57, 161), drug mechanisms, and supersensitivity denervation (237, 261, 262). The rich sympathetic innervation to the muscle of the membrane has been noted many times (292). Examination with the histofluorescence microscope of longitudinal sections shows fluorescent fibers parallel to muscle fibers, and in transverse section the nerve fibers are fluorescent points in close contact with the outside of smooth muscle cells. Fibers often run together, two or more in the same strands that go on to form a three-dimensional network. Several fibers reach one and the same cell, and the length of the terminals indicates that several cells are probably influenced by one and the same neuron, an example of the convergence principle of innervation of autonomic effectors (204).

The nictitans muscle isolated in the orbit of the cat (351, 404) is useful for the development of basic information about the effect of autonomic drugs (348, 413–416), acetycholine-mediated adrenergic transmission (76–78), and denervation supersensitivity (157, 413–416). Pharmacological analysis has shown that the muscle contains specific receptors for epinephrine and norepinephrine, for acetycholine, and for 5-hydroxytryptamine. The responses to nicotine and tetramethylammonium are explained by stimulation of fine postganglionic nerve fibers, which lie among the smooth muscle and innervate it. Stimulation of these fibers leads to the release of norepinephrine, which then causes contraction of the muscle.

A new observation about the nonmuscular portion of the nictitans is that, like the cornea, it has a stroma made up of uniform collagen fibrils interspersed in a mucinous matrix with some few cellular elements. The fibrils have twice the diameter of those found in the cornea (260). The nictitans is quite transparent, despite the presence of these fibrils. This feature is of interest because of the relation between microstructure and transparency (Fig. 11). It is apparent that only those fluctuations in the index of refraction having a spatial extent comparable with or larger than one-half the dimension of the light wavelength ($\sim$2,500 A) are important in the relation of the microstructure to transparency (181). This transparency makes possible the use of the nictitans as a lens. Then afferent stimuli resulting in the

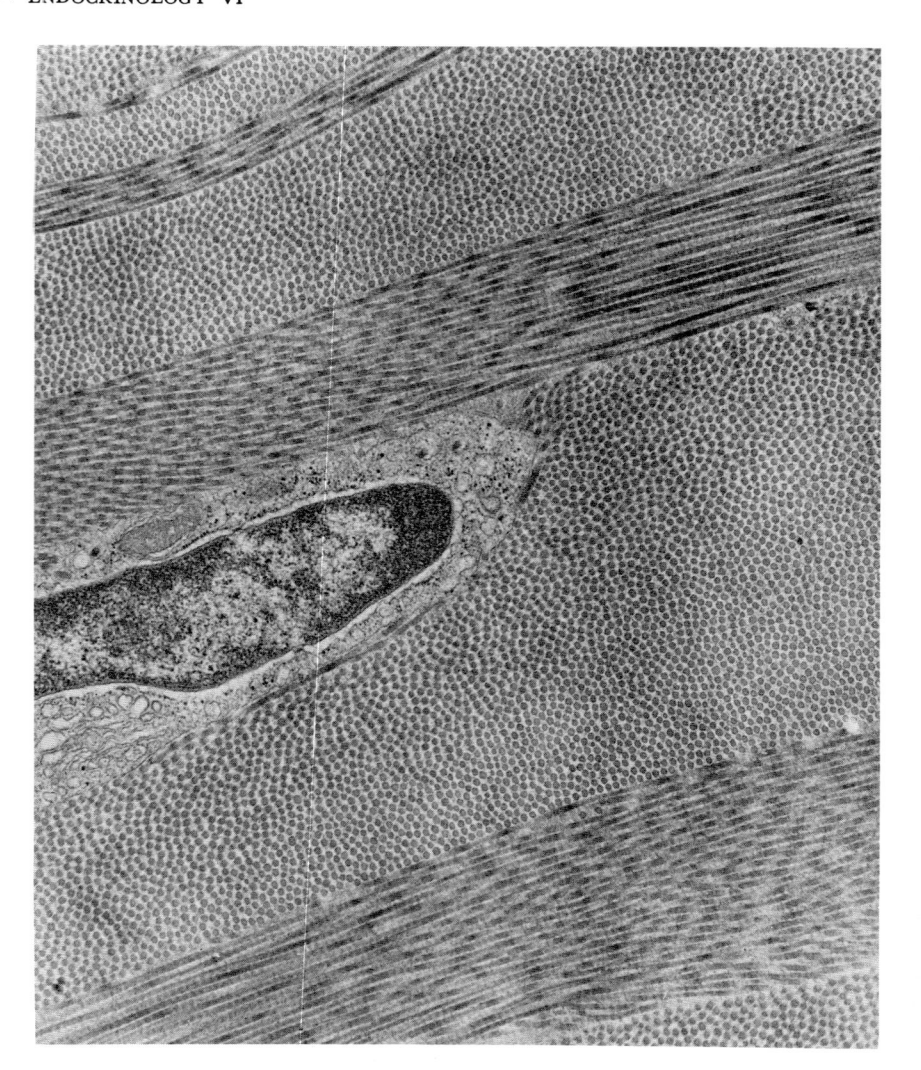

FIG. 11. Cross section through stroma or connective tissue layer of nictitating membrane. × 17,600. [From Lande & Zadunaisky (260).]

protrusion movement of the nictitans might serve a refractive or accommodative function. The movement would be analogous to the negative accommodation exerted by the sympathetic nerve in mammals.

EXTRINSIC MUSCLES. The extraocular muscles of mammals contain two distinct types of muscle fibers (86, 203, 316) similar to the twitch and slow fibers of the frog. The latter are multiply innervated by small nerves (402) and are smaller in size than the former. The two differ also in the disposition of the sarcoplasmic reticulum (113). Differences and similarities in their physiological responses during electrical stimulation have been reported.

Adrenergic innervation to the blood vessels of extraocular muscle is accepted, but some authors report a muscular innervation as well, especially of the outer surface layers (169, 419, 420), where the slow fibers predominate (203, 205). In pharmacological response, extraocular muscle behaves like chronically denervated mammalian muscle (68, 122, 233), amphibian or avian skeletal muscle, and the mammalian intrafusal muscle fibers of the muscle spindle. For example, epinephrine evokes a contracture and propagates conduction in chronically denervated skeletal muscle (65, 247). The response has been thought to be mediated by a beta receptor because it was most effectively produced by L-isoproterenol and blocked by dichloroisoproterenol and pronethalol. In the striated superior rectus muscle of the cat the response was clearly mediated by an alpha receptor, however (130, 233). In the rhesus monkey beta receptors were found (234).

Although the presence of small amounts of smooth muscle in the extraocular muscle has not been ruled out and might account for these adrenergic responses, it is likely that, similar to frog slow muscle, extraocular muscle has some of the physiological characteristics intermediate between smooth muscle and twitch skeletal muscle. Some effect from epinephrine might therefore be anticipated. The action of epinephrine might be indirect—in mobilizing acetylcholine from prejunctional storage sites and in giving rise to the well-known contracture, most probably from action on multiply innervated muscle fibers (253). Atropine blocks the contractile response caused by stimulation of sympathetic fibers but not by exogenous administration of epinephrine (364). This suggests that epinephrine has some direct effect on striated extraocular muscle. The maximum tension developing in an extraocular muscle after treatment with adrenergic agents is very small, however, compared to the tension elicited by cholinomimetic agents. The possibility that forces of this low magnitude, which develop in slow muscle and exhibit the electrical characteristics of a slow nonpropagated conduction, are related to tonic vergence movements of the eye has been considered (4).

LACRIMAL GLAND. The lacrimal gland is located in a fossa of the roof of the orbit. It is tubuloalveolar in type with numerous acini from which converging ducts emerge to drain into excretory ducts lined with myoepithelial cells. There is no regional differentiation of ducts. The gross innervation of the gland is parasympathetic and sympathetic. The former arises in the lacrimal nucleus in the floor of the fourth ventricle and runs with the facial nerve to the geniculate ganglion where some fibers leave the facial pathway to run with the greater superficial petrosal nerve to the sphenopalatine ganglion. Synapses are made here, and the postganglionic fibers pass either with the zygomatic nerve or alone directly to the lacrimal gland. Some adrenergic fibers pass by way of the superficial petrosal through the sphenopalatine ganglion for distribution to the gland along with the parasympathetic fibers. Some pass along the carotid plexuses to the gland by way of the lacrimal nerve or artery.

Histochemical (1), electron-microscopic (132, 360–362), and physiological studies (9, 62, 371, 453) have provided evidence confirming a dual innervation to the lacrimal gland. In animals like the turtle and bird that can produce a hypertonic secretion (1, 61, 63, 151, 371), the circulatory pattern of the gland exposes the most metabolically active cells to fresh arterial blood. The arterioles are located in an interlobular fashion and appear to be in close contact with cholinergic secretory fibers, whereas adrenergic fibers appear confined to perilobular connective tissue. This arrangement is carried further in sheep (452), monkeys (360), and other animals where adrenergic fibers may be seen in close proximity to perilobular tissue or near myoepithelial cells, but cholinergic fibers appear to penetrate the basement membrane and pass between acinar cells, especially those of a serous variety. The vascular innervation in these higher animals now may be of a dual sort, but the majority of all parenchymal and interstitial terminals are parasympathetic (361, 362).

Differentiation between sympathetic and parasympathetic functions has been attempted by denervation of the gland. Denervation supersensitivity to a variety of pharmacological agents occurs after surgical interruption of either parasympathetic (111, 378) or sympathetic (288) supplies or after chemical parasympatholysis (146). The lack of specificity of these changes prevents any inferences regarding the role of either innervational system. Interestingly a similar response occurs in patients with familial dysautonomia to methacholine (251, 389).

One specific change seen after parasympathetic denervation is a reduction in the proportion of serous granules (362).

Gross testing in human eyes with topically applied agents indicates that cholinomimetic drugs produce an increase in lacrimal flow, whereas cholinolytics reduce tear flow. Reflex secretion in humans and animals and weeping in humans have been assigned to parasympathetic control. In the cat and rabbit, records of lacrimal flow from a cannulated excretory duct after pharmacological stimuli show mixed effects from parenterally administered norepinephrine, whereas pilocarpine appeared to increase flow (184). The adrenergic effects on the blood circulation and on the contractility of the myoid structures in the gland could not be separated from secretion and obviously affect the gross measurement.

Further evidence for the dominance of cholinergic effects on glandular secretion is derived from electrophysiological records of secretory potentials (207). These have been obtained from the nasal salt gland (ductal potential changes), salivary glands, and the lacrimal gland. Although in the submaxillary gland, several groups of membrane potentials have been obtained after parasympathetic and sympathetic stimulation, a biphasic response related to excretory flow from the lacrimal gland could be obtained only with parasympathetic stimulation. These observations are compatible with those made in other glands. It is unlikely that any continuously secreting gland is directly innervated or controlled by noradrenergic fibers.

Although the tear film is vital to the protection and function of the cornea (305), very little is known about regulatory mechanisms for lacrimal secretion. Only the chemical composition (248) and rates of evaporation (298) and elimination of the tears have received prominent attention. The small tear volume, low rate of resting secretion, and evaporation of the tear film create technical problems for the measurement of lacrimal flow. Only one quantitative physiological study has been made in the intact eye of man. The dilution of a layer of fluorescein by the tears and the decay rate of its concentration can be determined fluorophotometrically. Tear volume was calculated by the construction and extrapolation to zero time of a semilogarithmic plot of the concentration decay of fluorescein after its application. A turnover rate of about 16% min^{-1} was calculated for normal human subjects. From tear volume and turnover rate an average tear flow of 1.2 μliter/min was found (306). Exploitation of the technique has not yet been reported for physiological studies of the lacrimal gland.

Eye

BLOOD FLOW. Proportionately the largest avascular mass of tissue in an organ anywhere in the body is contained in the eye. No blood vessels are found in the cornea, lens, vitreous, or chamber angle (the iridocorneal angle containing the trabecular meshwork and canal of Schlemm). Even those vessels found in the essentially avascular sclera are merely in transit. In sharp contrast to these tissues stands the retina with the highest metabolic rate of any tissue and demands for a large blood supply. Furthermore the eye is almost continually cooled by exposure to the atmosphere. For these reasons a very high rate of blood flow is maintained to ensure a constant composition of the interstitial tissues and fluids of the eye, as well as a constant workable temperature.

Two separate circulations supply the ocular tissues to accomplish these ends: the uveal and retinal systems (121). The names are misleading, however. The retinal circulation, in effect, supplies only the inner layer of the retinal tissue, whereas the uveal circulation supplies, without entering it, the largest volume of retinal tissue, as well as the rest of the eye.

The anatomy of the vascular systems is complex, and species differences are considerable. The following are some of the basic features in the mammal. The central retinal artery is an end artery (301), which supplies only a single tissue. Shunting of this circulation therefore occurs only between various portions of the retina. Very often therefore resistance may be located beyond the point of entry of significant collaterals. Shunt vessels may develop that trade resistance with parallel nutritional beds and vary the effectiveness of the circulation in disease states (Fig. 12). In health, however, except for the recent demonstration of arterial cushions at the extraocular bifurcation of ciliary and retinal circulation in the rat (310), no shunt devices, like precapillary sphincters, have been seen in either the choroidal or retinal vascular trees (11). The retinal capillaries themselves resemble cerebral ones. They have pericytes (12), also called periendothelial or mural cells (256), enclosed within a basement membrane in common with the endothelial cell proper. These cells are histamine resistant, whereas those of the uveal capillaries are not (434). Hence the effective "blood-retinal" barrier would appear to be at the retinal capillary level, whereas at the other extreme the uveal capillaries of the ciliary epithelium are fenestrated (215), like those of the kidney. Although ready access from the uveal side to the retina exists via the leaky choriocapillaris, tight junctions between the retinal pigment epithelia restrict the passage of large molecules into the retina proper from the leaky choroid. Similar junctions are found between adjacent cells of the inner, nonpigmented, ciliary epithelial layer (385).

The vascular system within the eye is affected by the pressure within its confines and therefore pressures within the veins and capillaries cannot be lower than the pressures to which they are subject (165). The venous pressure outside the eye is related to the low pressure in the large veins draining the orbit. Therefore a sudden drop in pressure occurs as blood moves from the intraocular to extraocular veins. The arterial pressure within the eye is roughly two-thirds of mean brachial artery pressure. If intraocular pressure rises sufficiently to reduce blood flow, the arterial pressure rises. The capillary pressures are then quite high to overcome the "tissue" or intraocular pressure. In the uvea, especially

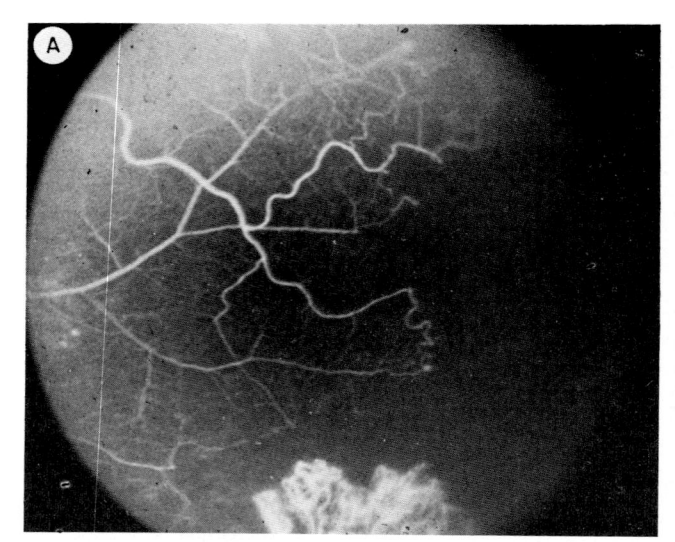

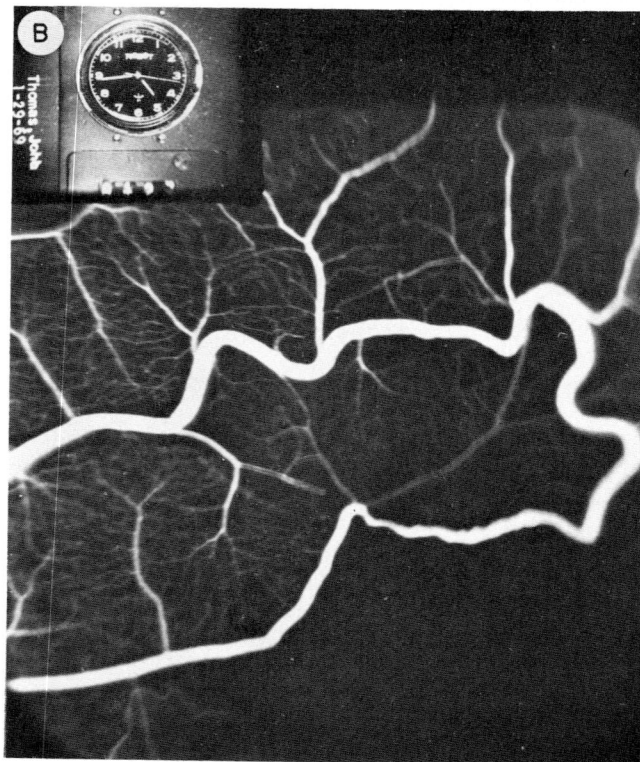

FIG. 12. *A*: fluorescein angiography of retinal vessels in patient with arteriolar occlusion, arteriovenous anastomosis, and neovascular proliferation (*below*). *B*: fluorescein angiography of retinal vessels in patient with arteriovenous shunt. (From M. F. Goldberg, unpublished observations.)

where arterioles abruptly change into capillaries, the pressure of the latter may be still higher. The effect of an increase in eye pressure is similar to the effect of a reduction in arterial pressure (94), however. In both instances a fall in the perfusion pressure of ocular tissues occurs (51).

In autoregulated systems, like the brain, when a fall in perfusion pressure takes place, vasodilation maintains blood flow. In the uvea, no such disproportion exists between pressure change and blood flow (48–50). Hence in the uvea the changes in the caliber of vessels are passive and can be said to be related almost directly to changes in transmural pressure. Although there is some evidence for autoregulation of retinal blood flow (115, 116), there does not appear to be any competent autoregulation of uveal blood flow (48). However, the pressure difference over the capillary wall falls when intraocular pressure is raised. This, in turn, may reduce the net fluid movement out of the vessel and lead to a reduction in net aqueous humor formation and tissue (intraocular) pressure (49). This mechanism, then, constitutes a form of local regulation. The demonstration of arteriovenous shunts in the ciliary circulation of the episclera operative at higher pressures is of interest here (170). Finally, when a degree of vasomotor tone is created in vessels of small diameter, the tension developed in the wall of the vessel may increase above transmural pressure. In this case complete closure of a vessel of small caliber may occur. This "critical closing pressure" is increased by norepinephrine administration (44, 45), is decreased by sympathectomy (3), and may be a factor in the responsiveness of the uveal circulation to the adrenergic impulses.

The blood vessels of the eye and adnexa do possess nonterminal axons of the sympathetic nervous system that give rise to abundant terminals, which themselves constitute a ground plexus (133–135, 291). The latter is a fine, widely meshed, two-dimensional network located on the border between the adventitia and smooth muscle. The choroid is extensively innervated, and numerous nerve terminals ramify in close relation to the capillary layer. Direct innervation of capillaries has not yet been substantiated, however. The central retinal artery and other vessels within the optic nerve are innervated by this nerve supply, which ceases abruptly when the retinal vessels penetrate the cribiform plate. On a very rare occasion a fluorescent twig may penetrate the papilla. The intraocular retinal vessels of the human, cat, rabbit, and rat do not appear to have an adrenergic innervation (270), but it is likely that sympathetic stimuli cause extraocular vasoconstriction of the retinal vascular tree (117, 163).

Stimulation of the cervical sympathetic chain produces intense uveal vasoconstriction (96, 97, 187, 446) in rabbits and cats and indicates the presence of alpha receptors (48, 51, 96, 97). These responses are blocked by Dibenzyline. These vessels also respond to injected norepinephrine (449) but not to isoproterenol (97). Hence there are no beta receptors and no sympathetic vasodilator nerves to the uvea. Acetylcholine, however, does lower uveal vascular resistance considerably, although no vascular effects from stimulation of the parasympathetic fibers to the eye are apparent (51). The source of the innervation for an acetylcholine-sensitive receptor is therefore not clear. Other vasodilators cause an increase in uveal blood flow only if they do not cause much fall in systemic arterial pressure. Carbon dioxide results in prominent vasodilation in the uveal circulation (449) and reduces vascular resistance (418). Although stimulation of the cervical sympathetic fibers increases uveal vascular resistance (50, 51) and reduces blood flow, an increase in ciliary artery pressure could occur with consequent increases in uveal blood flow, probably partly as a result of generalized vasoconstriction in the head and nearby structures of the neck and ears. Hence generalized afferent stimuli triggering sympathetic nervous responses of vasoconstriction would, for the most part, be expected to prevent sudden shifts in ocular blood volume but may well cause an increase in blood flow to the eye in some instances.

The purpose of a responsive vascular bed must be to maintain a high rate of nutrient flow to the retina via the choriocapillaris. Rates of 12 ml/g per minute have been estimated (168, 417, 418). The choriocapillaris is a rich, vascular bed located for the greatest part in a single plane that equilibrates with a small volume of (retinal) tissue having a Q_{O_2} of 31. The retina itself receives about 2 ml/g per minute; however, one group of investigators reported a flow rate of 8 ml/g per minute for combined retina and choroid (168).

The ciliary body has an even higher rate of flow (33, 51), 20 ml/g per minute, but extracts oxygen much less efficiently than the retina. Based on tests using the clearance of ascorbic acid (33), changes in the rate of blood flow through the ciliary processes after sympathetic stimulation and denervation have been estimated. The rate of secretion of ascorbic acid into the aqueous humor is so high that at low plasma levels the rate of supply of ascorbic acid to the ciliary processes by the plasma flowing through them is the limiting factor in its transport. Since extraction of ascorbic acid under these conditions is virtually complete, it can be used for estimates of blood flow (33, 277, 278) in a manner analogous to that of p-aminohippuric acid in renal blood flow measurements. Neurohumoral-directed shifts in the distribution of blood flow within the uvea (95, 200) could be of importance in the regulation of aqueous formation and intraocular pressure.

INTRAOCULAR PRESSURE. A pressure within the eye is required to maintain its structural integrity and the position of the refractive surfaces of the eye relative to each other. The development and maintenance of an intraocular pressure depend on blood flow, but it is the energy available from the cellular metabolism of the epithelia of the ciliary processes that largely accounts for the extraction and formation of the aqueous humor [(108, 109, 166); Fig. 13]. Whether any central (370)

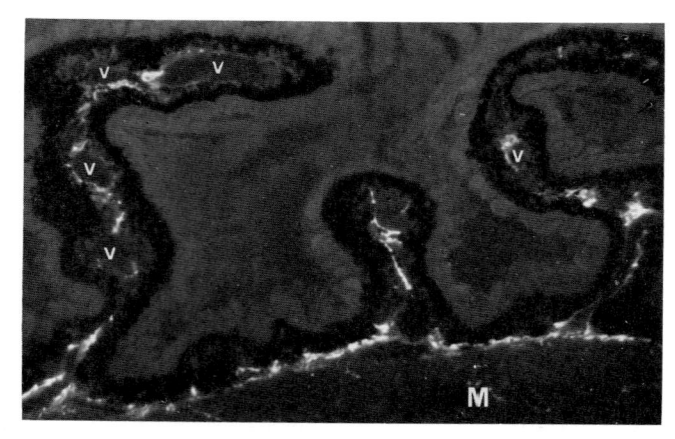

FIG. 13. Formaldehyde-induced fluorescence of adrenergic nerves in ciliary processes and ciliary body in vervet monkey, *Cercopithecus ethiops*. Adrenergic neurons appear as *bright strands* and *spots* in stroma of processes and in plexus under epithelium of ciliary body itself. V, blood vessels; M, ciliary muscle. × 157. (From B. Ehinger, unpublished observations.)

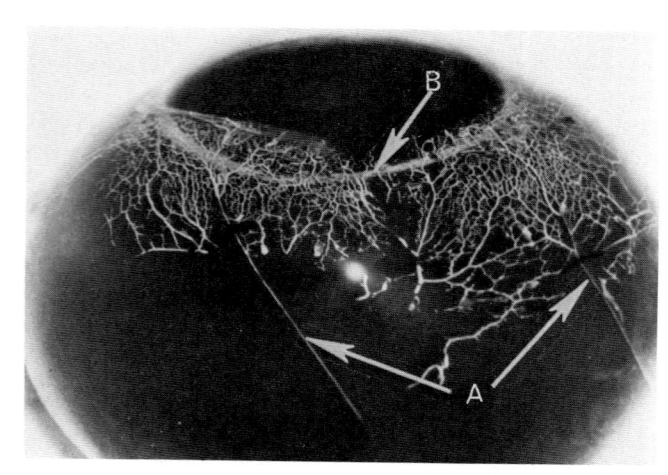

FIG. 14. Collector channels of human eye are injected with liquid silicone through fine-gauge cannulae (A), and later opaque scleral tissue is cleared with methylsalicylate. Schlemm's canal (B) and collector channels for outflow of aqueous humor are delineated. × 2.2. (From V. L. Jocson, unpublished observations.)

or humoral activators of this process can function independently of vasomotor influence (3) on the ciliary capillaries or independently of osmotic forces is a question still under investigation. The problem is not easily solved because of the difficulty in disentangling vascular effects on aqueous humor formation from the formation process itself (166). Studies of isolated ciliary processes lend some promise (36). In the intact eye, however, the techniques for measuring formation of aqueous humor are severely limited, demanding high technical skill to assure minimal disturbance of the eye. There is the usual requirement of intraocular cannulation for the purposes of perfusion and manometry. A complex accounting of the net movement of aqueous humor is necessary (55). Estimates of the formation of aqueous humor from manometric measurements of gross facility are approximate. An analysis must include components of gross facility, or true facility, as well as "pseudofacility," the pressure-sensitive part of aqueous formation (ultrafiltration) that appears as a facility in formulae for aqueous flow (19, 21, 55). When photofluorimetric techniques are used to determine aqueous formation (8, 183), values for the total turnover of fluorescein in the anterior chamber should include estimates of flow out of the anterior chamber by uveoscleral paths (21). Other techniques are useful but have different limitations (98, 149, 236).

Flow of aqueous humor through the trabecular meshwork and Schlemm's canal to the episcleral veins (Fig. 14) can be calculated from the equation

$$F_{trab} = (P_I - P_e)C_{out}$$

where P_I is the intraocular pressure; P_e, the venous pressure in the recipient episcleral veins at a point beyond influence of the intraocular pressure (zero point of Goldman); and C_{out}, the facility reciprocal of resistance of aqueous outflow. This equation should include uveoscleral flow, U, so that

$$F_{out} = (P_I - P_e)C_{out} + U$$

where F_{out} is total outflow of aqueous humor (315).

Uveoscleral flow. Particles injected into the anterior chamber make their way into the iris, ciliary body, and choroid. [Particles injected into the vitreous may enter and flow along the vessels of the optic nerve (162, 196).] Interest in this phenomenon was rekindled when a tracer substance introduced into the anterior chamber (52, 56) was recovered in the intraocular and episcleral tissues. The quantity of tracer was taken as an indication of the amount of water that must have gained access to this pathway. By this method it was shown in the monkey that a bulk flow of aqueous humor occurs from the anterior chamber into the stroma of the ciliary body and thereafter percolates or flows posteriorly toward the suprachoroid. [This process does not occur in the rabbit because the spaces of Fontana are lined with cells (349).] At least two uveoscleral exits for water are theoretically possible: *1*) out of the eye by way of the sclera (153); and *2*) reabsorption within the eye by the colloidal osmotic forces within the choroidal vessels. If the scleral path predominated, increased amounts of water would leave with increasing pressure. The phenomenon is independent of pressure, however. The juxtaposition of tissues with increases in intraocular pressure will have the effect of compacting the ciliary muscle and restricting posterior flow through its substance. Similarly uveoscleral flow is decreased by pilocarpine, but increased by atropine. Contraction (by pilocarpine) of the ciliary muscle may also close the interstices of the muscle to flow of water, whereas relaxation (by atropine) opens them (52). Uveoscleral flow may not exhibit pressure dependence because of this "artifact." The path is not known at present. Uveoscleral flow accounts for 4–14% of total flow in man (56).

Pseudofacility. The pressure-dependent trabecular outflow includes a pressure-sensitive part of aqueous humor formation (the ultrafiltration part) that appears as a facility of outflow with the manometric techniques usually employed for measurement of flow (19, 21). If raising intraocular pressure reduced the formation of fluid and if facility is determined by measuring, under an applied pressure, the flow of fluid from a cannula placed within the anterior chamber, more room would be available for inflow of fluid from the reservoir (109). The extra fluid entering for a given rise in pressure is expressed as a "pseudofacility" (i.e., the pressure-sensitive decrease in aqueous humor formation). When outflow measured manometrically in this way is compared with outflow determined by the clearance of ^{131}I from the anterior chamber both to the blood (trabecular outflow) and to scleral and episcleral tissues (uveoscleral flow), the net rate of secretion of fluid can be calculated from the differences found between the two methods (56). When this net secretion rate is calculated for different pressures, it decreases with increasing pressure. A rise in pressure causes a linear increase in trabecular outflow, but the uveoscleral flow does not change, so that a nonlinearity between pressure difference and inflow from the cannula develops. Under increased pressure the suppression of formation of aqueous humor, however, allows an "extra" influx of fluid from the cannula that may "compensate" for this and thereby leave the system with a linear relation between flow and pressure. True facility (C_{true}) and pseudofacility (C_{pseudo}) are related as follows

$$\frac{\Delta P_i}{\Delta P_e} = \frac{C_{true}}{C_{true} + C_{pseudo}}$$

where ΔP_i is a change in the steady-state intraocular pressure brought about by a change in episcleral venous pressure, ΔP_e. Various techniques have been developed to utilize this relationship (19, 21). Kupfer, who employed a neck cuff to elevate venous pressure, has had success in measuring pseudofacility in the human eye and in studying its pharmacological responses (255).

An expression of the relation of blood pressure, episcleral venous pressure, and uveoscleral flow to intraocular pressure is summarized (315)

$$P_I = P_a \frac{C_{in}}{C_{in} + C_{out}} + P_e \frac{C_{out}}{C_{in} + C_{out}} - U \frac{1}{C_{in} + C_{out}}$$

where P_I is intraocular pressure; P_a, ciliary artery blood pressure; C_{in}, facility of inflow (pseudofacility); C_{out}, trabecular facility of outflow; P_e, episcleral venous pressure; and U, uveoscleral outflow (see Table 1).

The process of formation has been studied and reviewed (95, 235, 236). The composition of the aqueous humor and the turnover of its constituents are largely known (29, 30, 95, 108, 109). The relation between colloidal osmotic and capillary pressures has been adequately summarized (19, 53). The secretory mechanism has been studied indirectly by mathematical treatment of time-concentration curves obtained from sam-

TABLE 1. *Representative Values in Expression of Relation of Blood and Episcleral Venous Pressures and Uveoscleral Flow to Intraocular Pressure*

Term	Definition	Value
B.P.	Brachial artery blood pressure	120/80 mmHg
P_a	Ciliary artery blood pressure*	60 mmHg
P_I	Intraocular pressure	15.5 mmHg
p_e	Episcleral venous pressure	8.0 mmHg
F_{in}	Rate of formation of aqueous humor†	2.1 µliter/min
U	Uveoscleral outflow	0.5 µliter/min
C_{in}	Facility of inflow	0.05 µliter/min per mmHg
C_{out}	Trabecular facility of outflow	0.21 µliter/min per mmHg
C_{total}	$C_{in} + C_{out}$	0.26 µliter/min per mmHg

* Equal to 0.6 mean B.P.   † At normal P_I.   [After Moses (315).]

ples of the posterior and anterior chambers. More direct approaches—perfusing the ciliary body or ocular chambers, as in cerebrospinal fluid studies—are frequently technically unsatisfactory, although supportive evidence for sodium as the primary secretate has been obtained (95).

The ciliary epithelia as glandular epithelia are unusual. Two layers of secretory cells are apposed apex-to-apex by embryogenesis. The base of the metabolically more active inner cell layer faces the posterior chamber. Extensive lateral interdigitations of this cell layer could represent the delivery site in the posterior chamber for a secretate. Movement of ions and water in this direction would then be comparable to the activity of the choroid plexus and perhaps some of the reabsorptive functions of the renal tubular epithelium (95). The ciliary epithelia do resemble these epithelia in several of their transporting properties. An outward-bound pump for anions has been studied in detail (29), but a study of the pharmacology of transport of substances into the eye, other than by use of conventional metabolic inhibitors, has not been made in detail.

Isolated preparations of ciliary processes were made years ago (166). A similar in vitro approach has been attempted to develop information about pharmacological receptors for secretion of aqueous humor by the ciliary processes. Planimetric measurements of photographs of optical sections of the processes may permit an estimate of the rate of shrinkage of the processes (36–38). Shrinkage is assumed to be a measure of transport across the processes. In this way vascular and other indirect effects on secretion are eliminated. Adrenergic compounds are among many that have been tested for their effects. Effects with epinephrine were unfortunately inconsistent. Norepinephrine and isoproterenol do not inhibit shrinkage (transport), but it is difficult in this in vitro system to tell whether stimulation occurs. Another approach to the preparation of the isolated ciliary processes has been to study the uptake and accu-

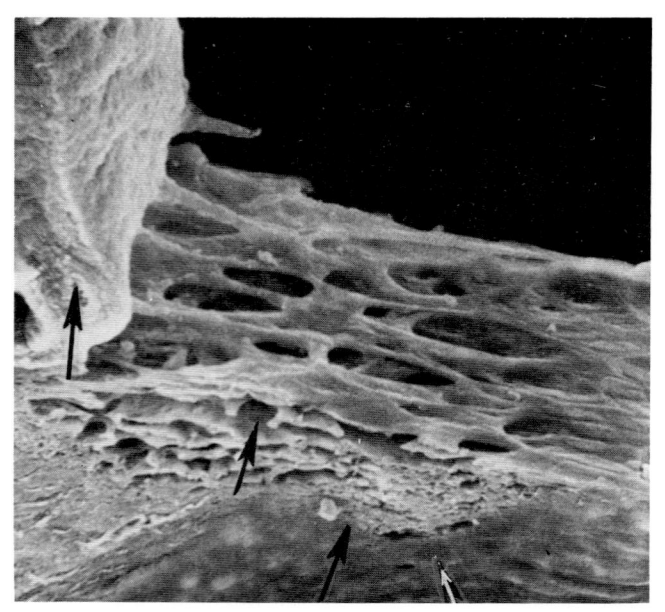

FIG. 15. Scanning photomicrograph of iridocorneal (chamber) angle. *Arrows* from left to right: iris; trabecular meshwork (large, 20–40-μ spaces); scleral spur; and canal of Schlemm, which is bifurcated by septa in this photo. × 89. [From Anderson (6a).]

mulation of substances by these processes (29, 30, 138). Here it is hoped that the accumulation of substances of the ciliary processes in vitro represents secretion of these substances in vivo. In the case of amino acids and amines, uptake was stimulated by low doses of norepinephrine and inhibited by high doses (435a). A start has been made, but data for the analysis of receptor mechanisms are far from sufficient.

The absence of nerves within the epithelial cell layers of the ciliary processes indicates that they are probably not under direct neural control, but neurohumoral reception may still be operative. Humoral influences on the process of secretion mediated by adenyl cyclase have not been fully studied (31, 217, 382, 448). One would expect to find such humoral activators for the secretory process linking in series the adenyl cyclase receptor with the system of Na-K-activated ATPases (95) present within the ciliary epithelia. The appropriate experiments have not yet been done.

Isolation of the outflow mechanism for study in vivo is also difficult. The use of the perfused, dead, enucleated eye has been very helpful, however, in developing important information about sites of resistance and other mechanical aspects of the outflow of aqueous humor through the trabecular meshwork and lumen of the canal of Schlemm and into the collector channels [see (144, 185) for review; Figs. 14 and 15].

The influence of the adrenergic nervous system on maintenance of intraocular pressure levels has been studied by *a*) electrical stimulation of the cervical sympathetic nerve, *b*) denervation (see section DENERVATION), *c*) degeneration release after denervation (see section DEGENERATION RELEASE), and *d*) exogenously administered adrenergic effectors and blocking agents. A clear picture of ordinary physiological receptor sites has not yet emerged, although studies of denervation and degeneration release have indicated the presence of an alpha receptor for the outflow of aqueous humor in the rabbit eye (353, 375, 380).

Electrical stimulation of the cervical sympathetic nerve of the rabbit causes a decrease in eye pressure (110, 321). Henderson & Starling (198) originally attributed this fall to constriction of the intraocular vessels so that the rate of ultrafiltration of aqueous humor was decreased. Even recent studies indicate that during and after prolonged stimulation the rate of blood flow through the ciliary processes may be decreased by as much as 50 % (265). A decrease in the rate of aqueous humor formation secondary to these vascular effects therefore is not unexpected. The vascular sites have alpha adrenergic receptors because the effects can be specifically blocked. Specific effects on aqueous formation have not been detected, however.

Electrical stimulation of the cervical sympathetic nerve in the rabbit causes a slight increase in outflow facility (decrease in outflow resistance) that is augmented by pretreatment of the animal with cocaine (330). These observations support data obtained from studies of denervation and degeneration release that alpha adrenergic reception mediates the outflow of aqueous humor. Stimulation of the cervical sympathetic nerve in the vervet monkey produces some slight increase in aqueous humor formation (54) but either no change or an increase in outflow resistance (83).

Studies of the effect of exogenously administered adrenergic effectors (208, 250), false transmitters (259, 332, 421), and blocking agents (69, 89, 99, 101, 232, 334) have produced a wide variety of results (186). Species differences, the use of both conscious and anesthetized animals and of different dosages with several routes of drug delivery, and delays in onset effects varying with the route have contributed to variation. Intrinsic activity of blocking agents (375) and nonadrenergic effects of some drugs, like the anesthetic properties of propranolol, have compounded the problem (224, 387). Other variations, especially in monkeys, are created by methods failing to distinguish between gross and true facility.

Systemic intravenous injections may have effects on distant organs with secondary effects on the eye that may either be transient or prolonged. Arterial injections close to the eye do not exclude vascular responses in these arteries. Topical application of adrenergic compounds requires penetration through a lipophilic layer, either the conjunctival or corneal epithelium. Furthermore topically applied drugs will affect both the arteries and veins over the surface of the eye, as well as internal structures. The extraocular vessels show strong alpha responses, but intraocular receptors for vessels (97), and especially ciliary epithelium and chamber angle, are poorly defined. Intraocular injections delivered by a single bolus or by perfusion can be made quantitatively and have the advantage of reaching the avascular chamber angle before affecting the vascular supply, especially if they are intracameral (i.e., injected into the anterior chamber). Intravitreal injections take a little longer and reach a wider variety of receptor sites. They more readily exert volumetric changes by diffuse effects on the choroidal vasculature and also affect both the ciliary processes and their blood supply and the chamber angle. Problems in the delivery system; the need to disentangle vascular from steady-state effects on aqueous humor formation; and the necessity to account for true facility, pseudofacility, pressure-dependent outflow (trabecular), and pressure-independent outflow (uveoscleral) make conclusions from in vivo studies hazardous, particularly when the pharmacological effects are small.

Some of the difficulties in interpreting data are apparent from the effects of topically applied adrenergic drugs in the human eye. The topical application of epinephrine, even in the presumably ordinarily innervated eyes of glaucomatous patients, is an effective method of reducing eye pressure (17, 32, 194, 239, 439, 440). Initial studies employing fluorescein turnover indicated that the pressure reduction was a consequence of decreased inflow (183). Later studies with tonographic techniques (similar to manometric methods in animals) showed that, 4–6 hr after administration of a single dose of epinephrine (245, 249) and even after 24 hr (340), an increase in outflow of aqueous humor occurred. But tonography measures gross facility only, and when these studies were repeated it was shown that a good part of this early facility increase is probably related to pseudofacility (255).

Minutes after topical application of epinephrine, the eye first becomes white and alpha effects may predominate and thus lead to a fall in ciliary blood flow. The effect on true outflow facility occurs hours to a day after topical epinephrine and takes place after the eye is no longer white. Often the eye is red at this time. Frequently the effect is greater in redder eyes. These intermediate effects, occurring after the eye is no longer white from vasoconstriction, are hard to explain but may involve the production and persistence of cyclic AMP in the aqueous humor. Topically administered adrenergic agonists increase cyclic AMP in the aqueous humor. This increase usually can be prevented by appropriate antagonists, and the direct intracameral injection of cyclic AMP in a final molar concentration (anterior chamber) of 4×10^{-4} mimics the decrease in intraocular pressure produced by these agents. Decreased responsiveness of the intraocular pressure to epinephrine due to prolonged daily treatment is accompanied by smaller increases in cyclic AMP in the aqueous humor (319a). Finally, after sympathetic denervation, a supersensitive response of the intraocular pressure to epinephrine is accompanied by an enhanced increase in the cyclic AMP content of the aqueous humor. The increase in outflow facility and increased cyclic AMP production are both two to three times normal. The idea that cyclic AMP is a mediator for increased outflow of aqueous humor seen several hours after topically applied adrenergic agents (16, 319b) is supported by the two- to threefold increase in outflow seen after direct intracameral injection of cyclic AMP. Whether aqueous cyclic AMP works directly on the trabecula as an extracellular intraocular messenger or acts to keep intracellular cyclic AMP of the trabecula elevated to produce a decrease in outflow resistance is not yet clear.

A biochemical explanation for these pharmacological actions of catecholamines on the aqueous outflow mechanism must await a better definition of the pharmacological receptor. Even in the rabbit eye, where adrenergic tone appears to be a primary regulator of outflow, questions remain unanswered. The adrenergic effect persists in the dead eye. It is therefore not vascular, nor is it likely to be mediated by the ciliary muscle. Besides, the ciliary muscle is sparse in the rabbit. In most species the endothelial cells of the meshwork and the canal of Schlemm are only occasionally innervated, yet the cells lining the canal have mitochondria, indented nuclei, and cytoplasmic, rodlike structures—all characteristic of cells with contractile properties. The augmented increase in outflow to alpha adrenergic agonists that occurs soon after ganglionectomy (379, 380) suggests true denervation supersensitivity of a contractile structure but does not specifically define the receptor or its mechanism.

The in vivo effects of the adrenergic compounds on intraocular pressure are tentatively outlined below.

a) Inflow. Adrenergic reception may influence inflow at either vascular or epithelial sites. Thus alpha receptors causing vasoconstriction may decrease inflow by reducing blood flow and ultrafiltration and thereby modifying or limiting the plasma filtrate (substrate) presented to the epithelia.

Alpha receptors are probably nonexistent in the ciliary epithelia themselves. Possibly there are beta receptors. After beta stimulation in the monkey an increase in inflow has been found (54). In the rabbit (126) and man (67, 352, 400) beta reception apparently suppresses formation of aqueous humor. The effects may be mediated by adenyl cyclase. In that case the results are unexpected in the sense that known catecholamine-activated beta receptors stimulate adenyl cyclase activity. It is possible that activities of Na-K-activated ATPase and adenyl cyclase in the ciliary epithelial cells are coupled in series, as in the renal tubule. The former may move sodium and water from the inner layer of the ciliary epithelia into the posterior chamber of the eye as the latter regulates the extraction of sodium from the stroma and outer epithelial layer for presentation to the sodium pump in the cell membrane of the inner epithelial layer. Topically applied isoproterenol apparently causes no tonographic change in outflow in the human eye, but the reported drop in pressure is presumably a result of decreased inflow (352, 440). In the rabbit, intraocularly administered isoproterenol apparently reduced pressure either by decreased inflow (126) or increased outflow (180). In the vervet monkey, stimulation of beta receptors by intraocular perfusion of isoproterenol can increase formation by 30% and increase outflow by 55% (54). [Beta blocking agents, whatever the route of administration, have poorly sustained effects (69, 426).]

b) Outflow. Alpha receptors in blood vessels may mediate arteriolar constriction and reduce episcleral venous pressure and thereby cause some slight increase in outflow (109, 373). These small effects may be prominent after intravenous, intraarterial, or topical administration of alpha adrenergic agents.

Major changes in outflow resistance at the level of Schlemm's canal and the trabecular meshwork, however, are caused by the ciliary muscle or by direct effects on the mesh (380). Muscular effects from the sparse ciliary body of the rabbit are unlikely with adrenergic agents, although there is speculation that the dilation of the iris might transmit mechanical pull onto the trabecula (22). Decreased resistance after intracameral (379, 380) and intravitreal (131) injections of alpha agonists indicates that the trabecular region of the rabbit does have prominent alpha receptors, but beta receptors are also present (180). This finding is not too surprising because alpha and beta receptors operate in the same direction in other ocular functions (164). In man, increases in outflow after treatment with beta stimulators have rarely been claimed (340), but decreased resistance is produced by isoproterenol in the vervet and other primates.

Finally, it is known that a puzzling progressive increase in outflow occurs over a period of weeks or even months with continued topical application of epinephrine (17, 32). The mechanism of these late or cumulative effects of adrenergics on outflow resistance (17) is not apparent. Concerning these delayed or cumulative effects, it is known that the meshwork is coated with a mucinous material: in the rabbit, hyaluronidase-sensitive hyaluronic acid; in man, perhaps another mucin. Such coating provides resistance to outflow and may be affected by adrenergic compounds. Experiments done in the aorta of rabbits indicate that epinephrine may decrease the production of mucoid substances (373). Similar effects in the trabecular meshwork could in time decrease resistance to aqueous outflow.

CORNEA AND LENS. The cornea is richly supplied with sensory fibers that form an annular plexus around its periphery. Fibers then pass into the cornea proper and ramify to form a plexus in the substantia propria from which fibers penetrate the elastic lamina to create a subepithelial plexus. Delicate fibers that branch between the epithelial cells emanate from the subepithelial plexus. Fibers from the annular and stromal plexuses may pass close to the corneal stromal cells. At least some of this innervation is sympathetic in the rat, rabbit, guinea pig, and cat. In embryonic cornea of primates a particularly rich, subepithelial adrenergic plexus adjacent to vessels exists (133, 134, 395). In rabbits the cornea of an eye deprived of its sympathetic innervation is less resistant to injury from quartz light than the cornea of the normally innervated fellow eye. Corneal defects produced by the quartz light also heal less promptly. These results were interpreted to indicate a trophic influence of the sympathetic nerve on tissue normally devoid of a blood circulation (87). The results of subsequent experiments suggested a similar trophic influence of the sympathetics on the corneal epithelial mitoses (167, 304). Tissue culture studies (72) of rabbit, dog, and human corneal epithelium indicated that epinephrine produced degenerative changes in the epithelial cells (244). Epinephrine applied topically also delays the epithelialization of a corneal wound. In this connection the reactivation of herpes limb paralysis (338) and herpes cornea (258) by the systemic and/or topical administration of epinephrine is interesting. Whether the failure of mitoses promotes the shedding of virus, however, is dubious because the mitotic rates of cells involved are so low anyway.

Nonetheless, even more recently, a role for epinephrine or norepinephrine as a mitotic control mechanism in the mammalian lens has been suggested (274, 435). In lens culture, epinephrine alone acts as a mitotic inhibitor. Norepinephrine is effective, but 10 times less so. Epinephrine, in conjunction with a water-soluble protein inhibitor of growth, has an interesting effect that norepinephrine does not have. In lenses cultured in vitro a chalone, very similar to one isolated from skin (71), exerts a mitotic inhibitory effect that is reversible but restored by washing the lens in epinephrine (2 μg/ml) but not in norepinephrine. On the contrary, lens epithelia taken from eyes of rabbits pretreated in vivo with atropine showed increases in mitoses and in the number of DNA-synthesizing cells (59). Although this latter study was designed to test the mechanical effect of accommodative movements of the lens on mitosis, there is the remote possibility of an autonomic regulatory effect on mitosis. The import of these studies for cell metabolism is not immediately apparent, particularly in light of the observation that the maximal depression in the mitotic rates for cornea and lens related to diurnal variation coincides with an elevated epinephrine concentration in blood, yet adrenalectomy has no effect on mitotic rate. Norepinephrine is not present within the aqueous humor under ordinary circumstances. Further any significant quantities would probably be liberated from the iris into the anterior, rather than the posterior, chamber. Finally the cellular activities carried out by a tissue should not be inferred from the content of enzymes within it. Although COMT and MAO activity are present in the lens (439), other transferases and oxidases are also. Their presence is somewhat analogous to the finding of acetylcholinesterase in the lens. The function of these enzymes in the lens is unknown. They may have come along with the lens as it pinched off from ectoderm during development.

INTRINSIC MUSCLE. *Pupillary movements.* The sympathetic nervous system is normally active at all times, and the degree of activity varies from moment to moment. In this manner, fine adjustments to a constantly changing environment can be accomplished. Dual innervations further provide for sensitive regulation because they may exert antagonistic effects. In the iris both the parasympathetic and sympathetic innervation are excitatory to their respective effectors, which then act antagonistically to regulate the diameter of the pupil.

The pupil serves three functions: *1)* it regulates the amount of light entering the eye; *2)* it increases the depth of focus of the eye by reducing the aperture of the optical system; and *3)* it decreases the effect of chromatic and spherical aberrations, especially in bright light when the pupil becomes small. One consequence of a reflex regulating the amount of light entering the eye might be to provide optimum apertures for visual acuity at varying light intensities (386). A large pupil admitting the maximum amount of light would appear to be advantageous at low luminance levels where acuity is limited by the rate at which light quanta activate retinal receptors. As luminance is increased into the photopic range, loss of image contrast resulting from optical aberrations, diffraction, and stray light limits acuity. The decrease in pupil size that normally accompanies increase of illumination should reduce the effect of optical aberrations on visual acuity. The idea of an optimum pupillary aperture for each luminance level can be supported by measurements of the relation among pupil size, luminance, and visual acuity (80). With an increase in pupil diameter the largest test objects are perceived at successively lower luminance levels up to a maximum pupil size of 8 mm, and with reduction of the test object size the optimum pupil diameter decreases progressively from 8 to 2 mm. For all test targets a rapid increase in threshold luminance occurs as the pupil diameter is decreased below 2 mm, because of diffraction effects. A good correspondence has been found between the natural pupil size at different luminance levels in fully adapted subjects and the mean values for optimum pupil size determined from the maxima of acuity curves (80).

The optimizing of visual acuity over a wide range of luminance by the pupillary light reflex is a major component in the response of man to sensory stimuli. At the same time the iris is an example of an autonomic neuroeffector strongly dominated by central nervous control. In other systems similarly dominated by the central nervous system, like the nictitans and the arteriovenous anastomosis of the foot pad, characteristics of the preganglionic sympathetic fibers to these effectors are their large diameter and low threshold (161). In some respects the functional characteristics of these neuroeffectors are related more to striated than to smooth muscle. It is not surprising to learn that the iris in nonmammalian vertebrates [e.g., turtle and bird (10, 35)] has a pupillary sphincter composed of striated muscle with the ordinary characteristics of a neuromuscular junction. In the fish (454) the dilator muscle is innervated by the oculomotor nerves, and the pupil dilates in response to acetylcholine and physostigmine, as well as to epinephrine.

The influence of the central nervous system on pupillary reflexes has created a need for a reproducible method of studying pupillary movements. The location of the pupillary reflex center for active dilation determined by pupillography (280) is placed cephalad to the midbrain but in a subcortical location effecting a pathway from the thalamus to the hypothalamus (280). The elements of the reflex are several (Fig. 16).

An interesting pupillary phenomenon is the residual dilation present after cervical sympathectomy (281). Although there may be a few ganglion cells in the iris, these exert effects of a very low order of magnitude. The phenomenon must therefore be ascribed to supranuclear inhibitory effects on the third nucleus. This concept has been supported by the finding that the iris fails to dilate after transection of the third nerve. Evidence for catecholamine-containing fibers specifically innervating and possibly modulating the Edinger-Westphal nucleus, but not the large-celled nuclei of the oculomotor complex, has been found. These fibers may play a role in the regulation of pupillary constriction.

The Argyll Robertson pupil of syphilis and other midbrain lesions is of interest (358). This pupil is miotic with a poor or absent pupillary reflex to light but preserved pupillary contraction to near vision. The pupillary light-near dissociation combined with miosis could be explained on the basis of a rostral midbrain lesion (281). The lesion should be located beyond the ventral hemidecussation of the light reflex path because impairment afferent to this decussation would involve both irises, and the pupil of Argyll Robertson may be unilateral. A small lesion just rostral to the Edinger-Westphal nucleus (i.e., a slightly dorsal location) would involve both crossed and uncrossed pretectal fibers and thus abolish the light reflex. The near vision fibers that approach the nucleus slightly more ventrally would be spared, and the pupillary light-near dissociation would be explained.

The mechanism of miosis in the Argyll Robertson pupil is cholinergically mediated sphincter contraction, because *a)* miosis is pronounced, *b)* the pupil does enlarge when the third nerve is subsequently blocked or damaged, and *c)* atropine, in the absence of iris damage, dilates the pupil.

Paralysis of the sympathetic nervous system has been dismissed as causal because *a)* miosis is more intense than that found in the usual Horner's syndrome, *b)* no other signs of sympathetic paralysis are seen, *c)* pupillary reflex dilation persists, and *d)* the conventional descending sympathetic fibers run lateral to the midline.

Compatible with these findings would be the hypothesis that a destructive lesion of a supranuclear inhibitory pathway to the Edinger-Westphal nucleus accounts for the mechanism of the Argyll Robertson pupil. The richly developed group of adrenergic fibers in the rat brain (106) that contain norepinephrine and 5-hydroxytryptamine in large amounts *a)* are supra-

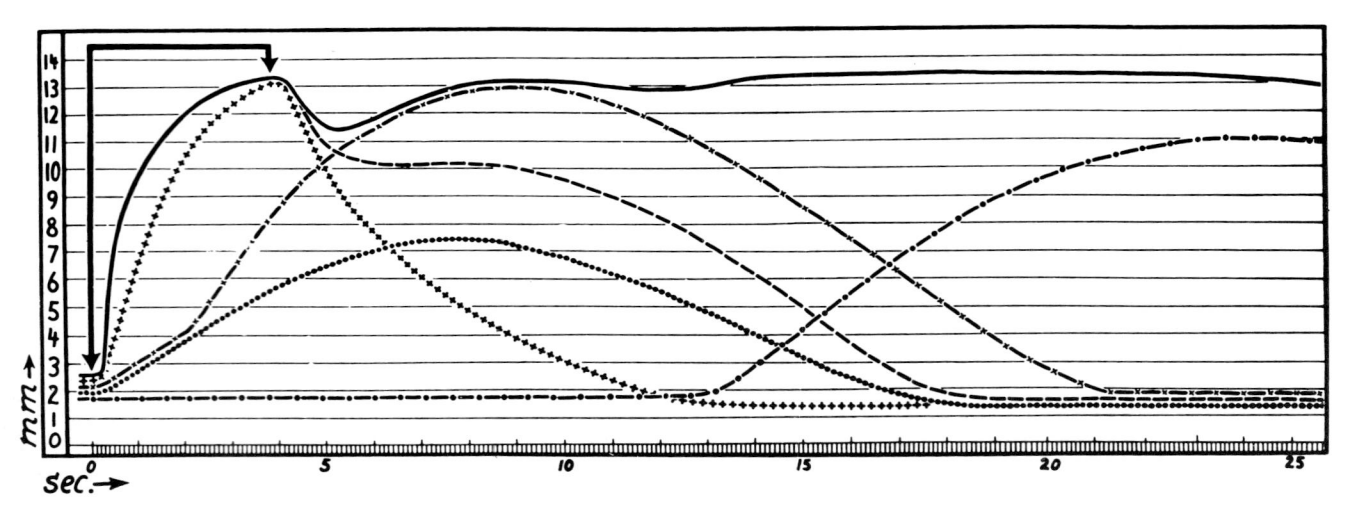

FIG. 16. Pupillary diameter is plotted on ordinate (in mm) against time on abscissa (in 0.1 sec). *Double arrow*, time of stimulation. *Solid line* represents complete response of normal pupil to strong stimulus of less than 5-sec duration (cortical, diencephalic, or sensory stimuli in non-narcotized cats, hypothalamic stimuli in narcotized animals). Pupil dilates with great rapidity and reaches maximal size within 3 to 4 sec. After initial contraction at end of stimulus, it dilates anew and may remain very large for several minutes. Analysis of this movement reveals the following component mechanisms.

1. Active innervation of dilator pupillae by sympathetic impulses that reach the eye via the cervical chain (*crosses*). This motion is characterized by relatively fast dilation and recontraction.

2. Inhibition of oculomotor nucleus (*dotted line*) leads to slower, longer-lasting pupillary dilation.

3. When iris has become hypersensitive to humoral substances after sympathetic denervation, acceleration of sympathectomized pupil's dilation becomes apparent within the second to third second of stimulation (*cross-dash line*). This acceleration is caused by adrenergic substances that reach the eye via the heart and/or arteries. Prolonged reaction causes "paradoxical" enlargement of sympathectomized pupil.

4. Epinephrine, reflexly poured out by adrenal glands and possibly other sources 12–15 sec after the start of stimulation, reaches the eye and may maintain maximal pupillary dilation for many minutes (*dash-dot line*).

5. *Dashed line* shows normal pupil's reaction to moderate sensory or central nervous stimulation. [From Loewenfeld (281).]

nuclear, *b*) contact specifically with the cells of the Edinger-Westphal group but not with those larger cells within the oculomotor complex, and therefore *c*) fit the requirement of a dorsomedial path (avoiding the ventral area described above). Interruption of this adrenergic pathway is compatible with the site required by the clinical and experimental data viewed to produce the Argyll Robertson pupil (281).

Whether the reserpine-induced miosis or enhanced light reflex is due to this sort of central mechanism is open to the same doubt that has been raised about the central induction of ptosis by reserpine. With low-to-ordinary doses of reserpine it is likely that these effects are the result of the peripheral action of the drug because of the parallel between the effector response, norepinephrine content of peripheral organs, and the temporal relation between changes of the two. Furthermore reserpine does not induce accommodation (407).

The miosis of sleep is open to similar speculation. During sleep the tone of both the ciliary muscle and iris is increased (39). It is not known whether the adrenergic pathway to the Edinger-Westphal nucleus is involved. Experiments indicating synchronization of the electro-encephalogram along with miosis (40, 75) as a result of the action of serotonin have been presented. The area postrema is thought to be involved with these actions associated with sleep. The smooth musculature of the eye itself is known to respond to serotonin (127, 241, 286, 372, 401). The connection between these central and peripheral effects of serotonin is not immediately apparent.

Although the reactions of the pupil are conditioned by the state of the whole nervous system and do not depend on the activity of an isolated reflex, valuable information regarding types of receptors and drug receptor mechanisms has been and will be obtained from studies of both the isolated perfused eye (28) and from isolated iris strips (27, 90, 125, 342, 359, 368, 437). In this way the influence of the whole organism on drug penetration, distribution, elimination, and changes related to adaptation is eliminated. A more precise quantitative study of the neuroeffector junction may be obtained.

Use of the isolated perfused eye (28) has the advantage of not injuring the intimate relation between the sphincter muscle fibers and Bruch's membrane (myo-epithelial contractile layer of the dilator muscle), as well as permitting the muscle to be suspended and to contract in an ordinary manner. Although drugs are not usually delivered from the arterial side, they could be delivered in such a manner, and artifacts of penetration avoided in this way, as well as by removal of the cornea. Furthermore information from these in vitro physiological studies can be correlated with the fiber anatomy. The thin-layered structure of the iris makes it ideal for study by the histologist (105, 135, 143), electron microscopist, and pharmacologist (70, 289, 290), as well as the clinician (60, 433, 445).

In the mammalian iris, there is a rich adrenergic innervation on the anterior surface of the dilator muscle (135). Often fluorescent fibers extend between muscle cells. In addition, the plexus of the pupillary edge is considered to form the adrenergic innervation of the sphincter. This plexus is especially well seen in transverse section. Cholinergic and adrenergic innervation to the sphincter has been demonstrated in the rat (291, 322) and cat (136), and this suggests the possibility of active innervation of the sphincter during dilation of the iris. How the postganglionic adrenergic fiber branches within the innervated tissue can be seen after partial denervation. A group of long preterminal axons extend to different parts of the iris (295). The systems of these terminals belonging to an individual neuron are distributed over large areas and support Hillarp's concept of convergence for the innervation of peripheral structures (204). Furthermore the same neuron can give excitatory and inhibitory innervation to antagonistic effectors. Although dual innervation provides for sensitive regulation, perhaps further fine regulation is provided by inhibitory sympathetic fibers that may be separate but are, on occasion, branches from one and the same neuron innervating the antagonistically acting muscles. Electron-microscopic studies of the innervation to the iris have shown a close intermingling of adrenergic and cholinergic axons in all parts of the iris plexuses (343, 345). With permanganate fixation the granular vesicles of the adrenergic nerves are better preserved and appear in greater numbers than with other modes of fixation (344). A side-by-side arrangement of cholinergic and adrenergic terminals is present within the strands of the autonomic ground plexus (323, 356). In the sphincter the former dominate, whereas in the dilator there is a considerably greater ratio of adrenergic to cholinergic axons even apart from vascular innervation. The suggestion that part of the cholinergic innervation comes from the superior cervical ganglion, based on histochemical evidence (221), is not supported by studies of fine structure of the iris (356), nor is the idea that acetylcholine and norepinephrine are released from the same axon terminal during stimulation. Although a close intermingling of adrenergic and cholinergic axons occurs, there are two distinct types of axons—those with agranular vesicles exclusively and those with predominantly granular vesicles (323, 356). The presence of agranular vesicles in axons with predominantly granular vesicles has been ascribed to preparation artifact. The side-by-side arrangement may still, however, have meaning for the hypothesis that norepinephrine release is mediated by acetylcholine.

The presence of adrenergic and cholinergic fibers in both sphincter (172, 324, 328) and dilator muscles (136, 148, 209–211, 291, 323, 345) complicates the pharmacological analysis of the pupillary muscles. Furthermore distribution of antagonistic alpha and beta adrenergic responses is unequal in both muscles (366–368). Quantitative aspects of these receptor activities have not been fully explored because of technical difficulties. The maximum tension developed by the iris muscles of smaller animals is less than 70 mg. A sphincter muscle strip from a larger animal has proved helpful (114, 331). Bovine iris sphincter appears to have a negligible number of excitatory alpha receptors and many beta adrenergic inhibitory receptors, which confirms the inhibitory effects of catecholamines found earlier (27, 339).

The presence of adrenergic inhibitory effects in the iris sphincter of cat (366, 429) and rabbit (428) has been well documented. These findings are consistent with the view that during mydriasis, in addition to active contraction of dilator fibers, there is active relaxation of sphincter muscle fibers (229).

Further studies of the neural control of the isolated iris from cats have been made in atropine-pretreated and in parasympathetically denervated preparations (368). The first and second peaks of electrically induced mydriasis were selectively suppressed by alpha and beta block, respectively. The first peak was attributed to active dilator contraction and the second to beta adrenergic sphincter relaxation. Pupillary width in the cat is controlled by beta-induced relaxation of the sphincter and contraction of the sphincter induced by acetylcholine and alpha reception. The beta effects are tuned to higher frequencies of stimulation than are the alpha effects. In the dilator muscle (367), beta activity and acetylcholine are found to cause relaxation, whereas alpha receptors mediate contraction of the dilator muscle. In the human it is generally believed that mydriatic action is largely mediated by alpha receptors (296, 422), whereas in the mouse both alpha and beta stimuli appear to act in the same direction (164).

A classification of the actions of sympathomimetic amines in various effectors, both denervated and normally innervated, led to the idea that the effects of certain amines might depend on the integrity of adrenergic nerve terminals, that is, the catecholamines may not act directly on adrenergic receptors (156–158, 257). A similar study (297) done in the iris of the cat indicated that after denervation *a*) the mydriatic action of nonphenolic phenylethylamines was lost; *b*) the threshold for the mydriatic dose was raised for substances with an OH group on either the phenyl ring or on the beta carbon atom of the side chain; *c*) an enhanced reaction with lowered threshold was found with substances having OH groups in the 3,4 position with or without a beta OH group on the side chain, or with substances having only one phenolic OH together with OH on the beta carbon atom of side chain.

Thus three groups of amines (with overlap) were distinguished: *1)* those potentiated by denervation and cocaine (direct-acting amines); *2)* those not much affected by either procedure (mixed-acting amines); and *3)* those definitely less effective after denervation or cocaine (indirect-acting amines). Examples of each category would be norepinephrine, ephedrine, and tyramine, respectively. In the case of the latter category, the hypothesis is advanced that tyramine and other similar compounds act by displacing norepinephrine from intraneuronal particles.

The clinical differentiation among lesions of the central, preganglionic, and postganglionic sympathetic fibers can be made, within certain limits, on the basis of the different reactions of the miotic pupil or ptotic lid, or both, to the topical application of compounds in the above categories. Topographic localization of lesions within the sympathetic fibers was attempted early in the 1900s (92, 160). The problems with the approach are the variables associated with penetration of the test drug through the intact cornea and inadequate knowledge of the precise degree of completeness of the destructive lesion. Positive reactions are helpful. Thus, for example, in a normal eye, cocaine will dilate the pupil because reuptake of endogenous norepinephrine present and tonically released from the nerve terminals of the iris will be blocked and amounts of norepinephrine will then be available to the iris muscle. Topically applied norepinephrine (except in large doses) will not dilate the normal pupil because not enough enters the iris. In the absence of endogenous norepinephrine stores (i.e., with postganglionic lesions), cocaine will have no effect, but topical norepinephrine may (depending on penetration) dilate the pupil, because a smaller amount is now required for a response. When the stores are intact, the indirect-acting amines, such as tyramine, hydroxyamphetamine (403), and amphetamine, will dilate the pupil. When the stores have been disrupted, only the direct-acting amines will dilate the pupil. Dopamine also acts on the human iris (394). In the course of treatment of Parkinsonian patients with L-dopa, a subtle postganglionic Horner's syndrome may become manifest by the dilating action of dopamine on the contralateral normal pupil (443). A more complete description of the actions of the amines, based on similar experiments, has been given by Trendelenburg (413).

Ciliary body and accommodation. The amplitude of accommodation is expressed by the number of diopters added to the refractive power of the eye by the action of the ciliary muscle. Accommodation is largely dependent on the dominant cholinergic innervation to that muscle. The nature of the adrenergic innervation to the ciliary muscle has long been a matter of debate, first as to its existence and later as to its specificity for muscular, as opposed to vascular, receptors. In the ciliary body, fluorescent adrenergic fibers form an uninterrupted layer under the basement membrane of ciliary epithelium (135, 271, 272, 395). The fibers are finely meshed around vessels and at the base of the ciliary processes themselves. Neither cholinergic fibers nor these fibers in the subepithelial plexus have been shown to penetrate the basal membrane of the ciliary epithelium, so there is no evidence for a direct sympathetic innervation of these glandular cells (Fig. 13). There is also a diffuse distribution of adrenergic fibers in the richly vascularized tissue of the muscle bundles themselves.

It had early been noted that a relaxation of the ciliary muscle occurs after application of cocaine to the eye (311). Later a flattening of the lens was observed after stimulation of the cervical sympathetic nerve (313). For these reasons it became interesting to consider whether adrenergic influences over accommodation were present and how they were exerted (312). Early theories of accommodation [see (311) for historical discussion] based on changes in length of the eyeball, in corneal curvature, or in position of the crystalline lens were easily dismissed by Young. Young, together with Helmholtz, proposed the theory of a decrease in forces working on the lens capsule, a hypothesis that displaced two earlier ideas. One of these, the hydraulic theory, was based on a transfer of fluid from the front of the lens to its circumference that caused increased lenticular refraction power. The second, the theory of increased tension, championed by Mannhardt and then Tscherning, stated that ciliary muscle contraction caused pressure on the vitreous body, which then forced the lens to assume a hyperbolic shape. The theory of decreased tension seemed more reasonable. The idea was that a neutralization of the pull of the suspensory ligaments (zonules) on the elastic capsule of the lens occurred as the ciliary muscle contracted and moved forward. This forward movement can actually be witnessed in the dead, enucleated cat eye through a scleral window (300). Now when nerve stumps of this eye preparation (that included sympathetic fibers) were stimulated, a radial inward (slightly posterior) movement of the ciliary muscle occurred. These findings tended to support Henderson's idea that the radial and longitudinal elements of the ciliary muscle caused negative accommodation, whereas circular elements caused positive (increased refractive power) accommodation. These experiments in the dead eye are supported by observations with the electron microscope that the human ciliary muscle consists of bundles of tightly packed muscle cells (384) with each bundle containing its own supply of nerve terminals (218). Independent functional units (346) have been found in vivo, and the macroscopic observations of focal areas of constriction and relaxation indicate further a lack of syncytial organization and the absence of spread of excitation (24).

Results of investigations in the dead eye have argued against a change in the vascular volume of the ciliary body as responsible for significant changes in accommodation amplitude. This idea gained favor before evidence for specific innervation to the ciliary muscle, apart from that to its blood vessels, was obtained (135,

159, 173). Its presence within muscle tissue is supported by physiological experiments, as well as by electron-microscopic observations (206, 424). In the monkey, stimulation of the sympathetic nerves decreases cholinergically induced accommodation, an effect blocked by guanethidine (409). Then it was shown that beta adrenergic blockade caused a complete elimination of the decrease in accommodative power induced by sympathetic stimulation (406). Atropine and alpha adrenergic blockade were without effect on the distance (decrease in) accommodation induced by sympathetic stimulation. These observations would indicate that changes in the vasculature play no part in regulating accommodation. Since the experiments were monitored for an overall change in ocular volume, however, it might be argued that local or specific changes in ciliary blood volume would not be detected. The merits of background vascular action versus specific muscular action could be pressed further because phenylephrine, an alpha-active agent, depressed the graded changes in accommodation elicited by electrical stimulation of the midbrain in the monkeys, *Macaca irus* and *Aotus trivigatus* (88). Additional factors that must be considered are the secondary influences on the ciliary muscle resulting from the equilibrium existing among intraocular pressure, blood circulation, and oxygenation (74, 407). Similar considerations apply to the pupil (85, 423). The uniqueness of the beta adrenergic response in the monkey (406, 408), however, taken together with the experiments made in the dead eye, indicate that the decreased amplitude of accommodation noted after sympathetic stimulation is related to specific muscular effects rather than to passive vascular influences.

In other species a variety of receptors may be involved. In the cat the influence of the adrenergics is mainly on beta receptors, but some alpha receptors appear to be present (400, 429). In the rabbit, on the other hand, a sparse ciliary muscle appears to have receptors of the alpha type (428). A flattening of the lens resulting from sympathetic stimulation causes only a small decrease in dioptric power in this animal (159) and could conceivably be related to changes in the vasculature (311, 312). In man the original observations, made in five patients with Horner's syndrome, of a small increase in accommodative amplitude (93) and later studies of drug-induced increases in negative accommodation indicate that an adrenergic influence, probably of the alpha type, on distance accommodation can be identified (47). Whether these changes in the human eye are of a vascular or muscular nature has not yet been completely clarified. They are likely the latter.

VITREOUS. No drugs have been reported to act selectively on the movement of the vitreous humor (185). The latter is a hydrophilic gel constituted by a matrix of fibrous collagen and hyaluronic acid. The water and solutes in the gel are in free exchange with the aqueous humor. The fibrous protein is known to have contractile properties influenced by the tonicity and pH of the media. The vitreous maintains the shape of the normal eye. Its forward movement after cataract surgery, however, can cause adherence to the cataract wound, iris, or cornea, or all three. Visual loss from such adhesions results from changes in the macula and sometimes from retinal detachment.

Attempts to influence the forward movement of the vitreous have been made by using hyperosmolar agents that act to dehydrate the gel. Recent experiments with cocaine indicate that the gel itself can be made to retreat posteriorly from the anterior segment. This retraction of the anterior hyaloid contour (face) occurs even in eyes with dilated pupils indicating that pupillary size alone is not responsible. The effect comes on within 10 min and lasts for several hours. A reduction in choroidal blood volume probably permits the retraction of the vitreous. This effect of cocaine relates to its ability to enhance the action of endogenously, as well as exogenously, applied adrenergic agonists by preventing their axonal uptake (376a).

ADRENERGICS AND OCULAR PIGMENT

Intraocular melanin is found in the pigment epithelium of the retina, iris, and ciliary body, and in the melanocytes of the uveal tract (302). The latter form a pseudosyncytium of branching cells, probably stimulated by the sympathetics (177). Other factors determining eye color are heredity (124, 347), melanocyte-stimulating hormone (355), and other biochemical factors governing the metabolism of melanin (299, 355).

Sympathetic cells and melanocytes originate from the neural crest. The pigmented cells of the posterior surface of the iris arise from those neuroectodermal cells that separate from the outer wall of the optic cup before pigment migration. The anterior portion of the iris arises from the mesoderm and cells that migrate from the neural crest. Under sympathetic influence these cells, stellate-shaped melanophores, travel into the iris and choroid. The trail they leave can be followed by a dopa staining technique (43, 314). The sympathetic nervous system influences the development of melanin pigment and therefore iris color. In the absence of sympathetic input the iris remains hypopigmented because the chromatophores fail to migrate.

Pigmentary anomalies result from section of the sympathetic fibers (e.g., injury to the brachial plexus during birth). It is generally believed that lack of pigmentation, rather than depigmentation, is associated with injury to sympathetic fibers. The evidence for this comes from the observation that pigmentation is recovered after injury. After 2 years of age, however, recovery is not usually seen. Depigmentation after injury to the cervical sympathetic chain in adults usually does not occur, although instances have been reported in man, adult cats, and pigmented rabbits (141). The depigmentation after an injury or lesion to sympathetic fibers suggests some kind of slowly acting trophic influence on the melanocytes. Interestingly no instance of choroidal or iris melanoma has been reported in eyes of patients with Horner's syndrome. It has been suggested that loss of control of tyrosinases may be related in some way to ocular melanoma. None of this enzyme is found in the retinal pigment epithelium of chicks on or after the 14th day (308). Malignant tumors of the choroid (melanocytes) are common, but tumors of the retinal pigment epithelium are most unusual. A preliminary study of the histofluorescence of ocular melanomas has not yet revealed any relation of fluorescent pattern or tyrosinase content to cell type or behavior (142, 354).

A rapid mechanism for color changing is lacking in mammals, but in lower animals rapid and often localized color changes are under neural control. Direct innervation has been seen in fish (222) and amphibians. Studies with electron microscopy (155) and fluorescence microscopy (139) indicate the presence of adrenergic terminals in close contact with melanophores in the choroid and iris. The appositions have the same appearance as synapses in peripheral tissues. In frogs, changes in skin color can be influenced by endocrine secretions (299). Thus lightening, the aggregation of melanophores, is mediated by an alpha receptor and provoked by melanotonin, phenylephrine, and acetylcholine. Darkening, the dispersion of melanophores, is mediated by a beta receptor and is provoked by melanocyte-stimulating hormone, adrenocorticotropin, caffeine, isoproterenol, and cyclic AMP. There is no evidence that the iris is under similar humoral controls.

Relation of Mydriasis to Iris Pigmentation

Clinical impressions that lightly colored irises respond differently from those that are dark in color to mydriatics has prompted a series of studies (327, 392). In isolated albino and pigmented guinea pig eyes with pupils constricted to a base line with methacholine, pigmented irises were one-third as sensitive to ephedrine mydriasis as were albinos (381). This did not occur with other mydriatics. The effect was not prevented by beta blockade; higher concentrations of ephedrine were antagonized only slightly by alpha blocking agents, but lower concentrations were not. It is likely therefore that ephedrine mydriasis is involved with other than alpha or beta adrenergic receptors (381).

Differences between the mydriatic response in darkly pigmented and lightly pigmented irises are therefore altogether not related to mechanical immobility of the former. Nor would the experiments described above support the suggestion that the sensitivity differences be attributed to a greater tyrosinase activity in the heavily pigmented iris (7). Although on occasion, selective absorption by pigment granules (331a) and the rates of penetration of the drugs tested may be important factors, in this instance they are ruled out by the selectivity of the phenomenon for molecular structure (i.e., the presence of a methyl group on the alpha carbon and of a hydroxyl group on the beta carbon of the phenylalkylamine).

Dilation of the pupil often causes an appearance of floaters (i.e., pigment granules having the same characteristics as the granules contained by the pigment epithelial cells of the iris) in the aqueous humor (189, 307). Sympathomimetic agents caused the most marked effect. The floaters appear within 30 min after application of the drug, and their duration depends on several factors, including the rate of exit of the aqueous humor from the eye. When the dilator contracts, a contraction of the pigment epithelium results because the dilator muscle of the iris is a thin membrane adherent to the pigment epithelium. With degenerative changes in the iris, release of granules from the cells on its posterior portion readily occurs. The effect with parasympatholytic agents is either absent or not nearly so marked because in this case the iris sphincter is affected, and thus the pupil is allowed to dilate more passively, possibly by virtue of the elastic stroma.

Pigment in Nuclear Portion of Crystalline Lens

The pigments in the crystalline lens have defied identification, probably because they are present in such small amounts (182, 337, 456). An early idea was that blood pigments or their degradation products accumulated in the lens and caused it to turn yellow. Even recently, comparisons of pigment from normal and cataractous human lenses with urochrome showed similarity. Another theory held that basic protein, protamine or histone, liberated from disintegrating fiber nuclei during "sclerosis," combined with cysteine to yield a precipitate that darkened in time. Free cysteine was not found in the lens, however.

The pigmentation in the vertebrate lens has been observed to occur only in strictly diurnal species. Within a group of related species the presence or absence of pigment was correlated with the animals' habits. Supporting this observation is the recent contention that the reaction of photo-oxidized compounds with proteins within the lens may cause some opacification. Brown fluorescent proteins accumulate in some forms of nuclear cataract in man. Similar proteins may be produced in vitro when bovine lens proteins are treated with tyrosine and its oxidizing systems, or when 1,2-naphthaquinine is formed in naphthalene-fed animals; 1,2-naphthaquinine has a yellow color, and its reaction with lens proteins leads to the formation of red-brown proteins. The finding that a compound of low molecular weight could alter the properties of protein gave rise to the idea that the gradual increase in color in some cataracts might be due to a similar reaction. The suggestion has been made that substances from the aqueous humor may diffuse into the lens to form a brown cataract. The rich supply of tyrosinase in the iris and ciliary body could oxidize tyrosine to form a dopaquinone that may link with lens protein. The finding of brown lenses in complete albinos, however, is compatible with the idea that tyrosine and other aromatic amino acids can be nonenzymatically photo-oxidized by light of near-ultraviolet wavelength (456). Indeed it has been shown that human lenses in vitro contain quantities of near-ultraviolet-sensitive substances sufficient to cause darkening of the lens from exposure to near-ultraviolet light at levels not in excess of those present in sunlight (337a). Direct exposure of lens proteins to sunlight (457) or exposure of the aromatic amino acids comprising them to near-ultraviolet light (337a) produces photoproducts that are bound to lens proteins and so alter them. So it appears that yellowing and browning of the lens may occur nonenzymatically in the laboratory. The entire reaction may protect the retina from toxic effects of light. In these connections the toxicity of phenothiazines in causing cataract is interesting. In this instance the cataracts are cortical and not nuclear. Evidence has been presented to indicate an effect of the drug in increasing membrane permeability to oxidizing enzymes of the tyrosinase group (431).

RETINA

Surprisingly, adrenergic neurons have been found in the inner part of the inner nuclear layer of the vertebrate retina, with synaptic terminals located in a well-defined zone of the outer portion of the inner plexiform layer (Fig. 17). The original description, in the retina of rats, of adrenergic perikaryra in the innermost cell rows of the inner cell area (289) was later supplemented by the finding of several tiers of fluorescent varicose terminals in the inner plexiform and ganglion cell layers (140). Dopamine, the amine responsible for the fluorescence, was first identified in the rabbit retina (190, 191) and later in the retina of the perch and trout (140), dog (365), and frog (369). At least some of the dopamine-containing cells appear to be amacrines, and these constitute about 5–10% of the total cell population. In the cichlid and perch, vertical fibers from these cells connect the inner and outer plexiform layers and thereby supplement the well-known bipolar synaptic connections (140).

To speculate on the function of these cells, it is necessary to consider the sites of interaction and major synaptic pathways that occur within the vertebrate retina (118, 333). The retina is constructed from five types of neurons and one type of glial cell. The cell bodies are organized into three nuclear layers. The synapses are largely confined to two areas, the outer and inner plexiform layers.

The outer plexiform layer is concerned mainly with the static or spatial aspects of illumination in the receptors. In the outer plexiform layer, processes from the bipolar and horizontal cells extend to the photoreceptor terminals. Horizontal cells generally have a much wider spread than do bipolar cells and probably mediate lateral interactions within the outer plexiform layer. The bipolar cells carry information from the outer to the inner plexiform layer. Here processes from bipolar, amacrine, and ganglion cells interact. The processes of some amacrine cells extend laterally for considerable distances. They are often the longest processes found anywhere in the vertebrate retina. Many conventional synapses of amacrine cells are seen in the inner plexiform layer as bipolar, ganglion, and other amacrine cell processes. Unconventional contacts by these amacrines include reciprocal synapses and serial synapses (118). Amacrine cells accentuate the changes in retinal illumination, and they respond briskly to moving stimuli. Amacrines therefore play an important role in the organization of receptive fields of the retina. Among vertebrate species, a spectrum of complexity exists with respect to receptive field organization. When receptive field organization is simple, bipolar terminals make numerous direct contacts with ganglion cells. When receptive field organization is complex, there are signifi-

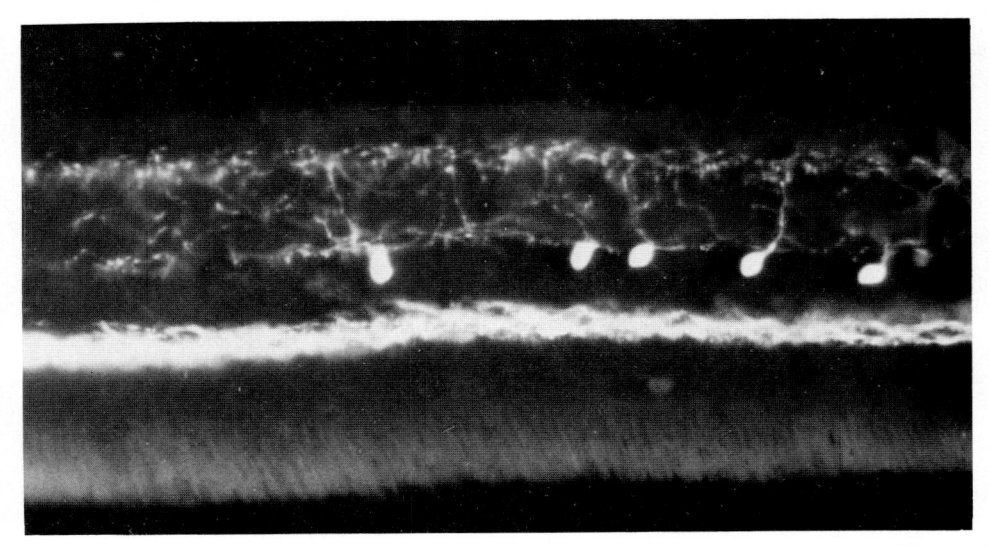

FIG. 17. Within inner plexiform layer of retina, 3 sublayers of varicose adrenergic fibers originate from adjoining fluorescent cells of the inner nuclear layer. Greatest fiber density is just beneath the ganglion cell layer. Fluorescent cell bodies seen here constitute 5–10% of total cell population of inner nuclear layer. Perch retina preparation. × 309. [From Ehinger et al. (140).]

cantly more amacrine synapses and amacrine interactions. These observations suggest that amacrines of the inner plexiform layer mediate complex interactions, such as motion detection and directional selectivity, and may provide primary input into the ganglion cells.

Ganglion cell recordings made in an isolated perfused retinal preparation (6, 397) do not yet permit the conclusion that dopamine contained within the amacrine system serves as a modulator of intraretinal synaptic transmission. Other circumstantial evidence bearing on this question includes the presence of an adenyl cyclase specifically activated by dopamine present in retinal tissue (68a) and the influences of light and dark on retinal dopamine (119, 120, 320). The parallelism to the dopamine-containing interneurons that modulate synaptic transmission in the superior cervical ganglion is intriguing, however.

ADRENAL MEDULLA

An eye deprived of the adrenal medullary secretion is apparently not very different from its normal counterpart. Inherent vascular tone is modified by changes in local neural and metabolic activity. Pupil size is largely determined by central mechanisms (280). Autonomic tone tends to minimize interindividual differences (between eyes) that exist with respect to the outflow of aqueous humor, but such tone is not medullary dependent. The bulk of evidence in a variety of experimental animals indicates that no local regulatory mechanisms for the control of the ocular (uveal) circulation exist (51), nor is there evidence that regulation or circulatory and other ocular parameters are significantly influenced by the adrenal medulla. Ordinarily one might imagine that the medullary secretion would produce a smooth homogenous response in tissues that might, for reason of point-to-point variation in density of innervation, otherwise exhibit some degree of heterogeneity. The richness of the adrenergic innervation to the uvea, however, is predominant. Sympathetic responses to a mass systemic stimulus (e.g., local intense vasoconstriction) "protect" the eye against a large rise in arterial pressure. [With reductions in arterial pressure, the uveal vascular bed behaves rather passively since the fall in uveal blood flow and pressure is proportional to the fall in arterial perfusion pressure (51).] After carotid occlusion the fall in carotid pressure tends to be determined by the impulse frequency (tone) in the fibers of the cervical sympathetic chain (50).

In instances of adrenergic denervation of the eye, the phenomenon of paradoxical pupillary dilation, supersensitivity secondary to the circulating medullary hormones, is well known.

REFERENCES

1. ABEL, J. H., JR., AND R. A. ELLIS. Histochemical and electron-microscopic observations on the salt-secreting lacrymal glands of marine turtles. *Am. J. Anat.* 118: 337–358, 1966.
2. ACHESON, G. H., A. ROSENBLUETH, AND P. F. PARTINGTON. Some afferent nerves producing reflex responses of the nictitating membrane. *Am. J. Physiol.* 115: 308–316, 1936.
3. ADLER, F. H., E. M. LANDIS, AND C. L. JACKSON. The tonic effect of the sympathetic on the ocular blood vessels. *Arch. Ophthalmol.* 53: 239–253, 1924.
4. ALPERN, M., AND J. R. WOLTER. The relation of horizontal saccadic and vergence movements. *Arch. Ophthalmol.* 56: 685–690, 1956.
5. AMBACHE, N., L. KAVANAGH, AND J. WHITING. Effect of mechanical stimulation on rabbit eyes: release of active substance in anterior chamber perfusates. *J. Physiol., London* 176: 378–408, 1965.
6. AMES, A., III, AND D. A. POLLEN. Neurotransmission in central nervous tissue: a study of isolated rabbit retina. *J. Neurophysiol.* 32: 424–442, 1969.
6a. ANDERSON, D. Experimental alpha chymotrypsin glaucoma studied by scanning electron microscopy. *Am. J. Ophthalmol.* 71: 470–476, 1971.
7. ANGENENT, W. J., AND G. B. KOELLE. A possible enzymatic basis for the differential action of mydriatics on light and dark irides. *J. Physiol., London* 119: 102–117, 1953.
8. ANSELMI, P., A. J. BRON, AND D. M. MAURICE. Action of drugs on the aqueous flow in man measured by fluorophotometry. *Exptl. Eye Res.* 7: 487–496, 1968.
9. ARENSON, M. S., AND H. WILSON. The peripheral parasympathetic innervation of the cat lacrimal gland. *Brit. J. Pharmacol.* 39: 242–243, 1970.
10. ARMSTRONG, P. B. Choline esterase at the nerve termination in the sphincter pupillae of the turtle. *J. Cell Comp. Physiol.* 22: 1–20, 1943.
11. ASHTON, N. Observations on the choroidal circulation. *Brit. J. Ophthalmol.* 36: 465–481, 1952.
12. ASHTON, N., AND F. DE OLIVEIRA. Nomenclature of pericytes. *Brit. J. Ophthalmol.* 50: 119–123, 1966.
13. ATKINSON, R. A., D. WITT, AND J. D. LONG. Mechanism of the sympathomimetic response of the cat's iris to nicotine. *J. Pharmacol. Exptl. Therap.* 147: 172–180, 1965.
14. AXELROD, J., G. HERTTING, AND L. POTTER. Effect of drugs on the uptake and release of ^{3}H-norepinephrine in the rat heart. *Nature* 194: 297, 1962.
15. BACQ, Z. M. Recherches sur la physiologie du système nerveux autonome. III. Les propriétés biologiques et physico-chimiques de la sympathine comparées à celles de l'adrénaline. *Arch. Intern. Physiol.* 36: 167–246, 1933.
16. BALDWIN, H. A., L. D. ZELEZNICK, AND F. E. LEADERS, JR. Effect of intraocular dibutyryl-cyclic AMP on outflow facility in the rabbit. *Pharmacologist* 12: 290, 1970.
17. BALLINTINE, E. J., AND L. L. GARNER. Improvement of the coefficient of outflow in glaucomatous eyes. Prolonged local treatment with epinephrine. *Arch. Ophthalmol.* 66: 314–317, 1961.
18. BÁRÁNY, E. H. Transient increase in outflow facility after superior cervical ganglionectomy in rabbits. *Arch. Ophthalmol.* 67: 303–311, 1962.
19. BÁRÁNY, E. H. A mathematical formulation of intraocular pressure as dependent on secretion, ultrafiltration, bulk outflow and osmotic reabsorption of fluid. *Invest. Ophthalmol.* 2: 584–590, 1963.
20. BÁRÁNY, E. H. Simultaneous measurement of changing intraocular pressure and outflow facility in the vervet monkey by constant pressure infusion. *Invest. Ophthalmol.* 3: 135–143, 1964.
21. BÁRÁNY, E. H. Pseudofacility and uveo-scleral outflow routes. Some non-technical difficulties in the determination of out-

flow facility and rate of formation of aqueous humour. In: *Glaucoma Symposium, Tutzing Castle, 1966*, edited by J. W. Rohen. New York: Karger, 1967, p. 27–51.
22. BÁRÁNY, E. H. Topical epinephrine effects on true outflow resistance and pseudofacility in vervet monkeys studied by a new anterior chamber perfusion technique. *Invest. Ophthalmol.* 7: 88–104, 1968.
23. BÁRÁNY, E. H., AND H. B. GASSMANN. The effect of death on outflow resistance in normal and sympathectomized rabbit eyes. *Invest. Ophthalmol.* 4: 206–210, 1965.
24. BÁRÁNY, E. H., AND J. W. ROHEN. Localized contraction and relaxation within the ciliary muscle of the vervet monkey, *Cercopithecus ethiops. Symp. Eye Structure, 2nd, 1965*, p. 287–311.
24a. BÁRÁNY, E. H., AND G. TREISTER. Release of smooth-muscle-active substance besides noradrenaline from degenerating terminals in the rabbit eye. *Acta Physiol. Scand.* 79: 287–288, 1970.
25. BÁRÁNY, E. H., AND G. TREISTER. Time relations of degeneration mydriasis and degeneration vasoconstriction in the rabbit ear after sympathetic denervation. Effect of bretylium. *Acta Physiol. Scand.* 80: 79–92, 1970.
26. BARLOW, C. M., AND W. S. ROOT. The ocular sympathetic path between the superior cervical ganglion and the orbit in the cat. *J. Comp. Neurol.* 91: 195–207, 1949.
27. BEAN, J. W., AND D. F. BOHR. Effects of adrenalin and acetylcholine on isolated iris muscle in relation to pupillary regulation. *Am. J. Physiol.* 133: 106–111, 1941.
28. BEAVER, W. T., AND W. F. RIKER. The quantitative evaluation of autonomic drugs on the isolated eye. *J. Pharmacol. Exptl. Therap.* 138: 48–56, 1962.
29. BECKER, B. The measurement of rate of aqueous flow with iodide. *Invest. Ophthalmol.* 1: 52–58, 1962.
30. BECKER, B. Ascorbate transport in guinea pig eyes. *Invest. Ophthalmol.* 6: 410–415, 1967.
31. BECKER, B., AND R. E. CHRISTENSEN. Beta hypophamine (vasopressin). Its effect upon intraocular pressure and aqueous flow in normal and glaucomatous eyes. *Arch. Ophthalmol.* 56: 1–9, 1956.
32. BECKER, B., AND A. P. LEY. Epinephrine and acetazolamine in the therapy of the chronic glaucomas. *Am. J. Ophthalmol.* 45: 639–643, 1958.
33. BECKER, B., AND E. LINNÉR. Ascorbic acid as a test substance for measuring relative changes in the rate of plasma flow through the ciliary processes. III. The effect of preganglionic section of the cervical sympathetic in rabbits on the ascorbic acid content of the aqueous humor at varying plasma levels. *Acta Physiol. Scand.* 26: 79–85, 1952.
34. BENMILOUD, M., AND U. S. VON EULER. Effects of bretylium, reserpine, guanethidine and sympathetic denervation on the noradrenaline content of the rat submaxillary gland. *Acta Physiol. Scand.* 59: 34–42, 1963.
35. BER, A., AND R. SINGER. Studies on the sensitivity of the iris of amphibians to epinephrine and norepinephrine. *Comp. Biochem. Physiol.* 29: 271–276, 1969.
36. BERGGREN, L. Direct observations of secretory pumping in vitro of the rabbit eye ciliary processes. Influence of ion milieu and carbonic anhydrase inhibition. *Invest. Ophthalmol.* 3: 266–272, 1964.
37. BERGGREN, L. Effect of parasympathomimetic and sympathomimetic drugs on secretion in vitro by the ciliary processes of the rabbit eye. *Invest. Ophthalmol.* 4: 91–97, 1965.
38. BERGGREN, L. Further studies on the effect of autonomous drugs on in vitro secretory activity of the rabbit eye ciliary processes. A. Inhibition of the pilocarpine effect by isopilocarpine, arecoline, and atropine. B. Influence of isoproterenol and norepinephrine. *Acta Ophthalmol.* 48: 293–302, 1970.
39. BERGGREN, L., AND P-E. WÄLINDER. Tonus of the ciliary muscle during sleep. *Acta Ophthalmol.* 47: 1149–1155, 1969.
40. BERLUCCHI, G., G. MORUZZI, G. SALVI, AND P. STRATA. Pupil behavior and ocular movements during synchronized and desynchronized sleep. *Arch. Ital. Biol.* 102: 230–244, 1964.

41. BERNARD, C. Expériences sur les fonctions de la portion céphalique du grand sympathique. *Compt. Rend. Soc. Biol.* 4: 155, 1852.
42. BERNARD, C. Sur les effets de la section de la portion céphalique du grand sympathique. *Compt. Rend. Soc. Biol.* 4: 168–170, 1852.
43. BERNHEIMER, H. Uber das Vorkommen von Katecholaminen und von 3,4-Dihydroxyphenylalanin (Dopa) im Auge. *Arch. Exptl. Pathol. Pharmakol.* 247: 202–213, 1964.
44. BEST, M., M. BLUMENTHAL, H. A. FUTTERMAN, AND M. A. GALIN. Critical closure of intraocular blood vessels. *Arch. Ophthalmol.* 82: 385–392, 1969.
45. BEST, M., M. BLUMENTHAL, S. MASKET, AND M. A. GALIN. Effect of sympathetic stimulation on critical closure of intraocular blood vessels. *Invest. Ophthalmol.* 9: 911–916, 1970.
46. BHATTACHERJEE, P. Uptake of [H^3]noradrenaline by the ocular tissues of rabbit. *Exptl. Eye Res.* 9: 73–81, 1970.
47. BIGGS, R. D., M. ALPERN, AND D. R. BENNETT. The effect of sympathomimetic drugs upon the amplitude of accommodation. *Am. J. Ophthalmol.* 48: 169–172, 1959.
48. BILL, A. Autonomic nervous control of uveal blood flow. *Acta Physiol. Scand.* 56: 70–81, 1962.
49. BILL, A. Intraocular pressure and blood flow through the uvea. *Arch. Ophthalmol.* 67: 336–348, 1962.
50. BILL, A. Effects of cervical sympathetic tone on the blood pressure and uveal blood flow after carotid occlusion. *Exptl. Eye Res.* 2: 203–209, 1963.
51. BILL, A. Uveal circulation, a review of methods and results. In: *Glaucoma Symposium, Tutzing Castle, 1966*, edited by J. W. Rohen. New York: Karger, 1967, p. 52–72.
52. BILL, A. Effects of atropine and pilocarpine on aqueous humor dynamics in cynomolgus monkeys (*Macaca irus*). *Exptl. Eye Res.* 6: 120–125, 1967.
53. BILL, A. Capillary permeability to and extravascular dynamics of myoglobin, albumin and gammaglobulin in the uvea. *Acta Physiol. Scand.* 73: 204–219, 1968.
54. BILL, A. Effects of norepinephrine, isoproterenol and sympathetic stimulation on aqueous humour dynamics in vervet monkeys. *Exptl. Eye Res.* 10: 31–46, 1970.
55. BILL, A. Early effects of epinephrine on aqueous humor dynamics in vervet monkeys (*Cercopithecus ethiops*). *Exptl. Eye Res.* 8: 35–43, 1969.
56. BILL, A., AND E. H. BÁRÁNY. Gross facility, facility of conventional routes, and pseudofacility of aqueous humor outflow in the cynomolgus monkey. *Arch. Ophthalmol.* 75: 665–673, 1966.
57. BISHOP, G. H., AND P. HEINBECKER. A functional analysis of the cervical sympathetic nerve supply to the eye. *Am. J. Physiol.* 100: 519–532, 1932.
59. BITO, L. Z., H. DAVSON, AND N. SNIDER. The effects of autonomic drugs on mitosis and DNA synthesis in the lens epithelium and on the composition of the aqueous humor. *Exptl. Eye Res.* 4: 54–61, 1965.
60. BONOMI, L. The effects of some sympathicolytic substances on the pupillary response to electric stimulation of the cervical sympathicus in the rabbit. *Boll. Oculist* 43: 55–68, 1964.
61. BORUT, A., AND K. SCHMIDT-NIELSEN. Respiration of avian salt-secreting gland in tissue slice experiments. *Am. J. Physiol.* 204: 573–581, 1963.
62. BOTELHO, S. Y., M. HISADA, AND N. FUENMAYOR. Functional innervation of the lacrimal gland in the cat. *Arch. Ophthalmol.* 76: 581–588, 1966.
63. BOTT, E., J. R. BLAIR-WEST, J. P. COGHLAN, D. A. DENTON, AND R. D. WRIGHT. Action of aldosterone on the lachrymal gland. *Nature* 210: 102, 1966.
64. BOUCHERON, C. R. Nerfs de l'hemisphère anterieur de l'oeil. *Compt. Rend. Soc. Biol.* 1: 71–78, 1889.
65. BOWMAN, W. C., AND C. RAPER. The effects of sympathomimetic amines on chronically denervated skeletal muscles. *Brit. J. Pharmacol. Chemotherap.* 24: 98–109, 1965.

66. BRODIE, B. B., E. COSTA, A. DLABAC, N. H. NEFF, AND H. H. SMOOKLER. Application of steady state kinetics to the estimation of synthesis rate and turnover time of tissue catecholamines. *J. Pharmacol. Exptl. Therap.* 154: 493-498, 1966.
67. BRON, A. J. Sympathetic control of aqueous secretion in man. *Brit. J. Ophthalmol.* 53: 37-45, 1969.
68. BROWN, G. L., AND A. M. HARVEY. Neuromuscular transmission in the extrinsic muscles of the eye. *J. Physiol., London* 99: 379-399, 1941.
68a. BROWN, J. H., AND M. H. MAKMAN. Influence of neuroleptic drugs and apomorphine on dopamine-sensitive adenylate cyclase of retina. *J. Neurochem.* 21: 477-479, 1973.
69. BUCCI, M. G., A. MISSIROLI, J. PECORI GIRALDI, AND M. VIRNO. Local administration of propranol in the glaucoma therapy. *Boll. Oculist* 47: 51-60, 1968.
70. BÜLBRING, E., AND I. N. HOOTON. Membrane potentials of smooth muscle fibres in the rabbit's sphincter pupillae. *J. Physiol., London* 125: 292-301, 1954.
71. BULLOUGH, W. S., AND E. B. LAURENCE. Mitotic control by internal secretion: the role of the chalone-adrenalin complex. *Exptl. Cell Res.* 33: 176-194, 1964.
72. BULOW, N., AND N. EHLERS. Morphology and dopa reaction of cultivated corneal epithelial cells. *Acta Ophthalmol.* 46: 749-756, 1968.
73. BURACK, W. R., AND P. R. DRASKOCZY. The turnover of endogenously labeled catecholamine in several regions of the sympathetic nervous system. *J. Pharmacol. Exptl. Therap.* 144: 66-75, 1964.
74. BURCH, P. G. Accommodation during general anesthesia. *Arch. Ophthalmol.* 81: 202-206, 1969.
75. BURFORD, G. E. Involuntary eyeball motion during anesthesia and sleep relationship to cortical rhythmic potentials. *Current Res. Anesthesia Analgesia* 20: 191-199, 1941.
76. BURN, J. H., E. M. LEACH, M. J. RAND, AND J. W. THOMPSON. Peripheral effects of nicotine and acetylcholine resembling those of sympathetic stimulation. *J. Physiol., London* 148: 332-352, 1959.
77. BURN, J. H., AND M. J. RAND. Sympathetic postganglionic mechanism. *Nature* 184: 163-165, 1959.
78. BURN, J. H., AND M. J. RAND. The cause of the sensitivity of smooth muscle to noradrenaline after sympathetic degeneration. *J. Physiol., London* 147: 135-143, 1959.
79. BURRI, C., AND E. R. WEIBEL. Effect of epinephrine on a specific organelle of endothelial cells of blood vessels. *Z. Zellforsch. Mikroskop. Anat.* 88: 426-440, 1968.
80. CAMPBELL, F. W., AND A. H. GREGORY. Effect of size of pupil on visual acuity. *Nature* 187: 1121-1123, 1960.
81. CANARY, J. J., M. SCHAAF, B. J. DUFFY, AND L. H. KYLE. Effects of oral and intramuscular administration of reserpine in thyrotoxicosis. *New Engl. J. Med.* 257: 435-442, 1957.
82. CANT, J. S., D. R. H. LEWIS, AND M. T. HARRISON. Treatment of dysthyroid ophthalmopathy with local guanethidine. *Brit. J. Ophthalmol.* 53: 233-238, 1969.
83. CASEY, W. J. Cervical sympathetic stimulation in monkeys and the effects on outflow facility and intraocular volume. *Invest. Ophthalmol.* 5: 33-41, 1966.
84. CHAPMAN, G. R., AND W. W. SPELSBERG. The occurrence of myelinated and unmyelinated nerves in the iris angle of man and rhesus monkey. *Exptl. Eye Res.* 2: 130-133, 1963.
85. CHARLES, S. T., AND D. I. HAMASAKI. The effect of intraocular pressure on the pupil size. *Arch. Ophthalmol.* 83: 729-733, 1970.
86. CHENG-MINODA, K., T. OZAWA, AND G. M. BREININ. Ultrastructural changes in rabbit extraocular muscles after oculomotor nerve section. *Invest. Ophthalmol.* 7: 599-616, 1968.
87. CHERVET, N. Untersuchungen über den trophischen Einfluss des Nervus sympathicus auf die Hornhaut der Kaninchen. *Z. Biol.* 97: 364-369, 1936.
88. CHIN, N. B., S. ISHIKAWA, H. LAPPIN, J. DAVIDOWITZ, AND G. M. BREININ. Accommodation in monkeys induced by midbrain stimulation. *Invest. Ophthalmol.* 7: 386-396, 1968.
89. CHRISTENSEN, L., K. C. SWAN, AND J. GOULD. Hypotensive action of dibenamine in glaucoma. *Northwest Med.* 47: 731-732, 1948.
90. CLARK, S. L. Innervation of the intrinsic muscles of the eye of the cat. *J. Comp. Neurol.* 66: 307-320, 1937.
91. COATS, D. A., AND N. EMMELIN. The short-term effects of sympathetic ganglionectomy on the cat's salivary secretion. *J. Physiol., London* 162: 282-288, 1962.
92. COBB, S., AND H. W. SCARLETT. A report of 11 cases of cervical sympathetic nerve injury causing the oculopupillary syndrome. *Arch. Neurol. Psychiat.* 3: 636-653, 1920.
93. COGAN, D. G. Accommodation and the autonomic nervous system. *Arch. Ophthalmol.* 18: 739-766, 1937.
94. COHAN, B. E., AND S. B. COHAN. Anterior ciliary venous blood flow and oxygen saturation at reduced arterial pressure. *Am. J. Physiol.* 205: 67-70, 1963.
95. COLE, D. F. Aqueous humor formation. *Doc. Ophthalmol.* 21: 116-238, 1966.
96. COLE, D. F., AND R. RUMBLE. Effects of catecholamines on circulation in the rabbit iris. *Exptl. Eye Res.* 9: 219-232, 1970.
97. COLE, D. F., AND R. RUMBLE. Responses of iris blood flow to stimulation of the cervical sympathetic in the rabbit. *Exptl. Eye Res.* 10: 183-191, 1970.
98. CONSTANT, M. A., AND B. BECKER. Experimental tonography. II. The effects of vasopressin, chlorpromazine, and phentolamine methanesulfonate. *Arch. Ophthalmol.* 56: 19-25, 1956.
99. CONSTANT, M. A., AND J. FALCH. Phosphate and protein concentrations of intraocular fluids. I. Effect of carbonic anhydrase inhibition in young and old rabbits. *Invest. Ophthalmol.* 2: 334-343, 1963.
100. CORRODI, H., T. MALMFORS, AND C. SACHS. Differences in the uptake of secondary catecholamines by the adrenergic nerves. *Acta Physiol. Scand.* 67: 358-362, 1966.
101. COTE, G., AND S. M. DRANCE. The effect of propranolol on human intraocular pressure. *Can. J. Ophthalmol.* 3: 207-212, 1968.
102. CROMBIE, A. L., AND E. D. HENDLEY. The 24-hour-ganglionectomy effect in rabbits. The influence of partial iridectomy and of acetazolamide. *Exptl. Eye Res.* 6: 309-315, 1967.
103. CROMBIE, A. L., AND A. LAWSON. Adrenergic blocking agents. A double blind trial in the treatment of the eye signs of thyroid disorder. *Brit. J. Ophthalmol.* 52: 616-620, 1968.
104. CSILLIK, B. Histochemical model experiments on the effect of various drugs on the catecholamine content of adrenergic nerve terminals. *J. Neurochem.* 11: 351-355, 1964.
105. CSILLIK, B., AND G. B. KOELLE. Histochemistry of the adrenergic and cholinergic autonomic innervation apparatus as represented by the rat iris. *Acta Histochem.* 22: 350-363, 1965.
106. DAHLSTRÖM, A., K. FUXE, N-A. HILLARP, AND T. MALMFORS. Adrenergic mechanisms in the pupillary light-reflex path. *Acta Physiol. Scand.* 62: 119-124, 1964.
107. DAHLSTRÖM, A., J. HÄGGENDAL, AND T. HÖKFELT. Noradrenaline content of the varicosities of sympathetic adrenergic nerve terminals in the rat. *Acta Physiol. Scand.* 67: 289-294, 1966.
108. DAVSON, H. *Physiology of the Ocular and Cerebrospinal Fluids.* Boston: Little, Brown, 1956.
109. DAVSON, H. *The Eye. Vegetative Physiology and Biochemistry* (2nd ed.). London: Acad. Press, 1969, vol. 1, p. 67-259.
110. DAVSON, H., AND P. A. MATCHETT. The control of intraocular pressure in the rabbit. *J. Physiol., London* 113: 387-397, 1951.
111. DE HAAS, E. B. H. Lacrimal gland response to parasympathicomimetics after parasympathetic denervation. *Arch. Ophthalmol.* 64: 64-73, 1960.
112. DENGLER, H. J., H. E. SPIEGEL, AND E. O. TITUS. Uptake of tritium-labeled norepinephrine in brain and other tissues of cat in vitro. *Science* 133: 1072-1073, 1961.
113. DIETERT, S. E. The demonstration of different types of muscle fibers in human extraocular muscle by electron microscopy and cholinesterase staining. *Invest. Ophthalmol.* 4: 51-63, 1965.

114. DJAHANGUIRI, B. Action d'amines dérivées du catéchol sur le muscle iridien de bovidé. *Arch. Intern. Pharmacodyn. Therap.* 142: 276-278, 1963.
115. DOLLERY, C. T. Dynamic aspects of the retinal microcirculation. *Arch. Ophthalmol.* 79: 536-539, 1968.
116. DOLLERY, C. T., P. HENKIND, E. M. KOHNER, AND J. W. PATERSON. Effect of raised intraocular pressure on the retinal and choroidal circulation. *Invest. Ophthalmol.* 7: 191-198, 1968.
117. DOLLERY, C. T., D. W. HILL, AND J. V. HODGE. The response of normal retinal blood vessels to angiotensin and noradrenaline. *J. Physiol., London* 165: 500-506, 1963.
118. DOWLING, J. E. Organization of vertebrate retinas. *Invest. Ophthalmol.* 9: 655-680, 1970.
119. DRUJAN, B. D., AND J. M. DÍAZ-BORGES. Adrenaline depletion induced by light in the dark-adapted retina. *Experientia* 24: 676-677, 1968.
120. DRUJAN, B. D., J. M. DÍAZ-BORGES, AND N. ALVAREZ. Relationship between the contents of adrenaline, noradrenaline and dopamine in the retina and its adaptational state. *Life Sci.* 4: 473-477, 1965.
121. DUKE-ELDER, W. S. The ocular circulation, its normal pressure relationships and their physiological significance. *Brit. J. Ophthalmol.* 10: 513-572, 1926.
122. DUKE-ELDER, W. S., AND P. M. DUKE-ELDER. The contraction of the extrinsic muscles of the eye by choline and nicotine. *Proc. Roy. Soc. London Ser. B* 107: 232-243, 1930.
123. DUNÉR, H., U. S. VON EULER, AND B. PERNOW. Catecholamines and substance P in the mammalian eye. *Acta Physiol. Scand.* 31: 113-118, 1954.
124. DURHAM, D. G. Congenital hereditary Horner's syndrome. *Arch. Ophthalmol.* 60: 939-940, 1958.
125. DUYFF, J. W. Kinetics of receptor occupation. *Acta Physiol. Pharmacol. Neerl.* 7: 239-254, 1958.
126. EAKINS, K. E. Effect of intravitreous injections of norepinephrine, epinephrine and isoproterenol on the intraocular pressure and aqueous humor dynamics of rabbit eyes. *J. Pharmacol. Exptl. Therap.* 140: 79-84, 1963.
127. EAKINS, K. E. Effect of angiotensin on intraocular pressure. *Nature* 202: 813-814, 1964.
128. EAKINS, K. E., E. COSTA, R. L. KATZ, AND C. L. REYES. Effect of pentobarbital anaesthesia on the turnover of [^{3}H]-noradrenaline in peripheral tissues of cats. *Life Sci., Part 1* 7: 71-76, 1968.
129. EAKINS, K. E., AND H. M. T. EAKINS. Adrenergic mechanisms and the outflow of aqueous humor from the rabbit eye. *J. Pharmacol. Exptl. Therap.* 144: 60-65, 1964.
130. EAKINS, K. E., AND R. L. KATZ. The effects of sympathetic stimulation and epinephrine on the superior rectus muscle of the cat. *J. Pharmacol. Exptl. Therap.* 157: 524-531, 1967.
131. EAKINS, K. E., AND S. J. RYAN. The action of sympathomimetic amines on the outflow of aqueous humour from the eye. *Brit. J. Pharmacol.* 23: 374-382, 1964.
132. EGEBERG, J., AND D. A. JENSEN. The ultrastructure of the acini of the human lacrimal gland. *Acta Ophthalmol.* 47: 400-410, 1969.
133. EHINGER, B. Adrenergic nerves to the eye and its adnexa in rabbit and guinea-pig. *Acta Univ. Lund., II* 20: 3-23, 1964.
134. EHINGER, B. Adrenergic nerves to the eye and to related structures in man and in the cynomolgus monkey (*Macaca irus*). *Invest. Ophthalmol.* 5: 42-52, 1966.
135. EHINGER, B. Ocular and orbital vegetative nerves. *Acta Physiol. Scand. Suppl.* 268, 1966.
136. EHINGER, B. Double innervation of the feline iris dilator. *Arch. Ophthalmol.* 77: 541-545, 1967.
137. EHINGER, B., AND B. FALCK. Uptake of some catecholamines and their precursors into neurons of the rat ciliary ganglion. *Acta Physiol. Scand.* 78: 132-141, 1970.
138. EHINGER, B., AND B. FALCK. Cellular uptake of some amino acids and amines in vitro into rabbit and monkey anterior eye segment preparations. *Exptl. Eye Res.* 10: 352-359, 1970.
139. EHINGER, B., AND B. FALCK. Innervation of iridic melanophores. *Z. Zellforsch. Mikroskop. Anat.* 105: 538-542, 1970.
140. EHINGER, B., B. FALCK, AND A. M. LATIES. Adrenergic neurons in teleost retina. *Z. Zellforsch. Mikroskop. Anat.* 97: 285-297, 1969.
141. EHINGER, B., B. FALCK, AND E. ROSENGREN. Adrenergic denervation of the eye by unilateral cervical sympathectomy. *Arch. Klin. Exptl. Ophthalmol.* 177: 206-211, 1969.
142. EHINGER, B., H. OLIVECRONA, AND H. RORSMAN. Malignant melanomas of the eye as studied with a specific fluorescence method. *Acta Pathol. Microbiol. Scand.* 69: 179-184, 1967.
143. EHINGER, B., AND B. SPORRONG. Adrenergic and cholinergic axons in the mouse iris. *Experientia* 22: 218, 1966.
144. EHLERS, N. The precorneal film. Biomicroscopical, histological and chemical investigations. *Acta Ophthalmol. Suppl.* 81: 1-136, 1965.
145. EMMELIN, N. Degeneration activity after sympathetic denervation of the submaxillary gland and the eye. *Experientia* 24: 44-45, 1968.
146. EMMELIN, N. G., AND B. C. R. STROMBLAD. Sensitization of the lachrymal gland by treatment with a parasympathicolytic agent. *Acta Physiol. Scand.* 36: 171-174, 1956.
147. ERÄNKÖ, O. Histochemistry of nervous tissues: catecholamines and cholinesterases. *Ann. Rev. Pharmacol.* 7: 203-222, 1967.
148. ERÄNKÖ, O., AND L. RÄISÄNEN. Fibers containing both noradrenaline and acetylcholinesterase in the nerve net of the rat iris. *Acta Physiol. Scand.* 63: 505-506, 1965.
149. ERICSON, L. A. Twenty-four hourly variation of the aqueous flow. Examinations with perilimbal suction cup. *Acta Ophthalmol. Suppl.* 50: 1-95, 1958.
150. FALCK, B. Observations on the possibilities of the cellular localization of monoamines by a fluorescence method. *Acta Physiol. Scand. Suppl.* 197: 1-25, 1962.
151. FANGE, R., K. SCHMIDT-NIELSEN, AND M. ROBINSON. The control of secretion from the avian salt gland. *Am. J. Physiol.* 195: 321-326, 1958.
152. FARNEBO, L-O., AND B. HAMBERGER. Release of norepinephrine from isolated rat iris by field stimulation. *J. Pharmacol. Exptl. Therap.* 172: 332-341, 1970.
153. FATT, I., AND B. O. HEDBYS. Flow of water in sclera. *Exptl. Eye Res.* 10: 243-249, 1970.
154. FEENEY, L. Ultrastructure of the nerves in the human trabecular region. *Invest. Ophthalmol.* 1: 462-473, 1962.
155. FEENEY, L., AND M. J. HOGAN. Electron microscopy of the human choroid. II. The choroidal nerves. *Am. J. Ophthalmol.* 51: 200-211, 1961.
156. FLECKENSTEIN, A., AND H. BASS. Die Sensibilisierung der Katzen-Nickhaut für Sympathomimetic der Brenzkatechen-Reihe. *Arch. Exptl. Pathol. Pharmakol.* 220: 143-156, 1953.
157. FLECKENSTEIN, A., AND J. H. BURN. The effect of denervation on the action of sympathomimetic amines on the nictitating membrane. *Brit. J. Pharmacol. Chemotherap.* 8: 69-78, 1953.
158. FLECKENSTEIN, A., AND D. STÖCKLE. Die Hemmung der Neuro-sympathomimetica durch Cocain. *Arch. Exptl. Pathol. Pharmakol.* 224: 401-415, 1955.
159. FLEMING, D. G., AND J. L. HALL. Autonomic innervation of the ciliary body. *Am. J. Ophthalmol.* 48: 287-293, 1959.
160. FOERSTER, O., AND O. GAGEL. Die Vorderseitenstrang-durchschneidung beim Menschen. Eine klinisch-pathophysiologische-anatomische Studie. *Z. Ges. Neurol. Psychol.* 138: 1-92, 1938.
161. FOLKOW, B., B. JOHANSSON, AND B. ÖBERG. The stimulation threshold of different sympathetic fibre groups as correlated to their functional differentiation. *Acta Physiol. Scand.* 44: 146-156, 1958.
162. FOWLKS, W. L., V. HAVENER, AND J. S. GOOD. Meridional flow from the corona ciliarie through the pararetinal zone of the rabbit vitreous. *Invest. Ophthalmol.* 2: 63-71, 1963.
163. FRAYSER, R., AND J. B. HICKAM. Effect of vasodilatator drugs in the retinal blood flow in man. *Arch. Ophthalmol.* 73: 640-642, 1965.

164. FRIEDENWALD, J. S. Retinal vascular dynamics. *Am. J. Ophthalmol.* 17: 387–395, 1934.
165. FRIEDENWALD, J. S., AND W. BUSCHKE. The role of epinephrine in the formation of intraocular fluid. *Am. J. Ophthalmol.* 24: 1105–1114, 1941.
166. FRIEDENWALD, J. S., AND W. BUSCHKE. The effects of excitement, of epinephrine, and of sympathectomy on the mitotic activity of the corneal epithelium. *Am. J. Physiol.* 141: 689–694, 1944.
167. FRIEDMAN, E., H. H. KOPALD, AND T. R. SMITH. Retinal and choroidal blood flow determined with krypton-85 in anesthetized animals. *Invest. Ophthalmol.* 3: 539–547, 1964.
168. FRIEDMAN, E., AND T. R. SMITH. Estimation of retinal blood flow in animals. *Invest. Ophthalmol.* 4: 1122–1128, 1965.
169. FUKUDA, M. Studies on the nerve endings in the extrinsic eye muscles of rabbit. *Acta Ophthalmol. Soc. Japan.* 61: 51–61, 1957.
170. GAASTERLAND, D. E., V. L. JOCSON, AND M. L. SEARS. Channels of aqueous outflow and related blood vessels. III. Episcleral arteriovenous anastomoses in the Rhesus monkey eye (*Macaca mulatta*). *Arch. Ophthalmol.* 84: 770–775, 1970.
171. GAY, A. J., AND M. A. WOLKSTEIN. Topical guanethidine therapy for endocrine lid retraction. *Arch. Ophthalmol.* 76: 364–367, 1966.
172. GELTZER, A. I. Autonomic innervation of the cat iris. An electron microscopic study. *Arch. Ophthalmol.* 81: 70–83, 1969.
173. GENIS-GALVEZ, J. M. Innervation of the ciliary muscle. *Anat. Record* 127: 219–224, 1957.
174. GILES, C. L., AND J. W. HENDERSON. Horner's syndrome: an analysis of 216 cases. *Am. J. Ophthalmol.* 46: 289–296, 1958.
175. GILLIS, C. N. Inactivation of norepinephrine released by electrical stimulation of rabbit aorta in a gaseous medium. In: *Physiology of Pharmacology of Neuroeffector Mechanisms in Blood Vessels*. Basel: Karger, 1971, p. 47–52.
176. GILLIS, C. N., F. H. SCHNEIDER, L. S. VAN ORDEN, AND N. J. GIARMAN. Biochemical and microfluorometric studies of norepinephrine redistribution accompanying sympathetic nerve stimulation. *J. Pharmacol. Exptl. Therap.* 151: 46–54, 1966.
177. GLADSTONE, R. M. Development and significance of heterochromia of the iris. *Arch. Neurol.* 21: 184–191, 1969.
178. GLOSTER, J. Responses of the intraocular pressure to diencephalic stimulation. *Brit. J. Ophthalmol.* 44: 649–664, 1960.
179. GLOSTER, J., AND D. P. GREAVES. The effect of cervical sympathectomy on an ocular response to hypothalamic stimulation. *Brit. J. Ophthalmol.* 42: 385–393, 1958.
180. GNÄDINGER, M. C., AND E. H. BÁRÁNY. Die Wirkung der B-adrenergischen Substanz Isoprenalin auf die Ausfluss Fazilitat des Kaninchenauges. *Arch. Klin. Exptl. Ophthalmol.* 167: 483–492, 1964.
181. GOLDMAN, J. N., AND G. B. BENEDEK. The relationship between morphology and transparency in the nonswelling corneal stroma of the shark. *Invest. Ophthalmol.* 6: 574–600, 1967.
182. GOLDMAN, H. Experimentelle Supranukleärkatarakt und Kernsklerose. *Klin. Monatsbl. Augenheilkunde* 83: 433–438, 1929.
183. GOLDSTEIN, A. M., A. DE PALAU, AND S. Y. BOTELHO. Inhibition and facilitation of pilocarpine-induced lacrimal flow by norepinephrine. *Invest. Ophthalmol.* 6: 498–511, 1967.
184. GRANT, W. M. Action of drugs on movement of ocular fluids. *Ann. Rev. Pharmacol.* 9: 85–94, 1969.
185. GRANT, W. M. *Toxicology of the Eye* (2nd ed.). Springfield, Ill: Thomas, 1973.
186. GREAVES, D. P., AND E. S. PERKINS. Influence of the sympathetic nervous system on the intraocular pressure and vascular circulation of the eye. *Brit. J. Ophthalmol.* 36: 258–264, 1952.
187. GRILLO, M. A. Electron microscopy of sympathetic tissues. *Pharmacol. Rev.* 18: 387–399, 1966.
188. HADDAD, N. J., N. J. MOYER, AND F. C. RILEY. Mydriatic effect of phenylephrine hydrochloride. *Am. J. Ophthalmol.* 70: 729–733, 1970.
189. HÄGGENDAL, J., AND T. MALMFORS. Evidence of dopamine-containing neurons in the retina of rabbits. *Acta Physiol. Scand.* 59: 295–296, 1963.
190. HÄGGENDAL, J., AND T. MALMFORS. Identification and cellular localization of the catecholamines in the retina and the choroid of the rabbit. *Acta Physiol. Scand.* 64: 58–66, 1965.
191. HAINING, C. G., J. L. HEYDON, AND L. R. MURRAY. Histochemical studies on the depletion of noradrenaline by adrenaline in adrenergic nerves of the rat iris. *J. Pharm. Pharmacol.* 21: 639–647, 1969.
192. HALLMAN, V. L. Effect of thyroid hormones on intraocular pressure. *Exptl. Eye Res.* 6: 219–226, 1967.
193. HAMBERGER, B., AND D. MASUOKA. Localization of catecholamine uptake in rat brain slices. *Acta Pharmacol. Toxicol.* 22: 363–368, 1965.
194. HAMBURGER, K. Experimentelle Glaukomtherapie. *Klin. Monatsbl. Augenheilkunde* 71: 810–811, 1923.
195. HARPER, J. Y., JR. Horner's syndrome and glaucoma. *Arch. Ophthalmol.* 83: 383, 1970.
196. HAYREH, S. S. Posterior drainage of the intraocular fluid from the vitreous. *Exptl. Eye Res.* 5: 123–144, 1966.
196a. HEDQVIST, P. Prostaglandin E compounds and sympathetic neuromuscular transmission. *Ann. NY Acad. Sci.* 180: 410–415, 1971.
197. HEDQVIST, P., AND L. STJARNE. The relative role of recapture and of de novo synthesis for the maintenance of neurotransmitter homeostasis in noradrenergic nerves. *Acta Physiol. Scand.* 76: 270–283, 1969.
198. HENDERSON, E. E., AND E. H. STARLING. The influence of changes in the intraocular circulation on the intraocular pressure. *J. Physiol., London* 31: 305–319, 1904.
199. HENDLEY, E. D., AND A. L. CROMBIE. The 24-hour ganglionectomy effect in rabbits. The influence of adrenergic blockade, adrenalectomy and carotid ligation. *Exptl. Eye Res.* 6: 152–164, 1967.
200. HENKIND, P. Circulation in the iris and ciliary processes. *Brit. J. Ophthalmol.* 49: 6–10, 1965.
201. HERR, B., AND E. COSTA. Normal rate of ³H norepinephrine uptake by isolated iris of rabbits injected with reserpine and pargyline. *Intern. J. Neuropharmacol.* 8: 463–469, 1969.
202. HERTTING, G., J. AXELROD, I. J. KOPIN, AND L. G. WHITBY. Lack of uptake of catecholamines after chronic denervation of sympathetic nerves. *Nature* 189: 66, 1961.
203. HESS, A., AND G. PILAR. Slow fibers in the extraocular muscles of the cat. *J. Physiol., London* 169: 780–798, 1963.
204. HILLARP, N. A. Construction and functional organization of the autonomic innervation apparatus. *Acta Physiol. Scand. Suppl.* 157: 1–38, 1959.
205. HINES, M. Studies on the innervation of skeletal muscle. III. Innervation of the extrinsic eye muscles of the rabbit. *Am. J. Anat.* 47: 1–54, 1931.
206. HIRANO, S. Electron microscopic study on ciliary muscle in regard to innervation. *Acta Soc. Ophthalmol. Japan.* 71: 948–950, 1967.
207. HISADA, M., AND S. Y. BOTELHO. Membrane potentials of in situ lacrimal gland in the cat. *Am. J. Physiol.* 214: 1262–1267, 1968.
208. HOFFMANN, F. Effect of noradrenalin on intraocular pressure and outflow in cynomolgus monkeys. *Exptl. Eye Res.* 7: 369–382, 1968.
209. HÖKFELT, T. Electron microscopic observations on nerve terminals in the intrinsic muscles of the albino rat iris. *Acta Physiol. Scand.* 67: 255–256, 1966.
210. HÖKFELT, T. Ultrastructural studies on adrenergic nerve terminals in the albino rat iris after pharmacological and experimental treatment. *Acta Physiol. Scand.* 69: 125–126, 1967.
211. HÖKFELT, T., AND O. NILSSON. The relationship between nerves and smooth muscle cells in the rat iris. II. The sphincter muscle. *Z. Zellforsch. Mikroskop. Anat.* 66: 848–853, 1965.
212. HOLLAND, M. G., AND J. L. MIMS, III. Anterior segment chemical sympathectomy by 6-hydroxydopamine. I. Effect on

intraocular pressure and facility of outflow. *Invest. Ophthalmol.* 10: 120–143, 1971.
213. HOLLAND, M. G., L. VON SALLMANN, AND E. M. COLLINS. A study of the innervation of the chamber angle. *Am. J. Ophthalmol.* 42: 148–161, 1956.
214. HOLLAND, M. G., L. VON SALLMANN, AND E. M. COLLINS. A study of the innervation of the chamber angle. II. The origin of trabecular axons revealed by degeneration experiments. *Am. J. Ophthalmol.* 44: 206–221, 1957.
215. HOLMBERG, A. The ultrastructure of the capillaries in the ciliary body. *Arch. Ophthalmol.* 62: 949–951; 1033–1036, 1959.
216. HORNER, F. Uber eine Form von Ptosis. *Klin. Monatsbl. Augenheilkunde* 7: 193–198, 1869.
217. HOULE, R. E., AND W. M. GRANT. Alcohol, vasopressin, and intraocular pressure. *Invest. Ophthalmol.* 6: 145–154, 1967.
218. ISHIKAWA, T. Fine structure of the human ciliary muscle. *Invest. Ophthalmol.* 1: 587–608, 1962.
219. IVERSEN, L. L. The uptake of noradrenaline by the isolated perfused rat heart. *Brit. J. Pharmacol.* 21: 523–537, 1963.
220. IVERSEN, L. L. Characteristics of noradrenaline uptake in the iris/ciliary body and other peripheral tissues of the rat. *Arch. Exptl. Pathol. Pharmakol.* 259: 179, 1968.
221. JACOBOWITZ, D., AND G. KOELLE. Histochemical correlations of acetylcholinesterase and catecholamines in postganglionic nerves of the cat, rabbit, and guinea pig. *J. Pharmacol. Exptl. Therap.* 148: 225–237, 1965.
222. JACOBOWITZ, D., AND A. M. LATIES. Direct adrenergic innervation of a teleost melanophore. *Anat. Record* 162: 501–504, 1968.
223. JAFFE, N. S. Sympathetic nervous system and intraocular pressure. *Am. J. Ophthalmol.* 31: 1597–1603, 1948.
224. JAJU, B. P., J. N. SINHA, AND R. C. SRIMAL. Local anesthetic activity of propranolol, a new β-adrenergic blocking agent. *J. Indian Med. Profess.* 12: 5663, 1966.
225. JONES, O. W., III. Toxic amblyopia caused by pheniprazine hydrochloride (JB-516, Catron). *Arch. Ophthalmol.* 66: 29–36, 1961.
226. JONNESCO, T. Die Resektion des Halssympathikus in der Behandlung der Epilepsie, des Morbue Basedowii und des Glaukoms. *Klin. Wochschr.* 12: 483–486, 1899.
227. JONSSON, G. Microfluorimetric studies on the formaldehyde-induced fluorescence of noradrenaline in adrenergic nerves of rat iris. *J. Histochem. Cytochem.* 17: 714–723, 1969.
228. JONSSON, G., B. HAMBERGER, T. MALMFORS, AND C. SACHS. Uptake and accumulation of ³H-noradrenaline in adrenergic nerves of rat iris. Effect of reserpine, monoamine oxidase and tyrosine hydroxylase inhibition. *European J. Pharmacol.* 8: 58–72, 1969.
229. JOSEPH, D. R. The inhibitory influence of the cervical sympathetic nerve upon the sphincter muscle of the iris. *Am. J. Physiol.* 55: 279–280, 1921.
230. KALSNER, S., AND M. NICKERSON. A method for the study of mechanisms of drug disposition in smooth muscle. *Can. J. Physiol. Pharmacol.* 46: 719–730, 1968.
231. KALSNER, S., AND M. NICKERSON. Disposition of norepinephrine and epinephrine in vascular tissue, determined by the technique of oil immersion. *J. Pharmacol. Exptl. Therap.* 165: 152–165, 1969.
232. KEATES, E., N. KRISHNA, AND I. H. LEOPOLD. *Symposium on Guanethidine.* Summit, N. J.: CIBA, 1960, p. 66.
232a. KEEN, W. W., G. R. MOREHOUSE, AND S. WEIR MITCHELL. 1864. [Cited by Kisch (238).]
233. KERN, R. A comparative pharmacologic-histologic study of slow and twitch fibers in the superior rectus muscle of the rabbit. *Invest. Ophthalmol.* 4: 901–910, 1965.
234. KERN, R. The adrenergic receptors of the extrinsic eye muscles of Rhesus monkeys, an in-vitro study. *Arch. Klin. Exptl. Ophthalmol.* 174: 278–286, 1968.
235. KINSEY, V. E. Transfer of ascorbic acid and related compounds across blood-aqueous barrier. *Am. J. Ophthalmol.* 30: 1262–1266, 1947.
236. KINSEY, V. E., AND D. V. N. REDDY. Chemistry and dynamics of aqueous humor. In: *The Rabbit in Eye Research*, edited by J. H. Prince. Springfield, Ill: Thomas, 1964, p. 218–319.
237. KIRPEKAR, S. M., P. CERVONI, AND R. F. FURCHGOTT. Catecholamine content of the cat nictitating membrane following procedures sensitizing it to norepinephrine. *J. Pharmacol. Exptl. Therap.* 135: 180–190, 1962.
238. KISCH, B. Horner's syndrome, an American discovery. *Bull. Hist. Med.* 25: 284–288, 1951.
239. KNAPP, A. The action of adrenalin on the glaucomatous eye. *Arch. Ophthalmol.* 50: 556–559, 1921.
240. KNYIHAR, E., K. RISTOVSKY, G. KÁLMÁN, AND B. CSILLIK. Chemical sympathectomy: histochemical and submicroscopical consequences of 6-hydroxy-dopamine treatment in the rat iris. *Experientia* 25: 518–520, 1969.
241. KOELLA, W., AND U. SCHAEPPI. The reaction of the isolated cat iris to serotonin. *J. Pharmacol. Exptl. Therap.* 138: 154–158, 1962.
242. KOJIMA, K., M. IIDA, Y. MAJIMA, AND S. OKADA. Histochemical studies on monoamine oxidase (MAO) of the human retina. *Japan. J. Ophthalmol.* 5: 205–210, 1961.
243. KRAMER, S. G., AND A. M. POTTS. Intraocular pressure and ciliary body norepinephrine uptake in experimental Horner's syndrome. *Am. J. Ophthalmol.* 68: 1076–1082, 1970.
244. KREJCI, L., AND R. HARRISON. Epinephrine effects on corneal cells in tissue culture. *Arch. Ophthalmol.* 83: 451–454, 1970.
245. KRILL, A. E., F. W. NEWELL, AND M. NOVAK. Early and long-term effects of levo-epinephrine. *Am. J. Ophthalmol.* 59: 833–839, 1965.
246. KRISHNA, N., V. J. DIANO, AND I. H. LEOPOLD. Manometric determination of monoamine oxidase in cat ocular tissues. *Arch. Ophthalmol.* 67: 488–489, 1962.
247. KRNJEVÍC, K., AND R. MILEDI. Some effects produced by adrenaline upon neuromuscular propagation. *J. Physiol., London* 141: 291–304, 1958.
248. KROGH, A., C. G. LUND, AND K. PEDERSEN-BJERGAARD. The osmotic concentration of human lacrymal fluid. *Acta Physiol. Scand.* 10: 88–90, 1945.
249. KRONFELD, P. C. Dose-effect relationships as an aid in the evaluation of ocular hypotensive drugs. *Invest. Ophthalmol.* 3: 258–265, 1964.
250. KRONFELD, P. C. The efficacy of combinations of ocular hypotensive drugs. *Arch. Ophthalmol.* 78: 140–146, 1967.
251. KROOP, I. G. The production of tears in familial dysautonomia. *J. Pediat.* 48: 328–329, 1956.
252. KUNTZ, A. Innervation of cephalic autonomic effectors. In: *Autonomic Nervous System.* Philadelphia: Lea & Febiger, 1945, chapt. XVI, p. 335–356.
253. KUPFER, C. Motor innervation of extraocular muscle. *J. Physiol., London* 53: 522–526, 1960.
254. KUPFER, C. Relationship of ciliary body meridional muscle and corneoscleral trabecular meshwork. *Arch. Ophthalmol.* 68: 132–136, 1962.
255. KUPFER, C., AND P. SANDERSON. Determination of pseudofacility in the eye of man. *Arch. Ophthalmol.* 80: 194–196, 1968.
256. KUWABARA, T., AND D. COGAN. Retinal vascular patterns. IV. Mural cells of the retinal capillaries. *Arch. Ophthalmol.* 69: 492–502, 1963.
257. LAGERCRANTZ, H. Potentiation of tyramine effect on the isolated iris muscle by cocaine. *Acta Physiol. Scand.* 73: 58–61, 1968.
258. LAIBSON, P. R., AND S. KIBRICK. Reactivation of herpetic keratitis by epinephrine. *Arch. Ophthalmol.* 75: 254–260, 1966.
259. LAIBSON, P. R., N. KRISHNA, AND I. H. LEOPOLD. Intraocular pressure studies with alpha-methyl-dopa. *Arch. Ophthalmol.* 68: 648–650, 1962.
260. LANDE, M. A., AND J. A. ZADUNAISKY. The structure and membrane properties of the frog nictitans. *Invest. Ophthalmol.* 9: 477–491, 1970.
261. LANGER, S. Z. The degeneration contraction of the nictitating

membrane in the unanesthetized cat. *J. Pharmacol. Exptl. Therap.* 151: 66–72, 1966.
262. LANGER, S. Z., AND U. TRENDELENBURG. The onset of denervation supersensitivity. *J. Pharmacol. Exptl. Therap.* 151: 73–86, 1966.
263. LANGHAM, M. E. The response of the pupil and intraocular pressure of conscious rabbits to adrenergic drugs following unilateral superior cervical ganglionectomy. *Exptl. Eye Res.* 4: 381–389, 1965.
264. LANGHAM, M. E., AND D. D. CARMEL. The action of protriptyline on adrenergic mechanisms in rabbit, primate and human eyes. *J. Pharmacol. Exptl. Therap.* 163: 368–378, 1968.
265. LANGHAM, M. E., AND A. R. ROSENTHAL. The role of cervical sympathetic nerve in regulation of the intraocular pressure and circulation. *Am. J. Physiol.* 210: 786–794, 1966.
266. LANGHAM, M. E., AND C. B. TAYLOR. The influence of pre- and postganglionic section of the cervical sympathetic on the intraocular pressure of rabbits and cats. *J. Physiol., London* 152: 437–446, 1960.
267. LANGHAM, M. E., AND C. B. TAYLOR. The influence of ganglionectomy on intraocular dynamics. *J. Physiol., London* 152: 447–458, 1960.
268. LANGHAM, M. E., AND G. W. WEINSTEIN. Horner's syndrome: ocular supersensitivity to adrenergic amines. *Arch. Ophthalmol.* 77: 462–469, 1967.
268a. LANGLEY, J. N. On the union of cranial autonomic (visceral) fibres with the nerve cells of the superior cervical ganglion. *J. Physiol., London* 23: 240–270, 1898.
269. LARSEN, G. Experimental uveitis. A histopathologic study with special reference to the mast cell. *Acta Ophthalmol.* 39: 231–258, 1961.
270. LATIES, A. M. Central retinal artery innervation. *Arch. Ophthalmol.* 77: 405–409, 1967.
271. LATIES, A., AND D. JACOBOWITZ. A histochemical study of the adrenergic and cholinergic innervation of the anterior segment of the rabbit eye. *Invest. Ophthalmol.* 3: 592–600, 1964.
272. LATIES, A. M., AND D. JACOBOWITZ. A comparative study of the autonomic innervation of the eye in monkey, cat, and rabbit. *Anat. Record* 156: 383–396, 1966.
273. LEE, W. Y., P. K. MORIMOTO, D. BRONSKY, AND S. S. WALDSTEIN. Studies of thyroid and sympathetic nervous system interrelationships. I. Blepharoptosis of myxedema. *J. Clin. Endocrinol.* 21: 1402–1412, 1961.
274. LEESON, S. J., AND M. J. VOADEN. A chalone in the mammalian lens. II. Relative effects of adrenaline and noradrenaline on cell division in the rabbit lens. *Exptl. Eye Res.* 9: 67–72, 1970.
275. LEVENE, R. Z. Mast cells and amines in normal ocular tissues. *Invest. Ophthalmol.* 1: 531–543, 1962.
276. LINKSZ, A. Der Einflus der Sympathicusausschaltung auf die blut-Kammerwasserschranke. *Klin. Wochschr.* 10: 839–840, 1931.
277. LINNÉR, A. A method for determining the rate of plasma flow through the secretory part of the ciliary body. *Acta Physiol. Scand.* 22: 83–86, 1951.
278. LINNÉR, A. Ascorbic acid as a test substance for measuring relative changes in the place of plasma flow through the ciliary processes. *Acta Physiol. Scand.* 26: 70–78, 1952.
279. LINNER, E., AND E. PRIJOT. Cervical sympathetic ganglionectomy and aqueous flow. *Arch. Ophthalmol.* 54: 831–833, 1955.
280. LIOTET, S., AND P. COCHET. Notions concernant les larmes humaines. Origine, physiologie et composition. *Arch. Ophthalmol. Paris* 27: 251–262, 1967.
281. LOEWENFELD, I. E. Mechanisms of reflex dilatation of the pupil. Historical review and experimental analysis. *Doc. Ophthalmol.* 12: 185–448, 1958.
282. LOEWENFELD, I. E. The Argyll-Robertson pupil, 1869–1969. A critical survey of the literature. *Surv. Ophthalmol.* 14: 199–299, 1969.
283. LORING, R. G. The present status of cervical sympathectomy for glaucoma simplex. *Arch. Ophthalmol.* 33: 529–544, 1904.

284. LUCO, J. V., AND K. LISSAK. Chemical mediators in the aqueous humor. *Am. J. Physiol.* 124: 271–278, 1938.
285. LUKÁŠ, Z., AND S. ČECH. Adrenergic nerve fibres and their relation to monoamine oxidase distribution in ocular tissues. *Acta Histochem.* 25: 133–140, 1966.
286. LUNDBERG, D. Adrenergic neuron blockers and transmitter release after sympathetic denervation studied in the conscious rat. *Acta Physiol. Scand.* 75: 415–426, 1969.
287. MACRI, F. J. The action of angiotensin on intraocular pressure. *Arch. Ophthalmol.* 73: 528–539, 1965.
288. MAES, J. P. The effect of the removal of the superior cervical ganglion on lachrymal secretion. *Am. J. Physiol.* 123: 359–363, 1938.
289. MALMFORS, T. Evidence of adrenergic neurons with synaptic terminals in the retina of rats demonstrated with fluorescence and electron microscopy. *Acta Physiol. Scand.* 58: 99–100, 1963.
290. MALMFORS, T. Studies of adrenergic nerves: the use of rat and mouse iris for direct observations on their physiology and pharmacology at cellular and subcellular levels. *Acta Physiol. Scand. Suppl.* 248: 1–93, 1965.
291. MALMFORS, T. The adrenergic innervation of the eye as demonstrated by fluorescence microscopy. *Acta Physiol. Scand.* 65: 259–267, 1965.
292. MALMFORS, T. Histochemical studies on the adrenergic innervation of the nictitating membrane of the cat. *Histochemie* 13: 203–206, 1968.
293. MALMFORS, T., AND L. OLSON. Adrenergic reinnervation of anterior chamber transplants. *Acta Physiol. Scand.* 71: 401–402, 1967.
294. MALMFORS, T., AND C. SACHS. Direct studies on the disappearance of the transmitter and changes in the uptake storage mechanism of degenerating adrenergic nerves. *Acta Physiol. Scand.* 64: 211–223, 1965.
295. MALMFORS, T., AND C. SACHS. Direct demonstration of the systems of terminals belonging to an individual adrenergic neuron and their distribution in rat iris. *Acta Physiol. Scand.* 64: 377–382, 1965.
296. MAPSTONE, R. Safe mydriasis. *Brit. J. Ophthalmol.* 54: 690–692, 1970.
297. MARLEY, E. Action of some sympathetic amines on the cats iris, in situ or isolated. *J. Physiol., London* 162: 193–211, 1962.
298. MASTMAN, G. J., E. J. BALDES, AND J. W. HENDERSON. The total osmotic pressure of tears in normal and various pathologic conditions. *Arch. Ophthalmol.* 65: 509–513, 1961.
299. MCGUIRE, J. Adrenergic control of melanocytes. *Arch. Dermatol.* 101: 173–180, 1970.
300. MELTON, C. E., E. W. PURNELL, AND G. A. BRECHER. The effect of sympathetic nerve impulses on the ciliary muscle. *Am. J. Ophthalmol.* 40: 155–162, 1955.
301. MICHAELSON, I. C. *Retinal Circulation in Man and Animals.* Springfield, Ill.: Thomas, 1954.
302. MIESCHER, G. Die Pigmentgenese im Auge nebst Bemerkungen über die Natur des Pigmentkorns. *Arch. Mikroskop. Anat. Entwicklungeschichte* 97: 326–396, 1923.
303. MILLER, S. J. H. Stellate ganglion block in glaucoma. *Brit. J. Ophthalmol.* 37: 70–76, 1953.
304. MISHIMA, S. The effects of the denervation and the stimulation of the sympathetic and the trigeminal nerve on the mitotic rate of the corneal epithelium in the rabbit. *Japan. J. Ophthalmol.* 1: 65–73, 1957.
305. MISHIMA, S. Some physiological aspects of the precorneal tear film. *Arch. Ophthalmol.* 73: 233–241, 1965.
306. MISHIMA, S., A. GASSET, S. D. KLYCE, JR., AND J. L. BAUM. Determination of tear volume and tear flow. *Invest. Ophthalmol.* 5: 264–276, 1966.
307. MITSUI, Y., AND Y. TAKAGI. Nature of aqueous floaters due to sympathomimetic mydriatics. *Arch. Ophthalmol.* 65: 626–631, 1961.
308. MIYAMOTO, M., AND T. B. FITZPATRICK. On the nature of the

pigment in retinal pigment epithelium. *Science* 126: 449–450, 1957.
309. MIZUNO, K. Studies on retinitis pigmentosa. 1. Monoamine oxidase and sulfate conjugation in the experimental degeneration of the retina. *Eye, Ear, Nose, Throat Monthly* 39: 493–499, 1960.
310. MOFFAT, D. B. Intra-arterial cushions in the arteries of the rat's eye. *Acta Anat.* 72: 1–11, 1969.
311. MORGAN, M. W., JR. A new theory for the control of accommodation. *Am. J. Optometry* 23: 99–108, 1946.
312. MORGAN, M. W., JR. The ciliary body in accommodation and accommodative-convergence. *Am. J. Optometry* 31: 219–229, 1954.
313. MORGAN, M. W., JR., J. M. D. OLMSTED, AND W. G. WATROUS. Sympathetic action in accommodation for far vision. *Am. J. Physiol.* 128: 588–591, 1940.
314. MORONE, G. Indagini sull' attivita' aminossidasica dell'iride dopo la resezione del simpatico cervicale. *Riv. Otoneurooftalmol.* 28: 317–322, 1953.
315. MOSES, R. A. *Adler's Physiology of the Eye* (5th ed.). St. Louis: Mosby, 1970.
316. MUKUNO, K. Fine structure of the human extraocular muscles. 2. Two distinct types of muscle fibers. *Acta Soc. Ophthalmol. Japan.* 71: 907–918, 1967.
317. MURRAY, J. G., AND J. W. THOMPSON. The occurrence and function of collateral sprouting in the sympathetic nervous system of the cat. *J. Physiol., London* 135: 133–162, 1957.
318. MUSTAKALLIO, A. Monoamine oxidase activity in the various structures of the mammalian eye. *Acta Ophthalmol. Suppl.* 93: 1–62, 1967.
319. NAGAI, M., T. BAN, AND T. KOROTSU. Studies on the changes of the intraocular pressure induced by electrical stimulation of the hypothalamus. *Med. J. Osaka Univ.* 2: 87–95, 1951.
319a. NEUFELD, A. H., R. M. CHAVIS, AND M. L. SEARS. Degeneration release of norepinephrine causes transient ocular hyperemia mediated by prostaglandins. *Invest. Ophthalmol.* 12: 167–175, 1973.
319b. NEUFELD, A. H., L. M. JAMPOL, AND M. L. SEARS. Cyclic-AMP in the aqueous humor: the effects of adrenergic agents. *Exptl. Eye Res.* 14: 242–250, 1972.
320. NICHOLS, C. W., D. JACOBOWITZ, AND M. HOTTENSTEIN. The influence of light and dark on the catecholamine content of the retina and choroid. *Invest. Ophthalmol.* 6: 642–646, 1967.
321. NIESEL, P. Zur Frage der nervösen Beeinflussung der Aderhautdurchblutung. *Ber. Deut. Ophthalmol. Ges.* 64: 86–90, 1961.
322. NILSSON, O. The relationship between nerves and smooth muscle cells in the rat iris. I. The dilatator muscle. *Z. Zellforsch. Mikroskop. Anat.* 64: 166–171, 1964.
323. NISHIDA, S., AND M. L. SEARS. Fine structural innervation of the dilator muscle of the iris of the albino guinea pig studied with permanganate fixation. *Exptl. Eye Res.* 8: 292–296, 1969.
324. NISHIDA, S., AND M. L. SEARS. Dual innervation of the iris sphincter muscle of the albino guinea pig. *Exptl. Eye Res.* 8: 467–469, 1969.
325. NISHIDA, S., J. TROTTER, AND M. L. SEARS. Innervation of the chamber angle of the guinea pig eye. *Exptl. Eye Res.* 8: 143–146, 1969.
326. NORBERG, K. A., AND B. HAMBERGER. The sympathetic adrenergic neuron. *Acta Physiol. Scand. Suppl.* 238, 1964.
327. OBIANWU, H. O., AND M. J. RAND. The relationship between the mydriatic action of ephedrine and the colour of the iris. *Brit. J. Ophthalmol.* 49: 264–270, 1965.
328. OCHI, J., M. KONISHI, H. YOSHIKAWA, AND Y. SANO. Fluorescence and electron microscopic evidence for the dual innervation of the iris sphincter muscle of the rabbit. *Z. Zellforsch. Mikroskop. Anat.* 91: 90–95, 1968.
329. O'STEEN, W. K. Retinal and optic nerve serotonin and retinal degeneration as influenced by photoperiod. *Exptl. Neurol.* 27: 194–205, 1970.
330. PATERSON, C. A. The effect of sympathetic nerve stimulation on the aqueous humor dynamics of the cocaine pretreated rabbit. *Exptl. Eye Res.* 5: 37–44, 1966.
331. PATIL, P. N. Adrenergic receptors of the bovine iris sphincter. *J. Pharmacol. Exptl. Therap.* 166: 299–307, 1969.
331a. PATIL, P. N. Cocaine-binding by the pigmented and nonpigmented iris and its relevance to the mydriatic effect. *Invest. Ophthalmol.* 11: 739–746, 1972.
332. PECZON, J. D. Effect of methyldopa on intraocular pressure in human eyes. *Am. J. Ophthalmol.* 60: 82–87, 1965.
333. PEDLER, C. M. H., AND D. A. YOUNG. Retinal ultrastructure and pattern recognition logic. *Brit. Med. Bull.* 26: 119–124, 1970.
334. PHILLIPS, C. I., G. HOWITT, AND D. J. ROWLANDS. Propranolol as ocular hypotensive agent. *Brit. J. Ophthalmol.* 51: 222–226, 1967.
335. PHILPOT, F. J. The inhibition of adrenaline oxidation by local anaesthetics. *J. Physiol., London* 97: 301–307, 1940.
336. PILLAT, B., AND M. M. POWERS. Epinephrine and arterenol determinations in aqueous humor and iris and ciliary body of cattle. *Arch. Ophthalmol.* 50: 323–330, 1953.
337. PIRIE, A. Color and solubility of the proteins of human cataracts. *Invest. Ophthalmol.* 7: 634–650, 1968.
337a. PIRIE, A. Formation of N'-formylkynurenine in proteins from lens and other sources by exposure to light. *Biochem. J.* 125: 203–208, 1971.
338. PLUMMER, G., P. H. CLEVELAND, AND C. STEVENS. Herpes simplex virus and paralysis of rabbits. Activation of the paralysis by adrenaline. *Brit. J. Exptl. Pathol.* 48: 390–394, 1967.
339. POOS, F. Pharmakologische und physiologische Untersuchungen an den isolierten Irismuskeln. *Arch. Exptl. Pathol. Pharmakol.* 126: 307–351, 1927.
340. PRIJOT, E. Contribution to the study of tonometry and tonography in ophthalmology. *Doc. Ophthalmol.* 15: 1–225, 1961.
341. QUAY, W. B. Retinal and pineal hydroxyindole-O-methyl transferase activity in vertebrates. *Life Sci.* 4: 983–991, 1965.
342. QUILLIAM, J. P. A quantitative method for the study of the reactions of the isolated cat's iris. *J. Physiol., London* 110: 237–247, 1949.
343. RICHARDSON, K. C. The fine structure of the albino rabbit iris with special reference to the identification of adrenergic and cholinergic nerves and nerve endings in its intrinsic muscles. *Am. J. Anat.* 114: 173–184, 1964.
344. RICHARDSON, K. C. Electron microscopic identification of autonomic nerve endings. *Nature* 210: 756, 1966.
345. RICHARDSON, K. C. Cholinergic and adrenergic axons in methylene blue-stained rat iris: an electron-microscopical study. *Life Sci., Part 1* 7: 509–604, 1968.
346. RIPPS, H., I. SIEGEL, AND W. B. GETZ. Functional organization of ciliary muscle in the cat. *Am. J. Physiol.* 203: 857–859, 1962.
347. ROBINSON, G. C., D. A. DIKRAINIAN, AND G. F. ROSEBOROUGH. Congenital Horner's syndrome and heterochromia iridum. Their association with congenital foregut and vertebral anomalies. *Pediatrics* 35: 103–107, 1965.
348. ROBINSON, J. Amine oxidase in the iris and nictitating membrane of the cat and the rabbit. *Brit. J. Pharmacol.* 7: 99–102, 1952.
349. ROHEN, J. W. Discussion. In: *Glaucoma Symposium, Tutzing Castle, 1966*, edited by J. W. Rohen. New York: Karger, 1967, p. 47.
350. RÖHMER, P. C. Quelques observations de sympathectomie dans le glaucome. *Ann. Oculist* 127: 328–378, 1902.
351. ROSENBLUETH, A., AND P. BARD. The innervation and functions of the nictitating membrane in the cat. *Am. J. Physiol.* 100: 537–544, 1932.
352. ROSS, R. A., AND S. M. DRANCE. Effects of topically applied isoproterenol on aqueous dynamics in man. *Arch. Ophthalmol.* 83: 39–46, 1970.
353. ROSSER, M. J., AND M. L. SEARS. Further studies on the mechanism of the increased outflow of aqueous humor from the eyes of rabbits twenty-four hours after cervical sympa-

thetic ganglionectomy. *J. Pharmacol. Exptl. Therap.* 164: 280–289, 1968.
354. ROST, F. W. D., AND J. M. POLAK. Fluorescence microscopy and microspectrofluorimetry of malignant melanomas, naevi and normal melanocytes. *Arch. Abt. A Pathol. Anat.* 347: 321–326, 1969.
355. ROST, F. W. D., J. M. POLAK, AND A. G. E. PEARSE. The melanocyte: its cytochemical and immunological relationship to cells of the endocrine polypeptide (APUD) series. *Arch. Abt. B Zellpathol.* 4: 93–101, 1969.
356. ROTH, C. D., AND K. C. RICHARDSON. Electron microscopical studies on axonal degeneration in the rat iris following ganglionectomy. *Am. J. Anat.* 124: 341–360, 1969.
357. ROTH, R. H., L. STJÄRNE, AND U. S. VON EULER. Factors influencing the rate of norepinephrine biosynthesis in nerve tissue. *J. Pharmacol. Exptl. Therap.* 158: 373–377, 1967.
358. RUCKER, C. W. Knowledge of the pupillary reactions in Argyll-Robertson's time. *Surv. Ophthalmol.* 14: 162–171, 1969.
359. RUEGG, J. C., AND W. R. HESS. Die Wirking von Adrenalin, Noradrenalin und Acetylcholin auf die isolierten Irismuskeln. *Helv. Physiol. Pharmacol. Acta* 11: 216–230, 1953.
360. RUSKELL, G. L. Vasomotor axons of the lacrimal glands of monkeys and the ultrastructural identification of sympathetic terminals. *Z. Zellforsch. Mikroskop. Anat.* 83: 321–333, 1967.
361. RUSKELL, G. L. The fine structure of nerve terminations in the lacrimal glands of monkeys. *J. Anat.* 103: 65–76, 1968.
362. RUSKELL, G. L. Changes in nerve terminals and acini of the lacrimal gland and changes in secretion induced by autonomic denervation. *Z. Zellforsch. Mikroskop. Anat.* 94: 261–281, 1969.
363. SALLMANN, L. VON, AND O. LOWENSTEIN. Responses of intraocular pressure, blood pressure, and cutaneous vessels to electric stimulation in the diencephalon. *Am. J. Ophthalmol.* 39: 11–28, 1954.
364. SALLMANN, L. VON, F. J. MACRI, T. WANKO, AND P. A. GRIMES. Some mechanisms of centrally induced eye pressure responses. *Am. J. Ophthalmol.* 42: 130–147, 1956.
365. SANGHVI, I. S. Effects of cholinergic and adrenergic agents and their antagonists at the neuromuscular junction of the cat extraocular muscles. *Invest. Ophthalmol.* 6: 269–276, 1967.
366. SCHAEPPI, U., AND W. P. KOELLA. Adrenergic innervation of cat iris sphincter. *Am. J. Physiol.* 207: 273–278, 1964.
367. SCHAEPPI, U., AND W. P. KOELLA. Innervation of the cat iris dilator. *Am. J. Physiol.* 207: 1411–1416, 1964.
368. SCHAEPPI, U., R. RUBIN, AND W. P. KOELLA. Electrical stimulation of the isolated cat iris. *Am. J. Physiol.* 210: 1165–1169, 1966.
369. SCHEIE, E., AND A. M. LATIES. Catecholamine-containing cells in the retinas of *Gekko gecko* and *Rana pipiens*. *Herpetologica* 27: 77–80, 1971.
370. SCHMERL, E., AND B. STEINBERG. Separation of diencephalic centers concerned with pupillary motility and ocular tension. *Am. J. Ophthalmol.* 33: 1379–1381, 1950.
371. SCHMIDT-NIELSEN, J., AND R. FANGE. Salt glands in marine reptiles. *Nature* 182: 783–784, 1958.
372. SCHUMACHER, H., AND H-G. CLASSEN. Der Einfluss von 5-hydroxytryptamin auf den Augenbinnendruck. *Arch. Klin. Exptl. Ophthalmol.* 164: 538–542, 1962.
373. SEARS, M. L. The mechanism of action of adrenergic drugs in glaucoma. *Invest. Ophthalmol.* 5: 115–119, 1966.
374. SEARS, M. L. Vitamin C as a requirement for the storage of norepinephrine by the iris. *Biochem. Pharmacol.* 18: 253–256, 1969.
374a. SEARS, M. L. Browning of the lens in generalized albinism. *Am. J. Ophthalmol.* 77: 819–823, 1974.
375. SEARS, M. L., AND E. H. BÁRÁNY. Outflow resistance and adrenergic mechanisms. Effects of sympathectomy, N-(2-chloroethyl) dibenzylamine hydrochloride (dibenamine) and dichloroisoproterenol on the outflow resistance of the rabbit eye. *Arch. Ophthalmol.* 64: 839–848, 1960.
376. SEARS, M. L., AND C. N. GILLIS. Mydriasis and the increase in outflow of aqueous humor from the rabbit eye after cervical ganglionectomy in relation to the release of norepinephrine from the iris. *Biochem. Pharmacol.* 16: 777–782, 1967.
376a. SEARS, M. L., E. B. MCLEAN, AND A. R. BELLOWS. Drug-induced retraction of the vitreous face after cataract extraction. *Trans. Am. Acad. Ophthalmol. Otolaryngol.* 76: 498–510, 1972.
377. SEARS, M., K. MIZUNO, C. CINTRON, A. ALTER, AND T. SHERK. Changes in outflow facility and content of norepinephrine in iris and ciliary processes of albino rabbits after cervical ganglionectomy. *Invest. Ophthalmol.* 5: 312–318, 1966.
378. SEARS, M. L., AND R. G. SELKER. Denervation supersensitivity of the lacrimal gland. *Am. J. Ophthalmol.* 63: 481–483, 1967.
379. SEARS, M. L., AND T. E. SHERK. Supersensitivity of the aqueous outflow resistance in rabbits after sympathetic denervation. *Nature* 197: 387–388, 1963.
380. SEARS, M. L., AND T. E. SHERK. The trabecular effect of noradrenalin in the rabbit eye. *Invest. Ophthalmol.* 3: 157–163, 1964.
381. SEIDEHAMEL, R. J., A. TYE, AND P. N. PATIL. An analysis of ephedrine mydriasis in relationship to iris pigmentation in the guinea pig eye in vitro. *J. Pharmacol. Exptl. Therap.* 171: 205–213, 1970.
382. SHANTA, T. R., W. D. WOODS, M. B. WAITZMAN, AND G. H. BOURNE. Histochemical method for localization of cyclic 3′,5′-nucleotide phosphodiesterase. *Histochemie* 7: 177–190, 1966.
383. SHANTHAVEERAPPA, T. R., AND G. H. BOURNE. Monoamine oxidase distribution in the rabbit eye. *J. Histochem. Cytochem.* 12: 281–288, 1964.
384. SHIOSE, Y. Electron microscopic studies on the ciliary muscle. *Acta Soc. Ophthalmol. Japan.* 65: 1267–1283, 1961.
385. SHLAER, S. The relation between visual acuity and illumination. *J. Gen. Physiol.* 21: 165–188, 1937.
386. SINGH, K. P., O. P. KULSHRESTHA, M. M. MAHAWAR, S. K. GAUTAM, AND M. M. SINGH. Propranolol for ocular anaesthesia. *Lancet* 2: 158, 1967.
387. SINGH, K. P., O. P. KULSHRESTHA, M. M. MAHAWAR, S. K. GAUTAM, AND M. M. SINGH. Propranolol as an ocular anaesthetic. *Orient. Arch. Ophthalmol.* 6: 159–160, 1968.
388. SMELSER, G. K., AND S. SILVER. The distribution of mast cells in the normal eye. A method of study. *Exptl. Eye Res.* 2: 134–140, 1963.
389. SMITH, A. A., J. DANCIS, AND G. BREININ. Ocular responses to autonomic drugs in familial dysautonomia. *Invest. Ophthalmol.* 4: 358–361, 1965.
390. SMITH, C. B., U. TRENDELENBURG, S. Z. LANGER, AND T. H. TSAI. The relation of retention of norepinephrine-H³ to the norepinephrine content of the nictitating membrane of the spinal cat during development of denervation supersensitivity. *J. Pharmacol. Exptl. Therap.* 151: 87–94, 1966.
391. SNEDDON, J. M., AND P. TURNER. Adrenergic blockade and the eye signs of thyrotoxicosis. *Lancet* 2: 525–527, 1966.
392. SNEDDON, J. M., AND P. TURNER. Ephedrine mydriasis in hypertension and response to treatment. *Clin. Pharmacol. Therap.* 10: 64–71, 1969.
393. SPIEGEL, E., AND I. SOMMER. *Neurology of the Eye, Ear, Nose and Throat.* New York: Grune & Stratton, 1944, p. 451–466.
394. SPIERS, A. S. D., AND D. B. CALNE. Action of dopamine on the human iris. *Brit. Med. J.* 4: 333–335, 1969.
395. STAFLOVA, J. Comparative study of the adrenergic innervation of the iris and ciliary structures in species in phylogenesis. *J. Morphol.* 128: 387–399, 1969.
396. STAFLOVA, J. Adrenergic innervation of the iris, ciliary body, and ciliary processes of the rabbit eye. *Johns Hopkins Med. J.* 125: 107–118, 1969.
397. STIBBE, E. P. A comparative study of the nictitating membrane of birds and mammals. *J. Anat.* 62: 159–176, 1928.
398. STRÖMBLAD, B. C. R., AND M. NICKERSON. Accumulation of epinephrine and norepinephrine by some rat tissues. *J. Pharmacol. Exptl. Therap.* 134: 154–159, 1961.

399. SWEGMARK, G. Aqueous humour dynamics in Horner's syndrome. *Trans. Ophthalmol. Soc. UK* 83: 255–261, 1963.
400. TAGAWA, S., K. FUKAE, T. NONAKA, K. FUZINO, AND K. NAKAI. Response of ciliary muscle to adrenergic agents. Adrenergic receptors of ciliary muscle. *Acta Soc. Ophthalmol. Japan.* 71: 984–988, 1967.
401. TAMMISTO, T. The effect of 5-hydroxytryptamine (serotonin) on retinal vessels of the rat. *Acta Ophthalmol.* 43: 430–433, 1965.
402. TARKHAN, A. A. The innervation of the extrinsic ocular muscles. *J. Anat.* 68: 293–317, 1934.
403. THOMPSON, J. W. Studies on the responses of the isolated nictitating membrane of the cat. *J. Physiol., London* 141: 46–72, 1958.
404. THOMPSON, H. S., AND J. H. MENSHER. Adrenergic mydriasis in Horner's syndrome. Hydroxyamphetamine test for diagnosis of postganglionic defects. *Am. J. Ophthalmol.* 72: 472–480, 1972.
405. TISSARI, A. 5-Hydroxytryptamine, 5-hydroxytryptophan decarboxylase and monoamine oxidase during foetal and postnatal development in the guinea pig. *Acta Physiol. Scand. Suppl.* 265: 1–80, 1966.
406. TÖRNQVIST, G. Effect of cervical sympathetic stimulation on accommodation in monkeys. An example of a beta-adrenergic, inhibitory effect. *Acta Physiol. Scand.* 67: 363–372, 1966.
407. TÖRNQVIST, G. Accommodation in monkeys. Some pharmacological and physiological aspects. *Acta Ophthalmol.* 45: 429–460, 1967.
408. TÖRNQVIST, G. The relative importance of the parasympathetic and sympathetic nervous system for accommodation in monkeys. *Invest. Ophthalmol.* 6: 612–617, 1967.
409. TÖRNQVIST, G. Effect of cervical sympathetic stimulation on accommodation in guanethidine-treated monkeys. *Invest. Ophthalmol.* 9: 765–768, 1970.
410. TREISTER, G., AND E. H. BÁRÁNY. Mydriasis and intraocular pressure decrease in the conscious rabbit after unilateral superior cervical ganglionectomy. *Invest. Ophthalmol.* 9: 331–342, 1970.
411. TREISTER, G., AND E. H. BÁRÁNY. The effect of bretylium on the degeneration mydriasis and intraocular pressure decrease in the conscious rabbit after unilateral cervical ganglionectomy. *Invest. Ophthalmol.* 9: 343–353, 1970.
412. TREISTER, G., AND E. H. BÁRÁNY. Degeneration mydriasis and hyperemia of the iris after superior cervical ganglionectomy in the rabbit. *Invest. Ophthalmol.* 9: 873–887, 1970.
413. TRENDELENBURG, U. Supersensitivity and subsensitivity to sympathomimetic amines. *Pharmacol. Rev.* 15: 225–276, 1963.
414. TRENDELENBURG, U. Time course of changes in sensitivity after denervation of the nictitating membrane of the spinal cat. *J. Pharmacol. Exptl. Therap.* 142: 335–342, 1963.
415. TRENDELENBURG, U. Mechanisms of supersensitivity and subsensitivity to sympathomimetic amines. *Pharmacol. Rev.* 18: 629–640, 1966.
416. TRENDELENBURG, U. Supersensitivity to norepinephrine induced by continuous nerve stimulation. *J. Pharmacol. Exptl. Therap.* 151: 95–102, 1966.
417. TROKEL, S. Measurement of ocular blood flow and volume by reflective densitometry. *Arch. Ophthalmol.* 71: 88–92, 1964.
418. TROKEL, S. Quantitative studies of choroidal blood flow by reflective densitometry. *Invest. Ophthalmol.* 4: 1129–1140, 1965.
419. TSUKAHARA, S. Histochemistry of catecholamine (CA) in the rabbit and human extraocular muscles. *Japan. J. Ophthalmol.* 12: 123–131, 1968.
420. TSUKAHARA, S. Distribution of catecholamine positive nerve fibers in the ocular tissue of rabbits. Effects of blocking agents on these nerve fibers. *Acta Soc. Ophthalmol. Japan.* 73: 982–990, 1969.
421. TUOVINEN, E., R. ESILÄ, AND M. LIESMAA. The effect of alpha-methyldopa on the intraocular pressure of the rabbit eye. *Acta Ophthalmol.* 44: 669–675, 1966.
422. TURNER, P., AND J. M. SNEDDON. Alpha receptor blockade by thymoxamine in the human eye. *Clin. Pharmacol. Therap.* 9: 45–49, 1968.
423. TYNER, G. S., AND H. G. SCHEIE. Mechanism of the miotic-resistant pupil with increased intraocular pressure. *Arch. Ophthalmol.* 50: 572–579, 1953.
424. UGA, S. Electron microscopy of the ciliary muscle. I. On six types of nerve endings in the ciliary muscle of human and monkey eyes. *Acta Soc. Ophthalmol. Japan.* 71: 951–961, 1967.
426. VALE, J., AND C. I. PHILLIPS. Effect of DL- and D-propranolol on ocular tension in rabbits and patients. *Exptl. Eye Res.* 9: 82–90, 1970.
427. VALU, L. New data concerning the innervation of the uveal-trabecular system. *Szemészet* 103: 65–69, 1966.
428. VAN ALPHEN, G. W. H., R. KERN, AND S. L. ROBINETTE. Adrenergic receptors of the intraocular muscles. *Arch. Ophthalmol.* 74: 253–259, 1965.
429. VAN ALPHEN, G. W. H., S. L. ROBINETTE, AND F. J. MACRI. The adrenergic receptors of the intraocular muscles of the cat. *Intern. J. Neuropharmacol.* 2: 259–272, 1964.
430. VAN ORDEN, L. S., III, K. G. BENSCH, S. Z. LANGER, AND U. TRENDELENBURG. Histochemical and fine structural aspects of the onset of denervation supersensitivity in the nictitating membrane of the spinal cat. *J. Pharmacol. Exptl. Therap.* 157: 274–283, 1967.
431. VAN WOERT, M. H. Effect of phenothiazines on melanoma tyrosinase activity. *J. Pharmacol. Exptl. Therap.* 172: 256–264, 1970.
432. VEGGE, T., AND A. RINGVOLD. Ultrastructure of the wall of human iris vessels. *Z. Zellforsch. Mikroskop. Anat.* 94: 19–31, 1969.
433. VELHAGEN, K. Ueber die Wirkungsweise der Cholinkörper auf die Irismuskeln, zugleich Beitrag zur Doppelinnervation derselben. *Arch. Augenheilkunde* 108: 126–136, 1934.
434. VILSTRUP, G. Studies on the vascular capacity and tissue fluid content of the choroid and their variation under treatment with histamine. *Acta Ophthalmol.* 30: 173–180, 1952.
435. VOADEN, M. J., AND S. J. LEESON. A chalone in the mammalian lens. I. Effect of bilateral adrenalectomy on the mitotic activity of the adult mouse lens. *Exptl. Eye Res.* 9: 57–66, 1970.
435a. WÅLINDER, P.-E. The accumulation of alpha aminoisobutyric acid by the rabbit ciliary body-iris preparations. *Invest. Ophthalmol.* 7: 67–76, 1968.
435b. WALLS, G. L., AND H. D. JUDD. The intra-ocular colour filters of vertebrates. *Brit. J. Ophthalmol.* 17: 641–695, 1933.
436. WALTER, W. G. Action of L-norepinephrine on the isolated rabbit iris. *Acta Physiol. Pharmacol. Neerl.* 7: 222–238, 1958.
437. WALTER, W. G., A. G. M. VAN GEMERT, AND J. W. DUYFF. Kinetics of pupillary dilation induced by administration of L-epinephrine. *Acta Physiol. Pharmacol. Neerl.* 3: 309–324, 1954.
438. WALTMAN, S., AND M. SEARS. Catechol-O-methyl transferase and monoamine oxidase activity in the ocular tissues of albino rabbits. *Invest. Ophthalmol.* 3: 601–605, 1964.
439. WEINER, N. Regulation of norepinephrine biosynthesis. *Ann. Rev. Pharmacol.* 10: 273–290, 1970.
440. WEINER, N., S. Z. LANGER, AND U. TRENDELENBURG. Demonstration by the histochemical fluorescence method of the prolonged disappearance of catecholamines from the denervated nictitating membrane of the cat. *J. Pharmacol. Exptl. Therap.* 157: 284–289, 1967.
441. WEINER, N., M. PERKINS, AND R. L. SIDMAN. Effect of reserpine on noradrenaline content of innervated and denervated brown adipose tissue of the rat. *Nature* 193: 137–138, 1962.
442. WEINSTEIN, G. W., AND M. E. LANGHAM. Horner's syndrome and glaucoma. *Arch. Ophthalmol.* 82: 483–486, 1969.
443. WEINTRAUB, M. I., D. GAASTERLAND, AND M. H. VAN WOERT. Pupillary effects of levodopa therapy. Development of anisocoria in latent Horner's syndrome. *New Engl. J. Med.* 283: 120–123, 1970.
444. WEISS, B. Effects of environmental lighting and chronic

denervation on the activation of adenyl cyclase of rat pineal gland by norepinephrine and sodium fluoride. *J. Pharmacol. Exptl. Therap.* 168: 146–152, 1969.
445. WERNER, G. Zur Innervation der Musculi sphincter und Dilatator pupillae. *Z. Mikroskop. Anat. Forsch.* 68: 61–78, 1962.
446. WIEDEMAN, M. P. Blood flow through terminal arterial vessels after denervation of the bat wing. *Circulation Res.* 22: 83–89, 1968.
447. WEISMAN, G. G., D. S. JONES, AND W. C. RANDALL. Sympathetic outflows from cervical spinal cord in the dog. *Science* 152: 381–382, 1966.
448. WOODS, W. D., AND M. B. WAITZMAN. Cyclic adenylic acid activity in ocular tissues. *Federation Proc.* 25: 574, 1966.
449. WUDKA, E., AND I. H. LEOPOLD. Experimental studies of the choroidal vessels. IV. Pharmacologic observations. *Arch. Ophthalmol.* 55: 857–885, 1956.
450. WURTMAN, R. J., J. AXELROD, AND D. E. KELLY. *The Pineal.* New York: Acad. Press, 1968.
451. WURTMAN, R. J., J. AXELROD, G. SEDVALL, AND R. Y. MOORE. Photic and neural control of the 24-hour norepinephrine rhythm in the rat pineal gland. *J. Pharmacol. Exptl. Therap.* 157: 487–492, 1967.
452. YAMAUCHI, A., AND G. BURNSTOCK. Nerve-myoepithelium and nerve-glandular epithelium contacts in the lacrimal gland of the sheep. *J. Cell Biol.* 34: 917–919, 1967.
453. YOSHIMURA, H., AND K. HOSOKAWA. Studies on the mechanism of salt and water secretion from the lacrimal gland. *Japan. J. Physiol.* 13: 303–318, 1963.
454. YOUNG, J. Z. Comparative studies on the physiology of the iris. I. Selachians. II. Uranoscopus and Lophius. *Proc. Roy. Soc. London Ser. B* 112: 228–249, 1933.
455. ZELLER, E. A., D. SHOCH, S. G. COOPERMAN, AND R. I. SCHNIPPER. Enzymology of the refractory media of the eye. IX. On the role of monoamine oxidase in the regulation of aqueous humor dynamics of the rabbit eye. *Invest. Ophthalmol.* 6: 618–623, 1967.
456. ZIGMAN, S. Eye lens color: formation and function. *Science* 171: 807–809, 1971.
457. ZIGMAN, S., J. SCHULTZ, AND T. YULO. Possible roles of near UV light in the cataractous process. *Exptl. Eye Res.* 15: 201–208, 1973.

CHAPTER 36

Catecholamines and control of sweat glands

D. ROBERTSHAW | *Department of Animal Physiology, University of Nairobi, Nairobi, Kenya*[1]

CHAPTER CONTENTS

Histology
Primates
   Man
   Other anthropoid primates
   Prosimian primates
Perissodactyla
   Equidae
   Rhinocerotidae
Artiodactyla
   Bovidae
   Suidae
   Camelidae
Carnivora
   Canidae
   Felidae
Rodentia
Conclusions

AS AMBIENT TEMPERATURES approach body temperature, the only means by which homeothermic mammals can lose the heat produced by metabolism or acquired by radiation (e.g., from the sun or surroundings) is by utilizing the latent heat of evaporation of water. For this purpose, two distinct mechanisms exist in terrestrial mammals: *1*) an increase in respiratory moisture loss by increased respiratory dead space ventilation variously described as panting, thermal tachypnea, and thermal polypnea; and *2*) an increase in cutaneous moisture loss by secretion of the sweat glands. A possible third mechanism, spreading of saliva over the fur, has been described in rats by Hainsworth (30). The degree to which mammals depend on panting or sweating varies; with the exception of man and possibly some of the anthropoid primates, all terrestrial mammals so far studied exhibit some panting on heat exposure. When and why man lost this ability, if he ever possessed it, in the course of his evolution, is a matter for interesting speculation. The prosimian primates certainly pant on heat exposure (5). Similarly there seems to be no teleological argument why, in some mammals, sweating has evolved as the principal evaporative heat loss mechanism. A clue to this may be found in the studies of Robertshaw & Taylor (65) who compared the sweating mechanism of eight species of East African bovid and noted that the smaller species utilized panting and the larger species sweating as their avenue of evaporative heat loss. Animals of intermediate size utilized both methods in nearly equal proportions. It would seem therefore that body size limits panting as a heat loss mechanism and necessitates the development of sweat glands as thermoregulatory structures. With the exception of the elephant, all the larger terrestrial mammals indigenous to tropical countries utilize sweating as their main heat loss mechanism. It seems probable therefore that thermoregulatory sweating has evolved independently in the various orders of Mammalia, an example of convergent evolution. Some sweat glands, such as the glands of the palm and sole of man and the foot pad of mammals, have no thermoregulatory function. Their secretion probably aids frictional contact (1) or improves tactile perception (85). Other glands are thought to produce an odoriferous secretion that has some social or sexual function (85).

With such diversity of function and possible phylogenetic background it is hardly surprising that there should be several modes of sudomotor control; thus cholinergic transmission, adrenergic transmission, and a humoral component have been described. They all have one feature in common—they can be stimulated by catecholamines. In man this appears to be of no physiological significance, but in other animals it reflects the adrenergic nature of sudomotor transmission.

Since sweating as a heat loss mechanism is most highly developed in man, primates are discussed first; a consideration of other orders of Mammalia follows.

HISTOLOGY

The classification of the sweat glands on anatomic grounds was originally made by Schiefferdecker (70, 71) and is still widely used today. He separated the sweat glands into two groups, eccrine and apocrine, on the basis of their mode of secretion. The secretory cells of eccrine glands elaborate their secretion without loss of the integrity of the cell membrane. Apocrine glands,

---

The unpublished observations of the author reported here were financially supported with a grant from the Wellcome Trust.

[1] Present address: Department of Anatomy and Physiology, Indiana University, Bloomington, Indiana

on the other hand, employ a necrobiotic process of secretion whereby the apical portion of the secretory cell is decapitated and constitutes the secretion; that is, it is a "semi-holocrine" process. Sweat gland classification and the existence of an apocrine secretory process have recently been questioned (42) because it has been suggested that the appearance of cellular configurations typical of a necrobiotic secretory cycle are merely artifacts of fixation. A physiological basis for sweat gland classification would be more appropriate, but, until the varied functions of sweat glands have been elucidated, the simple anatomic classification proposed by Bligh (10) is used. He suggested "epitrichial" glands, those associated with a hair follicle and having a duct that opens into the pilosebaceous orifice, and "atrichial" glands, those having a duct that opens independently onto the skin surface. This classification means, generally speaking, that the apocrine glands are epitrichial and the eccrine glands are atrichial, and it has the merit that controversy over the nature of the secretory process is avoided. The secretion of atrichial glands is a clear salt solution, whereas that of epitrichial glands is viscid, possibly because of admixture of sebaceous secretion. The secretory cells of all sweat glands possess spindle-shaped myoepithelial cells arranged with their long axes parallel to their basement membranes. The possible contractility of the secretory cells is suggested by fluctuations noted in continuous records of cutaneous evaporative loss (10) and by direct observation of the cells themselves (35). The appearance of moisture on the surface of the skin may therefore involve two distinct processes *1)* myoepithelial contraction and expulsion of preformed secretion; and *2)* stimulation of secretion and an overflow of the secretion. Alternatively a combination of both processes may occur.

PRIMATES

The order Primates contains some 80 genera, from the primitive tree shrews to man, the most advanced. The order is subdivided into two suborders, the Prosimii and Anthropoidea. Among the Prosimii are the tree shrews, lorises, lemurs, and tarsiers. All the others, including man, comprise the Anthropoidea. Unfortunately the functional activity of the sweat glands of species other than man has been little studied, although their anatomy has been described in great detail by Montagna and his colleagues at the Oregon Regional Primate Research Center.

Man

Man possesses epitrichial glands in certain regions of the body (e.g., axillary, inguinal, circumanal, and circumareolar). On the rest of the general body surface are atrichial glands, of which two distinct functional groups exist. The glands of the palms and sole are concerned not with thermoregulation, but with emotive responses. They respond to stimuli such as mental arithmetic, discussion of an embarrassing topic, or a sudden loud noise. The glands of the general body surface respond primarily to thermal stimulation. Sweating occurs in areas responsive to emotions only upon thermal stimulation at a higher temperature than that which stimulates the general body surface (53). It is well established that sweating by the atrichial glands of man is mediated through a cholinergic sympathetic innervation—atropine blocks the cholinergic response and anticholinesterases potentiate it and lower the threshold of stimulation (15, 16, 85). However, Ichibashi (37) demonstrated that iontophoretic administration of epinephrine caused sweating localized to the area of application. This observation has been confirmed on many occasions, and speculation on its physiological significance has resulted.

The sensitivity of the glands can be assessed by injecting intradermally various concentrations of drugs and determining the minimum effective concentration necessary to induce reaction.

The minimum effective concentration for epinephrine varies from 10^{-3} to 10^{-8} g/ml (14, 29, 52, 76, 78, 83). Norepinephrine seems to be effective at a similar range of concentrations, although the number of activated sweat glands and amount of sweating are less than that produced by epinephrine (29, 78). Isoproterenol will also stimulate the glands at the same range of concentrations, but the response cannot be obtained consistently (29, 76, 78). Sonnenschein et al. (76) make the interesting observation that one subject, who gave only a weak response to epinephrine and norepinephrine, manifested a strong response to isoproterenol. The relative sensitivities of the palmar and forearm sweat glands to epinephrine are in dispute. Haimovici (29) did not record any difference in sensitivity, whereas Sonnenschein et al. (76) reported that the palmar glands were less sensitive than the forearm glands to epinephrine. The reaction of the palmar glands is difficult to assess because the pain of intradermal injection itself may induce palmar sweating. Chalmers & Keele (15) abolished spontaneous palmar sweating by infiltration of the median nerve with local anesthetic. Under these conditions there appeared to be no difference in the sensitivity of the sweat glands of the two areas. Wada (83) noted that 80% of his subjects responded to intradermal epinephrine at a concentration of 10^{-7} g/ml and the remainder at a concentration of 10^{-6} g/ml (Fig. 1). The sensitivity is not affected by season, environmental temperature (83), or racial type (76), but is reduced in the age groups 1–12 years and 62–84 years (75, 83). Newborn children, however, show almost the same excitability as their mothers if tested within the first week of birth; sensitivity then declines. Thus the sensitivity to epinephrine is probably dependent on hormonal status, but in quite a different way from the effects that hormones have on the responsiveness of the glands to cholinergic stimulation. Intradermal mecholyl administration produces more sweat per gland in adult males than in females, but there is no sexual difference in the responsiveness to epinephrine administration (75). Equal

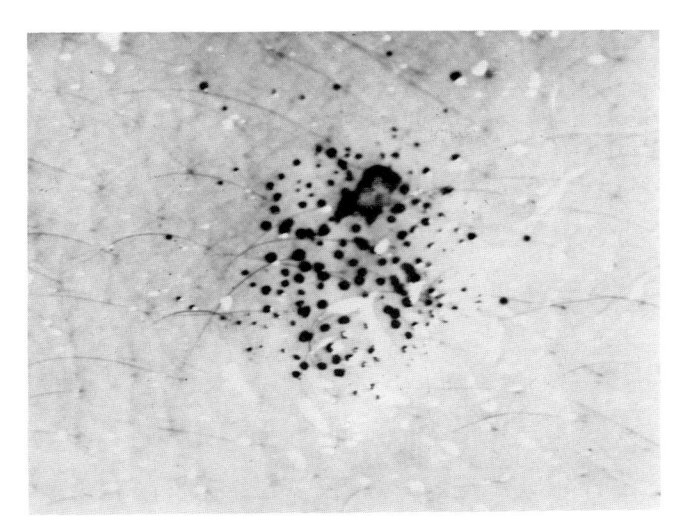

FIG. 1. Sweat spots at individual sweat gland openings of human forearm made visible by starch-iodine method of Wada (83). Effect of intradermal injection of epinephrine at a concentration of 10^{-7} g/ml. Photographed 18 min after injection. [Adapted from Wada (83).]

doses by weight of epinephrine and mecholyl in adult females stimulate approximately the same number of glands, and the amount of sweat secreted per gland is the same, the ratio of the epinephrine response to the mecholyl response being 1:1.15. In adult males the ratio is 1:7.67 (75). There seems to be divergence of opinion as to the numbers of sweat glands stimulated by epinephrine and mecholyl; Silver et al. (75) find that all glands are stimulated by both drugs, whereas Collins et al. (16) find that only half the sweat glands are stimulated by epinephrine. Both groups of workers used concentrations (10^{-4} to 10^{-5} g/ml) well above the threshold concentration. This discrepancy may be related to the relative sensitivities of the methods of sweat detection used; Silver et al. (75) used the starch-iodine method of Wada (83), and Collins et al. (16) used the plastic impression method of Thomson & Sutarman (81).

It is probable therefore that at concentrations above the threshold all the sweat glands are stimulated. This is suggested by the observation that the same gland is stimulated by epinephrine and acetylcholine and by heat (59).

Epinephrine and norepinephrine not only produce sweating at the site of injection, but also piloerection and vasoconstriction, the vasoconstriction usually outlasting the sweating effect (16, 76, 83). As the injected solution diffuses into the lymphatics, the area of sweating, piloerection, and vasoconstriction spreads with it to give a star-shaped appearance, radiating out from the injection weal. Suggestions that catecholamine-induced sweating is due to contraction of the myoepithelial cells are discounted because of the prolonged sweating response usually lasting over an hour (15, 53). This has been proved by injecting methylene blue intradermally and then stimulating the glands either with drugs or heat. The appearance of the dye in the sweat is taken as evidence of active sweat secretion; the dye is drawn from the extracellular fluid into the secretory cells and then secreted with the sweat. Epinephrine stimulation produces a dye-containing secretion, as do heat and cholinergic stimulation [(36); Fig. 2].

Atropine will block heat- and acetylcholine-induced sweating, as well as emotive sweating of the palms, but has no effect on catecholamine-induced sweating. The catecholamine-induced sweating can, however, be blocked by adrenergic-blocking drugs, and these have no effect on acetylcholine-induced sweating. The observation by Haimovici (29) that spontaneous sweating could be blocked by the adrenergic-receptor antagonist, N,N-dibenzyl-2-chloroethylamine (Dibenamine), led him to postulate a dual cholinergic and adrenergic innervation of the sweat glands. The drug was given intravenously in a large dose (5 mg/kg) that produced vomiting in some cases, and the anhidrotic effect may have been due to a central depression of sweating and not a direct action on the sweat glands. When Dibenamine is given locally, either intradermally (14) or iontophoretically (76), it has no effect on heat or acetylcholine-induced sweating but will block epinephrine-induced sweating. Other adrenergic antagonists that block catecholamine-induced sweating are dihydroergotamine (15, 76), ergotamine (76), dihydroergocristine (15), and tolazoline (15, 16, 50). No observa-

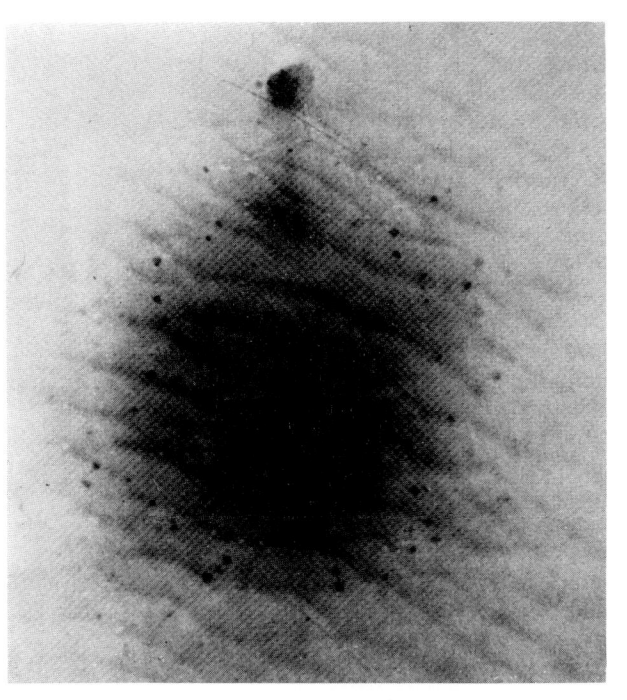

FIG. 2. Excretion of methylene blue after a previous intradermal injection of methylene blue in sweat that followed intradermal injection of epinephrine (0.3 ml of 10^{-3} g/liter) into skin of human forearm. Sweat droplets are shown. Since methylene blue must have been drawn into secretory cells of sweat glands from extracellular fluid, active secretion of sweat must have occurred during this process. *Large dark spot* at *upper part* of photograph represents reflux of dye from injection site. [Adapted from Hurley & Witkowski (36).]

tions have been made by using β receptor blocking drugs; all the drugs cited above block α receptor-mediated adrenergic effects. Until confirmatory evidence is forthcoming, it must be assumed that the receptors involved are of the α type. The inconsistent sudomotor effect of isoproterenol would support this general conclusion. The one individual, cited by Sonnenschein et al. (76), who showed a weak response to epinephrine and a strong one to isoproterenol, may have had receptors of the β variety.

Although the receptor sites for both cholinergic and adrenergic stimulation can be blocked by specific antagonists, which indicates that there may be a clear division of the effects of the two groups of drugs along the classic subdivisions of the autonomic nervous system, their responsiveness does appear to have certain features in common.

Intradermal injection of epinephrine suppresses spontaneous sweating, even though it may have no sudomotor effect of its own (76). Likewise, a second dose of epinephrine injected into an epinephrine-treated area will produce a considerably smaller response than the first dose (16). These effects are also observed with acetylcholine and cholinergic drugs (16, 80), and simultaneous injections of epinephrine and mecholyl enhance the depressing effects of mecholyl (16). The nature of this suppression, which may last from 1 or 2 days with a single injection to 2 or 3 weeks when repeated injections are made at the same site, is not known and may be similar with the two drugs since profuse and prolonged secretion does not seem to be a necessary prerequisite.

After denervation of the sweat glands of man, their responsiveness to intradermally administered acetylcholine declines and simultaneously their response to epinephrine diminishes. There is no evidence of supersensitivity to either drug (41). Arterial occlusion reduces the sudomotor effects of both epinephrine and acetylcholine (76).

In a search for the physiological significance of catecholamine-induced sweating in man, it might be postulated that catecholamines, particularly circulating epinephrine, may potentiate thermoregulatory sweating. There is evidence that the response to mecholyl "appeared more intense" when given with epinephrine (29). Sonnenschein et al. (76) believe that their results with subthreshold doses of each drug given simultaneously, which produce a positive sudomotor effect, suggest a true potentiating action. However, quantitative measurements show that, although the sweating produced by an intradermal mixture of epinephrine and acetylcholine is more prolonged than that produced by acetylcholine alone, the total output of sweat is usually less than that resulting from the sum of the separate sudorific responses of the two drugs (26). This is hard to reconcile with the results of Kennard (49) who has demonstrated that, when epinephrine or carbachol is introduced into the skin iontophoretically, the resulting rise in the ambient temperature can reduce the threshold of the thermoregulatory glands so that they are able to respond to emotive stimuli before the onset of thermoregulatory sweating. If it is assumed that, although thermal sweating areas can respond to emotive stimuli, thermal sudomotor stimuli are only distributed to the thermal sweating areas and that distribution of emotive sudomotor nerve fibers is generalized, the emotive sweating areas (i.e., palms, soles) may be subject to a high degree of sympathetic adrenergic influence, which may lower their threshold and make overt responses to emotive stimuli more likely. Although local adrenergic influences may be responsible for palmar sweating, severe stress, sufficient to induce adrenomedullary stimulation, will suppress palmar sweating (31). This is mediated through the central nervous system and is independent of any pituitary-adrenocortical activation (32). The physiological significance of this observation is difficult to assess unless one speculates on the significance of palmar sweating in man. If it be accepted that the palmar sweat glands represent a relic of man's arboreal existence and were adapted to enhance prehensibility, the observations of Adams & Hunter (1) might be relevant. Skin friction of the foot pad of the cat is increased by sweat gland activity until a level of sweating is reached above which skin friction progressively decreases and may be less than that for dry skin. Adrenomedullary secretion might therefore reduce the palmar sweat response so that prehensibility resulting from a high rate of sweat secretion is not reduced.

The generalized sweating in insulin hypoglycemia is not related to adrenomedullary release of catecholamines since it can occur in adrenalectomized subjects (28) and can be blocked by atropine (15). The profuse sweating observed during paroxysms of hypertension in pheochromocytoma may be due to high levels of circulating catecholamines acting directly on the sweat glands. With a ventilated capsule method of detecting cutaneous moisture loss, Foster et al. (26) have demonstrated a sweat response of the forearm during infusion of epinephrine (4–10 μg/min) and norepinephrine (5 μg/min) into the ipsilateral brachial artery, although intravenous infusion is without effect in doses up to 20 μg/min. This effect is blocked by phentolamine, but not by atropine. The failure of Chalmers & Keele (15) to produce sweating with rapid intraarterial injection of 20 μg epinephrine may have been due to the fact that sweat detection was by starch-iodine papers, which will only detect unevaporated water on the skin. Sweating occurs in both norepinephrine- and epinephrine-secreting tumors (W. S. Peart, personal communication). The question of whether or not the sweating of pheochromocytoma is due to a direct action of circulating catecholamines on the sweat glands can be easily determined; inhibition of sweating by intradermal phentolamine or Dibenamine would be indicative of such an action; blockade by atropine or hyoscine would suggest that sweating is due to central nervous stimulation. Prout & Wardell (63a) have, in fact, found that local application of hyoscine prevented two sweating attacks in two patients with pheochromocytoma.

In this context the mechanism of centrally induced sweating is of interest. Although there are major species differences in the response of the thermoregulatory systems to intrahypothalamic administration of catecholamines (9), epinephrine in monkeys causes a fall in body temperature presumably from stimulation of heat loss mechanisms. It is possible therefore that small amounts of epinephrine or norepinephrine can pass the blood-brain barrier in the region of the hypothalamus and centrally stimulate heat loss mechanisms. Severe hypertension may aid passage across the barrier because it is noted that sweating is only profuse in patients who have the severest hypertension (W. S. Peart, personal communication).

The epitrichial glands of man respond to emotive stimuli but are only active after puberty. They can be stimulated by epinephrine or norepinephrine given locally or systemically (73). Aoki (4) has demonstrated, contrary to earlier reports, that the epitrichial glands can be stimulated by cholinergic drugs, although atropine will not inhibit emotive sweating. A nerve supply to the glands that is positive for cholinesterase (13) has been demonstrated (4, 60). Since cholinesterase can be found in both adrenergic and cholinergic nerves its presence cannot be taken as indicative of cholinergic function. Unfortunately no studies have yet been made of the nerve supply to these glands with the formaldehyde-fluorescent technique of Falck & Owman (22) for detecting catecholamine-containing nerves. Denervation does not abolish the response to emotive stimuli (74), which suggests that the glands can be stimulated humorally, probably by circulating epinephrine or norepinephrine. There are still several problems to be answered with regard to the physiology of the epitrichial glands of man, but present evidence suggests that the glands may respond to emotive stimuli in the same manner as the atrichial glands on the palms and soles and that this response may be under cholinergic or adrenergic control. In addition, humoral stimulation by circulating catecholamines, epinephrine or norepinephrine, would appear to be important. Experiments with adrenergic blocking drugs would help to elucidate the nature of epitrichial sweat gland control in man.

Other Anthropoid Primates

It is generally assumed that the sweat glands of the anthropoid primates are similar to those of man and that sweating is the main evaporative heat loss mechanism, but this assumption has never been tested experimentally. The epitrichial glands of the chimpanzee (*Pan satyrus*) have a slightly wider distribution than those of man, but most of the glands of the general body surface and of friction surfaces are atrichial. The atrichial glands respond to cholinergic stimulation, whereas the epitrichial glands can be more readily stimulated by adrenergic drugs (61). The palmar glands of the green vervet monkey (*Cercopithecus aethiops*) are cholinergic but will respond to the local administration of epinephrine (68). There is considerable variation in the relative distribution of atrichial and epitrichial glands over the general body surface of Anthropoidea, and a study of their physiology would be of interest.

Prosimian Primates

The limited studies so far undertaken suggest that the atrichial sweat glands of the palm and sole are similar to those of man in that they are more readily stimulated by the local administration of cholinergic, rather than adrenergic, drugs (5, 69) and possess a cholinesterase-positive nerve supply. They do not, however, lose their responsiveness to methacholine after denervation (69), as do those of man. Only in the slow loris (*Nycticebus cougang*) are the glands of the general body surface surrounded by nerves that are demonstrable with the cholinesterase technique. However, in other species, except *Galago* sp., there are specialized aggregates of glands either on the flexor aspect of the arm or in the inguinal region, which have a readily demonstrable nerve supply (18). Thermal stimulation of these glands by raising the ambient temperature has not been demonstrated, but they will respond to radiant heating (5). The epitrichial glands of the slow loris and the potto (*Perodicticus potto*) can be stimulated by local administration of epinephrine and norepinephrine. Epinephrine is more potent than norepinephrine, the brachial glands of the slow loris being particularly sensitive and producing copious amounts of secretion. Isoproterenol is without effect, and the response can be annulled by dihydroergotamine, which would indicate an α receptor-mediated effect. Acetylcholine will also cause sweating but at a concentration 1,000 times greater than epinephrine. The epitrichial glands of the mongoose lemur (*Lemur mongoz*) cannot be stimulated either by epinephrine or acetylcholine (69).

The studies made so far are too meager for any conclusion to be drawn, but a comparison with man would suggest that the palmar glands of prosimians and man are similar, whereas those on the general body surface of prosimians appear to resemble more closely the epitrichial axillary glands of man, their response to pharmacological stimulation indicating an adrenergic, rather than cholinergic, mechanism of control.

PERISSODACTYLA

Equidae

The sweat glands of the general body surface of equids are epitrichial and respond to the intradermal administration of epinephrine at a concentration as low as 10^{-9} g/ml and norepinephrine at concentrations of 10^{-5} to 10^{-6} g/ml (6). They can also be stimulated by intravenous epinephrine administration (20). Norepinephrine given intravenously is without any sudorific effect in doses up to 12 µg/kg (20, 66). Isoproterenol given either intradermally or intravenously stimulates the glands to the same extent as epinephrine (6, 20). This observation would suggest that equine sweat gland receptors are of the β type, a conclusion supported by the fact that epinephrine-induced sweating cannot be blocked by phenoxybenzamine, dihydroergotamine (given intradermally or intravenously), phentolamine, tolazoline, or Dibenamine (given intradermally) but can be blocked by intravenous administration of the β receptor antagonist, propranolol (D. Robertshaw, unpublished observations). The α receptor antagonists (20), and to a small extent propranolol (D. Robertshaw, unpublished observations), have some sudorific action, probably resulting from some sympathomimetic effect. The β receptor antagonist, oxprenolol, has no such effect and completely inhibits epinephrine- and isoproterenol-induced sweating (D. Robertshaw, unpublished observations).

Parasympathomimetic compounds given intradermally can cause sweating but only at high concentrations relative to epinephrine (6, 20); the volume of sweat produced is small and of short duration when compared with that produced by epinephrine (Fig. 3). Atropine will block acetylcholine-induced but not epinephrine-induced sweating. Parasympathomimetic drugs given intravenously will produce sweating in horses when given in large doses or after inhibition of blood cholinesterase. This produces severe symptoms, such as intense salivation, muscle tremor, and defecation. These effects can be relieved by atropine, which does not suppress sweating (20). This would suggest that sweating is not due to the direct effect of the parasympathetic compounds on the sweat glands themselves but probably to epinephrine release from the adrenal medulla, the so-called "nicotinic" effect of parasympathetic compounds. Usenik (82) has verified this by showing that parasympathomimetic compounds do not produce sweating in adrenalectomized horses.

Contrary to the findings of Muto (62), Bell & Evans (8) were unable to produce sweating by stimulation of sympathetic nerves, and Evans et al. (21) demonstrated that plasma epinephrine levels are increased after exercise. On this evidence, Evans (19) suggested that sweating of the horse (*Equus equus*) is caused by blood-borne epinephrine of adrenomedullary origin and that no sudomotor nerve fibers exist. These conclusions were partially refuted by Usenik (82), who recorded sweating after exercise in adrenalectomized horses, although he noted that sweating was reduced. Jenkinson & Blackburn (46) have since demonstrated histologically a network of nerves around the sweat glands that are positive for specific cholinesterase. Equine sweat glands can be stimulated by heat (2, 72), as well as exercise. Robertshaw & Taylor (66) have examined the mechanism of heat- and exercise-induced sweating in the donkey (*Equus asinus*). They found that atropine has no effect on thermal sweating even at doses sufficient to cause stimulation of the central nervous system (i.e., 0.3 mg/kg body wt). The adrenergic neuron-blocking agent bethanidine will inhibit heat-induced, but not epinephrine-induced, sweating. Since bethanidine does not affect the release of adrenomedullary hormones, these findings suggest that thermal sweating is controlled by adrenergic neurons. The importance of sympathetic nerves to the sweat glands was further demonstrated when it was shown that thermal sweating does not occur on sympathetically decentralized skin (produced by preganglionic sympathectomy) although the glands will still respond to intravenous epinephrine administration. The decentralized glands also demonstrate the phenomenon of denervation supersensitivity. These observations do not, however, rule out the possibility of a humoral component in exercise-induced sweating. By using the technique of adrenomedullary denervation (splanchnicotomy), which reduces the levels of plasma epinephrine to undetectable amounts (67), it was possible to show that exercise may have a humoral component because denervated glands will sweat after exercise; however, this does not occur in animals that have undergone splanchnicotomy (Fig. 4). But there is also a neural component of exercise because sweating still occurs from the fully innervated skin of splanchnicotomized animals (see Fig. 4).

Since the decentralized glands are supersensitive to epinephrine a definite conclusion on the true physio-

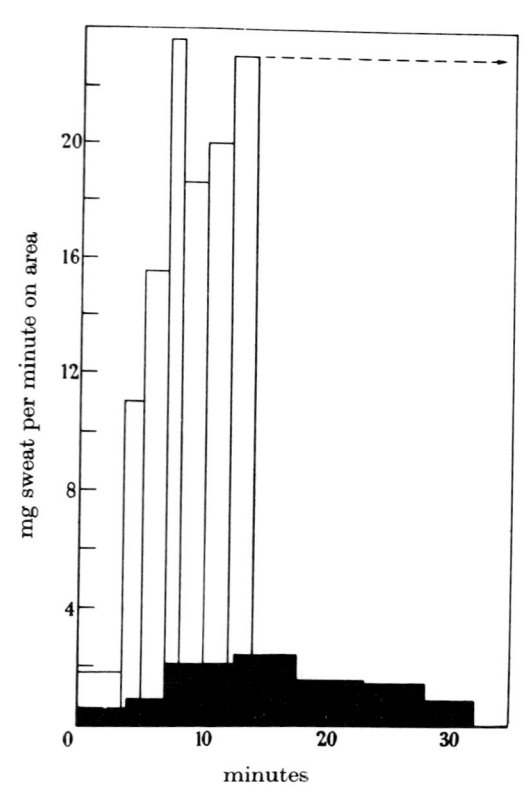

FIG. 3. Course of sweating in horses over a 5-cm² area after intradermal injection at center of area with 0.05 mg epinephrine (*open blocks*) and with 0.5 mg acetylcholine (*shaded blocks*). *Dashed line* and *arrow* indicate that sweating continued beyond the last measurement. [Adapted from Evans & Smith (20).]

logical significance of the adrenomedullary component of exercise-induced sweating is difficult to assess. Robertshaw & Taylor (66) examined this further by stimulating the adrenal medulla by means of insulin-induced hypoglycemia, under thermoneutral conditions (i.e., when there would be no thermal stimulus to sweating). Hypoglycemia produced sweating from the innervated glands in only two out of four cases, although the supersensitive decentralized glands always showed a sudomotor effect. The splanchnicotomized animals never showed any sign of sweating (see Fig. 4). This suggests that the humoral component might have little or no additive effect on the neural component. It is interesting to note that the sweating of insulin hypoglycemia in man is different from that in Equidae, the former being central in origin and the latter being of adrenomedullary origin; no central stimulation was observed. Sweating in Equidae would therefore appear to be truly adrenergic, involving β receptors. The nature of the transmitter substance at the sudomotor nerve endings awaits elucidation; it would seem unlikely that norepinephrine is the transmitter; epinephrine is certainly suggested by the evidence so far accrued. The sweat of horses contains a catecholamine-like substance that was identified by Brunaud & Pitre (11) as "adrenaline" (epinephrine) by using chemical and biological methods. However, no attempt was made to rule out other similar compounds; the existence of norepinephrine was not known at that time.

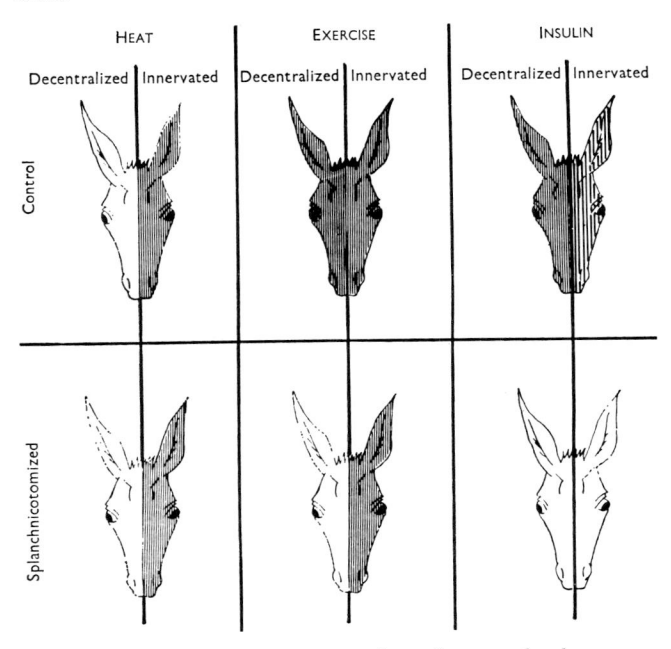

FIG. 4. Diagrammatic representation of sweat gland response of donkey (*Equus asinus*) to various stimuli. All animals were sympathetically decentralized on the right-hand side of the head (by section of right vagosympathetic trunk), and 1 group of animals also underwent bilateral splanchnicotomy, the control group of animals having an intact adrenomedullary nerve supply. *Heavy shading*, sweating occurred in all animals; *light shading*, sweating occurred in 2 out of 4 animals. [Adapted from Robertshaw & Taylor (66).]

The low-grade response of the glands to the local administration of relatively high doses of cholinergic drugs may be due to the nicotinic action of acetylcholine or may represent the cholinergic link that is purported to exist in adrenergic systems (12). The sudomotor nerve terminals may bear some similarity to the adrenomedullary cells in that intravenous tyramine does not cause the release of transmitter substance (D. Robertshaw, unpublished observations).

Rhinocerotidae

Rhinocerotidae is another family of the order Perissodactyla, and a few observations have been made on their mechanism of sweating. Game trappers report that the skin of the black rhinoceros (*Diceros bicornis*) becomes wet when they are being chased. The sweat glands can be stimulated equally by intradermal epinephrine and isoproterenol injections but not by carbachol (D. Robertshaw, unpublished observations). These findings suggest that the sweat gland mechanism may be similar to that of the horse and that at least two families of the Perissodactyla have a common sweat gland mechanism.

ARTIODACTYLA

Artiodactyla is another order of the ungulates and consists of the families Bovidae, Suidae, and Camelidae.

Bovidae

The most intensively studied members of this family are the domesticated species, such as cattle, sheep, and goats. Observations have also been made on some of the wild East African bovids (65).

The glands of the general body surface are epitrichial. Although Muto (62) reported that intravenous pilocarpine produced sweating in a calf (*Bos taurus*) and that 0.4 mg epinephrine per kilogram of body weight resulted in the death of a calf without any overt sweating, Ferguson & Dowling (23) observed the formation of sweat in response to intradermal injections of epinephrine and Taneja (79) showed that Dibenamine inhibited this response and in a hot environment reduced cutaneous moisture loss. Intravenous epinephrine, but not norepinephrine, administration results in an increase in cutaneous moisture loss (24). The glands can, however, be stimulated by the intradermal administration of norepinephrine or isoproterenol, but at a higher concentration than epinephrine. In contrast to the condition in the horse, parasympathomimetic drugs have no sudomotor effect in the ox (24). Heat-induced sweating is abolished after sympathetic denervation of the skin, but the denervated glands will still respond to intravenous or intradermal epinephrine administration, and the glands show no evidence of supersensitivity after denervation (24). The adrenal medulla plays no part in heat-induced sweating (24), and neither exercise nor insulin hypoglycemia can stimulate a sweat gland response of sympathetically denervated glands (D. Robertshaw, unpublished observations). Specific autonomic-blocking drugs verify these observations; bethanidine, an adrenergic neuron-blocking drug, which in effect produces a pharmacological sympathectomy, inhibits heat-induced, but not epinephrine-induced, sweating, and the α receptor antagonist, phenoxybenzamine, will completely block all forms of sweating (Fig. 5). The β receptor antagonist, propranolol, does not affect sweating. In contrast therefore to conditions in the horse, the sweat gland receptors are of the α type. Reserpine administration also abolishes heat-induced, but not epinephrine-induced, sweating (D. Robertshaw, unpublished observations), which confirms the adrenergic nature of sudomotor control. Although Findlay & Robertshaw (24) showed that a sympathetic innervation is necessary for thermal sweating in the ox, Jenkinson et al. (48) were unable to demonstrate histologically any nerve supply to the sweat glands. Ingram et al. (39) reported that arterial occlusion of a limb prevented sweating in that limb when the hypothalamus was heated, although sweating occurred elsewhere. They concluded therefore that sudomotor control is by humoral means. This apparent contradiction with the conclusions of Findlay & Robertshaw (24) may be interpreted as meaning that transmitter substance is released close to the sweat glands into the circulation and thus transported to the sweat glands, a neurohumoral type of transmission. Epinephrine would appear to be the most likely transmitter substance. Mabon (58) has isolated two catecholamine metabolites, 3-methoxy-4-hydroxymandelic acid and 3,4-dihydroxymandelic acid, from bovine skin washings. They were found only in washings from animals exposed to high ambient temperatures and were assumed to be associated with the sweating mechanism.

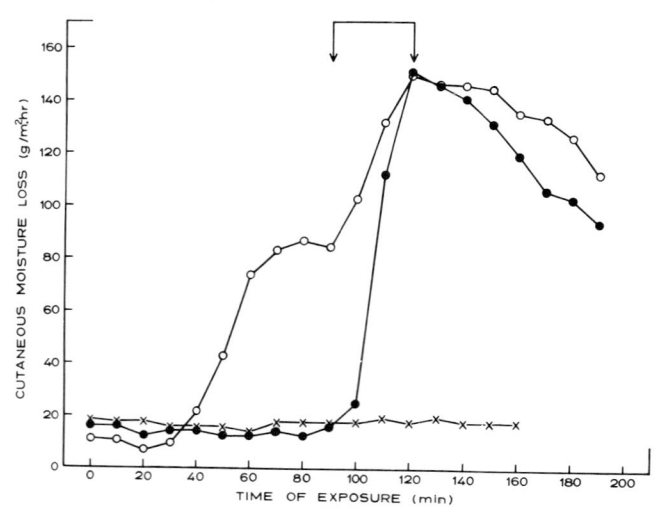

FIG. 5. Cutaneous moisture loss from the skin of an ox (*Bos taurus*) exposed to environment of 30 C. *Open circles*, control experiment; *closed circles*, after treatment with bethanidine (1 mg/kg); *crosses*, after treatment with phenoxybenzamine (3 mg/kg). Intravenous epinephrine infusion (0.25 µg/kg per min) at *arrows*. [Adapted from Findlay & Robertshaw (24).]

Of the other members of the family Bovidae, both the domestic sheep (*Ovis aries*) and goat (*Capra hircus*) and eight species of wild bovids have an adrenergic mechanism of sweat gland control involving α receptors (33, 51, 64, 65, 84). It has been suggested, however, that sheep may possess an adrenomedullary component of thermoregulatory sweating (33, 84). The evidence for this is that cutaneous sympathetic denervation by removal of the lumbar sympathetic chain does not completely abolish heat-induced sweating over the lower abdomen and inside of the thigh and that subsequent bilateral splanchnicotomy and adrenomedullectomy either partially or completely abolish the sweating of the sympathetically denervated areas. An alternative explanation of these results may be that incomplete cutaneous denervation produced by lumbar sympathectomy may be completed by splanchnicotomy. Robertshaw (64) concluded that there was no evidence of an adrenomedullary component of thermoregulatory sweating in sheep because the drug bethanidine, which does not reduce adrenomedullary secretion, but blocks adrenergic neurons, completely abolishes heat-induced sweating.

Kimura & Aoki (51) were able to demonstrate denervation supersensitivity to epinephrine in two out of three goats, but Hayashi (33) found no such evidence in the sweat glands of sheep. As in the ox, there is no histologically demonstrable nerve supply to the glands (44).

Suidae

Evans (19) examined the control of the atrichial sweat glands of the snout disk of pigs and was able to induce secretion by the intravenous administration of epinephrine (10 µg/kg). However, since atropine abolishes sweating from these glands he concluded that transmission is cholinergic. The epitrichial glands on the general body surface of the pig cannot be stimulated by heat or cholinergic compounds, but intravenous epinephrine and norepinephrine administration has a sudorific action, epinephrine being three times more potent than norepinephrine. Tolazoline will inhibit this response, which suggests an α receptor-mediated effect (38). Stimulation of the cervical sympathetic nerve produces sweating on the side of the head (38), but Jenkinson & Blackburn (45) have been unable to demonstrate histologically any nerve supply to the glands. The glands thus seem to resemble the sweat glands of Bovidae but possess no thermoregulatory function.

Camelidae

The single-humped camel (*Camelus dromedarius*) sweats on heat exposure, and the glands can be stimulated by intravenous epinephrine or isoproterenol administration; norepinephrine is without effect. The β receptor antagonist, propranolol, blocks the response to epinephrine and to isoproterenol. Bilateral splanchnicotomy does not affect the sweat response to heat exposure. Cholinergic compounds are without any sudorific action, and atropine does not abolish heat-induced sweating (D. Robertshaw and C. Taylor, unpublished observations). These results indicate that sweating in camels is also under adrenergic control but bears a greater resemblance to the sweating mechanism of equines than bovids in that it is mediated by β receptors.

The South American llama (*Lama peruana*) also sweats on heat exposure and in response to epinephrine administration (2).

CARNIVORA

The order Carnivora contains two families with species whose sweat glands have been studied, namely Canidae and Felidae.

Canidae

The dog (*Canis familiaris*) possesses atrichial glands on the foot pads and epitrichial glands on the general body surface. The glands on the foot pads have been shown to be cholinergic (77).

The glands of the general body surface respond to intradermal injections of both adrenergic and cholinergic compounds but are more sensitive to epinephrine and norepinephrine, epinephrine being more potent (3, 7). They also respond to intravenous epinephrine and norepinephrine administration (40). Cholinergic stimulation can be blocked by atropine and adrenergic stimulation by dihydroergotamine (3, 40). The physiological function of these glands appears uncertain; they cannot be stimulated by generalized heating, but localized heat application produces a sudomotor effect. This occurs in the absence of a nerve supply and even in excised skin (7). Asphyxiation can cause sweating that appears to have both neural and adrenomedullary components. There is no evidence of denervation supersensitivity (40).

Although a functional nerve supply is indicated, Jenkinson & Blackburn (47) were unable to demonstrate histologically any nerves around the sweat glands.

Felidae

The epitrichial glands on the general body surface of the cat (*Felis catus*) have not been investigated, but the atrichial glands on the cat's foot pad have been the subject of intensive study.

Dale & Feldberg (17) showed conclusively that the glands are supplied by sympathetic cholinergic fibers, but Lloyd (54) claimed that intravenous norepinephrine and epinephrine will stimulate sweating. Lloyd used the fluctuations in impedance as an index of sweating. Foster (25) measured the actual sweat output by means of a ventilated capsule (the moisture being detected by an infra-red analyzer), and in only one animal in five did intraarterial injection produce a sweat response; in actively secreting glands there was either an initial increase in sweating followed by a period of inhibition or inhibition without any stimulation. If an increase in secretion sufficient to fill the ducts but not to produce secretion at the skin surface is detected by the impedance method of Lloyd, epinephrine or norepinephrine probably always produces a sudomotor effect. Lloyd (55–57) has been able to block sweating produced by nerve stimulation with large doses of adrenergic blocking agents, such as phenoxybenzamine, guanethidine, and bretylium. However, Foster & Weiner (27) have demonstrated that this is due to a cholinergic blocking action that these drugs possess at high doses.

The denervated glands show an increase in sensitivity to intradermal epinephrine and methacholine that persists for about 2–3 weeks and then is followed by a diminution in responsiveness (63).

The catecholamine-stimulating action can be blocked by dihydroergotamine, which would indicate an α receptor-mediated effect.

RODENTIA

Rodentia have no sweat glands in the skin of the general body surface but have atrichial sweat glands on the foot pads. Only the sweat glands of the albino rat (*Rattus norvegicus*) have been investigated physiologically. Spontaneous sweating is inhibited by atropine; the glands can be stimulated by parasympathomimetic drugs (34). The glands have a cholinesterase-positive nerve supply (43), and this evidence therefore suggests that they have a cholinergic mode of transmission. However, they can be stimulated by intradermally administered epinephrine at a concentration of 10^{-6} g/ml, and this can be inhibited by the local administration of dihydroergotamine. There is a decline in responsiveness to all sudorific agents after denervation. They thus appear to be similar to the atrichial glands on the foot pads of Carnivora.

CONCLUSIONS

As information is gradually gathered on the physiology of sweat glands, a broad general picture concerning their common evolutionary origin and subsequent differentiation emerges. There appear to be two anatomic types; epitrichial and atrichial, depending on whether or not the skin is hairy or glabrous. Prosimians may have an intermediate type, in that the glands of the hairy skin open directly to the surface and not into the pilary canal. Physiologically the atrichial glands are cholinergic; the epitrichial glands and those on the general body surface of some prosimians are adrenergic. However, all cholinergic sweat glands can be stimulated by catecholamines, but there is no firm evidence that this has any physiological significance. It might therefore be a phylogenetic vestige and provide a clue as to the nature of the primitive form of sweat gland control. Since epinephrine is more potent than norepinephrine, control of the primitive gland may have been humoral rather than neural. Alternatively it may have been neural, with epinephrine as the transmitter substance; epinephrine is thought to be the adrenergic transmitter substance in Amphibia, and norepinephrine may therefore represent a phylogenetic development of the functional catecholamine in higher species.

Of the types of sweat gland in extant species, those of the hairy skin of the dog appear to be the least functionally developed. In these glands epinephrine is the most potent stimulus; they have no direct nerve supply; they can be stimulated by intravenous epinephrine or norepinephrine administration, by localized radiant heating of the skin, or by asphyxiation. Sweating therefore seems to be localized to the area stimulated by heating, except under emergency conditions, when all glands are activated by increased levels of circulating epinephrine, the effect being mediated by α receptors. This may be similar to the primitive type, but one cannot speculate as to its function.

With the development of sweat glands for thermoregulation, for moistening of friction surfaces, and possibly for the production of sexual attractants, certain changes in their control have become evident.

The glands on the general body surface of bovids, which possess to a varying extent a thermoregulatory function, have a nerve supply that releases its transmitter near, but not at, the secretory portion of the glands. The glands therefore come under the control of the central nervous system, but the functional adjustment is a relatively crude process; neural or humoral stimulation of sweat secretion of the ox may last for up to an hour (D. Robertshaw, unpublished observations). A large proportion of the termination of activity in other adrenergic systems depends on the reuptake of transmitter by the nerve terminals. This lack of a direct nerve supply to the glands of the bovids is probably reponsible for this prolonged secretory process.

The epitrichial glands of man have a nerve supply and are possibly adrenergic—the evidence so far suggests an α receptor-mediated effect. Those of prosiminan primates (with the exception of the slow loris) lack a nerve supply, except in certain specialized areas, and are also adrenergic. The prosimian primates may therefore display both the primitive form and a more developed type of gland.

The presence of a nerve supply, assuming that the nerve is motor in function, suggests a much closer control of secretion by the central nervous system. In animals such as the horse and camel where panting is a relatively minor form of evaporative heat loss, a finely modulated sweat gland control is required. These glands have a nerve supply, and the receptors are of the β variety. This is a fundamental difference between the two adrenergic systems, but the author knows of no evidence that β receptors represent an evolutionary advance on α receptors, or that only α receptors are associated with more primitive structures.

The thermoregulatory glands of man, which represent the sole means of evaporative heat loss, and the glands of friction surfaces require a very fine control of function, and this is associated with the development of a cholinergic mode of transmission. It is not generally considered that cholinergic transmission represents an evolutionary advance on adrenergic systems, but it is

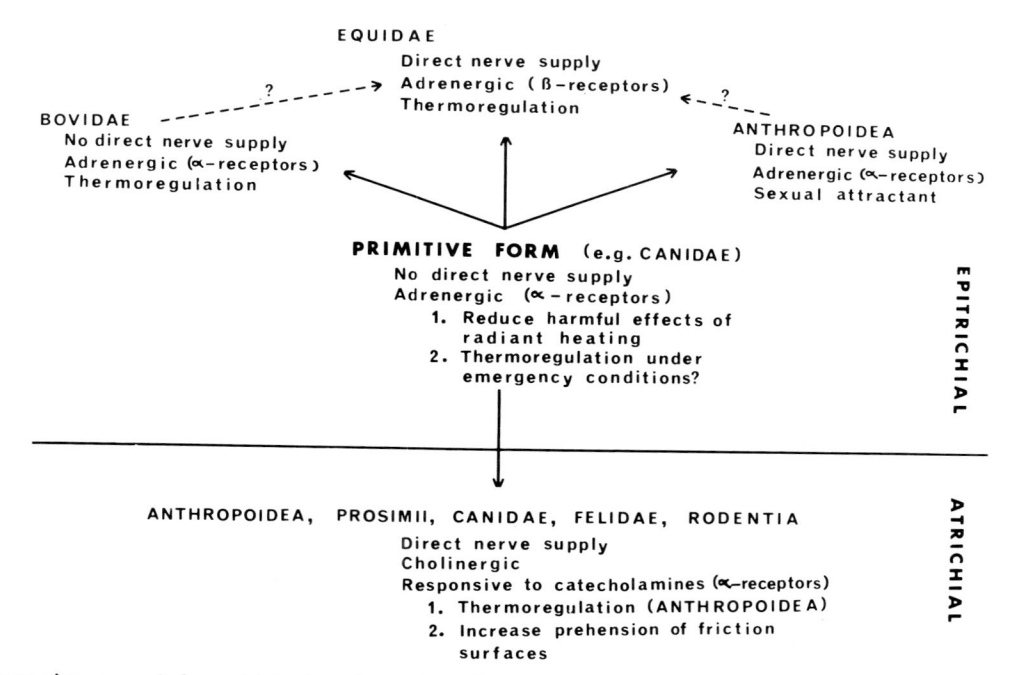

FIG. 6. Summary of an attempt to give some phylogenetic basis to the actions of catecholamines on sweat glands.

conceivable that the rapid hydrolysis of acetylcholine by acetylcholinesterase makes it particularly suitable for a delicately controlled system.

The cholinergic nature of sweat gland control of man is the commonly quoted example of the exception to the general rule that the parasympathetic nervous system is cholinergic and that the sympathetic nervous system is adrenergic. If one follows the thinking outlined above, this exception has some meaningful basis (Fig. 6).

The speculations outlined in Figure 6 provide a working hypothesis on which to base further investigations into this interesting field. A lot of the results appear to contradict classic autonomic physiology, for example, that epinephrine could be a neurotransmitter in mammals and that such a substance, which is thought to produce cutaneous vasoconstriction, should be released in the skin under conditions of heat exposure. An investigation into the nature of adrenergic sudomotor transmission should be approached with an open mind and without fear of contradicting classic concepts. It may be that such an investigation will reveal a unique and hitherto unknown neurotransmission system.

ADDENDUM

Recent evidence suggests that there may be a β receptor component of the response of human sweat glands to catecholamine stimulation. Allen and Roddie (Allen, J. A., and I. C. Roddie. The role of circulating catecholamines in sweat production in man. J. Physiol., London 227: 801–814, 1972) have shown that the intravenous infusion of isoproterenol, a catecholamine that predominantly stimulates β receptors, increases sweat production and is more potent in this respect than either epinephrine or norepinephrine. The response still occurs after the administration of atropine but is reduced by the β receptor antagonist, propranolol. Foster and co-workers (Foster, K. G., J. R. Haspineall, and C. L. Mollel. Effects of propranolol on the response of human eccrine sweat glands to acetylcholine. Brit. J. Dermatol. 85: 363–367, 1971) have shown that propranolol has no marked effect on either acetylcholine-induced sweating in man or the response of the sweat glands in the cat's pad to plantar nerve stimulation. Thus adrenergic receptor sites appear to be quite independent of cholinergic receptor sites.

An enhancement of sweating during exercise over the maximal sweat rate achieved at rest in a hot environment was demonstrated to occur in the stump-tail macaque (*Macaca speciosa*) by Robertshaw and colleagues (Robertshaw, D., C. R. Taylor, and L. M. Mazzia. Sweating in primates: secretion by adrenal medulla during exercise. Am. J. Physiol. 224: 678–681, 1973). This enhancement was shown to result from epinephrine released from the adrenal medulla in that it was abolished in splanchnicotomized animals and could be restored by epinephrine infusion. Sudomotor transmission in this species, as in man, is cholinergic so it would appear that epinephrine and acetylcholine have a synergistic effect on sweating and that the increased secretion of sweat during exercise results from the combined effects of acetylcholine, of neural origin, and epinephrine, of humoral origin, acting on different receptor sites of the secretory cell. This finding therefore demonstrates the possible functional significance of circulating catecholamines in the control of sweating in man and some other primates.

REFERENCES

1. ADAMS, T., AND W. S. HUNTER. Modification of skin mechanical properties by eccrine sweat gland activity. J. Appl. Physiol. 26: 417–419, 1969.
2. ALLEN, T. E., AND J. BLIGH. A comparative study of the temporal patterns of cutaneous water vapour loss from some domesticated mammals with epitrichial sweat glands. Comp. Biochem. Physiol. 31: 347–363, 1969.
3. AOKI, T. Stimulation of the sweat glands in the hairy skin of the dog by adrenaline, noradrenaline, mecholyl and pilocarpine. J. Invest. Dermatol. 24: 545–556, 1955.
4. AOKI, T. Stimulation of human axillary apocrine sweat glands by cholinergic agents. J. Invest. Dermatol. 38: 41–44, 1962.
5. AOKI, T. The skin of Primates. IX. Observations on the functional activity of the sweat glands in *Nycticebus coucang* and *Perodicticus potto*. J. Invest. Dermatol. 39: 115–122, 1962.
6. AOKI, T., S. KIMURA, AND M. WADA. On the responsiveness of the sweat glands in the horse. J. Invest. Dermatol. 33: 441–443, 1959.
7. AOKI, T., AND M. WADA. Functional activity of the sweat glands in the hairy skin of the dog. Science 114: 123–124, 1951.
8. BELL, F. R., AND C. L. EVANS. Sweating responses in the horse. J. Physiol., London 134: 421–426, 1956.
9. BLIGH, J. The thermosensitivity of the hypothalamus and thermoregulation in mammals. Biol. Rev. Cambridge Phil. Soc. 41: 317–367, 1966.
10. BLIGH, J. A thesis concerning the processes of secretion and discharge of sweat. Environ. Res. 1: 28–45, 1967.
11. BRUNAUD, M., AND J. PITRE. Existe-t-il de l'adrénaline dans la sueur du cheval? Bull. Acad. Vet. France 18: 339–347, 1945.
12. BURN, J. H., AND M. J. RAND. Sympathetic postganglionic mechanism. Nature 184: 163–165, 1959.
13. CAHN, M. M., AND W. B. SHELLEY. Hyaluronidase-methylene blue staining of nerve fibres about the human axillary apocrine sweat gland. J. Invest. Dermatol. 25: 63–66, 1955.
14. CHALMERS, T. M., AND C. A. KEELE. Physiological significance of the sweat response to adrenaline in man. J. Physiol., London 114: 510–514, 1951.
15. CHALMERS, T. M., AND C. A. KEELE. The nervous and chemical control of sweating. Brit. J. Dermatol. 64: 43–54, 1952.
16. COLLINS, K. J., F. SARGENT, AND J. S. WEINER. Excitation and depression of eccrine sweat glands by acetylcholine, acetyl-β-methylcholine and adrenaline. J. Physiol., London 148: 592–614, 1959.
17. DALE, H. H., AND W. FELDBERG. The chemical transmission of secretory impulses to the sweat glands of the cat. J. Physiol., London 82: 121–128, 1934.
18. ELLIS, R. A., AND W. MONTAGNA. The sweat glands of the Lorisidae. In: *Evolutionary and Genetic Biology of Primates*, edited by J. Buettner-Janusch. New York: Acad. Press, vol. I, p. 197–228, 1963.
19. EVANS, C. L. Sweating in relation to sympathetic innervation. Brit. Med. Bull. 13: 197–201, 1957.
20. EVANS, C. L., AND D. F. G. SMITH. Sweating responses in the horse. Proc. Roy. Soc. London Ser. B 145: 61–83, 1956.
21. EVANS, C. L., D. F. G. SMITH, AND H. WEIL-MALHERBE. The relation between sweating and the catechol content of the blood in the horse. J. Physiol., London 132: 542–552, 1956.
22. FALCK, B., AND C. OWMAN. A detailed methodological description of the fluorescence method for the cellular demonstration of biogenic monoamines. Acta Univ. Lund. 11(7): 1–23, 1965.
23. FERGUSON, K. A., AND D. F. DOWLING. The function of cattle sweat glands. Australian J. Agr. Res. 6: 641–644, 1955.
24. FINDLAY, J. D., AND D. ROBERTSHAW. The role of the sympathoadrenal system in the control of sweating in the ox (*Bos taurus*). J. Physiol., London 179: 285–297, 1965.
25. FOSTER, K. G. Response of the cats' pad eccrine sweat glands

to intravascular injections of catecholamines. *J. Physiol., London* 195: 331–337, 1968.
26. FOSTER, K. G., J. GINSBURG, AND J. S. WEINER. Role of circulating catecholamines in human eccrine sweat gland control. *Clin. Sci.* 39: 823–832, 1970.
27. FOSTER, K. G., AND J. S. WEINER. Effects of cholinergic and adrenergic blocking agents on the activity of the eccrine sweat glands. *J. Physiol., London* 210: 883–895, 1970.
28. GINSBURG, J., AND A. PATON. Effects in man of insulin hypoglycaemia after adrenalectomy. *J. Physiol., London* 133: 59–60P, 1956.
29. HAIMOVICI, H. Evidence for adrenergic sweating in man. *J. Appl. Physiol.* 2: 512–521, 1950.
30. HAINSWORTH, F. R. Evaporative water loss from rats in the heat. *Am. J. Physiol.* 214: 979–982, 1968.
31. HARRISON, J., AND P. C. B. MACKINNON. Central effect of epinephrine and norepinephrine on the palmar sweat index. *Am. J. Physiol.* 204: 785–788, 1963.
32. HARRISON, J., AND P. C. B. MACKINNON. Physiological role of the adrenal medulla in the palmar anhidrotic response to stress. *J. Appl. Physiol.* 21: 88–92, 1966.
33. HAYASHI, H. Functional activity of the sweat glands in the hairy skin of the sheep. *Tohoku J. Exptl. Med.* 94: 361–375, 1968.
34. HAYASHI, H., AND T. NAKAGAWA. Functional activity of the sweat glands of the albino rat. *J. Invest. Dermatol.* 41: 365–367, 1963.
35. HURLEY, H. J., AND W. B. SHELLEY. The role of the myoepithelium of the human apocrine gland. *J. Invest. Dermatol.* 22: 143–156, 1954.
36. HURLEY, H. J., AND J. A. WITKOWSKI. Mechanism of epinephrine-induced eccrine sweating in human skin. *J. Appl. Physiol.* 16: 652–654, 1961.
37. ICHIBASHI, T. Effect of drugs on the sweat glands by cataphoresis and effective method for suppression of local sweating. *J. Orient. Med.* 25: 1401, 1936.
38. INGRAM, D. L. Stimulation of cutaneous glands in the pig. *J. Comp. Pathol. Therap.* 77: 93–98, 1967.
39. INGRAM, D. L., J. A. MCLEAN, AND G. C. WHITTOW. The effect of heating the hypothalamus and the skin on the rate of moisture vaporization from the skin of the ox (*Bos taurus*). *J. Physiol., London* 169: 394–403, 1963.
40. IWABUCHI, T. General sweating on the hairy skin of the dog and its mechanisms. *J. Invest. Dermatol.* 49: 61–70, 1967.
41. JANOWITZ, H. D., AND M. I. GROSSMAN. The response of the sweat glands to some locally acting agents in human subjects. *J. Invest. Dermatol.* 14: 453–458, 1950.
42. JENKINSON, D. McE. On the classification of sweat glands and the question of the existence of an apocrine secretory process. *Brit. Vet. J.* 123: 311–316, 1967.
43. JENKINSON, D. McE. The distribution of nerves, monoamine oxidase and cholinesterase in the skin of the guinea pig, hamster, mouse, rabbit and rat. *Res. Vet. Sci.* 11: 60–70, 1970.
44. JENKINSON, D. McE., AND P. S. BLACKBURN. The distribution of nerves, monoamine oxidase and cholinesterase in the skin of the sheep and goat. *J. Anat.* 101: 333–341, 1967.
45. JENKINSON, D. McE., AND P. S. BLACKBURN. The distribution of nerves, monoamine oxidase and cholinesterase in the skin of the pig. *Res. Vet. Sci.* 8: 306–312, 1967.
46. JENKINSON, D. McE., AND P. S. BLACKBURN. The distribution of nerves, monoamine oxidase and cholinesterase in the skin of the horse. *Res. Vet. Sci.* 9: 165–169, 1968.
47. JENKINSON, D. McE., AND P. S. BLACKBURN. The distribution of nerves, monoamine oxidase and cholinesterase in the skin of the cat and dog. *Res. Vet. Sci.* 9: 521–528, 1968.
48. JENKINSON, D. McE., B. P. SENGUPTA, AND P. S. BLACKBURN. The distribution of nerves, monoamine oxidase and cholinesterase in the skin of cattle. *J. Anat.* 100: 593–613, 1966.
49. KENNARD, D. W. The nervous regulation of the sweating apparatus of the human skin, and emotive sweating in thermal sweating areas. *J. Physiol., London* 165: 457–467, 1963.
50. KERNEN, R., AND R. BRUN. Expériences sur la transpiration. v. Examens pharmacodynamiques au niveau de la gland sudoripare de l'homme. *Dermatologica* 106: 1–13, 1953.
51. KIMURA, S., AND T. AOKI. Functional activity of the apocrine sweat gland in the goat. *Tohoku J. Exptl. Med.* 76: 8–22, 1962.
52. KISIN, E. E. A method of pharmacological study of the sweating function of the skin *in situ*. *Vestn. Venerol. i Dermatol.* 5: 27–31, 1948.
53. KUNO, Y. *Human Perspiration*. Springfield, Ill.: Thomas, 1956.
54. LLOYD, D. P. C. Response of cholinergically innervated sweat glands to adrenaline and noradrenaline. *Nature* 184: 277–278, 1959.
55. LLOYD, D. P. C. Action of phenoxybenzamine on neural and humoral activation of sweat glands. *J. Physiol., London* 169: 116–117P, 1963.
56. LLOYD, D. P. C. Actions of guanethidine and bretylium on transmission to sweat glands in the cat. *J. Physiol., London* 175: 74P, 1964.
57. LLOYD, D. P. C. Effect of phenoxybenzamine on neural and humoral control of sweat glands. *Proc. Natl. Acad. Sci. US* 59: 816–820, 1968.
58. MABON, R. M. Two possible catecholamine metabolites in the secretion from ox skin. *Res. Vet. Sci.* 11: 287–288, 1970.
59. MELLINKOFF, S. M., AND R. R. SONNENSCHEIN. Identity of sweat glands stimulated by heat, epinephrine and acetylcholine. *Science* 120: 997–998, 1954.
60. MONTAGNA, W. Histology and cytochemistry of human skin. xxiv. Further observations on the axillary organ. *J. Invest. Dermatol.* 42: 119–129, 1963.
61. MONTAGNA, W., AND J. S. YUN. The skin of primates. xv. The skin of the chimpanzee (*Pan satyrus*). *Am. J. Phys. Anthropol.* 21: 189–204, 1963.
62. MUTO, K. Uber die Wirkung des Adrenalins auf die Schweissekretion; zugleich ein Beitrag zur Kenntnis der doppelsinnigen Innervation der Schweissdrüse. *Mitt. Med. Fak. K. Japon. Univ. Tokio* 15: 365–386, 1916.
63. NAKAMURA, Y., AND K. HATANAKA. The effect of denervation of the cat's sweat glands on their responsiveness to adrenaline, nicotine and mecholyl. *Tohoku J. Exptl. Med.* 68: 225–237, 1958.
63a. PROUT, B. J., AND W. M. WARDELL. Sweating and peripheral blood flow in patients with phaeochromocytoma. *Clin. Sci.* 36: 109–117, 1969.
64. ROBERTSHAW, D. The pattern and control of sweating in the sheep and the goat. *J. Physiol., London* 198: 531–539, 1968.
65. ROBERTSHAW, D., AND C. R. TAYLOR. A comparison of sweat gland activity in eight species of East African bovids. *J. Physiol., London* 203: 135–143, 1969.
66. ROBERTSHAW, D., AND C. R. TAYLOR. Sweat gland function of the donkey (*Equus asinus*). *J. Physiol., London* 205: 79–89, 1969.
67. ROBERTSHAW, D., AND G. C. WHITTOW. The effect of hyperthermia and localized heating of the anterior hypothalamus on the sympatho-adrenal system of the ox (*Bos taurus*). *J. Physiol., London* 187: 351–360, 1966.
68. SAKURAI, M., AND W. MONTAGNA. Experiments in the sweating on the palms of the green monkey (*Cercopithecus aethiops*). *J. Invest. Dermatol.* 43: 249–285, 1964.
69. SAKURAI, M., AND W. MONTAGNA. Observations on the eccrine sweat glands of Lemur mongoz after denervation. *J. Invest. Dermatol.* 44: 87–92, 1965.
70. SCHIEFFERDECKER, P. Die Hautdrüsen des Menschen und der Saugetiere, ihre biologische und rassenatomische Bedeutung, sowie die Muscularis sexualis. *Biol. Zentr.* 37: 534–562, 1917.
71. SCHIEFFERDECKER, P. Die Hautdrusen des Menschen und der Säugetiere, ihre biologische und rassenatomische Bedeutung, sowie die Muscularis sexualis. *Zoologica* 72: 1–154, 1922.
72. SCHMIDT-NIELSEN, K., B. SCHMIDT-NIELSEN, S. A. JARNUM,

AND T. R. HOUPT. Body temperature of the camel and its relation to water economy. *Am. J. Physiol.* 188: 103–112, 1957.
73. SHELLEY, W. B. Apocrine sweat. *J. Invest. Dermatol.* 17: 255, 1951.
74. SHELLEY, W. B., AND H. J. HURLEY. Methods of exploring human apocrine gland physiology. *Arch. Dermatol. Syphilol.* 66: 156–161, 172–179, 1952.
75. SILVER, A., W. MONTAGNA, AND I. KARACAN. Age and sex differences in spontaneous, adrenergic and cholinergic human sweating. *J. Invest. Dermatol.* 43: 255–266, 1964.
76. SONNENSCHEIN, R. R., H. KOBRIN, H. D. JANOWITZ, AND M. I. GROSSMAN. Stimulation and inhibition of human sweat glands by intradermal sympathomimetic agents. *J. Appl. Physiol.* 3: 573–581, 1951.
77. TAKAHASHI, Y. Functional activity of the eccrine sweat glands in the toe-pads of the dog. *Tohoku J. Exptl. Med.* 83: 205, 1964.
78. TANAKA, I., AND T. NAKAMURA. Action of adrenaline, noradrenaline, and isopropylnoradrenaline on the sweat glands in young healthy men. *Kumamoto Med. J.* 8: 26–28, 1955.
79. TANEJA, G. C. Sweating in cattle. IV. Control of sweat glands secretion. *J. Agr. Sci.* 52: 66–71, 1959.
80. THAYSEN, J. H., AND I. L. SCHWARTZ. Fatigue of the sweat glands. *J. Clin. Invest.* 34: 1719–1725, 1955.
81. THOMSON, M. L., AND SUTARMAN. The identification and enumeration of active sweat glands in man from plastic impressions of the skin. *Trans. Roy. Soc. Trop. Med. Hyg.* 47: 412–417, 1953.
82. USENIK, E. A. *Sympathetic Innervation of the Head and Neck of the Horse; Neuropharmacological Studies of Sweating in the Horse* (Ph.D. Thesis). Minneapolis: Univ. of Minnesota, 1957.
83. WADA, M. Sudorific action of adrenaline on the human sweat glands and determination of their excitability. *Science* 111: 376–377, 1950.
84. WAITES, G. M. H., AND J. K. VOGLMAYR. The functional activity and control of the apocrine sweat glands of the scrotum of the ram. *Australian J. Agr. Res.* 14: 839–851, 1963.
85. WEINER, J. S., AND K. HELLMAN. The sweat glands. *Biol. Rev. Cambridge Phil. Soc.* 35: 141–186, 1960.

CHAPTER 37

Effects of epinephrine on glycogenolysis and myocardial contractility

JOHN R. WILLIAMSON | *Johnson Research Foundation, University of Pennsylvania, Philadelphia, Pennsylvania*

CHAPTER CONTENTS

Metabolic Effects in Muscle
    In vitro studies on control of glycogenolysis
        Enzyme reactions involved in glycogenolysis
        Regulatory properties and interconversion of phosphorylase *b* and *a*
        Phosphorylase phosphatase
        Activation of phosphorylase kinase by cyclic AMP
        Activation of phosphorylase kinase by calcium ion
        Phosphorylase kinase phosphatase
        Integrated control of phosphorylase activity
    Control of glycogenolysis in intact muscle
        Skeletal muscle
        Cardiac muscle
Calcium and Muscle Contraction
    Calcium and contractile proteins
    Cellular calcium flux
    Role of calcium in excitation-contraction coupling
    Calcium release by sarcoplasmic reticulum
    Calcium uptake by sarcoplasmic reticulum
    Mitochondria and calcium sequestration
    Calcium transport by cell membrane
Cyclic AMP and Muscle Contraction
    Effects of cyclic AMP and hormones on cardiac contractility
    Hormone receptors and adenyl cyclase
    Effects of epinephrine on electromechanical properties of cardiac muscle
    Hormonal and cyclic AMP effects on isolated sarcoplasmic reticulum
    Effect of epinephrine on contractile proteins
Summary and Conclusions

A CONSIDERATION of the metabolic effects produced by catecholamines is inextricably involved with the formation, breakdown, and functions of cyclic 3′,5′-AMP in the various target organs. Numerous reviews provide detailed descriptions of the biological role of cyclic AMP in various tissues (21, 80, 246, 284–287, 289), and a number of recent monographs have been devoted to the subject (84, 247, 249). In addition, a collection of abstracts of papers related to cyclic AMP published over a 10-year period up to 1969 (plus extra volumes for succeeding years) has become available (265). The physiological role of catecholamines in metabolic regulation has been covered extensively in recent reviews (51, 61, 92, 103, 147, 167, 168, 297, 312) and in a Pharmacology Society Symposium (62), which should be consulted to supplement the present account. The reviews by Himms-Hagen (103) and Drummond (51) are particularly valuable for their detailed discussion of this complex subject and for extensive bibliographies of work published before 1967. Rather than providing yet another general account in this area, it has been decided to restrict the subject matter to the role of catecholamines in promoting glycogenolysis and cardiac contractility and to emphasize wherever possible the involvements of Ca^{2+} and cyclic AMP in these processes at the molecular level. This has necessitated the inclusion of a certain amount of basic descriptive material on the mechanism of cardiac contractility and the nature of the calcium cycle, which is used as a framework for considerations of the possible sites of action of cyclic AMP. The present account therefore is intended to provide a reasonably detailed, objective survey of this topic, which has interfaces with the areas of biochemistry, physiology, and pharmacology.

Until recently it has been accepted that both the metabolic effects of catecholamines and their stimulatory properties on cardiac contraction were exerted wholly or largely through the mediation of cyclic AMP, for which a role as second messenger has been proposed (287, 288). However, it is becoming increasingly clear that activation of adenyl cyclase and the resultant increase in the concentration of cyclic AMP may only be one expression of the changes that occur upon combination of catecholamines with the tissue receptors. Accumulating evidence indicates that an increase of intracellular Ca^{2+} concentration is intimately involved in the production of the final metabolic response, either as an alternative second messenger or as a third messenger triggered by the rise of cyclic AMP concentration (229, 230). Besides their inotropic effect on cardiac tissue, the most striking metabolic effects of catecholamines are

Research grants provided by the United States Public Health Service HE-14461 and NIH-71-2494 and the American Heart Association.

mobilization of glycogen via activation of the phosphorylase systems of liver and muscle and mobilization of lipid stores in adipose tissues by activation of intracellular triglyceride lipase. Of particular importance in the understanding of the diversity of the metabolic responses induced by cyclic AMP are recent findings showing that cyclic AMP causes activation of several protein kinases, which in turn modulate the activity of enzymes more directly concerned with fuel mobilization. In some instances, dual control by Ca^{2+} and cyclic AMP is exerted by direct effects of Ca^{2+} on the enzymes.

Alterations of the blood levels of glucose, lactate, ketone bodies, and free fatty acids as a result of these effects in turn influence the oxidative metabolism of different organs directly, or indirectly by altering the rate of secretion of key hormones such as insulin. Thus cycles of metabolic events are initiated that tend to correct for the initial overreaction caused by the release of catecholamines and serve to stabilize metabolism at a different level for the duration of the imposed stimulus. The chain of metabolic events is thereby controlled by strong negative feedback influences, each with a characteristic time constant. This means that experimentally the sequence of cause-and-effect relations can often only be elucidated by carefully designed kinetic measurements since biphasic changes of the concentrations of metabolites in tissues or blood may occur with time after the initial stimulus. Furthermore, because most of the metabolic consequences of catecholamine release result from changes in the concentration of tissue cyclic AMP and Ca^{2+}, it is clear that sensitivity and selectivity of response are determined at the level of the hormone action on the tissue adenyl cyclase and also at the level of the enzyme systems directly affected by cyclic AMP and Ca^{2+}. Very different results may therefore be obtained between small and large doses of epinephrine or norepinephrine or when the same dose is given to fed and fasted animals. Basically, however, each organ has a characteristic response to physiological concentrations of catecholamines, although additional effects may be seen at pharmacological levels.

METABOLIC EFFECTS IN MUSCLE

The classic metabolic response of muscle to the administration of catecholamines is increased glycogenolysis (39, 40). However, the physiological importance of glycogen as a reserve energy fuel depends on the type of muscle. The metabolic need for endogenous carbohydrate is greatest for fast-contracting skeletal muscle and least for cardiac muscle, which because of its high mitochondrial content and rich blood supply has a very high capacity for oxidative metabolism, with fatty acids and ketone bodies being the preferred substrates (16). Thus, whereas white skeletal muscle has a higher content of glycogen and enzymes of glycogenolysis than the slower-contracting red muscle, it also has a lower mitochondria and lipid content (57, 75, 218, 222, 281). The control mechanisms for activation of glycogen breakdown and subsequent conversion of glucose-1-P to lactate in white skeletal muscle are highly coordinated and respond rapidly to the initial electrical stimulus, so that energy is immediately made available to support fast anaerobic contractions, as so beautifully demonstrated by the work of Helmreich and co-workers (98, 100) with frog sartorius muscle. Most human skeletal muscles are of a type intermediate between white and red muscle and have a relatively high capacity for lipid oxidation, although glycogen represents a major fuel for short bursts of intense activity. For more moderate work, rapid glycogenolysis provides for a high rate of ATP production during the period of readjustment of blood flow from abdominal organs to the skeletal muscles. Clearly, sustained work must rely heavily on oxidative metabolism, with fatty acid oxidation representing a large portion (93). On the basis of the different sizes and thresholds for stimulation, it has been suggested that mainly red muscle fibers are activated in man at low work intensities. With increasing strength of the electrical stimuli, a greater number of white fibers having a more pronounced glycolytic metabolism are activated (133). Thus Hultman (109) has shown that the amount of high-intensity work a given human subject is capable of is proportional to the concentration of glycogen initially present in the muscle, with the rate of glycogen disappearance being linear over a wide range.

The effects of epinephrine on muscle differ both with the type of muscle and the nature of the preparation. In cardiac muscle the important physiological response is increased contractile force, and there appears to be little or no net change in the glycogen content of the hearts in vivo (179, 314). Increased oxidative metabolism is supported by an increased utilization of glucose (315) and free fatty acids (131) from the blood or perfusion fluid. Stimulation of glycogenolysis by epinephrine is more readily observed in isolated perfused rat heart preparations (216, 315, 317), but this effect is transient compared with the duration of the contractile response and is smaller when glucose is present in the perfusion medium. Slow-contracting red muscles are very sensitive to epinephrine, and their mechanical response is a decrease in twitch tension with a decrease in the duration of the twitch [(18); see the chapter by Tomita in this volume of the *Handbook*]. The physiological importance of this effect is obscure. Although glycogenolysis of red muscles is stimulated by catecholamines, the energy yield from glycogen metabolism represents only a portion of the energy expenditure required for sustained work. Probably stimulation of triglyceride lipase by epinephrine and increased fatty acid metabolism may be more important than carbohydrate mobilization in these muscles. The direct action of epinephrine on fast-contracting mammalian muscle involves an increase in twitch tension and in the total duration of the twitch with an augmentation of the amplitude of incomplete tetanic contractions (18). The physiological significance of this effect is not clear because of the relatively high concentrations of epinephrine needed. The metabolic effect of epinephrine on white skeletal muscle is very dependent on whether or not the muscles are stimulated. Epinephrine addition to quiescent anaerobic frog sartorii preparations causes an accumulation of hexose monophosphates, a decrease in inorganic phosphate, a decreased rate of glucose uptake, and only a small increase of lactate production. These effects are due to the absence of a coordinated stimulation of phosphorylase and phosphofructokinase, which is only observed when the muscles are stimulated to contract (98–100). Electrical stimulation increases lactate formation 50-fold, and at a given rate of stimulation epinephrine has no effect, which shows that electrical stimulation per se provides a sufficient stimulus to activate glycogenolysis (98). It thus appears that, even in white skeletal muscle, epinephrine has an ill-defined physiological function. One interesting response of epinephrine, which has been demonstrated in frog muscle but not in mammalian muscle, is delay in muscle fatigue (18). Epinephrine increases the responsiveness of the glycogenolytic activation system to repetitive stimulation apparently by maintenance of the phosphorylase a levels (99).

Besides activating glycogenolysis, catecholamines also have the reciprocal effect in skeletal muscle of inhibiting glycogen synthesis. The activity of glycogen synthetase, the rate-limiting step in glycogen formation, is higher in red than in white skeletal muscle (8), but again the physiological significance of the epinephrine effects on glycogen synthesis is probably rather minor. A number of recent reviews have been devoted to the control of glycogen metabolism in muscle and other tissues, and these should be consulted for details and important historical aspects (51, 71, 96, 98, 99, 130, 146, 147, 297, 298).

In Vitro Studies on Control of Glycogenolysis

ENZYME REACTIONS INVOLVED IN GLYCOGENOLYSIS. Activation of glycogenolysis by epinephrine has been likened to a reaction cascade that serves as a physiological amplifier whereby a low concentration of epinephrine (e.g., 10^{-6} to 10^{-7} M) can produce hexose phosphate units with an amplification factor of many orders of magnitude (19). Mobilization of glycogen is the result of a complex sequence of reactions, each of which involves the successive conversion of an enzyme from a less active to a more active form. Activation involves a phosphorylation of the intermediary enzyme if the initiating signal is cyclic AMP, whereas an increased Ca^{2+} concentration can activate the enzymes directly.

Control of glycogenolysis is exercised at the step of glycogen phosphorylase that catalyzes the formation of glucose-1-P from glycogen and P_i

$$P_i + \text{glucosyl}(\alpha\text{-}1,4)\text{-glycogen} \xrightleftharpoons{\text{phosphorylase}} \text{glucose-1-P} + \text{glycogen} \quad (1)$$

Although the equilibrium slightly favors glycogen synthesis ($K_{eq} = 0.28$ at pH 6.8), the enzyme functions physiologically in the direction of glycogen degradation. In resting skeletal muscle and cardiac muscle working under light loads, phosphorylase exists predominantly as a dimer of molecular weight 185,000, termed phosphorylase b. Phosphorylase b can be activated directly by allosteric interaction with AMP. Activation by epinephrine is achieved by phosphorylation with Mg-ATP and phosphorylase kinase to phosphorylase a (see Equation 2). Phosphorylase a exists in equilibrium between dimeric and tetrameric forms. The reverse reaction is catalyzed by phosphorylase phosphatase (see Equation 3).

$$\text{phosphorylase } b + 2 \text{ ATP} \xrightarrow{\text{phosphorylase kinase}} \text{phosphorylase } a + 2 \text{ ADP} \quad (2)$$

$$\text{phosphorylase } a + 2 H_2O \xrightarrow{\text{phosphorylase phosphatase}} \text{phosphorylase } b + 2 P_i \quad (3)$$

Phosphorylase kinase can also exist in phosphorylated and nonphosphorylated forms, both of which require Ca^{2+} for activity. The nonphosphorylated enzyme is essentially inactive at pH 6.8 but becomes active at higher pH values. The phosphorylated form, on the other hand, is active at pH 6.8, and the activity rises less steeply with increase of pH (127). Phosphorylation of phosphorylase kinase is achieved in a relatively slow autocatalytic reaction by incubating the enzyme with Mg-ATP or more rapidly by means of an enzyme originally called phosphorylase kinase kinase.

Dephosphorylation of phosphorylase kinase is accomplished by phosphorylase kinase phosphatase, an enzyme distinct from phosphorylase phosphatase. These interactions are summarized in Equation 4.

$$\begin{array}{c}
\text{phosphorylase kinase} \\
\text{(inactive at pH 6.8)}
\end{array} \xrightleftharpoons{Ca^{2+}} \begin{array}{c}
\text{phosphorylase kinase} \\
\text{(active at pH 6.8)}
\end{array}$$

$$\begin{array}{c}
\text{phosphorylase kinase} \\
\text{kinase + Mg-ATP}
\end{array} \Bigg\updownarrow \begin{array}{c} \text{phosphorylase} \\ \text{kinase} \\ \text{phosphatase} \end{array} \Bigg\updownarrow \text{Mg-ATP} \quad (4)$$

$$\begin{array}{c}
\text{P-phosphorylase kinase} \\
\text{(inactive at pH 6.8)}
\end{array} \xrightleftharpoons{Ca^{2+}} \begin{array}{c}
\text{P-phosphorylase kinase} \\
\text{(active at pH 6.8)}
\end{array}$$

Phosphorylase kinase kinase activity is only expressed in the presence of cyclic AMP, which itself is liberated by stimulation of adenyl cyclase by epinephrine (Equation 5). Cyclic AMP is removed by conversion to AMP by tissue phosphodiesterases.

$$\begin{array}{c} \text{epinephrine} \\ \downarrow \\ \text{adenyl cyclase} \longrightarrow \text{adenyl cyclase} \\ \text{(inactive)} \qquad \text{(active)} \\ \downarrow \\ \text{ATP} \longrightarrow \text{cyclic AMP} \xrightarrow{\text{phosphodiesterase}} \text{AMP} \\ \downarrow \\ \text{phosphorylase kinase kinase} \rightarrow \text{phosphorylase kinase kinase} \\ \text{(inactive)} \qquad\qquad \text{(active)} \end{array} \quad (5)$$

From the summary given above, it is apparent that Ca^{2+} is required for glycogenolysis mediated by phosphorylase a, whether or not epinephrine is involved in the activation process. Thus contractility and glycogenolysis have increased Ca^{2+} release in the sarcoplasm as a common denominator. Some details of the properties of the individual enzymes, together with an outline of the experimental evidence upon which the conclusions are drawn, are given below. Further details can be found in recent review articles (24, 68, 71, 96, 127, 130, 302).

REGULATORY PROPERTIES AND INTERCONVERSION OF PHOSPHORYLASE b AND a. Both forms of phosphorylase can be dissociated by treatment with p-chloromercuribenzoate into monomeric single polypeptide chains. These monomers have a number of different binding sites for a variety of ligands, all of which are involved in modulating the activity of the enzyme. Besides the catalytic site at which the three substrates (glycogen, P_i, glucose-1-P) and some inhibitors (e.g., glucose and UDP-glucose) are bound, there is a regulatory site for adenine nucleotides. Each monomer also contains one pyridoxal 5-phosphate site that is essential for activity (68, 96) and a phosphorylation site involved in stabilizing the active conformation of the protein. In addition, other secondary sites are involved in the subunit assembly of the molecule. The phosphorylation site of phosphorylase has been identified as a serine hydroxyl group (108, 210) in the amino acid sequence Lys-Glu-Ile-Ser-Val-Arg. This site must occupy an exposed position on the surface of the enzyme because of its ready reactivity with phosphorylase kinase and phosphatase and with proteolytic enzymes.

Both phosphorylated and unphosphorylated forms of phosphorylase have allosteric properties. Homotropic interactions are exhibited by substrates and allosteric effectors, and the catalytic and regulatory sites interact with one another to produce heterotropic effects (186). In general, the interactions cause large changes in the Michaelis-Menten constant (K_m) values for the substrate or effectors with little change in V_{max}. Thus AMP, which is essential for the activity of phosphorylase b ($K_a = 3 \times 10^{-5}$ M), greatly increases the affinity of the enzyme for its substrates (97). The stimulation of phosphorylase b by AMP is inhibited competitively by ATP [inhibitory constant (K_i) = 2 mM] and glucose-6-P (K_i = 0.3 mM), whereas UDP-glucose (K_i = 0.92 mM) is competitive with respect to glucose-1-P (173, 196). The tissue levels of these inhibitors are sufficiently high in aerobic tissues to overcome the activational effect of AMP at its normal tissue concentration of 0.2–0.5 mM. Inhibition by ADP is about equally as effective as that by ATP (100) but is of less importance as a physiological modulator because of its lower concentration in aerobic tissues. Phosphorylase a activity is also stimulated by AMP (162, 163) with a K_a of 2×10^{-6} M. It is not affected by ATP but is competitively inhibited by UDP-glucose and glucose. Glucose apparently alters the equilibrium between phosphorylase a tetramers and dimers in favor of inactive species (101, 305). The conformational transitions of muscle phosphorylase a have been summarized by Helmreich (96). The evidence indicates that both phosphorylase a dimers and tetramers can exist in active and inactive states, although the phosphorylase a dimer is the more active form. The inactive state is associated with weak binding of substrates and modifiers but strong binding of inhibitors, whereas in the active state the reverse occurs. Interconversions are effected by changes in ionic strength, pH, Mg^{2+}, and Ca^{2+}, in addition to glucose, glucose-1-P, and AMP.

Although it is difficult to assess the physiological significance of some of the methods of inducing allosteric transitions of muscle phosphorylase in vitro, it is clear that in resting muscle phosphorylase b is present in an inactive form and that glycogenolysis can be initiated either by a conversion of phosphorylase b to a or by a conversion of phosphorylase b to an active state. The partially phosphorylated forms of muscle phosphorylase that arise during the conversion of phosphorylase b to a in the presence of inorganic phosphate and glucose-1-P, but in the absence of glycogen (69, 110), and the strong inhibitory effect of glucose-6-P on the hybrids also may be important in providing a sensitive feedback control of glycogen utilization. Moreover glycogen itself appears to play an important role since it shifts the equilibrium between the different forms of phosphorylase a toward the more active phosphorylase a dimer (187). This effect provides another feedback control that regulates the amount of glycogenolysis, depending on the initial glycogen content, independently of dephosphorylation of phosphorylase a.

PHOSPHORYLASE PHOSPHATASE. Dephosphorylation of phosphorylase a accompanied by formation of the phosphorylase b dimer is catalyzed by a specific phosphorylase phosphatase. The enzyme-catalyzed dephosphorylation reaction is strongly inhibited by AMP with a K_i of 5×10^{-6} M (210). Apparently AMP causes a conformational change in phosphorylase a, which makes it less susceptible to reaction with the phosphatase (96). Of greater physiological significance is the recent discovery that phosphorylase phosphatase is inhibited by low concentrations of Ca^{2+} (89).

ACTIVATION OF PHOSPHORYLASE KINASE BY CYCLIC AMP. Phosphorylase kinase has been purified from rabbit skeletal muscle (45) and intensively investigated in the laboratories of Fischer and Krebs. As previously mentioned, it exists in two molecular forms, referred to as activated and nonactivated, which differ markedly in their affinity for phosphorylase b (128, 129). Activation is revealed by an increase in the ratio of activities measured at pH 6.8 and 8.2. Two mechanisms of physiological interest are capable of activating phosphorylase kinase: *1*) an increase of Ca^{2+} concentration above about 10^{-7} M; and *2*) phosphorylation induced by hormones. The latter mechanism is discussed first.

A series of studies (45, 303) have shown that activation by phosphorylation of the enzyme with Mg-ATP can occur by two separate processes: one involves a slow self-activation of Ca^{2+}-containing phosphorylase kinase, which is inhibited by the metal chelating agent, EGTA, whereas the other much faster reaction is mediated by a cyclic AMP-dependent protein kinase. This latter reaction is inhibited by a heat-stable protein isolated from skeletal muscle (301), but the physiological role of this inhibitor in vivo has not yet been elucidated. Unlike phosphorylation of phosphorylase b, a direct correlation between phosphorylation and activation of phosphorylase kinase has not been observed (45, 303). The phosphorylation sites with ^{32}P-labeled enzyme are alkali labile, and the phosphate is presumed bound to serine or threonine residues. The overphosphorylation of the enzyme observed in vitro, particularly when catalyzed by the cyclic AMP-dependent protein kinase, has not been explained (45) but is presumably due to nonspecific phosphorylation of sites unrelated to enzyme activation.

Cyclic AMP-dependent protein kinases active with phosphorylase kinase have been isolated from rabbit skeletal muscle (234, 275, 304) and heart (24, 252). The apparent K_m for Mg-ATP in the presence of excess Mg^{2+} is between 1 and 6×10^{-5} M, which is considerably lower than the corresponding apparent K_m of about 2×10^{-4} M observed with phosphorylase kinase in the phosphorylase b to a reaction (129). The highly purified enzyme (234) shows several peaks of activity upon column chromatography, each with a similar K_m for cyclic AMP ($1.5-3 \times 10^{-8}$ M) and maximum effect at 10^{-5} M cyclic AMP. Similar values were reported by Rubin et al. (252) for the beef heart enzyme. Cyclic AMP-dependent protein kinases have been demonstrated in many tissues, including trout testes (117), adipose tissue (38), brain (190), bacteria (135, 136), adrenal cortex (78, 79), frog bladder (116), and liver (139, 140). In general, the enzymes from different tissues exhibit a broad specificity toward protein substrates, which include protamine, histones, and casein. Of particular interest is the finding that highly purified cyclic AMP protein kinase from skeletal muscle and heart will phosphorylate both phosphorylase kinase and glycogen synthetase (234, 275). Cyclic AMP increases the V_{max} of the enzyme without affecting the apparent K_m for the substrate, and cooperativity has been observed with cyclic AMP but not with ATP when casein is used as substrate (275). Reimann et al. (234) report that the skeletal muscle protein kinase has been separated into a distinct cyclic AMP-binding regulatory subunit and a catalytic subunit, which upon reconstitution restores the dependence of the enzyme on cyclic AMP. A similar finding has been reported for the protein kinase from reticulocytes (291) and rat liver (290, 327). Cross reactivity of protein kinases and regulatory proteins capable of binding cyclic AMP from rat liver and rabbit skeletal muscle has also been demonstrated (326). A model for the mechanism of cyclic AMP action has been proposed (22, 24); it involves dissociation of the protein kinase by cyclic AMP into a regulatory subunit containing binding sites for cyclic AMP and an active catalytic subunit. An equilibrium between holo enzyme, free cyclic AMP, the regulatory subunit containing cyclic AMP, and the catalytic subunit has been suggested (22), which could account for sequestration of part of the tissue cyclic AMP in an inactive form.

ACTIVATION OF PHOSPHORYLASE KINASE BY CALCIUM ION. Of particular importance for understanding the mechanisms by which rates of energy production and energy expenditure are balanced in anaerobically contracting skeletal muscle is the finding that Ca^{2+} is required for activity of both the phosphorylated and nonphosphorylated forms of phosphorylase kinase. It has been known for some time that Ca^{2+} facilitates the conversion of phosphorylase b to a in crude muscle extracts (70). However, subsequent studies (189) failed to establish a clear-cut role for Ca^{2+} since, although phosphorylase kinase was shown to be activated by Ca^{2+}, another enzyme termed *kinase activating factor* [later shown to be a proteolytic enzyme (111)] was also required. The inhibition of phosphorylase kinase by ethylenediaminetetraacetate (EDTA) and ethylenebis(oxyethylenenitrilo)tetraacetic acid (EGTA) (189, 217) and reversal of inhibition by Ca^{2+} suggested a physiological role for Ca^{2+} at this enzyme step, particularly since only about 10^{-7} M Ca^{2+} was required for half-maximal activity (217). Recent work of Brostrom et al. (23), who studied the kinetics of phosphorylase kinase in the absence of Ca^{2+} contamination, has greatly clarified the effect of Ca^{2+} in the control of glycogenolysis. Activation by Ca^{2+} was found to be accompanied by a large increase in activity at pH 6.8 and a smaller increase at pH 8.2. This effect resulted from a decrease in the K_m for phosphorylase b, which in the absence of Ca^{2+} was 10 times higher than the estimated intracellular concentration of phosphorylase b. Phosphorylation of the enzyme also makes it more sensitive to low concentrations of Ca^{2+}. Thus apparent K_m values for Ca^{2+} were 2×10^{-7} M for phosphorylated phosphorylase kinase and 3×10^{-6} M for the nonphosphorylated form at pH 8.2, with similar values being obtained for the dissociation constants. Futhermore only the nonphosphorylated phosphorylase kinase could be completely inhibited by addition of skeletal muscle sarcoplasmic reticulum as a physiological Ca^{2+}-sequestering system. Therefore the phosphorylated enzyme may have residual activity at the intracellular free Ca^{2+} level of resting muscle, which is estimated to be somewhat greater than 10^{-7} M.

PHOSPHORYLASE KINASE PHOSPHATASE. A specific phosphorylase kinase phosphatase that catalyzes the dephosphorylation of activated phosphorylase kinase with resultant loss of activity has been isolated from rabbit skeletal muscle (242). This phosphatase is activated by metal ions and is inhibited by fluoride ions and glycogen. The occurrence of this enzyme, together with the ability of phosphorylase kinase to catalyze its own phosphorylation, raises the possibility of a relatively rapid phosphorylation-dephosphorylation cycle in muscle with consequent expenditure of ATP. This effect may account for the decreased efficiency of energy expenditure observed in cardiac muscle after catecholamine addition (35).

INTEGRATED CONTROL OF PHOSPHORYLASE ACTIVITY. A further contribution toward understanding the role of intracellular Ca^{2+} in the control of glycogenolysis in rabbit skeletal muscle has come from recent work in Fischer's laboratory (68, 89, 94, 188). This involved isolation of a protein-glycogen complex containing phosphorylase, phosphorylase kinase, phosphorylase phosphatase, and elements of the sarcoplasmic reticulum characterized by a strong ATPase. Phosphorylase was present in the b form because of an inactive kinase and active phosphatase. Addition of calcium to a reaction medium fortified with Mg^{2+} and ATP resulted in an immediate conversion of phosphorylase b to a and was followed by a reversal when all the added ATP was consumed. The phosphorylase interconversions were attributed to a cyclic AMP-independent, but Ca^{2+}-dependent, activation of phosphorylase kinase and simultaneous inhibition of phosphorylase phosphatase. No indication of phosphorylation of either phosphorylase kinase or phosphorylase phosphatase was obtained, and inhibitory effects of AMP on the phosphatase could be excluded. In several respects, the kinetic behavior of enzymes in the complex was different from that observed with purified enzymes, which possibly indicates that at high protein concentrations either glycogen itself or direct protein-protein interactions modify catalytic function, particularly of the phosphatase. Thus the affinity of phosphorylase kinase for Ca^{2+} decreased from about 2×10^{-7} M in the purified enzyme to about 2×10^{-6} M in the protein-glycogen complex. Since 1×10^{-6} M Ca^{2+} is the estimated intracellular concentration required for half-maximal activation of muscular contraction (59, 201, 255) and is also about the same as the binding constant of troponin for Ca^{2+} in effecting actomyosin interaction and muscle contraction, it is clear that alterations of the intracellular free Ca^{2+} concentration over the physiological range required to produce contraction and relaxation of skeletal muscle are also sufficient to trigger parallel pulses of glycogenolysis. Furthermore, unlike purified phosphorylase, which becomes activated to fully phosphorylated species that are insensitive to inhibition by glucose-6-P, activation of phosphorylase in the glycogen-protein complex is sensitive to glucose-6-P inhibition. This effect is indicative of partially phosphorylated hybrids (69), direct inhibition of phosphorylase kinase, or stimulation of the phosphatase. Another discrepancy between the kinetic behavior of the isolated enzyme and its presumed behavior in the tissue relates to the apparent lack of inhibition of phosphorylase phosphatase by AMP in the physiological state. Probably some factor in vivo protects phosphorylase phosphatase from inhibition by AMP, since the tissue level of AMP is 100 times greater than the inhibitory constant. Haschke et al. (89) postulate that the phosphatase may be buried in the protein-glycogen complex and suggest that it is more subject to protein-protein interactions than to control by AMP.

Control of Glycogenolysis in Intact Muscle

For many years, epinephrine administration either to intact animals or to isolated muscle preparations has been known to cause a rapid breakdown of muscle glycogen, and the history of the development of knowledge that led to understanding the role of cyclic AMP in this process has been extensively reviewed (245–249, 284–289). The present discussion is confined to a summary of the more recent literature and to the relation between findings with intact muscle preparations and the previously described studies with purified enzymes. Since the effects of epinephrine, particularly with skeletal muscle, are closely related to the state of activity of the muscle it is of interest to review also effects of electrical stimulation on carbohydrate metabolism and to contrast these effects with those obtained with epinephrine alone.

Muscle contains phosphodiesterases, which rapidly degrade cyclic AMP to AMP, and also specific phosphatases, which convert the phosphorylated forms of phosphorylase kinase and phosphorylase to the less active nonphosphorylated forms. Because of the high content of phosphodiesterases and phosphatases in tissue extracts, severe technical difficulties have been encountered in obtaining reliable estimates of the amount of the phosphorylated forms of phosphorylase and phosphorylase kinase present in tissues. Preservation of the enzyme forms during the fixation and extraction procedure has been achieved with partial success by means of rapid freezing techniques and extraction of the enzymes at low temperatures in the presence of EDTA and fluoride. It has thus been possible to follow on a kinetic basis changes in the percentage of phosphorylase a, activated phosphorylase kinase, and cyclic AMP levels in skeletal and heart muscle after addition of epinephrine or upon electrical stimulation of the muscle.

SKELETAL MUSCLE. From the work of Danforth et al. (42), it became evident that different mechanisms were responsible for initiating phosphorylase b to a interconversion with electrical stimulation and epinephrine. Resting frog sartorius muscle contained very low levels of phosphorylase a, and the values increased to nearly 100% of the total phosphorylase within 3 sec of the onset of tetanic contractions at 30 C under anaerobic conditions. After epinephrine addition, a maximum of 50% conversion to phosphorylase a required about 30 min. Likewise the decay of phosphorylase a was rapid after cessation of stimulation and slow after removal of epinephrine. Although no direct measurements were made, calculation of rate constants indicated that changes in the activity of phosphorylase kinase, rather than of phosphorylase phosphatase, were responsible for the increase and decrease of phosphorylase a. Another important difference between electrical stimulation and epinephrine addition in the phosphorylase b to a conversion was in the sensitivity of the latter effect to the β adrenergic blocking agent, dichloroisoproterenol. Further studies with isolated frog sartorius muscle (41, 98, 99) demonstrated that at low rates of stimulation (2 pulses/sec) there was a lag of about 25 sec before phosphorylase a levels started to increase. The lag phase decreased with increasing rates of stimulation and could be abolished by pretreatment of the muscle with low concentrations of epinephrine. The percentage of phosphorylase in the a form in the steady state increased with rates of stimulation up to 8 pulses/sec. These studies indicated that phosphorylase kinase activity was affected by the rate of contraction rather than by the work of the muscle, and the authors suggested that the lag period in phosphorylase a formation may represent the time required to activate phosphorylase kinase.

Direct measurements of cyclic AMP levels and of the ratio of phosphorylase kinase activity at pH 6.8 to that at pH 8.2 by other workers substantiated these conclusions and confirmed that different mechanisms were responsible for conversion of phosphorylase kinase to the activated form with epinephrine or electrical stimulation. Thus Posner et al. (225, 226) first showed that administration of epinephrine to rats in vivo, followed by rapid excision of the gastrocnemius muscle or addition of epinephrine to isolated frog skeletal muscle preparations, caused an increase of cyclic AMP concentration, phosphorylase kinase activity, and phosphorylase a levels within 60 sec. However, although electrical stimulation increased phosphorylase a levels and phosphorylase kinase activity, it had no effect on cyclic AMP levels, which suggested that during muscular contraction phosphorylase kinase is converted to an activated form by some process not involving the cyclic nucleotide. Subsequent studies by Drummond et al. (54) with improved analytical techniques confirmed that epinephrine caused a rapid increase of cyclic AMP, phosphorylase a, and activated phosphorylase kinase levels in isolated frog sartorius and in rat diaphragm and gastrocnemius. On the other hand, electrical stimulation increased phosphorylase a levels and caused no change of either cyclic AMP concentration or phosphorylase kinase activity (pH 6.8:8.2 ratio). Presumably under these conditions activity of nonphosphorylated phosphorylase kinase was increased directly by a rise of the Ca^{2+} concentration during electrical stimulation, with this activation not being detected after the extraction procedure.

Recent studies by Mayer & Krebs (182) were designed to show whether phosphorylations of phosphorylase b and phosphorylase kinase could be demonstrated in vivo in rabbit skeletal muscle after the administration of epinephrine followed by pretreatment of the animals with ^{32}P-inorganic phosphate. No ^{32}P was found in purified phosphorylase b, and the specific activity of the alkaline-labile ^{32}P-phosphate in purified phosphorylase a corresponded to that of the γ-phosphate of muscle ATP, which provided an elegant demonstration that the interconversion of phosphorylase b to a in vivo under the stimulus of epinephrine was consistent with the mechanisms proposed from experiments in vitro. However, phosphorylase kinase was found to contain bound phosphate irrespective of its degree of activation, and this phosphate exchanged in vivo with ^{32}P in the absence of epinephrine. The lack of stoichiometry between activation of phosphorylase kinase and its phosphorylation is similar to observations made with the enzyme in vitro (45).

CARDIAC MUSCLE. The effects of epinephrine on glycogen metabolism have also been intensively studied in cardiac muscle, which has lent itself to measurements of the time sequence of the various activation steps between administration of epinephrine and the appearance of the products of glycogen metabolism. After the initial observation of Hess & Haugaard (102) that epinephrine addition to perfused rat hearts caused an apparently simultaneous augmentation of contractile force and increased level of phosphorylase a, much work has been devoted to the question whether glycogenolysis was directly involved in the inotropic effect of epinephrine and related catecholamines (92). At first, the evidence seemed to support this suggestion, but the question was finally resolved in the negative on the basis of careful kinetic studies and dose-response relations, as well as dissociation of the effects by means of acetylcholine (17, 299). Although cyclic AMP levels increased to a maximum simultaneously with (36) or even before (53, 244) the full development of the contractile response after addition of epinephrine to perfused rat hearts, a distinct lag of a few seconds was observed before phosphorylase a levels started to increase. Maximal activation of phosphorylase was not observed until well after the peak of the inotropic response (36, 53, 56, 215, 244, 318). On the other hand, phosphorylase kinase was maximally activated within 1 sec of epinephrine addition, and its kinetics of activation could not be distinguished from the increase of tissue cyclic AMP levels (53). These basic findings were later confirmed by using rat hearts in situ after administration of epinephrine to the intact rat (198). Kinetic studies with isolated hearts therefore indicate that the lag period seen before the rise of phosphorylase a level is not caused by a delay in the activation of phosphorylase kinase, but rather to a slow interaction of activated phosphorylase kinase with phosphorylase b. A similar explanation probably accounts for the delay observed in phosphorylase a formation in skeletal muscle with low rates of stimulation (41). This explanation is to be preferred over the original one, namely, that the lag was due to the time required to activate phosphorylase kinase.

A second approach, which also indicates the absence of a cause-and-effect relation between the contractile response of cardiac muscle to epinephrine and activation of phosphorylase, is derived from measurements of the relative sensitivities of the two processes. Thus Mayer et al. (181), who used open chest dog heart preparations, found that, with suitably small doses of epinephrine, ventricular contractile force increased but phosphorylase *a* levels remained unaltered. Similar results have been obtained with different heart preparations by other workers (56). The objection that the sensitivity of the phosphorylase *a* assay in these studies was not sufficient to detect small changes can be raised. Williamson & Jamieson (318, 319) approached this problem by using the fluorescent properties of bound tissue NADH to detect whether more cytoplasmic NADH was being generated by glycolysis at the glyceraldehyde-3-P dehydrogenase step after addition of small doses of epinephrine to perfused rat hearts. This technique of measuring changes of reduced nicotinamide nucleotide levels by surface fluorometry is capable of great sensitivity and has the additional advantage that it provides a continuous in vivo kinetic recording (34). Two phases of the fluorescence response could be distinguished after addition of moderate doses of epinephrine: *1*) an initial oxidation of nicotinamide nucleotide that corresponds to the onset of the increased contractile response and increased respiratory activity; and *2*) a biphasic increase of fluorescence attributable to enhanced glycogenolysis. With small epinephrine doses (e.g., 0.002–0.02 μg) only the initial mitochondrial response was seen, together with a small increment of contractile force, which indicated the absence of glycogenolysis. However, Drummond et al. (53) found that phosphorylase kinase was activated in parallel with the augmentation of contractile force; so it is possible that this enzyme has to be activated above a threshold level before a net conversion of phosphorylase *b* to *a* is observed. The effects of epinephrine on the contractile response, on increases of cyclic AMP, phosphorylase kinase, and phosphorylase *a* levels, and on glycogenolysis in heart muscle are all prevented by β adrenergic blocking agents such as dichloroisoproterenol, nethalide, or propranolol; this suggests that all these events are secondary to the binding of epinephrine to specific receptor sites in the plasma membrane (see the chapter by Moran in this volume of the *Handbook*).

In summary, the earliest events observed after addition of epinephrine to normal heart preparations are increases in contractile force, cyclic AMP level, and phosphorylase kinase activity (pH 6.8:8.2 ratio). With the time resolution of available tissue freezing methods, the onset of these changes appears to be simultaneous, although peak changes of cyclic AMP and phosphorylase kinase levels have been observed well before maximum tension or work output is developed. Conversion of phosphorylase *b* to *a* and appearance of increased tissue levels of hexose phosphates occur at a later stage and with progressive delays (316).

Studies already alluded to with intact skeletal muscle or isolated enzyme preparations showed that phosphorylase kinase could be activated either by a cyclic AMP-dependent process or by an independent mechanism that appeared to be closely connected to increased availability of intracellular Ca^{2+}. The question arises therefore whether the Ca^{2+}-activated process is also operative in heart muscle after epinephrine stimulation, in addition to an activation of the cyclic AMP-dependent protein kinase. Several findings suggest that both processes are involved in the overall effect. Namm et al. (199) observed that, when contractions of the rat heart were stopped by using perfusion medium containing 56 mM K^+, the changes in cyclic AMP level, phosphorylase kinase activation, and phosphorylase *a* formation upon addition of epinephrine were all greatly decreased compared with effects obtained in normally contracting hearts; this suggests that K^+ was interfering with the action of epinephrine at or before the step of adenyl cyclase activation. Removal of Ca^{2+} from the perfusion medium also prevented heart contractions and greatly diminished the epinephrine-induced conversion of phosphorylase *b* to *a*. However, the rise of cyclic AMP level and activation of phosphorylase kinase were not greatly affected, except for a short delay in the onset of the latter effect. On the other hand, elevation of the Ca^{2+} concentration to three times normal (9.6 mEq/liter) increased phosphorylase *a* levels but produced only a small, statistically insignificant effect on phosphorylase kinase activity (pH 6.8:8.2 ratio) and no effect on cyclic AMP levels. These findings, together with the previously mentioned studies of Drummond et al. (54) and the in vitro properties of the enzymes, can be interpreted on the basis of a stimulatory effect of Ca^{2+} on the catalytic activity of both the nonphosphorylated and phosphorylated forms of phosphorylase kinase and an inhibitory effect on phosphorylase phosphatase activity. The cyclic AMP-mediated activation of phosphorylase kinase appears to be slower than the Ca^{2+} activation effect in both heart and skeletal muscle, so that the rapid responses obtained after addition of epinephrine to spontaneously contracting heart muscle can only be explained on the basis of a combined action of cyclic AMP and Ca^{2+}.

CALCIUM AND MUSCLE CONTRACTION

Data reviewed in previous sections have indicated that the glycogenolytic effect of epinephrine is mediated by the two chemical transmitters, cyclic AMP and Ca^{2+}. The remarkable interplay between these two agents on a wide variety of excitatory and secretory processes has been described by Rasmussen and associates (229, 230). It is important therefore to consider carefully whether a combined action of Ca^{2+} and cyclic AMP might also be involved in determining the dynamics and strength of cardiac contractility. However, before the possible involvement of cyclic AMP in the cardiac contraction cycle can be considered in more detail, it is appropriate first to review the considerable data on the relation between Ca^{2+} and muscular contraction. The interested reader should consult a number of recently published reviews on this topic (14, 58, 59, 87, 112, 122, 201, 202, 221a, 308, 311, 321).

Briefly, initiation of the action potential causes depolarization of the plasma membrane and increased permeability to Na^+, K^+, and Ca^{2+}. In heart, Ca^{2+} is made available by increased Ca^{2+} entry and release from internal storage sites, so that the intracellular free Ca^{2+} concentration rises possibly by as much as two orders of magnitude from a value in resting muscle of less than 10^{-7} M. The Ca^{2+} diffuses to the myofibrils and combines with a subunit of troponin, which causes an alteration of the configuration of the troponin-tropomyosin complex with the net result that inhibition of actomyosin ATPase is relieved. This allows combination of F-actin with myosin to produce shortening of the myofibril with utilization of energy from the hydrolysis of ATP. Relaxation occurs by a decrease of the free intracellular Ca^{2+} concentration and sequestration of calcium from its binding to troponin until the point is reached at which the troponin-tropomyosin complex reexerts an inhibitory effect on the actomyosin ATPase. The sarcoplasmic reticulum is thought to be the major system responsible for removal of free Ca^{2+} from the environment of the myofibrils. This is brought about by an ATP-dependent, active reaccumulation of Ca^{2+} followed by its redistribution in the sarcotubule system and sarcolemma membrane binding sites. The calcium balance is restored by transport of Ca^{2+} through the plasma membrane to the external medium during the interval between beats. In subsequent sections, the various events associated with the different phases of muscular contraction are described in some detail, so that possible interactions between Ca^{2+} and cyclic AMP at the molecular level can better be appreciated.

Calcium and Contractile Proteins

At least four proteins comprise the basic contractile element of muscle: myosin, actin, tropomyosin, and troponin. The properties of these proteins and their role in the biochemistry and physiology of muscular contraction in heart have been reviewed recently by Katz (122), whereas the mechanism of contraction of striated muscle has been reviewed by Huxley (112) and, with special emphasis on the role of Ca^{2+}, by Winegrad (321). Myosin is the chief constituent of the thick filament observed by microscopy, and the complex protein isolated from both cardiac and skeletal muscle has a molecular weight of about 500,000. It has a rodlike shape and is composed of two polypeptide chains arranged as a coiled coil. One end is enlarged forming a globular head, which is the site for both ATPase activity and actin binding. There are two types of skeletal muscle myosin: that obtained from white rabbit muscle has a higher ATPase activity than that prepared from the predominantly red fibers of dog skeletal muscle. This latter type is similar to that obtained from cardiac muscle. The K_m for ATP of cardiac myosin ATPase is about 10^{-4} M, whereas that for rabbit skeletal muscle is an order of magnitude lower. Actin is the major protein of the thin filament of striated muscle. It exists in two states, the monomeric form, G-actin (mol wt 47,000), which is polymerized to F-actin when a nucleotide and a divalent cation are bound, ATP and Ca^{2+} having the highest affinity. Polymerization of G-actin to F-actin occurs with dephosphorylation of ATP to ADP, and it has been estimated that most of the ADP present in skeletal muscle is bound to F-actin. The G-actin monomers are in a double-helical arrangement in F-actin, which is the normal form found in intact muscle. In certain features, the actomyosin ATPase extracted from muscle or reconstituted from purified actin and myosin is different from the myosin ATPase. Notably it is stimulated by low concentrations of Mg^{2+} and is affected by agents that influence the interaction between actin and myosin.

Two other proteins, tropomyosin and troponin, are associated with the thin filament. Tropomyosin from cardiac and skeletal muscle is a rodlike protein (mol wt 70,000) that binds stoichiometrically with actin. Its function, together with troponin, is to modulate the actin-myosin interaction. Troponin is essential for the Ca^{2+} sensitivity of actomyosin ATPase activity and also strengthens the binding of tropomyosin to F-actin (50). Originally it was thought that troponin consisted of two subunits: troponin A that binds Ca^{2+} in a molar ratio of 1:1, and troponin B that inhibits the actomyosin ATPase (88a). More recently up to four different proteins have been obtained from troponin of skeletal muscle by DEAE-Sephadex chromatography in 6 M urea (83a, 83b). Three of these have been extensively purified and together reconstitute an active troponin complex. According to Greaser & Gergely (83b), only one subunit, TN-C (mol wt 20,000) binds Ca^{2+} with high affinity (association constant of 1.4×10^6 M^{-1}), and is apparently identical with troponin A (88). Complicated interactions occur between the subunits of troponin, tropomyosin, and actin to control the actomyosin ATPase activity. A second subunit of troponin, TN-I (mol wt 24,000), inhibits actomyosin ATPase activity both in the presence and absence of Ca^{2+}. The third major subunit, TN-T (mol wt 37,000), interacts with tropomyosin and restores the original Ca^{2+}-sensitizing activity of troponin on actomyosin ATPase when added to TN-I and TN-C. The tropomyosin-troponin complex is distributed along the thin filaments at approximately 400-Å intervals and probably accounts for this periodicity observed in the muscle fiber.

Direct estimates of the concentration of Ca^{2+} required to elicit tension development have been made in crab muscle fibers by injection of calcium-EGTA buffers (224). These studies provided threshold values of Ca^{2+} between 3×10^{-7} and 1.5×10^{-6} M. Further studies with a variety of preparations from skeletal and cardiac muscle having different degrees of intactness (e.g., EGTA-treated ventricular strips, skinned fibers, glycerol extracted fibers, and myofibrils, in addition to natural or reconstituted actomyosin) provide a similar relation between tension development and ATPase activity and the variation of the Ca^{2+} concentration. However, some differences exist between the relative sensitivities of the preparations, half-maximum tension being produced by 0.6×10^{-6} M Ca^{2+} with EDTA-treated frog ventricular strips (323) and 1.6×10^{-6} M Ca^{2+} with skinned frog skeletal muscle fibers (95). Ebashi et al. (59), on the other hand, report a lower sensitivity to Ca^{2+} in which the threshold concentration of free Ca^{2+} for tension development was about 1×10^{-6} M. With purified actin and myosin in vitro, under suitable conditions of pH and ATP, Mg^{2+}, and KCl concentrations, calcium concentrations below 100 μM had little effect on ATPase activity or superprecipitation (the equivalent of contraction). However, with a reconstituted cardiac preparation containing tropomyosin and troponin, a sensitivity of the ATPase to Ca^{2+} over the range from 10^{-7} to 10^{-5} M was achieved with a half-maximum activation at about 1×10^{-6} M (123, 310), with revised values for the affinity constant of EGTA for Ca^{2+} being used (212). In view of the difficulties in calculating the true Ca^{2+} concentration because of changes in affinity of the Ca-EGTA complex with pH and ionic strength, the agreement between different preparations and muscle types is very good and contrasts strongly with similar calcium titrations with intact muscles or perfused hearts in which a half-maximal increase of tension is produced by external Ca^{2+} concentrations three orders of magnitude higher.

In his excellent review of the contractile proteins of heart, Katz (122) summarized estimates made by a number of investigators for the amount of Ca^{2+} required to fully activate contraction of skeletal and cardiac muscle. Calculations may be based either on the amount of exchangeable Ca^{2+} bound to myofibrils when ATPase activity or superprecipitation is maximal (310) or on the number of high-affinity Ca^{2+} binding sites on troponin and the troponin content per unit weight of muscle (74). Both methods agree in providing a value of 1 μmole of Ca^{2+} per gram of myofibrils in both heart and skeletal muscle for the amount of calcium required for the actin-myosin interaction to change from a state of complete inhibition to one of full activity of the Mg^{2+}-activated actomyosin ATPase. Since cardiac muscle contains about 50 g of actomyosin per kilogram wet weight, saturation of the troponin binding sites in the actomyosin complex will require approximately 50 μmoles Ca^{2+} per kilogram muscle. Katz (122) points out that, in addition to this bound Ca^{2+}, an extra 10 μmoles of Ca^{2+} per kilogram muscle will be needed to raise the free Ca^{2+} from 10^{-7} to 10^{-5} M. Various estimates (direct and indirect) for the calcium affinity of receptor sites on purified troponin or on the actomyosin complex provide values between 3.4×10^5 M^{-1} and 1.5×10^6 M^{-1} for cardiac muscle and between 6×10^5 M^{-1} and 2.5×10^6 M^{-1} for skeletal muscle (122). Apparently skeletal muscle troponin has two classes of binding sites (9.3×10^5 M^{-1} and 1.3×10^6 M^{-1}); so it is not clear that all the bound Ca^{2+} would be removed from troponin during the relaxation phase. Further measurements of the affinities of calcium binding sites to cardiac troponin are required. However, in general the calculated binding constants for the calcium site regulating actomyosin ATPase activity and tension development in glycerol-extracted fibers are similar to those of the high-affinity calcium binding site on troponin; so a value of about 1×10^{-6} M Ca^{2+} can be used for an estimated half-maximal effect on contractility.

In summary, it appears that Ca^{2+} plays the principal role in determining the interaction between actin and myosin. This is achieved by Ca^{2+} binding to a subunit of troponin; a conformational change is thereby produced in associated regulatory subunits, which through the mediation of tropomyosin releases an inhibition between the ATPase cross bridges of the myosin (thick) filaments and sites on the actin (thin) filaments. This allows ATP splitting with concomitant shortening of the myofibril. It may be noted that the active state of the muscle can be manifest either as chemical transformations correlating with shortening velocity or as the development of strong physiochemical attractions between the thick and thin filaments, which develop tension. These two conditions will be associated with different rates of ATP hydrolysis.

Cellular Calcium Flux

Both cardiac and skeletal muscle contain 2–4 mEq of total calcium per kilogram fat-free weight (47). Clearly very little of this is available in the form of free ionized Ca^{2+}. Disruption of the cell shows that calcium is associated with many subcellular structures, including the myofibrils, mitochondria, nuclei, myoplasm, sarcolemma, and sarcoplasmic reticulum (200). However, the absolute amounts that can be measured in these components after isolation from tissue homogenates probably bears little relation to the amounts of calcium they bind in the intact tissue. Consequently attention has been focused on methods for measuring calcium pool sizes that do not involve disruption of the tissue, such as rates of $^{45}Ca^{2+}$ exchangeability and autoradiographic and electron-microscopic techniques.

From studies in which muscle preparations are incubated with $^{45}Ca^{2+}$ followed by observation of the washout kinetics of the radioactivity, it has been possible to distinguish several intracellular compartments of calcium of different sizes and associated with different rates of $^{45}Ca^{2+}$ exchange. With the help of a number of assumptions, the complex curves of $^{45}Ca^{2+}$ washout can be analyzed into as many as five exponential components or phases, each of which can be assumed to represent a certain pool of exchangeable calcium in the tissue (142). However, the limitation of the kinetic analysis is such that Ca^{2+} arising from different sources with similar kinetics cannot be distinguished. Therefore, although certain phases can be tentatively assigned as originating from some anatomically identifiable structure, the calculated amount of Ca^{2+} associated with a specific phase cannot be associated accurately with any one type of calcium storage site. A number of studies with frog sartorius muscle (77), guinea pig atrium (324), dog papillary muscle (141, 143), and rabbit ventricular muscle (268) have provided evidence for at least three cellular compartments of calcium: *1*) a rapidly exchanging pool with a half-time of a few minutes assumed to originate largely from Ca^{2+} bound to surface membrane sites; *2*) a more slowly exchanging pool derived from metabolically active intracellular sites; and *3*) an essentially nonexchangeable pool representing calcium tightly bound to intracellular structures. The relative proportion of the total calcium assigned to each of these compartments was found to vary considerably with the preparation and method of perfusion, but each constituted about one-quarter to one-third of the total (142).

Measurements of the amounts of $^{45}Ca^{2+}$ taken up by cardiac muscle in experiments involving an increase of the external Ca^{2+}, decrease of external Na^+, increase of external K^+, or increase of stimulation rate have been made by a number of investigators (142, 201). In experiments with dog papillary muscle (141, 143) an increment in frequency of 27 beats/min was associated with an increment of tissue Ca^{2+} of 1.9 μmoles/kg per beat over a 10-min interval. In quiescent guinea pig atria, increasing external Ca^{2+} from 1.25 to 3.75 mM increased $^{45}Ca^{2+}$ uptake threefold (324), whereas electrical stimulation of guinea pig atria or frog ventricle at a given Ca^{2+} concentration produced a large extra influx of $^{45}Ca^{2+}$, which was quantitatively dependent on the frequency of contraction (207, 324). In general, conditions associated with an increased rate of Ca^{2+} flux in actively contracting cardiac muscle preparations (0.5–2.7 μmoles Ca^{2+} per kg per beat) are the same as those producing increased tension. This applies also to drugs having a positive inotropic effect on cardiac muscle. Thus, although epinephrine and norepinephrine have no effect on $^{45}Ca^{2+}$ exchange in quiescent guinea pig atria, $^{45}Ca^{2+}$ uptake in actively contracting preparations is significantly increased (85, 235). Most of the flux studies, with the exception of those with dog papillary muscle, show that increased Ca^{2+} flux is not associated with a net gain of tissue Ca^{2+}, which indicates that the increased influx with each beat is balanced by an equal efflux within the period of a contraction cycle. Since the amount of Ca^{2+} entering the cardiac cell with each contraction, as measured by these techniques, is much smaller than the amount of calcium needed to elicit maximum contraction through its binding to troponin, a secondary release of internally bound Ca^{2+} must be postulated (206).

Role of Calcium in Excitation-Contraction Coupling

The essential feature of excitation-contraction coupling is a rapid depolarization of the cell membrane during passage of the action potential followed by activation of contraction by a Ca^{2+}-dependent mechanism (20). The resting potential (-90 mv) is related to the K^+ gradient across the cell by the Nernst equations with a high $[K^+]_i$ being maintained by extrusion of Na^+ ions through activation of an asymmetrical Na^+-K^+-activated, Mg^{2+}-dependent ATPase in the sarcolemma membrane (274). This maintains the intracellular Na^+ concentration at 27–30 mM.

Electron-microscopic studies (67, 219, 272) show that the sarcolemma membrane of mammalian cardiac muscle is a multilayered structure 300–425 A in thickness. The thin plasma membrane (75 A) is separated from the basement membrane (75–200 A thick) by a space of approximately 150 A. The chemical composition of the cell membrane is about 65% protein, with the remainder being lipid and phospholipid. At approximately 2–3-μ intervals along the membrane in the region of the Z lines, the sarcolemma invaginates to form a tubular system (T tubules) that extends deep into the myoplasm. The lumen of the tubules communicates directly with the extracellular space, and depolarization of these membranes acts as a conducting mechanism for the spread of electrical activity from the surface to the interior of the cell (37a). Additional fine intracellular tubules (200–500 A in diameter) continuous across the Z lines and in close apposition to the myoplasmic surface of the sarcolemma have also been observed anatomically (219, 272) and may provide a locus for superficial rapid-release storage sites for Ca^{2+}.

Studies involving stepwise increases of the extracellular Ca^{2+} concentration (269) and inhibition studies in which La^{3+} was used to displace Ca^{2+} from superficial membrane sites (254) have provided evidence favoring a rapid equilibration of $^{45}Ca^{2+}$ between the interstitial space and sarcolemma binding sites, and its release during excitation to produce contraction of the myofibrils. A more slowly exchangeable Ca^{2+} pool (142) is now thought to represent a storage region accounted for by removal of Ca^{2+} by a fast unidirectional step into the sarcotubule space during relaxation, which is followed by a slower release through the sarcolemma binding sites into the interstitial space (269). In this model of calcium movements in mammalian cardiac muscle, the Ca^{2+} involved in excitation-contraction coupling passes essentially along a one-way path, and the main function of the sarcoplasmic reticulum system is in the sequestration of Ca^{2+} from the troponin binding sites.

In cardiac muscle the duration of the action potential (200–600 msec) is about the same as that of the contraction cycle (104), and unlike skeletal muscle, which has a very brief action potential (255), contraction is totally dependent on the presence of Ca^{2+} in the external medium. Studies with the voltage clamp technique in which Purkinje fibers, ventricular strips, or ventricular trabeculae muscles are used (10, 11, 195, 325) have established that the initial spike of the action potential is due to a rapid inward Na^+ current and that repolarization is caused by an outward K^+ flux (208, 209, 251). It has been postulated that, during the plateau phase of the action potential, Ca^{2+} may enter the myoplasm and that this small Ca^{2+} current may trigger the release of more Ca^{2+} from intracellular storage sites. The primary

Na$^+$ current is excited at membrane potentials more positive than the resting potential (e.g., -65 mv) and rises rapidly with a further decrease of the membrane potential (10). This initial, fast inward current has been characterized as a Na$^+$ current by its disappearance in the absence of external Na$^+$ and by its sensitivity to inhibition by tetrodotoxin (10^{-5} g/ml). A second much slower inward current, which becomes activated at about -35 mv and corresponds with tension development, has been investigated by a double-step voltage clamp technique that is thought to cause inactivation of the initial Na$^+$ current (237, 238). In these experiments, the secondary (i.e., calcium) current reached a peak at about -20 mv and was little affected by replacement of external Na$^+$ with choline or sucrose or by the presence of tetrodotoxin but was very sensitive to alterations of external Ca^{2+}. This current was inactivated rapidly at depolarizations in the range of -30 to 0 mv but more slowly with depolarization potentials in the positive region: a factor presumably of importance in causing the sudden collapse of the plateau phase of the action potential after onset of increased K$^+$ conductance.

Alteration in the duration and magnitude of the plateau phase of the action potential by voltage clamp techniques has provided considerable impetus to speculations concerning the relation between calcium influx and tension development by the muscle. However, a recent critical review by Johnson & Lieberman (119) should be consulted for a detailed discussion of the limitations of this technique as presently applied to cardiac muscle preparations. In studies with mammalian cardiac muscle (195), a minimum period of 1–5 msec of depolarization was required before any tension development could be elicited. Contraction strength developed rapidly with increasing duration of membrane depolarization up to about 200 msec, which was less than the normal duration of the action potential. After a long depolarization pulse, the contraction elicited by a subsequent stimulus was greater than normal for 5–6 beats. When the external Ca^{2+} concentration was increased, maximum tension was reached with progressively shorter periods of depolarization. Alteration of the strength of the depolarization potential of fixed duration showed that maintained tension appeared at -25 mv and increased steeply as the clamped membrane potential was made more positive. Similar studies with frog ventricular strips showed that membrane depolarization exerted continuous control over the contractile response, and relaxation only occurred with repolarization of the membrane (193). The apparent onset of tension development upon membrane depolarization occurred after about 100 msec, which is much longer than that observed with mammalian ventricle, but such depolarizations facilitated the tension response to subsequent depolarizations, provided the second stimulus was given within 500 msec. Furthermore membrane potential-tension relations were linear in the range from -10 to at least 120 mv and showed no tendency to decline at potentials more positive than the estimated calcium equilibrium potential (calculated from the Nernst equation to be about $+100$ mv), as was observed with mammalian heart preparations.

Various phenomena, such as latency, subthreshold stimulation, and poststimulation potentiation, imply that preceding electrical events influence the tension development for a given contraction, as well as the size and duration of the action potential. Difficulties arise in attempts to correlate the magnitude of the ^{45}Ca^{2+} influx per beat with the current required to hold the potential across the cell membrane at a depolarized level in voltage clamp experiments because of the impossibility of correcting for artifacts with both types of measurements. However, it is generally accepted that the amount of Ca^{2+} entering the cell during membrane depolarization is insufficient, possibly by as much as an order of magnitude, to account for the amount of Ca^{2+} required for troponin binding and elicitation of a contraction. Explanations for the many observations associated with excitation-contraction coupling therefore relate to possible mechanisms associated with the secondary release of Ca^{2+} induced by the primary activator calcium, which itself is controlled by the size and duration of the action potential. Thus Wood et al. (325) postulate that the presystolic level of intracellular Ca^{2+} bound to specific rapid release sites is influenced by preceding electrical events and is a major determinant of the concentration of free intracellular Ca^{2+} attained during the initial phase of the plateau of the action potential. With this model, the amount of Ca^{2+} dissociated from the rapid release sites by a given action potential is an approximately constant fraction of the total calcium stored at these sites. This calcium pool is clearly in a highly dynamic state, and unfortunately neither ^{45}Ca^{2+} flux studies, pyroantimonate staining techniques (149), nor autoradiographic studies with ^{45}Ca^{2+} have provided data that more than indirectly substantiate hypotheses consistent with the electrophysiological findings. However, comparative studies of mammalian and amphibian cardiac muscle have been useful in resolving the problem of identification of the rapid release binding sites for Ca^{2+} on membranes. Thus many of the differences between the electrophysiological responses of mammalian and frog myocardium can be accounted for on the basis of the less well-developed sarcotubular system in the frog ventricle (204, 278). Since the differences seem to be of degree rather than kind, various data are consistent in supporting the concept that, in cardiac muscle generally, the bulk of the storage Ca^{2+} is associated with rapid release sites present on membranes or in tubules located close to the sarcolemma and T tubule invaginations. Experiments with the ^{45}Ca^{2+} show that this calcium pool exchanges rapidly with external Ca^{2+}. These sites might be a possible locus of action for certain agents that modify cardiac contractile function, possibly by changing the affinity of anionic binding groups in the membrane for Ca^{2+}, and therefore altering their relative occupancy by Ca^{2+}. On this basis, effects produced by alterations of the pH or competition between cations for the same site are to be expected (142).

Calcium Release by Sarcoplasmic Reticulum

Skeletal muscle represents an example of a contractile tissue of a different nature from amphibian cardiac muscle since it is very rich in sarcoplasmic reticulum and has a brief action potential, with contraction being relatively independent of the external Ca^{2+} concentration. Evidence suggests that some details of the calcium cycle in skeletal muscle differ from those in cardiac muscle in several significant respects, which may explain differences in the mechanical response of the tissue to drugs and catecholamines. However, the basic mechanism of muscular contraction appears to be similar, and since much data is available concerning the role of Ca^{2+} in skeletal muscle contraction some extrapolation of findings between the tissues is justified. The biggest difference concerns the nature of membrane systems involved in Ca^{2+} release following membrane depolarization. Thus, whereas particularly in amphibian cardiac muscle a considerable body of evidence implicates the critical involvement of superficially located membranes as calcium release sites, the evidence obtained from skeletal muscle suggests that the better-developed sarcoplasmic reticulum serves a dual role, both as a storage site for Ca^{2+} release to troponin during contraction and as a Ca^{2+}-sequestering system during relaxation (59, 142, 256, 321). Probably these two processes occur in anatomically and functionally distinct regions of the membrane. In skeletal muscle, and to a lesser extent in mammalian cardiac muscle, the longitudinally oriented membranes of the sarcoplasmic reticulum envelop the thick and thin filaments of the sarcomere and make close contact with the T tubules in the region of the Z line and thereby form so-called "triads" (221a, 231, 232). In these end regions, the sarcoplasmic reticulum tubules of skeletal muscle enlarge to form structures called terminal cisternae. These appear to provide the bulk of the Ca^{2+} required to saturate the troponin binding sites after depolarization of the plasma membrane and spread of the excitation through the T tubules into the interior of the fiber. The data of Weber & Herz (310) indicate that between 100 and 200 μmoles of Ca^{2+} per kilogram of muscle is needed for production of a maximal contraction, a value two- to fourfold greater than that required for cardiac muscle because of the higher concentration of actomyosin in skeletal muscle.

Autoradiographic studies by Winegrad (320, 322), who used $^{45}Ca^{2+}$-labeled frog skeletal muscle, indicate that in resting muscle the exchangeable calcium content of the terminal cisternae is large, whereas it is smaller in the longitudinal tubules and practically absent in the thin filaments. During the peak of tetanus a redistribution of $^{45}Ca^{2+}$ was observed with a shift of about 200 μmoles/kg of muscle to the region of the thin filaments, an increase of about 400 μmoles/kg to the longitudinal tubules with a large depletion of the amount in the terminal cisternae. During recovery from tetanus, Ca^{2+} was lost from the tubules back to the terminal cisternae (322). The evidence from these studies indicates that exchanges of calcium within the different portions of the sarcoplasmic reticulum is considerably faster than Ca^{2+} exchange between the terminal cisternae and the transverse tubules. Clearly Ca^{2+} involved in the contractile response is in a highly dynamic state of turnover, but many details remain to be elucidated concerning the mechanism of calcium release and its control by potential changes across the membranes of the sarcolemma and T tubules. In skeletal muscle it has been suggested that Ca^{2+} itself acts as a trigger to release more Ca^{2+} from internal binding sites in a regenerative fashion (63, 72).

Direct evidence for the kinetics of the changes of intracellular Ca^{2+} following a contraction stimulus has been provided by the use of the calcium indicators, murexide, with toad sartorius muscle (118), and aequorin, with barnacle muscle (3, 4). These data showed that a rapid transient increase of intracellular Ca^{2+} occurred shortly after the onset of membrane depolarization and before any increase of tension. The peak of the Ca^{2+} transient coincided with the maximum rate of tension development and decayed exponentially with a time constant of 60–80 msec, so that peak tension together with relaxation occurred with the Ca^{2+} concentration virtually at resting levels. Increase of the intensity of stimulation in the barnacle muscle enhanced the rate of formation and peak of the Ca^{2+} transient, whereas an increase in the duration of the stimulus increased the peak and total amount of free Ca^{2+} released. These changes occurred in parallel with the degree and duration of membrane depolarization. For a brief tetanus, partial or complete summations of the Ca^{2+} transients were seen. Unfortunately no accurate in vivo calibration of the Ca^{2+} concentration was possible in these studies. Studies showing small Ca^{2+} transients obtained with membrane depolarizations too small to cause contraction (3), electrophysiological studies of Adrian et al. (1), as well as those discussed previously, and studies with low doses of caffeine (59, 63, 115, 308), K^+ (211, 293), and local anesthetics (91) suggest that there is no threshold for the coupling of an electrical membrane change to the release of Ca^{2+} (i.e., "trigger" calcium), unlike the clear threshold observed for the effect of Ca^{2+} on the contractile system (256). The triggering effect of free Ca^{2+} on calcium release is inhibited by Mg^{2+} (59, 63). Calcium release by isolated sarcoplasmic reticulum has recently been shown to be activated by ADP and P_i (9); however, it is not clear whether these effects are involved in the physiological regulation of Ca^{2+} release.

In cardiac muscle it is reasonable to suppose that Ca^{2+} entering the cell during the plateau phase of the action potential provides an increment of free Ca^{2+} to induce release of possibly a larger amount of Ca^{2+} from internal stores. However, the extent to which specific parts of the sarcoplasmic reticulum or other superficially located membranes contribute to this calcium store is unknown. Likewise the mechanism of Ca^{2+} release remains to be determined.

Calcium Uptake by Sarcoplasmic Reticulum

A considerable amount of information is available concerning the ability of isolated sarcoplasmic reticulum vesicles to accumulate Ca^{2+}, but again many questions concerning the basic mechanism remain (58, 59, 142, 256, 308, 311, 321). Reabsorption of calcium bound to troponin by the longitudinal tubules of the sarcoplasmic reticulum is considered to be the major mechanism of muscle relaxation. Among the many problems at present unresolved is the nature of the factors controlling the onset of calcium accumulation, particularly when this process appears to proceed after the termination of the free intracellular Ca^{2+} transient (4). On the other hand, the coordination of the Ca^{2+}-releasing and Ca^{2+}-absorbing properties of the sarcoplasmic reticulum may be determined by the relative occupancy of calcium binding sites and by anatomic considerations. For the sarcoplasmic reticulum to cause relaxation, it is clear that it must have an affinity for Ca^{2+} at least as great as that for troponin (approximately 10^6 M^{-1}) and an activity sufficient to reduce the amount of Ca^{2+} bound to troponin below the threshold level in the time taken for relaxation of the muscle.

The total calcium accumulation capacity of isolated sarcoplasmic reticulum both from heart (250 μmoles/kg of muscle) and skeletal muscle (600 μmoles/kg of muscle), calculated on the basis of 50 μmoles of Ca^{2+} per kilogram of muscle bound to cardiac troponin (122) and 100 μmoles of Ca^{2+} per kilogram of muscle bound to skeletal muscle troponin (308), is in each case about five times greater than that required to accomplish relaxation (142, 308). The affinity of microsomal membranes derived from sarcoplasmic reticulum for Ca^{2+} varies somewhat with different preparations, but values for high affinity Ca^{2+} binding sites are similar to those for Ca^{2+} binding to troponin. Likewise the rate of Ca^{2+} uptake by isolated sarcoplasmic reticulum from skeletal muscle (58, 114, 308) and possibly also from cardiac muscle (13, 264) appears adequate to effect relaxation in vivo. In a recent study in which an improved rapid mixing stopped flow apparatus and murexide were used to monitor the Ca^{2+} uptake (114), it was shown, contrary to earlier indications (214), that the rate of Ca^{2+} uptake by rabbit muscle sarcoplasmic reticulum fragments in the presence of ATP at room temperature was linear for the first 400–600 msec at a rate of 60–70 nmoles/mg protein per second. On the basis of a sarcoplasmic reticulum content of 4 mg/g muscle, which may be 50% too low (213), and a Q_{10} of 2.5, this corresponds to the removal of 120 μmoles Ca^{2+} per kilogram of muscle, which is equal to the estimated troponin-bound Ca^{2+} during contraction, in 100 msec at 37 C. Present estimates with cardiac sarcoplasmic reticulum (264) provide a value for Ca^{2+} uptake of 100 μmoles/kg of muscle in the 200 msec required for relaxation of mammalian ventricle, although further studies with the improved rapid mixing technique indicate a much lower rate of 5 μmoles/kg of muscle within the relaxation time (257).

Isolated sarcoplasmic reticulum vesicles, incubated under suitable conditions of ionic strength and pH and in the presence of Mg^{2+} and ATP, will accumulate Ca^{2+} down to 10^{-7} M Ca^{2+} in the medium. This Ca^{2+} uptake is associated with an increased rate of hydrolysis of ATP and exchange of phosphate between ATP and ADP. However, many details concerning the physiological mechanism of this process remain to be elucidated. Under appropriate conditions, 2 moles of Ca^{2+} are removed from the medium per mole of ATP hydrolyzed over the range of Ca^{2+} concentrations from 10^{-6} to 10^{-7} M (90, 311). However, from considerations of the energetics of the contraction and relaxation phases of the muscle twitch, there is considerable doubt that this stoichiometry can be obtained in vivo (122, 191). Probably the process of Ca^{2+} removal from the external medium by the sarcoplasmic reticulum in oxalate-free systems involves Ca^{2+} transport across the membrane followed by Ca^{2+} binding to fixed anionic sites. The studies of Carvalho and his associate (27–29) on the cation binding properties of isolated skeletal muscle sarcoplasmic reticulum suggest that about 80% of the maximal Ca-accumulating capacity can be accounted for in terms of Ca^{2+} interactions with fixed binding sites in the membrane for which normally Ca^{2+}, Mg^{2+}, K^+, and H^+ compete. The presence of ATP altered the relative affinities of the cation binding sites greatly in favor of Ca^{2+} and promoted the exchange of bound Ca^{2+} with free Ca^{2+} in the medium when this was greater than 10^{-8} M. This effect may be caused by an ATP-induced conformational change of the membrane structure (138), possibly associated with a high molar ratio of Ca^{2+} accumulation to ATP hydrolysis. The uptake of calcium by sarcoplasmic reticulum is a self-limiting process since the amount of calcium present in the interior of the vesicles has a negative feedback influence on Ca^{2+} uptake and ATP hydrolysis (309, 311).

An ATPase from skeletal muscle sarcoplasmic reticulum has been solubilized (175) and purified (170, 171); this enzyme catalyzes a Ca^{2+}- and Mg^{2+}-dependent hydrolysis of ATP. In the presence of Ca^{2+} and ATP, the enzyme is phosphorylated and the ATP-ADP exchange rate stimulated. The purified ATPase is a membrane-forming enzyme containing a single protein (mol wt 102,000) together with lipid, is estimated to comprise up to 70% of the total protein of the sarcoplasmic reticulum, and possibly represents a structural subunit of the membrane. It has 10 nmoles of high-affinity ($\sim 10^{-7}$ M) Ca^{2+} sites per milligram of protein, which is too small to account for more than a small percentage of the observed Ca^{2+} bound to sarcoplasmic reticulum and indicates that it probably functions as a Ca transport protein. MacLennan & Wong (172) report the isolation of a highly acidic protein that accounts for 7% of the sarcoplasmic reticulum protein and has a relatively low affinity for Ca^{2+} (0.25×10^5 M^{-1}) but is capable of binding about 1 μmole of Ca^{2+} per milligram of protein. They suggest that this protein can account for most of the Ca-binding sites of the sarcoplasmic reticulum and that it is hydrophobically bonded on the interior of the membranes. Possibly it serves to decrease the free Ca^{2+} concentration inside the sarcoplasmic reticulum to 1 mM or less from values that might otherwise be as high as 20 mM if the entire Ca^{2+} content were distributed in solution in the intratubular space (255). Other studies (91, 113, 174) have provided evidence suggesting that the membrane of sarcoplasmic reticulum vesicles is asymmetrical, with calcium transport proteins (possibly the ATPase) situated on the outside surface.

Mitochondria and Calcium Sequestration

In addition to the sarcoplasmic reticulum, mammalian mitochondria from many different tissues are able to remove Ca^{2+} from their incubation medium by an energy-dependent process (26, 151, 153). Hence the possibility arises that they may have a physiologically important role in the relaxation of cardiac muscle and red skeletal muscle, both of which contain a high proportion of mitochondria relative to sarcoplasmic reticulum. Interest in the ability of mitochondria to accumulate calcium arose principally as an outgrowth of studies on oxidative phosphorylation. Calcium uptake and phosphorylation of ADP are competitive processes, which suggests that mitochondria may have a dual role in ATP production and regulation of the Ca^{2+} concentration in the cell. Both effects are abolished by uncoupling agents, and this indicates that the energy is supplied by a common high-energy state generated by electron transport. Respiration-linked calcium uptake by mitochondria is not inhibited by oligomycin and has a Ca^{2+}:ADP ratio of about 2 (32). Calcium transport can also be driven by extramitochondrial ATP in the absence of respiration, but under these conditions it is sensitive to inhibition by oligomycin, which prevents formation of the energized state of the mitochondria. If phosphate or another permeant anion, such as acetate, is present, 400–600 μmoles of Ca^{2+} per gram of mitochondrial protein are removed from the medium, and swelling of the mitochondria occurs as calcium salts accumulate in the matrix. On the other hand, when Ca^{2+} is added in the absence of a permeant anion, about 100 μmoles of Ca^{2+} per gram of mitochondrial protein are taken up and the calcium becomes bound to the inner membrane. Interaction of calcium transport with the respiratory chain is observed by an increase of oxygen uptake and a change of the nicotinamide nucleotides and cytochrome *b* toward more oxidized states (32).

In the absence of energy, Ca^{2+} can also be bound to mitochondria. Two types of binding sites with different affinities for calcium have been recognized. One type is capable of binding up to 50 μmoles of Ca^{2+} per gram mitochondrial protein but has a rather low affinity, the apparent K_m being in the order of 10^{-4} M (241, 258). These sites may represent fairly nonspecific cation binding to phospholipids in the membrane (259), although participation of a glycoprotein has also been suggested (295) because of the sensitivity of Ca^{2+} binding to inhibition by ruthenium red. A second type of binding site has a much higher affinity for Ca^{2+} (apparent K_m 10^{-7} to 10^{-6} M), but the sites are less numerous and can account for the binding of between 0.2 and 1 μmole Ca^{2+} per gram mitochondrial protein with different types of mitochondria (26, 241). These and other studies (26, 33, 152) involving inhibition of respiration-dependent Ca^{2+} uptake and inhibition of high-affinity Ca^{2+} binding by micromolar amounts of La^{3+} have been interpreted in favor of a carrier mechanism for Ca^{2+} uptake by energy-linked translocation. With the murexide technique for measuring the concentration of extramitochondrial Ca^{2+}, Chance et al. (33) estimated that the initial rate of Ca^{2+} uptake by rat liver or pigeon heart mitochondria was 0.3 μmole/mg protein per minute or 60 μmoles/kg wet weight of tissue per 200 msec, with an external Ca^{2+} concentration of about 2×10^{-4} M. The rate of this process is just adequate to remove calcium from the troponin binding sites during relaxation of a cardiac contraction but may be expected to be much lower at physiological Ca^{2+} concentrations. The response of cytochrome *b* to Ca^{2+} addition is extremely rapid, with a half-time of 20–50 msec (185), and the oxidation transition of this internal indicator has been used to calculate the affinity of energy-linked transport for Ca^{2+}. On this basis, an apparent K_m of about 5×10^{-5} M has been obtained (32). It has also been shown that mitochondria can lower the Ca^{2+} concentration in the medium to below 10^{-7} M when aequorin is used as a calcium indicator (5, 33), although at rates considerably slower than with higher external Ca^{2+} concentrations. Using the murexide technique, Scarpa & Williamson (259a) obtained direct measurements of the rate of Ca^{2+} uptake by heart mitochondria from rat, guinea pig, and pigeon, which showed that the initial velocity was related to the Ca^{2+} concentration in a sigmoidal fashion such that the Ca^{2+} concentration required for half-maximal activation of Ca^{2+} uptake was between 50 and 100 μM. At an extramitochondrial Ca^{2+} concentration of 5 μM, initial rate measurements of Ca^{2+} uptake by mitochondria indicated that only 0.9–1.3 μmoles Ca^{2+}/kg wet weight of tissue could be removed at 37 C during the relaxation time, which is about two orders of magnitude lower than the value calculated to be required for relaxation.

In summary, the studies with isolated mitochondria show that their capacity to bind Ca^{2+} is adequate to account for calcium sequestration during the cardiac contraction cycle but that the rate of calcium uptake by mitochondria is insufficient to mediate Ca^{2+} transfer during the time of the relaxation phase at ranges of intracellular concentrations between 10^{-8} and 10^{-6} M. In fact, direct measurements of calcium uptake by mixed mitochondrial and microsomal fractions showed that mitochondria were relatively ineffective in the competition for Ca^{2+} uptake because of the considerably higher affinity of the sarcoplasmic reticulum system for Ca^{2+} transport (177, 307).

Several attempts have been made to determine whether energy-linked movements of Ca^{2+} occur in heart mitochondria in vivo and whether this process is involved in myocardial contractility. Two different approaches have been used: one involves a study of $^{45}Ca^{2+}$ distribution in subcellular fractions of the heart, and the other the use of various inhibitors in perfused heart preparations. Patriarca & Carafoli (220) injected rats intraperitoneally with 25 μc $^{45}CaCl_2$ per kilogram body weight 5 min before killing, and mitochondria and microsomes of heart muscle were isolated by differential centrifugation. A similar study was made by Horn et al. (106) who infused radioactive calcium for 10 sec into the perfusion fluid of isolated rat hearts and then homogenized the tissue. These studies showed that the isolated mitochondria contained most of the calcium in the heart and that the $^{45}Ca^{2+}$ was concentrated in the mitochondria rather than in the microsomes. Furthermore the amount of $^{45}Ca^{2+}$ in the heart mitochondria could be diminished by administration of an uncoupling agent to the rats before $^{45}Ca^{2+}$ injection, which suggested that calcium retention by the mitochondria in vivo was partially energy dependent (220). Epinephrine infusion, along with $^{45}Ca^{2+}$ administration, to isolated rat hearts increased the accumulation of isotope in the mitochondrial fraction (106). In other experiments, Patriarca & Carafoli (221) injected $^{45}Ca^{2+}$ (60 μc) into rabbits and isolated mitochondria and microsomes from rapidly excised samples of white muscle (adductor magnus) and red muscle (masseter). The yield of the separated organelles was low in these experiments since less than 10% of the total radioactivity of the homogenate with both preparations was found in either the mitochondria or the sarcoplasmic reticulum. The specific activity (cpm/mM Ca^{2+}) of the calcium in the mitochondria of red muscle was twice as high as that of white muscle, but whereas the specific activity of calcium in the microsomes of white muscle was almost as great as that of the mitochondria, very low counts were found in the microsomes of red muscle. These studies were interpreted as indicating an active role of the mitochondria in effecting relaxation of skeletal, as well as cardiac, muscle. However, it is very doubtful that the conclusions drawn by the authors are justified. The apparent finding that most of the calcium in the cell is associated with the mitochondrial fraction is at variance with the studies of Legato & Langer (149) who have described the subcellular localization of calcium in dog papillary muscles in electron micrographs by a potassium pyroantimonate staining technique following osmium tetroxide fixation through vascular perfusion. These latter authors found that electron-opaque granules, identified as calcium pyroantimonate deposits by their susceptibility to removal with EDTA or EGTA, were densely concentrated in the lateral sacs of the sarcoplasmic reticulum and over the I bands of the sarcomere, with relatively few in the mitochondria. In another study, Legato et al. (150) found that perfusion of dog papillary muscles with 12–27 mM Ca^{2+} produced mitochondrial swelling and vacuolization, together with electron-dense precipitates in the mitochondria, which suggested that the appearance of calcium deposits in mitochondria in vivo is associated with damage to the mitochondrial membrane and structure. From these and other studies in which autoradiographic techniques with $^{45}Ca^{2+}$ were employed (320), it may be concluded that in the intact muscle much of the cellular calcium is associated with the myofibrils and the sarcoplasmic reticulum rather than with the mitochondria. Since the nonspecific, low affinity anion binding sites of mitochondria can accommodate 3 μmoles of Ca^{2+} per gram wet weight of tissue (more than the tissue calcium content), the most reasonable explanation for the results of Patriarca & Carafoli (220, 221) and Horn et al. (106) would be that, upon disruption of the tissue, calcium is largely released from its binding sites on the myofibrils and sarcoplasmic reticulum and is rapidly taken up by the mitochondria (132). Possibly other distribution patterns for $^{45}Ca^{2+}$ would have been obtained if the pH and cation content of the homogenization medium (usually 0.4 M sucrose) had been altered.

The second approach used to assess the physiological importance of calcium-linked respiration by mitochondria relative to ADP-linked respiration has involved addition of specific inhibitors to perfused organ preparations. In perfused guinea pig livers, atractyloside (an inhibitor of adenine nucleotide exchange across the mitochondria membrane) inhibited mitochondrial respiration by 80%, which indicates a low contribution to the respiration by reactions involving hydrolysis of intramitochondrial ATP or dissipation of the high-energy state, as would be obtained with calcium-linked respiration (161). Perfused hearts are impermeable to atractyloside, but phosphorylation of intramitochondrial ADP in the intact tissue is susceptible to inhibition by oligomycin (30, 31, 107). With the rat heart preparation perfused in the manner of Langendorff, oligomycin impaired contractility, caused an increase in the state of reduction of the nicotinamide nucleotides, diminished ATP levels, and caused a 50% decrease of respiration from initial values of 2.1 matoms oxygen per gram dry weight per hour (30, 31). Oligomycin had no effect on the respiration of nonbeating K^+-arrested hearts, which consumed oxygen at the rate of less than 1 matom/g dry weight per hour. These results show that respiration associated with mechanical activity of the heart was essentially linked to ADP. Horn et al. (107) have reported that, in hearts perfused with 1 mM iodoacetate, pyruvate, and oligomycin, contraction ceased but could be started again by electrical stimulation or by administration of epinephrine, both treatments finally causing contracture. The failure of the heart to relax was interpreted as indicating a high intracellular Ca^{2+} concentration as a result of an oligomycin-induced inhibition of calcium uptake by the mitochondria. This viewpoint is untenable on the basis of the results, which may be explained either by energy deficiency or by deleterious effects of iodoacetate resulting from its nonspecific inhibition of SH groups [e.g., those involved in the troponin-tropomyosin interaction (328)].

Further attempts to define the role of mitochondria in Ca^{2+} sequestration during the cardiac contraction cycle have recently been made with the working rat heart preparation (261, 262). Because external work is greater than in the Langendorff retrograde perfusion system, oxygen consumption by the working heart is considerably higher (205). Furthermore cardiac performance is very sensitive to the Ca^{2+} concentration in the medium over the range from 0.3 to 1.0 mM. In a normal heart perfused with 10 mM glucose, a stepwise increase of external Ca^{2+} from 0.5 to 1.5 mM doubled heart work and increased oxygen uptake from 3.4 to 4.8 matoms/g dry weight per hour. Addition of oligomycin to hearts perfused with glucose and 0.5 mM Ca^{2+} decreased left ventricular pressure by 60% over a 15-min interval and decreased oxygen consumption to 1.3 matoms/g dry weight per hour. Under these conditions, contractility was maintained by glycolytically produced ATP. Increase of Ca^{2+} to 1.5 mM doubled left ventricular pressure, but no increase of oxygen consumption or change of flavin and pyridine nucleotide fluorescence (253) was observed. Hence, although increased intracellular Ca^{2+} was available to the contractile elements and presumably also to the mitochondria, it did not result in an increase of oligomycin-insensitive, Ca^{2+}-stimulated respiration. Clearly the mitochondria in vivo were unable to compete with other systems for calcium sequestration during the contraction cycle. The absence of an obligatory role of mitochondria for cardiac contraction was also shown by the lack of effect of oligomycin on left ventricular pressure in hearts perfused with glucose and 0.5 mM Ca^{2+} under anaerobic conditions, even though pressure development increased twofold upon raising the external Ca^{2+} concentration to 1.5 mM (261). Finally, no contracture was produced upon addition of norepinephrine to anaerobic hearts in the presence of oligomycin, although pressure development was augmented [cf. (107)].

Whether or not calcium uptake by mitochondria contributes to the basal oligomycin-insensitive respiration of the perfused rat heart cannot be deduced from presently available data, but it appears that the extra oxygen consumption associated with increased work of the heart is linked to ADP rather than to Ca^{2+}. It can be concluded therefore that uptake and release of Ca^{2+} by mammalian cardiac mitochondria plays only a minor role in cardiac excitation-contraction coupling. Preliminary data (259a, 261) indicate that a similar conclusion may not apply to amphibian cardiac muscle. An indirect effect of mitochondrial calcium on mammalian cardiac contractility and energy metabolism is not excluded, since the amount of Ca^{2+} bound to mitochondria represents one method of determining the overall calcium balance of the cell and therefore the amount of calcium available at the rapid release sites for excitation-contraction coupling.

Calcium Transport by Cell Membrane

Several different mechanisms probably are involved in effecting movements of Ca^{2+} across the cell membrane. Flux data for $^{45}Ca^{2+}$ show a slow calcium exchange in resting cardiac muscle, which is increased by an increase in the external Ca^{2+} concentration and by the rate of contractions. It is generally accepted that Ca^{2+} influx is greatly increased during the plateau phase of the action potential, with the calcium current contributing to membrane depolarization. Morad & Orkand (193) have suggested that some of this Ca^{2+} influx may be coupled with K^+ efflux via a carrier-mediated transport during membrane depolarization. Under these conditions the electrochemical gradient for K^+ increases; thus K^+ efflux from the cell is favored, whereas Ca^{2+} moves down a concentration gradient of about 10^4. Since cellular calcium does not accumulate under normal conditions in contracting cardiac muscle, a balanced efflux of Ca^{2+} from the cell must occur in the resting phase between action potentials. Reuter and co-workers (82, 239) found that Ca^{2+} efflux from guinea pig auricles depended to a large extent on the ratio of $[Ca^{2+}]$ to $[Na^+]^2$ in the external medium. The significance of this ratio for cardiac contractility of frog heart has previously been demonstrated by Lüttgau & Niedergerke (169). The Na^+-activated fraction of Ca^{2+} efflux was highly specific for Na^+ and had a low activation energy corresponding to a Q_{10} of 1.3. Reuter and associates proposed a carrier transport mechanism based on exchange diffusion in which the carrier had a high affinity for Ca^{2+} and a low affinity for Na^+ on the inner surface of the membrane and a high affinity for Na^+ and Ca^{2+} on the outer surface of the membrane (82, 239). A similar Na^+ and Ca^{2+} ouabain-insensitive exchange across the cell membrane of the giant axon of the squid has been described (7). If the carrier has at least four cation binding sites so that 3 or 4 Na^+ can exchange for one Ca^{2+}, an effective means of decreasing the intracellular Ca^{2+} concentration without a direct involvement of metabolic energy consumption would be provided. However, utilization of energy occurs indirectly since the Na^+ must eventually be pumped out of the cell on the Na^+-K^+ carrier. Calcium efflux from the cell may also occur by a separate energy-dependent mechanism. Schatzman (263) reported the presence of a Mg^{2+}-Ca^{2+}-activated ATPase associated with active Ca^{2+} transport in erythrocyte ghosts, and this finding led to the proposal that a similar mechanism may be operating at the sarcolemma membrane (142, 277, 280). More recently, Ca^{2+}-stimulated ATPase activity has been described in sarcolemma preparations from rat (48) and dog (283) heart, although whether this activity is associated with active Ca^{2+} transport remains to be demonstrated. Possibly the non-energy-linked exchange diffusion mechanism for Ca^{2+} efflux is associated with transport from the sarcoplasmic reticulum to the T tubule system, where the calcium concentration gradient may be much smaller than that across the sarcolemma, whereas transport across the cell membrane is more dependent on an energy-linked process.

CYCLIC AMP AND MUSCLE CONTRACTION

Effects of Cyclic AMP and Hormones on Cardiac Contractility

The following evidence [see (179, 180, 245, 248, 289) for reviews] directly implicates cyclic AMP in the positive inotropic effect of epinephrine on cardiac muscle: *a)* cyclic AMP levels appear to increase in parallel with or prior to the increased force of contraction after the addition of epinephrine to intact heart preparations; *b)* the relative potencies of a series of catecholamines in stimulating cyclic AMP production in vitro are similar to their relative effects as positive inotropic agents in vivo (isoproterenol > epinephrine > norepinephrine); *c)* drugs that stimulate (e.g., imidazole) or inhibit (e.g., theophylline) phosphodiesterases in vitro have parallel effects in potentiating or inhibiting the response of mechanical activity to catecholamines; and *d)* the effects of catecholamines on heart contractility and on cyclic AMP levels are prevented by β receptor blockade. Furthermore in some instances externally added cyclic AMP will mimic the effects of catecholamines (144, 160). However, not all workers have been successful in reproducing the positive inotropic effects of catecholamines by administration of exogenous cyclic AMP (44, 228, 244). More success has been achieved by using the N^6-$2'$-O-dibutyryl derivative of cyclic AMP, possibly because of its greater lipid solubility and increased resistance to degradation by phosphodiesterase. Effects of dibutyryl cyclic AMP have been obtained on isolated ventricular papillary muscle of the cat (273) and on perfused mammalian hearts (134). A positive chronotropic response on isolated cultured heart cells has also been observed (126). Skelton et al. (273) showed that dibutyryl cyclic AMP caused a concentration-dependent increase in isometric tension and rate of tension development in the cat papillary muscle. With maximum concentrations of dibutyryl cyclic AMP (3×10^{-3} M), the effects were similar to those observed with maximum norepinephrine concentrations (10^{-5} M). The inotropic response to dibutyryl cyclic AMP, unlike that to norepinephrine, was insensitive to blockade by propranolol. A notable difference between the effects of these two agents was that, whereas the contractile response to norepinephrine was maximal in 2–4 min, the dibutyryl cyclic AMP effect required 30–40 min. This may reflect either the slow diffusion time of dibutyryl cyclic AMP to reach its site of action or differences in mechanism. However, since the dibutyryl cyclic AMP effect was insensitive to inhibition by β blockade, it is clear that it was not caused by direct stimulation of the β receptor or by a secondary release of endogenous norepinephrine. Although problems arise in the interpretation of other data related to the relative sensitivities of epinephrine in provoking an inotropic response and increasing cyclic AMP levels and the different specificity of the two effects to blockade by agents such as N-isopropylmethoxamine (180, 267), the involvement of cyclic AMP in some phase of the cardiac contraction cycle appears well established.

Further insight into this problem and the relation between the β receptor site and adenyl cyclase has been obtained from studies with a variety of other hormones and drugs that affect myocardial contractility. Glucagon, for instance, also has a positive inotropic effect in cardiac muscle (60, 81, 164, 233) and causes an increased formation of cyclic AMP when added to particulate heart adenyl cyclase preparations (145, 158, 197) or to isolated perfused hearts (183). However, Mayer et al. (183) observed that a detectable increase of cyclic AMP levels in perfused rat hearts occurred at least 5 sec after the onset of increased contractility following addition of 3 μg of glucagon. Although by no means conclusive, this kinetic dissociation suggests that the hormone-induced increased contractility of cardiac muscle may not be mediated solely by increased cyclic AMP levels. The β blocking agent, propranolol, at concentrations that abolished the biochemical effects of epinephrine had no effect on the responses of hearts to glucagon. These data provide evidence that the catalytic moiety of adenyl cyclase is not the β receptor and that heart must contain at least two hormone binding sites responsible for activation of adenyl cyclase. Levey (154) found that combined maximal doses of norepinephrine and glucagon failed to produce an additive effect on cyclic AMP accumulation in cat heart, which suggested that the same adenyl cyclase enzyme of heart is responsive both to catecholamines and glucagon. On the other hand, some data suggest that heart may contain more than one adenyl cyclase. Thus L-thyroxine and L-triiodothyronine (5×10^{-6} M) increased the activity of particulate adenyl cyclase from cat heart (159), but although this effect, like that of glucagon, was not sensitive to inhibition by propranolol, a combination of maximum stimulatory doses of L-thyroxine and L-norepinephrine produced additive effects on adenyl cyclase activity. If this finding can be confirmed, it raises the possibility of a separate adenyl cyclase system responsive to thyroid hormone but not to norepinephrine or glucagon. However, it has not been possible to demonstrate a change in cardiac performance by acute exposure of cardiac muscle to thyroid hormones, and chronic treatment of rats with thyroxine failed to produce an increase of cardiac cyclic AMP levels or an activation of phosphorylase *b* kinase, although phosphorylase *a* levels were raised (73). Therefore whether thyroxine exerts its effects on the myocardium via cyclic AMP remains questionable.

Of considerable interest are recent reports (76, 137) showing that the negative inotropic agent, acetylcholine, caused a rapid increase of cyclic guanosine monophosphate (GMP) levels in perfused rat heart and rat ventricular slices. Furthermore acetylcholine inhibited the normal increase of cyclic AMP produced by catecholamines or glucagon, whereas these latter hormones reciprocally lowered the acetylcholine-induced increase of cyclic GMP levels. A separate guanyl cyclase specific for guanosine triphosphate (GTP) has been identified in most tissues, as have cyclic GMP-dependent protein kinases, which suggests a second messenger role for cyclic GMP analogous to that for cyclic AMP (86). With the exception of brain and lung, mammalian tissues contain up to 100-fold lower concentration of cyclic GMP than cyclic AMP, and separate phosphodiesterases exist for their degradation. However, at present the biological significance of cyclic GMP is unknown, although the data referred to above suggest a possible antagonistic relation with cyclic AMP at some stage of the cardiac contractile process (see ADDENDUM).

Hormone Receptors and Adenyl Cyclase

Evidence referred to above implicates cyclic AMP (and possibly also cyclic GMP) as a factor involved in affecting the overall sequence of events during the cardiac contraction cycle. The nature of the interaction and the effects of cyclic AMP at a more molecular level remain to be discussed. Because of the central role of Ca^{2+} in the cardiac contraction cycle, cyclic AMP is likely to exert an effect on contractility via an influence on the calcium cycle. Although the precise mechanism whereby the catecholamines and glucagon can augment the rate and force of contraction of cardiac muscle remains unknown, a consideration of the sequence of events initiated by the binding of the hormone to the receptor site, together with such fragmentary data as are available, permits certain conclusions on which a theory of the inotropic action of hormones that act via cyclic AMP can be based. However, it must be stressed that such considerations remain largely speculative in the absence of definitive experimental data.

The interaction of catecholamines with receptor sites is discussed in detail elsewhere in this volume of the *Handbook* (see the chapter by Moran); hence only salient features are mentioned here. Various models have been proposed for the so-called β adrenergic receptor (60, 245, 248), but it is generally agreed that binding of the hormone to specific groups on the membrane surface must lead to some kind of conformational perturbation and alteration of the catalytic activity of adenyl cyclase. Thus adenyl cyclase in the cell membrane may consist of two types of subunits: *1*) a regulatory subunit on the external surface; and *2*) a catalytic subunit with its active site facing the interior of the cell and accessible to intracellular ATP. The connection between the hormone receptor site and adenyl cyclase is probably complex, involving both proteins and phospholipid (60, 306). Lefkowitz & Haber (148) isolated a $78,000 \times g$ microsomal fraction from dog heart; it bound [^{3}H]norepinephrine tightly but lost the isotope upon addition of unlabeled catecholamines in the order of potency of their physiological effectiveness on contractility. Addition of the β blocking agent, propranolol (10^{-6} M), displaced bound [^{3}H]norepinephrine, but the α adrenergic blocking agent, phentolamine, was ineffective. The authors interpreted their results as indicating that the microsomal particles contained the β adrenergic receptor. The particles also contained adenyl cyclase activity (148a).

Adenyl cyclase from cardiac tissue has recently been solubilized with the nonionic detergent, Lubrol-PX (155). However, unlike the particulate adenyl cyclase, the soluble enzyme was unresponsive to hormone activation. In further experiments, Levey (156, 157) found that addition of phosphatidylserine to soluble, detergent-free adenyl cyclase restored responsiveness to glucagon and histamine, but not to norepinephrine, whereas addition of phosphatidylinositol restored the responsiveness to norepinephrine. This activation was abolished by propranolol. These results provide further evidence in favor of the postulate that norepinephrine activates cardiac adenyl cyclase by a receptor mechanism separate and distinct from the glucagon receptor and support the arguments that membrane lipids have an important role in maintaining the functional integrity of the hormone-receptor complex (223).

Various cations affect the activity of adenyl cyclase, but whether these effects are related to the inotropic action of catecholamines is not clear. Thus, although elevation of K^+ concentration from 5.6 to 56 mM in perfused rat hearts blocked the increase of cyclic AMP normally elicited by epinephrine (199), K^+ was found to have a stimulatory effect on a particulate preparation of adenyl cyclase from rat heart, which suggested that the effect in vivo was indirect and possibly associated with depolarization of the myocardial membrane (179). Isolated particulate adenyl cyclase from cardiac muscle has a K_m for ATP of about 0.08 mM, is activated by Mg^{2+} with a K_a of 2–3 mM, and is inhibited by Ca^{2+} with a K_i of about 0.3 mM (52). From further studies, Drummond et al. (55) concluded that epinephrine, like fluoride ions, stimulated the cardiac enzyme (increase of V_{max}) at all Mg^{2+} (or Mn^{2+}) concentrations and had little effect on the apparent K_a for Mg^{2+} or the K_m for the Mg-ATP substrate. Concentrations of ATP in excess of the Mg^{2+} concentration were inhibitory, presumably because of competition with Mg-ATP at the catalytic site or removal of free Mg^{2+}. These effects could have physiological significance if the availability of Mg^{2+} to adenyl cyclase changed relative to that of ATP. Likewise the role of membrane-bound Ca^{2+} in the modulation of adenyl cylcase activity requires further elucidation.

Effects of Epinephrine on Electromechanical Properties of Cardiac Muscle

A number of studies have shown that epinephrine (10^{-6} M) increases the amplitude and duration of the plateau phase of the action potential in cardiac muscle and increases the inward Ca^{2+} current during the plateau (2, 25, 120, 236, 296). This effect was independent of the initial fast depolarization due to increased Na$^+$ conductance and was relatively independent of external Na$^+$ concentration, but was critically dependent on the external Ca^{2+} concentration (25, 296). Partial depolarization of the membrane by increasing extracellular K$^+$ from 2.7 to 16.2 mM decreased the amplitude of the spike potential and also caused a fall in height and duration of the plateau phase. The presence of epinephrine abolished the latter but not the former effect of increasing external K$^+$, which indicated a fall of K$^+$ conductance (25). The influx of Ca^{2+} was clearly increased by epinephrine, as shown by the sensitivity of its effects on the plateau phase of the action potential to alterations of the external Ca^{2+} concentration and to inhibition by 0.5 mM Mn^{2+}. However, the increased amplitude of depolarization in the plateau phase of the action potential also appeared to be associated with an increased Na$^+$ current. The effects of catecholamines were blocked with propranolol (2×10^{-5} M), a β blocking agent, but not by phentolamine (1.7×10^{-5} M), an α blocking agent. Caffeine produced effects similar to epinephrine, but it is very doubtful that the positive inotropic effects of both types of compounds can be ascribed to a common effect via cyclic AMP. Thus inhibition of phosphodiesterases by caffeine or other xanthine derivatives with resultant increases of cyclic AMP levels requires such large concentrations of the drug that a depressant effect is produced on contractility (184). A stimulation of the exchange of Ca^{2+} across the plasma membrane induced by catecholamines is in accordance with earlier studies showing an increased uptake of ^{45}Ca^{2+} by contracting guinea pig atria after addition of norepinephrine (85, 240). The above studies clearly suggest that the increased force of contraction and rate of tension development induced by epinephrine is caused by an increased rate of availability of free Ca^{2+} to the myofibrils.

In accordance with the above postulate, Morad and co-workers (124, 194) in studies with mammalian papillary and trabecular muscles found that effects of epinephrine on the maximal tension and time to peak tension could be mimicked by increasing the external Ca^{2+} concentration and lowering the Na$^+$ concentration. However, a second effect induced by epinephrine, namely an early relaxation (276), which occurred before termination of the action potential, could not be duplicated by elevated Ca^{2+}. In fact, the rapid relaxing effect was antagonized by increasing the external Ca^{2+} concentration. An augmentation of contraction and relaxation induced by epinephrine was observed, despite rapid repolarization of the membrane at the onset of the plateau of the action potential by the voltage clamp procedure. Thus a major effect of epinephrine was to make the contraction cycle less dependent on the action potential, which indicated the involvement of mechanisms not directly controlled by the state of the membrane potential. The possibility that the effects of epinephrine on contraction and relaxation may be produced by separate effects on different systems was reinforced by further studies in which the relaxation effect of epinephrine was studied in KCl-induced contractures (83, 192, 194). The relaxation enhancement effect of catecholamines was independent of the membrane polarization but was strongly affected by temperature and rate of contraction and was most prevalent under conditions when the Ca^{2+}-sequestering system was overloaded or poorly developed, as in frog or neonatal cardiac tissue. Graham & Lamb (83) suggested that the relaxing effect of epinephrine on cardiac contracture was caused by a decreased permeability of the sarcolemma to Ca^{2+} in addition to an increased Na$^+$ permeability. However, this explanation would entail a rapid reversal of the Ca^{2+} current (P$_{CA}$) during the action potential since the increased rate of contraction induced by epinephrine correlates with an early increase of P$_{CA}$. An alternative possibility is that epinephrine increases the rate of Ca^{2+} sequestration by the sarcolemma and sarcotubule systems (194). This explanation is more in accordance with the observation that contractures develop more readily and are better maintained in frog cardiac muscle with its poorly developed sarcoplasmic reticulum than in mammalian myocardium.

There are very few reports concerning a direct action of cyclic AMP or its derivatives on the electrophysiological responses of cardiac muscle. Of interest is the report by Morad & Rolett (194) that, although 1 mM dibutyryl cyclic AMP potentiated the twitch tension in frog ventricle strips, it failed to enhance the rate of relaxation during either a single twitch or a KCl-induced contracture and therefore did not duplicate the effects of epinephrine. The effect of dibutyryl cyclic AMP in increasing the rate of tension development is similar to that observed by Skelton et al. (273) with cat papillary muscle. These studies raise the possibility that, whereas the increased rate and force of contraction induced by catecholamines appears to be mediated by cyclic AMP, potentiation of relaxation may not be a direct cyclic AMP effect. However, this conclusion is not in accordance with other data discussed below; hence the apparent discrepancy may involve the relative sensitivity of different systems to intracellular cyclic AMP.

Hormonal and Cyclic AMP Effects on Isolated Sarcoplasmic Reticulum

Although cardiac adenyl cyclase was initially found to be distributed mainly in a low-speed fraction containing nuclei and cell membranes (286), recent studies with a more sensitive assay have shown that the sarcoplasmic reticulum microsome fraction in the 100,000-g pellet also contains adenyl cyclase of the same specific activity as that of the low-speed pellet (64). Sarcoplasmic reticulum fractions from rabbit skeletal muscle have also been shown to contain adenyl cyclase (227). Shinebourne et al. (270) found that 10^{-3} M, but not 10^{-5} M, norepinephrine produced a small increase of calcium uptake by isolated cardiac sarcoplasmic reticulum. In a further study, Shinebourne & White (271) showed that calcium uptake could also be increased three- to fivefold by 10^{-3} M cyclic AMP. These results are unconvincing because of the high concentrations of norepinephrine and cyclic AMP needed to elicit effects. Better evidence for a physiological role of hormonal and cyclic AMP effects on calcium uptake by cardiac sarcoplasmic reticulum has been obtained by Entman et al. (65). A concentration-dependent stimulation of calcium uptake was produced by all three agents, with maximal effects being obtained at 10^{-6} M epinephrine, 3×10^{-8} M glucagon, and 5×10^{-6} M cyclic AMP. Considerably higher concentrations of the hormones were needed for maximal stimulation of adenyl cyclase. The effects produced by each agent on Ca^{2+} uptake were not additive, and the response to epinephrine, but not to glucagon or cyclic AMP, was inhibited by 10^{-5} M propranolol. The Ca^{2+}-stimulated ATPase activity of the vesicles, however, was not affected by the hormones or cyclic AMP, which showed the absence of a simple relation between Ca^{2+} transport and ATPase activity, as demonstrated by Martonosi et al. (176) in phospholipid-depleted sarcoplasmic reticulum. In contrast to the above results, other workers have failed to find an increased rate of Ca^{2+} uptake by cardiac sarcoplasmic reticulum in the presence of catecholamines (37, 46) or glucagon (203). In view of these discrepancies, which may be accounted for by contamination of the sarcoplasmic reticulum fraction with fragments of the sarcolemma, it remains uncertain whether a cyclic AMP-mediated stimulation of Ca^{2+} sequestration by the sarcoplasmic reticulum can account for the relaxation enhancement effect of catecholamines in intact cardiac muscle preparations (however, see ADDENDUM).

Of interest is a recent report (49) describing a stimulatory effect of 3×10^{-5} M cyclic AMP on the ATPase activity of the sarcoplasmic reticulum fraction of cardiac muscle and an inhibitory effect on the Ca^{2+}-activated ATPase of the sarcolemma fraction. This latter effect was dependent on the concentration of cyclic AMP over the range from 3×10^{-8} to 3×10^{-5} M and might relate to the control of the active transport of Ca^{2+} across the sarcoplasmic membrane.

Effect of Epinephrine on Contractile Proteins

Theoretically agents that alter myocardial contractility could do so by interfering with the interaction between the contractile proteins, particularly with the affinity of troponin for Ca^{2+}. A review of the literature showed that the data in this regard are inconclusive (122). Hypercapnia and metabolic acidosis result in depressed myocardial contractility, which apparently is not the result of an alteration of the cardiac action potential. The increased H^+ concentration may decrease the affinity of troponin for Ca^{2+} since a reduction of pH from 7 to 6 increased the Ca^{2+} concentration required for half-maximal activation of ATPase activity in glycerol-extracted fibers from cardiac muscle (260). A similar effect of H^+ on the Ca^{2+} affinity of troponin may also account in part for the rapid decrease of contractile force observed in ischemic hearts. Acidosis also depresses catecholamine release and the positive inotropic action of epinephrine (12, 43, 313). However, there is no clear evidence that catecholamines have a direct action on the contractile proteins, as measured by its effects on glycerol-extracted skeletal or cardiac muscle fibers (125, 282, 294), cardiac myofibrils (105, 279), cardiac myosin (121, 165, 166), or actomyosin preparations (105, 121, 243).

The lack of a consistent direct catecholamine effect in the above preparations may merely reflect the absence of functional adenyl cyclase. Thus cyclic AMP (10^{-4} to 10^{-3} M) was found to increase the rate of tension development by glycerol-extracted cardiac muscle (282). Of particular significance is a recent report (6) showing that the troponin subunit that confers inhibition on the ATPase activity of actomyosin can be phosphorylated by Mg-ATP in a reaction catalyzed by a cyclic AMP-dependent muscle protein kinase. Since the K_m for cyclic AMP was of the order of 10^{-8} M, this system has as great a sensitivity to cyclic AMP as phosphorylation of phosphorylase b kinase. In further studies, Stull and co-workers (281a) reported that phosphorylase kinase catalyzed the phosphorylation of the TN-I subunit of troponin in the presence of ATP and Mg^{2+}. The rate of phosphorylation was the same with nonactivated as with activated (phosphorylated) phosphorylase kinase, which suggests the absence of a direct interaction by cyclic AMP. Nevertheless since the activity of phosphorylase kinase is dependent on the Ca^{2+} concentration (23), it is possible that the positive inotropic action of catecholamines is due to Ca^{2+} stimulation of TN-I phosphorylation, secondary to an increased catecholamine-induced entry of Ca^{2+} across the sarcolemma. However, further studies are required to elucidate the role of phosphotroponin in the sequence of events resulting in activation of the actomyosin ATPase.

SUMMARY AND CONCLUSIONS

It is apparent from the previous discussion of the role of calcium in cardiac contraction and relaxation that this involves a complex sequence of coordinated events associated with the binding and release of Ca^{2+} from various membranes and vesicles. Because of the intimate relation between changes of Ca^{2+} concentration and the interaction between the actin and myosin filaments in the contractile process, it appears probable that the effects exerted by catecholamines on the myocardium will be mediated through local changes of Ca^{2+} concentration or changes in the affinity of receptor sites for Ca^{2+}. Moreover since catecholamines appear to exert separate effects on the contraction and relaxation phases, interaction at more than one location is to be expected.

Evidence obtained from *a*) comparisons between raising the external Ca^{2+} concentration and catecholamine effects, *b*) studies illustrating the increased exchangeability of $^{45}Ca^{2+}$ in the presence of epinephrine, and *c*) studies of effects of catecholamines in increasing the duration and magnitude of the plateau phase of the action potential, all suggest that the augmentation of the rate and extent of tension development induced by catecholamines is secondary to an increased availability of Ca^{2+} to the troponin binding sites of the actomyosin complex. This is probably achieved by an increased rate of delivery of activator Ca^{2+} to internal Ca^{2+} storage sites followed by a more complete filling of these sites and an augmentation of the speed and amount of Ca^{2+} released by the trigger of membrane depolarization. The interval for release of activator calcium appears to be primarily in the early phase of the action potential plateau, since membrane repolarization by the voltage clamp technique before termination of the normal action potential does not diminish the augmented rate of tension development induced by epinephrine (124, 194). Postulation of the above sequence of events implies *a*) an epinephrine-induced increase in the number of Ca^{2+} binding sites or increased permeability of superficial membranes to Ca^{2+}, or *b*) a decreased Ca^{2+} affinity at the rapid release sites. The similarity in response of frog and mammalian hearts to epinephrine suggests that rapid release sites on those sections of the sarcoplasmic reticulum adjacent to T tubules are not directly affected by epinephrine.

The following models are described to suggest how intracellular Ca^{2+} availability could be increased by catecholamines. The first is in accordance with the postulate of more than one second messenger with interdependent regulatory features, whereas the second illustrates the third messenger concept (229, 230). Each involves binding of catecholamine to a specific receptor on the cell surface followed by a conformational change of the phospholipid-protein structure of the membrane. However, in the first model it is proposed that the conformational change causes a displacement of bound Ca^{2+} (with possible replacement by Mg^{2+}) from the catalytic subunit of membrane-bound adenyl cyclase to effect an augmentation of Ca^{2+} release from internal rapid release sites upon membrane depolarization. Activation of adenyl cyclase could occur upon removal of enzyme-bound Ca^{2+}, so that cyclic AMP formation would occur in parallel with release of Ca^{2+} as the alternative second messenger. In contrast, as a second model, activation of adenyl cyclase could occur directly as a result of the conformation change, followed by formation of cyclic AMP and activation of a protein kinase effective in phosphorylating a membrane-bound protein. This process would have the effect of increasing the number of Ca^{2+} binding sites in the membranes available to extracellular Ca^{2+}, so that, with an increased filling of these sites with Ca^{2+}, an increment in the amount of trigger Ca^{2+} released by membrane depolarization would be achieved (325). This model differs from the first in that cyclic AMP is the direct causative agent in the sequence of events resulting in an increased speed and force of contraction, and therefore these effects should be mimicked by externally applied cyclic AMP or derivatives, as appears to be the case (194, 273).

A third model should also be mentioned because of its interesting implications, namely, modification of the ATPase inhibitory subunit of troponin by phosphorylation induced by a cyclic AMP-dependent protein kinase (6) or by Ca^{2+}-activated phosphorylase kinase (281a). Until further details are available, speculation is unwarranted, but clearly the change could make the subunit more sensitive to de-inhibition by the Ca^{2+}-binding troponin subunit TN-C. If so, an increased Ca^{2+} availability for troponin binding need not be postulated, in contrast to the above hypotheses.

Data reviewed in previous sections have shown that, besides an augmentation of the speed and force of cardiac muscle contraction, epinephrine has a separate relaxation enhancement effect. This latter response implies a stimulation of the rate of removal of Ca^{2+} from troponin. A cyclic AMP-induced increase in the rate of energy-linked Ca^{2+} accumulation by sarcoplasmic reticulum (65) provides a satisfactory theoretical basis for the observed enhancement of the rate of relaxation of cardiac muscle by catecholamines. Like other cyclic AMP-mediated effects, the mechanism for the postulated increased rate of Ca^{2+} removal by the sarcoplasmic reticulum could be via activation of a protein kinase and phosphorylation of sites on the membrane, which causes an increase in either the number or affinity of Ca^{2+} binding sites (see ADDENDUM).

Yet another effect of cyclic AMP in cardiac muscle that relates to Ca^{2+} availability is a partial inhibition of the sarcolemma Ca^{2+}-activated ATPase activity (49). Again this effect could be mediated via activation of a protein kinase, although involvement of this step has not yet been demonstrated. Inhibition of active Ca^{2+} efflux from the cell would tend to raise intracellular Ca^{2+}, as does inhibition of the Na^+-K^+ ATPase by digitalis. This effect could be transmitted as a positive inotropic stimulus if it resulted in a more complete filling of the rapid release sites with Ca^{2+}.

The models outlined above are presented merely as a stimulus to further thought and experimentation. Not all effects of cyclic AMP observed with in vitro systems are likely to have physiological significance, either because of their sensitivity or restricted accessibility of target enzymes to intracellular cyclic AMP. It should be stressed that, at present, no definite conclusions concerning the molecular mechanisms of the positive inotropic and relaxation-enhancement effects of epinephrine can be reached. Stimulation of adenyl cyclase and an increased rate of formation of intracellular cyclic AMP appear to be prerequisites for the effects. As a prognosis for future developments, one may speculate that the expression of cyclic AMP effects on cardiac contractility will be mediated by activation of protein kinases, as in the pathways of glycogenolysis and glycogen synthesis. Phosphorylation of specific membranes can be predicted to cause an alteration of the affinity or number of Ca^{2+} binding sites and therefore a modification of the basic calcium cycle, which controls muscular contraction and relaxation.

ADDENDUM

A number of important developments have occurred in the various fields covered in this review since the original writing, and although a complete updating of the literature published over the past 2 years is not feasible, a brief outline of some recent interesting papers is presented below. The general topic of excitation-contraction coupling in heart has been extensively covered from different points of view in several excellent reviews (2A, 17A, 21A, 25A, 37A). The role of Ca^{2+} as the major carrier of charge for the slow inward current is firmly established. The slow current is suppressed, whereas the initial rapid inward current is unaltered, by Mn^{2+}, La^{3+} (28A, 29A), and drugs such as verapamil and D 600 (16A, 33A). Recent studies with calf Purkinje fibers exposed to norepinephrine, N^6-monobutyryl cyclic AMP (35A), or after iontophoretic injection of cyclic AMP (34A) show directly that cyclic AMP closely mimics the electrical effects of catecholamines on the heart. In these studies catecholamines and cyclic AMP increased the initial plateau level of the action potential, indicating an increase in the magnitude of the slow inward current, but also shortened the duration of the plateau. This latter effect is attributable to activation of an outward K^+ current that is responsible for terminating the plateau. Both effects appear to be mediated by cyclic AMP, and whereas increased Ca^{2+} influx can account for the positive inotropic effect of catecholamine, the early repolarization may account for the chronotropic action.

An excellent review dealing principally with the mechanisms of Ca^{2+} release and uptake by sarcoplasmic reticulum, activation by Ca^{2+} of the contractile apparatus, and the molecular basis of cross-bridge activity in striated muscle with reference also to cardiac muscle has appeared recently (11A). The Cold Spring Harbor Symposium on the mechanism of muscular contraction (5A), held in 1972, provides an authoritative source of information on the biochemistry and biophysics of the contractile mechanism. Several specialized reviews on the mechanism of Ca^{2+} uptake by sarcoplasmic reticulum have been published (12A, 18A). Recent reviews on the energetics and control of muscle contraction (1A, 20A, 36A, 39A), cardiac metabolism (23A, 24A, 38A), and adrenergic mechanisms in myocardium (26A) are available. Further evidence has been forthcoming in favor of the concept of regenerative Ca^{2+} release promoted by a source of "trigger" Ca^{2+} (7A–10A), whereas in other reports release of Ca^{2+} from the sarcoplasmic reticulum has been demonstrated upon membrane depolarization (6A, 13A).

Noteworthy findings have recently been reported that are pertinent to possible mechanisms whereby cyclic AMP may modulate the rate of tension development and speed of relaxation in cardiac muscle. These findings in general provide experimental support to speculations raised in this review that changes of cyclic AMP levels regulate myocardial contractility through cyclic AMP-dependent protein kinase phosphorylation reactions, which in turn affect Ca^{2+} release and uptake by the intracellular organelles (22A). Brooker (4A) measured cyclic AMP levels in frog ventricle strips at different times during the contraction-relaxation cycle, and found that peak levels representing a 50% increase occurred in the early phase of the increased tension development during systole. A small increase of cyclic AMP content was observed at the peak of systole relative to diastole, and this difference was augmented along with the absolute levels after epinephrine administration. Further studies by Wollenberger et al. (40A), also with frog hearts, confirmed that cyclic AMP levels increased to a maximum during the early phase of the contraction cycle and showed in addition a reciprocal fall of cyclic GMP levels. The mechanisms responsible for an apparent activation of adenyl cyclase and inhibition of guanyl cyclase are not clear at present but would seem to be related to membrane depolarization during the early phase of the action potential, possibly via displacement of sarcolemma-bound Ca^{2+} from inhibitory sites on adenyl cyclase or alternatively resulting from a conformational change of the plasma membrane. No further evidence is available to resolve the question whether or not phosphorylation of membrane-bound proteins promotes increased Ca^{2+} influx during the early plateau phase of the action potential, but it is of interest that phosphorylation of a sarcolemma preparation from rabbit skeletal muscle by a cyclic AMP-dependent protein kinase has been reported (30A). The phosphorylated membranes accumulated Ca^{2+} at a greater rate than control membranes and had a higher Ca^{2+}-stimulated ATPase activity. If these findings do not represent contamination of the sarcolemma preparation with sarcoplasmic reticulum fragments, the data suggest that phosphorylation of specific sites on the sarcolemma may be functionally linked to an active Ca^{2+} transport system, although such a process is expected to be less significant in skeletal than in cardiac muscle.

Further evidence has been obtained that substantiates the previously postulated role of cyclic AMP in promoting Ca^{2+} sequestration by cardiac sarcoplasmic reticulum, thereby increasing the speed of relaxation. Isolated cardiac sarcoplasmic reticulum has been shown to contain adenyl cyclase and cyclic AMP-dependent protein kinase activity that catalyzed phosphorylation of a protein substrate in the membrane upon addition of cyclic AMP (22A, 41A). Half-maximal stimulation of phosphorylation was achieved with 8.5×10^{-8} M cyclic AMP (41A). Other extensive studies with purified preparations of cardiac sarcoplasmic reticulum (14A, 15A, 32A) showed a large specific phosphorylation of serine and threonine residues in membrane protein upon incubation of the vesicles with cyclic AMP-dependent protein kinase and cyclic AMP. Epinephrine stimulated the adenyl cyclase present in the preparation and also enhanced phosphorylation. The initial rates of Ca^{2+} uptake and Ca^{2+}-activated ATPase at micromolar Ca^{2+} concentrations were stimulated two- to threefold by addition of protein kinase, cyclic AMP, Mg^{2+}, and ATP. Solubilization of the phosphorylated vesicles in sodium dodecyl sulfate and fractionation by polyacrylamide gel electrophoresis allowed isolation of a single protein (mol wt approx. 22,000) that contained most of the ^{32}P label bound as a phosphoester (31A).

In an important paper, Scarpa & Graziotti (27A) measured the initial velocity of energy-dependent Ca^{2+} uptake by mitochondria isolated from the hearts of rats, guinea pigs, squirrels, pigeons, and frogs and concluded from the high apparent Michaelis-Menten (K_m) values of Ca^{2+} transport (30–90 μM) and low initial rates (below 10 μM Ca^{2+}) that Ca^{2+} sequestration by mitochondria is inadequate for regulation of the beat-to-beat Ca^{2+} cycle. However, a role for mitochondria in the overall Ca^{2+} homeostasis of the cell is not excluded by these results, and it is of interest that release of Ca^{2+} from Ca^{2+}-loaded isolated mitochondria has recently been demonstrated by the direct addition of low concentrations of cyclic AMP (3A, 19A). Nonetheless further data are required before the physiological significance of this observation can be evaluated. Clearly many new exciting developments can be anticipated in the next few years that will provide further confirmation and elucidation of the molecular mechanisms by which cyclic AMP and Ca^{2+} interact to modulate the complex series of events involved in the cardiac contraction-relaxation cycle. [See REFERENCES IN ADDENDUM, p. 635.]

REFERENCES

1. ADRIAN, R. H., W. K. CHANDLER, AND A. L. HODGKIN. The kinetics of mechanical activation in frog muscle. *J. Physiol., London* 204: 207–230, 1969.

2. ANTONI, H., AND W. DELIUS. Nachweis von zwei Komponenten in der Anstiegsphase des Aktionspotentials von Froschmyokardfasern. *Arch. Ges. Physiol.* 283: 187–202, 1965.

3. ASHLEY, C. C., AND E. B. RIDGWAY. Simultaneous recording of membrane potential, calcium transient and tension in single muscle fibres. *Nature* 219: 1168–1169, 1968.
4. ASHLEY, C. C., AND E. B. RIDGWAY. Aequorin—calcium luminescence and its application to muscle physiology. In: *A Symposium on Calcium and Cellular Function*, edited by A. W. Cuthbert. New York: St. Martin's, 1970, p. 42–53.
5. AZZI, A., AND B. CHANCE. The "energized state" of mitochondria: lifetime and ATP equivalence. *Biochim. Biophys. Acta* 189: 141–151, 1969.
6. BAILEY, C., AND C. VILLAR-PALASI. Cyclic AMP dependent phosphorylation of troponin (Abstract). *Federation Proc.* 30: 1147, 1971.
7. BAKER, P. F., M. P. BLAUSTEIN, A. L. HODGKIN, AND R. A. STEINHARDT. The influence of calcium on sodium efflux in squid axons. *J. Physiol., London* 200: 431–458, 1969.
8. BÄR, U., AND M. C. BLANCHAER. Glycogen and CO_2 production from glucose and lactate by red and white skeletal muscle. *Am. J. Physiol.* 209: 905–909, 1965.
9. BARLOGIE, B., W. HASSELBACH, AND M. MAKINOSE. Activation of calcium efflux by ADP and inorganic phosphate. *FEBS Letters* 12: 267–268, 1971.
10. BEELER, G. W., JR., AND H. REUTER. Voltage clamp experiments on ventricular myocardial fibres. *J. Physiol., London* 207: 165–190, 1970.
11. BEELER, G. W., JR., AND H. REUTER. The relation between membrane potential, membrane currents and activation of contraction in ventricular myocardial fibres. *J. Physiol., London* 207: 211–229, 1970.
12. BENDIXON, H. H., M. B. LAVER, AND W. E. FLACKE. Influence of respiratory acidosis on circulatory effect of epinephrine in dogs. *Circulation Res.* 13: 64–70, 1963.
13. BESCH, H. R., JR., AND A. SCHWARTZ. Initial calcium binding rates of canine cardiac relaxing system (sarcoplasmic reticulum fragments) determined by stopped-flow spectrophotometry. *Biochem. Biophys. Res. Commun.* 45: 286–292, 1971.
14. BIANCHI, P. *Cell Calcium*. London: Butterworths, 1968.
15. BIANCHI, C. P., AND T. C. BOLTON. Action of local anesthetics on coupling systems in muscle. *J. Pharmacol. Exptl. Therap.* 157: 388–405, 1967.
16. BING, R. J. Cardiac metabolism. *Physiol. Rev.* 45: 171–213, 1965.
17. BLUKOO-ALLOTEY, J. A., N. H. VINCENT, AND S. ELLIS. Interactions of acetylcholine and epinephrine on contractility, glycogen and phosphorylase activity of isolated mammalian hearts. *J. Pharmacol. Exptl. Therap.* 170: 27–36, 1969.
18. BOWMAN, W. C., AND M. W. NOTT. Actions of sympathomimetic amines and their antagonists on skeletal muscle. *Pharmacol. Rev.* 21: 27–72, 1969.
19. BOWNESS, J. M. Epinephrine: cascade reactions and glycogenolytic effect. *Science* 152: 1370–1371, 1966.
20. BRADY, A. J. Excitation and excitation-contraction coupling in cardiac muscle. *Ann. Rev. Physiol.* 26: 341–356, 1964.
21. BRECKENRIDGE, B. McL. Cyclic AMP and drug action. *Ann. Rev. Pharmacol.* 10: 19–34, 1970.
22. BROSTROM, C. O., J. D. CORBIN, C. A. KING, AND E. G. KREBS. Interaction of the subunits of adenosine 3′,5′-cyclic monophosphate dependent protein kinase of muscle. *Proc. Natl. Acad. Sci. US* 68: 2444–2447, 1971.
23. BROSTROM, C. O., F. L. HUNKELER, AND E. G. KREBS. The regulation of skeletal muscle phosphorylase kinase by Ca^{++}. *J. Biol. Chem.* 246: 1961–1967, 1971.
24. BROSTROM, M. A., E. M. REIMANN, D. A. WALSH, AND E. G. KREBS. A cyclic 3′,5′-AMP-stimulated protein kinase from cardiac muscle. *Advan. Enzyme Regulation* 8: 191–203, 1970.
25. CARMELIET, E., AND J. VEREECKE. Adrenaline and the plateau phase of the cardiac action potential. Importance of Ca^{++}, Na^+ and K^+ conductance. *Arch. European J. Physiol.* 313: 300–315, 1969.
26. CARAFOLI, E., P. GAZZOTTI, C. S. ROSSI, AND R. TIOZZO. Ca^{++} and mitochondrial membranes: evidence for specific enzymic carriers. In: *Membrane Bound Enzymes*, edited by G. Porcellati and F. Di Jeso. New York: Plenum Press, 1971, p. 63–85.
27. CARVALHO, A. P. Effects of potentiators of muscular contraction on binding of cations by sarcoplasmic reticulum. *J. Gen. Physiol.* 51: 427–442, 1968.
28. CARVALHO, A. P. Calcium-binding properties of sarcoplasmic reticulum as influenced by ATP, caffeine, quinine and local anesthetics. *J. Gen. Physiol.* 52: 622–642, 1968.
29. CARVALHO, A. P., AND B. LEO. Effects of ATP on the interaction of Ca^{++}, Mg^{++}, and K^+ with fragmented sarcoplasmic reticulum isolated from rabbit skeletal muscle. *J. Gen. Physiol.* 50: 1327–1352, 1967.
30. CHALLONER, D. R. Evidence for uncoupled respiration in thyrotoxic and epinephrine-stimulated myocardium. *Am. J. Physiol.* 214: 365–369, 1968.
31. CHALLONER, D. R., AND D. STEINBERG. Oxidative metabolism of myocardium as influenced by fatty acids and epinephrine. *Am. J. Physiol.* 211: 897–902, 1966.
32. CHANCE, B. The energy-linked reactions of calcium with mitochondria. *J. Biol. Chem.* 240: 2729–2748, 1965.
33. CHANCE, B., A. AZZI, AND L. MELA. Molecular interactions of calcium transport in mitochondrial membranes. In: *The Molecular Basis of Membrane Function*, edited by D. C. Testeson. Englewood Cliffs, N.J.: Prentice-Hall, 1969, p. 561–573.
34. CHANCE, B., J. R. WILLIAMSON, D. JAMIESON, AND B. SCHOENER. Properties and kinetics of reduced pyridine nucleotide fluorescence of the isolated and *in vivo* rat heart. *Biochem. Z.* 341: 357–377, 1965.
35. CHANDLER, B. M., E. H. SONNENBLICK, AND P. E. POOL. Mechanochemistry of cardiac muscle. III. Effects of norepinephrine on the utilization of high-energy phosphates. *Circulation Res.* 22: 729–735, 1968.
36. CHEUNG, W. Y., AND J. R. WILLIAMSON. Kinetics of cyclic adenosine monophosphate changes in rat heart following epinephrine administration. *Nature* 207: 979–981, 1965.
37. CHIMOSKY, J. E., AND J. GERGELY. Effect of norepinephrine, ouabain, and pH on cardiac sarcoplasmic reticulum. *Arch. Intern. Pharmacodyn.* 176: 289–297, 1968.
37a. CONSTANTIN, L. L., AND R. J. PODOLSKY. Depolarization of the internal membrane system in the activation of frog skeletal muscle. *J. Gen. Physiol.* 50: 1101–1124, 1967.
38. CORBIN, J. D., AND E. G. KREBS. A cyclic AMP-stimulated protein kinase in adipose tissue. *Biochem. Biophys. Res. Commun.* 36: 328–336, 1969.
39. CORI, C. F. Mammalian carbohydrate metabolism. *Physiol. Rev.* 11: 143–275, 1931.
40. CORI, C. F. Regulation of enzyme activity in muscle during work. In: *Enzymes—Units of Biological Structure and Function*, edited by O. H. Gaebler. New York: Acad. Press, 1956, p. 573–583.
41. DANFORTH, W. H., AND E. HELMREICH. Regulation of glycolysis in muscle. I. The conversion of phosphorylase *b* to phosphorylase *a* in frog sartorius muscle. *J. Biol. Chem.* 239: 3133–3138, 1964.
42. DANFORTH, W. H., E. HELMREICH, AND C. F. CORI. The effect of contraction and of epinephrine on the phosphorylase activity of frog sartorius muscle. *Proc. Natl. Acad. Sci. US* 48: 1191–1199, 1962.
43. DARBY, T. D., E. E. ALDINGER, R. H. GADSDEN, AND W. B. THROWER. Effects of metabolic acidosis on ventricular isometric systolic tension and the response to epinephrine and levarterenol. *Circulation Res.* 8: 1242–1253, 1960.
44. DE GUBAREFF, T., AND W. SLEATOR. Effects of caffeine on mammalian atrial muscle and its interaction with adenosine and calcium. *J. Pharmacol. Exptl. Therap.* 148: 202–214, 1965.
45. DE LANGE, R. J., R. G. KEMP, W. D. RILEY, R. A. COOPER, AND E. G. KREBS. Activation of skeletal muscle phosphorylase kinase by adenosine triphosphate and adenosine 3′,5′-monophosphate. *J. Biol. Chem.* 243: 2200–2208, 1968.

46. DHALLA, N. S., P. V. SULAKHE, R. L. KHANDELWAL, AND I. R. HAMILTON. Excitation contraction coupling in heart. II. Studies on the role of adenyl cyclase in the calcium transport by dog heart sarcoplasmic reticulum. *Life Sci.* 9: 625–632, 1970.
47. DIEM, K., AND C. LENTNER (editors). *Scientific Tables* (7th ed.). Basel: Geigy, 1970, p. 518.
48. DIETZE, G., AND K. D. HEPP. Calcium stimulated ATP-ase of cardiac sarcolemma. *Biochem. Biophys. Res. Commun.* 44: 1041–1049, 1971.
49. DIETZE, G., AND K. D. HEPP. Effect of 3′,5′-AMP on calcium-stimulated ATP-ase in rat heart sarcolemma. *Biochem. Biophys. Res. Commun.* 46: 269–278, 1972.
50. DRABIKOWSKI, W., D. R. KOMINZ, AND K. MARUYAMA. Effect of troponin on the reversibility of tropomyosin binding to F-actin. *J. Biochem., Tokyo* 63: 802–804, 1968.
51. DRUMMOND, G. I. Muscle metabolism. *Fortschr. Zool.* 18: 360–429, 1967.
52. DRUMMOND, G. I., AND L. DUNCAN. Adenyl cyclase in cardiac tissue. *J. Biol. Chem.* 245: 976–983, 1970.
53. DRUMMOND, G. I., L. DUNCAN, AND E. HERTZMAN. Effect of epinephrine on phosphorylase b kinase in perfused rat hearts. *J. Biol. Chem.* 241: 5899–5903, 1966.
54. DRUMMOND, G. I., J. P. HARWOOD, AND C. A. POWELL. Studies on the activation of phosphorylase in skeletal muscle by contraction and by epinephrine. *J. Biol. Chem.* 244: 4235–4240, 1969.
55. DRUMMOND, G. I., D. L. SEVERSON, AND L. DUNCAN. Adenyl cyclase, kinetic properties and nature of fluoride and hormone stimulation. *J. Biol. Chem.* 246: 4166–4173, 1971.
56. DRUMMOND, G. I., J. R. E. VALADARES, AND L. DUNCAN. Effect of epinephrine on contractile tension and phosphorylase activation in rat and dog hearts. *Proc. Soc. Exptl. Biol. Med.* 117: 307–309, 1964.
57. DUBOWITZ, V. *Developing and Diseased Muscle. A Histochemical Study* (Spastics Intern. Med. Publ. Res. Monogr.). New York: Wm. Heineman Med. Books, 1968.
58. EBASHI, S., AND M. ENDO. Calcium ion and muscle contraction. In: *Progress in Biophysics and Molecular Biology*, edited by J. A. V. Butler and D. Noble. New York: Pergamon Press, 1968, vol. 18, p. 123–183.
59. EBASHI, S., M. ENDO, AND I. OHTSUKI. Control of muscle contraction. *Quart. Rev. Biophys.* 2: 351–384, 1969.
60. EHRENPREIS, S., J. H. FLEISCH, AND T. W. MITTAG. Approaches to the molecular nature of pharmacological receptors. *Pharmacol. Rev.* 21: 131–181, 1969.
61. ELLIS, S. The effects of sympathomimetic amines and adrenergic blocking agents on metabolism. In: *Physiological Pharmacology*, edited by W. S. Root and F. G. Hofmann. New York: Acad. Press, 1967, vol. 4, p. 179–241.
62. ELLIS, S. Pharmacology society symposium: adrenergic receptors mediating metabolic responses. *Federation Proc.* 29: 1350–1425, 1970.
63. ENDO, M., M. TANAKA, AND Y. OGAWA. Calcium induced release of calcium from the sarcoplasmic reticulum of skinned skeletal muscle fibers. *Nature* 228: 34–36, 1970.
64. ENTMAN, M. L., G. S. LEVEY, AND S. E. EPSTEIN. Demonstration of adenyl cyclase activity in canine cardiac sarcoplasmic reticulum. *Biochem. Biophys. Res. Commun.* 35: 728–733, 1969.
65. ENTMAN, M. L., G. S. LEVEY, AND S. E. EPSTEIN. Mechanism of action of epinephrine and glucagon on the canine heart. Evidence for increase in sarcotubular calcium stores mediated by cyclic 3′,5′-AMP. *Circulation Res.* 25: 429–438, 1969.
66. FARAH, A., AND R. TUTTLE. Studies on the pharmacology of glucagon. *J. Pharmacol. Exptl. Therap.* 129: 49–55, 1960.
67. FAWCETT, D. W., AND N. S. MCNUTT. The ultrastructure of the cat myocardium. I. Ventricular papillary muscle. *J. Cell Biol.* 42: 1–45, 1969.
68. FISCHER, E. H., L. M. G. HEILMEYER, JR., AND R. H. HASCHKE. Phosphorylase and the control of glycogen degradation. *Current Topics Cellular Regulation* 4: 211–251, 1971.
69. FISCHER, E. H., S. S. HURD, P. KOH, V. L. SEERY, AND D. C. TELLER. Phosphorylase: relation of structure to activity. In: *Control of Glycogen Metabolism*, edited by W. J. Whelan. London: Acad. Press, 1968, p. 19–33.
70. FISCHER, E. H., AND E. G. KREBS. Conversion of phosphorylase b to phosphorylase a in muscle extracts. *J. Biol. Chem.* 216: 121–132, 1955.
71. FISCHER, E. H., A. POCKER, AND J. C. SAARI. The structure, function and control of glycogen phosphorylase. *Essays Biochem.* 6: 23–68, 1970.
72. FORD, L. E., AND R. J. PODOLSKY. Regenerative calcium release within muscle cells. *Science* 167: 58–59, 1970.
73. FRAZER, A., M. E. HESS, AND J. SHANFELD. The effects of thyroxine on rat heart adenosine 3′,5′-monophosphate, phosphorylase b kinase and phosphorylase a activity. *J. Pharmacol. Exptl. Therap.* 170: 10–16, 1969.
74. FUCHS, F., AND F. N. BRIGGS. The site of calcium binding in relation to the activation of myofibrillar contraction. *J. Gen. Physiol.* 51: 655–676, 1968.
75. GEORGE, J. C., AND C. L. TALESARA. Quantitative study of the distribution pattern of certain oxidizing enzymes and a lipase in the red and white fibers of the pigeon breast muscle. *J. Cellular Comp. Physiol.* 58: 253–260, 1961.
76. GEORGE, W. J., J. B. POLSON, A. G. O'TOOLE, AND N. D. GOLDBERG. Elevation of guanosine 3′,5′-cyclic phosphate in rat heart after perfusion with acetylcholine. *Proc. Natl. Acad. Sci. US* 66: 398–403, 1970.
77. GILBERT, D. L., AND W. O. FENN. Calcium equilibrium in muscle. *J. Gen. Physiol.* 40: 393–408, 1957.
78. GILL, G. N., AND L. D. GARREN. A cyclic-3′,5′-adenosine monophosphate dependent protein kinase from the adrenal cortex: comparison with a cyclic AMP binding protein. *Biochem. Biophys. Res. Commun.* 39: 335–343, 1970.
79. GILL, G. N., AND L. D. GARREN. Role of the receptor in the mechanism of action of adenosine 3′,5′-cyclic monophosphate. *Proc. Natl. Acad. Sci. US* 68: 786–790, 1971.
80. GILMAN, A. G., AND T. W. RALL. Adenosine 3′,5′-phosphate as a mediator of hormone action. In: *The Actions of Hormones: Genes to Population*, edited by P. P. Foà, N. L. Foà, and A. J. Whitty. Springfield, Ill.: Thomas, 1971, p. 87–128.
81. GLICK, G., W. W. PARMLEY, A. S. WECHSLER, AND E. H. SONNENBLICK. Glucagon: its enhancement of cardiac performance in the cat and frog and persistence of its inotropic action despite beta receptor blockade with propranolol. *Circulation Res.* 22: 789–799, 1968.
82. GLITSCH, H. G., H. REUTER, AND H. SCHOLZ. The effect of the internal sodium concentration on calcium fluxes in isolated guinea pig auricles. *J. Physiol., London* 209: 25–43, 1970.
83. GRAHAM, J. A., AND J. F. LAMB. The effects of adrenaline on the tension developed in contractures and twitches of the ventricle of the frog. *J. Physiol., London* 197: 479–509, 1968.
83a. GREASER, M. L., AND J. GERGELY. Reconstitution of troponin activity from three protein components. *J. Biol. Chem.* 246: 4226–4233, 1971.
83b. GREASER, M. L., AND J. GERGELY. Purification and properties of the components from troponin. *J. Biol. Chem.* 248: 2125–2133, 1973.
84. GREENGARD, P., AND E. COSTA (editors). *Role of Cyclic AMP in Cell Function*. New York: Raven Press, 1970.
85. GROSSMAN, A., AND R. F. FURCHGOTT. The effects of various drugs on calcium exchange in the isolated guinea-pig left auricle. *J. Pharmacol. Exptl. Therap.* 145: 162–172, 1964.
86. HARDMAN, J. G., G. A. ROBISON, AND E. W. SUTHERLAND. Cyclic nucleotides. *Ann. Rev. Physiol.* 33: 311–336, 1971.
87. HARRIS, P., AND L. H. OPIE (editors). *Calcium and the Heart*. New York: Acad. Press, 1971.
88. HARTSHORNE, D. J., AND H. Y. PYUN. Calcium binding by the troponin complex, and the purification and properties of troponin A. *Biochim. Biophys. Acta* 229: 698–711, 1971.
88a. HARTSHORNE, D. J., M. THEINER, AND H. MUELLER. Studies on troponin. *Biochim. Biophys. Acta* 175: 320–330, 1969.

89. HASCHKE, R. H., L. M. G. HEILMEYER, JR., F. MEYER, AND E. H. FISCHER. Control of phosphorylase activity in a muscle glycogen particle. III. Regulation of phosphorylase phosphatase. *J. Biol. Chem.* 245: 6657–6663, 1970.
90. HASSELBACH, W. Relaxing factor and the relaxation of muscle. *Progr. Biophys. Biophys. Chem.* 14: 167–222, 1964.
91. HASSELBACH, W., AND L-G. ELFVIN. Structural and chemical asymmetry of the calcium-transporting membranes of the sarcotubular system as revealed by electron microscopy. *J. Ultrastruct. Res.* 17: 598–622, 1967.
92. HAUGAARD, N., AND M. E. HESS. Actions of autonomic drugs on phosphorylase activity and function. *Pharmacol. Rev.* 17: 27–69, 1965.
93. HAVEL, R. J., A. NAIMARKS, AND C. F. BORCHGREVINK. Turnover rate and oxidation of free fatty acids of blood plasma in man during exercise: studies during continuous infusion of palmitate-1-C^{14}. *J. Clin. Invest.* 42: 1054–1063, 1963.
94. HEILMEYER, L. M. G., JR., F. MEYER, R. H. HASCHKE, AND E. H. FISHER. Control of phosphorylase activity in a muscle glycogen particle. II. Activation by calcium. *J. Biol. Chem.* 245: 6649–6656, 1970.
95. HELLAM, D. C., AND R. J. PODOLSKY. Force measurements in skinned muscle fibres. *J. Physiol., London* 200: 807–819, 1969.
96. HELMREICH, E. Control of synthesis and breakdown of glycogen, starch and cellulose. In: *Comprehensive Biochemistry: Carbohydrate Metabolism*, edited by M. Florkin and E. H. Stotz. Amsterdam: Elsevier, 1969, vol. 17, p. 17–92.
97. HELMREICH, E., AND C. F. CORI. The role of adenylic acid in the activation of phosphorylase. *Proc. Natl. Acad. Sci. US* 51: 131–138, 1964.
98. HELMREICH, E., AND C. F. CORI. Regulation of glycolysis in muscle. *Advan. Enzyme Regulation* 3: 91–107, 1965.
99. HELMREICH, E., AND C. F. CORI. The activation of glycolysis in frog sartorius muscle by epinephrine. *Pharmacol. Rev.* 18: 189–196, 1966.
100. HELMREICH, E., W. H. DANFORTH, S. KARPATKIN, AND C. F. CORI. The response of the glycolytic system of anaerobic frog sartorius muscle to electrical stimulation. In: *Control of Energy Metabolism*, edited by B. Chance, R. W. Estabrook, and J. R. Williamson. New York: Acad. Press, 1965, p. 299–312.
101. HELMREICH, E., M. C. MICHAELIDES, AND C. F. CORI. Effects of substrates and a substrate analog on the binding of 5′-adenylic acid to muscle phosphorylase a. *Biochemistry* 6: 3695–3710, 1967.
102. HESS, M., AND N. HAUGAARD. The effect of epinephrine and aminophylline on the phosphorylase activity of perfused contracting heart muscle. *J. Pharmacol. Exptl. Therap.* 122: 169–175, 1958.
103. HIMMS-HAGEN, J. Sympathetic regulation of metabolism. *Pharmacol. Rev.* 19: 367–461, 1967.
104. HOFFMAN, B. F., AND P. F. CRANEFIELD. *Electrophysiology of the Heart*. New York: McGraw-Hill, 1960, p. 1–20.
105. HONIG, C. R. Influence of catecholamines and their analogs on ATP-induced contraction of cardiac myofibrils and myosin B. In: *Factors Influencing Myocardial Contractility*, edited by R. D. Tanz, F. Kavaler, and J. Roberts. New York: Acad. Press, 1967, p. 373–383.
106. HORN, R. S., A. FYHN, AND N. HAUGAARD. Mitochondrial calcium uptake in the perfused contracting rat heart and the influence of epinephrine on calcium exchange. *Biochim. Biophys. Acta* 226: 459–466, 1971.
107. HORN, R. S., R. LEVIN, AND N. HAUGAARD. The influence of oligomycin on the actions of epinephrine and theophylline upon the perfused rat heart. *Biochem. Pharmacol.* 18: 503–509, 1969.
108. HUGHES, R. C., A. A. YUNIS, E. G. KREBS, AND E. H. FISCHER. Comparative studies on glycogen phosphorylase. III. The phosphorylated site in human muscle phosphorylase a. *J. Biol. Chem.* 237: 40–43, 1962.
109. HULTMAN, E. Muscle glycogen in man determined in needle biopsy specimens. *Scand. J. Clin. Invest.* 19: 209–217, 1967.
110. HURD, S. S., D. TELLER, AND E. H. FISCHER. Probable formation of partially phosphorylated intermediates in the interconversions of phosphorylase a and b. *Biochem. Biophys. Res. Commun.* 24: 79–84, 1966.
111. HUSTON, R. B., AND E. G. KREBS. Activation of skeletal muscle phosphorylase b kinase by Ca^{++}. *Biochemistry* 7: 2116–2122, 1968.
112. HUXLEY, H. E. The mechanism of muscular contraction. *Science* 164: 1356–1366, 1969.
113. IKEMOTO, N., F. A. SRETER, A. NAKAMURA, AND J. GERGELY. Tryptic digestion and localization of calcium uptake and ATPase activity in fragments of sarcoplasmic reticulum. *J. Ultrastruct. Res.* 23: 216–232, 1968.
114. INESI, G., AND A. SCARPA. Fast kinetics of adenosine triphosphate dependent Ca^{++} uptake by fragmented sarcoplasmic reticulum. *Biochemistry* 11: 356–359, 1972.
115. ISAACSON, A., AND A. SANDOW. Quinine and caffeine effects of ^{45}Ca movements in frog sartorius muscle. *J. Gen. Physiol.* 50: 2109–2128, 1967.
116. JARD, S., AND F. BASTIDE. A cyclic AMP-dependent protein kinase from frog bladder epithelial cells. *Biochem. Biophys. Res. Commun.* 39: 559–566, 1970.
117. JERGIL, B., AND G. H. DIXON. Protamine kinase from rainbow trout testis. *J. Biol. Chem.* 245: 425–434, 1970.
118. JOBSIS, F. F., AND M. J. O'CONNOR. Calcium release and reabsorption in the sartorius muscle of the toad. *Biochem. Biophys. Res. Commun.* 25: 246–252, 1966.
119. JOHNSON, E. A., AND M. LIEBERMAN. Heart: excitation and contraction. *Ann. Rev. Physiol.* 33: 479–532, 1971.
120. KASSEBAUM, D. G., AND A. R. VAN DYKE. Electrophysiological effects of isoproterenol on Purkinje fibers of the heart. *Circulation Res.* 19: 940–946, 1966.
121. KATZ, A. M. Absence of direct actions of norepinephrine on cardiac myosin and actomyosin. *Am. J. Physiol.* 212: 39–42, 1967.
122. KATZ, A. M. Contractile proteins of the heart. *Physiol. Rev.* 50: 63–158, 1970.
123. KATZ, A. M., D. I. REPKE, AND B. R. COHEN. Control of the activity of highly purified cardiac actomyosin by Ca^{2+}, Na$^+$ and K$^+$. *Circulation Res.* 19: 1062–1070, 1966.
124. KAVALER, F., AND M. MORAD. Paradoxical effects of epinephrine on excitation-contraction coupling in cardiac muscle. *Circulation Res.* 18: 492–501, 1966.
125. KOREY, S. Some factors influencing the contractility of a nonconducting fiber preparation. *Biochim. Biophys. Acta* 4: 58–67, 1950.
126. KRAUSE, E. G., W. HALLE, E. KALLABIS, AND A. WOLLENBERGER. Positive chronotropic response of cultured isolated rat heart cells to N^6,2′-O-dibutyryl-3′,5′ adenosine monophosphate. *J. Mol. Cellular Cardiol.* 1: 1–10, 1970.
127. KREBS, E. G., R. J. DELANGE, R. G. KEMP, AND W. D. RILEY. Activation of skeletal muscle phosphorylase. *Pharmacol. Rev.* 18: 163–171, 1966.
128. KREBS, E. G., J. D. GRAVES, AND E. H. FISCHER. Factors affecting the activity of muscle phosphorylase b kinase. *J. Biol. Chem.* 234: 2867–2873, 1959.
129. KREBS, E. G., D. S. LOVE, G. E. BRATVOLD, K. A. TRAYSER, W. L. MEYER, AND E. H. FISCHER. Purification and properties of rabbit skeletal muscle phosphorylase b kinase. *Biochemistry* 3: 1022–1033, 1964.
130. KREBS, E. G., AND D. A. WALSH. Studies on the mechanism of action of cyclic 3′,5′-AMP in the phosphorylase system. In: *Metabolic Regulation and Enzyme Action*, edited by A. Sols and S. Grisolía. New York: Acad. Press, 1970, vol. 19, p. 121–129.
131. KREISBERG, R. A. Effect of epinephrine on myocardial triglyceride and free fatty acid utilization. *Am. J. Physiol.* 210: 385–389, 1966.
132. KÜBLER, W., AND E. A. SHINEBOURNE. Calcium and the

mitochondria. In: *Calcium and the Heart*, edited by P. Harris and L. H. Opie. New York: Acad. Press, 1971, p. 93-123.
133. KUGELBERG, E., AND L. EDSTRÖM. Differential histochemical effects of muscle contractions on phosphorylase and glycogen in various types of fibres in relation to fatigue. *J. Neurol. Neurosurg. Psychiat.* 31: 415-423, 1968.
134. KUKOVETZ, W. R., AND G. PÖCH. Cardiostimulatory effects of cyclic 3',5' adenosine monophosphate and its acylated derivatives. *Arch. Exptl. Pharmakol. Pathol.* 266: 236-254, 1970.
135. KUO, J. F., AND P. GREENGARD. An adenosine 3',5'-monophosphate-dependent protein kinase from *Escherichia coli*. *J. Biol. Chem.* 244: 3417-3419, 1969.
136. KUO, J. F., AND P. GREENGARD. Cyclic nucleotide-dependent protein kinases. IV. Widespread occurrence of adenosine 3',5'-monophosphate-dependent protein kinase in various tissues and phyla of the animal kingdom. *Proc. Natl. Acad. Sci. US* 64: 1349-1355, 1969.
137. KUO, J. F., T-P. LEE, P. L. REYES, K. G. WALTON, T. E. DONNELLY, JR., AND P. GREENGARD. Cyclic nucleotide-dependent protein kinases. X. An assay method for the measurement of guanosine 3',5' monophosphate in various biological materials and a study of agents regulating its levels in heart and brain. *J. Biol. Chem.* 247: 16-22, 1972.
138. LANDGRAF, W. C., AND G. INESI. ATP dependent conformational change in "spin labelled" sarcoplasmic reticulum. *Arch. Biochem. Biophys.* 130: 111-118, 1969.
139. LANGAN, T. A. Histone phosphorylation: stimulation by adenosine 3',5'-monophosphate. *Science* 162: 579-580, 1968.
140. LANGAN, T. A. Action of adenosine 3',5'-monophosphate-dependent histone kinase *in vivo*. *J. Biol. Chem.* 244: 5763-5765, 1969.
141. LANGER, G. A. Kinetic studies of calcium distribution in ventricular muscle of the dog. *Circulation Res.* 15: 393-405, 1964.
142. LANGER, G. A. Ion fluxes in cardiac excitation and contraction and their relation to myocardial contractility. *Physiol. Rev.* 48: 708-757, 1968.
143. LANGER, G. A., AND A. J. BRADY. Calcium flux in the mammalian ventricular myocardium. *J. Gen. Physiol.* 46: 703-719, 1963.
144. LANGSLET, A., AND I. ØYE. The role of cyclic 3',5'-AMP in the cardiac response to adrenaline. *European J. Pharmacol.* 12: 137-144, 1970.
145. LA RAIA, P. J., AND W. J. REDDY. Hormonal regulation of myocardial adenosine 3',5'-monophosphate. *Biochim. Biophys. Acta* 177: 189-195, 1969.
146. LARNER, J., AND C. VILLAR-PALASI. Glycogen synthesis and its control. In: *Current Topics in Cellular Regulation*, edited by B. L. Horecker and E. R. Stadtman. New York: Acad. Press, 1971, vol. 3, p. 195-236.
147. LARNER, J., C. VILLAR-PALASI, N. D. GOLDBERG, J. S. BISHOP, F. HUIJING, J. I. WENGER, H. SASKO, AND N. B. BROWN. Hormonal and non-hormonal control of glycogen synthesis—control of transferase phosphatase and transferase I kinase. *Advan. Enzyme Regulation* 6: 409-423, 1967.
148. LEFKOWITZ, R. J., AND E. HABER. A fraction of the ventricular myocardium that has the specificity of the cardiac beta-adrenergic receptor. *Proc. Natl. Acad. Sci. US* 68: 1773-1777, 1971.
148a. LEFKOWITZ, R. J., G. W. C. SHARP, AND E. HABER. Specific binding of β-adrenergic catecholamines to a subcellular fraction from cardiac muscle. *J. Biol. Chem.* 248: 342-349, 1973.
149. LEGATO, M. J., AND G. A. LANGER. The subcellular localization of calcium ion in mammalian myocardium. *J. Cell Biol.* 41: 401-423, 1969.
150. LEGATO, M. J., D. SPIRO, AND G. A. LANGER. Ultrastructure alterations produced in mammalian myocardium by variations in perfusate ionic composition. *J. Cell Biol.* 37: 1-12, 1968.
151. LEHNINGER, A. L. Mitochondria and calcium ion transport. *Biochem. J.* 119: 129-138, 1970.
152. LEHNINGER, A. L., AND E. CARAFOLI. The interaction of La^{3+} with mitochondria in relation to respiration-coupled Ca^{2+} transport. *Arch. Biochem. Biophys.* 143: 506-515, 1971.
153. LEHNINGER, A. L., E. CARAFOLI, AND C. S. ROSSI. Energy-linked ion movements in mitochondrial systems. *Advan. Enzymol.* 29: 259-320, 1967.
154. LEVEY, G. S. Discussion remarks. *Ann. Internal Med.* 72: 561-578, 1970.
155. LEVEY, G. S. Solubilization of myocardial adenyl cyclase. *Biochem. Biophys. Res. Commun.* 38: 86-92, 1970.
156. LEVEY, G. S. Restoration of glucagon responsiveness of solubilized myocardial adenyl cyclase by phosphatidylserine. *Biochem. Biophys. Res. Commun.* 43: 108-113, 1971.
157. LEVEY, G. S. Restoration of norepinephrine responsiveness of solubilized myocardial adenylate cyclase by phosphatidyl-inositol. *J. Biol. Chem.* 246: 7405-7407, 1971.
158. LEVEY, G. S., AND S. E. EPSTEIN. Activation of adenyl cylase by glucagon in cat and human heart. *Circulation Res.* 24: 151-156, 1969.
159. LEVEY, G. S., AND S. E. EPSTEIN. Myocardial adenyl cyclase: activation by thyroid hormones and evidence for two adenyl cyclase systems. *J. Clin. Invest.* 48: 1663-1669, 1969.
160. LEVINE, R. A., L. M. DIXON, AND R. B. FRANKLIN. Effects of exogenous adenosine 3',5'-monophosphate in man. I. Cardiovascular responses. *Clin. Pharmacol. Therap.* 9: 168-179, 1968.
161. LIPTON, P., C. REFINO, AND J. R. WILLIAMSON. Respiration and active Na^+/K^+ transport in perfused liver (Abstract). *Federation Proc.* 31: 297, 1972.
162. LOWRY, O. H., D. W. SCHULZ, AND J. V. PASSONNEAU. Effects of adenylic acid on the kinetics of muscle phosphorylase a. *J. Biol. Chem.* 239: 1947-1953, 1964.
163. LOWRY, O. H., D. W. SCHULZ, AND J. V. PASSONNEAU. The kinetics of glycogen phosphorylases from brain and muscle. *J. Biol. Chem.* 242: 271-280, 1967.
164. LUCCHESI, B. R. Cardiac actions of glucagon. *Circulation Res.* 22: 777-787, 1968.
165. LUCHI, R. J., AND E. M. KRITCHER. Drug effects on cardiac myosin adenosine triphosphatase activity. *J. Pharmacol. Exptl. Therap.* 158: 540-545, 1967.
166. LUCHI, R. J., E. M. KRITCHER, AND H. L. CONN, JR. Modification of cardiac myosin adenosine triphosphatase activity by ions and cardiac drugs. *Circulation* 30, Suppl. III: 118, 1964.
167. LUNDHOLM, L., E. MOHME-LUNDHOLM, AND N. SVEDMYR. Introductory remarks. *Pharmacol. Rev.* 18: 255-272, 1966.
168. LUNDHOLM, L., E. MOHME-LUNDHOLM, AND N. SVEDMYR: Metabolic effects of catecholamines. In: *The Biological Basis of Medicine*, edited by E. E. Bittar and N. Bittar. New York. Acad. Press, 1968, vol. 2, p. 101-130.
169. LÜTTGAU, H. C., AND R. NIEDERGERKE. The antagonism between Ca and Na ions on the frog's heart. *J. Physiol., London* 143: 486-505, 1958.
170. MACLENNAN, D. H. Purification and properties of an adenosine triphosphatase from sarcoplasmic reticulum. *J. Biol. Chem.* 245: 4508-4518, 1970.
171. MACLENNAN, D. H., P. SEEMAN, G. H. ILES, AND C. C. YIP. Membrane formation by the adenosine triphosphatase of sarcoplasmic reticulum. *J. Biol. Chem.* 246: 2702-2710, 1971.
172. MACLENNAN, D. H., AND P. T. S. WONG. Isolation of a calcium-sequestering protein from sarcoplasmic reticulum. *Proc. Natl. Acad. Sci. US* 68: 1231-1235, 1971.
173. MADSEN, N. B. The inhibition of glycogen phosphorylase by uridine diphosphate glucose. *Biochem. Biophys. Res. Commun.* 6: 310-313, 1961.
174. MARTONOSI, A. Sarcoplasmic reticulum. V. The structure of sarcoplasmic reticulum membranes. *Biochim. Biophys. Acta* 150: 694-704, 1968.

175. MARTONOSI, A. Sarcoplasmic reticulum. IV. Solubilization of microsomal adenosine triphosphatase. *J. Biol. Chem.* 243: 71–81, 1968.
176. MARTONOSI, A., J. DONLEY, AND R. A. HALPIN. Sarcoplasmic reticulum. III. The role of phospholipids in the adenosine triphosphatase activity and Ca^{++} transport. *J. Biol. Chem.* 243: 61–70, 1968.
177. MARTONOSI, A., AND R. FERETOS. Sarcoplasmic reticulum. I. The uptake of Ca^{2+} by sarcoplasmic reticulum fragments. *J. Biol. Chem.* 239: 648–658, 1964.
178. MARTONOSI, A., M. A. GOUVEA, AND J. GERGELY. Studies on actin. III. G-F transformation of actin and muscular contraction (experiments *in vivo*). *J. Biol. Chem.* 235: 1707–1710, 1960.
179. MAYER, S. E. Regulation of cardiac and skeletal muscle glycogen metabolism by biogenic amines. In: *Biogenic Amines as Physiological Regulators*, edited by J. J. Blum. New York: Prentice-Hall, 1970, p. 139–159.
180. MAYER, S. E. Adrenergic receptors for metabolic responses in the heart. *Federation Proc.* 29: 1367–1372, 1970.
181. MAYER, S. E., M. DEV. COTTEN, AND N. C. MORAN. Dissociation of the augmentation of cardiac contractile force from the activation of myocardial phosphorylase by catecholamines. *J. Pharmacol. Exptl. Therap.* 139: 275–282, 1963.
182. MAYER, S. E., AND E. G. KREBS. Studies on the phosphorylation and activation of skeletal muscle phosphorylase kinase *in vivo*. *J. Biol. Chem.* 245: 3153–3160, 1970.
183. MAYER, S. E., D. H. NAMM, AND L. RICE. Effect of glucagon on cyclic 3′,5′-AMP, phosphorylase activity and contractility of heart muscle of the rat. *Circulation Res.* 26: 225–233, 1970.
184. MCNEILL, J. H., M. NASSER, AND T. M. BRODY. The effect of theophylline on amine-induced cardiac phosphorylase activation and cardiac contractility. *J. Pharmacol. Exptl. Therap.* 165: 234–241, 1969.
185. MELA, L., AND B. CHANCE. Spectrophotometric measurements of the kinetics of Ca^{2+} and Mn^{2+} accumulation in mitochondria. *Biochemistry* 7: 4059–4063, 1968.
186. METZGER, B. E., L. GLASER, AND E. HELMREICH. Purification and properties of frog skeletal muscle phosphorylase. *Biochemistry* 7: 2021–2036, 1968.
187. METZGER, B., E. HELMREICH, AND L. GLASER. The mechanism of activation of skeletal muscle phosphorylase *a* by glycogen. *Proc. Natl. Acad. Sci. US* 57: 994–1001, 1967.
188. MEYER, F., L. M. G. HEILMEYER, JR., R. H. HASCHKE, AND E. H. FISCHER. Control of phosphorylase activity in a muscle glycogen particle. I. Isolation and characterization of the protein-glycogen complex. *J. Biol. Chem.* 245: 6642–6648, 1970.
189. MEYER, W. L., E. H. FISCHER, AND E. G. KREBS. Activation of skeletal muscle phosphorylase *b* kinase by Ca^{2+}. *Biochemistry* 3: 1033–1039, 1964.
190. MIYAMOTO, E., J. R. KUO, AND P. GREENGARD. Cyclic nucleotide-dependent protein kinases. III. Purification and properties of adenosine 3′,5′-monophosphate-dependent protein kinase from bovine brain. *J. Biol. Chem.* 244: 6395–6402, 1969.
191. MOMMAERTS, W. F. H. M. Energetics of muscular contraction. *Physiol. Rev.* 49: 427–508, 1969.
192. MORAD, M. Contracture and catecholamines in mammalian myocardium. *Science* 166: 505–506, 1969.
193. MORAD, M., AND R. K. ORKAND. Excitation-contraction coupling in frog ventricle: evidence from voltage clamp studies. *J. Physiol., London* 219: 167–189, 1971.
194. MORAD, M., AND E. L. ROLETT. Relaxing effects of catecholamines on mammalian heart. *J. Physiol., London* 224: 537–558, 1972.
195. MORAD, M., AND W. TRAUTWEIN. The effect of the duration of the action potential on contraction in the mammalian heart muscle. *Arch. Ges. Physiol.* 299: 66–82, 1968.
196. MORGAN, H. E., AND A. PARMEGGIANI. Regulation of glycogenolysis in muscle. III. Control of muscle glycogen phosphorylase activity. *J. Biol. Chem.* 239: 2440–2445, 1964.
197. MURAD, F., AND M. VAUGHN. Effect of glucagon on rat heart adenyl cyclase. *Biochem. Pharmacol.* 18: 1053–1059, 1969.
198. NAMM, D. H., AND S. E. MAYER. Effects of epinephrine on cardiac cyclic 3′,5′-AMP, phosphorylase kinase, and phosphorylase. *Mol. Pharmacol.* 4: 61–69, 1968.
199. NAMM, D. H., S. E. MAYER, AND M. MALTBIE. The role of potassium and calcium ions in the effect of epinephrine on cardiac cyclic adenosine 3′,5′-monophosphate, phosphorylase kinase, and phosphorylase. *Mol. Pharmacol.* 4: 522–530, 1968.
200. NAYLER, W. G. Influx and efflux of calcium in the physiology of muscle contraction. *Clin. Orthoped. Related Res.* 46: 157–182, 1966.
201. NAYLER, W. G. Calcium exchange in cardiac muscle: a basic mechanism of drug action. *Am. Heart J.* 73: 379–394, 1967.
202. NAYLER, W. G. Ion movements in heart muscle. In: *Membranes and Ion Transport*, edited by E. E. Bittar. London: Wiley Interscience, 1970, vol. 2, p. 75–94.
203. NAYLER, W. G., I. MCINNES, D. CHIPPERFIELD, V. CORSON, AND P. DAILE. The effect of glucagon on calcium exchangeability, coronary blood flow, myocardial function and high energy phosphate stores. *J. Pharmacol. Exptl. Therap.* 171: 265–275, 1970.
204. NAYLER, W. G., AND N. C. R. MERRILLEES. Some observations on the fine structure and metabolic activity of normal and glycerinated ventricular muscle of toad. *J. Cell Biol.* 22: 533–550, 1964.
205. NEELY, J. R., H. LIEBERMEISTER, E. J. BATTERSBY, AND H. E. MORGAN. Effect of pressure development on oxygen consumption by isolated rat heart. *Am. J. Physiol.* 212: 804–814, 1967.
206. NIEDERGERKE, R. The rate of action of calcium ions on the contraction of the heart. *J. Physiol., London* 138: 506–515, 1957.
207. NIEDERGERKE, R. Movements of Ca in beating ventricles of the frog heart. *J. Physiol., London* 167: 551–580, 1963.
208. NIEDERGERKE, R., AND R. K. ORKAND. The dual effect of calcium on the action potential of the frog's heart. *J. Physiol., London* 184: 291–311, 1966.
209. NOBLE, D., AND R. W. TSIEN. Outward membrane currents activated in the plateau range of potentials in cardiac Purkinje fibers. *J. Physiol., London* 200: 205–231, 1969.
210. NOLAN, C., W. B. NOVA, E. G. KREBS, AND E. H. FISCHER. Further studies on the site phosphorylated in the phosphorylase *b* to *a* reaction. *Biochemistry* 3: 542–551, 1964.
211. NOVOTNÝ, I., AND F. VYSKOČIL. Possible role of Ca ions in the resting metabolism of frog sartorius muscle during potassium depolarization. *J. Cellular Physiol.* 67: 159–168, 1966.
212. OGAWA, Y. The apparent binding constant of glycoletherdiamine-tetraacetic acid for calcium at neutral pH. *J. Biochem., Tokyo* 64: 255–257, 1968.
213. OGAWA, Y. Some properties of fragmented frog sarcoplasmic reticulum with particular reference to its response to caffeine. *J. Biochem., Tokyo* 67: 667–683, 1970.
214. OHNISHI, T., AND S. EBASHI. The velocity of calcium binding of isolated sarcoplasmic reticulum. *J. Biochem., Tokyo* 55: 599–603, 1964.
215. ØYE, I. The action of adrenaline in cardiac muscle: dissociation between phosphorylase activation and inotropic response. *Acta Physiol. Scand.* 65: 251–258, 1965.
216. ØYE, I. The role of phosphorylase *a* and *b* for the control of glycogenolysis in the isolated working rat heart. *Acta Physiol. Scand.* 70: 229–235, 1967.
217. OZAWA, E., K. HOSOI, AND S. EBASHI. Reversible stimulation of muscle phosphorylase *b* kinase by low concentrations of calcium ions. *J. Biochem., Tokyo* 61: 531–533, 1967.
218. PADYKULA, H. A., AND G. F. GAUTHIER. Morphological and cytochemical characteristics of fiber types in normal mammalian muscle. In: *Exploratory Concepts in Muscular Dystrophy and Related Disorders*. Amsterdam: Excerpta Medica Foundation, 1967, p. 117–128.

219. PAGE, E. Tubular systems in Purkinje cells of the cat heart. *J. Ultrastruct. Res.* 17: 72–83, 1966.
220. PATRIARCA, P., AND E. CARAFOLI. A study of the intracellular transport of calcium in rat heart. *J. Cellular Physiol.* 72: 29–37, 1968.
221. PATRIARCA, P., AND E. CARAFOLI. A comparative study of the intracellular Ca^{2+} movements in white and red muscle. *Experientia* 25: 589–599, 1969.
221a. PEACHEY, L. D. Muscle. *Ann. Rev. Physiol.* 30: 401–440, 1968.
222. PETTE, D., AND T. BÜCHER. Proportionskonstante Gruppen in Beziehung zur Differenzierung der Enzymaktivitätsmuster von Skeletal Muskeln des Kaninchens. *Z. Physiol. Chem.* 331: 180–195, 1963.
223. POHL, S. T., H. M. J. KRANS, V. KOZYREFF, L. BIRNBAUMER, AND M. RODBELL. The glucagon-sensitive adenyl cyclase system in plasma membranes of rat liver. VI. Evidence for a role of membrane lipids. *J. Biol. Chem.* 246: 4447–4454, 1971.
224. PORTZEHL, H., P. C. CALDWELL, AND J. C. RÜEGG. The dependence of contraction and relaxation of muscle fibers from the crab *Maia Squinado* on the internal concentration of free calcium ions. *Biochim. Biophys. Acta* 79: 581–591, 1964.
225. POSNER, J. B., R. STERN, AND E. G. KREBS. In vivo response of skeletal muscle glycogen phosphorylase, phosphorylase b kinase and cyclic AMP to epinephrine administration. *Biochem. Biophys. Res. Commun.* 4: 293–296, 1962.
226. POSNER, J. B., R. STERN, AND E. G. KREBS. Effects of electrical stimulation and epinephrine on muscle phosphorylase, phosphorylase b kinase, and adenosine $3',5'$-phosphate. *J. Biol. Chem.* 240: 982–985, 1965.
227. RABINOWITZ, M., L. DESALLES, J. MEISLER, AND L. LORAND. Distribution of adenyl-cyclase activity in rabbit skeletal muscle fractions. *Biochim. Biophys. Acta* 97: 29–36, 1965.
228. RALL, T. W., AND T. C. WEST. The potentiation of cardiac inotropic responses to norepinephrine by theophylline. *J. Pharmacol. Exptl. Therap.* 139: 269–274, 1963.
229. RASMUSSEN, H. Cell communication, calcium ion, and cyclic adenosine monophosphate. *Science* 170: 404–412, 1970.
230. RASMUSSEN, H., AND N. NAGATA. Hormones, cell calcium and cyclic AMP. In: *A Symposium on Calcium and Cellular Function*, edited by A. W. Cuthbert. New York: St. Martin's, 1970, p. 199–213.
231. RAYNS, D. G., F. O. SIMPSON, AND W. S. BERTAUD. Surface features of striated muscle. I. Guinea-pig cardiac muscle. *J. Cell Sci.* 3: 467–474, 1968.
232. RAYNS, D. G., F. O. SIMPSON, AND W. S. BERTAUD. Surface features of striated muscle. II. Guinea-pig skeletal muscle. *J. Cell Sci.* 3: 475–482, 1968.
233. REGAN, T. L., P. H. LEHAN, D. H. HENNEMAN, A. BEHAR, AND H. K. HELLAMS. Myocardial metabolic and contractile response to glucagon and epinephrine. *J. Lab. Clin. Med.* 63: 638–647, 1964.
234. REIMANN, E. M., D. A. WALSH, AND E. G. KREBS. Purification and properties of rabbit skeletal muscle adenosine $3',5'$-monophosphate-dependent protein kinases. *J. Biol. Chem.* 246: 1986–1995, 1971.
235. REUTER, H. Über die Wirkung von Adrenalin auf den cellulären Ca-Umsatz des Meerschweinchenvorhofs. *Arch. Exptl. Pathol. Pharmakol.* 251: 401–412, 1965.
236. REUTER, H. The dependence of slow inward current in Purkinje fibres on the extracellular calcium-concentration. *J. Physiol., London* 192: 479–492, 1967.
237. REUTER, H. Kinetic aspects of calcium current in ventricular myocardial fibres. In: *A Symposium on Calcium and Cellular Function*, edited by A. W. Cuthbert. New York: St. Martin's, 1970, p. 261–269.
238. REUTER, H., AND G. W. BEELER, JR. Calcium current and activation of contraction in ventricular myocardial fibers. *Science* 163: 399–401, 1969.
239. REUTER, H., AND N. SEITZ. The dependence of calcium efflux from cardiac muscle on temperature and external ion composition. *J. Physiol., London* 195: 451–470, 1968.
240. REUTER, H., AND U. WOLLERT. Über die Wirkung verschiedener sympathomimetischer Amine auf Kontraktionskraft und ^{45}Ca-Aufrahm isolierter Meerschweinchenvorhofs. *Arch. Exptl. Pharmakol. Pathol.* 258: 288–296, 1967.
241. REYNAFARJE, B., AND A. L. LEHNINGER. High affinity and low affinity binding of Ca^{2+} by rat liver mitochondria. *J. Biol. Chem.* 244: 584–593, 1969.
242. RILEY, W. D., R. J. DELANGE, G. E. BRATVOLD, AND E. G. KREBS. Reversal of phosphorylase kinase activation. *J. Biol. Chem.* 243: 2209–2215, 1968.
243. ROBB, J. S., M. GRUBB, AND H. BRAUNFELDS. A spectrophotometric study of actomyosin. *Circulation Res.* 3: 525–531, 1955.
244. ROBISON, G. A., R. W. BUTCHER, I. ØYE, H. E. MORGAN, AND E. W. SUTHERLAND. The effect of epinephrine on adenosine-$3',5'$-phosphate levels in the isolated perfused rat heart. *Mol. Pharmacol.* 1: 168–177, 1965.
245. ROBISON, G. A., R. W. BUTCHER, AND E. W. SUTHERLAND. Adenyl cyclase as an adrenergic receptor. *Ann. NY Acad. Sci.* 139: 703–723, 1966.
246. ROBISON, G. A., R. W. BUTCHER, AND E. W. SUTHERLAND. Cyclic AMP. *Ann. Rev. Biochem.* 37: 149–174, 1968.
247. ROBISON, G. A., R. W. BUTCHER, AND E. W. SUTHERLAND (editors). *Cyclic AMP*. New York: Acad. Press, 1971.
248. ROBISON, G. A., J. W. DOBBS, AND E. W. SUTHERLAND. On the nature of receptor sites for biogenic amines. In: *Biogenic Amines as Physiological Regulators*, edited by J. J. Blum. Englewood Cliffs, N. J.: Prentice-Hall, 1970, p. 3–34.
249. ROBISON, G. A., G. G. NAHAS, AND L. TRINER (editors). Cyclic AMP and cell function. *Ann. NY Acad. Sci.* 185: 1–556, 1971.
251. ROUGIER, O., G. VASSORT, D. GARNIER, Y-M. GARGOÜIL, AND E. CORABOEUF. Données nouvelles concernant le rôle des ions Na^+ et Ca^{++} sur les propriétés électrophysiologiques des membranes cardiaques; existence d'un canal lent. *Compt. Rend.* 266: 802–805, 1968.
252. RUBIN, C. S., J. ERLICHMAN, AND O. M. ROSEN. Molecular forms and subunit composition of a cyclic adenosine $3',5'$-monophosphate-dependent protein kinase purified from bovine heart muscle. *J. Biol. Chem.* 247: 36–44, 1972.
253. SAFER, B., AND J. R. WILLIAMSON. Functional significance of the malate-aspartate shuttle for the oxidation of cytoplasmic reducing equivalents in rat heart. In: *Myocardiology: Recent Advances in Studies on Cardiac Structure and Metabolism*, edited by E. Bajusz and G. Rona. Baltimore: University Park Press, 1971, p. 34–43.
254. SANBORN, W. G., AND G. A. LANGER. Specific uncoupling of excitation and contraction in mammalian cardiac tissue by lanthanum: kinetic studies. *J. Gen. Physiol.* 56: 191–217, 1970.
255. SANDOW, A. Excitation-contraction coupling in skeletal muscle. *Pharmacol. Rev.* 17: 265–320, 1965.
256. SANDOW, A. Skeletal muscle. *Ann. Rev. Physiol.* 32: 87–138, 1970.
258. SCARPA, A., AND A. AZZI. Cation binding to submitochondrial particles. *Biochim. Biophys. Acta* 150: 473–481, 1968.
259. SCARPA, A., AND G. F. AZZONE. Effects of phospholipids in liver mitochondria osmotic properties and binding of cations. *Biochim. Biophys. Acta* 173: 78–85, 1969.
259a. SCARPA, A., AND J. R. WILLIAMSON. Calcium binding and calcium transport by subcellular fractions of hearts. In: *Calcium Binding Proteins*, edited by D. Drabikowsky and E. Carafoli. Amsterdam: Elsevier, 1974. In press.
260. SCHÄDLER, M. H. Proportionale Aktivierung von ATPase-Aktivität und Kontraktinononsspannung durch Calciumionen in isolierten contraktilen Strukturen verschiedener Muskelarten. *Arch. Ges. Physiol.* 296: 70–90, 1967.
261. SCHAFFER, S. W., B. SAFER, AND J. R. WILLIAMSON. Investigation of the role of mitochondria in the cardiac contraction-relaxation cycle. *FEBS Letters* 23: 125–130, 1972.
262. SCHAFFER, S. W., AND J. R. WILLIAMSON. The calcium cycle

and myocardial contractility (Abstract). *Federation Proc.* 31: 373, 1972.
263. SCHATZMAN, H. J. Ca-activated membrane ATP-ase in human red cells and its possible role in active Ca transport. *Proc. Protides Biol. Fluid Colloq., Bruges* 15: 251–255, 1967.
264. SCHWARTZ, A. Calcium and the sarcoplasmic reticulum. In: *Calcium and the Heart*, edited by P. Harris and L. H. Opie. New York: Acad. Press, 1971, p. 66–92.
265. SEMENUK, N. S., AND H. ZIMMERBERG. *Cyclic AMP: 1957–1969*. New Brunswick, N.J.: E. R. Squibb, 1970.
265a. SEMENUK, N. S., AND H. ZIMMERBERG. *Cyclic AMP: 1970*. New Brunswick, N.J.: E. R. Squibb, 1971.
266. SERAYDARIAN, K., W. F. H. M. MOMMAERTS, AND A. WALLNER. The amount and compartmentalization of adenosine diphosphate in muscle. *Biochim. Biophys. Acta* 65: 443–460, 1962.
267. SHANFELD, J., A. FRAZER, AND M. E. HESS. Dissociation of the increased formation of cardiac adenosine 3' 5'-monophosphate from the positive inotropic effect of norepinephrine. *J. Pharmacol. Exptl. Therap.* 169: 315–320, 1969.
268. SHELBURNE, J. C., S. D. SERENA, AND G. A. LANGER. Rate-tension staircase in rabbit ventricular muscle: relation to ionic exchange. *Am. J. Physiol.* 213: 1115–1124, 1967.
269. SHINE, K. I., S. D. SERENA, AND G. A. LANGER. Kinetic localization of contractile calcium in rabbit myocardium. *Am. J. Physiol.* 221: 1408–1417, 1971.
270. SHINEBOURNE, E. A., M. L. HESS, R. J. WHITE, AND J. HAMER. The effect of noradrenaline on calcium uptake of the sarcoplasmic reticulum. *Cardiovascular Res.* 3: 113–117, 1969.
271. SHINEBOURNE, E. A., AND R. WHITE. Cyclic AMP and calcium uptake of the sarcoplasmic reticulum in relation to increased rate of relaxation under the influence of catecholamines. *Cardiovascular Res.* 4: 194–200, 1970.
272. SIMPSON, F. O., AND D. G. RAYNS. The relationship between the transverse tubular system and other tubules at the Z disc levels of myocardial cells in the ferret. *Am. J. Anat.* 122: 193–208, 1968.
273. SKELTON, C. L., G. S. LEVEY, AND S. E. EPSTEIN. Positive inotropic effects of dibutyryl cyclic AMP. *Circulation Res.* 26: 35–44, 1970.
274. SKOU, J. C. Enzymatic basis for active transport of Na$^+$ and K$^+$ across cell membrane. *Physiol. Rev.* 45: 596–617, 1965.
275. SODERLING, T. R., J. P. HICKENBOTTOM, E. M. REIMANN, F. L. HUNKELER, D. A. WALSH, AND E. G. KREBS. Inactivation of glycogen synthetase and activation of phosphorylase kinase by muscle adenosine 3',5' monophosphate-dependent protein kinases. *J. Biol. Chem.* 245: 6317–6328, 1970.
276. SONNENBLICK, E. H. Active state in heart muscle. Its delayed onset and modification by inotropic agents. *J. Gen. Physiol.* 50: 661–676, 1967.
277. SONNENBLICK, E. H., AND A. C. STAM, JR. Cardiac muscle: activation and contraction. *Ann. Rev. Physiol.* 31: 647–674, 1969.
278. STALEY, N. A., AND E. S. BENSON. The ultrastructure of frog ventricular cardiac muscle and its relationship to mechanisms of excitation-contraction coupling. *J. Cell Biol.* 38: 99–114, 1968.
279. STAM, A. C., JR., AND C. R. HONIG. A biochemical mechanism by which adrenergic mediators modify cardiac contraction. *Am. J. Physiol.* 209: 8–16, 1965.
280. STAM, A. C., JR., W. B. WEGLICKI, JR., D. FELDMAN, J. C. SHELBURNE, AND E. H. SONNENBLICK. Canine myocardial sarcolemma—its preparation and enzymic activity. *J. Mol. Cellular Cardiol.* 1: 117–130, 1970.
281. STUBBS, S. ST. G., AND M. C. BLANCHAER. Glycogen phosphorylase and glycogen synthetase activity in red and white skeletal muscle of the guinea pig. *Can. J. Biochem.* 43: 463–468, 1965.
281a. STULL, J. T., C. O. BROSTROM, AND E. G. KREBS. Phosphorylation of the inhibitor component of troponin by phosphorylase kinase. *J. Biol. Chem.* 247: 5272–5274, 1972.

282. SU, J. Y., AND P. E. POOL. Effects of cyclic 3',5'-AMP (cAMP) on glycerol-extracted cardiac muscle. *Pharmacologist* 12: 267, 1970.
283. SULAKHE, P. V., AND N. S. DHALLA. Excitation-contraction coupling in heart. VI. Demonstration of calcium activated ATPase in the dog heart sarcolemma. *Life Sci., Part 1* 10: 185–191, 1971.
284. SUTHERLAND, E. W., I. ØYE, AND R. W. BUTCHER. The action of epinephrine and the role of the adenyl cyclase system in hormone action. *Recent Progr. Hormone Res.* 21: 623–646, 1965.
285. SUTHERLAND, E. W., AND T. W. RALL. The relation of adenosine 3',5'-phosphate and phosphorylase to the actions of catecholamines and other hormones. *Pharmacol. Rev.* 12: 265–299, 1960.
286. SUTHERLAND, E. W., T. W. RALL, AND T. MENON. Adenyl cyclase. I. Distribution, preparation, and properties. *J. Biol. Chem.* 237: 1220–1227, 1962.
287. SUTHERLAND, E. W., AND G. A. ROBISON. The role of cyclic 3',5'-AMP in responses to catecholamines and other hormones. *Pharmacol. Rev.* 18: 145–161, 1966.
288. SUTHERLAND, E. W., AND G. A. ROBISON. The Banting Memorial Lecture 1969. The role of cyclic AMP in the control of carbohydrate metabolism. *Diabetes* 18: 797–819, 1969.
289. SUTHERLAND, E. W., G. A. ROBISON, AND R. W. BUTCHER. Some aspects of the biological role of adenosine 3',5'-monophosphate (cyclic AMP). *Circulation* 37: 279–306, 1968.
290. TAKEDA, M., H. YAMAMURA, AND Y. OHGA. Phosphoprotein kinases associated with rat liver chromatin. *Biochem. Biophys. Res. Commun.* 42: 103–110, 1971.
291. TAO, M., M. L. SALAS, AND F. LIPMANN. Mechanism of activation by adenosine 3',5'-cyclic monophosphate of a protein phosphokinase from rabbit reticulocytes. *Proc. Natl. Acad. Sci. US* 67: 408–414, 1970.
292. VAN BREEMEN, D., AND C. VAN BREEMEN. Calcium exchange diffusion in a porous phospholipid ion-exchange membrane. *Nature* 223: 898–900, 1969.
293. VAN DER KLOOT, W. G. Potassium-stimulated respiration and intracellular calcium release in frog skeletal muscle. *J. Physiol., London* 191: 141–165, 1967.
294. VARGA, L. Observations on glycerinated muscle fibers. *Enzymologia* 14: 392–396, 1950.
295. VASSINGTON, F. D., P. GAZZOTTI, R. TIOZZO, AND E. CARAFOLI. The effect of ruthenium red in Ca^{2+} transport and respiration in rat liver mitochondria. *Biochim. Biophys. Acta* 256: 43–54, 1972.
296. VASSORT, G., O. ROUGIER, D. GARNIER, M-P. SAUVIAT, E. CORABOEUF, AND Y-M. GARGOUÏL. Effets de l'adrénaline sur les courants entrants transmembranaires au cours de l'activité cardiaque. *Compt. Rend.* 267: 1762–1765, 1968.
297. VILLAR-PALASI, C. The hormonal regulation of glycogen metabolism in muscle. *Vitamins Hormones* 26: 65–118, 1968.
298. VILLAR-PALASI, C., AND J. LARNER. Glycogen metabolism and glycolytic enzymes. *Ann. Rev. Biochem.* 39: 639–672, 1970.
299. VINCENT, N. H., AND S. ELLIS. Inhibitory effect of acetylcholine on glycogenolysis in the isolated guinea-pig heart. *J. Pharmacol. Exptl. Therap.* 139: 60–68, 1963.
300. WAKABAYASHI, T., AND S. EBASHI. Reversible change in physical state of troponin induced by calcium ion. *J. Biochem., Tokyo* 64: 731–732, 1968.
301. WALSH, D. A., C. D. ASHBY, C. GONZALEZ, D. CALKINS, E. H. FISCHER, AND E. G. KREBS. Purification and characterization of a protein inhibitor of adenosine 3',5'-monophosphate-dependent protein kinases. *J. Biol. Chem.* 246: 1977–1985, 1971.
302. WALSH, D. A., E. G. KREBS, E. M. REIMANN, M. A. BROSTROM, J. D. CORBIN, J. P. HICKENBOTTOM, T. R. SODERLING, AND J. P. PERKINS. The receptor protein for cyclic AMP in the control of glycogenolysis. In: *Advances in Biochemical Psychopharmacology: Role of Cyclic AMP in Cell Function*, edited by P. Greengard and E. Costa. New York: Raven Press, 1970, vol. 3, p. 265–285.
303. WALSH, D. A., J. P. PERKINS, C. O. BROSTROM, E. S. HO,

AND E. G. KREBS. Catalysis of the phosphorylase kinase activation reaction. *J. Biol. Chem.* 246: 1968–1976, 1971.
304. WALSH, D. A., J. P. PERKINS, AND E. G. KREBS. An adenosine 3′,5′-monophosphate-dependent protein kinase from rabbit skeletal muscle. *J. Biol. Chem.* 243: 3763–3774, 1968.
305. WANG, J. H., M. L. SHONKA, AND D. J. GRAVES. The effect of glucose on the sedimentation and catalytic activity of glycogen phosphorylase. *Biochem. Biophys. Res. Commun.* 18: 131–135, 1965.
306. WAUD, D. R. Pharmacological receptors. *Pharmacol. Rev.* 20: 49–88, 1968.
307. WEBER, A., R. HERZ, AND I. REISS. The regulation of myofibrillar activity by calcium. *Proc. Roy. Soc. London Ser. B* 160: 489–501, 1964.
308. WEBER, A. Energized calcium transport and relaxing factors. In: *Current Topics in Bioenergetics*, edited by D. R. Sanadi. New York: Acad. Press, 1966, vol. 1, p. 203–254.
309. WEBER, A. Regulatory mechanisms of the calcium transport system of fragmented rabbit sarcoplasmic reticulum. I. The effect of accumulated calcium on transport and adenosine triphosphate hydrolysis. *J. Gen. Physiol.* 57: 50–63, 1971.
310. WEBER, A., AND R. HERZ. The binding of calcium to actomyosin systems in relation to their biological activity. *J. Biol. Chem.* 238: 599–605, 1963.
311. WEBER, A., R. HERZ, AND I. REISS. Study of the kinetics of calcium transport by isolated fragmented sarcoplasmic reticulum. *Biochem. Z.* 345: 329–369, 1966.
312. WEINER, N. The catecholamines: biosynthesis, storage and release, metabolism and metabolic effects. In: *The Hormones*, edited by G. Pincus and K. Thimann. New York: Acad. Press, 1964, vol. 4, p. 403–479.
313. WILDENTHAL, K., D. S. MIERZWIAK, R. W. MYERS, AND J. H. MITCHELL. Effects of acute lactic acidosis on left ventricular performance. *Am. J. Physiol.* 214: 1352–1359, 1968.
314. WILLIAMS, B. J., AND S. E. MAYER. Hormonal effects on glycogen metabolism in the rat heart *in situ*. *Mol. Pharmacol.* 2: 454–464, 1966.
315. WILLIAMSON, J. R. Metabolic effects of epinephrine in the isolated perfused rat heart. I. Dissociation of the glycogenolytic from the metabolic stimulatory effect. *J. Biol. Chem.* 239: 2721–2729, 1964.
316. WILLIAMSON, J. R. Metabolic effects of epinephrine in the perfused rat heart. II. Control steps of glucose and glycogen metabolism. *Mol. Pharmacol.* 2: 206–220, 1966.
317. WILLIAMSON, J. R. Kinetic studies of epinephrine effects in the perfused rat heart. *Pharmacol. Rev.* 18: 205–210, 1966.
318. WILLIAMSON, J. R., AND D. JAMIESON. Dissociation of the inotropic from the glycogenolytic effect of epinephrine in the isolated rat heart. *Nature* 206: 364–367, 1965.
319. WILLIAMSON, J. R., AND D. JAMIESON. Metabolic effects of epinephrine in the perfused rat heart. I. Comparison of intracellular redox states, tissue PO_2 and force of contraction. *Mol. Pharmacol.* 2: 191–205, 1966.
320. WINEGRAD, S. Intracellular calcium movements of frog skeletal muscle during recovery from tetanus. *J. Gen. Physiol.* 51: 65–83, 1968.
321. WINEGRAD, S. Calcium and striated muscle. *Mineral Metab.* 3: 191–233, 1969.
322. WINEGRAD, S. The intracellular site of calcium activation of contraction in frog skeletal muscle. *J. Gen. Physiol.* 55: 77–88, 1970.
323. WINEGRAD, S. Studies of cardiac muscle with a high permeability to calcium produced by treatment with ethylenediaminetetraacetic acid. *J. Gen. Physiol.* 58: 71–93, 1971.
324. WINEGRAD, S., AND A. M. SHANES. Calcium flux and contractility in guinea pig atria. *J. Gen. Physiol.* 45: 371–394, 1962.
325. WOOD, E. H., R. L. HEPPNER, AND S. WEIDMANN. Inotropic effects of electric currents. I. Positive and negative effects of constant electric currents or current impulses applied during cardiac action potentials. II. Hypotheses: calcium movements, excitation-contraction coupling and inotropic effects. *Circulation Res.* 24: 409–445, 1969.
326. YAMAMURA, H., A. KUMON, AND Y. NISHIZUKA. Cross-reactions of adenosine 3′,5′ monophosphate dependent protein kinase systems from rat liver and rabbit skeletal muscle. *J. Biol. Chem.* 246: 1544–1547, 1971.
327. YAMAMURA, H., M. TAKEDA, A. KUMON, AND Y. NISHIZUKA. Adenosine 3′,5′-cyclic phosphate-dependent and independent histone kinases from rat liver. *Biochem. Biophys. Res. Commun.* 40: 675–682, 1970.
328. YASUI, B., F. FUCHS, AND F. N. BRIGGS. The role of the sulfhydryl groups of tropomyosin and troponin in the calcium control of actomyosin contractility. *J. Biol. Chem.* 243: 735–742, 1968.

REFERENCES IN ADDENDUM

1A. ABBOTT, B. C., AND J. V. HOWORTH. Heart studies in excitable tissues. *Physiol. Rev.* 53: 120–158, 1973.
2A. BASSINGTHWAIGHTE, J. B., AND H. REUTER. Calcium movements and excitation-contraction coupling in cardiac cells. In: *Electrical Phenomena in Heart*, edited by W. C. DeMello. New York: Acad. Press, 1972, p. 353–395.
3A. BORLE, A. B. Cyclic AMP stimulation of calcium efflux from kidney, liver, and heart mitochondria. *J. Membrane Biol.* 16: 221–236, 1974.
4A. BROOKER, G. Oscillation of cyclic adenosine monophosphate concentration during the myocardial contraction cycle. *Science* 182: 933–934, 1973.
5A. COLD SPRING HARBOR LABORATORY. The mechanism of muscle contraction. *Cold Spring Harbor Symp. Quant. Biol.* 37, 1972.
6A. ENDO, M., AND Y. NAKAJIMA. Release of calcium induced by 'depolarisation' of the sarcoplasmic reticulum membrane. *Nature New Biol.* 246: 216–218, 1973.
7A. FABIATO, A., AND F. FABIATO. Excitation-contraction coupling of isolated cardiac fibers with disrupted or closed sarcolemmas. Calcium dependent cyclic and tonic contractions. *Circulation Res.* 31: 293–307, 1972.
8A. FABIATO, A., AND F. FABIATO. Activation of skinned cardiac cells: subcellular effects of cardioactive drugs. *European J. Cardiol.* 1: 143–155, 1973.
9A. FORD, L. E., AND R. J. PODOLSKY. Calcium uptake and force development by skinned muscle fibres in EGTA buffered solutions. *J. Physiol., London* 223: 1–19, 1972.
10A. FORD, L. E., AND R. J. PODOLSKY. Intracellular calcium movements in skinned muscle fibres. *J. Physiol., London* 223: 21–33, 1972.
11A. FUCHS, F. Striated muscle. *Ann. Rev. Physiol.* 36: 461–502, 1974.
12A. INESI, G. Active transport of calcium ions in sarcoplasmic reticulum membranes. *Ann. Rev. Biophys. Bioenergetics* 1: 191–210, 1972.
13A. KASAI, M., AND H. MIYAMOTO. Depolarization induced calcium release from sarcoplasmic reticulum membrane fragments by changing ionic environment. *FEBS Letters* 34: 299–301, 1973.
14A. KIRCHBERGER, M. A., M. TADA, AND A. KATZ. Adenosine 3′,5′-monophosphate-dependent protein kinase catalysed phosphorylation reaction and its relationship to calcium transport in cardiac sarcoplasmic reticulum. *J. Biol. Chem.* In press.
15A. KIRCHBERGER, M. A., M. TADA, D. I. REPKE, AND A. M. KATZ. Cyclic adenosine 3′,5′-monophosphate-dependent protein kinase stimulation of calcium uptake by canine cardiac microsomes. *J. Mol. Cell. Cardiol.* 4: 673–680, 1972.
16A. KOHLHARDT, M., B. BAUER, H. KRAUSE, AND A. FLECKENSTEIN. Differentiation of the transmembrane Na^+ and Ca^{2+} channels in mammalian cardiac fibres by the use of specific inhibitors. *Arch. Ges. Physiol.* 335: 309–322, 1972.
17A. LANGER, G. A. Heart: excitation-contraction coupling. *Ann. Rev. Physiol.* 35: 55–86, 1973.

18a. MARTONOSI, A. Biochemical and clinical aspects of sarcoplasmic reticulum function. In: *Current Topics in Membranes and Transport*, edited by F. Bronner and A. Kleinzeller. New York: Acad. Press, 1972, vol. III, p. 83–197.
19a. MATLIB, A., AND P. J. O'BRIEN. Cyclic AMP stimulation of calcium efflux from mitochondria. *Biochem. Soc. Trans.* In press.
20a. MOMMAERTS, W. F. H. M. Energetics of contraction. In: *Muscle Biology*, edited by R. G. Cassens. New York: Dekker, 1972, vol. I, p. 1–12.
21a. MORAD, M., AND Y. GOLDMAN. Excitation-contraction coupling in heart muscle: membrane control of development of tension. *Progr. Biophys. Mol. Biol.* 27: 259–313, 1973.
22a. MORKIN, E., AND P. J. LA RAIA. Biochemical studies in the regulation of myocardial contractility. *Seminars Med. Beth Israel Hosp. Boston* 290: 445–451, 1974.
23a. NEELY, J. R., AND H. E. MORGAN. Relationship between carbohydrate and lipid metabolism and the energy balance of heart muscle. *Ann. Rev. Physiol.* 36: 413–459, 1974.
24a. NEELY, J. R., M. J. ROVETTO, AND J. F. ORAM. Myocardial utilization of carbohydrate and lipids. *Progr. Cardiovascular Diseases* 15: 289–329, 1972.
25a. REUTER, H. Divalent cations as charge carriers in excitable membranes. *Progr. Biophys. Mol. Biol.* 26: 1–43, 1973.
26a. ROLETT, E. L. Adrenergic mechanisms in mammalian myocardium. In: *The Mammalian Myocardium*, edited by G. A. Langer and A. Brady. New York: Wiley, 1974, p. 219–250.
27a. SCARPA, A., AND P. GRAZIOTTI. Mechanism for intracellular calcium regulation in heart. I. Stopped-flow measurements of Ca^{2+} uptake by cardiac mitochondria. *J. Gen. Physiol.* 62: 756–772, 1973.
28a. SHIGENOBU, K., AND N. SPERELAKIS. Calcium current channels induced by catecholamines in chick embryonic hearts whose fast sodium channels are blocked by tetrodotoxin or elevated potassium. *Circulation Res.* 31: 932–952, 1972.
29a. SHIGETO, N., AND H. IRISAWA. Slow conduction in the atrioventricular node of the cat: a possible explanation. *Experientia* 28: 1442–1443, 1972.
30a. SULAKHE, P. V., AND G. I. DRUMMOND. Protein kinase-catalysed phosphorylation of muscle sarcolemma. *Arch. Biochem. Biophys.* 161: 448–455, 1974.
31a. TADA, M., M. A. KIRCHBERGER, J-A. IORIO, AND A. KATZ. Effects of a cardiac adenosine 3',5'-monophosphate dependent protein kinase on the cardiac sarcoplasmic reticulum: role of a 22,000 dalton protein component. *J. Biol. Chem.* In press.
32a. TADA, M., M. A. KIRCHBERGER, D. I. REPKE, AND A. M. KATZ. The stimulation of calcium transport in cardiac sarcoplasmic reticulum by adenosine 3',5'-monophosphate-dependent protein kinase. *J. Biol. Chem.* In press.
33a. TRITTHART, H., R. VOLKMANN, R. WEISS, AND A. FLECKENSTEIN. Calcium-mediated action potentials in mammalian myocardium. *Arch. Exptl. Pathol. Pharmacol.* 280: 239–252, 1973.
34a. TSIEN, R. W. Adrenaline-like effects of intracellular iontophoresis of cyclic AMP in cardiac Purkinje fibres. *Nature New Biol.* 245: 120–122, 1973.
35a. TSIEN, R. W., W. GILES, AND P. GREENGARD. Cyclic AMP mediates the effects of adrenaline in cardiac Purkinje fibers. *Nature New Biol.* 240: 181–183, 1972.
36a. WEBER, A., AND J. M. MURRAY. Molecular control mechanisms in muscle contraction. *Physiol. Rev.* 53: 612–672, 1973.
37a. WEIDMANN, S. Heart: electrophysiology. *Ann. Rev. Physiol.* 36: 155–169, 1974.
38a. WILLIAMSON, J. R., B. SAFER, K. F. LA NOUE, C. M. SMITH, AND E. WALAJTYS. Mitochondrial-cytosolic interactions in cardiac tissue: role of the malate-aspartate cycle in the removal of glycolytic NADH from the cytosol. *Symp. Soc. Exptl. Biol.* 27: 241–281, 1973.
39a. WOLEDGE, R. C. Heat production and chemical change in muscle. *Progr. Biophys. Mol. Biol.* 22: 37–74, 1971.
40a. WOLLENBERGER, A., E. B. BABSKII, E-G. KRAUSE, S. GENZ, D. BLOHM, AND E. V. BOGDANOVA. Cyclic changes in levels of cyclic AMP and cyclic GMP in frog myocardium during the cardiac cycle. *Biochem. Biophys. Res. Commun.* 55: 446–452, 1973.
41a. WRAY, H. L., R. R. GRAY, AND R. A. OLSSON. Cyclic adenosine 3',5'-monophosphate stimulated protein kinase and a substrate associated with cardiac sarcoplasmic reticulum. *J. Biol. Chem.* 248: 1496–1498, 1973.

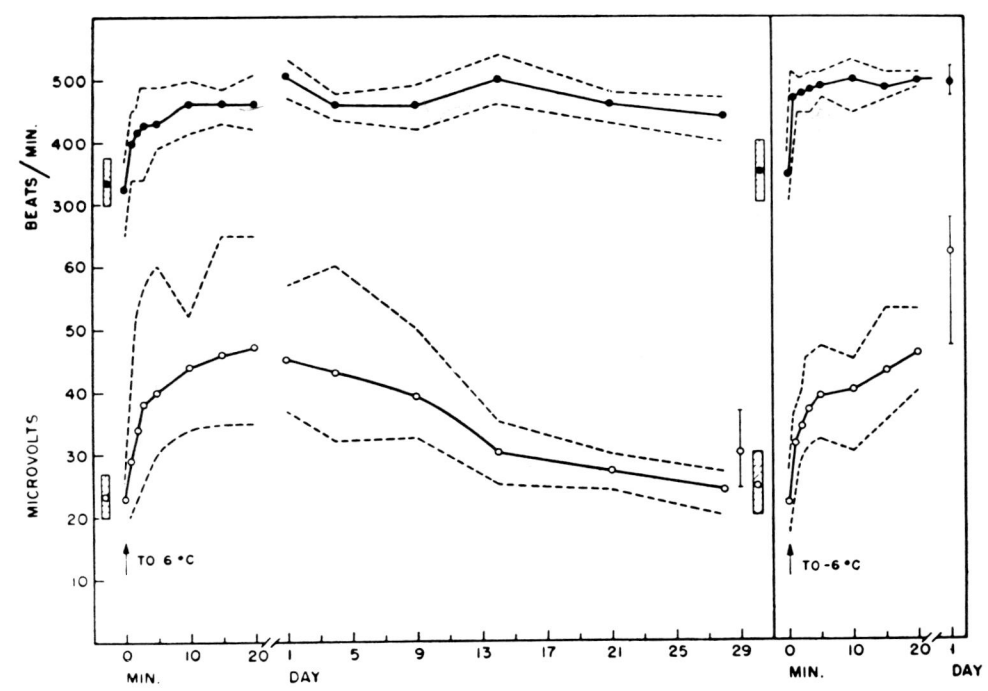

FIG. 5. Decrease in shivering, as measured by muscle electrical activity, during acclimation to cold. Muscle electrical activity and heart rate as related to time of exposure to 6 C and −6 C are shown. *Solid line* in *left-hand part* of diagram shows muscle electrical activity (*lower tracing*) and heart rate (*upper tracing*) in rats living at 6 C. *Broken lines* show range of variation. *Vertical bars* at 0 and 29 days show muscle electrical activity (*lower*) and heart rate (*upper*) in warm-acclimated rats living at 30 C. At 30 days cold-acclimated rats were moved to −6 C (*right-hand part* of diagram). [From Hart et al. (76).]

Role of Adrenal Medulla in Acclimation to Cold

The sympathetic nervous system is not only responsible for the switching on and off of nonshivering thermogenesis in cold-acclimated animals, but also, at least in part, for the development of the adaptation that allows nonshivering thermogenesis to occur. This role of the sympathetic nervous system is the least well understood of all the roles to be discussed in this chapter.

Experimental Approaches

The assessment of the relative roles of the adrenal medulla and of the remainder of the sympathetic nervous system in the metabolic responses of animals to cold is difficult to achieve experimentally. Three major questions can be asked about these roles:

1. To what extent is the sympathetic nervous system activated? Is enough epinephrine or norepinephrine, or both, secreted to produce the effects believed to be caused by the catecholamines?
2. What are the effects of epinephrine and norepinephrine?
3. How do epinephrine and norepinephrine exert those effects believed to be involved in the acclimation to cold?

The most common approach to Question 1 is the measurement in the urine, from animals exposed to cold or acclimated to cold, of epinephrine, norepinephrine, and certain of their metabolites, such as metanephrine, normetanephrine, 3,4-dihydroxyphenylglycol (DHPG), 3,4-dihydroxymandelic acid (DHMA), 3-methoxy-4-hydroxyphenylglycol (MHPG), and 3-methoxy-4-hydroxymandelic acid (MHMA). The major problems with this approach are *a*) the proportion of unchanged epinephrine and norepinephrine in the urine is exceedingly small compared with the total catecholamine metabolites, and unfortunately in many studies the unchanged catecholamines have been the only compounds measured; *b*) the major metabolites [MHPG or MHMA, depending on the species: MHPG is the major metabolite in the rat (109)] can be derived from both epinephrine and norepinephrine; and *c*) much of the norepinephrine that is secreted from nerve endings is taken up again into the same nerve endings so that a large part of it may not appear in the urine in any form. Thus this approach can yield information about changes in the activity of the sympathetic nervous system but cannot hope to measure them.

There are two approaches to Question 2. The first involves study of the extent to which administered catecholamines can mimic the effect of cold exposure and cold acclimation. The second involves inactivation, by surgical, immunological, or pharmacological means, of either one or both parts of the sympathetic nervous system. The major problem with this approach is that

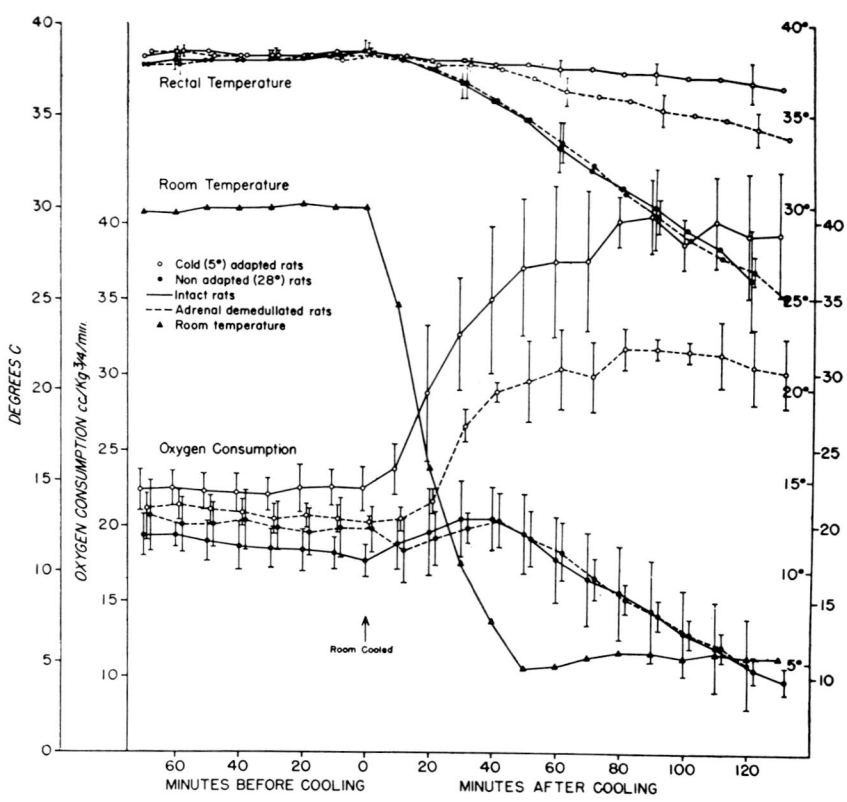

FIG. 6. Increased capacity for nonshivering thermogenesis in cold-acclimated rats. Metabolic response of curarized, warm- and cold-acclimated rats to lowered ambient temperature is shown. Mean oxygen consumption and rectal temperature of each group along with ambient temperature are plotted on *ordinate*, minutes before and after cooling on *abscissa*. Standard deviations are indicated by *vertical lines*. Effect of adrenal demedullation on nonshivering thermogenesis in warm-acclimated and cold-acclimated rats is shown. [From Cottle & Carlson (36).]

most animals are sufficiently adaptable so that other regulatory mechanisms can be brought into play when the regulatory mechanism normally subserved by the inactivated part of the sympathetic nervous system is missing, a phenomenon that has been recognized for many years (1). Thus the observation that removal of the adrenal medulla does not lead to a change in a particular metabolic response does not necessarily mean that the adrenal medulla played no part in the response when it was present in the animal; the adrenal medulla may have played a most important role when it was present, but this role may have been assumed by the remainder of the sympathetic nervous system when the adrenal medulla was absent.

Question 3 is by far the most difficult to answer. Although the advances in understanding of the nature and regulation of metabolic processes during recent years allow a fairly complete description of the metabolism of animals exposed to cold or subjected to stimulation by administered catecholamines, an elusive fundamental mechanism of the calorigenic effect of the catecholamines, and particularly of the enhanced calorigenic effect that occurs in cold-acclimated animals, remains to be explained.

The remainder of this chapter is divided into three major sections, each of which represents an attempt to answer, as far as is presently possible, the three questions posed above.

ACTIVATION OF SYMPATHETIC NERVOUS SYSTEM BY COLD

Excretion of Catecholamines and Their Metabolites

The excretion in the urine of both epinephrine and norepinephrine is increased in animals exposed to cold (see Table 1). The most commonly studied species has been the rat, but the other species studied similarly increase their excretion of catecholamines when stimulated by cold. The numerical values reported for the rate of excretion vary rather widely from one study to another, most probably because of differences in assay techniques used. However, there is no doubt that an increase in excretion of catecholamines does occur in the cold. The magnitude of the increase depends on the temperature of exposure [e.g., increase greater at lower temperatures (126)] and also on age, at least in the rat [e.g., increase greater in younger animals (126)]. The most complete study of the excretion of unchanged

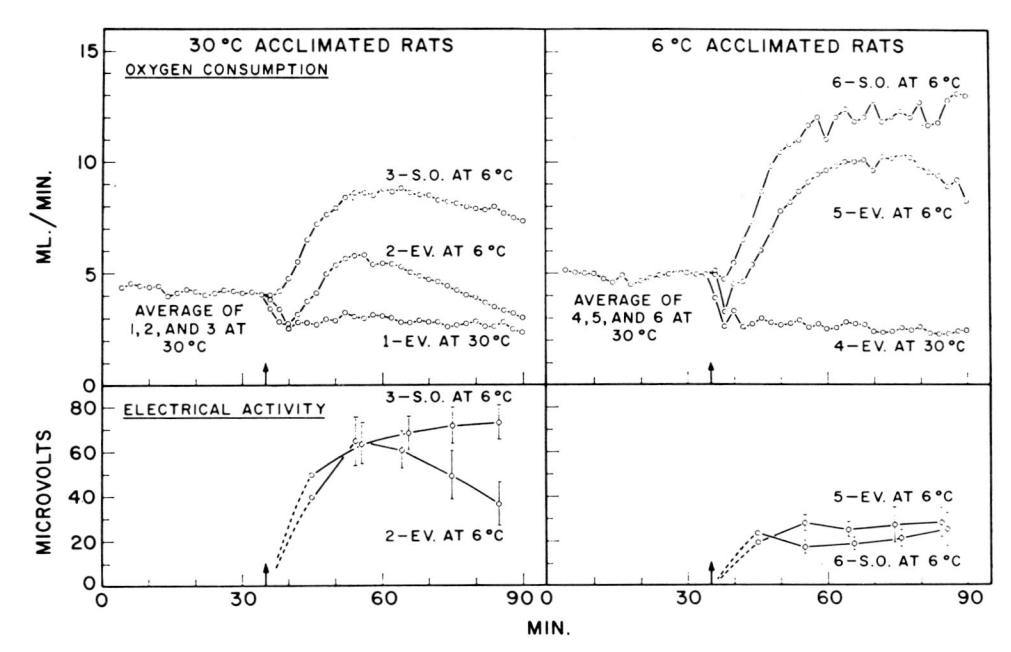

FIG. 7. Persistence of nonshivering thermogenesis in functionally eviscerated rats. Average O₂ consumption and muscle electrical activity of barbital-anesthetized, 30 C- and 6 C-acclimated rats at 30 C (average O₂ consumption of all similarly acclimated rats given for 0–35-min interval), at 30 C after evisceration (groups 1 and 4), at 6 C after evisceration (groups 2 and 5), and at 6 C after sham-operation (groups 3 and 6) are shown. *Arrow* indicates time of evisceration or transfer to 6 C, or both. All groups consisted of 5 animals, except group 3 in which there were 6. Evisceration consisted of tying off the rectal colon, celiac and superior mesenteric arteries, and the portal vein; this procedure effectively prevents blood flow through intestine and liver. *S.O*, sham-operated; *EV.*, eviscerated. [From Depocas (43), with permission of the National Research Council of Canada.]

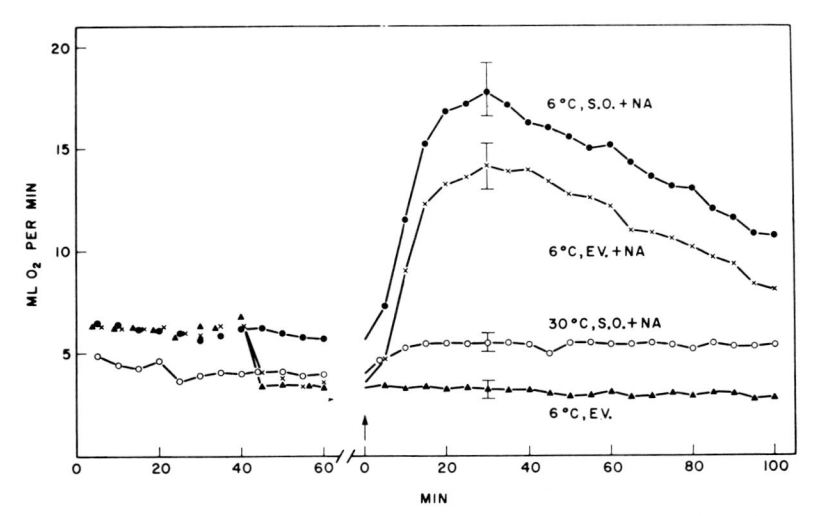

FIG. 8. Persistence of enhanced calorigenic response to norepinephrine in functionally eviscerated, cold-acclimated rats. Average oxygen consumption of barbital-anesthetized, cold-acclimated rats (3 rats per group) functionally eviscerated and infused with 0.1% sodium bisulphite in saline (*6°C, EV.*), functionally eviscerated and infused with norepinephrine (in 0.1% sodium bisulphite in saline) at a dose of 1 μg/min (*6°C, EV. + NA*), sham-operated and infused with norepinephrine at the same dose level (*6°C, S.O. + NA*). Average oxygen consumption of 2 warm-acclimated rats, sham-operated and infused with norepinephrine (*30°C, S.O. + NA*), is also given. *Arrow* indicates start of infusion that lasted 100 min. *Vertical bars* indicate total range of variation. *S.O.* sham-operated; *EV.*, eviscerated; *NA*, norepinephrine. [From Depocas (44), with permission of the National Research Council of Canada.]

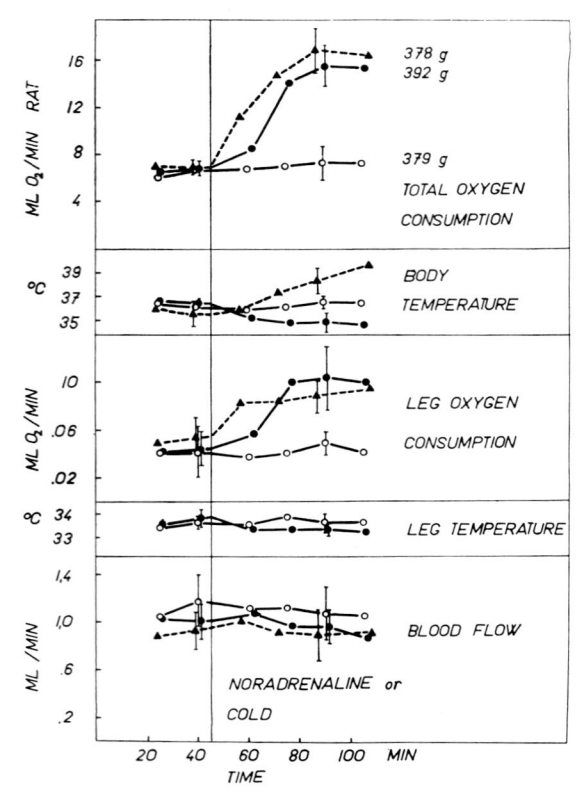

FIG. 9. Occurrence of nonshivering thermogenesis and of calorigenic response to norepinephrine in leg muscle of cold-acclimated rats. Comparison of responses in the leg and in the whole rat before and during norepinephrine infusion at 0.8 µg/min (▲) or exposure to 10 C (●). *Vertical line* at 45 min shows start of norepinephrine (*noradrenaline*) or cold. Untreated controls (○) are also indicated. *Vertical lines* denote SD. Results not corrected for change in body temperature during tests. [From Jansky & Hart (94), with permission of the National Research Council of Canada.]

catecholamines in the urine is that of Leduc (126); in this study the relations between age and temperature and the excretion of catecholamines in the rat are thoroughly documented.

The excretion of metabolites of the catecholamines has been studied in cold-exposed animals to only a limited extent (Table 1). However, in order to assess the significance of the changes in epinephrine and norepinephrine excretion, it is of importance to compare the excretion of the metabolites with the excretion of the unchanged catecholamines. In this way it might be possible to assess what proportion of the total catecholamines lost from the body is excreted unchanged. The following analysis is based on values presented in three papers (145, 168, 171). Before exposure to cold the average excretion of epinephrine was 0.021 µg/kg per hour and of norepinephrine, 0.075 µg/kg per hour. The methylated derivatives, metanephrine and normetanephrine, amounted to 0.19 and 0.32 µg/kg per hour, respectively, whereas the methylated and deaminated metabolites, MHPG and MHMA, amounted to 7.75 and 4.00 µg/kg per hour, respectively. The proportion of unchanged catecholamine is only 0.78 % of the total, of which 0.61 %

is represented by norepinephrine and 0.17% by epinephrine. Even if epinephrine and metanephrine are omitted from the calculation and it is assumed that all the MHPG and MHMA were derived from norepinephrine, the proportion of unchanged norepinephrine would be only 0.62%. When the rats were exposed to cold (3–4 C) for 1 day, the excretion of all these compounds increased but the relative proportions of un-

TABLE 1. *Increased Excretion of Catecholamines and Their Metabolites During Exposure of Warm-acclimated Animals to Cold*

Catecholamine or Metabolite	Species	Temperature of Exposure, C	Ref.
Norepinephrine	Rat	7	130
		5	9
		4	103, 104, 168, 171
		3	99, 126, 146
		−16	122
	Mouse	−10	123
	Pig	10	5
	Newborn human	20–27	176
		18–20	163
	Man	10–15	180
		6	4
		−5 to +2	203
	Sheep	−27 to −6	198
Epinephrine	Rat	7	130
		5	9
		4	103, 104, 168, 171
		3	99, 126, 145
		−16	122
	Mouse	−10	123
	Pig	10	5
	Newborn human	20–27	176
		18–20*	163
	Man	10–15	180
		6	4
		−5 to +2	203
	Sheep	−27 to −6	198
Normetanephrine	Rat	15	172
		7	130
		4	168, 171
Metanephrine	Rat	15*	172
		7	130
		4	171
MHPG	Rat	15	172
		4	104, 168, 171
MHMA	Rat	7	130
		3	145
	Newborn human	24	161
Dopamine	Rat, young	3	126
	Rat, old	3†	63, 126
	Man	−5 to +2	203
	Newborn human	18–20	163

MHPG, 3-methoxy-4-hydroxyphenylglycol; MHMA, 3-methoxy-4-hydroxymandelic acid. *No increase. †Very small change.

changed catecholamines changed very little. Of the increased excretion in the cold (above that which occurred in the warm), by far the largest component was MHPG (82.3%) and the next largest component was MHMA (15.8%); unchanged norepinephrine was still only 0.61% of the total.

Although the proportion of unchanged norepinephrine excreted appears to remain constant, it is so exceedingly small (about 0.6%) that the calculation of secretion rates of norepinephrine from the urinary excretion of norepinephrine itself is very difficult. Another difficulty is that much of the norepinephrine secreted from nerve endings is taken up into storage again at the same site and therefore may not appear in the urine either as free norepinephrine or as metabolites of norepinephrine. Thus calculation of secretion rate by the use of conversion factors based on the proportion of injected norepinephrine recovered unchanged in the urine [about 2.5% (126)] is not possible because injected norepinephrine is clearly handled by the body in a different way from norepinephrine secreted at nerve endings.

In theory a calculation of epinephrine secretion could be based on the excretion of unchanged epinephrine in the urine, by using a formula based on the recovery of epinephrine in the urine after its injection. Since epinephrine is normally secreted into the bloodstream, problems of local uptake do not arise. However, the adrenal medulla would normally secrete epinephrine into the blood in small but fairly constant amounts over prolonged periods, and the single injection of a large quantity of epinephrine, either subcutaneously or intramuscularly, as it is usually given, may bring into play degradative mechanisms that are not normally involved in handling the slow secretion by the adrenal medulla. For this reason, such a calculation may not be valid.

It is possible to calculate, from the values for excretion of catecholamine plus metabolites, a value that might be termed the minimum rate of catecholamine production (epinephrine plus norepinephrine); this value is approximately 12 µg/kg per hour for animals in the warm and 45.5 µg/kg per hour for animals in the cold. Such a value compares reasonably well with the minimal amount of norepinephrine needed (by intravenous infusion) to produce a calorigenic response in warm-acclimated and in cold-acclimated rats; the dose needed in either case to produce a maximal response is approximately 300 µg/kg per hour. Although it seems unlikely that the amount of epinephrine secreted by the adrenal medulla alone could ever be sufficiently high to produce a maximum calorigenic response (the sensitivity to epinephrine administered by intravenous infusion is almost exactly the same as the sensitivity to norepinephrine), it is clear that norepinephrine liberated at nerve endings, much of which, it must be remembered, never appears in the urine in any form, might be present at the appropriate receptors in sufficient concentration to produce a maximum calorigenic response, such as that produced by intravenous infusion of norepinephrine at a rate of approximately 300 µg/kg per hour. Most of the intravenously infused norepinephrine is probably metabolized very rapidly, and relatively little of it actually reaches the receptors. The rapidity with which the response ceases when the intravenous infusion is stopped supports the idea of rapid metabolism or uptake.

Once rats have become cold acclimated (i.e., once they have spent 4 or more weeks in the cold) the rate of excretion of the catecholamines and their metabolites is less than during the early phases of cold exposure. This phenomenon was first noted by Leduc (126) who observed that after 4 weeks in the cold the excretion of epinephrine returned to the low level seen in warm-acclimated rats; the amount of norepinephrine excreted was also much less after 4 weeks than during the first week of cold exposure, although it remained at an elevated level for as long as the rats continued to live in the cold (up to 6 months) (Fig. 10).

Increases in excretion of the metabolites of the catecholamines during the first 4 weeks of cold exposure have been reported by Shum et al. (171). The excretion of MHPG remains at a high level (24–28 µg/kg per hour) although not quite so high as during the first day, whereas the excretion of normetanephrine reaches a maximum after 2 weeks (1.2 µg/kg per hour) and decreases thereafter (to 0.38 µg/kg per hour). A rate of normetanephrine excretion much higher than this has also been reported for fully cold-acclimated rats (12 weeks in cold; 6.2 µg/kg per hour); the reason for this discrepancy is not clear (102).

The increase in catecholamine excretion caused by cold exposure of warm-acclimated rats is greater the lower the temperature to which they are exposed (126). During brief exposure to very low temperatures (−20 C) the excretion of epinephrine may be as high as that of norepinephrine (122). The excretion of MHPG and also of normetanephrine is directly related to ambient temperature over the range 4–30 C (171).

Cold-acclimated rats exposed to a temperature lower than the temperature of acclimation excrete more catecholamines in the urine than they do at the acclimation temperature (126). Cold-acclimated rats also excrete more catecholamines if the stress of cold exposure is increased, for example, by removing their hair but leaving them at the temperature of acclimation (126, 164); under these conditions the excretion of unchanged epinephrine in the urine is very high (0.25 µg/kg per hour), as is the excretion of unchanged norepinephrine (0.9–1.16 µg/kg per hour).

When rats have been acclimated to cold for 1 week or more, allowed to recover at room temperature, and then reexposed to the same low temperature, their excretion of norepinephrine and epinephrine is less than it would have been had they not been acclimated first (126). A similar reduction, particularly in epinephrine excretion, occurs in rats (119, 122) and mice (123) after short-term adaptation to cold.

There is, then, no doubt that the secretory activity of the adrenal medulla is increased when rats are exposed to cold, as judged by the increase in excretion of epineph-

FIG. 10. Urinary excretion of epinephrine (●) and norepinephrine (○) in rats (170–180 g) at 3 C (*solid line*) and 22 C (*dashed line*). Each point represents the mean of 6 individual rats. [From Leduc (126).]

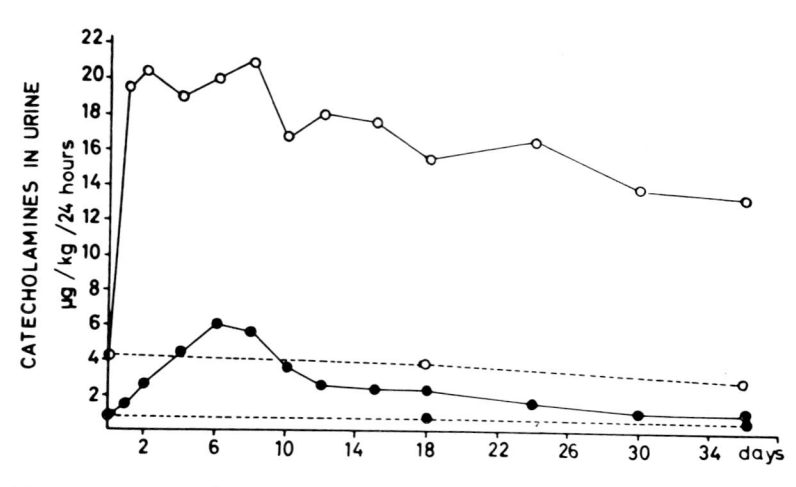

rine in the urine. During acclimation to cold this secretory activity gradually diminishes until, in the fully cold-acclimated rat, it is no greater than that of the medulla in a rat in the warm. The medulla is reactivated to secrete at a higher rate in the cold-acclimated animal if the stress of the cold exposure is further increased by lowering the temperature or by reducing the insulation of the rat by clipping its fur.

Sources of Catecholamines and Their Metabolites Excreted in Urine

The increased amount of epinephrine that appears in the urine of warm-acclimated rats exposed to cold comes almost entirely from the adrenal medulla since it does not appear in the urine of adrenalectomized (99, 100, 126) or adrenodemedullated (30, 164) rats. The increase in norepinephrine excretion is either unchanged (99) or accentuated (126) by adrenalectomy. Epinephrine is still detectable in the urine of adrenalectomized or adrenodemedullated rats and may increase slightly during exposure to cold (99, 100, 126). The source of the epinephrine has not been determined; it probably comes from extraadrenal chromaffin cells or from the brain. Once rats are fully acclimated to cold they may excrete only slightly more epinephrine than do warm-acclimated rats living in the warm (126), and adrenalectomy does not alter this small difference. However, if the basal epinephrine excretion is still much higher in the cold-acclimated rats than in the warm-acclimated rats, adrenalectomy reduces the elevated epinephrine excretion (120).

Content of Catecholamines in Adrenal Medulla

Cold exposure causes a reduction in the epinephrine content of the adrenal medulla of the warm-acclimated rats within 1 day (51, 126, 195). After 6 days in the cold the epinephrine content of the gland is greater than before exposure (126) and remains elevated throughout cold acclimation (31, 51, 126, 140). Since the excretion of epinephrine in the urine is at a maximum after 6 days in the cold it is clear that the resynthesis of epinephrine must be greatly accelerated during the early phases of cold exposure (126). Warm-acclimated rats exposed to severe cold (−7 C) have a progressive loss of epinephrine from the adrenal medulla and die within 5 to 7 days; the urinary excretion of epinephrine in these rats rises progressively to a maximum of 0.5 μg/kg per hour during the period of exposure to cold. In contrast, fully cold-acclimated rats (12 weeks at 3 C) increase their epinephrine excretion to only 0.09 μg/kg per hour and are able to maintain this rate of excretion for 12 days at −7 C; their adrenals do not become depleted; indeed they contain considerably more epinephrine at the end of 12 days exposure to −7 C than they do at the start (Fig. 11). The cold-acclimated rat therefore responds in a different way, with respect to epinephrine secretion, from the warm-acclimated rat; the capacity to do this depends on the period of acclimation to cold and appears to require at least 4 weeks. In warm-acclimated rats and in rats acclimated to the cold for only 1 or 2 weeks, death is associated with exceedingly high rates of epinephrine excretion in the urine (126). A similar very high rate of epinephrine excretion (approximately 0.4 μg/kg per hour) during exposure of warm-acclimated rats to −16 C is associated with death of the animals in hypothermia after about 4 hr (122). After short-term adaptation to cold, animals excreted much less epinephrine during exposure to −16 C and maintained their body temperature reasonably well for 4 hr (122).

Synthesis of Catecholamines

The rate of synthesis of epinephrine in the adrenal medulla during acclimation to cold can be calculated from the change in content of the gland and from the amount of the hormone excreted in the urine. Two assumptions must be made in order to permit this calculation: *1*) that the unchanged epinephrine excreted in the urine represents a constant proportion of the epinephrine secreted by the gland and that this proportion can be assumed to be the same as the proportion of subcutaneously injected epinephrine excreted unchanged in the urine; and *2*) that the proportion is constant regardless of the rate of secretion. Data reported by

content of the gland rises; after 36 days, by which time the rats would be considered cold acclimated, the rates of secretion and of synthesis have descended almost to the level seen in the warm-acclimated rat.

Although exposure to 3 C does not appear to alter synthesis during the first day of exposure to cold, a more severe cold stress (-7 C) not only elicits a considerably greater secretion, but also accelerates the resynthesis of epinephrine, the extent of both depending on the age of the rat and being greater in young rats (126).

There appear to be few reports of direct measurements of the rate of catecholamine turnover in the adrenal medulla during exposure to cold. Draskóczy and co-workers report no change in the adrenal medulla of cold-exposed mice (53); however, the method they used (decrease in specific activity of prelabeled catecholamines) would detect only resynthesis and not secretion, and, as mentioned above, there appears to be a lag phase during which resynthesis does not occur.

There do not appear to have been any direct estimates of the turnover of medullary catecholamines in cold-acclimated animals. From a number of different types of observations it is possible to conclude that the norepinephrine in the nerve endings turns over at an accelerated rate in animals acutely exposed to cold and in animals acclimated to cold. Acute cold exposure pro-

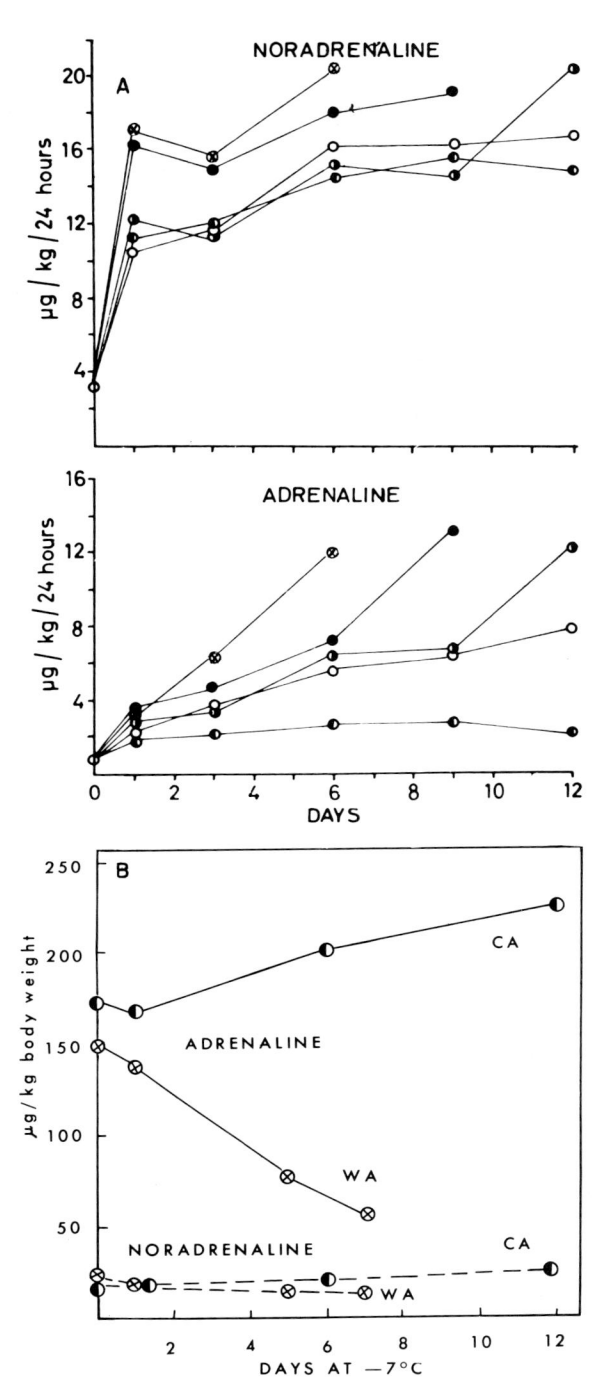

FIG. 11. Excretion of epinephrine (*adrenaline*) and norepinephrine (*noradrenaline*) (*A*) and the epinephrine (*adrenaline*) and norepinephrine (*noradrenaline*) content of adrenals (*B*) on prolonged exposure to -7 C in rats that have never been in the cold (⊗) or have been at 3 C for 1 (●), 2 (◐), 4 (○), or 12 (◉) weeks. There were 6 rats per group at beginning of experiments. Rats that have lived at 3 C for 4 and 12 weeks can be considered cold-acclimated rats. *CA*: cold-acclimated rats; *WA*: warm-acclimated rats. [From Leduc (126).]

Leduc (126) are plotted in Figure 12. It is apparent that the rate of synthesis lags behind the rate of secretion for 1 day, but then it exceeds the rate of secretion so that the

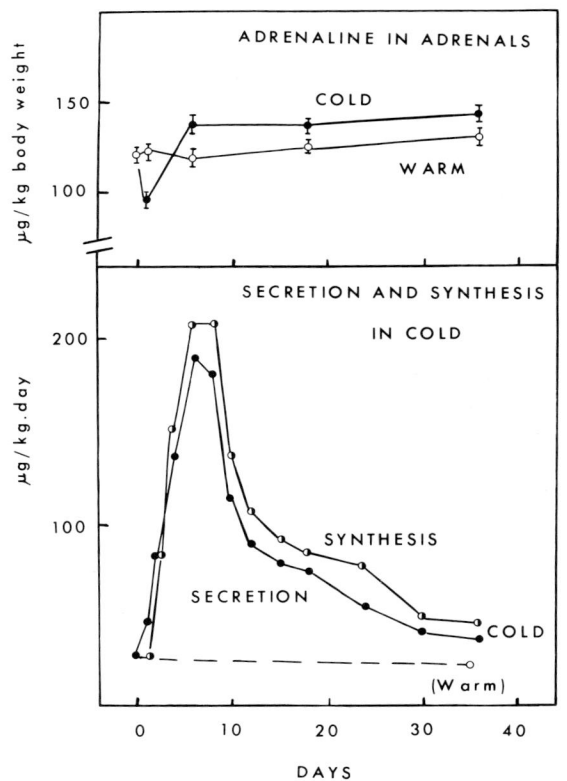

FIG. 12. Secretion and synthesis of epinephrine (*adrenaline*) and the epinephrine content of adrenals in rats during acclimation to cold (3 C). Values for rats that lived at room temperature (*warm*) are also shown. Calculation of these values is described in text. [Derived from Leduc (126).]

duces depletion of the norepinephrine content of many tissues, including heart (10, 37, 126), liver, muscle, spleen (126), and brown adipose tissue (37, 49). At the same time, in the urine there is a greatly elevated excretion of norepinephrine, which is not reduced by adrenalectomy (126) and must therefore originate from extraadrenal sources. Further evidence for its sympathetic origin comes from the observations that prior depletion of the nerve endings with reserpine reduces the excretion of norepinephrine in response to cold stress (126) and that ganglionic blockade (with mecamylamine) also prevents the rise in norepinephrine excretion in response to cold stress (126).

Direct measurements have shown that turnover of norepinephrine is increased in the heart of cold-exposed mice (150) and rats (10). Therefore release and synthesis of norepinephrine are increased under these conditions. That there may also be increased uptake of norepinephrine into the nerve endings is suggested by a greater uptake of labeled norepinephrine (61) and by the potentiation by cocaine, which inhibits uptake, of the depletion of norepinephrine that occurs in the heart of the cold-exposed rat (10).

Two observations imply an accelerated synthesis of norepinephrine in animals that are living in the cold for long periods. Cold-acclimated rats excrete far more norepinephrine than warm-acclimated rats (126). The norepinephrine content of the tissues of the cold-acclimated animals is either the same as or greater than normal (37, 126). Indeed direct measurements have shown that the turnover of norepinephrine in the brown adipose tissue of cold-acclimated rats (37) and hamsters (60) is increased. The nature of the innervation of brown adipose tissue is of great importance in the mechanism of cold acclimation, and for this reason it is discussed in more detail later.

Changes in Adrenal Medulla

Little is known about the activities of those enzymes involved in the synthesis of the catecholamines in the adrenal medulla during cold exposure and cold acclimation. The total amount of tyrosine hydroxylase has been shown to be increased in a group of rats that had lived at 3 C for up to 3 weeks (63). The increase starts within 1 day of exposure to cold and continues progressively thereafter (186).

The amount of phenylethanolamine N-methyltransferase (PNMT) is not altered in rats exposed to cold (5 C) for up to 1 day [(62, 114); R. W. Fuller, personal communication]: a small increase may occur between 1 and 3 weeks of exposure to cold (114), but PNMT levels in cold-acclimated rats are normal [(114); P. MacDonald and J. Himms-Hagen, unpublished results].

In rats adapted to a different kind of stress (immobilization for 2.5 hr/day), the content of tyrosine hydroxylase in the adrenal increases severalfold (116) by the seventh day of stress and remains at an elevated level for as long as the stress is continued; the increase in activity of this enzyme can be correlated with the ability of the rat to maintain normal (or supranormal) levels of epinephrine in its adrenal medulla during stress, an ability that appears to be acquired by adaptation to stress (115). However, with regard to the functioning of the adrenal medulla, the adaptation of rats to immobilization stress differs in two major respects from the adaptation of rats to cold: *1*) the excretion of epinephrine in the urine exceeds that of norepinephrine during the initial stress (115), whereas cold exposure causes the opposite pattern of catecholamine excretion (see Fig. 10); *2*) the excretion of epinephrine remains at a very high level for as long as the daily immobilization stress continues, and even after 1 year the daily excretion rate is 3 µg/kg per day compared with a basal rate of 1.2 µg/kg per day (115), whereas in cold-exposed rats the epinephrine excretion diminishes and is no greater than the basal level once the rats become adapted to cold [see Fig. 10; (126)]. Although a very high rate of epinephrine excretion can be provoked in rats by exposure to severe cold, as described above (see Fig. 11), it never exceeds the rate of norepinephrine excretion and it cannot be maintained for very long; the rats die when their adrenals are depleted of epinephrine and the excretion of epinephrine reaches the maximum of 12 µg/kg per day. The principal difference between the cold-exposed rats and the rats subjected to immobilization stress is that in the former the secreted epinephrine and norepinephrine serve a useful function (that of increasing heat production and therefore combating the effect of the stress), whereas in the latter the catecholamines do not exert any effect that allows the rats to adapt to the stress.

There is good evidence that PNMT of the adrenal medulla is a glucocorticoid-dependent enzyme, that is, that it requires the high levels of glucocorticoids present in the blood delivered from the adrenal cortex to the medullary cells for its optimal rate of synthesis [see (156) and the chapter by Weiner in this volume of the *Handbook*]. However, in the normal rat the amount of PNMT appears to be close to the maximum, and increased availability of glucocorticoids has little or no effect on the amount of enzyme (205). Thus, although increased adrenocortical activity does occur in the cold-exposed rat, as evidenced by the large but temporary rise in plasma corticosterone concentration (13, 136), this does not appear to markedly influence the synthesis of PNMT.

In contrast to PNMT, the amount of tyrosine hydroxylase in the adrenal medulla appears to be under neural control; if the gland is denervated no increase in tyrosine hydroxylase occurs in response to immobilization stress (116) or to cold stress (186).

An unexplained change in the adrenal medulla of rats that have been intermittently exposed to cold for a fairly long period is a decrease in the content of DNA per nucleus (191, 193). The DNA is lost during the exposure to cold and is resynthesized during recovery in the warm. The rats eventually appear to adapt so that resynthesis occurs during the cold-exposure period itself. There follows then a period during which the turnover of DNA is increased by the daily exposure to cold without any change in the amount of DNA present. The increased turnover ceases when the intermittent cold exposure is stopped (11, 153, 190, 192). Intermittent exposure to cold does induce a state of acclimation to cold similar to that induced by continuous exposure to cold. Thus these rats that have adapted to synthesizing more DNA while exposed to cold are presumably also cold acclimated. Pelc & Viola-Magni (153) consider that approximately 40–45% of the DNA of the adrenal medulla nuclei is "metabolic" DNA and is participating in the increased turnover. However, the significance of an accelerated turnover of DNA in the cells of the stimulated adrenal medulla is far from clear.

ROLE OF SECRETED CATECHOLAMINES
IN THERMOGENESIS

Mimicking Effects of Catecholamines

A major line of evidence for the participation of the catecholamines in nonshivering thermogenesis is the marked calorigenic action of these compounds, an action that is enhanced in cold-acclimated rats just as is the capacity for nonshivering thermogenesis. The initial observation of an enhanced calorigenic action of a catecholamine was made in 1942 by Ring (159) who subcutaneously administered epinephrine and then measured oxygen uptake; Ring was interested in the importance of the adrenal medulla in the responses of cold-acclimated rats to cold, but he was unable to devise any method of assessing this role of the medulla because of the problem of the replacement of epinephrine-induced calorigenesis by shivering thermogenesis when the medulla was removed (159). Subsequently, Swanson (181) also observed an enhanced calorigenic response to epinephrine in cold-acclimated rats; she concluded that epinephrine-induced calorigenesis might be important in heat production in the cold. Despite such early ideas about epinephrine as a calorigenic agent in cold-exposed and cold-acclimated rats—ideas originally formulated by Cannon (24) for dogs and cats exposed to cold—more attention has recently been given to the role of norepinephrine liberated from sympathetic nerve endings as a major calorigenic agent for the production of nonshivering thermogenesis in cold-acclimated rats. This change of emphasis dates back to the discovery of the presence of norepinephrine, rather than epinephrine, in sympathetic nerves [see (194)] and also to four papers by Carlson and co-workers published in 1956 and 1957 (36, 84–86). These important studies provided the first demonstration that the capacity of cold-acclimated rats for nonshivering thermogenesis was much greater than that of warm-acclimated rats [(36); see also Fig. 6] and the first demonstration that the calorigenic effect of norepinephrine was greatly enhanced in cold-acclimated rats (85). Although the calorigenic effect of epinephrine was also observed to be greater in the cold-acclimated animals (85), the authors presented several arguments in favor of norepinephrine as the mediator, rather than epinephrine (85). These arguments were based on the dissimilarity of the effects of injected epinephrine and the effects of cold exposure; first, epinephrine caused a hyperglycemia, whereas neither cold exposure nor norepinephrine caused hyperglycemia (85), and second, hypothyroidism caused a diminution of the calorigenic response to epinephrine (85) but a lesser diminution of the capacity for nonshivering thermogenesis (84). The large increase in the response to norepinephrine and the much weaker calorigenic response to epinephrine (given by intramuscular injection) led these authors to propose that norepinephrine was the mediator in nonshivering thermogenesis (85); norepinephrine was moreover shown to protect against the decrease in oxygen uptake and body temperature caused by hexamethonium, whereas epinephrine did not (86). More recently, research on the nature of nonshivering thermogenesis and the role of catecholamines in this process has involved almost exclusively the use of norepinephrine as a stimulating agent.

It is now apparent that cold-acclimated rats acquire an enhanced calorigenic response to epinephrine, as well as to norepinephrine (see Figs. 1 and 2). This enhanced response to epinephrine is not so clear when intramuscular administration is used (85, 92). The argument that epinephrine has a weaker calorigenic effect than norepinephrine in cold-acclimated animals (85) can therefore no longer be used. It is now also known that, although cold exposure of cold-acclimated rats does not cause hyperglycemia (85), it does nevertheless initiate a mobilization of glucose (via both glycogenolysis and gluconeogenesis) that is matched by an increased utilization of glucose; that is, glucose turnover is increased (46–48, 154). Thus a mobilization of glucose by epinephrine could well occur in these animals, but it is masked by the simultaneous increase in utilization of blood glucose. As far as the argument about hypothyroidism is concerned, it now seems likely that the calorigenic response to norepinephrine may also be decreased by hypothyroidism since it is known to be increased by hyperthyroidism (87); thus the argument used about the response to epinephrine being reduced by hypothyroidism could equally well be applied to the response to norepinephrine. The greater effectiveness of norepinephrine compared with epinephrine in maintaining oxygen uptake when nonshivering thermogenesis is inhibited by ganglionic blockade may be due to the inappropriate mode of administration of the epinephrine (intramuscular injection), since when given by intravenous infusion, norepinephrine and epinephrine are equally effective in raising metabolic rate in cold-acclimated rats. Thus, on these arguments alone, it cannot be concluded that epinephrine secreted from the adrenal medulla does not contribute to nonshivering thermogenesis. The principal argument that remains against such a role is the small quantity of epinephrine secreted, which would be only about one-hundredth of the amount required by intravenous infusion to produce a maximum calorigenic response.

Whether an increase in the secretion of epinephrine in the early stages of exposure to cold plays any role in the development of cold acclimation is still an open question. There is, however, evidence that the increased secretion of norepinephrine plays a role in the development of adaptation to cold. LeBlanc & Pouliot (121) first showed that prolonged treatment of rats with norepinephrine could produce an adaptive state similar to that of cold acclimation in that the calorigenic response to norepinephrine was enhanced and the resistance to cold was increased. This treatment also promotes the growth of the brown adipose tissue, just as does cold acclimation (124). The effect of norepinephrine is potentiated by guanethidine (125) and also by thyroid hormone (124). One report of no effect of prolonged treatment with norepinephrine on the development of cold acclimation (as measured by survival and maintenance of body temperature in the cold at −20 C) is most probably because the rats that were treated were already living in the cold, either continuously or intermittently (170); both treated and untreated rats appeared to possess a marked degree of adaptation, and any increase resulting from the norepinephrine was not apparent.

Consequences of Lack of Secretion and/or Action of Catecholamines

The secretion of catecholamines by the adrenal medulla is most readily eliminated by surgical removal of this organ. The remainder of the sympathetic nervous system continues to function in the demedullated animal. If it is desired to study an animal possessing only the medulla and lacking the remainder of the sympathetic nervous system or devoid of sympathetic function altogether, several techniques may be used, no one of which is entirely satisfactory, either because of lack of completeness or lack of specificity. These techniques may be surgical, immunological, or pharmacological, or combinations of techniques may be used. In order to determine what effect the lack of part of the sympathetic nervous system may have, some measure of the response to cold is required. Usually the maintenance of body temperature or the increase in oxygen uptake is measured in the animal exposed to cold. Since the maintenance of body temperature in the cold depends on both an increase in heat conservation and an increase in heat production, changes in either of these adjustment mechanisms may influence the results. The heat conservation mechanisms are catecholamine dependent and may therefore be disturbed in the animal that lacks part or all of its sympathetic nervous function. Mechanisms of heat production include both shivering and nonshivering thermogenesis; measurement of oxygen uptake alone does not distinguish between these two. Thus the measurements usually made give rather little information about the underlying mechanisms of adjustment. Measurements of the mobilization of energy resources [free fatty acid (FFA) and glucose] are also frequently made. Usually such a mobilization is deduced from the rise in concentration of these metabolites in the blood. It must, however, be remembered that an increased mobilization can occur without any change in the concentration of these metabolites in the blood if there should be a simultaneous increase in the rate of utilization resulting from an increase in metabolic rate.

DEMEDULLATION. Young rats lacking the adrenal medulla do not maintain their body temperature well when exposed to moderate cold (2–4 C) (8, 64, 132, 133, 159) and do not survive for very long (159). Injection of epinephrine can prevent the hypothermia during the first few hours of cold exposure (132, 133). Slightly older rats are able to survive in the cold (157, 166), even for several months (98), and their ability to maintain body temperature in the cold without appreciable shivering indicates that they have become cold acclimated (166).

The mobilization of triglyceride stores in rats exposed to cold appears to be uninfluenced by demedullation, as judged by the normal rise in concentration of plasma FFA (64, 132, 177) and the normal activation of adipose tissue lipase (135). However, demedullation prevents the normal rise in blood glucose concentration; such animals become slightly hypoglycemic in a few hours (64, 98, 177) and markedly hypoglycemic after 1 day (98). Although demedullated rats can survive for long periods in the cold, their blood glucose remains below the level of that of intact rats, and, in particular, the hyperglycemic phase normally seen during the first 3 weeks of cold acclimation is absent in the demedullated animals (98). The rise in plasma corticosterone is normal during the first few hours of cold exposure of adrenodemedullated rats (132); however, a marked hypertrophy of the adrenal cortex occurs in demedullated rats living in the cold for several weeks, and it seems likely that cortical activity is increased at this time (98). Adrenodemedullated rats show normal shivering and piloerection in response to cold (132, 137). Their oxygen uptake after only 1 hr in the cold is raised just as in normal rats (137).

The relatively minor effects of removal of the adrenal medulla on survival of rats in the cold and on acclimation of rats to cold might lead one to suppose that, except for the regulation of blood glucose concentration during the early phases of cold acclimation, the epinephrine secreted by the adrenal medulla is of little importance for adaptation to cold. However, the experiment of Cottle & Carlson (36) in 1956 on rats that were demedullated after acclimation to cold would suggest that epinephrine does have an effect when it is present, even though the rats are able to make other adjustments when it is not present. The results of this experiment are illustrated in Figure 6 and are described below. These authors exposed to 4 C curarized rats (which could not produce heat by shivering) that had been demedullated 10 days previously and compared their calorigenic response to cold with that of intact rats; they studied both warm-acclimated and cold-acclimated rats. The cold-acclimated rats had spent the 10 days immediately after the operation in the cold, so that they had had some time to readjust to the absence of the medulla. The intact cold-acclimated rats showed the usual large increase in metabolic rate on exposure to cold and maintained their body temperature fairly well during 2 hr; in contrast, the demedullated rats showed a much smaller increase in metabolic rate (about one-half the increase seen in the intact animals) and became somewhat hypothermic. The lack of the adrenal medulla made little or no difference in their metabolic rate at room temperature (29 C), but at the lower temperature it resulted in a definite disadvantage. Warm-acclimated, curarized rats cool quickly at 4 C, and their oxygen uptake decreases rapidly; this rapid rate of cooling is not altered by the removal of the adrenal medulla.

It may therefore be concluded that even in cold-acclimated rats the adrenal medulla plays a part in promoting thermogenesis. Rats are, however, sufficiently adaptable that they can survive perfectly well without their adrenal medulla and can even acquire some degree of acclimation to cold in its absence.

ADRENALECTOMY. An added complication of adrenalectomy as a means of removing the adrenal medulla is that the source of cortical hormones, as well as catecholamines, is removed. If the rats are provided with replacement amounts of these hormones, their response to cold is much like that of adrenodemedullated rats (132, 134): they can survive in the cold (100, 103, 126) and can become cold acclimated (72). If rats are adrenalectomized after they have become cold acclimated, maintained on corticosteroids, and reexposed to cold 4 days later, they excrete more norepinephrine in their urine than do intact rats. This observation suggests that an increased sympathetic activity is occasioned by the absence of the adrenal medulla (126). This difference between intact and adrenalectomized rats is not seen if the rats have been without their adrenals during the cold-acclimation period (126).

Thus it may be concluded that the response to cold of the cold-acclimated rats involves the adrenal medulla to some extent and that removal of the medulla sets in train a compensatory modification of the activity of the remainder of the sympathetic nervous system.

Adrenalectomized rats deprived of the cortical hormones become hypothermic and die very rapidly in the cold; they do not increase the concentration of either FFA or glucose in their blood, although they do not become hypoglycemic either. The lack of cortical and medullary hormones cannot be alleviated by the administration of epinephrine, as can the lack of adrenal medullary hormones alone; the reason for this appears to be that epinephrine is unable to exert its normal effects in the absence of adrenocortical hormones (132, 134). However, adrenalectomized rats have an additional defect which reduces their ability to withstand cold; these animals are unable to shiver and are unable to improve their insulation by piloerection and peripheral vasoconstriction. This defect is reversed by administration of the cortical hormones (132). Since prevention of shivering, as in the curarized, intact warm-acclimated rats (see Fig. 6), itself prevents survival of a rat in the cold (36) it is likely that this defect alone could account for the rapid death in hypothermia of untreated adrenalectomized rats subjected to cold exposure; the explanation for the lack of shivering is unknown, although lack of supply of substrate could be one possibility. A possible function of catecholamines in shivering, a function that presumably would be lacking in the corticoid-deprived animals, is discussed below.

Thus the essential role of the adrenal cortical hormones in the maintenance of body temperature would appear to be principally that of maintaining the capacity of the animals to respond to catecholamines (132). However, a supplementary role in shivering (i.e., in muscle metabolism) cannot be excluded.

IMMUNOSYMPATHECTOMY. The technique of immunosympathectomy usually requires the repeated administration to fetal or newborn animals, or both, of antiserum to nerve growth factor. This procedure prevents the development and subsequent normal functioning of those parts of the sympathetic nervous system that would normally appear at the time of administration. Some parts of the sympathetic nervous system are particularly resistant to damage by this treatment [e.g., the nerve endings in reproductive organs and intestine (65)]. The adrenal medulla is also unaffected by this treatment, possibly because it develops at a much later stage. The technique is therefore often used in combination with demedullation.

Normal infant rats tend to become hypothermic and die when exposed to moderate cold (33, 184, 188, 200); immunosympathectomized newborn rats cool much more rapidly than intact newborn rats under these conditions (200). By 16 days of age, intact rats are able to maintain their body temperature when exposed to 14–16 C, but immunosympathectomized rats still cool very rapidly (200). The capacity of newborn rats to raise their metabolic heat production in response to cold increases progressively during the first 3–4 weeks of life (184, 188), and the metabolic response to cold exposure during the first few days of life appears to result entirely from nonshivering thermogenesis. The relatively slow development of the capacity for heat production by any means other than nonshivering thermogenesis, for which the capacity is not very great, is one reason for the poor temperature regulation of the newborn rat. Another reason is the relatively slow development of heat conservation mechanisms (33). Also the adrenal medulla develops only toward the latter part of the first 3–4 weeks of life (32, 55). Thus during the first few days of life the newborn rat is entirely dependent on the nerve endings of its sympathetic nervous system for increasing its heat production in response to cold, and it is at this stage that the effects of immunosympathectomy are most marked.

Somewhat older immunosympathectomized rats (weighing less than 200 g) are able to maintain their body temperature when exposed to cold just as well as are untreated rats (8). Unlike the infant rats, these rats have a functioning adrenal medulla; if the adrenal medulla is removed, the immunosympathectomized rats cool very rapidly at 4 C and much more rapidly than untreated demedullated rats. Thus the adrenal medulla seems to have the capacity to play a major part in the calorigenic response to cold.

As the immunosympathectomized rats become still older they again become less dependent on their adrenal medulla. Immunosympathectomized rats, whether demedullated or not, can become cold acclimated [i.e., they can live at 4 C for several weeks (164)]. In fact, once acclimated, immunosympathectomized rats excrete as much epinephrine and norepinephrine in their urine as do untreated control rats; demedullated, immunosympathectomized rats excrete as much norepinephrine in their urine as do untreated demedullated rats. Only by means of a severe cold stress (e.g., clipping of fur and re-exposure to 4 C) is it possible to distinguish between untreated and immunosympathectomized rats by the amount of norepinephrine excreted; the latter excrete less norepinephrine under these conditions. Even so, the survival of these rats, demedullated or not, during such a severe cold stress is not impaired when compared with that of similar but untreated rats (164).

Thus the dependence of the rat on its adrenal medulla appears to vary with age. The newborn rat has no functioning adrenal medulla and therefore does not depend on this organ. Later the medulla appears to play an essential role, but later still this role, if it persists, is a dispensable one.

RESERPINE. Reserpine has been used extensively to deplete the sympathetic nervous system of its catecholamines. This drug depletes the adrenal medulla of its catecholamines only if large doses are given; smaller doses influence principally peripheral nerve endings. However, reserpine has other actions, which must be taken into consideration in interpreting studies of responses of reserpine-treated animals to cold exposure. Reserpine is known to deplete the brain of its amines and to deplete the pituitary gland of its hormones, actions resulting in disturbances of central nervous function and of hormonal regulation in the reserpinized animal [see (201)]; in addition, reserpine causes an initial liberation of large quantities of catecholamines, which may themselves be toxic under certain conditions.

If rats are exposed to cold shortly after the administration of reserpine, they become hypothermic and die (40, 126, 128, 136, 158, 166, 208). However, if rats are exposed to cold only 24–48 hr after administration of reserpine, at which time the tissues are still catecholamine depleted (126), they can survive at 4 C (126), and even their survival at −20 C is not impaired (158); these rats can indeed even become cold acclimated if allowed to remain at 4 C (126). The reason for the death of the animals that are exposed to cold shortly after reserpine may be the toxicity of the endogenously liberated catecholamines; cold exposure (128) and reserpine itself (117) have been observed to accentuate the toxicity of catecholamines.

That a functioning adrenal medulla may be necessary for the survival of reserpine-treated rats in the cold is indicated by the poor survival in the cold of adrenalectomized, reserpinized rats maintained on cortical hormones (100, 126). Newborn rats, which have an immature adrenal medulla, also cool rapidly after reserpine administration, even when exposed only to moderate cold (200), as do newborn guinea pigs of mothers that were treated with reserpine (89). In keeping with this suggestion is the rapid and large increase in excretion of epinephrine, but not of norepinephrine, in reserpine-treated rats on exposure to cold; the excretion of norepinephrine does not attain the normal level for a cold-acclimated rat until 4 weeks later, and the excretion of epinephrine remains higher than normal until this time (126).

Leduc (126) has calculated the rates of secretion and synthesis of epinephrine by the adrenal medulla in the reserpinized, cold-exposed rats (see previous section for description of assumptions made for the purposes of this calculation); his data are plotted in Figure 13 (cf. Fig. 12). The reserpinized animals, which started off in the cold with greatly depleted norepinephrine stores in their tissues and with a partially depleted adrenal medulla, increased their secretion of epinephrine about five times more than normal during the first day of cold exposure and continued to secrete more than the normal amount of epinephrine even after 5 weeks in the cold. Unlike normal rats, the reserpinized rats increased the rate of resynthesis of epinephrine immediately and continued to synthesize epinephrine at an accelerated rate for 5 weeks; the epinephrine content of the medulla also increased to about the same level as that seen in the untreated rats. Thus when the sympathetic nerves are nonfunctional or only partially functional the adrenal medulla appears to be able to compensate for the deficiency.

When administered to rats already acclimated to cold, reserpine does not have toxic effects in doses that would kill warm-acclimated rats exposed to cold immediately after the injection (166). A brief increase in epinephrine excretion occurs, and the norepinephrine excretion returns to normal more rapidly (within 2½ weeks) than in the rats exposed to cold for the first time (126).

Daily administration of a small dose of reserpine to cold-acclimated rats that continue to live in the cold has led to a large increase in excretion of epinephrine, which was maintained for as long as the treatment was continued (30 days), and a prolonged decrease in the excretion of norepinephrine (126). Peripheral tissues were depleted of their norepinephrine during this period, as was the adrenal medulla to some extent, but the epinephrine content of the adrenal medulla was maintained at a level higher than normal. This finding might lead one to suppose that the adrenal medulla substituted for the function of the depleted norepinephrine-containing nerves. However, cold-acclimated rats that were adrenalectomized before reserpine treatment survived in the cold without the accentuated epinephrine secretion and indeed without epinephrine secretion altogether; their excretion of norepinephrine was also reduced by the reserpine, but to no greater extent than the excretion of norepinephrine by intact rats was reduced by reserpine (126). This implies that the adrenal medulla was not absolutely essential to the reserpine-treated animals.

On the other hand, small daily doses of reserpine injected into previously cold-acclimated rats that are de-acclimating at room temperature hasten the deacclimation process; the enhanced metabolic response to norepinephrine is lost more rapidly in these animals (117). Thus although rats that continue to be stimulated by cold appear to retain their acclimation state, despite treatment with reserpine, once this stimulation is stopped the acclimation is similarly lost, presumably because sympathetic activity is reduced to a very low level.

GUANETHIDINE. The adrenergic neuron blocking agent, guanethidine, impairs the ability of warm-acclimated rats to survive in the cold when administered in large doses (131). Chronic treatment of rats with guanethidine during acclimation to cold does not, however, impair the acclimation process; in fact, these rats survive in the cold and develop a slightly greater cold resistance (at −20 C) than do untreated rats (158). Similarly hamsters are able to acclimate to cold and develop an enhanced calorigenic response to norepinephrine, despite continued administration of guanethidine (202). These animals would be expected to have a functioning adrenal medulla because guanethidine does not alter the functioning of the adrenal medulla. When demedullated rats are treated with guanethidine during exposure to cold they fail to increase their norepinephrine or epinephrine excretion and die fairly rapidly (157).

Thus it may be concluded that the adrenal medulla played an important part in those guanethidine-treated rats that were living in the cold: when it was absent the animals could not survive. However, once rats are acclimated to cold they appear to be unaffected by treatment with guanethidine, even in the absence of their adrenal medulla (166). As discussed above in relation to immunosympathectomy, once rats are cold acclimated, they appear to be able to maintain their acclimation state with the vestiges of sympathetic function left to them, whatever these might be; this is probably true also of the guanethidine-treated, demedullated, cold-acclimated rats that continue to live in the cold.

When warm-acclimated rats are treated for prolonged periods with guanethidine while continuing to live at room temperature, their calorigenic response to norepinephrine may (74) or may not (125) be enhanced; but, if guanethidine is administered together with norepinephrine for 3 weeks, a marked enhancement of the calorigenic effect of norepinephrine occurs (125). Even when the calorigenic response to norepinephrine is enhanced by guanethidine, the resistance to cold is not altered (74, 158), presumably because the rats are unable to secrete norepinephrine in response to cold.

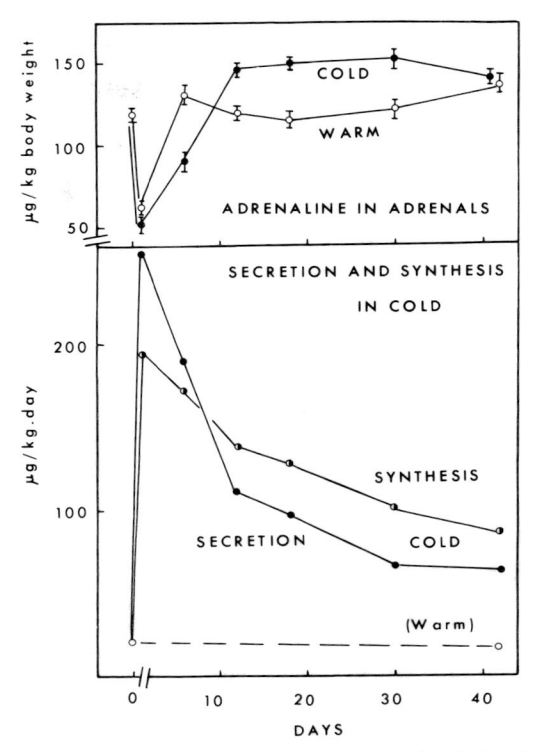

FIG. 13. Secretion and synthesis of epinephrine (*adrenaline*) and epinephrine content of adrenals in reserpine-treated rats during acclimation to cold (3 C). Values for rats that lived at room temperature (*warm*) are also shown. All rats received a single subcutaneous injection of reserpine (5 mg/kg) on day 0. They were kept at room temperature for 2 days, and some were then transferred to 3 C. Day 1 refers to first day in the cold; it is the third day after administration of reserpine. To see the effect of reserpine, compare with Fig. 12. [Derived from Leduc (126).]

GANGLIONIC BLOCKING AGENTS. If warm-acclimated rats are treated with chlorisondamine (64) or with mecamylamine (126) before they are exposed to cold, they become hypothermic and die very rapidly in the cold. These rats may (126) or may not (64) shiver, but shivering seems to make little difference to their survival; they may be demedullated (137) or not (64, 131), and this also seems to make little difference to their survival. The principal defect in these animals appears to be their inability to mobilize either lipid or glycogen stores, the former indicated by the lack of change of FFA concentration in plasma (64, 135, 177), which would normally increase in warm-acclimated rats exposed to cold, and by the lack of activation of adipose tissue lipase (135), the latter indicated by the lack of change of glucose concentration in blood (64, 177). The oxygen uptake of these rats treated with ganglionic blocking agents and exposed to cold is low, as might be expected from their hypothermic state (137). Treatment of the rats with epinephrine, but not with norepinephrine, can protect against the cold stress (64, 126, 137).

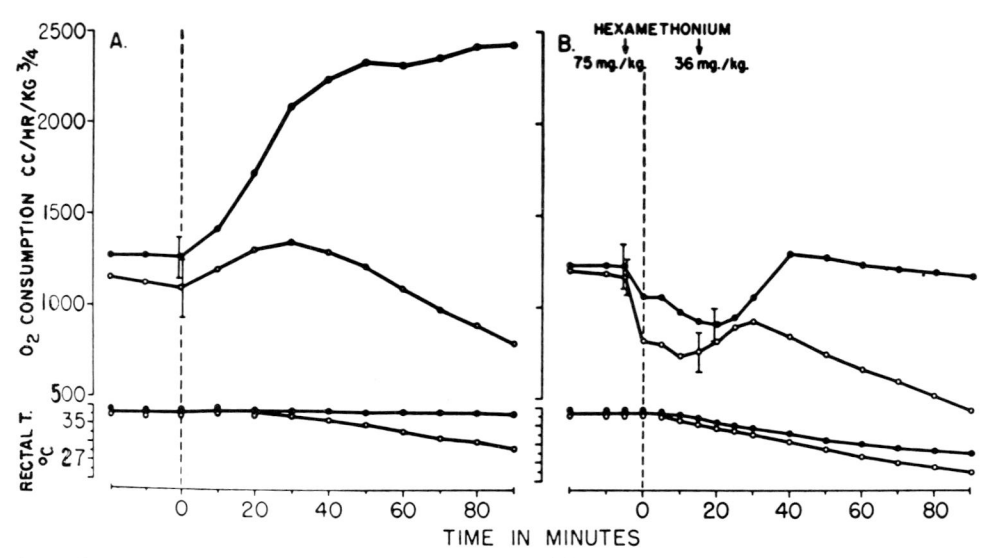

FIG. 14. Oxygen consumption and rectal temperature of curarized, cold-adapted rats (●) and warm-adapted rats (○) receiving hexamethonium. Room was cooled to 5 C at zero time. Hexamethonium was injected intravenously at points indicated by *arrows*. [From Hsieh et al. (86).]

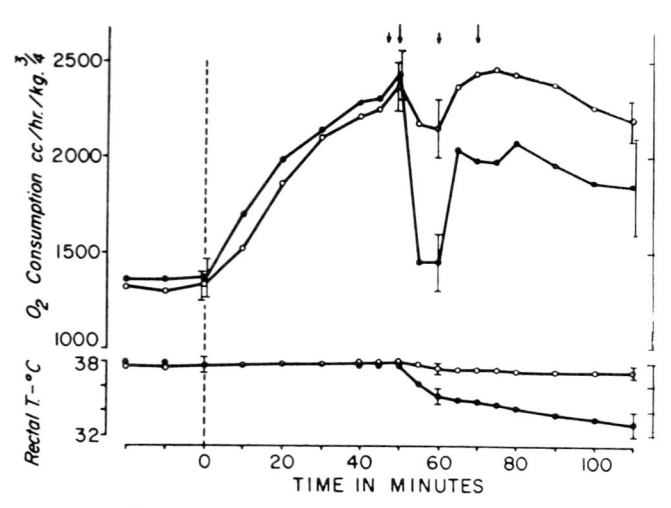

FIG. 15. Oxygen consumption and rectal temperature of curarized, cold-adapted rats receiving hexamethonium and epinephrine or norepinephrine. Room was cooled to 5 ± 1 C at zero time. Hexamethonium was injected intravenously at points indicated by *long arrows*. At points indicated by *short arrows*, epinephrine (0.2 mg/kg) was injected intramuscularly to group represented by *closed circles* and *l*-norepinephrine in the same dose given to group represented by *open circles*. T., temperature. [From Hsieh et al. (86).]

Rats already cold acclimated before treatment with mecamylamine survive slightly longer in the cold than do warm-acclimated rats; they do nevertheless die in hypothermia, despite very marked shivering (126); the presence of the adrenal medulla makes little difference to their survival. Treatment with norepinephrine can protect these cold-acclimated rats against the cold; epinephrine also has a protective action but appears to be less effective than norepinephrine (126).

Ganglionic blockade has also been demonstrated to promote cooling in newborn kittens (141, 142) and rats (200) and in rabbits and guinea pigs (42).

Thus ganglionic blockade, which inactivates the norepinephrine-secreting nerve endings and, if the dose is large enough, the adrenal medulla, exerts a deleterious effect on survival in the cold. As might be expected, the presence or absence of the adrenal medulla makes little difference to survival. Even if the rats are able to shiver (and even shivering may be inhibited by these drugs), they still do not survive. The warm-acclimated rats appear to suffer principally from lack of substrate to use for heat production.

Cold-acclimated rats treated with ganglionic blocking agents would be expected to suffer from lack of substrate for the increased heat production; in addition, they suffer from the lack of the calorigenic effect of the catecholamines. In the curarized cold-acclimated rat exposed to cold, in which any inhibition of shivering by the ganglionic blockade could not occur, hexamethonium inhibits the rise in oxygen uptake induced by exposure to cold [Fig. 14; (86)] and reverses the increase if it is administered after the increase has occurred [Fig. 15; (86)]. Norepinephrine, administered by intramuscular injection, can reverse the inhibitory effect of hexamethonium, whereas epinephrine is less effective [Fig. 15; (86)].

ADRENERGIC BLOCKING AGENTS. In rats (151, 178) and in newborn rabbits (70), β adrenergic blocking agents are known to inhibit the calorigenic effect of catecholamines. It would therefore be anticipated that these drugs would interfere with the calorigenic action of the catecholamines secreted in cold-exposed rats. It must, however, be remembered that these drugs might also be expected to interfere with the mobilization of FFA and glucose [see (78)], and this action could have the effect of cutting off the substrate supply necessary for the increase in metabolic rate.

That these drugs interfere with the calorigenic effect of the catecholamines in animals that possess the adaptation for nonshivering thermogenesis rather than with the supply of metabolizable substrate is indicated by the replacement of nonshivering thermogenesis by shivering thermogenesis in cold-acclimated rats treated with propranolol (165) and in newborn guinea pigs treated with pronethalol (17, 18); these agents do not interfere with shivering in warm-acclimated rats exposed to cold (165) or in older guinea pigs exposed to cold (17, 18). However, if the cold stress is severe enough (0 C), warm-acclimated animals (e.g., mice) die in hypothermia when exposed to cold after treatment with β adrenergic blocking agents, despite marked shivering (56, 58). Thus the principal defect caused by such drugs in animals that possess the adaptation for nonshivering thermogenesis appears to be in the response of the calorigenic process involved in nonshivering thermogenesis rather than in the substrate supply for the heat production. Unfortunately these agents do not allow any distinction to be made regarding the source of the secreted catecholamines. This conclusion is in keeping with the failure of antilipolytic agents, such as nicotinic acid (57) and 3′,5′-dimethylpyrazole (69), to alter survival in the cold. These agents are not adrenergic blocking agents, and nicotinic acid does not block the calorigenic effect of norepinephrine (151).

INHIBITION OF SYNTHESIS. When the formation of catecholamines is inhibited in warm-acclimated rats by drugs that inhibit one or more of the enzymes of the catecholamine biosynthetic pathway, these animals depend for survival on their store of catecholamines. Thus the phenylalanine hydroxylase inhibitor, trimethyldopa, does not prevent survival of warm-acclimated rats in the cold; rats treated with this drug increase their excretion of epinephrine when exposed to cold. However, demedullated rats treated with this same inhibitor die when exposed to cold (30). The tyrosine hydroxylase inhibitor, α-methyltyrosine, has effects similar to those of trimethyldopa (30). Studies with this drug have also shown that depletion of the catecholamines of the adrenal medulla, as well as of peripheral sympathetic nerve endings, occurs after long periods of its administration to rats living in the cold (30). This drug also blocks the arousal of hibernating hamsters, a process that is dependent on norepinephrine in nerve endings rather than on the adrenal medulla (59).

The dopa decarboxylase inhibitor, α-methyldopa, impairs the survival of rats exposed to severe cold (-20 C) even when the adrenal medulla is present (158). However, the adrenal medulla does serve to protect against less severe cold stress (4 C) in rats treated with the dopa decarboxylase inhibitors, Ro4-4602 [N-(DL-seryl)-N'-(2,3,4-trihydroxybenzyl)-hydrazine] (103, 105) and decaborane (99); adrenalectomized rats (maintained on glucocorticoids and/or mineralocorticoids) die rapidly when treated with these drugs and exposed to cold (99, 101).

Cold-acclimated rats appear to be less susceptible to the action of the dopa decarboxylase inhibitors; Ro4-4602 does not alter the urinary excretion of norepinephrine in adrenalectomized, cold-acclimated rats, and these rats survive in the cold (101, 103). Even when they are exposed to severe cold (-20 C), cold-acclimated rats treated with α-methyldopa are better able to maintain their body temperature than are warm-acclimated rats treated in a similar way (158).

CHEMICAL SYMPATHECTOMY. Chemical sympathectomy is a term describing the procedure in which animals are deprived of their sympathetic function by means of drugs. The drugs, which may be catecholamine-releasing agents, ganglionic blocking agents, or adrenergic neuron blocking agents, are usually used in combination with demedullation or adrenalectomy: this is a combined pharmacological and surgical approach. As noted above, these procedures markedly impair the ability of rats to survive in the cold (64, 131, 132, 137). However, the principal defect that contributes to the poor resistance to cold of these animals is their inability to shiver. Inhibition of shivering by itself causes an impairment of heat production sufficient to prevent the maintenance of body temperature by warm-acclimated rats exposed to cold [(36); see Fig. 6]. The observation that chemically sympathectomized rats are unable to shiver leads to the conclusion that the sympathetic nervous system plays some unknown role in the maintenance of shivering (16, 64, 132). This conclusion is strengthened by the observation that treatment of chemically sympathectomized rats with epinephrine during exposure to cold permits shivering to occur (132). The nature of the role of the catecholamines in shivering is discussed below.

MECHANISM OF ACTION OF SECRETED CATECHOLAMINES

Regardless of which catecholamine is the more important in the overall metabolic response of an animal to cold, there is no doubt that the metabolic and other effects of the catecholamines are of considerable importance in the defense against hypothermia. The metabolism of cold-acclimated animals, and particularly the metabolic effects of catecholamines in cold-acclimated animals, have been the subject of many extensive reviews [see (27–29, 45, 78, 82, 83, 91)]; this topic is not discussed in much detail here. A brief survey is given to provide some idea of current thinking about the actions of the catecholamines believed to underlie the various roles of these agents in cold-acclimated animals.

The catecholamines have roles in five fairly distinct adjustments that occur in response to cold: *1*) reduction in heat loss by causing piloerection and peripheral vasoconstriction; *2*) mobilization of substrates to support the elevated metabolic rate; *3*) shivering thermogenesis; *4*) nonshivering thermogenesis; and *5*) development and maintenance of the adaptation for nonshivering thermogenesis. Roles *1* and *2* are similar in warm-acclimated and cold-acclimated rats. Role *3* is involved principally in cold-exposed warm-acclimated rats, whereas Role *4* occurs principally in cold-exposed, cold-acclimated rats since the capacity for nonshivering thermogenesis in cold-exposed, warm-acclimated rats is limited. Role *5* is manifest only during the process of acclimation to cold; it persists in the rat that continues to live in the cold.

Reduction of Heat Loss

In the rat piloerection and peripheral vasoconstriction are important mechanisms, under sympathetic control, for the reduction of heat loss during exposure to cold. The extent to which an animal depends on these two mechanisms varies considerably from one species to another.

Mobilization of Substrates

Catecholamines appear to be of prime importance in the mobilization of both FFA and glucose, which are to be used as substrates for the increase in metabolic rate of cold-exposed animals. The concentrations of both these substrates usually rise in the blood of warm-acclimated rats on exposure to cold (64, 177). The prevention of the rise in blood glucose concentration by prior demedullation (64, 177) suggests that epinephrine from the medulla is important in the adjustment. The increased formation of glucose under the influence of epinephrine is due to both increased glycogenolysis and increased gluconeogenesis (46–48, 154). The hyperglycemic effect of epinephrine is known to be the net result of a variety of actions of this compound, not only on the liver but also on other tissues [see (78, 82)]. The extent to which the known action of epinephrine to inhibit insulin secretion [see (78, 82)] is involved in the production of hyperglycemia in the cold-exposed rat is unknown. The observation that diabetic rats can become acclimated to cold (155) indicates that insulin secretion and inhibition of insulin secretion do not play essential roles in the response to cold. However, in the cold these diabetic rats do appear to be under considerably greater stress than normal rats, as judged by their higher excretion of catecholamines (148) and their poorer survival rate (155).

Cold-acclimated rats living in the cold are not hyperglycemic (46–48, 77, 85), yet the glucose in their blood turns over much faster than in the same rats in the warm (46–48). Thus glucose mobilization is certainly accelerated in the cold-acclimated rat living in the cold; as might be expected, much of this glucose is derived from gluconeogenesis (47, 154).

The rise in the concentration of FFA in the blood of warm-acclimated rats exposed to cold appears to be a consequence principally of the activation of triglyceride lipase in white adipose tissue by norepinephrine liberated from sympathetic nerve endings (64, 135), an action known to be mediated by stimulation of adenyl cyclase and increased formation of cyclic AMP. Cold-acclimated rats do not have an elevated concentration of FFA in their blood while they are living in the cold and may indeed have a lower concentration than that seen in the same animals when they are living in the warm (77, 139). The turnover of the plasma FFA is, however, increased in the cold-acclimated rat living in the cold (139). Even infusion of norepinephrine raises the concentration of FFA in the plasma of cold-acclimated rats (transferred to the warm) only when the dose of norepinephrine administered is small enough not to produce a maximum calorigenic response; there is in fact a negative correlation between the size of the calorigenic response and the rise of FFA concentration in plasma (87), presumably because the maximum rate of output of FFA is achieved at a much lower concentration of norepinephrine (action on white adipose tissue) than the maximum rate of utilization of FFA (occasioned by the accelerated metabolic rate due to the action of norepinephrine on other tissues).

Shivering Thermogenesis

The provision of substrates is one important function of the catecholamines in promoting shivering thermogenesis. However, catecholamines may have another more direct role in shivering.

Shivering is not normally considered a function of the sympathetic nervous system (71), and indeed the original observations of Cannon and co-workers on the responses of surgically sympathectomized cats to cold (25, 162) did not suggest any role of the peripheral sympathetic nervous system or adrenal medulla in shivering; these sympathectomized cats shivered violently, indeed more so than intact cats, when they were exposed to cold. Although Britton (15) observed a failure of shivering in insulin-treated (and hypoglycemic) cats deprived of their adrenal medulla, this appears to have been due to lack of substrate (glucose) rather than lack of epinephrine since it could be rectified either by administration of glucose or by administration of epinephrine. Cats that are not made hypoglycemic are able to shiver in the absence of the adrenal medulla (108).

However, as discussed above (see section *Consequences of Lack of Secretion and/or Action of Catecholamines*), shivering is sometimes inhibited when the sympathetic nervous system is inactivated by "chemical sympathectomy" or by adrenalectomy. Such inhibition has been taken as evidence for a role of the sympathetic nervous system in shivering, a role that was not apparent in the earlier experiments of Cannon because of the incompleteness of the surgical sympathectomy (16, 131, 133). Other suggestions of involvement of catecholamines in shivering have been based on a potentiation of shivering by epinephrine or norepinephrine in cold-exposed, spinalized or pithed dogs (183) and in cold-exposed goats treated with ganglionic blocking agents (2, 3). Nothing is known concerning the way in which catecholamines can potentiate shivering or why in their absence shivering is sometimes inhibited. A direct action of the catecholamines on muscle (14, 138) may potentiate the effect of the nerve impulses that bring about the shivering (see the chapter by Tomita in this volume of the *Handbook*), but such potentiation would be expected to occur only with epinephrine and not with norepinephrine. Mott has described rather variable effects of the catecholamines on shivering (146) and has shown that baroreceptor stimulation by the catecholamines enhances shivering, whereas chemoreceptor stimulation inhibits shivering; thus the effect observed would seem to depend on the degree to which these two kinds of receptors are stimulated by the catecholamines. To some extent the lack of shivering in some of the situations mentioned above may be due to lack of, for example, baroreceptor stimulation, and it is this stimulation that is restored by the administration of catecholamines.

The role of catecholamines secreted by the brain in the regulation of shivering is too extensive a subject to be treated in any detail in this context. Recently, Zeisberger & Brück (206) have presented evidence for the existence of norepinephrine-sensitive cells in the anterior hypothalamus, the stimulation of which results in a raising of the threshold temperature for shivering and also for nonshivering thermogenesis in guinea pigs. An alteration in the function of these cells by depletion of hypothalamic catecholamines by some of the drugs studied (e.g., reserpine) might also lead to disturbances in the regulation of shivering.

Nonshivering Thermogenesis

The evidence that the catecholamines mediate the switching on of nonshivering thermogenesis has been presented in the section ADAPTATION TO COLD and the subsection *Mimicking Effects of Catecholamines*. The biochemical basis for the greatly increased capacity of the cold-acclimated rat to respond to norepinephrine and epinephrine in this way is still not understood. The sites of nonshivering thermogenesis appear to be principally skeletal muscle and brown adipose tissue. No mechanism for the calorigenic effect of catecholamines on muscle is known, and a major obstacle in the study of the mechanism of the calorigenic effect of catecholamines in the cold-acclimated rat is the inability to demonstrate such an enhanced effect in vitro. In contrast, the brown adipose tissue does respond calorigenically to catecholamines in vitro, and recent studies of the metabolism of this tissue have thrown some light on possible mechanisms of catecholamine-induced calorigenesis. It would not be appropriate to review all this work here because several recent reviews are available (82, 129, 175). At present it is only possible to conclude that a rather special loosening of the coupling of oxidative phosphorylation is brought about as a consequence of the rise in fatty acid concentration, which itself is a consequence of the lipolytic effect of the catecholamines on this tissue, an effect mediated by stimulation of adenyl cyclase and increased cyclic AMP production.

The evidence for a role of brown adipose tissue as a site of heat production under the control of the sympathetic nervous system in cold-exposed rats has been reviewed recently (29, 80, 129, 167, 175). There is no doubt that this tissue is a major heat-producing organ in animals, such as the newborn rabbit, that possess large quantities of brown adipose tissue relative to their size. The rat, however, even the cold-acclimated rat in which the amount of the tissue has increased, possesses relatively little brown adipose tissue (less than 1% of body wt), and calculations based on the observed blood flow through the tissue indicate that it cannot consume more than 8–12% of the oxygen consumed by the rat during nonshivering thermogenesis (80, 90, 95, 113). The proportion of the cardiac output going to the brown adipose tissue is only 0.2–0.4% in cold-exposed, warm-acclimated rats and not more than 2% in cold-exposed, cold-acclimated rats (95, 113). This is in marked contrast to the newborn rabbit in which almost 20% of the cardiac output is directed to the brown adipose tissue in the cold (97). The difference between these two species lies only in the relative proportions of brown adipose tissue present; the actual blood flow through the brown adipose tissue per unit weight of tissue is almost exactly the same in cold-exposed newborn rabbits (97) and cold-exposed, cold-acclimated rats (95, 113).

There is evidence that the brown adipose tissue participates in thermogenesis not only in cold-acclimated rats exposed to cold, but also in warm-acclimated rats exposed to cold. The temperature of the tissue rises, and its oxygen tension falls (52, 182). The blood flow of the tissue is also increased under these conditions, and this effect of cold is mimicked by norepinephrine (113). The brown adipose tissue has a rich sympathetic innervation whether the rat is warm-acclimated or cold-acclimated [see (35)]. This innervation includes a norepinephrine-containing supply to the parenchymal cells and a separate supply to the blood vessels (34, 50, 149). The norepinephrine content of the nerve supply to the parenchymal cells is resistant to depletion by procedures that normally deplete norepinephrine-containing nerves, such as immunosympathectomy (50) and denervation (50); it is depleted by reserpine (50, 149) and also by exposure of rats to cold (49). The parenchymal nerve supply appears to contain only a very small proportion of the total norepinephrine present in the tissue, because, although most of the norepinephrine in the tissue measured chemically disappears after surgical denervation (12, 173, 199), this procedure leaves intact the norepinephrine in the nerve endings on the parenchymal cells, as judged by the fluorescence histochemical procedure (50). A curious feature of the increase in blood flow caused by cold exposure is that it is not blocked by procedures or by drugs that would be expected to inactivate the sympathetic innervation. Hexamethonium does not block the cold-induced increase in blood flow in warm-acclimated rats (113), nor does denervation (112). Possibly increased norepinephrine secretion by the nerves to the parenchymal cells occurs in both these situations and is responsible for the increase in blood flow. Reserpine, which does deplete these nerves of their norepinephrine content, also prevents the cold-induced increase in blood flow (112).

As mentioned above, the contribution to nonshivering thermogenesis by brown adipose tissue in cold-acclimated rats would appear to have an upper limit of about 12%. Surgical removal of the interscapular brown adipose tissue (about one-third of the total amount of this rather diffusely distributed organ) has little or no immediate effect on the capacity of cold-acclimated rats (or of warm-acclimated rats) to respond calorigenically to norepinephrine or epinephrine (79). Thus the contribution of this tissue to nonshivering thermogenesis, as measured by the capacity of the animal to respond calorigenically to catecholamines, is small and nonessential. The significance of the heat-producing capacity of the interscapular brown adipose tissue may lie in its special anatomic location [see (175)], with the heat being directed specifically at the spinal cord receptors responsible for the suppression of shivering [see (20–22, 110, 111, 204)]. It should be noted that newborn species are more dependent on thermogenesis within the brown adipose tissue itself; removal of the interscapular brown adipose tissue in newborn rabbits results in almost complete and immediate loss of the calorigenic response to norepinephrine and to cold-exposure (88).

Development of Adaptation for Nonshivering Thermogenesis

The time course of the development of the enhanced calorigenic response to the catecholamines is illustrated in Figures 3 and 4 [see (44, 79, 93)]. Many endocrine adjustments presumably occur during the period of acclimation to cold; however, adjustments in neither adrenal cortical activity nor thyroid activity are necessary for cold-acclimation to be produced [see (75)].

Present evidence indicates that the principal agent that promotes the development of the adaptation is norepinephrine (121, 124, 125). However, the role of epinephrine, if any, seems not to have been studied. Brück (19, 23) has pointed out that certain species, notably the guinea pig and rabbit but also others, such as the rat (188) and sheep (187), are born in a state that resembles cold acclimation, in that they possess a large amount of brown adipose tissue and have a marked capacity for a calorigenic response to norepinephrine and for nonshivering thermogenesis. The newborn guinea pig retains this adaptive state if reared in the cold and regains it if returned to the cold after being reared in the warm (23, 207). Acclimation to cold therefore might be regarded as the reintroduction by the catecholamines of an adaptive state that existed at a certain stage of development during infancy. The development of this particular adaptive state before and immediately after birth is unlikely to be due merely to stimulation by catecholamines; it appears to be a normal stage of development in many species, including man.

In addition to its heat-producing function, the brown adipose tissue appears to have another function in the development and maintenance of adaptation to cold. The evidence for this function is that the surgical removal of the interscapular brown adipose tissue from cold-acclimated rats that subsequently live at room temperature causes a progressive loss of the enhanced capacity of the acclimated rat to respond to norepinephrine and epinephrine; as mentioned above there is no immediate loss of response [(79); Figs. 16 and 17] and no change in the sensitivity of the acclimated rat to norepinephrine (Fig. 18). There is also a progressive loss of cold resistance in these animals (127). Thus the rats lose their adaptive state more rapidly when the interscapular brown adipose tissue is removed. The conclusion to be drawn from these observations is that the interscapular brown adipose tissue influences the capacity of metabolic processes in other tissues to respond to the catecholamines; removal of this influence leads to the loss of the increased capacity of the other tissues to respond to epinephrine or norepinephrine. An endocrine function of the brown adipose tissue in the development of acclimation to cold has therefore been proposed (79) and has found some support in the observation that implantation of the interscapular brown adipose tissue in the peritoneal cavity of the rat from which it was removed delays the loss of the capacity to respond to norepinephrine [(80); Fig. 19]. The nature of the stimulus to this postulated function of the brown adipose tissue is unknown, but it would be logical to consider norepinephrine and epinephrine as likely stimulants. A major problem in studying the role of the brown adipose tissue is its diffuse distribution, which makes it impossible to surgically remove all the tissue; the remarkable

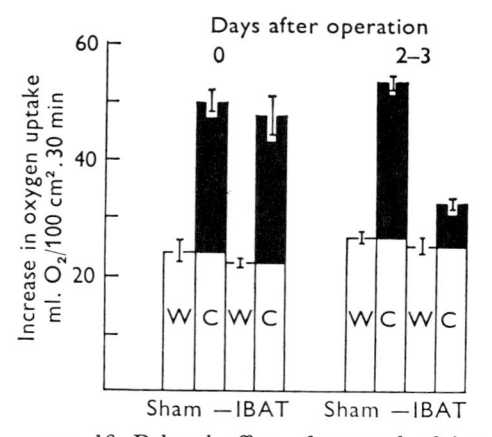

FIG. 16. Delayed effect of removal of interscapular brown adipose tissue on enhanced calorigenic response to epinephrine in cold-acclimated rats. Each *bar* represents mean of values from 10 rats; SE indicated by *vertical line*. Mean weight of cold-acclimated rats at the time they were removed from the cold was 265 g; they had lived in the cold for only 1–2 weeks. Mean weights of warm-acclimated rats at this time was 309 g. *W*, warm-acclimated rats; *C*, cold-acclimated rats. *Solid portion* of *bars* for cold-acclimated rats indicates difference in response between cold-acclimated rats and the corresponding warm-acclimated rats and represents enhancement of calorigenic response to epinephrine caused by acclimation to cold. Values obtained immediately after operation are shown on *left* (day 0); those obtained 2–3 days later are shown on *right*. *Sham*, sham-operated controls; *−IBAT*, rats with their interscapular brown adipose tissue removed. [From Himms-Hagen (79).]

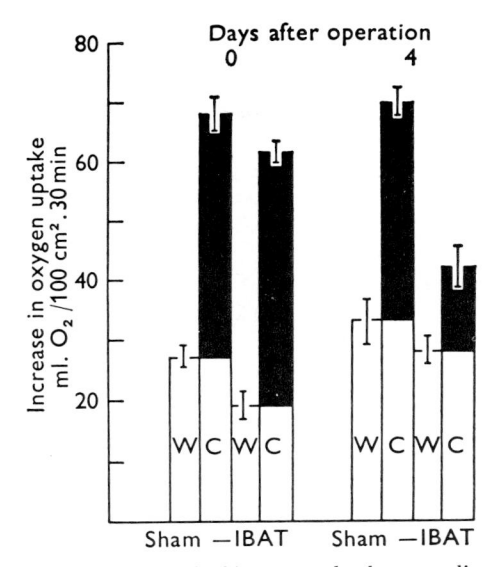

FIG. 17. Delayed effect of removal of interscapular brown adipose tissue on enhanced calorigenic response to norepinephrine in cold-acclimated rats. Each *bar* represents mean of values from 6 rats; SE indicated by *vertical line*. Mean weight of the cold-acclimated rats at time they were removed from the cold was 332 g; they had lived in the cold for 6-11 weeks. Mean weight of warm-acclimated rats at this time was 432 g. Other symbols as in Fig. 16. [From Himms-Hagen (79).]

adaptive ability of the rat to switch a function from one site to another when one is removed makes it impossible to study a rat from which all functioning brown adipose tissue has been removed. This situation is of course analogous to the problem of the function of the adrenal medulla and of the sympathetic nervous system; it is difficult to remove or inactivate either of these two components in a complete and specific manner, and the rat has a remarkable adaptive ability to switch from the use of one component of the sympathetic nervous system to another when one part is not functioning. It is perhaps not a coincidence that these two diffuse organs, sympathetic nervous system and brown adipose tissue, both involved in adaptive mechanisms, should also both possess this capacity to make one part do the work of the other when the latter is nonfunctional.

In the hope of finding a drug that would inactivate the brown adipose tissue throughout the body much as various drugs can inactivate the sympathetic nervous system, the antibiotic oxytetracycline has been used to inhibit mitochondrial biosynthesis in the brown adipose tissue of rats that were acclimating to cold (81). The rationale behind the choice of this drug was that in cold-acclimating rats the brown adipose tissue not only grows [see (175)] but also develops more mitochondria per cell, and each mitochondrion has more cristae (174, 179, 189). There is an accompanying marked increase in the total activity and specific activity of its cytochrome oxidase (7, 96, 174), an enzyme localized in the cristae of the mitochondria (6). It was considered likely that inhibition of this proliferation of mitochondria in the brown adipose tissue might impair the functioning of this tissue in the cold-acclimated rat. Since oxytetracycline is known to inhibit the synthesis of protein in mitochondria it was used in an attempt to inhibit the mitochondrial changes in the brown adipose tissue of cold-acclimating rats (81). The oxytetracycline-treated rats did not develop an enhanced calorigenic response to norepinephrine; nor did the normal proliferation of mitochondria occur in their brown adipose tissue, as judged by the lack of increase in the specific activity of cytochrome oxidase (81), under conditions where no effect of the antibiotic on the liver or muscle cytochrome oxidase was observed. More recent studies have shown that skeletal muscle mitochondria also proliferate in the cold-acclimated rat (7a). The mitochondria are more numerous but smaller, and the total mitochondrial mass does not change. The increase in number of mitochondria is prevented by treatment of the rats with oxytetracycline although, as noted above, this treatment does not alter the total mitochondrial mass. Thus mitochondrial changes that are dependent on mitochondrial protein synthesis occur in both brown adipose tissue and skeletal muscle of cold-acclimated rats. The relation between catecholamines and mitochondrial protein synthesis in acclimation to cold is at present unknown, but it is hoped that further investigations in this area will provide an insight into the nature of nonshivering thermogenesis and the mechanism of development of nonshivering thermogenesis.

CONCLUSIONS

Role of Adrenal Medulla in Acute Exposure to Cold

The transfer of rats or other animal species from a warm environment to a cold environment causes an in-

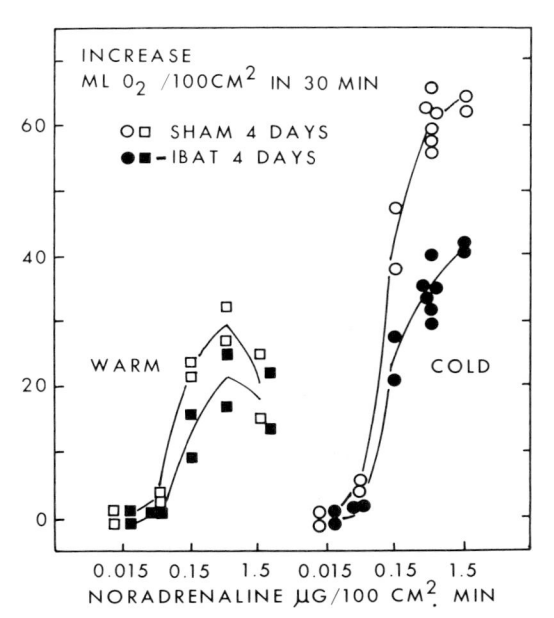

FIG. 18. Dose-response curve for the calorigenic response to norepinephrine (*noradrenaline*) by sham-operated rats and by rats with their interscapular brown adipose tissue removed 4 days previously (−IBAT). Cold-acclimated rats remained at room temperature during the 4 days following the operation.

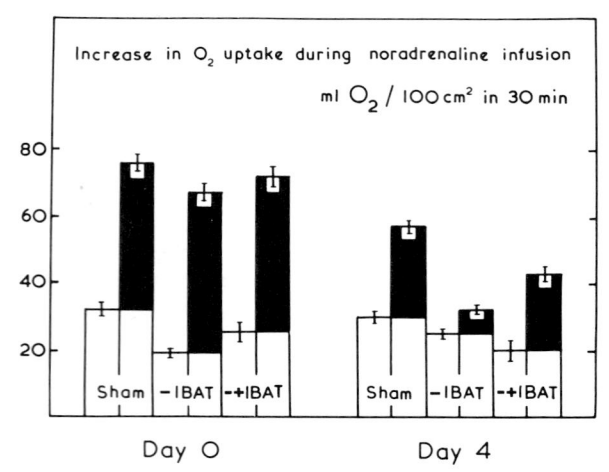

FIG. 19. Effect of removal and replacement of interscapular brown adipose tissue of warm-acclimated and cold-acclimated rats on calorigenic response to norepinephrine (*noradrenaline*). Values shown represent total increase in oxygen uptake during a 30-min infusion of norepinephrine. Each *bar* is mean of 4 experiments ± SEM. Cold-acclimated rats are represented by *bars* with *black upper portions* and warm-acclimated controls are represented by *open bar* to the *left*. *Blackened portion* of bar is difference between response of cold-acclimated rats and response of the corresponding control warm-acclimated rats; it is a measure of acclimation to cold. Cold-acclimated rats had lived in the cold for 10–13 weeks; warm-acclimated rats had lived at room temperature during this same period. Rats were removed from cold or warm rooms on day 0, anesthetized with ether, and operated on as follows: *a*) sham-operated (*Sham*); *b*) interscapular brown adipose tissue removed (*−IBAT*); and *c*) interscapular brown adipose tissue removed, cleaned and weighed, cut into 4 or 5 portions, and replaced in peritoneal cavity (*−+IBAT*); a similar laparotomy was performed also on rats in groups *a* and *b*. Rats remained at room temperature until infusion of norepinephrine. [From Himms-Hagen (80).]

crease in the secretion of epinephrine by the adrenal medulla.

During these early stages of exposure to cold, the principal role of the adrenal medulla appears to be the secretion of epinephrine sufficient to promote the acceleration of the formation of glucose via glycogenolysis and gluconeogenesis. This is not, however, an essential role. The rat can regulate its blood glucose concentration in the absence of the adrenal medulla, albeit in an impaired manner and at a hypoglycemic level; it has an alternate supply of substrate for the support of shivering thermogenesis, namely, the FFA mobilized under the influence of the norepinephrine liberated from sympathetic nerves. The rat appears to employ its adrenal medulla only as a second line of defense against the cold (126), so that this organ only becomes essential for survival if the remainder of the sympathetic nervous system is inactivated in some way. On the other hand, excessive secretion by the adrenal medulla occurs in severely cold-stressed rats and probably has a deleterious effect on survival in the cold; epinephrine is known to exert a toxic effect under such conditions.

Role of Adrenal Medulla in Adaptation to Cold

Certain species, notably the rat, become adapted (or acclimated) to cold when allowed to live at low temperatures for 4 weeks or more; this adaptation takes the form of a greatly enhanced capacity for a calorigenic response to epinephrine and norepinephrine, believed to be the basis of nonshivering thermogenesis, which in cold-acclimated animals replaces shivering as the main heat-producing process. During the development of adaptation to cold, after a brief initial period of a high rate of epinephrine secretion, the secretion of epinephrine by the adrenal medulla is gradually reduced, so that by the time the rats are fully acclimated (i.e., after several weeks) the secretory activity of the adrenal medulla is no longer much greater than that of the adrenal medulla of a rat living in the warm. These changes in the activity of the adrenal medulla might lead to the conclusion that this organ is playing an important role in the adaptation to cold. Although such a conclusion may be correct, it is not necessarily since the presence of the adrenal medulla is not essential for adaptation to take place. It is nevertheless possible to assign to the adrenal medulla certain functions in the regulation of metabolism of cold-acclimated rats living in the cold; these functions are taken over by other regulatory mechanisms when the adrenal medulla is missing. Two observations indicate that the medulla does play a part in nonshivering thermogenesis in cold-acclimated rats. First, removal of the adrenal medulla from rats already acclimated to cold reduces the capacity for nonshivering thermogenesis and impairs the ability to maintain body temperature in the cold. Second, removal of the adrenal medulla from rats already acclimated to cold leads to an upward adjustment in the activity of the remainder of the sympathetic nervous system. These observations suggest that the adrenal medulla, when present, does play some physiological role in cold-acclimated rats living in the cold. The nature of this role of the medulla is uncertain; it could be in substrate mobilization, in the reactions directly involved in calorigenesis, or in maintenance of the adaptive state. Whether epinephrine from the adrenal medulla plays any role in the development of the adaptive state of cold acclimation is unknown; if it does, this role is again a dispensable one. There is, however, no doubt that the sympathetic nervous system as a whole is deeply involved in the development of the adaptation.

The remarkable ability of the rat to substitute one regulatory mechanism for another to serve the same ends is at the same time a fascinating aspect of the regulation of metabolic processes and a difficult experimental problem. This adaptive capacity makes particularly difficult the study of the actual participation of the different parts of the sympathetic nervous system in animals in which no perturbation of function has been created experimentally. This adaptive capacity also interferes with the study of the actual participation of the different deposits of brown adipose tissue in the animal in which no perturbation of the function of this tissue has been made experimentally. The brown adipose tissue appears to play an important role in adaptation to cold, both in heat production and in the development and maintenance of the adaptation. The function of this tissue is regulated by the sympathetic nervous system, and the special sympathetic innervation of this tissue likely plays the major part in this control. Although the adrenal medulla undoubtedly participates in this regulation its precise role remains unknown.

REFERENCES

1. ABEL, J. J. Some recent advances in our knowledge of the ductless glands. *Bull. Johns Hopkins Hosp.* 38: 1–32, 1926.
2. ANDERSSON, B., A. H. BROOK, C. C. GALE, AND B. HÖKFELT. The effect of a ganglionic blocking agent on the thermoregulatory response to preoptic cooling. *Acta Physiol. Scand.* 61: 393–399, 1964.
3. ANDERSSON, B., L. EKMAN, B. HÖKFELT, M. JOBIN, K. OLSSON, AND D. ROBERTSHAW. Studies on the importance of the thyroid and the sympathetic nervous system in the defence to cold of the goat. *Acta Physiol. Scand.* 69: 111–118, 1967.
4. ARNETT, E. L., AND D. T. WATTS. Catecholamine excretion in men exposed to cold. *J. Appl. Physiol.* 15: 499–500, 1960.
5. BALDWIN, B. A., D. L. INGRAM, AND J. LEBLANC. The effects of environmental temperature and hypothalamic temperature on excretion of catecholamines in the urine of the pig. *Brain Res.* 16: 511–515, 1969.
6. BARNARD, T., B. A. AFZELIUS, AND O. LINDBERG. A cytochemical investigation into the distribution of cytochrome oxidase activity within the mitochondria of brown adipose tissue from the prenatal rat. *J. Ultrastruct. Res.* 34: 544–566, 1971.
7. BARNARD, T., J. SKÁLA, AND O. LINDBERG. Changes in interscapular brown adipose tissue of the rat during perinatal and early postnatal development and after cold acclimation. I. Activities of some respiratory enzymes in the tissue. *Comp. Biochem. Physiol.* 33: 499–508, 1970.
7a. BEHRENS, W., AND J. HIMMS-HAGEN. Association of altered skeletal muscle mitochondria with the enhancement of the metabolic response to noradrenaline in cold-acclimated rats. *Federation Proc.* 33: 424, 1974.
8. BERTI, F., R. LENTATI, AND M. M. USARDI. Effects of cold exposure on heart function in immunosympathectomized rats. *Med. Pharmacol. Exptl.* 13: 227–232, 1965.
9. BERTIN, R., AND L. CHEVILLARD. Elimination urinaire des catécholamines chez le rat ♂ Long Evans au cours de l'adaptation à diverses températures. *Compt. Rend. Soc. Biol.* 161: 248–251, 1967.
10. BHAGAT, B., AND E. FRIEDMAN. Factors involved in maintenance of cardiac catecholamine content: relative importance of synthesis and re-uptake. *Brit. J. Pharmacol.* 37: 24–33, 1969.
11. BIBBIANI, C., R. TONGIANI, AND M. P. VIOLA-MAGNI. I. Quantitative determination of the amount of DNA per nucleus by interference microscopy. *J. Cell Biol.* 42: 444–451, 1969.
12. BIECK, P., K. STOCK, AND E. WESTERMANN. Über die Bedeutung des Serotonins im Fettgewebe. *Arch. Pharmakol. Exptl. Pathol.* 256: 218–236, 1967.
13. BOULOUARD, R. Adrenocortical activity during adaptation to cold in the rat: role of Porter-Silber chromogens. *Federation Proc.* 25: 1195–1199, 1966.
14. BOWMAN, W. C., AND E. ZAIMIS. Effects of adrenaline, noradrenaline and isoprenaline on skeletal muscle contractions in the cat. *J. Physiol., London* 144: 92–107, 1958.
15. BRITTON, S. W. Studies on the conditions of activity in endocrine glands. XXII. Adrenin secretion on exposure to cold, together with a possible explanation of hibernation. *Am. J. Physiol.* 84: 119–131, 1928.
16. BRODIE, B. B., R. P. MAICKEL, AND D. N. STERN. Autonomic nervous system and adipose tissue. In: *Handbook of Physiology. Adipose Tissue*, edited by A. E. Renold and G. F. Cahill, Jr. Washington, D.C.: Am. Physiol. Soc., 1965, sect. 5, p. 583–600.
17. BRÜCK, K., AND B. WÜNNENBERG. Blockade der chemischen Thermogenese und Auslösung von Muskelzittern durch Adrenolytica und Ganglienblockade beim neugeborenen Meerschweinchen. *Arch. Ges. Physiol.* 282: 376–389, 1965.
18. BRÜCK, K., AND B. WÜNNENBERG. Untersuchungen über die Bedeutung des multilokulären Fettgewebes für die Thermogenese des neugeborenen Meerschweinchens. *Arch. Ges. Physiol.* 283: 1–16, 1965.
19. BRÜCK, K., AND B. WÜNNENBERG. Influence of ambient temperature in the process of replacement of nonshivering by shivering thermogenesis during postnatal development. *Federation Proc.* 25: 1332–1336, 1966.
20. BRÜCK, K., AND W. WÜNNENBERG. Beziehung zwischen Thermogenese im "braunen" Fettgewebe, Temperatur im cervicalen Anteil des Vertebralkanals und Kältezittern. *Arch. Ges. Physiol.* 290: 167–183, 1966.
21. BRÜCK, K., AND W. WÜNNENBERG. Die Steuerung des Kältezitterns beim Meerschweinchen. *Arch. Ges. Physiol.* 293: 215–225, 1967.
22. BRÜCK, K., AND W. WÜNNENBERG. Eine kälteadaptative Modifikation: Senkung der Schwellentemperaturen für Kältezittern. *Arch. Ges. Physiol.* 293: 226–235, 1967.
23. BRÜCK, K., W. WÜNNENBERG, AND E. ZEISBERGER. Comparison of cold-adaptive metabolic modifications in different species, with special reference to the miniature pig. *Federation Proc.* 28: 1035–1041, 1969.
24. CANNON, W. B. *The Wisdom of the Body.* New York: W. W. Norton Company, 1932.
25. CANNON, W. B., H. F. NEWTON, E. M. BRIGHT, V. MENKIN, AND R. M. MOORE. Some aspects of the physiology of animals surviving complete exclusion of sympathetic nerve impulses. *Am. J. Physiol.* 89: 84–107, 1929.
26. CANNON, W. B., A. QUERIDO, S. W. BRITTON, AND E. M. BRIGHT. Studies on the conditions of activity in endocrine glands. XXI. The role of adrenal secretion in the chemical control of body temperature. *Am. J. Physiol.* 79: 466–507, 1926.
27. CARLSON, L. D. Nonshivering thermogenesis and its endocrine control. *Federation Proc.* 19, Suppl. 5: 25–30, 1960.
28. CARLSON, L. D. The role of catecholamines in cold adaptation. *Pharmacol. Rev.* 18: 291–301, 1966.
29. CHAFFEE, R. R. J., AND J. C. ROBERTS. Temperature acclimation in birds and mammals. *Ann. Rev. Physiol.* 33: 155–202, 1971.
30. CHAN, W. C., AND G. E. JOHNSON. Influence of cold exposure on catecholamine depleting actions of hydroxylase inhibitors. *European J. Pharmacol.* 3: 40–46, 1968.
31. CHEVILLARD, L., AND R. BERTIN. Teneur des surrénales en catécholamines chez le rat ♂ Long Evans au cours de l'adaptation à diverses températures. *Compt. Rend. Soc. Biol.* 161: 279–283, 1967.
32. COMLINE, R. S., AND M. SILVER. Development of activity in the adrenal medulla of the foetus and new-born animal. *Brit. Med. Bull.* 22: 16–20, 1966.
33. CONKLIN, P., AND F. W. HEGGENESS. Maturation of tem-

perature homeostasis in the rat. *Am. J. Physiol.* 220: 333–336, 1971.
34. COTTLE, M. K. W., AND W. H. COTTLE. Adrenergic fibers in brown fat of cold-acclimated rats. *J. Histochem. Cytochem.* 18: 116–119, 1970.
35. COTTLE, W. H. The innervation of brown adipose tissue. In: *Brown Adipose Tissue*, edited by O. Lindberg. New York: Elsevier, 1970, p. 155–178.
36. COTTLE, W. H., AND L. D. CARLSON. Regulation of heat production in cold-adapted rats. *Proc. Soc. Exptl. Biol. Med.* 92: 845–849, 1956.
37. COTTLE, W. H., C. W. NASH, A. T. VERESS, AND B. A. FERGUSON. Release of noradrenaline from brown fat of cold-acclimated rats. *Life Sci.* 6: 2267–2271, 1967.
38. CRAMER, W. *Fever, Heat Regulation, Climate, and the Thyroid-Adrenal Apparatus.* London: Longmans, Green, 1928.
39. CROWDEN, G. P., AND M. G. PEARSON. The effect of cold on the adrenaline content of the suprarenal glands. *J. Physiol., London* 65: xxv, 1928.
40. DANDIYA, P. C., G. JOHNSON, AND E. A. SELLERS. Influence of variation in environmental temperature on the acute toxicity of reserpine and chlorpromazine in mice. *Can. J. Biochem. Physiol.* 38: 591–596, 1960.
41. DAVIS, T. R. A., D. R. JOHNSTON, F. C. BELL, AND B. J. CREMER. Regulation of shivering and non-shivering heat production during acclimation of rats. *Am. J. Physiol.* 198: 471–475, 1960.
42. DAWES, G. S., AND G. MESTYÁN. Changes in the oxygen consumption of new-born guinea pigs and rabbits on exposure to cold. *J. Physiol., London* 168: 22–42, 1963.
43. DEPOCAS, F. Chemical thermogenesis in the functionally eviscerated cold-acclimated rat. *Can. J. Biochem. Physiol.* 36: 691–699, 1958.
44. DEPOCAS, F. The calorigenic response of cold-acclimated white rats to infused noradrenaline. *Can. J. Biochem. Physiol.* 38: 107–114, 1960.
45. DEPOCAS, F. Calorigenesis from various organ systems in the whole animal. *Federation Proc.* 19, Suppl. 5: 19–24, 1960.
46. DEPOCAS, F. Glucose metabolism in warm- and cold-acclimated rats. *Federation Proc.* 19, Suppl. 5: 106–109, 1960.
47. DEPOCAS, F. Body glucose as fuel in white rats exposed to cold: results with fasted rats. *Am. J. Physiol.* 202: 1015–1018, 1962.
48. DEPOCAS, F., AND R. MASIRONI. Body glucose as fuel for thermogenesis in the white rat exposed to cold. *Am. J. Physiol.* 199: 1051–1055, 1960.
49. DERRY, D. M., J. RANSON, AND E. MORROW. Effect of isoproterenol on brown and white fat of the adult rat. *Can. J. Physiol. Pharmacol.* 49: 8–13, 1971.
50. DERRY, D. M., E. SCHÖNBAUM, AND G. STEINER. Two sympathetic nerve supplies to brown adipose tissue of the rat. *Can. J. Physiol. Pharmacol.* 47: 57–63, 1969.
51. DESMARAIS, A., AND L-P. DUGAL. Circulation périphérique et teneur des surrénales en adrénaline et en artérénol (noradrénaline) chez le rat blanc exposé au froid. *Can. J. Med. Sci.* 29: 90–99, 1951.
52. DONHOFFER, S., F. SÁRDY, AND G. SZEGVÁRI. Brown adipose tissue and thermoregulatory heat production in the rat. *Nature* 203: 765–766, 1964.
53. DRASKÓCZY, P. R., K. PULLEY, AND W. R. BURACK. The effects of cold environment on the endogenously labeled catecholamine stores. *Pharmacologist* 8: 178, 1966.
54. EKSTRÖM, T., N. LUNDGREN, AND C. G. SCHMITERLÖW. On the effect of local stimulation by cold on the adrenaline secretion. *Acta Physiol. Scand.* 6: 52–61, 1943.
55. ERÄNKÖ, O., AND L. RÄISÄNEN. Adrenaline and noradrenaline in the adrenal medulla during postnatal development of the rat. *Endocrinology* 60: 753–760, 1957.
56. ESTLER, C-J., AND H. P. T. AMMON. The importance of the adrenergic beta-receptors for thermogenesis and survival of acutely cold-exposed mice. *Can. J. Physiol. Pharmacol.* 47: 427–434, 1969.
57. ESTLER, C-J., H. P. T. AMMON, AND B. LANG. Ineffectiveness of nicotinic acid to impair thermoregulation in cold-exposed mice. *European J. Pharmacol.* 9: 257–260, 1970.
58. ESTLER, C-J., O. STRUBELT, AND H. P. T. AMMON. Der Einfluss adrenerger β-Blockade auf die Wärmebildung bei akuter Kälteexposition. *Arch. Ges. Physiol.* 289: 227–236, 1966.
59. FEIST, D. D. Blockade of arousal from hibernation by inhibition of norepinephrine synthesis in the golden hamster. *Life Sci., Part 1* 9: 1117–1125, 1970.
60. FEIST, D. D. Brown fat norepinephrine contents and turnover during cold acclimation and hibernation in the golden hamster. *Comp. Gen. Pharmacol.* 1: 299–315, 1970.
61. FRIEDMAN, E., AND B. BHAGAT. Uptake of (^{3}H) noradrenaline in the rat heart during increased sympathetic nervous activity associated with cold. *J. Pharm. Pharmacol.* 20: 963–965, 1968.
62. FULLER, R. W., AND J. M. HUNT. Inhibition of phenethanolamine N-methyl transferase by its product, epinephrine. *Life Sci.* 6: 1107–1112, 1967.
63. GIBSON, S., E. G. MCGEER, AND P. L. MCGEER. Metabolism of catecholamines in cold-exposed rats. *J. Neurochem.* 16: 1491–1493, 1969.
64. GILGEN, A., R. P. MAICKEL, O. NIKODIJEVIC, AND B. B. BRODIE. Essential role of catecholamines in the mobilization of free fatty acids and glucose after exposure to cold. *Life Sci.* 1: 709–715, 1962.
65. HAMBERGER, B., R. LEVI-MONTALCINI, K. A. NORBERG, AND F. SJÖQVIST. Monoamines in immunosympathectomized rats. *Intern. J. Neuropharmacol.* 4: 91–95, 1965.
66. HART, J. S., O. HÉROUX, AND F. DEPOCAS. Cold acclimation and the electromyogram of unanaesthetised rats. *J. Appl. Physiol.* 9: 404–408, 1956.
67. HARTMAN, F. A., AND W. B. HARTMAN. Influence of temperature changes on the secretion of epinephrine. *Am. J. Physiol.* 65: 612–622, 1923.
68. HARTMAN, F. A., H. A. MCCORDOCK, AND M. M. LODER. Conditions determining adrenal secretion. *Am. J. Physiol.* 64: 1–34, 1923.
69. HASHIMOTO, Y., T. NISHIMURA, Y. KUROBE, Y. KOHASHI, M. KAKIE, AND J. ANDO. Effect of 3′,5′-dimethylpyrazole on colonic temperature, plasma glucose, NEFA and corticosterone in the non-acclimated rat subjected to cold. *Japan. J. Pharmacol.* 20: 441–442, 1970.
70. HEIM, T., AND D. HULL. The effect of propranolol on the calorigenic response in brown adipose tissue of new-born rabbits to catecholamines, glucagon, corticotrophin and cold exposure. *J. Physiol., London* 187: 271–283, 1966.
71. HEMINGWAY, A., AND W. M. PRICE. The autonomic nervous system and regulation of body temperature. *Anesthesiology* 29: 693–701, 1968.
72. HÉROUX, O. Acclimation of adrenalectomized rats to low environmental temperature. *Am. J. Physiol.* 181: 75–78, 1955.
73. HÉROUX, O. The effect of intermittent indoor cold exposure on white rats. *Can. J. Biochem. Physiol.* 38: 517–521, 1960.
74. HÉROUX, O. Effect of guanethidine on metabolic response to noradrenaline and cold resistance in warm-acclimated rats. *Can. J. Physiol. Pharmacol.* 42: 265–267, 1964.
75. HÉROUX, O. Catecholamines, corticosteroids and thyroid hormones in nonshivering thermogenesis under different environmental conditions. In: *Physiology and Pathology of Adaptation Mechanisms*, edited by E. Bajusz. Oxford: Pergamon Press, 1969, p. 347–365.
76. HÉROUX, O., J. S. HART, AND F. DEPOCAS. Metabolism and muscle activity of anesthetized warm and cold acclimated rats on exposure to cold. *J. Appl. Physiol.* 9: 399–403, 1956.
77. HIMMS-HAGEN, J. Lipid metabolism in warm-acclimated and cold-acclimated rats exposed to cold. *Can. J. Physiol. Pharmacol.* 43: 379–403, 1965.
78. HIMMS-HAGEN, J. Sympathetic regulation of metabolism. *Pharmacol. Rev.* 19: 367–461, 1967.
79. HIMMS-HAGEN, J. The role of brown adipose tissue in the

calorigenic effect of adrenaline and noradrenaline in cold-acclimated rats. *J. Physiol., London* 205: 393–403, 1969.
80. HIMMS-HAGEN, J. Regulation of metabolic processes in brown adipose tissue in relation to nonshivering thermogenesis. In: *Advances in Enzyme Regulation*, edited by G. Weber. Oxford: Pergamon Press, 1970, vol. 8, p. 131–151.
81. HIMMS-HAGEN, J. Inhibition by oxytetracycline of the development of the enhanced response to noradrenaline in cold-acclimated rats: a new approach to the study of nonshivering thermogenesis. *Can. J. Physiol. Pharmacol.* 49: 545–553, 1971.
82. HIMMS-HAGEN, J. Effects of catecholamines on metabolism. In: *Handbuch der Experimentellen Pharmakologie. Catecholamines*, edited by H. Blaschko and E. Muscholl. Heidelberg: Springer, 1972, vol. 33, p. 363–462.
83. HIMMS-HAGEN, J., AND P. HAGEN. Actions of adrenalin and noradrenalin on metabolic systems. In: *Actions of Hormones on Molecular Processes*, edited by G. Litwack and D. Kritchevsky. New York: Wiley, 1964, p. 268–319.
84. HSIEH, A. C. L., AND L. D. CARLSON. Role of the thyroid in metabolic response to low temperature. *Am. J. Physiol.* 188: 40–44, 1957.
85. HSIEH, A. C. L., AND L. D. CARLSON. Role of adrenaline and noradrenaline in chemical regulation of heat production. *Am. J. Physiol.* 190: 243–246, 1957.
86. HSIEH, A. C. L., L. D. CARLSON, AND G. GRAY. Role of the sympathetic nervous system in the control of chemical regulation of heat production. *Am. J. Physiol.* 190: 247–251, 1957.
87. HSIEH, A. C. L., C. W. PUN, K. M. LI, AND K. W. TI. Circulatory and metabolic effects of noradrenaline in cold-adapted rats. *Federation Proc.* 25: 1205–1209, 1966.
88. HULL, D., AND M. M. SEGALL. The contribution of brown adipose tissue to heat production in the new-born rabbit. *J. Physiol., London* 181: 449–457, 1965.
89. HYMAN, A. I., AND M. E. TOWELL. Effects of catecholamine depletion on metabolic response to cold in the newborn guinea pig. *Am. J. Physiol.* 214: 691–694, 1968.
90. IMAI, Y., B. A. HORWITZ, AND R. E. SMITH. Calorigenesis of brown adipose tissue in cold-exposed rats. *Proc. Soc. Exptl. Biol. Med.* 127: 717–719, 1968.
91. JANSKÝ, L. Adaptability of heat production mechanisms in homeotherms. *Acta Univ. Carolinae Biol.* 1: 1–91, 1965.
92. JANSKÝ, L., R. BARTUŇKOVÁ, J. KOČKOVA, J. MEJSNAR, AND E. ZEISBERGER. Interspecies differences in cold adaptation and nonshivering thermogenesis. *Federation Proc.* 28: 1053–1058, 1969.
93. JANSKÝ, L., R. BARTUŇKOVÁ, AND E. ZEISBERGER. Acclimation of the white rat to cold: noradrenaline thermogenesis. *Physiol. Bohemoslov.* 16: 366–372, 1967.
94. JANSKÝ, L., AND J. S. HART. Participation of skeletal muscle and kidney during nonshivering thermogenesis in cold-acclimated rats. *Can. J. Biochem. Physiol.* 41: 953–964, 1963.
95. JANSKÝ, L., AND J. S. HART. Cardiac output and organ blood flow in warm- and cold-acclimated rats exposed to cold. *Can. J. Physiol. Pharmacol.* 46: 653–659, 1968.
96. JANSKÝ, L., Z. VOTÁPKOVÁ, AND E. FEIGLOVÁ. Total cytochrome oxidase activity of the brown fat and its thermogenetic significance. *Physiol. Bohemoslov.* 18: 443–451, 1969.
97. JÁRAI, I. The redistribution of cardiac output on cold exposure in new-born rabbits. *J. Physiol., London* 202: 559–567, 1969.
98. JARRATT, A. M., AND N. W. NOWELL. The effect of adrenal demedullation on the blood sugar level of rats subjected to long-term cold stress. *Can. J. Physiol. Pharmacol.* 47: 1–6, 1969.
99. JOHNSON, D. G. The effect of cold exposure on the catecholamine excretion of rats treated with decaborane. *Acta Physiol. Scand.* 68: 129–133, 1966.
100. JOHNSON, G. E. The effect of cold exposure on the catecholamine excretion of adrenalectomized rats treated with reserpine. *Acta Physiol. Scand.* 59: 438–444, 1963.
101. JOHNSON, G. E. Interrelationships of low environmental temperatures on the actions of drugs. In: *Physiology and Pathology of Adaptation Mechanisms*, edited by E. Bajusz. Oxford: Pergamon Press, 1969, p. 390–409.
102. JOHNSON, G. E., K. V. FLATTERY, AND E. SCHÖNBAUM. The influence of methimazole on the catecholamine excretion of cold-stressed rats. *Can. J. Physiol. Pharmacol.* 45: 415–421, 1967.
103. JOHNSON, G. E., AND K. PRITZKER. The influence of the dopa decarboxylase inhibitor Ro4-4602 on the urinary excretion of catecholamines in cold-stressed rats. *J. Pharmacol. Exptl. Therap.* 152: 432–438, 1966.
104. JOHNSON, G. E., AND T. A. PUGSLEY. The formation and release of metaraminol during exposure to warm or cold environments. *Brit. J. Pharmacol.* 34: 267–276, 1968.
105. JOHNSON, G. E., E. SCHÖNBAUM, AND E. A. SELLERS. Cold exposure: pharmacologic investigation of the compensatory mechanisms in the maintenance of normothermia. *Federation Proc.* 25: 1216–1219, 1966.
106. KAWAHATA, A., AND L. D. CARLSON. Role of rat liver in nonshivering thermogenesis. *Proc. Soc. Exptl. Biol. Med.* 101: 303–306, 1959.
107. KLEPPING, J., M. TANCHE, AND J. F. CIER. La sécrétion médullosurrénale dans la lutte contre le froid. *Compt. Rend. Soc. Biol.* 151: 1539–1541, 1957.
108. KOJIMA, S. A note on the calorigenic effect of cold in cats deprived of the suprarenal medulla. *Tohoku J. Exptl. Med.* 40: 353–370, 1941.
109. KOPIN, I. J., AND E. K. GORDON. Metabolism of norepinephrine-H^3 released by tyramine and reserpine. *J. Pharmacol. Exptl. Therap.* 138: 351–359, 1962.
110. KOSAKA, M., AND E. SIMON. Der zentralnervöse spinale Mechanismus des Kältezitterns. *Arch. Ges. Physiol.* 302: 357–373, 1968.
111. KOSAKA, M., E. SIMON, R. THAUER, AND O-E. WALTHER. Effect of thermal stimulation of spinal cord on respiratory and cortical activity. *Am. J. Physiol.* 217: 858–864, 1969.
112. KUROSHIMA, A., K. DOI, AND S. ITOH. Nervous and humoral influences on the blood flow response of brown adipose tissue to cold in the rat. *Japan. J. Physiol.* 19: 392–402, 1969.
113. KUROSHIMA, A., N. KONNO, AND S. ITOH. Increase in the blood flow through brown adipose tissue in response to cold exposure and norepinephrine in the rat. *Japan. J. Physiol.* 17: 523–537, 1967.
114. KVETŇANSKÝ, R., G. P. GEWIRTZ, V. K. WEISE, AND I. J. KOPIN. Catecholamine-synthesizing enzymes in the rat adrenal gland during exposure to cold. *Am. J. Physiol.* 220: 928–931, 1971.
115. KVETŇANSKÝ, R., AND L. MIKULAJ. Adrenal and urinary catecholamines in rats during adaptation to repeated immobilization stress. *Endocrinology* 87: 738–743, 1970.
116. KVETŇANSKÝ, R., V. K. WEISE, AND I. L. KOPIN. Elevation of adrenal tyrosine hydroxylase and phenylethanolamine-N-methyl transferase by repeated immobilization of rats. *Endocrinology* 87: 744–749, 1970.
117. LEBLANC, J. Effects of reserpine on increased sensitivity to noradrenaline of cold-adapted animals. *J. Appl. Physiol.* 21: 661–664, 1966.
118. LEBLANC, J. Adaptation to cold in three hours. *Am. J. Physiol.* 212: 530–532, 1967.
119. LEBLANC, J. Stress and interstress adaptation. *Federation Proc.* 28: 996–1000, 1969.
120. LEBLANC, J., AND G. NADEAU. Urinary excretion of adrenaline and noradrenaline in normal and cold-adapted animals. *Can. J. Biochem. Physiol.* 39: 215–217, 1961.
121. LEBLANC, J., AND M. POULIOT. Importance of noradrenaline in cold adaptation. *Am. J. Physiol.* 207: 853–856, 1964.
122. LEBLANC, J., C. ROBERGE, J. VALLIÈRE, AND G. OAKSON. The sympathetic nervous system in short-term adaptation to cold. *Can. J. Physiol. Pharmacol.* 49: 96–101, 1971.
123. LEBLANC, J., D. ROBINSON, D. F. SHARMAN, AND P. TOUSIGNANT. Catecholamines and short-term adaptation to cold in mice. *Am. J. Physiol.* 213: 1419–1422, 1967.
124. LEBLANC, J., AND A. VILLEMAIRE. Thyroxine and noradrena-

line on noradrenaline sensitivity, cold resistance, and brown fat. *Am. J. Physiol.* 218: 1742–1745, 1970.
125. LeBlanc, J., A. Villemaire, and J. Valliere. Simultaneous sensitization to metabolic and cardiovascular effects of noradrenaline. *Arch. Intern. Physiol. Biochem.* 77: 731–740, 1969.
126. Leduc, J. Catecholamine production and release in exposure and acclimation to cold. *Acta Physiol. Scand. Suppl.* 183, 1961.
127. Leduc, J., and P. Rivest. Effets de l'ablation de la graisse brune interscapulaire sur l'acclimatation au froid chez le rat. *Rev. Can. Biol.* 28: 49–66, 1969.
128. Lettau, H. F., E. A. Sellers, and E. Schönbaum. Modification of drug-induced hypothermia. *Can. J. Physiol. Pharmacol.* 42: 745–755, 1964.
129. Lindberg, O. (editor). *Brown Adipose Tissue.* New York: Elsevier, 1970.
130. Lutherer, L. O., M. J. Fregly, and A. H. Anton. An interrelationship between theophylline and catecholamines in the hypothyroid rat acutely exposed to cold. *Federation Proc.* 28: 1238–1242, 1969.
131. Maickel, R. P. Interaction of drugs with autonomic nervous function and thermoregulation. *Federation Proc.* 29: 1973–1979, 1970.
132. Maickel, R. P., N. Matussek, D. N. Stern, and B. B. Brodie. The sympathetic nervous system as a homeostatic mechanism. i. Absolute need for sympathetic nervous function in body temperature maintenance of cold-exposed rats. *J. Pharmacol. Exptl. Therap.* 157: 103–110, 1967.
133. Maickel, R. P., D. N. Stern, and B. B. Brodie. The role of autonomic nervous function in mammalian thermoregulation. In: *Biochemical and Neurophysiological Correlates of Centrally Acting Drugs,* edited by E. Trabucchi, R. Paoletti, and N. Canal. Oxford: Pergamon Press, 1964, p. 225–237.
134. Maickel, R. P., D. N. Stern, E. Takabatake, and B. B. Brodie. The sympathetic nervous system as a homeostatic mechanism. ii. Effect of adrenocortical hormones on body temperature maintenance of cold-exposed adrenalectomized rats. *J. Pharmacol. Exptl. Therap.* 157: 111–116, 1967.
135. Maickel, R. P., H. Sussman, K. Yamada, and B. B. Brodie. Control of adipose tissue lipase activity by the sympathetic nervous system. *Life Sci.* 3: 210–214, 1963.
136. Maickel, R. P., E. O. Westermann, and B. B. Brodie. Effects of reserpine and cold-exposure on pituitary-adrenocortical function in rats. *J. Pharmacol. Exptl. Therap.* 134: 167–175, 1961.
137. Manara, L., E. Costa, D. N. Stern, and R. P. Maickel. Effect of chemical sympathectomy on oxygen consumption by the cold-exposed rat. *Intern. J. Neuropharmacol.* 4: 301–307, 1965.
138. Marsden, C. D., and J. C. Meadows. The effect of adrenaline on the contraction of human muscle. *J. Physiol., London* 207: 429–448, 1970.
139. Masironi, R., and F. Depocas. Effect of cold exposure on respiratory $C^{14}O_2$ production during infusion of albumin-bound palmitate-1-C^{14} in white rats. *Can. J. Biochem. Physiol.* 39: 219–224, 1961.
140. Moore, K. E., D. N. Calvert, and T. M. Brody. Tissue catecholamine content of cold-acclimated rats. *Proc. Soc. Exptl. Biol. Med.* 106: 816–818, 1961.
141. Moore, R. E., and M. C. Underwood. Possible role of noradrenaline in control of heat production in the newborn mammal. *Lancet* 1: 1277–1278, 1960.
142. Moore, R. E., and M. C. Underwood. The thermogenic effects of noradrenaline in new-born and infant kittens and other small mammals. A possible hormonal mechanism in the control of heat production. *J. Physiol., London* 168: 290–317, 1963.
143. Morin, G. Medullo-surrénale et régulation thermique. ii. Action adrénalino-sécrétrice du froid. *Rev. Can. Biol.* 5: 388–399, 1946.
144. Morin, G. L'adrénaline, hormone de défense contre le froid. *Biol. Méd.* 37: 196–230, 1948.
145. Motelica, I. Urinary excretion of catecholamines and vanilmandelic acid in rats exposed to cold. *Acta Physiol. Scand.* 76: 393–395, 1969.
146. Mott, J. C. The effects of baroreceptor and chemoreceptor stimulation on shivering. *J. Physiol., London* 166: 563–586, 1963.
147. Nagakura, G. Influence of cold upon the heart and pupil, both denervated, in dogs, before and after demedullation of the suprarenals. *Tohoku J. Exptl. Med.* 50: 39–49, 1949.
148. Nathanielsz, P. W. Effect of cold (4°C) on catecholamine excretion in the diabetic rat and its relation to autonomic neuropathy. *Diabetes* 18: 625–626, 1969.
149. Ochi, J., M. Konishi, and H. Yoshikawa. Morphologischer Nachweis der sympathischen Innervation des braunen Fettgewebes bei der Ratte. *Z. Anat. Entwicklungsgeschichte* 129: 259–267, 1969.
150. Oliverio, A., and L. Stjärne. Acceleration of noradrenaline turnover in the mouse heart by cold exposure. *Life Sci.* 4: 2339–2343, 1965.
151. Opitz, K., and H. Chu. Zur stoffwechselsteigernden Wirkung der Brenzcatechinamine. *Arch. Pharmakol. Exptl. Pathol.* 259: 329–343, 1968.
152. Partington, P. P. The production of sympathin in response to physiological stimuli in the unanaesthetized animal. *Am. J. Physiol.* 117: 55–58, 1936.
153. Pelc, S. R., and M. P. Viola-Magni. iii. Decrease of labeled DNA in cells of the adrenal medulla after intermittent exposure to cold. *J. Cell Biol.* 42: 460–468, 1969.
154. Penner, P. E., and J. Himms-Hagen. Gluconeogenesis in rats during cold-acclimation. *Can. J. Biochem.* 46: 1205–1213, 1968.
155. Poe, R. H., and T. R. A. Davis. Cold exposure and acclimation in alloxan-diabetic rats. *Am. J. Physiol.* 202: 1045–1048, 1962.
156. Pohorecky, L. A., and R. J. Wurtman. Adrenocortical control of epinephrine synthesis. *Pharmacol. Rev.* 23: 1–35, 1971.
157. Pouliot, M. Catecholamine excretion in adreno-demedullated rats exposed to cold after chronic guanethidine treatment. *Acta Physiol. Scand.* 68: 164–168, 1966.
158. Pouliot, M., and J. Leblanc. Effets de la réserpine, guanethidine et alpha-methyl-dopa sur la resistance au froid. *Arch. Intern. Physiol. Biochem.* 71: 73–82, 1963.
159. Ring, G. C. The importance of the thyroid in maintaining an adequate production of heat during exposure to cold. *Am. J. Physiol.* 137: 582–588, 1942.
160. Saito, S. Influence of application of cold or heat to the dog's body upon the epinephrine output rate. *Tohoku J. Exptl. Med.* 11: 544–567, 1928.
161. Sandler, M., C. J. R. Ruthven, I. C. S. Normand, and R. E. Moore. Environmental temperature and urinary excretion of 3-methoxy-4-hydroxymandelic acid in the newborn. *Lancet* 1: 485–486, 1961.
162. Sawyer, M. E. M., and T. Schlossberg. Studies of homeostasis in normal, sympathectomized and ergotaminized animals. *Am. J. Physiol.* 104: 172–183, 1933.
163. Schiff, D., L. Stern, and J. Leduc. Chemical thermogenesis in newborn infants: catecholamine excretion and the plasma non-esterified fatty acid response to cold exposure. *Pediatrics* 37: 577–582, 1966.
164. Schönbaum, E., G. E. Johnson, and E. A. Sellers. Acclimation to cold and norepinephrine; effects of immunosympathectomy. *Am. J. Physiol.* 211: 647–650, 1966.
165. Schönbaum, E., G. E. Johnson, E. A. Sellers, and M. J. Gill. Adrenergic β-receptors and non-shivering thermogenesis. *Nature* 210: 426, 1966.
166. Schönbaum, E., E. A. Sellers, and G. E. Johnson. Noradrenaline and survival of rats in a cold environment. *Can. J. Biochem. Physiol.* 41: 975–983, 1963.
167. Schönbaum, E., G. Steiner, and E. A. Sellers. Brown adipose tissue and norepinephrine. In: *Brown Adipose Tissue,* edited by O. Lindberg. New York: Elsevier, 1970, p. 179–196.

168. Sellers, E. A., K. V. Flattery, A. Shum, and G. E. Johnson. Thyroid status in relation to catecholamines in cold and warm environment. *Can. J. Physiol. Pharmacol.* 49: 268–275, 1971.
169. Sellers, E. A., J. W. Scott, and N. Thomas. Electrical activity of skeletal muscle of normal and acclimatized rats on exposure to cold. *Am. J. Physiol.* 177: 372–376, 1954.
170. Sengupta, A. K., M. O. Prakesh, and A. Ghose. Noradrenaline and cold acclimation. *Japan. J. Physiol.* 18: 563–569, 1968.
171. Shum, A., G. E. Johnson, and K. V. Flattery. Influence of ambient temperature on excretion of catecholamines and metabolites. *Am. J. Physiol.* 216: 1164–1169, 1969.
172. Shum, A., G. E. Johnson, and K. V. Flattery. Influence of ganglionic blockade on catecholamine and metabolite excretion. *Am. J. Physiol.* 219: 58–61, 1970.
173. Sidman, R. L., M. Perkins, and N. Weiner. Noradrenaline and adrenaline content of adipose tissues. *Nature* 193: 36–37, 1962.
174. Skala, J., T. Barnard, and O. Lindberg. Changes in interscapular brown adipose tissue of the rat during perinatal and early postnatal development and after cold acclimation. II. Mitochondrial changes. *Comp. Biochem. Physiol.* 33: 509–528, 1970.
175. Smith, R. E., and B. A. Horwitz. Brown fat and thermogenesis. *Physiol. Rev.* 49: 330–425, 1969.
176. Stern, L., M. H. Lees, and J. Leduc. Environmental temperature, oxygen consumption, and catecholamine excretion in newborn infants. *Pediatrics* 36: 367–373, 1965.
177. Stock, K., and E. Westermann. Über die Bedeutung des Noradrenalingehaltes im Fettgewebe für die Mobilisierung unveresterter Fettsäuren. *Arch. Exptl. Pathol. Pharmakol.* 251: 465–487, 1965.
178. Strubelt, O. Die Bedeutung der adrenergischen β-Receptoren für die kalorigene Wirkung sympathicomimetischer Amine. *Arch. Exptl. Pathol. Pharmakol.* 251: 126–127, 1965.
179. Suter, E. R. The fine structure of brown adipose tissue. I. Cold-induced changes in the rat. *J. Ultrastruct. Res.* 26: 216–241, 1969.
180. Suzuki, M., T. Tonoue, S. Matsuzaki, and K. Yamamoto. Initial responses of human thyroid, adrenal cortex and adrenal medulla to acute cold exposure. *Can. J. Physiol. Pharmacol.* 45: 423–432, 1967.
181. Swanson, H. E. The effect of temperature on the potentiation of adrenalin by thyroxine in the albino rat. *Endocrinology* 60: 205–213, 1957.
182. Szelényi, Z. Effect of cold exposure on oxygen tension in brown adipose tissue in the non-cold-adapted adult rat. *Acta Physiol. Acad. Sci. Hung.* 33: 311–316, 1968.
183. Tanche, M., and A. Therminarias. Thyroxine and catecholamines during cold exposure in dogs. *Federation Proc.* 28: 1257–1261, 1969.
184. Taylor, P. M. Oxygen consumption in new-born rats. *J. Physiol., London* 154: 153–168, 1960.
185. Thibault, O. Les facteurs hormonaux de la régulation chimique de la température des homéothermes. *Rev. Can. Biol.* 8: 3–131, 1949.
186. Thoenen, H. Induction of tyrosine hydroxylase in peripheral and central adrenergic neurones by cold-exposure of rats. *Nature* 228: 861–862, 1970.
187. Thompson, G. E., and D. M. Jenkinson. Nonshivering thermogenesis in the newborn lamb. *Can. J. Physiol. Pharmacol.* 47: 249–253, 1969.
188. Thompson, G. E., and R. E. Moore. A study of newborn rats exposed to the cold. *Can. J. Physiol. Pharmacol.* 46: 865–871, 1968.
189. Thomson, J. F., D. A. Habeck, S. L. Nance, and K. L. Beetham. Ultrastructural and biochemical changes in brown fat in cold-exposed rats. *J. Cell Biol.* 41: 312–334, 1969.
190. Tongiani, R., and M. P. Viola-Magni. II. Differences in adrenal medulla nuclear DNA content among rats of different strains following intermittent exposure to cold. *J. Cell Biol.* 42: 452–459, 1969.
191. Viola-Magni, M. P. The incorporation of H^3-thymidine in the nuclei of the cells of adrenal medulla of rats. *Experientia* 21: 716–717, 1965.
192. Viola-Magni, M. P. A radioautographic study with H^3-thymidine on adrenal medulla nuclei of rats intermittently exposed to cold. *J. Cell Biol.* 28: 9–19, 1966.
193. Viola-Magni, M. P. An analysis of DNA loss and synthesis in the rat adrenal medulla nuclei upon cold stimulation. *J. Cell Biol.* 30: 213–225, 1966.
194. Von Euler, U. S. *Noradrenaline*. Springfield, Ill.: Thomas, 1956.
195. Von Euler, U. S. Exposure to cold and catecholamines. *Federation Proc.* 19, Suppl. 4: 79–81, 1960.
196. Wada, M., and K. Fuzuii. Effect of severe cold upon the rate of the denervated heart of non-anaesthetized dogs and the epinephrine secretion. *Tohoku J. Exptl. Med.* 37: 505–516, 1940.
197. Wada, M., M. Seo, and K. Abe. Further study of the influence of cold on the rate of epinephrine secretion from the suprarenals with simultaneous determination of the blood sugar. *Tohoku J. Exptl. Med.* 26: 381–411, 1935.
198. Webster, A. J. F., J. H. Heitman, F. L. Hays, and G. P. Olynyk. Catecholamines and cold thermogenesis in sheep. *Can. J. Physiol. Pharmacol.* 47: 719–724, 1969.
199. Weiner, N., M. Perkins, and R. L. Sidman. Effect of reserpine on noradrenaline content of innervated and denervated brown adipose tissue of the rat. *Nature* 193: 137–138, 1962.
200. Wekstein, D. R. Sympathetic function and development of temperature regulation. *Am. J. Physiol.* 206: 823–826, 1964.
201. Westermann, E. O. Cumulative effects of reserpine on the pituitary-adrenocortical and sympathetic nervous system. In: *Drugs and Enzymes*, edited by B. B. Brodie. Oxford: Pergamon, 1965, p. 381–392.
202. Williams, D. D. The effects of cold exposure and guanethidine on norepinephrine thermogenesis in the golden hamster. *Comp. Biochem. Physiol.* 27: 567–573, 1968.
203. Wilson, O., P. Hedner, S. Laurell, B. Nosslin, C. Rerup, and E. Rosengren. Thyroid and adrenal response to acute cold exposure in man. *J. Appl. Physiol.* 28: 543–548, 1970.
204. Wünnenberg, W., and K. Brück. Zur Funktionsweise thermoreceptiver Strukturen im Cervicalmark des Meerschweinchens. *Arch. Ges. Physiol.* 299: 1–10, 1968.
205. Wurtman, R. J., and J. Axelrod. Control of enzymatic synthesis of adrenaline in the adrenal medulla by adrenal cortical steroids. *J. Biol. Chem.* 241: 2301–2305, 1966.
206. Zeisberger, E., and K. Brück. Central effects of noradrenaline on the control of body temperature in the guinea-pig. *European J. Physiol.* 322: 152–166, 1971.
207. Zeisberger, E., K. Brück, W. Wünnenberg, and C. Wietasch. Das Ausmass der zitterfreien Thermogenese des Meerschweinchens in Abhängigkeit vom Lebensalter. *Arch. Ges. Physiol.* 296: 276–288, 1967.
208. Zilberstein, R. M. Effects of reserpine, serotonin and vasopressin on the survival of cold-stressed rats. *Nature* 185: 249, 1960.

Influence of circulating catecholamines on the central nervous system

MARTHE VOGT | *Institute of Animal Physiology, Babraham, Cambridge, England*

THE SUBJECTIVE FEELING of apprehension during intravenous infusions of epinephrine clearly demonstrates that this drug has an effect on the brain; since norepinephrine does not elicit such feelings, they cannot be the simple result of a rise in blood pressure. Nor is the effect confined to man. Thus rats given, from the age of 22–46 days, 25 µg epinephrine four times daily by subcutaneous injection became excited and difficult to handle by the end of the second week. They showed this behavior only at the third and fourth daily injection, the effect having again subsided by the next morning (15). This showed that the effect was not due to a resentment of the injections as such, but to a cumulative effect of doses of epinephrine that were not completely metabolized between the injections. The question to be answered is whether such effects are due to direct central effects of epinephrine or to peripheral actions that are transmitted to the brain by afferent impulses.

When Bonvallet et al. (4) demonstrated that intravenous injections of catecholamines into cats caused electroencephalographic arousal in doses sometimes as low as 1 µg/kg, they interpreted these effects as a direct action on the reticular formation. Rothballer (12) confirmed this view and showed that norepinephrine had approximately the same potency as epinephrine and that no clear correlation existed between arousal and hypertensive effect. However, in experiments (11) in which catecholamines were injected into both the carotid and the vertebral arteries of cats, no arousal was seen unless the dose was so high that enough amine escaped into the general circulation to cause a rise in blood pressure. [These experiments, like those of Bonvallet et al. (4), were done after denervation of the carotid sinuses, since pressure increases in the sinuses inhibit the ascending reticular-activating system and would mask any arousal.] Further evidence that vascular changes, and not direct central effects, are responsible for the arousal produced by injections of catecholamines was obtained by Baust et al. (3).

All the work so far discussed deals with doses of amines of about 1–10 µg/kg, and one may ask whether very much higher doses could have direct central effects. When doses of 100 µg/kg were infused into dogs (8), stupor and anesthesia resulted. These were most probably of direct central origin since they resembled the well-known effects on injecting catecholamines directly into the cerebral ventricles (2, 5, 9).

Whether it is possible for circulating catecholamines to exert direct central effects depends on the performance of the blood-brain barrier in preventing penetration of the amines into brain tissue. By using tritium-labeled catecholamines several authors have assessed the efficacy of this barrier. Cats were injected with the equivalent of 2.5 µg of epinephrine per kilogram per minute for 30 min and killed immediately after the end of the infusion or 2 hr later (1). The results were similar after both time intervals: the brain contained 0.7 or 0.8 ng/g tritiated epinephrine, whereas, for example, the heart had taken up 163 ng/g immediately after the infusion and had retained 87 ng/g after 2 hr. Rapid injections of large doses (71 µg/kg) led to similar figures and also showed that the pituitary gland, not protected by the blood-brain barrier, contained 327 ng/g, more than twice as much as the heart, which, in these experiments, took up 150 ng/g, whereas the brain concentration was 1.1 ng/g. In a more recent study of the penetration of epinephrine-^{3}H into rat tissues (13), an intravenous injection of about 6 µg/kg was followed by tissue analyses 10 and 60 min later. It was found that the pineal gland, which, like the pituitary, is not protected by the blood-brain barrier, contained, per gram of tissue, 150 times as much epinephrine as the brain.

Experiments with norepinephrine (about 10 µg/kg rapidly injected intravenously into cats) gave results that resembled those obtained with epinephrine (19). Thus 2 hr after the injection the cerebral cortex contained 0.1 ng/g, whereas the concentration in the pituitary was 300 times, and that in the heart 2,100 times, as high. Immediately after the injection the concentration in the cortex was 0.8 ng/g. When the same dose of norepinephrine was given by slow infusion over a period of 30 min, the results were essentially the same as after rapid injection. The postnatal development of the blood-brain barrier for norepinephrine was studied in the rat (6), and the barrier found to be fully effective as early as the fourth day of life.

Though this work has shown that little catecholamine enters the brain from the circulation, one might suspect that small, restricted regions might accumulate the compounds in sufficient quantity to account for some local action. Investigations into this possibility (17, 18) do not greatly favor such a view. The authors found that in most parts of the brain the catecholamine concentration could be accounted for by the blood content of the tissue. The exception was the hypothalamus, which contained five times as much as did the remainder of the brain. The absolute value for norepinephrine was 1.6 ng/g; this is still very much less than the 36 ng/g found in the pituitary. If one remembers that the median eminence is outside the blood-brain barrier, it is not at all unlikely that this region accounts for the whole of the radioactive catecholamines found in the hypothalamus. This view is supported by a recent investigation (10) in which the uptake of catecholamines into rat brain was studied by fluorescence microscopy. Fluorescence was found only in areas lacking the blood-brain barrier.

The protective performance of the blood-brain barrier is of necessity a function of the amine concentration in the blood. As shown by the experiments with injections of epinephrine (100 μg/kg) the barrier can be overcome (8), and a brief consideration of the highest naturally occurring concentrations of epinephrine in blood is required in order to assess whether central effects of circulating catecholamines are likely to be seen when amines have not been injected by the experimenter.

Insulin and hemorrhage are two of the most potent stimuli for the secretion of catecholamines by the adrenal medulla. However, the highest concentration of epinephrine found in venous blood of fasting man or dog after injection of insulin was 6.4 μg/liter, and it was usually much less (7). The same maximum was found in rat arterial blood collected during exsanguination in ether anesthesia (16). In view of the fact that the extraction method entailed a loss of 30% of the epinephrine, the maximum actual concentration ever (and rarely) found during these procedures was 10 μg/liter plasma, which is equivalent to 0.4 μg/kg body wt. Taking into account the half-life of the catecholamines in the circulation, which is about 20 sec (14), one can calculate that such a plasma concentration could be achieved artificially by an intravenous infusion of about 2 μg/kg per minute. As shown earlier, at such infusion rates the blood-brain barrier is fully effective.

In summary, catecholamines administered intravascularly in "moderate" doses (1–10 μg/kg), which may be given either per minute by slow infusion or in a single rapid injection, do not pass the blood-brain barrier; they penetrate only to those small regions of the brain in which this barrier is lacking. The same is true of concentrations of circulating catecholamines that may occur naturally in response to intense stimulation of the adrenal medulla; the amounts secreted are at the lower end of the scale of the "moderate" doses. Doses far in excess of these amounts overcome the blood-brain barrier and produce the same responses as injections of the amines into the cerebral ventricles.

REFERENCES

1. AXELROD, J., H. WEIL-MALHERBE, AND R. TOMCHICK. The physiological disposition of H^3-epinephrine and its metabolite metanephrine. *J. Pharmacol.* 127: 251–256, 1959.
2. BASS, A. Über eine Wirkung des Adrenalins auf das Gehirn. *Z. Ges. Neurol. Psychiat.* 26: 600–601, 1914.
3. BAUST, W., H. NIEMCZYK, AND J. VIETH. The action of blood pressure on the ascending reticular activating system with special reference to adrenaline-induced EEG arousal. *Electroencephal. Clin. Neurophysiol.* 15: 63–72, 1963.
4. BONVALLET, M., P. DELL, AND G. HIEBEL. Tonus sympathique et activité électrique corticale. *Electroencephal. Clin. Neurophysiol.* 6: 119–144, 1954.
5. FELDBERG, W., AND S. L. SHERWOOD. Injections of drugs into the lateral ventricles of the cat. *J. Physiol., London* 123: 148–167, 1954.
6. GLOWINSKI, J., J. AXELROD, I. J. KOPIN, AND R. J. WURTMAN. Physiological disposition of H^3-norepinephrine in the developing rat. *J. Pharmacol.* 146: 48–53, 1964.
7. HOLZBAUER, M., AND M. VOGT. The concentration of adrenaline in the peripheral blood during insulin hypoglycaemia. *Brit. J. Pharmacol.* 9: 249–252, 1954.
8. IVY, A. C., F. R. GOETZL, S. C. HARRIS, AND D. Y. BURRILL. The analgesic effect of intracarotid and intravenous injection of epinephrine in dogs and of subcutaneous injection in man. *Quart. Bull. Northwestern Univ. Med. School* 18: 298–306, 1944.
9. LEIMDORFER, A. The action of sympathomimetic amines on the central nervous system and the blood sugar. Mechanism of action. *J. Pharmacol.* 98: 62–71, 1950.
10. LOIZOU, L. A. Uptake of monoamines into central neurones and the blood brain barrier in the infant rat. *Brit. J. Pharmacol.* 40: 800–813, 1970.
11. MANTEGAZZINI, P., K. POECK, AND G. SANTIBAÑEZ-H. The action of adrenaline and noradrenaline on the cortical electrical activity of the "encéphale isolé" cat. *Arch. Ital. Biol.* 97: 222–242, 1959.
12. ROTHBALLER, A. B. Studies on the adrenaline-sensitive component of the reticular activating system. *Electroencephal. Clin. Neurophysiol.* 8: 603–621, 1956.
13. STEINMAN, A. M., S. E. SMERIN, AND J. D. BARCHAS. Epinephrine metabolism in mammalian brain after intravenous and intraventricular administration. *Science* 165: 616–617, 1969.
14. VANE, J. R. The release and fate of vaso-active hormones in the circulation. *Brit. J. Pharmacol.* 35: 209–242, 1969.
15. VOGT, M. The effect of chronic administration of adrenaline on the suprarenal cortex and the comparison of this effect with that of hexoestrol. *J. Physiol., London* 104: 60–70, 1945.
16. VOGT, M. Plasma adrenaline and release of ACTH in normal and demedullated rats. *J. Physiol., London* 118: 588–594, 1952.
17. WEIL-MALHERBE, H., J. AXELROD, AND R. TOMCHICK. Blood-brain barrier for adrenaline. *Science* 129: 1226–1227, 1959.
18. WEIL-MALHERBE, H., L. G. WHITBY, AND J. AXELROD. The blood-brain barrier for catecholamines in different regions of the brain. In: *Regional Neurochemistry*, edited by S. S. Kety and J. Elkes. Oxford: Pergamon Press, 1961, p. 284–291.
19. WHITBY, L. G., J. AXELROD, AND H. WEIL-MALHERBE. The fate of H^3-norepinephrine in animals. *J. Pharmacol.* 132: 193–201, 1961.

CHAPTER 40

Catechol-O-methyltransferase and other O-methyltransferases

JULIUS AXELROD | Laboratory of Clinical Science, National Institute of Mental Health, Bethesda, Maryland

CHAPTER CONTENTS

Catechol-O-methyltransferase
    Properties
    Substrate specificity
    Inhibitors
    Distribution
    Development and physiologically induced changes
    Assay
O-methylation of Catecholamines In Vivo
Enzymatic O-methylation of Iodophenols
Phenol-O-methyltransferase
Hydroxamic Acid O-methyltransferase
Hydroxyindole-O-methyltransferase

MACLAGAN AND WILKINSON first showed in 1951 that O-methylation can occur in animals (70). Later it was observed that the catechol flavinoids, rutin and quercitin, were excreted as homovanillic acid (3-methoxy-4-hydroxyphenylacetic acid) (41). At the same time it was found that homovanillic acid is a metabolite of dopa and occurs normally in the urine (4). Another O-methylated product, 3-methoxy-4-hydroxymandelic acid, was also demonstrated in the urine by Armstrong and co-workers (3). These investigators also found a marked elevation of the latter compound after the administration of norepinephrine and 3,4-dihydroxymandelic acid in patients with pheochromocytoma. From these observations it was concluded that norepinephrine is first deaminated and then O-methylated. This proposal stemmed from the demonstration that catecholamines are substrates for monoamine oxidase (31).

For many years it was believed that monoamine oxidase was the principal enzyme involved in the metabolism and inactivation of catecholamines. However, when potent monoamine oxidase inhibitors were introduced, it was found that in vivo these compounds potentiated physiological responses of administered phenylethylamines and tyramine, but the actions of epinephrine were not prolonged (48). All these observations suggested that catecholamine undergoes another metabolic pathway, possibly O-methylation.

Cantoni (35) showed that S-adenosylmethionine can methylate amino groups, and this suggested transmethylation similar to that occurring at the hydroxyl group of catecholamines. A rat liver preparation was incubated with epinephrine and S-adenosylmethionine and the reaction products examined so that this possibility could be tested (8). A new product was formed that was isolated by extraction into organic solvents and identified by paper chromatography. A likely metabolite was 3-O-methylated epinephrine. This compound, metanephrine (19), was synthesized and found to have an R_f value identical to that of the enzymatically formed product.

CATECHOL-O-METHYLTRANSFERASE

Properties

The initial studies of the properties of O-methylating enzyme, catechol-O-methyltransferase (COMT), were carried out on a partially purified preparation from rat liver (21). About a 30-fold purification of the enzyme was obtained by using ammonium sulfate precipitation and calcium phosphate gel adsorption and elution. The enzyme from this partially purified preparation required S-adenosylmethionine as the methyl donor. In addition, Mg^{2+} was necessary for the O-methylation to proceed. Other divalent cations, such as Mn^{2+}, Zn^{2+}, Co^{2+}, and Fe^{2+}, could be substituted for Mg^{2+}. Optimal enzyme activity occurred between pH 7.5 and 8.2 with phosphate buffers, at pH 9 with Tris buffer, and at pH 10 with glycine buffers (74).

The Michaelis-Menten constant (K_m) with respect to epinephrine is 1.2×10^{-4} and to S-adenosylmethionine is 3×10^{-6} (45). The enzyme was further purified about 180-fold with DEAE-cellulose and Biogel 60 (2). On the basis of its behavior on Sephadex, the molecular weight of the enzyme was calculated to be about 29,000. Several bands of activity were obtained using polyacrylamide gel electrophoresis. Two isozymes of COMT were found after starch block electrophoresis (22). Catechol-O-methyltransferase was also found in the livers of a number of mammalian species; the enzymes had different electrophoretic mobilities, heat stabilities, and K_m values (22). Recently about a 400-fold purification of COMT from rat liver to a purity of 70% has been achieved (74). The purified enzyme had two major bands of COMT activity on disc gel electrophoresis. The larger molecular weight component showed more enzyme activity. The molecular weights of these proteins were estimated by ultracentrifuge sedimentation, Sephadex chromatography, and acrylamide gel electrophoresis to be about 28,000 and 50,000 (C. R. Creveling and J. W. Daly, unpublished observations). Both COMT proteins were found to be glycoproteins containing galactose, glucose, and mannose (C. R. Creveling and J. W. Daly, unpublished observations). The recovery of amino acids on hydrolysis was low, which indicated that the carbohydrate portion of COMT is quite large. The glycoprotein component of COMT suggests a possible attachment of the enzyme to the cell wall. The purified COMT contained trace amounts of Mg^{2+}. Paramagnetic resonance studies showed that two to three Mn^{2+} are bound per mole of COMT, with a binding constant of 3×10^{-5} M. In the presence of S-adenosylmethionine, but not catechol substrate, the affinity of Mn^{2+} is increased (C. R. Creveling and J. W. Daly, unpublished observations).

Purification of COMT has been reported by several other investigators (7, 45). After purification, COMT loses activity and can be stabilized by dithiothreitol (45). Catechol-O-methyltransferase from human placenta has also been purified about 66-fold (49). Unlike the liver enzyme, placental COMT is active only in the presence of cysteine. The placental enzyme has a molecular weight of about 52,000. Its temperature optimum is 50 C, and it has an activation energy of 17.3 kcal/mole. An antibody to highly purified COMT from rat liver has been produced (6). This antibody cross reacts with enzyme from guinea pig, cat, and man, but not with that from rabbit, nor does it cross react with other O-methyltransferases, such as microsomal COMT, phenol-O-methyltransferase, or hydroxyindole-O-methyltransferase. It also cross reacts with all rat tissues except brain.

Substrate Specificity

A wide variety of catechols and monophenols were examined for their capacity to be O-methylated in the presence of rat liver COMT (21). All catechols examined, regardless of substituents, were O-methylated. None of the monophenols served as substrates. The enzyme lacked stereospecificity. Normally occurring catechols that are O-methylated by COMT are norepinephrine, epinephrine, dopamine, dopa, 3,4-dihydroxymandelic acid, 3,4-dihydroxyphenylacetic acid, 3,4-dihydroxyphenylethanol, and 3,4-dihydroxyphenylglycol. Other naturally occurring compounds O-methylated by COMT are 2-hydroxyestradiol, a metabolite of estradiol (59), and ascorbic acid (30). The enzyme can also O-methylate synthetic catechols, such as epinine, 3,4-dihydroxyephedrine, 3,4-dihydroxyamphetamine, and a variety of substituted catechols, including 7,8-dihydroxychlorpromazine (39). Polyphenols with three adjacent hydroxy groups, such as gallic acid and pyrogallol, are methylated on the middle hydroxy group whether this group is in the para or meta position (26). Also methylated by COMT on both the 5- and the 6-hydroxy group are 5,6-hydroxyindoles; methylation occurs mainly on the 6 position (16).

In vivo, methylation occurs almost exclusively on the meta position (19). Catechol-O-methyltransferase can also catalyze methylation on the para position in vitro (17). The extent of p-methylation in vitro is low, with substrate containing an ionized moiety on the ring. In the case of a completely nonpolar substituent, such as 4-ethyl catechol, there is an equal amount of para and meta O-methylation (38). With increasing pH, the extent of para O-methylation increases with catecholamines. Presumably, at a higher pH a greater portion of the less polar, nonprotonated amine would be available for binding and O-methylation. These observations suggest a nonpolar region in the catechol binding site of COMT that does not bind the polar substrate in the orientation necessary for para methylation. Nonpolar substrates, on the other hand, would bind in a random fashion and thus be available for para and meta methylation.

A novel type of para-to-meta intraconversion was observed in vivo, with 3-hydroxy-4-methoxyacetophenone forming 3-methoxy-4-hydroxyacetophenone (39). This intraconversion of the methyl group takes place in two steps: *1*) O-demethylation of the methoxy group by an NADPH-requiring microsomal enzyme; and *2*) remethylation on the para or meta hydroxy group by COMT.

Inhibitors

Catechol-O-methyltransferase is inhibited by p-chloromercuribenzoate, which suggests the presence of a sulfhydryl group in the region of the active site (21). In an early study pyrogallol and other polyphenols were shown to markedly increase the duration of response to epinephrine and to sympathetic nerve stimulation (24). This suggested that pyrogallol might prolong the responses to epinephrine by competing for COMT. In a series of experiments it was shown that pyrogallol inhibited COMT in vitro (14, 25) and in large doses slowed the metabolism of epinephrine and the reduced formation of its O-methylated metabolite, metanephrine, in vivo (14). Pyrogallol inhibits COMT in a competitive manner and is O-methylated itself. Pyrogallol was also found to augment briefly the pressor responses to sympathetic nervous stimulation (91) and to exogenous norepinephrine (92). Large and toxic amounts of pyrogallol are necessary to produce potentiation of responses to catecholamines in vivo. Other polyphenols, such as dihydroxyphenyl acetamides, gallic esters, and dimethyl papavarine (33), also inhibit COMT. In another class of COMT inhibitors are 3,5-dihydroxy-4-methoxy and

3-hydroxy-4,5-dimethoxybenzoic acids (74). These compounds exhibit a noncompetitive, mixed type of inhibition against various substrates and S-adenosylmethionine. They are relatively nontoxic and achieve effective inhibition of COMT in vivo. Tropolones, which act as chelating agents, are yet another type of COMT inhibitor (29). Tropolones are partially effective inhibitors in vivo, but they are toxic and short acting. Normally occurring inhibitors of COMT in vitro are 2-hydroxyestradiol (59) and pyridoxal-5′-phosphate (I. J. Black and J. Axelrod, unpublished observations). An effective inhibitor of the enzyme in vivo and in vitro is 2-hydroxyestradiol (59).

Distribution

Catechol-O-methyltransferase is widely distributed in all mammalian tissues. It is present in liver, kidney, spleen, intestine, salivary gland, aorta, vena cava (21), skin (27), skeletal muscle (5), pineal and pituitary (17), uterus (89), eye (86), neuroblastoma (64), adipose tissue (85), and red blood cells (11). The enzyme has also been found in all areas of the brain and peripheral nerves (39). An unequal distribution of COMT occurs in the brain; highest activity is found in the area postrema and lowest in the cerebellar cortex. In the brain COMT is highly localized in synaptic components (1). Catechol-O-methyltransferase is also present in the red cells of mammals (11) and has been found in fish (32), amphibian, and avian tissues (15).

Catechol-O-methyltransferase is present in the soluble fraction of the cell (21). However, enzyme activity has also been found in the microsomal fraction of the liver (53). Microsomal COMT in liver differs from the soluble COMT with respect to pH optima and distribution in the rat and rabbit. In addition, benzpyrene and cold stress increase microsomal COMT, but not the soluble enzyme. In the fat cell, COMT is present in the cell membrane (85). Procedures that cause a destruction of nerve terminals, such as denervation (86) or immunosympathectomy (55), do not result in a fall of COMT, which indicates that almost all the enzyme is present outside the neuron. However, COMT has been reported to be present in the sympathetic nerves of the nictitating membrane and vas deferens of rat and rabbit (57).

Catechol-O-methyltransferase enzymes have also been found in plants. In the flowering bulbs of *Narine bowdenii*, an enzyme that methylates the catechol norbelladine mainly on the para position has been described (71). In fruit plants another COMT-like enzyme is present that methylates mainly in the meta position (44). The latter enzyme does not require Mg^{2+}.

Development and Physiologically Induced Changes

In the newborn rat and chick embryo, COMT activity is very low and increases rapidly after birth (52). With advancing age in the rat, COMT activity increases in liver, decreases in kidney, and remains constant in the brain (76). During pregnancy there is a twofold elevation in COMT in the rat uterus (89). Hypophysectomy and large doses of thyroxine reduce COMT in the rat liver (65). Hypophysectomy or stress has little or no effect on adrenal COMT. In congestive heart failure, there is an increase in the total COMT in heart but not in its concentration (62). In a strain of genetically hypertensive rats COMT levels in the heart, kidney, and liver were found to be elevated during the development of hypertension (37). Depression results in a highly significant reduction of COMT in red blood cells of females (36).

Assay

In the initial procedure described for the assay of COMT, tissue homogenates were incubated with epinephrine, Mg^{2+}, and S-adenosylmethionine, and the metanephrine formed enzymatically was extracted into an organic solvent at pH 10 (21). The metanephrine was then returned to an acid phase and measured fluorometrically at 335 mμ after activation at 285 mμ. Methods based on the colorimetric determination of normetanephrine (29) or ultraviolet spectroscopy (46) after periodate cleavage have been described. A simple colorimetric procedure with pyrocatecholphthatalein as substrate has been reported (2).

The above assays, however, are not sufficiently sensitive to measure COMT in tissues with low activity. A more sensitive assay was introduced that used ^{3}H-epinephrine of high specific activity (9, 10). After incubation with tissue and S-adenosylmethionine, the ^{3}H-metanephrine is extracted into a mixture containing toluene and isoamyl alcohol and the radioactivity measured after the addition of phosphor. This method has the disadvantage of formation of other tritiated products, which are extracted into the solvent.

The most sensitive assay for COMT is the use of ^{14}C-methyl-S-adenosylmethionine and norepinephrine as the methyl acceptor (87). The ^{14}C-normetanephrine is extracted into a mixture of toluene and isoamyl alcohol, and the radioactivity is measured by the addition of phosphor. This assay can measure as little as 1 pmole of product. Other catechols, such as 3,4-dihydroxybenzoic acid (72) or 3,4-dihydroxypropiophenone, have been used as substrates. The latter is the more active and stable substrate (C. R. Creveling and J. W. Daly, personal communication). Assays involving ^{14}C-S-adenosylmethionine cannot be used to measure inhibition by catechols since they are themselves O-methylated.

The ability of COMT to form radioactive products with ^{14}C-S-adenosylmethionine and catecholamines make it possible to utilize this enzyme for highly sensitive assays of norepinephrine and epinephrine (43, 73).

O-METHYLATION OF CATECHOLAMINES IN VIVO

All normally occurring catecholamines are O-methylated by COMT in vivo. The major metabolic products of endogenous dopamine, norepinephrine, and epinephrine

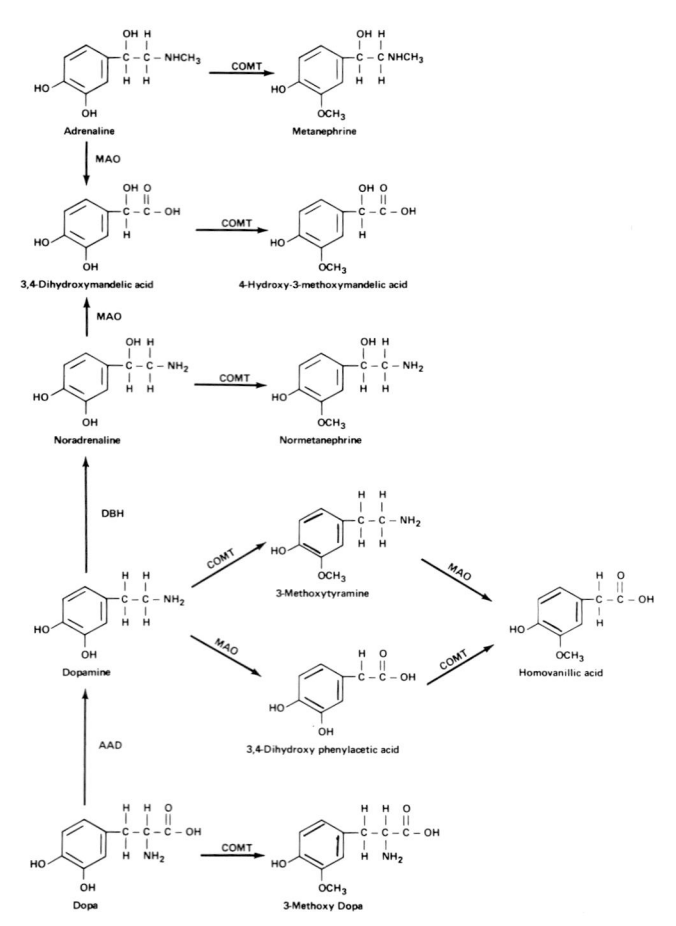

FIG. 1. O-methylation of catechols by catechol-O-methyltransferase. COMT, catechol-O-methyltransferase; MAO, monoamine oxidase; DBH, dopamine β-hydroxylase; AAD, aromatic amino acid decarboxylase.

lating epinephrine in man is O-methylated and 25% deaminated (60).

The catecholamine norepinephrine stored in sympathetic nerves is mainly deaminated in the sympathetic neuron by monoamine oxidase (MAO) (61), and the metabolite is then O-methylated either in the tissue or the liver. This is reflected in the relatively larger amounts of endogenous VMA found in urine as compared to normetanephrine and metanephrine.

The O-methylated products of catecholamines, normetanephrine, metanephrine, and 3-methoxytyramine, are also normally present in tissues (19).

The large amount of the amino acid, L-dopa, given for the treatment of Parkinson's disease is metabolized mainly by COMT to form 3-methoxydopa [(28, 34); Fig. 1]. The latter compound appears to be present in the brain. After dopa administration, about 10 times more 3-methoxydopa is present in cerebrospinal fluid than dopa (80). As a consequence of the O-methylation of large amounts of administered dopa, there is a considerable depletion of the methyl donor, S-adenosylmethionine, in the body (90).

The main mechanism for inactivation of catecholamines is reuptake into the sympathetic neuron (51). However, COMT plays a role in terminating the actions of catecholamines. Once the neurotransmitter is liberated from the sympathetic nerves, it is inactivated by COMT in the effector cell or in the liver and the kidney (Fig. 2). The extent of O-methylation of the neurotransmitter released from the nerves depends on the tissue and the species. For example, in the adventitia of blood vessels, which is rich in sympathetic nerve terminals, norepinephrine is mainly inactivated by reuptake into the nerves

excreted in the urine are both O-methylated and deaminated. These include homovanillic acid (4), 3-methoxy-4-hydroxyphenylglycol (13), and 3-methoxy-4-hydroxymandelic acid (VMA) (5). Other O-methylated metabolites of catecholamines excreted are normetanephrine, metanephrine (8), 3-methoxytyramine (19), N-acetylnormetanephrine (82), N-methylmetanephrine (54), 3-methoxydopa (83), 3-methoxy-4-hydroxyphenylethanol (4), and vanillic acid (78). The O-methylation of catecholamines and their metabolic products are shown in Figure 1. Another normally occurring O-methylated product is 2-methoxyestradiol (59).

The relative importance of O-methylation of circulating catecholamine was examined after an intravenous injection of physiological amounts of radioactive epinephrine (63). More than 80% of the administered epinephrine was excreted as O-methylated products: VMA (40%), metanephrine (free and conjugated, 40%), 3-methoxy-4-hydroxyphenylglycol sulfate (7%), and small amounts of unchanged epinephrine and 3,4-dihydroxymandelic acid. By the use of a double labeling technique it was calculated that about 70% of the circu-

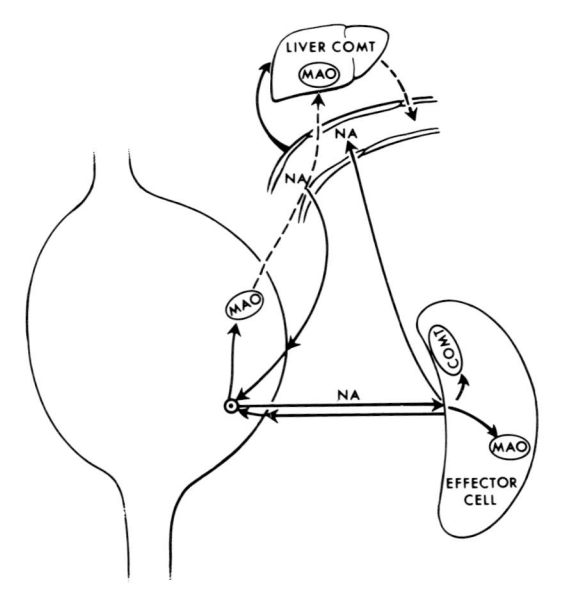

FIG. 2. Site of action of catechol-O-methyltransferase on norepinephrine (NA) after release from a varicosity of sympathetic nerve terminals. MAO, monoamine oxidase; COMT, catechol-O-methyltransferase.

(68). However, in media that have a sparse sympathetic innervation the catecholamine is inactivated mainly by COMT in the tissue.

An extraneural uptake mechanism for norepinephrine has been described (42). Catechol-O-methyltransferase has been found to be associated with this extraneural uptake site, and the enzyme might be an important mechanism for inactivation of norepinephrine in blood vessels. The COMT inhibitors, tropolone, acetamide, guanethidine, hydrocortisone, and bretylium, and phenoxybenzamine interfere with O-methylation in aortic strips, presumably at an extraneuronal uptake site (68). The norepinephrine is released by tyramine in a physiologically active form and is metabolized mainly by O-methylation (61). Procedures that destroy sympathetic nerves, such as denervation or immunosympathectomy, result in an increased O-methylation of norepinephrine (55).

ENZYMATIC O-METHYLATION OF IODOPHENOLS

An enzyme that O-methylates 3,5-diiodo-4-hydroxybenzoic acid was partially purified from the soluble fraction of rat liver (84). It requires S-adenosylmethionine as the methyl donor but, unlike COMT, divalent metals are not necessary. It is also more heat stable than COMT and can be separated from the latter enzyme by chromatography on DEAE-cellulose. The iodophenol-methylating enzyme can also O-methylate tetraiodothyroacetic acid but not triiodothyroacetic acid, thyroxine, or triiodothyronine.

PHENOL-O-METHYLTRANSFERASE

Phenol-O-methyltransferase, an enzyme that O-methylates monophenols and a wide variety of simple alkyl methoxy and halophenols, has been described (12). S-adenosylmethionine serves as the methyl donor but, unlike COMT, phenol-O-methyltransferase is mainly localized in the microsomes. The enzyme is widely distributed among various mammalian species and is present in all tissues examined except the heart. Liver and lung have the greatest activity. p-Hydroxyacetanilide is a good substrate for phenol-O-methyltransferase, and the enzyme can form the analgesic acetophenetidin with S-adenosylmethionine as the alkyl donor. Tyramine and 3-methoxy-4-hydroxyphenylethylamine are not O-methylated by the enzyme. Phenol-O-methyltransferase is inhibited by SKF 525 (β-diethylaminoethyl dipropylacetate), a compound that inhibits other enzymes present in the microsomes. The presence of an SH group in the enzyme is indicated since p-chloromercuribenzoate and N-ethylmaleimide also inhibit. In rats, hypophysectomy increases the activity of phenol-O-methyltransferase in the liver but not in lung or brain.

HYDROXAMIC ACID O-METHYLTRANSFERASE

An enzyme has been described that transfers the methyl group of S-adenosylmethionine to the O group of N-hydroxy-2-acetylaminofluorene to form an N-methoxy derivative (69). Hydroxamic acids, such as benzohydroxamic acid, N-hydroxy-4-acetylaminostilbene, and propionohydroxamic acid, are also O-methylated by the enzyme. The N,O-methylated metabolite of N-hydroxy-2-acetylaminofluorene is more carcinogenic than the parent compound. The enzyme has an absolute requirement for cysteine and is present in the cytoplasm of the liver of the rat and other species.

HYDROXYINDOLE-O-METHYLTRANSFERASE

An enzyme that O-methylates indoles has been isolated from the pineal gland (17). The search for such an enzyme was prompted by the identification of melatonin (5-methoxy-N-acetyl tryptamine) in the mammalian pineal gland (67). This compound was shown to have powerful skin-lightening actions in fishes and amphibians and to inhibit gonadal function in certain mammals (88). The O-methylating enzyme in the bovine pineal gland was partially purified and its properties studied. S-adenosylmethionine serves as the methyl donor but, in contrast to COMT, Mg^{2+} is not required by hydroxyindole-O-methyltransferase (HIOMT). By far the best substrate for HIOMT is N-acetylserotonin, but other 5-hydroxyindoles, such as serotonin, N-methylserotonin, bufotenine, 5-hydroxyindole, and 5,6-dihydroxyindoles, are also O-methylated, but to a much smaller extent. The avian HIOMT has a different substrate specificity in that it can methylate serotonin, as well as N-acetylserotonin (15). Recently HIOMT has been isolated as a homogenous protein from beef pineal (56). It has a molecular weight of 77,000 and has two identical subunits with molecular weights of 39,000. The purified HIOMT has a high leucine content. Hydroxyindole-O-methyltransferase has been shown to exhibit different electrophoretic mobilities among the different species (22).

In mammals HIOMT is exclusively localized in the pineal gland (17). It has been found in the pineals of birds, reptiles, amphibians, and fishes and in the western roach (18, 51, 77). Hydroxyindole-O-methyltransferase is also present in the brain of amphibians and the eyes of fishes, amphibians, reptiles, and some birds (77). It is present in pineal gland tumors of man and can be used as a marker to identify tumors of pineal origin (88).

Environmental lighting has an effect on pineal HIOMT activity. The enzyme increases when rats are kept in constant darkness (88). The effect of environmental lighting on HIOMT in mammals is mediated via the sympathetic nerves (88), but these nerves are not involved in mediating the effects of light on avian HIOMT (66). Hydroxyindole-O-methyltransferase activity can be maintained in pineal organ culture (81). Although norepinephrine stimulates the formation of melatonin (20) in organ culture, it acts mainly on the serotonin acetylating enzyme (58).

REFERENCES

1. ALBERICI, M., G. RODRIGUEZ DE LOREZ ARNAIZ, AND E. DE ROBERTIS. Catechol-O-methyltransferase in nerve endings of the rat brain. *Life Sci.* 4: 1951–1960, 1965.
2. ANDERSON, P. J., AND A. D'IORIO. Purification and properties of catechol-O-methyltransferase. *Biochem. Pharmacol.* 17: 1943–1949, 1968.
3. ARMSTRONG, M. D., A. MCMILLAN, AND K. N. F. SHAW. 3-Methoxy-4-hydroxy-d-mandelic acid, a urinary metabolite of norepinephrine. *Biochim. Biophys. Acta* 25: 422–425, 1957.
4. ARMSTRONG, M. D., K. N. F. SHAW, AND P. E. WALL. The phenolic acids of human urine. *J. Biol. Chem.* 218: 293–303, 1956.
5. ASSICOT, M., AND C. BOHUON. Catechol-O-methyl transferase activity in skeletal muscle. *Nature* 212: 861, 1966.
6. ASSICOT, M., AND C. BOHUON. Production of antibodies to catechol-O-methyltransferase of rat liver. *Biochem. Pharmacol.* 18: 1893–1898, 1969.
7. ASSICOT, M., AND C. BOHUON. Purification and studies of catechol-O-methyltransferase of rat liver. *European J. Biochem.* 12: 490–501, 1970.
8. AXELROD, J. O-methylation of epinephrine and other catechols in vitro and in vivo. *Science* 126: 400–401, 1957.
9. AXELROD, J. Catechol-O-methyl transferase in rat liver. In: *Methods in Enzymology*, edited by S. P. Colowick and N. O. Kaplan. New York: Acad. Press, 1962, vol. v, p. 748.
10. AXELROD, J., W. ALBERS, AND C. D. CLEMENTE. Distribution of catechol-O-methyl transferase in the nervous system and other tissues. *J. Neurochem.* 5: 68–72, 1959.
11. AXELROD, J., AND C. K. COHN. Methyltransferase enzymes in red blood cells. *J. Pharmacol. Exptl. Therap.* 176: 650–654, 1971.
12. AXELROD, J., AND J. W. DALY. Phenol-O-methyltransferase. *Biochim. Biophys. Acta* 159: 472–478, 1968.
13. AXELROD, J., I. J. KOPIN, AND J. D. MANN. 3-Methoxy-4-hydroxyphenylglycol sulfate, a new metabolite of epinephrine and norepinephrine. *Biochim. Biophys. Acta* 36: 576–577, 1959.
14. AXELROD, J., AND M. J. LAROCHE. Inhibition of O-methylation of epinephrine and norepinephrine in vitro and in vivo. *Science* 130: 800, 1959.
15. AXELROD, J., AND J. K. LAUBER. Hydroxyindole-O-methyltransferase in several avian species. *Biochem. Pharmacol.* 17: 828–830, 1968.
16. AXELROD, J., AND A. B. LERNER. O-methylation in the conversion of tyrosine to melanin. *Biochim. Biophys. Acta* 71: 650–655, 1963.
17. AXELROD, J., P. D. MACLEAN, R. W. ALBERS, AND H. WEISSBACH. Regional distribution of methyltransferase enzymes in the nervous system and glandular tissues. In: *Regional Neurochemistry*, edited by S. S. Kety and J. Elkes. Oxford: Pergamon Press, 1961, p. 307.
18. AXELROD, J., W. B. QUAY, AND P. C. BAKER. Enzymatic synthesis of the skin-lightening agent melatonin in amphibians. *Nature* 208: 386, 1965.
19. AXELROD, J., S. SENOH, AND B. WITKOP. O-methylation of catecholamines in vivo. *J. Biol. Chem.* 233: 697–701, 1958.
20. AXELROD, J., H. M. SHEIN, AND R. J. WURTMAN. Stimulation of C^{14}-melatonin synthesis from C^{14}-tryptophan by noradrenaline in the rat pineal in organ culture. *Proc. Natl. Acad. Sci. US* 62: 544–549, 1969.
21. AXELROD, J., AND R. TOMCHICK. Enzymatic O-methylation of epinephrine and other catechols. *J. Biol. Chem.* 233: 702–705, 1958.
22. AXELROD, J., AND E. S. VESELL. Heterogeneity of N- and O-methyltransferases. *Mol. Pharmacol.* 6: 78–84, 1970.
23. AXELROD, J., R. J. WURTMAN, AND S. H. SNYDER. Control of hydroxy indole-O-methyl transferase activity in the pineal gland by environmental lighting. *J. Biol. Chem.* 240: 949–954, 1965.
24. BACQ, Z. M. Sensibilization à l'adrénaline et à l'excitation des nerfs adrénergiques par les antioxygènes. *Bull. Acad. Roy. Med. Belg.* 15: 697–710, 1935.
25. BACQ, Z. M., L. GOSSELIN, A. DRESSE, AND J. RENSON. Inhibition of O-methyltransferase by catechol and sensitization to epinephrine. *Science* 130: 453–454, 1959.
26. BAKKE, O. M. O-methylation of simple phenols in the rat. *Acta Pharmacol. Toxicol.* 28: 28–38, 1970.
27. BAMSHAD, J., A. B. LERNER, AND J. S. MCGUIRE. Catechol-O-methyl transferases in skin. *J. Invest. Dermatol.* 43: 111–113, 1964.
28. BARTHOLINI, G., I. KURUMA, AND A. PLETSCHER. Distribution and metabolism of L-3-O-methyldopa in rats. *Brit. J. Pharmacol.* 40: 461–467, 1970.
29. BELLEAU, B., AND J. BURBA. Occupancy of adrenergic receptors and inhibition of catechol-O-methyl transferase by tropolones. *J. Med. Chem.* 6: 755–759, 1963.
30. BLASCHKE, E., AND G. HERTTING. Enzymatic methylation of L-ascorbic acid. *Arch. Exptl. Pathol. Pharmacol.* 266: 296, 1970.
31. BLASCHKO, H., D. RICHTER, AND H. SCHLOSSMAN. The oxidation of adrenaline and other amines. *Biochem. J.* 31: 2187–2196, 1937.
32. BRANDENBURGER-BROWN, A., AND E. G. TRAMS. Catecholamine metabolism in elasmobranch interrenal body. *Comp. Biochem. Physiol.* 25: 1099–1105, 1968.
33. BURBA, J. V., AND M. F. MURNAGHAN. Catechol-O-methyl transferase inhibition and potentiation of epinephrine responses by desmethylpapaverine. *Biochem. Pharmacol.* 14: 823–829, 1965.
34. CALNE, D. B., F. KAROUM, C. R. J. RUTHVEN, AND M. SANDLER. The metabolism of orally administered l-dopa in Parkinsonism. *Brit. J. Pharmacol.* 37: 57–68, 1969.
35. CANTONI, G. L. Methylation of nicotinamide soluble enzyme system from rat liver. *J. Biol. Chem.* 189: 203–216, 1951.
36. COHN, C. K., D. L. DUNNER, AND J. AXELROD. Reduced catechol-O-methyltransferase activity in red blood cells of women with primary affective disorder. *Science* 170: 1323–1324, 1970.
37. CREVELING, C. R., N. DALGARD, AND B. V. NIKODEJEVIC. Elevated catechol-O-methyltransferase activity in spontaneously hypertensive rats. *Federation Proc.* 23: 416, 1969.
38. CREVELING, C. R., N. DALGARD, H. SHIMIZU, AND J. W. DALY. Catechol-O-methyltransferase. III. m- and p-O-methylation of catecholamines and their metabolites. *Mol. Pharmacol.* 6: 691–696, 1970.
39. DALY, J. W., J. AXELROD, AND B. WITKOP. Dynamic aspects of enzymatic O-methylation and demethylation of catechols in vitro and in vivo. *J. Biol. Chem.* 235: 1155–1159, 1960.
40. DALY, J. W., AND A. MANION. The action of catechol-O-methyltransferase on 7,8-dihydroxychlorpromazine. *Biochem. Pharmacol.* 18: 1235–1238, 1969.
41. DE EDS, F., A. N. BOOTH, AND F. T. JONES. Methylation and dehydroxylation of phenolic compounds by rats and rabbits. *J. Biol. Chem.* 225: 615–621, 1957.
42. EISENFELD, A. J., L. LANDSBERG, AND J. AXELROD. Effect of drugs on the accumulation and metabolism of extraneuronal norepinephrine in the rat heart. *J. Pharmacol. Exptl. Therap.* 158: 378–385, 1967.
43. ENGELMAN, K., AND B. PORTNOY. A sensitive double isotope

derivative assay for norepinephrine and epinephrine. *Circulation Res.* 26: 53–57, 1970.
44. FINKLE, B. J., AND R. F. NELSON. Enzyme reaction with phenolic compounds by a meta-O-methyltransferase in plants. *Biochim. Biophys. Acta* 78: 747–749, 1963.
45. FLOHE, L., AND K. P. SCHWABE. Kinetics of purified catechol-O-methyltransferase. *Biochim. Biophys. Acta* 220: 469–476, 1970.
46. GARDIER, R. W., G. L. ENDAHL, AND W. HAMELBERG. Cyclopropane: effect on catecholamine biotransformation. *Anesthesiology* 28: 677–679, 1967.
47. GOLDSTEIN, M., A. J. FRIEDHOFF, S. POMERANTZ, AND J. F. CONTRERA. The formation of 3,4-dihydroxyphenylethanol and 3-methoxy-4-hydroxyphenylethanol from 3,4-dihydroxyphenylethylamine in the rat. *J. Biol. Chem.* 236: 1816–1821, 1961.
48. GRIESEMER, E. C., J. BARSKY, C. A. DRAGSTEDT, J. A. WELLS, AND E. A. ZELLER. Potentiating effect of iproniazid on the pharmacological action of sympathomimetic amines. *Proc. Soc. Exptl. Biol. Med.* 84: 699–701, 1953.
49. GUGLER, R., R. KNUPPEN, AND H. BREUER. Purification and characterization of human placenta catechol-O-methyltransferase. *Biochim. Biophys. Acta* 200: 10–21, 1970.
50. HAFEEZ, M. A., AND W. B. QUAY. Pineal acetylserotonin methyltransferase in the teleost fishes, *Hesperoleucus symmetricus* and *Salmo gairdneri*, with evidence for lack of effect of constant light and darkness. *Comp. Gen. Pharmacol.* 1: 257–262, 1970.
51. HERTTING, G., AND J. AXELROD. Fate of tritiated noradrenaline at the sympathetic nerve endings. *Nature* 192: 172–173, 1961.
52. IGNARRO, L. J., AND F. E. SHIDEMAN. Catechol-O-methyl transferase and monoamine oxidase activities in the heart and liver of the embryonic and developing chick. *J. Pharmacol. Exptl. Therap.* 159: 29–37, 1968.
53. INSCOE, J. K., J. W. DALY, AND J. AXELROD. Factors affecting the enzymatic formation of O-methylated dihydroxy derivatives. *Biochem. Pharmacol.* 14: 1257–1263, 1965.
54. ITOH, C., K. YOSHINAGA, T. SATO, N. ISHIDA, AND Y. WADA. Presence of N-methyl metadrenaline in human urine and tumor tissue of pheochromocytoma. *Nature* 193: 477, 1962.
55. IVERSEN, L. L., J. GLOWINSKI, AND J. AXELROD. The physiological disposition and metabolism of norepinephrine in immunosympathectomized animals. *J. Pharmacol.* 151: 273–284, 1966.
56. JACKSON, R. L., AND W. LOVENBERG. Isolation and characterization of multiple forms of hydroxyindole-O-methyltransferase. *J. Biol. Chem.* 246: 4280–4285, 1971.
57. JARROT, B. Occurrence and properties of catechol-O-methyltransferase in adrenergic neurons. *J. Neurochem.* 18: 17–27, 1971.
58. KLEIN, D. C., G. R. BERG, AND J. WELLER. Melatonin synthesis: adenosine 3′,5′-monophosphate and norepinephrine stimulate N-acetyltransferase. *Science* 168: 979, 1970.
59. KNUPPEN, V. R., M. HOLLER, D. TILMANN, AND H. BREUER. Wirkung von Ostrogenen auf den Abbau und die Methylerung von Adrenalin in der Maus. *Z. Physiol. Chem.* 350: 1301–1309, 1969.
60. KOPIN, I. J. Technique for the study of alternate pathways: epinephrine metabolism in man. *Science* 131: 372, 1960.
61. KOPIN, I. J., AND E. K. GORDON. Metabolism of H^3-norepinephrine released by tyramine and reserpine. *J. Pharmacol. Exptl. Therap.* 138: 351–359, 1962.
62. KRAKOFF, L. R., R. A. BUCCINO, J. F. SPANN, JR., AND J. DE CHAMPLAIN. Cardiac catechol-O-methyltransferase and monoamine oxidase activity in congestive heart failure. *Am. J. Physiol.* 215: 549–552, 1968.
63. LABROSSE, E. H., J. AXELROD, I. J. KOPIN, AND S. S. KETY. Metabolism of 7-H^3-epinephrine-d-bitartrate in normal young men. *J. Clin. Invest.* 40: 253–260, 1961.
64. LABROSSE, E. H., AND M. KARON. Catechol-O-methyltransferase activity in neuroblastoma tumor. *Nature* 196: 1222, 1962.
65. LANDSBERG, L., J. DE CHAMPLAIN, AND J. AXELROD. Increased biosynthesis of cardiac norepinephrine after hypophysectomy. *J. Pharmacol. Exptl. Therap.* 165: 102–107, 1969.
66. LAUBER, J. K., J. E. BOYD, AND J. AXELROD. Enzymatic synthesis of melatonin in avian pineal body: extraretinal response to light. *Science* 161: 489–490, 1968.
67. LERNER, A. B., J. D. CASE, AND R. V. HEINZELMAN. Structure of melatonin. *J. Am. Chem. Soc.* 81: 6084–6085, 1959.
68. LEVIN, J. A., AND R. F. FURCHGOTT. Interactions between potentiating agents of adrenergic amines in rabbit aortic strips. *J. Pharmacol. Exptl. Therap.* 172: 320–331, 1970.
69. LOTIKAR, P. D. Enzymatic N-O-methylation of hydroxamic acid. *Biochim. Biophys. Acta* 170: 468–471, 1968.
70. MACLAGAN, N. F., AND J. H. WILKINSON. Methylation of a phenolic hydroxy group in the human body. *Nature* 168: 251, 1951.
71. MANN, J. D., H. M. FALES, AND H. S. MUDD. Alkaloids and plant metabolism: O-methylation in vitro of norbelladine, a precursor of amaryllliaceae alkaloids. *J. Biol. Chem.* 238: 3820–3823, 1963.
72. MCCAMAN, R. E. Microdetermination of catechol-O-methyl transferase in brain. *Life Sci.* 4: 2353–2359, 1965.
73. NIKODEJEVIC, B., J. DALY, AND C. R. CREVELING. Catechol-O-methyltransferase. I. An enzymatic assay for norepinephrine. *Biochem. Pharmacol.* 18: 1577–1584, 1969.
74. NIKODEJEVIC, B., S. SENOH, J. W. DALY, AND C. R. CREVELING. Catechol-O-methyltransferase. II. A new class of inhibitors of catechol-O-methyl transferase. 3,5-Dihydroxy-4-methoxybenzoic acid and related compounds. *J. Pharmacol. Exptl. Therap.* 174: 83–93, 1970.
75. POTTER, L. T., T. COOPER, V. L. WILLMAN, AND D. E. WOLFE. Synthesis, binding, release and metabolism of norepinephrine in normal and transplanted dog hearts. *Circulation Res.* 16: 468–481, 1965.
76. PRANGE, A. J., JR., J. E. WHITE, M. A. LIPTON, AND A. M. KINKEAD. Influence of age on monoamine oxidase and catechol-O-methyltransferase in rat tissues. *Life Sci.* 6: 581–586, 1967.
77. QUAY, W. B. Retinal and pineal hydroxy-O-methyl transferase activity in vertebrates. *Life Sci.* 4: 983–991, 1965.
78. ROSEN, L., W. B. NELSON, AND MCC. GOODALL. Identification of vanillic acid as a catabolite of noradrenaline metabolism in the human. *Federation Proc.* 21: 363, 1962.
79. SENOH, S., J. DALY, J. AXELROD, AND B. WITKOP. Enzymatic p-O-methylation by catechol-O-methyltransferase. *J. Am. Chem. Soc.* 81: 6240–6245, 1959.
80. SHARPLESS, N. S., AND D. S. MCCANN. Dopa and 3-O-methyldopa in cerebrospinal fluid of Parkinsonian patients during treatment with oral L-dopa. *Clin. Chem. Acta* 31: 155–170, 1971.
81. SHEIN, H., R. J. WURTMAN, AND J. AXELROD. Synthesis of serotonin by pineal glands of the rat in organ culture. *Nature* 213: 730–731, 1967.
82. SMITH, A., AND S. B. WORTIS. Formation and metabolism of N-acetylnormetanephrine in the rat. *Biochim. Biophys. Acta* 60: 420–422, 1962.
83. STUDNITZ, W. Die Ausscheidung von Metaboliten des Dopa— und Dopaminstoffwechsels bei 2 Fällen mit Neuroblastom. *Scand. J. Clin. Lab. Invest.* 12, Suppl. 48: 58–65, 1960.
84. TOMITA, E., E. MACHA, AND C. A. LARDY. Enzymatic O-methylation of iodinated phenols and thyroid hormones. *J. Biol. Chem.* 239: 1202–1207, 1964.
85. TRAIGER, G. J., AND D. N. CALVERT. O-Methylation of ^{3}H-norepinephrine by epididymal adipose tissue. *Biochem. Pharmacol.* 18: 109–117, 1969.
86. WALTMAN, S., AND M. SEARS. Catechol-O-methyl transferase and monoamine oxidase activity in the ocular tissues of albino rabbits. *Invest. Ophthalmol.* 3: 601–605, 1964.
87. WURTMAN, R. J., AND J. AXELROD. Control of enzymatic synthesis of adrenaline in the adrenal medulla by adrenal cortical steroids. *J. Biol. Chem.* 241: 2301–2305, 1966.
88. WURTMAN, R. J., J. AXELROD, AND D. KELLY. *The Pineal.* New York: Acad. Press, 1968, p. 145–161.

89. WURTMAN, R. J., J. AXELROD, AND L. T. POTTER. The disposition of catecholamines in the rat uterus and the effect of drugs and hormones. *J. Pharmacol. Exptl. Therap.* 144: 150–155, 1964.
90. WURTMAN, R. J., C. CHOU, AND C. ROSE. The fate of C^{14}-dihydroxyphenylalanine (C^{14}-dopa) in the whole mouse. *J. Pharmacol. Exptl. Therap.* 174: 351–356, 1970.
91. WYLIE, D. W. Augmentation of the pressor response to guanethedine by inhibition of catechol-O-methyltransferase. *Nature* 189: 490–491, 1961.
92. WYLIE, D. W., S. ARCHER, AND A. ARNOLD. Augmentation of pharmacological properties of catecholamines by O-methyl transferase inhibitors. *J. Pharmacol. Exptl. Therap.* 130: 239–245, 1961.

CHAPTER 41

Monoamine oxidase

K. F. TIPTON | Department of Biochemistry, University of Cambridge, Cambridge, England

CHAPTER CONTENTS

Classification and Nomenclature
Distribution
Intracellular Localization
Reaction Catalyzed
Assay Methods
Properties of the Enzyme
  Flavin
  Metals
  Sulfhydryl groups
  Specificity
  Acceptors
  Kinetics
  Inhibitors
Multiple Forms
Monoamine Oxidase and Adrenal Gland
Function of Monoamine Oxidase

MUCH OF THE EARLIER LITERATURE on the properties and function of monoamine oxidase has been extensively reviewed (7, 21–24, 57, 84, 205, 240, 256, 257). This chapter does not attempt any detailed coverage of material that has been dealt with before but concentrates on more recent developments in our knowledge of this enzyme.

CLASSIFICATION AND NOMENCLATURE

The Enzyme Commission of the International Union of Biochemistry [see (62)] has listed three amine oxidases: monoamine oxidase [monoamine: O_2 oxidoreductase (deaminating); EC 1.4.3.4]; diamine oxidase [diamine: O_2 oxidoreductase (deaminating); EC 1.4.3.5]; and spermine oxidase [spermine: O_2 oxidoreductase (donor-cleaving); EC 1.5.3.3]. However, the distinction between these enzymes is not straightforward, and the trivial names, monoamine oxidase and diamine oxidase, are somewhat unsatisfactory. Monoamine oxidase has been shown to act on long-chain diamines, such as 1,10-decamethylene diamine and 1,12-dodecamethylene diamine (29), and both diamine oxidase and spermine oxidase are active toward monoamines [see (37, 258) for reviews concerning the specificities of these enzymes].
  Zeller (254, 255) originally suggested that sensitivity to inhibition by cyanide and carbonyl reagents, such as semicarbazide, could be used as a criterion for distinguishing between monoamine and diamine oxidases. He found that the histaminase from pig kidney was active toward putrescine (1,4-diaminobutane) and cadaverine (1,5-diaminopentane) and was inhibited by cyanide and carbonyl reagents, whereas the tyramine oxidase, originally discovered by Hare (108), would not act on these diamines and was resistant to the inhibitors (32). This criterion is generally used as the basis for distinguishing between these two types of enzymes. The distinction appears to be attributable to the coenzymes employed by the different oxidases since monoamine oxidase has been shown to be a flavoprotein (see below), whereas the diamine oxidases and spermine oxidase have been shown to contain pyridoxal phosphate [see (24, 37, 262) for reviews].
  Histamine has been generally considered not to be a substrate for monoamine oxidase; however, beef liver mitochondria oxidize histamine in the presence of semicarbazide at 0.07% of the rate at which they oxidize tyramine, although they are inactive toward cadaverine (264). The semicarbazide-insensitive oxidation of histamine and cadaverine by mitochondrial preparations from cat and mouse liver has also been reported (131, 132). The cyanide- and semicarbazide-insensitive histaminase from the cephalopod *Eledone cirrhosa* (33) would be classified as a monoamine oxidase by the criterion of Zeller. This enzyme, which is inactive toward short-chain aliphatic diamines, will also oxidize ω-N-methylhistamine (33), and although this compound is not a substrate for diamine oxidase (37, 127), it is a good substrate for monoamine oxidase (145, 261). Studies on the effect of pH on the activity of the cephalopod enzyme led Boadle (33) to suggest that the monocationic form of histamine (i.e., the form in which the imidazole ring does not carry a positive charge) represents the active form of the substrate. A similar conclusion has been reached concerning pig plasma benzylamine oxidase (a "diamine oxidase"), whereas pig kidney histaminase acts on the dicationic form of histamine (24, 26).
  An alternaet criterion for the recognition of monoamine oxidase is the ability of this enzyme to oxidize N-

methylated amines [(23); see also (37)]. By this criterion the amine oxidase from *Eledone cirrhosa* would also be classified as a monoamine oxidase (33). However, it is not clear whether the amine oxidase from *Sarcina lutea*, which has been shown to be insensitive to cyanide and semicarbazide (137, 246), is active toward *N*-methylated amines.

DISTRIBUTION

Monoamine oxidase is apparently universally distributed among vertebrates, and it has also been demonstrated in a number of invertebrates [see (21, 23, 57, 256) for reviews]. The enzyme is apparently absent from plants, but the previous conclusions that carbonyl reagent-insensitive amine oxidases do not exist in microorganisms (21, 256) must be modified in the light of the reported presence of such an enzyme in *Sarcina lutea* (137, 246).

The distribution of monoamine oxidase among different organs has been extensively reviewed (21, 23, 57). The enzyme has been found in all glandular tissue studied, the liver, parotid, and salivary glands being particularly rich sources. It also occurs in nervous tissue, smooth muscle, heart muscle, and gonads. It is absent or present only in very low concentrations in skeletal muscle, plasma, and erythrocytes, although monoamine oxidase activity is found in blood platelets (44, 186). In the adrenal gland the enzyme has been detected in both the cortex and the medulla (27, 28, 143, 191). In the brain the enzyme is widely distributed throughout the different regions, and the degree of variation is usually small, being much less than that found for some other enzymes (4, 20, 35, 225, 237).

Despite the wide distribution of the enzyme, there appear to be considerable differences in the activities and specificities of the enzyme among the same organs from different species [see (21, 57, 104)].

In brain the enzyme is present in glial cells (199a), as well as in synaptosomes (5), and it has been shown to be present both intra- and extraneuronally in a number of innervated tissues. Histochemical studies have demonstrated the presence of extraneuronal monoamine oxidase in rabbit ear artery (59a) and in parenchymal tissue, such as salivary gland and liver; the majority of the enzyme is extraneuronal (123a). Denervation of the vas deferens results in the loss of some 50% of the monoamine oxidase activity, and this has been interpreted as indicating that only about half of the enzyme is located in the sympathetic nerves with the remainder being in extraneuronal cells (120a). Similar results have been interpreted as indicating that the majority of the monoamine oxidase in rat heart and adrenergically innervated organs is extraneuronal (114a, 128a). Although the persistence of enzyme activity following denervation provides evidence for an extraneuronal location, quantitative estimates of the proportions of intra- and extraneuronal monoamine oxidase from such experiments may be open to doubt since a fall in the activity of an extraneuronal enzyme might be expected if it depended on an intact nerve supply for full activity (148a).

INTRACELLULAR LOCALIZATION

In brain homogenates almost all the monoamine oxidase activity is localized in the mitochondrial fraction (5, 148, 237), but in rat liver only some 70% of the monoamine oxidase activity was found to be associated with the mitochondrial fraction, with most of the remaining activity sedimenting with the microsomal fraction (49, 110). Oswald & Strittmatter (169) reported that rat liver mitochondria contained 76.7% of the monoamine oxidase activity of the total homogenate, whereas the microsomal fraction contained 12.6%; the respective figures for succinate dehydrogenase were 82.2% and 4.5%. These workers could find no more than traces of monoamine oxidase activity in the lysosomal fraction, and the absence of monoamine oxidase from this organelle and from peroxisomes has since been confirmed (13). A similar distribution of monoamine oxidase activity has been reported in rabbit liver (267); in rat heart muscle and salivary gland (58, 211) and in bovine thyroid gland (70) an even higher proportion of the total monoamine oxidase activity was associated with the microsomal fraction.

The monoamine oxidase activity in adrenal medulla is mainly mitochondrial with little activity associated with the chromaffin granules (27, 138, 139, 231), although a relatively high proportion of the activity (ca. 25%) is associated with the microsomal fraction. In bovine splenic nerve homogenates, however, some 30% of the monoamine oxidase activity was sedimented only by high-speed centrifugation (1,500,000 g-min) (187). The pellet that was produced appeared to contain no mitochondria but was rich in norepinephrine storage particles, and it has been suggested (210, 211) that part of the monoamine oxidase activity of splenic nerve was located in the norepinephrine storage particles. In the vas deferens, however, monoamine oxidase activity has been shown not to be associated with the norepinephrine storage particles (120).

Hawkins (110) discussed the possibility that the microsomal monoamine oxidase might be an artifact of the fractionation method employed, and elegant support for this view has come from electron-microscopic histochemical studies with guinea pig kidney cortex in which no extramitochondrial monoamine oxidase could be detected (34).

The relative ease with which a portion of the monoamine oxidase activity could be lost from the mitochondrion, compared with the much stronger retention of succinic dehydrogenase, has become rationalized with the development of techniques for mitochondrial fractionation. By treatment of rat liver mitochondria with digitonin followed by differential centrifugation, Schnaitman et al. (192) were able to separate the outer membrane from the remainder of the mitochondrion. They found that the monoamine oxidase activity was located primarily in the outer membrane fraction and suggested that monoamine oxidase could be used as an enzyme marker for this fraction. A similar conclusion concerning the localization of monoamine oxidase has been reached after the mitochondrial membranes have been separated by hypotonic treatment or by hypotonic treatment followed by sonic oscillation (204, 218). These results have since been confirmed by a number of workers (14, 36, 124, 168, 171, 193, 245).

Schnaitman et al. (192) have suggested that the apparent microsomal localization of some monoamine oxidase activity in rat liver may be an artifact of the fractionation procedure, the outer membrane of the rat liver mitochondrion being relatively easily broken, although the possibility of the extramitochondrial activity representing either a precursor of the mitochondrial enzyme or a distinct enzyme has recently been discussed (99a). In contrast, negligible microsomal monoamine oxidase activity has been observed in brain where the mitochondria are much more resistant to physical damage (217). With brain mitochondria the digitonin method was unsuccessful in separating the mitochondrial membrane fractions from ox and rat; digestion with phospholipase A (9) was also unsuccessful, although procedures involving hypotonic treatment did achieve some separation (53, 218). Boadle & Bloom (34) used a histochemical stain for enzyme activity combined with electron-microscopic examination to study the localization of monoamine oxidase in guinea pig cortex. They could only observe monoamine oxidase activity between the inner and outer membranes of the mitochondria. In the rat liver and vas deferens the origin of microsomal monoamine oxidase has been investigated by density gradient centrifugation (120). By differential centrifugation some 24% of the monoamine oxidase activity of rat liver homogenates and some 42% of that of vas deferens homogenates were found to sediment with the microsomal fraction. Density gradient centrifugation of the material from vas deferens indicated that the "microsomal" monoamine oxidase could be separated in a small particulate fraction that was distinct from either microsomes or norepinephrine storage particles [but see (58, 187, 210, 211)]. This particulate fraction also contained NADH-cytochrome c reductase activity, and since this enzyme is also present in the outer membrane of the mitochondrion, these particles were assumed to be broken mitochondrial outer membranes.

These conclusions have been strongly criticized by Green and his co-workers who have used a variety of different techniques, including digestion with phospholipase A, swelling induced by oleate followed by ATP-induced contraction, sonication in the presence of cholate, and extraction of an acetone powder with distilled water (2, 9, 98, 99), all of which are claimed to enable the separation of inner and outer mitochondrial membrane fractions. The results obtained from these methods indicate that, with the exception of succinate dehydrogenase, the enzymes of the citric acid cycle and those of fatty acid oxidation are associated with the outer mitochondrial membrane. These results are in sharp contrast with those obtained from digitonin treatment, hypotonic treatment, hypotonic treatment followed by sonic oscillation, or rapid freezing in a slightly hypertonic medium to separate the membranes (36, 172, 173, 192, 193, 204), all of which showed the enzymes of the citric acid cycle and fatty acid oxidation to be associated with the inner membrane fraction of the mitochondrion. Research relating to the localization of the enzymes of the citric acid cycle in the intact mitochondrion has recently been critically reviewed by Ernster & Kuylenstierna (64) who have concluded that the evidence is overwhelmingly against the localization of this system in the outer membrane. A comparison between the digitonin and phospholipase A treatments (36) has led to the conclusion that incubation with phospholipase A causes an opening of the intercristal space, as well as of the mitochondrial matrix.

Green's group found monoamine oxidase to be located within the inner membrane [(2, 98); see also (183)]. Because Green's techniques appear to be considerably more vigorous than those of other workers, release of the citric acid cycle and fatty acid oxidation enzymes from the inner membrane fraction is possible. Therefore the fact that monoamine oxidase remains with the inner membrane fraction is surprising. The observation that phospholipase treatment is less effective at releasing monoamine oxidase from the inner membrane fraction than it is at releasing malic dehydrogenase has been confirmed in a comparison of the large-amplitude swelling and phospholipase A digestion methods (218). The probability that the techniques used by Green's group do not achieve a clear separation of the membrane fractions of the mitochondrion has recently been critically examined [(64); see also (36)].

Green's group has criticized the results of other workers on two grounds: *1)* the rotenone-insensitive NADH-cytochrome c reductase, which has been used by other workers as an outer membrane marker, is not, in fact, a mitochondrial enzyme but represents a microsomal contaminant; and *2)* the monoamine oxidase assay system used by Schnaitman et al. (192) is inapplicable to crude mitochondrial systems.

In connection with the first postulate, Green and his co-workers (2, 98) reported that exhaustive washing of twice-washed liver mitochondria removes the rotenone-insensitive NADH-cytochrome c reductase activity from the mitochondria together with glucose 6-phosphatase (an enzyme known to be microsomal). However, Ernster & Kuylenstierna (63) found that extensive washing produced very little loss of rotenone-insensitive NADH-cytochrome c reductase, but the glucose-6-phosphate dehydrogenase activity declined exponentially; similar results have been reported by Beattie (14).

Although Schnaitman et al. (192) and Sottocasa et al. (204) used different methods for the separation of the membrane fractions, they used the same assay method for monoamine oxidase. This assay method (215) is based on the spectral change that occurs when benzylamine is oxidized to benzaldehyde. Green et al. (98) have pointed out that this assay method would not be valid if the benzaldehyde formed were further oxidized to benzoic acid or reduced to benzyl alcohol, and since aldehyde dehydrogenase is a mitochondrial enzyme, the further oxidation of the product cannot be excluded. Green's group therefore used an assay based on the disappearance of ^{14}C-labeled tyramine (150) in their studies. However, Beattie (14), in her studies with the digitonin method, found monoamine oxidase to be located in the outer mitochondrial membrane when the same assay method as that used by Green and co-workers was utilized; other workers have obtained similar results with a variety of other assay methods [(63, 218); see also (100, 181)].

Recently Greenawalt & Schnaitman (100) used five different assay methods to compare the apparent localization of monoamine oxidase in mitochondrial membrane fractions prepared by the digitonin method, and Racker & Proctor (181) used three different assay methods with membrane fractions prepared by a swelling technique (173). Both these groups found that the distribution of monoamine oxidase activity among the membrane fractions, which was primarily in the outer membrane, was unaffected by the assay method used. Greenawalt & Schnaitman (100) also studied the distribution of aldehyde dehydrogenase in liver mitochondria and found it to be largely associated with the inner membrane fraction. Thus further oxidation of the aldehyde would be likely to interfere with monoamine oxidase activity associated with the inner membrane fraction but not with that associated with the outer membrane fraction; however, the activity of monoamine oxidase in the outer membrane fraction, as measured by the spectrophotometric benzylamine assay, was unaffected when a sample of the inner membrane fraction was added to it. Racker & Proctor (181) have shown that the outer membrane fraction of kidney cortex mitochondria can be freed from monoamine oxidase by sonication at pH 9.6 followed by centrifugation at pH 6.0; fractions treated in this way will preferentially bind added monoamine oxidase.

Thus there is a considerable amount of experimental evidence in favor of monoamine oxidase activity being located in the outer membrane fraction of the mitochondrion, and it would appear that results to the contrary probably represent an artifact of the methods used to separate the mitochondrial membrane fractions.

REACTION CATALYZED

The overall reaction catalyzed by monoamine oxidase can be represented by the following equation

$$R \cdot CH_2 \cdot NH_2 + O_2 + H_2O \rightleftharpoons R \cdot CHO + NH_3 + H_2O_2$$

and in the presence of catalase the hydrogen peroxide formed will be decomposed to water and oxygen. The stoichiometry of this reaction has been demonstrated with a number of different preparations of the enzyme (65, 155, 180, 222).

Bernheim (16) was the first to propose that the reaction proceeded by way of an imine intermediate

$$R \cdot CH_2 \cdot NH_2 + O_2 \rightleftharpoons R \cdot CH{:}NH + H_2O_2$$
$$R \cdot CH{:}NH + H_2O \rightleftharpoons R \cdot CHO + NH_3$$

Richter (185) pointed out that, if such a scheme were to account for the oxidation of tertiary amines, such as hordenine (N,N-dimethyltyramine), the amino group must be protonated

$$R \cdot CH_2 \cdot \overset{+}{N}HR_1R_2 + O_2 \rightleftharpoons R \cdot CH{:}\overset{+}{N}R_1R_2 + H_2O_2$$
$$R \cdot CH{:}\overset{+}{N}R_1R_2 + H_2O \rightleftharpoons R \cdot CHO + NH_2R_1R_2$$

It has frequently been assumed that monoamine oxidases interact with the protonated forms of the amine [see (21, 203)]. However, Smith et al. (201) have proposed an alternative mechanism that does not involve the participation of the protonated form of the amine but does involve the removal of a hydride ion.

$$R - \underset{H}{\overset{H}{C}} - NR_1R_2 \rightleftharpoons R - \underset{H}{\overset{}{C}} = \overset{+}{N}R_1R_2$$
$$R - \underset{H}{\overset{}{C}} = \overset{+}{N}R_1R_2 + H_2O \rightleftharpoons RCHO + H_2\overset{+}{N}R_1R_2$$

The assumption that the nonprotonated form of the amine interacts with the enzyme is supported by studies on the effects of pH on the activity of human liver monoamine oxidase (154, 155). In these studies the Michaelis-Menten constants (K_m values) for the oxidation of three different substrates decreased, as the pH was increased, in a manner typical of a nonprotonated amine interacting with the enzyme. These results contrast with those reported for the rat liver enzyme in which no decrease in K_m with pH could be detected (48), although these latter results were obtained over a considerably more limited range of pH than those with the human liver enzyme.

Attempts to deduce the state of ionization of the amine substrate from the effect of pH on K_m should, however, be treated with caution since the kinetic mechanism proposed for monoamine oxidase is one in which K_m is a steady-state constant rather than the dissociation constant of the enzyme-amine complex (see below). The expression for the K_m for the amine includes the rate constant for the release of the product from the enzyme (221). Since release of the product may depend on the hydrolysis of the imine (229), a reaction involving the cationic form of the imine [see (122, 122a)], the relatively low pH optimum of this reaction could have a significant effect on the observed dependence of K_m on pH.

In an extensive study of the effects of pH on the kinetic parameters of the oxidation of benzylamine by beef liver monoamine oxidase, Oi et al. (167a) found no evidence for pronounced changes in the K_m or maximum velocity (V_{max}) of the reaction at the pK of the substrate. These results would indicate that the activity of the enzyme may be independent of the state of ionization of the amine substrate.

The theories of monoamine oxidase action discussed above involve the formation of an imine as an intermediate. This is analogous to the mechanism that has been proposed for the amino acid oxidases [see (156) for references]. Such a mechanism is supported by the observation that aromatic amines, such as aniline, which are not capable of undergoing carbon-nitrogen dehydrogenation, are not substrates for monoamine oxidase (21, 32). The fact that benzylamine is a substrate for the enzyme argues against a mechanism involving carbon-carbon bond dehydrogenation followed by rearrangement to form an imine, as was suggested to be a possible mechanism for diamine oxidase (256).

Indirect evidence in favor of the formation of an imine during the reaction comes from the observation that 2-phenylethylhydrazine is oxidized to the corresponding hydrazone by monoamine oxidase (228). A possible alternative mechanism in which an N-oxide is formed as an intermediate has been ruled out since the deamination of N,N-dimethyltryptamine-N-oxide by monoamine oxide appears to proceed by way of an imine intermediate (201). Although N-oxides can act as substrates for monoamine oxidase, this enzyme probably does not play an important role in the metabolism of these compounds (18).

ASSAY METHODS

Methods for assaying the activity of monoamine oxidase have been previously reviewed (19, 21, 84, 203). Activity may be followed by measuring the disappearance of oxygen manometrically (54) or polarographically (218, 224). The appearance of ammonia can be determined after microdiffusion (50, 51) or by a direct indophenol color reaction (160). The rate of hydrogen peroxide production has been measured by coupling it, by way of peroxidase, to the reduction of a dye that can be measured spectrophotometrically (151, 265) or fluorometrically [(202, 222); see also (102a, 103)], or its formation can be followed electrochemically in the presence of peroxidase (149). The aldehyde product can be measured spectrophotometrically after conversion to the dinitrophenylhydrazone (97) or by NAD$^+$ reduction in the presence of aldehyde dehydrogenase (153, 181, 213, 238).

Colorimetric assay methods that use specific substrates have been developed; serotonin and tryptamine disappearance can be followed spectrophotometrically by observing color reactions with the 1-nitro-2-naphthol and nitrous acid reagents (233). The changes in absorption that occur when benzylamine (215), m-iodobenzylamine (262), methoxy derivatives of benzaldehyde (153), p-dimethylaminobenzylamine (59), m-nitro-p-hydroxybenzylamine (88), and kynuramine (239) are oxidized have been used in assay methods. A modification of the kynuramine assay method allows the increase in fluorescence to be followed as the aldehyde produced spontaneously cyclizes to 4-hydroxyquinoline [(136); see also (41, 174)]; a similar method in which 5-hydroxykynuramine is used has been reported (216). Another fluorometric assay involves estimation of the indoleacetic acid that is formed from the product of tryptamine oxidation in the presence of NAD$^+$ and aldehyde dehydrogenase (146); a similar assay method in which serotonin is used as the substrate has been developed (112).

In addition a number of methods involving measurement of the disappearance of a radioactive substrate or the appearance of radioactive products have been developed (150, 170, 186, 207, 244); ^{14}C-labeled benzylamine, tyramine, tryptamine, dopamine, and serotonin have been used in such assays. A radiochemical method based on the release of tritium when 1,2-^{3}H-tyramine is oxidized has been reported (68).

Many of the assay methods mentioned above are restricted to measurements involving a single substrate, and a number of the others are restricted to a relatively small number of substrates. Methods based on the further utilization of hydrogen peroxide in the presence of peroxidase cannot be used with the catecholamines or with serotonin since these compounds are very powerful redox-acceptors in such a system (202, 222). The applicability of the methods involving the use of aldehyde dehydrogenase to form NADH is at present unknown and must await detailed studies on the substrate specificities of the aldehyde dehydrogenases. For a routine assay method that is not very restricted in choice of substrate, one of the oxygen uptake methods or, when primary amines are used, one of the ammonia detection methods can be used. With oxygen uptake measurements, endogenous oxygen uptake in crude preparations and further oxidation of the aldehyde product can be prevented by the presence of cyanide and semicarbazide (54). The use of cyanide in such systems should, however, be regarded with some caution since cyanide has been shown to cause a dramatic change in the sensitivity of the enzyme to some inhibitors [see (57)].

PROPERTIES OF THE ENZYME

Purified preparations of monoamine oxidase have been obtained from a number of sources. Great difficulty has been encountered in solubilizing the enzyme, and detergent treatment (10, 65, 71, 75, 76, 106, 130, 155, 161), sonication (102), sonication and freeze-thawing (157, 219), extraction with an organic solvent (113, 114, 168b), and a combination of sonication and detergent treatment (189, 252) have been used successfully in preparations from different sources. The vigor of the treatments necessary to obtain soluble preparations of the enzyme could lead to the generation of arti-

TABLE 1. *Some Properties of Monoamine Oxidase as Purified from Several Sources*

Source	Molecular Weight, $\times 10^5$ g	Flavin Content, mole/10^5 g	Flavin Fluorescence	Sulfhydryl Groups, per 10^5 g	Metal Content	Refs.
Beef kidney	2.9	1.0	Yes	7	Cu absent	65
Beef liver	4.2 and 12.5	1.0	No	8	Cu, Fe, Mn, Co, Mo absent	81, 82, 117, 247
Human brain	4.0		Yes			159a, 161
Pig brain	1.0	1.0	Yes		Cu, Fe absent	219, 220
Rat liver	1.5–3.0	0.7	Some preparations	8	Cu absent; Fe present	87, 206, 253
Pig liver	1.15 and aggregates	0.9	Yes		Cu, Mo, Mn absent; Fe present	168b
Sarcina lutea	1.3	1.5			Cu, Fe, Zn, Mn absent	137

facts, and a careful comparison of the properties of the purified enzyme with those of the enzyme in its more-or-less native state will be necessary before this possibility can be excluded.

Table 1 summarizes some of the molecular properties of monoamine oxidase preparations that have been studied in detail.

The molecular weights vary from about 1×10^5 to 1.28×10^6, the latter being the higher value for the beef liver enzyme that appears to exist in polymeric forms (81). The enzyme purified from pig liver has also been shown to form high molecular weight aggregates that can be dissociated by the detergent sodium cholate (113, 168b). A minor component of pig brain monoamine oxidase (<10%) was found to be eluted from Sephadex G-200 in a volume corresponding to a molecular weight of 4.35×10^5, and it was suggested that this higher molecular weight form might represent either a lipid complex or a polymeric form of the enzyme (219). In addition to the values given in Table 1, a molecular weight of about 3.0×10^5 (230) has been reported for the enzyme from beef adrenal medulla, 2.3×10^5 for the rat brain enzyme (249), 2.4×10^5 for the human platelet enzyme (44), and $2-3 \times 10^5$ for the enzyme from rabbit liver (75). Youdim & Collins (248) have reported that rat liver mitochondrial monoamine oxidase can be broken down by denaturation to subunits with a molecular weight of about 0.75×10^5.

Despite the wide differences in the molecular weights of monoamine oxidases from various sources, the minimum—or active site—molecular weight of each preparation, except the microbial enzyme, appears to be roughly similar from their flavin contents (see Table 1). In addition minimum molecular weight values of about 10^5 have been determined for the enzymes from beef kidney (111) and pig brain (221) by other methods. Hellerman & Erwin (111) calculated this value for the beef kidney enzyme from studies on the binding of the radioactive inhibitor pargyline (*N*-methyl-*N*-benzylpropylamine), although they did express some reservation concerning the homogeneity of the enzyme preparation they used. Tipton (221) calculated the value for the pig brain enzyme by determining the amount of aldehyde released when the enzyme was incubated with tyramine in the absence of oxygen; recently similar results have been reported with the beef liver enzyme (167).

Flavin

Information on the mode of attachment of the flavin to the enzyme is obscure. The enzymes prepared from beef kidney (65), pig liver (168b) and brain (220), human brain (161), and beef brain (106) exhibit flavin fluorescence at about 520 nm when excited by light at 450 nm, but no flavin fluorescence could be detected with the enzyme from beef liver (117, 163). The absence of flavin fluorescence from the rat liver enzyme has also been reported (252), but recently it has been found that some preparations of this enzyme do fluoresce, whereas others do not (253). A similar situation has been reported in the beef kidney enzyme (65) in which less pure preparations do not show flavin fluorescence; it is only after a considerable degree of purification that flavin fluorescence could be detected. It may be therefore that the lack of fluorescence with the beef liver enzyme and some preparations of the rat liver enzyme could result from quenching by impurities, although the possibility of species and organ differences cannot be ruled out with the beef liver enzyme.

The flavin is covalently bound to the beef liver enzyme, and a flavopeptide has been isolated after proteolytic digestion of the enzyme (81, 117, 127a, 163). The flavin component has been shown to be FAD, which is joined from its 8α position to a cysteine residue in a thioether linkage [(127a, 236a); see also (77b)]. Covalent binding also appears likely in the cases of the beef liver and pig liver enzymes (65, 110a, 168b), and a flavopeptide has been isolated from the former (110a). In contrast, flavin can be relatively easily removed from the pig brain enzyme (220) and from the bacterial tyramine oxidase (137, 246). Some flavin was removed from partly purified preparations of the beef and human brain enzymes (106, 159a, 161), but because these preparations were not homogeneous it is not possible to decide whether this flavin was extracted from monoamine oxidase or from another component of the mixture.

The situation regarding the attachment of flavin to rat liver monoamine oxidase is more complex, in that some 50% of the total flavin can be removed by treatment with trichloroacetic acid, whereas the remainder is tightly and probably covalently bound (206, 253, 253a). Since the rat liver enzyme has been reported to be composed of a number of isoenzymes (see below) it may be that some of the isoenzyme species contain covalently bound flavin, whereas in others the flavin is more loosely bound.

The flavin has been identified as FAD in the enzymes from beef liver (236a), pig brain (220), and *Sarcina lutea* (137, 246). The loosely bound flavin material associated with the rat liver (253a), human brain (159a, 161), and beef brain (106, 159a) enzymes has also been shown to be FAD. The nature of the tightly bound flavin component of the pig liver enzyme is unknown (168b). Digestion of the enzymes from rat liver (253a), beef kidney (65), and beef liver (117) with the bacterial proteinase, pronase, liberated a flavin that could be shown to be associated with amino acids by its positive reaction with ninhydrin, and the flavin in the beef kidney enzyme and the tightly bound component of the rat liver enzyme may be bound in the same way as that in the beef liver enzyme (236a). Indeed the absorption spectrum of the flavin component isolated from the beef kidney enzyme is similar to that of the oxidized form of cysteinyl-8α-FAD [(110a); see also (77b, 236a)]. In contrast, pronase treatment of the pig liver enzyme yielded a flavin material that did not give a color reaction with ninhydrin (168b). Since pronase digestion would not be expected to cleave a thio-ether linkage, the attachment of the flavin to the pig liver enzyme may be different from that demonstrated with the enzyme from beef liver. The flavin component isolated from the pig liver enzyme was chromatographically distinct from FAD, and the possibility that it may be a modified form of this coenzyme has been discussed (168b).

The fluorescence of the flavin component of monoamine oxidase has been shown to be quenched by its environment since digestion of the beef liver and kidney, pig brain, and rat liver enzymes with the bacterial proteolytic enzyme, pronase, causes a large increase in flavin fluorescence (65, 117, 206, 220). The addition of substrate to monoamine oxidase preparations results in a decrease in the flavin fluorescence (65, 106, 161, 220, 253) and absorption (65, 137, 163). These results indicate that the flavin component of the enzyme becomes reduced or partially reduced in the presence of an amine. With the pig brain enzyme a small reduction of the flavin fluorescence was observed when the enzyme, in an atmosphere of nitrogen, was treated with hydrogen peroxide; this decrease in fluorescence was reversed by the addition of catalase or by shaking the sample in air (220).

Metals

The extent of the involvement of a metal in the activity of monoamine oxidase is not clear. Monoamine oxidase preparations from a number of sources have been shown to be inhibited by chelating agents [see (10, 21, 65, 90, 142, 157, 161, 162, 206, 219, 246)]. These results indicate that a metal may be involved in the activity of the enzyme, but there is no clear indication of what that metal may be. Earlier reports that copper was involved in the activity of the beef liver enzyme (162, 164) were modified when it was later found possible to obtain highly purified preparations of the enzyme containing only traces of copper (247). No significant amounts of copper could be found in purified preparations of the enzyme from rat liver (252), beef kidney (65), pig liver (113, 168b), and pig brain (220). A report that copper might be present in the microbial tyramine oxidase (246) has subsequently been shown to be incorrect (137).

Approximately 2 moles of iron per 150,000 g of protein has been reported in rat liver monoamine oxidase (252), and iron was also shown to be present in the pig liver enzyme in amounts ranging from 0.5–2.0 moles/115,000 g, although there was no correlation between the iron content and the activity of the enzyme preparation (168b). In contrast, only traces of iron could be found in the beef liver and pig brain enzymes (162, 220), and none could be detected in the microbial enzyme (137). Chronic iron deficiency in the diets of rats has been shown to cause an 18–31% decrease in the liver monoamine oxidase activity, whereas copper deficiency had little effect (212). In this connection the failure of cyanide, carbon monoxide, and azide to irreversibly inhibit monoamine oxidase does not necessarily rule out the involvement of iron (or copper) in this enzyme since these reagents have been shown not to inhibit all iron- and copper-containing enzymes [see (61)].

For the enzyme from rabbit liver it has been reported that the chelating agent, 1,10-phenanthroline, inhibits at relatively high concentrations (1–5 mM) but activates at lower concentrations (23–330 μM), and similar effects were observed with neocuproine (2,9-dimethyl-1,10-phenanthroline) (75). The observations that 1,10-phenanthroline, 2,2′-dipyridyl, and 8-hydroxyquinoline are potent inhibitors of the rat liver enzyme, although the copper chelating agent cuprizone (bicyclohexanone oxalyldihydrazone) is a relatively weak inhibitor, have been taken to support the involvement of iron in the activity of this enzyme (206). Cuprizone was also found to be a poor inhibitor of the enzyme from human brain (161), although it is a potent inhibitor of the beef liver and thyroid enzymes (71, 247). Gorkin & Romanova (90) did not find 1,10-phenanthroline and 2,2′-dipyridyl to be strong inhibitors of less highly purified preparations of rat liver monoamine oxidase, although 8-hydroxyquinoline was a potent inhibitor. Although it does appear to be a relatively good inhibitor of the beef and pig brain enzymes (159, 219), 1,10-phenanthroline has also been shown to be a relatively poor inhibitor of the beef liver and kidney and pig liver enzymes (65, 168a, 247). Preincubation of the pig brain enzyme with 1,10-phenanthroline or theonyltrifluoroacetone prevents the reduction of flavin fluorescence caused by substrate but not that caused by H_2O_2 (220), which suggests that this agent acts at the stage of conversion of the amine to the aldehyde rather than at the stage of reoxidation of the reduced enzyme (see below).

In relatively impure preparations of rat liver monoamine oxidase, 8-hydroxyquinoline has been found to inhibit the oxidation of tyramine but to be without effect on the oxidation of benzylamine (194). However, 2-hydroxyquinoline, which is a much less powerful chelating agent, will inhibit the deamination of both these substrates, although with different potencies (195). The inhibition of tyramine oxidation by 8-hydroxyquinoline can be reversed by addition of a number of metal ions (Co^{2+}, Ni^{2+}, Zn^{2+}, and Fe^{2+}), whereas inhibition by 2-hydroxyquinoline could not be reversed at all in this way, and the inhibition of benzylamine oxidation by this latter compound could be reversed only by Co^{2+} ions. These results have been interpreted as evidence for the existence of multiple forms of monoamine oxidase (194, 195). Severina & Sheremet'evskaya (197) have compared the effects of 8-hydroxyquinoline with those of a number of quinoline and naphthalene derivatives that are poor metal complexing agents. The observation that these derivatives can be more powerful selective inhibitors of rat liver monoamine oxidase than 8-hydroxyquinoline has led these authors to suggest that quinoline and naphthalene derivatives may exert their effects by means other than metal chelation. Similar suggestions have been made with respect to the beef kidney and microbial enzymes that are inhibited by 8-hydroxyquinoline and α- and β-naphthols (65, 137), and phenolic compounds of this type are known to inhibit other flavoenzymes [see (65) for references].

Thus the possible involvement of a metal in the action of monoamine oxidase remains obscure, and it may be that some of the conflicting results obtained with chelating agents may, to some extent, reflect the degree of purity of the preparations, since it has been suggested that metal ions may be involved in maintaining the structure of particles containing monoamine oxidase (235).

Sulfhydryl Groups

Monoamine oxidases from various sources have been reported to be inhibited by sulfhydryl reagents (10, 72, 111, 130, 142, 159, 161, 162, 200, 205, 206, 219). Belleau & Moran (15) suggested that the inhibitor pargyline (*N*-methyl-*N*-benzylpropylamine) inhibited monoamine oxidase by reacting with sulfhydryl groups in the enzyme. Determination of the sulfhydryl group content of the enzyme before and after treatment with pargyline has, however, revealed no significant difference (111, 236).

The beef liver enzyme contains seven (82) and the beef kidney eight sulfhydryl groups per 10^5 g of protein (85a, 111), and a similar value has been reported for preparations of the rat liver enzyme [(87); see also (129)]. Denaturation did not cause an increase in the detectable sulfhydryl groups of the beef liver (82) and kidney (111) enzymes.

With a less pure preparation of the rat liver enzyme the activity toward serotonin was completely inhibited when three sulfhydryl groups per 10^5 g of protein had reacted with *p*-chloromercuribenzoate, although the oxidation of tyramine was totally inhibited only when five sulfhydryl groups had reacted (129). Gorkin's group has attempted to correlate the oxidation of sulfhydryl groups in the enzyme with changes in its specificity (87, 94). The reduction of the flavin fluorescence of the pig brain enzyme and of the flavin absorption spectrum of the beef liver enzyme that occurs when substrate is added has been shown to be abolished by preincubation of these enzymes with *p*-chloromercuribenzoate (117, 220). In contrast, gradual reaction of all the sulfhydryl groups in the beef liver enzyme with *p*-chloromercuribenzoate has been reported to result in a loss of only some 20–30% of the initial activity when benzylamine was used as the substrate (82).

The role of sulfhydryl groups in the activity of monoamine oxidase must await further clarification. It would appear that one or more of the sulfhydryl groups may be essential in some preparations of the enzyme, although there is no evidence that a sulfhydryl group is involved at the active site. However, in the beef liver enzyme sulfhydryl groups are apparently not essential for activity of the enzyme (82), and they presumably play a structural role.

Specificity

The substrate specificity of monoamine oxidase has been reviewed in considerable detail elsewhere (21, 23, 24), and the data collected in these reviews are only briefly summarized. The enzyme acts on a variety of primary monoamines and also on secondary and tertiary amines provided the substituents are methyl groups, although the oxidation of *N*,*N*-dimethyltryptamine-*N*-oxide has also been shown to occur (201). The amino group must be attached to an unsubstituted methylene group (32); aniline and amphetamine, for example, are not substrates (15, 32). In the case of aliphatic amines, methylamine is not oxidized and ethylamine is oxidized only in some species (1, 32, 179, 180). For straight-chain aliphatic amines the optimum chain length for oxidation has been shown to be C_5 or C_6 (1), although the apparent decrease in oxidation rates when higher homologues are used may be due, in part, to the relative insolubility of these compounds (21, 23).

Short-chain aliphatic diamines are normally not oxidized, but longer-chain members of the homologous series $H_2N(CH_2)_nNH_2$ are oxidized when n is greater than 7; the maximum rate of oxidation is obtained when n equals 13 (29). Similar results have been reported with ω-amino acids (31) and with quaternary compounds of the general formula $H_2N(CH_2)_nN(CH_3)_3$ (11).

Monoamine oxidase will oxidize benzylamine, 2-phenylethylamine and its derivatives, and indolealkylamines, these latter two classes of compounds providing the natural substrates. The 2-phenylethylamine derivatives include tyramine, dopamine, epinephrine, norepinephrine, m-O-methyladrenaline (metanephrine), and m-O-methylnoradrenaline (normetanephrine). In a study of the effects of substituents on the benzene ring on the oxidation of benzylamine derivatives by preparations of beef liver mitochondria, it was found that a variety of groups (chloro, iodo, methoxy, nitro, and methyl) could be substituted in the meta position to yield good substrates for the enzyme. However, ortho or para substitution produced poor substrates (259). Since these substituents are widely different in nucleophilic or electrophilic character it was concluded that the position of the substituent, rather than the distribution of electrons on the aromatic nucleus, was most important in forming a good substrate. This view is supported by the report that both rat and guinea pig monoamine oxidases only have significant activity toward the meta isomer of xylidene diamine (25). With 2-phenylethylamines, however, ring substitution of methyl, hydroxy, or methoxy groups has a considerably smaller and less consistent effect (1, 184).

Multiple substitution in the benzene ring has shown that 3,4-dimethoxybenzylamine is a substrate for monoamine oxidase, whereas 3,4,5-trimethoxybenzylamine is not (259). Of the three dimethoxy derivatives, Randall (184) showed that the 2,3-isomer was oxidized by both guinea pig and cat liver monoamine oxidase more rapidly than the 3,4 and 4,5 derivatives. Mescaline (3,4,5-trimethoxyphenylethylamine) is not a substrate for monoamine oxidase but can be oxidized by an enzyme of the diamine oxidase type (116, 260).

Monoamine oxidase shows some optical specificity for its substrates. Thus, with crude preparations of the enzyme, the *l* forms of epinephrine and norepinephrine appear to be oxidized to a greater extent than the *d* forms (32, 78, 178). In guinea pig liver preparations, however, no evidence of optical specificity could be detected (144). It has been shown that monoamine oxidase exhibits absolute stereospecificity for the configuration around the α carbon atom, by the use of deuterated derivatives of tyramine in which one or both of the hydrogen atoms on this atom are replaced by deuterium (15).

The amount of kinetic data that has accumulated for the oxidation of the natural substrates of monoamine oxidase is unfortunately sparse. The K_m and V_{max} values for some such substrates are listed for a number of preparations in Table 2.

As well as amines, monoamine oxidase has been shown to oxidize the inhibitory hydrazine, 2-phenylethylhydrazine (42, 43, 228, 229). Also the ability of beef and mouse liver mitochondria to very slowly oxidize histamine has been reported (131, 132, 264), and the enzyme from *Eledone cirrhosa* is, as mentioned earlier, active toward histamine (33). Some preparations of the enzyme have considerably narrower specificities. The beef thyroid enzyme is inactive toward benzylamine, epinephrine, and norepinephrine (71), and the *Sarcina lutea* enzyme also appears to have a restricted specificity (246).

Any discussion of the specificity of monoamine oxidase must take account of a remarkable series of experiments reported by Gorkin and his co-workers. They have reported that treatment of crude preparations of rat liver or beef liver monoamine oxidase with oxidizing agents, such as cupric ions, oxidized oleic acid, or benzoyl peroxide, decreases the ability of the enzyme to oxidize monoamines but results in the appearance of an ability of the enzyme to oxidize some diamines (86, 91, 94). This phenomenon has been termed *transformation* and has recently been repeated with purified preparations of the rat and beef liver enzymes and of the tyramine oxidase from *Sarcina lutea* (85a, 87).

TABLE 2. *Oxidation of Some Natural Substrates by Monoamine Oxidase*

Source	Oxygen	Tyramine	Tryptamine	Serotonin	Dopamine	Epinephrine	m-O-Metanephrine	pH	Refs.
Rat liver[†]		2,000 (100)	4,800 (21)	(37)	7,400 (27)			7.4	94
		1,300	2,000	22,000	1,600			7.0	130
Beef liver[†]	175	(100)	(53)	(46)				7.4	162, 167
Pig brain	234	120 (100)	115 (62)	28 (35)		85 (20)	20 (34)	7.2	221, 224a
Human brain									
Isoenzyme 1		42 (100)	15 (50)		19 (126)				
Isoenzyme 2		61 (100)	18 (82)		26 (348)				
Isoenzyme 3		92 (100)	43 (114)		20 (2,880)			7.4	45
Isoenzyme 4		40 (100)	67 (149)		2.7 (12,900)				
Beef thyroid	120	150				Inactive		7.4	71
Beef adrenal medulla		840 (100)		65 (16)		1,300 (35)	160 (10)	7.2	230
Human blood platelet		31 (100)	8.0 (63)		1.9 (42)			7.4	44

Values in parentheses indicate V_{max} relative to tyramine. * Expressed as K_m value (μM). [†] Velocity measurements are not V_{max} values, but are initial velocities determined at a single substrate concentration.

The substrates that "transformed" liver monoamine oxidases will oxidize include histamine, cadaverine, L-lysine, spermine, and AMP. As well as treatment with oxidizing agents, transformation has been reported to occur slowly in mitochondria that are stored at room temperature (86); this process is enhanced by the presence of oxidized glutathione but inhibited by reduced glutathione. After radiation injury, hypervitaminosis D_2, or parenteral administration of oxidized oleic acid, a marked decrease in the ability of liver mitochondria to oxidize monoamines, together with an increased ability to oxidize histamine and diamines, has been reported (87).

The transformation of monoamine oxidase may be reversed by treatment with reducing agents, such as sodium borohydride, H_2S, or glutathione (87), and an attempt has been made to correlate the "transformation state" with the sulfhydryl group content of the enzyme (85a, 87, 94). In addition the transformation of purified diamine oxidase into an enzyme that will not oxidize putrescine but will oxidize tyramine and tryptophan has been reported to occur when the enzyme is treated with reducing agents (85a, 87).

Perhaps the most provocative results to come from these studies are those demonstrating that transformation alters the inhibitor sensitivites of the enzymes. Thus transformed monoamine oxidase is inhibited by KCN and hydroxylamine (91), whereas transformed diamine oxidase is insensitive to carbonyl reagents (87). Since the difference in the inhibitor sensitivities of these two enzymes is believed to be a function of their cofactor requirements it is difficult to understand how this effect comes about.

Acceptors

There have been no reports indicating the ability of purified preparations of monoamine oxidase to use artificial electron acceptors. With crude preparations of liver monoamine oxidase, Philpot (175) demonstrated the reduction of o-bromophenolindophenol and o-cresolindophenol by tyramine under anaerobic conditions, but a number of the other dyes were found not to be acceptors, and methylene blue was found to be a strong inhibitor of the enzyme (175, 176). This latter observation has been confirmed with a purified preparation of the beef liver enzyme (247). However, other workers have reported that at low oxygen concentrations methylene blue causes an increase in oxygen uptake (96, 133).

Crude preparations from rabbit liver are able to reduce triphenyltetrazolium chloride in the presence of tyramine and under anaerobic conditions. This activity was, however, lost more rapidly than the ability to oxidize tyramine in the presence of oxygen. Well-washed acetone powders of liver yielded extracts that would oxidize substrate in the presence of oxygen but would not reduce the tetrazolium derivative (21). These results led Blaschko (21) to suggest that an additional enzyme system was required for the anaerobic reduction of the tetrazolium derivative. Lagnado and Sourkes observed that in rat brain and liver suspensions the anaerobic reduction of tetrazolium salts required the presence of an unidentified, heat-stable, dialyzable cofactor (141).

In a highly purified preparation of beef liver monoamine oxidase, no reduction of 2,6-dichlorophenolindophenol, cytochrome c, or tetrazolium salts could be observed in the presence of substrate (247). This observation is at first surprising since tetrazolium salts have been used widely to stain for monoamine oxidase in histochemical (34, 52, 79, 141) and electrophoretic studies (46, 128). However, the reduction of tetrazolium salts in the presence of monoamine oxidase and tryptamine results from the reaction of the indoleacetaldehyde formed with the tetrazolium salt rather than from an enzymatic electron transport mechanism (80), although further reaction of the aldehyde product could also play a part in color formation. These results implicating the aldehyde in the color reaction are consistent with earlier observations in which the process of pigment formation was shown to be inhibited by carbonyl reagents (30).

The anaerobic reduction of tetrazolium salts by monoamine oxidase obviously cannot be explained in the above way. Although bacterial amine oxidizing systems that reduce acceptors, other than oxygen, have been known for some time (158, 214), no reports of such a system in animal tissues had been reported until recently when Guha & Ghosh (101) detected a monoamine dehydrogenase system in rat brain that is apparently capable of reducing neotetrazolium chloride in the presence of tyramine under anaerobic conditions. This reaction did not cause the formation of ammonia. Lagnado et al. (140, 251) have, however, reported that the reaction of purified rat liver monoamine oxidase with tetrazolium salts and substrates causes inhibition of the enzyme without the release of detectable quantities of ammonia or aldehyde.

Several workers have reported that the activity of monoamine oxidase is increased when the oxygen concentration is increased above air saturation (133, 166, 175), and this has since been borne out by the relatively high K_m values for oxygen that have been reported for a number of preparations of the enzyme [see Table 2; (267)]. These results imply that the enzyme will be working at only about half its maximum efficiency at air-saturated oxygen concentrations. Blaschko (21) has suggested this to imply that in the living cell the enzyme uses some other, as yet unidentified, acceptor rather than oxygen. However, it should be pointed out that the relatively high K_m of monoamine oxidase for oxygen is by no means unique, similar values having been reported for other oxidases, such as D-amino acid oxidase and uricase (60, 147).

Kinetics

The kinetics of the enzymes prepared from pig brain (221), beef thyroid gland (71), and beef liver (167) have been studied in some detail. Kinetic analyses of the reaction catalyzed by the pig brain and beef liver enzymes indicate that the reaction proceeds by way of a number of binary complexes between the enzyme and one of its substrates without the formation of kinetically significant amounts of any ternary complex, but with the formation of a free modified form of the enzyme as an intermediate. The kinetic reaction pathways proposed for the pig brain and beef liver enzymes differ in detail, but the general pathway followed can be illustrated by that proposed for the pig brain enzyme

$$\begin{array}{ccc} & E \cdot S \longrightarrow E' \cdot P & \\ E & & E' \\ & E \cdot H_2O_2 \leftarrow E' \cdot O_2 & \end{array}$$

In this scheme S and P represent the amine substrate and the product derived from it, respectively, and the free modified form of the enzyme, designated E', presumably represents the form of the enzyme in which the flavin component is in the reduced state. This mechanism is consistent with the reduction of flavin fluorescence observed when substrate is added to the enzyme in the absence of oxygen. Further evidence in favor of such a scheme is supplied by the demonstration that stoichiometric quantities of aldehyde are produced when the enzymes from pig brain and beef liver are incubated with substrate in the absence of oxygen (167, 221).

This kinetic mechanism can be illustrated in terms of the following reaction pathway

$$E + RCH_2NH_2 \rightleftharpoons E \cdot RCH_2NH_2 + EH_2 \cdot RCH:NH$$
$$\rightleftharpoons EH_2 + RCH:NH$$
$$EH_2 + O_2 \rightleftharpoons EH_2 \cdot O_2 \rightleftharpoons E \cdot H_2O_2 \rightleftharpoons E + H_2O_2$$
$$RCH:NH + H_2O \rightleftharpoons RCHO + NH_3$$

For the thyroid enzyme the kinetic results were similar to those reported for the liver and brain enzymes, but a somewhat different pattern of inhibition by the products of the reaction was observed. These data were interpreted in terms of a mechanism involving a ternary complex between the enzyme and two of the reactants. Since in this case product inhibition data are available only with respect to one substrate (the amine) it is not possible to draw firm conclusions from these results.

The kinetics of the oxidation of a hydrazine by the pig brain enzyme have also been studied (229). The kinetic patterns are considerably different from those obeyed by amine oxidation. The results are consistent with either the formation of a ternary complex or the direct displacement of the hydrazone product from the enzyme by oxygen. It is suggested that the difference between the mechanism of hydrazine and amine oxidation may lie in the ability of the product to be hydrolyzed. If the imine produced by amine oxidation were hydrolyzed on the enzyme surface, this hydrolysis could facilitate the release of product from the enzyme by weakening the chelate effect. The oxidation of hydrazines, however, results in the formation of a hydrazone

$$RCH_2NHNH_2 \xrightarrow{(2H)} RCH:NNH_2$$

Such compounds are less readily hydrolyzed than imines, and this could result in the product not being released from the enzyme before the binding of oxygen.

Inhibitors

In addition to chelating agents and sulfhydryl group reagents, a large number of monoamine oxidase inhibitors have been synthesized, some of which have found clinical use as antidepressant drugs. These inhibitors include derivatives of hydrazine, cyclopropylamines, propargylamines, derivatives of aminopyrazine, carbolines related to the harmala alkaloids, and some indole-alkylamines. There have been a number of extensive reviews on monoamine oxidase inhibitors [(19, 21, 57, 177, 266); see also (242, 243)].

Pharmacological aspects are outside the scope of this review, but selective inhibitors of monoamine oxidase, which is a topic that has developed considerably since the above reviews were written, are discussed briefly in the following section.

MULTIPLE FORMS

A considerable amount of evidence suggests that, in some species at least, there may be more than one enzyme with monoamine oxidase activity. A number of investigators report that the effects of inhibitors on monoamine oxidase preparations varied according to the substrate used to measure the activity [see (38, 84, 107, 115, 196, 208, 234, 263)]. The temperature stabilities (169, 196, 208, 234) and pH optima (1, 10, 175, 194, 196) of monoamine oxidase preparations have also been shown to vary with the substrate used.

Werle & Röwer (241) briefly reported the separation of monoamine oxidase activity into two distinct entities, one of which oxidized tyramine and the other oxidized aliphatic amines; Gorkin (83) has reported the chromatographic separation of monoamine oxidases deaminating *p*-nitrophenylethylamine from that oxidizing *m*-nitro-*p*-hydroxybenzylamine. More recently electrophoresis has been used to separate different forms of monoamine oxidase. Polyacrylamide disc gel electrophoresis has been used to separate the multiple forms of monoamine oxidase from human liver (46), brain (45), placenta, and cerebellum (250); from chick brain (198); and from rat liver (46, 199), uterus (190), and brain (249); whereas cellulose acetate electrophoresis has been used to separate the different forms of the enzyme from rat liver, brain, and kidney (128). Marked differences between the substrate specificities, temperature stabilities, and pH optima of the electrophoretically separated forms of monoamine oxidase have been reported (45, 46, 199, 249, 250).

The majority of the monoamine oxidase activity migrates toward the anode when the enzyme is subjected to polyacrylamide disc gel electrophoresis at pH 9.1. A species that migrates toward the cathode has, however, been separated from a number of sources, including rat and human brain [see (247a)], rat liver (247a, 250) and uterus (45a), and beef adrenal medulla (224a, 230). This species differs from the other forms of the enzyme in pH optimum and temperature stability (247a, 250) and is less sensitive to a number of monoamine oxidase inhibitors, including the substituted hydrazine derivatives [see (224a, 247a)]. The activity of this species toward dopamine has been shown to be considerably higher than the activities of the other multiple forms of monoamine oxidase although it has a relatively low activity toward tyramine, kynuramine, benzylamine, or tryptamine [see (247a)]. The name "dopamine monoamine oxidase" has been suggested for this species (247a), but this may be a misnomer since no studies have yet been reported on its activity toward other catecholamines.

The partial separation of the activities from rat, beef, and rabbit liver monoamine oxidase preparations toward different substrates by gel filtration on Sephadex G-200 has been reported (182) although the isoenzymes of the rat liver enzyme that had been separated by electrophoresis have been reported not to differ significantly in their molecular weights (248). Three different forms of the beef liver enzyme have been separated by hydroxylapatite chromatography, and two of these have been studied in detail (81). These two enzymes differ in molecular weight and in electrophoretic mobility but have very similar substrate and inhibitor specificities. Gomes et al. (81) suggested that these multiple forms represented species of the enzyme that existed in different polymeric states, although they did not rule out the possibility of attachment of the enzyme to fragments of the mitochondrial membrane. Pig liver monoamine oxidase has been shown to exist in a number of aggregated forms (168b), and a high molecular weight form of the pig brain enzyme has also been detected (219). No antigenic difference could be detected between the different forms of the beef liver enzyme, which implies a close similarity (109, 109a). A specific antibody to the beef liver enzyme was found to react with some 80% of the monoamine oxidase in beef brain (108a, 109a). The remaining 20% of beef brain activity has been shown to differ in substrate specificity and inhibitor sensitivities from the major portion of the monoamine oxidase activity in beef brain and from the enzyme from beef liver (108a, 109a).

Just as there appear to be species and organ differences in the substrate specificities and molecular properties of monoamine oxidase, there appears to be a considerable difference in the occurrence of isoenzymes. Rat and human liver and beef adrenal medulla monoamine oxidase have been separated into five species by electrophoresis (224a, 247a, 250); human brain monoamine oxidase can be resolved into four bands (247a), whereas the enzyme from human placenta can only be separated into two forms [see (250)]. The number of forms of rat liver, brain, and heart, and of chick brain monoamine oxidase appears to increase with the development of the organ (62a, 200a), and as many as seven forms have been separated from adult rats (62a, 200a). In a number of species monoamine oxidase appears to exist in a single form. The enzyme from pig brain mitochondria appears to be homogeneous by a number of enzymatic criteria (223, 226) and by electrophoresis on polyacrylamide gel (223, 224a). The enzyme from platelets was shown to be homogeneous on polyacrylamide disc gel electrophoresis (44), and similar results have been obtained with the enzyme from monkey intestine (157). The inhibitor, N-methyl-N-propargyl-3-(2,4-dichlorophenoxy)propylamine hydrochloride (Clorgyline), which has been shown to be able to selectively inhibit the monoamine oxidase activities of brain and liver of a number of species (123, 105) toward different substrates, was found to be unable to distinguish multiple activities in the livers of cat, dog, pig, ox, or rabbit or from pig brain [(105); see also (208a)].

It has been suggested that the multiple forms of monoamine oxidase might result from a single enzyme that had various amounts of membrane material bound to it (235). The small fraction of monoamine oxidase activity that can be relatively easily extracted from mitochondria appears to differ from the remainder in substrate specificity (126, 238); such an observation would, on this view, result from alteration in the specificity of the enzyme by the membrane material bound to it. Mitochondria subjected to sonic disintegration have been shown to yield particles varying from 50 to 200 A in diameter (235), and these particles may be partially separated by density gradient electrophoresis into fractions differing in substrate specificity (85). The electrophoretic separation of the multiple forms of monoamine oxidase from rat tissues or chick brain was, however, found to be unchanged if sonication rather than detergent treatment was used to solubilize the enzyme (128, 198).

The separated forms of monoamine oxidase from rat liver and beef adrenal medulla have been shown to contain different amounts of phospholipid material (224a, 230). Only a single band of monoamine oxidase could be separated when rat liver monoamine oxidase was subjected to polyacrylamide disc gel electrophoresis in the presence of the detergent Triton X-100 at a concentration of 1.25%, although this treatment caused no inhibition of the enzyme activity (230). The five different isoenzymes from rat liver monoamine oxidase have, however, been shown to be dissociable into subunits of molecular weight 75,000, which appear to be identical in electrophoretic mobility and could be reassociated into the native isoenzymes (248). The purified pig liver monoamine oxidase has been shown to have an extremely high affinity for cardiolipin (168a, 168d), and a comparison between the soluble and membrane-bound forms of that enzyme indicated that the soluble enzyme was considerably more thermolabile (168c).

A number of studies have indicated the possible existence of multiple forms of monoamine oxidase in vivo.

When sympathetically innervated tissues, such as salivary glands (3, 73), vas deferens (120a), and nictitating membrane (121), are denervated, a fall in monoamine oxidase activity occurs; this has been interpreted as resulting from a loss of the enzyme activity that was located in the synaptic nerves (121). The extent of the apparent fall in activity depends on the substrate used to assay monoamine oxidase (3, 73, 119, 121), which suggests that there may be differences in the specificities of neuronal and extraneuronal monoamine oxidases. Mitochondria and synaptosomes separated from rat brain by sucrose density gradient centrifugation have been shown to form an extremely heterogeneous population, and Kroon & Veldstra (136a) have reported the presence of distinct populations of mitochondria with different specificities in this organ. When rats were injected with monoamine oxidase inhibitors 2 hr before monoamine oxidase was prepared from them the activities of the separated isoenzymes were shown to be affected to different extents by the prior treatment with the inhibitors although the differing degrees to which the isoenzymes were inhibited did not correspond to the results obtained when the separated isoenzymes were treated with the same inhibitors in vitro (46a).

With the development of the idea that there may be multiple forms of monoamine oxidase, each having a different substrate specificity, a number of monoamine oxidase inhibitors have been investigated for possible selective action. Inhibitors that have been shown to exert a differential effect toward different substrates include pargyline (74, 208a, 236), harmine and some related compounds (74, 93), tranylcypromine (*trans*-2-phenyl-cyclopropylamine) (74), some α-substituted tryptamine derivatives (95), Clorgyline (105, 123, 208a), 2-bromo-2-phenylacetaldehyde (227), and γ-morpholinebutyrophenone (209). The differential action of a number of monoamine oxidase inhibitors toward separated isoenzymes from a number of sources has been demonstrated (190, 249, 250). Considerable species and organ differences in the sensitivity of monoamine oxidase to harmine (92, 93) have also been reported. In addition the monoamine dehydrogenase of rat brain has been shown to have a considerably different inhibitor specificity from that of monoamine oxidase in the same organ (101).

MONOAMINE OXIDASE AND ADRENAL GLAND

Monoamine oxidase has been detected in both the adrenal cortex and medulla (17, 28, 143, 191). The enzyme is localized largely in the mitochondria in the adrenal medulla (27, 138), rather than in the chromaffin granules (138, 139, 231). In the cortex the enzyme has been shown to be localized in the outer membrane fraction of mitochondria (245). The enzyme has recently been partly purified from adrenal medulla, and its substrate specificity has been studied [Table 2; (230)].

Adrenalectomy has been shown to cause an increased turnover of norepinephrine (39) and a hypersensitivity to histamine and serotonin [see (77) for references]. These effects are accompanied by an elevation of the amount of monoamine oxidase activity in the heart (6, 39) and, to a lesser extent, in other tissues (39). These changes can be reversed by the administration of hydrocortisone (39, 77). The elevated amount of monoamine oxidase activity in the heart, which has been observed by using several substrates, was shown to be accompanied by a somewhat smaller rise in the activity of another enzyme located in the outer mitochondrial membrane, whereas the activities of inner membrane and cytoplasmic markers were found to be unchanged (40).

FUNCTION OF MONOAMINE OXIDASE

The function of monoamine oxidase has been discussed in detail in a number of review articles (7, 21, 23, 57, 84, 118, 118a, 134, 135, 156a, 205, 224b, 257), but the physiological role of the enzyme is not yet fully understood. The three catecholamines, epinephrine, norepinephrine, and dopamine, can be oxidized by monoamine oxidase in vivo to produce the corresponding aldehydes, which are then further metabolized to the corresponding acid or alcohol. Axelrod [see (7, 8) for references] has shown that methylation of epinephrine and norepinephrine to *m-O*-methyladrenaline (metanephrine) and *m-O*-methylnoradrenaline (normetanephrine) can occur; these *O*-methylated compounds can then act as substrates for monoamine oxidase. The possibility of oxidative deamination preceding methylation has been discussed (8, 135). It is worth noting in this connection that, with both pig brain and beef adrenal medulla monoamine oxidases, the K_m values for the methylated derivative have been shown to be considerably lower than the values obtained for epinephrine, which indicates that the enzyme will be more efficient at oxidizing small concentrations of the methylated derivatives.

There has been much discussion as to the relative importance of these two pathways (see reviews above). The major metabolic route for the inactivation of circulating amines appears to be *O*-methylation (7, 8, 135). Monoamine oxidase probably plays an important role in the destruction of potentially toxic amines that are ingested, and the relatively high levels of activity in the liver, stomach, and intestine may be important in this respect. The severe hypertensive reaction that can occur when patients who have been treated with monoamine oxidase inhibitors eat food with a high tyramine content [see (130a)] is in accord with such a function. In contrast, neither monoamine oxidase nor catechol-*O*-methyl-transferase activities appear to be essential for termination of the activities of the catecholamines in vivo since inhibitors of both these enzymes do not greatly potentiate the action of administered epinephrine and norepinephrine (55). It has been suggested that uptake of epinephrine by nerve terminals may be an important mechanism for terminating the action of this hormone [see (156a)].

In neural tissue the function of presynaptically localized monoamine oxidase may be to metabolize transmitter amines after reuptake into the nerve endings or after leakage from intraneuronal storage vesicles. It appears that reuptake by the nerve endings is the principal mechanism by which the action of released transmitter amines is terminated [see (156a)]. However, there is evidence that this uptake process may depend on the presence of monoamine oxidase in the nerve terminals. There appears to be an equilibrium between free and bound amines in the nerve terminals [see (77a)], and this will obviously be affected by the oxidation of the free amines by the action of monoamine oxidase. Administration of the monoamine oxidase inhibitor pargyline has been shown to result in an increase in the concentrations of free amines in the nerve terminals (207a, 230a) and in an impairment of the ability of these terminals to take up amines (230b). Trendelenburg et al. (230b) have proposed that the uptake process is governed by the relative concentrations of free amines inside and outside the neurons and that inhibition of monoamine oxidase results in an impairment of the capacity of the nerve endings to take up amines as the storage vesicles become saturated and the concentration of free intraneuronal amines rises.

The function of postsynaptic (or postjunctional) monoamine oxidase is less clear. An extraneuronal uptake mechanism for norepinephrine has been observed in rat brain (111a), and presumably monoamine oxidase would deaminate norepinephrine that had been taken up in this way.

5-Hydroxyindole acetic acid has been identified as the principal product of serotonin metabolism (232). Evidence from observations of rat brain indicates that amine oxidation represents the principal pathway of inactivation in vivo (165), and a similar conclusion applies to rat pineal gland in vitro (67). O-methylation of serotonin and N-acetyl-5-hydroxytryptamine can also occur in the pineal gland, but this represents a synthetic process for the production of melatonin (N-acetyl-5-methoxytryptamine) (8). 5-Methoxytryptamine is probably a substrate for monoamine oxidase in the pineal gland since both 5-methoxytryptophol and 5-methoxyindoleacetic acid have been detected [see (67) for references]. In nervous tissues histochemical studies have shown that monoamine oxidase inhibitors appear to have a considerably greater effect on the serotonin-containing neurons than on those containing catecholamines (56).

Although histamine appears not to be a substrate for monoamine oxidase in many species, N-methylation can occur to produce biologically inactive N-methylhistamine (1,4-methylhistamine). This compound is a substrate for monoamine oxidase (145, 261). Histamine-N-methylase has a widespread distribution in tissues and is particularly active in the brain (8). This latter finding may be significant since diamine oxidase appears to be absent from the brain and N-methylation followed by the action of monoamine oxidase may represent the major pathway of histamine degradation in this tissue (258).

In addition to its role in the oxidative deamination of the biogenic amines, other functions for monoamine oxidase have been suggested. Bovine thyroid gland monoamine oxidase does not appear to act on epinephrine or norepinephrine, but tyramine is a good substrate, and it has been suggested that thyroidal monoamine oxidase may function as a hydrogen peroxide-generating system for iodothyronine synthesis (69). It has also been suggested that the metabolites produced by monoamine oxidase action may function as regulators of cellular oxidation reactions (89).

Although monoamine oxidase plays a central role in the inactivation of biogenic amines, the view that oxidation completely terminates their action has to be revised in view of the recent findings that the aldehydes derived from the catecholamines and indolealkylamines may have some pharmacological activity in the brain (188). Indirect evidence has also been presented to indicate a role of deaminated amines in the mechanism of sleep (125), and deaminated metabolites of serotonin have been implicated in temperature regulation and sleep induction in mice (12, 66).

REFERENCES

1. ALLES, G. A., AND E. V. HEEGAARD. Substrate specificity of amine oxidase. *J. Biol. Chem.* 147: 487–503, 1943.
2. ALLMANN, D. W., E. BACHMANN, N. ORME-JOHNSON, W. C. TAN, AND D. E. GREEN. Membrane systems of mitochondria. VI. Membranes of liver mitochondria. *Arch. Biochem. Biophys.* 125: 981–1012, 1968.
3. ALMGREN, O., N. W. ANDÉN, J. JONASON, K. A. NORBERG, AND L. OLSON. Cellular localization of monamine oxidase in rat salivary glands. *Acta Physiol. Scand.* 67: 21–26, 1966.
4. APRISON, M. H., R. TAKAHASHI, AND T. L. FOLKERTH. Biochemistry of the avian central nervous system. I. The 5-hydroxytryptophan decarboxylase-monoamine oxidase and cholineacetylase-acetylcholinesterase systems in several discrete areas of the pigeon brain. *J. Neurochem.* 11: 341–350, 1964.
5. ARNAIZ, G. R. DE L., AND E. D. P. DE ROBERTIS. Cholinergic and non-cholinergic nerve endings in the rat. II. Subcellular localization of monoamine oxidase and succinate dehydrogenase. *J. Neurochem.* 9: 503–508, 1962.
6. AVAKIAN, V. M., AND B. A. CALLINGHAM. An effect of adrenalectomy upon catecholamine metabolism. *Brit. J. Pharmacol.* 33: 211P, 1968.
7. AXELROD, J. Metabolism of epinephrine and other sympathomimetic amines. *Physiol. Rev.* 39: 751–776, 1959.
8. AXELROD, J. Methylation reactions in the formation and metabolism of catecholamines and other biogenic amines. *Pharmacol. Rev.* 18: 95–112, 1966.
9. BACHMANN, E., D. W. ALLMANN, AND D. E. GREEN. The membrane systems of the mitochondrion. 1. The S fraction of the outer membrane of beef heart mitochondria. *Arch. Biochem.* 115: 153–164, 1966.
10. BARBATO, L. M., AND L. G. ABOOD. Purification and proper-

ties of monoamine oxidase. *Biochim. Biophys. Acta* 67: 531–541, 1963.
11. BARLOW, R. B., H. BLASCHKO, J. M. HIMMS, AND U. TRENDELENBURG. Observations on ω-amino polymethylene trimethylammonium compounds. *Brit. J. Pharmacol.* 10: 116–123, 1955.
12. BAROFSKY, I., AND A. FELDSTEIN. Serotonin and its metabolites, their respective roles in the production of hypothermia in the mouse. *Experientia* 26: 990–991, 1970.
13. BAUDHUIN, P., H. BEAUFAY, Y. RAHMAN-LI, O. SELLINGER, R. WATTIAUX, P. JACQUES, AND C. DE DUVE. Tissue fractionation studies. 17. Intracellular distribution of monoamine oxidase, aspartate amino transferase, alanine amino transferase, D-amino acid oxidase and catalase in rat liver tissue. *Biochem. J.* 92: 179–184, 1964.
14. BEATTIE, D. S. Enzyme localization in the inner and outer membranes of rat liver mitochondria. *Biochem. Biophys. Res. Commun.* 31: 901–907, 1968.
15. BELLEAU, B., AND J. MORAN. Deuterium isotope effects in relation to the chemical mechanism of monoamine oxidase. *Ann. NY Acad. Sci.* 107: 822–839, 1963.
16. BERNHEIM, M. L. C. Tyramine oxidase. II. The course of the oxidation. *J. Biol. Chem.* 93: 299–309, 1931.
17. BHAGVAT, K., H. BLASCHKO, AND D. RICHTER. Amine oxidase. *Biochem. J.* 33: 1338–1341, 1939.
18. BICKEL, M. H. The pharmacology and biochemistry of N-oxides. *Pharmacol. Rev.* 21: 325–355, 1969.
19. BIEL, L., A. HORITA, AND A. E. DRUKKER. Monoamine oxidase inhibitors (hydrazines). In: *Psychopharmacological Agents*, edited by M. Gordon. New York: Acad. Press, 1964, p. 359–443.
20. BIRKHÄUSER, H. Fermente im gehirn geistig normaler Menschen. (Cholin-esteraser mono-und diamin-oxydase, cholin-oxydase). *Helv. Chim. Acta* 23: 1071–1086, 1940.
21. BLASCHKO, H. Amine oxidase and amine metabolism. *Pharmacol. Rev.* 4: 415–453, 1952.
22. BLASCHKO, H. Enzymic oxidation of amines. *Brit. Med. Bull.* 9: 146–149, 1953.
23. BLASCHKO, H. Amine oxidase. In: *The Enzymes*, edited by P. D. Boyer, H. Lardy, and K. Myrbäck. New York: Acad. Press, 1963, vol. 8, p. 337–351.
24. BLASCHKO, H. Amine oxidases. In: *Molecular Basis of Some Aspects of Mental Activity*, edited by O. Walaas. New York: Acad. Press, 1966, vol. 1, p. 403–413.
25. BLASCHKO, H., AND T. L. CHRUŚCIEL. Observations on the substrate specificity of amine oxidases. *Brit. J. Pharmacol.* 14: 364–367, 1959.
26. BLASCHKO, H., P. J. FRIEDMAN, R. HAWES, AND K. C. NILSSON. The amine oxidases of mammalian plasma. *J. Physiol., London* 145: 384–404, 1959.
27. BLASCHKO, H., J. M. HAGEN, AND P. HAGEN. Mitochondrial enzymes and chromaffin granules. *J. Physiol., London* 139: 316–322, 1957.
28. BLASCHKO, H., P. HAGEN, AND A. D. WELCH. Observations on the intracellular granules of the adrenal medulla. *J. Physiol., London* 129: 27–49, 1955.
29. BLASCHKO, H., AND J. HAWKINS. Enzymic oxidation of aliphatic diamines. *Brit. J. Pharmacol.* 5: 625–632, 1950.
30. BLASCHKO, H., AND K. HELLMANN. Pigment formation from tryptamine and 5-hydroxytryptamine in tissues: a contribution to the histochemistry of amine oxidase. *J. Physiol., London* 122: 403–408, 1953.
31. BLASCHKO, H., S. M. KIRPEKAR, AND S. D. PHIPPS. The enzymic oxidation of ω-amino acids. *Arch. Intern. Pharmacodyn. Therap.* 139: 120–122, 1962.
32. BLASCHKO, H., D. RICHTER, AND H. SCHLOSSMANN. The oxidation of adrenaline and other amines. *Biochem. J.* 31: 2187–2196, 1937.
33. BOADLE, M. C. Observations on a histaminase of invertebrate origin: a contribution to the study of cephalopod amine oxidases. *Comp. Biochem. Physiol.* 30: 611–620, 1969.
34. BOADLE, M. C., AND F. E. BLOOM. A method for the fine structural localization of monoamine oxidase. *J. Histochem. Cytochem.* 17: 331–340, 1969.
35. BOGDANSKI, D. F., H. WEISSBACH, AND S. UDENFRIEND. The distribution of serotonin, 5-hydroxytryptophan decarboxylase, and monoamine oxidase in brain. *J. Neurochem.* 1: 272–278, 1957.
36. BRDICZKA, D., D. PETTE, G. BRUNNER, AND F. MILLER. Kompartimentierte Verteilung von Enzymen in Rattenlebermitochondrien. *European J. Biochem.* 5: 294–304, 1968.
37. BUFFONI, F. Histaminase and related amine oxidases. *Pharmacol. Rev.* 18: 1163–1199, 1966.
38. BURGER, A., AND S. NARA. In vitro inhibition studies with homogeneous monoamine oxidases. *J. Med. Chem.* 8: 859–862, 1965.
39. CAESAR, P. M., G. G. S. COLLINS, AND M. SANDLER. Catecholamine metabolism and monoamine oxidase activity in adrenalectomized rats. *Biochem. Pharmacol.* 19: 921–926, 1970.
40. CALLINGHAM, B. A., AND L. DELLA CORTE. Effect of adrenalectomy upon some rat heart enzymes. *Brit. J. Pharmacol.* 41: 392P, 1971.
41. CENTURY, B., AND K. L. RUPP. Comment on microfluorometric determination of monoamine oxidase. *Biochem. Pharmacol.* 17: 2012–2013, 1968.
42. CLINESCHMIDT, B. V., AND A. HORITA. The monoamine oxidase catalyzed degradation of phenelzine-1-^{14}C, an irreversible inhibitor of monoamine oxidase. I. Studies *in vitro*. *Biochem. Pharmacol.* 18: 1011–1020, 1969.
43. CLINESCHMIDT, B. V., AND A. HORITA. The monoamine oxidase catalyzed degradation of phenelzine-1-^{14}C, an irreversible inhibitor of monoamine oxidase. II. Studies *in vivo*. *Biochem. Pharmacol.* 18: 1021–1028, 1969.
44. COLLINS, G. G. S., AND M. SANDLER. Human blood platelet monoamine oxidase: purification and characterization. *Biochem. Pharmacol.* 20: 289–296, 1971.
45. COLLINS, G. G. S., M. SANDLER, E. D. WILLIAMS, AND M. B. H. YOUDIM. Multiple forms of human brain mitochondrial monoamine oxidase. *Nature* 225: 817–820, 1970.
45a. COLLINS, G. G. S., AND J. SOUTHGATE. The effect of progesterone and oestradiol on rat uterine monoamine oxidase activity. *Biochem. J.* 117: 38P, 1970.
46. COLLINS, G. G. S., M. B. H. YOUDIM, AND M. SANDLER. Isoenzymes of human and rat liver monoamine oxidase. *FEBS Letters* 1: 215–218, 1968.
46a. COLLINS, G. G. S., M. B. H. YOUDIM, AND M. SANDLER. Multiple forms of monoamine oxidase. Comparison of *in vitro* and *in vivo* inhibition patterns. *Biochem. Pharmacol.* 21: 1995–1998, 1972.
47. COQ, M. H., AND C. BARON. Solubilisation de la monoamineoxydase des mitochondries de foie de rat. *Experientia* 20: 374–375, 1964.
48. COQ, H., AND C. BARON. Étude cinétique de l'activité monoamineoxydasique de mitochondries de foie de rat. *Bull. Soc. Chim. Biol.* 50: 163–178, 1968.
49. COTZIAS, G. C., AND V. P. DOLE. Metabolism of amines. II. Mitochondrial localization of monoamine oxidase. *Proc. Soc. Exptl. Biol.* 78: 157–160, 1951.
50. COTZIAS, G. C., AND V. P. DOLE. Metabolism of amines. I. Microdetermination of monoamine oxidase in tissues. *J. Biol. Chem.* 190: 665–672, 1951.
51. COTZIAS, G. C., AND J. J. GREENOUGH. Quantitative estimation of amine oxidase. *Nature* 183: 1732–1733, 1959.
52. COUTEAUX, R., C. BOUCHAUD, AND J. GAUTRON. Données histochimiques sur l'inhibition *in vitro* et *in vivo* des monoamine oxydases. *Actualites Pharmacol.* 18: 33–68, 1965.
53. CRAVEN, P. A., P. J. GOLDBLATT, AND R. E. BASFORD. Brain hexokinases. The preparation of inner and outer mitochondrial membranes. *Biochemistry* 8: 3525–3532, 1969.
54. CREASEY, N. H. Factors which interfere in the manometric assay of monoamine oxidase. *Biochem. J.* 64: 178–183, 1956.
55. CROUT, J. R. Effect of inhibiting both catechol-O-methyltransferase and monoamine oxidase on cardiovascular re-

sponses to norepinephrine. *Proc. Soc. Exptl. Biol. Med.* 108: 482–484, 1961.
56. DAHLSTRÖM, A., AND K. FUXE. Evidence for the existence of monoamine-containing neurones in the central nervous system. I. Demonstration of monoamines in the cell bodies of brain stem neurones. *Acta Physiol. Scand. Suppl.* 232, 1964.
57. DAVISON, A. N. Physiological role of monoamine oxidase. *Physiol. Rev.* 38: 729–747, 1958.
58. DE CHAMPLAIN, J., R. A. MUELLER, AND J. AXELROD. Subcellular localization of monoamine oxidase in rat tissues. *J. Pharmacol. Exptl. Therap.* 166: 339–345, 1969.
59. DEITRICH, R. A., AND V. G. ERWIN. A convenient spectrophotometric assay for monoamine oxidase. *Anal. Biochem.* 30: 395–402, 1969.
59a. DE LA LANDE, I. S., B. D. HILL, L. B. JELLET, AND J. M. MCNEIL. The role of monoamine oxidase in the response of the isolated central artery of the rabbit ear to tyramine. *Brit. J. Pharmacol.* 40: 249–256, 1970.
60. DIXON, M., AND K. KLEPPE. D-Amino acid oxidase. II. Specificity, competitive inhibition and reaction sequence. *Biochim. Biophys. Acta* 96: 368–382, 1965.
61. DIXON, M., AND E. C. WEBB. *Enzymes.* London: Longmans, Green, 1964, p. 337–341.
62. DIXON, M., AND E. C. WEBB. *Enzymes.* London: Longmans, Green, 1964, p. 671–785.
62a. EIDUSON, S. Ontogenetic development of monoamine oxidase. *Advan. Biochem. Psychopharmacol.* 5: 271–287, 1972.
63. ERNSTER, L., AND B. KUYLENSTIERNA. Structure, composition and function of mitochondrial membranes. In: *Mitochondria—Structure and Function,* edited by L. Ernster and Z. Drahota. London: Acad. Press, 1969, p. 5–31.
64. ERNSTER, L., AND B. KUYLENSTIERNA. Outer membrane of mitochondria. In: *Membranes of Mitochondria and Chloroplasts,* edited by E. Racker. New York: Van Nostrand Reinhold, 1970, p. 172–212.
65. ERWIN, V. G., AND L. HELLERMAN. Mitochondrial monoamine oxidase. I. Purification and characterization of the bovine kidney enzyme. *J. Biol. Chem.* 242: 4230–4238, 1967.
66. FELDSTEIN, A., F. H. CHANG, AND J. M. KUCHARSKI. Tryptophol, 5-hydroxytryptophol and 5-methoxytryptophol induced sleep in mice. *Life Sci. Part 1* 9: 323–329, 1970.
67. FELDSTEIN, A., AND O. WILLIAMSON. Serotonin metabolism in pineal homogenates. *Advan. Pharmacol.* 6A: 91–96, 1968.
68. FELLMAN, J. H., E. S. ROTH, AND R. F. MOLLICA. A radiochemical method for monoamine oxidase assay. *Anal. Biochem.* 30: 339–345, 1969.
69. FISCHER, A. G., A. R. SCHULZ, AND L. OLINER. The possible role of thyroid monoamine oxidase in iodothyronine synthesis. *Life Sci.* 5: 995–1002, 1966.
70. FISCHER, A. G., A. R. SCHULZ, AND L. OLINER. Distribution of monoamine oxidase in the thyroid gland. *Endocrinology* 82: 1098–1102, 1968.
71. FISCHER, A. G., A. R. SCHULZ, AND L. OLINER. Thyroidal biosynthesis of iodothyronines. II. General characteristics and purification of mitochondrial monoamine oxidase. *Biochim. Biophys. Acta* 159: 460–471, 1968.
72. FRIEDENWALD, J. S., AND H. HERRMANN. The inactivation of amine oxidase by the enzymatic oxidative products of catechol and adrenaline. *J. Biol. Chem.* 146: 411–419, 1942.
73. FUJIWARA, M., C. TANAKA, H. HIKOSAKA, AND T. OKAGAWA. Cytological localization of noradrenaline, monoamine oxidase and acetylcholinesterase in salivary glands of dog. *J. Histochem. Cytochem.* 14: 483–490, 1966.
74. FULLER, R. W., B. J. WARREN, AND B. B. MOLLOY. Selective inhibition of monoamine oxidase in rat brain mitochondria. *Biochem. Pharmacol.* 19: 2934–2936, 1970.
75. GABAY, S., AND A. J. VALCOURT. Studies on monoamine oxidases. I. Purification and properties of the rabbit liver mitochondrial enzyme. *Biochim. Biophys. Acta* 159: 440–450, 1968.
76. GANROT, P. O., AND E. ROSENGREN. Isolation of a mitochondrial fraction containing monoamine oxidase. *Med. Exptl.* 6: 315–319, 1962.
77. GARATTINI, S., AND L. VALZELLI. *Serotonin.* Amsterdam: Elsevier, 1965, p. 111–114.
77a. GEFFEN, L. B., AND B. G. LIVETT. Synaptic vesicles in synaptic neurones. *Physiol. Rev.* 51: 98–157, 1971.
77b. GHISLA, S., AND P. HEMMERICH. Synthesis of the flavocoenzyme of monoamine oxidase. *FEBS Letters* 16: 229–232, 1971.
78. GIACHETTI, A., AND P. A. SHORE. Optical specificity of monoamine oxidase. *Life Sci.* 5: 1373–1378, 1966.
79. GLENNER, G. C., H. T. BURTNER, AND G. W. BROWN. The histochemical demonstration of monoamine oxidase activity by tetrazolium salts. *J. Histochem. Cytochem.* 5: 591–600, 1957.
80. GLENNER, G. C., H. WEISSBACH, AND B. G. REDFIELD. The histochemical demonstration of enzymatic activity by a nonenzymatic redox reaction. Reduction of tetrazolium salts by indolyl-3-acetaldehyde. *J. Histochem. Cytochem.* 8: 258–261, 1960.
81. GOMES, B., I. IGAUE, H. KLOEPFER, AND K. T. YASUNOBU. Amine oxidase. XIV. Isolation and characterization of the multiple beef liver amine oxidase components. *Arch. Biochem.* 132: 16–27, 1969.
82. GOMES, B., G. NAGUWA, H. G. KLOEPFER, AND K. T. YASUNOBU. Amine oxidase. XV. The sulphydryl groups of beef liver mitochondrial amine oxidase. *Arch. Biochem.* 132: 28–33, 1969.
83. GORKIN, V. Z. Partial separation of rat liver mitochondrial amine oxidases. *Nature* 200: 77, 1963.
84. GORKIN, V. Z. Monoamine oxidases. *Pharmacol. Rev.* 18: 115–120, 1966.
85. GORKIN, V. Z. Separation of rat liver mitochondrial amine oxidases. *Experientia* 25: 1142, 1969.
85a. GORKIN, V. Z. Qualitative alterations in enzymatic properties of amine oxidase. *Advan. Biochem. Psychopharmacol.* 5: 55–65, 1972.
86. GORKIN, V. Z., ZH. I. AKOPYAN, I. V. VERYOVKINA, L. I. GRIDNEVA, AND L. N. STRESINA. Deamination of some biogenic amines and other nitrogenous compounds by liver mitochondria. *Biokhimiya* 35: 140–151, 1970.
87. GORKIN, V. Z., ZH. I. AKOPYAN, I. V. VERYOVKINA, L. N. STRESINA, AND M. M. A. SAMED. Effects of monoamine oxidase inhibitors on qualitative alterations ('transformation') of the catalytic properties of amine oxidases. *Biochem. J.* 121: 31–33P, 1971.
88. GORKIN, V. Z., N. A. KITROSSKII, L. B. KLYASHTORIN, N. V. KOMISSAROVA, G. A. LEONT'EVA, AND V. A. PUCHKOV. Substrate specificity of amine oxidases. *Biokhimiya* 29: 88–96, 1964.
89. GORKIN, V. Z., AND W. N. OREKHOVITCH. Monoamine oxidases: new data on their nature, possible biological role and specific inhibition by pharmaceutical preparations. *Biochim. Appl.* 14: 343–358, 1967.
90. GORKIN, V. Z., AND L. A. ROMANOVA. Some properties of the mitochondrial monoamine oxidase of the rat liver and brain. *Biokhimiya* 24: 826–832, 1959.
91. GORKIN, V. Z., AND L. V. TATYANENKO. "Transformation" of monoamine oxidase into a diamine oxidase-like enzyme *in vitro. Biochem. Biophys. Res. Commun.* 27: 613–617, 1967.
92. GORKIN, V. Z., AND L. V. TATYANENKO. On the inhibition by harmine of oxidative deamination of biogenic amines. *Life Sci.* 6: 791–795, 1967.
93. GORKIN, V. Z., L. V. TATYANENKO, D. M. KRASNOKUTSKAYA, E. V. PRONINA, AND L. N. YAKHONTOV. Selective inhibition of the enzymatic deamination of serotonin by harmine and related tricyclic compounds. *Biokhimiya* 32: 510–519, 1967.
94. GORKIN, V. Z., L. V. TATYANENKO, AND T. A. MOSKVITINA. On the conversion *in vitro* of monoamine oxidase into an enzyme resembling diamine oxidase. *Biokhimiya* 33: 393–402, 1968.
95. GORKIN, V. Z., L. V. TATYANENKO, N. N. SUVOROV, AND A. D. NEKLYUDOV. Selective inhibition of the enzymatic

deamination of serotonin by α-substituted tryptamine derivatives. *Biokhimiya* 32: 1036–1046, 1967.

96. GOVIER, W. M., M. E. GRELLIS, N. S. YANZ, AND K. H. BEYER. Studies on the mechanism of action of sympathomimetic amines. III. The oxidation of tyramine by rat liver homogenates. *J. Pharmacol. Exptl. Therap.* 87: 149–158, 1946.

97. GREEN, A. L., AND T. M. HAUGHTON. A colorimetric method for the estimation of monoamine oxidase. *Biochem. J.* 78: 172–175, 1961.

98. GREEN, D. E., D. W. ALLMANN, R. A. HARRIS, AND W. C. TAN. Enzyme localization in the inner and outer mitochondrial membranes. *Biochem. Biophys. Res. Commun.* 31: 368–378, 1968.

99. GREEN, D. E., E. BACHMANN, D. W. ALLMANN, AND J. F. PERDUE. The membrane systems of the mitochondrion. III. The isolation and properties of the outer membrane of beef heart mitochondria. *Arch. Biochem. Biophys.* 115: 172–180, 1966.

99a. GREENAWALT, J. W. Localization of monoamine oxidase in rat liver. *Advan. Biochem. Psychopharmacol.* 5: 207–226, 1972.

100. GREENAWALT, J. W., AND C. SCHNAITMAN. An appraisal of the use of monoamine oxidase as an enzyme marker for the outer membrane of rat liver mitochondria. *J. Cell Biol.* 46: 173–179, 1970.

101. GUHA, S. R., AND S. K. GHOSH. Inhibition of monoamine oxidation in brain by monoamine oxidase inhibitors. *Biochem. Pharmacol.* 19: 2929–2932, 1970.

102. GUHA, S. R., AND C. R. KRISHNA MURTI. Purification and solubilization of monoamine oxidase of rat liver mitochondria. *Biochem. Biophys. Res. Commun.* 18: 350–354, 1965.

102a. GUILBAULT, G. G. *Enzymatic Methods of Analysis.* Oxford: Pergamon Press, 1970, p. 77–92.

103. GUILBAULT, G. G. *Enzymatic Methods of Analysis.* Oxford: Pergamon Press, 1970, p. 128–129.

104. HAGEN, P., AND N. WEINER. Enzymic oxidation of pharmacologically active amines. *Federation Proc.* 18: 1005–1012, 1959.

105. HALL, D. W. R., B. W. LOGAN, AND G. H. PARSONS. Further studies on the inhibition of monoamine oxidase by M & B 9302 (Clorgyline). I. Substrate specificity in various mammalian species. *Biochem. Pharmacol.* 18: 1447–1454, 1969.

106. HARADA, M., AND T. NAGATSU. Identification of the flavin in the purified beef brain mitochondrial monoamine oxidase. *Experientia* 25: 583–584, 1969.

107. HARDEGG, W., AND E. HEILBRON. Oxydation von Serotonin und Tyramin durch Rattenlebermitochondrien. *Biochim. Biophys. Acta* 51: 553–560, 1961.

108. HARE, M. L. C. Tyramine oxidase. 1. A new enzyme system in liver. *Biochem. J.* 22: 968–979, 1928.

108a. HARTMAN, B. K. The discovery and isolation of a new monoamine oxidase from brain. *Biol. Psychiat.* 4: 147–155, 1972.

109. HARTMAN, B. K., H. KLOEPFER, AND K. YASUNOBU. Demonstration of antigenic identity of several forms of monoamine oxidase prepared from bovine liver mitochondria. *Federation Proc.* 28: 857, 1969.

109a. HARTMAN, B. K., AND S. UDENFRIEND. The use of immunological techniques for the characterization of bovine monoamine oxidase from liver and brain. *Advan. Biochem. Psychopharmacol.* 4: 119–128, 1972.

110. HAWKINS, J. The localization of amine oxidase in the liver cell. *Biochem. J.* 50: 577–581, 1952.

110a. HELLERMAN, L., H. Y. K. CHUANG, AND D. C. DE LUCA. Approaches to the catalytic mechanism of mitochondrial monoamine oxidase. *Advan. Biochem. Psychopharmacol.* 5: 327–337, 1972.

111. HELLERMAN, L., AND V. G. ERWIN. Mitochondrial monoamine oxidase. II. Action of various inhibitors for the bovine kidney enzyme. Catalytic mechanism. *J. Biol. Chem.* 243: 5234–5243, 1968.

111a. HENDLEY, E. D., K. M. TAYLOR, AND S. H. SNYDER. ³H-normetanephrine uptake in rat brain slices. Relationship to extraneuronal accumulation of norepinephrine. *European J. Pharmacol.* 12: 167–179, 1970.

112. HIDAKA, H., T. NAGATSU, AND K. YAGI. Micro-determination of monoamine oxidase using serotonin as substrate. *J. Biochem.* 62: 621–623, 1967.

113. HOLLUNGER, G., AND L. ORELAND. Solubilization and purification of pig liver mitochondrial monoamine oxidase. *Acta Pharmacol. Toxicol.* 25, Suppl. 4: 11, 1967.

114. HOLLUNGER, G., AND L. ORELAND. Preparation of soluble monoamine oxidase from pig liver mitochondria. *Arch. Biochem.* 139: 320–328, 1970.

114a. HORITA, A., AND M. C. LOWE. On the extraneuronal nature of cardiac monoamine oxidase in the rat. *Advan. Biochem. Psychopharmacol.* 5: 227–242, 1972.

115. HUSZTI, Z., AND J. BORSY. The effect of dimethyltryptamine and its derivatives on monoamine oxidase. *Biochem. Pharmacol.* 13: 1151–1156, 1964.

116. HUSZIT, Z., AND J. BORSY. Differences between amine oxidases deaminating mescaline and the structurally related 3,4-dimethoxyphenylethyl amine. *Biochem. Pharmacol.* 15: 475–480, 1966.

117. IGAUE, I., B. GOMES, AND K. T. YASUNOBU. Beef mitochondrial monoamine oxidase, a flavin dinucleotide enzyme. *Biochem. Biophys. Res. Commun.* 29: 562–570, 1967.

118. IVERSEN, L. L. *The Uptake and Storage of Noradrenaline in Sympathetic Nerves.* London: Cambridge Univ. Press, 1967, p. 62–74.

118a. IVERSEN, L. L. *The Uptake and Storage of Noradrenaline in Sympathetic Nerves.* London: Cambridge Univ. Press, 1967, p. 227–233.

119. JARROTT, B. Occurrence and properties of monoamine oxidase in adrenergic neurones. *J. Neurochem.* 18: 7–16, 1971.

120. JARROTT, B., AND L. L. IVERSEN. Subcellular distribution of monoamine oxidase activity in rat liver and vas deferens. *Biochem. Pharmacol.* 17: 1619–1625, 1968.

120a. JARROTT, B., AND L. L. IVERSEN. Noradrenaline metabolizing enzymes in normal and sympathetically denervated vas deferens. *J. Neurochem.* 18: 1–6, 1971.

121. JARROTT, B., AND S. Z. LANGER. Changes in monoamine oxidase and catechol-O-methyl transferase activities after denervation of the nictitating membrane of the cat. *J. Physiol., London* 212: 549–559, 1971.

122. JENKS, W. P. *Catalysis in Chemistry and Enzymology.* New York: McGraw-Hill, 1969, p. 182–191.

122a. JENKS, W. P. *Catalysis in Chemistry and Enzymology.* New York: McGraw-Hill, 1969, p. 490–497.

123. JOHNSTON, J. P. Some observations upon a new inhibitor of monoamine oxidase in brain tissue. *Biochem. Pharmacol.* 17: 1285–1297, 1968.

123a. JONASON, J. Metabolism of catecholamines in the central and peripheral nervous system. *Acta Physiol. Scand. Suppl.* 320: 1–50, 1969.

124. JONES, M. S., AND O. T. G. JONES. Evidence for the location of ferrochelatase on the inner membrane of rat liver mitochondria. *Biochem. Biophys. Res. Commun.* 31: 977–982, 1968.

125. JOUVET, M. Biogenic amines and the states of sleep. *Science* 163: 32–41, 1969.

126. KALIMAN, P. A. The role of mitochondrial monoamine oxidase of some rabbit organs in the oxidation of catecholamines and tyramine. *Biokhimiya* 30: 1194–1203, 1965.

127. KAPELLER-ADLER, R., AND B. IGGO. Histamine and its derivatives in human urine. *Biochim. Biophys. Acta* 25: 394–402, 1957.

127a. KEARNEY, E. B., J. I. SALACH, W. H. WALKER, R. L. SENG, W. KENNEY, E. ZESZOTEK, AND T. P. SINGER. The covalently-bound flavin peptide of hepatic monoamine oxidase. 1. Isolation and sequence of a flavin peptide and evidence for binding at the 8α position. *European J. Biochem.* 24: 321–327, 1971.

128. KIM, H. C., AND A. D'IORIO. Possible isoenzymes of monoamine oxidase in rat tissues. *Can. J. Biochem. Physiol.* 46: 295–297, 1968.

128a. KLINGMAN, G. I. Monoamine oxidase activity of peripheral

organs and sympathetic ganglia of the rat after immunosympathectomy. *Biochem. Pharmacol.* 15: 1729–1736, 1966.
129. KLYASHTORIN, L. B., AND L. I. GRIDNEVA. Sulphydryl groups of mitochondrial monoamine oxidase. *Biokhimiya* 31: 831–839, 1966.
130. KLYASHTORIN, L. B., L. I. GRIDNEVA, AND V. Z. GORKIN. Chromatographic purification and some properties of the monoamine oxidase of liver mitochondria. *Biokhimiya* 31: 167–173, 1966.
130a. KNOLL, J., AND K. MAGYAR. Some puzzling pharmacological effects of monoamine oxidase inhibitors. *Advan. Biochem. Psychopharmacol.* 5: 393–408, 1972.
131. KOBAYASHI, Y. A histamine metabolizing enzyme system of mouse liver. *Arch. Biochem.* 71: 352–357, 1957.
132. KOBAYASHI, Y. Histamine catabolism by cat liver homogenates. *Arch. Biochem.* 77: 275–285, 1958.
133. KOHN, H. I. Tyramine oxidase. *Biochem. J.* 31: 1693–1704, 1937.
134. KOPIN, I. J. Storage and metabolism of catecholamines: the role of monoamine oxidase. *Pharmacol. Rev.* 16: 179–191, 1964.
135. KOPIN, I. J. Biosynthesis and metabolism of catecholamines. *Anesthesiology* 29: 654–660, 1968.
136. KRAML, M. A rapid microfluorimetric determination of monoamine oxidase. *Biochem. Pharmacol.* 14: 1683–1685, 1965.
136a. KROON, M. C., AND H. VELDSTRA. Multiple forms of rat brain mitochondrial monoamine oxidase. Subcellular localization. *FEBS Letters* 24: 173–176, 1972.
137. KUMAGI, H., H. MATSUI, K. OGATA, AND H. YAMADA. Properties of crystalline tyramine oxidase from *Sarcina lutea*. *Biochim. Biophys. Acta* 171: 1–8, 1969.
138. LADURON, P., AND F. BELPAIRE. Tissue fractionation and catecholamines. II. Intracellular distribution patterns of tyrosine hydroxylase, dopa decarboxylase, dopamine-β-hydroxylase, phenylethanolamine N-methyltransferase and monoamine oxidase in adrenal medulla. *Biochem. Pharmacol.* 17: 1127–1140, 1968.
139. LAGERCRANTZ, H., B. KUYLENSTIERNA, AND L. STJÄRNE. On the origin of adenosine triphosphatase in chromaffin granules. *Experientia* 26: 479–480, 1970.
140. LAGNADO, J. R., A. OKAMOTO, AND M. B. H. YOUDIM. The effect of tetrazolium salts on monoamine oxidase activity. *FEBS Letters* 17: 117–120, 1971.
141. LAGNADO, J. R., AND T. L. SOURKES. Enzymatic reduction of tetrazolium salts by amines. *Can. J. Biochem. Physiol.* 34: 1095–1106, 1956.
142. LAGNADO, J. R., AND T. L. SOURKES. Inhibition of amine oxidase by metal ions and by sulphydryl compounds. *Can. J. Biochem. Physiol.* 35: 1185–1194, 1956.
143. LANGEMANN, H. Enzymes and their substrates in the adrenal gland of the ox. *Brit. J. Pharmacol.* 6: 318–325, 1951.
144. LEEPER, L. C., H. WEISSBACH, AND S. UDENFRIEND. Studies on the metabolism of norepinephrine, epinephrine and their O-methyl derivatives by partially purified enzyme preparations. *Arch. Biochem. Biophys.* 77: 417–427, 1958.
145. LINDELL, S. E., AND H. WESTLING. Enzymic oxidation of some substances related to histamine. *Acta Physiol. Scand.* 39: 370–384, 1957.
146. LOVENBERG, W., R. J. LEVINE, AND A. SJOERDSMA. A sensitive assay of monoamine oxidase activity *in vitro*: application to heart and sympathetic ganglia. *J. Pharmacol. Exptl. Therap.* 135: 7–10, 1962.
147. MAHLER, H. R. Uricase. In: *The Enzymes* edited by P. D. Boyer, H. Lardy, and K. Myrback. New York: Acad. Press, 1963, vol. 8, p. 285–296.
148. MARCHBANKS, R. M. Serotonin binding to nerve ending particles and other preparations from rat brain. *J. Neurochem.* 13: 1481–1493, 1966.
148a. MARSDEN, C. A., O. J. BROCK, AND H. C. GULDBERG. Catechol-O-methyl transferase and monoamine oxidase activities in rat submaxillary gland: effects of ligation, sympathectomy and some drugs. *European J. Pharmacol.* 15: 335–342, 1971.
149. MASON, W. O., AND C. L. OLSON. Differential amperometric measurement of monoamine oxidase activity at tubular carbon electrodes. *Anal. Chem.* 42: 488–492, 1966.
150. McCAMAN, R. E., M. W. McCAMAN, J. M. HUNT, AND M. S. SMITH. Microdetermination of monoamine oxidase and 5-hydroxytryptophan decarboxylase activities in nervous tissues. *J. Neurochem.* 12: 15–23, 1965.
151. McEWEN, C. M. Human plasma monoamine oxidase. I. Purification and identification. *J. Biol. Chem.* 240: 2003–2010, 1965.
152. McEWEN, C. M. Human plasma monoamine oxidase. II. Kinetic studies. *J. Biol. Chem.* 240: 2011–2018, 1965.
153. McEWEN, C. M., K. T. CULLEN, AND A. J. SOBER. Rabbit serum monoamine oxidase. *J. Biol. Chem.* 241: 4544–4556, 1966.
154. McEWEN, C. M., G. SASAKI, AND D. C. JONES. Human liver mitochondrial monoamine oxidase. II. Determination of substrate and inhibitor specificities. *Biochemistry* 8: 3953–3962, 1970.
155. McEWEN, C. M., G. SASAKI, AND W. R. LENZ. Human liver mitochondrial monoamine oxidase. I. Kinetic studies and model interactions. *J. Biol. Chem.* 243: 5217–5225, 1968.
156. MEISTER, A., AND D. WELLNER. Flavoprotein amino acid oxidases. In: *The Enzyme*, edited by P. D. Boyer, H. Lardy, and K. Myrbäck. New York: Acad. Press, 1963, vol. 7, p. 609–648.
156a. MOLINOFF, P. B., AND J. AXELROD. Biochemistry of catecholamines. *Ann. Rev. Biochem.* 40: 465–500, 1971.
157. MURALI, D. K., AND A. N. RADHAKRISHNAN. Preparation and properties of an electrophoretically homogeneous monoamine oxidase from monkey intestine. *Biochim. Biophys. Acta* 206: 61–70, 1970.
158. MURAOKA, S., A. HOSHIKA, H. YAMASAKI, H. YAMADA, AND A. OSAO. Reduction of cytochrome c by amine oxidase from *Aspergillus niger*. *Biochim. Biophys. Acta* 122: 544–546, 1966.
159. NAGATSU, T. Partial separation and properties of mitochondrial monoamine oxidase in brain. *J. Biochem.* 59: 606–612, 1966.
159a. NAGATSU, T., G. NAKANO, M. KIMIKO, AND M. HARADA. Purification and properties of amine oxidases in brain and connective tissue (dental pulp). *Advan. Biochem. Psychopharmacol.* 5: 25–36, 1972.
160. NAGATSU, T., AND K. YAGI. A simple assay of monoamine oxidase and D-amino acid oxidase by measuring ammonia. *J. Biochem.* 60: 219–221, 1966.
161. NAGATSU, T., T. YAMAMOTO, AND M. HARADA. Purification and properties of human brain mitochondrial monoamine oxidase. *Enzymologia* 39: 15–25, 1969.
162. NARA, S., B. GOMES, AND K. T. YASUNOBU. Amine oxidase. VII. Beef liver mitochondrial monoamine oxidase, a copper containing protein. *J. Biol. Chem.* 241: 2774–2780, 1966.
163. NARA, S., I. IGAUE, B. GOMES, AND K. T. YASUNOBU. The prosthetic groups of animal amine oxidases. *Biochem. Biophys. Res. Commun.* 23: 324–328, 1966.
164. NARA, S., AND K. T. YASUNOBU. Some recent advances in the field of amine oxidases. In: *The Biochemistry of Copper*, edited by J. Peisach, P. Aisen, and W. E. Blumberg. New York: Acad. Press, 1966, p. 423–436.
165. NEFF, N. H., AND T. N. TOZER. *In vivo* measurement of brain serotonin turnover. *Advan. Pharmacol.* 64: 97–109, 1968.
166. NOVICK, W. J. Effect of oxygen tension on monoamine oxidase activity. *Biochem. Pharmacol.* 15: 1009–1012, 1966.
167. OI, S., K. SHIMADA, M. INAMASU, AND K. T. YASUNOBU. Mechanistic studies of beef liver mitochondrial amine oxidase. XVIII. Amine oxidase. *Arch. Biochem.* 139: 28–37, 1970.
167a. OI, S., K. T. YASUNOBU, AND J. WESTLEY. The effect of pH on the kinetic parameters and mechanism of beef liver monoamine oxidase. *Arch. Biochem. Biophys.* 145: 557–564, 1971.
168. OKAMOTO, H., S. YAMAMOTO, M. NOZAKI, AND O. HAYAISHI.

On the submitochondrial localization of L-kynurenine-3-hydroxylase. *Biochem. Biophys. Res. Commun.* 26: 309–314, 1967.

168a. OLIVECRONA, T., AND L. ORELAND. Reassociation of soluble monoamine oxidase with lipid-depleted mitochondria in the presence of phospholipids. *Biochemistry* 10: 332–340, 1971.

168b. ORELAND, L. Purification and properties of pig liver mitochondrial monoamine oxidase. *Arch. Biochem. Biophys.* 146: 410–421, 1971.

168c. ORELAND, L., AND B. EKSTEDT. Soluble and membrane-bound pig liver mitochondrial monoamine oxidase: thermostability, tryptic digestibility and kinetic properties. *Biochem. Pharmacol.* 21: 2479–2488, 1972.

168d. ORELAND, L., AND T. OLIVECRONA. The role of acidic phospholipids in the binding of monoamine oxidase to the mitochondrial structure. *Arch. Biochem. Biophys.* 146: 710–714, 1971.

169. OSWALD, E. O., AND C. F. STRITTMATTER. Comparative studies in the characterization of monoamine oxidase. *Proc. Soc. Exptl. Biol. Med.* 114: 668–673, 1963.

170. OTSUKI, S., AND Y. KOBAYASHI. A radioisotopic assay for monoamine oxidase determination in human plasma. *Biochem. Pharmacol.* 13: 995–1006, 1964.

171. PARKES, J. G., AND W. THOMPSON. The composition of phospholipids in outer and inner mitochondrial membranes from guinea-pig liver. *Biochim. Biophys. Acta* 196: 162–169, 1970.

172. PARSONS, D. F., G. R. WILLIAMS, AND B. CHANCE. Characteristics of isolated and purified preparations of the outer and inner membranes of mitochondria. *Ann. NY Acad. Sci.* 137: 643–666, 1966.

173. PARSONS, D. F., G. R. WILLIAMS, W. THOMPSON, D. WILSON, AND B. CHANCE. Improvements in the procedure for purification of mitochondrial outer and inner membrane. Comparison of the outer membrane with smooth endoplasmic reticulum. In: *Round Table Discussion on Mitochondrial Structure and Compartmentation*, edited by E. Quagliariello, S. Papa, E. C. Slater, and J. M. Tayer. Bari: Adriatica Editrice, 1967, p. 29–70.

174. PFEFFER, M., M. SEMMEL, AND J. M. SCHOR. Rat brain monoamine oxidase inhibition by β-diethylaminoethyl diphenylpropylacetate (SKF-525A). *Enzymologia* 34: 299–303, 1968.

175. PHILPOT, F. J. Some observations on the oxidation of tyramine in the liver. *Biochem. J.* 31: 856–861, 1937.

176. PHILPOT, F. J., AND G. CANTONI. Adrenaline destruction and methylene blue. *J. Pharmacol. Exptl. Therap.* 71: 95–103, 1941.

177. PLETSCHER, A. Monoamine oxidase inhibitors. *Pharmacol. Rev.* 18: 121–129, 1966.

178. PRATESI, P., AND H. BLASCHKO. Specificity of amine oxidase for optically active substrates and inhibitors. *Brit. J. Pharmacol.* 14: 256–260, 1959.

179. PUGH, C. E. M., AND J. H. QUASTEL. Oxidation of aliphatic amines by brain and other tissues. *Biochem. J.* 31: 286–291, 1937.

180. PUGH, C. E. M., AND J. H. QUASTEL. Oxidation of amines by animal tissues. *Biochem. J.* 31: 2306–2321, 1937.

181. RACKER, E., AND H. PROCTOR. Reconstitution of the outer mitochondrial membrane with monoamine oxidase. *Biochem. Biophys. Res. Commun.* 39: 1120–1125, 1970.

182. RAGLAND, J. B. Multiplicity of mitochondrial monoamine oxidases. *Biochem. Biophys. Res. Commun.* 31: 203–208, 1968.

183. RAGLAND, J. B., AND R. J. MITCHELL. Sub-mitochondrial localization of monoamine oxidase. *Federation Proc.* 26: 842, 1967.

184. RANDALL, L. O. Oxidation of phenethylamine derivatives by amine oxidase. *J. Pharmacol. Exptl. Therap.* 83: 216–220, 1946.

185. RICHTER, D. Adrenaline and amine oxidase. *Biochem. J.* 31: 2022–2028, 1937.

186. ROBINSON, D. S., W. LOVENBERG, H. KEISER, AND A. SJOERDSMA. Effect of drugs on human blood platelet and plasma amine oxidase activity in vitro and in vivo. *Biochem. Pharmacol.* 17: 109–119, 1968.

187. ROTH, R. H., AND L. STJÄRNE. Monoamine oxidase activity in the bovine splenic nerve granule preparation. *Acta Physiol. Scand.* 68: 342–346, 1966.

188. SABELLI, H. C., W. J. GIARDINA, S. G. A. ALIVISATOS, P. K. SETH, AND F. UNGAR. Indoleacetaldehydes: serotonin-like effects on the central nervous system. *Nature* 223: 73–74, 1969.

189. SAKAMOTO, Y., Y. OGAWA, AND K. HYASHI. Studies on monoamine oxidase. *J. Biochem.* 54: 292–294, 1963.

190. SANDLER, M., G. G. S. COLLINS, AND M. B. H. YOUDIM. Inhibition patterns of monoamine oxidase isoenzymes: clinical implications. In: *Mechanisms of Toxicity*, edited by W. N. Aldridge. London: MacMillan, 1971, p. 3–11.

191. SCHAPIRA, G. Répartition de l'amine-oxydase et métabolisme de l'adrénaline. *Compt. Rend. Soc. Biol.* 139: 36–37, 1945.

192. SCHNAITMAN, L., V. G. ERWIN, AND J. W. GREENAWALT. The submitochondrial localization of monoamine oxidase. *J. Cell Biol.* 32: 719–735, 1967.

193. SCHNAITMAN, L., AND J. W. GREENAWALT. Enzymatic properties of the inner and outer membranes of rat liver mitochondria. *J. Cell Biol.* 38: 158–175, 1968.

194. SEVERINA, I. S., AND V. Z. GORKIN. On the nature of mitochondrial monoamine oxidases. *Biokhimiya* 28: 896–902, 1963.

195. SEVERINA, I. S., AND V. Z. GORKIN. Selective inhibition by various hydroxyquinolines of the activity of monoamine oxidases of rat liver mitochondria. *Biokhimiya* 29: 1093–1102, 1964.

196. SEVERINA, I. S., AND T. N. SHEREMET'EVSKAYA. Concerning substrate specificity of mitochondrial monoamine oxidase from rat liver and binding of enzyme and substrate into enzyme-substrate complex. *Biokhimiya* 32: 843–853, 1967.

197. SEVERINA, I. S., AND T. N. SHEREMET'EVSKAYA. Relation between substrate structure and mitochondrial monoamine oxidase activity. *Biokhimiya* 34: 125–135, 1969.

198. SHIH, J-H. C., AND S. EIDUSON. Multiple forms of monoamine oxidase in the developing brain. *Nature* 224: 1309–1310, 1969.

199. SIERENS, L., AND A. D'IORIO. Multiple monoamine oxidases in rat liver mitochondria. *Can. J. Biochem. Physiol.* 48: 659–663, 1970.

199a. SILBERSTEIN, S. D., H. M. SHEIN, AND K. R. BERV. Catechol-O-methyl transferase and monoamine oxidase activity in cultured rodent astrocytoma cells. *Brain Res.* 41: 245–248, 1972.

200. SINGER, T. P., AND E. S. G. BARRON. Studies on biological oxidations. XX. Sulfhydryl enzymes in fat and protein metabolism. *J. Biol. Chem.* 157: 241–253, 1945.

200a. SHIH, J-H., AND S. EIDUSON. Multiple forms of monoamine oxidase in developing brain: tissue and substrate specificities. *J. Neurochem.* 18: 1221–1227, 1971.

201. SMITH, T. E., H. WEISSBACH, AND S. UDENFRIEND. Studies on the mechanism of action of monoamine oxidase: metabolism of N,N-dimethyltryptamine and N,N-dimethyltryptamine-N-oxide. *Biochemistry* 1: 137–143, 1962.

202. SNYDER, S. H., AND E. D. HENDLEY. A simple and sensitive fluorescence assay for monoamine oxidase and diamine oxidase. *J. Pharmacol. Exptl. Therap.* 163: 386–392, 1968.

203. SOEP, H. The determination of monoamine oxidase activity. *Pure Appl. Chem.* 3: 481–489, 1961.

204. SOTTOCASA, G. L., B. KUYLENSTIERNA, L. ERNSTER, AND A. BERGSTRAND. Separation and some enzymatic properties of the inner and outer membranes of rat liver mitochondria. In: *Methods in Enzymology*, edited by S. P. Colowick and N. O. Kaplan. New York: Acad. Press, 1967, vol. 10, p. 448–463.

205. SOURKES, T. L. Oxidative pathways in the metabolism of biogenic amines. *Rev. Can. Biol.* 17: 328–366, 1958.

206. SOURKES, T. L. Properties of the monoamine oxidase of rat liver mitochondria. *Advan. Pharmacol.* 6A: 61–69, 1968.

207. SOUTHGATE, J., AND G. G. S. COLLINS. The estimation of monoamine oxidase using ^{14}C-labelled substrates. *Biochem. Pharmacol.* 18: 2285–2287, 1969.

207a. SPECTOR, S., R. GORDON, A. SJOERDSMA, AND S. UDENFRIEND. End-product inhibition of tyrosine hydroxylase as a possible

mechanism for regulation of norepinephrine synthesis. *Mol. Pharmacol.* 3: 549–555, 1963.
208. SQUIRES, R. F. Additional evidence for the existence of several forms of mitochondrial monoamine oxidase in the mouse. *Biochem. Pharmacol.* 17: 1401–1409, 1968.
208a. SQUIRES, R. F. Multiple forms of monoamine oxidase in intact mitochondria as characterized by selective inhibitors and thermal stability: a comparison of eight mammalian species. *Advan. Biochem. Psychopharmacol.* 5: 355–370, 1972.
209. SQUIRES, R. F., AND J. B. LASSEN. Some pharmacological and biochemical properties of γ-morpholino-butyrophenone (NSD 2023), a new monoamine oxidase inhibitor. *Biochem. Pharmacol.* 17: 369–384, 1968.
210. STJÄRNE, L. Studies of noradrenaline biosynthesis in nerve tissue. *Acta Physiol. Scand.* 67: 411–454, 1966.
211. STJÄRNE, L., R. H. ROTH, AND N. J. GIARMAN. Microsomal monoamine oxidase in sympathetically innervated tissues. *Biochem. Pharmacol.* 17: 2008–2012, 1968.
212. SYMES, A. L., T. L. SOURKES, M. B. H. YOUDIM, G. GREGORIADIS, AND H. BIRNBAUM. Decreased monoamine oxidase activity in liver of iron deficient rats. *Can. J. Biochem. Physiol.* 47: 999–1002, 1969.
213. TABOR, H. Diamine oxidase. *J. Biol. Chem.* 188: 125–136, 1951.
214. TABOR, C. W., AND P. D. KELLOGG. Identification of flavin adenine dinucleotide and heme in a homogeneous spermidine dehydrogenase from *Serratia marcescens*. *J. Biol. Chem.* 245: 5429–5433, 1970.
215. TABOR, C. W., H. TABOR, AND S. M. ROSENTHAL. Purification of amine oxidase from beef plasma. *J. Biol. Chem.* 208: 645–661, 1954.
216. TAKAHASHI, H., AND S. TAKAHARA. A sensitive fluorometric assay for monoamine oxidase based on the formation of 4,6-quinolinediol from 5-hydroxykynuramine. *J. Biochem.* 64: 7–11, 1968.
217. TAPLEY, D. F., AND C. COOPER. Effect of thyroxine on the swelling of mitochondria isolated from various tissues of the rat. *Nature* 178: 1119, 1956.
218. TIPTON, K. F. The sub-mitochondrial localization of monoamine oxidase in rat liver and brain. *Biochim. Biophys. Acta* 135: 910–920, 1967.
219. TIPTON, K. F. The purification of pig brain mitochondrial monoamine oxidase. *European J. Biochem.* 4: 103–107, 1968.
220. TIPTON, K. F. The prosthetic groups of pig brain mitochondrial monoamine oxidase. *Biochim. Biophys. Acta* 159: 451–459, 1968.
221. TIPTON, K. F. The reaction pathway of pig brain mitochondrial monoamine oxidase. *European J. Biochem.* 5: 316–320, 1968.
222. TIPTON, K. F. A sensitive fluorometric assay for monoamine oxidase. *Anal. Biochem.* 28: 318–325, 1969.
223. TIPTON, K. F. Monoamine oxidases and their inhibitors. In: *Mechanisms of Toxicity*, edited by W. N. Aldridge. London: MacMillan, 1971, p. 13–27.
224. TIPTON, K. F. (Pig brain mitochondrial) monoamine oxidase. In: *Methods in Enzymology*, edited by S. P. Colowick and N. O. Kaplan. New York: Acad. Press, 1971, vol. 17B, p. 717–722.
224a. TIPTON, K. F. Some properties of monoamine oxidase. *Advan. Biochem. Psychopharmacol.* 5: 11–24, 1972.
224b. TIPTON, K. F. Biochemical aspects of monoamine oxidase. *Brit. Med. Bull.* 29: 116–119, 1973.
225. TIPTON, K. F., AND A. P. DAWSON. The distribution of monoamine oxidase and α-glycerophosphate dehydrogenase in pig brain. *Biochem. J.* 108: 95–99, 1968.
226. TIPTON, K. F., AND I. P. C. SPIRES. The homogeneity of pig brain mitochondrial monoamine oxidase. *Biochem. Pharmacol.* 17: 2137–2144, 1968.
227. TIPTON, K. F., AND I. P. C. SPIRES. The inhibition of rat liver mitochondrial monoamine oxidase by 2-bromo-2-phenylacetaldehyde. *Biochem. Pharmacol.* 18: 2559–2561, 1969.
228. TIPTON, K. F., AND I. P. C. SPIRES. Oxidation of 2-phenylethylhydrazine by monoamine oxidase. *Biochem. Pharmacol.* 21: 268–270, 1972.
229. TIPTON, K. F., AND I. P. C. SPIRES. The kinetics of 2-phenylethylhydrazine oxidation by monoamine oxidase. *Biochem. J.* 125: 521–524, 1971.
230. TIPTON, K. F., M. B. H. YOUDIM, AND I. P. C. SPIRES. Beef adrenal medulla monoamine oxidase. *Biochem. Pharmacol.* 21: 2197–2204, 1972.
230a. TOZER, T. N., N. H. NEFF, AND B. B. BRODIE. Application of steady-state kinetics to the synthesis rate and turnover time of serotonin in the brain of normal and reserpine-treated rats. *J. Pharmacol. Exptl. Therap.* 153: 177–182, 1962.
230b. TRENDELENBURG, U., P. R. DRASKÓCZY, AND K. H. GRAEFE. The influence of intraneuronal monoamine oxidase on neuronal net uptake of noradrenaline and on sensitivity to noradrenaline. *Advan. Biochem. Psychopharmacol.* 5: 371–377, 1972.
231. TRIFARÓ, J. M., AND J. DWORKIND. A new simple method for isolation of adrenal chromaffin granules by means of an isotonic density gradient. *Anal. Biochem.* 34: 403–412, 1970.
232. UDENFRIEND, S. Metabolism of 5-hydroxytryptamine. In: *5-Hydroxytryptamine*, edited by G. P. Lewis. London: Pergamon Press, 1958, p. 43–49.
233. UDENFRIEND, S., H. WEISSBACH, AND B. B. BRODIE. Assay of serotonin and related metabolites, enzymes, and drugs. *Methods Biochem. Anal.* 6: 95–130, 1958.
234. VAN WOERT, M. H., AND G. C. COTZIAS. Anion inhibition of monoamine oxidase. *Biochem. Pharmacol.* 15: 275–285, 1966.
235. VERYOVKINA, I. V., V. Z. GORKIN, V. M. MITYUSHIN, AND I. E. ELPINER. On the effect of ultrasonic waves on monoamine oxidase connected with the submicroscopical structures of mitochondria. *Biophysics* 9: 503–506, 1964.
236. VINA, I., V. Z. GORKIN, L. I. GRIDNEVA, AND L. B. KLYASHTORIN. On the mechanism of the inhibition of the activity of mitochondrial monoamine oxidase by pargyline. *Biokhimiya* 31: 282–290, 1965.
236a. WALKER, W. H., E. B. KEARNEY, R. SENG, AND T. P. SINGER. The covalently-bound flavin of hepatic monoamine oxidase. 2. Identification and properties of cysteinyl riboflavine. *European J. Biochem.* 24: 328–331, 1971.
237. WEINER, N. The distribution of monoamine oxidase and succinic oxidase in brain. *J. Neurochem.* 6: 79–86, 1960.
238. WEISSBACH, H., B. G. REDFIELD, AND S. UDENFRIEND. Soluble monoamine oxidase; its properties and actions on serotonin. *J. Biol. Chem.* 229: 953–963, 1957.
239. WEISSBACH, H., T. E. SMITH, J. W. DALY, B. WITKOP, AND S. UDENFRIEND. A rapid spectrophotometric assay of monoamine oxidase based on the rate of disappearance of kynuramine. *J. Biol. Chem.* 235: 1160–1163, 1960.
240. WERLE, E. Aminoxydasen. In: *Hoppe Seyler Thierfelder Handbuch der physiologisch- und pathologisch-chemischen Analyse*. Berlin: Springer, 1964, vol. A, p. 653–704.
241. WERLE, E., AND F. RÖWER. Uber tierische und pflanzliche Monoaminoxydasen. *Biochem. Zeit.* 322: 320–326, 1952.
242. WHIPPLE, H. G. (editor). New reflections on monoamine oxidase inhibition. *Ann. NY Acad. Sci.* 107: 809–1158, 1963.
243. WHITELOCK, O. V. ST. Amine oxidase inhibitors. *Ann. NY Acad. Sci.* 80: 551–1045, 1959.
244. WURTMAN, R. J., AND J. AXELROD. A sensitive and specific assay for the estimation of monoamine oxidase. *Biochem. Pharmacol.* 12: 1439–1440, 1963.
245. YAGO, N., AND S. ICHII. Submitochondrial distribution of components of the steroid 11-beta hydroxylase and cholesterol side chain-cleaving enzyme systems in hog adrenal cortex. *J. Biochem.* 65: 215–224, 1969.
246. YAMADA, H., T. UWAJIMA, H. KUMAGI, M. WATANBE, AND K. OGATA. Crystalline tyramine oxidase from *Sarcina lutea*. *Biochem. Biophys. Res. Commun.* 27: 350–355, 1967.
247. YASUNOBU, K. T., I. IGAUE, AND B. GOMES. The purification and properties of beef liver mitochondrial monoamine oxidase. *Advan. Pharmacol.* 6A: 43–59, 1968.
247a. YOUDIM, M. B. H. Multiple forms of monoamine oxidase

and their properties. *Advan. Biochem. Psychopharmacol.* 5: 67–77, 1972.
248. YOUDIM, M. B. H., AND G. G. S. COLLINS. The dissociation and reassociation of rat liver mitochondrial monoamine oxidase. *European J. Biochem.* 18: 73–78, 1971.
249. YOUDIM, M. B. H., G. G. S. COLLINS, AND M. SANDLER. Multiple forms of rat brain monoamine oxidase. *Nature* 223: 626–628, 1969.
250. YOUDIM, M. B. H., G. G. S. COLLINS, AND M. SANDLER. Isoenzymes of soluble mitochondrial monoamine oxidase. In: *Enzymes and Isoenzymes. Structure, Properties and Function*, edited by D. Shugar. New York: Acad. Press, 1970, p. 281–289.
251. YOUDIM, M. B. H., AND J. LAGNADO. The effects of tetrazolium salts on monoamine oxidase activity. *Advan. Biochem. Psychopharmacol.* 5: 289–292, 1972.
252. YOUDIM, M. B. H., AND T. L. SOURKES. Properties of purified, soluble monoamine oxidase. *Can. J. Biochem. Physiol.* 44: 1397–1400, 1966.
253. YOUDIM, M. B. H., AND T. L. SOURKES. Rat liver mitochondrial monoamine oxidase a flavin-containing enzyme. *Biochem. J.* 121: 20P, 1970.
253a. YOUDIM, M. B. H., AND T. L. SOURKES. The flavin prosthetic group of purified rat liver mitochondrial monoamine oxidase. *Advan. Biochem. Psychopharmacol.* 5: 45–53, 1972.
254. ZELLER, E. A. Uber den enzymatischen Abbau von Histamin und Diaminen. *Helv. Chim. Acta* 21: 880–890, 1938.
255. ZELLER, E. A. Diamin-oxydase. *Advan. Enzymol.* 2: 93–112, 1942.
256. ZELLER, E. A. Oxidation of amines. In: *The Enzymes. Chemistry and Mechanism of Action*, edited by J. B. Sumner and K. Myrbäck. New York: Acad. Press, 1951, vol. 2, part 1, p. 536–558.
257. ZELLER, E. A. The role of amine oxidases in the destruction of catecholamines. *Physiol. Rev.* 11: 387–393, 1959.
258. ZELLER, E. A. Diamine oxidases. In: *The Enzymes*, edited by P. D. Boyer, H. Lardy, and K. Myrbäck. New York: Acad. Press, 1963, vol. 8, p. 313–335.
259. ZELLER, E. A. A new approach to the analysis of the interaction between monoamine oxidase and its substrates and inhibitors. *Ann. NY Acad. Sci.* 107: 811–820, 1963.
260. ZELLER, E. A., J. BARSKY, E. R. BERMAN, M. S. CHERKAS, AND J. R. FOUTS. Degradation of mescaline by amine oxidases. *J. Pharmacol. Exptl. Therap.* 124: 282–289, 1958.
261. ZELLER, E. A., J. BARSKY, L. A. BLANKSMA, AND J. C. LAZANAS. Reactive site of amine oxidases. *Federation Proc.* 16: 276, 1957.
262. ZELLER, V., G. RAMACHANDER, AND E. A. ZELLER. Amine oxidases. XXI. A rapid method for the determination of the activity of monoamine oxidase and monoamine oxidase inhibitors. *J. Med. Chem.* 8: 440–450, 1965.
263. ZELLER, E. A., AND S. SARKER. Amine oxidases. XIX. Inhibition of monoamine oxidase by phenylcyclopropylamines and iproniazid. *J. Biol. Chem.* 237: 2333–2336, 1962.
264. ZELLER, E. A., P. STERN, AND L. A. BLANKSMA. Degradation of histamine by monoamine oxidase. *Naturwissenschaften* 43: 157, 1956.
265. ZELLER, E. A., R. STERN, AND M. WENK. Über die diamindiaminoxydase Reaktion. *Helv. Chim. Acta* 23: 3–17, 1940.
266. ZIRKLE, C. L., AND C. KAISER. Monoamine oxidase inhibitors (non-hydrazines). In: *Psychopharmacological Agents*, edited by M. Gordon. New York: Acad. Press, 1964, p. 445–554.
267. ZUBRZYCKI, V. Z., AND H. STAUNDINGER. Kinetik, intrazelluläre Lokalisation und Induziebarkeit der Monoaminoxydase. *Z. Physiol. Chem.* 348: 639–644, 1967.

CHAPTER 42

The metabolism of circulating catecholamines

D. F. SHARMAN | *Agricultural Research Council, Institute of Animal Physiology, Babraham, Cambridge, England*

CHAPTER CONTENTS

Metabolic Transformations
Disappearance of Catecholamines from Blood
Sites of Removal of Catecholamines from Blood
Quantitative Aspects of Metabolism of Circulating Catecholamines
    Metabolism of epinephrine
    Metabolism of norepinephrine
    Metabolism of dopamine
Disposition of Catecholamines in Blood
Conclusion

THIS CHAPTER is concerned with the metabolism of those catecholamines that have been demonstrated to be present in mammalian blood. These are epinephrine [l-α-(3,4-dihydroxyphenyl)-β-methylaminoethanol], norepinephrine [l-α-(3,4-dihydroxyphenyl)-β-aminoethanol], and dopamine [β-(3,4-dihydroxyphenylethylamine)].

The disposal of the physiologically active principle of the adrenal medulla was discussed by Oliver & Schäfer (109) in 1895. They obtained evidence that neither the kidneys nor the adrenal glands were major sites for the removal of the active substance from the body and also showed that canine arterial blood had little or no tendency to destroy the active principle in vitro. The experiments of Langlois (93) and of Battelli (24) led to the conclusion that the liver was important in the removal of the active substance from the circulation. Langlois (93) also showed that the active principle disappeared from the blood of a dog as the pressor effect of an injection of adrenal extract declined. By 1901 epinephrine had been isolated from the adrenal gland (1, 3, 135). Four years later Elliott (55) described his investigations with this substance and showed that, following an intravenous injection into the cat, no pressor activity was present in the blood after a few minutes. He further found that the lungs did not remove epinephrine from the blood but that, when blood containing epinephrine was passed through the liver, the intestine, or the tissues of the leg, the epinephrine disappeared. It was concluded that epinephrine disappears in the tissues which it excites. Two conditions were known to prolong the response of a tissue to epinephrine: cooling (93) and decentralization or denervation of the tissue (55). Elliott concluded that the data were not sufficient for a clear statement of the manner in which epinephrine was removed from the blood but discussed physical disappearance by diffusion and possible biochemical conversion in the tissues, processes that might be affected by temperature. He also suggested that the disappearance of epinephrine was concerned in its physiological function and that epinephrine might be involved with the transference of a sympathetic nerve impulse and might be stored for such a purpose in the region of the myoneural junction. In 1949 Bacq (22) reviewed what was known of the metabolism of epinephrine. By this time it was thought that both epinephrine and norepinephrine might be present in the blood (58). Holtz et al. (78) had suggested, on the basis of biological tests, that "urosympathin" in the urine was a mixture of epinephrine, norepinephrine, and dopamine. The components of urosympathin were excreted mostly as acid-hydrolyzable, pharmacologically inactive forms. Richter (119) had demonstrated that epinephrine could be excreted in the urine as a sulfate conjugate, and Blaschko et al. (31) had described the presence of an enzyme in the liver that would oxidize epinephrine. This enzyme was shown to be identical with other monoamine oxidases (32) that had been found in the liver. The possibility that 3,4-dihydroxymandelic acid might be a metabolite of epinephrine was considered but was somewhat obscured by the observation that a substance reacting like 3,4-dihydroxybenzoic acid could be detected in the urine of rabbits given large doses of epinephrine (142). In man no 3,4-dihydroxybenzoic acid could be detected in the urine after the ingestion of epinephrine (119). Much thought was given to the possibility that adrenochrome or a related substance was a major metabolite of epinephrine, but the presence of such oxidation products of epinephrine in the tissues could not be established.

The key to the metabolism of catecholamines was provided by the separate studies of Armstrong and of De Eds and their co-workers. Armstrong et al. (9) made a detailed investigation into the phenolic acids of human urine. They found that organic acids containing a 4-hydroxy-3-methoxyphenyl group occurred normally in human urine.

The methylation of a phenolic hydroxyl group in animal tissues was not observed until 1951 (102). Booth et al. (33) later found that, after the administration of the catechol derivatives rutin and quercetin to rabbits, 4-hydroxy-3-methoxyphenylacetic acid (homovanillic acid, HVA; vanylacetic acid, VAA) was excreted in the urine. A similar result was obtained when other catechol derivatives, including 3,4-dihydroxyphenylacetic acid (homoprotocatechuic acid; DOPAC) and 3,4-dihydroxyphenylalanine (DOPA), the amino acid precursor of the catecholamines, were given orally to rabbits (51, 52). These workers did not detect the presence of HVA or DOPAC in normal rabbit urine. However, in man Shaw et al. (130) demonstrated the presence of HVA in normal urine and estimated its concentration. They also observed an increased urinary excretion of HVA after oral administration of DOPAC or L-DOPA.

The methylation of a phenolic hydroxyl group was shown to be important in the metabolism of epinephrine and norepinephrine by Armstrong et al. (8). After the parenteral administration of norepinephrine or the ingestion of 3,4-dihydroxymandelic acid (DOMA), the urinary excretion of 4-hydroxy-3-methoxymandelic acid (vanillylmandelic acid, VMA; vanylglycollic acid, VGA) increased. The concentration of this acid was higher in the urine of patients with pheochromocytoma than in the urine of normal humans. The presence of the methoxylated amine metabolites of norepinephrine, epinephrine, and dopamine, intermediates in the formation of HVA and VMA, together with the distribution of the enzyme responsible for the transformation, catechol-O-methyltransferase (COMT), in both tissue and urine was demonstrated by Axelrod and his co-workers (11, 14, 16, 18, 20). It is of interest to recall that in 1905 Abel & Taveau (2) obtained vanillin (4-hydroxy-3-methoxybenzaldehyde) when they oxidized samples of epinephrine obtained by extracting adrenal glands. The presence of both metanephrine [1-(4-hydroxy-3-methoxyphenyl)-2-methylaminoethanol] and normetanephrine [1-(4-hydroxy-3-methoxyphenyl)-2-aminoethanol] in the adrenal gland (18) affords an explanation for this finding.

The detailed quantitative analysis of the metabolism of the catecholamines awaited the preparation of radioactively labeled compounds. Schayer (124, 125) in 1951 prepared two labeled forms of epinephrine, one of which had ^{14}C at the N-methyl group and the other ^{14}C at the β carbon atom. These two substances were used to study the metabolism of epinephrine; at least five metabolites were found in the urine, and some of the carbon of the N-methyl group was excreted as carbon dioxide in the expired air. The ready availability of catecholamines specifically labeled with ^{14}C and ^{3}H and with high specific activities has enabled a clearer picture of the metabolism of circulating catecholamines to be drawn.

METABOLIC TRANSFORMATIONS

The main changes in the structures of the catecholamine molecules that can occur during their metabolism by animal tissues are illustrated in Figure 1, which was derived from experiments in several different species. A detailed discussion of the enzymes involved is beyond the scope of this chapter, but some of them are covered in detail elsewhere in this volume of the *Handbook*.

That dopamine can be metabolized to norepinephrine and epinephrine was proposed by Blaschko (28) in 1939 and demonstrated by Goodall & Kirshner (70) in 1957. The enzyme dopamine β-hydroxylase [3,4-dihydroxyphenylethylamine ascorbate:oxygen oxidoreductase, hydroxylating (EC 1.14.2.1)] (95, 96) converts dopamine to norepinephrine, which can then be metabolized to epinephrine by the enzyme phenylethanolamine N-methyltransferase [noradrenalin-N-methyltransferase (EC 2.1.1.28)]. Some epinephrine might be methylated to N-methylepinephrine (12).

The two enzymes monoamine oxidase [MAO; monoamine:oxygen oxidoreductase, deaminating (EC 1.4.3.4)] and catechol-O-methyltransferase [COMT; S-adenosylmethionine: catechol-O-methyltransferase (EC 2.1.1.6)] are responsible for most of the chemical inactivation of the catecholamines. Oxidative deamination by MAO gives rise to an aldehyde. Metabolites of the catecholamines that possess this aldehyde group are rarely detected in tissues or urine but may be observed in in vitro experiments (94). The action of MAO is immediately followed by further metabolism either by the enzyme aldehyde dehydrogenase (EC 1.2.1.3), which gives rise to an acid metabolite, or by the not yet clearly defined enzyme aldehyde reductase, which results in the formation of an alcohol and in the case of the phenylethanolamine derivatives is a 1,2-glycol. The introduction of a methyl group at the 3 position of the benzene ring by COMT is an important step in the chemical inactivation of the catecholamine molecule. The methoxy derivatives of the catecholamines—4-hydroxy-3-methoxyphenylethylamine (methoxytyramine) from dopamine, 1-(4-hydroxy-3-methoxyphenyl)-2-aminoethanol [normetanephrine, normetadrenaline (NMN)] from norepinephrine, and 1-(4-hydroxy-3-methoxyphenyl)-2-methylaminoethanol [metanephrine, metadrenaline (MN)] from epinephrine—are also substrates for MAO. The enzyme COMT can also methylate the acids that have a catechol group in their structure.

Phenols are detoxicated in animals mainly by two reactions: conjugation of the hydroxyl group with glucuronic acid or with sulfuric acid. Catecholamines and many of their metabolites are phenolic, and both glucuronides and ethereal sulfates of these substances are formed. The pattern of conjugation appears to differ between species.

Most of the evidence for the pathways of metabolism of circulating catecholamines is derived from the presence of the different metabolites in the urine and the demonstration of an increased excretion after the infusion of the parent amine. Some metabolites have been demonstrated only after the injection of radioactively labeled catecholamines.

In addition to free dopamine, norepinephrine, and

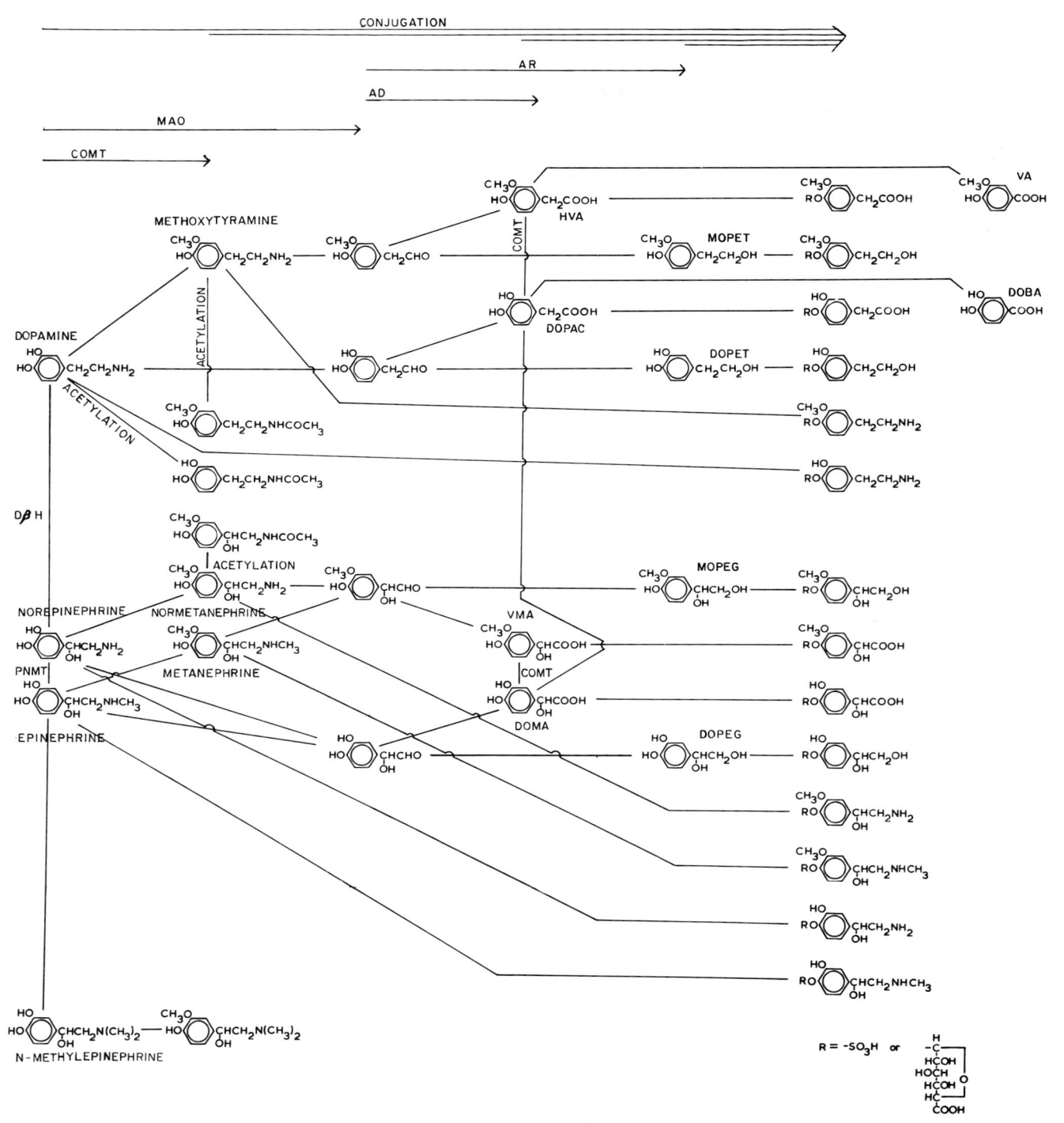

FIG. 1. Metabolic transformations of circulating catecholamines. Enzymes concerned in transformations are indicated by *arrows* at top of diagram. Some transformations that do not correspond with arrows are indicated on diagram where they occur. Enzymes: *COMT*, catechol-*O*-methyltransferase; *MAO*, monoamine oxidase; *AD*, aldehyde dehydrogenase; *AR*, aldehyde reductase; *DβH*, dopamine β-hydroxylase; *PNMT*, phenylethanolamine *N*-methyltransferase. Compounds: *MOPEG*, 1-(4-hydroxy-3-methoxyphenyl)ethane-1,2-diol; *DOPEG*, 1-(3,4-dihydroxyphenyl)-ethane-1,2-diol; *MOPET*, 1-(4-hydroxy-3-methoxyphenyl)ethan-2-ol; *DOPET*, 1-(3,4-dihydroxyphenyl)ethan-2-ol; *VMA*, 4-hydroxy-3-methoxymandelic acid; *DOMA*, 3,4-dihydroxymandelic acid; *HVA*, 4-hydroxy-3-methoxyphenylacetic acid (homovanillic acid); *DOPAC*, 3,4-dihydroxyphenylacetic acid; *VA*, 4-hydroxy-3-methoxy benzoic acid (vanillic acid); *DOBA*, 3,4-dihydroxybenzoic acid.

epinephrine, conjugates of these amines also appear in the urine. Conjugation of epinephrine to form the ethereal sulfate in man (119) and the glucuronide in rabbit (43) has been reported. In the rat, Schayer (125) has shown that a large excretion of an epinephrine conjugate only occurred when the catecholamine was administered orally. This suggests that conjugation can take place to a great extent in the intestine. However, conjugates of catecholamines are normally excreted in human urine.

The presence of normetanephrine and of metanephrine in rat urine was demonstrated by Axelrod et al. (18) who also found, after the intraperitoneal injection of dopamine, norepinephrine, or epinephrine into rats, an increase in the urinary excretion of the methoxylated amine metabolites, mainly in the form of glucuronic acid conjugates. In man normetanephrine and metanephrine, derived from an intravenous infusion of norepinephrine or epinephrine, respectively, are excreted mainly as ethereal sulfates (68, 90). The glycol metabolite of epinephrine and norepinephrine, 1-(4-hydroxy-3-methoxyphenyl)-1,2-ethanediol (MOPEG, MHPG), is present in human urine as the sulfate conjugate (17), and the alcohol metabolite of dopamine, 2-(4-hydroxy-3-methoxyphenyl)ethanol (MHPE, MOPET, MOPOL), has also been detected (61). When either of the enzymes COMT or aldehyde dehydrogenase is inhibited, increased amounts of 2-(3,4-dihydroxyphenyl)ethanol (DHPE, DOPET, DOPOL) and 1-(3,4-dihydroxyphenyl)-1,2-ethanediol (DHPG, DOPEG) are formed (61, 87). The acid metabolites of dopamine, homovanillic acid and 3,4-dihydroxyphenylacetic acid, and of epinephrine and norepinephrine, 4-hydroxy-3-methoxymandelic acid and 3,4-dihydroxymandelic acid (DOMA), are also present in the urine (9, 56, 57, 130). Radioactive homovanillic acid and 3,4-dihydroxyphenylacetic acid are found in the urine after the intraperitoneal (145) or intravenous (66) administration of radioactively labeled dopamine, and radioactive 3,4-dihydroxymandelic acid and 4-hydroxy-3-methoxymandelic acid are excreted after radioactive norepinephrine or epinephrine is injected (63, 85). The acid metabolites are present in the urine also as conjugates. In man they appear to be conjugated mainly with sulfuric acid at the 4 position on the benzene ring (66).

The catecholamines may undergo other metabolic conversions. These appear to be of minor importance in the normal metabolism of circulating catecholamines, but their possible involvement in abnormal states should not be overlooked. The metabolic changes described above are all theoretically reversible reactions. The use of radioactively labeled compounds with high specific activities has shown that the reverse reactions can also take place. These include O- and N-demethylation and dehydroxylation of the ring and of the β carbon atom in the side chain of the molecule (19, 116, 127). For example, radioactive homovanillic acid and 3,4-dihydroxyphenylacetic acid occur in the urine after the administration of radioactively labeled epinephrine (65), and both m- and p-hydroxyphenylacetic acids are formed in vivo from 3,4-dihydroxyphenylacetic acid (127).

4-Hydroxy-3-methoxybenzoic acid [vanillic acid (VA)] and 3,4-dihydroxybenzoic acid [protocatechuic acid (DOBA)] are metabolites of epinephrine and norepinephrine (54, 114, 120), of 3,4-dihydroxyphenylacetic acid (5), and thus presumably of dopamine, and they are also metabolites of 3,4-dihydroxymandelic acid (67). 4-Hydroxy-3-methoxybenzaldehyde (vanillin) can be formed from norepinephrine and epinephrine by the liver (136), and 4-hydroxy-3-methoxyphenylglyoxylic acid is a possible minor metabolite (137). The nitrogen of the amino group can be acetylated (62, 131). The normal process in the adrenal gland is the formation of epinephrine from norepinephrine by the enzyme phenylethanolamine N-methyltransferase. Further methylation of the amino nitrogen to form N-methylepinephrine can occur in this tissue (12), and the metabolite 1-(4-hydroxy-3-methoxyphenyl)-2-dimethylaminoethanol (N-methylmetanephrine) is present in human urine (81).

Another possible metabolite of dopamine is the very labile 2,3,5-trihydroxyphenylethylamine (6-hydroxydopamine) (129). The implications of the possible formation of this substance, which destroys noradrenergic sympathetic nerve terminals, are too wide to be discussed here. The methylation of the catechol moiety in the catecholamines at positions other than the 3 position has been shown to take place (128), and the possibility that substances like mescaline (3,4,5-trimethoxyphenylethylamine) could be formed can be mentioned only in passing. The catecholamines can also be oxidized by an enzyme found in most tissues of certain species (13). This enzyme oxidizes epinephrine to adrenochrome and is found to be particularly active in the cat.

DISAPPEARANCE OF CATECHOLAMINES FROM BLOOD

Catecholamines are rapidly removed from the circulating blood. In 1895 Oliver & Schäfer (109) reported that the pressor effect of a single injection of an adrenal gland extract lasted for, at most, 4 min in the dog and 6 min in the rabbit, whereas, if the extract was allowed to flow continuously into a vein, the blood pressure was maintained for as long as the flow continued. In the absence of positive evidence to show the site where the active substance disappeared from the blood, it was suggested that it was taken up into the muscular system. Cybulski (48, 134a) in 1895 showed that vasopressor activity was to be found in the urine of dogs that had received an injection of an extract of adrenal glands, but could detect no, or very little, activity in the urine of normal dogs.

By 1898 Langlois (93) had shown that adrenal venous blood that contained the active principle retained its pressor activity in vitro for 30 or 40 min when kept at 38 C. He was further able to demonstrate the rapid disappearance of the active substance from the circulation.

Blood was taken from a dog that had been given an injection of adrenal gland extract and was tested for its pressor activity on another dog. The pressor activity in the blood of the first dog declined as the blood pressure, which increased in response to the adrenal extract, returned to its initial value. None of the active substance could be detected in the blood 1 min after the blood pressure returned to baseline level. These observations were confirmed by Elliott (55) in the cat and Jackson (82) in the dog with epinephrine rather than the glandular extract.

The rapid disappearance of epinephrine from the blood was observed many times by workers who used bioassay and chemical methods of analysis [for review, see (113)]. With the development of more sensitive fluorimetric methods for the estimation of catecholamines, the rapid disappearance of epinephrine and norepinephrine from the circulation was among the first of the results to be reported (98, 113). Cohen et al. (45) concluded that the removal of both epinephrine and norepinephrine was associated with first-order kinetics since the steady-state concentration of the amine in the plasma during an intravenous infusion in man showed a linear relation to the rate of infusion. They also observed that epinephrine appeared to be removed from the circulation at a faster rate than norepinephrine.

Cahen (39) investigated the disappearance of epinephrine from the blood after an injection, and the results suggested that the fall in concentration followed a hyperbolic curve. However, studies with radioactively labeled catecholamines showed that the disappearance of epinephrine and norepinephrine from the blood appeared to follow a time course that might be represented by two curves—an initial fast phase that is followed by a slow exponential removal of radioactive catecholamine from the blood. The earlier experiments, because of their limited sensitivity, were only able to trace the first, faster phase. The two phases of removal of epinephrine and norepinephrine from the blood of the cat are illustrated in Figure 2. The rapid phase reflects the passage of the amines into the tissues where it can be stored or metabolized. The uptake of catecholamines into tissues is discussed elsewhere in this volume (see the chapter by Iversen in this volume of the *Handbook*). Figure 2 also demonstrates the differences in the relative amounts of epinephrine and norepinephrine that are stored or metabolized. After the injection of a dose of 25 µg/kg of ^{3}H-norepinephrine or a dose of 70 µg/kg of ^{3}H-epinephrine, the plasma concentrations of the two amines are similar, which indicates a more rapid removal of epinephrine. This is further illustrated by the half-lives for the two catecholamines during the slow exponential phase of removal from the blood of humans. The half-life of epinephrine is 75.3 min (91) and of norepinephrine 240 min (60). The much higher concentration of metanephrine, formed from epinephrine by the action of COMT, compared with that of normetanephrine, the congener from norepinephrine (see Fig. 2), demonstrates that metabolism plays a greater part in the removal of

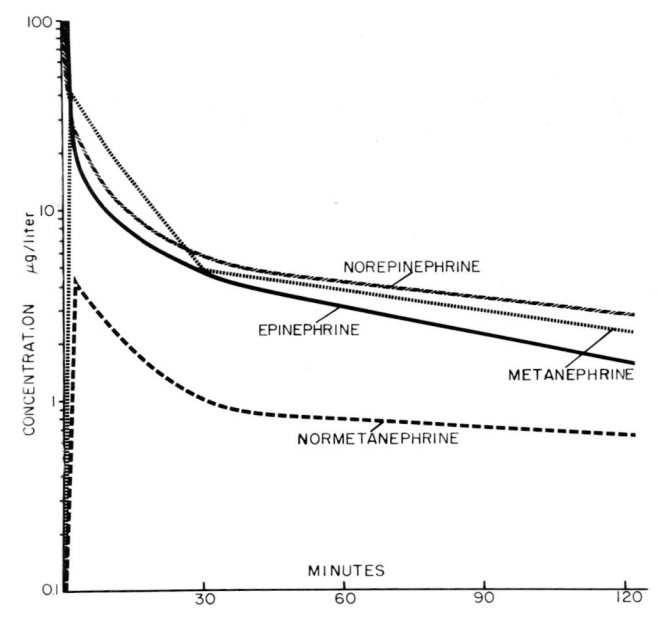

FIG. 2. Concentrations of epinephrine and metanephrine and of norepinephrine and normetanephrine in blood plasma of cat. Rapid intravenous administration of ^{3}H-epinephrine (70 µg/kg) preceded measurement of epinephrine and metanephrine; rapid intravenous administration of ^{3}H-norepinephrine (25 µg/kg) preceded measurement of norepinephrine and normetanephrine. [Adapted from Axelrod et al. (21) and Whitby et al. (144).]

epinephrine from the circulation than it does in the removal of norepinephrine, whereas tissue binding of unchanged amine is more important for the removal of norepinephrine from the blood than it is for epinephrine (144).

The slow phase of removal of catecholamines from the circulation reflects the release into the bloodstream of the catecholamines that had been taken up by the tissues. It should be noted that the portion of the circulating catecholamines removed in any given tissue in the intact animal might be different, when the concentration of catecholamine is high enough to produce an alteration in blood flow through the tissue, from the portion removed when the concentration of catecholamines is low. When injected intravenously into sheep, dopamine rapidly disappears from the blood (84).

SITES OF REMOVAL OF CATECHOLAMINES FROM BLOOD

Early experiments showed that the liver was capable of removing epinephrine from the blood. An infusion of adrenal gland extract or epinephrine through the hepatic portal vein produces a vasopressor response smaller than that produced by a similar infusion into the jugular vein (92, 105), and the exclusion of the hepatic circulation prolongs the vasopressor response to an adrenal gland extract (10). Elliott (55) demonstrated that epinephrine disappeared from blood passing through the intestine but that it did not disappear in the lungs. Sundberg (134)

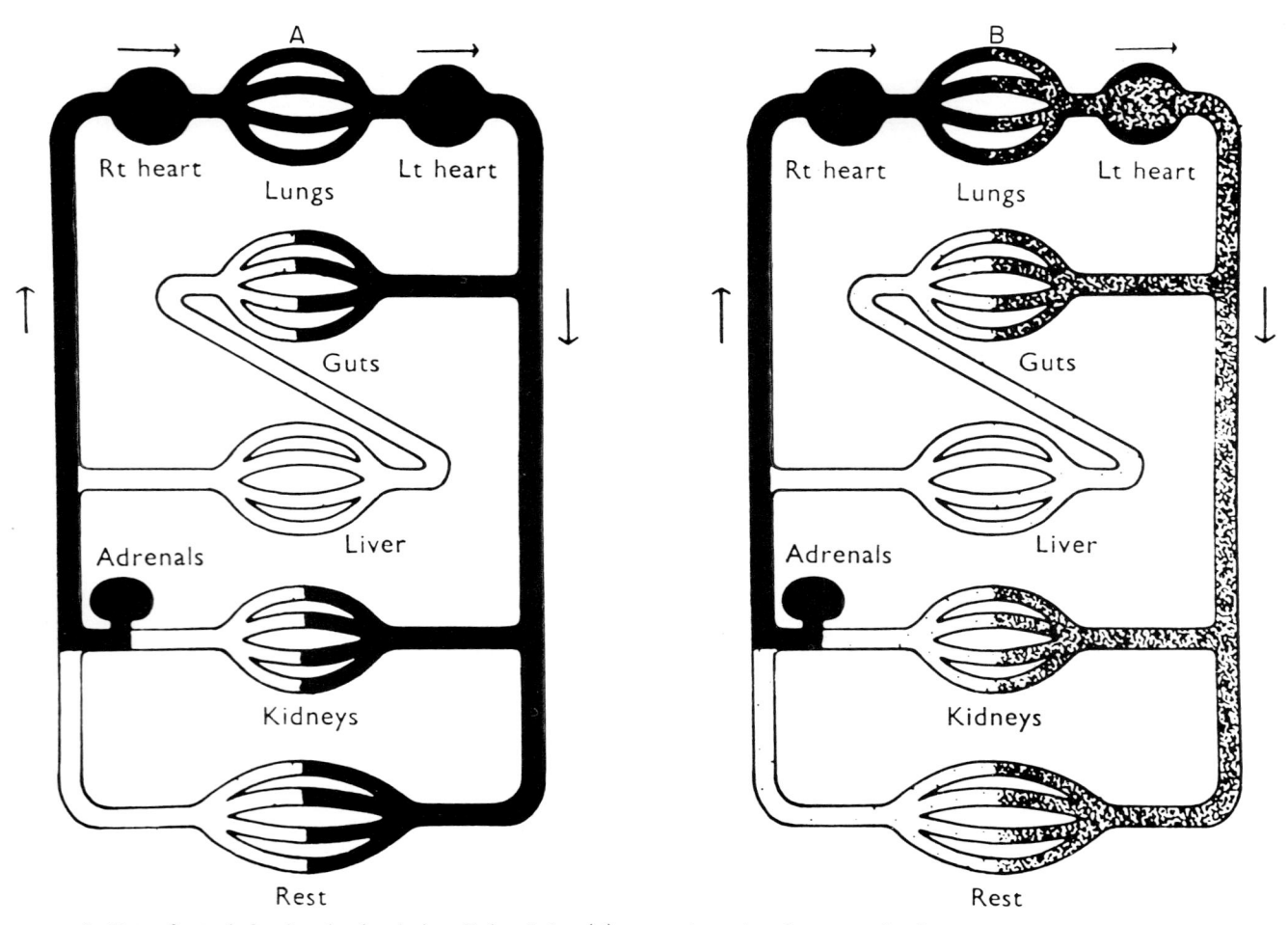

FIG. 3. Fate of catecholamines in circulation. Epinephrine (A) passes through pulmonary circulation unchanged, but up to one-third of norepinephrine (B) is removed. Both catecholamines disappear in peripheral vascular beds. Rt, right; Lt, left. [From Vane (139).]

extended these observations and concluded that, in the cat, more than 80% of an infusion of epinephrine could be removed by the liver, but he could find little evidence for the removal of epinephrine from the blood during its passage through the hind leg. However, Markowitz & Mann (105) showed that the eviscerated dog was still able to destroy injected epinephrine albeit at a slightly slower rate. Celander & Mellander (41) investigated the disappearance of both epinephrine and norepinephrine from the circulation of the cat and found that, when either of these catecholamines was infused in low doses (3 µg/kg per min) into the abdominal aorta, up to 90% of the amine was lost in the skin and skeletal muscle through which the blood passed before reaching the general circulation. When higher concentrations of the catecholamines were infused, proportionately higher amounts reached the venous side of these tissues. The disappearance of the catecholamines was unaffected when the animals were treated with MAO-inhibiting drugs. These authors found that other tissues, including spleen, kidneys, and intestine, were able to remove epinephrine and norepinephrine from the blood. They

also showed (42) that lymph did not destroy catecholamines and concluded that the metabolism of norepinephrine was strictly bound up with the tissue cells. Ginn & Vane (59) have examined the removal of epinephrine and norepinephrine from the circulation in different tissues, and their results are summarized in Figure 3. It can be seen that epinephrine passes through the pulmonary circulation unchanged but that up to one-third of the norepinephrine is removed in this tissue. From these observations it would appear that the liver is not usually presented with high concentrations of catecholamines but may be more important when there is a high concentration of catecholamine in the blood. The liver is also important in the metabolism of catecholamines after their intraperitoneal administration (40). There is some difficulty in reconciling the above results with those obtained after the infusion of radioactive catecholamines. For example, Axelrod et al. (21) and Whitby et al. (144) have found that skeletal muscle contains very little epinephrine or metanephrine after an infusion of radioactively labeled epinephrine, whereas the experiments of Celander & Mellander (41) and Ginn

& Vane (59) show that this tissue is capable of inactivating a large proportion of the catecholamine presented to it. The results of experiments with radioactively labeled epinephrine give an indication of the ability of the tissue to take up and retain the amine or its metabolites and do not necessarily give any indication of the rate at which the amine is taken up and released from the tissue either unchanged or after metabolism.

QUANTITATIVE ASPECTS OF METABOLISM
OF CIRCULATING CATECHOLAMINES

Metabolism of Epinephrine

The first quantitative studies of the metabolism of intravenously administered, radioactive epinephrine were made by Schayer (124, 125) in 1951 on rats and rabbits. A difference in the pattern of the metabolites excreted in the urine was seen after the administration of epinephrine labeled with ^{14}C at the β carbon of the ethanolamine side chain or epinephrine labeled with ^{14}C at the carbon of the N-methyl group. All the radioactivity of the epinephrine labeled at the β carbon was excreted in the urine, whereas only 55–77% of the radioactivity of the derivative labeled on the methyl group was excreted by this route. A significant amount of the radioactivity in the latter case was excreted as carbon dioxide. It was also shown that some radioactivity could be extracted into ether from acidified urine of animals given epinephrine-β-^{14}C but that none could be extracted into ether from the urine of animals injected with the methyl-labeled derivative. It was concluded that cleavage between the β carbon and the N-methyl group constituted a major pathway for the metabolism of epinephrine. The difference in the excretion of the radioactivity of the two labeled derivatives was confirmed in man by Resnick & Elmadjian (118). Schayer et al. (126) further showed that some of the radioactivity of the N-methyl-labeled derivative could be transferred to creatinine in the body and that there was no significant difference in the metabolism of the *dl* and *l* forms of epinephrine.

Since the discovery of the pathways for the metabolism of the catecholamines there have been many studies of the quantitative excretion of the metabolites of radioactively labeled epinephrine, norepinephrine, and dopamine after intravenous administration. Some of the results obtained are summarized in Table 1. This shows that, for epinephrine, 4-hydroxy-3-methoxymandelic acid and the sulfate conjugate of metanephrine are the major excretion products. It has been found (64) that the proportions of the different metabolites excreted change with time after the administration of radioactively labeled epinephrine. Immediately after injection the major metabolite excreted is free metanephrine, which reflects the high concentrations of this amine in plasma, but after 30 min most of the radioactivity excreted is associated with 4-hydroxy-3-methoxymandelic acid and the conjugates of metanephrine. The changes in the proportions of the metabolites excreted reflect both the rates and the pathways of the metabolism of the catecholamine at different sites in the body, but it is not yet possible to relate these to one another in more than general terms. Table 1 also shows that, when epinephrine is infused over a long period so that the various metabolic compartments come into equilibrium, the pattern of the excreted metabolites does not differ greatly from that seen for the total metabolism of a single injection. The studies of Kopin and his colleagues (86, 88) have given us an elegant method for determining the fractions of an injected dose of epinephrine or any other substance metabolized by alternate pathways, such as those involved in the metabolism of the catecholamines. The analysis is made for the metabolism of epinephrine by the enzymes MAO and COMT and the conjugation of the metabolic products. It is based on the fact that the fraction of a substance entering into a given metabolic reaction is equal to the rate constant for that reaction divided by the sum of the rate constants for all the reactions by which the substance leaves its metabolic pool. By intravenously infusing [^{3}H] *l*-epinephrine and ^{14}C-metanephrine simultaneously into humans (86) it was possible to calculate the proportions of the catecholamine metabolized through the different pathways from the ratio of the amounts of the two isotopes present in the different metabolites isolated from the urine. It was estimated that 67% of the injected epinephrine was methylated to form metanephrine. Approximately 21% of the epinephrine was further metabolized, after conversion to metanephrine, to form 4-hydroxy-3-methoxymandelic acid. A total of 45% of the epinephrine was converted to 4-hydroxy-3-methoxymandelic acid, so that about 24% must have been deaminated before methylation. Approximately 2.5% of the injected catecholamine was recovered as 1-(4-hydroxy-3-methoxyphenyl)ethane-1,2-diol formed by methylation followed by deamination, and a similar fraction was formed by deamination followed by methylation. A total of 97% of the injected epinephrine could be accounted for in the urine as metabolites formed by methylation and deamination and as free and conjugated epinephrine. A detailed analysis of the metabolism of circulating epinephrine in the rat has been made by Kopin et al. (88).

Metabolism of Norepinephrine

Many of the studies on the metabolism of radioactively labeled norepinephrine after its intravenous administration have been directed toward the metabolism of that fraction taken up by the sympathetic nerve endings in the tissues in order to study the metabolism of the norepinephrine released from these nerves. This might be reflected by the metabolites that appear some time after the injection of the norepinephrine.

Table 1 shows the proportions of the metabolites of norepinephrine appearing in human urine after a single injection of the catecholamine and during a long-term infusion. The proportion of the injected dose appearing

TABLE 1. *Relative Amounts of Catecholamines and Their Metabolites in Human Urine After Intravenous Administration of Catecholamines*

Catecholamine Infused																		Total Recovered	Ref.
	Epinephrine	Metanephrine	Metanephrine-O-SO₃H	Metanephrine Glucuronide	MOPEG	DOPEG	MOPEG-O-SO₃H	DOPEG-O-SO₃H	MOPET	DOPET	VMA	DOMA	HVA	DOPAC	VA				
Epinephrine	2	12		42							37							88	89
	6.8	4.5	33	1.3	7.1[a]		6.3	2.1			30.2	1.6	0.8	1.7	1.8			77.2	64
		5.2	29.5	6.0							41.2	0.66 free; 0.93 conj						93	90
	4.5	3.0	39.4	1.4	1.7		3.4	IA			24.7	1.8	2.5		1.3			91.2	4
	6.0[b]	3.5[b]	35.6[b]	1.7[b]	1.8[b]		3.5[b]	IA[b]			28.2[b]	2.0[b]	2.7[b]		1.5[b]				4
	Norepinephrine	Normetanephrine	Normetanephrine-O-SO₃H	Normetanephrine-glucuronide															
Norepinephrine	4	3	19								32	Present	5 other unidentified metabolites = 40					67	71
	5.3	3.0	12.7	5.3	13.39[a,c]		9.7	7.9			31.9[c]	1.6			3.8			83.21[c]	69
	11.27 free;[c] 8.86 conj[c]		13.03[c]								35.17[c]	Nonamine catechols: 0.67 free; 0.77 conj[c]							101
	16.2 free;[d] 8.19 conj[d]		13.58[d]		10.35[a,d]						32.66[d]	Nonamine catechols: 0.65 free; 0.75 conj[d]						82.43[d]	101
	Epinephrine	Norepinephrine	Normetanephrine	Dopamine	Methoxytyramine														
Dopamine	Trace	1.49 free;[c] 2.41 conj	0.23 free; 4.47 conj	3.35 free; 1.53 conj	Trace free; 6.30 conj		MOPEG and MOPET conjugates = 4.24			0.69	7.7 free; 2.1 conj	0.63	27.5 free; 4.77 conj	2.02 free; 5.85 conj				87.6	66

Values expressed as percentages of radioactivity of administered radioactively labeled catecholamine excreted during periods 24–54 hr after administration. MOPEG, 1-(4-hydroxy-3-methoxyphenyl)ethane-1,2-diol; DOPEG, 1-(3,4-dihydroxyphenyl)ethane-1,2-diol; MOPET, 1-(4-hydroxy-3-methoxyphenyl)ethan-2-ol; DOPET, 1-(3,4-dihydroxyphenyl)ethan-2-ol; VMA, 4-hydroxy-3-methoxymandelic acid; DOMA, 3,4-dihydroxymandelic acid; HVA, 4-hydroxy-3-methoxyphenylacetic acid (homovanillic acid); DOPAC, 3,4-dihydroxyphenylacetic acid; VA, 4-hydroxy-3-methoxybenzoic acid (vanillic acid); IA, insignificant amount; conj, conjugated. [a] Includes MHPG-O-SO₃H. [b] Percentage of radioactivity present in urine excreted during last 2 hr of an 8-hr intravenous epinephrine infusion. [c] Percentage of radioactivity present in urine excreted during an infusion of norepinephrine over 48 hr and for 48 hr after cessation of infusion. Total recovered is the mean percentage of radioactivity present in the urine associated with the compounds noted. [d] Percentage of radioactivity present in urine during the third 12-hr period of a 48-hr infusion of norepinephrine. Total recovered is the mean percentage of radioactivity present in the urine associated with the compounds noted.

as normetanephrine is slightly lower than the proportion of epinephrine appearing as metanephrine, but the fraction converted to 4-hydroxy-3-methoxymandelic acid is similar to that formed from epinephrine. As with epinephrine, the metabolites appearing in the urine change with time after the injection of norepinephrine. Goodall & Rosen (72) have shown that initially norepinephrine and normetanephrine are excreted in the largest amounts and, as seen after the injection of epinephrine, 4-hydroxy-3-methoxymandelic acid is the major metabolite 30 min after the injection of norepinephrine. The sulfate conjugate of normetanephrine was excreted at a constant rate for 70 min after the administration of norepinephrine. There appears to be a linear relation between the concentration of norepinephrine in the plasma and the norepinephrine excreted in the urine (99, 110).

Maas and his co-workers (99–101, 112) have carried out a detailed kinetic analysis of the disposition of circulating norepinephrine to obtain solutions for a kinetic model that represents the disposition of the norepinephrine released from the sympathetic nerve endings into the circulation. They have concluded that the norepinephrine normally excreted in the urine by man represents 2–3% of the norepinephrine released into the circulation from the nerve endings and that 75% of the catecholamine metabolites present in the urine are derived from the metabolism of epinephrine or from norepinephrine that has not been released from nerve endings. Crout (47) has drawn attention to the fact that the ratio of the amount of radioactive catecholamines to their metabolites that appear in the urine after an injection is different from the ratio of the amount of catecholamines to their metabolites that is normally excreted in urine in which 4-hydroxy-3-methoxymandelic acid constitutes over 90% of the total excretion. Maas & Landis (101) have obtained evidence from which they concluded that all the free norepinephrine, conjugated norepinephrine, and normetanephrine excreted in the urine could be accounted for by the metabolism of circulating norepinephrine and those pools of the catecholamine that are in equilibrium with the circulating norepinephrine. In contrast, most of the urinary 4-hydroxy-3-methoxymandelic acid and 1-(4-hydroxy-3-methoxyphenyl)ethane-1,2-diol appears to be derived from pools that, relative to their size or their rates of norepinephrine synthesis, are poorly penetrated by the circulating norepinephrine. These pools might represent the brain, adrenal medulla, or intraaxonal norepinephrine.

Metabolism of Dopamine

Table 1 shows the proportions of the metabolites excreted after an intravenous injection of radioactive dopamine into humans. The results obtained by Goodall & Alton (66) show that dopamine is further metabolized to norepinephrine and epinephrine. Approximately 75% of the infused dopamine was metabolized directly to products of dopamine and 25% to norepinephrine and its metabolic products. Only a trace of epinephrine was formed, and no metanephrine could be detected in the urine. This suggests that dopamine was taken up by the sympathetic nervous system and converted to norepinephrine, which was then released with the endogenous catecholamine. Much of the infused dopamine was converted to homovanillic acid. These authors were unable to identify all the metabolites formed from dopamine, but it would appear that, if tetrahydropapaveroline (79, 140) is a product of the metabolism of dopamine, then the amount formed is small.

Some of the metabolites from infused catecholamines are excreted in the bile. Hertting & La Brosse (73) have examined the excretion of the metabolites of radioactive epinephrine into the bile in the rat. Both the glucuronide conjugate of metanephrine and the sulfate conjugate of 1-(4-hydroxy-3-methoxyphenyl)ethane-1,2-diol were found in the bile. After an intrajugular injection, excretion in the bile accounted for 10% of the dose, whereas after injection into the hepatic portal vein 31% of the injected radioactivity appeared in the bile. The formation of the metabolites of norepinephrine has been studied by Zimon et al. (148) who used the isolated rat liver perfused with blood. They showed that normetanephrine glucuronide and the sulfate conjugate of 1-(4-hydroxy-3-methoxyphenyl)ethane-1,2-diol were the major metabolites produced from norepinephrine by this tissue.

DISPOSITION OF CATECHOLAMINES IN BLOOD

The early observations that blood is able to delay the inactivation of epinephrine in vitro were confirmed by Wiltshire (146) and Bain et al. (23). The latter authors used bioassay to investigate the apparent disappearance of epinephrine from cat blood in vitro. They found about 50% of epinephrine added to blood to be inactivated in 4–5 hr after which the apparent epinephrine concentration remained constant for up to 24 hr. However, when added to serum or plasma, the epinephrine was slowly inactivated and had completely disappeared in 8–13 hr. It was found that much of the epinephrine inactivated in whole blood was in fact associated with the red corpuscles and that it could be released from them by laking. Other reports have confirmed that epinephrine and norepinephrine are comparatively stable in plasma. Jones & Blake (83) observed little, if any, loss of epinephrine from dog plasma after 24 hr at 20–26 C; Cohen et al. (44) reported that 2.5% of epinephrine and norepinephrine added to human plasma disappeared in 1 hr at 37 C, and after 3 hr only 5% had been destroyed. The more rapid initial apparent disappearance of catecholamines added to whole blood can be seen in the observations of Mangan & Mason (103) and Manger et al. (104), which confirmed the results of Bain et al. (23). The uptake of organic bases by human red corpuscles has been studied by Schanker et al. (123) who found that the rate of uptake was related to the lipid solubility and to the degree of ionization of the base. They showed that the uptake of epinephrine into red cells was faster than that of norepinephrine. The rapid movement of epinephrine and norepinephrine into human erythrocytes has been studied with radioactively labeled catecholamines (121); it was suggested that active transport might be responsible for the rapid penetration of small amounts of catecholamines into erythrocytes whereas diffusion is responsible for the entry of large amounts (123).

Bryson & Bischoff (37) have examined the distribution of dopamine between human red blood cells and blood plasma. They conclude that about half of the dopamine added to their system was distributed according to its water solubility and the remainder was associated with the red cells and the plasma proteins.

Catecholamines have been reported to be present in and taken up by the blood platelets (34, 106, 122, 141). The uptake takes place against a concentration gradient; more epinephrine is taken up than norepinephrine (34), and the amount of epinephrine taken up by the platelets is proportional to their content of adenosine triphosphate. Born & Smith (35) have studied the metabolism of epinephrine in human blood platelets and described the formation of a hydrolyzable acidic conjugate of the catecholamine. The amines are stored in organelles within the platelet (49), and it has been found that dopamine is taken up by these organelles at a rate 68% that of 5-hydroxytryptamine (serotonin), the monoamine normally present in high concentration in the platelets. Epinephrine and norepinephrine are taken up by these organelles at a rate approximately one-third that of 5-hydroxytryptamine (50, 115).

The uptake of dopamine by blood platelets has been investigated because of the treatment of Parkinson's disease with L-3,4-dihydroxyphenylalanine (L-DOPA), the amino acid precursor of dopamine. Soloman et al. (133) examined the kinetics of the uptake of dopamine by human blood platelets and demonstrated a linear relation between the reciprocals of the initial velocity of uptake of ^{14}C-dopamine and the concentration of the amine in the surrounding medium. They also reported that no norepinephrine was formed from the dopamine taken up by the blood platelets and that dopamine was not a very good substrate for the MAO in the platelets. Boullin & O'Brien (36) have reported that the intact human platelet can accumulate dopamine to an extent equal to that of 5-hydroxytryptamine and concluded that, although both 5-hydroxytryptamine and dopamine can form micelles with adenosine triphosphate (25, 26), it would seem that dopamine has a lower affinity for adenosine triphosphate.

Epinephrine and norepinephrine appear to be bound to plasma proteins, although there are some conflicting reports. Antoniades et al. (7) reported that epinephrine was completely bound to albumin in human plasma and that norepinephrine was bound to a lesser extent. Bickel & Bovet (27) were unable to demonstrate any interaction between dog plasma albumin and epinephrine or norepinephrine. However, it has been reported that epinephrine will bind to bovine (97) and rabbit (46) serum albumin. A detailed analysis of the in vitro binding of epinephrine to bovine serum albumin has been made by Zia et al. (147) who conclude that the side chain of the epinephrine molecule is directly involved in the binding process. It also appears that the bound epinephrine is rapidly exchanging with unbound catecholamine.

The classic monoamine oxidase [monoamine:O_2 oxidoreductase, deaminating (EC 1.4.3.4)] is apparently absent from blood plasma (29) but is present in the blood platelets where it is associated with the mitochondria (111, 132). There are monoamine oxidases in the blood plasma, but their activity with different substrates varies. In the ruminant mammals the enzyme has been named *spermine oxidase* (74), whereas the blood plasma of the horse, the pig, man, and many other nonruminant mammals contains an enzyme that has been called *benzylamine oxidase* (30). The latter enzyme will not deaminate spermine and spermidine, whereas spermine oxidase will metabolize many of the substrates oxidized by benzylamine oxidase. Both enzymes can be inhibited by carbonyl reagents in contrast to the classic monoamine oxidase. The plasma monoamine oxidases are unable to oxidize N-substituted (secondary) amines (30), and thus epinephrine is not a substrate for these enzymes. They are also inactive against β-phenylethanolamine derivatives (108), including norepinephrine. However, dopamine is a good substrate for the benzylamine oxidase found in pig, rat, and human plasma (38, 53, 107), and it has been suggested that this catecholamine is a physiological substrate for the plasma monoamine oxidase. The methoxy metabolite of dopamine, 4-hydroxy-3-methoxyphenylethylamine (methoxytyramine), is also metabolized by the plasma enzymes, including that from the steer (108). The metabolism of dopamine by the plasma enzyme might be of particular importance in the ruminant mammals where the mast cells contain very high concentrations of dopamine, but as yet there is little information in this respect.

The other enzyme that plays a major role in the metabolism of the catecholamines, catechol-O-methyltransferase (COMT) is apparently also absent from the plasma (138). However, this enzyme is present in the red corpuscles (15, 80). The activity of COMT in the red cells is reduced during treatment with L-DOPA (143). Other enzymes present in the plasma that can metabolize catecholamines are ceruloplasmin (75, 76, 77) and an enzyme that can bring about the cyclization of epinephrine to adrenochrome (6, 13). Although these enzymes appear to metabolize a very small proportion of the catecholamines under normal conditions, the possibility that they are important in abnormal states should not be ignored.

CONCLUSION

The knowledge of the fate of catecholamines in the bloodstream is extensive, but a few gaps remain to be filled, particularly concerning the way different animals metabolize circulating catecholamines. These differences are more likely quantitative than qualitative since, for example, the chicken (117) appears to excrete the same metabolic end products as the mammals.

REFERENCES

1. ABEL, J. J., AND A. C. CRAWFORD. On the blood pressure raising constituent of the suprarenal capsule. *Bull. Johns Hopkins Hosp.* 8: 151–157, 1897.
2. ABEL, J. J., AND R. DE M. TAVEAU. On the decomposition products of epinephrine hydrate. *J. Biol. Chem.* 1: 1–32, 1905.
3. ALDRICH, T. B. A preliminary report on the active principle of the suprarenal gland. *Am. J. Physiol.* 5: 457–461, 1901.
4. ALTON, H., AND McC. GOODALL. Metabolic products of adrenaline (epinephrine) during long-term constant rate intravenous infusion in the human. *Biochem. Pharmacol.* 17: 2163–2169, 1968.
5. ALTON, H., AND McC. GOODALL. Metabolism of 3,4-dihydroxyphenylacetic acid (DOPAC) in the human. *Biochem. Pharmacol.* 18: 1373–1379, 1969
6. ALTSCHULE, M. D., AND U. NAYAK. Epinephrine-cyclizing enzyme in schizophrenic serum. *Diseases Nervous System* 32: 51–52, 1971.
7. ANTONIADES, H. N., A. GOLDFIEN, S. ZILELI, AND F. ELMADJIAN. Transport of epinephrine and norepinephrine in human plasma. *Proc. Soc. Exptl. Biol. Med.* 97: 11–12, 1958.
8. ARMSTRONG, M. D., A. McMILLAN, AND K. N. F. SHAW. 3-Methoxy-4-hydroxy-D-mandelic acid, a urinary metabolite of norepinephrine. *Biochim. Biophys. Acta* 25: 422–423, 1957.
9. ARMSTRONG, M. D., K. N. F. SHAW, AND P. E. WALL. The phenolic acids of human urine. *J. Biol. Chem.* 218: 293–303, 1956.
10. ATHANASIU, H., AND P. LANGLOIS. Du rôle du foie dans la destruction de la substance active des capsules surrénales. *Compt. Rend. Soc. Biol.* 575–576, 1897.
11. AXELROD, J. O-methylation of epinephrine and other catechols in vitro and in vivo. *Science* 126: 400–401, 1957.
12. AXELROD, J. N-methyladrenaline, a new catecholamine in the adrenal gland. *Biochim. Biophys. Acta* 45: 614–615, 1960.
13. AXELROD, J. Enzymic oxidation of epinephrine to adrenochrome by the salivary gland. *Biochim. Biophys. Acta* 85: 247–254, 1964.
14. AXELROD, J., W. ALBERS, AND C. D. CLEMENTE. Distribution of catechol-O-methyltransferase in the nervous system and other tissues. *J. Neurochem.* 5: 68–72, 1959.
15. AXELROD, J., AND C. K. COHN. Methyltransferase enzymes in red blood cells. *J. Pharmacol. Exptl. Therap.* 176: 650–654, 1971.
16. AXELROD, J., J. K. INSCOE, S. SENOH, AND B. WITKOP. O-methylation, the principal pathway for the metabolism of epinephrine and norepinephrine in the rat. *Biochim. Biophys. Acta* 27: 210–211, 1958.
17. AXELROD, J., I. J. KOPIN, AND J. D MANN. 3-Methoxy-4-hydroxyphenylglycol sulfate, a new metabolite of epinephrine and norepinephrine. *Biochim. Biophys. Acta* 36: 576–577, 1959.
18. AXELROD, J., S. SENOH, AND B. WITKOP. O-methylation of catecholamines in vivo. *J. Biol. Chem.* 233: 697–701, 1958.
19. AXELROD, J., AND S. SZARA. Enzymic conversion of metanephrine to epinephrine. *Biochim. Biophys. Acta* 30: 188–189, 1958.
20. AXELROD, J., AND R. TOMCHICK. Enzymatic O-methylation of epinephrine and other catechols. *J. Biol. Chem.* 233: 702–705, 1958
21. AXELROD, J., H. WEIL-MALHERBE, AND R. TOMCHICK. The physiological disposition of H³-epinephrine and its metabolite metanephrine. *J. Pharmacol. Exptl. Therap.* 127: 251–256, 1959.
22. BACQ, Z. M. The metabolism of adrenaline. *Pharmacol. Rev.* 1: 1–26, 1949.
23. BAIN, W. A., W. E. GAUNT, AND S. F. SUFFOLK. Observations on the inactivation of adrenaline by blood and tissues in vitro. *J. Physiol., London* 91: 233–253, 1937.
24. BATTELLI, M. F. Transformation de l'adrénaline dans l'organisme. *Compt. Rend. Soc. Biol.* 1518–1520, 1902.
25. BERNEIS, K. H., M. DA PRADA, AND A. PLETSCHER. Micelle formation between 5-hydroxytryptamine and adenosine triphosphate in platelet storage organelles. *Science* 165: 913–914, 1969.
26. BERNEIS, K. H., M. DA PRADA, AND A. PLETSCHER. Metal dependent aggregation of biogenic amines: a hypothesis for their storage and release. *Nature* 224: 281–282, 1969.
27. BICKEL, M. H., AND D. BOVET. Relationships between structure and albumin binding of amines tested with crossing paper electrophoresis. *J. Chromatog.* 8: 466–474, 1962.
28. BLASCHKO, H. The specific action of l-dopa decarboxylase. *J. Physiol., London* 96: 50–51P, 1939.
29. BLASCHKO, H. Amine oxidase. In: *The Enzymes* (2nd ed.), edited by P. D. Boyer, H. Lardy, and K. Myrbäck. New York: Acad. Press, 1963, vol. 8, p. 337–351.
30. BLASCHKO, H., AND R. BONNEY. Spermine oxidase and benzylamine oxidase. Distribution, development and substrate specificity. *Proc. Roy. Soc. London, Ser. B* 156: 268–279, 1962.
31. BLASCHKO, H., D. RICHTER, AND H. SCHLOSSMAN. The inactivation of adrenaline. *J. Physiol., London* 90: 1–17, 1937.
32. BLASCHKO, H., D. RICHTER, AND H. SCHLOSSMAN. The oxidation of adrenaline and other amines. *Biochem. J.* 31: 2187–2196, 1937.
33. BOOTH, A. N., C. W. MURRAY, F. DE EDS, AND F. T. JONES. Metabolic fate of rutin and quercetin. *Federation Proc.* 14: 321, 1955.
34. BORN, G. V. R., O. HORNYKIEWICZ, AND A. STAFFORD. The uptake of adrenaline and noradrenaline by blood platelets of the pig. *Brit. J. Pharmacol. Chemotherap.* 13: 411–414, 1958.
35. BORN, G. V. R., AND J. B. SMITH. Uptake, metabolism and release of [³H]adrenaline by human platelets. *Brit. J. Pharmacol.* 39: 765–778, 1970.
36. BOULLIN, D. J., AND R. A. O'BRIEN. Accumulation of dopamine by blood platelets from normal subjects and Parkinsonian patients under treatment with L-dopa. *Brit. J. Pharmacol.* 39: 779–788, 1970.
37. BRYSON, G., AND F. BISCHOFF. Dopamine transport in human blood. *Clin. Chem.* 16: 312–317, 1970.
38. BUFFONI, F., AND L. DELLA CORTE. Plasma amine oxidases: their substrates and inhibitors. *Soc. Pharmacol. Hung. Conf. Hung. Therap. Invest. Pharmacol., 4th,* 1966, p. 485–488.
39. CAHEN, A. Vitesse de disparition de l'adrénaline dans le sang. Modifications apportées par l'injection préable de substances synergiques (cocaine et ephedrine). *Compt. Rend. Soc. Biol.* 139: 22–36, 1945.
40. CARLSSON, A., AND B. WALDECK. Role of the liver catechol-O-methyltransferase in the metabolism of circulating catecholamines. *Acta Pharmacol. Toxicol.* 20: 47–55, 1963.
41. CELANDER, O., AND S. MELLANDER. Elimination of adrenaline and noradrenaline from the circulating blood. *Nature* 176: 973–974, 1955.
42. CELANDER, O., AND S. MELLANDER. The rate of elimination of catecholamines in lymph. *Acta Physiol. Scand.* 37: 84–90, 1956.
43. CLARK, W. G., AND W. DRELL. Isolation of epinephrine monoglucuronide. *Federation Proc.* 13: 343, 1954.
44. COHEN, G., B. HOLLAND, AND M. GOLDENBERG. The stability of epinephrine and arterenol (norepinephrine) in plasma and serum. *Arch. Neurol. Psychiat.* 80: 484–487, 1958.
45. COHEN, G., B. HOLLAND, J. SHA, AND M. GOLDENBERG.

Plasma concentrations of epinephrine and norepinephrine during intravenous infusions in man. *J. Clin. Invest.* 38: 1935–1941, 1959.
46. COHEN, Y., J. BRALET, AND J-P. ROUSSELET. Liason de l'adrénaline ^{14}C et de la noradrénaline ^{14}C aux protéines sériques de lapin in vitro. *Compt. Rend. Soc. Biol.* 162: 62–67, 1968.
47. CROUT, J. R. Phaeochromocytoma. *Pharmacol. Rev.* 18: 651–657, 1966.
48. CYBULSKI, N. [Cited by Szymonowicz (134a).]
49. DA PRADA, M., AND A. PLETSCHER. Storage of exogenous monoamines and reserpine in 5-hydroxytryptamine organelles of blood platelets. *European J. Pharmacol.* 7: 45–48, 1969.
50. DA PRADA, M., AND A. PLETSCHER. Differential uptake of biogenic amines by isolated 5-hydroxytryptamine organelles of blood platelets. *Life Sci., Part 1* 8: 65–72, 1969.
51. DE EDS, F., A. N. BOOTH, AND F. T. JONES. Methylation of phenolic hydroxyl groups by rabbit. *Federation Proc.* 14: 332, 1955.
52. DE EDS, F., A. N. BOOTH, AND F. T. JONES. Methylation and dehydroxylation of phenolic compounds by rats and rabbits. *J. Biol. Chem.* 225: 615–621, 1957.
53. DELLA CORTE, L., AND I. PERRINO. Il ruolo della aminossidasi plasmatiche nel metabolismo della dopamina. *Il Farmaco* 23: 204–209, 1968.
54. DIRSCHERL, W., H. THOMAS, AND H. SCHREIFERS. Vanillinsäure als Endprodukt des Abbaues von Adrenalin und Noradrenalin. *Acta Endocrinol.* 39: 385–394, 1962.
55. ELLIOTT, T. R. The action of adrenalin. *J. Physiol., London* 32: 401–467, 1905.
56. EULER, U. S. VON. Distribution and metabolism of catechol hormones in tissues and axones. *Recent Progr. Hormone Res.* 14: 483–512, 1958.
57. EULER, U. S. VON, I. FLODING, AND F. LISHAJKO. The presence of free and conjugated 3,4-dihydroxyphenylacetic acid (DOPAC) in urine and blood plasma. *Acta Soc. Med. Upsalien.* 64: 217–225, 1959.
58. EULER, U. S. VON, AND C. G. SCHMITERLÖW. Sympathomimetic activity in extracts of normal human and bovine blood. *Acta Physiol. Scand.* 13: 1–8, 1947.
59. GINN, R., AND J. R. VANE. Disappearance of catecholamines from the circulation. *Nature* 219: 740–742, 1968.
60. GITLOW, S. E., M. MENDLOWITZ, E. K. WILK, S. WILK, R. L. WOLF, AND N. E. NAFTCHI. Plasma clearance of dl-β-H^3-norepinephrine in normal human subjects and patients with essential hypertension. *J. Clin. Invest.* 43: 2009–2015, 1964.
61. GOLDSTEIN, M., A. J. FRIEDHOFF, S. POMERANTZ, AND J. F. CONTRERA. The formation of 3,4-dihydroxyphenylethanol and 3-methoxy-4-hydroxyphenylethanol from 3,4-dihydroxyphenylethylamine in the rat. *J. Biol. Chem.* 236: 1816–1821, 1961.
62. GOLDSTEIN, M., AND J. M. MUSACCHIO. Formation in vivo of N-acetyldopamine [N-acetyl-3,4-dihydroxyphenylethylamine] and N-acetyl-3-methoxydopamine. *Biochim. Biophys. Acta* 58: 607–608, 1962.
63. GOODALL, McC. Metabolic products of adrenaline and noradrenaline in human urine. *Pharmacol. Rev.* 11: 416–425, 1959.
64. GOODALL, McC, AND H. ALTON. Urinary excretion of adrenaline metabolites in man during intervals of 2 minutes, 5 minutes and 10 minutes after intravenous injection of adrenaline. *Biochem. Pharmacol.* 14: 1595–1604, 1965.
65. GOODALL, McC., AND H. ALTON. Preliminary identification of 3,4-dihydroxyphenylacetic acid and 3-methoxy-4-hydroxyphenylacetic acid in human urine as metabolites of epinephrine. *Texas Rep. Biol. Med.* 26: 107–115, 1968.
66. GOODALL, McC., AND H. ALTON. Metabolism of 3-hydroxytyramine (dopamine) in human subjects. *Biochem. Pharmacol.* 17: 905–914, 1968.
67. GOODALL, McC., AND H. ALTON. Metabolism in the human of 3,4-dihydroxymandelic acid, one of the metabolites of noradrenaline and adrenaline. *Biochem. Pharmacol.* 18: 295–302, 1969.
68. GOODALL, McC., H. ALTON, AND M. HENRY. Noradrenaline and normetadrenaline metabolism in portal cirrhosis. *Am. J. Physiol.* 207: 1087–1094, 1964.
69. GOODALL, McC., W. R. HARLAN, JR., AND H. ALTON. Noradrenaline release and metabolism in orthostatic (postural) hypotension. *Circulation* 36: 489–496, 1967.
70. GOODALL, McC., AND N. KIRSHNER. Biosynthesis of adrenaline and noradrenaline in vitro. *J. Biol. Chem.* 226: 213–221, 1957.
71. GOODALL, McC., N. KIRSHNER, AND L. ROSEN. Metabolism of noradrenaline in the human. *J. Clin. Invest.* 38: 707–714, 1959.
72. GOODALL, McC., AND L. ROSEN. Urinary excretion of noradrenaline and its metabolites at 10 minute intervals following intravenous injection of dl-noradrenaline. *J. Clin. Invest.* 42: 1578–1588, 1963.
73. HERTTING, G., AND E. H. LA BROSSE. Biliary and urinary excretion of metabolites of 7-H^3-epinephrine in the rat. *J. Biol. Chem.* 237: 2291–2295, 1962.
74. HIRSCH, J. G. Spermine oxidase: an amine oxidase with specificity for spermine and spermidine. *J. Exptl. Med.* 97: 345–355, 1953.
75. HOLMBERG, C. G., AND C-B. LAURELL. Investigations in serum copper. II. Isolation of the copper containing protein and a description of some of its properties. *Acta Chem. Scand.* 2: 550–556, 1948.
76. HOLMBERG, C. G., AND C-B. LAURELL. Investigations into serum copper. III. Coeruloplasmin as an enzyme. *Acta Chem. Scand.* 5: 476–480, 1951.
77. HOLMBERG, C. G., AND C-B. LAURELL. Oxidase reactions in plasma caused by coeruloplasmin. *Scand. J. Clin. Lab. Invest.* 3: 103–107, 1951.
78. HOLTZ, P., K. CREDNER, AND G. KRONEBERG. Über das sympathicomimetische pressorische Prinzip des Harns ("Urosympathin"). *Arch. Pharmakol. Exptl. Pathol.* 204: 228–243, 1947.
79. HOLTZ, P., K. STOCK, AND E. WESTERMANN. Pharmakologie des Tetrahydropapaverolins und seine Entstehung aus Dopamin. *Arch. Pharmakol. Exptl. Pathol.* 248: 387–405, 1964.
80. HORST, W. D., P. GATTANELL, S. URBANO, AND H. SHEPPARD. Catechol-O-methyltransferase in erythrocytes and fat cells. *Life Sci., Part 2* 8: 473–476, 1969.
81. ITOH, C., K. YOSHINAGA, T. SATO, N. ISHIDA, AND Y. WADA. The presence of N-methylmetadrenaline in human urine and tumour tissue of phaechromocytoma. *Nature* 193: 477–478, 1962.
82. JACKSON, D. E. The prolonged existence of adrenaline in the blood. *Am. J. Physiol.* 23: 226–245, 1909.
83. JONES, R. T., AND W. D. BLAKE. Dynamics of epinephrine distribution in the dog. *Am. J. Physiol.* 193: 365–370, 1958.
84. KELLY, M., D. F. SHARMAN, AND P. TEGERDINE. Dopamine in the blood of the ruminant. *J. Physiol., London* 210: 130P, 1970.
85. KIRSHNER, N., McC. GOODALL, AND L. ROSEN. Metabolism of dl-adrenaline in the human. *Proc. Soc. Exptl. Biol. Med.* 98: 627–630, 1958.
86. KOPIN, I. J. Technique for the study of alternate metabolic pathways; epinephrine metabolism in man. *Science* 131: 1372–1374, 1960.
87. KOPIN, I. J., AND J. AXELROD. 3,4-Dihydroxyphenylglycol, a metabolite of epinephrine. *Arch. Biochem. Biophys.* 89: 148, 1960.
88. KOPIN, I. J., J. AXELROD, AND E. GORDON. The metabolic fate of H^3-epinephrine and C^{14} metanephrine in the rat. *J. Biol. Chem.* 236: 2109–2113, 1961.
89. LA BROSSE, E. H., J. AXELROD, AND S. S. KETY. O-methylation, the principal route of metabolism of epinephrine in man. *Science* 128: 593–594, 1958.
90. LA BROSSE, E. H., J. AXELROD, I. J. KOPIN, AND S. S. KETY.

Metabolism of 7-H³-epinephrine-d-bitartrate in normal young men. *J. Clin. Invest.* 40: 253–259, 1961.
91. LA BROSSE, E. H., J. D. MANN, AND S. S. KETY. Metabolism of epinephrine-7-H³ as determined on blood and urine. *J. Psychiat. Res.* 1: 68–75, 1961.
92. LANGLOIS, P. Du foie comme organe destructeur de la substance active des capsules surrénales. *Compt. Rend. Soc. Biol.* 571–575, 1897.
93. LANGLOIS, P. Le mécanisme de destruction du principe actif des capsules surrénales dans l'organisme. *Arch. Physiol.* 10: 124–137, 1898.
94. LEEPER, L. C., H. WEISSBACH, AND S. UDENFRIEND. Studies on the metabolism of norepinephrine, epinephrine and their O-methyl analogs by partially purified enzyme preparations. *Arch. Biochem. Biophys.* 77: 417–427, 1958.
95. LEVIN, E. Y., AND S. KAUFMAN. Studies on the enzyme catalysing the conversion of 3,4-dihydroxyphenylethylamine to norepinephrine. *J. Biol. Chem.* 236: 2043–2049, 1961.
96. LEVIN, E. Y., B. LEVENBERG, AND S. KAUFMAN. The enzymatic conversion of 3,4-dihydroxyphenylethylamine to norepinephrine. *J. Biol. Chem.* 235: 2080–2086, 1960.
97. LITT, G. J. The interaction of epinephrine with bovine serum albumin and related studies (Abstract). *Dissertation Abstr.* 23: 1936–1937, 1962.
98. LUND, A. Elimination of adrenaline and noradrenaline from the organism. *Acta Pharmacol. Toxicol.* 7: 297–308, 1951.
99. MAAS, J. W. A kinetic model for the study of the disposition of circulating norepinephrine. *J. Pharmacol. Exptl. Therap.* 174: 369–378, 1970.
100. MAAS, J. W., H. BENENSOHN, AND D. H. LANDIS. A kinetic study of the disposition of circulating norepinephrine in normal male subjects. *J. Pharmacol. Exptl. Therap.* 174: 381–387, 1970.
101. MAAS, J. W., AND D. H. LANDIS. The metabolism of circulating norepinephrine by human subjects. *J. Pharmacol. Exptl. Therap.* 177: 600–612, 1971.
102. MACLAGAN, N. F., AND J. H. WILKINSON. Methylation of a phenolic hydroxyl group in the human body. *Nature* 168: 251, 1951.
103. MANGAN, G. F., JR., AND J. W. MASON. Fluorimetric measurement of exogenous and endogenous epinephrine and norepinephrine in peripheral blood. *Am. J. Physiol.* 194: 476–480, 1958.
104. MANGER, W. M., K. G. WAKIM, AND J. L. BOLLMAN. *Chemical Quantitation of Epinephrine and Norepinephrine in Plasma.* Springfield, Ill.: Thomas, 1959.
105. MARKOWITZ, J., AND F. C. MANN. The role of the liver and other abdominal viscera in the destruction of epinephrine in the body. *Am. J. Physiol.* 89: 176–181, 1929.
106. MARKWARDT, F. Studies on the release of biogenic amines from blood platelets. In: *Biochemistry of Blood Platelets,* edited by E. Kowalski and S. Niewiarowski. New York: Acad. Press, 1967, p. 105–114.
107. MCEWEN, C. M., JR. Human plasma monoamine oxidase. I. Purification and identification. *J. Biol. Chem.* 240: 2003–2010, 1965.
108. MCEWEN, C. M., JR., K. T. CULLEN, AND A. J. SOBER. Rabbit serum monoamine oxidase. Purification and characterisation. *J. Biol. Chem.* 241: 4544–4556, 1966.
109. OLIVER, G., AND E. A. SCHÄFER. The physiological effects of extracts of the suprarenal capsules. *J. Physiol., London* 18: 230–276, 1895.
110. OVERY, H. R., R. PFISTER, AND C. A. CHIDSEY. Studies on the renal excretion of norepinephrine. *J. Clin. Invest.* 46: 482–489, 1967.
111. PAASONEN, M. K., E. SOLATUNTURI, AND E. KIVALO. Monoamine oxidase activity of blood platelets and their ability to store 5-hydroxytryptamine in some mental deficiencies. *Psychopharmacologia* 6: 120–124, 1964.
112. PATEL, M., AND J. W. MAAS. A least squares approach to the solution of a nonlinear model. *J. Pharmacol. Exptl. Therap.* 174: 379–380, 1970.

113. PEKKARINEN, A. Studies on the chemical determination, occurrence and metabolism of adrenaline in the animal organism. *Acta Physiol. Scand. Suppl.* 54: 1948.
114. PESKAR, B., G. HELLMANN, AND G. HERTTING. Demonstration of 3,4-dihydroxy[¹⁴C]benzoic acid and [¹⁴C]vanillic acid after administration of [¹⁴C]noradrenaline in the rat. *J. Pharm. Pharmacol.* 23: 270–275, 1971.
115. PLETSCHER, A., M. DA PRADA, AND J. P. TRANZER. Transfer and storage of biogenic monoamines in subcellular organelles of blood platelets. *Progr. Brain Res.* 31: 47–52, 1969.
116. POTTER, W. DE, Z. M. BACZ, G. CRIEL, A. F. DE SCHAEPDRYVER, AND J. RENSON. O- and N-demethylation of metanephrine-7-³H in vivo. *Biochem. Pharmacol.* 12: 661–667, 1963.
117. RENNICK, B., M. PRYOR, AND B. BASCH. Urinary metabolites of epinephrine and norepinephrine in the chicken. *J. Pharmacol. Exptl. Therap.* 148: 270–276, 1965.
118. RESNICK, O., AND F. ELMADJIAN. The metabolism of epinephrine containing isotopic carbon in man. *J. Clin. Endocrinol. Metab.* 18: 28–35, 1958.
119. RICHTER, D. The inactivation of adrenaline in vivo in man. *J. Physiol., London* 98: 361–374, 1940.
120. ROSEN, L., AND MCC. GOODALL. Identification of vanillic acid as a catabolite of noradrenaline metabolism in the human. *Proc. Soc. Exptl. Biol. Med.* 110: 767–769, 1962.
121. ROSTON, S. Rapid movement of epinephrine and norepinephrine into human erythrocytes. *Nature* 215: 432–433, 1967.
122. SANO, I., Y. KAKIMOTO, K. TANIGUCHI, AND M. TAKESADA. Active transport of epinephrine into blood platelets. *Am. J. Physiol.* 197: 81–84, 1959.
123. SCHANKER, L. S., P. A. NAFPLIOTIS, AND J. M. JOHNSON. Passage of organic bases into human red cells. *J. Pharmacol. Exptl. Therap.* 133: 325–331, 1961.
124. SCHAYER, R. W. Studies of the metabolism of β-C¹⁴-dl-adrenalin. *J. Biol. Chem.* 189: 301–306, 1951.
125. SCHAYER, R. W. The metabolism of adrenalin containing isotopic carbon. *J. Biol. Chem.* 192: 875–881, 1951.
126. SCHAYER, R. W., R. L. SMILEY, AND E. H. KAPLAN. Metabolism of epinephrine containing isotopic carbon II. *J. Biol. Chem.* 198: 545–551, 1952.
127. SCHELINE, R. R., R. T. WILLIAMS, AND J. G. WIT. Biological dehydroxylation. *Nature* 188: 849–850, 1960.
128. SENOH, S., J. DALY, J. AXELROD, AND B. WITKOP. Enzymatic p-O-methylation by catechol-O-methyl transferase. *J. Am. Chem. Soc.* 81: 6240–6245, 1959.
129. SENOH, S., B. WITKOP, C. R. CREVELING, AND S. UDENFRIEND. 2,4,5-Trihydroxyphenylethylamine, a new metabolite of 3,4-dihydroxyphenylethylamine. *J. Am. Chem. Soc.* 81: 1768–1769, 1959.
130. SHAW, K. N. F., A. MCMILLAN, AND M. D. ARMSTRONG. The metabolism of 3,4-dihydroxyphenylalanine. *J. Biol. Chem.* 226: 255–266, 1957.
131. SMITH, A. A., AND S. B. WORTIS. Formation and metabolism of N-acetyl normetanephrine in the rat. *Biochim. Biophys. Acta* 60: 420–422, 1962.
132. SOLATUNTURI, E., AND M. K. PAASONEN. Intracellular distribution of monoamine oxidase, 5-hydroxytryptamine and histamine in blood platelets of rabbit. *Ann. Med. Exptl. Biol. Fenniae* 44: 427–430, 1966.
133. SOLOMON, H. M., N. M. SPIRT, AND W. B. ABRAMS. The accumulation and metabolism of dopamine in the human platelet. *Clin. Pharmacol. Therap.* 11: 838–845, 1970.
134. SUNDBERG, C. G. Über das Verschwinden des Adrenalins aus dem zirkulierenden Blute. *Acta Soc. Med. Upsalien.* 33: 301–325, 1928.
134a. SZYMONOWICZ, L. Die Funktion der Nebennieren. *Arch. Ges. Physiol.* 64: 97–164, 1896.
135. TAKAMINE, J. The isolation of the active principle of the suprarenal gland. *J. Physiol., London* 27: xxix–xxx, 1901.
136. THOMAS, H., AND W. DIRSCHERL. 3-Methoxy-4-hydroxybenzaldehyde (Vanillin) als Metabolit von Adrenalin und Noradrenalin. *Acta Endocrinol.* 47: 69–75, 1964.

137. Thomas, H., and W. Dirscherl. 4-Hydroxy-3-methoxyphenylglyoxylsäure als Metabolit von Adrenalin und Noradrenalin. *Z. Physiol. Chem.* 339: 115–121, 1964.
138. Truhaut, R., A. Amar, and C. Bohuon. Recherche d'une activité monoamine oxydase et catéchol O-méthyl transférase dans le plasma de rats intoxiqués par le tétrachlorure de carbone. *Ann. Biol. Clin.* 22: 1055–1065, 1964.
139. Vane, J. R. The release and fate of vasoactive hormones in the circulation. *Brit. J. Pharmacol.* 35: 209–242, 1969.
140. Walsh, M. J., V. E. Davis, and Y. Yamanaka. Tetrahydropapaveroline: an alkaloid metabolite of dopamine in vitro. *J. Pharmacol. Exptl. Therap.* 174: 388–400, 1970.
141. Weil-Malherbe, H., and A. D. Bone. The association of adrenaline and noradrenaline with blood platelets. *Biochem. J.* 70: 14–22, 1958.
142. Weinstein, S. S., and R. J. Manning. The disappearance of injected epinephrine in the animal body. *Science* 86: 19–20, 1937.
143. Weiss, J. L., C. K. Cohn, and T. N. Chase. Reduction of catechol-O-methyl transferase activity by chronic L-dopa therapy. *Nature* 234: 218–219, 1971.
144. Whitby, L. G., J. Axelrod, and H. Weil-Malherbe. Fate of H^3-norepinephrine in animals. *J. Pharmacol. Exptl. Therap.* 132: 193–201, 1961.
145. Williams, C. M., A. A. Babuscio, and R. Watson. In vivo alteration of the pathways of dopamine metabolism. *Am. J. Physiol.* 199: 722–726, 1960.
146. Wiltshire, M. O. P. The influence of tissues and amino acids on the oxidation of adrenaline. *J. Physiol., London* 72: 88–109, 1931.
147. Zia, H., R. H. Cox, and L. A. Luzzi. In vitro binding study of epinephrine and bovine serum albumin. *J. Pharm. Sci.* 60: 89–92, 1971.
148. Zimon, R. P., G. M. Tyce, E. V. Flock, S. G. Sheps, and C. A. Owen, Jr. Effect of monoamine oxidase inhibition on biliary excretion of metabolites of norepinephrine by isolated rat liver. *J. Pharmacol. Exptl. Therap.* 157: 89–95, 1967.

CHAPTER 43

Uptake of circulating catecholamines into tissues

L. L. IVERSEN | MRC Neurochemical Pharmacology Unit, Department of Pharmacology, University of Cambridge, Cambridge, England

CHAPTER CONTENTS

Inactivation of Circulating Catecholamines
Uptake of Circulating Catecholamines by Peripheral Tissues
Properties of Catecholamine Uptake Processes in Peripheral Tissues
    Uptake$_1$—uptake of catecholamines by sympathetic nerves
    Uptake$_2$—extraneuronal uptake of catecholamines
Role of Uptake Processes in Inactivation of Circulating Catecholamines
    Role of uptake$_1$
    Role of uptake$_2$ and other extraneuronal uptake systems
    Conclusions

INACTIVATION OF CIRCULATING CATECHOLAMINES

From the earliest studies of the biological effects of epinephrine by Oliver & Schafer (77) in 1895 it was apparent that the actions of this substance in vivo are evanescent. The rapid inactivation of circulating epinephrine was also described by Elliott (29) who showed that the substance was stable when added to blood in vitro but that biological activity disappeared rapidly from blood in vivo. Many other studies have confirmed that the pharmacological actions of epinephrine and norepinephrine are of only brief duration when these substances are administered by intravenous injection or infusion. In most cases the time course of disappearance of catecholamines from circulation has been inferred by the indirect method of observing some pharmacological response, such as a change in blood pressure or contraction of the cat nictitating membrane, evoked by the circulating amine. Such methods are clearly less precise than direct measurements of the catecholamine content of blood, which have more recently been employed; sensitive bioassay, fluorimetric, or radiochemical techniques have been used to measure the small amounts of catecholamines present in blood (see the chapter by Callingham in this volume of the Handbook). With sensitive bioassay techniques, Ferreira & Vane (32) have provided perhaps the most reliable information on the rates of removal of catecholamines from circulation after intravenous administrations. In the cat,

Ferreira & Vane observed that, after injections of small amounts of epinephrine or norepinephrine, most of the injected dose disappeared from the blood in one circulation time. The estimated half-lives were 0–10 sec for epinephrine and 0–15 sec for norepinephrine. Several studies have shown a removal of up to 90% of the catecholamine content from blood during a single passage through various peripheral capillary beds, such as the perfused hind limb preparation (18, 32, 43, 69).

Although a rapid metabolism of circulating catecholamines occurs in the liver and other visceral organs, this is not an essential factor for the rapid disappearance of catecholamines from blood. Markowitz & Mann (71), for example, observed that the inactivation of injected epinephrine occurred rapidly in the dog, even after exclusion of the liver and abdominal viscera from the circulation. The inactivation of circulating catecholamines thus seems to be a general property of most tissues; catecholamines are rapidly inactivated as blood passes through the various peripheral capillary beds. This inactivation does not seem to depend on the metabolic conversion of the active amines to inactive derivatives, but rather on the ability of various peripheral tissues to remove circulating amines by specific uptake processes. Monoamine oxidase and catechol-O-methyltransferase (COMT), the two enzymes involved in the catecholamines, are widely distributed in peripheral tissues, but neither enzyme appears to be crucial for the inactivation of circulating norepinephrine and epinephrine. The administration of inhibitors of either enzyme or a combination of inhibitors of both enzymes generally has only a modest effect in potentiating and prolonging the actions of injected catecholamines (8, 18, 19, 21, 36, 44, 60, 72).

UPTAKE OF CIRCULATING CATECHOLAMINES BY PERIPHERAL TISSUES

That circulating catecholamines might be taken up into storage sites in peripheral tissues was suggested by Burn (14). After the administration of large doses of

TABLE 1. *Tissue Distribution of ³H-Epinephrine and ³H-Norepinephrine in the Cat*

Tissue	Concentration, μg/kg*			
	³H-NE	³H-NMN	³H-Epinephrine	³H-MN
Plasma	35	5	40	44
Heart	156	44	190	383
Spleen	229	37	230	148
Lung	126	124	12	122
Liver	48	65	40	432
Small intestine	36	11	17	66
Skeletal muscle	10	8	4	32
Kidney	83	39	28	306
Salivary gland	46	12	67	73
Pancreas	46	13	40	51
Adrenal gland	150	16	192	80

Values are means for 3 experiments in each case. In comparing results for epinephrine and norepinephrine (NE), note that the dose of DL-³H-epinephrine used was 70 μg/kg, and the dose of DL-³H-norepinephrine was 25 μg/kg. NMN, normetanephrine; MN, metanephrine. * Measured 2 min after intravenous injection. [Data from Axelrod et al. (5) and Whitby et al. (96).]

epinephrine or norepinephrine to cats and dogs, Raab and co-workers (81–83) were the first to demonstrate an accumulation of exogenous catecholamines in the heart. Nickerson and colleagues (76) also described an accumulation of epinephrine in the rat heart after the administration of large doses of epinephrine in vivo. With smaller doses of norepinephrine and epinephrine, however, von Euler (30) failed to detect any increase in the catecholamine content of various cat tissues. Early studies with relatively large doses of ¹⁴C-labeled epinephrine showed that the radioactive catecholamine accumulated in the adrenal medulla and in several other tissues after intravenous injection (23, 87, 94).

Only when tritium-labeled catecholamines of high specific activity became available could similar studies be performed in which the injected doses were comparable to the minute amounts likely to be released into the circulation under physiological conditions. The first demonstration of the importance of tissue uptake in the disposition of circulating catecholamines was made by Axelrod et al. (5). They showed that, after intravenous injections of small doses of DL-³H-epinephrine (0.1 mg/kg) to mice, the unchanged hormone disappeared in two phases. In the first 5 min after injection about 70 % of the injected dose was metabolized, largely by O-methylation. The remaining 30 %, however, disappeared only slowly thereafter; detectable amounts of unchanged epinephrine were still present in animals killed several hours after injection. Studies of the fate of ³H-epinephrine after intravenous injections or infusions in cats showed that unchanged epinephrine accumulated rapidly in various peripheral tissues, particularly heart, spleen, lung, and kidney (Table 1). These results suggested that after the intravenous administration of epinephrine a substantial proportion of the injected dose was inactivated by a rapid transfer from the circulation into peripheral tissues. Whitby et al. (96) subsequently performed similar experiments with DL-³H-norepinephrine. Again it was found that intravenously administered norepinephrine was rapidly removed from circulation into peripheral tissues (see Table 1). The uptake of norepinephrine from circulation was greater for norepinephrine than for epinephrine; in the mouse about 60 % of the injected dose of norepinephrine, as opposed to about 30–35 % of the injected dose of epinephrine, persisted in the tissues for prolonged periods after injection. In similar studies in which a wide range of doses of injected ³H-norepinephrine and ³H-epinephrine were used, Iversen & Whitby (56) extended and confirmed these observations (Figs. 1 and 2).

Muscholl (73, 74) used sensitive bioassay and fluorimetric assay techniques to demonstrate an accumulation of norepinephrine in the rat heart after the intravenous administration of small doses of norepinephrine (0.08 mg/kg). With fluorimetric techniques, Strömblad & Nickerson (90) also found accumulations of norepinephrine or epinephrine in the heart and salivary glands of rats after the administration of approximately 4 mg/kg of either amine. These authors suggested that the uptake of circulating catecholamines by tissue might represent an important mechanism for the physiological inactivation of the catecholamines. Increases in the catecholamine content of peripheral tissues after the administration of catecholamines in vivo were also observed in other studies (10, 22, 47, 79). The ability of many peripheral

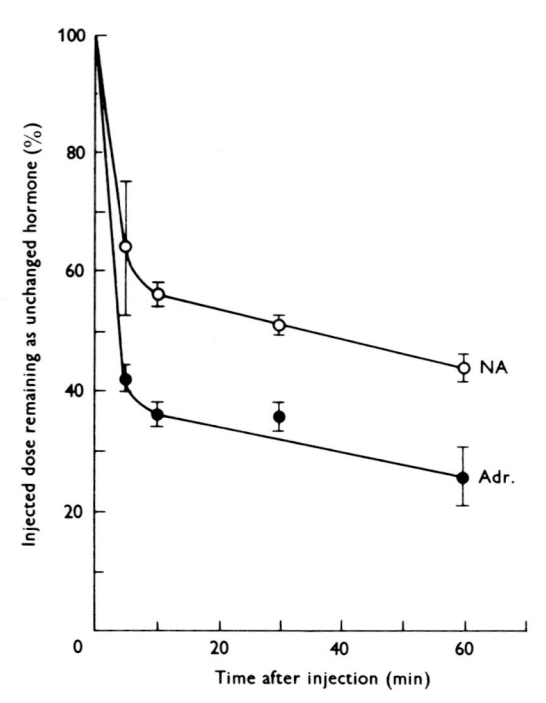

FIG. 1. Disappearance of ³H-norepinephrine (*NA*; *NE* in text) and ³H-epinephrine (*Adr.*) in mice after intravenous injection of 1 μg of either compound. Each point is mean ± SEM for 3–8 animals. [Adapted from Iversen & Whitby (56).]

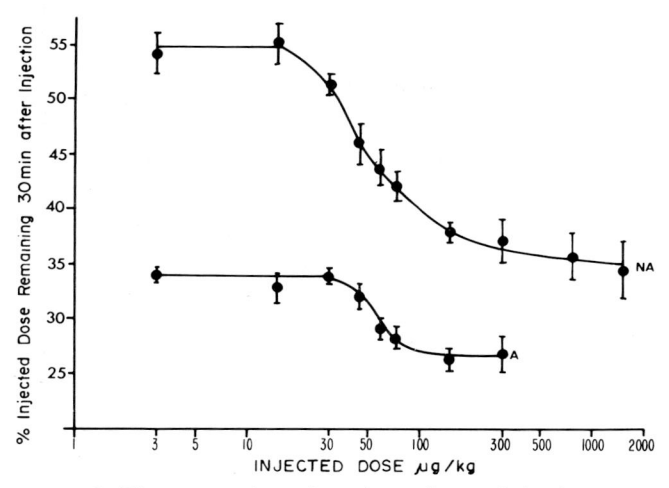

FIG. 2. Tissue retention of unchanged catecholamines as a function of injected dose in mouse. Amount of unchanged catecholamine remaining in mice was measured 30 min after intravenous injections of various doses of ^{3}H-norepinephrine (*NA; NE* in text) and ^{3}H-epinephrine (*A*). Values are means ± SEM for 5–8 animals at each point. [Adapted from Iversen & Whitby (56).]

tissues to take up exogenous catecholamines has subsequently been studied in a variety of isolated organ or tissue slice preparations.

PROPERTIES OF CATECHOLAMINE UPTAKE
PROCESSES IN PERIPHERAL TISSUES

Studies of the uptake of catecholamines by isolated mammalian tissues have revealed the existence of at least two distinct uptake systems for the catecholamines. These have been termed *uptake*$_1$ and *uptake*$_2$ (52), and their properties have been reviewed in detail in recent publications (53, 54). The properties of these two uptake systems are described only briefly here, and their possible functions in the inactivation of circulating catecholamines are then discussed.

Uptake$_1$—*Uptake of Catecholamines by Sympathetic Nerves*

Postganglionic neurons of the sympathetic nervous system possess the ability to take up and retain exogenous catecholamines (53, 54). Briefly it has been shown that *a*) exogenous norepinephrine (NE) is avidly accumulated by organs with a sympathetic innervation but that this accumulation is markedly reduced or absent in the same organs if the sympathetic innervation is destroyed by surgical, immunologic, or chemical means; *b*) radioactively labeled NE accumulated by normally innervated organs appears to be localized almost exclusively in the sympathetic nerve terminals, when the tissues are examined autoradiographically with both light and electron microscopy; *c*) exogenous NE is taken up by sympathetic nerves and can be visualized with the formaldehyde fluorescence histochemical technique; *d*) radioactive NE taken up by peripheral tissues can be released in response to stimulation of the sympathetic innervation.

The uptake of exogenous norepinephrine into sympathetic nerves is thought to be mediated by an active transport process, probably located in the axonal membrane of such neurons (54). The following evidence favors this interpretation.

1. The rate of NE uptake is temperature dependent; Q_{10} is approximately 2.0.
2. Rate of uptake is very severely reduced if sodium ions are removed from the external medium, although uptake is not markedly impaired by the removal of calcium ions. Low concentrations of potassium ion (about 5 mM) are required to maintain normal rates of NE uptake, whereas higher concentrations of potassium (> 50 mM) are inhibitory.
3. The initial rates of NE uptake at various amine concentrations are expressed by Michaelis-Menten kinetics.
4. Norepinephrine uptake is inhibited by ouabain.
5. Norepinephrine uptake is inhibited by metabolic poisons.

All these properties are characteristic of active transport processes, such as those responsible for the uptake of amino acids or sugars in other tissues (20, 62). The ionic requirements of such processes and their sensitivity to cardiac glycosides suggest that they depend on the maintenance of the normal ionic imbalance between the intracellular and extracellular spaces in which a low internal sodium concentration is maintained, despite the high extracellular concentration of this ion. Conditions that inhibit the sodium pump and lead to a running down of the normal sodium gradient inhibit the uptake of NE and other actively transported substrates. This may result from the action of cardiac glycosides, such as ouabain, which inhibit the sodium pump, or from the absence of potassium ions from the external medium—the sodium pump is a coupled system requiring external potassium because sodium efflux is associated with potassium influx. Bogdanski & Brodie (11) have based a model for NE uptake on similar suggestions by other authors for the active transport of sugars and amino acids.

The NE uptake system in adrenergic nerves exhibits stereochemical and structural specificity. In the rat heart, for example, the kinetic parameters K_m (affinity constant) and V_{max} (maximum rate of transport) for various substrates (Table 2) indicate that the uptake system has a higher affinity for (−)-NE than for (+)-NE and a higher affinity for NE than for epinephrine (51). In other species there are appreciable quantitative differences in the kinetic parameters of the uptake system, but the specificity appears to be similar to that seen in the rat heart [Table 3; (58)]. In the rabbit heart, however, NE uptake has been reported to lack stereochemical specificity (24).

In the amphibian heart, an interesting reversal of specificity is seen (Table 3), in that epinephrine has a

TABLE 2. *Kinetic Constants for Catecholamine Uptake in Sympathetic Innervation of the Rat Heart*

Substrate	K_m, µM	V_{max}, nmole/g per min
(±)-Norepinephrine	0.67	1.36
(+)-Norepinephrine	1.39	1.70
(−)-Norepinephrine	0.27	1.18
(+)-Epinephrine	1.40	1.04
Dopamine	0.68	1.45
(±)-Isoproterenol*		

* Not a substrate. [After Iversen (54).]

TABLE 3. *Catecholamine Uptake in Perfused Hearts of Various Vertebrates*

Species	IC 50, µM (−)-Norepinephrine	IC 50, µM (−)-Epinephrine
Rat	0.28	1.02
Mouse	0.65	1.08
Guinea pig	0.98	2.72
Pigeon	1.15	2.96
Toad (*Bufo marinus*)	2.34	0.96

IC 50, concentration required to produce 50% inhibition of ³H-NE uptake. [Data from Jarrott (58).]

higher affinity for the catecholamine uptake system than NE (58). In amphibians epinephrine, rather than NE, is the naturally occurring catecholamine in adrenergic nerves.

A wide variety of amines that are structurally related to NE can be transported by the catecholamine uptake system in adrenergic neurons. These amines also act as competitive inhibitors of NE uptake. An interesting situation is found, however, with certain β-phenylethylamine derivatives that lack phenolic hydroxyl groups, such as β-phenylethylamine, β-phenylethanolamine, ephedrine, and amphetamine. These amines act as potent competitive inhibitors of NE uptake (13) but are not themselves transported into the adrenergic nerves (85, 91). This suggests that it may be possible to distinguish between those structural features that are required for interaction with the uptake sites on the external surface of the adrenergic nerve membrane and additional structural features that are required if a molecule is also to be subsequently transported through the membrane. Results obtained on the potency of sympathomimetic amines as inhibitors of NE uptake (13) give a clear picture of the structure-activity relations for interaction with the uptake sites at the external nerve surface: *a*) β-hydroxylation decreases affinity, with the (−)-isomer having a higher affinity than the (+)-isomers; *b*) phenolic hydroxyl groups in para and meta positions increase affinity; *c*) α-methylation increases affinity, with the (+)-isomer having a much higher affinity than the (−)-isomer; *d*) N-substitution or methoxylation of phenolic hydroxyl decreases affinity; and *e*) the aromatic ring may be replaced without great loss of affinity by saturated five- or six-membered ring structures. The structural features that seem to be necessary, on the other hand, for a substance to be a substrate for the transport mechanism are *a*) presence of phenolic hydroxyl groups in para and/or meta positions; *b*) absence of bulky N-substituents (isoproterenol); and *c*) absence of ring methoxy groups (normetanephrine, metanephrine). If one of the latter conditions is not fulfilled, the substance will not be transported at any appreciable rate, even though it may have a high affinity for the uptake sites [e.g., (+)-amphetamine].

After an exogenous amine has been taken up into the adrenergic neuron by the membrane transport system, a further redistribution of the accumulated substance occurs into the storage vesicles that abound in the axoplasm of such neurons. Accumulated catecholamines are rapidly sequestered by such vesicles (57, 80, 89). The entry of the catecholamines into the vesicle binding sites takes place by a mechanism quite distinct from the membrane transport process in the axonal membrane. Amine binding in the vesicle does not appear to involve a transport of the external amine across the vesicle membrane, which seems to be permeable to catecholamines. The binding of amine in particles in the storage vesicles involves a hydrolysis of ATP and requires Mg^{2+} ions, but not sodium or potassium ions. The vesicle binding system is not potently inhibited by ouabain or by active inhibitors of the membrane transport system, such as (−)-metaraminol or cocaine. Vesicle uptake is, however, very potently inhibited by prenylamine (Segontin) and reserpine (17). The amine storage vesicles have a definite structural and stereochemical specificity—a high affinity for 5-hydroxytryptamine and for the (−)-isomers of the catecholamines. Studies of the uptake of various sympathomimetic amines into intact adrenergic nerves have shown that the presence of either a catechol grouping or a side-chain β-hydroxyl group is essential for vesicle binding. An interesting corollary is the finding that only those amines that were bound by the storage vesicles could be released from adrenergic nerves by stimulation (75, 80). Adrenergic nerve storage vesicles play an important role in the overall process of catecholamine uptake in these neurons. The accumulated amines are in this way protected from metabolic degradation or from passive diffusional leakage and are held in a form from which they can subsequently be released by nerve activity.

Apart from the wide range of structural analogues of NE that inhibit the uptake of catecholamines across the neuronal membrane, this uptake is also inhibited by several drugs that are not structural analogues of NE. Some of the most potent of these drugs are listed in Table 4. The tricyclic antidepressant drugs, imipramine and amitriptyline, and especially their N-desmethyl derivatives, are the most potent inhibitors of catecholamine uptake so far described, with K_i values (dissociation

TABLE 4. *Some Potent Inhibitors of Catecholamine Uptake in Isolated Rat Heart*

Drug	IC 50, μM
Desipramine	0.01
Imipramine	0.04
Nortriptyline	0.02
(−)-Metaraminol	0.08
Amitriptyline	0.11
Promazine	0.07
(+)-Amphetamine	0.18
Cocaine	0.38
p-Tyramine	0.45
Phenoxybenzamine	0.75
β-Phenylethylamine	1.10
Tranylcypromine	1.30
Dichloroisoproterenol	2.00
Guanethidine	3.30
Phenelzine	3.80

IC 50, concentration required to produce a 50% inhibition of ^{3}H-NE uptake. [Data from Callingham (15) and Iversen (53).]

TABLE 5. *Kinetic Constants for Uptake$_2$ in Isolated Rat Heart*

Substrate	K_m, μM	V_{max}, nmole/g per min
(±)-NE	252.0	100.0
(±)-Epinephrine	52.0	64.4
(±)-Isoproterenol	23.0	15.5

NE, norepinephrine. [Data from Callingham & Burgen (16) and Iversen (52).]

constant for binding to uptake sites) of the order of 0.1 μM (15).

Uptake$_2$—Extraneuronal Uptake of Catecholamines

In addition to the uptake of exogenous catecholamines into adrenergic neurons, an uptake of these substances also occurs into a variety of nonneuronal tissues. Histochemical studies have shown that when cardiac muscle or various types of smooth muscle are exposed to high concentrations of NE (> 5 μg/ml), unchanged NE accumulates in the muscle cells (31, 39). The uptake of NE was blocked by normetanephrine and by phenoxybenzamine. This histochemically demonstrated uptake probably represents the accumulation of NE by a process first described in biochemical studies of catecholamine uptake in the isolated rat heart (52). At high perfusion concentrations, NE and epinephrine were found to accumulate very rapidly in the heart, which resulted in tissue-to-medium ratios as high as 4:1. The process mediating this uptake only became apparent at amine concentrations of greater than 0.75 μg/ml for epinephrine and greater than 2.5 μg/ml for NE. The uptake under these conditions was clearly different in its specificity and drug sensitivity from the uptake of the amines into the sympathetic nerves. This uptake at high concentrations of amines was termed uptake$_2$ to distinguish it from the neuronal uptake system (uptake$_1$). Uptake$_2$ was not stereochemically specific and had a higher affinity for epinephrine than for NE. Isoproterenol was later found to be an even better substrate than epinephrine [(16); Table 5]. Uptake$_2$ was potently inhibited by the O-methylated catecholamine metabolites, normetanephrine and metanephrine, and was insensitive to inhibition by (−)-metaraminol, which had previously been found to be a potent inhibitor of uptake$_1$ (13). The structure-activity relations for uptake$_2$ inhibition are in fact almost precisely the converse of those previously described for inhibition of uptake$_1$. For uptake$_2$ inhibition, for example, potency was increased by para- or meta-O-methylation and by the presence of bulky N-substituents. Despite the clear differences in the sensitivity of the neuronal and extraneuronal uptake processes to inhibition by various catecholamine analogues, no completely selective inhibitor of uptake$_2$ was found among this group of compounds. Normetanephrine was the compound with the greatest selectivity, being approximately 50 times more potent as an inhibitor of uptake$_2$ [concentration required to produce 50% inhibition of ^{3}H-NE uptake (IC 50) = 4 μM] than as an inhibitor of uptake$_1$. On the other hand, (−)-metaraminol was almost completely selective for uptake$_1$; this drug produced no measurable inhibition of uptake$_2$ even at concentrations more than 5,000 times higher than its IC 50-inhibiting uptake$_1$ (13). The search for more selective inhibitors of uptake$_2$ has continued. We have found that phenoxybenzamine is a very potent inhibitor of uptake$_2$ (IC 50 = 2.5 μM) (67), but this compound is also active as an inhibitor of uptake$_1$. It has recently been found that several steroid hormones are active as inhibitors of uptake$_2$ [(55); Table 6]. Some of these compounds (testosterone, corticosterone), at concentrations that almost completely inhibited uptake$_2$, produced no detectable inhibition of the neuronal uptake process, and they are thus of potential interest for further studies (86a). It was originally considered unlikely that uptake$_2$ and the other forms of extraneuronal uptake that have been demonstrated histochemically were of physiological importance because of the very high amine concentrations needed to demonstrate such processes. In the rat, however, it is now apparent that uptake$_2$ operates even at very low amine concentrations (67). At NE con-

TABLE 6. *Inhibition of Uptake$_2$ in Rat Heart by Steroids*

Inhibitor	IC 50, μM
Estradiol-17β	1.84
Corticosterone	2.60
Deoxycorticosterone	5.30
Progesterone	34.98
Diethylstilbestrol	137.90

IC 50, concentration required to produce 50% inhibition of ^{3}H-NE uptake. [After Iversen & Salt (55).]

centrations below 2.5 µg/ml, however, no accumulation of unchanged NE in the cardiac muscle occurs, because all the catecholamine taken up by uptake$_2$ is rapidly degraded by monoamine oxidase and COMT. Only when uptake$_2$ accumulates catecholamine more rapidly than it can be metabolized does any accumulation of unchanged catecholamine occur. If the degradative enzymes are inhibited, it is possible to demonstrate that uptake$_2$ occurs even at low concentrations of NE. An accumulation of unchanged NE was found, for example, in rat hearts perfused with 0.5 µg NE per milliliter in the presence of a combination of enzyme inhibitors and metaraminol, which selectively inhibits uptake$_1$. This accumulation of NE could be prevented by a low concentration of normetanephrine, a potent uptake$_2$ inhibitor. The uptake and extraneural metabolism of ^{3}H-NE in rat hearts perfused with very low concentrations of NE (10 ng/ml) in the presence of cocaine to block uptake$_1$ could also be prevented by normetanephrine and by various other inhibitors of uptake$_2$, such as phenoxybenzamine (27, 28), which again suggests the operation of uptake$_2$ even at low catecholamine concentrations. From the kinetic constants previously determined for uptake$_1$ and uptake$_2$ in the rat heart, it is possible to calculate the predicted rates of uptake of catecholamines by these two processes at various amine concentrations (67). Uptake$_2$ is predicted to operate as rapidly as uptake$_1$ even at relatively low NE concentrations (about 0.5 µg/ml); in the case of epinephrine, uptake$_2$ is more rapid than uptake$_1$ throughout the range of 0.01–1.00 µg/ml.

The relative importance of uptake$_1$ and uptake$_2$, however, can be expected to vary in different tissues, since the number of uptake sites depends on the density of the sympathetic innervation and the relative abundance of postsynaptic cells capable of transporting catecholamines by the uptake$_2$ mechanism. The latter mechanism appears to be widely distributed in peripheral tissues. Histochemical and radiochemical studies have shown an accumulation of catecholamine in arterial smooth muscle (3), in splenic smooth muscle (40), in atrial muscle (86), in salivary gland parenchymal tissue (2), in tracheal smooth muscle (34), in the cat nictitating membrane (25), and in vas deferens and colonic smooth muscle (42). The comparative studies of Gillespie & Muir (42) showed considerable variation in the accumulation of NE by various peripheral tissues in the mouse, rabbit, rat, and guinea pig; in general, arterial smooth muscle exhibited the most prominent uptake ability. Although it is not clear that all the extraneural accumulations of catecholamine described above are due to the operation of a mechanism identical to uptake$_2$ in the rat heart, this seems likely since the accumulation of NE is inhibited in most cases by normetanephrine, metanephrine, and phenoxybenzamine (34, 39, 40).

The ability of vascular smooth muscle to take up and metabolize catecholamines may be of particular importance to the fate of circulating catecholamines. In most arterial smooth muscles there is only a sparse sympathetic innervation of the adventitial layers of the tissue. There is thus only a minor uptake$_1$ component in comparison with the large numbers of uptake$_2$ sites in the bulk of such muscle tissues. It might be expected therefore that uptake$_2$, followed by intracellular metabolism, could be an important mechanism for the disposition of circulating catecholamines.

ROLE OF UPTAKE PROCESSES IN INACTIVATION OF CIRCULATING CATECHOLAMINES

Role of Uptake$_1$

As described above, the uptake and retention of circulating catecholamines by sympathetic nerves (uptake$_1$) appears to be one of the major mechanisms involved in the disposition of circulating catecholamines. After the intravenous injection of small doses of epinephrine and NE, a substantial proportion of the injected dose (approximately 35 and 55%, respectively) is inactivated in this way (5, 96). This rapid removal of amines from the circulation by neuronal uptake explains the relative ineffectiveness of metabolic inhibitors in potentiating the pharmacological actions of intravenously administered catecholamines (see above). The importance of uptake$_1$ seems to be greatest for NE, less for epinephrine, and hardly effective at all for isoproterenol (16, 48). This is also consistent with the observations that inhibition of monoamine oxidase or COMT, or both, usually has no effect on the pharmacological actions of injected NE but may sometimes potentiate and prolong the actions of epinephrine and particularly those of isoproterenol. On the other hand, inhibition of uptake$_1$ by, for example, cocaine has a marked potentiating action on the effects of NE, less for those of epinephrine, and usually does not affect those of isoproterenol (38, 46, 63). The "uptake hypothesis" to account for the potentiating actions of cocaine on catecholamine effects (70, 74, 96) is now generally accepted. The drug appears to have relatively specific actions on uptake$_1$—it does not inhibit catecholamine metabolism and is only a weak inhibitor of uptake$_2$ (53). Related compounds, such as tetracaine, which do not potentiate the actions of catecholamines, also fail to block the uptake of NE (74). Several other inhibitors of uptake$_1$, such as imipramine and sympathomimetic amines, also have the effect of potentiating the actions of circulating catecholamines, although some uptake$_1$ inhibitors have other activities, such as adrenergic receptor blockade (phenoxybenzamine, chlorpromazine), which obscure their potentiating actions on adrenergic responses. The most direct evidence for the role of uptake$_1$ in the inactivation of circulating catecholamines comes from the observations that inhibitors of this process can prolong the disappearance of catecholamines from circulation. Trendelenburg (92) found that pretreatment with cocaine significantly delayed the disappearance of NE from cat plasma during the first 3 min after an intravenous injection of 25 µg NE. Hertting et al. (49) found that pretreatment with cocaine, amphetamine, tyramine, chlorpromazine, imipramine, or phenoxybenzamine delayed the disappearance of ^{3}H-NE from cat plasma during the first 5 min after an intravenous injection of the labeled amine; compounds such as pyrogallol, pheniprazine, or dichloroisoproterenol, however, which were not potent inhibitors of uptake$_1$, failed to influence the disappearance of circulating ^{3}H-NE. Eble et al. (26) reported that pretreatment with desipramine increased the peak plasma concentration of NE in the dog by up to 50% after a rapid intravenous injection; the concentration of NE recirculating as a "tail" was increased three- to fourfold, and the duration of the tail increased more than fivefold. In isolated perfused organs or limb preparations, uptake$_1$ inhibitors significantly reduce the removal of catecholamines from the perfusing medium during passage through the tissues (41, 45, 68, 95).

In the mouse, inhibition of uptake$_1$ by pretreatment with amines, such as amphetamine, phenylethylamine, or ephedrine, reduced the amount of injected ^{3}H-NE or ^{3}H-epinephrine retained by tissue uptake to less than 20% of the total injected dose, instead of the normal 40–60% (4).

Role of Uptake$_2$ and Other Extraneuronal Uptake Systems

The importance of uptake$_2$ or other extraneuronal uptake systems in the disposition of circulating catecholamines is far more difficult to evaluate, largely because specific inhibitors of the uptake$_2$ mechanism have not been available. Nevertheless it seems useful to consider the working hypothesis that uptake$_2$, or some similar mechanism, may be of major importance in the inactivation of circulating amines, in particular epinephrine. Uptake$_2$ sites are widely and strategically distributed in cardiovascular tissues, especially in the vascular smooth muscle of capillary beds. Although the affinity for catecholamines is not high, the abundance of uptake$_2$ sites constitutes a large "sink" into which circulating amines may be removed. This removal would be followed rapidly by the intracellular catabolism of the catecholamines into pharmacologically inactive products by the combined actions of the enzymes, monoamine oxidase and COMT. Inactivation would thus be achieved by the sequence of uptake followed by metabolism. Since epinephrine is removed by uptake$_2$ with a considerably higher affinity than NE this mechanism might be expected to be particularly important for the removal of epinephrine released into circulation from the adrenal medulla. Since the metabolic degradation of catecholamines is involved in this postulated inactivation system, inhibitors of catecholamine metabolism and inhibitors of uptake$_2$ would be expected to interfere with the overall process and cause a potentiation and prolongation of the actions of circulating epinephrine. Such effects have been observed. Thus, whereas inhibition of monoamine oxidase or COMT generally has little effect on the actions of administered NE, the actions of epinephrine and, particularly, isoproterenol have often been found to be increased and prolonged (6, 8, 18, 19, 21, 44, 60, 72, 84). In isolated arterial or venous muscle preparations the actions of exogenous catecholamines can be potentiated by inhibitors of monoamine oxidase or COMT (59, 78). Similar effects are observed after COMT inhibition in the isolated nictitating membrane (93) and in dog papillary muscle (61). In most cases the potentiation was greater for epinephrine than for NE. Evidence for a potentiating action of uptake$_2$ inhibitors is also available; in tracheal muscle, Foster (33, 34) found that the potentiating actions of various drugs on isoproterenol responses correlated well with the ability of these compounds to inhibit the accumulation of ^{3}H-isoproterenol. In the cat nictitating membrane the responses to catecholamines were increased by metanephrine (7), although Langer et al. (64) later showed this to be due to an increase in basal tone of the preparations rather than to a true potentiating action. Similarly pressor responses to catecholamines are selectively augmented by metanephrine by a similar mechanism. There is considerable evidence that various steroids potentiate and prolong the effects of catecholamines on effector tissues, and many of these substances are inhibitors of uptake$_2$. Adrenal corticoids increased the responsiveness of the vasculature to NE in adrenalectomized dogs (37); Schayer (88) reported that corticoids potentiated the constrictor actions of catecholamines on vascular smooth muscle; Lecompte et al. (65) found that hydrocortisone potentiated the actions of epinephrine on blood pressure in the cat and rabbit and on the contraction of isolated aortic strips in the rabbit. Similar effects on catecholamine responses in aortic strips have been observed with other steroids (9, 12, 35, 54, 66). The rank order of effectiveness of steroids in the studies of Kalsner (59) agrees well with the actions of these compounds as uptake$_2$ inhibitors in the isolated rat heart reported by Iversen & Salt (55). Furthermore corticosterone potentiated the inotropic actions of catecholamines in the isolated rat heart, whereas hydrocortisone, which does not inhibit uptake$_2$ in this preparation, had no potentiating effect (P. J. Salt, unpublished observations). Kalsner (59) and Levin & Furchgott (66) found that the potentiating actions of COMT inhibitors and steroids were not additive; the presence of one compound reduced the potentiation otherwise produced by the other. This is also consistent with the "uptake$_2$-and-metabolism" hypothesis, and these authors suggested that the steroids might act by preventing access of the catecholamine substrate to the metabolizing enzymes. The possible involvement of steroids in enhancing tissue responses to circulating catecholamines has important physiological implications and clearly needs further investigation.

If catecholamines are removed from the circulation into peripheral tissues where they are metabolized, one would expect to find catecholamine metabolites in such tissues shortly after intravenous administration of the amines. This is indeed the case. In the cat substantial

TABLE 7. *Tissue Distribution of ³H-Norepinephrine and ³H-Isoproterenol and Their Methoxylated Metabolites in the Rat*

Tissue	Concentration, nmole/kg wet wt*			
	³H-NE	³H-NMN	³H-ISO	³H-MISO
Blood	3.0	0.5	0.3	1.1
Heart	89.6	5.4	1.7	4.8
Spleen	5.8	1.9	1.3	9.0
Liver	1.6	1.1	1.4	1.8
Kidney	12.8	4.3	9.4	16.9
Lung	6.0	7.6	1.8	9.7
Uterus	3.4	1.4	1.2	4.9

Values are mean results from 6 animals. NE, norepinephrine; NMN, normetanephrine; ISO, isoproterenol; MISO, 3-methoxy-isoproterenol. Injected dose for each amine was 17.4 nmole/kg of the racemic labeled forms. * Measured 10 min after intravenous injection. [After Hertting (48).]

amounts of labeled metabolites were observed 2 min after the intravenous injection of labeled NE or epinephrine (see Table 1). It may also be noted that after injection of ³H-epinephrine there were relatively more labeled metabolites and less unchanged catecholamine in all tissues than after NE injection (see Table 1). This is even more striking after ³H-isoproterenol injection, as shown in Table 7 [cf. Table 1; (48)], and is also consistent with the view that uptake$_2$ followed by local metabolism may be more important for the disposition of circulating epinephrine and isoproterenol than for NE.

Conclusions

It is impossible to assess the precise quantitative importance of uptake$_1$, uptake$_2$, and other mechanisms in the inactivation of circulating catecholamines. However, it seems likely that uptake$_1$ is an important mechanism for the disposition of circulating NE and may be less important for epinephrine. Uptake$_2$ followed by metabolism may well be of major importance in the inactivation of epinephrine after its release into circulation from the adrenal. However, other possible mechanisms exist, including the uptake and metabolism of catecholamines in visceral organs, such as the liver, and the uptake and metabolism of amines in the lungs during passage of the blood through the pulmonary circulation (43, 50); whether the uptake systems in these tissues are similar to uptake$_2$ is not known. It seems that the various fates of circulating catecholamines are able to compensate readily for the loss or blockade of any one mechanism; there is thus no single answer to the question of which mechanism is the more important, since this may vary according to the experimental conditions and possibly to the physiological or pathological state of the organism.

REFERENCES

1. ALLEN, D. O., D. N. CALVERT, AND B. K. B. LUM. Selective augmentation of the pressor responses to catecholamines by metanephrine. *J. Pharmacol. Exptl. Therap.* 167: 309–318, 1969.
2. ALMGREN, O., AND J. JONASON. Relative importance of neuronal and extraneuronal mechanisms for the uptake and retention of noradrenaline in different tissues of the rat. *Arch. Exptl. Pathol. Pharmakol.* 270: 289–309, 1971.
3. AVAKIAN, O. V., AND J. S. GILLESPIE. Uptake of noradrenaline by adrenergic nerves, smooth muscle and connective tissue in isolated perfused arteries and its correlation with the vasoconstrictor response. *Brit. J. Pharmacol.* 32: 168–184, 1968.
4. AXELROD, J., AND R. TOMCHICK. Increased rate of metabolism of epinephrine and norepinephrine by sympathomimetic amines. *J. Pharmacol. Exptl. Therap.* 130: 367–369, 1960.
5. AXELROD, J., H. WEIL-MALHERBE, AND R. TOMCHICK. The physiological disposition of ³H-epinephrine and its metabolite metanephrine. *J. Pharmacol. Exptl. Therap.* 127: 251–256, 1959.
6. BACQ, Z. M., L. GOSSELIN, A. DRESSE, AND J. RENSON. Inhibition of O-methyltransferase by catechol and sensitization to epinephrine. *Science* 130: 453–454, 1959.
7. BACQ, Z. M., AND J. RENSON. Actions et importance physiologique de la metanephrine et de la normetanephrine. *Arch. Intern. Pharmacodyn. Therap.* 130: 385–402, 1961.
8. BALZER, H., AND P. HOLZ. Beeinflussung der Wirkung biogener Amine durch Hemmung der Aminoxydase. *Arch. Exptl. Pathol. Pharmakol.* 227: 547–558, 1956.
9. BESSE, J. C., AND A. D. BASS. Potentiation by hydrocortisone of responses to catecholamines in vascular smooth muscle. *J. Pharmacol. Exptl. Therap.* 154: 224–238, 1966.
10. BHAGAT, B. Effect of various monoamine oxidase inhibitors on the catecholamine content of rat heart. *Arch. Intern. Pharmacodyn. Therap.* 146: 65–72, 1963.
11. BOGDANSKI, D. F., AND B. B. BRODIE. The effects of inorganic ions on the storage and uptake of ³H-norepinephrine by rat heart slices. *J. Pharmacol. Exptl. Therap.* 165: 181–189, 1969.
12. BOHR, D. F., AND G. CUMMINGS. Comparative potentiating action of various steroids on contraction of vascular smooth muscle. *Federation Proc.* 17: 17, 1958.
13. BURGEN, A. S. V., AND L. L. IVERSEN. The inhibition of noradrenaline uptake by sympathomimetic amines in the rat isolated heart. *Brit. J. Pharmacol.* 25: 34–49, 1965.
14. BURN, J. H. The action of tyramine and ephedrine. *J. Pharmacol. Exptl. Therap.* 46: 75–95, 1932.
15. CALLINGHAM, B. A. The effects of imipramine and related compounds on the uptake of noradrenaline into sympathetic nerve endings. In: *First International Symposium on Antidepressant Drugs*. Amsterdam: Excerpta Medica Foundation. *Excerpta Med. Found. Intern. Congr. Ser.* 122, 1967, p. 35–43.
16. CALLINGHAM, B. A., AND A. S. V. BURGEN. The uptake of isoprenaline and noradrenaline by the perfused rat heart. *Mol. Pharmacol.* 2: 37–42, 1966.
17. CARLSSON, A., N. A. HILLARP, AND B. WALDECK. Analysis of the Mg^{++} ATP dependent storage mechanisms in the amine granules of the adrenal medulla. *Acta Physiol. Scand. Suppl.* 215, 1963.
18. CELANDER, O., AND S. MELLANDER. Elimination of adrenaline and noradrenaline from the circulating blood. *Nature* 176: 973–974, 1955.
19. CORNE, S. J., AND J. D. GRAHAM. The effect of inhibition of amine oxidase in vivo on administered adrenaline, noradrenaline, tyramine and serotonin. *J. Physiol., London* 135: 339–349, 1957.
20. CRANE, R. K. Na$^+$-dependent transport in the intestine and other animal tissues. *Federation Proc.* 24: 1000–1006, 1965.
21. CROUT, J. R. Effect of inhibiting both catechol-O-methyl transferase and monoamine oxidase on cardiovascular re-

sponses to norepinephrine. *Proc. Soc. Exptl. Biol. Med.* 108: 482–484, 1961.
22. CROUT, J. R. The uptake and release of ³H-norepinephrine by the guinea pig heart in vivo. *Arch. Exptl. Pathol. Pharmakol.* 248: 85–98, 1964.
23. DE SCHAEPDRYVER, A. F., AND N. KIRSHNER. Metabolism of DL-adrenaline-2-C¹⁴ in the cat. II. Tissue metabolism. *Arch. Intern. Pharmacodyn. Therap.* 131: 433–449, 1961.
24. DRASKÓCZY, P. R., AND U. TRENDELENBURG. The uptake of l- and d-norepinephrine by the isolated perfused rabbit heart in relation to the stereospecificity of the sensitizing action of cocaine. *J. Pharmacol. Exptl. Therap.* 159: 66–73, 1968.
25. DRASKÓCZY, P. R., AND U. TRENDELENBURG. Intra- and extraneuronal accumulation of sympathomimetic amines in the isolated nictitating membrane of the cat. *J. Pharmacol. Exptl. Therap.* 174: 290–306, 1970.
26. EBLE, J. N., C. W. GOWDEY, AND J. R. VANE. Blood concentration of noradrenaline in the dog after intravenous administration and the effects of desipramine. *Nature* 231: 181–182, 1971.
27. EISENFELD, A. J., J. AXELROD, AND L. KRAKOFF. Inhibition of the extraneuronal accumulation of norepinephrine by adrenergic blocking agents. *J. Pharmacol. Exptl. Therap.* 156: 107–113, 1966.
28. EISENFELD, A. J., L. LANDSBERG, AND J. AXELROD. Effect of drugs on the accumulation and metabolism of extraneuronal norepinephrine in the rat heart. *J. Pharmacol. Exptl. Therap.* 158: 378–385, 1967.
29. ELLIOTT, T. R. The action of adrenaline. *J. Physiol., London* 32: 401–467, 1905.
30. EULER, U. S. VON. The catechol amine content of various organs of the cat after injections and infusions of adrenaline and noradrenaline. *Circulation Res.* 4: 647–652, 1956.
31. FARNEBO, L. O., AND T. MALMFORS. Histochemical studies on the uptake of noradrenaline and α-methylnoradrenaline in the perfused rat heart. *European J. Pharmacol.* 5: 313–320, 1969.
32. FERREIRA, S. H., AND J. R. VANE. Half-lives of peptides and amines in the circulation. *Nature* 215: 1237–1240, 1967.
33. FOSTER, R. M. The potentiation of the responses to noradrenaline and isoprenaline of the guinea pig isolated tracheal chain preparation by desipramine, phentolamine, guanethidine, metanephrine and cooling. *Brit. J. Pharmacol.* 31: 466–482, 1967.
34. FOSTER, R. W. An uptake of radioactivity from DL-³H-isoprenaline and its inhibition by drugs which potentiate the responses to L-isoprenaline in the guinea pig isolated trachea. *Brit. J. Pharmacol.* 35: 418–427, 1969.
35. FOWLER, N. O., AND D. H. CHOU. Potentiation of smooth muscle contraction by adrenal steroids. *Circulation Res.* 9: 153–156, 1961.
36. FRIEND, G., M. S. ZILELI, J. R. HAMILIN, AND F. W. FEUTTER. The effect of iproniazid on the inactivation of norepinephrine in the human. *J. Clin. Psychopathol. Psychotherap.* 19: 61–68, 1959.
37. FRITZ, I., AND R. LEVINE. Action of adrenal cortical steroids and norepinephrine on vascular responses of stress in adrenalectomized rats. *Am. J. Physiol.* 165: 456–465, 1951.
38. FURCHGOTT, R. F. The pharmacology of vascular smooth muscle. *Pharmacol. Rev.* 7: 183–265, 1955.
39. GILLESPIE, J. S. The role of receptors in adrenergic uptake. In: *Adrenergic Neurotransmission*, edited by G. E. W. Wolstenholme. London: Churchill, 1968, p. 61–72.
40. GILLESPIE, J. S., D. N. H. HAMILTON, AND R. J. A. HOSIE. The extraneuronal uptake and localization of noradrenaline in the cat spleen and the effects of some drugs, of cold and of denervation. *J. Physiol., London* 206: 563–590, 1970.
41. GILLESPIE, J. S., AND S. M. KIRPEKAR. The inactivation of infused noradrenaline by the cat spleen. *J. Physiol., London* 176: 205–227, 1965.
42. GILLESPIE, J. S., AND T. C. MUIR. Species and tissue variation in extraneuronal and neuronal accumulation of noradrenaline. *J. Physiol., London* 206: 591–604, 1970.

43. GINN, R., AND J. R. VANE. Disappearance of catecholamines from the circulation. *Nature* 219: 740–742, 1968.
44. GRIESEMER, E. C., J. BARSKY, C. A. DRAGSTEDT, J. A. WELLS, AND E. A. ZELLER. Potentiating effects of iproniazid on the pharmacological actions of sympathomimetic amines. *Proc. Soc. Exptl. Biol. Med.* 84: 699–701, 1953.
45. GRYGLEWSKI, R., AND J. R. VANE. The inactivation of noradrenaline and isoprenaline in dogs. *Brit. J. Pharmacol.* 39: 573–584, 1970.
46. HARDMAN, J. G., J. E. MAYER, AND B. CLARK. Cocaine potentiation of the cardiac inotropic and phosphorylase responses to catecholamines as related to the uptake of ³H-catecholamines. *J. Pharmacol. Exptl. Therap.* 150: 341–348, 1965.
47. HARVEY, J. A., AND J. N. PENNEFATHER. Effect of adrenaline infusions on the catechol amine content of cat and rat tissues. *Brit. J. Pharmacol.* 18: 183–189, 1962.
48. HERTTING, G. The fate of ³H-iso-proterenol in the rat. *Biochem. Pharmacol.* 13: 1119–1128, 1964.
49. HERTTING, G., J. AXELROD, AND L. G. WHITBY. Effect of drugs on the uptake and metabolism of H³-norepinephrine. *J. Pharmacol. Exptl. Therap.* 134: 146–153, 1961.
50. HUGHES, J., C. N. GILLIS, AND F. E. BLOOM. The uptake and disposition of dl-norepinephrine in perfused rat lung. *J. Pharmacol. Exptl. Therap.* 169: 237–248, 1969.
51. IVERSEN, L. L. The uptake of noradrenaline by the isolated perfused rat heart. *Brit. J. Pharmacol.* 21: 523–537, 1963.
52. IVERSEN, L. L. The uptake of catecholamines at high perfusion concentrations in the rat isolated heart: a novel catecholamine uptake process. *Brit. J. Pharmacol.* 25: 18–33, 1965.
53. IVERSEN, L. L. *The Uptake and Storage of Noradrenaline in Sympathetic Nerves.* London: Cambridge Univ. Press, 1967.
54. IVERSEN, L. L. The uptake of biogenic amines. In: *The Role of Biogenic Amines and Physiological Membranes in Modern Drug Therapy*, edited by J. Biel. New York: Dekker, 1971, p. 259–327.
55. IVERSEN, L. L., AND P. J. SALT. Inhibition of catecholamine uptake₂ by steroids in the isolated rat heart. *Brit. J. Pharmacol.* 40: 528–530, 1970.
56. IVERSEN, L. L., AND L. G. WHITBY. Retention of injected catechol amines by the mouse. *Brit. J. Pharmacol.* 19: 355–364, 1962.
57. IVERSEN, L. L., AND L. G. WHITBY. The subcellular distribution of catecholamines in normal and tyramine-depleted mouse hearts. *Biochem. Pharmacol.* 12: 582–584, 1963.
58. JARROTT, B. Uptake and metabolism of ³H-noradrenaline by the perfused hearts of various species. *Brit. J. Pharmacol.* 38: 810–821, 1970.
59. KALSNER, S. Steroid potentiation of responses to sympathomimetic amines in aortic strips. *Brit. J. Pharmacol.* 36: 582–593, 1969.
60. KAMIJO, J., B. G. KOELLE, AND H. H. WAGNER. Modification of the effects of sympathomimetic amines and of adrenergic nerve stimulation by 1-isonicotinyl-2-isopropylhydrazine and isonicotinic acid hydrazide. *J. Pharmacol. Exptl. Therap.* 117: 213–227, 1955.
61. KAUMANN, A. J. Adrenergic receptors in heart muscle: relations among factors influencing the sensitivity of the cat papillary muscle to catecholamines. *J. Pharmacol. Exptl. Therap.* 173: 383–393, 1970.
62. KIPNIS, D. M., AND J. E. PARRISH. Role of Na⁺ and K⁺ in sugar (2-deoxyglucose) and amino acid (α-aminoisobutyric acid) transport in striated muscle. *Federation Proc.* 24: 1051–1959, 1965.
63. KOERKER, R. L., AND N. C. MORAN. An evaluation of the inability of cocaine to potentiate the responses to cardiac nerve stimulation in the dog. *J. Pharmacol. Exptl. Therap.* 178: 482–496, 1971.
64. LANGER, S. Z., M. G. BOGAERT, AND A. F. DE SCHAEPDRYVER. Influence of metanephrine on responses of the nictitating membrane of the pithed cat to sympathomimetic amines. *J. Pharmacol. Exptl. Therap.* 157: 517–523, 1967.
65. LECOMPTE, J., J. GREVISSE, AND M. L. BEAUMARIAGE. Poten-

tiation par l'hydrocortisone des effets moteurs de l'adrenaline. *Arch. Intern. Pharmacocyn. Therap.* 119: 133–141, 1959.
66. LEVIN, J. A., AND R. F. FURCHGOTT. Interactions between potentiating agents of adrenergic amines in rabbit aortic strips. *J. Pharmacol. Exptl. Therap.* 172: 320–331, 1970.
67. LIGHTMAN, S., AND L. L. IVERSEN. Role of uptake₂ in the extraneuronal uptake and metabolism of catecholamines in the isolated rat heart. *Brit. J. Pharmacol.* 37: 638–649, 1969.
68. LINDMAR, R., AND E. MUSCHOLL. Die Wirkung von Pharmaka auf die Elimination von Noradrenalin aus der Perfusionsflussigkeit und die Noradrenalin-Aufnahme in das isolierte Herz. *Arch. Exptl. Pathol. Pharmakol.* 247: 469–492, 1964.
69. LUND, A. Elimination of adrenaline and noradrenaline from the organism. *Acta Pharmacol. Toxicol.* 7: 297–308, 1951.
70. MACMILLIAN, W. H. A hypothesis concerning the effect of cocaine on the action of sympathomimetic amines. *Brit. J. Pharmacol.* 14: 385–391, 1959.
71. MARKOWITZ, J., AND F. C. MANN. The role of the liver and other abdominal viscera in the destruction of epinephrine in the body. *Am. J. Physiol.* 89: 176–181, 1929.
72. MURNAGHAN, M. F., AND I. M. MAZURKIEWICZ. Some pharmacological properties of 4-methyltropolone. *Rev. Can. Biol.* 22: 99–102, 1963.
73. MUSCHOLL, E. Die Hemmung der Noradrenaline-Aufnahme des Herzens durch Reserpin und die Wirkung von Tyramin. *Arch. Exptl. Pathol. Pharmakol.* 240: 234–241, 1960.
74. MUSCHOLL, E. Effect of cocaine and related drugs on the uptake of noradrenaline by heart and spleen. *Brit. J. Pharmacol.* 16: 352–359, 1961.
75. MUSSACHIO, J. M., I. J. KOPIN, AND V. K. WEISE. Subcellular distribution of some sympathomimetic amines and their β-hydroxylated derivatives in the rat heart. *J. Pharmacol. Exptl. Therap.* 148: 22–28, 1965.
76. NICKERSON, M., J. BERGHOUT, AND R. N. HAMMERSTROM. Mechanism of the acute lethal effect of epinephrine in rats. *Am. J. Physiol.* 160: 479–484, 1950.
77. OLIVER, G., AND E. A. SCHAFER. The physiological effects of extracts of the suprarenal capsules. *J. Physiol., London* 18: 230–276, 1895.
78. OSSWALD, W., S. GUIMARAES, AND A. COIMBRA. The termination of action of catecholamines in the isolated venous tissue of the dog. *Arch. Exptl. Pathol. Pharmakol.* 269: 15–31, 1971.
79. PENNEFATHER, J. N., AND M. J. RAND. Increase in noradrenaline content of tissues after infusion of noradrenaline, dopamine and L-DOPA. *J. Physiol., London* 154: 277–287, 1960.
80. POTTER, L. T. Role of intraneuronal vesicles in the synthesis, storage and release of noradrenaline. *Circulation Res.* 20, Suppl. III: 13–24, 1967.

81. RAAB, W., AND W. GIGEE. Die Katecholamine des Herzens. *Arch. Exptl. Pathol. Pharmakol.* 219: 248–262, 1953.
82. RAAB, W., AND W. GIGEE. Specific avidity of heart muscle to adsorb and store epinephrine and norepinephrine. *Circulation Res.* 3: 553–558, 1955.
83. RAAB, W., AND R. J. HUMPHREYS. Drug action upon myocardial epinephrine-sympathin concentration and heart rate (nitroglycerine, papaverine, priscol, dibenaminehydrochloride). *J. Pharmacol. Exptl. Therap.* 89: 64–76, 1957.
84. ROSS, S. B. In vivo inactivation of catechol amines in mice. *Acta Pharmacol. Toxicol.* 20: 267–273, 1963.
85. ROSS, S. B., A. L. RENYI, AND B. BRUNFELTER. Cocaine-sensitive uptake of sympathomimetic amines in nerve tissue. *J. Pharm. Pharmacol.* 20: 283–288, 1968.
86. SACHS, CH. Noradrenaline uptake mechanisms in the mouse atrium. A biochemical and histochemical study. *Acta Physiol. Scand. Suppl.* 341: 1–67, 1970.
86a. SALT, P. J. Inhibition of noradrenaline uptake₂ in the isolated rat heart by steroids, clonidine and methoxylated phenylethylamines. *European J. Pharmacol.* 20: 329–340, 1972.
87. SCHAYER, R. W. Studies of the metabolism of β-C¹⁴-DL-adrenaline. *J. Biol. Chem.* 189: 301–306, 1951.
88. SCHAYER, R. W. Histidine decarboxylase in mast cells. *Ann. NY Acad. Sci.* 103: 164–178, 1963.
89. STJARNE, L. Studies of catecholamine uptake, storage and release mechanisms. *Acta Physiol. Scand. Suppl.* 228, 1964.
90. STRÖMBLAD, B. C. R., AND M. NICKERSON. Accumulation of epinephrine and norepinephrine by some rat tissues. *J. Pharmacol. Exptl. Therap.* 134: 154–159, 1961.
91. THOENEN, H., A. HURLIMANN, AND W. HAEFELY. Mechanism of amphetamine accumulation in the isolated perfused heart of the rat. *J. Pharm. Pharmacol.* 20: 1–11, 1968.
92. TRENDELENBURG, U. The supersensitivity caused by cocaine. *J. Pharmacol. Exptl. Therap.* 125: 55–65, 1959.
93. TRENDELENBURG, U., D. HOHN, K. H. GRAEFE, AND S. PLUCHINO. The influence of block of catechol-O-methyl transferase on the sensitivity of isolated organs to catecholamines. *Arch. Exptl. Pathol. Pharmakol.* 271: 59–92, 1971.
94. UDENFRIEND, S., AND J. B. WYNGAARDEN. Precursors of adrenal epinephrine and norepinephrine in vivo. *Biochim. Biophys. Acta* 20: 48–52, 1956.
95. VANE, J. R. The release and fate of vasoactive hormones in the circulation. *Brit. J. Pharmacol.* 35: 209–242, 1969.
96. WHITBY, L. G., J. AXELROD, AND H. WEIL-MALHERBE. The fate of H³-norepinephrine in animals. *J. Pharmacol. Exptl. Therap.* 132: 193–201, 1961.
97. WHITBY, L. G., G. HERTTING, AND J. AXELROD. Effect of cocaine on the disposition of noradrenaline labelled with tritium. *Nature* 187: 604–605, 1960.

INDEX

Index

Acetylcholine
  depolarizing effect on adrenal chromaffin cells, 373
  evocation of adrenal medullary secretion, ionic influences, 374–379
    Ca, essential and sufficient for responses, 375–376
    Ca itself as secretagogue, 376–377
    K lack and potentiation of basal and evoked secretion, 378
    K stimulates and also requires Ca, 376
    Mg inhibition of responses to acetylcholine, K, Ca, Sr, and Ba, 377–378
    Na lack and potentiation of basal and evoked secretion, 378
    prolonged Na deprivation causing inhibition, 379
    Sr and Ba as Ca substitutes and stimulants, 377
    stimulant effects of ouabain, 378–379
  receptors in mechanism of adrenal medullary secretion, 371–372
  role in controlling adrenal medullary secretion, 309, 315
ACTH: *see* Corticotropin
Addison's disease
  historical aspects, 231, 245
  salt appetite and sensitivity in, effect of corticosteroids on, 184
Adenosine monophosphate, cyclic
  activation of phosphorylase kinase, 608–609
  as mediator of glucocorticoid action in muscle, 255–256
  direct activation of adrenal cortical mitochondrial enzymes, 75
  exogenous, effects in gluconeogenesis in perfused livers from normal and adrenalectomized rats, 153
  levels in adipose tissue, effects of glucocorticoids on, 174–176
  levels in perfused livers of normal and adrenalectomized rats, effects of glucagon and epinephrine on, 153
  role in muscle contraction, 622–625
    effects on cardiac contractility, 622–623
    effects on isolated cardiac sarcoplasmic reticulum, 624–625
    hormone receptors and adenyl cyclase, 623
  role in regulation of adrenal tyrosine hydroxylase activity, 361–362
Adenosine triphosphatase
  Na-K ATPase activity in kidney, effect of corticosteroids on, 184
Adenosine triphosphate
  role in storage of catecholamines in chromaffin granules, 328, 330–334
Adenylate cyclase
  activity in fat cell ghosts, effects of glucocorticoids on, 174–176
  increased norepinephrine-sensitivity activity in fat cell ghosts after fat cell incubation with growth hormone and dexamethasone, 174, 175
Adipose tissue
  adenylate cyclase, cyclic AMP, and phosphodiesterase levels, effects of glucocorticoids on, 174–176
  fatty acid release and lipolysis stimulated by glucocorticoids in vitro, 173–174
  glucose metabolism in, inhibition by glucocorticoids, 169–172
  lipid deposition changes in Cushing's syndrome during treatment with glucocorticoids, 172
  metabolism in, model for glucocorticoid action on, 17
  recovery of glucose oxidation from dexamethasone inhibition, effect of dactinomycin on, 171

Adrenal cortex
  see also Adrenocortical zonation
  ACTH-increased cellular permeability to glucose as mode of action of ACTH in stimulating cortical secretory activity, 70
  anatomic relationship to adrenal medulla and biosynthesis of epinephrine, 357–358
  arteriae corticis and cortical capillaries, 287
  enzymes involved in corticosteroid biosynthesis, distribution of, 60
  history of, 1–12
    adrenal-gonad relations, 7
    adrenal-pituitary relations, 8
    as essential for life, 3
    chemistry of cortex, 5
    early work with cortex extracts, 4–5
    endocrine role, 4
    functions of, 3–4
    role in carbohydrate metabolism, 6–7
    role in electrolyte and water metabolism, 5–6
    role in inflammation, 9–10
    role in stress, 8–9
  in fetus, 107–115
    effect of fetal adrenocortical insufficiency on postnatal survival, 113
    effect of hypophysectomy on development and function, 108–109
    effects on maturation of adrenal medulla, 112
    effects on parturition, 112–113
    effects on thymus and hematopoietic tissue, 112
    extreme development in humans, 110–111
    functional development, 107–109
    functions, 111–113
    hypophysial control of adrenal development and function, 108–109
    hypothalamic control of hypophysial corticostimulating activity, 109
    in human anencephalic monsters, 109
    maturational changes, 107–108
    metabolic pathways of pregnenolone and progesterone in human fetuses, 110
    response of pituitary-adrenal system to stresses, 109
    role in glycogen deposition in fetal liver, 111–112
  metabolism of pregnenolone in, 57
  mitoses in, distribution, 14
  regeneration of, 15
  regulation of adrenal dopamine β-hydroxylase activity, 362–363
  regulation of adrenal tyrosine hydroxylase activity, 361
  secretion of androgens, role of zona reticularis, 19
  secretion of estrogens, 19–20
  ultrastructural changes with functional activity, 32–36
    organelles in relation to steroidogenesis, 28–32
    zona fasciculata and zona reticularis changes, 34–36
    zona glomerulosa changes, 33–34
  ultrastructure in mammals, 25–32
    lipid droplets, 26–28, 30, 31, 33
    mitochondria, 25–26, 27, 28, 29, 31, 35, 36

Adrenal cortex (continued)
    other organelles, 28
    smooth endoplasmic reticulum, 25, 26, 27, 28, 30, 31
Adrenal cortex diseases
    see also Adrenal cortex hyperfunction; Adrenal cortex hypofunction; Adrenal cortex neoplasms
    taste acuity in patients with, 216
Adrenal cortex extracts
    early work with, 4–5
    effects on urinary nitrogen excretion in fasted rats, 138
Adrenal cortex hormones
    see also Glucocorticoids; Mineralocorticoids
    administration to replace adrenal secretion and vital functions disturbed by adrenalectomy, 136
    as inhibitors of biosynthesis of corticosteroids, 63
    binding by plasma proteins, 117–125
        association constants for hormone complexes with α_1-acid glycoprotein, 117–118
        binding phenomenon, 117–118
        complexes in human serum, 118–119
        corticosteroid-binding globulin levels, influence of corticosteroids on, 122–123
        development of, high-affinity binding in sera of different species, 120–121
        endocrine influences on serum levels of corticosteroid-binding globulin, 121–123
        influence of gonadal hormones on, 121–122
        influence of thyrotropin and thyroxine on, 123
        physicochemical properties of complexes of CBG, 119–120
        significance of, 123–124
    biosynthesis of, 55–68
        by inner zones of adrenal cortex in vitro, 17–18
        by zona glomerulosa in vitro, 16–17
        C_{19} and C_{18} steroids, 58
        conversion of pregnenolone to glucocorticoids and aldosterone, 56–58
        dehydrogenases in, 59–60
        early steps in, 55–56
        enzymes in, distribution in adrenal cortex, 60
        fetal-placental activities, 60–61
        genetic blocks in hydroxylation of corticosteroids, 62
        hydroxylation pathway in, 58–59
        in nonmammalian vertebrates, 61–62
        isomerases in, 60
        relation to adrenocortical organelles, 28–32
        simplified scheme and intracellular pathways in mammals, 32
    biosynthesis of, inhibitors, 62–64
        amphenone, 62
        cyanoketone, 63
        o,p'-DDD, 63
        17α-hydroxylase inhibitors, 63
        18-hydroxylase and 18-oxidase inhibitors, 63
        inhibitors of cholesterol biosynthesis and metabolism, 63
        inhibitors of protein biosynthesis, 63–64
        metyrapone, 62–63
        ouabain, 64
        steroids, 63
    cardiac effects of, 195–197
        electrocardiographic effects, 197
        in whole animals, 196–197
        inotropic effects in intact animals, 197
        inotropic effects in isolated cardiac tissue, 195–196
        myocardial metabolic effects, 197
    effect on bone electrolytes, 183
    effect on gastrointestinal tract electrolytes, 183–184
    effect on kidney, 179–182
        K excretion, 180–181
        Mg, Ca, and acid-base balance, 181–182
        Na excretion, 179–180
        Na-K ATPase activity, 184
    effect on muscle electrolytes, 182–183
    effect on salivary gland electrolytes, 182
    effect on salt appetite and sensitivity, 184
    effect on sweat sodium concentration, 182
    effect on water and electrolyte metabolism, 179–189
    influence on protein and carbohydrate metabolism, 135–167
    influence on serum levels of corticosteroid-binding globulin, 122–123
    inhibition of ACTH secretion, 46–49
        concentration of corticosteroid and degree of inhibition of ACTH secretion, 48
        kinetics of, 48–49
        relation between structure of corticosteroid and inhibitory potency, 49
        sites of inhibitory actions, 47–48
    interaction with connective tissue, 267–268
    interaction with other agents in regulation of circulatory function, 199–202
        cardiac glycosides, 201–202
        catecholamines, 200–201
        kinins, 202
        renin and angiotensin II, 201
    localization in inflamed or injured tissue area, 265
    peripheral vascular effects of, 197–199
        blood pressure and vascular resistance, 197–198
        effects on isolated vascular smooth muscle, 198–199
        microcirculation, 198
    pituitary-adrenal secretion, circadian rhythm of, 128–129
    plasma 11-hydroxycorticosteroids, circadian rhythm of, 129
    plasma 11-hydroxycorticosteroids in circadian periodicity, effect of dexamethasone administration on, 131–132
    plasma 17-hydroxycorticosteroids, circadian rhythm of, 128
    relation to skeletal muscle function, 245–261
        steroid myopathy, 252–254
    relative thymolytic and glycogenic activities of, 233–234
    role in blood volume regulation, 199
    role in function of visual system, 225
    role in gustation, 209–217, 225–227
        detection and recognition in states of corticosteroid excess, 216–217
        detection thresholds in adrenal cortical insufficiency, 210–213
        recognition-detection relationships, 216
        recognition of tastes in adrenal cortical insufficiency, 214–216
    role in hearing, 221–225
        detection and recognition in Cushing's syndrome, 224–225
        detection thresholds in adrenal cortical insufficiency, 221–223
    role in olfaction, 218–221
        detection in Cushing's syndrome, 220–221
        detection thresholds in adrenal cortical insufficiency, 218–220
    role in sensory processes, 209–230
    role in touch and pain stimuli, 225
    secretion of, regulation of, 41–53
    secretion of, ultrastructural changes in adrenal cortex in relation to, 32–36
    secretion stimulated by ACTH, theories on mode of action of, 69–76
        activation of glucose 6-phosphate dehydrogenase, 70–71
        availability of energy, 70–71
        control of cofactor entrance into mitochondria, 72–73
        control of product removal from mitochondria, 73–74
        control of substrate entrance into mitochondria, 72
        direct activation of mitochondrial enzymes by cyclic AMP, 75
        increased permeability of cells to glucose, 70
        increased permeability of mitochondria, 71–74
        phosphorylase activation, 70
        substrate utilization by mitochondria, 71

synthesis of protein related to stimulation of secretion by ACTH, 74–75
structure-activity relations of, 264, 265
Adrenal cortex hyperfunction
see also Cushing's syndrome
relation to resting rate of glucocorticoid secretion, 137–138
taste detection and recognition in, 216–217
Adrenal cortex hypofunction
see also Addison's disease
auditory detection thresholds in, 221–223
chronic, cardiovascular consequences of, 191–195
blood volume reduction, 194–195
cardiac changes, 192–194
peripheral vasculature changes, 194
olfactory detection thresholds in, 218–220
speech discrimination ability in patients with, 223–224
taste detection thresholds in, 210–213
taste recognition thresholds in, 214–216
Adrenal cortex neoplasms
causing cortisol excess, 276–277
Adrenal gland
see also Adrenal cortex; Adrenal medulla
as essential for life, 2–3
development of, relation to control of medullary epinephrine biosynthesis by cortex, 358–359
monoamine oxidase in, 689
Adrenal gland vasculature
capsular and intracapsular vessels, 286–291
arteriae corticis and cortical capillaries, 287
arteriae medullae and medullary capillaries, 287–289
arterial and venous plexuses, 286, 287
central vein and medullary veins, 289–291
stereogram models of central vein of human adrenal, 290
venogram of human adrenal, 289
venous tree, 288, 289
extraglandular blood vessels, 283–286
adrenal vein, 289
in cat, 284
in dog, 284, 285
in macaque, 284–285
in man, 285–286
in rabbit, 283–284
in rat, 283
factors affecting adrenal blood flow, 291–292
regional distribution of blood in medulla, functional significance of, 292
Adrenal medulla
see also Chromaffin cells
arteriae medullae and medullary capillaries, 287–289
as essential for life, 3
biosynthesis of catecholamines, control by adrenal cortex, 357–366
anatomic relationship between cortex and medulla in, 357–358
catecholamine content in warm-acclimated rats exposed to cold, 646
enzyme changes during cold exposure and cold acclimatization, 648–649
intracellular recording with microelectrodes in, 372–374
depolarization in response to acetylcholine, 373
inward Na and Ca currents, 374
resting transmembrane potentials, 373
maturation in fetus, effects of fetal adrenal cortex on, 112
medullary veins, 289–291
regional distribution of blood in, functional significance of, 292
Adrenal medullary secretion
see also Catecholamines; Epinephrine secretion; Norepinephrine secretion
basal secretion, splanchnic denervation, and supersensitivity, 370
deprivation of, effects on eye, 580
excitation-secretion coupling, 401–418
chromaffin cell energy metabolism in relation to secretion, 407
chromaffin cell motility, 402
effects of drugs on secretion, 407–411
electrophysiology of adrenomedullary cell in relation to secretion, 402–403
factors that may determine amount of material secreted in response to stimulus, 401–402
general hypotheses for, 415–418
ionic requirements for secretion, 403–407
mechanism of, adaptability to homeostatic demands, 418
mechanism of membrane fusion, 414–415
relevance of catecholamine release from isolated storage vesicles to study of chromaffin cell secretion, 411–414
hormone discharge, functional significance of, 311–312
hormone discharge, stimulation of, 312–316
by asphyxia and anoxia, 313–314
by cold, heat, and pH, 313
by emotional stress, 312–313
by glucagon, 315
by hypoglycemia, 314–315
by hypotension, 314
by naturally occurring substances, 315–316
by physical stress, 313
in acclimatization to cold, 641–642
ions and stimulus-secretion coupling, 374–379
Ca, essential and sufficient for responses to acetylcholine, 375–376
Ca itself as secretagogue, 376–377
K lack and potentiation of basal and evoked secretion, 378
K stimulates and also requires Ca, 376
Mg inhibition of responses to acetylcholine, K, Ca, Sr, and Ba, 377–378
Na lack and potentiation of basal and evoked secretion, 378
prolonged Na deprivation causing inhibition, 379
Sr and Ba as Ca substitutes and stimulants, 377
stimulant effect of ouabain, 378–379
lack of secretion produced by various methods, consequences in animals exposed to cold, 650–655
effects of adrenalectomy, 651
effects of adrenergic blocking agents, 654–655
effects of demedullation, 650–651
effects of ganglionic-blocking agents, 653–654
effects of guanethidine, 653
effects of immunosympathectomy, 651–652
effects of reserpine, 652–653
mechanism of, 389–426
by increased amine outflow from storage vesicle into cytoplasm, 391–392
by increased permeability of plasma membrane to catecholamines, 391
direct extrusion of catecholamine storage vesicle content into extracellular space, 392–397
physiological mechanisms of control of, 309–319
central nerve pathway, 310–311
epinephrine and norepinephrine levels at various ages, 310
peripheral nerve pathway, 309
selective release, 310
quantal secretion of catecholamines, 399–400
release of newly synthesized catecholamines, 400–401
response of animals to exposure to cold, 639–640
responses to stimulation of splanchnic nerves, 368–370
frequency-response relations, 369
preferential secretion of epinephrine and norepinephrine, 370, 371–372
spatial recruitment, overlap, and convergence, 369
splanchnic-adrenal fatigue, 369–370

Adrenal medullary secretion (continued)
  role in thermogenesis, 649–655
  role of depolarization in, 379–380
  secretomotor control of, 367–388
    acetylcholine receptors, 371–372
    Ca inactivation and termination of secretory responses, 380–381
    cholinergic nature of secretomotor fibers, 370–371
    historical background, 367–368
    membrane and ionic events in, 381–382
    nicotinic and muscarinic receptors, 371
    secretagogues other than acetylcholine, 372
    stimulus-secretion coupling, parallels with excitation-contraction coupling, 382–383
  subcellular origin of, 390–401
    apocrine or holocrine secretion, 390–391
    fate of storage vesicle membrane, 397–399
Adrenalectomy
  carbohydrate stores in rats after, effects of cortisol treatment on, 136–137
  causing decrease in urinary glucose and urinary nitrogen in fasting depancreatized cats, 138
  causing disturbance in vital functions, replacement of adrenal secretion by administered corticosteroids, 136
  causing reduction in blood volume, 194–195
  circulatory changes in cats 10 days after, 191–192
  effect on animals exposed to cold, 651
  effect on body composition of rats fed ad libitum or force-fed, 141
  effect on glycine incorporation into protein of isolated diaphragm, 148
  effect on histidine incorporation into protein fraction of diaphragms, 147
  effect on responses of livers from fed rats to gluconeogenic agents, 156, 157
  effect on urinary nonprotein nitrogen excretions and body weights of rats fed medium carbohydrate diet, 139
  glucose turnover in postabsorptive state in dogs after, 142
Adrenaline: see Epinephrine
Adrenergic receptors
  attempts at chemical definition of, 448–449
  classification of, 450–452
    in selected tissues, 452, 453
  in cardiovascular system, 455–461
    blood vessels, 458–461
    coronary arteries, 459–460
    heart, 455–458
    pulmonary vessels, 460–461
    veins, 459
  in central nervous system, 464–465
  in nonvascular smooth muscle, 461–463
    gastrointestinal, 461–462
    iris, 462
    nictitating membrane, 462
    respiratory tract, 463
    spleen, 462
    uterus, 462–463
  in skeletal muscle, 463–464
  mediation of action of catecholamines on skeletal muscles, 540–541
  mediation of skin gland secretions in amphibians, 465
  role in action of catecholamines on gastrointestinal motility, 517–519
  role in melanophore responses of skin, 465
  role in sympathoadrenal responses, 466–467
  that subserve metabolic responses, 452–455
    calorigenesis, 455
    carbohydrate metabolism, 453–454
    lipid metabolism, 454–455
Adrenocortical insufficiency: see Adrenal cortex hypofunction
Adrenocortical-stimulating hormone: see Corticotropin

Adrenocortical zonation
  see also Zona fasciculata; Zona glomerulosa; Zona reticularis
  cell migration theory of, 14–15
    adrenal regeneration, 15
    distribution of mitoses within adrenal cortex, 14
    migration of labeled cells, 15
    origin of glomerulosa cells from capsular fibroblasts, 14–15
    site of cell death, 15
  theories of, 13–14
  transformation field theory, 20
  zonal theory of, 15–20
    ACTH effect on zones, 18–19
    histochemical evidence, 18–19
    morphological bases for considering inner zones as distinct functional unit, 17
    morphological bases for considering zona glomerulosa as distinct functional unit, 15–16
    role of zona reticularis in androgen secretion, 19
    steroid production by inner zones, 17–18
    steroid production by zona glomerulosa, 16–17
Adrenocorticotropic hormone: see Corticotropin
Adrenomedullary secretion: see Adrenal medullary secretion
Aldosterone
  biosynthesis from pregnenolone, 56–58
  complexes with human serum proteins, 118–119
  direct effects on skeletal muscle, 248–249
  effect on body weight and on Na and K excretion in normal humans, 180–181
  effect on muscle electrolytes, 182–183
  effect on renal Na transport, mechanism of action, 185–186
  research use only, 10
Aldosterone secretion
  altered electrolyte metabolism and, 89–95
    effects of altered plasma Na level, 93
    effects of K intake and altered plasma K levels, 93–95
    effects of Mg deficiency, 95
    effects of Na intake and depletion, 89–93
  anterior pituitary gland and, 95–97
    effect of ACTH administration, 81
    effects of hypophysectomy, 95
    possible role of adenohypophysial hormones other than ACTH, 97
    role of ACTH, 95–97
  circadian rhythm of, 132–133
  regulation of, 77–106
    effects of estrogens, progesterone, oral contraceptives, and erythropoietin, 97–98
    evidence for humoral mechanism in, 78
    possible neural mechanisms, 98–99
    role of possible hepatic hormone, 98
  regulation of, role of renin-angiotensin system, 78–89
    early evidence of relation of adrenal cortex to kidney, 80
    effect of angiotensin II injection, 80–82
    evidence as primary control mechanism, 80–83
    factors regulating renin secretion, 85–88
    in lower vertebrates, 83–84
    juxtaglomerular apparatus, 84–85
    locus of secretion and chemical nature of aldosterone-stimulating agent, 78–80
    negative feedback mechanism in, 88–89
    renin origin from juxtaglomerular cells, 85
Amino acids
  composition of chromaffin granule proteins, 325
  net transfer from peripheral tissues to liver in rats with glucocorticoid excess, 145–151
Amphenone
  inhibition of biosynthesis of corticosteroids, 62
Androgens
  see also Testosterone
  secretion by adrenal cortex, role of zona reticularis in, 19

Anencephalus
  human anencephalic monsters, adrenal gland size in, 109
Anesthetics
  effects on plasma catecholamines, 436–437
Angiotensin II
  see also Renin-angiotensin system
  injection of, effect on adrenal cortex hormone secretion, 80–82
  interaction with corticosteroids in regulation of circulatory function, 200, 201
  stimulation of adrenal cortical secretory activity, 43
Anoxia
  hypoxia causing changes in plasma catecholamines, 432–433
  hypoxia causing stimulation of catecholamine release from adrenals, 438–439
  of respiratory center as possible explanation for epinephrine-induced apnea, 491–492
  stimulation of adrenal medullary secretion, 314
Ascorbic acid
  role in biosynthesis and catabolism of adrenal catecholamines, 363
Asphyxia
  stimulation of adrenal medullary secretion, 313–314
ATPase: see Adenosine triphosphatase
Audition: see Hearing

Barium
  as Ca substitute and stimulant in adrenal medullary secretion, 377
Biological assay
  of catecholamines in blood, 428
  of corticotropin-releasing factor, 43–44
  of glucocorticoids by measurement of effect on carbohydrate metabolism, 136–137
Blood cells
  see also Blood platelets; Lymphocytes
  responses to inflammation, effects of glucocorticoids on, 266
Blood chemical analysis
  assay of catecholamines, 427–428
Blood circulation
  adrenal blood flow, factors affecting, 291–292
  hemodynamic changes in cats 10 days after bilateral adrenalectomy, 191–192
  microcirculatory effects of corticosteroids, 198
  regional distribution of blood in adrenal medulla, functional significance of, 292
Blood platelets
  role in inflammation, effect of cortisone on, 268
Blood pressure
  effect of corticosteroid administration on, 197–198
  hypotension causing change in plasma catecholamines, 433–434
  hypotension causing increase in adrenal medullary secretion, 314
  hypotension causing stimulation of catecholamine release from adrenals, 439
  in relation to resting plasma norepinephrine levels in man, 429, 430
Blood proteins
  binding of corticosteroids, 117–125
    association constants for hormone complexes with α_1-acid glycoprotein, 117–118
    binding phenomenon, 117–118
    complexes in human serum, 118–119
    concentration of binding sites and apparent association constants of steroid-CBG complexes in mammalian sera, 120
    corticosterone-binding activity and corticosterone levels in developing rats, 121
    endocrine influences on, 121–123
    high-affinity binding of cortisol in sera of different species, 120
    influence of corticosteroids on corticosteroid-binding globulin levels, 122–123
    influence of gonadal hormones on, 121–122
    influence of thyrotrophin and thyroxine on, 123
    significance of, 123–124
Blood sugar
  see also Hypoglycemia
  level in fasting rats, effect of prednisolone injection on, 144
  level in sheep, effect of cortisol on, 144
Blood vessels
  see also Adrenal gland vasculature; Gastrointestinal vasculature
  adrenergic receptors in, 458–461
  permeability in inflammation, effect of glucocorticoids on, 265–266
  regional vascular beds, effects of catecholamines on, 476–480
    cerebral vessels, 478
    coronary vessels, 479
    cutaneous vessels, 478
    muscle vessels, 476–478
    pulmonary vessels, 479–480
    renal vessels, 478–479
    splanchnic and hepatic vessels, 479
    veins, 480
Blood volume
  reduction in adrenal insufficiency, 194–195
  regulation of, role of corticosteroids in, 199
Body composition
  changes in normal and adrenalectomized rats fed ad libitum or force-fed, 141
Body temperature
  acclimatization to cold, role of adrenal medulla in, 641–642
  adrenal medulla role in exposure to cold, 639–640
  in cold-acclimated animals, 649–650
  regulation on exposure to cold, 637–642
  thermogenesis, role of secreted catecholamines in, 649–655
    calorigenic effect of catecholamines, 455, 649–650
    consequences of lack of secretion or lack of action of catecholamines, 650–655
    shivering and nonshivering thermogenesis, 637, 638, 639, 641, 642, 643, 644, 656–659
Bone and bones
  electrolyte metabolism in, effect of corticosteroids on, 183
Brain
  blood vessels of, effects of catecholamines on, 478
Bronchi
  effects of α-adrenoceptor stimulant drugs on, 509–510
  effects of β-adrenoceptor stimulant drugs on, 509
  effects of catecholamines on smooth muscle of, 507–513
    actions of blood-borne catecholamines, 510
    direct in vivo methods of study, 508
    in vitro methods of study, 508
    indirect in vivo methods of study, 508–509
  innervation of smooth muscle of, 507–508
  nature of sympathetic nervous transmitters to smooth muscle of, 510–511

Calcium
  activation of phosphorylase kinase, 609
  as secretagogue on adrenal medulla, 376–377
  essential and sufficient for adrenal medullary secretion in response to acetylcholine, 375–376
  inactivation of, in termination of adrenal medullary secretory responses, 380–381
  renal excretion of, effect of corticosteroids on, 181–182
  requirements for adrenomedullary secretion of catecholamines, 403–407
  role in muscle contraction, 612–622
    Ca and contractile proteins, 613–614
    Ca release by sarcoplasmic reticulum, 617–618
    Ca transport by cell membrane, 621–622
    Ca uptake by sarcoplasmic reticulum, 618–619
    cellular Ca flux, 614–615
    mitochondria and Ca sequestration, 619–621

Calcium (continued)
　role in excitation-contraction coupling, 615–617
Carbohydrate metabolism
　see also Gluconeogenesis; Glycogen metabolism; Glycogenolysis
　influence of corticosteroids on, 135–167
　　carbohydrate stores of fasted adrenalectomized rats after treatment with cortisol, 136–137
　　glucocorticoids and skeletal muscle, 249–251
　　gross interrelationship of whole-animal carbohydrate and protein metabolism in glucocorticoid effects, 138–141
　　urinary nonprotein N excretions and body weights of rats fed medium carbohydrate diet, effect of adrenalectomy, 139
　　use in bioassay of glucocorticoids, 136–137
　　modifications caused by glucocorticoid deficiency and excess, physiological mechanisms for, 141–163
　　　changes in secretion of epinephrine, 141–142
　　　changes in secretion of insulin, 142–145
　　　consequences of decreased appetite in glucocorticoid deficiency, 141
　　　oxidative decarboxylation of pyruvate, 162–163
　role of adrenal cortex in, 6–7
Carbon dioxide
　hypercapnia causing change in plasma catecholamines, 433
Cardiac glycosides
　interaction with corticosteroids in regulation of circulatory function, 200, 201–202
Cardiovascular system
　see also Blood vessels; Heart; Myocardium
　adrenergic receptors in, 455–461
　consequences of chronic adrenocortical insufficiency, 191–195
　　blood volume reduction, 194–195
　　cardiac changes, 192–194
　　peripheral vasculature changes, 194
　effects of catecholamines on, 473–489
　　on cardiac function, 480–486
　　on regional vascular beds, 476–480
　　relative importance of circulating catecholamines and of sympathetic innervation, 475–476
　effects of corticosteroids on, 197–203
　　blood pressure and vascular resistance, 197–198
　　effects on isolated vascular smooth muscle, 198–199
　　interaction with catecholamines, renin, angiotensin II, cardiac glycosides, and kinins in regulation of circulatory function, 199–202
　　peripheral vascular effects, 197–199
　　role in blood volume regulation, 199
　hemodynamic changes in cats 10 days after bilateral adrenalectomy, 191–192
Catechol-O-methyltransferase
　activity during periods of development and during physiologically induced changes, 671
　assays of, 671
　distribution of, 671
　inhibitors of, 670–671
　O-methylation of catecholamines in vivo, 671–673
　properties of, 669–670
　substrate specificity of, 670
Catecholamine biosynthesis
　see also Epinephrine biosynthesis; Norepinephrine biosynthesis
　by adrenal medulla, control by adrenal cortex, 357–366
　by adrenal medulla, role of ascorbic acid, 363
　inhibitors of, effects on animals exposed to cold, 655
　pathway of, 341–342
　　changes in enzymes of pathway during cold exposure and cold acclimatization, 648–649
　　enzymes of pathway, 342–346
　role of chromaffin granules, 334–335

Catecholamine secretion
　see also Epinephrine secretion; Norepinephrine secretion
　excitation-secretion coupling, 401–418
　　chromaffin cell energy metabolism in relation to secretion, 407
　　chromaffin cell motility, 402
　　effects of drugs on secretion, 407–411
　　electrophysiology of adrenomedullary cell in relation to secretion, 402–403
　　factors that may determine amount of material secreted in response to stimulus, 401–402
　　general hypotheses for, 415–418
　　ionic requirements for secretion, 403–407
　　mechanism of, adaptability to homeostatic demands, 418
　　mechanism of membrane fusion, 414–415
　　relevance of catecholamine release from isolated storage vesicles to study of adrenal chromaffin cell secretion, 411–414
　in fetus and chemoreceptor stimulation of respiration at birth, 501–502
　mechanism of, 389–426
　　by increased amine outflow from storage vesicle into cytoplasm, 391–392
　　by increased permeability of plasma membrane to catecholamines, 391
　　direct extrusion of catecholamine storage vesicle content into extracellular space, 392–397
　quantal secretion from adrenal medulla, 399–400
　release of newly synthesized catecholamines from adrenal gland, 400–401
　subcellular origin of, 390–401
　　apocrine or holocrine secretion, 390–391
　　fate of storage vesicle membrane, 397–399
Catecholamines
　see also Dopamine; Epinephrine; Norepinephrine
　calorigenic effect of, 455
　　in cold-acclimated animals, 649–650
　catabolism of, role of ascorbic acid in, 363
　content and distribution in rabbit adrenals, effect of insulin treatment on, 397
　content in adrenal medulla of warm-acclimated rats exposed to cold, 646
　content in extraadrenal chromaffin tissue of fetus, 359
　direct action on skeletal muscle fibers, 537–545
　　changes in electrical properties, 542–544
　　in excess K environment, 539–540
　　in fast muscles, 537–538
　　in low-K environment, 540
　　in normal ionic environment, 537–539
　　in slow muscles, 538–539
　　influence of low temperature on, 541–542
　　influence of ouabain on, 541
　　mechanism of action, 544–545
　　mediation by adrenoreceptors, 540–541
　effects on bronchial smooth muscle, 507–513
　　actions of blood-borne catecholamines, 510
　　direct in vivo methods of study, 508
　　in vitro methods of study, 508
　　indirect in vivo methods of study, 508–509
　effects on cardiac function, 480–486
　　inotropic effects on heart-lung preparation, 484–485
　　inotropic effects on isolated papillary muscle preparation, 482–484
　　on conduction velocity, 482
　　on heart rate, electrophysiological studies, 480–482
　　on myocardial oxygen usage, 485–486
　effects on cardiovascular system, 473–489
　　on cerebral vessels, 478
　　on coronary vessels, 479
　　on cutaneous vessels, 478
　　on muscle blood vessels, 476–478
　　on pulmonary vessels, 479–480

on regional vascular beds, 476–480
on renal vessels, 478–479
on splanchnic and hepatic vessels, 479
on veins, 480
relative importance of circulating catecholamines and of sympathetic innervation, 475–476
effects on gastric acid secretion and on mucous secretion, 521
effects on gastrointestinal absorption, 521–522
effects on gastrointestinal motility, 516–519
general considerations, 516
on muscularis mucosae, 517
on nonsphincter muscle, 516
on receptor sites, 517–519
on sphincter muscle, 516–517
effects on gastrointestinal vasculature, 519–521
dilator effects, 520
duration of action, 520–521
general observations, 519
local reactions, 520
effects on neuromuscular transmission, 545–550
facilitatory action, 545–546
inhibitory action, 546
mechanism of increase of transmitter release, 548–549
on end-plate potential, 546–547
on miniature end-plate potential, 547–548
effects on respiratory reflexes, 500
excretion in animals exposed to cold, 642–646
sources of, 646
extraneuronal uptake of, 717–718
role in inactivation of circulating catecholamines, 719–720
factors causing change in plasma levels of, 431–435
disease, 435
hemorrhage and hypotension, 433–434
hypercapnia and acidemia, 433
hypoglycemia, 432
hypoxia, 432–433
mental activity and emotional stress, 434–435
muscular work, 434
myocardial infarction, 435
temperature changes, 434
function of monoamine oxidase in relation to, 689–690
in adrenal venous blood, resting secretion, 437
in adrenal venous blood, stimulated release of, 437–440
by cholinergic drugs, 438
by electrical stimulation, 438
by histamine, 439
by hypoglycemia, 438
by hypoxia, 438–439
by polypeptides and other substances, 439–440
in blood, 427–445, 699–712
adrenergic nerves as source of, 525
assay methods, 427–428
disappearance from blood, 702–703
disposition of, 707–708
effects of anesthetics on, 436–437
effects of drugs on, 435–437
effects of nicotine on, 436
inactivation of, 713
inactivation of, role of uptake processes in, 718–720
influence on central nervous system, 667–668
metabolic transformations, 700–702
origination from all parts of body by virtue of sympathetic innervation to various organs and to vascular smooth muscle, 440
peripheral plasma concentrations, 428–430
plasma concentrations after administration of catecholamines, 431
plasma levels and relation to sensitivity of gastrointestinal structures, 526–528
properties of catecholamine uptake processes in peripheral tissues, 715–718
quantitative aspects of metabolism of, 705–707

role in relation to role of locally-released catecholamines, 525–526
sites of removal from blood, 703–705
uptake by peripheral tissues, 713–715
in lung tissue, 510
increased circulating levels in various conditions, effect on gut, 522–524
exercise, 523–524
intense emotion, 523
pheochromocytoma, 524
shock, 522–523
interaction with corticosteroids in regulation of circulatory function, 200–201
locally released and circulating catecholamines, relative roles of, 525–526
mechanism of action in animals exposed to cold, 655–659
development of adaptation for nonshivering thermogenesis, 658–659
mobilization of substrates, 656
nonshivering thermogenesis, 657–658
reduction of heat loss, 656
shivering thermogenesis, 656–657
O-methylation by COMT in vivo, 671–673
possible involvement in peptic ulceration, 524
relation to eye, 553–590
metabolism, uptake, storage, and release by eye, 555–557
role in control of sweat glands, 592–601
in Bovidae, 597–598
in Camelidae, 598–599
in Canidae, 599
in Equidae, 595–597
in Felidae, 599
in man, 592–595
in other anthropoid primates, 595
in prosimian primates, 595
in Rhinocerotidae, 597
in rodents, 599
in Suidae, 598
phylogenetic basis for, 599–601
stimulation of respiration, physiological significance of, 500–501
storage in chromaffin granules, possible mechanisms of, 328–334
active uptake into granules, 331–333
formation of high-molecular-weight aggregates, 330
macromolecular storage complex, 329–331
maintenance of store, 333–334
permeability of granule membrane, 328–329
role of ATP, 328, 330–334
uptake by sympathetic nerves, 715–717
role in inactivation of circulating catecholamines, 718–719
CBG: see Corticosteroid-binding globulin
Cell division
distribution of mitoses within adrenal cortex, relation to cell migration theory of zonation, 14
Central nervous system
see also Brain
adrenergic receptors in, 464–465
central adrenergic pathway inhibiting ACTH secretion, 49–50
central effects of epinephrine and norepinephrine as possible explanation for their induction of hyperpnea, 494–495
central pathway in control of adrenal medullary secretion, 310–311
influence of circulating catecholamines on, 667–668
possible neural mechanisms in regulation of aldosterone secretion, 98–99
Cholesterol
biosynthesis and metabolism of, inhibitors causing inhibition of biosynthesis of corticosteroids, 63
biosynthesis from squalene, 55–56

Cholesterol (continued)
  biosynthesis in placenta, 60–61
  conversion to pregnenolone, 56, 57
Cholinergic drugs
  stimulation of catecholamine release from adrenals, 438
Chromaffin cells
  see also Chromaffin granules
  as model system for stimulus-secretion coupling, 383
  depolarizing effect of acetylcholine on, 373
  electrical properties of, 374
  energy metabolism in relation to adrenomedullary
      secretion of catecholamines, 407
  extraadrenal tissue in fetus, catecholamine content of, 359
  function of, 336
  motility in relation to excitation-secretion coupling, 402
  secretion by, relevance of catecholamine release from isolated
      storage vesicles to study of, 411–414
  subcellular dynamics of, 335–336
  subcellular fractions of, centrifugation scheme for
      obtaining of, 322
  ultrastructure of, 295–308
    endoplasmic reticulum, 295, 297, 298
    epinephrine-storing cells, 296, 297, 299–301
    exocytosis profiles at cell-to-cell apposed surface,
        302–306
    exocytosis profiles at free cell surface, 301, 302, 303
    exocytosis profiles, schematic representation of, 307
    general organization of cell, 295–297
    norepinephrine-storing cells, 297–300
    presence of coated pits in granule membrane fused with
        plasma membrane, 301, 302, 303, 305–306
    secretory vesicles, 297–302
Chromaffin granules
  catecholamine storage in, possible mechanisms of, 328–334
    active uptake of catecholamines into granules,
        331–333
    formation of high-molecular-weight aggregates, 330
    macromolecular storage complex, 329–331
    maintenance of store, 333–334
    permeability of granule membrane, 328–329
    role of ATP, 328, 330–334
  composition of, 323–327
    adenine nucleotides in granules from different species,
        324, 330
    amino acid composition of proteins in granules, 325
    characteristic constituents of microsomal fraction, 323
    chromogranins and chrommembrins, 324–327
    lipids, 327
    nucleotides, 324
    phospholipids, 327
    proteins, 324–327
    specific constituents of bovine granules, 324
  dynamic role of, 334–336
    biosynthesis of catecholamines, 334–335
    secretion of its products, 335–336
    storage of secretory products, 334
  heterogeneity of, 327–328
    differences between amine storage pools in
        bovine granules, 328
  isolation from adrenal chromaffin cells, 321–323
    components of large granule fraction, 321–323
    components of microsomal fraction, 323
Circadian rhythm
  of aldosterone secretion, 132–133
  of cortisol secretion, 127–128
    alterations in circadian rhythm, 130–132
    relation to activity-sleep cycle, 130–131
  of pituitary-adrenal secretion, 128–129
  of plasma ACTH and cortisol in normal subjects, 128
  of plasma 11-hydroxycorticosteroids and ACTH, 129
  of plasma 11-hydroxycorticosteroids, effect of
      dexamethasone administration on, 131–132
  of plasma 17-hydroxycorticosteroids, 128
  of testosterone and estrogen plasma levels, 133
Coenzymes
  acetyl coenzyme A, conversion to squalene, 55, 56
Cold
  adaptation to, 637–642
    adrenal medulla role in acclimatization, 641–642, 660–661
    enzyme changes in adrenal medulla during,
        648–649
    mechanisms on exposure to cold, 637
    nature of acclimatization, 637–639
  effect on catecholamine action on skeletal muscles, 541–542
  exposure to, mechanism of action of secreted
      catecholamines in, 655–659
    development of adaptation for nonshivering thermogenesis,
        658–659
    mobilization of substrates, 656
    nonshivering thermogenesis, 657–658
    reduction of heat loss, 656
    shivering thermogenesis, 656–657
  exposure to, role of adrenal medulla in, 639–640, 659–660
    consequences of lack of secretion or lack of action of
        catecholamines, 650–655
    enzyme changes in adrenal medulla during,
        648–649
  stimulation of hormone discharge from adrenal medulla,
      313
Compound E: see Cortisone
COMT: see Catechol-O-methyltransferase
Connective tissue
  interaction with corticosteroids, 267–268
Contraceptives, oral
  effect on aldosterone secretion, 98
Coronary vessels
  adrenergic receptors in, 459–460
  effects of catecholamines on, 479
Corticosteroid-binding globulin
  association constants of steroid complexes with, 118, 119–120
  concentration of binding sites and apparent association
      constants of steroid-CBG complexes in mammalian
      sera, 120
  endocrine influences on serum levels of, 121–123
    corticosteroids, 122–123
    gonadal hormones, 121–122
    thyrotrophin and thyroxine, 123
  physicochemical properties of corticosteroid complexes of,
      119–120
Corticosteroids: see Adrenal cortex hormones
Corticosterone
  binding activity and levels in sera of developing
      rats, 121
  complexes with human serum proteins, 118–119
  preincubation of intact diaphragms of adrenalectomized rats
      with, effect on methionine incorporation
      into protein, 148
Corticosterone secretion
  stimulation by ACTH, 41–43
    mode of action of ACTH, 42
    receptor reserve and sensitivity of adrenal cortex
        cells, 42
    regulatory role of adenohypophysis, 41
    response to graded doses of ACTH, 128
    structure-activity relationships of ACTH, 42–43
    temporal aspects of secretory response of adrenal cortex, 42
  stimulation by factors of questionable physiological
      significance, 43
Corticotropin
  see also Corticotropin secretion
  administration of, effect on aldosterone secretion, 80
  effect on zones of adrenal cortex, 18–19
  graded doses of, effect on corticosterone secretion, 128

role in epinephrine biosynthesis by adrenal medulla, 359–361
role in regulation of aldosterone secretion, 95–97
stimulation of corticosterone and hydrocortisone secretion, 41–43
  mode of action of, 42
  receptor reserve and sensitivity of adrenal cortex cells, 42
  regulatory role of adenohypophysis, 41
  structure-activity relationships of ACTH, 42–43
  temporal aspects of secretory response of adrenal cortex, 42
stimulation of secretory activity of adrenal cortex, theories on mode of action of, 69–76
  activation of glucose 6-phosphate dehydrogenase, 70–71
  availability of energy, 70–71
  control of cofactor entrance into mitochondria, 72–73
  control of product removal from mitochondria, 73–74
  control of substrate entrance into mitochondria, 72
  direct activation of mitochondrial enzymes by cyclic AMP, 75
  increased permeability of cells to glucose, 70
  increased permeability of mitochondria, 71–74
  phosphorylase activation, 70
  substrate utilization by mitochondria, 71
  synthesis of protein related to stimulation of secretion by ACTH, 74–75
Corticotropin-releasing factor
  ACTH secretion inhibition by short-loop feedback of ACTH on, 49
  bioassay of, 43–44
  hypothalamic CRF, 44–45
  neurohypophysial CRF, 45–46
  regulation of ACTH secretion, 129–130
  tissue CRF, extrahypothalamic production of, 46
Corticotropin secretion
  diurnal variation in plasma levels in relation to cortisol levels, 128
  inhibition by central inhibitory adrenergic pathway, 49–50
  inhibition by corticosteroids, 46–49
    concentration of corticosteroid and degree of inhibition of ACTH secretion, 48
    kinetics of, 48–49
    relation between structure of corticosteroid and inhibitory potency, 49
    sites of inhibitory actions, 47–48
  inhibition by short-loop feedback of ACTH on corticotropin-releasing factor, 49
  physiologically inappropriate secretion, causing syndrome of cortisol excess in man, 271–272
  plasma levels, circadian periodicity of, 129
  regulation by corticotropin-releasing factor, 129–130
  stimulation of, 43–46
    by corticotropin-releasing factors, 43–46
    by hypothalamic corticotropin-releasing factor, 44–45
    by tissue extrahypothalamic corticotropin-releasing factor, 46
    by vasopressin, 45–46
Cortisol: see Hydrocortisone
Cortisol excess syndromes: see Hydrocortisone secretion
Cortisone
  early use of, 9, 10
  effect on histidine incorporation into protein fraction of diaphragms from adrenalectomized rats, 147
  effect on lysosomes during inflammatory process, 268
  effect on nitrogen distribution in organs and in blood and liver constituents of adrenalectomized, protein-depleted rats, 145–146
  effect on platelet role in inflammatory process, 268
  long-term effects on liver composition in fed rats, 146, 147
  short-term effects on liver composition in fed rats, 146
CRF: see Corticotropin-releasing factor

Cushing's syndrome
  auditory detection and recognition in, 224–225
  lipid deposition changes in adipose tissue during treatment with glucocorticoids, 172
  olfactory detection in, 220–221
Cyanoketone
  inhibition of biosynthesis of corticosteroids, 63
Cyclic AMP: see Adenosine monophosphate, cyclic

Dactinomycin
  effect on recovery of glucose oxidation from dexamethasone inhibition in adipose tissue, 171
o,p'-DDD
  inhibition of biosynthesis of corticosteroids, 63
Dehydrogenases
  in biosynthesis of corticosteroids, 59–60
Depolarization
  role in evocation of adrenal medullary secretion, 379–380
Dexamethasone
  effect on circadian periodicity of plasma 11-hydroxycorticosteroids, 131–132
  effect on incorporation of lactate carbon into glucose by perfused livers from adrenalectomized rats, 153
  inhibition of glucose oxidation in adipose tissue, effect of dactinomycin on recovery of, 171
  ketogenic effects in pancreatectomized, hypophysectomized rats, 172, 173
Dihydropteridine reductase
  in pathway of epinephrine biosynthesis, 344
L-Dopa
  inhibition of ACTH secretion, 49–50
Dopa decarboxylase
  in pathway of epinephrine biosynthesis, 344–345
  inhibitors of, effects on animals exposed to cold, 655
Dopamine
  content in blood, 430
  in mammalian lung, 510
  quantitative aspects of metabolism of, 706, 707
Dopamine β-hydroxylase
  adrenal activity, regulation by adrenal cortex, 362–363
  content and distribution in rabbit adrenals, effect of insulin treatment on, 397
  in pathway of epinephrine biosynthesis, 345–346, 348, 350–351
Drugs
  effects on adrenomedullary secretion of catecholamines, 407–411

Electric potentials
  resting transmembrane potentials in adrenal medulla, intracellular recording of, 373
Electrical stimulation
  of catecholamine release from adrenal gland, 438
Electrocardiography
  effects of corticosteroids on, 197
Electrolyte metabolism
  adrenal cortex role in, history of, 5–6
  altered metabolism, effects on aldosterone secretion, 89–95
  effect of corticosteroids on, 179–189
    in bone, 183
    in gastrointestinal tract, 183–184
    in kidney, 179–182
    in muscle, 182–183, 247–248
    in salivary glands, 182
    in sweat glands, 182
Emotional stress
  causing changes in plasma catecholamines, 434–435
  intense situations causing increased levels of circulating catecholamines, effects on gut, 523
  stimulation of hormone discharge from adrenal medulla, 312–313

Endoplasmic reticulum
  of adrenal cortex, electron microscopy of, 25, 26, 27, 28, 30, 31
    changes in relation to hormone secretion, 32–36
  of chromaffin cells, 295, 297, 298
Enzymes
  involved in corticosteroid biosynthesis, distribution in adrenal cortex, 60
Epinephrine
  content in normal human plasma, 428–430
  content in plasma of various experimental animals, 430
  control of glycogenolysis in intact cardiac muscle, 611–612
  control of glycogenolysis in intact skeletal muscle, 610–611
  control of glycogenolysis in muscle, in vitro studies, 607–610
    activation of phosphorylase kinase by Ca^{2+}, 609
    activation of phosphorylase kinase by cyclic AMP, 608–609
    enzyme reactions involved in, 607–608
    integrated control of phosphorylase activity, 610
    phosphorylase kinase phosphatase, 609–610
    phosphorylase phosphatase, 608
    regulatory properties and interconversion of phosphorylase b and a, 608
  disappearance after iv injection of, 714
  effects on cyclic AMP levels in perfused livers of normal and adrenalectomized rats, 153
  effects on electromechanical properties of cardiac muscle, 623–624
  effects on fast-contracting skeletal muscles, 537–538
  effects on isolated cardiac sarcoplasmic reticulum, 624–625
  effects on myocardial contractile proteins, 625
  effects on myocardial contractility, role of cyclic AMP, 622–623
  effects on soleus muscle of cat, 538
  epinephrine-storing cells in adrenal gland, ultrastructure, 296, 297, 299–301
    exocytosis profiles at cell-to-cell apposed surface, 302–306
    exocytosis profiles at free cell surface, 301, 302, 303
  induction of apnea, possible explanations of, 491–493
    acute anoxia of respiratory center, 491–492
    direct depression of respiratory center, 492
    increased blood supply to respiratory center, 492
    reflex inhibition of respiration, 492–493
  induction of hyperpnea, possible explanations of, 493–500
    central effects of epinephrine, 494–495
    effects on arterial chemoreceptors, 497–499
    metabolic effects of epinephrine, 495–497
  levels in adrenal medulla in relation to norepinephrine levels at various ages, 310
  metabolic effects in muscle, 606–612
  quantitative aspects of metabolism of, 705, 706
  stimulation of arterial chemoreceptors, mechanism of, 499–500
  tissue distribution of, 714
  urinary excretion of, in animals exposed to cold, 642–646
Epinephrine biosynthesis
  anatomic relationship between adrenal cortex and medulla in, 357–358
  development of adrenal gland and, 358–359
  enzymes of pathway, 342–346
    dihydropteridine reductase, 344
    dopa decarboxylase, 344–345
    dopamine β-hydroxylase, 345–346
    phenylethanolamine N-methyltransferase, 346, 358–361, 363
    tyrosine hydroxylase, 342–344
  pathway of, 341–342
  rate in adrenal medulla during acclimatization to cold, 646–648
  role of glucocorticoids and ACTH in, 359–361
Epinephrine secretion
  during exposure to cold, 639–640

functional significance of, 311–312
  relation to effects of glucorticoids in hypophysectomized animals, 141–142
Erythropoietin
  effect on aldosterone secretion, 98
Estrogens
  circadian variation in plasma levels of, 133
  complexes with human CBG, apparent association constants of, 119
  effect on aldosterone secretion, 97–98
  influence on corticosteroid-binding globulin levels, 121–122
  secretion by adrenal cortex, 19–20
Exercise
  as systemic stress, role of glucocorticoids in, 254–256
  blood glucocorticoid levels in relation to, 251–252
  causing changes in plasma catecholamines, 434
  increased circulating catecholamines during, effect on gut, 523–524
  sympathoadrenal responses to, mediation by adrenergic receptors, 466–467
Eye
  adnexal functions, 562–565
    eyelids, 562–563
    lacrimal gland, 565
    nictitating membrane, 563–564
    oculomotor muscles, 564–565
  adrenergic neurons in retina, 579–580
  adrenergic pathways to, 553–555
  adrenergic receptors in smooth muscle of iris, 462
  blood flow of, 565–567
  catecholamines in relation to, 553–590
    effect of deprivation of adrenal medullary secretion, 580
    metabolism, uptake, storage, and release of catecholamines, 555–557
  cornea and lens, 572
  intraocular pigment, 577–579
    pigment in nuclear portion of crystalline lens, 578–579
    relation of mydriasis to iris pigmentation, 578
  intraocular pressure, 567–572
    effects of adrenergic compounds on, 571–572
    pseudofacility, 568–571
    uveoscleral flow, 568
  intrinsic muscle, 572–577
    ciliary body and accommodation, 576–577
    pupillary movements, 572–576
  sympathetic denervation of, degeneration release of transmitter after, 560–562
  sympathetic denervation of, in study of adrenergic compounds, 557–560

Fatty acids
  release from adipose tissue in vitro stimulated by glucocorticoids, 173–174
Fatty tissue: see Adipose tissue
Feedback
  negative feedback mechanism in control of aldosterone secretion, 88–89
  regulation of cortisol secretion, 130
  regulation of sensory detection and integration, 227
  short-loop feedback of ACTH on CRF causing inhibition of ACTH secretion, 49
Fetus
  adrenal cortex in, 107–115
    biosynthesis of corticosteroids, 60–61
    effect of adrenocortical insufficiency on postnatal survival, 113
    effect of hypophysectomy on development and function, 108–109
    effects on maturation of adrenal medulla, 112

effects on parturition, 112–113
effects on thymus and hematopoietic tissue, 112
extreme development in humans, 110–111
functional development, 107–109
functions, 111–113
hypophysial control of adrenal development and function, 108–109
hypothalamic control of hypophysial corticostimulating activity, 109
in human anencephalic monsters, 109
maturational changes, 107–108
metabolic pathways of pregnenolone and progesterone in human fetuses, 110
response of pituitary-adrenal system to stresses, 109
role in glycogen deposition in fetal liver, 111–112
catecholamine content of extraadrenal chromaffin tissue in, 359
catecholamine secretion and chemoreceptor stimulation of respiration at birth, 501–502

Fibroblasts
  changes in inflammation, effects of cortisol on, 267

Ganglionic blockaders
  effects on animals exposed to cold, 653–654
Gastrointestinal motility
  effects of catecholamines on, 516–519
    general considerations, 516
    on muscularis mucosae, 517
    on nonsphincter muscle, 516
    on receptor sites, 517–519
    on sphincter muscle, 516–517
Gastrointestinal system
  absorption in, effects of catecholamines on, 521–522
  adrenergic receptors in smooth muscle of, 461–462
  effects of circulating catecholamines from adrenergic nerve source on, 525
  electrolyte transport in, effect of corticosteroids on, 183–184
  gastric acid secretion and mucous secretion, effects of catecholamines on, 521
  relative effects of circulating and locally released catecholamines on, 525–526
  response to conditions of increased levels of circulating catecholamines, 522–524
    exercise, 523–524
    intense emotion, 523
    pheochromocytoma, 524
    shock, 522–523
  sensitivity to catecholamines in relation to plasma levels of catecholamines, 526–528
Gastrointestinal vasculature
  effects of catecholamines on, 519–521
    dilator effects, 520
    duration of action, 520–521
    general observations, 519
    local reactions, 520
    on splanchnic blood vessels, 479
Glucagon
  effect on cyclic AMP levels in perfused livers of normal and adrenalectomized rats, 153
  stimulation of adrenal medullary secretion, 315
Glucocorticoids
  see also Corticosterone; Cortisone; Dexamethasone; Hydrocortisone; Prednisolone
  biosynthesis from pregnenolone, 56–58
  deficiency and excess causing modifications of carbohydrate and protein metabolism, physiological mechanisms for, 141–163
    altered facility for glucose utilization by peripheral tissues, 159–163
    changes in rate of gluconeogenesis, 151–156
    changes in rates of glycogen breakdown and deposition, 156–159
    changes in secretion of epinephrine, 141–142
    changes in secretion of insulin, 142–145
    consequences of decreased appetite in glucocorticoid deficiency, 141
    early effects on gluconeogenesis of glucocorticoid administration in steroid-deficient rat, 151–155
    execution of order for increased gluconeogenesis, 154–155
    later effects on gluconeogenesis of glucocorticoid administration, 155–156
    net gain in liver protein in steroid-treated animals, 149–151
    net transfer of amino acids from peripheral tissues to liver in glucocorticoid excess, 145–151
    oxidative decarboxylation of pyruvate, 162–163
    possibility that glucocorticoids convey direct message for increased gluconeogenesis, 155
  effect on adenylate cyclase, cyclic AMP, and phosphodiesterase in adipose tissues, 174–176
  effect on adipose tissue metabolism, model for, 176
  effect on cellular response to inflammation, 266
  effect on lymphatic tissue responses in inflammation, 266–267
  effect on vascular permeability in inflammatory process, 265–266
  general effects and chemical structure of, 264–265
  influences on protein and carbohydrate metabolism, 135–167
    as means for bioassay of glucocorticoids, 136–137
    carbohydrate stores of fasted adrenalectomized rats after treatment with cortisol, 136–137
    gross interrelationship of whole-animal carbohydrate and protein metabolism, 138–141
  inhibition of glucose metabolism in adipose tissue, 169–172
  inotropic effects in isolated cardiac tissue, 196
  interaction with lymphoid tissue, 231–243
    actions on lymphoid tissues, specificity of, 233–234
    effects on lymphocyte morphology and lymphoid tissue organization and function, 234–236
    glucocorticoid receptors and initial steps in actions of glucocorticoids on lymphoid cells, 237–239
    metabolic effects, 236–237
    physiological significance of actions, 239–240
    relative activities on glucose uptake in rat thymus cells in vitro, 237–238
    thymus gland responses, 234–236
  involvement in development of ketosis and fatty livers, 172–173
  relation to skeletal muscle function, 249–252
    blood levels in relation to exercise, 251–252
    carbohydrate metabolism, 249–251
    cyclic AMP and prostaglandins as second messengers in, 255–256
    exercise as systemic stress, 254–256
    protein metabolism, 251
    regulation of lysosome function, 254–255
  relative anti-inflammatory potency of, 264–265
  resting rate of secretion of and meaning of hypercorticalism, 137–138
  role in epinephrine biosynthesis by adrenal medulla, 359–361
  skeletal structure of, 135–136
  stimulation of fatty acid release and lipolysis in adipose tissue in vitro, 173–174
  treatment of Cushing's syndrome causing changes in lipid deposition in adipose tissues, 172
Gluconeogenesis
  changes in rate of, in response to glucocorticoid deficiency and excess, 151–156
    early effects of glucocorticoid administration in steroid-deficient rat, 151–155
    execution of order for increased gluconeogenesis, 154–155

Gluconeogenesis (continued)
  later effects of glucocorticoid administration, 155–156
  possibility that glucocorticoids convey direct message for increased gluconeogenesis, 155
  from alanine, pyruvate, or lactate, proposed carbon path for, 154
  in kidneys from normal and adrenalectomized rats in vitro, effect of ad libitum feeding, force-feeding, or pair-feeding on, 141, 142
  in perfused livers from normal and adrenalectomized rats, effects of exogenous cyclic AMP on, 153
  response of livers of fed rats to gluconeogenic agents, effects of adrenalectomy on, 156, 157

Glucose
  see also Blood sugar
  ACTH-increased permeability of adrenal cortex cells to, as mode of action of ACTH in stimulating secretory activity of adrenal cortex, 70
  decreased urinary level in fasting depancreatized cats caused by adrenalectomy, 138
  incorporation of ^{14}C from lactate by perfused livers from adrenalectomized rats, effects of dexamethasone on, 153
  metabolism in adipose tissue, inhibition by glucocorticoids, 169–172
  oxidation inhibition in adipose tissue by dexamethasone, effect of dactinomycin on recovery of, 171
  turnover in postabsorptive state in normal, hypophysectomized, and adrenalectomized dogs, 142
  uptake and glycogen synthesis by liver in adrenalectomized rats, 157–159
  uptake and phosphorylation by isolated heart from hypophysectomized, diabetic rats, effect of growth hormone and hydrocortisone on, 160
  uptake by isolated rat diaphragm, effect of adrenalectomy, cortisol, and insulin on, 161
  uptake by isolated rat diaphragm, effect of hypophysectomy, growth hormone, and insulin on, 161
  uptake in rat thymus cells in vitro, relative activities of steroids in, 237–238
  utilization by peripheral tissues, altered facility under conditions of glucocorticoid deficiency or excess, 159–163

Glucose 6-phosphate dehydrogenase
  activation by ACTH as possible mode of action of ACTH in stimulating secretory activity of adrenal cortex, 70–71

Glycine
  incorporation into protein of isolated diaphragm, effect of adrenalectomy and cortisone on, 148

Glycogen metabolism
  biosynthesis by liver of adrenalectomized rats after glucose administration, 157–159
  deposition in fetal liver, role of fetal adrenocortical hormones, 111–112
  glycogenic activities of various steroids, 233–234

Glycogenolysis
  control in intact cardiac muscle, effects of epinephrine, 611–612
  control in intact skeletal muscle, effects of epinephrine, 610–611
  control in muscle, in vitro studies of epinephrine effects on, 607–610
    activation of phosphorylase kinase by Ca^{2+}, 609
    activation of phosphorylase kinase by cyclic AMP, 608–609
    enzyme reactions involved in, 607–608
    integrated control of phosphorylase activity, 610
    phosphorylase kinase phosphatase, 609–610
    phosphorylase phosphatase, 608
    regulatory properties and interconversion of phosphorylase b and a, 608
  in adrenalectomized rats, 156–157
  role of adrenergic receptor in, 453–454

Growth hormone: see Somatotrophin

Guanethidine
  effects on animals exposed to cold, 653

Gustation: see Taste

Hearing
  role of corticosteroids in, 221–225
    detection and recognition in Cushing's syndrome, 224–225
    detection thresholds in adrenal cortical insufficiency, 221–223
    speech discrimination ability in adrenal cortical insufficiency, 223–224

Heart
  see also Myocardium
  adrenergic receptors in, 455–458
  changes in chronic adrenal insufficiency, 192–194
  effects of corticosteroids on, 195–197
    electrocardiographic effects, 197
    in whole animals, 196–197
    inotropic effects in intact animals, 197
    inotropic effects of glucocorticoids in isolated cardiac tissue, 196
    inotropic effects of mineralocorticoids in isolated cardiac tissue, 195–196
  function of, effects of catecholamines, 480–486
    inotropic effects on heart-lung preparation, 484–485
    inotropic effects on isolated papillary muscle preparation, 482–484
    on conduction velocity, 482
    on heart rate, electrophysiological studies, 480–482

Heat
  stimulation of hormone discharge from adrenal medulla, 313

Hemorrhage
  causing change in plasma catecholamines, 433–434
  effects on renin secretion, 86

Histamine
  stimulation of catecholamine release from adrenals, 439

Histidine
  incorporation into protein of diaphragms, effect of adrenalectomy, steroid replacement, and cortisone excess, 147

Horner's syndrome
  characteristics of, 557, 562
  effect of supersensitivity denervation in, 559, 560

Hydrocortisone
  complexes with human serum proteins, 118–119
  effect of treatment of thymocytes with physiological amounts in vitro, 149
  effect on carbohydrate stores of adrenalectomized rats, 136–137
  effect on fibroblasts involved in inflammatory process, 267
  effect on glucose uptake by isolated diaphragm from adrenalectomized and insulin-treated rats, 161
  effect on glycine incorporation into protein of isolated diaphragm from normal or from adrenalectomized rats, 148
  effect on plasma glucose and plasma insulin in sheep, 144
  effect on uptake and phosphorylation of glucose by isolated heart from hypophysectomized, diabetic rats, 160
  high-affinity binding in sera of different species, 120–121

Hydrocortisone secretion
  circadian rhythm of, 127–132
    alterations in circadian rhythm, 130–132
    diurnal variation in plasma levels in relation to ACTH levels, 128
    relation to activity-sleep cycle, 130–131
  effect of exogenously administered substances on, 131–132
  effect of stress on, 131
  excess secretion syndromes, pathophysiology in man, 271–282
    adrenal tumor-dependent excess, 276–277

extrapituitary, extraadrenal, tumor-dependent excess, 275–276, 277
  pituitary-dependent excess, 271–275, 277
 feedback regulation of, 130
 stimulation by ACTH, 41–43
  mode of action of ACTH, 42
  receptor reserve and sensitivity of adrenal cortex cells, 42
  regulatory role of adenohypophysis, 41
  structure-activity relationships of ACTH, 42–43
  temporal aspects of secretory response of adrenal cortex, 42
 stimulation by factors of questionable physiological significance, 43
Hydrogen-ion concentration
 acid-base balance, effect of corticosteroids on, 181–182
 hypercapnia and acidemia causing change in plasma catecholamines, 433
 metabolic acidosis and alkalosis causing increases in adrenal medullary secretion, 313
Hydroxylases
 17α-hydroxylase inhibitors and 18-hydroxylase inhibitors causing inhibition of biosynthesis of corticosteroids, 63
Hypercorticalism: see Adrenal cortex hyperfunction
Hypoglycemia
 causing change in plasma catecholamines, 432
 causing increase in adrenal medullary secretion, 314–315
 causing stimulation of catecholamine release from adrenals, 438
Hypophysectomy
 effect on adrenal development and function in fetuses and newborns, 108
 effect on aldosterone secretion, 95
 effect on glucorticoid production and epinephrine secretion, 141–142
 glucose turnover in postabsorptive state in dogs after, 142
Hypothalamus
 control of hypophysial corticostimulating activity in fetuses, 109
  in human anencephalic monsters, 109
  pituitary-adrenal system responses to stresses, 109
 corticotropin-releasing factor in, 44–45
  neural paths to release of, 45
 stimulation causing increase in adrenal medullary secretion, 311
Hypoxia: see Anoxia

Immunity
 role of lymphoid system in, 232–233
Inborn errors of metabolism
 genetic blocks in hydroxylation of corticosteroids, 62
Infant, newborn
 postnatal survival of fetuses with adrenocortical insufficiency, 113
Inflammation
 anti-inflammatory effects of adrenal cortex hormones, 9–10
 anti-inflammatory potency of therapeutic corticosteroids, 264–265
 cellular response to, effect of glucocorticoids on, 266
 fibroblast changes in, effects of cortisol on, 267
 localization of corticosteroids in areas of, 265
 lymphatic tissue involvement in, effects of glucocorticoids on, 266–267
 lysosome role in, effect of cortisone on, 268
 platelet role in, effect of cortisone on, 268
 process of, 263–264
 vascular permeability in, effect of glucocorticoids on, 265–266
Insulin
 effect on dopamine β-hydroxylase and catecholamine content and distribution in rabbit adrenals, 397
 plasma levels in sheep, effect of cortisol on, 144
 serum levels in fasting rats, effect of prednisolone injection on, 144
Insulin secretion
 effect of glucocorticoid deficiency or excess on, 142–145
 in postabsorptive state in normal, hypophysectomized, and adrenalectomized dogs, 142
Iodophenols
 enzymatic O-methylation of, 673
Ions
 requirements for adrenomedullary secretion of catecholamines, 403–407
Isomerases
 in biosynthesis of corticosteroids, 60

Juxtaglomerular apparatus
 factors regulating renin secretion, 85–88
  effects of hemorrhage, 86
  effects of papaverine infusion, 86–87
 origin of renin from juxtaglomerular cells, 85
 renin secretion and role in regulation of aldosterone secretion, 84–85

Ketosis
 involvement of glucocorticoids in development of, 172–173
 ketogenic effects of somatotropin and dexamethasone in pancreatectomized, hypophysectomized rats, 172, 173
Kidney
 effect of corticosteroids on, 179–182
  aldosterone mechanism of action on Na transport, 185–186
  K excretion, 180–181
  Mg, Ca, and acid-base balance, 181–182
  Na excretion, 179–180
  Na-K ATPase activity, 184
 from adrenalectomized rats fed in different ways, influence on gluconeogenesis in vitro, 141, 142
Kinins
 interaction with corticosteroids in regulation of circulatory function, 200, 202

Lipids
 changes in deposition in Cushing's syndrome during treatment with glucocorticoids, 172
 droplets in adrenal cortex, electron microscopy of, 26–28, 30, 31, 33
  changes in relation to hormone secretion, 32–36
 lipolysis in adipose tissue stimulated by glucocorticoids in vitro, 173–174
 lipolysis, role of adrenergic receptors, 454–455
 mobilization of, effects of glucocorticoids on, 169–178
 phospholipid composition of chromaffin granules, 327
Liver
 blood vessels of, effects of catecholamines on, 479
 composition of, long-term effects of cortisone regimen in fed rats, 146, 147
 composition of, short-term effects of cortisone regimen in fed rats, 146
 cyclic AMP levels in perfused livers of normal and adrenalectomized rats, effects of glucagon and epinephrine on, 153
 fatty liver development, involvement of glucocorticoids in, 172–173
 gain of protein in animals treated with excess glucocorticoids, 149–151
 gluconeogenesis in perfused livers from normal and adrenalectomized rats, effects of exogenous cyclic AMP on, 153
 glucose uptake and glycogen synthesis in adrenalectomized rats, 157–159
 glycogen deposition in fetuses, role of fetal adrenocortical hormones, 111–112

Liver (continued)
    hematopoietic tissue of, effects of fetal adrenocortical hormones on, 112
    net transfer of amino acids from peripheral tissues to liver in rats with glucocorticoid excess, 145–151
    response to gluconeogenic agents, effects of adrenalectomy in fed rats, 156, 157
    role of possible hepatic hormone in regulation of aldosterone secretion, 98
Lung
    dopamine in, 510
    heart-lung preparation, inotropic effects of catecholamines on, 484–485
Lymphocytes
    effects of glucocorticoids on morphology of, 234–236
Lymphoid tissue
    functional relationships among major compartments of lymphoid system, 232–233
    interactions of glucocorticoids with, 231–243
        effects on lymphocyte morphology and lymphoid tissue organization and function, 234–236
        glucocorticoid receptors and initial steps in actions of glucocorticoids on lymphoid cells, 237–239
        metabolic effects, 236–237
        physiological significance of actions, 239–240
        specificity of actions on lymphoid tissues, 233–234
    involvement in inflammatory process, effects of glucocorticoids on, 266–267
    lymphoid system and immune responses, 232–233
    stress influence on, mediation by adrenal glands, 231
Lysosomes
    in chromaffin cells, components of, 323
    muscle lysosomal activity, role of glucocorticoids, 254–255
    role in inflammation, effect of cortisone on, 268

Magnesium
    deficiency of, effect on aldosterone secretion, 95
    inhibition of adrenal medullary secretion in response to acetylcholine, K, Ca, Sr, and Ba, 377–378
    renal excretion of, effect of corticosteroids on, 181–182
Metals
    involvement in activity of monoamine oxidase, 683–684
Methionine
    incorporation into protein of intact diaphragms from adrenalectomized rats, effect of preincubation with corticosterone, 148
O-Methyltransferases
    see also Catechol-O-methyltransferase
    hydroxamic acid O-methyltransferase, 673
    hydroxyindole-O-methyltransferase, 673–674
    O-methylation of iodophenols, 673
    phenol-O-methyltransferase, 673
Metyrapone
    inhibition of biosynthesis of corticosteroids, 62–63
Microscopy, electron
    of adrenal cortex in relation to secretory function, 25–39
        lipid droplets, 26–28, 30, 31, 33
        mitochondria, 25–26, 27, 28, 29, 31, 35, 36
        other organelles, 28
        smooth endoplasmic reticulum, 25, 26, 27, 28, 30, 31
        zona fasciculata and zona reticularis changes with functional activity, 34–36
        zona glomerulosa changes with functional activity, 33–34
    of chromaffin cells, 295–308
        endoplasmic reticulum, 295, 297, 298
        epinephrine-storing cells, 296, 297, 299–301
        exocytosis profiles at cell-to-cell apposed surface, 302–306
        exocytosis profiles at free cell surface, 301, 302, 303
        general organization of cell, 295–297
        norepinephrine-storing cells, 297–300

presence of coated pits in granule membrane fused with plasma membrane, 301, 302, 303, 305–306
secretory vesicles, 297–302
Mineralocorticoids
    see also Aldosterone; Corticosterone
    inotropic effects in isolated cardiac tissue, 195–196
    relation to skeletal muscle function, 246–249
        direct muscle-aldosterone effects, 248–249
        work capacity and electrolyte balance, 247–248
Mitochondria
    in adrenal cortex, direct activation of their enzymes by cyclic AMP, 75
    in adrenal cortex, electron microscopy of, 25–26, 27, 28, 29, 31, 35, 36
        changes in relation to hormone secretion, 32–36
    in adrenal cortex, increased permeability induced by ACTH as possible mode of action in stimulating secretory activity, 71–74
    in adrenal cortex, substrate utilization increased by ACTH as possible mode of action in stimulating secretory activity, 71
    in chromaffin cells, components of, 323
Monoamine oxidase
    assay methods for, 681
    classification and nomenclature of, 677–678
    detection in adrenal cortex and medulla, 689
    distribution in animals and in tissues, 678
    function of, 689–690
    inhibitors of, 687
    intracellular localization of, 678–680
    multiple forms of, 687–689
    oxidation of natural substrates by, 685
    properties of, 681–687
        acceptors, 686
        attachment of flavin, 682–683
        involvement of metal in activity of, 683–684
        kinetics of, 686–687
        substrate specificity, 684–686
        sulfhydryl groups of, 684
    reaction catalyzed by, 680–681
Muscle, cardiac: see Myocardium
Muscle contraction
    Ca ions and relation to, 612–622
        Ca and contractile proteins, 613–614
        Ca release by sarcoplasmic reticulum, 617–618
        Ca transport by cell membrane, 621–622
        Ca uptake by sarcoplasmic reticulum, 618–619
        cellular Ca flux, 614–615
        mitochondria and Ca sequestration, 619–621
        role of Ca in excitation-contraction coupling, 615–617
Muscle, skeletal
    adrenergic receptors in, 463–464
    blood vessels of, effects of catecholamines on, 476–478
    direct action of catecholamines on, 537–545
        changes in electrical properties, 542–544
        in excess potassium environment, 539–540
        in fast muscles, 537–538
        in low potassium environment, 540
        in normal ionic environment, 537–539
        in slow muscles, 538–539
        influence of low temperature on, 541–542
        influence of ouabain on, 541
        mechanism of action, 544–545
        mediation by adrenoreceptors, 540–541
    effect of corticosteroids on, 245–261
        steroid myopathy, 252–254
    effect of glucocorticoids on, 249–252
        carbohydrate metabolism, 249–251
        cyclic AMP and prostaglandins as second messengers in, 255–256

protein metabolism, 251
regulation of lysosomes, 254–255
effect of mineralocorticoids on, 246–249
  direct muscle-aldosterone effects, 248–249
  electrolyte metabolism, 182–183
  work capacity and electrolyte balance, 247–248
glycogenolysis in, in vitro studies of epinephrine effects on, 607–610
  activation of phosphorylase kinase by Ca^{2+}, 609
  activation of phosphorylase kinase by cyclic AMP, 608–609
  enzyme reactions involved in, 607–608
  integrated control of phosphorylase activity, 610
  phosphorylase kinase phosphatase, 609–610
  phosphorylase phosphatase, 608
  regulatory properties and interconversion of phosphorylase b and a, 608
glycogenolysis in intact muscle, epinephrine effects on, 610–611
Muscle, smooth
  adrenergic receptors in, 461–463
    gastrointestinal, 461–462
    iris, 462
    nictitating membrane, 462
    respiratory tract, 463
    spleen, 462
    uterus, 462–463
  bronchial, effects of β-adrenoceptor stimulant drugs and α-adrenoceptor stimulant drugs on, 509–510
  bronchial, effects of catecholamines on, 507–513
    actions of blood-borne catecholamines, 510
    direct in vivo methods of study, 508
    in vitro methods of study, 508
    indirect in vivo methods of study, 508–509
  bronchial, innervation of, 507–508
  bronchial, nature of sympathetic nervous transmitters to, 510–511
  gastrointestinal sphincters, effects of catecholamines on, 516–517
  muscularis mucosae of digestive tract, effects of catecholamines on, 517
  nonsphincter muscle of gastrointestinal system, effects of catecholamines on, 516
Myocardial infarction
  plasma catecholamine levels in, 435
Myocardium
  see also Heart
  contractile proteins of, effect of epinephrine on, 625
  contractility of, effects of cyclic AMP and epinephrine on, 622–623
  electromechanical properties of, effects of epinephrine on, 623–624
  glycogenolysis in intact muscle, effects of epinephrine on, 611–612
  isolated sarcoplasmic reticulum of, hormonal and cyclic AMP effects on, 624–625
  metabolic effects of corticosteroids on, 197
  oxygen usage of, effects of catecholamines on, 485–486

Neoplasms
  extrapituitary, extraadrenal tumors causing cortisol excess in man, 275–276, 277
Neurohypophysial CRF: see Vasopressin
Neuromuscular junction
  effects of catecholamines on, 545–550
    effects on end-plate potential, 546–547
    effects on miniature end-plate potential, 547–548
    facilitatory action, 545–546
    inhibitory action, 546
    mechanism of increase of transmitter release, 548–549
Nicotine
  effects on plasma catecholamines, 436

Nictitating membrane
  adrenergic receptors in smooth muscle of, 462
  function of, 563–564
Nitrogen
  daily excretion in humans at 2 levels of protein intake, 139
  decreased urinary excretion in fasting depancreatized cats caused by adrenalectomy, 138
  distribution in organs and in blood and liver constituents of adrenalectomized protein-depleted rats treated with cortisone, 145–146
  urinary excretion in fasted rats, effects of injected adrenocortical extract on, 138
Noradrenaline: see Norepinephrine
Norepinephrine
  content in normal human plasma, 428–430
    age in relation to, 430
    resting blood pressure and, 430
  content in plasma of various experimental animals, 430
  disappearance after iv injection of, 714
  induction of hyperpnea, possible explanations of, 493–500
    central effects of norepinephrine, 494–495
    effects on arterial chemoreceptors, 497–499
    metabolic effects of norepinephrine, 495–497
  interaction with corticosteroids in regulation of circulatory function, 200–201
  level in adrenal medulla in relation to epinephrine levels at various ages, 310
  norepinephrine-storing cells in adrenal gland, 297–300
    exocytosis profiles at cell-to-cell apposed surface, 302, 306
    exocytosis profiles at free cell surface, 302, 303
  overflow into circulation from sympathetically innervated organs, 440
  quantitative aspects of metabolism of, 705–707
  stimulation of arterial chemoreceptors, mechanism of, 499–500
  tissue distribution of, 714
  urinary excretion of, in animals exposed to cold, 642–646
Norepinephrine biosynthesis
  enzymes of pathway, 342–346
    dihydropteridine reductase, 344
    dopa decarboxylase, 344–345
    dopamine β-hydroxylase, 345–346, 348, 350–351
    tyrosine hydroxylase, 342–344, 346–347, 349–351
  pathway of, 341–342
  rate in adrenal medulla during acclimatization to cold, 646–648
  regulation of, 346–351
    in adrenal medulla in response to immediate demands, 348–349
    in response to prolonged stimulation, 349–351
    in sympathetic nerves in response to stimulation, 346–347
Norepinephrine secretion
  functional significance of, 311–312
Nucleotides
  see also Adenosine monophosphate, cyclic; Adenosine triphosphate
  in adrenal chromaffin granules, 324, 330

Olfaction: see Smell
Ouabain
  effects on catecholamine action on skeletal muscles, 541
  inhibition of biosynthesis of corticosteroids, 64
  stimulant effects on adrenal medullary secretion, 378–379
Ovary
  adrenal-gonad relations, historical aspects, 7
Oxidases
  18-oxidase inhibitors causing inhibition of biosynthesis of corticosteroids, 63
Oxygen consumption
  myocardial, effects of catecholamines on, 485–486

Papaverine
  effect on renin secretion, 86–87
Parabiosis
  cross-circulation experiments on regulation of aldosterone secretion in dogs, 78
Peptic ulcer
  possible involvement of catecholamines in, 524
Peptides
  polypeptides, stimulation of catecholamine release from adrenals, 439–440
Peripheral nerves
  pathway for control of secretory activity of adrenal medulla, 309
Phenylethanolamine N-methyltransferase
  in adrenal medulla, changes during cold exposure and cold acclimatization, 648–649
  in pathway of epinephrine biosynthesis, 346, 358–361, 363
Pheochromocytoma
  increased circulating catecholamines in, effect on gut, 524
Phosphodiesterase
  activity in adipose tissue, effects of glucocorticoids on, 174–176
Phosphorylase kinase
  activation by Ca ion, 609
  activation by cyclic AMP, 608–609
Phosphorylases
  activation by ACTH as possible mode of action of ACTH in stimulating secretory activity of adrenal cortex, 70
  in glycogenolysis, 607–610
Pineal body
  extracts and pinealectomy, effect on aldosterone secretion, 79
Pituitary gland
  see also Hypophysectomy
  adrenal-pituitary relations, historical aspects, 8
  corticostimulating activity in fetuses, hypothalamic control of, 109
    in human anencephalic monsters, 109
    pituitary-adrenal system responses to stresses, 109
  pituitary-adrenal secretion, circadian rhythm of, 128–129
  pituitary-dependent cortisol excess in man, 271–275, 277
  role in control of adrenal development and function in fetus, 108–109
  role in regulation of aldosterone secretion, 95
    possible role of adenohypophysial hormones other than ACTH, 97
    role of ACTH, 95–97
Placenta
  steroid biosynthesis in, 60–61
PNMT: see Phenylethanolamine N-methyltransferase
Potassium
  excess and low external K concentrations, effects of catecholamines on skeletal muscles in, 539–540
  excess causing stimulation of adrenal medullary secretion, requirement of Ca, 376
  lack of, potentiation of basal and evoked adrenal medullary secretion, 378
  level of intake and altered plasma levels, effects on aldosterone secretion, 93–95
  renal excretion of, effect of corticosteroids on, 180–181
  salivary concentrations, effect of corticosteroids on, 182
Prednisolone
  injection of, effect on blood sugar and serum insulin in fasting rats, 144
Pregnancy
  role of fetal adrenal cortex in parturition, 112–113
Pregnenolone
  conversion to glucocorticoids and aldosterone, 56–58
  formation from cholesterol, 56, 57
  metabolic pathways in human fetal adrenal gland, 110
  metabolism in human adrenal cortex, 57
Progesterone
  complexes with human CBG, apparent association constants of, 119
  effect on aldosterone secretion, 97
  metabolic pathways in human fetal adrenal gland, 110
Prostaglandins
  as mediators of glucocorticoid action in muscle, 256
Protein biosynthesis
  by aldosterone action on renal Na transport, 185–186
  inhibitors of as inhibitors of corticosteroid secretion, 63–64
  relation to ACTH stimulation of secretion by adrenal cortex, 74–75
Protein metabolism
  influence of corticosteroids on, 135–167
  daily nitrogen excretion in humans at 2 levels of protein intake, 139
  decreased urinary nitrogen excretion caused by adrenalectomy in fasting depancreatized cats, 138
  effects of injected adrenocortical extracts on nitrogen excretion in fasted rats, 138
  glucocorticoids and skeletal muscle, 251
  gross interrelationship of whole-animal carbohydrate and protein metabolism in glucocorticoid effects, 138–141
  modifications caused by glucocorticoid deficiency and excess, physiological mechanisms for, 141–163
    changes in secretion of epinephrine, 141–142
    consequences of decreased appetite in glucocorticoid deficiency, 141
    glycine incorporation into protein of isolated diaphragm, effect of adrenalectomy and cortisol on, 148
    histidine incorporation into protein of diaphragms, effect of adrenalectomy, steroids, and cortisone excess, 147
    methionine incorporation into protein of intact diaphragms of adrenalectomized rats, effect of preincubation with corticosterone, 148
    net gain in liver protein in steroid-treated animals, 149–151
    net transfer of amino acids from peripheral tissues to liver in glucocorticoid excess, 145–151
    nitrogen distribution in organs and in blood and liver constituents of adrenalectomized protein-depleted rats treated with cortisone, 145–146
Proteins
  chromogranins and chromomembrins isolated from chromaffin granules, 324–327
  in chromaffin granules, 324–327
    amino acid composition of, 325
Pulmonary blood vessels
  adrenergic receptors in, 460–461
  effects of catecholamines on, 479–480

Receptors
  see also Adrenergic receptors
  arterial chemoreceptors, mechanism of stimulation by catecholamines, 499–500
  arterial chemoreceptors, stimulation by catecholamines as possible explanation for their induction of hyperpnea, 497–499
  chemoreceptor stimulation of respiration at birth by catecholamine secretion, 501–502
  development of concept of, 447–450
    classification of, 450
    definition of, 448
    operational concept of, 449–450
  glucocorticoid receptors and initial steps in glucocorticoid actions on lymphoid cells, 237–239
  receptor reserve and sensitivity of adrenal cortex cells to ACTH, 42
Reflex
  respiratory reflexes, effects of catecholamines on, 500

Renin
  interaction with corticosteroids in regulation of circulatory function, 201
  plasma activity in relation to aldosterone excretion, diurnal variations in, 132–133
Renin-angiotensin system
  role in regulation of aldosterone secretion, 78–89
    early evidence of relation of adrenal cortex to kidney, 80
    effect of angiotensin II injection, 80–82
    evidence as primary control mechanism, 80–83
    factors regulating renin secretion, 85–88
    in lower vertebrates, 83–84
    juxtaglomerular apparatus, 84–85
    locus of secretion and chemical nature of aldosterone-stimulating agent, 78–80
    negative feedback mechanism in, 88–89
    renin origin from juxtaglomerular apparatus, 85
Reserpine
  effects on animals exposed to cold, 652–653
Respiration
  apnea induced by epinephrine, possible explanations of, 491–493
    acute anoxia of respiratory center, 491–492
    direct depression of respiratory center, 492
    increased blood supply to respiratory center, 492
    reflex inhibition of respiration, 492–493
  chemoreceptor stimulation at birth by catecholamine secretion, 501–502
  hyperpnea induced by epinephrine and norepinephrine, possible explanations of, 493–500
    central effects of epinephrine and norepinephrine, 494–495
    effects on arterial chemoreceptors, 497–499
    metabolic effects of catecholamines, 495–497
  respiratory reflexes, effects of catecholamines on, 500
  stimulation by catecholamines, physiological significance of, 500–501
Respiratory tract
  see also Bronchi; Lung
  adrenergic receptors in smooth muscle of, 463

Skin
  blood vessels of, effects of catecholamines on, 478
  melanophore responses to catecholamines, 465
  skin gland secretions in amphibians, mediation by adrenergic receptors, 465
Salivary glands
  Na and K concentrations, effect of corticosteroids on, 182
Sensory processes
  role of corticosteroids in, 209–230
Shock
  increased circulating catecholamines in, effect on gut, 522–523
Smell
  role of corticosteroids in, 218–221
    detection in Cushing's syndrome, 220–221
    detection thresholds in adrenal cortical insufficiency, 218–220
  role of nonadrenal steroid hormones in, 221
Sodium
  altered plasma level of, effect on aldosterone secretion, 93
  concentration in saliva, effect of corticosteroids on, 182
  concentration in sweat, effect of corticosteroids on, 182
  depletion of, effects on aldosterone secretion, 89–93
  lack of, potentiation of basal and evoked adrenal medullary secretion, 378
  metabolism in bone, effect of corticosteroids on, 183
  prolonged deprivation causing inhibition of adrenal medullary secretion, 379
  renal excretion of, effect of corticosteroids on, 179–180
  renal transport of, mechanism of action of aldosterone on, 185–186
  sodium-retaining effect of various therapeutic corticosteroids, 264–265
Sodium chloride
  salt appetite and sensitivity, effect of corticosteroids on, 184
Somatotrophin
  effect on glucose uptake by isolated diaphragm from hypophysectomized and insulin-treated rats, 161
  effect on uptake and phosphorylation of glucose by isolated heart from hypophysectomized, diabetic rats, 160
  ketogenic effects in pancreatectomized, hypophysectomized rats, 172, 173
Speech discrimination
  ability in patients with adrenal cortex insufficiency, 223–224
Splanchnic nerves
  acetylcholine receptors and mechanism of adrenal medullary secretion, 371–372
    nicotinic and muscarinic receptors, 371
  denervation of, effect on adrenal medullary secretion, 370
  secretomotor fibers, cholinergic nature of, 370–371
  stimulation of, responses of adrenal medullary secretion to, 368–370
    frequency-response relations, 369
    preferential secretion of epinephrine and norepinephrine, 370, 371–372
    spatial recruitment, overlap, and convergence, 369
    splanchnic-adrenal fatigue, 369–370
Spleen
  adrenergic receptors in, 462
Squalene
  biosynthesis of cholesterol from, 55–56
  conversion of acetyl coenzyme A to, 55, 56
Steroids
  inhibition of biosynthesis of corticosteroids, 63
  nonadrenal steroid hormones, role in olfaction, 221
  nonadrenal steroid hormones, role in taste acuity, 217
  relative activities on glucose uptake in rat thymus cells in vitro, 237–238
  relative thymolytic and glycogenic activities of, 233–234
Stress
  see also Emotional stress
  adrenal role in, historical aspects, 8–9
    influence on lymphoid tissue, 231
  effect on cortisol secretion, 131
  effect on pituitary-adrenal system of fetuses, 109
  exercise as systemic stress, role of glucocorticoids in, 254–256
  physical stress stimulating hormone discharge from adrenal medulla, 313
Strontium
  as Ca substitute and stimulant in adrenal medullary secretion, 377
Suprarenal glands: see Adrenal gland
Sweat
  sodium concentration in, effect of corticosteroids on, 182
Sweat glands
  histology of, 591–592
  stimulation by catecholamines, 592–601
    in Bovidae, 597–598
    in Camelidae, 598–599
    in Canidae, 599
    in Equidae, 595–597
    in Felidae, 599
    in man, 592–595
    in other anthropoid primates, 595
    in prosimian primates, 595
    in Rhinocerotidae, 597
    in rodents, 599
    in Suidae, 598
    phylogenetic basis for, 599–601

Sympathetic nervous system
  activation by exposure to cold, 642–649
    excretion of catecholamines and their metabolites, 642–646
    sources of catecholamines and their metabolites excreted in urine, 646
  adrenergic nerves as source of circulating catecholamines, 525
  adrenergic pathways to eye and ocular structures, 553–555
  chemical sympathectomy, effects on animals exposed to cold, 655
  denervation of eye, degeneration release of transmitter after, 560–562
  denervation of eye in study of adrenergic compounds, 557–560
  immunosympathectomy, effects on animals exposed to cold, 651–652
  norepinephrine biosynthesis in, 341, 346–347
    acute regulation in response to stimulation, 346–347
  sympathetic nervous transmitters to bronchial smooth muscle, nature of, 510–511
  sympathetically innervated organs, origin of plasma catecholamines from, 440

Taste
  role of corticosteroids in, 209–217, 225–227
    acuity in patients with various adrenal cortex diseases, 216
    detection and recognition in states of corticosteroid excess, 216–217
    detection thresholds in adrenal cortical insufficiency, 210–213
    recognition-detection relationships, 216
    recognition of tastes in adrenal cortical insufficiency, 214–216
  role of nonadrenal steroid hormones in, 217
Temperature
  see also Body temperature; Cold; Heat
  changes causing variations in plasma catecholamines, 434
  influence on catecholamine storage in chromaffin granules, 328–329
Testis
  adrenal-gonad relations, historical aspects, 7
Testosterone
  circadian variation in plasma levels of, 133
  complexes with human CBG, apparent association constants of, 119
  influence on corticosteroid-binding globulin levels, 121–122
Thymus gland
  effect of fetal adrenocortical hormones on, 112
  glucose uptake in vitro, relative activities of steroids in, 237–238
  response to glucocorticoids, 234–236
  thymocyte treatment with cortisol in vitro, effects, 149
  thymolytic activities of various steroids, 233–234

Thyrotrophin
  influence on serum levels of corticosteroid-binding globulin, 123
Thyroxine
  influence on serum levels of corticosteroid-binding globulin, 123
Touch
  role of corticosteroids in, 225
Transcortin: see Corticosteroid-binding globulin
Tyrosine hydroxylase
  adrenal activity, regulation by adrenal cortex, 361
  adrenal activity, role of cyclic AMP in regulation of, 361–362
  in pathway of epinephrine biosynthesis, 342–344, 346–347, 349–351

Uterus
  adrenergic receptors in, 462–463

Vasopressin
  stimulation of ACTH secretion, 45–46
  stimulation of adrenal cortical secretory activity, 43
Veins
  adrenergic receptors in, 459
  effects of catecholamines on, 480
Vertebrates
  lower vertebrates, renin-angiotensin-aldosterone system in, 83–84
  nonmammals, corticosteroid biosynthesis in, 61–62
Vision
  corticosteroid role in function of, 225

Water metabolism
  adrenal cortex role in, history of, 5–6
  effect of corticosteroids on, 184–185

Zona fasciculata
  steroid production by, 17–18
  transformation of zona glomerulosa into, 20
  ultrastructural changes with functional activity, 34–36
Zona glomerulosa
  cell origin from capsular fibroblasts, 14–15
  consideration as distinct functional unit, morphological bases, 15–16
  steroid production by, 16–17
  transformation into zona fasciculata, 20
  ultrastructural changes with functional activity, 33–34
Zona reticularis
  region of cell death and removal, 15
  role in androgen secretion by adrenal cortex, 19
  steroid production by, 17–18
  ultrastructural changes with functional activity, 34–36